CHINESE HERBAL MEDICINE

Formulas & Strategies

2ND EDITION

CHINESE
HERBAL
MEDICINE

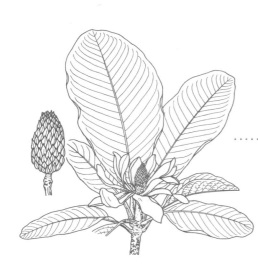

Formulas & Strategies

2nd EDITION

COMPILED AND TRANSLATED BY

Volker Scheid   Dan Bensky
Andrew Ellis   Randall Barolet

International Standard Book Number: 978-0-939616-67-1
Library of Congress Control Number: 2008943299
Printed in the United States of America

4   6   8   10   9   7   5

Brush calligraphy by Kou Hoi-Yin
Indexes by Sybil Ihrig
Cover design by Patricia O'Connor
Front cover photo © 2009 by Lilian Lai Bensky
Back cover photo © 2009 by Clare O'Connor

Book design and typesetting by Gary Niemeier

General Contents

Preface to 2nd Edition

STUDYING CHINESE HERBAL medicine is an arduous task that is similar to learning a language. The first step, familiarizing yourself with the medicinal substances, corresponds to accumulating a sufficient vocabulary. But words alone are not enough. Before you can speak a language, you must understand the rules of syntax and grammar. And before you can 'talk' to the body with Chinese herbal medicine, you must understand the formulas and the strategies that underlie them. This is the syntax and grammar of Chinese herbal medicine. Just as individual words are rarely used outside of their context in a sentence, it is rare in Chinese herbal medicine to prescribe individual substances outside of their context in a formula.

This book is the companion volume to *Chinese Herbal Medicine: Materia Medica,* which provides basic information about the medicinal substances or 'vocabulary' of traditional Chinese herbal medicine. Our goal here is to provide a similar level of information about the formulas so that they can be used in a responsible and effective manner.

The impetus behind both of these works is the same: to contribute to a deeper understanding, utilization, and investigation of China's medical tradition in the West. In this effort we have been motivated by several, sometimes conflicting, intentions:

- First, we wanted to create a textbook that closely reflects the understanding of contemporary Chinese practitioners. The usual way of doing this is to translate the textbooks that are used in Chinese medical colleges and universities. However, not only do these textbooks change over time (the current 6th edition is significantly different from the experimental texts of the late 1950s), they are also complemented by an ever-increasing range of specialist books and articles by individuals who have their own idiosyncratic understandings.

- Second, we felt that the time had come to provide readers with a more in-depth understanding of Chinese medicine as a living tradition. By this we mean a tradition that continuously grows, develops, adapts, and changes and that is able to do so precisely because it is intrinsically diverse and heterogeneous. Tradition, as the philosopher Alasdair MacIntyre has so poignantly remarked, dies the moment it degenerates into traditionalism; and traditionalism is primarily recognized by an absence of disagreement and conflict. Facilitating the development of Chinese medicine in the West thus means enabling practitioners to join a two-thousand-year-old debate about formulas and strategies.

- Third, it is becoming increasingly obvious that the development of Chinese medicine in China, Asia, and the West cannot be detached from its development in Japan, Korea, and other countries. This means that, even as we focus on Chinese medicine, we must give some attention to non-Chinese, primarily Japanese, sources.

- Fourth, above all we wanted to write a book that is clinically useful. Here, although seasoned practitioners find that an ability to draw from a diversity of sources allows them to develop their own style, novices generally prefer the clear structure that textbooks provide and not the complex reality described in case studies.

Our attempt to reconcile the sometimes different directions in which we were pulled by these intentions is reflected in the content and composition of this book. In the writing of the main sections, we have drawn on some of the most important formula textbooks in contemporary China: *Formulas,* edited by Li Fei; *Contemporary Interpretations of Ancient Formulas* by Ding Xue-Ping; *Dictionary of Chinese Medicine Formulas Grouped in Categories,* edited by Duan Ku-Han; *Guide to Medical Formulas for Clinical Patterns* by Huang Rong-Zong, Chen Huan-Hong, and Wu Da-Zhen; *A New Edition of Formulas,* edited by Ni Cheng; *Chinese Medicine Treatment Strategies and Formulas* by Chen Chao-Zu; and *Elaboration of Medical Formulas,* edited by Fu Yan-Kui and You Rong-Ji.

By and large, our selection of formulas, the manner in which we have grouped them into chapters, and the sequence of chapters follow these works. The vast majority of the formulas included in this book were listed in most of our sources, although some can be found in only one or two. Where we had to choose among different formulas, our decision was governed by considerations of the utility of a certain formula in the clinic, or its value in illuminating an important aspect of traditional Chinese medicine.

Compared to the first edition of this book, we discuss a significantly larger number of principal formulas—340 compared to 254—along with around 460 variations and associated formulas, for a total of about 800 formulas. This moves the current edition closer to the best contemporary Chinese reference books and away from simple textbooks. However, we have maintained the original organization of grouping formulas into principal and secondary formulas to make the amount of information provided more manageable. Some formulas have been moved to different chapters in the current edition; for instance, Jade Windscreen Powder (*yù píng fēng sǎn*), which was previously listed as an astringent formula, is now included in the chapter on qi-tonifying formulas. This reflects changes in some contemporary Chinese textbooks, but also shows that there is more than one way of doing things. Finally, the sequence of chapters has also been rearranged from the first edition to bring it in line with our main source texts.

In writing the commentary sections for each formula, we have drawn on a far wider range of sources. These include the source texts, all of the major works in the commentarial tradition of formulas, and the contemporary literature. In order to avoid adding even more words to what is already a very large text, we have not provided individual references, as would be the practice in a strictly scholarly work. We have, however, attributed all ideas to their sources and it would not be too difficult for anyone wishing to do so to trace these in the originals. In addition to the list of cited sources in Appendix III, and the bibliography of modern sources in Appendix IV, a bibliography of premodern texts that we consulted in writing the commentary sections can be found on the Resources page of the Eastland Press website (*www. eastlandpress.com*).

Another significant change from the first edition is the importance we have accorded to non-Chinese sources, specifically those from Japan. There are several reasons for this. First, Japanese and Korean interpretations of Chinese medicine are becoming increasingly popular in the West. Second, these interpretations often provide useful information regarding the use of specific formulas in clinical practice, so much so that it has become openly integrated once more into the practices of leading Chinese physicians. In fact, in compiling this information we have drawn on both primary sources and Chinese language secondary texts. Third, while only about a dozen of the formulas in our book originated outside of China, many of the remainder are currently not that popular in China but are very commonly used in Korea or Japan as well as in some Western countries.

We have attempted in this book to provide a clear, readable translation that is faithful both to the spirit of the medicine and the realities of the clinic. This goal is an elusive one, and the best that we can hope is that we have come closer to reaching it. In the meantime, we appreciate the reader's patience.

Technical terms have been translated literally in most cases, as this generally gives the best sense of the word. For example, we use 'sudden turmoil disorder' for 霍亂 *huò luàn,* instead of the 'cholera,' not only because it is more historically accurate, but also because it gives a better sense of what the disorder is about. On the other hand, for some disorders, there appears to us to be no alternative to translating them by reference to semi-equivalent biomedical diseases, for example, 'dysenteric disorder' for 痢疾 *lì jí.* The translation of symptoms and traditional disorders also requires a flexible approach that is both faithful to the original and accessible to the practitioner. We usually translate these literally, but have sometimes felt obliged to perhaps overtranslate in order to make the meaning as clear as possible. One example is 'frigid extremities' instead of 'four rebellions' for the term 四逆 *sì nì.* This is often a question of taste for which there is no one right approach. We have included the Chinese for most problematic technical terms in the text for the purpose of making cross reference easier. For readers who would like to find out more about our choices of terminology, the present Eastland Press draft glossary is available on the Resources page of our website at *www.eastlandpress.com.*

The only significant change in terminology between this book and the most recent edition of *Chinese Herbal Medicine: Materia Medica* is our translation of 六經 *liù jīng* as 'six warps' rather than 'six stages.' In the context of the cold damage (傷寒 *shāng hán*) approach to medicine, the term 經 *jīng* refers to the six main categories of a disorder. Although rendering 經 *jīng* as 'stage' captures the temporal nature of cold damage disorders associated with the concept of transmission (傳 *chuán*), it simultaneously de-emphasizes the other meanings associated with the Chinese term. These include the location of the disorder in specific areas of the body, the association of these with the six main channel systems, and the idea of a constancy of reaction that may be related to a pathogen getting stuck somewhere, or even to a person's constitution or type. We believe that these multiple connotations of 經 *jīng* are better captured by its original meaning in Chinese, which is that of a warp in a loom. The silk threads of the warp provide the basic structure around which a textile is woven, just as the 六經 *liù jīng* provide the basic framework for all cold damage disorders, as well as the organization of the healthy body.

We have put much thought and work into making this book accessible and useful for both students and practitioners. This has involved making many choices, not only relating to presentation, but also to the selection and organization of content. Indeed, for us, one of the most important aspects of writing and editing this book has been to bring clarity about these choices and why they were made. As clinicians and scholars, we could not avoid, for instance, having opinions about some of the issues raised among commentators. Yet we decided to do our best not to add our own voices to the existing commentary. And yet even the manner in which the commentary section has been written and organized is, nevertheless, also a kind of commentary. There exists, in fact, no way in which one might avoid taking up some kind of position in the writing of a text such as this. Even the decision to translate a particular Chinese text implies a choice for disseminating the position taken by that text over another one that is not included. We thus do not claim to present to our readers the definitive understanding of Chinese medical knowledge on formulas and strategies. All we can claim to have done is to provide what we hope is a useful and interesting tool with which to gain a better understanding of this knowledge and its utilization in contemporary clinical practice.

We have profited enormously from the time and talents of many different people in completing this book. First and foremost are the many Chinese and other East Asian scholars and practitioners through the ages on whose works we draw and whose words we are privileged to translate for an English-speaking audience.

Several people contributed their technical expertise to this project. We would like to thank our colleagues Charles Chace, James Flowers, Craig Mitchell, and Wang Kui for their helpful criticism of the manuscript. Michael Fitzgerald helped us with the alternate names of the formulas. Whenever we had a question about the materia medica, Erich Stöger graciously answered them. Anne Harper, with the assistance of Cyong Jong-Chol, contributed the majority of the background information for the section on Japanese herbal medicine in the introduction. Prof. Kenji Watanabe of Keio University, Tokyo, was always at hand when we needed to know something we could not find in our sources. Professor Makoto Mayanagi, Shinjiro Kanazawa, and David Engstrom graciously helped us with the *romanji* and other aspects of our work, and Nigel Dawes helped fill in some of the other lacunae in our knowledge of herbal medicine in Japan. Soyoung Suh was kind enough to write the section in the introduction on herbal medicine and formulas in Korea. All errors in this book are due to our own deficiencies and limitations.

We deeply appreciate the patience and enthusiasm of our students who helped us on this project, particularly Mary Beddoe, who contributed to this work in many ways. Engaged and interested students are the primary audience that makes our work in this area worthwhile. We would also like to acknowledge the editorial skill of John O'Connor at Eastland Press, who made this book as clear and understandable as possible, along with contributions from Louis Poncz. We also appreciate the proofreading by Lilian Bensky and James Flowers.

Volker would especially like to thank all of the students he has been privileged to teach over the years. They have provided him with the space to explore the often contradictory interpretations of many formulas, and through their patience and questioning, to develop his own understanding. He is indebted to both Dan Bensky and Andy Ellis for their scholarship, persistence, and team spirit despite the distances involved, and for keeping him on the straight and narrow throughout. Most of all he says thank you to Cinzia for her love and support.

Dan would like to thank Volker and Andy for taking this book to another level and having a good time doing it. He also thanks Lilian for her tireless love and support, and expresses his appreciation for the patience of just about everyone he has known during this long project, particularly his patients.

Andy would like to thank Dan and Volker for inviting him to participate in such a rewarding project and for their patience and camaraderie during the process. He would also like to acknowledge his family, Sheng-Jing, Sara, Rebeca, and Jesse, for allowing him to trade many of his family responsibilities for time spent on this book. Thanks also go to Barbara Seymour for entering all of Andy's scribble into Word so many years ago.

Randall would like to thank all the healing teachers over the years for sharing their collective insights, guidance, and generous care and affection, which remains a blessing and inspiration. Much gratitude to Ted Kaptchuk for care and introductions, to Dan Bensky for the invitation to be a part of the original work and its continuing creation, to John O'Connor for keeping the channels open, and for Volker and Andy's important contributions to the new edition.

How to Use this Book

THIS BOOK IS designed for both students and practitioners of Chinese herbal medicine. However, each group will use the book in a different way. Students can use it as a textbook in conjunction with lectures to learn the basics about herbal formulas. Practitioners, on the other hand, are more likely to use it as a reference for finding particular formulas in the clinic. For this reason, we have tried as much as possible to make each formula stand on its own. Nevertheless, we still recommend that practitioners read at least the introduction to the chapter and section in which any given formula appears.

The discussion of each of the over 340 principal formulas in the book is divided into ten sections or categories. The 'core' sections are concerned with the most basic information about the formula: its name, source, ingredients, method of preparation, actions, indications, and an analysis of how the individual ingredients fit together in the formula. Students will primarily be concerned with these aspects of the formulas, and we therefore suggest that they read these sections carefully to prepare for class. The remaining sections will likely be of more interest to experienced practitioners: commentary, cautions and contraindications, and modifications. In addition, information about related or secondary formulas is provided in over 460 variations and associated formulas.

Like all other aspects of Chinese medicine, formulas and strategies undergo constant change and transformation. This holds true for every aspect outlined in this book, from formula names to ingredients, from methods of preparation to debates about indications, usage, and formula composition.

The authors and editors of contemporary Chinese medicine textbooks on formulas—most of which use the name *Formulas* (方劑學 *fāng jì xué)* as their title—have done an admirable job in collating this material, sorting through different interpretations, and providing their readers with relatively clear descriptions of indications and actions. At the same time, from a historical perspective, such editing constitutes one aspect of the state-directed process of modernization that has shaped the development of Chinese medicine in the late 20th and early 21st centuries. It thus adds merely one more interpretation to the many other interpretations that already exist. In the best Chinese texts, readers are able to compare such interpretations by adding to the discussion of formulas extensive sections from source texts. If we had followed this practice, an already large text would have doubled or even tripled in size. We have attempted to resolve this dilemma by adhering to modern formula textbooks from mainland China in the description of actions, indications, and analysis of formula composition. In the commentary section, on the other hand, we present a historically-informed account that places each formula in the context of its original usage, charts changes of usage over time, and presents commentaries with many citations to original sources.

We wish to remind readers that the subject of this book is herbal formulas, and that it is not intended as a substitute for learning other aspects of traditional Chinese medicine. One should not assume that he or she can competently treat a patient by simply prescribing a formula from this book. The information in these pages will only be useful to a practitioner who has a good foundation in traditional theory and practice. Moreover, accurate diagnosis is of paramount importance. Should you experience less than optimal success in treating a patient, first review the diagnosis.

Below is a discussion of the information contained under each of the headings in this book.

NAME: The name of each formula is provided in Chinese (both regular and simplified characters, when there is a difference), English, and *pinyin* transliteration. Where the formula is known by more than one name in Chinese, we have chosen the name that is most frequently used in our sources. Where the meaning of the name is not obvious, we have included a brief section that explains its derivation, to the best of our abilities.

Translating the name of a formula can be difficult because there sometimes exist several acceptable solutions. Bearing in mind that this book is a reference text, our choices reflect as closely as possible the meaning and syntax of the original Chinese. Where a plant is part of the name, we used the most common English name from the companion text, *Chinese Herbal Medicine: Materia Medica*. The part of the plant is noted only if more than one part of the plant is commonly used in Chinese medicine and is specified in the name. For example, because both the fruit and leaves of perilla are commonly used, we translate *su zi jiang qi tang* as Perilla Fruit Decoction for Directing Qi Downward.

Where our understanding has grown, we have revamped and changed some of the names of the formulas that were listed in the first edition of this book. Where there is a difference, a cross reference to those names is posted in the Resources section of the Eastland Press website at *www.eastlandpress.com*. In addition, many readers will not be familiar with our translations of the formula names, so we have included, in Appendix 2 to this book, a *pinyin* to English cross reference of the formula names.

SOURCE: This is the title of the book in which the formula, as it is presently recognized, was first described. Generally speaking, this would be a book authored by the composer of the formula or his disciples, but in some cases is a compilation of the formulas of many practitioners, past and present. Those readers seeking more information about the source texts are referred to the List of Cited Sources in Appendix 3 to this book. This includes the characters of the book titles as well as the authors and dates of publication.

INGREDIENTS: In this section we have used, as much as possible, the original name and dosage of each of the substances in the formula. We have usually taken the liberty of translating measurements that were expressed in terms of volume or number of pieces into comparable weights, while also providing the original terms of measurement. This is because measurement by weight is now the form of measurement used by pharmacies and other vendors for most medicinal substances. Where the source text did not identify the particular substance in the manner in which it is now identified (e.g., Paeoniae Radix *[sháo yào]*, we have followed the original. We feel this is important, as it gives readers a sense of the original formula. When there is a discrepancy between the original dosages and those that are commonly used at present, we have added the latter in brackets. We have also included any preparations of the ingredients noted in the source texts that are still commonly used today. Regarding the import of these preparations, see *Chinese Herbal Medicine: Materia Medica*.

METHOD OF PREPARATION: This section describes the practical aspects of preparing the formula. When the common form of decoction is used, no special instructions are provided. (The reader is referred to the introduction for additional information about decoctions.) When there is a significant difference between the original ingredients, dosage, or method of preparation and those used at present, it will be noted in this section. It is not unusual that, while the original formulation was a pill or a powder, the more common method of preparation at present is a decoction. In such cases, we usually refer to the change by noting that the ingredients should be used with an appropriate reduction in dosage. We do not include the original method of preparation when it was extremely complex and no longer used; nor do we usually include any industrial methodology for making pills. If you are unfamiliar with the normal range of dosage for a particular substance, we suggest that you consult our companion volume, *Chinese Herbal Medicine: Materia Medica*.

ACTIONS: These are the strategies embodied by the formulas as defined in modern textbooks from mainland China. They represent the link between the clinical indications and the ingredients according to mainstream contemporary Chinese medicine.

INDICATIONS: These are the signs and symptoms of the condition for which the formula is indicated. Such constellations of signs and symptoms constitute what is known as a pattern or syndrome (證 *zhèng*) in Chinese medicine. Sometimes a formula may treat more than one pattern. This may be because the same pathodynamic may manifest with different patterns, or because the formula is capable of addressing a variety of different pathodynamics.

The information provided in this section is what one generally finds in contemporary formula textbooks. This may be drawn from the source text or a later interpretation, but in any case will correspond to mainstream contemporary usage in mainland China. Following a list of the signs and symptoms is an explanation of what this information tells you about the patient, that is, how and why the diagnosis fits this presentation. Occasionally, there is a discussion of how a patient develops this type of problem. The importance of this information is that it allows the reader to grasp the essence of the pathodynamic(s) underlying the disorder and the resulting formation of patterns. With this understanding, the formula can be used to treat a wide variety of problems.

There is a considerable difference among the formulas with respect to the amount of information provided about the indications. Sometimes there is very little information, and sometimes it is quite comprehensive. These differences are reflected in almost all of the source texts. When little information could be found in our principal sources, we turned to supplementary works to flesh out the indications and discussion. However, we refrained from adding anything of our own to the signs and symptoms. No matter how scanty the information in this section appears, it should be enough to use the formula responsibly.

ANALYSIS OF FORMULA: This section discusses the makeup of the formula, that is, why particular substances were chosen to treat the disorder for which the formula is indicated. The discussion is arranged in accordance with the hierarchy of the ingredients, starting with the chief ingredients and working down to the envoys. It should be apparent to the reader that the relationships among the constituent ingredients are quite complex, and that the formulation of the whole is more than merely the sum of the ingredients' individual functions or actions. Some actions will only occur when particular ingredients are combined. This information supplements the basic information about the functions of individual substances found in materia medica textbooks, and should be particularly helpful to students seeking a greater understanding of the materia medica.

For a considerable number of formulas in this book there exists no consensus as to which herbs occupy which role or function in the formula. In these cases, we have selected what appeared to us to be the most sensible contemporary interpretation, and recorded different views in the commentary.

CAUTIONS AND CONTRAINDICATIONS: This section provides cautionary advice about using the formulas. We have generally omitted advice from our sources that we believe to be self-evident, for example, a formula for treating a heat-induced disorder should not be used for treating a cold-induced disorder. Obviously, the cautionary advice in this section is not the *only* thing to be concerned about when prescribing the formula, but is certainly worth bearing in mind.

COMMENTARY: Contributions to this section, which have been considerably expanded from the first edition of this book, fulfill different yet integrated functions. They deepen the reader's understanding of a formula's genealogy, provide an overview of debates regarding composition, usage, or other controversial issues, describe expansion of usage, and list key clinical pointers to facilitate use of the formula in contemporary practice.

As outlined above, the information presented in most other sections such as actions, indications, and analysis corresponds to what is available in mainstream formularies in mainland China today. These formularies, in turn, provide the foundation of what is taught about formulas in Chinese and Western schools, colleges, and universities of Chinese medicine. The way this knowledge is presented ties in seamlessly with other key subjects in the Chinese medicine curriculum today, from basic theory to diagnosis and internal medicine. For instance, patterns and treatment strategies are, wherever possible, linked to the dysfunction of organ systems or otherwise integrated into the mainstream understandings of physiology and pathology as taught in Chinese medical schools. The systematic and integrated nature of this presentation facilitates learning and has contributed greatly to the dissemination of Chinese medicine around the world. At the same time, however, it is best viewed not as an end point in the linear development of the Chinese medical tradition, but rather as yet another layer of interpretation in the many layers that already exist and on which it builds.

At times, such interpretations radically change a formula's usage. At other times, they extend it in new directions. Yet again, interpreters may agree on indications but offer radically different views regarding a formula's mode of action or composition. Subsequent layers of interpretation may help us better understand earlier ones. They may also, however, obscure the intentions of the original author and make it more difficult to effectively use the formula. One example would be when, for the sake of fitting into a system, a formula that helps emotional constraint is described as resolving Liver qi stagnation yet contains no herbs that enter the Liver channel. Another example would be when a formula for the treatment of night sweats is said to tonify the yin (because nights sweats are supposedly due to yin deficiency), but in terms of its composition mainly focuses on the qi. In cases like these, to use the formula effectively it is very helpful to understand it on its own terms.

The task we set ourselves in this section, therefore, was that of an archeology that would allow readers with no access to original Chinese sources to see how layers of interpretation build up over the course of a formula's long history. Because this is first and foremost a book for clinicians, we have aimed to focus only on those discussions and debates that are immediately relevant to clinical practice. We generally present these in the form of a narrative interspersed with quotations from original sources. Our intention in doing so was to create a text that is readily accessible yet still provides some of the flavor of the language in which Chinese physicians and scholars have given voice to their ideas over time. To keep the narrative flowing, we naturally had to be selective in our quotations. However, we believe that we have captured for each formula the main arguments, disputes, and contested issues.

In order to counterbalance the dispersing tendency of controversy and debate (which leaves especially students and beginners wondering which view, if any, makes sense), we have added wherever possible clinical pointers drawn from the literature that should help the reader select formulas for given patterns. This is further facilitated by the next section, that of comparisons.

COMPARISONS: This is a new section added to the 2nd edition that is intended to help students and practitioners focus on the distinguishing characteristics of a formula by contrasting it with other formulas that are similar in terms of composition or indication. While we have attempted to include as many of these comparisons as possible, some formulas are so distinctive that adducing comparisons was simply deemed unhelpful. Where a particularly succinct comparison could be found in the classical literature, we translated it. At other times, we have drawn on modern sources or constructed the comparisons ourselves. To avoid needlessly copying information, we have listed each comparison just once, and then provided cross references to comparisons elsewhere in the text where appropriate.

Comparative tables at the end of each chapter reinforce these comparisons by comparing formulas across a wider range.

BIOMEDICAL INDICATIONS: In most cases we have included a section that notes the biomedically-defined disorders for which the formula has been used. These were gleaned from our Chinese sources and sometimes the terminology used is inconsistent, as it is in our sources. These are not in any way meant to be all-inclusive or exclusive. Their significance simply lies in showing that, depending on the presentation, not only can a single formula be used for treating a variety of biomedically-defined disorders, but each disorder can be treated by a variety of formulas.

ALTERNATIVE NAMES: Standardization and systematization only occur where institutions exist that are sufficiently powerful to enforce them. For most of the history of Chinese medicine this has not been the case. As a result, many formulas exist under different names. Alternatively, the same name may be used for formulas that contain very different ingredients and have different indications. Today some of these names are only of historical interest, although even then a formula's other names may open up new windows on their intended usage or the effects that physicians attrib-

uted to it over time. Sometimes, even today a formula might be known by several different names. This section lists the alternative names of each formula and the texts in which they first occur.

MODIFICATIONS: In Chinese medicine it is very important that the practitioner adjust or fine tune the formula to the specific requirements of the patient. The modifications provided in this section are examples taken from our sources that illustrate how this can be done. There are many different ways in which a formula can be modified, and such differences reflect the experiences and viewpoints of the individual practitioners. To make the information in this section more accessible, we have generally arranged the modifications in the following order: 1) those that accommodate changes in the symptoms; 2) those that combine the principal formula with other formulas; and 3) those that focus the formula on treating a biomedically-defined disorder.

VARIATIONS: Sometimes merely adding or subtracting a few ingredients in a formula will change it enough to warrant a different name. This type of modification is called a variation. The dosage of the remaining ingredients, and the method of preparation, are basically the same as those of the principal formula. The dosage of the additional ingredients is also in line with those of the ingredients in the principal formula. For this reason, only the names of the additional ingredients are identified, together with the name of the formula and its source.

ASSOCIATED FORMULAS: These are formulas that are related to the principal formulas either because they contain many of the same ingredients, or because they are used in treating similar disorders. However, their differences with the principal formulas are more pronounced than is the case with variations. At the very least, the dosage of ingredients or method of preparation is quite different from the principal formula with which each it is associated. Thus, we often compare them with their principal formulas.

APPENDICES: At the back of the book are a number of appendices to assist the reader in understanding and using the material in this book. Appendix 1 is a guide to the *pinyin* transliteration system. This will help the reader pronounce the names of the formulas. Appendix 2 is the *pinyin* to English cross reference of formula names. Appendix 3 is a list of sources cited in the text, which provides basic information about our sources. Appendix 4 is a bibliography of modern sources. And Appendix 5 is a formulary of symptoms and disorders, a summary table of the various disorders treated by the formulas in this book. Arranged alphabetically by symptom and disorder, it is designed to serve as a handy shortcut for finding an appropriate formula. However, this is intended only as a starting point and reference; it is no substitute for a firm grounding in internal medicine.

INDICES: At the very back of the book are two indices. The first is for the formulas themselves while the second is a general index.

WEB RESOURCES: In order to make the book easier to handle, we have put some of the reference material on the web. This includes the bibliography of premodern sources, a cross reference of formula names that have changed from the first to the second edition of this book, and a Japanese-English cross reference of formula names. All of these files are in the Resource section of our publisher's website, *www. eastlandpress.com.*

Introduction

IN CHINESE THE term meaning formulas (also known as prescriptions or recipes) consists of two words, 方劑 *fāng jì*. Since the Han and pre-Han eras these words have referred to separate but complementary aspects of medical as well as other types of practices. The word 方 *fāng* generally refers to the technique in an abstract or written form, and most commonly to the written recipe. The word 劑 *jì* generally refers to the practice of the technique itself, that is, the act of preparing and administering the written recipe. Thus, *fāng jì* are formulas that are put into practice, and not merely concepts or intellectual exercises. It is this functional aspect of the formulas that is at the heart of traditional Chinese herbal medicine.

The process of treating disease in traditional Chinese medicine is defined as differentiating patterns and determining treatment (辨證論治 *biàn zhèng lùn zhì*). As an integral part of this process, the formulas are specific groupings or configurations of medicinal substances that serve as tools for instituting treatment. The focus of this book is understanding how the particular configurations of substances in the formulas work together to effectively treat disease. This introduction will explain the relationship between the traditional descriptions of pathological conditions in Chinese medicine (i.e., the patterns of disharmony) and the strategies or methods underlying the formulas that treat them.

In the 1930s, the scholar-physician Xie Guan in *On the Origins and Development of Medicine in China* summed up the nature of the practice of Chinese medicine in four terms: principles, strategies, formulas, and medicinals (理法方藥 *lǐ fǎ fāng yào*). This means that once one identifies the pathodynamic principles underlying the patient's problem, the strategy of treatment, the formula that incorporates that strategy, and the specific herbs that constitute the formula for that particular patient will naturally follow. Conversely, the pattern of disharmony itself can be defined in terms of the treatment strategy, and, even more precisely, by the formula used to treat it. In other words, it is often possible to diagnose a pattern via a formula (辨方 *biàn fāng*). This identification of a formula with a particular disorder dates back at least to the 3rd-century classic, *Discussion of Cold Damage*. As we shall see below, since the very beginning, a thorough understanding of the formulas has been essential to the practice of traditional Chinese herbal medicine.

A BRIEF HISTORY OF HERBAL FORMULAS IN CHINA

Like all other aspects of the Chinese medical tradition, the art of formulas has developed and changed through history and continues to do so today. While it is common in medical texts to interpret such development in purely naturalist terms (i.e., as a response to newly-occurring diseases or to the gradual accumulation of experience), historical and ethnographic research reveals a more complex interplay of social, cultural, economic, political, technological, and epidemiological factors. If, at different times in the history of Chinese medicine, or at different places, physicians used formulas with more or less ingredients, with higher or lower dosages, emphasized

Zhou 周	1066–221 B.C.E.
Warring States 戰國	475–221 B.C.E.
Qin 秦	221–206 B.C.E.
Western (Former) Han 西漢	206 B.C.E.–23 C.E.
Eastern (Later) Han 東漢	25–220
Three Kingdoms 三國	220–280
Jin 晉	265–420
North and South Kingdoms 南北朝	420–589
Sui 隋	589–618
Tang 唐	618–907
Five Dynasties 五代	907–960
Song 宋	960–1279
Southern Song 南宋	1127–1279
Jin 金	1115–1234
Yuan 元	1279–1368
Ming 明	1368–1644
Qing 清	1644–1911

Table 1 Chinese Dynasties

adherence to classical precedent or pushed for innovation, then the precise reasons for these differences require careful examination of the context of practice that goes well beyond the scope of what is possible, or indeed necessary, in this book.

Nevertheless, each formula does have its own history. It was composed at a certain time for a specific purpose, and its composition was guided by certain ideas about the nature of pathology, treatment strategy, and formula composition. Later physicians often reinterpreted the formula in the light of their own context of practice, or according to different ideas about illness causation and treatment. Sometimes these changes were discussed explicitly, sometimes not. An older usage might continue to exist side-by-side with newer ones, or it might be completely forgotten. In the COMMENTARY section of most formulas we have tried to briefly outline the history of the formula in order to facilitate its use in the clinic. In this introduction, by contrast, we will briefly focus on the history of Chinese medicine at large insofar as it relates to the development of formulas.

Qin and Han Dynasties
(3rd Century B.C.E. to 3rd Century C.E.)

Among the earliest of the Chinese formularies extant are those found among the silk manuscripts in the Mawangdui tomb in Hunan, originally sealed in 168 B.C.E. and discovered in the early 1970s. This tomb contained the mummified body of an aristocratic woman, many household items, and a number of manuscripts on both silk and bamboo. Among these were several medical texts.

One of these texts, named *Prescriptions for Fifty-Two Ailments* (五十二病方 *Wǔ shí èr bìng fāng*) by its discoverers, is a silk manuscript. While it cites various methods of treatment including moxibustion, cupping, massage, and internal and external applications of herbs, the use of herbs is paramount. The format of the text is straight forward: a disorder is listed and the treatment is given. No theoretical discussions are found. This leaves us to surmise that either the author assumed that the reader would understand the medical theories underlying the treatments or that the treatments themselves were simply pragmatic, with no particular theoretical underpinnings. The following excerpt from *Prescriptions for Fifty-Two Ailments* is more detailed than many sections, but does provide us with an idea of one aspect of medical practice during the Western Han:

> Deep-lying abscess disease, treat [with] Ampelopsis Radix (*bái liàn*), Astragali Radix (*huáng qí*), Paeoniae Radix (*sháo yào*), Cinnamomi Cortex (*ròu guì*), Zingiberis Rhizoma (*shēng jiāng*) [may be fresh or dried], Zanthoxyli Pericarpium (*huā jiāo*), and Evodiae Fructus (*wú zhū yú*), these seven items. For bone abscess, double the Ampelopsis Radix (*bái liàn*). For flesh abscess, double the Astragali Radix (*huáng qí*), and for Kidney abscess, double the Paeoniae Radix (*sháo yào*)…

The use of pungent, warm herbs to treat a deep-lying abscess is consistent with treatment methods found in later eras. This parallel, along with the manner in which the formula is modified based on the depth of the abscess, can be seen as implying an underlying strategy and theoretical assumptions similar to those found in medical literature of the Eastern Han, though no details are provided. The formulas themselves are not given names and are very simple in structure. The nature of the text is quite shamanistic and includes incantations and exorcistic practices. Many of the formulas have a distinct air of sympathetic magic. The text does contain rather specific instructions for preparing the formulas, among which are decoctions, drafts, and pills.

The other medical texts found in this tomb deal with various aspects of Chinese medicine. While some of them can be clearly related to later classics, there are obvious differences, some of which are difficult to explain. For example, one text, named *Moxibustion Classic of the Eleven Vessels of the Foot and Arm* (足臂十一脈灸經 *Zú bì shí yī mài jiǔ jīng*), describes eleven vessels that are similar in the course of their pathways and associated symptoms to those described in the *Inner Classic*. Yet the symptoms in the Mawangdui text relate directly to the pathways of the vessels, with no mention of either acupuncture or acupuncture points. This is quite different from the *Inner Classic*, which often relates symptoms of the vessels to systemic issues, and also discusses acupuncture points and needles at some length. While it is clear that these archeological treasures are important in aiding our understanding of the foundations of Chinese medicine, they also make it clear that the early stages of this medicine contained many currents of practice and lacked a straightforward A-B transmission of information from that period.

The contents of the Mawangdui tombs, as well as other recently excavated Western Han tombs, contribute to the idea that Chinese culture during this period was one that supported artisans and craftspeople and encouraged intellectual exchange. It would appear that rationality in medical thought became more prominent during this period, although shamanistic aspects continued, as they do to the present day.

This rationalism continues in the writings that comprise the *Inner Classic,* which is now believed to have been primarily compiled during the Eastern Han, as well as in the theories that appear to underpin the clinically oriented writings of Zhang Zhong-Jing, such as *Discussion of Cold Damage.*

Another recently excavated set of medical texts, thought to date from the first century C.E., is known as *Han Dynasty Medical Bamboo Strips from Wuwei* (武威漢代醫簡 *Wǔwēi Hàn dài yī jiǎn).* This is more developed than *Prescriptions for Fifty-Two Ailments,* and certain aspects resemble the works of Zhang Zhong-Jing, although it is not nearly as organized or detailed as his writings. It contains decoctions, pills, powders, syrups, and many external applications as well.

By the time of the *Yellow Emperor's Inner Classic,* which is comprised of *Basic Questions* and *Divine Pivot,* the theoretical foundations of traditional Chinese medicine were in place. In terms of therapeutic techniques, this text is almost exclusively concerned with acupuncture. Thirteen formulas are described, one of which is noted in our text. More importantly for our purposes, there is an outline of the rudiments of a therapeutic strategy that is based on the tastes of the substances. For example, in Chapter 22 of *Basic Questions* there is a discussion about the actions of the different tastes: "Acrid [taste] disperses, sour retains, sweet moderates, bitter strengthens, and salty softens."

In addition, many of the basic treatment strategies that have since become medical adages, for example, "For fire from constraint, discharge it", can be traced back to discussions in Chapters 71 or 74 of *Basic Questions.* While it is generally agreed that these chapters were added to the text in the 7th century by Wang Bing, they were probably written during the Eastern Han dynasty and so are reflective of that era's medical thought. By the Jin-Yuan period a thousand years later, these statements had come to be accepted as the foundation of treatment strategies. It is during this period, too, that the theories of the *Inner Classic* began to be more

fully integrated into the practice of herbal medicine.

The true ancestor of all formularies is the *Discussion of Cold Damage and Miscellaneous Diseases,* written at the end of the Eastern Han dynasty by Zhang Zhong-Jing. This book was edited about 50 years later by Wang Shu-He, author of the *Pulse Classic.* In the course of his editing, Wang divided the book into two parts: *Discussion of Cold Damage,* which deals with externally-contracted diseases, and *Essentials from the Golden Cabinet,* which is primarily concerned with internally-generated disorders. While the principles of the five phases are not of primary importance in these works, there is a detailed system of diagnosis in *Discussion of Cold Damage* that focuses on the six warps (or stages) of disease, and a well-developed taxonomy of disease in *Essentials from the Golden Cabinet.* In addition, each of the formulas is given a name, and the dosage and method of preparation of the herbs are specifically described. These books have had a tremendous influence on Chinese herbal medicine, and on traditional medicine throughout East Asia, to the present day. In fact, over 150 (about one-quarter) of the formulas in our book, which were selected from texts written during the past 1,800 years, are drawn directly from these works by Zhang Zhong-Jing. They are far and away the greatest single source of formulas in traditional Chinese medicine.

Zhang, who described himself primarily as a collector rather than as a composer of formulas, was the first person we know of to identify the condition of a patient (the diagnosis) with a particular formula used to treat that condition. In other words, the name of the formula itself is another way of expressing the diagnosis. For example, instead of saying that a patient is suffering from a lesser yang pattern, one could also describe it as a Minor Bupleurum Decoction *(xiǎo chái hú tāng)* pattern. Note that while Zhang's works did not have wide-spread influence until the Song period, they remain extremely influential today.

Jin, Sui, and Tang Dynasties (3rd to 10th Centuries)

The most important formulary of the Jin dynasty was written by Ge Hong and is entitled *Emergency Formulas to Keep Up One's Sleeve.* This book features the use of simple and inexpensive, yet effective, formulas. A very important medical work of the early 7th century is the encyclopedic *Discussion of the Origins of the Symptoms of Disease.* This work, which describes the etiology, pathodynamic, and natural history of over 1,700 symptoms and disorders, had a great impact on the physicians of the Tang dynasty, even though it did not often discuss treatment directly (see Timeline 1 on page *xlix).*

The leading medical figure of the Tang dynasty was Sun Si-Miao. His two books, *Important Formulas Worth a Thousand Gold Pieces* and *Supplement to Important Formulas Worth a Thousand Gold Pieces,* have had a major impact on later generations of physicians. Many of the formulas in these books are still in use (ten are included in our text), and many other commonly-used formulas are variations on those which were first devised by him. Later in the eighth century, Wang Tao compiled *Arcane Essentials from the Imperial Library,* which is based on previously-published Chinese works as well as some foreign texts. Wang categorized the formulas according to the type of disorder they were designed to treat. Eleven of these formulas are included in our text.

All of these works are notable for the sheer volume of formulas they contain, and the relative lack of discrimination. In part this is due to the fact that they are compilations, and in part because a certain level of knowledge was presumed of the readers. This is an era of medical proliferation on many levels. The focus of treatments were diseases (病 *bìng*) rather than patterns (證 *zhèng),* of which there were hundreds, and in these texts under each disease up to 20 formulas could be listed, without any indication as to which of them is most effective in a particular situation. Furthermore, many of the formulas from this era contained a large number of herbs. And even at this date there were many competing currents of thought, some of which disparaged what they saw as loosely constructed formulas in the service of an overly symptomatic treatment. For example, the early Tang-dynasty physician Xu Yin-Zong wrote:

> Nowadays people are unable to differentiate the pulses, nor do they recognize the origins of disease. They base decisions on their feelings and use many medicinal substances. This is like hunting for rabbits by sending out many men and horses to surround the area in the hope that, by luck, one of them will stumble upon the rabbit. Treating like this is really negligent.

Measures that moved herbal medicine in a more systematic direction began to appear at this time. One aspect of reform, which did not really pick up steam until much later, was the categorization of substances and formulas. This was first done by the 8th-century writer Chen Cang-Qi in *Omissions from the [Classic of the] Materia Medica.* Chen's system of categorization later came to be known as the ten types of formulas (十劑 *shí jì).*

Song, Jin, and Yuan Dynasties (10th to 14th Centuries)

This period was one of intense turmoil in China, politically, socially, and economically. As part of the process of growth in state power, literacy, trade and industry, and the rise of educated officialdom (versus the largely hereditary aristocracies of previous periods), the state, perhaps for the first time in the world, took a strong interest in the organization and practice of medicine. It was during this period that all aspects of Chinese culture, including medicine, were both catalogued and reexamined. Of at least equal importance, this era marked the ascendancy (in terms of the written

record) of the scholar-physicians who compiled formularies and other medical texts and then began adapting medicine to their own needs. In the northern Song dynasty a state dispensary was established and compilations of formulas and other medical texts were published under imperial auspices. The most famous of these, *Formulary of the Pharmacy Service for Benefiting the People in the Taiping Era,* was compiled between 1078 and 1107. This book contains 16,834 entries, approximately 40 of which are included in our book (see Timeline 2, page *l*).

The compilation of formularies containing great numbers of formulas had many consequences. The plethora of formulas for different complaints had a tendency to stretch or even break the connection between the formulas and the theoretical understanding of the conditions for which they were indicated. This encouraged the practice of symptomatic medicine in which there was no theoretical structure to enable the practitioner to adapt and fine tune the formulas for a particular patient. It also led to some confusion, as more than one formula often shared the same name.

During the latter part of the 12th century, an attempt was made to correct this tendency by devising schemes that would help make disease processes more understandable, and methods of treatment more practical, yet still grounded in theory. This consisted of refining and simplifying the theoretical understanding of disease and its treatment. For example, in *Extension of the Materia Medica,* Kou Zong-Shi devised a system of categories called the 'eight essentials' (八 要 *bā yào)* into which the various aspects and stages in the progression of disease could be placed. These included deficiency, excess, cold, heat, pathogenic (qi), normal (qi), internal, and external. In a similar vein, Chen Yan, in *Discussion of Illnesses, Patterns, and Formulas Related to the Unification of the Three Etiologies,* classified the causes of disease into three categories: internally-generated, externally-generated, and miscellaneous.

This shift toward a more rational and systematic understanding of herbal therapeutics in general, and formulas in particular, was representative of the ferment in medicine that occurred during the Jin and Yuan dynasties. For example, Zhang Yuan-Su in *Pouch of Pearls* was the first to discuss the concept of herbs entering specific channels as a means of understanding and classifying their functions.

This period came to be viewed as pivotal in the development of Chinese medicine as several currents of thought emerged, centered around four great figures. Each current emphasized a particular etiology of disease and its corresponding strategy of treatment. These were the cooling current (寒涼派 *hán liáng pài*) of Liu Wan-Su; the purging current (攻下派 *gōng xià pài)* of Zhang Cong-Zheng; the earth-tonifying current (補土派 *bǔ tǔ pài)* of one of Zhang Yuan-Su's students, Li Dong-Yuan (also known as Li Gao);

and the yin-enriching current (滋陰派 *zī yīn pài*) of Zhu Dan-Xi (also known as Zhu Zhen-Heng). Each of these currents made a significant contribution to the literature on formulas, especially the latter two because of their bias toward tonification. In our book, approximately seven formulas are attributed to Liu Wan-Su, five to Zhang Cong-Zheng, 30 to Li Gao, and 14 to Zhu Zhen-Heng. Many other formulas were composed by disciples of these currents.

The emergence of these currents can be attributed to a number of factors, many of them socioeconomic rather than medical in nature. As more and more scholars took up the practice of medicine, competing with each other in a competitive marketplace, associating oneself with a distinctive current bestowed both authenticity and a certain cachet to one's practice. Focusing on the treatment of distinctive organ systems, for instance, or on purgation or tonification, allowed for the definition of social groups and created distinctions among physicians. From a purely medical point of view, there were at least as many connections and overlaps among these currents as there were differences. All four of the medical masters of the Jin-Yuan period, for example, concerned themselves with the role of fire in the body and its associated pathologies; they all increasingly focused on the qi dynamic and the upward- and downward-directing actions of different herbs and formulas facilitated by Zhang Yuan-Su's innovations. For example, Zhang Yuan-Su is said to have studied with Liu Wan-Su before going on to become the teacher of Li Dong-Yuan. And not only did Zhu Dan-Xi borrow many theoretical concepts from the earth-tonifying current, he also studied with a disciple in the line of Liu Wan-Su. As the reader will see, these physician-scholars figure prominently in the COMMENTARY sections of many formulas (see Timeline 3, page *li*).

Ming and Qing Dynasties (14th to 19th Centuries)

In terms of understanding the formulas, this period was one in which the theories and achievements of the past were built upon and taken in new directions. Owing to developments in medical theory, the understanding of treatment strategies became inseparable from diagnostics. The idea that differentiation of the pattern required that the nature (cold, hot, excessive, or deficient) and location (organ, qi, or blood) of the disease be ascertained became firmly established as the basis of treatment in traditional Chinese medicine. The treatment principle is likewise based on these findings.

The impact of these developments on the practice of traditional Chinese medicine in modern times cannot be overstated. Most of the works discussed in the following section which detail the relationship between strategies and formulas date from this period, as do the major categorization schemes for the formulas. Over one-third of the formulas in our book are derived from this period in history.

One of the most influential books from the 16th century is *Restoration of Health from the Myriad Diseases* by Gong Ting-Xian, a large collection of formulas categorized by illness. In this text, Gong, who was later to become an imperial physician, combined the learning of the physicians of the Jin-Yuan period with his collected clinical experience and that of his father, the well-know physician Gong Xin. This book is still extremely important, especially to practitioners in Taiwan and Japan, and 16 of its formulas appear in our book.

Another of the important figures of this era was Wang Ken-Tang, who lived in the late 16th and early 17th centuries. In *Indispensable Tools for Pattern Treatment*, Wang developed a synthesis of the approaches of the various currents by utilizing concepts from both *Yellow Emperor's Inner Classic* and *Discussion of Cold Damage.* This book contains rather detailed differentiations of patterns. Twenty of the formulas in our book are derived from this text. Another very important figure was the early-17th-century physician Zhang Jie-Bin, also known as Zhang Jing-Yue. Zhang was a representative of the warming and tonifying current and was a great force in compiling and integrating the knowledge of previous ages. He wrote two books: *Classified Classic,* in which he organized and classified the information from *Yellow Emperor's Inner Classic,* and *Collected Treatises of [Zhang] Jing-Yue,* which covers all aspects of internal medicine. Over 20 formulas from the latter text are included in our collection. Zhang's contributions are discussed at greater length below.

The late-17th-century writer Wang Ang is another individual who had a strong influence on the course of traditional Chinese medicine. While not a practitioner himself, the books he wrote about materia medica and formulas became favorites among many clinicians for their easily-applied knowledge and systems of classification, although there are those who found his work to be too rigid. Wang's writings emphasized the relationship between medicinal substances and the organs and channels. Fifteen formulas that were first mentioned in his *Medical Formulas Collected and Analyzed* appear in our book (see Timeline 4, page *lii*).

Perhaps the most important development in traditional Chinese medicine during the Qing dynasty was the emergence of the warm pathogen disease current (溫病派 *wēn bìng pài*). Until the Ming dynasty, the treatment of externally-contracted disorders was dominated by cold-damage (傷寒 *shāng hán*) discourse. This held that all feverish disorders—even those that occurred in the summer or where chills or other signs of cold were absent—were nevertheless at their root caused by cold. While Zhang Zhong-Jing's *Discussion of Cold Damage* had provided the most influential approach to the treatment of these disorders, later physicians found it increasingly difficult to match this approach to many of the patterns they observed in their practices. From the Song onward, cold damage treatment formulas had thus been modified, and new formulas added to practitioners' repertoires, in order to deal with newly emergent disorders, particularly the epidemics that periodically swept through China. In terms of core treatment strategies, however, sweating (to resolve heat from constraint in the exterior) and draining downward (to remove clumping, knotting, and constraint of heat in the interior) continued to function as the core around which all formulas for the treatment of these problems were constructed. This is because symptoms of heat were always interpreted as arising from the transformation of more fundamental cold damage. It was only during the late Ming and early Qing that a truly new understanding of feverish diseases gradually took shape in the Yangzi River delta. This held that heat (but also other pathogens such as dryness or even miscellaneous pestilential qi) could enter the body directly, and that these pathogens required entirely new strategies of treatment. For instance, heat at the surface was now treated with cooling, toxicity-resolving, and opening formulas rather than with acrid and warming ones. Heat in the interior could require sweet, cooling treatments rather than just draining, and so forth.

The most important exponents of this new current came from Suzhou, which was then the center of Chinese cultural life. They included the 17th-century physician Wu You-Ke, who developed highly innovative theories regarding the etiology of epidemic disorders; the early-18th-century physician Ye Tian-Shi, who developed the four-level system of differentiating disease; and Ye's contemporary Xue Sheng-Bai, who is famous for an approach to the treatment of damp-warmth disorders that focuses on the Triple Burner. The late-eighteenth-century physician Wu Ju-Tong expanded on these works by developing the three-burner system of diagnosis. Over 45 formulas from his book *Systematic Differentiation of Warm Pathogen Diseases* are included in ours.

The ferment and reexamination of the medical tradition that occurred during the Qing dynasty led to the formation of two broad currents of thought: the classical formula (經方 *jīng fāng*) current and the modern formula (時方 *shí fāng*) current, although both currents can be traced back to at least the Song. 'Classical' refers to the formulas in the books of Zhang Zhong-Jing, *Discussion of Cold Damage* and *Essentials from the Golden Cabinet*. 'Modern' refers to formulas which were devised from the Song dynasty onward, and particularly those developed by practitioners of the warm pathogen disease current.

Partisans of the classical formula current believe that the formulas of Zhang Zhong-Jing are more focused in their effect because they contain fewer ingredients, each with a relatively large dosage. As long as the diagnosis is correct,

they say, these formulas will be effective. They criticize the modern formulas for being overly complicated and somewhat disorganized. They also believe that such formulas consist of so many ingredients that it is difficult to distinguish the effect of any one, or to tell whether the effect is the result of the formula as a whole. Practitioners of the modern current reply that diseases and clinical standards have changed during the 18 centuries since *Discussion of Cold Damage* was written. Trying to force modern diseases to fit the pattern of ancient ones is like trying to fit round pegs into square holes, and is doomed to failure. Not only will such formulas fail to help patients, but if they are used in the wrong circumstances, they may actually cause them serious harm. Suffice to say that both of these currents of practice have their strong and weak points, and that many practitioners combine both approaches in their practices.

It would be a mistake, however, to limit a discussion of developments in the late imperial period to just these two currents. This was a time when Chinese intellectuals critically examined the very foundations of their intellectual traditions, a movement that extended also to the domain of medicine. A typical example is the late-18th-century physician Wang Qing-Ren, who critically examined traditional concepts of anatomy, replacing them with insights drawn from his own examination of dead bodies. This led Wang to revise older concepts regarding the interplay of qi and blood, and the role of blood stasis in the causation of disease. His innovative approach to understanding blood stasis became particularly influential in the 20th century, and eight of his formulas are included in our book.

Another very important influence during this time is the encounter with Western medicine. Although this had entered China several centuries earlier, it was only around the turn of the 20th century that Chinese medicine physicians were forced to redefine themselves in relation to this powerful import. This led initially to the definition of qi transformation (氣化 *qì huà*) as the core characteristic of Chinese medicine, even as scholars like Zhou Xue-Hai sought to move the body of Chinese medicine closer to that of Western medicine. This produced highly innovative therapeutic strategies, such as those developed by Zhang Xi-Chun, who combined Western pharmaceuticals such as aspirin with Chinese formulas such as White Tiger Decoction (*bái hǔ tāng*). Zhang also utilized what he knew of Western pathophysiology as an input to the composition of new but very traditional Chinese medical formulas. The composition of Sedate the Liver and Extinguish Wind Decoction (*zhèn gān xī fēng tāng*), discussed in Chapter 14, is a typical example of this approach. Eight formulas from Zhang's influential *Essays on Medicine Esteeming the Chinese and Respecting the Western* are included in our book.

During the early 20th century, Japan functioned as an important model for Chinese medical modernization. This led to a renewed emphasis on cold damage therapeutics, much utilized in Japanese Kampō medicine, because it was believed that this form of medicine was closest to the empiricism that had produced Western science. An enduring legacy of this approach has been the emphasis on patterns (證 *zhèng*) in contemporary Chinese medicine, which matches the role of *shō* in Japanese Kampō. Pharmacological knowledge about the effects of individual herbs is also now entering formula composition, as reflected in the COMMENTARY to Gastrodia and Uncaria Drink *(tiān má gōu téng yǐn)*, also discussed in Chapter 14. These examples demonstrate the continued vitality of the Chinese medical tradition and its ability to assimilate multiple external influences that, in turn, reshape the medicine itself.

RELATIONSHIP OF FORMULAS TO STRATEGIES

As previously noted, the practice of traditional Chinese herbal medicine can be seen as consisting of a chain linking theoretical principles, treatment strategies, medical formulas, and medicinal substances. A formula is comprised of substances, the particular configuration of which is dictated by the organizing principles of the treatment strategy. If the pattern of a disorder is misdiagnosed, the treatment strategy will be incorrect, and its derivative formula will be ineffective. For example, a patient presents with fever, irritability, thirst, a red face, and a flooding, big pulse. If the practitioner ignores the fact that the fever is low, the thirst is for warm beverages, and the pulse is also deficient, he could misdiagnose the pattern as a yang brightness channel-warp (stage) disorder and prescribe White Tiger Decoction *(bái hǔ tāng)*, a formula used for clearing heat from the qi level. No matter how cleverly the formula is modified, the results will be disappointing because the patient is really suffering from consumptive fatigue. For this condition, an appropriate formula would be Tangkuei Decoction to Tonify the Blood *(dāng guī bǔ xuè tāng)*, which tonifies the qi in order to augment the blood.

Similarly, the formula chosen must be consistent with the strategy of treatment. If it is not, the condition will not improve and may even worsen. It is helpful to remember the adage, "The formula is derived from the strategy, and the strategy arises from the pattern."

Principles of Treatment

Before discussing strategies that are specific to Chinese herbal medicine, we should review some of the fundamental principles of treatment in Chinese medicine as a whole. These principles, in turn, are based on a certain understanding of how people get sick (i.e., the etiology and pathogenesis of disease), which is shared by other therapeutic modalities in traditional Chinese medicine such as acupuncture.

Root and Branch of Disease

To maximize the benefit of a treatment and minimize its side effects it is vital to identify which aspects of a disorder in a particular patient are most important. In traditional Chinese medicine, this is known as distinguishing the branch manifestation of a problem (標 *biāo*) from its root cause (本 *běn*). The following distinctions are useful in making this determination:

- The strength of the patient's normal qi is the root and that of the pathogenic influence is the branch.
- The etiology (cause) of a disease is the root and its presentation (symptoms) is the branch.
- During the course of a disease the underlying, primary disorder is the root and any secondary complications are the branch.
- With respect to the location of a disease, the internal aspect is the root and the external aspect is the branch.

Clinically, it is important to distinguish the root from the branch of a disease so that treatment can be directed accordingly and fine tuned to the precise needs of the patient at a particular time. The basic rules governing treatment of the root and branch are as follows:

- For acute disorders, treat the branch. Examples include acute bleeding or vomiting where it is vitally important to promptly alleviate the symptoms irrespective of their cause. The branch is also the focus of treatment for a recently-contracted acute disorder in a patient with an underlying chronic condition. In such cases, the treatment strategy is a bit more complex, as discussed below.
- For chronic disorders, treat the root. Examples include lower back pain due to Kidney deficiency, and edema due to yang deficiency. Sometimes the root cause of a chronic problem can be some form of stagnation; in other words, the root is not always deficiency. In such cases, the symptoms will disappear only when the root cause has been effectively treated. However, it is a relatively rare case where treatment is directed only at the root without regard to the symptoms.
- Simultaneous treatment of the root and branch. There are many examples of this approach, the most common of which occur in cases where the constitution of the patient is weak and the pathogenic influence is strong. In such cases, although both the root and branch are treated simultaneously, the focus of treatment is still on one or the

other aspect. Take, for example, the coughing and wheezing associated with cold-phlegm obstructing the Lungs in a patient suffering from underlying Kidney deficiency, which leads to rebellious qi. To be successful, treatment must both direct the rebellious qi downward (branch) and restore the Kidneys' ability to grasp the qi (root). However, in acute conditions such as this, the focus of treatment is clearly on the branch. (For further discussion of this process, see Perilla Fruit Decoction for Directing Qi Downward *[sū zǐ jiàng qì tāng]* in Chapter 9.) Another example is heat from yin deficiency. Depending on the intensity of the heat, the appropriate strategy would either be to focus almost entirely on enriching the yin (root) or directly draining the heat from deficiency (branch). More commonly, however, both the root and branch are addressed.

Another aspect of root and branch revolves around the most basic strategy of treatment: whether the nature of the disorder requires that the normal qi (the constitutional strength of the person) be supported, which is called tonification (補 *bǔ*), or that the pathogenic influence be eliminated, which is called attacking (攻 *gōng*). For example, when both the normal qi and pathogenic influence are weak, one can eliminate the pathogenic influence by tonifying the normal qi; conversely, by eliminating the pathogenic influence through a strategy of attack, one can indirectly support the normal qi by allowing it to rest and recuperate. Which strategy treats the root and which the branch will depend on the specific presentation of the patient, as well as the perspective of the practitioner. In some circumstances, a strategy of simultaneous attack and support is required, as in the case of a weak patient who requires purging (see Chapter 3). Distinguishing between the root and branch in such cases can be difficult.

Normal and Contrary Treatment

The treatment of disease in traditional Chinese medicine is generally said to be antagonistic to the disease process, that is, it utilizes strategies and substances that are opposite in nature to the disease. For example, heat is treated with cold, cold is treated with heat, stagnation is treated by promoting movement, leakage is treated by stabilizing and binding. This is known as normal treatment (正治 *zhèng zhì*).

There are, however, occasions when treatment is characterized as being contrary (反治 *fǎn zhì*) because it appears to depart from the general rule of direct treatment. Contrary treatment in herbal medicine is of two types. The first consists of using a formula whose nature appears to be similar to that of the disease. This would include, for example, prescribing a formula composed primarily of hot ingredients for treating a disorder which is apparently due to heat that displays symptoms of heat, or one composed of cold ingredients for treating a disorder apparently due to cold that displays symptoms of cold. Although the nature of such formulas would appear to be contrary to the disorders for which they are prescribed, this is not the case when the disorders themselves are characterized by false or misleading symptoms. For example, a warming strategy is appropriate in treating a patient with 'false' fire and 'true' cold. In this case, there are signs of irritability, flushed face, and sometimes a sore throat, which on first glance appear to be due to heat. In fact, however, the patient is actually suffering from cold, which is evidenced by the 'true' signs of cold extremities, watery diarrhea, and a faint pulse. Thus, an appropriate warming formula such as Frigid Extremities Decoction *(sì nì tāng)* would be directed at the underlying cold nature of the disorder, rather than at the apparent but false symptoms of heat.

A similar problem arises at the extremes of excess and deficiency. The patient may present with symptoms that appear to be excessive, but in fact are indicative of severe deficiency, and vice versa. For example, distention, a stifling sensation, and pain in the abdomen accompanied by irritability, restlessness, and constipation might lead the practitioner to think that the condition is one of excess. On further examination, however, it is noted that all the symptoms improve when the patient is rested, the pain responds favorably to warmth and pressure, the tongue is pale and swollen, and the pulse is frail and forceless. In this case, there is true deficiency and false excess.

The second type of contrary treatment does not involve false or misleading symptoms, but simply represents an apparent departure from the norm of antagonistic treatment. For example, one generally disperses obstruction, but when the obstruction is due to deficiency (usually of the Spleen), it is treated by tonification (which normally causes blockage). When the deficiency is rectified, this type of obstruction will resolve itself. This approach is known as 'using blockage when the cause is blockage.' (塞因塞用 *sāi yīn sāi yòng*). Similarly, one generally stabilizes or binds up diarrhea or loss of blood. However, when the leakage is due to retention of a pathogenic influence in the body, the diarrhea is treated by purging, and the loss of blood by a strategy that invigorates the blood. An example is the use of Peony Decoction *(sháo yào tāng)* or Aucklandia and Betel Nut Pill *(mù xiāng bīng láng wán)* for treating dysenteric diarrhea. This is known as 'facilitating flow when the cause is too much flow' (通因通用 *tōng yīn tōng yòng*).

At first glance, such strategies would appear to violate the normal principles of treatment, but appearances can be deceiving. As is always the case in traditional Chinese medicine, when the underlying cause of a disorder is understood, the proper treatment is instituted even if the major symptoms suggest otherwise. Thus, in the example above, the type of diarrhea for which Aucklandia and Betel Nut Pill (*mù xiāng bīng láng wán*) is indicated is marked by various signs of stagnation such as pain, distention, and tenesmus. It is therefore entirely 'normal' to treat this problem with a formula that facilitates flow. Because at the heart of Chinese medicine—if we follow the writings and practices of some of its most outstanding physicians, from Zhang Zhong-Jing to Ye Tian-Shi and Fei Bo-Xiong—is a concern with facilitating movement, flow, and transformation. Hence, although Chinese medicine is sometimes described as allopathic in nature with the aim of creating homeostasis, the use of such terms originates within Western medical discourse and thus inevitably distorts what it tries to translate.

By examining what is perhaps the most famous formula in the history of Chinese medicine, Cinnamon Twig Decoction (*guì zhī tāng*), we can gain an understanding of these most fundamental principles of Chinese medicine. Although this formula eliminates a pathogen, it does not do so by focusing on the pathogen itself, but rather on harmonizing (和 *hé*) the nutritive and protective qi, that is, between yin and yang. In ancient usage, 和 *hé* was equivalent to the contemporary term 治 *zhì*, or treatment. Harmonization thus might be said to be the ultimate goal of Chinese medicine. But, as the composition of Cinnamon Twig Decoction (*guì zhī tāng*) makes clear, such harmonization is not limited to producing equal amounts of nutritive and protective qi, qi and blood, yin and yang. Rather, it consists of allowing yang to interpenetrate yin so as to facilitate harmonious movement and transformation. If that occurs, there is no space for a pathogen and no place for disorder. By extension, anything that facilitates flow and transformation—and sometimes this can be purgation, sweating, or vomiting—is able to produce harmony and thus serves as effective treatment.

Different Treatments for the Same Disease, Same Treatment for Different Diseases

Treatment in traditional Chinese medicine is not disease oriented, but is strategy oriented. The treatment strategy, in turn, is based upon the underlying cause of a disease. Whether defined in traditional terms or as a biomedical entity, the same disease will be treated in different ways depending on the particular pathogenic mechanisms involved. For example, dysenteric disorders are variously due to wind-cold-dampness, wind-heat, heat toxin, damp-heat, or cold of the Kidneys and Spleen from deficiency. Each of these etiologies requires a completely different treatment strategy, even though the disease (a dysenteric disorder) is the same.

Conversely, whenever the same pathogenic mechanisms are involved, the treatment will be similar no matter how different the diseases and their symptoms appear to be. For example, Pulsatilla Decoction (*bái tóu wēng tāng*) is used for treating acute damp-heat in the lower burner. Although orig-

inally designed for treating dysenteric disorders, it can be used for treating any problem associated with acute damp-heat in the lower burner, including urogenital disorders.

Treating Disease According to the Season, Environment, and Individual

The effective practice of Chinese herbal medicine requires more than simply selecting the proper treatment strategy and formula. Treatment must also be adapted to the time of year, the environment in which the patient lives, and the particular characteristics of the individual. Otherwise, not only might the treatment fail to help the patient, it may actually cause further harm. The use of formulas that induce sweating to release an exterior disorder is a good illustration of this problem. The type and dosage of herbs used during the summer, in a hot climate, and for a weak or debilitated patient should be considerably less potent than those used for treating the same disorder during the winter, in a cold climate, and for a strong or robust patient.

Traditional Strategies

The use of particular strategies or methods of treatment has been an integral part of traditional Chinese medicine for at least two-thousand years. Like other aspects of traditional medicine in China, these strategies have undergone considerable change and development during that time. While they are not identical, the categorization of treatment strategies serves as the basis for the categorization of the formulas.

In *Awakening of the Mind in Medical Studies*, the early 18th-century physician Cheng Guo-Peng organized the various strategies into a relatively simple scheme that he called the eight methods (八法 *bā fǎ*). Cheng is also credited with giving final form to the eight parameters of diagnosis (八綱 *bā gāng*), and thus had a tremendous influence on traditional Chinese medicine. The eight methods of treatment serve as the foundation for all present discussion of herbal strategies, and while they do not include every possible strategy, they are the building blocks for other strategies. As Cheng himself observed, "The eight methods exist in any single method. Likewise, a myriad of methods exist within the eight methods."

The salient features of each of the eight methods of treatment are summarized on the next four pages. All of these methods are still commonly used today, with the exception of vomiting. As previously noted, writers through the centuries have described the various treatment strategies in different ways. Nonetheless, all of these strategies can be incorporated within the broad framework of the eight methods. It should be emphasized, however, that many disorders are too complex to be effectively treated with one method alone. Sometimes two, three, or even four methods are used concurrent-

MECHANISM	REFERENCE IN *INNER CLASSIC*	APPLICATIONS
Sweating (汗法 *hàn fǎ*)		
Induces sweating by stimulating and disseminating the Lung qi and regulating and facilitating the interaction between the nutritive and protective qi so that the pores open and pathogenic influences in the exterior or other superficial levels of the body can be released with the sweat.	"When it is at [the level of] the skin, use sweating to discharge it." *(Basic Questions, Chapter 5)*	• Externally-contracted exterior excess conditions • Measles and similar rashes • Acute edema that is more severe above the waist • Early-stage pain and swelling from wind-dampness • Skin disorders caused by wind (with itching) • Diseases which are working their way out from the interior
Vomiting (吐法 *tù fǎ*)		
Stimulates the Stomach so that phlegm, stagnant food, or toxic matter stuck in the throat, chest, or stomach cavity can be expelled through the mouth.	"When it is at the upper [levels], lead it up and out." *(Basic Questions, Chapter 74)*	• Phlegm stuck in the throat • Phlegm accumulating in the chest • Food stagnating in the Stomach • Ingestion of poisons
Draining downward (下法 *xià fǎ*)		
Induces defecation to cleanse the bowels and expels pathogens with form through the rectum.	"When it is at the lower [levels], lead and draw it down. ...When the middle is full, drain internally." *(Basic Questions, Chapter 74)*	• Constipation • Dried feces in the Intestines • Hot accumulations • Cold accumulations • Water build-up • Blood build-up
Harmonizing (和法 *hé fǎ*)		
Harmonizes or regulates the functions of different levels or organs.	None	• Half-exterior, half-interior (lesser yang) disorders • Malarial disorders • Depression • Dysmenorrhea • Epigastric focal distention
Warming (温法 *wēn fǎ*)		
Warms the interior and unblocks the channels to dispel cold from the interior or the channels, thereby restoring the functions of the yang qi.	"Warm that which is cold. ...Treat cold [disorders] with warmth." *(Basic Questions, Chapter 74)*	• Cold in the channels • Cold attacking the middle burner • Cold with devastated yang
Clearing (清法 *qīng fǎ*)		
Clears heat and drains fire to eliminate heat, fire, and their associated toxicity from the body.	"Clear that which is warm. ... Treat hot [disorders] with cold." *(Basic Questions, Chapter 74)*	• Interior heat • Heat in any organ

TREATMENT STRATEGIES	COMBINED STRATEGIES	COMMENTS
• Acrid and warming to release the pathogen from the exterior • Acrid and cooling to release the pathogen from the exterior	• Benefit the qi and release the pathogen from the exterior • Warm the yang and release the pathogen from the exterior • Nourish the yin and release the pathogen from the exterior • Drive out fluids and release the pathogen from the exterior • Release the pathogen from the exterior and cool the pathogen in the interior	Remember that sweating itself is not the goal of this strategy. Rather, it is a sign that tells the practitioner that the pores have opened, the nutritive and protective qi are harmonized, and the pathogens have been dispelled. This strategy must be combined with tonification if used in treating weak patients.
Induce vomiting to reduce phlegm	None	This is a strong strategy used for ejecting pathogens that have form from the body. The inducement of vomiting usually causes sweating, and easily injures the Stomach qi (in part because it can be regarded as iatrogenic rebellious Stomach qi). It should therefore only be used for treating acute disorders in relatively robust patients.
• Purge heat accumulation • Warm the yang and guide out accumulation • Moisten the Intestines and unblock the bowels • Drive out excess water	• Simultaneously purge and tonify • Invigorate the blood and drain downward	This is a strong strategy used for ejecting pathogens with form from the body, such as heat with form (有形之熱 *yǒu xíng zhī rè*).
• Harmonize the lesser yang • Vent the membrane source • Harmonize the Liver and Spleen • Regulate the Stomach and Intestines	• Harmonize and release • Harmonize and purge	On one level, this category has today become a grab bag of methods that do not fit anywhere else. The term harmonizing (or mediating) is fitting because it doesn't focus solely on attacking or tonifying, but rather on aspects of both, while harmonizing those functions which are at odds with one another. At another level, the term harmonizing has a more narrow and specific meaning, which was discussed previously.
• Warm the channels and disperse cold • Warm the middle and dispel cold • Restore and revive the yang	• Warm the yang and guide out accumulation • Warm and transform cold-phlegm • Warm and transform water and dampness	The cold disorders for which warming is appropriate usually have some aspect of deficiency, generally of the yang. For that reason, this method is often combined with tonification.
• Clear heat from the qi level • Clear the nutritive level and cool the blood • Clear heat and resolve toxicity • Clear heat from the organs	• Clear heat and augment the fluids • Clear heat and benefit the qi • Clear heat and enrich the yin	The clearing method is used only for interior heat without any sign of clumping or accumulation, that is, for heat without form (無形之熱 *wú xíng zhī rè*).

cont. ↘

MECHANISM	REFERENCE IN *INNER CLASSIC*	APPLICATIONS
Reducing (消法 *xiāo fǎ*)		
Gradually reduces or eliminates clumping or accumulation due to the stagnation of food or other causes.	"Pare away that which is firm. ... Disperse that which is clumped." *(Basic Questions,* Chapter 74)	• Qi stagnation • Blood stasis • Food stagnation • Phlegm • Parasites • Abscesses
Tonifying (補法 *bǔ fǎ*)		
Tonifies by enriching, nourishing, augmenting, or replenishing those aspects of the body that are weak or deficient.	"Tonify that which is deficient." *(Basic Questions,* Chapter 20) "Augment that which is injured." *(Basic Questions,* Chapter 74)	• Deficiency of qi, blood, yin, or yang • Deficiency of any organ

ly. Take the case of a patient whose long-standing deficiency leads to stagnation and eventually to acute accumulation. In this case, the concurrent use of tonifying, reducing, and downward-draining methods would be appropriate. To be effective in the clinic, the practitioner must carefully discern the underlying mechanism of a disorder and be flexible in selecting the appropriate methods of treatment.

Although the eight methods of treatment were broad enough, they did not describe with specificity all of the strategies that were actually used in practice. Specifically, the scope of the reducing method was thought to be too broad, and other dispersing strategies were therefore added to amplify this category. These include regulating the qi, regulating the blood, eliminating dampness, and expelling phlegm. Although formulas which incorporate these strategies date back to at least the 3rd-century works of Zhang Zhong-Jing, it was not until the Ming and Qing dynasties that they came into full flower. For example, Wang Qing-Ren's 19th-century *Correction of Errors among Physicians* was the first book to clearly articulate the manifold uses of invigorating the blood.

Categorization of the Formulas

Over the past two-thousand years, East Asians have devised a variety of systems for classifying the combination of medicinal substances that we call formulas. There are systems based upon the nature of the disease, pattern, etiology, form of application, branch of medicine, organ, treatment strategy (now the most widely used), as well as various combinations of these systems.

Although, as noted earlier, the *Inner Classic* does not focus on herbal medicine, there is some discussion about the types of formulas in Chapter 74 of *Basic Questions.* This dis-

cussion revolves primarily around the number of substances in the formulas. For example, "One chief and two deputies comprise a small formula. ... One chief, three deputies, and nine assistants comprise a large formula. ... Two chiefs and four deputies comprise an even-numbered formula. ... Two chiefs and three deputies comprise an odd-numbered formula." Other passages in this chapter describe the nature of the formulas: "Tonifying the upper to treat the upper [part of the body] requires a slow-acting or mild (緩 *huǎn*) formula; tonifying the lower to treat the lower [part of the body] requires a quick-acting or urgent (急 *jí*) formula."

In *Discussion Illuminating the Principles of Cold Damage,* the 12th-century writer Cheng Wu-Ji devised a system based in part on these passages, which he called the seven types of formulas (七方 *qī fāng*): large, small, mild, urgent, odd-numbered, even-numbered, and composite. This is regarded as the earliest system for classifying the formulas. However, a careful examination of the passages from *Basic Questions* upon which this system is based reveals some problems. It is true that this book alludes to many different aspects of disease including the strength of the pathogenic influence, the location and progression of the disease, the constitutional strength of the patient, and the need for treatment. But while each of these aspects is important, they are not presented in a manner which is either comprehensive or directly related to a particular type of formula. There is also some inconsistency in the number of substances which the formulas should contain. For example, in one passage it says that there are many substances in a large formula, and few in a small; yet in another passage it says that there are few substances in a large formula, and many in a small. Furthermore, some of the instructions are not thought to be useful from a contemporary perspective and have not been followed in formulas

TREATMENT STRATEGIES	COMBINED STRATEGIES	COMMENTS
• Eliminate food stagnation • Reduce accumulation • Transform phlegm • Eliminate childhood nutritional impairment • Kill parasites • Reduce sores and disperse abscesses	• Reduce stagnation and drain downward • Simultaneously reduce and tonify	In contrast to the downward-draining method, reducing is a gradual reduction in the accumulation or clumping, and also involves transformation instead of just expulsion. Even parasites are transformed into something relatively harmless (i.e., killed) before they are eliminated from the body.
• Tonify the qi • Nourish the blood • Tonify the yang • Enrich the yin	• Tonify the qi, blood, yin, or yang, and release the exterior • Support the normal and purge • Enrich the yin and moisten dryness • Tonify the qi and invigorate the blood	Generally speaking, one should avoid using this method by itself in treating disorders with an active pathogenic influence, as this may aggravate the disorder.

through the centuries. For example, "To induce sweating, do not use an even-numbered [formula]; to drain downward, do not use an odd-numbered [formula]."

The forerunner of the classification system that has been used for the past few hundred years was devised by the Tang-dynasty writer Chen Cang-Qi. (It was mistakenly attributed by Li Shi-Zhen to the 6th-century physician Xu Zhi-Cai.) This is the first system to group the medicinal substances and formulas by functional categories tied to specific types of clinical presentations. Chen organized the substances and formulas into ten categories and then provided instructions for the use of each category. While the book itself was subsequently lost, that portion which described the ten categories was preserved in Li Shi-Zhen's *Comprehensive Outline of the Materia Medica*. Cheng Wu-Ji referred to these categories as the ten types of formulas (十劑 *shí jì*), which are listed together with their functions in Table 2.

Because the ten categories do not fully encompass the variety of formulas used in the clinic, other categories were added later. In *Extension of the Materia Medica*, the Song-dynasty writer Kou Zong-Shi added heating and cooling. In the Ming dynasty, Liao Zhong-Chun added ascending and descending, and over time, more and more categories were added such as regulating, harmonizing, releasing, facilitating, warming, cooling, pacifying, guiding, calming, and clearing. By the late Qing, most formularies settled on around twenty categories.

In the earliest books, such as *Prescriptions for Fifty-Two Ailments* and most of the works recorded in the 2nd-century history *Book of the Han*, formulas were arranged according to disease. This practice was continued for a long time. Such important works as *Formulary of the Pharmacy Service for Benefiting the People in the Taiping Era*, *Formulas of Uni-*

Formulas that:	Eliminate:
disseminate (宣 *xuān*)	clogging
unblock (通 *tōng*)	stagnation
tonify (補 *bǔ*)	weakness
drain (泄 *xiè*)	obstruction
clear (清 *qīng*)	excess
weigh down (重 *zhòng*)	anxiety
bind (澀 *sè*)	abandoned disorders
lubricate (滑 *huá*)	sticky retentions in the body
dry (燥 *zào*)	dampness
moisten (濕 *shī*)	dryness

Table 2 Ten Types of Formulas

versal Benefit from My Practice, and *Investigations of Medical Formulas* adopted this system. Where the formulas were arranged according to a branch of medicine, the most common categories were those dealing with diseases of women and children. This occurs as early as *Book of the Han*. *Important Formulas Worth a Thousand Gold Pieces* and *Arcane Essentials from the Imperial Library* classified the formulas based upon the affected organ. None of these systems was all-encompassing, and most of the books ended up using a mixture of systems.

Each of these systems was found to be either too complex and unwieldy or overly simplified. Over time there was a demand for an approach that was easy to learn, convenient to reference, and that placed similar formulas within the same category for comparison. Classifying the formulas according to their underlying actions or strategies is such a method. As with any method, this one has its problems, and all systems based upon it (including that used in this book) involve some inconsistencies.

The problem of categorization became most acute during the Ming dynasty. The popularization of books during this era was reflected in the large number of works published in the field of herbal medicine. Physicians had access to more information than ever before, but they lacked a convenient method of finding what they needed. A representative figure of this era was Zhang Jie-Bin. Zhang's background was in the military, and he had a very organized mind. He observed that in older books where the formulas were arranged by disease, it was often difficult to find a particular formula. This is because most formulas can be used for treating a variety of diseases. If each formula were listed under every disease it could treat, there would be a tremendous amount of repetition. However, if it was only listed under the most important disease, it would often be difficult to find the formula.

In *Collected Treatises of [Zhang] Jing-Yue*, Zhang sought to resolve this problem by organizing the formulas into eight categories, which he called the "eight battle arrays" (八陣 *bā zhèn*). A variation on the ten types of formulas, he classified 1,516 ancient and 186 contemporary formulas under the headings of those that tonify (補 *bǔ*), harmonize (和 *hé*), attack (攻 *gōng*), disperse (散 *sǎn*), cool (寒 *hán*), heat (熱 *rè*), stabilize (固 *gù*), and pattern-specific (因 *yīn*). However, even Zhang was unable to completely dispense with the previous systems. His book also contains categories for women's disorders (186 formulas), pediatric disorders (171 formulas), rashes (174 formulas), and external medicine (391 formulas).

During the early part of the Qing dynasty, another comprehensive classification scheme was devised by Wang Ang. Like Zhang Jie-Bin, Wang's system also combined categories based on the actions or treatment strategies underlying the formulas with other categories that focus on specific branches of medicine. In *Medical Formulas Collected and Analyzed*, Wang divided the formulas into the following twenty-two categories:

Tonify and nourish	(補養 *bǔ yǎng*)
Discharge the exterior	(發表 *fā biǎo*)
Induce vomiting	(涌吐 *yǒng tù*)
Attack the interior	(攻裡 *gōng lǐ*)
Simultaneous treatment of the exterior and interior	(表裡 *biǎo lǐ*)
Harmonize and resolve	(和解 *hé jiě*)
Regulate the qi	(理氣 *lǐ qì*)
Regulate the blood	(理血 *lǐ xuè*)
Dispel wind	(祛風 *qū fēng*)

Dispel cold	(祛寒 *qū hán*)
Clear summerheat	(清暑 *qīng shǔ*)
Resolve dampness	(利濕 *lì shī*)
Moisten dryness	(潤燥 *rùn zào*)
Drain fire	(瀉火 *xiè huǒ*)
Eliminate phlegm	(除痰 *chú tán*)
Reduce and guide out	(消導 *xiāo dǎo*)
Preserve and bind	(收澀 *shōu sè*)
Kill parasites	(殺蟲 *shā chóng*)
Improve the eyes	(明目 *míng mù*)
Abscesses and sores	(癰瘍 *yōng yáng*)
Menstruation and childbirth	(經產 *jīng chǎn*)
Emergencies	(救急 *jiù jí*)

This book had a major influence on subsequent formularies and was the basis for such important works as *Practical Established Formulas* by Wu Yi-Luo in the late 18th century, and *Convenient Reader of Established Formulas* by Zhang Bing-Cheng in the early 20th century. Although this system has undergone some modification, it still serves as the model for the classification of formulas in modern times.

The formularies used in contemporary China list around twenty major categories. In general, these parallel the categories under which the actions of individual medicinal substances are organized. Although there is no officially-sanctioned standardization, the books usually differ in only a few categories. However, the order in which the categories are presented varies from book to book. The reader is referred to the table of contents for the order of chapters in our book. Additional information about particular treatment strategies is provided in the introduction to each chapter.

COMPOSITION OF THE FORMULAS

The formulas in Chinese medicine are not mere collections of medicinal substances in which the actions of one herb are simply added to those of another in a cumulative fashion. They are complex recipes of interrelated substances, each of which affects the actions of the others in the formula. It is this complex interaction which makes the formulas so effective, but also makes them more difficult to study.

Every medicinal substance has its strengths and its shortcomings. An effective formula is one in which the substances are carefully balanced to accentuate the strengths and reduce the side effects. The combination of substances in a formula creates a new therapeutic agent that can treat much more effectively and completely than can a single substance.

To understand how the substances interact with each

other, one must first understand the actions and other characteristics of the individual substances. One must also become familiar with particular combinations, which can be viewed as the building blocks of the formulas. For example, the combination of Cinnamomi Ramulus (*guì zhī*) and Paeoniae Radix *(sháo yào)* regulates the relationship between the protective and nutritive qi in treating exterior cold from deficiency; in other circumstances, it also warms and tonifies the middle burner. This combination is an important building block in both Cinnamon Twig Decoction (*guì zhī tāng*) and Minor Construct the Middle Decoction *(xiǎo jiàn zhōng tāng)*. A knowledge of herbal combinations also implies an awareness of when a particular combination would be inappropriate, that is, would lead to mutual counteraction, mutual suppression, mutual antagonism, or mutual incompatibility. For this type of information, the reader should consult a basic textbook of materia medica such as the companion volume to this book, *Chinese Herbal Medicine: Materia Medica.*

Hierarchy of Ingredients

Constructing an effective formula involves more than simply putting ingredients together to obtain a certain effect. One needs an organizing principle to guide the construction so that the ingredients are combined in an optimal fashion. The orderly arrangement of ingredients in a formula is called a hierarchy. The concept of hierarchy was first suggested in a passage from Chapter 74 of *Basic Questions:* "That [ingredient] which primarily treats the disease is the chief, that which aids the chief is the deputy, and that which is bound to the deputy is the envoy." This was amplified by later practitioners. Zhang Yuan-Su, one of the great physicians of the Jin-Yuan era who had a tremendous influence on the course of Chinese herbal medicine, noted that "The [ingredient] with the greatest power is the chief." Another renowned physician of that period, Zhang's student Li Gao, observed in *Discussion of the Spleen and Stomach:* "That [ingredient] which treats the primary disorder is called the chief. When other disorders are present, their treatment is divided between the assistant and the envoy. This is an essential part of constructing a formula." Li also noted that: "The dosage of the chief herb is the greatest, the deputy next, and the assistant and envoy follow. The [dosage of the] deputy cannot be allowed to exceed that of the chief."

Traditional Chinese society was always very conscious of rank, which revolved in the first instance around the emperor and his court. For this reason, the terms used to signify the importance or rank of the ingredients in a formula reflect those used at court. In this book we have used slightly different terms to make things a bit clearer and perhaps less 'feudal.' The four ranks of ingredients in the hierarchy of a formula are the chief (君 *jūn)*, deputy (臣 *chén)*, assistant (佐 *zuǒ)*, and envoy (使 *shǐ)*. We will discuss each of these in turn.

Chief (also known as monarch, ruler, king, emperor, principal). The ingredient that is directed against, and has the greatest effect upon, the principal pattern or disease. This ingredient is absolutely indispensable to the formula.

Deputy (also known as minister, adjutant, associate). Refers to two different functions: 1) aids the chief ingredient in treating the principal pattern or disease; and 2) serves as the main ingredient directed against a coexisting pattern or disease.

Assistant (also known as adjutant). Refers to three different functions: 1) reinforces the effect of the chief or deputy ingredients, or directly treats a less important aspect of the pattern or disease. In this capacity, it is known as a helpful assistant (佐助 *zuǒ zhù)*. 2) Moderates or eliminates the toxicity of the chief or deputy ingredients, or moderates their harsh properties. This is known as a corrective assistant (佐制 *zuǒ zhì)*. 3) Has an effect that is opposite that of the chief ingredient and is used in very serious and complex disorders. This is known as an opposing assistant (佐反 *zuǒ fǎn)*.

Envoy (also known as messenger, guide, conductant). Refers to two different functions: 1) focuses the actions of the formula on a certain channel or area of the body; and 2) harmonizes and integrates the actions of the other ingredients.

Not all formulas contain the full hierarchy of ingredients. In fact, it would be quite unusual for a formula to include all the various types of deputies, assistants, and envoys. Many formulas consist of only a chief and one or two deputy ingredients. If the chief and deputies are not toxic, there is no need for corrective assistants. Sometimes the chief ingredient itself focuses on the level and location of the disorder, obviating the need for an envoy.

The classic example of how the hierarchy of ingredients works in a formula is Ephedra Decoction (*má huáng tāng*) from *Discussion of Cold Damage.* This formula is used for externally-contracted wind-cold which leads to a presentation of exterior excess cold characterized by chills, fever, head and body aches, an absence of sweating, wheezing, a thin, white tongue coating, and a floating, tight pulse. The chief ingredient is warm, acrid Ephedrae Herba (*má huáng*), a particularly strong diaphoretic that also disseminates the Lungs and treats wheezing. This potent herb directly attacks the disorder. One of the deputies is Cinnamomi Ramulus (*guì zhī)*, another diaphoretic that releases the exterior (especially the muscle layer) and warms and facilitates the flow of qi in the channels. It assists the chief ingredient in releasing the exterior. The other deputy, Armeniacae Semen *(xìng rén),* unblocks the flow of Lung qi. It assists the chief ingredient in treating one of the secondary symptoms, wheezing, and helps the chief and first deputy expel the pathogenic influence. Glycyrrhizae Radix praeparata *(zhì gān cǎo)* harmonizes the actions of the other herbs. It serves as a corrective assistant by moderating the diaphoretic actions of the chief and deputy ingredients. This disorder affects the Lungs and outer layer of the body. Because both Ephedrae Herba *(má huáng)* and Armeniacae Semen *(xìng rén)* enter the Lungs, there is no need in this formula for an envoy to guide the actions of the ingredients toward the locus of the disorder.

Another, not quite so classic example is a formula from *Systematic Differentiation of Warm Pathogen Diseases* called Sweet Wormwood and Soft-Shelled Turtle Shell Decoction (Version 1) *(qīng hāo biē jiǎ tāng).* This formula is indicated for a condition of heat from deficiency where the heat has settled in the body. The only proper course of treatment is to simultaneously nourish the yin and vent the heat. One of the chief ingredients is salty, cold Trionycis Carapax *(biē jiǎ),* which enriches the yin and thereby reduces the fever from deficiency. The other chief ingredient is aromatic Artemisiae annuae Herba *(qīng hāo),* which vents the heat through the yang or external aspects of the body. There are two chief ingredients in this formula because both of their actions are indispensable in treating the disorder. The deputy ingredients, Rehmanniae Radix *(shēng dì huáng)* and Anemarrhenae Rhizoma *(zhī mǔ),* assist in nourishing the yin and thereby clearing the heat from deficiency. This tells us that while both of the chief ingredients are indispensable, the actions of Trionycis Carapax *(biē jiǎ),* which enriches the yin, are of primary importance. The assistant ingredient, Moutan Cortex *(mǔ dān pí),* drains heat from the blood and assists Artemisiae annuae Herba *(qīng hāo)* in venting the heat from the body. That this ingredient is regarded as an assistant means that its actions are less important than those of the deputies. Because the chief ingredients focus directly on the diseased aspect of the body, there is no need in this formula for an envoy.

In practice, the hierarchy of ingredients is not always so clear-cut. While all formulas require a chief ingredient, sometimes the formula is so well balanced that it is difficult to distinguish the function served by each of its ingredients. Examples are Five-Ingredient Drink to Eliminate Toxin *(wǔ wèi xiāo dú yǐn)* and Five-Peel Powder *(wǔ pí sǎn)* in which all of the ingredients are accorded equal status. In other cases, the position of an ingredient in the hierarchy will vary depending on the particular circumstances for which the formula is used. An example is Four-Substance Decoction *(sì wù tāng),* in which the relative dosage of the ingredients varies depending on whether its tonifying or invigorating actions are emphasized.

In addition, for several of the formulas in our book there has been intense debate over the centuries regarding which of the herbs is the chief ingredient. Such disagreement arises from different understandings of the underlying mechanism of the formula, or even the condition for which the formula is indicated. An example is Cinnamon Twig, Peony, and Anemarrhena Decoction *(guì zhī sháo yào zhī mǔ tāng).* There has been strong disagreement over whether the formula was intended primarily for hot or cold disorders. As a result, Cinnamomi Ramulus *(guì zhī),* Ephedrae Herba *(má huáng),* Atractylodis macrocephalae Rhizoma *(bái zhú),* Anemarrhenae Rhizoma *(zhī mǔ),* and Aconiti Radix lateralis praeparata *(zhì fù zǐ)* have each been identified as the chief herb in the formula.

The dosage of the individual ingredients in a formula also plays a part in determining its hierarchy. However, this too can be problematic. It is often said that the chief ingredient must have the largest dosage, but this refers to its dosage relative to its own normal dosage. Take, for example, two herbs for which the normal dosage of the first is 3-6g and that of the second is 18-24g. If 9g of the first and 18g of the second are used in a particular formula, the relative dosage of the first would be greater than the second, and it would therefore more likely be the chief ingredient. An example is Clear the Nutritive Level Decoction *(qīng yíng tāng)* where the dosage of the original chief ingredient, Rhinocerotis Cornu *(xī jiǎo),* is much less in absolute terms than the other ingredients because of its potency.

On the other hand, there are a few formulas where the dosage of the ingredient generally considered to be the chief is less than that of other ingredients in the formula. Sometimes this occurs because of different interpretations of the underlying mechanism of the formula. An example is Chuanxiong Powder to be Taken with Green Tea *(chuān xiōng chá tiáo sǎn).* Many commentators designate the herb with the largest dosage, Menthae haplocalycis Herba *(bò hé),* as a deputy. In other cases, although the chief ingredients as a group may dominate the formula, one of the deputy or assistant ingredients may nonetheless have the largest dosage. An example is Platycodi Radix *(jié gěng)* in Five-Accumulation Powder *(wǔ jī sǎn).*

When any of these issues are relevant, they are discussed in the COMMENTARY section of the formula in question.

Modifications in Composition

The art of constructing a formula requires more than a good grasp of the hierarchical principles discussed above. It also requires considerable flexibility in tailoring the formula to fit the specifications of the patient. Adjustments must be made for changes in the pattern, the strength of the patient, the season, climate, and other environmental factors. This may involve altering the selection of herbs or their relative dosage, the method of preparation, or the means of administration. This ability to modify a formula to fit a particular patient at a particular time is what separates the distinguished practitioner from the mediocre.

In the discussion which follows, the reader should note that most of the formulas used as examples are drawn from *Discussion of Cold Damage*. This is a reflection of the tremendous influence that this book has exerted on traditional Chinese medicine.

Modification of the Dosage

By modifying the dosage of ingredients, the strength of a formula and even its indications may be altered. In some cases, the modification may be significant enough to warrant being considered a different formula. An example in which modifying the dosage affects the strength of a formula is reflected in the difference between Frigid Extremities Decoction (*sì nì tāng*) and Unblock the Pulse Decoction for Frigid Extremities (*tōng mài sì nì tāng*). Both formulas contain 6g of Glycyrrhizae Radix praeparata (*zhì gān cǎo*) together with Aconiti Radix lateralis praeparata (*zhì fù zǐ*) and Zingiberis Rhizoma (*gān jiāng*). However, the dosage of the latter two ingredients is less in Frigid Extremities Decoction (*sì nì tāng*), which is used for a condition in which the yang is deficient and the yin is ascendant with internal cold. The dosage of these ingredients in Unblock the Pulse Decoction for Frigid Extremities (*tōng mài sì nì tāng*) is approximately twice as much, and that formula is accordingly used for the more severe condition in which the yang has separated from the yin.

Cinnamon Twig Decoction plus Peony (*guì zhī jiā sháo yào tāng*) is an example of modifying the dosage of an herb to alter the scope of a formula's indications. This formula is identical to Cinnamon Twig Decoction (*guì zhī tāng*) except that the dosage of Paeoniae Radix (*sháo yào*) has been doubled. Because one of this herb's major functions is to alleviate abdominal pain, by doubling its dosage the modified

formula can be used in treating the same presentation for which Cinnamon Twig Decoction (*guì zhī tāng*) is indicated, with the addition of abdominal fullness and pain.

Modifying the relative dosage of the ingredients can also have a more radical effect on a formula by changing its entire therapeutic scope, and thus the hierarchy of its ingredients. For example, both Minor Order the Qi Decoction (*xiǎo chéng qì tāng*) and Three-Substance Decoction with Magnolia Bark (*hòu pò sān wù tāng*) are composed of Rhei Radix et Rhizoma (*dà huáng*), Magnoliae officinalis Cortex (*hòu pò*), and Aurantii Fructus immaturus (*zhǐ shí*). However, because the dosage of these ingredients in the two formulas is different, both the indications of the formulas and the hierarchy of their ingredients are also quite different (see Table 3).

Modification of the Ingredients

This is the most common type of modification. The adage "Formulas are composed of medicinal substances" is a simple truism, yet it conveys an important message. The formulas are effective in treating disease precisely because of the nature and composition of their ingredients. When one changes the ingredients, one changes the actions of the formula. There are three types of ingredient modifications.

The first type occurs when the chief ingredient in the formula and the formula's primary action do not change, but minor ingredients are added or subtracted to fine tune the formula for a specific condition. Most of the modifications and variations listed in our text are of this type. For example, if a patient presents with symptoms for which Cinnamon Twig Decoction (*guì zhī tāng*) is indicated (aversion to drafts, fever, headache, sweating, a floating and lax pulse), but also presents with wheezing, then Magnoliae officinalis Cortex (*hòu pò*) and Armeniacae Semen (*xìng rén*) would be added. In this case, another formula is created which is called Cinnamon Twig Decoction plus Magnolia Bark and Apricot

Formula	Chief	Deputy	Assistant/Envoy	Indications
Minor Order the Qi Decoction (*xiǎo chéng qì tāng*)	Rhei Radix et Rhizoma (*dà huáng*) 12g	Aurantii Fructus immaturus (*zhǐ shí*) 3 pieces	Magnoliae officinalis Cortex (*hòu pò*) 6g	Relatively mild yang brightness organ-warp disorder (heat clumping) with tidal fever, constipation, focal distention, and abdominal fullness, abdominal pain that does not increase with pressure, an 'old-looking' (dirty and dry), yellow tongue coating, and a slippery, rapid pulse
Three-Substance Decoction with Magnolia Bark (*hòu pò sān wù tāng*)	Magnoliae officinalis Cortex (*hòu pò*) 24g	Aurantii Fructus immaturus (*zhǐ shí*) 5 pieces	Rhei Radix et Rhizoma (*dà huáng*) 12g	Qi stagnation causing constipation and unremitting pain and fullness in the epigastrium and abdomen

Table 3 Effects of Modifying the Relative Dosage of Ingredients

Kernel (guì zhī jiā hòu pò xìng zǐ tāng). Usually, however, this type of modification does not change the name of the formula. For example, if a patient with a Cinnamon Twig Decoction (guì zhī tāng) presentation also has marked nasal congestion, Saposhnikoviae Radix (fáng fēng) and Magnoliae Flos (xīn yí) could be added without changing the name of the formula.

This type of modification can also take the form of subtracting an ingredient, rather than adding one. For example, if a patient with a Cinnamon Twig Decoction (guì zhī tāng) presentation was improperly treated by purging, the primary signs and symptoms of the disorder would persist, but would now be accompanied by an irregular pulse and fullness in the chest. In this case, because the yang qi has been injured and has become listless, Paeoniae Radix alba (bái sháo), which is a slightly cool and sour substance, would be removed from the formula. This resulting formula is accordingly named Cinnamon Twig Decoction minus Peony (guì zhī qù sháo yào tāng).

In the second type of modification, the chief ingredient remains the same, but all or most of the other ingredients are changed so that the action of the formula is also changed. Take, for example, the two-ingredient formulas in which Coptidis Rhizoma (huáng lián) is the chief ingredient. If this herb is combined with acrid, warm Evodiae Fructus (wú zhū yú), which directs rebellious qi downward, the result is Left Metal Pill (zuǒ jīn wán). This formula clears and drains fire from the Liver, and thereby stops vomiting. It is used for constrained fire in the Liver channel with nausea, vomiting, and hypochondriac pain and distention. On the other hand, if it is combined with Aucklandiae Radix (mù xiāng), which promotes the movement of qi, the result is Aucklandia and Coptis Pill (xiāng lián wán). This formula clears and dries damp-heat and promotes the movement of qi, and is therefore used for dysenteric disorders due to damp-heat. Finally, if Coptidis Rhizoma (huáng lián) is combined with acrid, hot Cinnamomi Cortex (ròu guì), which warms the yang, the result is Grand Communication Pill (jiāo tài wán). This formula opens up communication between the Heart and Kidneys and is used for persistent palpitations and insomnia due to lack of communication between the Heart and Kidneys.

The third type of modification occurs when an alteration in the ingredients (sometimes only one ingredient) changes the formula so fundamentally that its character, hierarchy, and actions are completely altered. One of the best examples is the transformation of Ephedra Decoction (má huáng tāng), which is indicated for cold in the exterior, into Ephedra, Apricot Kernel, Gypsum, and Licorice Decoction (má xìng shí gān tāng), which is indicated for heat in the Lungs. In this transformation, Gypsum fibrosum (shí gāo) is substituted for Cinnamomi Ramulus (guì zhī) as the dep-

uty ingredient. In addition, the dosages of Ephedrae Herba (má huáng) and Glycyrrhizae Radix praeparata (zhì gān cǎo) are increased, while that of Armeniacae Semen (xìng rén) is reduced.

Another example is the addition of Maltosum (yí táng) to Cinnamon Twig Decoction plus Peony (guì zhī jiā sháo yào tāng). This addition forms Minor Construct the Middle Decoction (xiǎo jiàn zhōng tāng), which is indicated for spasmodic, hypertonic pain in the abdomen due to overwork deficiency, a disorder without a trace of exterior symptoms.

Modification in the Form of Administration

The form in which a formula is administered is also often of some consequence. Decoctions usually have a stronger effect than drafts, which in turn are usually stronger than pills. For example, when taken as a pill, Regulate the Middle Pill (lǐ zhōng wán) is used for treating cold from deficiency of the Spleen and Stomach, particularly when it is a long-term problem such as chronic epigastric pain. If the same herbs are taken as a decoction, however, the effect is much stronger and more immediate. It is therefore administered as a decoction for relatively acute problems such as oral sores due to cold in the middle burner. Of course, there are many counter-examples to these general rules, as in the use of pills for quick results in food stagnation, or powders for trauma.

The form of administration is an important factor in the practice of traditional Chinese herbal medicine in the West. It is difficult, if not impossible, to persuade many of our patients to use decoctions, and we must therefore resort to other forms such as powders and prepared medicines. As long as we are aware of those types of problems that truly require a particular form of administration, we can still practice effectively. This problem is discussed at greater length in the following section.

PRACTICAL ASPECTS

Understanding the pattern of disharmony and prescribing an appropriate formula is not, unfortunately, the end of the practitioner's responsibility. How to administer the medicine in the most effective manner is also an important consideration. Such practical aspects must be handled carefully. If, for example, the wrong form of medicine is used or the patient does not prepare the formula correctly or even refuses to take it, even the most skillful practitioner will not obtain good clinical results.

Types of Formulations for Ingestion or Injection

Over the course of the past two-thousand years medical practitioners in East Asia have developed many different types of formulations to administer herbal medicines. Matching the appropriate type of formulation to the patient and disease is an important aspect of good practice. The development of new types of formulations has continued down to the present day. In fact it is here, perhaps more than in any other aspect of traditional Chinese medicine, that the influence of modern technology has been felt, as modern formulations and means of extraction are now used on a wide scale. In this section we will discuss the more common types of formulations and their applications in the clinic.

Decoctions (湯劑 *tāng jì*): The ingredients are placed in water, or a mixture of wine and water, and then boiled for a specified period of time. The liquid is strained from the dregs and ingested through the mouth. One of the primary advantages of a decoction is that it is rapidly absorbed by the body; its effects are strong and immediately perceived by the patient. In addition, it is easy to modify the formulation to fit a particular patient at a given time. Until recently, these advantages have made decoctions the preferred method of dispensing Chinese herbal medicine. It is not, however, without drawbacks: decoctions are relatively expensive, time-consuming, difficult to prepare, and usually bad-tasting. (The preparation and administration of decoctions is discussed in the following section.)

Powders (散劑 *sǎn jì*): The ingredients are ground up and sifted into a relatively uniform powder, then either ingested or applied externally. Powders can be finely or coarsely ground. They can be taken directly, followed by a liquid, or as a draft (煮散 *zhǔ sǎn*). Taking a powder as a draft means to boil the powder for a short time in a relatively small amount of water (usually one to one-and-a-half cups) and ingesting the liquid that is strained from the dregs. Powders can be applied externally for treating skin conditions. They can also be blown into the nose or throat for treating localized disorders or as a means of reviving a patient from a coma (e.g., Open the Gate Powder [*tōng guān sǎn*]). The advantages of powders over decoctions include convenience in preparation, ability to store for long periods of time, and lower cost. Compared with pills and other forms of prepared medicines, powders are relatively easy to prepare and can be formulated specifically for a particular patient. This enables the practitioner to adjust the formula to fit the individual.

Pills (丸劑 *wán jì*): The ingredients are finely ground or pulverized, a liquid or other viscous medium is added, and round pills are formed. In general, pills are absorbed slowly and over a long period of time. The size of pills is specified as either large, medium, or small, or is described in terms of a common edible substance such as mustard seeds or soybeans. Pills are more easily stored and ingested than decoctions, and are less expensive. They are most commonly used for treating chronic disorders associated with deficiency, but can also be stored for quick use in treating acute disorders when there is little time to prepare decoctions or powders. Pills are also the formulation of choice when a formula calls for ingredients that should not be decocted. These include extremely aromatic substances such as those used in Calm the Palace Pill with Cattle Gallstone (*ān gōng niú huáng wán*), and very toxic ones such as those used in Vessel and Vehicle Pill (*zhōu chē wán*). The most common types of pills are those made with honey, water, or paste, or from concentrate.

• PILLS MADE WITH HONEY (蜜丸 *mì wán*): These are made of ground herbs and processed honey. The honey is heated to a temperature that preserves its adhesive characteristics, but makes it easier to work with. A mixture of beeswax and sesame oil is often added to the honey to prevent it from sticking to the utensils. Honey makes the pills moist and lubricating, and has a moderating effect on the actions of other ingredients in the formulas. Honey itself is a tonic, and pills made from honey are usually tonics. They are traditionally rather large in size, ranging between 1-2cm in diameter. This type of pill is sometimes referred to as a 'bolus.'

• PILLS MADE WITH LIQUIDS (水丸 *shuǐ wán*): These are made of ground herbs and a liquid, usually water, wine, vinegar, or a strained decoction. Compared with other types of pills, these are small (usually 2-5mm in diameter). They are easy to swallow, quickly digested, and are the most common type of prepared medicine from China.

• PILLS MADE WITH PASTES (糊丸 *hú wán*): These are composed of ground herbs and a paste made from either rice or wheat flour. Pastes are extremely viscous, and pills made with pastes break up in the digestive tract and are absorbed more slowly than any other type. This prolongs the effect of a formula (in a 'time-release' manner) and reduces irritation to the digestive tract.

• PILLS MADE FROM CONCENTRATES (濃縮丸 *nóng suō wán*): These are made of a concentrate from the strained decoction of a formula with the addition of a filler, usually starch, the dried and powdered dregs from the decoction, or ground up raw herbs. Depending on the particular formulation, water or wine may be added at certain times during the processing. These pills have the advantage of containing a relatively large amount of the active ingredients per volume. This makes them very convenient to use.

Soft Extracts (膏劑 *gāo jì*): The ingredients are simmered with water or vegetable oil until a concentrate with a syrupy or gummy consistency forms. Soft extracts can be used internally or externally. They are applied externally as plasters for skin disorders or the effects of trauma. (These are discussed in the section on external applications below.) When taken internally, the three most common types of soft extracts are those made from prolonged decoction, liquid extraction, and semi-solid extraction.

• SYRUPS FROM PROLONGED DECOCTION (煎膏 *jiān gāo*): These are made by repeatedly decocting the ingredients to a specified concentration, further concentrating the strained liquid, and finally cooking with the addition of honey or sugar to make into a syrup or gel-like extract. These are easy to take, sweet in flavor, and have the effect of enriching and tonifying. For this reason, they are also known as 'enriching soft extracts' (膏滋 *gāo zī*).

• LIQUID EXTRACTIONS (流浸膏 *liú jìn gāo*): These are made by soaking the ingredients in a solvent (usually alcohol) to extract the active ingredients, and then heating the result to dispose of a specified percentage of the solvent. Usually 1ml of a liquid extraction contains the active ingredients of 1g of a normal ingredient. Liquid extracts are similar to tinctures; they are, however, more concentrated so that less alcohol needs to be ingested to get the same amount of active ingredient.

• SEMI-SOLID EXTRACTS (浸膏 *jìn gāo*): These are made in the same manner as liquid extracts, except that they are heated until all of the solvent is gone. Usually 1g of an extract contains the active ingredients of 2-5g of a normal ingredient. The extracts are either fashioned into tablets or pills, or are put into capsules. This is an effective and convenient way to dispense medicine and does not have the side effects associated with the solvent.

Syrups (糖漿劑 *táng jiāng jì*): These are made by taking the strained liquid from a decoction and adding a specified quantity of cane sugar and then cooking for a prolonged period. Syrups are sweet and are principally used in treating children and chronic disorders.

Special Pills (丹劑 *dān jì*): These are not a distinct type of formulation, but instead are a form of pill. The ingredients are ground into a fine powder, mixed with water, paste, or the strained liquid from a decoction, and then formed into pills. Most of the formulas whose names include this term contain specially processed and/or expensive ingredients, and are thus called special pills. The term is also used in Taoist alchemy where different metals are made into pills to promote longevity or spiritual attainment. It is for this reason that this type of formulation is also called an 'elixir.'

Medicinal Wines (酒劑 *jiǔ jì* or 藥酒 *yào jiǔ*): These are made by soaking the ingredients in rice or sorghum wine or other spirits, using the alcohol as a solvent. The wine is warmed, the dregs are discarded, and the resulting liquid can be used internally or externally. Wine itself is considered to nourish, invigorate the blood, and unblock the channels. This type of formulation is therefore most commonly used in treating chronic deficiency, or pain associated with wind-dampness or trauma. When used externally as a liniment, often the herbs are simply soaked in the wine for an extended period of time and then the liquid is strained out. Most liniments treat wind-dampness in the joints and channels and traumatic injury.

Lozenges (錠劑 *dìng jì*): These are made by grinding the ingredients into a powder which is formed into ingot-shaped tablets, sometimes with the addition of paste, honey, or other excipient. Before taking, the lozenge is ground into a thick liquid in a similar way that ink is ground. Lozenges can be ingested or applied externally.

Tablets (片劑 *piàn jì*): These are made by processing or otherwise extracting the active parts of the ingredients, adding a filler, and forming the result into tablets (usually under pressure). The tablets are a relatively standardized formulation and can be easily coated. For example, if the ingredients are especially bitter or malodorous, a sugar coating can be added; if the ingredients are adversely affected by the acidic environment of the stomach, an enteric coating can be added. This type of preparation is becoming increasingly popular in China.

There is another type of formulation that is also called a tablet. These are finely ground herbs that are pressed together in tablet form. This type of formulation is actually a variant of the powders discussed above.

Injections (針劑 *zhēn jì*): These are made by extracting the active ingredients with modern methods and preparing a sterile solution that can be administered by injection. These are injected subcutaneously, intramuscularly, or intravenously. The advantage of this method is that the delivery of the active ingredients is precise, fast, and unaffected by any interaction with the digestive system or foods. One disadvantage is that the solutions focus on what is commonly believed to be the active ingredients and so may not have the full spectrum of effects that cruder extraction methods may have. In addition, this method of administration contains none of the empirical evidence of the two-thousand-year history of Chinese medicine and thus it should not be assumed that the functions will be similar to those of ingested herbs. It is used especially often in hospital settings.

Herb Concentrates

A particularly important form of herbal preparation are the various types of granules (沖服劑 *chōng fú jì* in Chinese; 和漢藥 *wakanyaku* in Japanese). This is also referred to as concentrated powders or granules (濃縮藥粉 *nóng suō yào fěn*) and scientific Chinese medicine (科學中藥 *kē xué zhōng yào*).

This is a modern formulation that is based upon the decoction and syrup. There are many different types of granules, but most are made by decocting the ingredients until a thick, concentrated semi-liquid remains. Then a carrier, which can be starch, ground up raw herbs (such as Dioscoreae Rhizoma [*shān yào*]), or the dregs of the decoction, is added and thoroughly mixed with the concentrate. The resulting mixture is made into granules or powder by heating it in a low-heat oven and ground into a powder. If properly packaged and stored, granules can retain their potency for long periods of time, commonly 12-18 months. They are more quickly absorbed and stronger-acting than most pills and tablets, and are more convenient and require less medicine per volume than decoctions or syrups. Another advantage is that, like powders, they can be chewed into a paste in the mouth before swallowing. This allows for partial direct absorption through the membranes of the oral cavity, bypassing the digestive tract.

The procedures are certainly more sophisticated in herbal factories. Industrial approaches to granule production were developed in Japan after WWII and then became popular in Taiwan, Korea, the People's Republic of China, and the United States. In Japan and Taiwan these formulations are recognized by the ministries of health and are part of the national health insurance system. For this reason, they have become by far the most popular form of herbal medicines in these countries. In Japan, pharmacists are licensed to dispense these products in response to client requests and may do so using any diagnostic approach except palpatory examination (pulse and abdomen), which is reserved for licensed physicians. While the information presented here is current with the Good Manufacturing Practices (GMP) of Taiwan, it should be broadly congruent with the method of production in other countries with similar regulations.

- INSPECTION OF INCOMING MEDICINALS: Each lot of incoming herbs is quarantined, inspected, and assigned a source herb number upon arrival. After passing inspection for herb quality, herb identification, heavy metal levels, presence of bugs and other contaminants – and, in specific instances, active constituents – the items are removed from quarantine and allowed to enter the storage facility. Agents are then cleaned by hand, and all extraneous material is removed in preparation for further processing. Where needed, herbs are further prepared (dry-fried, wine-fried, etc.) according to the traditional tenets of Chinese medicine.

- EXTRACTION: The ingredients for a formula are gathered together and placed in a large stainless steel vat filled with water. The water is heated to a set temperature. The herbs are cooked for an optimal length of time to extract the most ingredients without overcooking and destroying the constituents. Cooking duration and temperatures are thus unique to each product. At various intervals, the volume and temperature of the solution are recorded in the batch record. At the beginning of the heating process, many companies collect volatile oils in a volatile oil retrieval system installed on each extraction vat. These oils are reintroduced into the product during the granulation process.

- CONCENTRATION: When the optimal extraction strength is reached, the herbs are removed from the extraction vat and the liquid is piped directly into the condensing vat. Here it is condensed through evaporation in a relative vacuum under low temperature.

- FLOW COATING: After vacuum evaporation, the thickened liquid, similar in consistency to molasses, is piped into a vacuum dryer and flow-coating chamber. At this time, a base powder of either starch (corn or potato are most common) or a powder of the raw herbs or a sugar such as maltodextrine is sprayed into the chamber. This material mixes with the liquid spray to form a powder. The addition of methylcellulose will produce a granule. Toward the end of this process, if volatile oils have been collected earlier in the extraction phase they are introduced into the chamber and absorbed into the powder.

- PACKAGING: The granules are then packaged and sealed in bottles by machine. The labels for each lot are accounted for and printed with the expiration date and lot number. In Japan, the most common form of packaging of formulas is in 2g sachets. Typically, the sachets are arranged in strips of three with the standard adult dose being 1 sachet, 3x per day (6g total). While this form of packaging allows for maximum shelf life and convenience, it does make formula modification more complicated. All of the procedures that occur after extraction are done in a cleanroom atmosphere where all employees adhere to cleanroom requirements and the air is filtered and conditioned to approved standards.

- TRACKING: GMP standards demand that each step of production is tracked through meticulous bookkeeping. For example, batch numbers of the source herbs are recorded in the batch record so each final product can be traced back to its source material. Because of these strict operating and tracking measures, one can quickly see the details of each procedure applied to a product during the production process.

- TESTING: The goal of testing is to insure the quality, purity, and consistency of each product. Samples from each lot are kept on site so that any lot can be checked at a later time. Each lot is checked to insure that it meets the manufacturer's acceptable levels for heavy metals and plate count. Thin-layer chromatography and HPLC are performed on products for which those tests are appropriate and meaningful. Further, each lot is tested to make certain it contains no dangerous microbes such as *E. coli* and *Salmonella*.

Frequently Asked Questions about Herb Concentrates

What is the concentration ratio of herb concentrates?

There are several ways to answer this question. The simplest is to reply that 250–500g of raw herbs are used to produce 100g of concentrate. This yields a concentration ratio of 2.5:1 to 5:1 depending on the specific formula or single herb. Regardless of any claims to the contrary, most formulas are in the range of 3:1 to 4:1. Formulas of a very glutinous nature require more starch in order to be prepared into a dry form and thus tend to lower concentration.

These figures are misleading, however, because the highly controlled environment in which the concentrates are produced and the reintroduction of captured volatile oils result in a product superior to what would be produced on one's kitchen stove. Thus, the 250–500g of herbs produce a more potent product than they would if cooked in a less efficient method. For this reason, it is not accurate to think that 10g of a raw herb equals 2–4g of a concentrate. (See the following section on how to use herb concentrates for more information on dosing.)

Are all single-herb products concentrates?

No, it is not possible to concentrate minerals, saps, or most animal products since their constituents are not very soluble in water. These items are sold as ground powders when in single-herb form. In formulas, they are generally cooked with the rest of the herbs and are part of the base onto which the concentrate is sprayed in the flow-coating process.

What dose of concentrated granules should I give a patient per day?

In Japan, the standard recommended adult dose is usually 6g per day, normally divided into three doses. Most practitioners in Taiwan, where concentrated granules have been in use for over 40 years, give between 10 and 12g per day. Naturally, children get considerably less (about half) and infants and toddlers are usually given about one-half gram or less per dose, four to five times a day.

What is the best way to take the granules?

Most patients mix the granules with warm water and drink this between meals. For children, it is sometimes best to mix the granules with a food such as applesauce. In Japan, the standard practice is to put the granules straight into the mouth and chew them into a paste. This allows for immediate absorption prior to swallowing the remaining paste with or without water. This approach meets with varying degrees of cooperation in Western patients.

How to Use Herb Concentrates

In some traditions that utilize herb concentrates, notably Japan, formulas are primarily used as defined in the source texts, so the issue of modification does not commonly arise. If modification is deemed necessary (usually by one or two herbs at most), a standard rule of thumb is to do this at a ratio of 1:10, modifying herb to formula. For example, a commonly used prescription for dermatological problems in Japan would be 50g of Tangkuei and Peony Powder *(dāng guī sháo yào sǎn)* with the addition of 5g of Coicis Semen *(yì yǐ rén)*.

In Taiwan, combining herb concentrates is often more complex. Prescribing and dosing granular herb concentrates requires a slightly different reasoning process and different mathematics from those used for crude herbs, for two reasons. First, the concentrated herb granules are available in both formula and single-herb form. Thus, one must consider how to combine and dose these two forms. Second, experience has shown that, for herb concentrates, 10g per day (approximately three grams, three times a day) is generally an effective dose. Thus, the prescribed herbs and formulas must be fit into a 10g-per-day dose.

Dosage determination

As discussed above, the efficient extraction process used in producing concentrates differs considerably from the process of decocting crude herbs in a patient's home. Thus, calculating the dosage of herb concentrates demands a unique method, quite unlike that used for crude herbs. The system described here is based on observation of prescription methods in Taiwan, where concentrated granules have long been an accepted form of herbal therapy. Appropriate dosages of each component of combinations, such as those discussed above, can be determined through a four-step process:

Step 1. Calculate the total number of grams to be dispensed by multiplying the grams per day times the number of days the formula will be taken. For example, if 10g of herbs per day are to be prescribed for a 10-day period, the total amount of herbs to be dispensed is 100g.

Step 2. Dose the single herbs in the prescription at 0.5-2g per day. Herbs that are typically prescribed in small doses, such as Polygalae Radix *(yuǎn zhì)* and Aconiti Radix lateralis praeparata *(zhì fù zǐ)*, should be dosed at about 0.5g per day; herbs that are typically prescribed in large doses, such as Polygoni multiflori Caulis *(yè jiāo téng)* and Coicis Semen *(yì yǐ rén)*, should be prescribed at 1.5-2g per day. Most herbs should be dosed at about 1g per day.

Step 3. After dosing the single herbs, find the sum of all single-herb dosages and deduct that number from the total grams to be dispensed, as determined in Step 1. This is the number of grams left for formulas in the prescription.

Step 4. Divide the amount determined in Step 3 among the formulas in the prescription, giving a larger amount to the formula or formulas that you wish to emphasize.

When prescribing an unmodified formula, dosing 10g per day is simple and straightforward. However, if more than one formula is used, or if single herbs are added to the prescription, there are three possible strategies:

1. *One or two formulas, with or without single herbs:* In this case, the 4-step procedure described above is usually used to construct the formula. For example, for a wind-heat exterior pattern with sore throat and thirst, one could construct the following for a 2-day treatment (20g total, since 10g per day is standard):

Honeysuckle and Forsythia Powder (*yín qiáo sǎn*) 16g
Isatidis/Baphicacanthis Radix (*bǎn lán gēn*) 2g
Trichosanthis Radix (*tiān huā fěn*) 2g

> Dosage   10g per day divided into 3 doses

2. *Three or more formulas, with or without single herbs:* Some practitioners regard the formulas that are cooked together as a functional unit and often combine several formulas together. This strategy usually combines formulas for root and branch together. For example, treatment of acute nasal congestion in a patient with chronic rhinitis attributable to qi deficiency might have a formula as follows:

Clear the Nose Decoction (*qīng bí tāng*) 40g
Xanthium Powder (*cāng ěr zǐ sǎn*) 40g
Tonify the Middle to Augment the Qi Decoction
    (*bǔ zhōng yì qì tāng*) 20g

> Dosage   10g per day divided into 3 doses

This would be a 10-day formula that emphasizes treatment of the branch. Should symptoms decrease in severity, the practitioner may wish to change the proportions to attend more to the root disharmony as follows:

Clear the Nose Decoction (*qīng bí tāng*) 25g
Xanthium Powder (*cāng ěr zǐ sǎn*) 25g
Tonify the Middle to Augment the Qi Decoction
    (*bǔ zhōng yì qì tāng*) 50g

> Dosage   10g per day divided into 3 doses

3. *Combining only single herbs:* There are instances when no formula exists in concentrated granule form that is appropriate for the case at hand. One then usually constructs a formula using reasoning similar to that applied to traditionally decocted formulas. For example, a patient with angina owing to blood stasis and underlying qi deficiency could be treated with the following formula:

Persicae Semen (*táo rén*) 12g
Carthami Flos (*hóng huā*) 10g
Cyathulae Radix (*chuān niú xī*) 10g
Paeoniae Radix rubra (*chì sháo*) 10g
Chuanxiong Rhizoma (*chuān xiōng*) 6g
Glycyrrhizae Radix (*gān cǎo*) 6g

Notoginseng Radix (*sān qī*) 8g
Daemonoropis Resina (*xuè jié*) 6g
Salviae miltiorrhizae Radix (*dān shēn*) 16g
Ginseng Radix (*rén shēn*) 10g
Schisandrae Fructus (*wǔ wèi zǐ*) 6g

> Dosage   10g per day divided into 3 doses. Note also that herbs such as Schisandrae Fructus (*wǔ wèi zǐ*), Chuanxiong Rhizoma (*chuān xiōng*), and Daemonoropis Resina (*xuè jié*), which are generally given in smaller doses when in decoction, are in smaller percentage in this formula. Likewise, Salviae miltiorrhizae Radix (*dān shēn*), which is often used in a dosage as large as 30-60g in decoctions for treatment of angina, is given a large dose in this concentrated-powder formula.

In summary, some adjustments in thinking must be made to accommodate the difference in form of concentrated powders. Treatment principals and theory, however, remain the same as for prescribing with traditional decoctions.

Unresolved Issues

One important issue affecting the utilization of herb concentrates relates to the efficacy of making a formula based on combining concentrates of single herbs versus that of using formulas that are prepared by the manufacturer in which all the herbs are combined and (with the exceptions noted above) cooked together. Many practitioners, particularly in Japan, believe that the synergy of this process, though not well understood, is nonetheless very important. To these practitioners, combining individually granulated single herbs into a formula will produce an inferior clinical effect.

Types of Formulations for External Applications

Modern texts on the subject of external applications of herbs use various categorization schemes to break down the numerous methods into groups that can be discussed succinctly. Some use the methods of application as rubrics and others use the state and nature of the substance (powder, liquid, syrup, etc.) as the basis for their system. For our purposes, we use a combination of these categories to introduce the reader to the scope of this treatment modality. In Chapter 21, Formulas for External Application, we present examples of the most commonly used methods of application of herbs, namely, soft plasters, ointments, powders and wash-steam-soak-compresses. We also include a few examples of less-commonly used external application methods.

Solids Used as External Applications

- SOFT PLASTERS AND OINTMENTS (軟膏 *ruǎn gāo*): An ointment is generally made by soaking and then cooking herbs in oil or lard, and, after removing the cooked herbs, solidifying the oil by adding beeswax, paraffin, or some other hardening agent. Soft plasters are assembled from powdered herbs mixed with an adjuvant. The most common adjuvants are vegetable oil, lard, water, rice wine, rice vinegar, or egg white. The choice of adjuvant is sometimes dependent on the function desired. For example, wine helps to move the blood, vinegar softens hardness, and vegetable oil moistens the skin. In some cases, fresh herbs such as Taraxaci Herba *(pú gōng yīng)* or Portulacae Herba *(mǎ chǐ xiàn)* are pounded together with herb powders to make a plaster. In modern times, materials such as petroleum jelly, isopropyl alcohol, and glycerin are sometimes substituted for the natural adjuvants used in earlier times.

A soft plaster is applied directly to the affected area or can be spread on a gauze pad and secured with tape. The general rule is to change a plaster once a day. Ointments are applied as needed and can be put on a gauze pad or massaged into the site of the lesion. The scope of treatment for plasters and ointments is quite wide-ranging. Customary functions include resolving toxicity, dispersing stasis, relieving pain, clearing heat, dispelling wind, moistening skin, and softening hardness. While most plasters and ointments are used for the treatment of traumatic injury or skin disorders, they can also be used to treat tumors and swellings, inflamed lymph nodes, hemorrhoids, and internal disorders such as headache, menstrual pain, and constipation.

• HARD PLASTERS (硬膏 *yìng gāo*): These are made by cooking herbs in vegetable oil for long periods of time, and, after removing the herbs, adding a hardening agent, usually Minium *(qiān dān)*, while the liquid is hot. The hot liquid is spread onto a cloth backing where it sets into a hard plaster. To apply the plaster, one heats the herb face of the plaster until it softens and then applies it to the affected area. Most hard plasters are used in the treatment of painful obstruction or other stubborn, painful disorders, but some are used to disperse toxic swellings.

• POWDERS AND DAUBS (搽粉 *chá fěn*, 塗藥 *tú yào*): Powders are made by grinding medicinal agents into a powder, which is usually sifted through a fine-meshed sieve. A daub is made by mixing the powder with a liquid adjuvant such as water, vegetable oil, rice vinegar, rice wine, egg white, or tea water.

Powders can dry dampness, relieve itching, close sores, abate sweating, resolve toxicity, clear heat, and kill parasites. Daubs have similar functions, but with their paste-like consistency, they are more suitable for small areas. Powders are used to treat disorders such as heat rash, athlete's foot, weeping eczema, and excessive sweating of the hands or feet. Sprinkled into sores, they can stop bleeding, generate flesh, and help wounds to close. Daubs can be dabbed onto small sores such as those associated with herpes zoster, impetigo, or poison ivy rash. In addition, some powders can be blown into body orifices or snorted into the nose.

Liquids and Gases Used as External Applications

• STEAMS, SOAKS, WASHES, AND COMPRESSES (蒸 *zhēng*, 浸 *jìn*, 洗 *xǐ*, 熱敷 *rè fū*): These are all made in a similar manner. Herbs are put in water, soaked, and brought to a boil. They are simmered 20-40 minutes and the strained decoction is used as a wash or soak or to moisten a compress. The hot vapor is also used to steam the affected area when applicable.

Large areas where soaking or applying a compress is impractical are usually washed with the decoction. This is allowed to dry. Washes are applied 2-4 times a day. A soak is the ideal method for applying the decoction to hands, feet, elbows, and other areas that can fit in a small container. Instructions vary, but soaking for 20-30 minutes twice a day is typical. Compresses can be made by soaking a washcloth in the decoction. The moist washcloth is also usually applied for 20-30 minutes twice a day. For some hot skin disorders, compresses are applied at room temperature, but for most disorders it is important to keep the compress hot.

Steams, soaks, washes, and compresses serve various functions depending on the herbs in the formula. Common functions include resolving toxicity, relieving itching, killing parasites, relieving pain, dispelling cold, invigorating the collaterals, and promoting the expression of rashes. They are applied to skin rashes, small sores, wind-cold painful obstruction, and areas of trauma (usually after inflammation has receded), and are used for eye, mouth, and genital and rectal disorders. Sitz baths are best for rectal and genital disorders, and whole body baths are suitable for rashes that cover a large portion of the body. Soaks, for example foot soaks, can also used to treat internal disorders in addition to local problems.

• FUMIGATION (熏 *xūn*): This is the burning of a medicinal agent while directing the smoke to waft over the area to be treated. For example, in ancient times, Realgar *(xióng huáng)* fumigation was used in this manner to treat scabies. Nowadays, various fumigation formulas are used to treat a variety of disorders including eczema, athlete's foot, painful obstruction, and rectal prolapse. A variation of this treatment is inhalation of the smoke of burning herbs.

• LINIMENTS (搽劑 *chá jì*): These are an external application made by soaking herbs in rice wine, sorghum liquor, or vinegar for a period of several days to several months. The liquid is strained out and used to rub into the skin. Most liniments move the blood, dispel stasis, and relieve pain and are used to relieve the pain of painful obstruction disorders.

Other Methods of Topical Application

• ADHERING HERBS (貼法 *tiē fǎ* or 敷法 *fū fǎ*): This method involves placing plasters, ointments, herb cakes, herb powders, or freshly pounded herbs on specific acupuncture points, most commonly CV-8 *(shèn quē)* or KI-1 *(yōng quán)*. This method is applied to a large number of internal disorders.

• HOT PRESSING (熨法 *yùn fǎ*): This is a method of dispelling cold, moving blood and qi, and relieving pain. It consists of heating coarsely ground herbs and putting them in a cloth bag that is pressed, while the herbs are still warm, to the painful spot. Hot pressing is mostly used to treat menstrual pain or painful obstruction due to cold.

• BLISTERING (發泡法 *fā pào fǎ*): For this method, caustic herbs are applied to specific locations on the body (usually acupuncture points) in order to cause blistering. One common example is a combination of herbs, including Sinapis Semen *(bái jiè zǐ)*, placed on points on the back in summertime to treat asthma that is usually worse in the winter. This method causes a slight scarring of the skin.

• MEDICATED THREADS OR HERB STICKS (藥線 *yào xiàn*, 藥撚 *yào niǎn*): This type of application is made by mixing the powder of caustic agents with a liquid to form a thread or stick. Threads are placed on toxic swellings to perforate the skin and allow the lesion to suppurate. Herb sticks are applied at a later stage of treatment where they are placed into the open lesion to eat away at dead flesh and the core of the sore to set the stage for successful wound closing.

Preparation and Administration of Decoctions

Once one has decided which formula to use and the form in which it is to be administered, the practitioner must prepare and administer the formula. Except for decoctions, the method for preparing and administering the different types of formulations was described above. Because the preparation of decoctions is a rather complex task, we will discuss it at length here.

Through the centuries, practitioners have always stressed the importance of correctly decocting the formulas. This is not unusual because, like all types of cooking, the results depend in large measure on the way in which it is actually done. In *On the Origins and Development of Medicine*, the 18th-century writer Xu Da-Chun observed, "It is most appropriate to discuss the method of decoction in depth; whether the medicine is effective or not completely depends on this."

Equipment: The pots used for decocting should be ceramic or earthenware. This is because metals, particularly iron or aluminum, can cause unknown chemical reactions when herbs are decocted in them. In the West it is not uncommon to find households in which there are no nonmetallic pots. It is the experience of many practitioners that stainless steel pots can be used without any untoward effects because there is no reaction between the metal and the ingredients of the formulas. Whatever the material, the pots must have a tight-fitting lid and be clean.

Proper water: At present, unless the formula requires some special type of water, tap water is usually good enough for decoctions. In areas where the tap water is polluted or has high mineral content, distilled or clean bottled water may be substituted. Where special types of water are required, they are specifically noted under the method of preparation for the particular formula.

Amount of water: This varies depending on how the formula is to be decocted and the type of ingredients used. The water should generally cover the herbs by about one-half inch. This translates into anywhere from 200-300ml of water for 30g of herbs. Minerals and shells absorb very little water, while roots, leaves, and flowers will absorb more. When instructing a patient on how to make a decoction at home, remember that one cup of water is approximately 200ml.

Type of heat: The Chinese traditionally distinguish two types of heat for cooking herbs: the high flame or 'military fire' (武火 *wǔ huǒ*) and the low flame or 'civilian fire' (文火 *wén huǒ*). Usually, the decoction is brought to a boil over a high flame, and then cooked over a lower flame. This was succinctly stated by Li Shi-Zhen in *Comprehensive Outline of the Materia Medica:* "Start with a military [fire] and then use a civilian [fire]. If [decoctions are] prepared in this manner, none will be ineffective."

Method of decoction: When the herbs have been put in the pot and covered with an appropriate amount of water, allow them to soak for awhile. This will facilitate the extraction of the active ingredients during the process of decoction. Once the herbs have come to a boil, turn the heat down. Do not lift the lid to look at the herbs too often, as this may diminish their effect by allowing the 'flavor' of the herbs to escape.

Most formulas are cooked for 20-30 minutes. However, to be most effective, formulas that release the exterior, clear heat, or contain herbs with volatile oils should be cooked over a relatively high flame for a shorter period of time (10-15 minutes). This is particularly true of cool, acrid formulas that treat exterior wind-heat such as Mulberry Leaf and Chrysanthemum Drink *(sāng jú yǐn)*. This idea was originated by Wu Ju-Tong and is at some variance with the methods of decoction described in *Discussion of Cold Damage*. Tonics and other formulas that contain rich, cloying substances should be cooked over a relatively low flame for a longer period of time (45-60 minutes) to extract as much from them as possible. Toxic substances such as Aconiti Radix lateralis praeparata *(zhì fù zǐ)* should be cooked for at least 45 minutes to reduce their toxicity.

The most common method is to decoct the ingredients twice, using slightly less water the second time. Both times the herbs are boiled down until only one cup (about 200ml) of liquid remains. After the second cooking, the herbs are discarded. The two cups of liquid are then combined, and one cup is taken twice a day (usually morning and evening), or two-thirds of a cup is taken three times a day (upon awakening, and then an hour before lunch and dinner). Decoctions are generally taken before meals. This permits the maximum absorption to occur quickly. There are times when this is impractical, or when the ingredients may irritate the digestive tract. In such cases, the formulas should be taken after meals.

There are many different ways in which decoctions are prepared in China. Some are regional variations, but other differences are related to the nature of what is being decocted. For example, tonic formulas are often cooked only once, but in relatively more water and for a longer period of time. The liquid is then divided into three doses and taken on an empty stomach, usually right before meals. For children or the seriously ill, the decoction is generally divided into smaller doses and taken frequently throughout the day. This is also a good practice for anyone who has trouble taking a full cup of the decoction at a time. An example of a regional variation is the practice in Guangdong of cooking *all* decoctions just once for 30-40 minutes, and then taking the resulting cup of strained liquid on an empty stomach before a meal.

If a formula is overcooked or burnt, never add water to cook it again. Some herbs must be specially treated during the decocting process (see Table 4). When these special treatments are required, they should be noted on the prescription that is given to the pharmacist.

• DECOCTED FIRST (先煎 *xiān jiān):* There are three types of substances that should be decocted first before adding the other ingredients. The first are some toxic herbs that are cooked for 30-45 minutes before adding the other ingredients in order to make them safe. The second are minerals and shells that must be cooked longer to obtain any effect. They are cooked 10-20 minutes before adding the other ingredients. The third are the lightweight substances when they are used in large dosages. There is simply no room in most pots to decoct them with the other ingredients. For this reason, they are decocted first for about 20 minutes, and the resulting liquid is used to decoct the other ingredients.

• ADDED NEAR END (後下 *hòu xià):* Aromatic herbs such as Menthae haplocalycis Herba *(bò hé)* should be added to the decoction 4-5 minutes before the end. This prevents their volatile oils from wafting away instead of remaining in the strained decoction. Some herbs will have a much stronger effect if added near the end, but can be decocted with the other ingredients if the practitioner wants to mute this particular effect. For example, the purgative action of Rhei Radix et Rhizoma *(dà huáng)* is much greater when it is added near the end. If this is not desired, the herb should be decocted together with the other ingredients.

• DECOCTED IN GAUZE (包煎 *bāo jiān):* Some ingredients should be packaged in a gauze or cheesecloth sack before cooking. Otherwise they will stimulate the throat or digestive tract, with adverse effect. Included are herbs with cilia (fine, hair-like structures) such as Inulae Flos *(xuán fù huā)*, small seeds such as Plantaginis Semen *(chē qián zǐ)*, and some minerals. In addition, some formulas which are ground before they are decocted are also prepared in this manner.

Decocted first	Aconiti Radix lateralis praeparata *(zhì fù zǐ)*, Aconiti Radix praeparata *(zhì chuān wū)*, Aconiti kusnezoffii Radix praeparata *(zhì cǎo wū)*, Haliotidis Concha *(shí jué míng)*, Fossilia Ossis Mastodi *(lóng gǔ)*, Ostreae Concha *(mǔ lì)*, Magnetitum *(cí shí)*, Margaritiferae Concha usta *(zhēn zhū mǔ)*, Haematitum *(dài zhě shí)*, Testudinis Plastrum *(guī bǎn)*, Trionycis Carapax *(biē jiǎ)*, Gypsum fibrosum *(shí gāo)*, Bubali Cornu *(shuǐ niú jiǎo)*, Luffae Fructus Retinervus *(sī guā luò)*
Added near end	Menthae haplocalycis Herba *(bò hé)*, Aucklandiae Radix *(mù xiāng)*, Amomi Fructus *(shā rén)*, Amomi Fructus rotundus *(bái dòu kòu)*, Artemisiae annuae Herba *(qīng hāo)*, Uncariae Ramulus cum Uncis *(gōu téng)*, Houttuyniae Herba *(yú xīng cǎo)*, Rhei Radix et Rhizoma *(dà huáng)* [when desired]
Decocted in gauze	Inulae Flos *(xuán fù huā)*, Plantaginis Semen *(chē qián zǐ)*, Halloysitum rubrum *(chì shí zhī)*, Talcum *(huá shí)*
Separately decocted or simmered	Ginseng Radix *(rén shēn)*, Panacis quinquefolii Radix *(xī yáng shēn)*, Cervi Cornu pantotrichum *(lù róng)*
Dissolved in the strained decoction	Asini Corii Colla *(ē jiāo)*, Maltosum *(yí táng)*, Cervi Cornus Colla *(lù jiǎo jiāo)*, Daemonoropis Resina *(xuè jié)*
Taken with the strained decoction	Fritillariae cirrhosae Bulbus *(chuān bèi mǔ)*, Notoginseng Radix *(sān qī)*, Bovis Calculus *(niú huáng)*

Table 4 Commonly Used Substances Requiring Special Treatment for Decocting

• SEPARATELY DECOCTED OR SIMMERED (另煎 *lìng jiān* or 另燉 *lìng dùn*): Some rare and very expensive substances such as Ginseng Radix *(rén shēn)* must be separately decocted or simmered to obtain the maximum effect. These are often sliced very thin and then cooked in a double boiler for a long time (usually 2-3 hours) so that every last drop of active ingredient can be extracted.

• DISSOLVED IN THE STRAINED DECOCTION (溶化 *róng huà*): Highly viscous or sticky substances such as Asini Corii Colla *(ē jiāo)* cannot be decocted with the other ingredients. This is because they themselves will stick to the pot and burn, or they may stick to the other ingredients and thereby reduce the effect of decocting. These substances are therefore separately dissolved in a small bowl, and the solution is then added to the strained decoction.

• TAKEN WITH THE STRAINED DECOCTION (沖服 *chōng fú*): Some expensive, aromatic substances such as Fritillariae cirrhosae Bulbus *(chuān bèi mǔ)* are ground into a powder and then taken first, followed (or 'chased') by the strained decoction. Precious horns are often shaved or filed into a powder and ingested, followed by the strained decoction.

Administration

The manner and timing of administration also influences the effect of the formula on the body. Formulas should generally be taken about an hour before meals. Formulas that contain ingredients that irritate the stomach should be taken after meals. Rich, cloying tonics should be taken on an empty stomach. Formulas that calm the spirit should be taken before going to bed. Formulas for malarial conditions should be taken two hours before an attack, if the timing is regular. In an emergency, however, the formulas should be taken irrespective of the time. When taking prepared medicines, it is important that they be taken at a specified time for maximum effect. Some formulas can be taken many times a day, or over the course of the day, like a tea. Certain formulas have special times for administration. For example, Powder to Take at Cock's Crow *(jī míng sǎn)* should be taken on an empty stomach as soon as one awakens for maximum effect.

Decoctions are usually taken warm. This is especially true for exterior cold disorders since taking the decoction warm helps stimulate sweating. Even when a disorder is due to heat, the decoction is usually taken warm. The exception is when taking the medicine warm causes nausea or vomiting, in which case it should be taken cool. Other solutions to this problem include having the patient take a small amount of Citri reticulatae Pericarpium *(chén pí)* or ground ginger before drinking the decoction, or take smaller amounts of the decoction more frequently throughout the day, instead of the normal amount in just two or three doses.

Great care must be exercised in administering very toxic formulas. This means starting with a small dose, then slowly increasing the dosage until the desired effect is obtained. When this occurs, administration of the formula should be discontinued.

Standards of Measurement

In this book, measurements are expressed in the metric system (grams, milliliters, etc.) instead of the traditional Chinese style (錢 *qiǎn*, 兩 *liǎng*, 升 *shēng*, etc.). There are two reasons for this. One is that this book is a compilation of modern Chinese sources, all of which since the early 1980s have been based on the metric system. This was done so that the measurement of medicinal substances would be consistent with all other measurements used in medicine. While there was considerable debate about this issue at the time, it seems to have been settled for now.

The other reason is that using the traditional measurements of weight and volume can be confusing because they have changed over time. For example, before the Jin dynasty (265-420) the measures of weight were the 黍 *shǔ*, 銖 *zhū*, 兩 *liǎng*, and 斤 *jīn*. At that time, the measure 分 *fēn* was added and the ratios of one measure to another were as follows: 10 *shǔ* = 1 *zhū*; 6 *zhū* = 1 *fēn*; 4 *fēn* = 1 *liǎng*; 16 *liǎng* = 1 *jīn*. By the Song dynasty (960-1279) some different measures were introduced, including the *qián*. The system established during the Song has been followed until recently. The ratios among these measures are: 10 毫 *háo* = 1 釐 *lí*; 10 *lí* = 1 分 *fēn*; 10 *fēn* = 1 錢 *qián*; 10 *qián* = 1 兩 *liǎng*; and 16 *liǎng* = 1 斤 *jīn*. Similar changes have occurred in the measurements for volume. The major unit was the 升 *shēng*, the actual volume of which changed over the course of imperial history.

By the Ming dynasty (1368-1644) there was definite confusion about the meaning of traditional measurements. Li Shi-Zhen, for example, noted that "The *liǎng* of the ancients is the *qián* of today; the *shēng* of the ancients equals two-and-a-half *liǎng* today." Another physician of this period, Zhang Jie-Bing, wrote that "The *liǎng* of the ancients equals six of today's *qián*." It should therefore be obvious that the measure for *liǎng* in a 3rd-century work like *Discussion of Cold Damage* is a different unit of measurement than the *liǎng* in a 17th-century work such as *Medical Formulas Collected and Analyzed*. Moreover, the standards of measurement used in medicine were always slightly different than those used in the market. For example, the *liǎng* used in medicine since Song times is roughly 1.2 times the size of the *liǎng* used in the market. In addition, the tools used to weigh herbs have been fairly primitive, and studies have shown that they were far from standardized.

To simplify and standardize this aspect of traditional medicine, the Chinese government in 1979 promulgated a rule that all standards of measurement be expressed in the metric system. It was declared that 1 *jīn* would equal 500g and that all other measurements would follow accordingly: 1 *liǎng* = 31.25g; 1 *qián* = 3.125g; and 1 *fēn* = 0.3125g. In this book we have followed the convention used in our sources of rounding off these numbers so that 1 *liǎng* = 30g and 1 *qián* = 3g. In addition, while there is still quite a bit of discussion about the metric equivalents of ancient units of measurement, we have followed the majority view and assigned a value of 3g to 1 *liǎng,* based on *Discussion of Cold Damage.* Other views of the Han dynasty *liǎng* vary from less than 1.5g to over 15g. The difference of opinion is even more striking when applied to measurements of volume. For example, according to most of our sources, 1 *shēng* at the time of *Discussion of Cold Damage* would equal about 200ml or one cup today. However, there are modern specialists who believe that 1 *shēng* in *Discussion of Cold Damage* equals only 60-80ml.

Although the metric system is now the standard within China, the traditional standards of measurement are still often used in pharmacies outside of China. For that reason, if you write a prescription that is to be filled in the herbal pharmacies of North America or Europe, you should use the traditional measurements. To determine these measurements, simply divide the number of grams by 3 or 30. For example, if the dosage in our book specifies 18g, you should write 6 *qián;* if it specifies 60g, you should write 2 *liǎng.*

JAPANESE HERBAL MEDICINE: HISTORY AND CURRENT USE[*]

The Japanese variation of Chinese herbal medicine is known as Sino-Japanese herbal medicine, or Kampō (a shortened form of 漢方薬 *kampōyaku).* Herbal medicine entered Japan in part directly from China, and in part from Korea. It has undergone continuous transformation as it has been adapted to the character and culture of the Japanese people, and in its present form is a unique medical system that has had a significant impact on the West. Some of the formulas in this book are included not because they are commonly used in China, but because they are considered important in Japan and therefore often used in the West. We hope that this discussion of the background and development of Sino-Japanese herbal medicine, however brief, will be helpful to our readers.

There are two major branches of traditional herbal medicine in present-day Japan. The first of these is the Gosei ('later development' 後世) current, which is based on the theories presented in the *Inner Classic* and incorporated into

[*] We would like to thank Anne Harper for her contribution to this section, which is based on the book by Otsuka Keisetsu, *Sino-Japanese Herbal Medicine (Kampō igaku),* Tokyo: Sogensha Publishing Company (1956), and her discussions with Cyong Jong-Chol of the Kitasato Institute in Tokyo.

Chinese herbal medicine during the 12th-14th centuries and later imported into Japan. The other is the Kohō ('ancient formulas' 古方) current, which looks to the 3rd-century *Discussion of Cold Damage* as its principal text. The Gosei current bears a closer resemblance to traditional Chinese medicine as practiced in modern China, as it extensively utilizes the theories of the five phases and the channels. The Kohō current, although based on an ancient Chinese book, is more distinctively Japanese and represents the break which occurred between the medical systems of China and Japan.

The two Japanese currents do have several points in common which distinguish them from Chinese herbal medicine. First, there is a simplification of the theories with an emphasis on the empirical knowledge of practitioners. Abdominal diagnosis is favored over pulse diagnosis, as it is considered easier to learn, more direct, accurate, and possessing less theoretical entanglements. There are fewer commonly-used medicinal substances and formulas than in China. This may be due to the penchant for simplification, as well as the relative difficulty in obtaining herbs, many of which are imported from China. Finally, the dosage for individual substances in the formulas is only one-third to one-half the amount used in China. There are many different conjectures about the reasons for these differences, ranging from constitutional differences to an array of social factors, but there is no generally accepted understanding.

Before the Nara period (710-794), medical knowledge was largely transmitted to Japan via Korea. Beginning in this period, it was increasingly imported through direct contacts with China. This influx of knowledge culminated in the compilation during the Heian period (794-1185) of the *Ishimpo,* which Yasuyori Tamba presented to the emperor in 984. This text summarized the essentials of Chinese medical knowledge during the Sui (581-618) and Tang (618-907) dynasties. During the Kamakura period (1185-1333), the more dense, theoretical medicine of the Song (960-1279) dynasty was imported to Japan, primarily by Buddhist monks. It was during this period that Chinese medicine became popularized in Japan, as during the previous eras its use had been restricted to the nobility.

It was not until the Muromachi period (1336-1573) that Japanese medicine began to assume a distinct character of its own. Sanki Tashiro (1465-1537), who studied in China, brought back the theories of the Jin-Yuan currents of medicine, particularly those of the warming and tonifying current associated with Li Ao. Sanki's student, Dōsan Manase, actively promulgated this form of medicine and founded a current of medical thought in Japan which was known as the Gosei current. The disciples of this current, who were versed in the Chinese medical classics (especially the *Inner Classic* and *Classic of Difficulties),* did not merely imitate Chinese herbal medicine, but simplified it. Fewer medicinal substances were used, in part because fewer herbs were available in Japan, and in part because the deep influence of Buddhism gave the Japanese a distaste for formulas which utilized animal products. While there are many references to abdominal palpation (腹診 *fukushin*) prior to this time, Dōsan Manase is generally considered the person primarily responsible for its popularization as a major form of diagnosis. Although this current maintained the theoretical basis of Jin-Yuan medicine, which incorporated the theories of the five phases and the channels into herbal medicine, it offered practical, easily-applied treatments and therefore became a very popular current. The books came to Japan via a monk from the Hangzhou area. These monk-physicians were apparently very much involved in the transmission of medical knowledge at the time.

The rise of the Kohō current during the Tokugawa or Edō period (1603-1867) truly marked the emergence of a new and unique system of herbal medicine in Japan. This current advocated a return to the 3rd-century text *Discussion of Cold Damage* as the basis for herbal medicine. The return to the classics affected segments of educated society in China as well as Japan. However, in terms of medicine, the movement in Japan was much more radical than that in China, and led to a major split between the two forms of herbal medicine. This radical philosophical movement was contemporaneous with the seclusionist policies of the Tokugawa shogunate. The severe restrictions on foreign trade led to a marked reduction in the availability of herbs from China and other countries.

The founders of the Kohō current understood the *Discussion of Cold Damage* in the following way. There are five causes of disease: wind, cold, heat, dampness, and improper diet or overwork. When the body is affected by one or more of these influences, the movement of qi, blood, or water (which includes the fluids in traditional Chinese medical parlance) is in turn affected. The qi is particularly important because stagnation of the qi impedes the circulation of blood and water. Symptoms of disease arise when any of these stagnate. Depending on where in the body the stagnation occurs and the strength of the body's resistance, disease is divided into six warps (or stages), the names of which correspond to the six categories of acupuncture channels. *Discussion of Cold Damage* is accordingly divided into six sections, three for the yang warps of disease, and three for the yin warps. It is only in this classification system that the words yin and yang are used. Notable for their absence is any vestige of the five-phase theory, or the theory of the yin and yang organs. Diagnosis was performed by observation and inquiry concerning the presenting symptoms, palpation of the abdomen, and palpation of the pulse (to determine the location and nature of the disease, not to evaluate the affected organs). An appropriate formula was selected based upon the warp or stage of the disease, the nature of the disease-causing agent, the strength of the body, and the aspect of the body which was affected (qi, blood, or water). Also at this time empiricism in Japanese medicine was strongly influenced by the Dutch doctors who practiced in Nagasaki, known as *Oranda-ryu* or the 'Dutch school.'

The founders of the Kohō current held the *Discussion of Cold Damage* in high esteem. Although their view of this book is considered by some to be overly simplistic, they simplified its system even more. Many disciples of the Kohō current regarded the five disease-causing agents in *Discussion of Cold Damage* as one. For example, one of the founders of the current, Gen-i Nagoya (1628–1696), regarded wind, cold, and dampness as forms of cold. This tendency was taken a step further by Tōdō Yoshimasu (1702–1773). In *Myriad Diseases—One Toxin*, he asserted that all diseases stem from toxin in the body. He grandly dismissed the five disease-causing agents as well as the role of qi, blood, and water. He stated that knowing how to treat disease was simply a matter of learning the formulas in *Discussion of Cold Damage*, as they enabled one to treat all ailments. When the pattern (証 *shō*; *zhèng* in Chinese) of signs and symptoms associated with a disease disappears, the disease is cured. He advocated his method of abdominal diagnosis as a means of streamlining the diagnostic process. Skeptical of pulse diagnosis, he believed that while some pulse qualities (such as floating, submerged, slow, rapid, slippery, and irregular) could be discerned, it was impossible to determine the state of the five yin organs through the pulse. These ideas had an enormous impact on the world of Sino-Japanese herbal medicine which can still be felt today.

Tōdō Yoshimasu's ideas were amplified by his students. Yōdō Odai (1799-1870) in particular is credited for having further developed Tōdō's teachings. Nangai Yoshimasu (1750-1813) reinstated the theory of the qi, blood, and water, and many practitioners of the Kohō current today classify the formulas according to their effectiveness in relieving stagnation of these factors. For example, Cinnamon Twig Decoction (*guì zhī tāng*) is used for stagnant qi, Peach Pit Decoction to Order the Qi (*táo hé chéng qì tāng*) for stagnant blood, and Five-Ingredient Powder with Poria (*wǔ líng sǎn*) for stagnant water.

It is important to remember that there are other aspects to herbal medicine in Japan besides the Kohō current. For example, there are many adherents of the Gosei current in Japan today, especially among those practitioners who use both acupuncture and herbal medicine. This is because the theories of the five phases and the channels are considered to be integral to the practice of acupuncture, although some Kohō practitioners have adapted *Discussion of Cold Damage* to acupuncture.

In addition, as evidenced by our book, not only do many Japanese practitioners use formulas that were developed in Japan, but many of them also favor the 16th century Chinese book *Restoration of Health from the Myriad Diseases*. This is likely to have been transmitted to Japan by monk-physicians from the Hangzhou area; in turn, this text is held in particularly high regard in Taiwan, due to the Japanese colonization of Taiwan during the first part of the 20th century.

The above is evidence that many different theories coexist within Japanese herbal medicine today. Perhaps the most common method, however, is a blending of both currents that utilizes the formulas and approaches of each. There has also been a recent surge in translations of current Chinese texts into Japanese. This has given the modern practice of traditional Chinese medicine a direct influence on Sino-Japanese herbal medicine.

Herbal extracts (usually in the form of powders) are by far the most common form of herbal medicine in Japan today. Crude herbs are used less frequently, and are prepared in a somewhat different manner than in China. They are usually cooked in 600ml of water for a period of 30-40 minutes until it is reduced to 300ml. The resulting liquid is divided into three 100ml doses, which is taken before meals.

KOREAN HERBAL MEDICINE: HISTORY AND CURRENT USE*

It is well known that recorded traditional medicine in Korea began with the sharing of Chinese textual traditions. The Koreans have continued to catch up with the latest medical discourses and precious medicinal herbs from China while attempting to fully utilize the locally available medical resources. Herbal medicine in Korea has developed in line with Korea's dual position in both importing and modifying Chinese medicine. Koreans regarded the latest Chinese materia medica as an advanced form of textual knowledge and material entities, yet simultaneously altered foreign medicinals to use them as a foundation for an indigenous tradition of medicine. The development of 'local botanicals' (鄉藥 *hyang-yak*) demonstrates well how Koreans have pursued the management of materia medica for their own use.

Not many records about Korean herbs are found before the Goryeo dynasty (高麗 918-1392). Records available now indicate that Tao Hong-Jing's *Collection of Commentaries on the Classic of the Materia Medica* and *Newly Improved Materia Medica* were transmitted to Korea before the 7th century, and medical texts, materia medica, and even famous medical practitioners themselves moved between Korean and Chi-

nese territories before the Goryeo dynasty. One of the most notable aspects of this traffic was the trade in Ginseng Radix (*rén shēn*). Most ginseng from the Silla Kingdom (新羅 57 B.C.E.–935 C.E.) was valued as high in quality, such that from the Song onward it was common to use the term 'Silla ginseng' to identify its local habitat. This distinction, made by the combination of a species and a particular habitat, shows how botanicals from Korea gained a name and place within the Chinese classification system.

During the Goryeo dynasty, publications about locally available Korean herbs increased, reflecting Goryeo's cultural pride and the prevalence of in-depth knowledge about the classics of Chinese medicine. Paralleling the influx of foreign materia medica from China, Japan, and Arabia, major texts about local botanicals flourished in line with other orderly, planned state publications of medicine. *Prescriptions of Local Botanicals for Emergency Use* (鄉藥救急方 *Hyangyak guge-upbang*, c. 1236), which survives today, provides a list of local botanicals (方中鄉藥目草部 *Bangjung hyangyak mokcho-bu*) representing 180 species. Here the local name, attributes, toxicity, and method of collecting each herb are described. Other major texts about local herbs from this period include *San Hezi's Prescriptions Using Local Botanicals* (三和子鄉藥方 *Samhwaja hyangyakbang*), *Old Prescriptions Based on Local Botanicals* (鄉藥古方 *Hyangyak gobang*), *Tested Prescriptions Using Local Botanicals to Benefit the People* (鄉藥惠民經驗方 *Hyangyak hyemin kyeongheombang*), and *Easy Prescriptions Using Local Botanicals* (鄉藥簡易方 *Hyang-yakganibang*). Although most of these texts are lost, titles and dozens of formulas from each text are found in later publications. Using locally available herbs, the prescriptions in these texts show minor modifications in dosage, therapeutic methods, and herbal entities, while the accounts of symptoms and the course of diseases follow the significant medical texts of Tang China.

Local botanicals continued to be valued during the 15th century as the newly-founded Joseon dynasty (朝鮮, 1392-1910) sought to display its cultural authority and confidence in the knowledge of indigenous medical resources. *Standard Prescriptions of Local Botanicals* (鄉藥集成方 *Hyangyak jipseongbang*, 1433) listed more than 700 species under the category of local materia medica. Composed of 57 nosological categories and 959 subsections, *Standard Prescriptions of Local Botanicals* increased the number of previously known nosological categories from 338 to 959, expanded the number of formulas from 2,803 to 10,706, and added 1,416 new items about acupuncture, thus distinguishing itself from its predecessors. The bibliography of *Standard Prescriptions of Local Botanicals* listed 160 medical texts overall, mostly transmitted from China. Yet local botanicals were grouped as a thematic framework through which Koreans defined their location not as a marginalized backwater left behind by

---

*We would like to thank Soyoung Suh, Ph.D. (UCLA) for contributing this section of the introduction. She is at present a post-doctoral fellow in the Department of East Asian Languages and Civilizations, Harvard University.

medical novelties, but as a unique location for the creation of its own medicinal arts.

As texts about local botanicals were planned as a dynastic project, it became more important to distinguish locally grown botanicals from foreign botanicals. This was done by identifying the names, shapes, and attributes of local botanicals and comparing them with Chinese botanicals. Articulating those characteristics was crucial, since some botanicals of the same species had different names, or different species were sometimes called by the same name. All of these circumstances complicated the elaboration of the categories of local botanicals and their medical effects. Confusion in identifying botanicals was a significant issue in medical prescription and treatment.

During King Sejong's reign (1418-1450), medical officials were dispatched to China to resolve this problem. In 1423, for instance, envoys to Ming China examined 62 Korean species in collaboration with Chinese scholars and found that 14 of them were different from the Chinese varieties. Dozens of botanicals turned out to be different from Chinese products and were banned from use in medical preparations. Additionally, in 1430 and 1431, the dynasty attempted to discriminate between the qualities of domestic botanicals, hoping to substitute them for the Chinese botanicals that were named in prescriptions.

In conjunction with these efforts at identification and comparison, the dynasty continued to localize foreign botanicals, particularly those in high demand. A few remarks in *Veritable Records of the Joseon Dynasty* (朝鮮王朝實錄 *Joseon wangjo sillok*, 1392-1863) indicate that Glycyrrhizae Radix (*gān cǎo*), Piperis Fructus (*hú jiāo*), Ephedrae Herba (*má huáng*), and Alpiniae officinarum Rhizoma (*gāo liáng jiāng*) were some of the plants that Koreans tried to naturalize on Korean soil.

Heo Jun's (許 浚, 1546-1615) *Precious Mirror of Eastern Medicine* (東醫寶鑑 *Dongui bogam*, 1610), which has received more scholarly and popular attention than any other pre-modern medical text in Korea, also reveals a need to categorize local botanicals succinctly. Heo Chun appended characters like 'Chinese' (唐, literally 'Tang') and 'local' (鄉 *hyang*) to the name of each botanical and provided local names, places of production, appropriate times for collecting, and processes of management so that people could obtain indigenous herbs easily without having to seek medicines from remote places. Accumulated knowledge about local herbs helped Heo Jun to produce more single ingredient prescriptions.

Koreans' continual interest in indigenous herbs, however, should be viewed in light of the growing eclecticism and commercialism in medicine that occurred during the 18th and 19th centuries. The growth of private publications in the late Joseon dynasty (朝鮮, 1392-1910), the influx of practical and professional medical texts from Qing China, and the attempts by Joseon scholars to synthesize various Chinese medical trends are the major characteristics of medicine during the 18th and 19th centuries. For instance, Qing scholar Wang Ang's *Medical Formulas Collected and Analyzed* and *Essentials of the Materia Medica*, which were already well-known as practical and appropriate summaries of Li Shi-Zhen's *Comprehensive Outline of the Materia Medica*, served as a reference for Hwang To-yeon's (黃度淵, 1807-1884) *Compendium of Prescriptions* (方藥合編 *Bangyak happyeun*, 1885), one of the most popular medical texts in 19th-century Korea.

During the period of Japanese colonialism (1910-1945), the Japanese investigated locally specific Korean herbs as a part of a broader project of mapping fauna and flora in northeastern Asia. Korean herbs, particularly Ginseng Radix (*rén shēn*), gained Japanese pharmacists' attention. Moreover, during the late 1930s and the early 1940s, a couple of Japanese pharmaceutical companies explored the possibility of commercializing botanicals that were mainly produced in Korea. The Shionogi (鹽野義) company investigated the nature of Cheju Island to cultivate foxglove (*digitalis purpurea*), which is acknowledged as a cardiotonic in both traditional and biomedicine.

From a practitioner's point of view, it is difficult to generalize about any explicitly indigenous attribute of herbal medicine in contemporary Korea. Herbs are chosen according to different schools of traditional medicine, practitioners' preferences, family traditions, and the situation in the market. For instance, a school that follows the tradition of Lee Je-ma's (李濟馬, 1838-1900) 'constitutional medicine' (四象醫學 *Sasang uihak)*, which systematically classified human beings into four categories, regards Ginseng Radix (*rén shēn*), Astragali Radix (*hung qí*), Atractylodis macrocephalae Rhizoma (*bái zhú*), Citri reticulatae Pericarpium (*chén pí*), Angelicae sinensis Radix (*dāng guī*), Chuanxiong Rhizoma (*chuān xiōng*), Paeoniae Radix (*sháo yào*), Polygoni multiflori Radix (*hé shǒu wū*), Cinnamomi Cortex (*ròu guì*), Cyperi Rhizoma (*xiāng fù*), Zingiberis Rhizoma recens (*shēng jiāng*), and Pinelliae Rhizoma praeparatum (*zhì bàn xià*) as the twelve most popular herbs that are well-suited to the most common constitutional types among Koreans. In addition, in 1997, Korea traded with China for more than 37 percent of her entire imports of herbs. Glycyrrhizae Radix (*gān cǎo*), an indispensable constituent of formulas from *Discussion of Cold Damage*, is the most commonly imported herb from China. Although there was no Korean parallel to the Japanese Kohō ('ancient formulas') current, formulas from *Discussion of Cold Damage* have been frequently used by most Korean doctors of traditional medicine.

As these examples reflect, herbal medicine in Korea developed alongside Koreans' interest in local botanicals and

xlviii   Introduction

their incessant desire to indigenize foreign materia medica for their own use. Simple and convenient prescriptions based on a single ingredient were constantly pursued, yet precious medicinals from overseas were also in high demand. Traditional medicine in Korea piggybacked on the post-colonial nationalist agenda, while research on herbs that are native to or available in Korea still remains popular in contemporary Korea.

CHINESE HERBAL MEDICINE IN THE WEST

The widespread availability of Chinese herbal medicine in the West outside of the Chinese diaspora is still a very young phenomenon. Unlike acupuncture, which has long stimulated Western curiosity because of its difference to indigenous forms of therapy, herbal medicine was perceived at best as offering new herbs such as ginseng to the materia medica. It was thus on the back of the increasing popularity of acupuncture and the opening up of China in the 1980s that Chinese herbal medicine started to become more widely available. While the amount and quality of information available to Western audiences unable to directly access primary sources has greatly increased over the last quarter century, the development of traditional Chinese herbal medicine here is still in its infancy. Only a handful of the key texts of the tradition have been translated, while issues regarding the availability and quality of herbal products as well as the regulation of professional practice present considerable challenges for the foreseeable future. It is hoped that this text will contribute to that process.

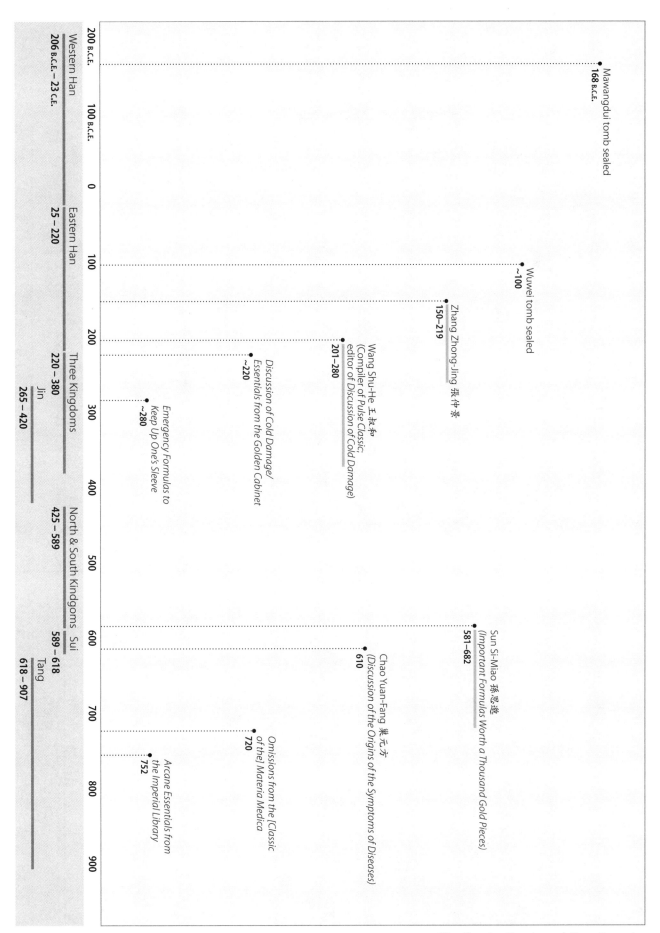

Timeline 1　Han through Tang Dynasties

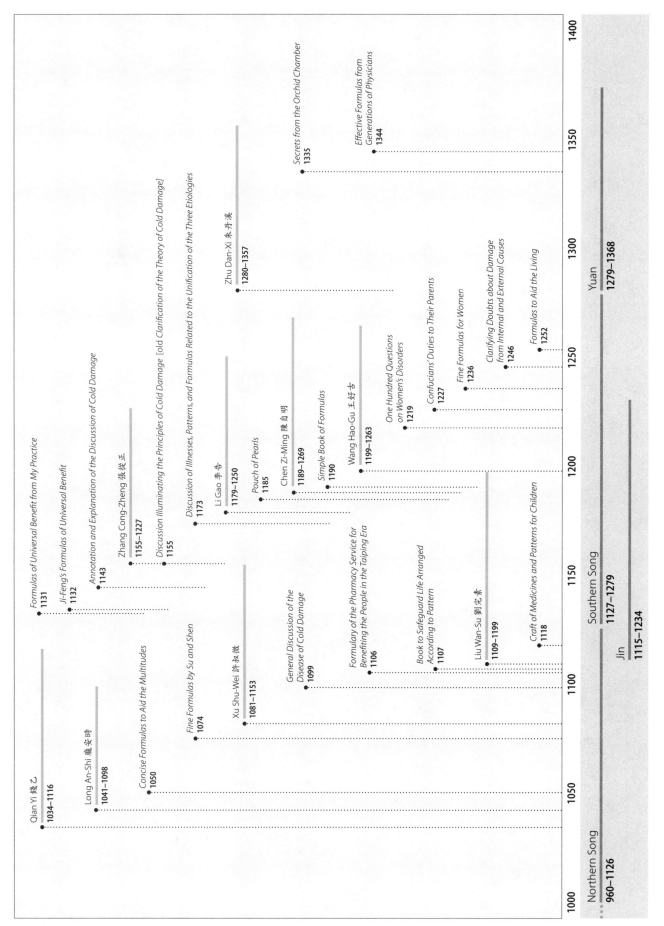

Timeline 2 Song through Yuan Dynasties

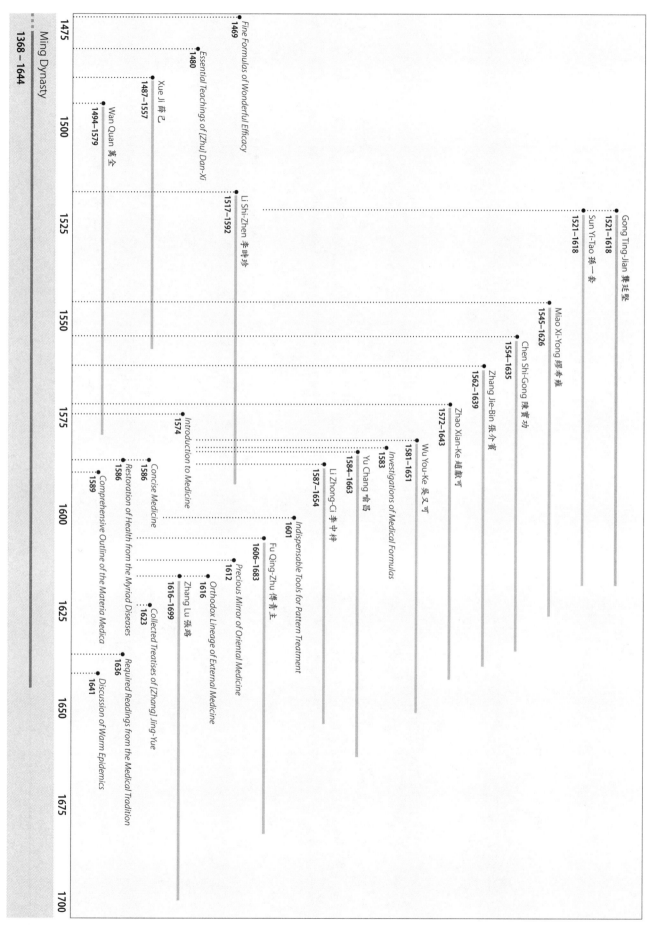

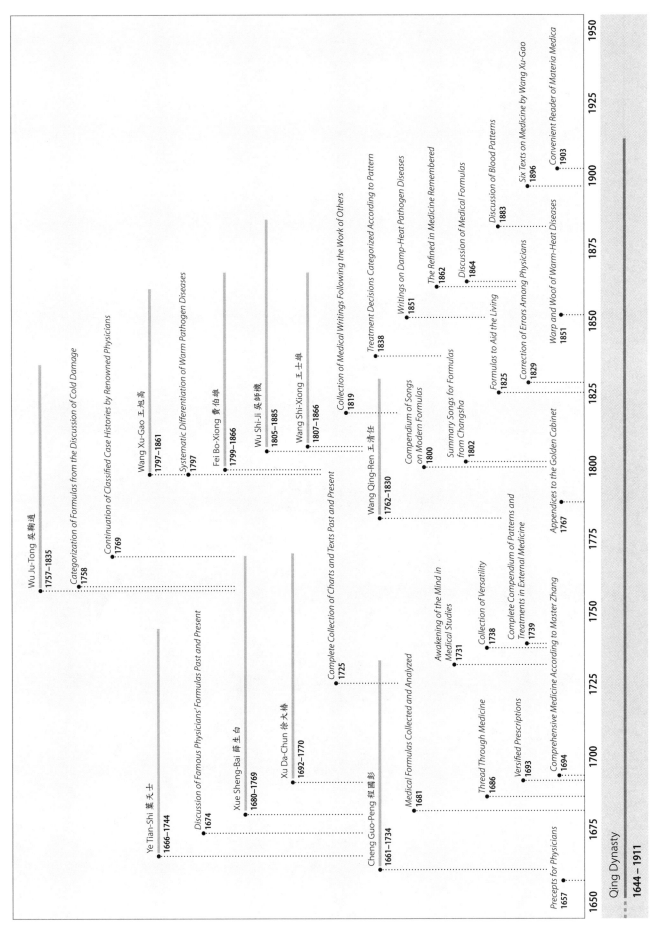

Timeline 4 Qing Dynasty

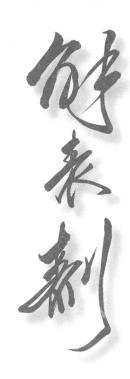

Chapter 1 Contents

Formulas that Release the Exterior

Formulas that Release the Exterior

WHEN A PATHOGENIC influence first penetrates the body, it tends to cause a disorder of the exterior. In this context, the term exterior (表 biǎo) denotes the superficial layers of the body comprised of the skin and muscles. These are perfused by the body's protective qi, which is fierce and hot in nature and whose task it is to warm and defend against penetration into the body by external pathogens. If a pathogenic influence lodges in this aspect of the body it not only obstructs the normal physiological diffusion of qi and fluids there, but encourages the body to move more protective qi toward the exterior in an attempt to push out the invading pathogen. For this reason, exterior disorders are characterized by fever and chills (indicating obstruction of normal physiological warming, even as protective yang in the exterior tends toward excess), head and body aches (indicating obstruction of qi and fluids in the most yang, i.e., exterior, portions of the body), and a floating pulse (indicating the movement of protective yang toward the exterior).

The following are also regarded as exterior disorders: early-stage measles and incompletely expressed rashes, the initial stage of carbuncles and sores accompanied by fever and chills, and acute, superficial edema. Since wind is the vehicle by which other external pathogenic influences enter the body via the exterior, it is involved in most exterior disorders, especially those involving cold and heat. Thus, it is said that "wind is the leader of the hundred diseases" (風為百病之長 fēng wéi bǎi bìng zhī zhǎng).

The symptoms associated with an exterior disorder indicate that the body is actively trying to overcome obstruction of the qi dynamic by one or more of the six pathogenic influences. Treatment in Chinese medicine seeks to support these physiological reactions through strategies that release the pathogenic influence from the exterior (解表 jiě biǎo). For this purpose, one deploys light, acrid, moving herbs that unblock obstruction, diffuse the protective qi, and disseminate fluids to vent pathogenic influences back toward the outside. No other strategy will prevent the pathogenic influence from penetrating more deeply into the body. Often, but not always, this results in sweating. This type of sweating indicates that an obstruction has been overcome and that the qi and fluids can once again stream to the surface of the body. Like the flow of water that breaks through a dam, the sweating may initially be pronounced, especially if a very acrid and warming formula is used. However, the profuse sweating should quickly abate as the body finds its physiological balance. For this reason, releasing the exterior is often equated with inducing sweating. Yet in many contexts where formulas to release the exterior are used, the sweating may hardly be noticeable, or strong pathological sweating may evolve into a milder physiological sweat. This is because the ultimate goal of these formulas is not to promote sweating, but to unblock and restore order to the flow of qi and fluids.

The term 'release [from the] exterior' was first described in Chapter 5 of *Basic Questions:* "If a person harbors a pathogen the body becomes soaked as [the movement of protective qi to the exterior] transforms [fluids] into sweat. Hence, when [the pathogen] is at [the level of] the skin, use sweating to discharge it." The first known text to list herbal formulas that embody this strategy is the early 3rd-century work *Discussion of Cold Damage*, which provides some of the most influential formulas in this category such as Ephedra Decoction (*má huáng tāng*), Cinnamon Twig Decoction (*guì zhī tāng*), and their variants. Its focus on acrid, warming herbs to overcome obstruction from wind, cold, and dampness dominated medical practice until the Jin-Yuan dynasties of the 12th to 14th centuries. Innovation, until then, consisted of extending the range of substances used to promote sweating rather than in seeking new areas of application. This changed in the 12th century with Liu Wan-Su's focus on heat pathogens, which led to the idea that heat in the exterior can occur there directly, rather than being due to constraint caused by cold. Venting such heat requires the use of acrid, cooling substances, which do not necessarily promote noticeable sweating. The treatment strategies and formulas composed by 17th- and 18th-century physicians like Ye Tian-Shi and Wu Ju-Tong, who are associated with the warm pathogen current, are most emblematic of this approach. Other innovations stemming from the Jin-Yuan era are the combination of exterior venting with tonifying herbs to treat exterior excess combined with deficiency of qi, blood, or fluids in the interior, and the use of herbs to dispel pathogens from specific channels and their associated surface regions.

Reflecting these historical developments, the present chapter is divided into three main sections: formulas for exterior cold disorders, formulas for wind-heat disorders, and formulas for exterior disorders with interior deficiency. A fourth section, formulas for early-stage exterior disorders, discusses strategies that are useful when a pathogenic influence begins to penetrate the body, but a clear diagnosis regarding its precise nature is difficult to render. Other chapters in this book include further examples of formulas that can be used to vent pathogens from the exterior. These include Formulas that Dispel Summerheat to Resolve the Exterior (Chapter 5), Formulas for Exterior-Interior Excess (Chapter 6), Formulas that Release Wind from the Skin and Channels (Chapter 14), Formulas that Gently Disperse and Moisten Dryness (Chapter 15), and Formulas that Expel Dampness (Chapter 16). While the basic principles underlying the venting of pathogens from the exterior apply, the formulas discussed in these chapters often combine those principles with others that are specific to the relevant pathology. For this reason, they are conventionally not listed as purely exterior-releasing formulas, and we have followed this practice.

Sweating is the first of the eight methods of treatment formulated by the 18th-century physician Cheng Guo-Peng, underlining its importance in clinical practice. Yet many practitioners continue to underrate this method. This is unfortunate, because the odds of preventing the development of a serious condition are always better when intervention occurs at the early stage of an illness:

> It is best to treat [diseases at the level of] the skin and hair; the next best is to treat [them at the level of] the muscles and flesh; the next best is to treat [them at the level of] the sinews and vessels; the next best is to treat [them at the level of] the six yang organs; the next best is to treat [them at the level of] the five yin organs. When treating [at the level of] the five yin organs, half the patients die and the other half survive. (*Basic Questions*, Chapter 5)

Successful use of the formulas discussed in this chapter will be aided by paying attention to the following principles:

First, accurate diagnosis is essential. If an interior disorder develops before the exterior has been released, the practitioner must choose between releasing the exterior first or treating the exterior and interior simultaneously. The formulas in this chapter are inappropriate for treating disorders solely of the interior, expressed rashes, or edema due to deficiency. Likewise, it is important to be clear about the precise nature of the pathogenic influence to be released, as this determines the choice of formula. One must also be cognizant of the type of sweating to expect from a particular formula.

Second, most of these formulas should be cooked briefly. They treat acute disorders and are prepared as decoctions or powders. They contain substances that are light and volatile in nature, which, if subjected to too much heat, lose their efficacy.

Third, formulas taken hot after meals will provide the best results. Sweating is further encouraged by instructing the patient to bundle up after taking the medicine. As the goal of sweating is not sweating itself but to assist the function of the protective qi, only a slight sweat over the entire body is needed to release the exterior. Excessive sweating dissipates the qi and fluids.

Fourth, the formula and dosage should be adjusted to the individual's constitution, local climate, and season. For example, a person who sweats easily, lives in a warm climate, and contracts an illness during the spring or summer requires only mild treatment. On the other hand, a person who does not sweat easily, lives in a cold climate, and contracts an illness in the autumn or winter requires stronger treatment.

Section 1

FORMULAS THAT RELEASE EARLY-STAGE EXTERIOR DISORDERS

In the first stage of an externally-contracted disorder, a person will feel as if the outer layer of protection has been "stripped off," making them feel very vulnerable to drafts.

This sensation is called aversion to wind (惡風 *wù fēng*) and can be treated by a simple infusion of Allii fistulosi Bulbus (*cōng bái*). Stronger chills indicate that the condition has progressed slightly and that it requires one or another of the formulas discussed in this section. These formulas should be prescribed for one or two doses only. If ineffective, a stronger formula is needed.

蔥豉湯 (葱豉汤)

Scallion and Prepared Soybean Decoction

cōng chǐ tāng

Source *Emergency Formulas to Keep Up One's Sleeve* (3rd century)

Allii fistulosi Bulbus (*cōng bái*) . . . . .3-5 stalks (9-12g)
Sojae Semen praeparatum (*dàn dòu chǐ*) 12-30g

Method of Preparation   Decoction. Dosage is adjusted depending on whether the diagnosis is one of wind-cold or wind-heat. Cook no more than 5-10 minutes.

Actions   Unblocks the yang (protective) qi in the exterior and induces sweating

Indications

Mild fever and slight chills without sweating, headache, stuffy nose, a thin, white tongue coating, and a floating pulse.

This is the earliest stage of an externally-contracted wind-cold or wind-heat disorder. The Lungs govern the exterior as well as the skin and nasal passages. When wind-cold attacks the exterior or wind-heat attacks the Lungs directly, the first symptoms are fever and chills, an indication that the protective qi and the pathogenic influences are struggling with each other in the exterior. As a consequence, the protective qi cannot fulfill its normal function of warming the exterior, causing chills; meanwhile, the constraint of yang qi in the exterior leads to an accumulation of heat, and thus fever. Since this is the earliest stage of the disorder, all of the signs and symptoms are mild.

Analysis of Formula

Wind-cold or wind-heat in the exterior of the body is dispersed with acrid herbs. A mild condition in its early stages can be treated with light and gentle herbs that induce gentle sweating. Allii fistulosi Bulbus (*cōng bái*) is a warm, acrid herb that unblocks the flow of yang (protective) qi in the exterior and induces sweating. Sojae Semen praeparatum (*dàn dòu chǐ*) releases both externally-contracted pathogenic factors from the exterior and constrained yang qi in the interior. Together, these herbs gently release the exterior, which is all that is needed to resolve this pattern.

Commentary

This is a rather neutral formula that will not dry out or injure the fluids. It is useful for the treatment of mild exterior conditions, especially those marked by headache and nasal congestion. Most modern textbooks prescribe this formula primarily for wind-cold externally-contracted disorders. However, typically in such cases, the individual will rarely seek attention until after the condition has worsened; the formula is therefore usually prescribed with additional herbs. Yet some practitioners recommend it for treating any kind of pathogenic qi in the exterior. Historically, it was certainly a very popular formula among leading physicians associated with the warm pathogen disease current, such as Ye Tian-Shi and Wang Shi-Xiong. These physicians recommended it for feverish diseases arising from both newly-contracted and lurking pathogens. Scallion and Prepared Soybean Decoction is especially suited for early stage external invasion, when it may be difficult to judge whether one is dealing with a cold damage or warm pathogen disease.

Although the basic formula contains only two simple ingredients, their combined effect provides a significant potency. Accordingly, the Qing-dynasty physician Fei Bo-Xiong, who favored the use of such gentle formulas wherever possible, noted: "[This formula] is exceptionally good at releasing the exterior and unblocking the yang. Do not neglect its use merely because [it is composed] of herbs with a mild flavor."

Biomedical Indications

With the appropriate presentation, this formula may be used to treat a variety of biomedically-defined disorders including upper respiratory tract infections and the very early stages of many respiratory infections.

Alternate names

Scallion Whites and Prepared Soybean Decoction (*cōng bái chǐ tāng*) in *Book to Safeguard Life Arranged According to Pattern*

Modifications

- If this formula fails to induce sweating, add Puerariae Radix (*gé gēn*) and Cimicifugae Rhizoma (*shēng má*). If there is still no sweating, add Ephedrae Herba (*má huáng*). (source text)
- For pronounced chills and headache, add Notopterygii Rhizoma seu Radix (*qiāng huó*), Saposhnikoviae Radix (*fáng fēng*), and Schizonepetae Herba (*jīng jiè*).
- For pronounced cold with abdominal pain, add Zingiberis Rhizoma recens (*shēng jiāng*) and brown sugar.
- For pronounced fever with a sore and swollen throat, add Scutellariae Radix (*huáng qín*), Gardeniae Fructus (*zhī zǐ*), and Forsythiae Fructus (*lián qiáo*).

- For pronounced coughing and hoarseness, add Cicadae Periostracum (*chán tuì*), Platycodi Radix (*jié gěng*), and Arctii Fructus (*niú bàng zǐ*).

- For concurrent turbid dampness with nausea, a stifling sensation in the chest, loss of taste, and a thick, greasy tongue coating, add Pogostemonis/Agastaches Herba (*huò xiāng*) and Eupatorii Herba (*pèi lán*).

- For a common cold occurring in the spring or summer as a result of a lurking pathogen with aversion to wind, chills and fever, headache, sweating or an absence of sweating, irritability, and thirst, add Saposhnikoviae Radix (*fáng fēng*), Platycodi Radix (*jié gěng*), Citri reticulatae Pericarpium (*chén pí*), and Armeniacae Semen (*xìng rén*). (*Discussion of Seasonal Disorders*)

Variations

活人蔥豉湯 (活人葱豉汤)
Scallion and Prepared Soybean Decoction from *Book to Safeguard Life*
huó rén cōng chǐ tāng

SOURCE *Book to Safeguard Life Arranged According to Pattern* (1108)

Add Ephedrae Herba (*má huáng*) and Puerariae Radix (*gé gēn*) for a one-to-two day old wind-cold disorder with no chills or sweating, but with headache, neck pain, upper and lower back pain, and a tight pulse. Compared to the original formula, Scallion and Prepared Soybean Decoction from *Book to Safeguard Life* is indicated for a more severe penetration of wind-cold into the exterior. This is a good example of how the original formula can be adapted to treat cold damage disorders in the greater yang.

Associated Formulas

蔥豉桔梗湯 (葱豉桔梗汤)
Scallion, Prepared Soybean, and Platycodon Decoction
cōng chǐ jié gěng tāng

SOURCE *Revised Popular Guide to the Discussion of Cold Damage* (Qing dynasty)

Allii fistulosi Bulbus (*cōng bái*) . . . . .3-5 pieces (9-12g)
Platycodi Radix (*jié gěng*) 3-4.5g
Sojae Semen praeparatum (*dàn dòu chǐ*) 9-15g
scorched Gardeniae Fructus (*jiāo zhī zǐ*) 6-9g
Menthae haplocalycis Herba (*bò hé*) 3-4.5g
Forsythiae Fructus (*lián qiáo*) 3-4.5g
Glycyrrhizae Radix (*gān cǎo*) 1.8-2.4g
Lophatheri Herba Recens
    (*xiān dàn zhú yè*) . . . . 30 leaves (1.5-3g)

Scatters wind, releases the exterior, and clears heat from the Lungs. For the early stages of a warm pathogen disease characterized by fever, headache, a slight aversion to wind, coughing, sore throat, thirst, a red-tipped tongue with a white coating, and a floating, rapid pulse.

Compared to the original formula, Scallion and Platycodon Decoction contains more herbs to clear heat both from the exterior and the qi aspect. This heat has not yet acquired any form, but its deeper penetration, indicated by the cough and perhaps by a reddening of the tip of the tongue, makes it advisable to vent it not only through the skin, but also through the urine. It is a good example of how the original formula can be adapted to treat warm pathogen disorders.

杏前蔥豉湯 (杏前葱豉汤)
Apricot Kernel, Peucedanum, Scallion, and Prepared Soybean Decoction
xìng qián cōng chǐ tāng

SOURCE *Selected Formulas for Warm-Heat Pathogen Diseases* (c. 1900)

Armeniacae Semen (*xìng rén*) 9g
Sojae Semen praeparatum (*dàn dòu chǐ*) 6g
Peucedani Radix (*qián hú*) 4.5g
fresh Aurantii Fructus (*xiān zhǐ ké*) 3g
immature Perillae Caulis (*nèn sū gěng*) 4.5g
Platycodi Radix (*jié gěng*) 2.1g
honey-fried Citri reticulatae Exocarpium rubrum (*zhǐ jú hóng*) . 2.4g
Allii fistulosi Bulbus (*cōng bái*) . . . . .3 pieces (9g)

This formula was orginally formulated to treat sudden wind-dryness disorders caused by a sudden and violent westerly wind that occurs in the autumn when the weather begins to turn cold. The signs and symptoms of this type of disorder are fever, headache, nasal congestion, an aversion to wind, chills without sweating, dry skin, a continuous dry cough, chest fullness, qi rebellion, and a pain that penetrates to the back. The pulse is floating and rough on the right, and floating and wiry or tight on the left. Although the disease dynamic of wind-cold fettering the yang qi in the exterior is the same in autumn or winter, the cold of autumn is less severe while the dryness more directly constrains the qi dynamic in the chest. To address this condition, Ye Tian-Shi, the author of this formula, combined bitter and warm herbs that facilitate the dispersing and downward-directing functions of Lung qi, with light and acrid herbs that dispel wind-cold from the exterior.

Comparison

➤ Vs. APRICOT KERNEL AND PERILLA LEAF POWDER (*xìng sū sǎn*)

The textbook formula for cold-dryness, Apricot Kernel and Perilla Leaf Powder (*xìng sū sǎn*) (see Chapter 15), is warmer and focuses on conditions with very clear constraint from phlegm. By contrast, Apricot Kernel, Peucedanum, Scallion, and Soybean Decoction (*xìng qián cōng chǐ tāng*) is lighter and is suitable for conditions that, according to Ye Tian-Shi, resemble wind-warmth disorders occurring in the spring, that is, marked by sudden onset and rapid development.

Alternate names

Another common name for this formula is Scallion and Platycodon Decoction (蔥桔梗湯 *cōng jié gěng tāng*).

Section 2

....

FORMULAS THAT RELEASE EXTERIOR WIND-COLD

Wind-cold disorders are marked by fever and chills (chills predominant), head and body aches, clear or white secretions (nasal discharge, sputum), and a floating pulse. There are many types of wind-cold disorders and all require the use of formulas that release pathogenic influences from the exterior by inducing sweating. By definition, all exterior cold disorders are excessive in nature. Depending on the body's defensive reaction, two major types can be differentiated in practice: cold damage (傷寒 *shāng hán*) and wind attack (中風 *zhòng fēng*). Cold damage is characterized by a strong defensive reaction to a strong pathogen. Cold blocks the circulation of protective qi and fluids in the outer layers of the body, and closes up the interstices and pores, which prevents sweating; meanwhile, internally, the constraint of protective and nutritive qi causes high fever and severe body aches. Patients displaying this pattern require a formula that strongly induces sweating.

If the defensive reaction is characterized by disorder and disruption rather than complete obstruction, it is termed wind attack. In this case, although there is sweating, the condition does not improve. This is because the protective qi is unable to expel the pathogen. Treatment still requires sweating, but it must be accompanied by appropriate regulation and harmonization of the relationship between the protective and nutritive qi so that the sweating will achieve the goal of expelling the pathogen.

The core ingredients of these formulas are acrid, warming herbs that release the exterior such as Ephedrae Herba (*má huáng*), Cinnamomi Ramulus (*guì zhī*), Notopterygii Rhizoma seu Radix (*qiāng huó*), Perillae Folium (*zǐ sū yè*), Saposhnikoviae Radix (*fáng fēng*), and Schizonepetae Herba (*jīng jiè*). The Lungs focus on the skin and surface of the body and govern the dissemination and clarification of qi. Cold, externally-contracted diseases often enter through the skin and disrupt the downward-directing functions of the Lungs with such symptoms as cough and nasal congestion. For this reason, herbs that help the Lungs disseminate and direct qi downward, such as Armeniacae Semen (*xìng rén*), are often included in these formulas. Because cold has a tendency to congeal, which can lead to headaches and body pain from constraint and stagnation of the nutritive aspect, often warm, acrid, exterior-releasing herbs are matched with those that invigorate the blood and unblock the vessels, such as Chuanxiong Rhizoma (*chuān xiōng*). The tendency of cold to cause contraction also affects the fluids, transforming them into

dampness or phlegm. For this reason, herbs that dry dampness and transfrom phlegm, such as Pinelliae Rhizoma praeparatum (*zhì bàn xià*), Citri reticulatae Pericarpium (*chén pí*), and Perillae Fructus (*zǐ sū zǐ*), are also included.

麻黃湯 （麻黄汤）

Ephedra Decoction

má huáng tāng

Source   *Discussion of Cold Damage* (c. 220)

Ephedrae Herba (*má huáng*)...............................9g
Cinnamomi Ramulus (*guì zhī*)..........................6g
Armeniacae Semen (*xìng rén*).............70 pieces (9-12g)
Glycyrrhizae Radix praeparata (*zhì gān cǎo*)..........3g

Method of Preparation   The source text advises to first decoct Ephedrae Herba (*má huáng*) in approximately 9 cups of water until 7 cups remain. The froth is removed, the other ingredients are added, and the result is decocted until approximately 2.5 cups remain. The strained decoction is taken warm in 3 doses. At present, however, all of the ingredients are decocted together, and it is thought that they should not be cooked for more than 20 minutes. The decoction is taken hot to induce significant sweating. Once sweating occurs, the formula should not be taken again.

Actions   Releases exterior cold and arrests wheezing

Indications

Fever and chills (chills predominant) without sweating, headache, generalized body aches, wheezing, a thin, white tongue coating, and a floating, tight pulse.

    This is wind-cold attacking the exterior where it fetters, constrains, or 'bottles up' the protective qi. This inhibits the flow of the yang qi in the exterior, which produces chills. The struggle between the external pathogenic influence and the normal qi causes fever and makes the skin warm to the touch. The head is the meeting place of the yang channels, and an attack of wind-cold on the superficial (yang) aspects of the body gives rise to headache. Cold causes the interstices and pores to close and prevents sweating. It also interferes with the flow of nutritive qi in the muscle layer and channels, which produces generalized body aches. The bottling-up of the exterior constrains the normal dissemination of Lung qi. This results in rebellious Lung qi that manifests as a harsh, barking cough or wheezing. Since this is an exterior condition only, the tongue is not affected. The floating pulse indicates that the pathogenic influence is in the exterior, and the tight pulse indicates the presence of cold.

Analysis of Formula

The pattern treated by this formula is caused by severe wind-cold fettering the protective yang in the exterior, which constrains the dissemination of Lung qi. This requires the use of a strategy that focuses on resolving the exterior with acrid and strongly warming herbs, while secondarily supporting the dissemination and downward-directing of Lung qi.

The chief herb, warm, acrid Ephedrae Herba *(má huáng),* is a particularly strong diaphoretic that also disseminates the Lung qi and treats wheezing. The deputy, Cinnamomi Ramulus *(guì zhī),* is also a diaphoretic that releases the exterior (especially the muscle layer) and warms and facilitates the flow in the channels. When combined with the chief herb, it strengthens the diaphoretic effect of the formula. This combination is very effective in releasing the exterior. The assistant, Armeniacae Semen *(xìng rén),* is bitter and slightly warm. It directs Lung qi downward to help the chief ingredient arrest wheezing and expel the pathogenic influence. Its oily nature simultaneously moderates the acrid quality of the two main diaphoretic herbs to protect the Lung, which is averse to dryness. The envoy, Glycyrrhizae Radix praeparata *(zhì gān cǎo),* harmonizes the actions of the other herbs, moderates the diaphoretic action of Ephedrae Herba *(má huáng),* and protects against the slight toxicity of Armeniacae Semen *(xìng rén).*

Commentary

This is the classic formula for treating cold excess in the exterior. Its primary focus is to stimulate sweating. It appears at least nine times in *Discussion of Cold Damage* for treatment of greater yang-warp disorders where the presentation is referred to as cold damage. This is the narrow meaning of the term 傷寒 *shāng hán,* the broader meaning of which encompasses all types of cold damage disorders.

Commentators differ in their explanation of why Zhang Zhong-Jing, the author of the formula, chose for his chief herb Ephedrae Herba *(má huáng)* rather than another diaphoretic herb indicated for *taiyang* disorders. The early 20th-century physician Zhang Xi-Chun argues that, of all these herbs, only Ephedrae Herba *(má huáng)* combines all the actions needed to address the various aspects of a cold damage pathology. Besides inducing sweating and opening up Lung constraint, Ephedrae Herba *(má huáng)* also enters the Bladder and functions as a diuretic. This allows it to push out cold that has already penetrated deeper into the greater yang.

Other commentators focus their attention on the interaction of the chief and deputy herbs in the prescription. The most common view is that Ephedrae Herba *(má huáng)* relieves the constraint of protective qi in the exterior to open the pores and interstices, while Cinnamomi Ramulus *(guì zhī)* penetrates deeper into the muscle layer and channels to open up areas of stagnation of the nutritive qi, so that pathogens can also be vented to the outside from there. Fang You-Zhi, the influential Qing-dynasty commentator on the *Discussion of Cold Damage,* goes one step further to argue that the deputy not only enhances the diaphoretic effect of the chief herb, but also checks and controls it. Likening both

herbs to generals in battle, Fang notes that Ephedrae Herba *(má huáng)* "is like a powerful general who smashes through the enemy lines in order to detain the foe." By contrast, Cinnamomi Ramulus *(guì zhī)* acts "like a military advisor who plans strategies from within his command tent." Viewed from this perspective, ensuring the harmonious interaction of protective and nutritive qi emerges as the ultimate objective of Ephedra Decoction, just as it does for the better known Cinnamon Twig Decoction, discussed below.

Harmonious and balanced, however, does not mean mild, and the *Golden Mirror of the Medical Tradition* calls Ephedra Decoction "[Zhang] Zhong-Jing's fiercest medicine for opening the exterior and driving out pathogens by inducing sweating." Another famous commentator on the works of Zhang Zhong-Jing, Ke Qin, likewise explains that "[this] is a purely yang formula, which only discharges and disperses. Like a commander who comes straight to the point, it does only what is appropriate and [thereby] achieves victory with one single battle. … Therefore, one can use it to release the exterior, but one must [use it only once] and not repeatedly." Given the potentially adverse effects of such a potent formula, a healthy respect gradually turned into outright suspicion and fear among physicians and patients in late imperial China, who increasingly avoided its use. This attitude was especially prevalent among the proponents of the warm pathogen disease current and the population of the lower basin of the Yangzi River, where this style of practice was most influential. In view of some of the problems facing practitioners in many Western countries regarding the use of Ephedrae Herba *(má huáng),* alternative formulas composed in the wake of such anxieties—particularly Augmented Cyperus and Perilla Leaf Powder, discussed later in this chapter—are of undoubted value. They should not distract, however, from the real value of Ephedra Decoction in the treatment of cold damage disorders.

Contemporary Usage

The modern physician Niu Yuan-Qi provides important pointers for how key signs and symptoms that define the classical cold damage pattern (absence of sweating, chills, and high fever) may manifest in contemporary practice. In his experience, the self-prescription of biomedical antipyretics like aspirin, which from a Chinese medical perspective are acrid and cold, often produce some sweating. If this sweating does not resolve the fever, or if the fever actually increases, this indicates the presence of a wind-cold pathogen. Similarly, a predominance of chills need not be present in every single case for which Ephedra Decoction may be indicated. One can make a diagnosis of cold damage if the chills are particularly pronounced at the onset of the disorder or if they persist for a relatively long period of time even as the fever rises. Finally, while many textbooks present fever accompanied by thirst and a rapid pulse to be a distinguishing feature of warm pathogen disorders, Niu notes that they can also occur with wind-cold invasion. In these cases, however, a sensation of dryness in the mouth will not be accompanied by much thirst, or the thirst will be for warm rather than cold drinks. The pulse, although rapid when measured against a normal resting pulse, will be less fast than one would expect given the oftentimes high fever.

Besides wind-cold fevers without sweating, the most common contemporary applications of this formula are for cough and wheezing due to cold, and painful obstruction due to wind-cold-dampness. It is also used for nosebleeds with an absence of sweating and a floating, tight pulse. This is a specific type of nosebleed due to cold. In this case, wind-cold 'bottles up' the exterior and constrains the yang, which surges upward and causes the nosebleed. Less well-known is its usage in gynecology. Both the Chinese and Japanese case history literature documents the successful treatment of painful periods and difficult labor with Ephedra Decoction (*má huáng tāng*). This can be explained by the formula's ability to unblock obstruction due to cold, and by the fact that in the classical texts, the word Bladder (膀胱 *páng guāng*) is a term that can refer to the pelvic organs in general, and not just the bladder. Contemporary writers, like Huang Huang in *One Hundred Classic Formulas*, thus recommend Ephedra Decoction (*má huáng tāng*) with the addition of herbs such as Poria (*fú líng*), Moutan Cortex (*mǔ dān pí*), Persicae Semen (*táo rén*), Artemisiae argyi Folium (*ài yè*), Paeoniae Radix (*sháo yào*), and Chuanxiong Rhizoma (*chuān xiōng*) for the treatment of dysmenorrhea, abdominal masses, pelvic inflammatory disease, and similar disorders, provided that the overall symptom pattern matches the formula's presentation.

Ephedra Decoction (*má huáng tāng*) is the foundation for a number of other formulas that are used in treating disorders associated with wind affecting the Lungs, including Minor Bluegreen Dragon Decoction (*xiǎo qīng lóng tāng*), discussed later in this section, and Ephedra, Apricot Kernel, Gypsum, and Licorice Decoction (*má xìng shí gān tāng*), discussed in Chapter 4.

Comparisons

➢ Vs. Kudzu Decoction (*gé gēn tāng*); *see* page 20

➢ Vs. Inula Powder (*jīn fèi cǎo sǎn*); *see* page 33

➢ Vs. Licorice and Ginger Decoction (*gān cǎo gān jiāng tāng*); *see* page 271

Biomedical Indications

With the appropriate presentation, this formula may be used to treat a wide variety of biomedically-defined disorders. These can be divided into the following groups:

- Acute externally-contracted diseases such as the common cold, influenza, rheumatic fever, pneumonia, rhinitis, pharyngitis, otitis media, and the early stages of mastitis
- Disorders marked by pain such as traumatic arthropathy, cervical spine disease, lumbar strain, periarthritis of the shoulder, rheumatoid arthritis, ankylosing spondylitis, Raynaud's disease, sciatica, trigeminal neuralgia, migraine, sinusitis, and scleroderma
- Disorders marked by wheezing such as asthma, chronic bronchitis, chronic obstructive pulmonary disease, hay fever, and pericardial effusions
- Dermatological diseases marked by dry skin such as some forms of eczema, urticaria, and chilblains
- Other disorders such as glomerulonephritis, pylenonephritis, benign prostatic hypertrophy, ascites, phlebitis, and solar dermatitis

Cautions and Contraindications

In *Discussion of Cold Damage*, this formula is contraindicated for patients with debility and copious urination, and for patients who are prone to bleeding (especially from the nose). Because of the adrenergic effects of Ephedrae Herba (*má huáng*), this formula should be used with caution in cases with hypertension. In addition, it is designed only to be used for very short periods of time.

Alternate names

Ephedra Decoction to Release the Muscle Layer (*má huáng jiě jī tāng*) in *Arcane Essentials from the Imperial Library*

Modifications

- For exterior cold with interior heat, add Gypsum fibrosum (*shí gāo*), Anemarrhenae Rhizoma (*zhī mǔ*), or Scutellariae Radix (*huáng qín*).
- For concurrent qi and blood deficiency, add Astragali Radix (*huáng qí*), Ginseng Radix (*rén shēn*), Angelicae sinensis Radix (*dāng guī*), and Rehmanniae Radix praeparata (*shú dì huáng*).
- For sore throat, reduce the dosage of Cinnamomi Ramulus (*guì zhī*) by half, and add Trichosanthis Radix (*tiān huā fěn*) and Belamcandae Rhizoma (*shè gān*).
- For external wind-cold invasion accompanied by dampness, combine with Saposhnikoviae Radix (*fáng fēng*), Notopterygii Rhizoma seu Radix (*qiāng huó*), and Atractylodis macrocephalae Rhizoma (*bái zhú*).
- To disseminate and direct Lung qi downward in cases with wheezing, cough, and phlegm, add Perillae Fructus (*zǐ sū zǐ*), Mori Cortex (*sāng bái pí*), Poria (*fú líng*), and Citri reticulatae Pericarpium (*chén pí*).
- Where trauma is accompanied by contraction of wind-cold, add Persicae Semen (*táo rén*) and Carthami Flos (*hóng huā*) to invigorate the blood and open the collaterals.

Variation

麻黃加朮湯 （麻黄加术汤）

Ephedra Decoction plus Atractylodes

má huáng jiā zhú tāng

SOURCE *Essentials from the Golden Cabinet* (c. 220)

Add Atractylodis macrocephalae Rhizoma *(bái zhú)* for pronounced body aches with irritability due to damp-cold in the exterior or invasion of wind-dampness in patients with chronic dampness, usually due to Spleen deficiency.

Associated Formulas

三拗湯 （三拗汤）

Three-Unbinding Decoction

sān ǎo tāng

SOURCE *Formulary of the Pharmacy Service for Benefiting the People in the Taiping Era* (1107)

Ephedrae Herba *(má huáng)*. . . . . (6-9g)
Armeniacae Semen *(xìng rén)* . . . . (6-9g)
Glycyrrhizae Radix *(gān cǎo)* . . . . (3-6g)

The source text advises to coarsely grind equal amounts of the ingredients and take 15g as a draft with 5 slices of Zingiberis Rhizoma recens *(shēng jiāng)*. At present, however, it is usually prepared as a decoction with the dosage specified in parentheses above. After taking the formula, the patient should go to bed and stay under the covers until there is slight sweating. Disseminates the Lung qi and releases the exterior. For externally-contracted wind-cold characterized by head and body aches, nasal congestion, coughing, wheezing, copious white, thin sputum, and a sensation of fullness in the chest. May also be used for coughing and loss of voice due to wind-cold. Its diaphoretic action is not as strong as that of the principal formula.

新加三拗湯 （新加三拗汤）

Newly Augmented Three-Unbinding Decoction

xīn jiā sān ǎo tāng

SOURCE *Revised Popular Guide to the Discussion of Cold Damage* (Qing dynasty)

Ephedrae Herba *(má huáng)*. . . . . [entire stalks with nodes] 1.8g

This formula was composed by the Ming-dynasty physician Yu Gen-Chu to treat greater yang-warp cold damage that is accompanied by pronounced Lung signs and symptoms such as headache, chills, fever, absence of sweating, wheezing, nasal resonance, a hacking cough, and copious thin, white phlegm. Massa Fortunellae Fructus *(jīn jù bǐng)* is a cake made out of kumquats or mandarin oranges. Its properties include the ability to resolve stagnation of qi due to harbored food, and more specifically the ability to unblock the collaterals and to disperse knotting. Its use in this formula suggests that the pattern treated occurs against a background of constitutional phlegm-dampness. The formula is also a typical example for how physicians sought to influence the therapeutic action of a formula by specifying how herbs were to be used or prepared. Ephedrae Herba *(má huáng)* is to be used with the nodes because these are thought to add some astringency to its powerful dispersing action. Armeniacae

Semen *(xìng rén)* is to be used unpeeled and with the tips left on (both are usually removed) to make the herb milder in action. Glycyrrhizae Radix *(gān cǎo)* is used unprepared to add heat-clearing to its tonifying action. Overall, this formula is milder than Ephedra Decoction *(má huáng tāng)* and is therefore very suitable for children and other patients with a weaker constitution.

華蓋散 （华盖散）

Canopy Powder

huá gài sǎn

SOURCE *Formulary of the Pharmacy Service for Benefiting the People in the Taiping Era* (1107)

Ephedrae Herba *(má huáng)*. 30g
Mori Cortex *(sāng bái pí)* 30g
Perillae Fructus *(zǐ sū zǐ)* 30g
Armeniacae Semen *(xìng rén)* 30g
Poria rubra *(chì fú líng)* 30g
Citri reticulatae Pericarpium *(chén pí)* 30g
Glycyrrhizae Radix *(gān cǎo)* 15g

Grind into powder and take in 9g doses as a draft. Disseminates the Lung qi, releases the exterior, expels phlegm, and stops coughing. For wind-cold attacking the Lungs characterized by coughing with copious sputum and a stifling sensation in the chest. This is often seen in patients who have phlegm and then suffer an attack of wind-cold. Replacing Cinnamomi Ramulus *(guì zhī)* with herbs that direct Lung qi downward and disperse phlegm focuses the action of this formula on the Lungs rather than the exterior of the body. In the opinion of most commentators, the addition of the cold herb Mori Cortex *(sāng bái pí)* does not indicate that cold has transformed into heat or that the sputum has become yellow. Combined with herbs that are warm and acrid, Mori Cortex *(sāng bái pí)* focuses on directing qi downward and eliminating excess fluid via the Bladder.

There are several different formulas bearing the name Canopy Powder that all treat the same basic pattern but differ in the details of their composition. The formula listed above should therefore be modified to match the precise manifestation of the person being treated. With appropriate modifications to match the patient's presentation, it is especially effective for the treatment of chronic bronchitis and bronchial asthma where wind-cold often presents as a lurking pathogen.

麻黃杏仁薏苡甘草湯 （麻黄杏仁薏苡甘草汤）

Ephedra, Apricot Kernel, Coicis, and Licorice Decoction

má huáng xìng rén yì yǐ gān cǎo tāng

SOURCE *Essentials from the Golden Cabinet* (c. 220)

Ephedrae Herba *(má huáng)*. 1.5g
Armeniacae Semen *(xìng rén)* 3g
Coicis Semen *(yì yǐ rén)* 1.5g
Glycyrrhizae Radix *(gān cǎo)* 3g

Releases the exterior and dispels wind-dampness. For externally-contracted wind-dampness characterized by mild, generalized body aches, slight aversion to wind, and fever that worsens in the afternoon. The reduced dosage of the herbs, except for Glycyrrhizae Radix *(gān cǎo)*, reflects the mild nature of the disorder. Note that while the dosages given here are based on those in the source text, other texts list different dosages for this formula. These reflect the personal interpretations of the authors as well as changes in the usage of certain herbs. For example, if the exterior symptoms are pronounced, the dosage of both Ephedrae Herba (*má huáng*) and Armeniacae Semen (*xìng rén*) could be increased to 6g each. If dampness predominates, the dosage of Coicis Semen (*yì yǐ rén*) could be increased up to 12g.

大青龍湯 (大青龙汤)

Major Bluegreen Dragon Decoction

dà qīng lóng tāng

The name of this formula is thought to be derived from ancient Chinese symbolic associations. The wood spirit from the east, known as the bluegreen dragon, is present in the billowing ocean waves and is responsible for generating clouds, and for stimulating them to produce rain. This formula produces sweating like the dragon produces rain. It is one of the strongest diaphoretic formulas in *Discussion of Cold Damage*, and is thus referred to as 'major.' Minor Bluegreen Dragon Decoction (*xiǎo qīng lóng tāng*), discussed below, transforms thin mucus and expels pathogenic influences, much like the dragon manifests in the power of the waves. Its effect on the qi and fluids is milder, hence it is referred to as 'minor.'

Source   *Discussion of Cold Damage* (c. 220)

Ephedrae Herba (*má huáng*). 18g
Armeniacae Semen (*xìng rén*). . . . . 60 pieces (6-9g)
Cinnamomi Ramulus (*guì zhī*). 6g
Glycyrrhizae Radix praeparata (*zhì gān cǎo*) 6g
Gypsum fibrosum (*shí gāo*). . . .1 piece the size of an egg (12-30g)
Zingiberis Rhizoma recens (*shēng jiāng*) 9g
Jujubae Fructus (*dà zǎo*). . . . . .12 pieces

Method of Preparation   Decoction. The source text advises to first boil Ephedrae Herba (*má huáng*) separately and decant the froth that forms on the surface of the decoction before adding the other ingredients. Once the decoction has been prepared, it should be taken gradually in several doses. As soon as a sweat is produced, administration should stop. At present, the dosage of Ephedrae Herba (*má huáng*) and Jujubae Fructus (*dà zǎo*) is reduced.

Actions   Promotes sweating, releases the exterior, and clears interior heat

Indications

For exterior cold with heat from constraint in the interior characterized by severe fever and chills without sweating, body aches, thirst, irritability, and a floating, tight pulse. The formula may also be used for overflowing thin mucus (溢飲 *yì yǐn*) patterns defined by heaviness and aching of the entire body or by superficial edema in the extremities, in addition to the other signs and symptoms outlined above.

Individuals who possess a strong constitution react to the invasion of pathogens with a forceful mobilization of yang qi.

If wind-cold fetters the protective qi in the exterior, the yang qi that rises to battle the pathogen will become constrained in the interior, complicating a pattern of exterior cold with signs and symptoms of interior heat. This disease dynamic is cogently summed up by Zhang Bin-Cheng in *Convenient Reader of Established Formulas*: "When wind-cold is suddenly added to the exterior of a person with an abundance of yang, their yang qi is constrained in the interior because it cannot extend. Therefore, one sees a pattern [characterized by] irritability and unease." This formula strongly disperses the exterior while simultaneously clearing heat from constraint in the interior, and calms unease without inhibiting the qi dynamic, thereby facilitating the complete discharge of pathogenic qi.

The second major pattern treated by this formula is overflowing thin mucus, which is defined in *Essentials from the Golden Cabinet*: "The fluids flow [throughout the entire body] and come together in the four limbs. They should issue as sweat, and when they do not, the entire body aches and [feels] heavy." This is a description of superficial edema with the fluids constraining yang qi in the interior leading to a sensation of heaviness and aching that is accompanied by generalized irritability and restlessness. By promoting physiological sweating, the formula disperses superficial edema, even as it clears and discharges interior heat from constraint.

Analysis of Formula

Treating a pattern characterized by wind-cold in the exterior complicated by constrained heat in the interior requires a strategy that resolves the exterior while simultaneously clearing heat constraint in the interior. This is achieved by an ingenious modification of Ephedra Decoction (*má huáng tāng*). The dosages of Ephedrae Herba (*má huáng*) and Glycyrrhizae Radix praeparata (*zhì gān cǎo*) have been doubled, while that of Armeniacae Semen (*xìng rén*) has been reduced. Three more herbs—Gypsum fibrosum (*shí gāo*), Zingiberis Rhizoma recens (*shēng jiāng*), and Jujubae Fructus (*dà zǎo*)—have been added, making the structure of its composition and range of indications distinctly different from its parent formula.

Ephedrae Herba (*má huáng*) remains the chief herb. The increase in dosage implies, however, that the fettering of the exterior by wind-cold is even more pronounced. For the same reason, the diaphoretic action of Ephedrae Herba (*má huáng*) is assisted not only by Cinnamomi Ramulus (*guì zhī*), but also by Zingiberis Rhizoma recens (*shēng jiāng*). Together, these three herbs strongly open the pores, induce sweating, and scatter wind-cold. Two other assistants, the sweet and warm Jujubae Fructus (*dà zǎo*) and Glycyrrhizae Radix praeparata (*zhì gān cǎo*), tonify the middle burner qi and provide the essence from which the fluids can be replenished. They actively facilitate sweating in a context where fluids may have been damaged by internal heat, while also moderating the drying action of the acrid and warming diaphoretic herbs. Glycyrrhizae Radix praeparata *(zhì gān cǎo)* also functions as a harmonizing herb that pulls the different actions of the formula into a coherent whole. The combination of Zingiberis Rhizoma recens *(shēng jiāng)* and Jujubae Fructus *(dà zǎo)* tonifies the Spleen and Stomach and harmonizes the nutritive and protective qi.

Gypsum fibrosum *(shí gāo)*, the deputy herb in this formula, is acrid, sweet, and cold. It clears internal heat without inhibiting the dispersing action of the diaphoretics or further damaging the yin fluids. Armeniacae Semen *(xìng rén)* is the final assistant. Its dosage has been reduced because the cough and wheezing are not pronounced aspects of the presentation treated by this formula. It has not been dropped entirely, however, because the synergism that it develops with Ephedrae Herba *(má huáng)* is still important. Its bitter flavor directs Lung qi downward and balances the dispersive action of Ephedrae Herba *(má huáng)*, while its oily nature moderates the damage to the Lungs by the latter's drying effect.

This formula's ability to treat the superficial edema of overflowing thin mucus patterns is due to its ability to unblock the qi dynamic of the Lungs, the upper source of water, and to promote sweating, rather than to any direct effect on the water metabolism. Ephedrae Herba *(má huáng)*, Cinnamomi Ramulus *(guì zhī)*, and Zingiberis Rhizoma recens *(shēng jiāng)* open the pores and interstices and thereby provide an outlet for excess fluids. Zingiberis Rhizoma recens *(shēng jiāng)* warms the Stomach and disperses fluids. In combination with Jujubae Fructus *(dà zǎo)* and Glycyrrhizae Radix *(gān cǎo)*, it reinforces the movement and transformation of middle burner qi. Thus, as Li Fei notes in the modern textbook *Formulas*, "Although the formula does not contain herbs that [directly] treat thin mucus [by way of diuresis], its effects in treating thin mucus patterns are [nevertheless] reliable."

Commentary

This formula is exemplary for realizing a treatment strategy first advocated in the *Inner Classic*: "For fire [due to] constraint, discharge it" (火鬱發之 *huǒ yù fā zhī*). The fire referred to in this maxim is the body's own yang qi (also known as the ministerial fire or the fire at the gate of vitality), which has become constrained and thereby changed from physiological qi into pathological fire. Under normal circumstances, ministerial fire warms and disperses body fluids, which in the exterior manifests as physiological sweating. It follows that promoting sweating can therefore also be used to discharge from the body a pathological accumulation or build-up of yang qi. This is what is meant when Zhang Xi-Chun speaks of "transforming heat that has accumulated and built up in the chest into sweat." This strategy is particularly indicated where

the accumulation is due to cold. Acrid warming, in this case, not only increases the diffusion of yang qi toward the exterior, it also actively disperses the pathogen from the body.

Irritability and restlessness due to yang qi constraint in the interior is thus one of the most important clinical markers for selecting this formula. Symptomatically, such constraint may also be reflected in skin that is burning hot to the touch, up-flushing of heat, a dry nasal passage, or thirst.

Sweating and Edema

Given the prominence of such heat signs, it may seem odd that the formula is also able to treat superficial edema, that is, water excess. This apparent contradiction is easily resolved by remembering that, from a yin/yang perspective, the excess of fluids (water) in the exterior necessarily implies a deficiency of physiological heat (fire). By mobilizing yang qi toward the exterior while simultaneously opening the pores, the formula restores a more physiological balance between water and fire, relieving the edema even if it does not directly treat the fluids. The commentators therefore agree that inducing sweating is the main goal of this formula and that unblocking the pores and interstices is the necessary means for achieving this end.

Zhang Zi-He, famous for his focus on eliminating pathogens from the body, argues in *Confucians' Duties to Their Parents* that in a wider sense, the sweating method denotes not just the actual production of sweat at the body surface, but an "opening of the 'mysterious mansions' (玄府 *xuān fǔ*) in order to drive out pathogenic qi." The term 'mysterious mansions' is commonly understood as referring to the sweat pores. Some physicians, however, most notably the 19th-century writer Zhou Xue-Hai, define them as points of entry and exit for the qi and body fluids that can be found throughout the tissues and organs of the body. This gives a useful perspective on how we might best understand the complex composition of this formula, especially the functions of what we regard as the two deputy herbs, Gypsum fibrosum *(shí gāo)* and Zingiberis Rhizoma recens *(shēng jiāng)*.

While Gypsum fibrosum *(shí gāo)* is cooling, it is also acrid and sweet and thereby facilitates the movement of qi and fluids through the pores. In *Essays on Medicine Esteeming the Chinese and Respecting the Western*, Zhang Xi-Chun describes the action of Gypsum fibrosum *(shí gāo)* in this formula: "Its acrid-dispersing and cooling-moistening character can help Ephedrae Herba *(má huáng)* and Cinnamomi Ramulus *(guì zhī)* thrust out the pathogen from the exterior. It is also excellent for transforming heat that has accumulated and built up in the chest into sweat, which is emitted as it follows Ephedrae Herba's *(má huáng)* and Cinnamomi Ramulus' *(guì zhī)* venting of the exterior."

The relatively large dose of Zingiberis Rhizoma recens *(shēng jiāng)*, on the other hand, unblocks the flow of qi and blood throughout the entire body and facilitates the expulsion of pathogenic cold from the deepest to the most superficial regions. According to Zhang, "its pungency opens up obstructions, while its heat is able to disperse. Therefore, it is capable of warming the muscles and flesh, yet also deeply vents from the sinews and bones so as to dispel congealing, stubborn cold, causing the water to flow again as the ice disappears."

Key Strategy

In practice, focusing on this ability to unblock the qi dynamic is thus key to the successful use of Major Bluegreen Dragon Decoction (*dà qīng lóng tāng*). Paragraph 39 of *Discussion of Cold Damage* is explicit in distinguishing a pattern characterized by a floating and relaxed pulse, and a sensation of heaviness in the body that sometimes becomes better and sometimes worse and that responds to Major Bluegreen Dragon Decoction (*dà qīng lóng tāng*), from a similar presentation in lesser yin stage disorders. In both cases, the circulation of yang qi through the body is impeded by the presence of yin excess. This is experienced as heaviness of the body, accompanied by sensations of heat, chills, and an absence of sweating. However, because in lesser yin patterns the yang qi is deficient, the patient will be primarily cold, and any heat signs will be due to weak yang floating toward the surface. In the present pattern, however, the yang qi is strong, and the constraint—and thus the irritability and restlessness—are pronounced.

Historically, this formula has been enormously influential in establishing a strategy for releasing the exterior while simultaneously clearing heat from the interior. Formulas like Nine-Herb Decoction with Notopterygium (*jiǔ wèi qiāng huó tāng*) and Saposhnikovia Powder that Sagely Unblocks (*fáng fēng tōng shèng sǎn*) employ new herbs and treat new patterns. Their authors, the famous Jin-Yuan master physicians Zhang Yuan-Su and Liu Wan-Su, can be seen as honoring Zhang Zhong-Jing by following the path he blazed.

Comparison

➢ Vs. Gypsum Decoction (*shí gāo tāng*); see PAGE 295

Biomedical Indications

With the appropriate presentation, this formula may be used to treat a wide variety of biomedically-defined disorders, primarily infectious in origin, such as upper respiratory tract infections, influenza, suppurative keratitis, acute infectious conjunctivitis, sinusitis, bronchial asthma, viral pneumonia, lobar pneumonia, pulmonary gangrene, septicemia, scarlet fever, and erisypelas.

In addition, it has been used in dermatology for such conditions as contact dermatitis, drug dermatitis, exfoliative dermatitis, sebaceous cysts, and psoriasis. This formula has also been used to treat a miscellany of biomedically-defined problems, among them drug fevers, acute stage of leukemia, nephritis, brain trauma, hypertension, cerebrovascular disease, and strokes.

Alternate names

Licorice Decoction (*gān cǎo tāng*) in *Comprehensive Recording of Sagely Beneficence*

Cautions and Contraindications

This formula is strongly diaphoretic. It should be administered gradually and stopped once sweating has been induced. The formula is contraindicated in lesser yin patterns, in cases of yang deficiency, in wind-stroke patterns with deficiency of the exterior, and in all cases where sweating is associated with an increase in irritability, restlessness, and heat (i.e., cases of yin or blood deficiency). It is also inappropriate for wind-cold fettering the exterior with severe accumulation of fluids in the interior.

Modifications

- For less severe cold in the exterior, reduce the dosage of Ephedrae Herba (*má huáng*).
- For more pronounced signs of heat in the interior with severe irritability and restlessness and pronounced thirst, increase the dosage of Gypsum fibrosum (*shí gāo*).
- For cough and wheezing with thin mucus, increase the dosage of Armeniacae Semen (*xìng rén*) and add Pinelliae Rhizoma (*bàn xià*), Perillae Fructus (*zǐ sū zǐ*), and Mori Cortex (*sāng bái pí*).
- For superficial edema with reduced urination, add Poria (*fú líng*), Polyporus (*zhū líng*), Mori Cortex (*sāng bái pí*), and Lepidii/ Descurainiae Semen (*tíng lì zǐ*).

桂枝湯（桂枝汤）

Cinnamon Twig Decoction

guì zhī tāng

Source *Discussion of Cold Damage* (c. 220)

Cinnamomi Ramulus (*guì zhī*) 9g
Paeoniae Radix (*sháo yào*) 9g
Zingiberis Rhizoma recens (*shēng jiāng*) .9g
Jujubae Fructus (*dà zǎo*) . . . . .12 pieces
Glycyrrhizae Radix praeparata (*zhì gān cǎo*) 6g

Method of Preparation The source text advises to coarsely grind the ingredients and decoct over a low flame in about 7 cups of water until about 3 cups of liquid remain. One cup is taken hot with hot rice gruel to induce sweating. If the first cup is successful, do not administer a second cup. If there is little sweating, repeat once or twice, progressively reducing the interval between doses.

At present, however, this formula is prepared as a decoction and is cooked no more than 20 minutes, then taken hot. The patient should bundle up to help induce mild sweating. Once sweating occurs, stop administering the formula.

According to the source text, the consumption of alcohol and raw, cold, spicy, or greasy foods is prohibited during medication.

At present, only 4 pieces of Jujubae Fructus *(dà zǎo)* are used. Paeoniae Radix alba *(bái sháo)* is the type of Paeoniae Radix *(sháo yào)* that is generally used, but see the COMMENTARY below for a detailed discussion.

Actions   Releases pathogenic influences from the muscle layer and regulates the nutritive and protective qi

Indications

Fever and chills unrelieved by sweating, headache, aversion to wind, stiff neck, nasal congestion, dry heaves, no particular thirst, a thin, white, and moist tongue coating, and a floating pulse that is either lax or frail. May also be used for a similar presentation in patients not suffering from an external invasion.

This is externally-contracted wind-cold or wind attack (中風 *zhòng fēng*), a condition characterized by disharmony between the nutritive and protective qi. Under normal circumstances, the two regulate and support each other. The protective qi (associated with yang) guards the exterior and prevents leakage of nutritive qi to the outside. The nutritive qi (associated with yin) nourishes and stabilizes the interior, regulating the function of protective qi as well as constituting a reservoir for it. In case of wind attack, this mutual regulation and support is lost. When the protective qi rises to the surface to fend off the invading pathogenic qi, fever and chills are produced. Agitated by the externally-contracted wind, it is unable to adequately perform its other functions, such as guarding the nutritive qi. The nutritive qi thereupon becomes unstable and is unable to contain the fluids. The resulting sweating does not have the full force of the protective qi behind it, and thus does not lead to any improvement in the condition.

The opening of the interstices and pores (during sweating) makes one more sensitive to the environment, which leads to an aversion or sensitivity to wind. When wind-cold invades the muscles and the exterior, it impedes the flow of qi in the channels (especially the greater yang channels), which leads to headache and stiff neck. The Lungs control the qi and are associated with the skin, body hair, and nose. Wind-cold, which fetters or 'bottles up' the exterior, also impairs the qi mechanism of the Lungs, which causes nasal congestion. The impaired qi mechanism of the Lungs and the loss of mutual regulation between the nutritive and protective qi disrupts the Stomach qi, which leads to dry heaves.

As is typical of fever due to exterior cold, there is no particular thirst. The thin, white tongue coating and floating pulse are also characteristic of exterior wind-cold. Sweating 'opens up' the superficial levels of the body, which is reflected in a relaxation of the pulse. The pulse is lax in that it is not as tight as the tight pulse associated with exterior cold excess; this reflects the general state of the exterior.

Loss of mutual regulation between the nutritive and protective qi can also occur after a serious illness, childbirth, or in patients with a weak constitution. In such cases, even though there may be no externally-contracted wind-cold, there may still be fever, sweating, and an aversion to wind.

Analysis of Formula

The strategy guiding the composition of this formula is known in Chinese medicine as the 'harmonization of nutritive and protective qi.' This refers to a two-pronged approach that attends to the dispersal of wind-cold excess at the level of the protective qi and the restoration of normal flow at the level of the nutritive qi in such a manner as to facilitate their harmonious physiological interaction and interpenetration. In *Discussion of Cold Damage,* the objective of this strategy is highlighted by means of a well-known rhetorical question: "When the protective qi does not act together with the nutritive qi, how can [the organism function] in a harmonious manner?"

The chief herb, warm, acrid Cinnamomi Ramulus *(guì zhī),* releases externally-contracted wind-cold from the muscle layer. It is combined with the deputy, Paeoniae Radix alba *(bái sháo),* which benefits the yin and contains the weak nutritive qi. Together, they simultaneously enhance the ability of the protective qi to dispel pathogenic influences while strengthening the nutritive qi. For this reason, the formula is said to regulate both the protective and nutritive qi as well as harmonize their interactions. One of the assistants, Zingiberis Rhizoma recens *(shēng jiāng),* helps the chief ingredient release the exterior while also treating the nausea and vomiting by warming the middle and directing qi downward. The other assistant, sweet Jujubae Fructus *(dà zǎo),* helps the sour deputy nourish and harmonize the nutritive qi and the blood. Together, these assistants benefit the middle qi (Spleen), which rises to regulate the nutritive and protective qi. Glycyrrhizae Radix praeparata *(zhì gān cǎo),* the envoy, harmonizes the actions of the other ingredients, combining with Cinnamomi Ramulus *(guì zhī)* and Zingiberis Rhizoma recens *(shēng jiāng)* to transform the yang aspects of the condition and with Paeoniae Radix alba *(bái sháo)* and Jujubae Fructus *(dà zǎo)* to transform the yin. Thus, the formula elegantly regulates and harmonizes the protective and nutritive in such a way as to disperse wind and release the muscle layer.

Commentary

This is one of the most important formulas in *Discussion of Cold Damage.* As many as twenty variations and associated formulas are described in that text alone. Later generations of physicians not only widely extended its indications, but also used it as the foundation for many other formulas to treat an ever-expanding array of disorders. For example, some of the formulas that treat interior cold (Chapter 7), such as Minor Construct the Middle Decoction *(xiǎo jiàn zhōng tāng)* and Tangkuei Decoction for Frigid Extremities *(dāng guī sì nì tāng),* as well as formulas that restrain abnormal leakage (Chapter 12), such as Cinnamon Twig Decoction Plus Dragon Bone and Oyster Shell *(guì zhī jiā lóng gǔ mǔ lì tāng),* are variations of this formula.

Key Symptoms

Clinically, the single most important symptom for the use of this formula is sweating. Because the sweating here is due to disharmony between the nutritive and protective qi and not to a specific organ pathology, it is not limited to specific body regions, climates, or other organ correspondences. It may occur in any season, and during the day or at night. It may be more or less pronounced, limited to the hands and feet, one side of the body, or the back or head, yet it may also occur all over the body. It may appear in the context of specific illnesses but also independently of specific causes. Thus, not only does the source text discuss the use of Cinnamon Twig Decoction *(guì zhī tāng)* in the context of a typical wind-cold disorder, but also, for instance, for "patients who generally have spontaneous sweating" (paragraph 53), or who exhibit "severe leakage of sweat [accompanied by] a flooding, large pulse" (paragraph 25). In all of these cases, sweating represents a loss of the body's essences and an inability to control yang functions. This occurs more frequently in patients who are constitutionally weak and easily overstimulated, that is, in those with a 'nervous disposition.' A characteristic sign of such a reaction is increased tension of the rectus abdominus muscles upon palpation. Furthermore, the pathological sweating observed before a patient takes Cinnamon Twig Decoction *(guì zhī tāng)* is categorically different from the physiological sweating induced by this formula. Whereas the former is a type of uncontrolled leakage, the latter signifies that the body has reestablished control over its yang qi. Physiological sweating induced by Cinnamon Twig Decoction *(guì zhī tāng)* will thus only occur when a pathogen is being expelled and not necessarily when the formula is used to treat chronic internal medicine disorders.

The second most important symptoms are aversion to wind or drafts, and the occurrence of heat-type reactions in response to cold. This may be fever in the course of a wind-cold disorder, but also a rash caused by exposure to cold water when swimming in the summer. Other important symptoms include body aches and pain, and up-flushing of qi, discussed in more detail below. Due to the chronic loss of fluids caused by sweating, patients for whom Cinnamon Twig Decoction *(guì zhī tāng)* is indicated may sometimes suffer from thirst and constipation. If thirsty, they will prefer warm drinks, unlike patients with a White Tiger plus Ginseng Decoction *(bái hǔ jiā rén shēn tāng)* presentation (discussed in Chapter 4),

who also sweat easily but favor cold drinks. The constipation in patients with a Cinnamon Twig Decoction *(guì zhī tāng)* presentation will not be accompanied by signs of internal dryness or obstruction of the gastrointestinal system. If these signs are observed, other formulas such as Minor or Major Bupleurum Decoction *(xiǎo dà chái hú tāng)* are indicated.

Exterior Deficiency

Given its importance and wide range of application, this formula has been extensively discussed in the literature. Not surprisingly, commentators differ considerably in their understanding of its actions and indications, and on issues relating to dosage and formula composition. Claims by some commentators that exterior deficiency refers to a relative weakness of protective qi are difficult to reconcile with the original definition of wind attack (中風 *zhòng fēng)* in paragraph 95 of the *Discussion of Cold Damage,* where it is characterized as being "due to nutritive [qi being] frail and protective [qi being] strong." Likewise, if strengthening the protective qi is the main objective of this formula, why does it rely on a chief ingredient that, down to its red color, has a closer affinity to nutritive qi and blood than to the protective qi? Finally, how does this kind of exterior deficiency differ from the deficiency of protective qi treated by formulas like Jade Windscreen Powder *(yù píng fēng sǎn),* discussed in Chapter 8?

One way of resolving these questions is to remember that, while both of these formulas treat patterns produced by the simultaneous invasion of wind and cold, in the pattern for which Cinnamon Twig Decoction *(guì zhī tāng)* is indicated, wind is predominant. For the cold damage pattern treated by Ephedra Decoction *(má huáng tāng),* the predominance of cold is such that, while wind is presumed to be present as a disease vector, it does not contribute much to the actual symptomatology.

Wind, by definition, describes a pathological condition where the forces of yang that manifest through motion and transformation are no longer controlled by the constraining nature of yin. In patterns of wind attack, this pathology is produced by two interrelated processes. External wind penetrates into the greater yang warp of the body where it stirs up the activity of yang protective qi. Because external wind and protective qi are of similar natures, this moves the balance of yin and yang within the greater yang warp toward an excess of yang. This condition is exacerbated by the simultaneous penetration of cold. As a yin pathogen, cold attaches to nutritive yin, contracting its substance, slowing down its movement, and diminishing its ability to control the protective yang. The result is an excessive outward and upward movement of protective qi that manifests in increased sweating and fever, but also in dry retching or similar symptoms of upward-surging, while the stagnation of nutritive qi in the channels leads to head and body aches.

In *Commentary on the Classic of the Materia Medica*, the Qing dynasty physician Zou Shu describes this pathology with great clarity. He also explains why it does not resolve by itself. "[When] the nutritive yin clumps in the interior, the protective yang can [no longer] enter into it; … the interpenetration of nutritive and protective qi is abandoned; … [and they] finally oppose each other [to such an extent] that they completely part from each other, hence sweat comes out."

Discussion of Ingredients

Although the condition requires the discharge of pathogens to the outside, this cannot be achieved by the simple use of warm, acrid herbs to promote sweating. Such herbs would add even more yang to the already excessive yang in the exterior, aggravating the existing imbalance. Furthermore, the stasis of nutritive qi needs to be resolved as well, which cannot be achieved by merely mobilizing protective qi. For this reason, Zhang Zhong-Jing has composed what is widely regarded to be a harmonizing (和 *hé*) formula that focuses on the nutritive yin rather than on the protective yang. Its chief herb, warm, acrid, and sweet Cinnamomi Ramulus (*guì zhī*), enters the nutritive qi and blood in the channels and muscle layer, facilitating their flow and dispersing cold to the outside. In this way, it strengthens the regulatory function of nutritive qi even as its acrid nature promotes sweating and dispels wind-cold. Ke Qin, the famous Qing commentator on classical formulas, underlines this intention when he argues that Cinnamomi Ramulus (*guì zhī*) "internally assists the chief; it induces the dispersion of Heart yin fluids as sweat." The term 'chief' here refers to the Heart because of its resonance with not only the nutritive blood, but also the greater yang warp. As stated in Chapter 9 of *Basic Questions*, the Heart "constitutes the greater yang in the yang" (為陽中之太陽 *wéi yáng zhōng zhī tài yáng*). Dispersing its yin fluids as sweat implies an activation of Heart yang functions, which encompass flow and movement, focus and concentration, the transformation of yang fire into yin essence, and a guarding against their inherent potential to separate. Grasping this aspect of Heart yang activity allows us to understand how the promotion of physiological sweating (indicating strong Heart yang) can control pathological sweating (indicating separation of yin and yang).

Ke Qin also extends this line of reasoning—identifying Heart function as the key fulcrum to which the formula attaches—to the action of its deputy. He argues that this "lies primarily in stopping irritability. For when irritability has been stopped, sweating also stops." Irritability arises when Heart qi is constrained, and Radix Paeoniae (*sháo yào*) is seen here as assisting Cinnamomi Ramulus (*guì zhī*) in breaking through this stasis. It does so because of its ability to relax spasms, although some commentators emphasize its bitter opening and draining qualities as being more important.

Note that this interpretation more closely matches the action of Paeoniae Radix rubra (*chì sháo*) and not the more commonly used Paeoniae Radix alba (*bái sháo*).

The modern preference for Paeoniae Radix alba (*bái sháo*) can be traced to the Song dynasty and, in particular, to the influence of the scholar-physician Xu Shu-Wei. Although Xu categorically rejected the use of Paeoniae Radix rubra (*chì sháo*) in this formula, he never emphasized the sour, astringent properties of Paeoniae Radix alba (*bái sháo*) when advocating its use. Rather, he argued that it strengthened the frail nutritive yin, ensuring that it would not be invaded again by pathogens from the outside, and making it sufficiently strong to support protective yang. The modern physician Zhang Ci-Gong likewise points out that the function of the deputy in a flagship formula like Cinnamon Twig Decoction (*guì zhī tāng*) cannot be that of antagonistic control, for that would be far too inelegant. Instead, the deputy must support and assist the chief herb. Zhang thus follows Zou Shu's view that Radix Paeoniae (*sháo yào*) has the function of ensuring that the nutritive yin is sufficiently strong, yet also soft enough to receive the protective yang and thereby ensure their mutual interpenetration. This also explains why the choice of assistant herbs is weighted toward sweet and warm tonification rather than acrid dispersal, even though expelling wind-cold is the ultimate goal of the formula. The sweetness of Jujubae Fructus (*dà zǎo*) and Glycyrrhizae Radix praeparata (*zhì gān cǎo*) softens and relaxes the yin and allows the yang to penetrate into it again, counteracting any latent disposition to separate. In this way, too, even though the formula focuses almost entirely on nutritive yin, it controls the harmonious unfolding of protective yang.

The reduction in dosage of Jujubae Fructus (*dà zǎo*), which has also occurred with many of the other formulas listed in the books of Zhang Zhong-Jing, is due to a change in the understanding of how best to utilize this herb. It has always been thought to tonify the normal qi. However, for the past thousand years, it has also been regarded as a very cloying herb, that is, one that causes fullness and distention in the middle burner. Because of this, its dosage has been reduced.

Usage

Once the harmonization of nutritive and protective qi is understood as facilitating their harmonious movement and interpenetration, the use of Cinnamon Twig Decoction (*guì zhī tāng*) can be readily extended to a wide range of conditions where the protective yang is unable to enter into the nutritive yin and instead exits, ascends, or accumulates pathologically. Symptomatically, such conditions are characterized by yang excess (wind, heat, upward-gushing of qi) in the exterior of the body (the greater yang warp) that occurs in conjunction with stagnation due to cold (irrespective of whether this is due to external invasion or internal deficiency) at the level of the nutritive qi or Heart yang.

Cinnamon Twig Decoction *(guì zhī tāng)* patterns are differentiated from Ephedra Decoction *(má huáng tāng)* patterns, where cold pathogens completely fetter the movement of qi and fluids, by the presence of sweating or other signs indicating that the protective yang is separating from the nutritive yin. They are differentiated from early stage warm pathogen disorders, where pathogenic heat is lodged in the protective aspect, by the simultaneous presence of heat (fever, rashes, irritability) and cold (chills, exacerbation in the winter or after exposure to cold). From the perspective of the organ systems, Cinnamon Twig Decoction *(guì zhī tāng)* patterns imply constraint—and with appropriate modifications, even deficiency—of the Heart qi and yang. As the early 18th-century text *Personal Standards for the Essentials from the Golden Cabinet* notes: "In exterior patterns, one uses [this formula] to release the muscles and harmonize the nutritive and protective; in interior patterns, one uses it to transform qi and regulate yin and yang."

The famous Shanghai physician Zhang Yao-Qing, cited in *Contemporary Explanations of Classical Formulas,* sums up the many uses of this formula under twelve headings:

1. Harmonization of nutritive and protective qi
2. Releasing the muscle layer to promote sweating
3. Yang deficiency with spontaneous sweating
4. Insufficiency of Stomach yang
5. Running piglet qi with wheezing
6. Deficiency cold pain in the lower abdomen, causing cramping pains
7. Wind-dampness painful obstruction
8. Deficiency wheezing
9. Chronic Spleen wind in children
10. Enriching yin and harmonizing yang
11. Frostbite
12. Yin-type patterns in external medicine

The modifications listed below provide further examples of the wide range of applications for which this formula may be indicated. Readers should study them carefully in order to grasp the sophistication, and also the beauty, of formula composition. Cinnamon Twig Decoction *(guì zhī tāng)* is, after all, universally acknowledged to be the "crown (冠 *guàn*) of Zhang Zhong-Jing's formulas" and therefore of Chinese herbal medicine in general.

Comparisons

➤ Vs. Jade Windscreen Powder *(yù píng fēng sǎn)*; see PAGE 328

➤ Vs. Minor Construct the Middle Decoction *(xiǎo jiàn zhōng tāng)*; see PAGE 266

Biomedical Indications

With the appropriate presentation, this formula may be used to treat a wide variety of biomedically-defined disorders. These can be divided into the following groups:

- Febrile diseases, including the common cold, influenza, postpartum fevers, and fever of unknown origin
- Problems marked by an upward-gushing or surging sensation in the trunk, including cardiovascular disease, myocarditis, premature ventricular contractions, paroxysmal atrial tachycardia, sick sinus syndrome, and functional cardiac disorders
- Allergic disorders such as allergic rhinitis, allergic purpura, food allergies, asthma, recalcitrant urticaria, and eczema
- Miscellaneous disorders such as hemiplegia, neutropenia, hyperactivity, enuresis, perimenopausal syndrome, hypotension, and diffuse esophageal spasms.

Cautions and Contraindications

Contraindicated in most cases with exterior cold and interior heat, characterized by fever and thirst or sore throat with a rapid pulse. It should not be given to patients with internal heat, as nosebleeds may result. It is also contraindicated in patients with internal damp-heat. It should be used with caution during the summer or spells of hot weather. If incorrectly prescribed, or if the dosage is too strong, profuse sweating, high fever, severe thirst, palpitations, and irritability may result. In such cases, White Tiger plus Ginseng Decoction *(bái hǔ jiā rén shēn tāng)* should be prescribed to cope with the side effects.

Alternate names

Yang Dawn Decoction *(yáng dàn tāng)* in *Essentials from the Golden Cabinet*

Modifications

- For marked nasal congestion with sneezing, add Saposhnikoviae Radix *(fáng fēng)* and Magnoliae Flos *(xīn yí huā)*.
- For shortness of breath and rough breathing or other signs of qi stagnation, add qi-regulating herbs like Magnoliae officinalis Cortex *(hòu pò)*, Aurantii Fructus *(zhǐ ké)*, or Citri reticulatae Pericarpium *(chén pí)*.
- For a swollen, heavy sensation in the head indicating the presence of heat that prevents the yang from directing downward, add Chrysanthemi Flos *(jú huā)* and Cicadae Periostracum *(chán tuì)*.
- For simultaneous presence of internal heat, add herbs such as Gypsum fibrosum *(shí gāo)*, Anemarrhenae Rhizoma *(zhī mǔ)*, and Scutellariae Radix *(huáng qín)* to clear the heat or Cimicifugae Rhizoma *(shēng má)* to vent the exterior.

- For profuse sweating, increase the dosage of Paeoniae Radix alba (bái sháo) and reduce by one-third that of Cinnamomi Ramulus (guì zhī), Zingiberis Rhizoma recens (shēng jiāng), and Glycyrrhizae Radix praeparata (zhì gān cǎo). In case of qi deficiency, also add Astragali Radix (huáng qí) and Saposhnikoviae Radix (fáng fēng).

- For severe headache, substitute Paeoniae Radix rubra (chì sháo) for Paeoniae Radix alba (bái sháo) and add Ligustici Rhizoma (gǎo běn).

- For severe vomiting, increase the dosage of Paeoniae Radix alba (bái sháo) and Zingiberis Rhizoma recens (shēng jiāng) and add Citri reticulatae Pericarpium (chén pí) and Magnoliae officinalis Cortex (hòu pò).

- For joint pain in the extremities accompanied by fatigue (symptoms of dampness), add Notopterygii Rhizoma seu Radix (qiāng huó) and Saposhnikoviae Radix (fáng fēng).

- For diarrhea due to wind-cold accompanied by summer-heat-dampness, add Poria (fú líng) and Alismatis Rhizoma (zé xiè).

- For wind attack in women, menstrual pain, or ulcers and sores indicating blood stasis, use Paeoniae Radix rubra (chì sháo) instead of Paeoniae Radix alba (bái sháo) and add Persicae Semen (táo rén), Carthami Flos (hóng huā), or Angelicae sinensis Radix (dāng guī).

- For Spleen yang deficiency reducing the Spleen's ability to control the blood, add Terra flava usta (zào xīn tǔ) and Asini Corii Colla (ē jiāo).

- For low grade fever of unknown etiology, add Artemisiae annuae Herba (qīng hāo) and Cynanchi atrati Radix (bái wēi).

Variations

桂枝加桂湯 （桂枝加桂汤）

Cinnamon Twig Decoction plus Cinnamon

guì zhī jiā guì tāng

SOURCE   *Discussion of Cold Damage* (c. 220)

Increase the dosage of Cinnamomi Ramulus (guì zhī) to 15g for greater yang-warp disorders that were improperly treated by use of the fire needle or where excessive sweating has provoked running piglet disorder. This is characterized by qi rushing upward from the lower abdomen to the chest and Heart. The patient is uncomfortable both standing up and lying down, and the symptoms tend to occur in recurrent attacks. At present, this formula is used for a wide variety of diseases with symptoms of an upward-surging of qi and chest discomfort. Some commentators recommend the addition of Cinnamomi Cortex (ròu guì) rather than increasing the dosage of Cinnamomi Ramulus (guì zhī).

After listing the composition of the formula, the source text observes: "The reason for adding Cinnamomi Ramulus (guì zhī) is to drain running piglet qi." Although it may at first appear counterintuitive to use an acrid, warm, and ascend-ing herb to control uncontrolled up-rushing of qi, once the transformative function of the Heart has been grasped, the strategic logic at the heart of Cinammon Twig Decoction (guì zhī tāng) and its modifications is easily understood. In the present case, inapporpriate treatment has not only caused the Heart yang to disperse, but has also accelerated the physiological ascent of yang from the lower to the upper burner, and from inside to outside. As the yang in the chest becomes deficient, it can no longer control this ascent, and thus running piglet qi results. Depending on whether this deficiency is strictly local or stems from a more systemic deficiency of the fire at the gate of vitality, one should use either Cinnamomi Ramulus (guì zhī) or Cinnamomi Cortex (ròu guì) to strengthen the Heart yang. Thus, when the source text speaks of draining, it is referring to a secondary effect rather than to a primary strategy.

桂枝加芍藥湯 （桂枝加芍药汤）

Cinnamon Twig Decoction plus Peony

guì zhī jiā sháo yào tāng

SOURCE   *Discussion of Cold Damage* (c. 220)

Double the dosage of Paeoniae Radix (sháo yào) for greater yang-warp disorders that have been improperly treated with purgatives and thus advanced to the greater yin, characterized by abdominal fullness and occasional pain.

This is a good example of how the basic strategy implicit in a formula can be employed to treat a similar problem in a different context. Doubling the dosage of Radix Paeoniae (sháo yào) redirects the focus of the formula from the upper to the middle burner, from the Heart to the Spleen, from warming the nutritive qi to dealing with its constraint.

桂枝去芍藥湯 （桂枝去芍药汤）

Cinnamon Twig Decoction minus Peony

guì zhī qù sháo yào tāng

SOURCE   *Discussion of Cold Damage* (c. 220)

Remove Paeoniae Radix (sháo yào) for greater yang-warp disorders improperly treated with purgatives with subsequent injury to the yang of the chest, manifesting in an irregular pulse and a feeling of fullness in the chest.

桂枝加厚樸杏子湯 （桂枝加厚朴杏子汤）

Cinnamon Twig Decoction plus Magnolia Bark and Apricot Kernel

guì zhī jiā hòu pò xìng zǐ tāng

SOURCE   *Discussion of Cold Damage* (c. 220)

Add Magnoliae officinalis Cortex (hòu pò) and Armeniacae Semen (xìng rén) for a Cinnamon Twig Decoction (guì zhī tāng) presentation plus wheezing, or where improper treatment with purgatives has failed to release an exterior disorder, which is then accompanied by slight wheezing.

Comparison

➤ Vs. Ephedra, Apricot Kernel, Gypsum, and Licorice Decoction (*má xìng shí gān tāng*); see PAGE 184

桂枝加附子湯（桂枝加附子汤）

Cinnamon Twig plus Aconite Accessory Root Decoction

guì zhī jiā fù zǐ tāng

Source *Discussion of Cold Damage* (c. 220)

Add Aconiti Radix lateralis praeparata (*zhì fù zǐ*) for a condition where the over-induction of sweating has damaged the yang of the exterior without releasing the pathogen. This is characterized by incessant sweating along with a continuation of the other signs and symptoms of wind attack, including a floating pulse and painful obstruction due to pathogenic influences battling in the channels, characterized by generalized aches and pains, difficulty in rotating the trunk, and a floating, deficient, and rough pulse. Because this disorder has not affected the interior, there is no thirst or nausea.

Comparison

➤ Vs. White Atractylodes and Aconite Accessory Root Decoction (*bái zhú fù zǐ tāng*); see PAGE 273

桂枝加葛根湯（桂枝加葛根汤）

Cinnamon Twig Decoction plus Kudzu Root

guì zhī jiā gé gēn tāng

Source *Discussion of Cold Damage* (c. 220)

Add Puerariae Radix (*gé gēn*) to release the muscle layer and relax and moisten the sinews. For greater yang-warp disorders characterized by stiff neck and upper back, sweating, and sensitivity to wind.

Associated Formulas

桂枝麻黄各半湯（桂枝麻黄各半汤）

Half Cinnamon Twig and Half Ephedra Decoction

guì zhī má huáng gè bàn tāng

Source *Discussion of Cold Damage* (c. 220)

Cinnamomi Ramulus (*guì zhī*) 5g
Paeoniae Radix alba (*bái sháo*) 3g
Ephedrae Herba (*má huáng*) 3g
Armeniacae Semen (*xìng rén*) . . . . .24 pieces (3-6g)
Glycyrrhizae Radix praeparata (*zhì gān cǎo*) 3g
Zingiberis Rhizoma recens (*shēng jiāng*) 3g
Jujubae Fructus (*dà zǎo*) . . . . 4 pieces

Regulates the nutritive and protective qi, induces sweating, and releases the exterior. For persistent greater yang-warp disorders in which the pathogenic influences have not been fully released and the normal qi has become slightly weakened. This condition is characterized by a flushed face and generalized itching.

桂枝二越婢一湯（桂枝二越婢一汤）

Two-Parts Cinnamon Twig Decoction and One-Part Maidservant from Yue's Decoction

guì zhī èr yuè bì yī tāng

Source *Discussion of Cold Damage* (c. 220)

Cinnamomi Ramulus (*guì zhī*) 3g
Paeoniae Radix alba (*bái sháo*) 3g
Ephedrae Herba (*má huáng*) 3g
Glycyrrhizae Radix praeparata (*zhì gān cǎo*) 3g
Zingiberis Rhizoma recens (*shēng jiāng*) 3g
Gypsum fibrosum (*shí gāo*) 3g
Jujubae Fructus (*dà zǎo*) . . . . 4 pieces

Induces sweating and clears interior heat. For persistent exterior disorders that have become constrained and are accompanied by mild interior heat. This is characterized by fever and chills (fever predominant), thirst, slight irritability, and a floating, big, and forceful pulse.

烏頭桂枝湯（乌头桂枝汤）

Aconite and Cinnamon Twig Decoction

wū tóu guì zhī tāng

Source *Essentials from the Golden Cabinet* (c. 220)

Cinnamomi Ramulus (*guì zhī*) 9g
Aconiti Radix praeparata (*zhì chuān wū*) 6g
Paeoniae Radix alba (*bái sháo*) 9g
Glycyrrhizae Radix praeparata (*zhì gān cǎo*) 6g
Zingiberis Rhizoma recens (*shēng jiāng*) 9g
Jujubae Fructus (*dà zǎo*) . . . . 4 pieces

Warms the interior, reinforces the yang, and releases the exterior. For interior cold due to yang deficiency accompanied by wind-cold that gives rise to a cold bulging disorder. This is characterized by abdominal pain, cold extremities, numb hands and feet, and generalized body aches. The source text notes that this condition will not respond to acupuncture, moxibustion, or other herbal remedies. Because of the potency of this formula, administration should cease as soon as it takes effect. This will prevent the development of toxicity from Aconiti Radix praeparata (*zhì chuān wū*).

葛根湯（葛根汤）

Kudzu Decoction

gé gēn tāng

Source *Discussion of Cold Damage* (c. 220)

Puerariae Radix (*gé gēn*) 12g
Ephedrae Herba (*má huáng*) 9g
Cinnamomi Ramulus (*guì zhī*) 6g
Paeoniae Radix (*sháo yào*) 6g
Zingiberis Rhizoma recens (*shēng jiāng*) 9g
Jujubae Fructus (*dà zǎo*) . . . . .12 pieces
Glycyrrhizae Radix praeparata (*zhì gān cǎo*) 6g

Method of Preparation The source text advises to place Puerariae Radix (*gé gēn*) and Ephedrae Herba (*má huáng*) in about 10 cups of water and decoct until 8 cups remain, then add the other herbs and decoct until 3 cups remain. However, this practice is rarely followed at the present time, and the formula is decocted in the normal manner. Also, only 4 pieces of Jujubae Fructus (*dà zǎo*) are used at present. Paeoniae Radix alba (*bái sháo*) is the type of Paeoniae Radix (*sháo yào*) that is generally used.

Actions   Releases the exterior and muscle layer, and generates fluids

Indications

Fever and chills without sweating, stiff and rigid neck and upper back, a thin, white tongue coating, and a floating, tight pulse.

This is one type of externally-contracted wind-cold affecting the greater yang warp. The distinguishing feature is the stiff and rigid neck and upper back, the appearance of which the source text likens to "a small bird that strains its neck and upper back in an attempt to fly." This is caused by wind-cold, which binds the upper portion of the greater yang channel and prevents the fluids from reaching the area.

Analysis of Formula

This formula disperses wind-cold from the greater yang warp that is constraining the movement of fluids and qi in the yang brightness channel. For this reason, it modifies a formula that disperses wind-cold from the exterior by adding a substance that releases constraint from the yang brightness channel.

The chief herb, Puerariae Radix (*gé gēn*), releases the muscle layer (especially of the upper back and neck) by drawing fluids to the affected area, and releases the exterior. Ephedrae Herba (*má huáng*), one of the deputies, induces sweating. It is the most powerful herb for releasing excess cold from the exterior. The other deputy, Cinnamomi Ramulus (*guì zhī*), helps the chief herb release the exterior and muscle layer.

Paeoniae Radix alba (*bái sháo*), one of the assistants, preserves the yin by preventing the exterior-releasing herbs from causing excessive sweating. Together with Cinnamomi Ramulus (*guì zhī*), it regulates the protective and nutritive qi and assists in the expulsion of the pathogenic influences. The other assistants, Zingiberis Rhizoma recens (*shēng jiāng*) and Jujubae Fructus (*dà zǎo*), regulate the protective and nutritive qi and harmonize the Stomach, protecting that organ from injury. The envoy, Glycyrrhizae Radix praeparata (*zhì gān cǎo*), harmonizes the actions of the other herbs. Together with Paeoniae Radix alba (*bái sháo*), it also relieves muscle spasms and is therefore useful in the treatment of neck and back stiffness.

Commentary

In *Discussion of Cold Damage* (paragraph 32) it is noted that this formula can also be used for a simultaneous greater yang and yang brightness-warp disorder with diarrhea. This is usually explained by the formula's ability to help the Stomach qi rise while simultaneously releasing the exterior. In *Essentials from the Golden Cabinet* this formula is indicated for a greater yang-warp disorder in the absence of sweating and scanty urination. This is a condition of exterior excess in a person with deficient fluids. In this case, the qi pours upward into the chest and prevents one from opening the mouth to speak.

This formula may also be used in treating the transitional stage between acute and chronic rhinitis or sinusitis characterized by mucosal swelling, congestion, and sensitivity to dust and cold drafts. For this reason, some practitioners use the formula as a foundation in formulas that treat allergic rhinitis. Deng Shao-Xian, a prominent modern physician from Chengdu, uses this decoction for chronic pediatric diarrhea with considerable success. It is also very effective for acute stiff neck.

Comparisons

➤ Vs. Ephedra Decoction (*má huáng tāng*)

Both formulas treat greater yang patterns caused by wind-cold fettering protective yang in the exterior. The difference is that Ephedra Decoction (*má huáng tāng*) treats patterns where this constraint is affecting the dispersion and downward-directing of Lung qi, leading to coughing and wheezing. Kudzu Decoction (*gé gēn tāng*), on the other hand, treats patterns where the constraint is affecting the dispersion of qi and blood in the yang brightness channel, manifesting as stiff and rigid neck or other yang brightness channel symptoms.

➤ Vs. Kudzu, Scutellaria, and Coptis Decoction (*gé gēn huáng qín huáng lián tāng*)

Both formulas are used for treating acute diarrhea. However, Kudzu Decoction (*gé gēn tāng*) releases cold from the exterior while it is still in the greater yang warp, while Kudzu, Scutellaria, and Coptis Decoction (*gé gēn huáng qín huáng lián tāng*) clears heat after the pathogenic influence has advanced into the interior.

Biomedical Indications

With the appropriate presentation, this formula may be used to treat a wide variety of biomedically-defined disorders. These can be divided into the following groups:

- Problems characterized by neck and back pain, including the common cold, cervical spine disease, torticollis, periarthritis of the shoulder, lumbar disc disease, lumbar strain

- Problems affecting the head, including trigeminal neuralgia, cerebral vascular insufficiency, hypertension, cerebrovascular disease, otitis media, gingivitis, sinusitis, allergic rhinitis, tonsilitis, and iritis

- Acute digestive problems, including acute enteritis and bacillary dysentery.

Modifications

- For severe nasal blockage, add Chuanxiong Rhizoma (*chuān xiōng*), Scutellariae Radix (*huáng qín*), Magnoliae Flos (*xīn yí huā*), and Platycodi Radix (*jié gěng*).
- For urticaria, add Cicadae Periostracum (*chán tuì*).
- For severe facial pain, add Angelicae pubescentis Radix (*dú huó*) and Peach Pit Decoction to Order the Qi (*táo hé chéng qì tāng*).

Variation

葛根加半夏湯 (葛根加半夏汤)

Kudzu Decoction plus Pinellia

gé gēn jiā bàn xià tāng

Source *Discussion of Cold Damage* (c. 220)

Add Pinelliae Rhizoma praeparatum (*zhì bàn xià*) for a simultaneous greater yang and yang brightness-warp disorder with vomiting, but no diarrhea.

Associated Formulas

清鼻湯 (清鼻汤)

Clear the Nose Decoction

qīng bí tāng

Source *Nakakura Pharmacy in Japan* (19th century)

Puerariae Radix (*gé gēn*) 12g
Coicis Semen (*yì yǐ rén*) 10g
Platycodi Radix (*jié gěng*) 9g
Magnoliae Flos (*xīn yí*) 8g
Ephedrae Herba (*má huáng*) 7g
Paeoniae Radix alba (*bái sháo*) 7g
Cinnamomi Ramulus (*guì zhī*) 7g
Gypsum fibrosum (*shí gāo*) 4g
Zingiberis Rhizoma recens (*shēng jiāng*) 3.5g
Chuanxiong Rhizoma (*chuān xiōng*) 3.5g
Rhei Radix et Rhizoma (*dà huáng*) 3.5g
Glycyrrhizae Radix praeparata (*zhì gān cǎo*) 2g

The dosages here are estimates for decoctions based on the percentages found in the concentrated extract form in which the formula is commonly prepared. Releases pathogens from the exterior, clears heat, resolves toxicity, and unblocks the nasal passages. The formula treats nasal congestion, rhinitis, or sinusitis if they result from an invasion of wind or remain after the signs of a wind invasion have disappeared. With modifications, the formula is also used for allergic rhinitis that is not associated with an exterior pattern. Like the principal formula, Clear the Nose Decoction (*qīng bí tāng*) can treat wind-cold patterns and also wind-cold that enters the yang brightness warp and begins to transform into heat. For the principal formula, the yang brightness symptom is diarrhea, or vomiting with the addition of Pinelliae Rhizoma praeparatum (*zhì bàn xià*); for this formula, the yang brightness symptom is heat in the sinuses, which are traversed by the yang brightness channels.

Because this is a balanced formula, it is generally amended when heat or cold signs predominate:

- Signs of cold include clear nasal discharge, chills, and a tight pulse; remove Gypsum fibrosum (*shí gāo*) and Rhei Radix et Rhizoma (*dà huáng*) and add Angelicae dahuricae Radix (*bái zhǐ*) and Xanthii Fructus (*cāng ěr zǐ*).
- Signs of heat include thick yellow nasal discharge, thirst, a hot sensation in the nose, and a rapid pulse; reduce the dosage of Ephedrae Herba (*má huáng*), remove Cinnamomi Ramulus (*guì zhī*), and add Scutellariae Radix (*huáng qín*) and Paeoniae Radix rubra (*chì sháo*).
- For the acute stages of allergic rhinitis, often Xanthii Fructus (*cāng ěr zǐ*), Scutellariae Radix (*huáng qín*), and Paeoniae Radix rubra (*chì sháo*) are added.

小青龍湯 (小青龙汤)

Minor Bluegreen Dragon Decoction

xiǎo qīng lóng tāng

The name of this formula is discussed under the entry for Major Bluegreen Dragon Decoction (*dà qīng lóng tāng*).

Source *Discussion of Cold Damage* (c. 220)

Ephedrae Herba (*má huáng*) 9g
Cinnamomi Ramulus (*guì zhī*) 9g
Zingiberis Rhizoma (*gān jiāng*) 9g
Asari Radix et Rhizoma (*xì xīn*) 9g
Schisandrae Fructus (*wǔ wèi zǐ*) 9g
Paeoniae Radix alba (*bái sháo*) 9g
Pinelliae Rhizoma praeparatum (*zhì bàn xià*) 9g
Glycyrrhizae Radix praeparata (*zhì gān cǎo*) 9g

Method of Preparation Decoction. Should be taken hot. At present, the dosage of Zingiberis Rhizoma (*gān jiāng*) and Asari Radix et Rhizoma (*xì xīn*) is reduced to 3g because of their extremely hot natures.

Actions Releases the exterior, transforms thin mucus, warms the Lungs, and directs rebellious qi downward

Indications

Fever and chills (chills predominant) without sweating, cough, wheezing, sputum that is copious, white, stringy, and difficult to expectorate, stifling sensation in the chest, generalized sensation of heaviness and body aches, no particular thirst, moist tongue coating, and a floating, tight pulse. In severe cases, there may be floating edema or considerable difficulty in breathing when lying down.

From an organ systems perspective, chronic water metabolism problems and thin mucus are associated with a disposition toward weakness of the Lungs, Spleen, or Kidneys. When such persons contract external wind-cold, these problems are further exacerbated by closure of the interstices and pores at the surface. Wind-cold fettering the exterior hinders the protective (yang) qi and constrains the nutritive (yin) qi, resulting in fever and chills without sweating. The Lungs control the qi and the exterior and facilitate flow in the water pathways. When Lung qi is constrained by wind-cold, the qi mechanism is further impeded. Thin mucus readily attacks the Lungs from the epigastric area, where it accumulates due to a failure of the Spleen's transportive and transformative functions. This process leads to coughing and wheezing (with copious, white, stringy sputum that is difficult to expectorate), a stifling sensation in the chest, and, in very severe cases, difficulty in breathing while lying down. Fluids entering the superficial levels of the body can cause floating edema, a generalized sensation of heaviness, and body aches. Thin mucus accumulating in the Stomach prevents its qi from directing downward, leading to dry retching. The absence of thirst and the moist tongue coating indicate a surfeit of fluids. The floating nature of the pulse indicates an exterior condition, while tightness reflects the presence of cold.

Analysis of Formula

The efficacy of this formula is attributed to its ability to simultaneously release wind-cold from the exterior and transform thin mucus in the interior. If the exterior is not resolved, the fluids cannot be moved. If thin mucus constrains the interior, protective yang cannot penetrate to the exterior. Only a strategy that focuses on both dispersing the protective yang and transforming the yin excess can overcome this vicious circle.

One of the chief herbs, Ephedrae Herba *(má huáng)*, releases the exterior, arrests wheezing, and promotes urination. The other chief ingredient, Cinnamomi Ramulus *(guì zhī)*, also combines three interrelated functions. It releases the exterior, opens the blood vessels, and promotes qi transformation. Together, the two herbs disperse wind-cold from the exterior, promote water metabolism to remove thin mucus, disseminate Lung qi, and open the vessels to treat wheezing and body aches. The deputies, Zingiberis Rhizoma *(gān jiāng)* and Asari Radix et Rhizoma *(xì xīn)*, warm the interior, transform thin mucus, and help the chief herbs release the exterior. Zingiberis Rhizoma *(gān jiāng)* is particularly effective in warming the Spleen, the deficiency of which is the primary cause of the thin mucus. Asari Radix et Rhizoma *(xì xīn)* also stops the coughing by facilitating the flow of qi throughout the body.

Employing only warm, acrid herbs whose function is to scatter and dry might easily injure the qi and fluids and adversely affect Lung function. For this reason, the assistant herbs Schisandrae Fructus *(wǔ wèi zǐ)*, which prevents the leakage of Lung qi, and Paeoniae Radix alba *(bái sháo)*, which nourishes the blood and nutritive qi, are added.

Pinelliae Rhizoma praeparatum *(zhì bàn xià)*, another assistant, transforms thin mucus and harmonizes the Stomach. The envoy, Glycyrrhizae Radix praeparata *(zhì gān cǎo)*, augments the qi and harmonizes the interaction of the acrid and sour herbs.

Commentary

This formula is basically a combination of two formulas that release the exterior, Ephedra Decoction *(má huáng tāng)* and Cinnamon Twig Decoction *(guì zhī tāng)*, together with Poria, Licorice, Schisandra, Ginger, and Asarum Decoction *(líng gān wǔ wèi jiāng xīn tāng)* (see Chapter 16). It acts to warm the interior and transform thin mucus, and is most often used for acute attacks of wind-cold in cases with chronic thin mucus.

Water Metabolism

However, *Essentials from the Golden Cabinet* explicitly uses this formula for problems of water metabolism that are not associated with exterior disorders. These include seeping thin mucus (溢飲 *yì yǐn*), coughing with rebellious qi that makes it impossible for the patient to lie down, and vomiting of frothy saliva during pregnancy. The efficacy of the formula in these cases is due to its ability to remove constraints to qi circulation that impede the transformation and elimination of fluids. Sometimes the image of a teapot is used to illustrate this function. In order for tea to pour from its spout, a teapot needs a second hole in the lid that allows air in as liquid flows out. Minor Bluegreen Dragon Decoction opens both holes (the pores in the skin and the urinary passageways) when they have become blocked due to either external wind-cold or insufficient penetration of yang qi from the gate of vitality to the body's surface.

This formula is thus an early example of the importance attached to regulating the qi mechanism in treating disorders of water metabolism. Here, this is partly achieved by regulating the ascending and descending aspects of the qi dynamic, primarily through the synergism between Cinnamomi Ramulus *(guì zhī)* and Pinelliae Rhizoma *(bàn xià)*. The latter herb, focused on the Stomach, eliminates water and dampness, both by drying and dispersing and through its ability to direct qi downward. The former herb, on the other hand, facilitates the ascending of qi and transformation of fluids via the Liver, as discussed by Tang Zong-Hai in *Discussion of Blood Patterns*:

> Cinnamomi Ramulus *(guì zhī)* is a Liver herb that transforms water. The Liver is the child of the Kidneys. When in a state of excess, the child drains the mother. Furthermore, the Liver also governs dredging and draining and thus has the ability to transform water. [The herb] also tonifies the Heart. In case of deficiency, one tonifies the mother. The Liver is the mother of Heart fire. Furthermore, Cinnamomi Ramulus *(guì zhī)* is red and enters the Heart [directly]. To promote sweating, one can therefore also use Cinnamomi Ramulus *(guì zhī)*. [In this case], one borrows the warmth of wood qi in order to disperse and facilitate dissemination toward the exterior.

Just as important is the formula's focus on ensuring unhindered entering and exiting. This is why acrid, warm herbs that promote exiting are combined with sour, astringent herbs that facilitate holding and entering. Paeoniae Radix alba (*bái sháo*) and Schisandrae Fructus (*wǔ wèi zǐ*) thereby contribute actively to the effect of the formula, rather than merely counteracting the potential side effects of the main herbs.

Key Indicators

In summary, this is one formula that should be considered for any condition characterized by an excess of water that cannot be transformed by the body's yang qi and that, in turn, constrains the qi dynamic. In clinical practice, this will most often involve conditions characterized by coughing and wheezing, although it may extend to other symptoms of water excess such as nausea, diarrhea, or edema. However, given the harsh nature of the formula, it is important to be certain that its use is, in fact, indicated in a particular case. Paying attention to the following four indicators will greatly assist in making the correct diagnosis.

1. **Complexion:** Cold, thin mucus obstructing the dispersion of yang to the exterior is often reflected in some degree of puffiness, especially around the eyes, but also the occurrence of dark spots, indicating constraint due to cold, at the temples, under the eyes, on the cheeks, or at the neck.

2. **Pulse:** Textbooks describe the typical pulse accompanying this pattern as wiry (indicating constraint due to thin mucus), or floating and tight (indicating cold fettering the exterior). In practice, however, the pulse can also be deep and slow, or frail, at the distal or proximal positions, indicating that the yang qi cannot penetrate to the exterior because it is constrained by yin fluids.

3. **Tongue:** The typical tongue in this pattern will be wet with a slippery white coating. The tongue body itself will not be abnormal, unlike patterns marked by dampness due to Kidney or Spleen deficiency.

4. **Secretions:** Visible mucus in this pattern will be thin, watery, and bubbly. Sputum expectorated from the Lungs will resemble egg white in consistency and be clear and transparent.

Furthermore, once the acute symptoms have abated, it is advisable to switch to a milder formula, like those built around the combination of Cinnamomi Ramulus (*guì zhī*) and Poria (*fú líng*), in order to promote the transformation of qi and water.

Comparisons

➤ Vs. FIVE-INGREDIENT POWDER WITH PORIA (*wǔ líng sǎn*)

Both formulas treat accumulation of water excess in the interior with cold in the exterior. However, this formula focuses on the upper burner (chest and Lungs) and is used primarily for patterns characterized by wheezing. Secondary symptoms are an absence of sweating and no thirst. Five-Ingredient Powder with Poria (*wǔ líng sǎn*), on the other hand, focuses on the lower burner and the Bladder and is used primarily for patterns characterized by inhibited urination. Both thirst and sweating are important secondary symptoms.

➤ Vs. EPHEDRA, APRICOT KERNEL, GYPSUM, AND LICORICE DECOCTION (*má xìng shí gān tāng*); see PAGE 184

➤ Vs. DREDGING AND CUTTING DRINK (*shū záo yǐn zi*); see PAGE 96

➤ Vs. PERILLA FRUIT DECOCTION FOR DIRECTING QI DOWNWARD (*sū zǐ jiàng qì tāng*); see PAGE 540

➤ Vs. ARREST WHEEZING DECOCTION (*dìng chuǎn tāng*); see PAGE 541

➤ Vs. PORIA, LICORICE, SCHISANDRA, GINGER, AND ASARUM DECOCTION (*líng gān wǔ wèi jiāng xīn tāng*); see PAGE 807

Biomedical Indications

With the appropriate presentation, this formula may be used to treat a wide variety of biomedically-defined disorders. These can be divided into the following groups:

- Disorders marked by coughing and/or wheezing, including upper respiratory tract infections, acute and chronic bronchitis, bronchial asthma, emphysema, and cardiopulmonary disease
- Disorders marked by discharges from the nose and/or eyes, including hay fever, allergic rhinitis, viral conjunctivitis, and dacryosolenitis
- Disorders marked by hiccups or retching, including enteritis, peptic ulcer, atrophic gastritis, cirrhosis, and chronic bacillary dysentery
- Miscellaneous diseases such as nephritis, rheumatic heart disease, pleuritis, epilepsy, enuresis, and periarthritis of the shoulder.

Cautions and Contraindications

This formula should not be used long term, nor for conditions with heat, coughing of blood, or coughing due to yin deficiency. Use with caution in cases with hypertension. In such cases, prepared Ephedrae Herba (*zhì má huáng*) is often substituted for Ephedrae Herba (*má huáng*).

Modifications

- For severe exterior cold disorders, increase the dosage of Ephedrae Herba (*má huáng*) and Cinnamomi Ramulus (*guì zhī*).

- For marked congestion, copious sputum, breathing difficulty while lying down, a slippery and wet tongue coating, and a wiry and tight or wiry and slippery pulse, increase the dosage of Asari Radix et Rhizoma (*xì xīn*) and Pinelliae Rhizoma praeparatum (*zhì bàn xià*) and add Zingiberis Rhizoma recens (*shēng jiāng*).

- For pronounced nasal congestion, runny nose, and headache, substitute Zingiberis Rhizoma recens (*shēng jiāng*) for Zingiberis Rhizoma (*gān jiāng*), substitute Paeoniae Radix rubra (*chì sháo*) for Paeoniae Radix alba (*bái sháo*), and add Saposhnikoviae Radix (*fáng fēng*) and Schizonepetae Herba (*jīng jiè*).

Variation

小青龍加石膏湯 （小青龙加石膏汤）

Minor Bluegreen Dragon Decoction plus Gypsum

xiǎo qīng lóng jiā shí gāo tāng

SOURCE   *Essentials from the Golden Cabinet* (c. 220)

Add Gypsum fibrosum (*shí gāo*) for coughing, chest and abdominal distention, wheezing, and irritability.

Associated Formula

射干麻黃湯 （射干麻黄汤）

Belamcanda and Ephedra Decoction

shè gān má huáng tāng

SOURCE   *Essentials from the Golden Cabinet* (c. 220)

Belamcandae Rhizoma (*shè gān*) 9g
Ephedrae Herba (*má huáng*) 12g
Asteris Radix (*zǐ wǎn*) 9g
Farfarae Flos (*kuǎn dōng huā*) 9g
Pinelliae Rhizoma praeparatum (*zhì bàn xià*). 9g
Asari Radix et Rhizoma (*xì xīn*) 9g
Schisandrae Fructus (*wǔ wèi zǐ*) 3g
Zingiberis Rhizoma recens (*shēng jiāng*) 12g
Jujubae Fructus (*dà zǎo*) . . . . .3 pieces

Warms the Lungs, transforms cold and thin mucus lingering in the chest, redirects rebellious qi downward, and stops coughing. For pronounced coughing and wheezing with a rattling sound. In contrast to the principal formula, its focus is on treating a more severe cough with mild or no exterior symptoms.

麻黃等十味丸

Ephedra Pill with Ten Ingredients

má huáng děng shí weì wán

SOURCE   *Arcane Essentials from the Imperial Library* (752)

Ephedrae Herba (*má huáng*). 60g
Cynanchi stauntonii Rhizoma (*bái qián*) 60g
Mori Cortex (*sāng bái pí*) 120g
Belamcandae Rhizoma (*shè gān*) 120g
Cynanchi atrati Radix (*bái wēi*) 90g
Stemonae Radix (*bǎi bù*) 150g

Rehmanniae Radix (*shēng dì huáng*) 180g
Lycii Cortex (*dì gǔ pí*) 180g
Citri reticulatae Pericarpium (*chén pí*) 90g

The source text advises to take 10-15 very small pills with a decoction made from Mori Cortex (*sāng bái pí*), which, when added to the number of herbs in the pills, makes it ten ingredients altogether. This is a further development of Belamcanda and Ephedra Decoction (*shè gān má huáng tāng*) and indicated for the treatment of cough in patients with an accumulation of phlegm-heat in the interior who suffer an invasion of wind-cold. Even though the fettering of the exterior may be relatively mild, it readily disrupts the qi dynamic of the Lungs, leading to cough that does not respond to treatment with more common formulas. In this formula, Ephedrae Herba (*má huáng*), with its acrid taste, opens up the Lungs and disperses wind-cold. Belamcandae Rhizoma (*shè gān*) and Cynanchi stauntonii Rhizoma (*bái qián*) are acrid but slightly cooling and are especially useful for directing qi downward and transforming phlegm. Lycii Cortex (*dì gǔ pí*) is sweet, bland, and cold, and clears lurking heat from the Lungs. Stemonae Radix (*bǎi bù*), sweet, bitter, and slightly warming, moistens the Lungs and stops coughing. Rehmanniae Radix (*shēng dì huáng*) and Cynanchi atrati Radix (*bái wēi*) are sweet, bitter, and cold. Together, they enrich the yin and drain internal heat. The overall effect of the formula is to remove the heat and constraint that are the root causes of this pathology. The formula is taken as a pill because the condition has most likely existed for some time and can therefore only be resolved slowly.

九味羌活湯 （九味羌活汤）

Nine-Herb Decoction with Notopterygium

jiǔ wèi qiāng huó tāng

Source   *Hard-Won Knowledge* (1308)

Notopterygii Rhizoma seu Radix (*qiāng huó*). 4.5g
Saposhnikoviae Radix (*fáng fēng*) 4.5g
Atractylodis Rhizoma (*cāng zhú*). 4.5g
Asari Radix et Rhizoma (*xì xīn*). 1.5g
Chuanxiong Rhizoma (*chuān xiōng*). 3g
Angelicae dahuricae Radix (*bái zhǐ*). 3g
Scutellariae Radix (*huáng qín*) 3g
Rehmanniae Radix (*shēng dì huáng*) 3g
Glycyrrhizae Radix (*gān cǎo*) 3g

Method of Preparation   Decoction. The source text advises to coarsely grind the herbs.

Actions   Induces sweating and dispels dampness while simultaneously draining interior heat

Indications

Fever and chills (chills predominant) without sweating, headache, stiff neck, generalized aches and pain, slight thirst, a bitter taste in the mouth, a white tongue coating, and a floating pulse.

This is externally-contracted wind-cold-dampness with concurrent internal accumulation of heat characterized by fever and chills (chills predominant), an absence of sweating, headache, and a stiff neck. The predominance of chills and the generalized aches and pains are the primary markers of externally-contracted cold-dampness. Heat accumulating internally produces slight thirst and a bitter taste in the mouth. The white tongue coating and floating pulse indicate that the pathogenic influences remain in the exterior.

Analysis of Formula

This formula uses a strategy of simultaneously resolving the exterior and dispelling dampness. It is characterized by a combination of ascending and dispersing herbs with heat-clearing herbs intended to facilitate the unobstructed movement of the qi dynamic and by the use of herbs that enter all of the channels of the head and neck. The choice of herbs can be altered in the clinic to match the precise location of the symptoms in each case.

The chief herb, aromatic Notopterygii Rhizoma seu Radix *(qiāng huó)*, is the principal substance in the materia medica for dispersing exterior wind-cold-dampness. Two of the deputies, Saposhnikoviae Radix *(fáng fēng)* and Atractylodis Rhizoma *(cāng zhú)*, assist the chief herb in releasing the exterior and eliminating dampness. The other deputies, Asari Radix et Rhizoma *(xì xīn)*, Chuanxiong Rhizoma *(chuān xiōng)*, and Angelicae dahuricae Radix *(bái zhǐ)*, assist the chief herb in releasing the exterior and treating the head and body aches. The assistants, Scutellariae Radix *(huáng qín)* and Rehmanniae Radix *(shēng dì huáng)*, clear qi- and blood-level interior heat, respectively, treating the thirst and bitter taste in the mouth and also preventing the dry nature of the other herbs from injuring the fluids. The envoy, Glycyrrhizae Radix *(gān cǎo)*, harmonizes the middle burner and the actions of the other herbs.

Commentary

History

Although this formula was not recorded until the Yuan dynasty, many commentators attribute its composition to the Song dynasty physician Zhang Yuan-Su, the founder of the Yishui (易水 *Yì shuǐ*) current in Chinese medicine, named after his native district in what is now Hebei province. He was the teacher of Li Dong-Yuan and Wang Hao-Gu. All of these physicians belonged to a movement that rejected many of the pre-Song assumptions in medicine. This formula is typical of their style of prescribing, which encompassed three important innovations: first, a focus on the ascending and descending movement of the qi dynamic; second, a concern with the action of herbs on particular channels; and third, a moving away from the use of fixed formulas for given conditions toward the idea of formulas as constituting models that could be flexibly adapted to the actual presenting signs and symptoms in clinical practice.

Herb Combinations

Prior to the Song, seasonal feverish diseases were generally understood as cold damage disorders that, in the first instance, were to be treated by either Ephedra Decoction *(má huáng tāng)* or Cinnamon Twig Decoction *(guì zhī tāng)*. Both of these formulas focus on the greater yang. The present formula accepts that wind-cold-dampness can invade any channel. Although its chief herb, Notopterygii Rhizoma seu Radix *(qiāng huó)*, still focuses on the greater yang channel, the remaining herbs all focus on other channels. Angelicae dahuricae Radix *(bái zhǐ)* enters into the yang brightness channel and treats frontal headaches; Atractylodis Rhizoma *(cāng zhú)* dispels dampness from the foot greater yin, allowing the clear qi to ascend and the turbid to descend; Chuanxiong Rhizoma *(chuān xiōng)* enters into the foot terminal yin channel and treats headaches at the crown of the head; Asari Radix et Rhizoma *(xì xīn)* enters into the foot lesser yin channel and opens the collaterals, while Saposhnikoviae Radix *(fáng fēng)* is considered to be a generalized wind herb that can enter into any channel to treat pain in the entire body; Scutellariae Radix *(huáng qín)* enters the hand greater yin to drain heat accumulation from the chest; and Rehmanniae Radix *(shēng dì huáng)*, depending on which text one follows, clears heat from the blood aspect of either the hand or foot greater yin. In this way, the formula extends its indications to all types of headache, as well as to painful obstruction patterns in any of these channels.

In practice, the precise composition of the formula must be adjusted according to the location of the problem and the predominance of one pathogen over others. In Chinese medicine, this type of prescribing is referred to as 'discussing treatment on the basis of channel distribution' (分經論治 *fēn jīng lùn zhì*). As the source text notes: "One should examine the difference in the channels in the front and the back, on the left and right. Depending on differences in occurrence, intensity, and severity [of symptoms], one increases or decreases [the amount of individual herbs. If one sticks to] this, one achieves miraculous results."

A precedent for the use of acrid, warm medicinals that induce sweating to resolve the exterior with cold herbs to treat internal heat accumulation already existed in Zhang Zhong-Jing's Major Bluegreen Dragon Decoction *(dà qīng lóng tāng)*. The disease mechanism, treatment strategy, and herbs used differ, however, in each case. Major Bluegreen Dragon Decoction *(dà qīng lóng tāng)* treats heat from constraint caused by cold fettering the exterior, which manifests as irritability and restlessness. In order to open this constraint, it relies on the cold and acrid herb Gypsum fibrosum *(shí gāo)*. In the reasoning underlying Zhang Yuan-Su's formula, it is assumed that dampness predominates, generating damp-heat in the interior, particularly in persons with preexisting dampness.

For this reason, Zhang uses the bitter, cold herb Scutellariae Radix (huáng qín), which dries dampness and drains heat. The very acrid nature of the formula—necessary in order to promote sweating, dry dampness, and open the channels—readily injures the fluids, making the inclusion of a cold, moistening herb like Rehmanniae Radix (shēng dì huáng) advisable.

Influential commentators like Xu Da-Chun, Wang Xu-Gao, and Fei Bo-Xiong argue, however, that the use of such a thick and cloying herb is only necessary if the heat is severe and the dryness is pronounced. In all other cases, they suggest the use of either Angelicae sinensis Radix (dāng guī) or Radix Paeoniae (sháo yào). When treating patients with a disposition toward damp-phlegm retention, modern practitioners go one step further and remove Rehmanniae Radix (shēng dì huáng), substituting herbs that move the qi and transform dampness, such as Magnoliae officinalis Cortex (hòu pò) and Citri reticulatae Pericarpium (chén pí).

The combination of acrid, warm herbs thought to have an ascending nature with bitter, cold herbs that direct qi downward must also be viewed against the increased importance that the Jin-Yuan innovators attached to the qi dynamic. These physicians reasoned that herbs like Notopterygii Rhizoma seu Radix (qiāng huó), Saposhnikoviae Radix (fáng fēng), or Atractylodis Rhizoma (cāng zhú) raise the clear qi, a dynamic that not only corresponds to that of the Spleen, but also to that of the lesser yang, and, by implication, to spring. This ascending movement dries dampness in the same manner that the warm spring winds dry the earth. It is for this reason that these herbs are also known as 'wind herbs' (風藥 fēng yào).

Comparisons

➤ Vs. Other Formulas that Treat Exterior Conditions

Although Nine-Herb Decoction with Notopterygium (jiǔ wèi qiāng huó tāng) was specifically composed to treat exterior disorders irrespective of the season, great care should be taken to distinguish its indications from those of Ephedra Decoction (má huáng tāng) and Cinnamon Twig Decoction (guì zhī tāng), which do not treat dampness. In fact, it is the close association between dampness and the middle burner as the fulcrum of the qi dynamic that makes the focus on ascending and directing downward so important in understanding this formula. Its use should also be distinguished from formulas like Three-Seed Decoction (sān rén tāng), discussed in Chapter 16. Whereas these formulas treat the simultaneous invasion of dampness and heat from the outside, Nine-Herb Decoction with Notopterygium (jiǔ wèi qiāng huó tāng) drains heat that accumulates in the interior because cold-dampness inhibits the qi dynamic.

➤ Vs. Notopterygium Decoction to Overcome Dampness (qiāng huó shèng shī tāng); see page 756

Biomedical Indications

With the appropriate presentation, this formula may be used to treat a wide variety of biomedically-defined disorders including the common cold, migraine, urticaria, sinusitis, facial nerve palsy, torticollis, fibromyalgia, torticollis, tenosynovitis, lumbar strain, erysipelas, acute myocarditis, and rheumatoid arthritis.

Alternate names

Major Notopterygium Decoction (dà qiāng huó tāng) in Secret Empirical Formulas; Notopterygium Flush and Harmonize Decoction (qiāng huó chōng hé tāng) in Complete Compendium of Cold Damage; Flush and Harmonize Decoction (chōng hé tāng) in Systematic Great Compendium of Medicine Past and Present; Miraculous Release Powder (shén jiě sǎn) in Achieving Longevity by Guarding the Source; Notopterygium Powder (qiāng huó sǎn) in Complete Treatise on Respecting Life from the Lofty Precipice

Cautions and Contraindications

Due to its acrid and drying nature, this formula is contraindicated in warm pathogen diseases (including damp-warmth disorders). It should be used with great care in patients who tend toward yin deficiency.

Modifications

- For upper back and shoulder pain, add Gentianae macrophyllae Radix (qín jiāo).
- Where there is an absence of thirst or bitter taste in the mouth, remove Scutellariae Radix (huáng qín) and Rehmanniae Radix (shēng dì huáng).
- For pronounced thirst and irritability, add Gypsum fibrosum (shí gāo) and Anemarrhenae Rhizoma (zhī mǔ).
- For a dry or sore throat, add Platycodi Radix (jié gěng), Arctii Fructus (niú bàng zǐ), and Menthae haplocalycis Herba (bò hé).
- For epigastric discomfort and distention with a greasy tongue coating, remove Rehmanniae Radix (shēng dì huáng) and add Pogostemonis/Agastaches Herba (huò xiāng) and Pinelliae Rhizoma praeparatum (zhì bàn xià).
- For coughing up of thick sputum, add Armeniacae Semen (xìng rén) and Peucedani Radix (qián hú).

Variations

沖和湯 (冲和汤)

Penetrating and Harmonizing Decoction
chōng hé tāng

Source   Versified Prescriptions (1694)

Add 3 slices of Zingiberis Rhizoma recens (shēng jiāng) and 3 stalks of Allii fistulosi Bulbus (cōng bái) to strengthen the formula's power of unblocking the yang and releasing the exterior.

Associated Formulas

大羌活湯 (大羌活汤)

Major Notopterygium Decoction

dà qiāng huó tāng

SOURCE *Hard-Won Knowledge* (1308)

Notopterygii Rhizoma seu Radix (*qiāng huó*) 9g
Angelicae pubescentis Radix (*dú huó*) 9g
Saposhnikoviae Radix (*fáng fēng*) 9g
Asari Radix et Rhizoma (*xì xīn*) 9g
fáng jǐ (Stephaniae/Cocculi/etc. Radix) 9g
Scutellariae Radix (*huáng qín*) 9g
Coptidis Rhizoma (*huáng lián*) 9g
Atractylodis Rhizoma (*cāng zhú*) 9g
Glycyrrhizae Radix praeparata (*zhì gān cǎo*) 9g
Atractylodis macrocephalae Rhizoma (*bái zhú*) 9g
Anemarrhenae Rhizoma (*zhī mǔ*) 30g
Chuanxiong Rhizoma (*chuān xiōng*) 30g
Rehmanniae Radix (*shēng dì huáng*) .30g

Coarsely grind the ingredients, prepare as a decoction, and take in 15g doses. Scatters wind-cold, expels dampness, and clears heat. For exterior wind-cold-dampness with interior heat characterized by fever and chills (fever predominant), headache, dry mouth, thirst, and irritability. In contrast to the principal formula, the focus here is on clearing more severe interior heat and expelling dampness.

加味香蘇散 (加味香苏散)

Augmented Cyperus and Perilla Leaf Powder

jiā wèi xiāng sū sǎn

Source *Awakening of the Mind in Medical Studies* (1732)

Perillae Folium (*zǐ sū yè*) 4.5g
Cyperi Rhizoma (*xiāng fù*) 3.6g
Citri reticulatae Pericarpium (*chén pí*) 3.6g
Glycyrrhizae Radix praeparata (*zhì gān cǎo*) 2.1g
Schizonepetae Herba (*jīng jiè*) 3g
Saposhnikoviae Radix (*fáng fēng*) 3g
Gentianae macrophyllae Radix (*qín jiāo*) 3g
Viticis Fructus (*màn jīng zǐ*) 3g
Chuanxiong Rhizoma (*chuān xiōng*) .1.5g
Zingiberis Rhizoma recens
  (*shēng jiāng*) . . . . 3 slices added to each prescription

Method of Preparation Decoction. The source text advises that the decoction should be taken warm and that its consistency should be thin, resembling sweat. This implies that the herbs should not be cooked very long.

Actions Promotes sweating and releases the exterior

Indications

For the common cold year-round, headache and stiffness of the neck, nasal obstruction or runny nose, aches and pains in the body or extremities, fever with chills or aversion to wind but without sweating, a thin, white tongue coating, and a floating pulse.

This is wind-cold in the exterior, where the battle between the pathogenic and the normal qi produces relatively mild symptoms. This may be because the pathogen itself is not strong and has only penetrated relatively superficially, or because the person's constitution is not strong enough to engage in such a battle. The formula is therefore particularly suitable for patients with a weak constitution, children, and the elderly.

Analysis of Formula

This formula is a variation of Cyperus and Perilla Leaf Powder (*xiāng sū sǎn*), discussed below. Its strategy is to disperse wind-cold from the exterior, while simultaneously facilitating the proper movement of qi in the interior. Resolving the exterior allows the qi in the interior to flow more freely. Opening qi constraint in the interior facilitates its movement to the surface, where it helps disperse pathogenic influences.

The chief ingredients are the warm, acrid, and light herbs Perillae Folium (*zǐ sū yè*) and Schizonepetae Herba (*jīng jiè*), which facilitate the movement of qi in the exterior, open up the skin and interstices, and dispel wind-cold. The deputies are three herbs that focus on releasing pathogens from the muscles, channels, and collaterals: Saposhnikoviae Radix (*fáng fēng*) and Gentianae macrophyllae Radix (*qín jiāo*) dispel wind-cold and alleviate pain, while Viticis Fructus (*màn jīng zǐ*) is particularly indicated for headaches. Three assistants regulate the qi and blood in the interior, promoting the qi dynamic to enable the normal qi to ascend and spread throughout the exterior. Cyperi Rhizoma (*xiāng fù*) releases constraint and disperses stagnation from all twelve channels. Together with Chuanxiong Rhizoma (*chuān xiōng*), an essential herb in the treatment of headaches, it focuses particularly on the Liver, which governs ascension and dispersal. If qi and blood can move unobstructed in the interior, external pathogens are more easily dispersed from the exterior. Citri reticulatae Pericarpium (*chén pí*) regulates the qi, directs downward, and drys dampness. Together with the acrid and dispersing Zingiberis Rhizoma recens (*shēng jiāng*), it focuses on the Lungs, facilitating its control of the pores and interstices. The envoy, Glycyrrhizae Radix praeparata (*zhì gān cǎo*), harmonizes the actions of the other herbs, strengthens the Stomach, and prevents the qi-regulating herbs from depleting the qi.

Commentary

The composition of this formula reflects widespread concerns among physicians and patients in late imperial China regarding the potential side effects associated with improper use of strong diaphoretic formulas like Ephedra Decoction (*má huáng tāng*) and Cinnamon Twig Decoction (*guì zhī tāng*). These fears arose against the background of cultural beliefs that attributed a weaker constitution to southern Chinese, due primarily to climatic factors. The cold climate in the north forced people to develop strong qi in the exterior in order to regulate the opening and closing of the pores and interstices. In the humid climate of the south, by contrast, the pores and interstices tended to be open, causing the qi in the exterior to become weak, while the qi dynamic itself was constrained by dampness. In the south, an aesthetic of prescribing developed that favored the use of mild and harmonizing herbs and formulas. The intention was to regulate the qi dynamic and rely on the body's own defenses rather than expel pathogens forcefully. Augmented Cyperus and Perilla Leaf Powder (*jiā wèi xiāng sū sǎn*) is a prime example of this style of medicine.

Historical Background

Another theory based on perceived climatic differences held that pathogenic qi in the north and south were substantially different. Rather than leading to proper cold damage disorders, the milder climate of the south was thought to cause more superficial invasions known as the 'common cold' (感冒 *gǎn mào*). Wind rather than cold was presumed to be the main pathogen with manifestations that were more varied and more difficult to affix to any specific one of the six warps. Wu Kun, a Ming-dynasty physician from Anhui, cogently summed up this line of thought: "[The pathogenic qi] contracted by a person enters through the nose. It is really located in the upper portion [of the body] and not in any one of the six warps. Therefore, it causes headache and fever, and not much else." For this reason, it was necessary to find formulas that specifically treated this kind of common cold. Wu Kun suggested Cyperus and Perilla Leaf Powder (*xiāng sū sǎn*), a formula used for wind-cold in the exterior accompanied by qi stagnation in the interior. Cheng Guo-Peng, another physician from Anhui, who is more famous for systematizing treatment strategies into eight methods (八法 *bā fǎ*), followed Wu Kun's lead but developed a more specific alternative.

In his own commentary to this formula, Cheng Guo-Peng states that the use of classical cold damage formulas not only readily leads to potentially dangerous side effects, but also that many physicians find it difficult to differentiate accurately between the various exterior patterns. He therefore offers one single formula to replace their usage: "Its herbs are safe yet effective, and it also embodies superb methods [of treatment from previous generations] of physicians."

Usage

To the foundation of Cyperus and Perilla Powder (*xiāng sū sǎn*) discussed below, Cheng Guo-Peng added a number of herbs aimed specifically at the dispersion of wind from the exterior and the head. This directs the forces of the qi dynamic toward this area, allowing it to dispel wind and relieve headaches without forcefully promoting sweating. The formula is thus ideally suited for the treatment of common colds in Western medical practice as well and can be used as a standard formula for this purpose. Physicians, however, should follow Cheng's advice and make appropriate adjustments based on the local climate and culture, on individual constitution, and the precise location of the pathogen. His personal suggestions are listed under MODIFICATIONS below.

Even though the formula achieves some of its power by opening the qi dynamic and thereby releasing the body's own potential for expelling pathogenic qi, its focus is nevertheless entirely on releasing the exterior. Thus, Chen Guo-Peng himself advises against its use in patients who are constitutionally very deficient. To treat these patients, one should select from the formulas that tonify interior deficiency and release the exterior, discussed in section 4 of this chapter. In such cases, the pulse will be deficient in spite of very clear signs indicating external invasion.

Comparison

➤ Vs. TEN DIVINE DECOCTION (*shí shén tāng*); *see* PAGE 32

Biomedical Indications

With the appropriate presentation, this formula may be used to treat biomedically-defined disorders such as the common cold, influenza, upper respiratory tract infections, acute gastroenteritis, and globus pharyngeus.

Modifications

- For severe headaches, add 2.4g of Notopterygii Rhizoma seu Radix (*qiāng huó*) and 2 stalks of Allii fistulosi Bulbus (*cōng bái*). (source text)

- For spontaneous sweating and aversion to wind, add 3g each of Cinnamomi Ramulus (*guì zhī*) and Paeoniae Radix alba (*bái sháo*). If these symptoms occur toward the end of spring or beginning of summer, one should be cautious about the simultaneous invasion of warm-summerheat pathogens. It is not advisable to use Cinnamomi Ramulus (*guì zhī*), which should be replaced by 4.5g of Atractylodis macrocephalae Rhizoma (*bái zhú*). (source text)

- For food stagnation, focal distention, and fullness in the chest or diaphragm, add 4.5g of Crataegi Fructus (*shān zhā*), Hordei Fructus germinatus (*mài yá*), and Raphani Semen (*lái fú zǐ*). (source text)

- For greater yang channel pathology that has not been resolved but is accompanied by thirst and rough urination indicating a Bladder organ pattern, add 4.5g of Poria (*fú líng*) and Akebiae Caulis (*mù tōng*). (source text)
- For wheezing and coughing, add 4.5g each of Platycodi Radix (*jié gěng*) and Peucedani Radix (*qián hú*), and 7 pieces (1g) of Armeniacae Semen (*xìng rén*). (source text)
- For nosebleeds or spitting of blood, remove Zingiberis Rhizoma recens (*shēng jiāng*) and add 4.5g each of Rehmanniae Radix (*shēng dì huáng*), Paeoniae Radix rubra (*chì sháo*), Salviae miltiorrhizae Radix (*dān shēn*), and Moutan Cortex (*mǔ dān pí*). (source text)
- For swelling and pain in the throat, add 4.5g each of Platycodi Radix (*jié gěng*) and Arctii Fructus (*niú bàng zǐ*) and 1.5g of Menthae haplocalycis Herba (*bò hé*). (source text)
- For constipation, add Raphani Semen (*lái fú zǐ*) and Aurantii Fructus (*zhǐ ké*). (source text)
- For inversion with frigid extremities and cold breath from the mouth and nose indicating simultaneous cold in the middle burner, add herbs like Zingiberis Rhizoma (*gān jiāng*) and Cinnamomi Cortex (*ròu guì*), and only use one or two of the herbs that release the exterior. (source text)
- For simultaneous invasion by summerheat pathogen, add herbs like Anemarrhenae Rhizoma (*zhī mǔ*) and Scutellariae Radix (*huáng qín*). (source text)
- For dry retching, fever, and coughing indicating that there is water qi in the exterior, add 4.5g of Pinelliae Rhizoma (*bàn xià*) and Poria (*fú líng*). (source text)
- For plum-pit qi with a sensation of something being stuck in the throat that can neither be spit out nor swallowed, add 2.4g of both Platycodi Radix (*jié gěng*) and Perillae Caulis (*sū gěng*). (source text)
- For occurrence of symptoms during menstruation, add Angelicae sinensis Radix (*dāng guī*) and Salviae miltiorrhizae Radix (*dān shēn*). (source text)
- For contraction of wind-cold after giving birth, add Zingiberis Rhizoma praeparatum (*páo jiāng*), Zingiberis Rhizoma (*gān jiāng*), and Angelicae sinensis Radix (*dāng guī*) and reduce the herbs that release the exterior by more than half. (source text)

Associated Formulas

香蘇散 （香苏散）

Cyperus And Perilla Leaf Powder

xiāng sū sǎn

SOURCE *Formulary of the Pharmacy Service for Benefiting the People in the Taiping Era* (1107)

Perillae Folium (*zǐ sū yè*). 120g (6-9g)
Cyperi Rhizoma (*xiāng fù*) 120g (6-9g)
Citri reticulatae Pericarpium (*chén pí*) 60g (3-6g)
Glycyrrhizae Radix praeparata (*zhì gān cǎo*) 30g (3-6g)

Method of Preparation Grind into powder and take as a draft in 3-6g doses three times a day. May also be prepared as a decoction with the dosage indicated in parentheses.

This is the original formula, which was later modified by Cheng Guo-Peng to construct the principal formula. In contrast to this later modification, the original formula focuses equally on regulating the qi and releasing the exterior. It is therefore indicated for treating exterior wind-cold that occurs in conjunction with qi constraint in the interior. This can occur when exterior wind-cold obstructs the spreading of Lung qi, which in turn obstructs the qi mechanism of the Spleen and Stomach. It can also occur when patients with preexisting constraint of the qi dynamic encounter a wind-cold pathogen but fail to engage with it forcefully because of the constraint. This produces such symptoms as lack of appetite, belching, and focal distention and a stifling sensation in the chest and epigastrium. The thin, white tongue coating and floating pulse reflect the presence of cold in the exterior.

香蘇蔥豉湯 （香苏葱豉汤）

Cyperus, Perilla Leaf, Scallion, and Prepared Soybean Decoction

xiāng sū cōng chǐ tāng

SOURCE *Revised Popular Guide to the Discussion of Cold Damage* (Qing dynasty)

Perillae Folium (*zǐ sū yè*) 4.5-9g
processed Cyperi Rhizoma (*zhì xiāng fù*) 4.5-6g
Citri reticulatae Pericarpium (*chén pí*) 4.5-6g
Glycyrrhizae Radix praeparata (*zhì gān cǎo*) 1.8-2.4g
Allii fistulosi Bulbus recens (*xiān cōng bái*) . . . . 2-3 pieces
Sojae Semen praeparatum (*dàn dòu chǐ*) 9-12g

Releases the exterior, regulates the qi, and calms the fetus. Used in pregnant women with exterior wind-cold. In contrast to the principal formula, here even lighter herbs are used for releasing the exterior. This is necessary because stimulating excessive sweating in pregnant women can readily damage their fluids and blood. The chief herb, Perillae Folium (*zǐ sū yè*), is able to calm the fetus, making this formula especially useful during pregnancy.

杏蘇飲 （杏苏饮）

Apricot Kernel and Perilla Drink

xìng sū yǐn

SOURCE *Golden Mirror of the Medical Tradition* (1742)

Perillae Folium (*zǐ sū yè*) 6-9g
bran-fried Aurantii Fructus (*fū chǎo zhǐ ké*) 4-6g
Platycodi Radix (*jié gěng*) 4-6g
Puerariae Radix (*gé gēn*) 4-6g
Peucedani Radix (*qián hú*) 6-9g
Citri reticulatae Pericarpium (*chén pí*) 4-6g
Glycyrrhizae Radix (*gān cǎo*) 2-4g
ginger-fried Pinelliae Rhizoma praeparatum (*jiāng bàn xià*) 6-9g
dry-fried Armeniacae Semen (*chǎo xìng rén*) 6-9g
Poria (*fú líng*) 6-9g
Zingiberis Rhizoma recens (*shēng jiāng*) . . . . 2-3 slices

Note: No dosages are listed in the source text; the amounts shown here reflect modern usage.

Disperses pathogens and releases them from the exterior. Directs qi downward and transforms phlegm. In the source text, this formula is said to treat the onset of pox disorders that present with wheezing due to "a wind-cold pathogen visiting the Lung." At present, this formula is applied to wind-cold exterior patterns that present with cough, nasal congestion, low-grade fever, headache, and wheezing. It is primarily used to treat the initial stage of this pattern and to specifically address chills as well as cough or wheezing; it can be thought of as a mild Ephedra Decoction (*má huáng tāng*) that is appropriate for weak patients or mild conditions. It is also often combined with some or all of the ingredients of Arrest Wheezing Decoction (*dìng chuǎn tāng*), discussed in Chapter 12, to treat cold asthmatic episodes that are brought on by a wind-cold attack. Biomedical disease categories to which this formula can be applied include bronchitis, asthma, and influenza where wheezing, cough, and chills are present.

Note that one of the major formulas to treat dryness, discussed in Chapter 15, has the similar name of Apricot Kernel and Perilla Leaf Powder (*xìng sū sǎn*). That formula first appeared in *Systematic Differentiation of Warm Pathogen Diseases* and was written approximately 50 years after this one, in 1798.

寧嗽丸 (宁嗽丸)

Calm Coughing Pill

níng sòu wán

<small>Source</small>　*Selected Chinese Patent Medicines* (1994)

Fritillariae thunbergii Bulbus (*zhè bèi mǔ*) 60 (6-9g)
Platycodi Radix (*jié gěng*) 60 (6-9g)
Dendrobii Herba (*shí hú*) 30g (6-9g)
Pinelliae Rhizoma praeparatum (*zhì bàn xià*) 60 (6-9g)
Perillae Fructus (*zǐ sū zǐ*) 60 (9g)
Poria (*fú líng*) 60 (9g)
Menthae haplocalycis Herba (*bò hé*) 60 (6g)
Armeniacae Semen (*xìng rén*) 60 (6-9g)
Mori Cortex (*sāng bái pí*) 60 (6-9g)
Citri reticulatae Exocarpium rubrum (*jú hóng*) 30 (6g)
Glycyrrhizae Radix (*gān cǎo*) 15g (3g)
Setariae (Oryzae) Fructus germinatus (*gǔ yá*) 60 (6-9g)

Directs Lung qi downward, disseminates Lung qi, eases coughs, transforms phlegm, and nourishes the Lung. For wind-cold exterior patterns that present with nasal congestion, runny nose, headache, fever, cough with thin sputum, or wheezing and thoracic fullness. It is also used for patients who complain of sneezing and aversion to drafts.

This formula can be seen as a variation of Apricot and Perilla Drink (*xìng sū yǐn*). Both formulas treat wind-cold patterns that present with cough or wheezing. Calm Coughing Pill (*níng sòu wán*) contains fewer herbs to release pathogens from the exterior and also contains Poria (*fú líng*) to supplement the Spleen. This makes it better suited for lingering coughs, while Apricot and Perilla Drink (*xìng sū yǐn*) is better for acute conditions. Both formulas use the perilla plant, but Calm Coughing Pill (*níng sòu wán*) uses the seed, Perillae Fructus (*zǐ sū zǐ*), and thus focuses on rebellious Lung qi rather than on the exterior wind-cold pathogen.

As a prepared medicine, the ground herbs are mixed with a de-

coction of Setariae (Oryzae) Fructus germinatus (*gǔ yá*) and made into a pill. The dosages above reflect the common amounts used at present for decoctions.

Note: This is a modification of a formula that was first published in *Revised Popular Guide to the Discussion of Cold-induced Disorders.* That formula included Coicis Semen (*yì yǐ rén*) and Adenophorae Radix (*nán shā shēn*) and used Fritillariae cirrhosae Bulbus (*chuān bèi mǔ*) instead of Fritillariae thunbergii Bulbus (*zhè bèi mǔ*).

This formula, when not used in pill form, is often modified as follows:

- For chronic cough, add Adenophorae Radix (*nán shā shēn*) and Coicis Semen (*yì yǐ rén*).
- For wind-cold patterns that are beginning to engender Lung heat, add Scutellariae Radix (*huáng qín*) and Anemarrhenae Rhizoma (*zhī mǔ*).
- For acute wind-cold with strong chills and lack of sweating, add Ephedrae Herba (*má huáng*) or combine with Canopy Powder (*huá gài sǎn*).
- For copious sputum, remove Dendrobii Herba (*shí hú*) and increase the dosage of Pinelliae Rhizoma praeparatum (*zhì bàn xià*) and Citri reticulatae Exocarpium rubrum (*jú hóng*).
- For chronic painful coughing, add Persicae Semen (*táo rén*).

十神湯 (十神汤)

Ten-Miracle Decoction

shí shén tāng

Source　*Formulary of the Pharmacy Service for Benefiting the People in the Taiping Era* (1107)

Ephedrae Herba (*má huáng*) 149g (6g)
Cimicifugae Rhizoma (*shēng má*) .149g (6-9g)
Paeoniae Radix rubra (*chì sháo*) 149g (6-9g)
Angelicae dahuricae Radix (*bái zhǐ*) 149g (6g)
Chuanxiong Rhizoma (*chuān xiōng*) 149g (6g)
Glycyrrhizae Radix praeparata (*zhì gān cǎo*) 149g (6g)
Citri reticulatae Pericarpium (*chén pí*) 149g (6-9g)
Perillae Folium (*zǐ sū yè*) 149g (6-9g)
Cyperi Rhizoma (*xiāng fù*) 149g (6-9g)
Puerariae Radix (*gé gēn*) 522g (12-18g)

Method of Preparation　Grind to a coarse powder and use 10g each time. Decoct with a large cup of water and 5 slices of Zingiberis Rhizoma recens (*shēng jiāng*) until 70% of the liquid remains. Remove the dregs and drink while hot.

Note: the dosages in parentheses are the common range for decoctions at present.

Actions　Releases pathogens from the exterior, regulates the qi, disseminates the Lung qi, and relieves cough

Indications

Epidemic disorders and wind-cold patterns that present with internal qi stagnation. Symptoms include headache, stifling oppression and focal distention in the chest, absence of sweating, fever, cough, nasal congestion, and a low voice. The tongue coating is thin and white. It is also sometimes applied to the treatment of wind-cold-damp painful obstruction.

Headache, fever, chills, and the absence of sweating are all due to exterior wind. Focal distention and a stifling oppression in the chest reflect qi stagnation and damp obstruction. The qi and fluids both rely on the free flow in the Triple Burner to properly ascend and descend. The ability of the protective qi to move in the Triple Burner is dependent on the Lung's ability to clarify and descend, the Liver's capacity to dredge and drain, and the Spleen-Stomach's functions of raising, ascending, and transporting. In patients who already suffer from a tendency toward qi stagnation, an externally-contracted pathogen immediately hinders the Lung's ability to disseminate, the Spleen's ability to transport, and the Liver's ability to dredge. The resulting stagnation of qi hinders the flow of fluids, and the obstruction of qi and fluids further adds to the stagnation. The result is a situation where one suffers simultaneously from externally-contracted wind-cold and internal qi stagnation. Stifling oppression in the chest and focal distention are signs of the stagnant obstruction of qi and fluids. The tongue coating being thin and white, rather than greasy, shows that the root cause is primarily qi stagnation and not dampness.

Analysis of Formula

This is another formula built on the basis of Cyperus and Perilla Leaf Powder (*xiāng sū sǎn*), which aims at simultaneously dispersing wind-cold from the exterior while opening stagnant qi in the interior. The chief ingredient, Perillae Folium (*zǐ sū yè*), is acrid and warm. It opens obstructed Lung qi, disseminates qi in the body's exterior, and warms and disperses the cold pathogen that fetters the exterior. By dispersing the cold pathogen and opening the interstices, Perillae Folium (*zǐ sū yè*) frees the Lung qi, fluids, and protective qi to discharge naturally to the body's exterior and thus relieves the symptoms of exterior patterns such as chills and fever and the absence of sweating. In addition, Perillae Folium (*zǐ sū yè*) arouses the Spleen and transforms dampness, thus helping to eliminate focal distention and the stifling oppression in the chest. One deputy, Citri reticulatae Pericarpium (*chén pí*), assists Perillae Folium (*zǐ sū yè*) in moving the qi and transforming dampness. Another deputy, Cyperi Rhizoma (*xiāng fù*), supported by Citri reticulatae Pericarpium (*chén pí*), regulates the qi and dredges the Liver, allowing it to return to its preferred state of orderly reaching. Perillae Folium (*zǐ sū yè*), Citri reticulatae Pericarpium (*chén pí*), and Cyperi Rhizoma (*xiāng fù*) as a group promote the free flow of qi through the three burners.

The last two deputies, Ephedrae Herba (*má huáng*) and Puerariae Radix (*gé gēn*), work with Perillae Folium (*zǐ sū yè*) to release pathogens from the body's exterior. One assistant, Cimicifugae Rhizoma (*shēng má*), works with Puerariae Radix (*gé gēn*) to ascend and disperse; they release the muscle layer. The deputies, Chuanxiong Rhizoma (*chuān xiōng*), which moves the qi within the blood, and Angelicae dahuricae Radix (*bái zhǐ*), work together with the ascending herbs, Puerariae Radix (*gé gēn*) and Cimicifugae Rhizoma (*shēng má*), to treat wind-cold headache and nasal congestion. The final deputy, Paeoniae Radix rubra (*chì sháo*), adjusts and connects yin and yang, allowing the heat from internal stasis to move to the exterior where it is released. This herb and Chuanxiong Rhizoma (*chuān xiōng*) also move the blood.

The remaining ingredients are envoys. Acrid and warm Zingiberis Rhizoma recens (*shēng jiāng*) helps Ephedrae Herba (*má huáng*) and Perillae Folium (*zǐ sū yè*) dispel the wind-cold pathogen from the exterior. Glycyrrhizae Radix praeparata (*zhì gān cǎo*) tonifies and harmonizes the middle and also harmonizes the various groups of ingredients. With the exception of this herb, every ingredient fills one or more of three roles: releasing wind-cold from the exterior; regulating the qi in the upper, middle, or lower burner; and relieving specific symptoms such as headache or nasal congestion.

Commentary

Formulary of the Pharmacy Service for Benefiting the People in the Taiping Era groups Ten-Miracle Decoction (*shí shén tāng*) with others that treat damage from cold. It is specifically listed to "treat unseasonable weather that brings on fast spreading epidemics which affect many people. [It treats these] without [the need of] inquiring into [whether] the affliction [belongs to] yin or yang. Also, it can treat wind-cold-damp painful obstruction." The text goes on to say that the formula is safe for the treatment of cold damage in pregnant women as well as the old and young, irrespective of whether the disorder is internal or external.

Since this formula has been on record since the Song dynasty, there has been ample time for practitioners to develop other uses for it and to refine the uses set forth in the source text. The most common use for the formula is in the treatment of wind-cold patterns that occur in the presence of internal qi stagnation. *Golden Mirror of the Medical Tradition* suggests this use when it notes that the formula can "discharge external cold and soothe internal qi constraint to treat a condition termed cold qi disease. [It] has the ability to warm the channels and enable the free flow of qi."

The Ming-dynasty text *Achieving Longevity by Guarding the Source*, and others, list Ten-Miracle Decoction (*shí shén tāng*) for epidemic pox disorders, to express papules. Puerariae Radix (*gé gēn*) and Cimicifugae Rhizoma (*shēng má*) are used for this purpose, as in Cimicifuga and Kudzu Decoction (*shēng má gé gēn tāng*). The formula is also mentioned in several texts for the treatment of febrile epidemic disorders, such as massive head febrile disorder.

The source text's advice that the formula is safe for children and pregnant women prompted its recommendation in *Posthumous Manuscript from [Bian Que in] Handan* for treating serious wind-cold disorders during pregnancy, and in *Guide to Pediatrics* for pediatric fevers due to wind-cold with body aches, headache, chills, and the absence of sweating.

Although references to Ten-Miracle Decoction (*shí shén tāng*) fill the classical literature, its use seems to have lost popularity in modern China. This is reflected in its omission from modern teaching textbooks in the Peoples Republic. This loss of esteem may be related to the sentiments expressed by the Ming-dynasty physician Wu Shou, who urged caution when using this formula because he felt that its yang brightness herbs, Cimicifugae Rhizoma (*shēng má*) and Puerariae Radix (*gé gēn*), when used to treat greater yang disorders, would lead wind-cold pathogens deeper, into the yang brightness. However, the formula is still frequently used in Taiwan and Japan for initial-stage wind-cold patterns. Interestingly, a key use of Ten-Miracle Decoction (*shí shén tāng*) in those places as well as in the Peoples Republic is as a preventative to epidemic disorders. The formula's ability to promote the free flow of qi in the interior and exterior of the body is viewed as an effective way to enhance the body's protective qi and ward off illness. For this purpose, sources generally suggest a smaller dose of 3-6g per day of the decocted powder.

Comparison

➤ Vs. Augmented Cyperus and Perilla Leaf Powder (*jiā wèi xiāng sū sǎn*)

Both formulas regulate the qi and release pathogens from the exterior. However, because Augmented Cyperus and Perilla Leaf Powder (*jiā wèi xiāng sū sǎn*) does both of these things in a milder fashion, it is appropriate for less severe patterns.

Modifications

- For middle burner fullness with excess qi, add Aurantii Fructus (*zhǐ ké*). (source text)
- For fever and headache, add Allii fistulosi Bulbus (*cōng bái*) with fine roots intact. (source text)
- For tidal fevers, add Scutellariae Radix (*huáng qín*) and Ophiopogonis Radix (*mài mén dōng*). (*Achieving Longevity by Guarding the Source*)
- For cough, add Platycodi Radix (*jié gěng*), Mori Cortex (*sāng bái pí*), and Pinelliae Rhizoma praeparatum (*zhì bàn xià*). (*Achieving Longevity by Guarding the Source*)
- For headache, add Asari Radix et Rhizoma (*xì xīn*), Gypsum fibrosum (*shí gāo*), and Allii fistulosi Bulbus (*cōng bái*). (*Achieving Longevity by Guarding the Source*)
- For lack of appetite, add Amomi Fructus (*shā rén*) and Atractylodis macrocephalae Rhizoma (*bái zhú*). (*Achieving Longevity by Guarding the Source*)

- For vomiting, add Caryophylli Flos (*dīng xiāng*) and Amomi Fructus (*shā rén*). (*Achieving Longevity by Guarding the Source*)
- For incessant nosebleed, add Mume Fructus (*wū méi*) and Scutellariae Radix (*huáng qín*). (*Achieving Longevity by Guarding the Source*)
- For abdominal pain, add wine-fried Paeoniae Radix alba (*jiǔ chǎo bái sháo*).

金沸草散
Inula Powder
jīn fèi cǎo sǎn

Source *Formulary of the Pharmacy Service for Benefiting the People in the Taiping Era* (1107)

Inulae Flos (*xuán fù huā*) . . . . .90g (9g) (wrap separately)
Ephedrae Herba (*má huáng*). 90g (3-6g)
Peucedani Radix (*qián hú*) .90g (9g)
Schizonepetae Herba (*jīng jiè*) 120g (6-9g)
Glycyrrhizae Radix praeparata (*zhì gān cǎo*) 30g (3g)
Pinelliae Rhizoma praeparatum (*zhì bàn xià*) 30g. . . . . . . (5-9g)
Paeoniae Radix rubra (*chì sháo*). 30g (3-6g)
Zingiberis Rhizoma recens (*shēng jiāng*) . . . . 3 slices
Jujubae Fructus (*dà zǎo*). . . . . .1 piece

Method of Preparation   The source text recommends that the herbs, excluding Zingiberis Rhizoma recens (*shēng jiāng*) and Jujubae Fructus (*dà zǎo*), be ground to a powder. Decoct 9g (Zhu Dan-Xi recommends 15g) for each dose with Zingiberis Rhizoma recens (*shēng jiāng*) and Jujubae Fructus (*dà zǎo*). Cook 1.5 cups down to 0.8 cups. At present, it is commonly taken as a decoction with the dosages listed in parentheses.

Actions   Discharges and disperses wind-cold, disseminates and directs the Lung qi downward, transforms phlegm, stops cough, and calms wheezing

Indications

Wind-cold exterior patterns with chills, fever, cough with copious sputum, nasal congestion, deep and low voice, headache, clouded vision, fullness and oppression in the chest and diaphragm, a puffy tongue with tooth marks and a greasy, white coating, and a floating pulse. It is also specifically indicated for toothache with a swollen tongue due to wind-cold invasion.

Wind-cold exterior patterns present with chills because the protective level is compromised. Fever results from the struggle between the normal qi and the pathogen. The disruption to the flow of Lung qi that results from the fettering of the Lungs by wind-cold gives rise to a deep and low voice, as well as fullness and oppression in the chest and diaphragm. The nose is the opening of the Lung and thus becomes congested as the Lung qi is fettered. Headache and clouded vision result from the obstruction in the Lung that blocks the flow of clear qi to the upper body.

Analysis of Formula

The indications for this formula are the result of an external pathogen invading and fettering the Lung and causing it to lose its ability to clarify and direct qi downward. This is complicated by the presence of phlegm, which itself accumulates because the fettered Lung fails to disseminate the fluids and send them downward. To address this complicated pattern, the formula utilizes a strategy of discharging wind-cold from the exterior while simultaneously unblocking the Lung collaterals that are obstructed by phlegm and thin mucus.

The formula's chief herbs, Inulae Flos (*xuán fù huā*) and Ephedrae Herba (*má huáng*), help the Lung qi to flow smoothly and in a downward direction, thus relieving the cough and wheezing. These two herbs disperse the wind-cold pathogenic qi and phlegm and direct the qi downward, thereby treating the external wind-cold and internal collection of phlegm. Schizonepetae Herba (*jīng jiè*) aids the chief herbs in releasing the wind-cold pathogen from the exterior; it is the deputy herb. Pinelliae Rhizoma praeparatum (*zhì bàn xià*) transforms phlegm, dries dampness, directs the qi downward, and relieves the cough, while Peucedani Radix (*qián hú*) disseminates the Lung qi, eliminates phlegm, relieves the cough, and directs the qi downward. Paeoniae Radix rubra (*chì sháo*) cools the blood and clears heat; coupled with Jujubae Fructus (*dà zǎo*), it nourishes and cools the yin and nutritive level and thereby prevents them from being damaged by the formula's acrid and warm herbs, as well as the yang wind pathogen. It also resolves the pathogenic heat in the channels and collaterals that results from wind-cold stagnation. These are the three assistant herbs. Glycyrrhizae Radix (*gān cǎo*) harmonizes the middle, augments the qi, and harmonizes the various actions of the herbs in the formula. As is often the case, Zingiberis Rhizoma recens (*shēng jiāng*) and Jujubae Fructus (*dà zǎo*) are intended to harmonize the nutritive and protective levels. In addition, Zingiberis Rhizoma recens (*shēng jiāng*) helps Ephedrae Herba (*má huáng*) and Schizonepetae Herba (*jīng jiè*) release the wind-cold pathogen from the exterior. These last three herbs serve as envoys.

Commentary

This formula is named Inula Powder (*jīn fèi cǎo sǎn*) because originally, Inulae Herba (*jīn fèi cǎo*) was used as the lead ingredient. Nowadays, however, Inulae Flos (*xuán fù huā*), the flower portion of the same plant, is used because it is considered to have a stronger action. We have placed the formula in this section of the book because it is commonly used to treat the early stages of externally-contracted wind-cold leading to a productive cough. Other texts place it in the category of dispelling phlegm. This implies that it can be used in both the acute stages of a wind-cold invasion as well as later, when the acute symptoms have abated and cough becomes the main symptom.

Paeoniae Radix rubra (chì sháo)

One of the interesting aspects of this formula is its use of Paeoniae Radix rubra (*chì sháo*). There are no obvious signs of blood stasis or heat, which delimit the modern parameters of its usage. An answer is provided by the Qing-dynasty physician Wang Fu, in *Collectanea of Investigations from the Realm of Medicine*: "Paeoniae Radix rubra (*chì sháo*) is a sour herb used in draining the Liver and astringing yin. In the present context [it checks] excessive dispersing by Ephedrae Herba (*má huáng*). The red [variety of the herb] is used here because it moves the water aspect and absorbs phlegm-dampness." This explanation can be extended to the use of Radix Paeoniae (*sháo yào*) in many formulas that drain dampness and regulate the fluids, such as True Warrior Decoction (*zhēn wǔ tāng*), discussed in Chapter 16; and it helps us understand the synergism between Poria (*fú líng*) and Radix Paeoniae (*sháo yào*) in formulas such as Cinnamon Twig and Poria Pill (*guì zhī fú líng wán*), discussed in Chapter 13. It may even shed new light on the use of Radix Paeoniae (*sháo yào*) in Cinnamon Twig Decoction (*guì zhī tāng*), discussed above.

Composition

Wang Fei also provides a useful analysis of the formula's composition as a whole, and specifically its use of Inulae Flos (*xuán fù huā*) as chief herb. He argues that the light herbs in the formula, all of which are used in relatively high doses, help to focus the action of the formula on the upper burner. The heavier, downward-draining herbs, such as Pinelliae Rhizoma (*bàn xià*) and Paeoniae Radix rubra (*chì sháo*), however, are necessary to guide excessive fluids to the lower burner for elimination. This combined action is embodied in the chief herb Inulae Flos (*xuán fù huā*). Although it is light and floating, it is also bitter and thus able to direct downward. Its salty nature, furthermore, prevents its acridity from damaging the physiological fluids, making it an important herb for dislodging accumulations from the collaterals. This usage is discussed in more detail under Inula Decoction (*xuán fù huā tāng*) in Chapter 13.

Comparisons

➤ Vs. Ephedra Decoction (*má huáng tāng*)

Ephedra Decoction (*má huáng tāng*) is better at dispelling wind-cold, while Inula Powder (*jīn fèi cǎo sǎn*) treats a wider range of symptoms and is better able to deal with coughs with copious sputum.

➤ Vs. Stop Coughing Powder (*zhǐ sòu sǎn*)

Both formulas treat wind-cold cough with phlegm. However, Stop Coughing Powder (*zhǐ sòu sǎn*) mostly contains herbs that aim to regulate the qi, eliminate phlegm, and relieve cough; it has little ability to release pathogens from the exterior. It is thus best for cough that remains after the overt signs of an external pathogen have receded. Inula Powder (*jīn fèi cǎo sǎn*), on the other hand, addresses cough with phlegm at the onset of an attack from an exterior wind-cold pathogen.

Modifications

- When the contemporary practitioner Jiao Shu-De uses this formula to treat wind-cold cough, he often adds Perillae Fructus (*zǐ sū zǐ*), Armeniacae Semen (*xìng rén*), Asteris Radix (*zǐ wǎn*), Eriobotryae Folium (*pí pá yè*), and Raphani Semen (*lái fú zǐ*).
- If headache accompanies the invasion of wind-cold, add Chuanxiong Rhizoma (*chuān xiōng*) and Angelicae dahuricae Radix (*bái zhǐ*).
- If nasal congestion is prominent, add Xanthii Fructus (*cāng ěr zǐ*), Angelicae dahuricae Radix (*bái zhǐ*), and Magnoliae Flos (*xīn yí*).

Variations

金沸草散

Inula Powder from *Book to Safeguard Life*

jīn fèi cǎo sǎn

SOURCE   *Book to Safeguard Life Arranged According to Pattern* (1108)

Replace Ephedrae Herba (*má huáng*) and Paeoniae Radix rubra (*chì sháo*) with Asari Radix et Rhizoma (*xì xīn*) and Poria rubra (*chì fú líng*) to reduce the formula's ability to release pathogens from the exterior while increasing its capacity to dispel yin-fluids that have accumulated in the Lung.

Associated Formula

杏蘇飲［幼科］（杏苏饮［幼科］）

Apricot and Perilla Drink [pediatric version]

xìng sū yǐn [yòu kē]

SOURCE   *Golden Mirror of the Medical Tradition* (1742)

Perillae Folium (*zǐ sū yè*) 6-9g
bran-fried Aurantii Fructus (*fū chǎo zhǐ ké*) 6-9g
Platycodi Radix (*jié gěng*) 6-9g
Scutellariae Radix (*huáng qín*) 6-9g
Ophiopogonis Radix (*mài mén dōng*) 6-9g
Peucedani Radix (*qián hú*) 6-9g
Citri reticulatae Exocarpium rubrum (*jú hóng*) 2-3g
Mori Cortex (*sāng bái pí*) 6-9g
Fritillariae thunbergii Bulbus (*zhè bèi mǔ*) 6-9g
Glycyrrhizae Radix (*gān cǎo*) 2-3g
Armeniacae Semen (*xìng rén*) (dry-fried) 6-9g
Zingiberis Rhizoma recens (*shēng jiāng*) 2-3g

Dispels wind, promotes the proper movement of qi, reduces phlegm, and transforms stagnation. For a form of the common cold known as 'wind damage' (傷風 *shāng fēng*) in children, where pathogenic wind attacks the superficial level of the body that affects the Lung. According to the source text:

The skin and body hair [which is] governed by the Lung are affected by pathogenic wind. The body becomes hot [with fever] with [symptoms of] abhorrence of cold, headache, sweating, sneezing, runny nose, a floating and moderate pulse, nasal congestion, a low and deep voice, and intermittent cough. Apricot and Perilla Drink [pediatric version] (*xìng sū yǐn [yòu kē]*), like Inula Powder (*jīn fèi cǎo sǎn*), dredges wind and releases [pathogens from] the exterior without [causing] agitation.

Because this is a formula for children and is for a mild condition, its ingredients are gentler than the pox-treating version of Apricot and Perilla Drink (*xìng sū yǐn*) from the same source. Fritillariae Bulbus (*bèi mǔ*) replaces the harsher Pinelliae Rhizoma praeparatum (*zhì bàn xià*), and the addition of Mori Cortex (*sāng bái pí*) and Ophiopogonis Radix (*mài mén dōng*) protect a child's fragile yin. The inclusion of bitter and cold Scutellariae Radix (*huáng qín*) addresses heat that arises from wind fettering the exterior and the Lung. Though originally intended for the treatment of children, it can be used for adults as well. This is especially true for older adults or for patients in whom one fears damaging the yin with more bitter and acrid formulas.

Modifications

- For Lung-heat cough, add Trichosanthis Fructus (*guā lóu*) and increase the dosage of Scutellariae Radix (*huáng qín*).
- For nasal congestion with yellow discharge, add Magnoliae Flos (*xīn yí*), Menthae haplocalycis Herba (*bò hé*), Xanthii Fructus (*cāng ěr zǐ*), Paeoniae Radix rubra (*chì sháo*), and Gypsum fibrosum (*shí gāo*).

Section 3

. . . .

FORMULAS THAT RELEASE EXTERIOR WIND-HEAT

Externally-contracted wind-heat disorders are characterized by fever, sweating, a slight aversion to wind or slight chills, headache, thirst, and sore throat. There may also be a cough or redness of the eyes. The tongue coating is white or slightly yellow (indicating that heat has not penetrated deeply enough to cause a purely yellow coating), and the tip of the tongue may be slightly red (indicating that heat is already entering and damaging the fluids). The pulse tends to be floating and rapid. Among the four-level differentiation of the patterns of disease, this presentation corresponds to the protective level, which is the most superficial.

The core ingredients for these formulas are light, acrid, and cooling herbs that release the exterior, such as Mori Folium (*sāng yè*), Chrysanthemi Flos (*jú huā*), Menthae haplocalycis Herba *(bò hé)*, and Arctii Fructus *(niú bàng zǐ)*. Because warm-heat pathogen diseases can develop suddenly and quickly enter the deeper levels of the body, these formulas commonly include herbs that clear heat, such as Lonicerae Flos *(jīn yín huā)*, Forsythiae Fructus *(lián qiáo)*, and Lophatheri Herba *(dàn zhú yè)*, to interrupt this process. These diseases first attack the Lungs and disrupt its disseminating and descending functions, so the formulas often contain herbs that treat these problems, such as Platycodi Radix *(jié gěng)* and Armeniacae Semen *(xìng rén)*. Warm pathogens also have a tendency to injure the fluids, and herbs that generate fluids and also clear heat, such as Trichosanthis Radix *(tiān huā fěn)* and Phragmitis Rhizoma *(lú gēn)*, are therefore frequently used in formulas to release exterior wind-heat.

桑菊飲 (桑菊饮)

Mulberry Leaf and Chrysanthemum Drink

sāng jú yǐn

Source *Systematic Differentiation of Warm Pathogen Diseases* (1798)

Mori Folium *(sāng yè)*. 7.5g
Chrysanthemi Flos *(jú huā)*. 3g
Forsythiae Fructus *(lián qiáo)*. 4.5g
Menthae haplocalycis Herba *(bò hé)*. . . . . [add near end] 2.4g
Platycodi Radix *(jié gěng)*. 6g
Armeniacae Semen *(xìng rén)*. 6g
Phragmitis Rhizoma *(lú gēn)* 6g
Glycyrrhizae Radix *(gān cǎo)* 2.4g

Method of Preparation Decoction. Do not cook for more than 20 minutes as the source text says to cook down to 1 cup from 2. Because, at present, 'drinks' (飲 *yǐn*) are thought to be most effective when transparent, followers of the warm pathogen disease school commonly cook this formula for only 10 minutes.

Actions Disperses wind and clears heat, stops coughing by facilitating the flow of Lung qi

Indications

Slight fever, cough, slight thirst, a thin, white tongue coating, and a floating, rapid pulse.

This is the early, superficial stage of a warm pathogen disease. This type of disorder enters through the nose and mouth and thus most readily damages the Lungs. In the initial stages, the pathogen penetrates and obstructs the collaterals of the Lungs, inhibiting its clarifying and descending function. Coughing is thus the main symptom. The mild fever and slight thirst reflect the presence of mild exterior heat. The floating, rapid pulse also reflects exterior heat. The normal tongue coating indicates that the condition is still in the exterior.

Analysis of Formula

When heat lodges in the Lungs and causes coughing, the appropriate strategy is to clear the heat and disseminate the Lung qi. Because the heat is externally contracted and located primarily at the protective level, equal attention must be paid to venting wind-heat from the exterior. Following the adage that in treating the upper burner the medicine must be as light a feather, all of the key herbs are extremely light and floating in nature.

Mori Folium *(sāng yè)* and Chrysanthemi Flos *(jú huā)*, the chief herbs, are cool and light and can clear heat from the exterior. Mori Folium *(sāng yè)* has a sweet and bitter flavor. It clears heat from the lungs and stops the coughing. Chrysanthemi Flos *(jú huā)* disperses upper burner wind-heat, including that which affects the eyes. Two of the deputies, Forsythiae Fructus *(lián qiáo)* and Menthae haplocalycis Herba *(bò hé)*, strengthen the formula's exterior-releasing properties. Two other deputies, Platycodi Radix *(jié gěng)*, which has an ascending action, and Armeniacae Semen *(xìng rén)*, which has a descending action, assist the chief herbs by facilitating the flow of Lung qi to stop the coughing. The assistant, Phragmitis Rhizoma *(lú gēn)*, clears heat and generates fluids, thereby reducing thirst. Glycyrrhizae Radix *(gān cǎo)*, the envoy, helps clear the heat and harmonizes the actions of the other herbs.

Commentary

This is the classic formula for early-stage warm pathogen diseases or other mild exterior heat disorders in which coughing is the main symptom. It is also used for eye disorders due to wind-heat and hacking cough due to exterior dryness. According to its author, Wu Ju-Tong, the famous systematizer of warm pathogen disorder therapeutics, it can address these different disorders because they all require a dispersing formula that releases obstruction in the exterior without injuring the fluids. For this reason, Wu selected as chief herbs Mori Folium *(sāng yè)* and Chrysanthemi Flos *(jú huā)*, a synergistic combination that relies on subtle manipulation of the qi dynamic rather than merely on acrid opening. Mori Folium *(sāng yè)* specifically acts on the Lung collaterals, which are implicated in the superfical penetration of pathogens into an organ. Both of the chief herbs enter the Liver and Lung channels. While heat pathogens obstruct the clarifying and downward-directing function of the Lung qi, the fire of Liver yang ascends uncontrolled. By clearing heat from both channels, this formula treats root and branch simultaneously. In addition, both of the chief herbs combine sweet moistening with their clearing and dispersing actions. Chrysanthemi Flos *(jú huā)*, in particular, protects the fluids, and by gently nourishing the yin helps to control the excess of yang that is the root of the pathology.

Comparisons

➤ Vs. Honeysuckle and Forsythia Powder
(*yín qiáo sǎn*)

While these formulas share many of the same ingredients, Mulberry Leaf and Chrysanthemum Drink (*sāng jú yǐn*) is lighter in nature and, through its effect on the qi dynamic of the Lungs, more effective in treating cough. Honeysuckle and Forsythia Powder (*yín qiáo sǎn*) is a stronger formula for releasing the exterior and clearing heat and is therefore more suitable for the early stage of warm pathogen disorders presenting with fever and sore throat.

➤ Vs. Mulberry Leaf and Apricot Kernel Decoction
(*sāng xìng tāng*); see page 666

Biomedical Indications

With the appropriate presentation, this formula may be used to treat a variety of biomedically-defined disorders primarily involving acute respiratory tract infections including the common cold, influenza, bronchitis, pneumonia, tonsilitis, and conjunctivitis.

Modifications

- For qi-level dryness, add Gypsum fibrosum (*shí gāo*) and Anemarrhenae Rhizoma (*zhī mǔ*). (source text)
- For nutritive-level heat with a dark-red tongue, add Scrophulariae Radix (*xuán shēn*) and Rhinocerotis Cornu (*xī jiǎo*). (source text)
- For heat entering the blood, remove Phragmitis Rhizoma (*lú gēn*) and Menthae haplocalycis Herba (*bò hé*) and add Ophiopogonis Radix (*mài mén dōng*), Rehmanniae Radix (*shēng dì huáng*), Polygonati odorati Rhizoma (*yù zhú*), and Moutan Cortex (*mǔ dān pí*). (source text)
- For severe Lung heat, add Scutellariae Radix (*huáng qín*). (source text)
- For pronounced thirst, add Trichosanthis Radix (*tiān huā fěn*). (source text)
- For viscous, yellow sputum that is difficult to expectorate, add Trichosanthis Pericarpium (*guā lóu pí*) and Fritillariae thunbergii Bulbus (*zhè bèi mǔ*).
- For labored breathing or slight wheezing, add Gypsum fibrosum (*shí gāo*) and Anemarrhenae Rhizoma (*zhī mǔ*).
- For blood-streaked sputum, add Moutan Cortex (*mǔ dān pí*), Imperatae Rhizoma (*bái máo gēn*), and Nelumbinis Nodus rhizomatis (*ǒu jié*).
- For sore throat, add Lasiosphaera/Calvatia (*mǎ bó*) and Arctii Fructus (*niú bàng zǐ*).
- For wind-heat affecting the eyes, add Tribuli Fructus (*cì jí lí*), Cassiae Semen (*jué míng zǐ*), and Prunellae Spica (*xià kū cǎo*).

銀翹散 （银翘散）

Honeysuckle and Forsythia Powder

yín qiáo sǎn

Source   *Systematic Differentiation of Warm Pathogen Diseases* (1798)

Lonicerae Flos (*jīn yín huā*)	30g (9-15g)
Forsythiae Fructus (*lián qiáo*)	30g (9-15g)
Platycodi Radix (*jié gěng*)	18g (3-6g)
Arctii Fructus (*niú bàng zǐ*)	18g (9-12g)
Menthae haplocalycis Herba (*bò hé*)	18g (3-6g)
Sojae Semen praeparatum (*dàn dòu chǐ*)	15g (3-6g)
Schizonepetae Spica (*jīng jiè suì*)	12g (6-9g)
Lophatheri Herba (*dàn zhú yè*)	12g (3-6g)
Phragmitis Rhizoma recens (*xiān lú gēn*)	15-30g
Glycyrrhizae Radix (*gān cǎo*)	15g (3-6g)

Method of Preparation   The source text advises to prepare a decoction of Phragmitis Rhizoma recens (*xiān lú gēn*), which is cooked just long enough for the aroma to become strong. The other herbs are then ground into powder and taken in 9g doses with the decoction. Three doses (or four in more serious cases) are to be taken over the course of a day. At present, the formula is usually prepared as a decoction with the dosage indicated in parentheses and generally not cooked for more than 20 minutes. Menthae haplocalycis Herba (*bò hé*) should be added 5 minutes before the end.

Actions   Disperses wind-heat, clears heat, and resolves toxicity

Indications

Fever, slight chills or chills lasting for only a very brief period of time before aversion to heat develops, headache, thirst, cough, sore throat, a red-tipped tongue, a thin, white or thin, yellow tongue coating, and a floating, rapid pulse.

In *Discussion of Warm Pathogen Heat [Disorders]*, Ye Tian-Shi notes that "Warm pathogens are contracted [through] the upper [burner and] first attack the Lungs." Yang in nature, wind-heat tends to enter the body via the nose and mouth, allowing it to directly damage the superficial aspect of the Lungs. It also constrains the diffusion of protective qi in the skin and muscle layer. The conjunction of these pathologies explains the characteristic signs and symptoms of the pattern for which this formula is indicated. Constraint of protective yang qi causes fever and, at least initially, also chills. In contrast to wind-cold disorders, these chills are relatively mild, or, if the pathogen rapidly moves into the qi aspect, noticeable only at the very onset of the disease. The level of penetration also determines whether or not the patient will sweat: sweating indicates involvement of the qi aspect. If the dissemination of Lung qi is blocked, a cough will develop. When heat damages the fluids, it causes thirst. Because the throat is 'the door of the Lungs,' heat from constraint will first cause itching and soreness or, if it transforms into toxin, more severe pain and inflammation. If the pathogenic influence is lodged mainly in the exterior, the tongue coating will be normal (thin and white). If it penetrates into the the superficial aspect of the Lungs, one may see a red-tipped tongue and a white or yellow coating. A floating, rapid pulse reflects the presence of superficial heat.

Analysis of Formula

Being purely yang in nature, wind-heat disorders tend to develop rapidly, with a quick penetration of the pathogen from the protective to the qi and then blood levels, and progressive exhaustion of yin fluids. Furthermore, the foul turbidity that is traditionally associated with warm pathogen epidemics readily causes knotting of the qi dynamic and the transformation of heat into toxin. The composition of this formula is thus aimed not only at releasing the exterior, clearing heat from the Lungs, and resolving toxicity, but also at interrupting the progression of the disorder from the Lungs to the Pericardium, from the upper to the middle burner.

All of the herbs in this formula are light and unfold their actions in the upper burner. The chief herbs, Lonicerae Flos *(jīn yín huā)* and Forsythiae Fructus *(lián qiáo)*, are acrid, cool, and fragrant; they release the exterior, clear heat from the Lungs, and resolve toxicity. Their dosage is greatest because their actions are the focus of the formula. Two of the deputies, Platycodi Radix *(jié gěng)* and Arctii Fructus *(niú bàng zǐ)*, spread the Lung qi and improve the throat. The other deputies, Menthae haplocalycis Herba *(bò hé)* and Sojae Semen praeparatum *(dàn dòu chǐ)*, help the chief herbs to release exterior heat.

Although it is a warm, acrid diaphoretic, Schizonepetae Spica *(jīng jiè suì)* is used here to boost the exterior-releasing action of the formula without producing dryness. The combination of three other assistants, Lophatheri Herba *(dàn zhú yè)*, Phragmitis Rhizoma recens *(xiān lú gēn)*, and Glycyrrhizae Radix *(gān cǎo)*, generates fluids and alleviates thirst. The combination of Glycyrrhizae Radix *(gān cǎo)* and Platycodi Radix *(jié gěng)* is very effective for treating sore throat.

Commentary

This is the classic formula for treating protective-level warm pathogen diseases. Its unique value lies in its integration of three distinctly different strategies: vent wind-heat from the exterior; clear heat from the Lung collaterals and resolve toxicity; and prevent the sinking inward of pathogens into the Pericardium or middle burner. This may appear unproblematic to us now. But a look at the formula's genealogy shows that its composition marked a distinctive breakthrough in the treatment of warm pathogen disorders by Chinese medicine; so much so, in fact, that its precise structure and mode of action is still being debated today.

History

Although physicians began to question the usefulness of the established cold damage doctrine for the treatment of febrile disorders from the late Song onward, their understanding of pathology remained tied to existing intellectual frameworks for several more centuries. For example, the physician Liu Wan-Su, widely regarded as the first ancestor of the warm pathogen disease current in Chinese medicine, thought that fire could be traced to the invasion of a cold pathogen that underwent a process of constraint and transformation. The efforts of Wan and others in treating warm pathogen diseases by clearing or draining heat from the interior thus constituted an extension of existing cold damage therapeutics, rather than a radical departure. Cool the Diaphragm Powder *(liáng gé sǎn)*, discussed in Chapter 4, is an important and influential example of this approach.

It was only from the late Ming onward that new theories gradually emerged that posited the invasion of foul turbidity (穢濁 *huì zhuó*) and warm pathogens directly into the body. In this new context, where the goal was to arrest the disease process as early as possible before heat entered the interior, the traditional cold damage therapeutics became much more problematic. In the first place, while bitter, cold herbs were useful for draining interior heat and resolving fire toxin, they also inhibited the qi dynamic and thereby prevented the venting of pathogens to the outside. Second, bitter herbs that eliminated pathogens via the bowels and urine would also push pathogens from the exterior into the interior and thereby accelerate the natural progression of warm pathogen diseases. Finally, the acrid and warm herbs that had heretofore been used to release the exterior were inappropriate for treating direct invasion of heat. A solution to these problems was offered by physicians like Yu Chang and Ye Tian-Shi, who proposed to combine herbs into formulas that were simultaneously acrid, cool, light, and aromatic.

Wu Ju-Tong's composition of Honeysuckle and Forsythia Powder *(yín qiáo sǎn)* clearly reflects this influence, as he was at pains to point out:

> The [composition] of this formula painstakingly honors the teachings of the *Yellow Emperor's Inner Classic* [that had recently been placed at the heart of Ye Tian-Shi's approach to the treatment of early stage warm pathogen heat disorders] … It also follows the doctrine advocated by Yu Chang of expelling foulness by means of fragrant and aromatic herbs. I have utilized Li Gao's [i.e., Li Dong-Yuan's] formula Clear the Heart and Cool the Diaphragm Powder *(qīng xīn liáng gé sǎn)*, which employs acrid, cold, bitter, and sweet [ingredients]. However, [because of what I have said regarding] the early stage of a [warm pathogen heat] disorder, I have taken out Scutellariae Radix *(huáng qín)*, which enters the interior, so as not to attack the middle burner [and guide pathogens inward]. I have added the acrid and cool Lonicerae Flos *(jīn yín huā)* and the aromatic and fragrant Schizonepetae Spica *(jīng jiè suì)* to disperse heat

and resolve toxicity. [I have also added] Arctii Fructus *(niú bàng zǐ)*, which is acrid, balanced, and moistens the Lungs. It resolves heat and disperses clumps, eliminates wind and improves the condition of the throat. All of these [additional] herbs [have been selected because they] enter the hand greater yin.

Controversies

Wu Ju-Tong's intention was thus clear. Nevertheless, later commentators still disputed precisely how this was realized within the structure of the formula. The modern physician Qin Bo-Wei represents one distinctive perspective. To Qin, it seemed logical that since the focus of the formula was on the exterior, the chief herbs should be those that release the exterior, namely Sojae Semen praeparatum *(dàn dòu chǐ)*, Menthae haplocalycis Herba *(bò hé)*, and Schizonepetae Spica *(jīng jiè suì)*. Yet it was Lonicerae Flos *(jīn yín huā)* and Forsythiae Fructus *(lián qiáo)* for which the formula was named. Qin believed that Wu Ju-Tong did this to alert practitioners to the fact that cold herbs should be the primary constituents of formulas that treat the early stages of warm pathogen disease.

Most other commentators think that the herbs which gave the formula its name are also its chief ingredients. Yet the issue raised by Qin Bo-Wei is more profound. It addresses not only the question of why Wu Ju-Tong thought it necessary to add acrid and warm herbs to a formula that seeks to resolve fire toxicity, but also whether—as in cold damage disorders—sweating is a desired and, indeed, necessary outcome of treating warm pathogen disorders at the protective level.

In *Discussion of Warm Pathogen Heat [Disorders]*, Ye Tian-Shi stated that a pathogen "at the protective [level] can be [resolved] by sweating." Some commentators take this to indicate that sweating is the actual goal of treatment at the protective level. It dispels pathogens to the outside, explains Wu Ju-Tong's inclusion of Schizonepetae Spica *(jīng jiè suì)* and Sojae Semen praeparatum *(dàn dòu chǐ)*, and even supports Qin Bo-Wei's analysis. Others, like Qin's contemporary Zhao Shao-Qin, a well-known expert on warm pathogen diseases from Beijing, dispute this view. He argues that the real goal of treatment at this level is to reestablish the unhindered circulation of protective yang throughout the exterior through a combination of acrid and aromatic dispersal and cool clearing. Sweating may occur as a result of this process, as the protective qi is released from its constraint, but it is not necessary for the treatment to be successful.

These apparently opposing views can be reconciled in the clinic by paying close attention to the precise conjunction of signs and symptoms and adjusting the formula accordingly. Where the constraint of protective yang by wind-heat is marked—indicated by chills, an absence of sweating, and itching in the throat—Schizonepetae Spica *(jīng jiè suì)* ensures that the pathogen is vented to the outside, a pro-

cess usually accompanied by sweating. If, on the other hand, chills are completely absent, the patient is already perspiring, there is thirst, and the throat is visibly inflamed—all signs that the heat has already entered the qi or even the nutritive level—Schizonepetae Spica *(jīng jiè suì)* should be used with more circumspection. Scrophulariae Radix *(xuán shēn)* is one herb that was already recommended in some passages of the source text to be added for just this type of problem.

To achieve the best results from using this formula, it is advisable, in any case, to modify and adjust it to the multitude of permutations with which early stage warm pathogen diseases present in the clinic. If physicians belonging to the warm pathogen disease current in Chinese medicine had one thing in common, it was this style of practice: to think of formulas as models of action rather than prescriptions that had to be followed.

Comparison

➤ Vs. Mulberry Leaf and Chrysanthemum Drink *(sāng jú yǐn)*; see page 36

Biomedical Indications

With the appropriate presentation, this formula may be used to treat a variety of biomedically-defined disorders, primarily involving acute respiratory tract infections like the common cold, influenza, bronchitis, pneumonia, and tonsilitis, but also measles, mumps, meningitis, and encephalitis B.

Alternate names

Honeysuckle and Forsythia Powder to Resolve Toxicity *(yín qiáo jiě dú sǎn)* in *Nationwide Collection of TCM Patent Formulas*

Cautions and Contraindications

This formula will be ineffective in cases with damp-heat, unless significantly modified. Proper treatment of wind-dampness requires leaching out the dampness and dispelling the heat through the lower burner (urine or stool). Based on the discussion above, it follows that this is precisely what this formula does *not* do.

Modifications

- For a stifling sensation in the chest, add Pogostemonis/Agastaches Herba *(huò xiāng)*. (source text)
- For severe thirst, add Trichosanthis Radix *(tiān huā fěn)*. (source text)
- For severe sore throat, add Lasiosphaera/Calvatia *(mǎ bó)* and Scrophulariae Radix *(xuán shēn)*. (source text)
- For pronounced cough, add Armeniacae Semen *(xìng rén)*. (source text)
- For heat entering the interior with scanty urine, add Rehmanniae Radix *(shēng dì huáng)*, Ophiopogonis Radix *(mài*

mén dōng), Scutellariae Radix *(huáng qín)*, Anemarrhenae Rhizoma *(zhī mǔ)*, and Gardeniae Fructus *(zhī zǐ)*. (source text)

- For nosebleed, remove Schizonepetae Herba *(jīng jiè)* and Sojae Semen praeparatum *(dàn dòu chǐ)* and add Imperatae Rhizoma *(bái máo gēn)* and Gardeniae Fructus *(zhī zǐ)*. (source text)
- For dampness causing a tight, stifling sensation in the chest and epigastrium, add Pogostemonis/Agastaches Herba *(huò xiāng)* and Curcumae Radix *(yù jīn)*.
- For early-stage measles with incomplete expression of rash, add Cicadae Periostracum *(chán tuì)* and Spirodelae Herba *(fú píng)*.
- For early-stage carbuncles, add Taraxaci Herba *(pú gōng yīng)* and Isatidis Folium *(dà qīng yè)*.
- For a yellow tongue coating and diarrhea, combine with Kudzu, Scutellaria, and Coptis Decoction *(gé gēn huáng qín huáng lián tāng)*.
- For acute endometritis, remove Glycyrrhizae Radix *(gān cǎo)* and Lophatheri Herba *(dàn zhú yè)* and add Gardeniae Fructus *(zhī zǐ)*, Saposhnikoviae Radix *(fáng fēng)*, and Rehmanniae Radix *(shēng dì huáng)*.

Associated Formulas

銀翹湯 （银翘汤）

Honeysuckle and Forsythia Decoction

yín qiáo tāng

SOURCE *Systematic Differentiation of Warm Pathogen Diseases* (1798)

Lonicerae Flos *(jīn yín huā)* 15g
Forsythiae Fructus *(lián qiáo)* .9g
Lophatheri Herba *(dàn zhú yè)* 6g
Glycyrrhizae Radix *(gān cǎo)* .3g
Ophiopogonis Radix *(mài mén dōng)* 12g
Rehmanniae Radix *(shēng dì huáng)* 12g

Enriches the yin and vents exterior heat. For the remnants of a yang brightness-warp warm pathogen disease that has been incompletely purged. Although purging has eliminated the accumulation, some of the pathogen remains in the exterior and the yin has been damaged. This causes a lack of sweating and a floating pulse. It follows that if the pulse is floating but also overflowing (indicating continued qi level excess), or rapid but not superficial (indicating heat remaining in the interior), this formula is contraindicated.

銀翹馬勃散 （银翘马勃散）

Honeysuckle, Forsythia, and Puffball Powder

yín qiáo mǎ bó sǎn

SOURCE *Systematic Differentiation of Warm Pathogen Diseases* (1798)

Lonicerae Flos *(jīn yín huā)* 15g
Forsythiae Fructus *(lián qiáo)* 30g

Arctii Fructus *(niú bàng zǐ)* 18g
Belamcandae Rhizoma *(shè gān)* 9g
Lasiosphaera/Calvatia *(mǎ bó)* 6g

The method of preparation is the same as for the main formula. Clears heat, resolves toxicity, and drains heat from the Lungs to improve the functioning of the throat. For severe sore throat with great difficulty in swallowing, a red tongue with a thick white or yellow coating, and a rapid, slippery, and possibly floating pulse. This is painful obstruction of the throat (喉痹 *hóu bì*) due to damp-heat collecting in the Lungs. A damp-heat invasion often begins by an attack on the Lungs. Damp-heat constrains the qi level of the Lungs, which results in obstruction of the throat; when it attacks the blood level of the Lungs, there is a sore throat. The red tongue and rapid pulse reflect the presence of heat, while the thick tongue coating and slippery pulse indicate dampness. If the damp-heat is relatively superficial, the tongue coating will be white and the pulse will float; if it penetrates deeper, the tongue coating will turn yellow and the pulse will no longer float.

For no pain but severe obstruction, the source text recommends adding 18g of Talcum *(huá shí)*, 15g of Platycodi Radix *(jié gěng)*, and 15g of Phragmitis Rhizoma *(lú gēn)*. At present, Isatidis Folium *(dà qīng yè)* and Isatidis/Baphicacanthis Radix *(bǎn lán gēn)* are commonly added for signs of heat toxin.

柴葛解肌湯 （柴葛解肌汤）

Bupleurum and Kudzu Decoction to Release the Muscle Layer

chái gé jiě jī tāng

Source *Six Texts on Cold Damage* (1445)

Bupleuri Radix *(chái hú)* 3-9g
Puerariae Radix *(gé gēn)* 6-12g
Notopterygii Rhizoma seu Radix *(qiāng huó)* 3-6g
Angelicae dahuricae Radix *(bái zhǐ)* 3-6g
Scutellariae Radix *(huáng qín)* 6-9g
Gypsum fibrosum *(shí gāo)* 4.5-15g
Platycodi Radix *(jié gěng)* 3-6g
Paeoniae Radix alba *(bái sháo)* 6-9g
Glycyrrhizae Radix *(gān cǎo)* .3-6g
Zingiberis Rhizoma recens *(shēng jiāng)* 3-6g
Jujubae Fructus *(dà zǎo)* . . . . .2-3 pieces

Method of Preparation Decoction. Do not cook for more than 20 minutes. The source text does not specify dosage, except that 3g of Gypsum fibrosum *(shí gāo)* should be used. In modern texts, the dosage of this substance ranges from 3-30g. The deeper the level of penetration of the pathogenic influence, the larger the recommended dosage.

Actions Releases pathogenic influences from the muscle layer and clears interior heat

Indications

An exterior wind-cold presentation characterized by increasing fever and decreasing chills accompanied by headache, stiffness of the extremities, orbital and eye pain, dry nasal passages, irritability, insomnia, a thin, yellow tongue coating, and a floating, slightly flooding pulse.

This is unresolved, exterior wind-cold that has become constrained and is transforming into heat. It is also known as 'simultaneous greater yang and yang brightness-warp disorder,' reflected in the increasing fever and decreasing chills. The pathogenic influence that remains in the exterior (greater yang) causes headache, stiffness of the extremities, and a floating pulse. The interior heat (yang brightness) causes irritability, insomnia, orbital and eye pain, dry nasal passages, and a slightly flooding pulse.

Analysis of Formula

This condition requires the use of cool, acrid herbs to release the pathogenic influence from the muscle layer while concurrently clearing heat. The chief ingredients, Bupleuri Radix (chái hú) and Puerariae Radix (gé gēn), accomplish this task. Two of the deputies, Notopterygii Rhizoma seu Radix (qiāng huó) and Angelicae dahuricae Radix (bái zhǐ), help the chief ingredients release the exterior and alleviate pain. They enter into the greater yang and yang brightness channels and thereby assist in focusing the formula on this territory. The other deputies, Scutellariae Radix (huáng qín) and Gypsum fibrosum (shí gāo), focus on the other aspect of the problem, clearing interior heat: Scutellariae Radix (huáng qín) clears heat from the Lungs and upper burner, while Gypsum fibrosum (shí gāo) clears heat from the yang brightness channel. The modest dosage of the latter ingredient indicates that the pathogenic influence has just entered the yang brightness channel.

Platycodi Radix (jié gěng), an assistant, facilitates the flow of Lung qi and helps scatter the pathogenic influence from the exterior. The other assistant, sour and cold Paeoniae Radix alba (bái sháo), preserves the yin by preventing the exterior-releasing herbs from causing excessive sweating. One of the envoys, Glycyrrhizae Radix (gān cǎo), harmonizes the actions of the other herbs. In concert with Platycodi Radix (jié gěng), this herb helps clear heat from the upper burner, especially from the throat. The other envoys, Zingiberis Rhizoma recens (shēng jiāng) and Jujubae Fructus (dà zǎo), regulate the protective and nutritive qi to facilitate the release of the pathogenic influence.

Commentary

In the source text, the author Tao Hua refers to this formula as Kudzu Decoction (gé gēn tāng). The present name is used to avoid confusion with the more well-known formula by the same name from Discussion of Cold Damage, which was discussed earlier in this chapter. Whereas Kudzu Decoction (gé gēn tāng) treats greater yang-warp disorders, Tao Hua emphasized that his new formula was designed "to treat pathogens picked up by the yang brightness Stomach

channel." However, because the formula's indications differ substantially from the classical definition of a yang brightness channel-warp disorder, discussed in detail in Chapter 4 under the heading of White Tiger Decoction (bái hǔ tāng), and because many herbs in the formula enter into the greater and lesser yang channels, the formula's composition and the precise pathology it addresses became the subject of much debate by later generations of physicians.

Controversies

The inclusion of Bupleuri Radix (chái hú) in a formula designed for treating a disorder without any obvious lesser yang-warp signs or symptoms caused particular concern. Fei Bo-Xiong in Discussion of Medical Formulas even argued that this formula should not be used at all because it was so poorly formulated. Other commentators, instead, resolved these difficulties by extending the formula's original indication or by readjusting its composition. According to Wang Ang, for instance, it treats a combined greater yang and yang brightness disorder. Wu Qian, in the Golden Mirror of the Medical Tradition, reasoned instead that Bupleuri Radix (chái hú) should be regarded as the chief herb because the formula resolves a combined disorder of all three yang channels.

Many modern Chinese and Japanese commentators believe that such controversy can be avoided by differentiating between interior and exterior yang brightness channel patterns. The former is characterized by systemic heat from excess. This is treated by clearing, for which White Tiger Decoction (bái hǔ tāng) is indicated. The latter, instead, is characterized by heat from constraint, because the presentation of heat (i.e., fever and inflammation) is closely tied to that of stagnation (i.e., pain and irritability). The manifestation of these symptoms in the mucous membranes of the sensory orifices, 'the interior of the exterior,' defines this constraint to be located in the yang brightness channel. Following the therapeutic principle that 'for fire from constraint, discharge it,' this heat must be vented to the outside through the use of acrid and cool herbs.

Viewed from this perspective, Bupleuri Radix (chái hú) has the function of supporting Puerariae Radix (gé gēn) in discharging this constraint, rather than in resolving the lesser yang channel. In fact, Bupleuri Radix (chái hú) is "an essential herb for releasing the muscle layer" (Displays of Enlightened Physicians) because it has the ability to vent heat from below the immediate surface of the exterior. This is clearly explained in Rectification of the Meaning of Materia Medica:

> Bupleuri Radix (chái hú) has a bitter flavor and thus specifically focuses on pathogenic heat. … It grows in the early spring, its qi is fragrant, and its character light and clear. With both a light qi and flavor, and an ascending, discharging nature constitutionally received in the spring, it is thus completely different, in both character and function, from other bitter, cooling,

draining, and downward-directing herbs. ... When pathogenic qi gradually enters into the interior and is no longer located just at the muscle layer and surface [of the body] from where all other exterior dispersing herbs can no longer vent it, only Bupleuri Radix (*chái hú*) with its clear and light qi and aromatic fragrance is able to dredge and drain it, guiding and lifting out the pathogenic qi to be resolved via the exterior. This is why Bupleuri Radix (*chái hú*) is [included among the herbs that] resolve the exterior, even if its action is different from other herbs focusing on resolving the exterior such as Ephedrae Herba (*má huáng*), Cinnamomi Ramulus (*guì zhī*), Saposhnikoviae Radix (*fáng fēng*), and Schizonepetae Herba (*jīng jiè*).

For this reason, some physicians in contemporary China routinely add Bupleuri Radix (*chái hú*) to any formula that resolves heat from constraint in the exterior, irrespective of its precise cause.

If Puerariae Radix (*gé gēn*) and Bupleuri Radix (*chái hú*) are excellent for venting heat, they are less useful for opening stagnation and stopping pain. This requires the use of more acrid, moving herbs like Angelicae dahuricae Radix (*bái zhǐ*) and Notopterygii Rhizoma seu Radix (*qiāng huó*), which explains their addition to the formula. Finally, because heat from constraint at the yang brightness level is, by definition, a condition of excess that tends to occur in patients with a strong constitution and an exuberance of yang, interior heat frequently occurs before the emergence of acute symptoms, or, if not, is rapidly generated once the exterior becomes constrained. The inclusion of herbs that clear and drain interior heat is thus not only a wise precaution, but almost always a necessity.

The continued use of this formula for more than seven centuries and, indeed, the ongoing debates regarding its indications and mode of action underline its value in clinical practice. Over time, its indications were extended to include toothache due to wind-heat and inflammation of the gums. It may also be considered as a basic formula for venting lurking pathogens from the muscle layer.

Biomedical Indications

With the appropriate presentation, this formula may be used to treat a variety of biomedically-defined infectious disorders including the common cold, influenza, gingivitis, and conjunctivitis.

Alternate names

Kudzu Decoction to Release the Muscle Layer (*gé gēn jiě jī tāng*) in *Mirror of Medicine Past and Present*; Bupleurum Decoction to Release the Muscle Layer (*chái hú jiě jī tāng*) in *Restoration of Health from the Myriad Diseases*

Cautions and Contraindications

This formula is inappropriate for simple exterior wind-heat disorders.

Modifications

- For severe chills without sweating, substitute Ephedrae Herba (*má huáng*) for Scutellariae Radix (*huáng qín*), increasing the dosage in the winter and reducing it in the spring. During the summer and fall, substitute Perillae Folium (*zǐ sū yè*) instead. (source text)

- For cases without chills, headache, or pain, remove Notopterygii Rhizoma seu Radix (*qiāng huó*) and Angelicae dahuricae Radix (*bái zhǐ*).

- For cases without chills but with more severe heat, fever, irritability and restlessness, and a red tongue, add Forsythiae Fructus (*lián qiáo*) and Lonicerae Flos (*jīn yín huā*) and increase the dosage of Gypsum fibrosum (*shí gāo*).

- For a dry mouth and tongue, add Anemarrhenae Rhizoma (*zhī mǔ*) and Trichosanthis Radix (*tiān huā fěn*).

- For coughing of viscous sputum, add Trichosanthis Pericarpium (*guā lóu pí*) and Fritillariae thunbergii Bulbus (*zhè bèi mǔ*).

Associated Formula

柴葛解肌湯 (柴葛解肌汤)

Bupleurum and Kudzu Decoction to Release the Muscle Layer from *Awakening of the Mind in Medical Studies*

chái gé jiě jī tāng

Source *Awakening of the Mind in Medical Studies* (1732)

Bupleuri Radix (*chái hú*) 6g
Puerariae Radix (*gé gēn*) 9g
Paeoniae Radix rubra (*chì sháo*) 6g
Scutellariae Radix (*huáng qín*) 9g
Anemarrhenae Rhizoma (*zhī mǔ*) 6g
Rehmanniae Radix (*shēng dì huáng*) 12g
Moutan Cortex (*mǔ dān pí*) 9g
Fritillariae Bulbus (*bèi mǔ*) 6g
Glycyrrhizae Radix (*gān cǎo*) 3g

Releases the muscle layer and clears heat. For externally-contracted warm pathogen disease with constrained interior heat characterized by fever with no chills, headache, and thirst. This condition is common in those warm pathogen diseases that are contracted in the spring but surface in the summer. If there is delirious speech, add 9g of Gypsum fibrosum (*shí gāo*). In contrast to the principal formula that focuses on releasing the muscle layer, this formula focuses on clearing interior heat. It is a good example of how physicians approached the problem of lurking pathogens prior to the emergence of warm pathogen disease therapeutics.

升麻葛根湯 (升麻葛根汤)

Cimicifuga and Kudzu Decoction

shēng má gé gēn tāng

Source *Craft of Medicines and Patterns for Children* (1119)

Cimicifugae Rhizoma (*shēng má*) 3-6g

Puerariae Radix *(gé gēn)*. 3-9g
Glycyrrhizae Radix praeparata *(zhì gān cǎo)* 3g
Paeoniae Radix rubra *(chì sháo)*. 6-9g

Method of Preparation   The source text advises to grind equal amounts of the herbs into powder and take in 12g doses. At present, it is usually prepared as a decoction with the dosage indicated. Do not cook for more than 20 minutes. Glycyrrhizae Radix *(gān cǎo)* is generally substituted for Glycyrrhizae Radix praeparata *(zhì gān cǎo)*.

Actions   Releases the muscle layer and vents rashes

Indications

Early-stage measles or rashes that do not surface evenly, fever and chills, headache, generalized body aches, sneezing, coughing, red eyes, tearing, thirst, a red and dry tongue, and a floating, rapid pulse.

The premodern Chinese medical tradition contained diverse ideas regarding the cause of measles and similar rashes. Some physicians attributed them to the release of fetal toxins triggered in the course of an external invasion. Others posited the collection of heat in the Lungs and Spleen, or the presence of epidemic seasonal toxins. Contemporary physicians identify the measles virus as one such epidemic toxin that combines with or leads to heat collecting in the Lungs and Stomach. Venting the rash is seen as a way of releasing heat, making it spread out from the muscle layer and interstices toward the skin and exterior, from inside to outside. Heat attacking the Lungs produces fever and chills, headache, sneezing, coughing, and a floating, rapid pulse. Heat attacking the Stomach injures the fluids and produces thirst and a dry, red tongue. The fever and headache will be severe if the heat is not released smoothly, which is reflected in an uneven surfacing of the rash.

Analysis of Formula

The focus of this formula is to enable the expression of rashes in the early stages of measles and similar conditions in order to provide heat toxin with an exit route from the body, while also protecting yin in the interior. The chief herb, Cimicifugae Rhizoma *(shēng má)*, disperses wind in the yang brightness channel, raises the clear yang of the Stomach, and vents rashes. The deputy, Puerariae Radix *(gé gēn)*, disperses and stimulates activity in the superficial levels of the body, thereby unblocking the interstices and pores to help vent the rash; it also raises the fluids to expel heat. The assistant, Glycyrrhizae Radix praeparata *(zhì gān cǎo)*, augments the qi and resolves toxicity, and thereby helps the chief and deputy herbs to clear heat and vent the rash. The substitution of untreated Glycyrrhizae Radix *(gān cǎo)* is common because its ability to resolve toxicity is much greater than that of the honey-fried variety. Paeoniae Radix rubra *(chì sháo)* cools the blood and attacks the problem from the interior. The combination of

Glycyrrhizae Radix *(gān cǎo)* and Paeoniae Radix rubra *(chì sháo)* prevents the dispersing properties of the chief and deputy herbs from injuring the qi and yin.

Commentary

Measles and similar rashes are relatively superficial disorders caused by heat in the Lungs, Stomach, and blood. Drawing out the heat by venting the rash is the most effective method of treatment. Otherwise, the disease will become troublesome or even dangerous. This formula ensures a smooth resolution of early-stage measles and similar rashes. It is also useful when the rash does not develop smoothly.

This formula is representative of how measles and similar rashes were treated prior to the advent of warm pathogen disease theory in the 17th century. In fact, physicians like Ye Tian-Shi and Wu Ju-Tong, who formulated this theory, specifically warned not to use ascending herbs like Puerariae Radix *(gé gēn)* or Cimicifugae Rhizoma *(shēng má)* when treating maculas and papules in the course of warm pathogen diseases. According to warm pathogen disease theory, maculas and papules represent disorders at the nutritive or blood level when the yin fluids have already been damaged. In such cases, moving the qi and fluids toward the exterior would further damage the yin and exacerbate the underlying pathology.

Thus, although the indications for this formula have been expanded by some commentators to include all early-stage feverish diseases, the noted modern physician Pu Fu-Zhou recommends that its use be limited to patients in which the presence of wind-cold in the exterior can be clearly established. In such cases, Pu Fu-Zhou also advises to add Perillae Folium *(zǐ sū yè)*, Saposhnikoviae Radix *(fáng fēng)*, Arctii Fructus *(niú bàng zǐ)*, and Chuanxiong Rhizoma *(chuān xiōng)* to the original formula in order to strengthen its exterior-releasing properties. This advice follows the recommendation by the 18th-century author Wang Fu, who, in *Collectanea of Investigations from the Realm of Medicine*, added coriander and Zingiberis Rhizoma recens *(shēng jiāng)* in order to facilitate the opening of pores and interstices.

Because of the ascending action of its chief ingredients, the formula is also used to treat diarrhea and dysenteric disorders in the early stages of a yang brightness disorder where heat has shifted into the Spleen. This usage was first suggested by Ke Qin, a famous Ming-dynasty commentator on *Discussions of Cold Damage*. He recommends that for diarrhea, one should add herbs that transform dampness, and for dysenteric disorders, herbs that regulate the qi and invigorate the blood.

Comparison

➢ Vs. Lophatherum and Tamarisk Decoction *(zhú yè chēng liǔ tāng)*; see PAGE 44

Biomedical Indications

With the appropriate presentation, this formula may be used to treat a variety of biomedically-defined disorders, primarily those involving rashes such as measles, herpes zoster, herpes simplex, and chickenpox. It has also been used for bacillary dysentery and sinusitis.

Alternate names

Cimicifuga Powder(*shēng má sǎn*) in *Discussion of Emergency Formulas for Pediatric Macules and Rashes*; Cimicifuga Decoction (*shēng má tāng*) in *Book to Safeguard Life Arranged According to Pattern*; Four-Substance Cimicifuga and Kudzu Decoction *(sì wèi shēng má gé gēn tāng)* in *Discussion of Formulas for Pediatric Pox and Rashes*; Calm the Blood Drink *(píng xuè yǐn)* in *Tranquil Hut Collection of Experiential Secret Formulas*; Release the Muscle Layer Decoction *(jiě jī tāng)* in *Formulas of Universal Benefit*; Kudzu and Cimicifuga Decoction *(gé gēn shēng má tāng)* in *Subtle Import of the Jade Key*; Kudzu Decoction *(gé gēn tāng)* in *Wan Family Tradition Jade Tablets on Pox and Rashes*; Cimicifuga Drink *(shēng má yǐn)* in *Complete Collection of Red Water and Dark Pearls*; Dried Kudzu Decoction *(gān gé tāng)* in *Symptom, Cause, Pulse, and Treatment*; Four-Substance Cimicifuga Decoction *(sì wèi shēng má tāng)* in *Great Compendium of Medicine for Sores*

Cautions and Contraindications

Contraindicated for rashes that surface evenly, as this may cause exterior deficiency. Also inappropriate in cases of measles toxin sinking internally with shortness of breath, rough breathing, coughing, and wheezing. Should be used with caution in warm pathogen heat diseases.

Modifications

- To assist venting pathogens from the exterior, add herbs like Menthae haplocalycis Herba *(bò hé)*, Cicadae Periostracum *(chán tuì)*, Schizonepetae Herba *(jīng jiè)*, or Arctii Fructus *(niú bàng zǐ)*.
- To strengthen the heat-clearing and detoxifying properties of the formula, add herbs like Forsythiae Fructus *(lián qiáo)* and Lonicerae Flos *(jīn yín huā)*.
- To regulate and direct Lung qi downward in cases with pronounced cough and wheezing, add herbs like Platycodi Radix *(jié gěng)*, Aurantii Fructus *(zhǐ ké)*, Peucedani Radix *(qián hú)*, and Armeniacae Semen *(xìng rén)*.
- To prevent damage to the fluids by heat toxin, add herbs like Ophiopogonis Radix *(mài mén dōng)* and Radix Adenophorae seu Glehniae *(shā shēn)*.
- For swollen and sore throat, add Platycodi Radix *(jié gěng)*, Scrophulariae Radix *(xuán shēn)*, and Lasiosphaera/Calvatia *(mǎ bó)*.
- If the rash is dark-red, add Arnebiae/Lithospermi Radix *(zǐ cǎo)* and Moutan Cortex *(mǔ dān pí)*.
- For exterior yang brightness-warp disorders characterized by fever, thirst, and dry nasal passages, or for dysenteric diarrhea, substitute Paeoniae Radix alba *(bái sháo)* for Pae-oniae Radix rubra *(chì sháo)*.
- For viral rashes, especially herpes zoster, add Arnebiae/Lithospermi Radix *(zǐ cǎo)*.

Associated Formula

宣毒發表湯（宣毒发表汤）

Dissipate Toxin and Release the Exterior Decoction
xuān dú fā biǎo tāng

SOURCE   *Golden Mirror of the Medical Tradition* (1742)

Cimicifugae Rhizoma *(shēng má)* 3-6g
Puerariae Radix *(gé gēn)* 3-9g
Peucedani Radix *(qián hú)* 3-6g
Armeniacae Semen *(xìng rén)* 6g
Platycodi Radix *(jié gěng)* 3-6g
Aurantii Fructus *(zhǐ ké)* 3g
Schizonepetae Herba *(jīng jiè)* 3g
Saposhnikoviae Radix *(fáng fēng)* 3g
Menthae haplocalycis Herba *(bò hé)* 3g
Akebiae Caulis *(mù tōng)* 3-6g
Forsythiae Fructus *(lián qiáo)* 6g
dry-fried Arctii Fructus *(chǎo niú bàng zǐ)* 6g
dry-fried Lophatheri Herba *(chǎo dàn zhú yè)* 3-6g
Glycyrrhizae Radix *(gān cǎo)* 1.5-3g

Releases the exterior, vents rashes, stops coughing, and improves the functioning of the throat. For early-stage measles in which the surfacing of the rash is blocked, characterized by fever, absence of sweating, cough, sore throat, irritability, thirst, and dark urine. In contrast to the principal formula, this is a stronger, less balanced formula for more severe exterior symptoms with sore throat.

竹葉桎柳湯（竹叶桎柳汤）

Lophatherum and Tamarisk Decoction
zhú yè chēng liǔ tāng

Source   *Extensive Notes on Medicine from the First-Awakened Studio* (1613)

Tamaricis Cacumen *(chēng liǔ)* 15g
Schizonepetae Spica *(jīng jiè suì)* 3g
Puerariae Radix *(gé gēn)* 4.5g
Cicadae Periostracum *(chán tuì)* 3g
Menthae haplocalycis Herba *(bò hé)* 3g
Arctii Fructus *(niú bàng zǐ)* 4.5g
honey-prepared Anemarrhenae Rhizoma *(mì zhì zhī mǔ)* 3g
Scrophulariae Radix *(xuán shēn)* 6g
Glycyrrhizae Radix *(gān cǎo)* 3g
Ophiopogonis Radix *(mài mén dōng)* 9g
Lophatheri Herba *(dàn zhú yè)* 9g

Method of Preparation   Decoction. The source text advises to add 15g of Gypsum fibrosum *(shí gāo)* and one pinch of winter rice if the heat symptoms are severe.

Actions   Releases the exterior, vents rashes, clears heat, and generates fluids

Indications

Early-stage measles, scarlet fever, or similar diseases that present with unevenly distributed rashes, cough, wheezing, nasal obstruction and runny nose, slight chills and a sustained high fever, irritability, a stifling sensation in the chest, restlessness or even confusion, swollen and painful throat, thirst with dryness of the mouth, a thin yellow and dry tongue coating, and a floating, rapid pulse.

This is heat collecting in the Stomach and Lungs due to yang toxins (variously conceived of as fetal toxins, endemic warm pathogen toxins, or the measles virus) that have already damaged the fluids, along with simultaneous obstruction of the exterior by wind-heat. Heat, together with constraint in the exterior, causes slight chills and high fever and prevents the venting of yang toxins and heat to the outside. This becomes visible as a rash that does not surface evenly. Heat collecting in the Lungs obstructs the dissemination and downward-directing of qi, leading to cough, wheezing, nasal obstruction and discharge, and a painful, swollen throat. Heat collecting in the Stomach readily enters the blood and disturbs the spirit, causing irritability, restlessness, confusion, and a stifling sensation in the chest. This heat also damages the fluids, as reflected in thirst along with dry mouth and tongue. The pulse is floating because the protective qi in the exterior is obstructed, and rapid because this obstruction is due to heat that has accumulated in the interior.

Analysis of Formula

To facilitate the complete expression of rashes in early-stage measles and similar disorders, it is important to release the exterior while simultaneously facilitating the venting of toxins to the outside. Tamaricis Cacumen (*chēng liǔ*), the formula's chief herb, is acrid in taste, balanced in temperature, and ascending in action. It enters the yang brightness channel and is used specifically for discharging and dispersing measle-like rashes. Its action is supported by two different deputy herbs. Arctii Fructus (*niú bàng zǐ*) is acrid, cool, and moist. It opens up areas of constraint in the exterior and the Lung collaterals, soothes the throat, resolves toxicity, vents rashes, and stops itching. Lophatheri Herba (*dàn zhú yè*) clears heat from the Heart via the urine. It thereby eliminates irritability but without damaging the fluids, and prevents heat toxins from sinking into the Pericardium. The various assistant herbs support the actions of these three herbs. Puerariae Radix (*gé gēn*), Cicadae Periostracum (*chán tuì*), Schizonepetae Spica (*jīng jiè suì*), and Menthae haplocalycis Herba (*bò hé*) release the exterior, disperse fire from constraint, and facilitate the venting of toxins. Anemarrhenae Rhizoma (*zhī mǔ*), Scrophulariae Radix (*xuán shēn*), and Ophiopogonis Radix (*mài mén dōng*) drain heat from the interior, generate fluids, and thereby facilitate the venting of toxin from the nutritive into the qi and protective qi aspects. Glycyrrhizae Radix (*gān cǎo*) clears heat, resolves toxicity, and harmonizes the actions of the other herbs in the formula.

The addition of Gypsum fibrosum (*shí gāo*) and winter rice for severe cases is patterned on White Tiger Decoction (*bái hǔ tāng*) and is intended to protect the fluids from damage by qi level heat.

Commentary

The author of this formula is Miao Xi-Yong, who lived in southern China during the late Ming dynasty. His works strongly influenced the thinking of chief proponents of warm pathogen disease theory, like Ye Tian-Shi. The development of the present formula is a prime example of the transition from cold damage to warm pathogen therapeutics that took place during the Ming. In his writings, Miao Xi-Yong claims to have had good results in treating wheezing caused by heat pathogens clogging the Lungs using Lophatherum and Gypsum Decoction (*zhú yè shí gāo tāng*)—a heat-clearing formula from *Discussion of Cold Damage*, discussed in more detail in Chapter 4—to which he added Scrophulariae Radix (*xuán shēn*), Menthae haplocalycis Herba (*bò hé*), and Tamaricis Cacumen (*chēng liǔ*). As measle-like rashes, too, were thought to be caused by heat collecting in the Lungs, adapting the formula to this purpose was a logical next step.

Miao Xi-Yong described the treatment strategy underlying the composition of his new formula as "[combining] acrid cold, sweet cold, and bitter cold herbs to raise out and discharge [rashes]." Two generations later, Ye Tian-Shi recommended the use of acrid cool herbs like Menthae haplocalycis Herba (*bò hé*) and Arctii Fructus (*niú bàng zǐ*) in order to vent heat from the protective level and prevent it from sinking into the Pericardium. He emphasized that augmenting the Stomach in order to protect the fluids was the key to treating warm pathogen diseases at the qi level. And when wind-heat pathogens threatened to enter into the nutritive level, he used Lophatheri Herba (*dàn zhú yè*) as one of the main herbs for clearing this heat and suggested that it be combined with herbs to cool the blood and nourish the fluids. All of these strategies are represented in the present formula, which thus embodies much of Ye Tian-Shi's theory of warm pathogen heat diseases before the theory formally existed.

Comparisons

➢ Vs. Cimicifuga and Kudzu Decoction
  (*shēng má gé gēn tāng*)

This formula is a good example of how one might treat early-stage measles and similar disorders from a warm pathogen rather than the cold damage disorder perspective used in Cimicifuga and Kudzu Decoction (*shēng má gé gēn tāng*). In both cases, it is essential to disperse constraint in the exterior in order to facilitate the complete venting of heat toxin from the Lungs and Stomach. However, where a newly-contracted warm pathogen combines with lurking heat toxins in the interior, it is just as important to also protect the fluids and to prevent the adverse possibility of heat sinking into the Pericardium. This is achieved through the addition of bitter, cold herbs that clear qi-aspect heat and sweet, cold herbs that nourish the fluids.

Biomedical Indications

With the appropriate presentation, this formula may be used to treat a variety of biomedically-defined disorders marked by rashes including measles, chicken pox, and herpes.

Alternate names

Bamboo Leaf and Gypsum Decoction (*zhú yè shí gāo tāng*) in *Selected Annotations to Ancient Formulas from the Garden of Crimson Snow*

Cautions and Contraindications

Because of the strong heat-clearing properties of this formula, it should only be used where heat from excess is actively damaging the fluids. For this purpose, it contains bitter, cold, and sweet herbs that inhibit the qi dynamic. This may prevent the venting of toxins and rashes to the outside, if prescribed inappropriately. In cases with less heat, one might use Honeysuckle and Forsythia Powder (*yín qiáo sǎn*) with the addition of Cicadae Periostracum (*chán tuì*) and Isatidis Folium (*dà qīng yè*).

Modifications

- For severe coughing and wheezing, add Eriobotryae Folium (*pí pá yè*), Peucedani Radix (*qián hú*), and Cynanchi stauntonii Rhizoma (*bái qián*) to disseminate the Lung qi and stop coughing.

- For inflammation of the throat with severe pain and swelling, add Isatidis Radix (*bǎn lán gēn*) and Isatidis Folium (*dà qīng yè*) to clear the heat and resolve toxins.

- For dark red rashes, indicating that heat has entered the blood aspect, add Moutan Cortex (*mǔ dān pí*) and Paeoniae Radix rubra (*chì sháo*) to cool and invigorate the blood.

- For severe qi-aspect heat with sweating and thirst, add Gypsum fibrosum (*shí gāo*) and Forsythiae Fructus (*lián qiáo*) to clear the heat and resolve toxins.

荊芥連翹湯（荆芥连翘汤）
Schizonepeta and Forsythia Decoction

jīng jiè lián qiáo tāng

Source *Wondrous Lantern for Peering into the Origin and Development of Miscellaneous Diseases* (1773)

Schizonepetae Herba (*jīng jiè*) 3g
Forsythiae Fructus (*lián qiáo*). 3g
Saposhnikoviae Radix (*fáng fēng*). 3g
Angelicae sinensis Radix (*dāng guī*) 3g
Chuanxiong Rhizoma (*chuān xiōng*) 3g
Paeoniae Radix alba (*bái sháo*) .3g
Bupleuri Radix (*chái hú*) 3g
Aurantii Fructus (*zhǐ ké*) 3g
Scutellariae Radix (*huáng qín*) .3g
Gardeniae Fructus (*zhī zǐ*). 3g
Angelicae dahuricae Radix (*bái zhǐ*). 3g
Platycodi Radix (*jié gěng*) 3g
Glycyrrhizae Radix (*gān cǎo*) .1.5g

Preparation The amounts listed above are from a modern textbook and are an interpretation of the ratios listed in *Restoration of Health from the Myriad Diseases*. The source text prescribes 2g (7 *fēn*) of each herb, with 1.5g (5 *fēn*) of Glycyrrhizae Radix (*gān cǎo*). The formula is taken as a decoction.

Actions Dispels wind, clears heat, disperses stagnation, and resolves toxicity

Indications

Wind-heat patterns that give rise to symptoms such as earache, rhinitis, tonsillitis, and nosebleeds. The formula is also used in dermatology to treat the acute stage of facial acne and other upper-body toxic swellings.

Analysis of Formula

While the source text does not explicitly divide the ingredients by rank, we can deduce that the chief herbs in this formula are Schizonepetae Herba (*jīng jiè*) and Forsythiae Fructus (*lián qiáo*). Together, they release pathogens from the exterior and dispel wind. Forsythiae Fructus (*lián qiáo*) also clears heat, resolves toxicity, and disperses the accumulation of toxin. These herbs direct the main function of the formula to the body's exterior. Two of the deputies, Paeoniae Radix alba (*bái sháo*) and Bupleuri Radix (*chái hú*), which are the core of Frigid Extremities Powder (*sì nì sǎn*), help the formula treat heat disorders that center around the lesser yang channels. The other two deputies, Scutellariae Radix (*huáng qín*) and Gardeniae Fructus (*zhī zǐ*), help the chief herbs clear heat and resolve toxicity. Given the context of this formula, their focus is near the surface of the body.

Two of the assistants, Chuanxiong Rhizoma (*chuān xiōng*) and Angelicae sinensis Radix (*dāng guī*), move and nourish the blood and are used here because sores tax the blood and disrupt its flow. The other assistants are Angelicae dahuricae Radix (*bái zhǐ*), Platycodi Radix (*jié gěng*), and Aurantii Fructus (*zhǐ ké*), which disperse accumulations and thrust out pus. The envoy is Glycyrrhizae Radix (*gān cǎo*), which harmonizes the effects of the other ingredients.

In summary, this formula disperses wind and clears heat and stagnation from the Liver channel, thrusts out pus, releases wind-heat from the exterior, and resolves toxicity. Its upward nature tracks to the head and neck and is thus best suited for toxic heat patterns that affect the upper body.

Commentary

In the source text, this combination of herbs is intended to treat wind-heat attacking the upper body and giving rise to swelling and pain in the ear. *Restoration of Health from the Myriad Diseases* suggests that this combination be used to treat wind-heat in the Kidney channel that results in pain and swelling in the ears. Inclusion of Frigid Extremities Powder (*sì nì sǎn*), however, implies involvement of the Liver and Gallbladder. Since those channels circumscribe the ear, it is not uncommon for them to be included in the treatment of ear disorders.

Both the source text and *Restoration of Health from the Myriad Diseases* mention this formula for pain and swelling in the ears; ear infections are thus the most common disorder that this formula is called upon to treat. Still, it is also used in the treatment of nasal polyps, nosebleed, tonsillitis, and other upper body inflammatory disorders.

Restoration of Health from the Myriad Diseases also mentions a modified version of this formula, adding Menthae haplocalycis Herba (*bò hé*) and Rehmanniae Radix (*shēng dì huáng*). This is intended to treat "patients with deep-source nasal congestion [as a result of] Gallbladder heat that has shifted to the brain." This is a use of the formula that directly draws on its Frigid Extremities Powder (*sì nì sǎn*) ingredients to guide the formula's heat-clearing agents to the Liver-Gallbladder. Deep-source nasal congestion is recognized nowadays as overlapping significantly with the biomedical disorders of chronic rhinitis and sinusitis.

Because it contains several agents to release pathogens from the exterior, Schizonepeta and Forsythia Decoction (*jīng jiè lián qiáo tāng*) is ideal for treating the above conditions when they occur during the course of a wind-heat exterior pattern. If the symptoms of an exterior pattern have subsided or do not exist, Schizonepetae Herba (*jīng jiè*) can be removed or reduced, thus making the formula more suitable for treating the internal pattern.

Aside from clearing heat, resolving toxicity, moving blood, and releasing pathogens from the exterior, the formula also contains Angelicae dahuricae Radix (*bái zhǐ*) and Platycodi Radix (*jié gěng*) to thrust out pus, Saposhnikoviae Radix (*fáng fēng*) and Schizonepetae Herba (*jīng jiè*) to bring the actions of the formula to the skin, and Forsythiae Fructus (*lián qiáo*) to disperse accumulation of heat toxin. Thus, Schizonepeta and Forsythia Decoction (*jīng jiè lián qiáo tāng*) also treats suppurating skin disorders of the upper body such as the acute phase of facial acne or toxic swellings on the chest, upper back, neck, or head.

Comparisons

➢ Vs. Coptis Pill to Clear the Upper [Burner] (*huáng lián shàng qīng wán*) and Clear the Upper [Burner] Decoction with Saposhnikovia (*qīng shàng fáng fēng tāng*)

All these formulas address pus-producing infections in the upper body. Schizonepeta and Forsythia Decoction (*jīng jiè lián qiáo tāng*) is the mildest of the three. Because it contains Angelicae sinensis Radix (*dāng guī*) and Paeoniae Radix alba (*bái sháo*), it is better for weaker patients and relatively long-standing disorders. Coptis Pill to Clear the Upper [Burner] (*huáng lián shàng qīng wán*) is the most bitter and cold of the three, and is best for treating extremely hot and acute conditions.

Cautions and Contraindications

This formula contains herbs that drain and disperse qi and is thus for short-term use only. In addition, for patients with deficiency patterns, the formula must be modified to avoid injuring the qi and blood.

Modifications

- For acute middle ear infections, add Paeoniae Radix rubra (*chì sháo*) and Puerariae Radix (*gé gēn*) and increase the dosage of Scutellariae Radix (*huáng qín*).

- For sore throat or tonsillitis, add Isatidis/Baphicacanthis Radix (*bǎn lán gēn*), Lasiosphaera/Calvatia (*mǎ bó*), or Paridis Rhizoma (*chóng lóu*).

- For rhinitis or sinusitis, add Puerariae Radix (*gé gēn*), Xanthii Fructus (*cāng ěr zǐ*), and Magnoliae Flos (*xīn yí*). Also, include Menthae haplocalycis Herba (*bò hé*) and Rehmanniae Radix (*shēng dì huáng*) as per *Restoration of Health from the Myriad Diseases*.

- For facial acne or other toxic swellings, add Hedyotis diffusae Herba (*bái huā shé shé cǎo*) and Taraxaci Herba (*pú gōng yīng*).

Section 4

· ·

FORMULAS THAT RELEASE EXTERIOR DISORDERS WITH INTERIOR DEFICIENCY

The formulas in this section address those cases in which a person suffering from interior deficiency contracts a disease of external origin and where the ensuing disorder is characterized by symptoms of both excess and deficiency. The complexity of these disease patterns requires the use of formulas that are themselves complex, in that they combine herbs that release the excess from the exterior with herbs that tonify the deficiency in the interior. This is one example of using the method of supporting the normal with dispelling the pathogen (扶正祛邪 *fú zhèng qū xié*). With the exception of the patterns discussed here, these two classes of herbs would rarely be used together; tonifying herbs are ordinarily contraindicated for exterior conditions, as are exterior-releasing herbs in cases of interior deficiency.

The particular formulation of herbs in these prescriptions is based on whether the underlying deficiency is one of qi, blood, yin, or yang. Qi and yang deficient patients will tend to be those invaded by wind, cold, and dampness. For this reason, formulas that treat these conditions combine acrid, warming herbs that disperse pathogens from the exterior such as Ephedrae Herba (má huáng), Notopterygii Rhizoma seu Radix (qiāng huó), Saposhnikoviae Radix (fáng fēng), or Perillae Folium (zǐ sū yè) with qi tonics such as Astragali Radix (huáng qí) and Ginseng Radix (rén shēn), or herbs that warm the interior such as Aconiti Radix lateralis praeparata (fù zǐ) and Asari Radix et Rhizoma (xì xīn). Blood and yin deficient patients, on the other hand, are more prone to invasion by wind-heat, or if wind-cold invades, require strategies that do not emphasize sweating as this would further damage the essences. For that reason, the formulas used to treat such patterns combine herbs that enrich the yin and nourish the blood, such as Rehmanniae Radix (shēng dì huáng), Ophiopogonis Radix (mài mén dōng), and Polygonati odorati Rhizoma (yù zhú), with acrid, cooling, or slightly warming herbs that gently vent pathogens from the exterior, such as Menthae haplocalycis Herba (bò hé), Sojae Semen praeparatum (dàn dòu chǐ), or Allii fistulosi Bulbus (cōng bái).

人參敗毒散 (人参败毒散)

Ginseng Powder to Overcome Pathogenic Influences

rén shēn bài dú sǎn

The word 毒 *dú* in the name of this formula, although generally rendered as toxin, refers here to externally-contracted pathogenic influences. The name suggests the ability of this formula to strengthen the normal qi and thereby enable the body to overcome pathogenic influences.

Source *Craft of Medicines and Patterns for Children* (1119)

Notopterygii Rhizoma seu Radix (qiāng huó) 30g
Angelicae pubescentis Radix (dú huó) 30g
Chuanxiong Rhizoma (chuān xiōng) .30g
Bupleuri Radix (chái hú) 30g
Platycodi Radix (jié gěng) 30g
bran-fried Aurantii Fructus (fū chǎo zhǐ ké) 30g
Peucedani Radix (qián hú) 30g
Ginseng Radix (rén shēn) 30g
Poria (fú líng) 30g
Glycyrrhizae Radix (gān cǎo) 15g

Method of Preparation The source text advises to grind the ingredients into a fine powder and cook 6g together with a small amount of Zingiberis Rhizoma recens (shēng jiāng) and Menthae haplocalycis Herba (bò hé). Codonopsis Radix (dǎng shēn) is usually substituted for Ginseng Radix (rén shēn) at 2-3 times its dosage. At present, this formula is often prepared as a decoction, with the dosage of the ingredients reduced by about 80 percent.

Actions Releases the exterior, dispels wind and dampness, and augments the qi

Indications

High fever accompanied by severe chills and shivering, absence of sweating, pain and stiffness of the head and neck, soreness and pain of the extremities, focal distention and fullness of the chest, nasal congestion with sonorous breathing, a productive cough, a greasy, white tongue coating, and a floating, soggy pulse.

This is externally-contracted wind-cold-dampness battling the body's deficient normal qi, which is unable to expel the pathogenic influences. This produces a high fever, severe chills with shivering, an absence of sweating, and pain and stiffness of the head and neck. Lingering dampness causes focal distention and fullness in the chest. The deficiency of qi allows dampness to penetrate rather quickly, producing a greasy, white tongue coating. (If the qi were strong, the tongue coating would remain thin and white.) The attack of wind-cold on the Lungs disrupts the circulation of qi, causing nasal congestion, sonorous breathing, and a productive cough. The presence of wind, cold, and dampness at the level of the muscles produces generalized soreness and pain and a floating pulse. The floating, soggy quality of the pulse reflects the deficiency of qi, which is the salient aspect of this disorder.

Analysis of Formula

The herbs in this formula reflect the twin strategies of expelling the pathogenic influences and strengthening the deficient qi. Because the formula is designed for acute, externally-contracted disorders, the emphasis is on expelling the pathogenic influences.

The chief herbs, Notopterygii Rhizoma seu Radix (qiāng huó) and Angelicae pubescentis Radix (dú huó), dispel wind-cold from the exterior, dispel dampness, and alleviate pain. These herbs address the primary symptoms of fever and chills without sweating, headache, and generalized pain and soreness. Chuanxiong Rhizoma (chuān xiōng), one of the deputies, helps the chief herbs release the exterior, moves the blood, and dispels wind, which enhances the pain-relieving action of the formula, especially in the head and neck. The other deputies, Bupleuri Radix (chái hú) and Menthae haplocalycis Herba (bò hé), release the exterior, reduce the fever, and expel the pathogenic influences. Together, they are particularly effective in releasing pathogenic influences from the muscle layer.

The ascending action of Platycodi Radix (jié gěng) and the descending action of Aurantii Fructus (zhǐ ké) is a very effective combination for regulating the flow of qi in the chest, thereby relieving the symptoms of discomfort in the chest. These two herbs also interact with Peucedani Radix (qián hú) to improve the circulation of Lung qi, expel phlegm, and stop the coughing. The phlegm that collects in the Lungs is produced in the Spleen. For this reason, Peucedani Radix (qián hú) is used with Poria (fú líng), which transforms phlegm and strengthens the Spleen, and Zingiberis Rhizoma recens (shēng jiāng) to treat both the branch and root of this disorder. Zingiberis Rhizoma recens (shēng jiāng) also helps release the exterior. All of these herbs serve as assistants.

The tonifying herbs in this formula include Ginseng Radix (rén shēn), Poria (fú líng), and Glycyrrhizae Radix (gān cǎo). These are three of the four herbs in Four-Gentlemen Decoction (sì jūn zǐ tāng), discussed in Chapter 8. Ginseng Radix (rén shēn), an assistant, serves three functions here: it strengthens the normal qi to expel the pathogenic influences, generates fluids so that sweating becomes possible, and strengthens the body's resistance to invasion, which prevents a relapse. Another assistant, Poria (fú líng), leaches out dampness, promotes urination, transforms phlegm, and strengthens the Spleen. It tonifies without causing stagnation or retention of pathogenic influences, unlike the tonic herb Atractylodis macrocephalae Rhizoma (bái zhú). The envoy, Glycyrrhizae Radix (gān cǎo), assists Ginseng Radix (rén shēn) in tonifying the qi, and also harmonizes the actions of the other ingredients.

Commentary

This formula was originally devised for children suffering from externally-contracted wind-cold-dampness. Because the source qi in children is not fully developed, a strategy was required that would tonify the qi in order to expel the pathogenic influences. Later, the application of this formula was expanded to include all cases of wind-cold-dampness in patients with underlying qi deficiency and phlegm-dampness obstructing the qi dynamic, including the elderly, postpartum women, and those recovering from a debilitating illness.

Controversies

Most of the debate surrounding this formula has focused on the precise function of Ginseng Radix (rén shēn). Its use in formulas designed to expel external pathogens can be traced back to several formulas in Discussion on Cold Damage, including Cinnamon Twig and Ginseng Decoction (guì zhī rén shēn tāng) and Minor Bupleurum Decoction (xiǎo chái hú tāng). However, whereas the role of Ginseng Radix (rén shēn) in these formulas is generally regarded as merely strengthening the source qi and the middle burner, influential Qing-era physicians like Yu Chang, Zhang Lu, and Zhang Bing-Cheng

extended its role here to include the active enhancement of the function of the chief ingredients in pushing pathogens back to the outside. Wu Ju-Tong, the famous systematizer of warm pathogen disease therapeutics, even went so far as to designate Ginseng Radix (rén shēn) as the chief herb in this formula. However, these interpretations were criticized by Fei Bo-Xiong, who generally favored ordering the qi dynamic in all disorders, and therefore viewed Ginseng Radix (rén shēn) as addressing any deficiency.

A clear and useful understanding of the formula is provided by Zhao Yu-Huang in Discussion of Famous Physicians' Formulas Past and Present. He thought of this formula as a complement to Nine-Herb Decoction with Notopterygium (jiǔ wèi qiāng huó tāng), discussed earlier in this chapter. Both formulas were composed during the same period, have the same chief herb, and treat an invasion of wind-cold-dampness or unseasonable qi that relies on sweating in order to expel the pathogen. Zhao Yu-Huang notes that such sweating can only be produced if the body has sufficient fluids and qi. Nine-Herb Decoction with Notopterygium (jiǔ wèi qiāng huó tāng) uses Rehmanniae Radix (shēng dì huáng) to increase the fluids where they are deficient. The present formula similarly employs Ginseng Radix (rén shēn) to tonify the qi.

The Qing physician Yu Chang extended the indication of this formula to treat early-stage, wind-cold-damp dysenteric disorders with exterior symptoms, which he believed were caused by a sinking of the pathogenic influences into the Intestines. This approach, known as 'hauling the boat upstream' (nì liú wǎn zhōu 逆流挽舟), remains popular today, but at the time represented a major departure from standard practice. Unlike diarrhea, which is a pathology of middle burner qi transformation, dysenteric disorders are thought to be due to pathogens (mainly damp-heat toxin) obstructing the flow of qi in the Intestines. The preferred treatment strategy for resolving this pathology is to follow the inherent dynamic of the disorder (where pathogens move inward and downward) and the physiology of the organ systems involved (the qi of the bowels moves downward) by draining the damp-heat and regulating the qi and blood. Yu Chang's approach moves in the opposite direction, employing herbs that are ascending and that dispel pathogens from the surface. This ascending movement is what 'hauling the boat upstream' refers to.

Examined more closely, however, Yu Chang's treatment strategy also facilitates the physiological movement of qi in the Intestines by removing obstruction from both the Lungs (tied to the Large Intestine via an interior/exterior relationship) and the qi dynamic. It represents a further development in an approach to the treatment of early-stage dysenteric disorders already embodied in Kudzu Decoction (gé gēn tāng), which stops diarrhea by dispelling pathogens from the exterior of the greater yang and yang brightness channels. Both formulas treat early-stage dysentery characterized by fever and chills. However, Kudzu Decoction (*gé gēn tāng*) supplements the fluids and stops spasms in the bowels, and is thus indicated where wind symptoms predominate. Ginseng Powder to Overcome Pathogenic Influences (*rén shēn bài dú sǎn*), on the other hand, opens the qi dynamic and promotes water metabolism and is thus indicated where dampness predominates.

The principal formula is also used for very early-stage measles (before the rash has begun to surface) characterized by moderate fever and chills, no significant thirst, loose stools, a white tongue coating, and a thin, weak pulse. The modern physician Yue Mei-Zhong has extended this application and uses the formula in the treatment of deep-seated sores and boils in cases with qi deficiency.

Biomedical Indications

With the appropriate presentation, this formula may be used to treat a variety of biomedically-defined disorders, primarily acute infections, including the common cold, influenza, mumps, bronchitis, dysentery, and the early stages of boils. It has also been used for allergic dermatitis, urticaria, and eczema.

....

Alternate names

Overcome Pathogenic Influences Powder (*bài dú sǎn*) in *Book to Safeguard Life Arranged According to Pattern*; Notopterygium Decoction (*qiāng huó tāng*) in *Comprehensive Recording of Sagely Beneficence*; Ten Season Decoction (*shí shí tāng*) in *Comprehensive Recording of Sagely Beneficence*; Ginseng and Peucedanum Powder (*rén shēn qián hú sàn*) in *Jing-Feng's Formulas of Universal Formulas of Universal Benefit*

....

Cautions and Contraindications

Because of the warm, drying properties of many of the ingredients, it is important to remember that this formula is indicated only for externally-contracted wind-cold-dampness and is contraindicated for cases due to heat or damp-heat.

Modifications

- If the normal qi is not weak and exterior cold symptoms are very pronounced, remove Ginseng Radix (*rén shēn*) and add Schizonepetae Herba (*jīng jiè*) and Saposhnikoviae Radix (*fáng fēng*) or use the associated formula Schizonepeta and Saposhnikovia Powder to Overcome Pathogenic Influences (*jīng fáng bài dú sǎn*).
- If qi deficiency is severe, increase the dosage of Ginseng Radix (*rén shēn*) or add Astragali Radix (*huáng qí*).
- If dampness obstructs the muscle layer with pronounced aching, soreness, and pain in the muscles and joints, add Clematidis Radix (*wēi líng xiān*), Mori Ramulus (*sāng zhī*), Gentianae macrophyllae Radix (*qín jiāo*), or Stephaniae tetrandrae Radix (*hàn fáng jǐ*).

- If coughing is severe, add Armeniacae Semen (*xìng rén*) and Cynanchi stauntonii Rhizoma (*bái qián*).
- For malarial disorders, increase the dosage of Bupleuri Radix (*chái hú*) and add Scutellariae Radix (*huáng qín*) and Arecae Semen (*bīng láng*).
- For dysenteric disorders characterized by abdominal pain, blood or pus in the stools, and tenesmus, add Aucklandiae Radix (*mù xiāng*) and Paeoniae Radix alba (*bái sháo*).
- For wind toxin dormant papules, add Cicadae Periostracum (*chán tuì*) and Sophorae flavescentis Radix (*kǔ shēn*).
- For early-stage sores, remove Ginseng Radix (*rén shēn*) and add Forsythiae Fructus (*lián qiáo*) and Lonicerae Flos (*jīn yín huā*).

Variations

銀翹敗毒散 （银翘败毒散）

Honeysuckle and Forsythia Powder to Overcome Pathogenic Influences

yín qiáo bài dú sǎn

SOURCE *Medical Formulas Collected and Analyzed* (1682)

Add Lonicerae Flos (*jīn yín huā*) and Forsythiae Fructus (*lián qiáo*) for early-stage abscesses and sores which are red, swollen, and painful accompanied by symptoms of an exterior condition.

Associated Formulas

荊防敗毒散 （荆防败毒散）

Schizonepeta and Saposhnikovia Powder to Overcome Pathogenic Influences

jīng fáng bài dú sǎn

SOURCE *Multitude of Marvelous Formulas for Sustaining Life* (1550)

Schizonepetae Herba (*jīng jiè*)	4.5g
Saposhnikoviae Radix (*fáng fēng*)	4.5g
Bupleuri Radix (*chái hú*)	4.5g
Peucedani Radix (*qián hú*)	4.5g
Chuanxiong Rhizoma (*chuān xiōng*)	4.5g
Notopterygii Rhizoma seu Radix (*qiāng huó*)	4.5g
Angelicae pubescentis Radix (*dú huó*)	4.5g
Poria (*fú líng*)	4.5g
Platycodi Radix (*jié gěng*)	4.5g
Aurantii Fructus (*zhǐ ké*)	4.5g
Glycyrrhizae Radix (*gān cǎo*)	1.5g
Zingiberis Rhizoma recens (*shēng jiāng*)	3 pieces

Grind the ingredients into powder and take as a draft, usually with the addition of 1.5-3g of Menthae haplocalycis Herba (*bò hé*). Induces sweating, releases the exterior, dispels wind, and alleviates pain. For externally-contracted wind-cold-dampness characterized by fever and chills without sweating, pain and stiffness of the head and neck, generalized body aches and pain, a thin, white tongue coating, and a floating pulse. This is a more severe presentation than that for which the principal formula is indicated, and occurs in those with no underlying qi deficiency. Also for early-stage abscesses or sores that are red, swollen, and painful and accompanied by fever, chills, absence of sweating, thirst, a thin white tongue coating, and a floating, rapid pulse.

Comparison

➤ Vs. Support the Interior and Eliminate Toxin Drink (tuō lǐ xiāo dú yǐn); see page 868

_____

參蘇飲 (参苏饮)

Ginseng and Perilla Leaf Drink

shēn sū yǐn

Source　*Formulary of the Pharmacy Service for Benefiting the People in the Taiping Era* (1107)

Ginseng Radix (rén shēn). 22.5g
Perillae Folium (zǐ sū yè) 22.5g
Puerariae Radix (gé gēn) 22.5g
ginger-fried Pinelliae Rhizoma praeparatum (jiāng bàn xià). . . .22.5g
Peucedani Radix (qián hú) 22.5g
Poria (fú líng) 22.5g
Aucklandiae Radix (mù xiāng). 15g
bran-fried Aurantii Fructus (fū chǎo zhǐ ké) 15g
Platycodi Radix (jié gěng) 15g
Glycyrrhizae Radix praeparata (zhì gān cǎo) 15g

The source text advises to grind the ingredients into a coarse powder and cook 12g with 7 pieces of Zingiberis Rhizoma recens (shēng jiāng) and 1 piece of Jujubae Fructus (dà zǎo). At present, it is prepared as a decoction with a proportionate reduction in dosage and with the addition of 3 pieces of Zingiberis Rhizoma recens (shēng jiāng) and 3 pieces of Jujubae Fructus (dà zǎo).

Augments the qi, releases the exterior, harmonizes the Stomach, and transforms phlegm. For externally-contracted wind-cold with phlegm and thin mucus in the interior in patients with a qi deficient constitution, characterized by fever and chills, headache, nasal congestion, productive cough, stifling sensation in the chest, a white tongue coating, and a frail pulse. Compared to Ginseng Powder to Overcome Pathogenic Influences (rén shēn bài dú sǎn), this formula treats patterns with more pronounced qi deficiency and obstruction of the qi dynamic by phlegm and thin mucus.

Comparison

➤ Vs. Apricot Kernel and Perilla Leaf Powder (xìng sū sǎn); see page 664

麻黃細辛附子湯 (麻黄细辛附子汤)

Ephedra, Asarum, and Aconite Accessory Root Decoction

má huáng xì xīn fù zǐ tāng

Source　*Discussion of Cold Damage* (c. 220)

Ephedrae Herba (má huáng). 6g
Aconiti Radix lateralis praeparata (zhì fù zǐ) 9g
Asari Radix et Rhizoma (xì xīn). 6g

Method of Preparation　The source text advises to first decoct Ephedrae Herba (má huáng) in about 10 cups of water until 8 cups remain. Remove the froth, add the other ingredients, and cook until 3 cups remain. The strained decoction is taken warm in 3 doses over the course of a day. At present, Aconiti Radix lateralis praeparata (zhì fù zǐ) is cooked for 30-60 minutes (at least until there is no numbing of the tongue upon tasting), and then the other ingredients are added to the decoction.

Actions　Assists the yang and releases the exterior

Indications

Slight fever with severe chills that is not relieved by wearing more clothing or adding covers, exhaustion with an almost constant desire to sleep, and a submerged, faint pulse.

This is exterior cold in a patient with preexisting yang deficiency. In terms of the six warps of disease, this is a simultaneous greater yang (exterior cold) and lesser yin (interior yang deficiency) warp disorder. A sensation of extreme cold may be attributed to either internal cold or externally-contracted wind-cold. In this case, the presence of fever indicates an externally-contracted pathogenic influence. The chills are due to both interior cold (which in other circumstances can be reduced by adding layers of clothes) and exterior cold (for which additional layers are of no use). Normally, people with yang deficiency have a hard time staying warm, much less developing a fever; the presence of even a slight fever here is evidence of externally-contracted wind-cold. However, the pulse in an exterior condition should be floating; here it is submerged, which (along with the exhaustion and desire to sleep) shows that the interior is deficient.

Analysis of Formula

Wind-cold in the exterior is treated by sweating. However, in cases of yang deficiency, the use of this method readily leads to devastated yang because sweating also disperses the already deficient yang in the exterior. Therefore, the appropriate strategy in such cases is to combine discharging the exterior (greater yang) with assisting the yang in the interior (lesser yin). For this reason, the chief herb is warm, acrid Ephedrae Herba (má huáng), which induces sweating, releases the exterior, and disperses cold. The deputy is the very acrid and warm Aconiti Radix lateralis praeparata (zhì fù zǐ), which warms the Kidneys and assists the yang. This is an excellent pairing for this condition because, in the interior, Aconiti Radix lateralis praeparata (zhì fù zǐ) activates the yang qi to help it push out the pathogen, while in the exterior, Ephedrae Herba (má huáng) opens up the skin and pores so that the pathogen can be dispersed. The Qing-dynasty physician Ke Qin cogently summed up the interaction between these two herbs:

Ephedrae Herba *(má huáng)* opens the pores and interstices. … Without Aconiti Radix lateralis praeparata *(fù zǐ)* securing the primal qi, the fluids [stored by] the lesser yin would be extruded and the weak yang of the greater yang would be totally lost to the outside. How could the end of life be far away? Only if Ephedrae Herba *(má huáng)* and Aconiti Radix lateralis praeparata *(fù zǐ)* are employed together can one succeed in regulating both the interior and exterior in such a manner that wind-cold is dispersed while yang naturally returns [to its source], that essence is stored and yin is not troubled.

The assistant, Asari Radix et Rhizoma *(xì xīn)*, helps the chief herb to release the exterior, and the deputy herb to scatter interior cold. It also serves as the envoy by entering the lesser yin Kidney channel where it helps focus the actions of the formula on the lesser yin-warp symptoms.

Together, these three herbs tonify in the midst of discharging and discharge in the midst of tonifying. This allows the wind-cold pathogens in the exterior to be dispersed and the interior yang qi to be protected. In this way, the externally-contracted disease in a patient with underlying yang deficiency can be treated effectively, which makes this the classic formula for treating cold in both the exterior and the interior.

Commentary

Key Indicators

Exhaustion, slight fever and severe chills, and a submerged pulse have traditionally been defined as the chief indications for this formula. The modern physician Wang Yi-Yi extends this list to six key signs and symptoms that signal the use of Ephedra, Asarum, and Aconite Accessory Root Decoction *(má huáng xì xīn fù zǐ tāng)* in the clinic:

1. Soreness, aching, and chills in the lower back
2. Generalized chills or cold extremities
3. Chills and fever, or simultaneous cold and heat signs and symptoms, with cold being predominant
4. A sensation of cold in the exterior of the body
5. A pale and puffy tongue that often has indentations, and a white or wet and greasy coating
6. A submerged pulse

The simultaneous occurrence of external cold and internal yang depletion that underlies these signs and symptoms gives rise to a wide variety of problems, and thus the use of this formula has accordingly been extended to many different internal medicine disorders. According to *Indispensable Tools for Pattern Treatment*, for instance, this formula can be used in treating Kidney coughing characterized by pain penetrating to the back, or cold attacking the brain and teeth, where it causes headache and toothache.

Expanded Usage

In *Treatment Strategies and Formulas in Chinese Medicine*, Chen Chao-Zu, a contemporary writer from Chengdu, prescribes this formula for edema due to constraint of the protective qi, which impairs the Lung function of disseminating and directing downward, and causes the Kidney yang (the source of the protective qi) to weaken and become sluggish. This can be viewed as a disorder of both the greater yang and lesser yin, or as a disorder of both the Lungs and Kidneys. Ephedrae Herba *(má huáng)* focuses on disseminating the Lung qi and directing it downward; Aconiti Radix lateralis praeparata *(zhì fù zǐ)* fortifies the Kidney yang so that it can transform the pathogenic water that is stopped internally; and Asari Radix et Rhizoma *(xì xīn)* unblocks both the exterior and the interior, both above and below. Chen also recommends this formula for treating obstruction of the body's orifices and disorders of the sensory orifices, as well as throat obstruction arising from combined Lung and Heart disorders. For the same reasons, the formula may also be used for headache due to cold deficiency with sore throat and a raspy voice, laryngitis, and chronic coughing or wheezing. Modern Chinese physicians use it to treat skin disorders, allergies, arthritis, connective tissue disorders, and diseases of the blood vessels and nerves, including sick sinus syndrome.

Dosage

Note that the dosage of Asari Radix et Rhizoma *(xì xīn)* in this formula is twice as high as the maximum dosage of 3g generally recommended in the materia medica. Although the source text advises to boil Asari Radix et Rhizoma *(xì xīn)* together with the other herbs, many modern physicians only add it during the last 5 minutes of boiling to prevent excessive loss of the volatile oils on which much of the pharmacological action of this herb is based.

Comparison

➤ Vs. Renewal Powder *(zài zào sǎn)*; *see* page 53

➤ Vs. Rhubarb and Aconite Accessory Root Decoction *(dà huáng fù zǐ tāng)*; *see* page 73

Biomedical Indications

With the appropriate presentation, this formula may be used to treat a variety of biomedically-defined disorders, particularly infectious and allergic diseases in the debilitated, such as the common cold, bronchial asthma, allergic rhinitis, chronic bronchitis, pertussis, measles, pneumonia, and viral pneumonia.

It is also used for a variety of painful disorders including trigeminal neuralgia, migraine, sciatica, and renal colic. Finally, it has been used to stimulate normal functioning in such disorders as sick sinus syndrome, erectile dysfunction, myasthenia gravis, and chronic fatigue syndrome.

Alternate names

Ephedra, Aconite Accessory Root, and Asarum Decoction *(má huáng fù zǐ xì xīn tāng)* in *Annotation and Explanation of the Discussion of Cold Damage*; Aconite and Asarum Decoction *(fù zǐ xì xīn tāng)* in *Discussion of Illnesses, Patterns, and Formulas Related to the Unification of the Three Etiologies*

Cautions and Contraindications

This formula may safely be used to release the exterior only in those cases where the underlying yang deficiency is mild. Where the deficiency is more severe (characterized by undigested food in the stool and a faint, almost imperceptible pulse), this formula is contraindicated, as its use could devastate the yang.

Modifications

- For more pronounced yang and qi deficiency, add Astragali Radix *(huáng qí)* and Ginseng Radix *(rén shēn)*.

- For wind-cold headache, add Chuanxiong Rhizoma *(chuān xiōng)* and Zingiberis Rhizoma recens *(shēng jiāng)*.

- For chronic wheezing due to cold deficiency, combine with Two Aged [Herb] Decoction or Semen Sinapis Albae *(bái jiè zǐ)*, Armeniacae Semen *(xìng rén)*, and Perillae Fructus *(zǐ sū zǐ)*.

- For more severe cold obstructing the circulation of blood with pain in the extremities and joints, add Angelicae sinensis Radix *(dāng guī)*, Saposhnikoviae Radix *(fáng fēng)*, and Angelicae pubescentis Radix *(dú huó)*.

- For dampness obstructing the channels and collaterals with heavy body and muscle aches, add Atractylodis Rhizoma *(cāng zhú)* and Angelicae pubescentis Radix *(dú huó)*.

Variations

麻黃附子甘草湯（麻黄附子甘草汤）

Ephedra, Aconite Accessory Root, and Licorice Decoction
má huáng fù zǐ gān cǎo tāng

SOURCE   *Discussion of Cold Damage* (c. 220)

Substitute Glycyrrhizae Radix *(gān cǎo)* for Asari Radix et Rhizoma *(xì xīn)* for milder exterior conditions (less severe fever and chills). May also be used for mild edema with shortness of breath, urinary difficulty, and a small, submerged pulse.

再造散
Renewal Powder
zài zào sǎn

This formula was designed by Tao Hua for treating 'yang-less' (無陽 *wú yáng*) conditions, which are those in which the defi-

ciency of yang is so severe that the use of strong diaphoretics could prove fatal. Its name refers to a passage in the *New History of the Tang*: "The renewal of the country depends on the power of its most senior officials." This reference implies that the appropriate use of this formula can bring a person back from the edge of death, and that this change is dependent on mobilizing the body's primal qi.

Source   *Six Texts on Cold Damage* (1445)

Astragali Radix *(huáng qí)* 6g
Ginseng Radix *(rén shēn)* 3g
Aconiti Radix lateralis praeparata *(zhì fù zǐ)* 3g
Cinnamomi Ramulus *(guì zhī)* 3g
Asari Radix et Rhizoma *(xì xīn)* 3g
Notopterygii Rhizoma seu Radix *(qiāng huó)* 3g
Chuanxiong Rhizoma *(chuān xiōng)* .3g
Saposhnikoviae Radix *(fáng fēng)* 3g
dry-fried Radix Paeoniae *(chǎo sháo yào)* 3g
Glycyrrhizae Radix *(gān cǎo)* 1.5g
baked Zingiberis Rhizoma recens *(wēi shēng jiāng)* 3g
Jujubae Fructus *(dà zǎo)* . . . . .2 pieces

Method of Preparation   Note that the source text does not provide dosages and states that preparation should be done by boling all of the ingredients with the exception of Radix Paeoniae *(sháo yào)* in 2 cups of water until half has been boiled off. Use this to decoct the pounded herbs with an additional pinch of dry-fried Paeoniae Radix alba *(chao bái sháo)*, divide into three portions, and take warm. Paeoniae Radix alba *(bái sháo)* is the type of Paeoniae Radix *(sháo yào)* that is generally used. Note that some formulations delete Jujubae Fructus *(dà zǎo)* and dry-fried Radix Paeoniae *(sháo yào)*.

Actions   Tonifies the yang, augments the qi, induces sweating, and releases the exterior

Indications

Slight fever with strong chills, absence of sweating, headache, cold extremities, fatigue with a constant desire to lie down, pallid complexion, weak voice, a pale tongue with a white coating, and a submerged, forceless or a floating, big, and forceless pulse.

This is externally-contracted wind-cold with preexisting qi and yang deficiency. The slight fever and strong chills, absence of sweating, and headache are signs of exterior wind-cold. The cold extremities, fatigue, weak voice, and pallid complexion are signs of qi and yang deficiency. The forceless pulse reflects the debilitated state of the patient and the body's inability to rally against the invasion of wind-cold.

Analysis of Formula

The source text prescribes this formula for treating patterns characterized by deficiency of true yang with externally-contracted cold that has been treated with the sweating method but has failed to produce a sweat. According to the adage that 'yang added to yin is called sweating,' this implies that there is insufficient yang to push out the sweat—and thereby the pathogens—from the pores. In order to promote sweating, this formula thus combines acrid, warming herbs that disperse wind-cold from the exterior with those that tonify and warm the original qi.

Astragali Radix (*huáng qí*) and Ginseng Radix (*rén shēn*), the chief herbs, tonify the source qi and stabilize the exterior. They provide the yang force to drive out the pathogenic influences and prevent the exterior-releasing herbs from causing the collapse of yang. The deputies, Aconiti Radix lateralis praeparata (*zhì fù zǐ*), Cinnamomi Ramulus (*guì zhī*), and Asari Radix et Rhizoma (*xì xīn*), release the exterior by unblocking and activating the yang and scattering cold. The assistants, Notopterygii Rhizoma seu Radix (*qiāng huó*), Chuanxiong Rhizoma (*chuān xiōng*), and Saposhnikoviae Radix (*fáng fēng*), reinforce the formula's exterior-releasing, cold-dispersing actions. Another assistant, dry-fried Paeoniae Radix alba (*chǎo bái sháo*), is added for the purposes of regulating the protective and nutritive qi, similar to its use in Cinnamon Twig Decoction (*guì zhī tāng*). It moderates the warm, drying properties of the other herbs without hindering their ability to induce sweating. Glycyrrhizae Radix (*gān cǎo*) also moderates the sweat-inducing actions of the other ingredients. The envoys, baked Zingiberis Rhizoma recens (*shēng jiāng*) and Jujubae Fructus (*dà zǎo*), nourish and revive the Spleen and Stomach qi and regulate the nutritive and protective qi.

Commentary

The composition of this formula, which may be viewed as a combination of Ephedra, Asarum, and Aconite Accessory Root Decoction (*má huáng xì xīn fù zǐ tāng*) and Cinnamon Twig Decoction (*guì zhī tāng*), is well-balanced. Ephedrae Herba (*má huáng*) has been removed because its yang-dispersing properties are considered too strong in the present context. Noteworthy, too, is the use of baked Zingiberis Rhizoma recens (*wēi shēng jiāng*), which is roasted to enhance its Stomach-warming actions while reducing its acrid, qi-dispersing quality, as well as Paeoniae Radix alba (*bái sháo*), which is dry-fried to moderate the drying properties of the other substances without impairing their ability to resolve the exterior. It is a very effective formula for treating externally-contracted wind-cold with underlying qi and yang deficiency. In clinical practice, this is indicated by the presence of severe chills yet only mild fever, and a forceless pulse that may be either sinking or floating.

Comparisons

➤ Vs. Ephedra, Asarum, and Aconite Accessory Root Decoction (*má huáng xì xīn fù zǐ tāng*)

While both formulas focus on mobilizing the body's yang qi, Renewal Powder (*zài zào sǎn*) also tonifies the Spleen and Stomach as the source of blood and sweat in the body, and

harmonizes the nutritive and protective qi. In clinical practice, a differentiation can be made by means of signs and symptoms that indicate the need for such additional tonification. These include a lusterless, somber, pallid complexion, weak voice, and a pale tongue with a white coating that reflects the presence of dampness, which is absent in a lesser yin pattern. The pulse may be weak and forceless, but it can also be large and empty, whereas the pulse in lesser yin patterns tend to be submerged and thin.

Biomedical Indications

With the appropriate presentation, this formula may be used to treat a variety of biomedically-defined disorders, primarily the common cold in the elderly and rheumatic fever.

....

Alternate names

Renewal Drink (*zài zào yǐn*) in *Complete Collection of Red Water and Dark Pearls*

....

Modifications

- For a presentation where exterior cold is less pronounced, replace Saposhnikoviae Radix (*fáng fēng*) and Notopterygii Rhizoma seu Radix (*qiāng huó*) with Schizonepetae Herba (*jīng jiè*), Allii fistulosi Bulbus (*cōng bái*), and Sojae Semen praeparatum (*dàn dòu chǐ*).

- For joint pain and muscle aches, add Angelicae pubescentis Radix (*dú huó*), Clematidis Radix (*wēi líng xiān*), and Taxilli Herba (*sāng jì shēng*).

- For nasal obstruction, runny nose, and cough with white phlegm, add Peucedani Radix (*qián hú*), Platycodi Radix (*jié gěng*), Aurantii Fructus (*zhǐ ké*), Perillae Folium (*zǐ sū yè*), and Cynanchi stauntonii Rhizoma (*bái qián*).

蔥白七味飲（葱白七味饮）
Scallion Drink with Seven Ingredients
cōng bái qī wèi yǐn

Source *Arcane Essentials from the Imperial Library* (752)

Allii fistulosi Bulbus (*cōng bái*)....................9-12g
Puerariae Radix (*gé gēn*)........................9-12g
Zingiberis Rhizoma recens (*shēng jiāng*)...............6-9g
Ophiopogonis Radix (*mài mén dōng*)..................9-12g
Rehmanniae Radix (*shēng dì huáng*).................9-15g

Method of Preparation Decoction. The source text advises to cook the ingredients in special aerated or 'worked water' (撈水 *lāo shuǐ*), which is prepared by repeatedly ladling water in and out of a pail until bubbles cover the surface. Only the water near the surface is used. This was regarded as the seventh ingredient. At present, the water used to make this decoction is not prepared in any special manner.

Actions Nourishes the blood and releases the exterior

Indications

Headache, fever, and slight chills without sweating following a long-term illness or significant blood loss.

This is an exterior wind-cold disorder with simultaneous blood or yin deficiency due to a long-term illness or significant blood loss. The headache, fever, and chills are the classic presentation of wind-cold. The body is debilitated and therefore does not have the strength to produce strong chills. There is an absence of sweating not only because of the nature of this exterior disorder (wind-cold), but also because it is more difficult for the body to sweat when the blood or yin is deficient.

Analysis of Formula

Although exterior disorders require sweating to release the exterior, the presence of blood deficiency complicates the situation since blood and sweat share the same source (see COMMENTARY below). Traditionally, the sweating method was contraindicated in cases of blood deficiency. For this reason, the relatively mild, exterior-releasing Allii fistulosi Bulbus *(cōng bái)*, Sojae Semen praeparatum *(dàn dòu chǐ)*, Puerariae Radix *(gé gēn)*, and Zingiberis Rhizoma recens *(shēng jiāng)*, and the blood- and yin-nourishing Rehmanniae Radix *(shēng dì huáng)* and Ophiopogonis Radix *(mài mén dōng)*, are used. The 'worked water' was said to gently focus the formula on the upper burner and assist in releasing the exterior. The mild, exterior-releasing herbs also generate fluids; the yin- and blood-nourishing herbs are also relatively light and therefore noncloying. This formula is carefully balanced to avoid excessive releasing action (which would exhaust the blood or yin) and excessive tonification (which would cause retention of the pathogenic influences).

Commentary

The close connection between blood and sweat (both of which are fluids associated with yin) and the problems of treating conditions that involve their intertwining relationship were recognized very early in Chinese medicine. In Chapter 18 of the *Divine Pivot*, it is noted that "Those from whom blood flows [i.e., lose blood] do not have sweat, and those from whom sweat flows [i.e., sweat profusely] do not have blood." *Discussion of Cold Damage* also states that "The sweating [method] is forbidden in those with exhaustion of blood; the bleeding [method] is forbidden in those with exhaustion of sweat."

However, the blood that is tonified in the present formula is not blood in a narrow sense (i.e., the essences that turn red as they are transformed by the Heart), but rather blood in a wider sense as encompassing the body fluids. Both of the yin-tonifying herbs—Rehmanniae Radix *(shēng dì huáng)* and Ophiopogonis Radix *(mài mén dōng)*—enrich these fluids but do not tonify the blood. This correlates

with the view of the much later Qing physician Ye Tian-Shi, who emphasized in *Discussion of Warm Pathogen Heat [Disorders]* that in the course of treating these illnesses, "one assists yin not by focusing on the blood, but by focusing on the yang fluids and the sweat."

When using this formula, it is important to ensure that any sweating that occurs as the result of administering the formula not be excessive and to guard against the renewed contraction of pathogens as the pores begin to open. For this reason, the source text advises that the patient be covered once they become aware that a sweat is developing. Given the patient's constitution (i.e., their deficiency of fluids), this will not occur immediately but some time after the formula has been taken. Lack of sweating, or difficulty in producing a sweat, can thus be read as one of the key signs of this pattern.

Comparisons

➢ Vs. MODIFIED SOLOMON'S SEAL DECOCTION
    (jiā jiǎn wēi ruí tāng)

Differentiation of the proper use of these two formulas should not be made on the basis that one supplements blood and the other yin. Rather, the present formula focuses on early stage invasion of wind-cold pathogens in patients with preexisting deficiency of fluids (which may, in turn, be an aspect of blood deficiency), whereas Modified Solomon's Seal Decoction *(jiā jiǎn wēi ruí tāng)* is more suited to treating early-stage warm pathogen disorders against a similar constitutional background.

Biomedical Indications

With the appropriate presentation, this formula may be used to treat a variety of biomedically-defined disorders, primarily perimenstural or postpartum common colds.

Cautions and Contraindications

Only the slightest amount of sweating is desirable. Pronounced sweating will aggravate the condition. For this reason, the source texts advises to administer the decoction very slowly and only after it has been determined that the patient is definitely not sweating.

Modifications

- For strong chills, add Perillae Folium *(zǐ sū yè)* and Schizonepetae Herba *(jīng jiè)*.
- For sustained high fevers, add Lonicerae Flos *(jīn yín huā)* and Forsythiae Fructus *(lián qiáo)*.
- For accompanying indigestion, add Citri reticulatae Pericarpium *(chén pí)*.
- For continuous bleeding with an exterior condition, add Bletillae Rhizoma *(bái jí)*, Imperatae Rhizoma *(bái máo*

gēn), Nelumbinis Nodus rhizomatis (ŏu jié), and Asini Corii Colla (ē jiāo).

加減葳蕤湯（加減葳蕤汤）
Modified Solomon's Seal Decoction

jiā jiǎn wēi ruí tāng

Polygonati odorati Rhizoma (yù zhú), the chief herb in this formula, is also known as *wēi ruí*.

Source　*Revised Popular Guide to the Discussion of Cold Damage* (Qing dynasty)

Polygonati odorati Rhizoma (yù zhú)..................6-9g
Allii fistulosi Bulbus (cōng bái)..........................6g
Platycodi Radix (jié gěng)...........................3-4.5g
Sojae Semen praeparatum (dàn dòu chǐ) 9-12g
Menthae haplocalycis Herba (bò hé)................3-4.5g
Cynanchi atrati Radix (bái wēi) 1.5-3g
Glycyrrhizae Radix praeparata (zhì gān cǎo) 1.5g
Jujubae Fructus (dà zǎo)...........................2 pieces

Method of Preparation　Decoction

Actions　Nourishes the yin, clears heat, induces sweating, and releases the exterior

Indications

Fever and slight chills, little or no sweating, headache, dry throat, cough, sputum which is difficult to expectorate, thirst, irritability, a dark-red tongue, and a rapid pulse.

This is externally-contracted wind-heat in a patient with underlying yin deficiency. The headache, fever, slight chills, little or no sweating, and cough are signs of wind-heat. The dry throat, irritability, dark-red tongue, and rapid pulse indicate that the externally-contracted condition has begun to transform into internal heat. This relatively quick transformation is due to the underlying yin deficiency, a condition which usually involves some degree of injury to the fluids; when combined with wind-heat, thick sputum is produced that is difficult to expectorate. Although most cases of wind-heat are characterized by considerable sweating, there is little or no sweating in cases with yin deficiency.

Analysis of Formula

Generally, it is not advisable to use yin-tonifying substances when venting a pathogen from the exterior because their cloying nature readily obstructs the qi dynamic. In the present pattern, however, the body's yin fluids are depleted and need to be enriched in order to produce a sweat. For this reason, this formula employs a strategy of simultaneously tonifying the yin and venting wind-heat by means of acrid, cooling herbs.

The chief herb, Polygonati odorati Rhizoma (yù zhú), nourishes the yin of the Lungs and Stomach, clears heat, and generates fluids. It is especially useful for its ability to tonify without causing stagnation and thus can begin to restore the fluids without getting in the way of the elimination of the pathogens, which more cloying yin tonics might do. The deputies, Allii fistulosi Bulbus (cōng bái), Platycodi Radix (jié gěng), Sojae Semen praeparatum (dàn dòu chǐ), and Menthae haplocalycis Herba (bò hé), mildly release the exterior and dispel wind-heat. Cynanchi atrati Radix (bái wēi), one of the assistants, cools the blood and clears heat without injuring the yin, thereby treating the irritability and thirst. The other assistant, Platycodi Radix (jié gěng), disseminates the Lung qi to stop the coughing and expel the phlegm. The envoys, Glycyrrhizae Radix praeparata (zhì gān cǎo) and Jujubae Fructus (dà zǎo), assist Polygonati odorati Rhizoma (yù zhú) in moistening dryness and harmonizing the actions of the other ingredients.

Commentary

The principal indications for this formula are fever with slight chills, dry mouth, thirst, irritability, and a rapid pulse. Because the pathogen is still in the exterior and has not yet penetrated into the nutritive or blood levels, the tongue may still have a thin or even white coating. If the tongue is peeled due to the constitutional yin deficiency, it is not yet dark red.

Although this formula enriches the body fluids, its primary purpose is to vent the pathogen from the exterior, and it is for this purpose (i.e., to produce a physiological sweat) that body fluids are required. Wu Ju-Tong sums up this treatment principle in Chapter 4 of *Systematic Differentiation of Warm Pathogen Diseases*:

> Sweat as a substance depends on yang qi for its movement and on yin essence for its material basis. … Those with a surplus of yang qi and insufficient yin fluids, whose [fluids] are consumed by the rising and discharging qi of warm-heat [pathogen disorder], regardless of whether they spontaneously sweat [caused by the surplus of yang qi] or not [because of the lack of yin fluids], must have acrid and cool herbs [which disperse the yang excess] used to stop the spontaneous sweating. Sweet, cool and sweet, moistening herbs are used to nourish the yin fluids which serve as the material basis [of sweat] in order to prepare the ground for correct sweating.

The formula embodies this strategy inasmuch as the herbs that nourish the yin and clear internal heat do not impede the release of the exterior, while those that release the exterior do not injure the yin.

This formula is based on Solomon's Seal Decoction (*wēi ruí tāng*) from the Tang-dynasty classic, *Important Formulas Worth a Thousand Gold Pieces* (see ASSOCIATED FORMULAS below).

Comparison

➤ Vs. SCALLION DRINK WITH SEVEN INGREDIENTS (*cōng bái qī wèi yǐn*); *see* PAGE 54

Biomedical Indications

With the appropriate presentation, this formula may be used to treat a variety of biomedically-defined disorders such as the common cold postpartum or in the elderly, acute tonsilitis, and pharyngitis.

Modifications

- For more severe exterior disorders, add Saposhnikoviae Radix (fáng fēng) and Puerariae Radix (gé gēn).

- For cough, dry throat, and sputum that is difficult to expectorate, add Arctii Fructus (niú bàng zǐ) and Trichosanthis Pericarpium (guā lóu pí).

- For more pronounced thirst and irritability, add Trichosanthis Radix (tiān huā fěn) and Lophatheri Herba (dàn zhú yè).

Associated Formula

葳蕤湯 （葳蕤汤）

Solomon's Seal Decoction

wēi ruí tāng

Source   *Important Formulas Worth a Thousand Gold Pieces* (650)

Polygonati odorati Rhizoma (yù zhú) 60g
Cynanchi atrati Radix (bái wēi) 60g
Ephedrae Herba (má huáng) 60g
Allii fistulosi Bulbus (cōng bái) 6g
Angelicae pubescentis Radix (dú huó) 60g
Armeniacae Semen (xìng rén) 60g
Chuanxiong Rhizoma (chuān xiōng) 60g
Glycyrrhizae Radix (gān cǎo) 60g
Aristolochiae Radix (qīng mù xiāng) 60g
Gypsum fibrosum (shí gāo) 90g

The source text advises to grind the herbs into a coarse powder and take as a draft three times a day. At present, however, it is prepared as a decoction with a proportionate reduction in dosage. Scatters wind, releases the exterior, clears heat, and nourishes the yin. For a warm pathogen wind disease (溫風之病 *wēn fēng zhī bìng*) characterized by sweating, a sensation of heaviness in the body, wheezing, a sullen demeanor, no desire to sleep, and a floating pulse at both the proximal and distal positions. This formula is stronger than the principal formula and is indicated for a pattern of excess where the pathogen has invaded both the qi and blood. For Sun Si-Miao, the author of this formula, a warm pathogen disease was caused by a cold pathogen that invaded the body in winter and then lurked in the interior until the spring, when the raising yang qi would become sufficiently strong to engage it in battle and cause an acute illness. It was widely assumed that patients whose yin essence was depleted were particularly prone to this type of disease. For treatment, Sun composed a formula that dispersed cold from the exterior as well as the blood, cleared heat from excess, and augmented the fluids.

Because the formula contains many acrid, warm herbs, later physicians felt that it was inappropriate for treating true warm pathogen disorders. In *Developing the Meaning of Prescriptions Worth a Thousand*, the late-Ming dynasty scholar-physician Zhang Lu thus made the following recommendations:

> For [treating cases] with severe fever that has damaged the fluids or with thirst in spite of a mild fever, it does no harm to remove Ephedrae Herba (má huáng) and Armeniacae Semen (xìng rén) and replace them with Allii fistulosi Bulbus (cōng bái) and Sojae Semen praeparatum (dàn dòu chǐ) in order to unblock constraint of the yang, and Trichosanthis Radix (tiān huā fěn) in order to enrich the fluids. [In cases] with wheezing and rising qi, Chuanxiong Rhizoma (chuān xiōng) and Angelicae pubescentis Radix (dú huó) should also not be used lightly. Deficient [patients] cannot overcome cold [damage, and using] Gypsum fibrosum (shí gāo) makes it [even more] unlikely that this can be carried out. It should be replaced with Lophatheri Herba (dàn zhú yè) to clear the Heart and Poria (fú líng) to secure the middle [burner] in order to provide for tonification. In this manner, one supplies something that was not yet attained [by Sun Si-Miao] in *Important Formulas Worth a Thousand Gold Pieces*.

It was this suggestion that was later picked up by Yu Gen-Chu and further developed into Modified Solomon's Seal Decoction (jiā jiǎn wēi ruí tāng).

Comparative Tables of Principal Formulas

■ FORMULAS THAT RELEASE EARLY-STAGE EXTERIOR DISORDERS AND EXTERIOR WIND-COLD

Common symptoms: fever and chills (chills predominant), floating pulse, normal tongue

Formula Name	Diagnosis	Indications	Remarks
Scallion and Prepared Soybean Decoction (cōng chǐ tāng)	Early stages of exterior conditions	Mild fever and slight chills without sweating, headache, stuffy nose, a thin, white tongue coating, floating pulse	For either wind-cold or wind-heat.
Ephedra Decoction (má huáng tāng)	Exterior cold excess conditions	Absence of sweating, headache, generalized body aches, wheezing, tight pulse	This is the classic cold damage condition. Also for cold causing wheezing or nosebleeds, as well as painful obstruction due to wind-cold-dampness.

CONT. ↘

Formula Name	Diagnosis	Indications	Remarks
Major Bluegreen Dragon Decoction (*dà qīng lóng tāng*)	Wind-cold in the exterior with heat constraint in the interior	Absence of sweating, headache, generalized body aches, wheezing, irritability, tight pulse	This is cold fettering the exterior with heat constraint in the interior; presence of irritability is the key clinical marker.
Cinnamon Twig Decoction (*guì zhī tāng*)	Exterior cold deficient conditions	Sweating that does not lead to improvement of the condition, headache, aversion to wind, stiff neck, nasal congestion, dry heaves, no particular thirst, moderate or frail pulse	This is the classic attack by wind. May also be used for a similar presentation in patients recovering from serious illness or after childbirth.
Kudzu Decoction (*gé gēn tāng*)	Externally-contracted wind-cold at the greater yang warp	Fever and chills without sweating, stiff and rigid neck and upper back, thin and white tongue coating, tight pulse	Also used for greater yang/yang brightness patterns with diarrhea.
Minor Bluegreen Dragon Decoction (*xiǎo qīng lóng tāng*)	External wind-cold conditions with the addition of thin mucus	Absence of sweating, cough, wheezing, sputum that is copious, white, stringy, and difficult to expectorate, stifling sensation in the chest, generalized sensation of heaviness and body aches, no particular thirst, moist tongue coating, tight pulse	In severe cases, there may be floating edema or considerable difficulty in breathing when lying down.
Nine-Herb Decoction with Notopterygium (*jiǔ wèi qiāng huó tāng*)	Externally-contracted wind-cold-dampness with concurrent internal accumulation of heat	Absence of sweating, headache, stiff neck, generalized aches and pain, slight thirst, bitter taste in the mouth	Also for toothache with exterior symptoms.
Augmented Cyperus and Perilla Leaf Powder (*jiā wèi xiāng sū sǎn*)	Exterior wind-cold together with qi constrained in the interior	Absence of sweating, headache, focal distention and a stifling sensation in the chest and epigastrium, poor appetite, belching	Also for wind-cold conditions during pregnancy.
Ten-Miracle Decoction (*shí shén tāng*)	Epidemic disorders and wind-cold patterns with internal qi stagnation	Headache, stifling oppression and focal distention in the chest, absence of sweating, fever, cough, nasal congestion, low voice, thin and white tongue coating	Also sometimes applied to the treatment of wind-cold-damp painful obstruction.
Inula Powder (*jīn fèi cǎo sǎn*)	Early stages of externally-contracted wind-cold with a productive cough	Cough with copious sputum, nasal congestion, deep and low voice, headache, clouded vision, fullness and oppression in the chest, puffy tongue with tooth marks and greasy, white coating, floating pulse	Also indicated specifically for toothache with a swollen tongue due to invasion of wind-cold.

■ FORMULAS THAT RELEASE EXTERIOR WIND-HEAT

Common symptoms: fever, sweating, floating and rapid pulse

Formula Name	Diagnosis	Indications	Remarks
Mulberry Leaf and Chrysanthemum Drink (*sāng jú yǐn*)	Early, superficial stage of a warm pathogen disease	Slight fever, cough, slight thirst, thin and white tongue coating	Focuses on the Lungs and is especially useful for coughs. Also used for eye disorders due to wind-heat.
Honeysuckle and Forsythia Powder (*yín qiáo sǎn*)	Protective level warm pathogen disease	Headache, thirst, cough, sore throat, red-tipped tongue, thin and white or thin and yellow tongue coating, floating and rapid pulse	Relatively strong at releasing the exterior and clearing heat.

CONT. ↘

Formula Name	Diagnosis	Indications	Remarks
Bupleurum and Kudzu Decoction to Release the Muscle Layer (chái gé jiě jī tāng)	Exterior wind-cold (greater yang) that is just beginning to transform into interior heat (yang brightness)	Increasing fever and decreasing chills accompanied by headache, stiffness of the extremities, orbital and eye pain, dry nasal passages, irritability, insomnia, thin and yellow tongue coating, slightly flooding pulse	Also for toothache due to wind-heat.
Cimicifuga and Kudzu Decoction (shēng má gé gēn tāng)	Externally-contracted heat collecting in the Lungs and Stomach	Early-stage measles or rashes that do not surface evenly, headache, generalized body aches, sneezing, coughing, red eyes, tearing, thirst, red and dry tongue	
Lophatherum and Tamarisk Decoction (zhú yè chēng liǔ tāng)	Heat collecting in the Stomach and Lungs due to toxins that have damaged the fluids with simultaneous obstruction of the exterior by wind-heat	Early-stage disease with rashes that do not surface evenly, cough, slight chills and a sustained high fever, stifling sensation in the chest, swollen and painful throat, thirst, thin, yellow, and dry tongue coating, floating and rapid pulse	
Schizonepeta and Forsythia Decoction (jīng jiè lián qiáo tāng)	Wind-heat attacking the upper body	Acute earache, rhinitis, tonsillitis, nosebleeds	Also for acute upper body toxic swellings such as acne.

■ FORMULAS THAT RELEASE EXTERIOR DISORDERS WITH INTERIOR DEFICIENCY

Common symptoms: none listed

Formula Name	Diagnosis	Indications	Remarks
Ginseng Powder to Overcome Pathogenic Influences (rén shēn bài dú sǎn)	External wind-cold-dampness with preexisting deficient qi	High fever and severe chills with shivering, absence of sweating, pain and stiffness of the head and neck, soreness and pain of the extremities, focal distention and fullness of the chest, nasal congestion, productive cough, greasy and white tongue coating, soggy pulse	Also used for early-stage dysenteric disorders from wind-cold-dampness and measles.
Ephedra, Asarum, and Aconite Accessory Root Decoction (má huáng xì xīn fù zǐ tāng)	Exterior excessive cold in a patient with preexisting yang deficiency	Extreme cold and chills, slight fever, absence of sweating, exhaustion, submerged and faint pulse	Also used for Kidney coughing and cold deficiency headache.
Renewal Powder (zài zào sǎn)	Exterior wind-cold in a patient with qi and yang deficiency	Slight fever with strong chills, absence of sweating, headache, cold extremities, fatigue with a constant desire to lie down, pallid complexion, weak voice, pale tongue with white coating, submerged and forceless or floating, big, and forceless pulse	
Scallion Drink with Seven Ingredients (cōng bái qī wèi yǐn)	Exterior wind-cold with simultaneous deficient blood and/or yin	Fever, slight chills, and absence of sweating after a prolonged illness or blood loss	This condition requires great delicacy in treatment.
Modified Solomon's Seal Decoction (jiā jiǎn wēi ruí tāng)	Exterior wind-heat in a patient with deficient blood and yin	Headache, fever, slight chills with little or no sweating, thirst, irritability, dark-red tongue, rapid pulse	Usually follows a long-term illness or significant blood loss.

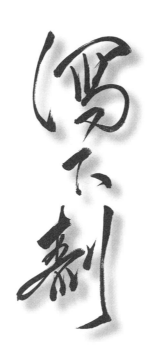

Chapter 2 Contents

Formulas that Drain Downward

Formulas that Drain Downward

AMONG THE EIGHT methods of treatment, the formulas in this chapter utilize the downward-draining method (下法 *xià fǎ*) to break up and expel accumulations of heat, cold, or fluids (including water) and other matter (e.g., buildup of blood or dry stools) in the interior. Many of the formulas contain ingredients that unblock the bowels, thereby serving as laxatives to remove the accumulation through the stool. Others contain ingredients that have a cathartic effect upon the accumulation of fluids. Given the harsh effects of some of the more drastic purgatives, physicians throughout the course of Chinese medicine's long history have been cautious about their use. Yet, downward draining also constitutes one of the cornerstones of the therapeutic arsenal that, if correctly deployed, holds the key to resolving many otherwise intractable problems. This is aptly summarized by Sun Si-Miao in *Important Formulas Worth a Thousand Gold Pieces*: "Any accumulation in the yin and yang organs that needs to be drained has to be drained, no matter how old or young [the patient]."

The type of formula discussed in this chapter can be traced back at least to the *Inner Classic,* which mentions downward draining many times, including this statement from Chapter 21 of *Basic Questions*: "Fullness for three days will be stopped if [the patient] is drained." As with most other strategies, the basic formulas for downward draining were collected by Zhang Zhong-Jing in the late Han dynasty. Purging is one of the core strategies for treating yang brightness disorders in *Discussion of Cold Damage* and is used alone or in combination in treating patterns of all other warps as well. The formulas listed in that text became the models for almost all of the later developments in this field.

Among the earliest of these developments were the concepts developed by Liu Wan-Su, one of the four great masters of the Jin-Yuan period. He argued that any kind of pathogenic influence could transform into internal heat as a result of constraint and emphasized the clearing, draining, and purging of such heat by means of substances such as Coptidis Rhizoma *(huáng lián),* Rhei Radix et Rhizoma *(dà huáng),* or Talcum *(huá shí).* Liu believed that externally-contracted disorders with heat clumping in the interior, characterized by symptoms such as unclear vision, abdominal fullness and pain, irritability, raving, and a submerged, excessive pulse, should be purged even if the exterior has not yet been released. He also recommended the use of Major Order the Qi Decoction *(dà chéng qì tāng)* with Coptis Decoction to Resolve Toxicity *(huáng lián jiě dú tāng),* discussed in Chapter 4, for deep-lying heat toxin where pathogens are entering the blood aspect with such symptoms as cold extremities and pains throughout the body, a dry or painful throat, abdominal fullness and pain, confusion, wheezing, and a submerged, thin pulse. His follower, Zhang Cong-Zheng, advocated the use of downward draining for a wide range of situations, including recurrent bouts of fever even after the use of strong diaphoretics, indicating that the heat was not being cleared; internal medicine disorders characterized by unremitting abdominal fullness and pain, indicating interior excess; alternating chills and fever accompanied by bouts of productive coughing; trauma resulting in swellings and pain that gets worse at night; and certain types of sores and swellings. Translated into contemporary theories, these indications suggest the use of downward-draining strategies not just for accumulations of heat in the interior, but also for blood stasis, excess phlegm, or damp obstruction.

The Ming physician Wu You-Xing emphasized the use of downward-draining strategies in the treatment of seasonal epidemic disorders. He admonished against delaying the use of purgation due to unwarranted reservations about their side effects and also suggested that doctors "not remain stuck [in considering their use merely] for patterns characterized by clumping of stools."

Downward-draining strategies also have a prominent place in Kampo medicine. Prominent members of the Kohō-hā or 'ancient formula current' that developed in Japan during the Edo period (1602-1868), such as Yoshimasu Tōdō, Yoshimasu Nangai, and Yumoto Kyushin, focused on the elimination of toxins as a central aspect of medical practice and naturally looked to downward draining as one means to achieve this.

Summing up the experiences and doctrines of these and other physicians, we can say that the formulas discussed in this chapter are mainly indicated for patterns characterized by interior excess. These can be divided into two large groups. The first comprises excess conditions of the bowels (often summarily referred to as the Stomach) caused by externally-contracted heat that moves into the interior. Typically, such patterns are characterized by high fever, irritability, thirst, abdominal pain, and constipation. The second group comprises patterns caused by constraint and clumping of qi and blood, stopped up fluids, harbored food, or parasitic accumulations in the interior. Such interior excess patterns arise when strong normal qi contends with strong pathogenic influences. In certain contexts, however, internal accumulations arising in deficient patients may become so pronounced that they, too, need to be drained downward.

Generally speaking, the formulas in this chapter should not be used when there is an exterior condition, as their downward-draining actions will have the effect of dragging the pathogen internally. With the exception of those that moisten and lubricate the intestines, all of these formulas contain harsh ingredients that must be prescribed with care. They are contraindicated during pregnancy and should only be used when absolutely necessary after childbirth or loss of blood, or in the weak or elderly. Because their harshness can easily injure the Stomach qi, their use should be discontinued as soon as they take effect and should never be used on a prolonged basis. Foods that are greasy or otherwise difficult to digest increase the risk of injuring the Stomach qi and should therefore be avoided when taking these formulas.

Note that purging itself is an important aspect of some formulas that are grouped in other chapters. This includes Chapter 4, which specifically discusses formulas for conditions where there is excess simultaneously in the exterior and the interior; Chapter 13, where they play a significant role in treating some types of blood stasis; Chapters 18 and 19, where they are used in treating food stagnation and parasites; and Chapter 20, where they are used in treating some types of internal abscesses.

Section 1

. . . .

FORMULAS THAT PURGE
HEAT ACCUMULATION

Heat accumulation is a condition of interior excess characterized by fever, abdominal pain that increases upon pressure, constipation, a yellow tongue coating, and a pulse that is strong, excessive, and usually submerged. The core ingredients in these formulas are cold purgatives (also known as downward-draining medicinals) such as Rhei Radix et Rhizoma (*dà huáng*) and Natrii Sulfas (*máng xiāo*). Because the clumped dry stool disrupts the qi dynamic and leads to stagnation, this increases the severity of the clumping. For this, herbs that promote movement of the qi are added, such as Magnoliae officinalis Cortex (*hòu pò*), Aurantii Fructus immaturus (*zhǐ shí*), and Aucklandiae Radix (*mù xiāng*). While the act of purgation treats heat by 'removing the fuel from beneath the pot,' for intense internal heat, this is insufficient, and herbs that clear heat must be added, such as Scutellariae Radix (*huáng qín*), Patriniae Herba (*bài jiàng cǎo*), and Gardeniae Fructus (*zhī zǐ*). Sometimes, pathogenic heat gets tied up with pathogenic water in the trunk. When this occurs, it is necessary to add herbs that drive out excess water, such as Kansui Radix (*gān suì*), Genkwa Flos (*yuán huā*), and Pharbitidis Semen (*qiān niú zǐ*). Excess heat accumulating and stagnating in the Stomach and Intestines readily leads to problems with the circulation of blood and can cause blood stasis. When this occurs, it is necessary to add herbs that dispel static blood, such as Persicae Semen (*táo rén*), Paeoniae Radix rubra (*chì sháo*), and Moutan Cortex (*mǔ dān pí*). Occasionally, long-standing interior heat from excess can sap the yang qi leading to cold presentations; in these cases, the formulas must include herbs that warm the yang and disperse cold, such as Aconiti Radix lateralis praeparata (*zhì fù zǐ*) and Zingiberis Rhizoma (*gān jiāng*). Finally, as the locus of disorders treated by cold purgatives is often the middle burner (Spleen and Stomach), which can be damaged by cold purgatives, sometimes it is necessary to add herbs that harmonize the middle burner and nourish the Stomach to ameliorate this damage. Most commonly, Glycyrrhizae Radix (*gān cǎo*) and Jujubae Fructus (*dà zǎo*) are used for this purpose.

大承氣湯（大承气汤）
Major Order the Qi Decoction
dà chéng qì tāng

This formula treats heat accumulation in the Stomach and Intestines by directing the Stomach qi downward, thereby forcing open the obstruction to the orderly flow of qi. The word 'major' indicates that it is the strongest of the formulas in this group.

Source *Discussion of Cold Damage* (c. 220)

Rhei Radix et Rhizoma (*dà huáng*) . . . . [add near end] 12g
Natrii Sulfas (*máng xiāo*) . . [dissolve in strained decoction] 9-12g
prepared Aurantii Fructus immaturus
   (*zhì zhǐ shí*) . . . . 5 pieces (12-15g)
prepared Magnoliae officinalis Cortex (*zhì hòu pò*) 24g

Method of Preparation The source text advises to cook Aurantii Fructus immaturus (*zhǐ shí*) and Magnoliae officinalis Cortex (*hòu pò*) in 10 cups of water until 5 cups remain, then add Rhei Radix et Rhizoma (*dà huáng*) and continue cooking until 2 cups remain. Natrii Sulfas (*máng xiāo*) is added to the strained decoction, which is brought to a boil for a few seconds and then removed from the heat.

At present, it is generally prepared as a decoction with the ingredients treated as described in brackets above. The listed dosages are based on the source text, while at present the textbook dosages are 6-12g of Rhei Radix et Rhizoma (*dà huáng*) and 12-15g of Magnoliae officinalis Cortex (*hòu pò*), unless there is severe focal distention; in that case, the original dosage of Magnoliae officinalis Cortex (*hòu pò*) is indicated. Once loose stools have been induced, the use of this formula should be discontinued.

Actions Vigorously purges heat accumulation

Indications

This formula is indicated for three different patterns: heat excess in the yang brightness organs, heat clumping with circumfluence (熱結旁流 *rè jié páng liú*), and heat inversion (熱厥 *rè jué*).

Heat excess in the yang brightness organs manifests with severe constipation and flatulence, focal distention and abdominal fullness, abdominal pain that increases upon pressure, a tense and firm abdomen, a dry, yellow or dry, black tongue coating with prickles, and a submerged, excessive pulse. In severe cases, there may be tidal fevers, delirious speech, and profuse sweating from the palms and soles.

Heat clumping with circumfluence manifests with green, watery, and foul-smelling diarrhea accompanied by the same abdominal signs and symptoms outlined above. The tongue body and coating are dry, and the pulse is rapid and slippery.

Internal heat excess manifesting with heat inversion presents with fever, cold extremities, thirst, sweating from the head, constipation, scanty and dark urine, disorientation, delirious speech, cracked lips, a red tongue, and a submerged, excessive, and forceful pulse. This formula is also for tetany and mania with a similar presentation.

Yang brightness organ-warp disorders are characterized by heat accumulating in the interior and 'taking on form' (有形 *yǒu xíng*). This heat can have different sources. It can be due to externally-contracted cold that has transformed into heat; to a heat pathogen that enters the body directly via the nose or mouth; or to an internal disturbance of the yin and yang organs. Whatever the cause, heat in the yang brightness organ injures the fluids, which become viscous and turbid. The heat and turbidity of the fluids cause the stool to dry out. The heat and dry stool then combine to form clumps, which obstruct the orderly, downward movement of qi through the Stomach and Intestines. This results in severe constipation and flatulence, focal distention, a sensation of fullness in the abdomen, and the other abdominal symptoms mentioned.

These symptoms can also be viewed as four types of abdominal disharmony: focal distention, fullness, dryness, and excess, each of which is treated primarily with one of the ingredients in the formula.

1. Focal distention (痞 *pǐ*) refers to the sensation of obstruction, distention, and heaviness that is focused in the epigastrium and treated with Aurantii Fructus immaturus (*zhǐ shí*).

2. Fullness (滿 *mǎn*) refers to the visible distention that is resistant to palpation and treated with Magnoliae officinalis Cortex (*hòu pò*).

3. Dryness (燥 *zào*) refers to the dry stool that accumulates in the Intestines and causes parts of the abdomen to become tense and firm. This is treated with Natrii Sulfas (*máng xiāo*).

4. Excess (實 *shí*) refers to the heat that accumulates and takes form, resulting in constipation and abdominal pain that increases upon pressure. This is treated with Rhei Radix et Rhizoma (*dà huáng*).

The other signs and symptoms are also associated with severe heat. Upward-blazing interior heat disturbs the spirit and causes delirious speech. There are two explanations for the tidal fever, which appears in relatively serious cases. The first is that the dry stool absorbs and thus depletes the fluids, thereby injuring the yin. The second explanation is suggested by a passage in *Discussion of Cold Damage* (paragraph 193), where it is noted that pathogenic influences at the yang brightness warp tend to be released between 3 and 9 P.M. This has been interpreted to mean that because the qi in the yang brightness level of the body is strongest during this time, it is then that the body's normal qi and the pathogenic influence struggle for dominance; thus, the fever is strongest during this time. Heat in the yang brightness warp can transform the fluids into steam, which is forced out as profuse sweating through the palms and soles.

A red tongue is associated with heat while a dry, yellow tongue coating indicates dryness in the interior, as does cracked lips. In severe cases, the coating becomes black with prickles. The submerged, excessive pulse indicates that an excess pathogen is located in the interior.

Heat clumping with circumfluence is caused by an overabundance of heat drying out the fluids within the stools and causing them to become clogged in the Intestines. The breakdown of physiological qi transformation also, however, disables the process of fluid resorption normally carried out by the Intestines. Instead of being transmitted to the Bladder and Kidneys, this fluid, which carries with it some of the pathogenic heat, flows around the clogged stools and manifests as green watery diarrhea with an intensely offensive odor. Pathogenic heat and failure of resorption rapidly deplete the body's own physiological fluids, leading to dryness of the mouth, throat, and tongue. The slippery and rapid pulse indicates that this insufficiency of fluids is secondary to the presence of excess heat in the interior.

The same excess can also constrain the dispersal of yang qi toward the exterior and lead to a pattern known as 'heat inversion.' Here, the heat constraint becomes so pronounced that the four extremities are no longer supplied with yang qi and turn icy cold. At the same time, severe internal heat damages the fluids. Deprived of moisture and nourishment, the muscles and sinews stiffen and contract.

Mania is caused by excess interior heat harassing the clear spirit, while turbidity and dryness combine to block the orifices. Xu Da-Chun elucidates this process in *Categorization of Formulas from the Discussion of Cold Damage*: "Delirious speech arises from constipation. Constipation arises from dryness. Dryness arises from sweating. Sweating arises from lack of body fluids. Each one of these causes the other, making the nature of the disorder clear."

Analysis of Formula

In Chinese medicine, the constipation associated with conditions of interior excess should be treated by purging, and the heat should be treated by cooling. For this reason, Rhei Radix et Rhizoma (dà huáng) serves as the chief ingredient in the formula. Its function is succinctly described in *Divine Husbandman's Classic of the Materia Medica*: "breaks up abdominal masses, accumulations, lingering fluids, and harbored food by flushing them from the Stomach and Intestines, pushing out the old so that the new [can enter], unblocking [the passages for] food and drink, regulating the middle [burner so that it can again] transform food and the

five yin organs are calmed." Its propulsive purgation is aided by the stool-softening action of salty, cold Natrii Sulfas (máng xiāo), the deputy ingredient. Together, they moisten dryness as they drain downward.

One assistant ingredient, Aurantii Fructus immaturus (zhǐ shí), dissipates clumps and reduces focal distention. The other, Magnoliae officinalis Cortex (hòu pò), disseminates the qi and relieves the sensation of fullness. Both herbs assist in the expulsion of stool by moving the qi. Even though the root of the condition is heat, the resultant clumping leads to severe stagnation of qi. Moving the qi is thus an important aspect of the formula. This is outlined by Ke Qin in *Further Appendices to the Discussion of Cold Damage*:

> All diseases have their cause in the qi. Foul matter not being eliminated is due to qi not flowing normally. Therefore, formulas that purge accumulation must use herbs that move the qi to govern this. Hyperactivity [of qi] leads to harm. Ordering [the qi] controls it. [The term] ordering the qi [in the formula's name] is based on this [principle]. The [real] intention of ordering the qi [however] is to eliminate the disorder without damaging the primal qi.

Cautions and Contraindications

Because this is a powerful formula, it has always been used with caution and only when necessary. The early-modern physician He Lian-Chen lists eight contraindications that serve as a helpful guide to the use of this formula:

1. Conditions where *a pathogen remains in the protective level and exterior*. This is indicated by aversion to cold and by urine that remains normal in both color and amount. In such cases, pathogens should be vented and dispersed.

2. *Hardness in the epigastric area*, indicating that the pathogen remains above the diaphragm and has not yet penetrated into the Intestines. In such cases, one should use Gardenia and Prepared Soybean Decoction (zhī zǐ chǐ tāng) or a similar method.

3. A *flushed face*, indicating that heat is not yet bound in the interior but still floats in the exterior. This requires the use of a strategy to clear heat.

4. Patients who *habitually eat only small amounts*, indicating deficiency of Spleen and Stomach qi. In such cases, constipation requires tonification.

5. Patients who *stop eating* as the disorder develops. This implies there is nothing to produce stools with which the heat may bind. In such cases, heat should be drained rather than purged.

6. *Frequent vomiting*, indicating that the disorder remains at the lesser yang warp. Here, the harmonizing method is indicated.

7. A *slow pulse*, indicating cold in the interior. This is treated by the simultaneous use of warming and purging strategies.

8. *Spontaneous sweating and normal urination*, indicating that the fluids in the interior are expended and that one must use a moistening formula to drain downward.

In addition, this is a very strong formula that may cause vomiting or severe diarrhea. For weak patients, it should be used only when absolutely necessary, and then with the addition of tonic herbs. Contraindicated during pregnancy.

Commentary

The principal pattern for which this formula is indicated includes focal distention, abdominal fullness, dry stools, and symptoms of yang brightness-type interior excess heat. Although the formula is mentioned nineteen times in *Discussion of Cold Damage* for a variety of conditions, it is most frequently discussed in connection with this pattern. In addition to the other patterns listed under INDICATIONS, the formula has also been used for lesser yin-warp disorders that present with similar signs and symptoms. In *Essentials from the Golden Cabinet,* it is recommended for internal blood stasis accompanied by spasms as well as some types of diarrhea and other disorders. Although the indications vary considerably, each of these presentations shares the same underlying mechanism: heat excess accumulating in the Stomach and Intestines where it injures the fluids and forms clumps that obstruct the downward flow of qi. It can thus be used, for instance, to regulate menstruation in women with heat excess. Once this is eliminated, the flow of qi becomes regular, and once the flow of qi is regular, its control over the flow of blood and menstruation will normalize. This formula is also used to treat such problems as visual disturbances, dizziness, and wheezing with inability to lie down when the pathological dynamic is the same. Following the same rationale, this formula is used to treat closed-type wind-stroke.

Throughout the history of Chinese herbal medicine, this formula has served as a model for the development of new formulas. The new formulas have extended the scope of purgative treatment strategies to warm pathogen disorders, deficiency conditions, and modern emergency Chinese medicine. Some of the new formulas appear later in this chapter, while others are found in Chapter 13 on regulating the blood and Chapter 15 on treating dryness.

There has been considerable debate among physicians regarding the chief herb in this formula. Ke Qin, who emphasized its qi-regulating aspects, argued that Magnoliae officinalis Cortex (*hòu pò*) and Aurantii Fructus immaturus (*zhǐ shí*) were the most important herbs. This, he believed, explained the large dosage of these herbs in the formula. The opposite view is represented by the Qing-dynasty physician Zou Shu, who argued in *Commentary on the Classic of Materia Medica* that because Rhei Radix et Rhizoma (*dà huáng*) is the only herb contained in all of the various Order the Qi Decoctions (*chéng qì tāng),* it must be the chief herb.

Qi is the leader of blood, thus blood follows the movement of qi. This includes [becoming static] when qi stagnates. If qi stagnates and blood does not follow this stagnation [to become static too], then this is because [to begin with] qi is insufficient rather than excessive. In cases of [true] qi stagnation, [such stagnation always] spreads to the blood. The qi then uses the blood like an underground lair [where it escapes attack from qi-regulating herbs], while the blood uses the qi [at which treatment is directed, like a shield for] resisting attack [on itself]. If [such stagnation] is further connected to harbored food, it steams the body fluids, completely transforming [qi into] fire. At such a time, only Rhei Radix et Rhizoma (*dà huáng*) can directly purge the core of the disorder, pouring out [the problem from] the underground cave [in which it was hiding]. Once the clumping of qi has been dispersed from the blood, Aurantii Fructus immaturus (*zhǐ shí*) and Magnoliae officinalis Cortex (*hòu pò*) can successfully carry out their task of opening the qi [dynamic]. This is how Rhei Radix et Rhizoma (*dà huáng*) orders the qi.

Many commentators furthermore suggest that although the formula orders the qi, its most important purpose is to preserve the fluids, which are threatened by the severe heat in the interior. Yang is generated from yin. Thus, if heat is eliminated and the fluids are preserved, qi will automatically return. This logic allows a physician to forcefully drain qi in the process of purgation without, over the long run, damaging the body's normal qi. The alternative, avoiding purgation for fear of damaging the qi, would in fact end up doing much more harm to the qi. Still, one must take recourse to purgation only when the circumstances demand such a course of action. The following basic rules, and the contraindications listed below, provide clinicians with clear guidelines.

First, it is important to distinguish the principal pattern for which this formula is indicated from that of a yang brightness channel or White Tiger Decoction (*bái hǔ tāng*) pattern, discussed in Chapter 4. In such a pattern, the momentum of the heat is to move outward, and it is better to follow rather than fight this movement. Thus, the heat should be cleared rather than purged. One of the most important markers for making this differentiation is the relationship between pulse and abdominal symptoms. In a White Tiger Decoction (*bái hǔ tāng*) pattern, the heat has not acquired form and thus follows its natural tendency to expand outward. This is reflected in a flooding pulse. In all of the Order the Qi Decoction (*chéng qì tāng*) patterns, the heat binds with matter in the interior and thus acquires form. This is reflected in a pulse that is submerged, excessive, and forceful. If the normal qi is completely blocked, the pulse may become confined or even disappear altogether.

In cold damage patterns, where transformation of cold into heat is slow and the main objective is to prevent damage to the yang qi, it is considered essential to wait until the pulse becomes submerged before using a purging formula. In warm pathogen disorders, where the main consideration is to prevent damage to the yin fluids, one should consider using a purgative formula as soon as abdominal signs indicate that heat is acquiring form, even if the pulse is still flooding.

For maximum effectiveness, it is also important to adhere to the directions for preparation and only decoct Rhei Radix et Rhizoma (*dà huáng*) for a short period of time. Ke Qin notes that when it is used "fresh, its [own] qi is fast and therefore it moves the qi. When it is decocted, its qi is blunted and it becomes balanced and moderate."

Comparisons

➤ Differentiation of Order the Qi Decoctions (*chéng qì tāng*)

All of the formulas that 'order the qi' use Rhei Radix et Rhizoma (*dà huáng*) to cleanse heat accumulation from the Stomach and Intestines. Major Order the Qi Decoction (*dà chéng qì tāng*), the strongest of the group, treats focal distention, fullness, dryness, and hardness. Minor Order the Qi Decoction (*xiǎo chéng qì tāng*), not as strong as the former, treats focal distention, fullness, and hardness without dryness. Regulate the Stomach and Order the Qi Decoction (*tiáo wèi chéng qì tāng*), which has the mildest purgative action, treats cases without focal distention or fullness.

The famous modern physician Cheng Men-Xue presents the following differentiation. Regulate the Stomach and Order the Qi Decoction (*tiáo wèi chéng qì tāng*) can be used to purge a greater yang-warp disorder that is beginning to transmit to the yang brightness warp, with dryness but no clumping. Major Order the Qi Decoction (*dà chéng qì tāng*) treats a yang brightness-organ warp that is centered on the Large Intestine with heat, excess, and clumping. Minor Order the Qi Decoction (*xiǎo chéng qì tāng*) treats a yang brightness-organ warp that is centered on the Small Intestine with a pattern marked by more pronounced qi stagnation.

➤ Vs. Major Bupleurum Decoction (*dà chái hú tāng*)

Both formulas treat heat excess patterns characterized by abdominal distention, pain, and constipation. To distinguish their usage, it is helpful to pay attention to the precise location of the abdominal symptoms. Major Bupleurum Decoction (*dà chái hú tāng*) treats combined lesser yang and yang brightness patterns and is thus specific for pain and distention in the flanks and upper abdomen. Major Order the Qi Decoction (*dà chéng qì tāng*) focuses solely on yang brightness patterns, which are characterized by pain and distention centered around the umbilicus.

➤ Vs. Major Decoction [for Pathogens] Stuck in the Chest (*dà xiàn xiōng tāng*); see page 69

➤ Vs. Coptis Decoction to Relieve Toxicity (*huáng lián jiě dú tāng*); see page 168

➤ Vs. Cool the Diaphragm Powder (*liáng gé sǎn*); see page 177

➤ Vs. Rhubarb and Moutan Decoction (*dà huáng mǔ dān tāng*); see page 882

Biomedical Indications

With the appropriate presentation, this formula may be used to treat a wide variety of biomedically-defined disorders. These can be divided into three main categories:

1. Acute abdominal conditions marked by pain, including various forms of intestinal obstruction, pancreatitis, appendicitis, cholecystitis, as well as postoperative problems

2. Febrile infectious diseases, including bacterial dysentery, acute icteric hepatitis, encephalitis, influenza, lobar pneumonia, and purulent tonsillitis

3. Any condition marked by intense abdominal fullness, high fevers, and a submerged, excessive, and slippery pulse. These include cardiopulmonary disease, asthma, enuresis, urinary tract stones, hemorrhoids, stroke, hypertension, and schizophrenia.

Modifications

• For high fever, severe thirst, and a rapid and forceful pulse (concurrent yang brightness channel and organ disorders), add Anemarrhenae Rhizoma (*zhī mǔ*) and Gypsum fibrosum (*shí gāo*).

• For a yang brightness organ disorder with damage to the yin fluids characterized by dry lips, a burnt yellow, dry tongue coating, and a thin and rapid pulse, add Rehmanniae Radix (*shēng dì huáng*), Scrophulariae Radix (*xuán shēn*), and Ophiopogonis Radix (*mài mén dōng*).

• For severe abdominal distention, add Raphani Semen (*lái fú zǐ*).

• For signs of blood stasis, add Persicae Semen (*táo rén*), Paeoniae Radix rubra (*chì sháo*), and Angelicae sinensis Radix (*dāng guī*).

Associated Formulas

小承氣湯（小承气汤）

Minor Order the Qi Decoction
xiǎo chéng qì tāng

Source   *Discussion of Cold Damage* (c. 220)

wine-washed Rhei Radix et Rhizoma (*jiǔ xǐ dà huáng*) 12g
prepared Magnoliae officinalis Cortex (*zhì hòu pò*) 6g
prepared Aurantii Fructus immaturus (*zhì zhǐ shí*) . . . . 3 pieces (6-9g)

Cook in 4 cups of water until slightly over 2 cups remain, and take in two divided doses. Moderately purges clumped heat. For relatively mild yang brightness organ-warp disorders characterized by tidal fever, constipation, focal distention, and abdominal fullness, abdominal pain that does not increase upon pressure, an 'old-looking' (dirty and dry) yellow tongue coating, and a slippery, rapid pulse. Also for early-stage dysenteric disorders. Because the dryness and clumping in the Intestines are relatively mild, the formula focuses on moving the qi without breaking up and eliminating heat that has acquired form. In clinical practice, this means that the obstruction will be less severe compared to the principal formula, and all core symptoms are thus less pronounced. For this reason, Natrii Sulfas (*máng xiāo*) is removed, as no softening of hardness is required. Furthermore, Rhei Radix et Rhizoma (*dà huáng*), the chief substance, is cooked here together with the other ingredients in order to moderate the harshness of its downward-draining action. Finally, the dosage of Magnoliae officinalis Cortex (*hòu pò*) and Aurantii Fructus immaturus (*zhǐ shí*) is reduced because the qi stagnation is not as pronounced.

Several passages in the source text describe use of this formula in order to determine whether purgation is appropriate. For example, paragraph 209 states that if one is unclear as to the diagnosis after six or seven days of no bowel movements, a small amount of this formula can be administered. If there are dried-up feces in the Large Intestine, this will cause them to shift and the patient will pass gas, whereupon Major Order the Qi Decoction (*dà chéng qì tāng*) should be given. No passing of gas means that only the tip of the fecal mass is hard and the rest is loose, so purging will not only be ineffective in treating the problem, it will damage the Spleen and Stomach. It is important to note that if all the manifestations of a Major Order the Qi Decoction (*dà chéng qì tāng*) presentation are present, time should not be wasted for this type of testing. It should be used, and not a weaker alternative.

Comparisons

➤ Vs. Hemp Seed Pill (*má zǐ rén wán*); *see* page 82

調胃承氣湯 (调胃承气汤)
Regulate the Stomach and Order the Qi Decoction
tiáo wèi chéng qì tāng

Source   *Discussion of Cold Damage* (c. 220)

Rhei Radix et Rhizoma (*dà huáng*) 12g
Glycyrrhizae Radix (*gān cǎo*) 6g
Natrii Sulfas (*máng xiāo*) 9-12g

Cook Rhei Radix et Rhizoma (*dà huáng*) with Glycyrrhizae Radix (*gān cǎo*), and dissolve Natrii Sulfas (*máng xiāo*) in the strained decoction. Mildly purges clumped heat. For mild constipation due to yang brightness-warp heat characterized by the absence of focal distention and abdominal fullness, but with irritability and a slippery, rapid pulse. Also for nosebleed, swollen gums and throat, and petechiae (subcutaneous bleeding) due to heat in the Stomach and Intestines. As the name of the formula indicates, it is intended to regulate and harmonize Stomach qi by removing obstructions. For this reason, Glycyrrhizae Radix (*gān cǎo*) is substituted for the potent qi-moving herbs Aurantii Fructus immaturus (*zhǐ shí*) and Magnoliae officinalis Cortex (*hòu pò*). The 18th-century physician Wang Zi-Jie explains: "[The formula] uses Glycyrrhizae Radix (*gān cǎo*) to moderate [the actions] of Rhei Radix et Rhizoma (*dà huáng*) and Natrii Sulfas (*máng xiāo*). It drains lingering heat from the middle [burner] and therefore is said to regulate the Stomach."

This gives the formula a very wide range of clinical applications. It is used, for example, to address the side effects or complications arising from the inappropriate use of warming substances, including excessive alcohol consumption. It is able to direct rebellious stomach qi downward and thus treats hiccup or retching due to excess Stomach heat. It can also be used to consolidate the effect of purgation once a dose of Major Order the Qi Decoction (*dà chéng qì tāng*) has opened the bowels, but the excess heat has not been entirely eliminated. When excess heat in the yang brightness has already damaged the yin, characterized by a faint or thin pulse, the modern physician Zhang Xi-Chun combines this formula with substances such as Haematitum (*dài zhě shí*), Asparagi Radix (*tiān mén dōng*), and Ginseng Radix (*rén shēn*) to order the qi while simultaneously tonifying the qi and blood.

大黃甘草湯 (大黄甘草汤)
Rhubarb and Licorice Decoction
dà huáng gān cǎo tāng

Source   *Essentials from the Golden Cabinet* (c. 220)

Rhei Radix et Rhizoma (*dà huáng*) 12g
Glycyrrhizae Radix (*gān cǎo*) 3g

Unblocks the bowels, purges, harmonizes the Stomach, and stops vomiting. For heat clumping in the Intestines (indicated by constipation) and fire rising to disturb the Stomach (indicated by vomiting). In contrast to the 'order the qi' formulas, this is not indicated for severe symptoms such as delirious speech, nor for pronounced abdominal distention or pain. It is, however, very useful for guiding excess fire downward and eliminating it via the bowels. Such patterns are characterized by facial flushing, red eyes, a red tongue with prickles, irritability, a bitter taste in the mouth, and an excessive, forceful pulse.

厚樸三物湯 (厚朴三物汤)
Three-Substance Decoction with Magnolia Bark
hòu pò sān wù tāng

Source   *Essentials from the Golden Cabinet* (c. 220)

Magnoliae officinalis Cortex (*hòu pò*) 24g
Aurantii Fructus immaturus (*zhǐ shí*) . . . . 5 pieces (12-15g)
Rhei Radix et Rhizoma (*dà huáng*) 12g

The source text says to cook the first two ingredients in approximately 12 cups of water until 5 cups remain. Then add the last herb, cook down until 3 cups remain, and take in three divided doses. At present, it is usually decocted in the normal manner, with the Rhei Radix et Rhizoma (*dà huáng*) added near the end.

Drains qi downward and unblocks the bowels. For qi stagnation causing constipation and unrelenting pain and fullness in the epigastrium and abdomen.

The source text states that this formula treats patients suffering "from pain with blockage (痛而閉 *tòng ér bì*)." Later commentators read this as indicating that constipation here is secondary to qi stagnation, unlike in Minor Order the Qi Decoction (*xiǎo chéng qì tāng*)—which contains the same ingredients but with a different dosage—where qi stagnation is secondary to clumping of heat and stools. This difference is explained in *Personal Standards for the Essentials from the Golden Cabinet*:

> Pain with blockage [implies] that the qi of the six yang organs does not move. Three-Substance Decoction with Magnolia Bark (*hòu pò sān wū tāng*) and Minor Order the Qi Decoction (*xiǎo chéng qì tāng*) are the same [in terms of their ingredients]. However, the intention of Minor Order the Qi Decoction (*xiǎo chéng qì tāng*) is to flush out excess, so its chief is Rhei Radix et Rhizoma (*dà huáng*). The intention of Three-Substance Decoction with Magnolia Bark (*hòu pò sān wū tāng*) is to move qi, so its chief is Magnoliae officinalis Cortex (*hòu pò*).

Alternate names

Magnolia Bark Decoction (厚樸湯 *hòu pò tāng*) in *Important Formulas Worth a Thousand Gold Pieces*; Three Substance Decoction (三物湯 *sān wù tāng*) in *Discussion of Blood Patterns*

三化湯 （三化汤）

Three-Transformation Decoction

sān huà tāng

SOURCE   *Collection of Writings on the Mechanism of Disease, Suitability of Qi, and the Safeguarding of Life as Discussed in Basic Questions* (1186)

Rhei Radix et Rhizoma (*dà huáng*) . . . .
Magnoliae officinalis Cortex (*hòu pò*) . . . .
Aurantii Fructus immaturus (*zhǐ shí*) . . . .
Notopterygii Rhizoma seu Radix (*qiāng huó*) . . . .

The source text advises to grind equal amounts of the four herbs into powder and then to prepare a draft by decocting 9g with 3 cups of water until half of the liquid has evaporated. The draft is then taken over the course of the day to produce a slight bowel movement and induce urination. Unblocks the bowels and dispels wind. For wind-stroke entering into the Intestines where pathogenic qi accumulates in the interior and the momentum of the heat is overwhelming. This leads to constipation and urinary blockage, mania with yang brightness characteristics, and delirious speech.

In contrast to Minor Order the Qi Decoction (*xiǎo chéng qì tāng*), on which this formula is based, it also dispels wind. *Supplemental Formulas Omitted from the Inner Classic* explains its action and name:

> Three [refers to] wind, stagnation, and phlegm. Transformation refers to the changes brought about by clearing and dispersal. The formula uses Notopterygii Rhizoma seu Radix (*qiāng huó*) to transform wind, Magnoliae officinalis Cortex (*hòu pò*) and Rhei Radix et Rhizoma (*dà huáng*) to transform stagnation, and Aurantii Fructus immaturus (*zhǐ shí*) to transform phlegm. Therefore, it is called Three Transformation [Decoction].

Investigations of Medical Formulas offers a slightly different explanation:

> Fullness of the upper burner is treated by Magnoliae officinalis Cortex (*hòu pò*). Fullness of the middle burner is broken up by Aurantii Fructus immaturus (*zhǐ shí*). Fullness of the lower burner is conducted out by Rhei Radix et Rhizoma (*dà huáng*). Notopterygii Rhizoma seu Radix (*qiāng huó*) is used so as not to forget the wind [that causes this condition]. Administration promotes slight movement of the bowels and urination. Accordingly, the qi of the three burners is no longer obstructed and takes up its charge of transmission and transformation once more. Therefore, it is called Three Transformation [Decoction].

At present, the formula is mainly used to treat wind-stroke due to external wind penetrating with a pattern dominated by constipation and abdominal fullness.

宣白承氣湯 （宣白承气汤）

Disseminate the White and Order the Qi Decoction

xuān baí chéng qì tāng

SOURCE   *Systematic Differentiation of Warm Pathogen Diseases* (1798)

Gypsum fibrosum (*shí gāo*) 15g
Rhei Radix et Rhizoma (*dà huáng*) 9g
Armeniacae Semen (*xìng rén*) 6g
Trichosanthis Pericarpium (*guā lóu pí*) 5g

The source text advises to decoct with 5 cups of water until 2 cups remain. The patient then drinks 1 cup. The second cup is administered only if the first does not cause the bowels to move. Drains heat clumping downward, disseminates the Lung qi, and transforms phlegm. Indicated for a yang brightness warm pathogen disorder where heat clumping in the Intestines is accompanied by phlegm-heat clogging the Lungs. This is characterized by afternoon tidal fever, constipation, acute wheezing, a stifling sensation in the chest, overabundance of sputum and oral mucus, a thick, greasy, yellow tongue coating, and a submerged, slippery, and rapid pulse.

White is the color of the Lungs. The name of the formula therefore refers to its ability to disseminate Lung qi. If diffusion of Lung qi is clogged up by phlegm, it can impede the downward movement of qi in the Intestines because the Lungs and Large Intestine are connected as yin and yang organs in an interior/exterior relationship. In a similar manner, heat clumping in the Intestines can impinge on the dissemination of Lung qi. The formula effectively addresses both aspects of this pattern.

導赤承氣湯 （导赤承气汤）

Guide Out the Red and Order the Qi Decoction

dǎo chì chéng qì tāng

SOURCE   *Systematic Differentiation of Warm Pathogen Diseases* (1798)

Paeoniae Radix rubra (*chì sháo*) 9g
Rehmanniae Radix (*shēng dì huáng*) 15g
Rhei Radix et Rhizoma (*dà huáng*) 9g
Coptidis Rhizoma (*huáng lián*) 6g
Phellodendri Cortex (*huáng bǎi*) 6g
Natrii Sulfas (*máng xiāo*) 3g

The source text advises to decoct the herbs with 5 cups of water until 2 cups remain. The patient then drinks 1 cup. A second cup is administered only if the first does not cause the bowels to open. Indicated for a yang brightness warm pathogen disease where use of a purgative formula has not been effective. The pattern is characterized by fever, irritability, thirst, abdominal fullness, constipation, reduced urination or urine that is darkish or red in color, rough urination accompanied by a burning sensation, a dry yellow tongue coating, and a submerged, rapid pulse that is wiry and powerful at the left distal position.

This is heat in the yang brightness organ that has been transmitted to the Small Intestine and Bladder. There it causes clumping of water and heat that, in turn, obstructs the movement and transformation of qi. Such a pattern is more likely to occur in patients who already have heat in the Heart that drains via the Small Intestine. The formula addresses this complex pathology by purging heat from the yang brightness with the help of Rhei Radix et Rhizoma (*dà huáng*) and Natrii Sulfas (*máng xiāo*), as well as draining it from the upper and lower burners with the help of Coptidis Rhizoma (*huáng lián*) and Phellodendri Cortex (*huáng bǎi*). In addition, it enriches the yin fluids with Rehmanniae Radix (*shēng dì huáng*), while Paeoniae Radix rubra (*chì sháo*) is used to promote urination and clear heat from the blood level.

復方大承氣湯 (复方大承气汤)

Revised Major Order the Qi Decoction

fù fāng dà chéng qì tāng

SOURCE *Integrated Chinese and Western Medical Treatment of the Acute Abdomen* (1973)

Magnoliae officinalis Cortex (*hòu pò*) 15g
dry-fried Raphani Semen (*chǎo lái fú zǐ*) 30g
Aurantii Fructus immaturus (*zhǐ shí*) 9g
Persicae Semen (*táo rén*) 9g
Paeoniae Radix rubra (*chì sháo*) 15g
Rhei Radix et Rhizoma (*dà huáng*) . . . . [add near end] 9g
Natrii Sulfas (*máng xiāo*) . . . . . [dissolve in strained decoction] 9-15g

The first dose is usually administered by nasogastric tube, and the second by enema 1-2 hours later. Purges the interior, promotes the movement of qi, and invigorates the blood. For uncomplicated intestinal obstruction with yang brightness organ-warp symptoms and relatively severe signs of qi stagnation. Also used to prevent adhesions after abdominal surgery. By adding Raphani Semen (*lái fú zǐ*) to open areas of constraint and move the qi, as well as Persicae Semen (*táo rén*) and Paeoniae Radix rubra (*chì sháo*) to invigorate the blood, the formula focuses more directly than the original formula on blood stasis and phlegm caused by the combination of qi stagnation, heat, and dryness.

大陷胸湯 (大陷胸汤)

Major Decoction [for Pathogens] Stuck in the Chest

dà xiàn xiōng tāng

The formula treats a pattern caused by the clumping of heat and internal accumulation of water and fluids in the chest. Although the literal term for this condition is 'chest clumping' (結胸 *jié xiōng*), the term 陷胸 *xiàn xiōng*, referring to something that has become 'stuck in the chest,' has the same meaning. In the source text, two types of this disorder are described. This formula is used for the more severe type, thus its designation as 'major.'

Source *Discussion of Cold Damage* (c. 220)

Kansui Radix (*gān suì*) 0.3-0.6g
Rhei Radix et Rhizoma (*dà huáng*) 18g
Natrii Sulfas (*máng xiāo*) 9-12g

Method of Preparation Decoction. Cook Rhei Radix et Rhizoma (*dà huáng*) separately, dissolve Natrii Sulfas (*máng xiāo*) in the strained decoction, and take warm with powdered Kansui Radix (*gān suì*). At present, 9-12g of Rhei Radix et Rhizoma (*dà huáng*) and 1.0-1.5g of Kansui Radix (*gān suì*) are generally used.

Actions Drains heat and drives out water by flushing downward

Indications

Fullness and hardness of the epigastrium or the entire abdomen with severe pain that becomes unbearable upon even the slightest amount of pressure, tidal fever at dusk, severe constipation, thirst, a very dry tongue coating, and a submerged, tight, and forceful pulse. There may also be shortness of breath and irritability.

This pattern is referred to as clumping in the chest (結胸 *jié xiōng*). It arises when heat and internal accumulation of water and fluids clump in the chest, interrupting the flow of qi in the trunk. Its etiology is most commonly attributed to the improper use of purgatives in the treatment of an exterior disorder. This disease dynamic is described by Ke Qin:

> The chest is the meeting place for all the greater yang and is where the gathering qi is focused, so it is called the sea of qi. The greater yang governs the qi for all the yang, and qi is the mother of water. If the qi is clear, the fluid essences are spread to the four extremities. When the qi becomes hot, water becomes turbid, leading to clogging and stasis.

In relatively mild cases, there is fullness, hardness, and pain in the epigastrium; in more severe cases, these symptoms may extend to the lower abdomen, and the pain becomes unbearable upon even the slightest pressure. Tidal fever at dusk is a sign of heat clumping in the interior. Clumping inhibits the distribution of fluids throughout the body. This manifests as severe constipation below and as thirst and a very dry tongue coating above. In this condition, the pathogenic influence is vigorous in the interior (indicated by the submerged, tight pulse), but the normal qi is strong (indicated by the forceful pulse).

Analysis of Formula

This formula combines two strategies to treat a pattern characterized by the clumping of water and heat: the cooling of heat and the downward draining of excess water via the bowels. The chief ingredient, cathartic and toxic Kansui Radix (*gān suì*), drives out the accumulation of water and fluids in the chest and abdomen by flushing downward. It is taken as a powder together with the decoction because this form of application further enhances the purgative actions of this herb. The deputies, Rhei Radix et Rhizoma (*dà huáng*) and Natrii Sulfas (*máng xiāo*), form a particularly powerful combination for flushing out the Intestines while draining and dispersing the clumps due to heat in the trunk. They moisten and soften hard, dry stool and assist the chief ingredient in driving out the heat and fluids clumped in the chest by way of the stool.

Cautions and Contraindications

Because of the strength of this formula and the toxicity of its chief ingredient, it should only be used for acute conditions. It should be taken just long enough to obtain results, and never for more than a few doses. Contraindicated during pregnancy or for very weak patients.

Commentary

Besides the improper use of purgatives, other etiologies for clumping in the chest have been identified over the centuries. As early as the *Discussion of Cold Damage,* it was indicated for externally-contracted disorders of over six days duration in which pathogenic heat enters the interior and clumps in the chest.

Clinically, the following signs and symptoms taken from the modern Japanese physician Nakamura Kensuke may be helpful in differentiating the pattern for which this formula is indicated. He finds that the pulse should also be wiry in addition to being submerged and excessive. The wiry quality reflects obstruction due to phlegm fluids and is not generally seen in similar patterns due to clumping of heat. The tongue coating may be white, which is also not seen in pure heat excess patterns, and dryness—indicating stagnation of fluids—rather than the color is the most important sign. The entire abdomen may be hard and resistant to pressure, but this will be most pronounced in the epigastric region where fluids most readily accumulate.

Commentators have debated the composition of the formula with respect to its chief herb. The majority view—represented by commentators like Cheng Wu-Ji and Wang Hu—is that Kansui Radix (*gān suì*) is the chief ingredient. However, Xu Hong, a well-known early Ming commentator on *Discussion of Cold Damage,* disagrees. He argues that while the pattern is caused by heat and water clumping in the chest, the most effective strategy for treating such clumping is to flush it out via the bowels. Thus, the chief herb must be Rhei Radix et Rhizoma (*dà huáng*). A third view is that of Lü Cha-Cun in *Seeking the Source of Cold Damage.* He succinctly sums up the interaction between the three ingredients in the formula and thereby resolves the tension between previous authors:

> [The action of the entire formula] completely hinges on the one ingredient Kansui Radix (*gān suì*). From the diaphragm, it causes the pathogen that has sunk downward to the yang brightness along with the pathogenic water that has risen upward to be separated and resolved. [Only then] can Natrii Sulfas (*máng xiāo*) and Rhei Radix et Rhizoma (*dà huáng*) begin to complete their action of conducting down and out.

Cheng Wu-Ji, the famous commentator on *Discussion of Cold Damage,* has an interesting understanding of this formula's name. He argues that the word 陷 *xiàn,* which also means 'sinking,' refers to the purgative action of this formula: "Chest clumping refers to a pathogen that is [lodged] high, one sinks it downward in order to [restore] balance."

Comparison

➢ Vs. Major Order the Qi Decoction (*dà chéng qì tāng*)

Major Decoction [for Pathogens] Stuck in the Chest (*dà xiàn xiōng tāng*) has a stronger purgative effect and drives out fluids instead of breaking up clumping of heat and stools. A clinically useful comparison of the two formulas is provided by You Yi in *String of Pearls from the [Discussion] of Cold Damage*:

> Major Decoction [for Pathogens] Stuck in the Chest (*dà xiàn xiōng tāng*) and Major Order the Qi Decoction (*dà chéng qì tāng*) differ in their action on the epigastrum (心下 *xīn xià*) and Stomach center (胃中 *wèi zhōng*) [respectively]. In my humble opinion, what [Zhang] Zhong-Jing calls the epigastrium really refers to the Stomach proper, and what he calls Stomach center really refers to the Large and Small Intestines. The Stomach is the great meeting place where food and drink stay together and the clear and turbid are not yet separated. When a pathogen enters and clumps together with residual phlegm and diverse foods without this being resolved, it turns into clumping of the chest. The Large and Small Intestines are places where only the dregs remain after the essences have been moved out. When a pathogen enters, it only clumps together with this foul matter, turning it into dry stools.
>
> Major Order the Qi Decoction (*dà chéng qì tāng*) focuses on dry stools in the Intestines. Major Decoction [for Pathogens] Stuck in the Chest (*dà xiàn xiōng tāng*) focuses on food and drink in the Stomach. [Treating] dry stools in the Intestines depends on [sufficient] power to drive them out, thus [the formula] needs Magnoliae officinalis Cortex (*hòu pò*) and Aurantii Fructus immaturus (*zhǐ shí*). [Treating] water and thin mucus in the Stomach requires an additional force to break up fluids, thus [the formula] uses Kansui Radix (*gān suì*). Furthermore, Major Order the Qi Decoction (*dà chéng qì tāng*) first decocts Magnoliae officinalis Cortex (*hòu pò*) and Aurantii Fructus immaturus (*zhǐ shí*) and then adds Rhei Radix et Rhizoma (*dà huáng*). Major Decoction [for Pathogens] Stuck in the Chest (*dà xiàn xiōng tāng*) first decocts Rhei Radix et Rhizoma (*dà huáng*) before taking all the herbs together. In treating the upper burner, mild control is appropriate, while in treating the lower burner, forceful control is appropriate. Raw Rhei Radix et Rhizoma (*dà huáng*) moves fast, while prepared Rhei Radix et Rhizoma (*dà huáng*) moves slowly. Although it is the same substance, its uses differ according to [its method of preparation].

Biomedical Indications

With the appropriate presentation, this formula may be used to treat a wide variety of biomedically-defined disorders, primarily acute abdominal diseases such as pancreatitis, cholecystitis, obstructive cholangitis, adhesive ileus, paralytic ileus, peritonitis, and upper GI perforations. This formula has also been used for acute exudative pleurisy, severe pneumonia, pericardial effusions, acute gastritis, pediatric meningitis, and psychiatric disorders.

Alternate name

Decoction [for Pathogens] Stuck in the Chest (*xiàn xiōng tāng*) in *Confucians' Duties to Their Parents*

Modification

- For acute pancreatitis or intestinal obstruction, combine with Major Order the Qi Decoction (*dà chéng qì tāng*).

Associated Formula

大陷胸丸

Major Pill [for Pathogens] Stuck in the Chest

dà xiàn xiōng wán

SOURCE   *Discussion of Cold Damage* (c. 220)

Rhei Radix et Rhizoma (*dà huáng*) 250g
Lepidii/ Descurainiae Semen (*tíng lì zǐ*) 175g
Natrii Sulfas (*máng xiāo*) 175g
Armeniacae Semen (*xìng rén*) 175g
Kansui Radix (*gān suì*) 30g

Grind the ingredients into powder, form into pills with 250g of honey, and take in 6-12g doses with warm water. Drains heat and drives out accumulation of water. For clumping in the chest with hardness, fullness, and pain, stiffness of the upper back and neck, and sweating. In contrast to the principal formula, which focuses on manifestations below the diaphragm, this formula focuses on manifestations above the diaphragm by incorporating herbs that aid the Lungs. Furthermore, by taking the herbs in pill form rather than as a decoction, the forceful action of the original formula is moderated. In the words of You Yi, author of *String of Pearls from the [Discussion] of Cold Damage*, it becomes a formula "that employs the nature of flushing out but turns it into a harmonized and moderate usage." Moderate usage, however, does not imply suitability for a deficient condition. In all cases, it is important before using this formula to ensure that the symptoms and pulse really reflect a pattern of excess. In terms of practical applications, Li Dong-Yuan's disciple Wang Hao-Gu expanded the indications of the formula to the treatment of yang-type hot wheezing, while the Ming-dynasty physician Ke Qin used it for the early stages of edema and dysenteric disorders.

Section 2

FORMULAS THAT WARM AND PURGE

The formulas in this section are used in treating accumulation due to cold excess in the interior characterized by constipation, abdominal fullness and distention, abdominal pain that responds favorably to warmth, cold in the extremities, and a submerged, tight pulse. For these conditions, purging

substances are still the most crucial ingredients, the most common ones being Rhei Radix et Rhizoma (*dà huáng*) and Crotonis Fructus (*bā dòu*). Because the conditions are due to internal cold, it is important to add herbs that warm the interior and dispel cold, such as Aconiti Radix lateralis praeparata (*zhì fù zǐ*), Asari Radix et Rhizoma (*xì xīn*), and Zingiberis Rhizoma (*gān jiāng*). Sometimes a significant part of the pathology is insufficiency of Spleen yang, where the Spleen qi and yang have been injured (perhaps by chronic diarrhea). If only purgatives are used, this will further damage the middle qi and any improvement will be temporary. In these cases, one should add herbs that tonify the middle qi, such as Ginseng Radix (*rén shēn*) and Codonopsis Radix (*dǎng shēn*).

大黃附子湯 (大黄附子汤)

Rhubarb and Aconite Accessory Root Decoction

dà huáng fù zǐ tāng

Source   *Essentials from the Golden Cabinet* (c. 220)

baked Aconiti Radix lateralis (*bāo fù zǐ*) . . . . 3 pieces (9-12g)
Rhei Radix et Rhizoma (*dà huáng*) 9g
Asari Radix et Rhizoma (*xì xīn*) 6g

Method of Preparation   Decoction. Cook Rhei Radix et Rhizoma (*dà huáng*) with the other herbs.

Actions   Warms the interior, disperses cold, unblocks the bowels, and alleviates pain

Indications

Abdominal pain, constipation, hypochondriac pain, chills, low-grade fever, cold hands and feet, a white, greasy tongue coating, and a submerged, tight, and wiry pulse.

This is a cold pathogen and accumulation from stagnation that clump together in the interior. Cold is a yin pathogen. When it enters into the interior, it obstructs and constrains the flow of qi and blood, causing abdominal or hypochondriac pain, the province of the terminal yin (Liver) channel. Cold excess impeding the Intestines manifests as constipation. It also interferes with the spreading of yang qi through the body, producing a feeling of cold, especially in the hands and feet. This is different from the chills due to an exterior condition in which all parts of the body are equally cold. When the yang is constrained, it may also produce a low-grade fever. The white, greasy tongue coating and the submerged, tight, and wiry pulse are indicative of cold excess in the interior.

Analysis of Formula

This formula uses a combination of warming and purging substances: warming substances for interior cold and draining substances for accumulation. The chief herb, acrid and hot Aconiti Radix lateralis praeparata *(zhì fù zǐ),* is the most effective substance in the materia medica for warming the yang and dispelling cold. In this case, because the cold is severe and because it is combined with a cooling substance, its dosage is higher than usual.

The deputy herb, Rhei Radix et Rhizoma *(dà huáng),* is used here to flush the Intestines and purge stagnant accumulation. It also enters the Liver channel at the blood level where it assists in the treatment of hypochondriac pain and directs the actions of the other herbs into the Intestines. This is a more subtle and complex action than merely draining fire through the stool. For this reason, the dosage of this herb is much lower than in formulas in which it serves as the chief herb, such as Major Order the Qi Decoction *(dà chéng qì tāng).* It is also cooked with the other herbs. The cold, bitter nature of Rhei Radix et Rhizoma *(dà huáng)* is counterbalanced by the acrid, warm nature of the other herbs.

Asari Radix et Rhizoma *(xì xīn),* the assistant, is a powerful substance for expelling cold and dispersing accumulation or clumping. Zhang Zhong-Jing regularly combined this herb with Aconiti Radix lateralis *(fù zǐ)* to treat pathogenic cold that lurks deeply in the yin portion of the body.

Cautions and Contraindications

Because the formula is warming, it is contraindicated in patterns of interior heat excess. Furthermore, if application of the formula is followed by a bowel movement, the prognosis is generally good. If, on the other hand, it causes vomiting, increased chills, or the appearance of a thin pulse, it indicates a worsening of the condition that requires urgent attention.

Commentary

This formula is the model for all other formulas that warm the yang and purge. It was first listed in Chapter 10 of *Essentials from the Golden Cabinet,* which deals with the differential diagnosis and treatment of abdominal fullness, bulging disorders, and harbored food. All of these disorders are due to accumulation or stagnation, with pain as the most prominent symptom. The present formula treats a pattern that is characterized by "stubborn pain under the ribs, fever, and a tight and wiry pulse."

Because the ribs correspond to the Liver and the terminal yin, several commentators interpret this pattern as reflecting a Liver disorder. The Qing-dynasty physician Wu Ju-Tong is representative of this group:

> This [formula treats] a pathogen residing in the terminal yin, where both exterior and interior need urgent attention. … A wiry pulse indicates Liver constraint, a tight [pulse] interior cold. Stubborn pain under the ribs, [the area traversed by] the channels and collaterals of the Liver and Gallbladder, indicates cold and dampness contending. This [leads to] constraint within the blood aspect that manifests as pain. Fever is due to the Liver being constrained. Thus, one employs Aconiti Radix

lateralis *(fù zǐ)* to warm the interior and unblock the yang, and Asari Radix et Rhizoma *(xì xīn)* to warm the water organ and disperse cold and damp pathogens. The Liver and Gallbladder have no exit passage [of their own]. Therefore, one uses Rhei Radix et Rhizoma *(dà huáng)* to supply them with an exit passage via the Stomach [from which accumulation can be eliminated].

Other commentators, such as the compilers of the *Golden Mirror of the Medical Tradition,* argue that the primary disease dynamic is cold in the Spleen and Liver. Unlike the source text, they therefore regard the main symptoms to include abdominal fullness and pain (Spleen) as well as stubborn pain in the ribs (Liver). Accordingly, they interpret the dynamic of the formula differently. They suggest that Rhei Radix et Rhizoma *(dà huáng)* is used to drain accumulation from the Spleen and abdomen, and Asari Radix et Rhizoma *(xì xīn)* to relieve pain in the Liver and ribs. While they do not specify the precise dynamic of the Asari Radix et Rhizoma *(xì xīn)* action, one can presume it works by warm dispersal of water and dampness to open the collaterals.

Yet another interpretation is advanced by the early 20th-century expert of classical formulas, Cao Ying-Fu. In *Elaborating on the Subtleties of the Golden Cabinet,* Cao argues that the underlying problem is one of water qi or thin mucus accumulating under the ribs:

> How does one know that stubborn pain under the ribs is [due to] cold water congealing and clumping? Fever [makes this problem] resemble a pattern [where the pathogen resides in the] exterior. How does one know that one must drain downward? Anyone diagnosing such a disorder must know [the answer] for certain. [The area] below the ribs pertains to the Kidneys. It is a key point [of transmission] for the waterways in the middle and lower burner [because the fluids return from the Lungs in the upper burner via the Stomach and Intestines located below the ribs to the Bladder and Kidneys] …
> If the waterways are obstructed at this key point, there is pain below the ribs. … If yin cold seizes the interior, floating yang oversteps [its bounds] in the exterior. If yin cold is not broken, the solitary yang [in the exterior] cannot return to its source in the gate of vitality [causing fever]. … The formula employs Aconiti Radix lateralis *(fù zǐ)* and Asari Radix et Rhizoma *(xì xīn)* to dispel cold and direct rebellious [yang] downward, to move water, and stop pain. Furthermore, it relies on Rhei Radix et Rhizoma *(dà huáng)* to facilitate [this downward movement]. In this manner, the congealing and stasis of water is broken up and the waterways below the ribs are unblocked. The *Inner Classic* says: pain indicates that something is blocked. Is this [not always] so?

The apparent disagreement among commentators regarding all aspects of the formula's indication and functions—of which the above is but a small selection—should not distract us from the underlying consensus: that the formula opens the qi dynamic, which is obstructed by cold; that this obstruction is severe and involves binding of qi and fluids or blood; that obstruction of the qi dynamic in the lower burner, the dwelling place of Liver and Kidneys, often manifests with rebellion; and that the bowels are used as a pathway to conduct the pathogens out of the body.

This allows us to understand the many directions in which use of this formula has been developed over subsequent centuries. *Comprehensive Medicine According to Master Zhang* recommends it for "jaundice with slight sweating of the forehead, [unobstructed] urination, black stools, and pain in the lower abdomen extending to the back." Lu Yuan-Lei, in *Modern Explanation of the Golden Cabinet,* uses it to treat cold-type bulging disorders, gripping pain in the chest and abdomen, swelling of the testicles, occasional water sounds in the abdomen, and severe aversion to cold. More recently, the formula has become a standard in the treatment of uremia, where it is frequently applied as an enema with the intention of conducting toxins out of the body. This can be seen as an extrapolation of the disease dynamic described by Cao Ying-Fu and others above.

Comparisons

➤ Vs. Ephedra, Asarum, and Aconite Accessory Root Decoction (*má huáng xì xīn fù zǐ tāng*)

The combination of Aconiti Radix lateralis praeparata (*fù zǐ*) and Asari Radix et Rhizoma (*xì xīn*) is frequently used in formulas that seek to dispel lurking cold from the interior. Both this formula and Rhubarb and Aconite Accessory Root Decoction (*dà huáng fù zǐ tāng*) use Aconiti Radix lateralis praeparata (*fù zǐ*) to warm the channels and support the yang, and Asari Radix et Rhizoma (*xì xīn*) to dispel cold from the interior in a manner that mutually accentuates their action. Combining them with bitter and downward-draining Rhei Radix et Rhizoma (*dà huáng*), the present formula is able to dislodge cold excess accumulating in the interior and purge it via the bowels. Combining them with acrid and light Ephedrae Herba (*má huáng*), Ephedra, Asarum, and Aconite Accessory Root Decoction (*má huáng xì xīn fù zǐ tāng*) focuses their action on warming the channels in order to resolve the exterior.

➤ Vs. Warm the Spleen Decoction (*wēn pí tāng*); see page 74

Biomedical Indications

With the appropriate presentation, this formula may be used to treat a wide variety of biomedically-defined disorders. These can be divided into three categories:

1. Acute pain anywhere in the body that primarily occurs on one side, including trigeminal neuralgia, periarthritis of the shoulder, gallstones, kidney stones, appendicitis, inguinal hernia, orchitis, sciatica, and phlebitis

2. Acute inflammatory processes affecting the head that can be seen as 'cold enclosing fire' (寒包火 *hán bāo huǒ*), such as sties, keratitis, conjunctivitis, tonsillitis, and purulent gingivitis

3. A variety of other diseases including chronic renal failure, lumbar disc disease, recalcitrant skin diseases such as urticaria or eczema, dermatitis from allergies to drugs, and bacillary dysentery.

Alternate name

Rhubarb, Aconite Accessory Root, and Asarum Decoction (*dà huáng fù zǐ xì xīn tāng*) in *Notes from Random Wandering*

Modifications

- For severe abdominal pain, add Cinnamomi Ramulus (*guì zhī*) and Paeoniae Radix alba (*bái sháo*).
- For severe distention and a thick, dirty tongue coating, add Aurantii Fructus immaturus (*zhǐ shí*) and Massa medicata fermentata (*shén qū*).
- For more severe qi stagnation and accumulation, add Magnoliae officinalis Cortex (*hòu pò*) and Aucklandiae Radix (*mù xiāng*).
- For cold hernial disorders with severe back and groin pain, add Cinnamomi Cortex (*ròu guì*) and Foeniculi Fructus (*xiǎo huí xiāng*).
- For general debility or rather mild accumulation, use prepared Rhei Radix et Rhizoma (*zhì dà huáng*).
- For patients with a weak constitution, add Codonopsis Radix (*dǎng shēn*) and Angelicae sinensis Radix (*dāng guī*).

Associated Formula

降氮湯 （降氮汤）

Direct Nitrogen Downward Decoction

jiàng dàn tāng

Source　Fang Shu-Yuan, *Shanghai Journal of Chinese Medicine and Pharmacology* 上海中醫藥雜誌 (1987) 3: 19

Rhei Radix et Rhizoma (*dà huáng*) 20g
Aconiti Radix lateralis praeparata (*zhì fù zǐ*) 15g
Scutellariae Radix (*huáng qín*) 50g
Ostreae Concha (*mǔ lì*) 50g

Decoction. Apply 150ml as an enema two to three times per day. Drains downward, pushes out toxins, and expels turbidity. This is one of a number of similar formulas composed during the 1980s to treat uremia.

温脾湯 （温脾汤）

Warm the Spleen Decoction

wēn pí tāng

Source　*Important Formulas Worth a Thousand Gold Pieces* (650)

Rhei Radix et Rhizoma *(dà huáng)* 12g
Ginseng Radix *(rén shēn)* 6g
Glycyrrhizae Radix *(gān cǎo)* 6g
Zingiberis Rhizoma *(gān jiāng)* 6g
Aconiti Radix lateralis praeparata *(zhì fù zǐ)* 9g

Method of Preparation   Decoction. Rhei Radix et Rhizoma *(dà huáng)* is added near the end.

Actions   Warms and tonifies Spleen yang and purges cold accumulation

Indications

Constipation or chronic red-and-white dysenteric disorders (i.e., those with both pus and blood in the stool) associated with abdominal pain, cold extremities, a white tongue coating, and a submerged, wiry pulse.

This is Spleen cold from yang deficiency with accumulation impeding the Intestines. If the Spleen yang is insufficient to fulfill its functions of transportation and transformation, cold accumulates in the Intestines, impeding their downward-directing of qi and the movement of stools. This leads to abdominal pain and constipation. Alternatively, chronic accumulation that is not transformed exhausts the Spleen qi and yang. This results in dysentery with both pus and blood as the Spleen's retaining function is impaired. Insufficiency of Spleen yang implies failure of yang qi to reach the extremities, which manifests in hands and feet that are difficult to keep warm. The white tongue coating indicates cold accumulation. A submerged pulse reflects an interior disorder, while a wiry pulse is associated with stagnation and pain.

Analysis of Formula

Treating insufficiency of Spleen yang accompanied by accumulation of cold in the interior presents the physician with a dilemma. Merely tonifying a deficiency does not eliminate severe stagnation. Attacking the accumulation by draining downward, on the other hand, risks further damaging the body's yang qi. Thus, it is necessary to combine the strategy of warming and tonifying the Spleen yang with that of purging the accumulation. This formula accordingly has two chief herbs, Aconiti Radix lateralis praeparata *(zhì fù zǐ)* and Rhei Radix et Rhizoma *(dà huáng)*. Aconiti Radix lateralis praeparata *(zhì fù zǐ)* is acrid and strongly warming. It invigorates the Spleen yang in order to disperse the congealed cold. Rhei Radix et Rhizoma *(dà huáng)* flushes the Stomach and Intestines to eliminate accumulation. Zingiberis Rhizoma *(gān jiāng)* functions as deputy by focusing the action of the formula on the Spleen yang. It is acrid and warming and enters into the Spleen and Stomach channels. Together with Aconiti Radix lateralis praeparata *(zhì fù zǐ)*, it supports the Spleen yang so as to eliminate the cold pathogen. As early as the *Divine Husbandman's Classic of the Materia Medica*, it was indicated for the treatment of dysenteric disorders. Ginseng

Radix *(rén shēn)* and Glycyrrhizae Radix *(gān cǎo)* are the assistants. Together with Aconiti Radix lateralis praeparata *(zhì fù zǐ)* and Zingiberis Rhizoma *(gān jiāng)*, they warm the Spleen yang following the principle that, in order to assist the yang, one must first augment the qi. Glycyrrhizae Radix *(gān cǎo)* also functions as an envoy to harmonize the contradictory functions of the different herbs in the formula, accommodating heating with cooling and tonification with draining.

Cautions and Contraindications

This formula treats accumulations of interior cold. It is contraindicated in cases of constipation due to interior heat with clumping and damage to the body fluids.

Commentary

The source text lists a number of different formulas under the name Warm the Spleen Decoction *(wēn pí tāng)*. The present formula is from Chapter 15 of that text. The same chapter contains a second formula that uses Cinnamomi Cortex *(ròu guì)* instead of Glycyrrhizae Radix *(gān cǎo)* and is indicated for "chronic accumulations of heat and cold [leading to] red-and-white dysentery." Chapter 13 of the same text, which deals with abdominal and epigastric pain, lists a formula that contains two additional substances, Angelicae sinensis Radix *(dāng guī)* and Natrii Sulfas *(máng xiāo)*. It treats chronic gripping abdominal pain with accumulations below the umbilicus.

Based on an analysis of the similarities and differences among these formulas, the Qing-dynasty commentators Zhang Lu and Xu Da-Chun argue that over time, accumulations in the Intestines that are not drained exhaust the body's yang qi. This accounts for the chronic nature of the disorders. However, even if the external manifestation is one of insufficiency of yang, there will invariably be some heat in the Intestines. This may be residual damp-heat, which predominates in the early, acute stages of dysenteric disorders, or it may be heat that arises from stagnation of yang qi and mixes with the stools. Because this heat takes on form, it must be drained. However, the chronic nature of these disorders indicates that this can only be achieved by simultaneously fortifying the yang.

Comparison

➤ Vs. Rhubarb and Aconite Accessory Root
   Decoction *(dà huáng fù zǐ tāng)*

Both formulas warm the yang to disperse cold and purge cold accumulations. For this reason, they combine strongly warming Aconiti Radix lateralis praeparata *(zhì fù zǐ)* with cold and bitter but downward-draining Rhei Radix et Rhizoma *(dà huáng)*. Rhubarb and Aconite Accessory Root Decoction *(dà huáng fù zǐ tāng)* is indicated for conditions of cold excess accumulating below the flanks or in the lower abdomen. The site of the accumulation will be visibly tense with pain increasing on palpation. As a variation of Frigid Extremities Decoction with Ginseng *(sì nì jiā rén shēn tāng)*, the present formula focuses primarily on Spleen deficiency and only secondarily flushes out accumulations from the Intestines. Although patients may experience a sensation of fullness in the lower abdomen, pressure will reduce rather than increase any such discomfort. Warmth brings relief in both patterns.

Biomedical Indications

With the appropriate presentation, this formula may be used to treat a variety of biomedically-defined disorders, primarily digestive, such as ulcerative colitis, chronic bacillary dysentery, intestinal adhesions, and intestinal obstruction. It has also been used for uremia following chronic renal disease.

Modifications

- For more severe abdominal pain, add Cinnamomi Cortex *(ròu guì)*, Aucklandiae Radix *(mù xiāng)*, and Magnoliae officinalis Cortex *(hòu pò)*.
- For vomiting, add Pinelliae Rhizoma praeparatum *(zhì bàn xià)* and Amomi Fructus *(shā rén)*.
- For chronic dysentery with more severe heat in the Intestines, add Coptidis Rhizoma *(huáng lián)*, Scutellariae Radix *(huáng qín)*, and Lonicerae Flos *(jīn yín huā)*.
- For relatively mild cases of accumulation, reduce the dosage of Rhei Radix et Rhizoma *(dà huáng)*.

Associated Formula

溫脾湯 （温脾汤）

Warm the Spleen Decoction from *Formulas of Universal Benefit*

wēn pí tāng

SOURCE   *Formulas of Universal Benefit from My Practice* (1132)

Magnoliae officinalis Cortex *(hòu pò)* 15g
Zingiberis Rhizoma praeparatum *(páo jiāng)* 15g
Glycyrrhizae Radix *(gān cǎo)* 15g
Cinnamomi Cortex *(ròu guì)* 15g
Aconiti Radix lateralis praeparata *(zhì fù zǐ)* 15g
Rhei Radix et Rhizoma *(dà huáng)* 12g

Grind the herbs into a powder and prepare as a draft. Rhei Radix et Rhizoma *(dà huáng)* is added near the end. Warms and tonifies the Spleen yang and purges cold accumulation. For Spleen cold from deficiency with accumulation of cold characterized by constipation or diarrhea. The diarrhea here has no pattern and is not relieved by the use of warming herbs alone. The source text recommends this formula for draining the accumulation from the Intestines; once this has been achieved, it should be followed with tonifying formulas to regulate the underlying deficiency. Compared with the principal formula, this modification is more warming.

三物備急丸 （三物备急丸）

Three-Substance Pill Prepared for Emergencies

sān wù bèi jí wán

According to Wang Zi-Jie in *Selected Annotations to Ancient Formulas from the Garden of Crimson Snow*:

> The term 'prepared' refers to a previously [readied] tool waiting to be used. 'Urgent' (及 *jí*) means just in time, referring to a pressing situation. *Essentials from the Golden Cabinet* uses this formula to help where obnoxious guest qi in the middle [burner leads to] distention and fullness in the heart [chest] and abdomen, sudden pain as if being stabbed by an awl, urgent breathing, and trismus. If one does not have prepared herbs ready in a situation where one must break the teeth to irrigate [the mouth] for immediate revival, then [treatment does not] come in time.

Source   *Essentials from the Golden Cabinet* (c. 220)

Crotonis Fructus *(bā dòu)* 30g
Zingiberis Rhizoma *(gān jiāng)* 30g
Rhei Radix et Rhizoma *(dà huáng)* 30g

Method of Preparation   Grind the ingredients into powder and take in 0.6-1.5g doses (reduce for children) with rice water or warm, boiled water. The source text advises to take in either powdered or pill form (made with honey). Administer with a nasogastric tube for those patients who are unable to open their mouths.

Actions   Harshly purges cold accumulation

Indications

Sudden epigastric and abdominal pain and distention with pain so intense that it feels "as if an awl is piercing the abdomen," rough, uneven breathing, a cyanotic complexion, no bowel movements, a bluish-purple tongue with a white coating, and a submerged, tight pulse. In severe cases, there may also be loss of consciousness with the mouth tightly closed.

This is sudden onset of severe cold accumulation, which is attributed to cold food stagnating in the Stomach and Intestines where it completely obstructs the flow of qi. This leads to a sudden, excruciatingly sharp pain in the epigastrium and abdomen, and obstruction of the bowels. The qi dynamic becomes rebellious and chaotic, which is manifested in the abdominal distention and the rough, uneven breathing. The combination of cold and severe stagnation produces a cyanotic complexion and a bluish-purple tongue. In extreme cases, there may be loss of consciousness with the mouth tightly closed, which is a life-threatening condition. Both the bluish-purple tongue and the submerged, tight pulse are indicative of cold excess in the interior.

Analysis of Formula

In this condition, only very hot, acrid substances can disperse the accumulation of cold, and only harsh purgatives can expel the excess. The chief herb, Crotonis Fructus *(bā dòu)*, is a hot, acrid, and harsh purgative. The deputy, warm and acrid Zingiberis Rhizoma *(gān jiāng)*, assists the chief herb in dispelling cold. It also revives the Spleen yang. The assistant, cold and bitter Rhei Radix et Rhizoma *(dà huáng)*, flushes the Stomach and Intestines and moderates the hot, acrid, and toxic properties of the chief herb.

Cautions and Contraindications

Crotonis Fructus *(bā dòu)* is a toxic substance that should be used with extreme caution. It is contraindicated in weak and pregnant patients and in cases of acute abdominal pain due to heat or summerheat.

Commentary

This is an extremely harsh formula that will induce diarrhea and often vomiting. It should only be used in true emergencies. If the diarrhea becomes severe, it may be stopped by taking cool rice porridge.

Commentators have debated the precise function of Rhei Radix et Rhizoma *(dà huáng)* in the formula. One good explanation is offered by Wang Zi-Jie in *Selected Annotations to Ancient Formulas from the Garden of Crimson Snow*:

- Crotonis Fructus *(bā dòu)* is acrid, warming, and severely toxic. Used fresh, it has an urgent nature that opens obstructions to the pathways of food and drink and flushes yin haze from the five yin organs and six yang organs. Its nature and taste and that of Rhei Radix et Rhizoma *(dà huáng)* are antagonistic to one another. When used together, their draining [effect] on a person is moderated.

Comparisons

The classic indication of this formula is 'yin clumping' (陰結 *yīn jié*), denoting that cold pathogens have penetrated into the Stomach and Intestines. This is differentiated from 'yang clumping' (陽結 *yáng jié*) caused by heat pathogens, for which the various Order the Qi Decoctions *(chéng qì tāng)* or Pill Requiring a Change of Clothing *(gēng yī wán)* are indicated. However, because the present formula contains both warming and cooling substances, it can also be used for mixed patterns, provided that cold is dominant.

Both White Powder *(bái sǎn)*, discussed as an associated formula below, and the present formula use Crotonis Fructus *(bā dòu)* in order to drain yin clumping from the body. White Powder *(bái sǎn)* drains yin clumping from the chest. It contains Platycodi Radix *(jié gěng)*, which focuses the action of the formula on the upper burner. The present formula drains yin clumping from the Stomach and Intestines. It contains Rhei Radix et Rhizoma *(dà huáng)*, which focuses the action of the formula on the middle and lower burners.

➢ Vs. Pinellia and Sulphur Pill *(bàn liú wán)*; *see* PAGE 77

Biomedical Indications

With the appropriate presentation, this formula may be used to treat a variety of biomedically-defined disorders, including postoperative adhesions, intestinal obstruction, acute cholecystitis, and recalcitrant constipation.

Alternate names

Pill Prepared for Emergencies *(beì jí wán)* in *Supplement to Important Formulas Worth a Thousand Gold Pieces*; Sagely Support Pill Prepared for Emergencies *(dǐ shèng beì jí wán)* in *Monthly Ordinances Worth a Thousand Gold Pieces*; Croton Seed Three Ingredients Pill *(bā dòu sān wèi wán)* in *Xu Ren-Ze's Formulas*; Three-Substance Pill Prepared for Emergencies *(beì jí sān wù wán)* in *Comprehensive Recording of Sagely Beneficence*; Return the Ethereal Soul Pill *(fǎn hún dān)* in *Ji-Feng's Formulas of Universal Benefit*; Rhubarb Pill Prepared for Emergencies *(beì jí dà huáng wán)* in *Clarifying Doubts about Damage from Internal and External Causes*; Pill Prepared for Emergencies *(beì jí dān)* in *Precious Mirror of Health*; Emergency Preparedness Rhubarb Pill *(beì jí dà huáng wán)* in *Introduction to Medicine*; Three Immortals Strung Together *(sān xiān chuàn)* in *Supplement to the Elegant Lexicon of Itinerant Physicians*; and Three Sages Pill *(sān shèng dān)* in *Collection Picked by Immortals*

Associated Formula

白散

White Powder

bái sǎn

SOURCE *Discussion of Cold Damage* (c. 220)

Platycodi Radix *(jié gěng)* . . . . 3 parts
Crotonis Fructus *(bā dòu)* . . . . 1 part
Fritillariae Bulbus *(bèi mǔ)* . . . . 3 parts

Grind the ingredients into powder and take in 0.5-1.0g doses with warm water. The source text advises to give the patient warm rice gruel if taking the formula does not induce diarrhea, or cold rice gruel if the diarrhea does not stop. Warmly drains downward, expels water, transforms phlegm, and disperses clumping. For cold-phlegm leading to cold excess clumping in the chest characterized by a sensation of extreme fullness and hardness in the chest (possibly extending to the lower abdomen), constipation, and coughing up of turbid, fishy-smelling sputum. It is less harsh a purgative than the principal formula, and is more effective in treating phlegm and those conditions localized in the chest.

Comparison

➢ Vs. Pinellia and Sulphur Pill *(bàn liú wán)*; *see* PAGE 77

半硫丸

Pinellia and Sulphur Pill

bàn liú wán

Source *Formulary of the Pharmacy Service for Benefiting the People in the Taiping Era* (1107)

Pinelliae Rhizoma praeparatum *(zhì bàn xià)*
processed Sulphur *(zhì liú huáng)*

Method of Preparation   The source text advises to prepare pills by using equal amounts of both substances, grinding them into a fine powder, and mixing this with the juice extracted from Zingiberis Rhizoma recens *(shēng jiāng)* to form pills. Men should take 15-20 pills the size of a Chinese parasol tree fruit (comparable to the small size pills in which Chinese herbal formulas are sold commercially) with warm wine or a decoction of Zingiberis Rhizoma recens *(shēng jiāng)* on an empty stomach. Women should take the same amount with a vinegar decoction. At present, no distinction is made between men and women, and the normal dosage is to take as a powder, starting at 0.5g a day and increasing up to 3g a day if necessary.

Actions   Fortifies the fire at the gate of vitality, expels cold, unblocks the yang, and drains turbidity

Indications

Habitual constipation or chronic diarrhea, increased urination with urine that is clear in color, a pale complexion, cold extremities, abdominal pain that is aggravated by cold, a heavy or cold sensation in the lower back and spine, a pale tongue with a white coating, and a submerged, slow pulse.

This is deficiency cold manifesting as habitual constipation or chronic diarrhea, a pattern found most frequently in older people. Although the symptoms of constipation and diarrhea appear to be contradictory, the underlying disease dynamic in both cases is declining fire at the gate of vitality, which leads to cold and turbid yin congealing and accumulating internally. If the yang qi in the yang brightness channels is insufficient, downward movement of qi and matter in the Intestines slows down, the stools become difficult to push out, and habitual constipation results. The Kidneys govern storage and the two yin openings (the anus and the urethra). They are the 'gate of the Stomach.' If Kidney yang becomes insufficient, this gate does not close securely and the two yin openings leak. Chronic diarrhea and urination with large amounts of clear urine ensue. The pale complexion and cold extremities both indicate that the fire at the gate of vitality is failing. A pale tongue with a white coating are manifestations of debilitated yang with yin cold accumulating internally. The submerged and slow pulse also reflects this condition.

Analysis of Formula

In order to dispel turbid yin accumulating in the Intestines due to yang deficiency and leading to constipation or diarrhea, one should warm the interior, dispel cold, unblock the yang, and discharge turbidity. To this end, the formula employs sour, warming, and toxic processed Sulphur *(zhì liú huáng)* as the chief. It strongly fortifies the fire at the gate of vitality and promotes the dynamic of yang qi. Its action, however, is gentle. Its sour taste, furthermore, secures the yin, keeping physiological fluids in the Intestines to facilitate bowel movement. Wang Ken-Tang aptly notes, "Warming

herbs mostly cause constipation. Only Sulphur *(liú huáng)* is gentle and can unblock [the Intestines]."

Pinelliae Rhizoma praeparatum *(zhì bàn xià)* is the deputy. It is acrid and warm, harmonizes the Stomach, and directs its qi downward, while its bitterness also dries turbid yin. It thereby focuses the action of the chief herb on the yang brightness. Zingiberis Rhizoma recens *(shēng jiāng)* juice, used in the preparation of the pills, acts as assistant and envoy. It reduces the toxicity of the two main ingredients, warms the middle burner, disperses cold, and facilitates the movement of qi by unblocking the interstices.

All of the substances in this formula are warming in nature and facilitate the movement of qi. Nevertheless, by fortifying the function of the Kidney yang, they also assist the body in containing the essence. Thus, even as the formula promotes bowel movement and expels cold, it also has the ability to stop chronic diarrhea.

Cautions and Contraindications

Although this formula is indicated for habitual constipation in the eldery, it must not be used in cases with yin or blood deficiency.

Commentary

Although this formula contains two potentially toxic substances, the toxicity is moderated by their preparation with the juice of Zingiberis Rhizoma recens *(shēng jiāng)* The form of processed Sulphur *(zhì liú huáng)* preferred is the so-called sinuous sulphur (倭硫磺 *wō liú huáng*), which are small, crystalline, light yellow, translucent pieces. Although the substance is referred to as very toxic in the older materia medica, modern pharmacological research suggests that this is not the case and that it is very safe to use. Due caution should be exercised in patients with heart, liver, or kidney disease. The prepared form of Pinelliae Rhizoma praeparatum *(zhì bàn xià)* should be used in contemporary practice.

The indications of this formula have been expanded by later generations of physicians. Wu Ju-Tong used it to treat interior cold leading to 'dampness obstructing the qi without form' in the Triple Burner, causing constipation and reduced urination or urinary blockage. In *Compendium of China's Medicine and Medicinals,* the early modern physician Cai Lu-Xian argues that the formula also is useful in treating phlegm patterns manifesting with constipation because it contains Pinelliae Rhizoma praeparatum *(zhì bàn xià)*.

Comparisons

➤ Vs. THREE-SUBSTANCE PILL PREPARED FOR EMERGENCIES *(sān wù bèi jí wán)* OR WHITE POWDER *(bái săn)*

Both Crotonis Fructus *(bā dòu)* and Sulphur *(liú huáng)* are toxic substances that can be used in the treatment of cold-type constipation and bowel obstruction. However, Crotonis Fructus (*bā dòu*) has a very harsh action. Formulas containing Crotonis Fructus (*bā dòu*), such as Three-Substance Pill Prepared for Emergencies (*sān wù bèi jí wán*) or White Powder (*bái sǎn*), are therefore used to treat acute conditions from excess. Processed Sulphur (*zhì liú huáng*) acts gently. Formulas like Pinellia and Sulphur Pill (*bàn liú wán*) are thus indicated to treat chronic conditions associated with deficiency.

➤ Vs. Benefit the River [Flow] Decoction (*jì chuān jiān*); *see* PAGE 85

Biomedical Indications

With the appropriate presentation, this formula may be used to treat a wide variety of biomedically-defined disorders, such as constipation in the elderly, chronic diarrhea, and impotence.

Alternate Names

Pinellia Pill (*bàn xià wán*) in *Discussion of Illnesses, Patterns, and Formulas Related to the Unification of the Three Etiologies*; Sulphur and Pinellia Pill (*liú bàn wán*) in *Good Friend Compilation*

Section 3

FORMULAS THAT MOISTEN THE INTESTINES AND UNBLOCK THE BOWELS

The formulas in this section induce bowel movements by lubricating the Intestines. They contain substances of a sweet, bland, and oily nature such as Cannabis Semen (*huǒ má rén*), Armeniacae Semen (*xìng rén*), and Pruni Semen (*yù lǐ rén*). This makes them particularly useful for treating constipation due to dryness, which can be caused by febrile disease, debility, old age, childbirth, or as a side effect of various medications. Often they are combined with herbs that enrich the yin and nourish the blood, such as Paeoniae Radix alba (*bái sháo*), Rehmanniae Radix (*shēng dì huáng*), or Angelicae sinensis Radix (*dāng guī*), to aid in moistening the Intestines and treating the underlying damage to the fluids and yin. When deficiency of the Kidney qi is partially responsible for constipation, it is important not only to use herbs that warm the Kidneys and moisten the Intestines, such as Cistanches Herba (*ròu cōng róng*) or Achyranthis bidentatae Radix (*niú xī*), but also to combine these with herbs that help raise the clear and direct the turbid downward, such as Cimicifugae Rhizoma (*shēng má*), Alismatis Rhizoma (*zé xiè*), and Aurantii Fructus (*zhǐ ké*).

In comparison to the formulas in the next group (i.e., those that simultaneously tonify and purge), moistening formulas focus on enabling movement that has been inhibited by dryness. Tonifying formulas, on the other hand, aim to directly increase the amount of body fluids and thereby increase the volume of the stools.

五仁丸
Five-Seed Pill
wǔ rén wán

Source *Effective Formulas from Generations of Physicians* (1345)

dry-fried Persicae Semen (*chǎo táo rén*) 30g
dry-fried Armeniacae Semen (*chǎo xìng rén*) 30g
Platycladi Semen (*bǎi zǐ rén*) 15g
Pini Semen (*sōng zǐ rén*) 3.8g
dry-fried Pruni Semen (*chǎo yù lǐ rén*) 3g
Citri reticulatae Pericarpium (*chén pí*) 120g

Method of Preparation The source text advises to make a paste from the seeds and roll in a powder made from Citri reticulatae Pericarpium (*chén pí*). Form into small pills with honey, and take 50 pills with rice gruel on an empty stomach. At present, all the ingredients are ground into powder and formed into pills with honey. The normal dosage is 12g taken with warm water on an empty stomach.

Actions Moistens the Intestines and unblocks the movement of stools

Indications

Constipation with dry stools that are difficult to pass. The tongue is dry, the pulse thin and rough.

This is constipation due to desiccated Intestines (腸枯 *cháng kū*). It is seen most frequently in old age or after childbirth, but can occur in other situations where yin or blood are damaged. This may be a chronic illness, prolonged dehydration, or the inappropriate use of medicinals (including biomedical drugs) that induce sweating, urination, or are otherwise drying. When the fluids in the Intestines are damaged or lacking, the stools become dry and their passage difficult. The dryness of the tongue, and the thin and rough pulse, are manifestations of blood deficiency and reduced body fluids.

Analysis of Formula

This formula treats a situation in which the stools have become dry because the body fluids are dessicated. Using harsh purgation would be inappropriate because it would further damage the yin. Therefore, the formula relies on seeds that are rich in oils to lubricate the Intestines. The sinking nature attributed to seeds in Chinese medicine further facilitates their ability to move the qi downward.

The two chief herbs are bitter and oily Armeniacae Semen *(xìng rén)* and Persicae Semen *(táo rén)*. According to *Thoroughly Revised Materia Medica*, Armeniacae Semen *(xìng rén)* unblocks qi-aspect constipation due to its association with the Lungs, while Persicae Semen *(táo rén)* unblocks blood-aspect constipation due to its association with the Liver. Platycladi Semen *(bǎi zǐ rén)*, Pruni Semen *(yù lǐ rén)*, and Pini Semen *(sōng zǐ rén)* act as deputies that increase the formula's capacity to moisten the Intestines. Citri reticulatae Pericarpium *(chén pí)*, used in a high dosage, functions as the assistant. Its ability to move the qi and unblock the Intestines transforms the moistening action of the five seeds into bowel movement. The honey, which is used to make the pills, serves as the envoy and uses sweetness to harmonize the actions of the other ingredients while further adding to the overall moistening effect of the formula.

Cautions and Contraindications

This formula contains Persicae Semen *(táo rén)*, which breaks up blood stasis, and Pruni Semen *(yù lǐ rén)*, which has a strong laxative effect. During pregnancy, one should only use the formula after careful consideration.

Commentary

This formula can be safely used over long periods of time without the habit-forming side effects that attach to the use of laxatives containing anthraquinone glycosides, such as Rhei Radix et Rhizoma *(dà huáng)*, Sennae Folium *(fān xiè yè)*, and Aloe *(lú huì)*. It is well-suited for use in the elderly, or for constipation following blood loss, such as after giving birth or major surgery. It is also suited for patients with a yin deficient constitution who suffer from habitual constipation and for stools that become dry following the use of diaphoretic, diuretic, or strongly warming formulas.

There are many other formulas for constipation that combine the ingredients of this formula in different combinations. Some of these are listed below under ASSOCIATED FORMULAS.

Comparisons

➢ Vs. HEMP SEED PILL *(má zǐ rén wán)*; see PAGE 83

➢ Vs. MOISTEN THE INTESTINES PILL FROM MASTER SHEN'S BOOK *(rùn cháng wán)*; see PAGE 80

Biomedical Indications

With the appropriate presentation, this formula may be used to treat a variety of biomedically-defined disorders marked by constipation, including those involving hemorrhoids.

Modifications

• For more severe dessication of body fluids, add Trichosan-

this Semen *(guā lóu rén)*, Cannabis Semen *(huǒ má rén)*, Rehmanniae Radix *(shēng dì huáng)*, Scrophulariae Radix *(xuán shēn)*, or Ophiopogonis Radix *(mài mén dōng)*.

• For blood deficiency after childbirth, add Angelicae sinensis Radix *(dāng guī)* and Polygoni multiflori Radix *(hé shǒu wū)*.

• For deficiency constipation in the elderly, add Cistanches Herba *(ròu cōng róng)* and Sesami Semen nigrum *(hēi zhī má)*.

• For abdominal distention and bloating, add Aurantii Fructus *(zhǐ ké)* and Raphani Semen *(lái fú zǐ)*.

Associated Formulas

橘杏丸

Tangerine and Apricot Pill

jú xìng wán

SOURCE *Effective Formulas from Generations of Physicians* (1345)

Citri reticulatae Pericarpium *(chén pí)*
Armeniacae Semen *(xìng rén)*

Grind equal amounts of both ingredients into powder and form into pills with honey. Moistens the Intestines and regulates the qi. For constipation due to qi stagnation.

三仁丸

Three-Seed Pill

sān rén wán

SOURCE *Fine Formulas of Wonderful Efficacy* (1470)

Platycladi Semen *(bǎi zǐ rén)* 30g
Pini Semen *(sōng zǐ rén)* 30g
Cannabis Semen *(huǒ má rén)* 30g

Grind equal amounts of all ingredients into powder and form into pills with yellow beeswax. Moistens the intestines and unblocks the stool. For constipation due to heat injuring the fluids in the Intestines associated with tenesmus.

二仁丸

Two-Seed Pill

èr rén wán

SOURCE *Treatment Decisions Categorized According to Pattern* (1839)

Armeniacae Semen *(xìng rén)*
Cannabis Semen *(huǒ má rén)*
Aurantii Fructus *(zhǐ ké)*
Chebulae Fructus *(hē zǐ)*

Grind equal amounts of all ingredients into powder and form into pills. Moistens the Intestines, unblocks the stool, regulates the qi, and eases the Intestines. For constipation in the elderly associated with dryness and qi stagnation.

潤腸丸（润肠丸）

Moisten the Intestines Pill from Master Shen's Book

rùn cháng wán

Source   *Shen's Book for Revering Life* (1773)

Cannabis Semen (*huǒ má rén*) 15g
Persicae Semen (*táo rén*) 9g
Angelicae sinensis Radix (*dāng guī*) 9g
Rehmanniae Radix (*shēng dì huáng*) 30g
Aurantii Fructus (*zhǐ ké*) 9g

Method of Preparation   Grind the ingredients into powder and form into pills with honey. Take 15g daily.

Actions   Moistens the Intestines and unblocks the bowels

Indications

Constipation, lusterless skin and nails, dry mouth with an unquenchable thirst, a dry tongue, and a thin pulse.

This is constipation due to desiccated Intestines (腸枯 *cháng kū*), a common condition among the elderly and debilitated. It is also frequently seen after childbirth when the loss of blood injures the yin and depletes the fluids. The other signs and symptoms are characteristic of yin deficiency with depleted fluids.

Analysis of Formula

This formula combines herbs that nourish the blood, enrich the yin, and moisten the Intestines. Cannabis Semen (*huǒ má rén*) and Persicae Semen (*táo rén*) contain an abundance of oils that moisten the Intestines and unblock the bowels. The combination of these herbs is especially effective in cases of constipation with yin deficiency. Angelicae sinensis Radix (*dāng guī*) nourishes the blood and moistens the desiccated Intestines. Rehmanniae Radix (*shēng dì huáng*) nourishes the yin, the root of this condition. The qi-moving action of Aurantii Fructus (*zhǐ ké*) reinforces the laxative effect of the formula and prevents the cloying nature of the other herbs from injuring the Spleen and Stomach.

Commentary

This formula may be used in treating many types of constipation associated with debility. Key symptoms suggesting its use are dry stools that are not difficult to pass and a thin tongue with little or no coating. Because its actions are mild, it does not always work quickly but may require extended use for maximum effect. It should not be prescribed in cases that require purging.

Comparisons

➢ Vs. Five-Seed Pill (*wǔ rén wán*) and Moisten the Intestines Pill from *Discussion of the Spleen and Stomach* (*rùn cháng wán*)

All of these formulas treat habitual constipation. Of the three, Moisten the Intestines Pill from *Discussion of the Spleen and Stomach* (*rùn cháng wán*) is the strongest. It focuses specifically on nourishing the blood and eliminating wind-heat clumping in the Intestines (風結 *fēng jié*). Five-Seed Pill (*wǔ rén wán*) moistens the Intestines and moves the qi with a relatively large dosage of Citri reticulatae Pericarpium (*chén pí*). It is thus inappropriate where the yin and blood have been severely damaged and the qi is already excessive. Moisten the Intestines Pill from Master Shen's Book (*rùn cháng wán*) is the most strongly moistening and least moving formula of the three. It is thus indicated for cases of blood and yin deficiency but does not work as well in moving the qi.

Biomedical Indications

With the appropriate presentation, this formula may be used to treat a variety of biomedically-defined disorders with long-standing constipation.

Modifications

• For heat signs, add Anemarrhenae Rhizoma (*zhī mǔ*) and Polygonati odorati Rhizoma (*yù zhú*).

Associated Formulas

潤腸丸（润肠丸）

Moisten the Intestines Pill from
Discussion of the Spleen and Stomach

rùn cháng wán

Source   *Discussion of the Spleen and Stomach* (13th century)

Rhei Radix et Rhizoma (*dà huáng*) 15g
Angelicae sinensis radicis Cauda (*dāng guī wěi*) 15
Notopterygii Rhizoma seu Radix (*qiāng huó*) 15g
Persicae Semen (*táo rén*) 30g
Cannabis Semen (*huǒ má rén*) 37.5g

Grind the ingredients into powder and form into pills with honey. Moistens dryness, harmonizes the blood, and disperses wind. For constipation (usually severe) from injury to the Spleen and Stomach due to wind-heat entering the Intestines or from improper diet or overwork. This type of constipation includes aspects of blood deficiency, blood stasis, and wind (due to blood deficiency). The generation of wind further desiccates the Intestines, thereby aggravating the constipation. This formula is stronger than the principal formula, and is indicated for more severe conditions.

五子湯（五子汤）

Five-Seed Decoction

wǔ zǐ tāng

Source   *Therapeutic Experiences of Pu Fu-Zhou* (1976)

Cistanches Herba (*ròu cōng róng*) 12g
Ligustri lucidi Fructus (*nǚ zhēn zǐ*) 9g
Ecliptae Herba (*mò hàn lián*) 9g

Platycladi Semen (*bǎi zǐ rén*) 9g
Cannabis Semen (*huǒ má rén*) 12g
Cassiae Semen (*jué míng zǐ*) 6g
Sesami Semen nigrum (*hēi zhī má*) 9g

Decoction. The source text advises to decoct the herbs over low heat for about one hour until about 200ml remain, then add one teaspoon of honey to this decoction, and drink in two portions. Enriches the Kidneys and augments the Spleen, moistens the Intestines, and unblocks the passage of stools. For habitual constipation with dry stools that resemble small pellets, accompanied by discomfort in the lower abdomen, as well as difficulty in falling asleep at night. The tongue will have little coating and the pulse is submerged, thin, and rough on the right and submerged, wiry, thin, and slightly rapid on the left. Application of the decoction should result in a bowel movement that improves all the symptoms.

Comparison

➤ Vs. Hemp Seed Pill (*má zǐ rén wán*); see page 83

宣肺潤腸湯 （宣肺润肠汤）

Disseminate the Lungs and Moisten the Intestines Decoction

xuān fèi rùn cháng tāng

Source *Case Histories of Cheng Men-Xue (2002)*

Cistanches Herba (*ròu cōng róng*) 9g
Angelicae sinensis Radix (*dāng guī*) 9g
Cannabis Semen (*huǒ má rén*) 9g
Paeoniae Radix alba (*bái sháo*) 9g
Bupleuri Radix (*chái hú*) 3g
Aurantii Fructus (*zhǐ ké*) 2.4g
Mume Flos (*méi huā*) 3g
Citri reticulatae Semen (*jú hé*) 12g
Chaenomelis Fructus (*mù guā*) 3g
Citri reticulatae Folium (*jú yè*) 4.5g
Platycladi Semen (*bǎi zǐ rén*) 9g
honey-fried Asteris Radix (*zǐ wǎn*) 9g

Decoction. Nourishes the blood, softens the Liver, moistens dryness, and unblocks the passage of stool. For constipation accompanied by lower abdominal distention, lack of appetite, fatigue, and muscle twitching. This formula was composed by the renowned modern physician from Shanghai, Cheng Men-Xue. Its special characteristic is the use of honey-fried Asteris Radix (*zǐ wǎn*), a strategy borrowed from the Song-dynasty physician Shi Zai. The intention is to direct the Lung qi downward so that it may facilitate the movement of qi in the Intestines. This is assisted by herbs like Bupleuri Radix (*chái hú*), Aurantii Fructus (*zhǐ ké*), and Citri reticulatae Semen (*jú hé*), all of which focus the action of the formula on the lower abdomen in different ways. In this manner, the moistening of blood facilitates movement of the bowels.

Note: Mume Flos (*méi huā*) is bitter, slightly sweet, slightly sour, and cold. It enters the Liver, Stomach, and Lung channels and dredges the Liver and resolves constraint, opens the Stomach and generates fluids, and transforms phlegm. The normal dosage in decoctions is 2-6g.

麻子仁丸

Hemp Seed Pill

má zǐ rén wán

Source *Discussion of Cold Damage* (c. 220)

Cannabis Semen (*huǒ má rén*) 500-600g
Armeniacae Semen (*xìng rén*) 250g
Paeoniae Radix (*sháo yào*) 250g
prepared Aurantii Fructus immaturus (*zhì zhǐ shí*) 250g
prepared Magnoliae officinalis Cortex (*zhì hòu pò*) 250g
Rhei Radix et Rhizoma (*dà huáng*) .500g

Method of Preparation Grind the herbs into powder and form into pills with honey. Take in 9g doses one to three times a day with warm water. Paeoniae Radix alba (*bái sháo*) is the type of Paeoniae Radix (*sháo yào*) most commonly used today. May also be prepared as a decoction with a proportionate reduction in dosage.

Actions Moistens the Intestines, drains heat, promotes the movement of qi, and unblocks the bowels

Indications

Constipation with hard stool that is difficult to expel, normal to frequent urination, a dry, yellow tongue coating, and a submerged, rapid or floating, choppy pulse.

This is a 'Spleen bind' (脾約 *pí yuē*) pattern, as defined in *Discussion of Cold Damage*. Its cause is heat-dryness blocking the physiological movement of fluids in the Spleen. The Spleen is unable to distribute fluids to the extremities and upward into the Lungs and, by association, the Intestines. This causes the stools to become hard. Instead, the fluids seep downward into the Bladder. Thus, urination is normal or even increased. The dry, yellow tongue coating reflects the depletion of fluids and slight heat in the interior. The submerged, rapid pulse indicates heat in the interior. A floating, choppy pulse may also appear, indicating dryness as an external pathogen causing stagnation of fluid movement in the body.

Analysis of Formula

To address the problems of heat-dryness causing stagnation of qi, the formula focuses on moistening dryness in the Intestines, draining the heat, and moving the qi. This is achieved with a variation of Minor Order the Qi Decoction (*xiǎo chéng qì tāng*) in which the dosage of those herbs that strongly disperse and purge has been reduced, while herbs that nourish and moisten have been added as chief and deputies.

The chief herb, Cannabis Semen (*huǒ má rén*), is rich in oils that moisten the Intestines and unblock the bowels. One of the deputies, Armeniacae Semen (*xìng rén*), directs the qi downward and moistens the Intestines. It, too, contains oils that facilitate bowel movement. The other deputy, Paeoniae Radix (*sháo yào*), is bitter, sour, and slightly cold. It enters the Spleen, nourishes the yin, and harmonizes the interior.

Aurantii Fructus immaturus *(zhǐ shí)*, an assistant, breaks up accumulation (especially in the Intestines). Magnoliae officinalis Cortex *(hòu pò)*, another assistant, removes fullness and distention. The third assistant, Rhei Radix et Rhizoma *(dà huáng)*, is a purgative. Honey, used as a medium in forming the pills, plays an active role by moistening the Intestines, but mainly acts as the envoy whose sweetness harmonizes the actions of the other herbs.

Cautions and Contraindications

Because most of the herbs in this formula possess draining, dispersing, or purgative properties, it should not be used without modification for treating the very weak or for constipation due solely to blood deficiency. Contraindicated during pregnancy.

Commentary

The definition of the 'Spleen bind' pattern in paragraph 247 of *Discussion of Cold Damage* is extremely brief: "When the dorsal pedis pulse is floating and choppy along with frequent urination and hard bowel movements, the Spleen is bound. Hemp Seed Pill *(má zǐ rén wán)* masters it." Given the limited nature of this passage, successive generations of commentators have added their own interpretations.

The earliest commentator on this book was Cheng Wu-Ji. In *Discussion Illuminating the Principles of Cold Damage*, he defined the word binding (約 *yuē*) as "being bound by a contract or pact" (結約 *jié yuē*) or "being controlled or dominated" (約束 *yuē shù*). He went on to say that here:

> The Stomach is strong and the Spleen is weak. [As the Spleen] governs the [movement of] fluids, they are not distributed to the four extremities but transported to the Bladder. As a consequence, urination is frequent and the stool is hard. Therefore, one says that the Spleen [in such a case] is bound.

While this clearly states that the pathology is one of the problems with fluid transportation due to Stomach excess, his unfortunate insertion of the notion of a weak Spleen caused much confusion among later writers. Some physicians—foremost among them Zhu Dan-Xi—took this to mean that dry-heat had damaged the Spleen, or even that blood or yin had become deficient. As a result, some physicians have prescribed this formula for the treatment of chronic constipation in the weak and elderly. However, the emphasis of the formula is clearly on removing excess. Even the moistening herbs in the formula are primarily intended to move stagnation and not to enrich yin or generate fluids. In *Writings on the Esteemed Discussion*, the Ming-dynasty physician Yu Chang therefore severely criticized this mistake:

> Should not a weak Spleen be tonified? Why then does Hemp Seed Pill *(má zǐ rén wán)* contain herbs contrary [to this intention] like Rhei Radix et Rhizoma *(dà huáng)*, Aurantii Fructus immaturus *(zhǐ shí)*, and Magnoliae officinalis Cortex *(hòu*

> *pò)*? … [Zhang] Zhong-Jing said 'strong Stomach.' The original text never mentioned a 'weak Spleen.' The fact is that when [the original] talks about a strong Stomach, what it really means by strong is that the Spleen is strong. To bind [means] to economize. If the Spleen qi is excessively strong, it will economize by expelling the food taken in by the Stomach over three to five days in only one or two pellets. Altogether, [this pattern] is one where earth is excessively dry causing the fluids within the Stomach and Intestines to become daily more dessicated, hence the stools become difficult [to expel]. If the Spleen qi were weak, this would cause diarrhea. What could be the reason for making such stools difficult to expel?

The manner in which this formula modifies Minor Order the Qi Decoction *(xiǎo chéng qì tāng)*, and the preference for prescribing it in pill form, make it a relatively mild laxative. Nevertheless, it is inappropriate for all types of chronic constipation. As the early 20th-century physician Yun Tie-Qiao stated in *Notated Discussion of Cold Damage Edited for Meaning*: "Compared to the Order the Qi Decoctions *(chéng qì tāng)*, Hemp Seed Pill *(má zǐ rén wán)* is relatively mild. However, one [still] must use it [only to treat] yang patterns. If one mistakenly employs it for yin patterns, its mildness turns into violence."

Drawing on these discussions as well as his own clinical experience, Chen Zhao-Zu, the modern physician and writer of formula textbooks, suggests three main uses of this formula in contemporary practice:

1. Constipation in the elderly, debilitated, or postpartum or other contexts involving loss of blood or essence, characterized by signs of excess in the yang brightness, but where strong purgation is contraindicated

2. Patients suffering from hemorrhoids who require laxative treatment that does not aggravate the condition

3. Patients who do not exercise but who are neither excessively deficient nor have pronounced signs of damp-heat in the Intestines. Another important indication in contemporary practice is postoperative constipation due to heat and dryness.

The early 20th-century physician Cao Ying-Fu used this formula for constipation that is accompanied by sweating or a moist skin. In these cases, such sweating constitutes the equivalent of relatively excessive urination rather than the heat-type sweating associated with yang brightness organ-warp patterns. However, the inclusion of moistening herbs such as Cannabis Semen *(huǒ má rén)*, Armeniacae Semen *(xìng rén)*, and Paeoniae Radix *(sháo yào)* in this formula indicates that, irrespective of the presence of sweat, the skin itself may also be dry.

Comparison

➤ Vs. Minor Order the Qi Decoction *(xiǎo chéng qì tāng)*

Compared to patterns of heat excess in the yang brightness organs with clumping of the stools, which is treated by Minor Order the Qi Decoction *(xiǎo chéng qì tāng)*, the Spleen bind pattern treated by Hemp Seed Pill *(má zǐ rén wán)* is milder and often more chronic. Nevertheless, it is a pattern of excess.

Yang brightness organ patterns are due to severe heat causing clumping of the stools and stagnation of qi. Dryness is secondary to this obstruction. Thus, it can be resolved by simply flushing the Stomach and Intestines and breaking the qi stagnation. In a Spleen bind pattern, dryness is the primary pathogen. This inhibits the movement of stool in the bowels and leads to qi stagnation, but does not cause acute clumping. Thus, it is resolved by a strategy of moistening the Intestines combined with mild purgation.

➢ Vs. Five-Seed Pill *(wǔ rén wán)*

On the other hand, the 'dessicated Intestines' patterns treated by Five-Seed Pill *(wǔ rén wán)* and its modifications, including Moisten the Intestines Pill from *Master Shen's Book (rùn cháng wán)*, and also by Benefit the River [Flow] Decoction *(jì chuān jiān)*, are patterns where dryness of the stools is caused by deficiency of blood, essence, or body fluids.

Biomedical Indications

With the appropriate presentation, this formula may be used to treat a wide variety of biomedically-defined disorders, primarily those affecting the digestive system such as incomplete intestinal obstruction, postoperative ileus, atrophic gastritis, reflux gastritis, hemorrhoids, bleeding post-hemorrhoidectomy, habitual constipation, constipation in the elderly, or postpartum constipation. It has also been used to treat cardiopulmonary disease, asthma, cystitis, coronary heart disease, and diabetes.

Alternate names

Hemp Seed Pill *(má rén wán)* in *Arcane Essentials from the Imperial Library*; Spleen Bind Hemp Seed Pill *(pí yuē má rén wán)* in *Formulary of the Pharmacy Service for Benefiting the People in the Taiping Era*; Spleen Bind Pill *(pí yuē wán)* in *Discussion of Formulas from Straight Directions from [Yang] Ren-Zhai*; Hemp Seed Spleen Bind Pill *(má rén pí yuē wán)* in *Complete Book on Treating Pox and Rashes*; Hemp Seed Enrich the Spleen Pill *(má rén zī pí wán)* in *Nationwide Collection of TCM Patent Formulas*

Modifications

• For severe injury to the fluids, add Platycladi Semen *(bǎi zǐ rén)* and Trichosanthis Semen *(guā lóu rén)*.

• For severe heat accumulation with a yellow tongue coating and a rapid pulse, increase the dosage of Rhei Radix et Rhizoma *(dà huáng)* and add Natrii Sulfas *(máng xiāo)*.

• For severe debility, omit Rhei Radix et Rhizoma *(dà huáng)* and add a small amount of Sennae Folium *(fān xiè yè)*.

• For hemorrhoids, add Persicae Semen *(táo rén)* and Angelicae sinensis Radix *(dāng guī)*.

• For bleeding hemorrhoids, add Sophorae Flos immaturus *(huái mǐ)* and Sanguisorbae Radix *(dì yú)*.

• For deficiency of the middle qi, combine with Tonify the Middle to Augment the Qi Decoction *(bǔ zhōng yì qì tāng)*.

• For intestinal obstruction from roundworms, add Mume Fructus *(wū méi)*, Arecae Semen *(bīng láng)*, and Citri reticulatae Pericarpium *(chén pí)*.

Associated Formulas

搜風順氣丸 （搜风顺气丸）

Track Down Wind and Smooth the Flow of Qi Pill

sōu fēng shùn qì wán

SOURCE *Fine Formulas for Women with Annotations and Commentary* (16th century)

Plantaginis Semen *(chē qián zǐ)* 45g
Rhei Radix et Rhizoma *(dà huáng)* . . . (half prepared, half fresh) 15g
Cannabis Semen *(huǒ má rén)* 6g
Achyranthis bidentatae Radix *(niú xī)* 6g
Pruni Semen *(yù lǐ rén)* 6g
Cuscutae Semen *(tù sī zǐ)* 6g
Aurantii Fructus *(zhǐ ké)* 6g
Dioscoreae Rhizoma *(shān yào)* 6g

Grind the ingredients into a fine powder, form into pills with a small amount of honey, and take in 13.5g doses on an empty stomach. Moistens the Intestines, unblocks the passage of stool, drains heat, and disperses clumping. For hemorrhoids and constipation caused by the penetration of wind-heat into the Intestines. In comparison to the principal formula, this modification treats dampness, wind, and heat accumulating in the Intestines and causing stagnation that manifests in constipation and hemorrhoids.

––––––––––––––––

更衣丸

Pill Requiring a Change of Clothing

gēng yī wán

SOURCE *Extensive Notes on Medicine [from the First-Awakened Studio]* (1613)

Cinnabaris *(zhū shā)* 15g
Aloe *(lú huì)* 21g

Grind the ingredients into a fine powder, form into pills with a small amount of wine, and take in 3.6g doses. Drains fire and unblocks the bowels. For constipation due to accumulation of dryness and heat in the Intestines with disturbance of the spirit (indicated by restlessness, short temper, and insomnia). The formula's name is derived from its strong purgative properties: when taken at night, its effects will be felt before morning (and vice versa), thus requiring a change of clothing. Due to the unacceptable toxicity of Cinnabaris *(zhū shā)*, use of this formula is no longer recommended.

濟川煎 (济川煎)

Benefit the River [Flow] Decoction

jì chuān jiān

The name of this formula is derived from its function of warming and moistening in order to move the stool. *Jì* (濟) means to aid or relieve and suggests the action of tonifying or increasing. *Chuān* (川) means river. It is sometimes taken to refer to the fluids flowing through the body. More specifically, however, it refers to the six warps that order and regulate the distribution of qi and blood in the body. Drawing on a statement in Chapter 5 of *Basic Questions* that likens the six warps to rivers, Zhang Jie-Bin, the author of this formula, observes: "The three yin and the three yang [warps] function together to [manage] the flow of qi and blood. Thus, they function as the rivers of a person." Tonifying the Kidneys and Liver facilitates the distribution of fluids, thereby helping to move the stool.

Source   *Collected Treatises of [Zhang] Jing-Yue* (1624)

wine-prepared Cistanches Herba *(jiǔ cōng róng)* 6-9g
Angelicae sinensis Radix *(dāng guī)* 9-15g
Achyranthis bidentatae Radix *(niú xī)* 6g
Alismatis Rhizoma *(zé xiè)* 4.5g
Aurantii Fructus *(zhǐ ké)* 3g
Cimicifugae Rhizoma *(shēng má)* 1.5-3g

Method of Preparation   Decoction.

Actions   Warms the Kidneys, nourishes the blood, augments the essence, moistens the Intestines, and unblocks the bowels

Indications

Constipation, clear and copious urine, lower back pain, and a cold sensation in the back.

This can be considered constipation due to Kidney deficiency. The Kidneys are the foundation of the body's yang qi. Their functions include controlling the process that transforms and circulates water through the body. When Kidney yang and qi are deficient, the processes of warming and transforming the water are weakened. The water is not moved from the Bladder, resulting in clear and copious urine. This same disruption in the normal circulation of water in the lower burner dries out the Intestines and leads to constipation. Deficiency of Kidney yang also deprives the Kidneys of proper nourishment and warmth. Because the lower back is the residence of the Kidneys, there is pain and a sensation of cold in that part of the body.

Analysis of Formula

Treating a pattern characterized by dry stools in the context of cold and deficiency requires the simultaneous use of a tonifying and moistening strategy. The chief herb, Cistanches Herba *(ròu cōng róng)*, is ideally suited for this condition as it warms and tonifies the Kidney yang, warms the lower back, and moistens the Intestines to unblock the bowels. Angelicae sinensis Radix *(dāng guī)*, a deputy herb, nourishes and har-

monizes the blood and moistens the Intestines. Achyranthis bidentatae Radix *(niú xī)*, the other deputy, strengthens the lower back and Kidneys. It also has a descending nature that focuses the actions of the formula on the lower burner. Alismatis Rhizoma *(zé xiè)*, the assistant herb, has a descending nature that drains turbidity from the Kidneys. Together with Achyranthis bidentatae Radix *(niú xī)*, it facilitates movement and guides the actions of the other herbs downward. It also prevents the moistening property of the chief herb from causing stagnation.

Aurantii Fructus *(zhǐ ké)*, an envoy, relaxes the Intestines and directs the qi downward, thus helping to unblock the bowels. A small amount of Cimicifugae Rhizoma *(shēng má)*, the other envoy, is used to raise the clear yang as a subtle inducement to the descent of the turbid yin. In combination with Aurantii Fructus *(zhǐ ké)*, one ascending and the other descending, the regulation of the Kidney qi mechanism is enhanced.

Commentary

The analysis of the formula's indications and actions above follows that of modern Chinese textbooks. Given the emphasis on organ systems of functions in contemporary Chinese medicine, this analysis defines the formula as primarily strengthening the Kidneys. However, neither the source text nor later premodern commentators view this as a Kidney formula. A more thorough understanding of its actions, indications, and functions can be gained by taking into account these other interpretations.

In the source text, Zhang Jie-Bin simply notes that constipation due to deficiency should not be treated with harsh purgatives like Natrii Sulfas *(máng xiāo)* and Rhei Radix et Rhizoma *(dà huáng)*. He then says: "As the general momentum [of deficiency disorders] cannot but have a lack of unobstructed passage, it is appropriate to govern [such a disorder] by means of the present [strategy]. This is to employ unblocking within a tonifying formula." Clearly, Zhang Jie-Bin's main concern is the process of qi transformation as a whole and not the function of individual organs. In *Revised Popular Guide to the Discussion of Cold Damage*, He Lian-Chen underlines this perspective by focusing on the complementary roles of the Kidneys and Liver, substance (yin) and function (qi):

> Benefit the River [Flow] Decoction *(jì chuān jiān)* mainly emphasizes the Liver and Kidneys and uses [the fact that] the Kidneys govern urination and defecation. Accordingly, it uses Cistanches Herba *(ròu cōng róng)* and Achyranthis bidentatae Radix *(niú xī)* as chiefs. They enrich the Kidney yin to unblock the passage of stool. The Liver governs dredging and draining. Accordingly, it uses Angelicae sinensis Radix *(dāng guī)* and Aurantii Fructus *(zhǐ ké)* as deputies. The first is acrid and moistening [and focuses on] Liver yin. The second is bitter and draining [and focuses on] Liver qi. The marvel [of the formula's

composition, however, lies in its combination of] Cimicifugae Rhizoma *(shēng má)*, which raises the clear qi to contribute to Spleen [qi transformation], and Alismatis Rhizoma *(zé xiè)*, which directs the turbid qi downward to contribute to the Bladder [qi transformation]. They assist Cistanches Herba *(ròu cōng róng)* in realizing its power of facilitating [passage of the stools] by means of moistening.

Precisely because this formula uses tonification as a means of facilitating movement, it is listed in almost all fomularies as a formula that moistens the Intestines and not as one that simultaneously tonifies and purges.

The formula can thus be used to treat constipation that arises from Liver blood problems as well as Kidney qi deficiency, or where the essences are too depleted to enable bowel movement. Zhang Jie-Bin also suggested a number of modifications, which are listed below.

Comparison

➢ Vs. Pinellia and Sulphur Pill *(bàn liú wán)*

Both formulas are indicated for treating constipation from Kidney deficiency in the elderly and in weak patients. Pinellia and Sulphur Pill *(bàn liú wán)* invigorates the fire at the gate of vitality, tonifies the Stomach yang, and drains turbid accumulations from the Intestines. Its nature is warming and drying, and it only directs qi downward. Benefit the River [Flow] Decoction *(jì chuān jiān)* is more balanced. It tonifies both essence and yang, Liver and Kidneys, and regulates the qi dynamic by supporting both uplifting and directing downward. In clinical practice, one uses Pinellia and Sulphur Pill *(bàn liú wán)* where there are clear signs of internal cold due to deficiency of fire. Once the bowels have been opened, one can switch to a more balanced formula to treat the underlying deficiency. Benefit the River [Flow] Decoction *(jì chuān jiān)*, on the other hand, can be used more long term because it combines opening with tonification, moistening with draining. It is not strong enough, however, to remove cold accumulations.

Biomedical Indications

With the appropriate presentation, this formula may be used to treat a variety of biomedically-defined disorders marked by constipation, including constipation in the elderly, habitual constipation, and postpartum constipation.

Modifications

- For pronounced qi deficiency, add Ginseng Radix *(rén shēn)*. (source text)
- For fire, add Scutellariae Radix *(huáng qín)*. (source text)
- For severe Kidney deficiency, add Rehmanniae Radix praeparata *(shú dì huáng)*. (source text)
- For severe deficiency, omit Aurantii Fructus *(zhǐ ké)*. (source text)

- To increase the moistening action in the Intestines, add Cannabis Semen *(huǒ má rén)*.
- For severe lower back pain, omit Alismatis Rhizoma *(zé xiè)* and add Lycii Fructus *(gǒu qǐ zǐ)* and Eucommiae Cortex *(dù zhòng)*.

Associated Formulas

通幽湯 （通幽汤）

Unblock the Pylorus Decoction

tōng yōu tāng

Source *Discussion of the Spleen and Stomach* (13th century)

Persicae Semen *(táo rén)* 0.3g
Carthami Flos *(hóng huā)* 0.3g
Rehmanniae Radix *(shēng dì huáng)* 1.5g
Rehmanniae Radix praeparata *(shú dì huáng)* 1.5g
Angelicae sinensis Radix *(dāng guī)* 3g
Glycyrrhizae Radix praeparata *(zhì gān cǎo)* 3g
Cimicifugae Rhizoma *(shēng má)* 3g

Grind the herbs into a powder and prepare as a draft. Take before meals. *Secrets from the Orchid Chamber*, by the same author, says to add 1.5g of very finely ground Arecae Semen *(bīng láng)* to the draft before taking it. Nourishes the blood, moistens dryness, lifts the clear qi upward, and directs the turbid downward. For pyloric obstruction, up-rushing of qi, dysphagia, qi that can move neither up nor down, and constipation. Although its name suggests that the formula is indicated for pyloric obstruction, in practice it is usually used for constipation due to blood deficiency and dessicated fluids.

Li Dong-Yuan, the author of the formula, describes the underlying disease dynamic as follows:

> The Kidneys open the two yin orifices. The *[Inner] Classic* states: If the bowels [move] with difficulty, select the lesser yin [for treatment]. The Kidneys govern the five yin fluids. If the body fluids are sufficient, the bowels are normal. Those who eat too much and exhaust themselves damage and harm the Stomach qi. Eating acrid and warming things that have a strong flavor assists the fire pathogen. Fire lurking within the blood consumes [the fluids] and damages the true yin. The body fluids become dessicated, therefore the stools become dry and clump.

Zhang Jie-Bin was a great admirer of Li Dong-Yuan. The Ming dynasty current of warming and supplementation—of which Zhang Jie-Bin is a main representative—was a direct outgrowth of Li Dong-Yuan's emphasis on tonifying the Spleen and Stomach yang, known at the time as the 'royal path' (王道 *wāng dào*) in medicine. Anyone aware of this connection will be able to perceive the strong influence of the present formula on Zhang Jie-Bin's Benefit the River [Flow] Decoction *(jì chuān jiān)*. In comparison to that formula's emphasis on water metabolism, Li Dong-Yuan's formula focuses more strongly on the physiology of blood transformation.

養正通幽湯（养正通幽汤）

Nourish the Normal and Unblock the Pylorus Decoction

yǎng zhēng tōng yōu tāng

SOURCE *Fu Qing-Zhu's Women's Disorders* (1826)

Chuanxiong Rhizoma *(chuān xiōng)* .7.5g
Angelicae sinensis Radix *(dāng guī)* 18g
Glycyrrhizae Radix praeparata *(zhì gān cǎo)* 1.5g
Persicae Semen *(táo rén)* . . . . .15 pieces
Cannabis Semen *(huǒ má rén)* 6g
Cistanches Herba *(ròu cōng róng)* 3g

Decoction. Nourishes blood and moves the stools. For constipation following childbirth with other signs and symptoms of any one of the three yin warps (in six-warp diagnostics). This is a synthesis of Li Dong-Yuan's and Zhang Jie-Bin's original formulas that only focuses on nourishing the blood and essence and does not attempt to regulate the qi dynamic. The source text advises the following modifications: for severe sweating, add 3g each of Scutellariae Radix *(huáng qín)* and Ophiopogonis Radix *(mài mén dōng)*; for abdominal distention, add 3g each of Ophiopogonis Radix *(mài mén dōng)* and Cistanches Herba *(ròu cōng róng)*, 1.8g of Aurantii Fructus *(zhǐ ké)*, and 6g of Ginseng Radix *(rén shēn)*; for severe blood deficiency with sweating, raving, and the spirit failing in its functions, add 3g each of Poriae Sclerotium pararadicis *(fú shén)*, Polygalae Radix *(yuǎn zhì)*, Cistanches Herba *(ròu cōng róng)*, Astragali Radix *(huáng qí)*, Angelicae dahuricae Radix *(bái zhǐ)*, and Platycladi Semen *(bǎi zi rén)*, and 6g each of Ginseng Radix *(rén shēn)* and Atractylodis macrocephalae Rhizoma *(bái zhú)*.

Section 4

. . . .

FORMULAS THAT SIMULTA-NEOUSLY ATTACK AND TONIFY

The formulas in this section induce bowel movement by tonifying qi and generating fluids while simultaneously attacking the clumping of heat and stools within the Intestines by way of purgation. For this reason, they combine substances that increase the amount of body fluids (and thereby the volume of the stools) such as Rehmanniae Radix *(shēng dì huáng)*, Scrophulariae Radix *(xuán shēn)*, and Ophiopogonis Radix *(mài mén dōng)*, with those that tonify the qi (and thereby increase the body's ability to move stools) such as Ginseng Radix *(rén shēn)*, Codonopsis Radix *(dǎng shēn)*, and Glycyrrhizae Radix *(gān cǎo)*, together with those that flush the Intestines, such as Rhei Radix et Rhizoma *(dà huáng)* and Natrii Sulfas *(máng xiāo)*. This makes them particularly useful for treating blockage of bowel movement occurring in the course of febrile disorders where the qi and yin have been severely damaged. Often these are serious and life-threatening conditions.

黃龍湯（黄龙汤）

Yellow Dragon Decoction

huáng lóng tāng

The color yellow corresponds to the earth and refers to this formula's effect on the central digestive processes controlled by the earth organs, the Stomach and Spleen. The dragon is said to stimulate the clouds and produce rain. According to the 17th- century writer Zhang Lu, the dragon in the formula's name refers to its effect in stimulating the Stomach qi and promoting the distribution of fluids. The dragon's ability to generate rain is closely linked to its ability to fly freely between heaven and earth. The slightly later Qing-dynasty physician Wang Xu-Gao alludes to this function in his explanation:

> In calling it Yellow Dragon [the author emphasized] Rhei Radix et Rhizoma *(dà huáng)*, taking Ginseng Radix *(rén shēn)* as its assistant. Because of this, it obtains the same magical powers of movement possessed by the dragon. Leaping up and down, its transformations become visible everywhere.

Source *Six Texts on Cold Damage* (1445)

Rhei Radix et Rhizoma *(dà huáng)* 9-12g
Natrii Sulfas *(máng xiāo)* 9-12g
Aurantii Fructus immaturus *(zhǐ shí)* 6-9g
Magnoliae officinalis Cortex *(hòu pò)* 3-12g
Ginseng Radix *(rén shēn)* 6-9g
Angelicae sinensis Radix *(dāng guī)* 9-12g
Platycodi Radix *(jié gěng)* 3-6g
Zingiberis Rhizoma recens *(shēng jiāng)* 9g
Jujubae Fructus *(dà zǎo)* . . . . .2 pieces
Glycyrrhizae Radix *(gān cǎo)* 3g

Method of Preparation Decoction. Some sources recommend adding Platycodi Radix *(jié gěng)* near the end. The source text does not specify dosages.

Actions Purges heat from the interior and supports the normal qi

Indications

Green, watery, and foul-smelling diarrhea, abdominal pain that increases upon pressure, fever, thirst, a dry tongue and mouth, shortness of breath, lethargy, delirious speech, a dry, yellow or black tongue coating, and a deficient pulse. Some patients present with constipation or firm, painful abdominal distention. In severe cases, there may be hallucinations and 'grabbing at the air' or impaired consciousness with frigid, contracted extremities.

This is heat excess in the interior with qi and blood deficiency. As heat (due to cold transforming into heat or the direct penetration of a heat pathogen) accumulates in the interior, it intensifies and injures the fluids. This leads to internal clumping of heat and fluids, which disrupts the qi mechanisms of the yang organs. Green, watery, and foul-smelling diarrhea reflects the body's unsuccessful attempt to eliminate the accumulation. In Chinese medicine, this is referred to as 'heat clumping with circumfluence' (熱結旁流 *rè jié páng liú).* The clumping is also reflected in the abdominal distention, fullness, and firmness, with pain that increases upon pressure. Vigorous yang brightness-warp heat causes fever and delirious speech.

Injury to the fluids results in a dry tongue and mouth with thirst. Dryness with vigorous heat in the interior is reflected in the dry, yellow or dry, black tongue coating. Qi and blood deficiency (due to constitutional weakness or clumping of heat left untreated) is reflected in the lethargy, shortness of breath, and deficient pulse. Delirious speech is a sign of a yang brightness-warp disorder and is also a manifestation of heat injuring the spirit. As the condition worsens, there may be hallucinations and, in the most severe cases (when the normal qi is near exhaustion), impaired consciousness and cold, contracted extremities.

Analysis of Formula

This formula is designed to drain heat accumulation while preventing further injury to the normal qi. The chief ingredients, Rhei Radix et Rhizoma *(dà huáng)* and Natrii Sulfas *(máng xiāo),* are an especially powerful combination for draining heat and unblocking the bowels. The deputies, Aurantii Fructus immaturus *(zhǐ shí),* which reduces distention and fullness, and Magnoliae officinalis Cortex *(hòu pò),* which disseminates the qi, aid the chief ingredients in expelling stool by moving the qi. The other deputies, Ginseng Radix *(rén shēn)* and Angelicae sinensis Radix *(dāng guī),* protect the normal qi. The former tonifies the source qi while the latter tonifies the blood.

The assistant ingredient, Platycodi Radix *(jié gěng),* unblocks the flow of qi in the Lungs and thus the Large Intestine (paired organs). In addition, this herb possesses an uplifting action that helps to counteract the downward-draining action of the chief ingredients. This allows the clumping to be eliminated without causing a collapse of the middle qi. The other assistants, Zingiberis Rhizoma recens *(shēng jiāng)* and Jujubae Fructus *(dà zǎo),* adjust and regulate the nutritive and protective qi, regulate the disparate actions of the other ingredients, and thereby hasten recovery. The envoy, Glycyrrhizae Radix *(gān cǎo),* assists the other tonifying ingredients in supporting the normal qi and strengthening the Spleen and Stomach. It also harmonizes the actions of the other ingredients.

Commentary

This formula, a variation of Major Order the Qi Decoction *(dà chéng qì tāng),* treats a form of yang brightness organ-warp disorder. The distinguishing characteristics of this condition are severe, acute indications of heat accompanied by signs and symptoms of qi and blood deficiency such as fatigue, shortness of breath, the dry, yellow, or black tongue coating, and the deficient pulse. This is a very acute condition, and the most important aspect of the formula is the draining of heat accumulation. The tonifying herbs serve an auxiliary function by preventing further injury to the normal qi.

In practice, this pattern is most often seen in elderly or debilitated patients whose qi is already deficient before they contracted a cold damage or warm pathogen disorder. Following this line of thought, the 20th-century physician Chen Dao-Long routinely combined Ginseng Radix *(rén shēn)* and Rhei Radix et Rhizoma *(dà huáng)* in treating constipation in the elderly. His contemporary, Cheng Men-Xue, roots this practice in interpretations of the present formula:

> This formula [treats] excess in deficient and debilitated patients. It is one of the formulas to learn by heart for use [in clincal practice]. Once one has understood its way of combining Ginseng Radix *(rén shēn)* and Rhei Radix et Rhizoma *(dà huáng)* and the [underlying] principle of supporting the normal while eliminating the pathogenic [qi], there is no need to adhere to the original formula. One should also not overlook that in using Yellow Dragon Decoction *(huáng lóng tāng)* in the elderly [it is advisable] to omit Natrii Sulfas *(máng xiāo).*

Modification

- For elderly or very weak patients, omit Natrii Sulfas *(máng xiāo).*

Biomedical Indications

With the appropriate presentation, this formula may be used to treat a variety of biomedically-defined disorders including acute infectious diseases such as typhoid, paratyphoid, meningitis, and encephalitis, along with intestinal obstruction in the elderly.

Associated Formula

新加黃龍湯（新加黄龙汤）

Newly Augmented Yellow Dragon Decoction

xīn jiā huáng lóng tāng

SOURCE *Systematic Differentiation of Warm Pathogen Diseases* (1798)

Rehmanniae Radix *(shēng dì huáng)* 15g
Glycyrrhizae Radix *(gān cǎo)* 6g
Ginseng Radix *(rén shēn)* 4.5g
Rhei Radix et Rhizoma *(dà huáng)* 9g
Natrii Sulfas *(máng xiāo)* 3g
Scrophulariae Radix *(xuán shēn)* 15g
Ophiopogonis Radix *(mài mén dōng)* 15g
Angelicae sinensis Radix *(dāng guī)* 4.5g
Stichopus *(hǎi shēn)* 2

Decoction. Add ginger juice before taking. Enriches the yin, augments the qi, drains heat, and purges. For heat accumulation in the interior with qi and yin deficiency characterized by constipation, abdominal distention, hardness, and fullness, fatigue, shortness of breath, dry mouth and throat, cracked lips, and a dry, yellow or black tongue coating with cracks. In contrast to the principal formula, it has a weaker purgative effect, and focuses more on nourishing the yin, qi, and fluids.

The pattern for which it is indicated—marked by the combination of yang brightness excess and deficiency of qi, blood, and yin—is a severe condition with little hope of success. This is because purging will further aggravate the deficiency while tonification feeds the excess. Wu Ju-Tong, the author of this formula, admits as much in his own preamble: "The composition of this formula addresses an insurmountable problem by exerting all possible strength. It is a strategy aimed at avoiding the slightest regret [for having failed by way of not trying]."

增液承氣湯 (增液承气汤)

Increase the Fluids and Order the Qi Decoction

zēng yè chéng qì tāng

Source   *Systematic Differentiation of Warm Pathogen Diseases* (1798)

Scrophulariae Radix *(xuán shēn)* 30g
Ophiopogonis Radix *(mài mén dōng)* 24g
Rehmanniae Radix *(shēng dì huáng)* 24g
Rhei Radix et Rhizoma *(dà huáng)* .9g
Natrii Sulfas *(máng xiāo)* 4.5g

Method of Preparation   Decoction. The source text advises to add Rhei Radix et Rhizoma *(dà huáng)* near the end and dissolve Natrii Sulfas *(máng xiāo)* in the strained decoction.

Actions   Enriches the yin, generates fluids, drains heat, and unblocks the bowels

Indications

Dry stools that cannot be expelled even with a purging formula, distention and fullness of the epigastrium and abdomen, dry mouth and lips, a dry tongue with a thin yellow or burnt yellow coating, and a rapid, thin pulse.

This is a yang brightness organ-warp pattern that develops in the course of a warm pathogen disorder with heat clumping in the Stomach and Intestines burning up the body fluids. The same pattern can also develop in yin deficient patients that contract a warm pathogen disorder. When heat clumping and yin deficiency occur together, the Intestines lose all of their moisture. The stools become so hard and dry that even a purgative formula can no longer expel them. This disease dynamic was analyzed by Wu Ju-Tong, the formula's author, using a simple analogy: "When the body fluids are insufficient, there is no water so the boat [i.e., the stool] gets stuck." In this situation, one cannot merely push the boat but must provide water to float it.

Clumping in the Stomach and Intestines is experienced as distention and bloatedness. The dry lips and mouth, the dry

tongue, and the thin pulse all reflect damage to the body fluids. The thin and yellow or burnt-yellow tongue coating and the rapid pulse denote the presence of a heat pathogen.

Analysis of Formula

This is a variation of Increase the Fluids Decoction *(zēng yè tāng)*, discussed in Chapter 15, to which Rhei Radix et Rhizoma *(dà huáng)* and Natrii Sulfas *(máng xiāo)*, that is, Regulate the Stomach and Order the Qi Decoction *(tiáo wèi chéng qì tāng)*, have been added.

The three yin-nourishing substances in the formula clear heat and increase the body fluids to address the severe dryness at the root of this condition. The traditional materia medica attributes laxative effects to all three herbs, making them especially useful for this purpose. Scrophulariae Radix *(xuán shēn)* is described in *Divine Husbandman's Classic of the Materia Medica* as "governing hot and cold accumulations in the abdomen." *Comprehensive Outline of the Materia Medica* notes that Ophiopogonis Radix *(mài mén dōng)* "governs clumping of qi in the epigastrium, damage to the middle [burner], damage due to overeating, … It [helps to] digest food and regulates the middle [burner]." *Miscellaneous Records of Famous Physicians* states that Rehmanniae Radix *(shēng dì huáng)* "promotes urination and defecation, [and] eliminates harbored food from the Stomach." In combination, these three substances thus enrich the yin without being excessively cloying, to generate fluids and promote bowel movement.

Rhei Radix et Rhizoma *(dà huáng)* and Natrii Sulfas *(máng xiāo)* soften hardness, drain heat, and flush the Stomach and Intestines. If Increase the Fluids Decoction *(zēng yè tāng)* increases the water in this formula, then the combination of these two substances provides the power to 'move the boat' that has become stuck. Wu Ju-tong describes the overall effect: "The marvel [of this formula} resides in the draining within the tonification. It employs the tonifying herbs as a foundation for the draining substances [to accomplish their] function. In this manner, one can attack the excess while preventing deficiency."

Cautions and Contraindications

Although this formula is mild compared to the strong formulas that purge heat accumulation, it still must be used with circumspection. The formula is only indicated for a pattern combining deficiency of yin fluids with accumulation of dry stools in the Intestines.

Commentary

Historically, this formula is modeled on Raw Rhemannia Decoction *(shēng dì huáng tāng)*, which was first listed in the Tang-dynasty work by Sun Si-Miao, *Important Formulas Worth a Thousand Gold Pieces*. This formula is made up of 1500g of Rehmanniae Radix *(shēng dì huáng)*, 120g of Rhei

Radix et Rhizoma (dà huáng), 2 pieces of Jujubae Fructus (dà zǎo), 30g of Glycyrrhizae Radix (gān cǎo), and 40ml of Natrii Sulfas (máng xiāo). It is indicated for cold damage disorders with yin and qi deficiency and constipation. Over subsequent centuries, it became the model for the treatment strategy called 'adding water to move the boat' (zēng shuǐ xíng chuán 增水行船) outlined above.

Although the formula was developed for treatment of constipation that occurs in the course of acute feverish disorders, deficiency of yin fluids, and yang brightness excess, is a commonly seen pattern in clinical practice. Physicians have thus used this formula to treat toothache, skin diseases, dryness of the mucous membranes, hemorrhoids, anal fissures, and similar problems.

The combination of downward-draining and yin-enriching herbs in the treatment of warm pathogen disorders is widely considered to be an important innovation by physicians associated with the warm pathogen disorder current in Chinese medicine. The logic underlying this combination has been severely criticized, however, by the famous Qing dynasty scholar-physician Fei Bo-Xiong. Fei argues that the intention of downward draining is to preserve yin by eliminating a pathogen. This is inhibited by the addition of moistening herbs such as Rehmanniae Radix (shēng dì huáng) or Ophiopogonis Radix (mài mén dōng), which have the tendency to retain pathogenic heat in the interior. The use of this formula should thus be carefully considered.

Comparison

➢ Vs. Increase the Fluids Decoction (zēng yè tāng); see PAGE 678

Biomedical Indications

With the appropriate presentation, this formula may be used to treat a variety of biomedically-defined disorders, including any acute infectious disease marked by high fever and constipation, as well as severe hemorrhoids. It has also been used for renal failure.

Associated Formula

承氣養榮湯 (承气养荣汤)

Order the Qi and Nourish the Nutritive Decoction
chéng qì yǎng róng tāng

SOURCE *Discussion of Warm-Heat Pathogen [Disorders]* (early 18th century)

Anemarrhenae Rhizoma (zhī mǔ)	9g
Angelicae sinensis Radix (dāng guī)	6g
Rehmanniae Radix (shēng dì huáng)	12g
Rhei Radix et Rhizoma (dà huáng)	3g
Aurantii Fructus immaturus (zhǐ shí)	9g
Magnoliae officinalis Cortex (hòu pò)	9g
Paeoniae Radix alba (bái sháo)	15g

Decoct with Zingiberis Rhizoma recens (shēng jiāng). The source text does not specify dosages. Clears heat, unblocks the bowels, enriches the yin, and moistens dryness. For warm pathogen disorders where the repeated administration of purging formulas has caused devastated yin characterized by dryness of the mouth, cracked lips, thirst, unresolved fever, a hard, distended, painful abdomen, and constipation. This is a combination of Minor Order the Qi Decoction (xiǎo chéng qì tāng) and Four-Substance Decoction (sì wù tāng) in which Anemarrhenae Rhizoma (zhī mǔ) has been substituted for Chuanxiong Rhizoma (chuān xiōng). Compared with Increase the Fluids and Order the Qi Decoction (zēng yè chéng qì tāng), this formula is indicated for a more severe problem, where not only the fluids, but also the blood has been damaged by repeated purgation.

Alternate name

Nourish the Nutritive and Order the Qi Decoction (yǎng róng chéng qì tāng) in *Revised Popular Guide to the Discussion of Cold Damage*

Section 5

FORMULAS THAT DRIVE OUT EXCESS WATER

The formulas in this section are used in treating conditions of excess due to accumulation of water and fluids that obstruct the interior and gather in the chest and abdominal cavities, characterized by difficulty in urination and defecation. They reduce and eliminate accumulation by unblocking the passage of urine and stool. In doing so, their key ingredients are harsh, purgative substances that are toxic, such as Knoxiae Radix (hóng dà jǐ), Kansui Radix (gān suì), Pharbitidis Semen (qiān niú zǐ), or Phytolaccae Radix (shāng lù). With this degree of blockage, the qi dynamic is always affected and so these formulas commonly include herbs that move the qi, such as Citri reticulatae viride Pericarpium (qīng pí), Citri reticulatae Pericarpium (chén pí), Aucklandiae Radix (mù xiāng), and Arecae Semen (bīng láng). Because the main herbs are so harsh, it is common to ameliorate these side effects and improve the overall results by adding herbs that augment the qi and nourish the Stomach, such as Jujubae Fructus (dà zǎo). Also, when the internal stoppage of water has either turned to heat or increased the internal stagnation, it is useful to add regular purgative herbs, such as Rhei Radix et Rhizoma (dà huáng), or those that leach out dampness and promote urination, such as Alismatis Rhizoma (zé xiè) and Akebiae Caulis (mù tōng).

Note that all of these formulas are contraindicated during pregnancy and should be used with extreme caution in treating weak or debilitated patients.

十棗湯 (十枣汤)

Ten-Jujube Decoction

shí zǎo tāng

The name of this formula is a tribute to the importance of the ten jujubes, which are taken to moderate the harsh, downward-draining action of the other herbs, and thereby protect the Stomach qi.

Source   *Discussion of Cold Damage* (c. 220)

Kansui Radix *(gān suì)*
Euphorbiae pekinensis Radix *(jīng dà jǐ)*
Genkwa Flos *(yuán huā)*

Method of Preparation   Grind equal measures of each herb into powder. Take in 0.5-1g doses (may be placed in gelatin capsules) in the early morning (i.e., between 3-5 A.M.) on an empty stomach with a warm decoction made from 10 pieces of Jujubae Fructus *(dà zǎo)*. Begin with a low dosage. This should produce discomfort in the epigastrium about one hour after administration, followed by borborygmus and abdominal pain that diminishes after a watery bowel movement. There are generally five to six bowel movements after each dose. If there are fewer (one to two), another dose may be taken a day or two later. If the patient becomes weak from the effects of the formula, prescribe easily-digested foods (such as rice gruel or oatmeal) and tonics.

Actions   Purges and drives out thin mucus

Indications

Cough with pain in the chest and hypochondria, hard focal distention in the epigastrium, dry heaves, shortness of breath, headache, vertigo, a white, slippery tongue coating, and a submerged, wiry pulse. There may also be chest pain extending to the back that makes breathing difficult.

This is suspended, thin mucus (懸飲 *xuán yǐn*) clogging up the chest and hypochondriac regions. This causes the qi to rebel, producing cough and shortness of breath. Obstruction of the flow of qi also produces chest and hypochondriac pain that, in severe cases, may extend to the back. Thin mucus is yin in nature and follows the qi. When the qi is halted in the epigastrium, the thin mucus collects into clumps, manifested as hard focal distention in this region. Obstruction of the middle burner causes the Stomach qi to rebel, producing dry heaves. The rising of thin mucus disturbs the clear yang and causes headache and vertigo. The white, slippery tongue coating is a sign of thin mucus, and the submerged, wiry pulse indicates accumulation in the interior and pain.

This formula is also used for edema due to obstruction from accumulation of thin mucus, a condition of excess characterized by generalized edema that is worse in the lower part of the body, abdominal distention, wheezing, fullness in the chest, and difficult urination and defecation.

Analysis of Formula

Because this condition is due to a clogging up of the entire interior of the body, it cannot be effectively treated with herbs ordinarily used to transform and leach out thin mucus. Harsh purgatives are required to purge the thin mucus from the body. There are three such ingredients in this formula: Kansui Radix *(gān suì)* expels fluids and dampness from the channels and collaterals, Euphorbiae pekinensis Radix *(jīng dà jǐ)* drains fluids and dampness from the organs, and Genkwa Flos *(yuán huā)* reduces and eliminates thin mucus from the chest and hypochondria. Since these are toxic substances that readily injure the normal qi, Jujubae Fructus *(dà zǎo)* is added to augment the qi, protect the Stomach, and moderate the harshness and toxicity of the other ingredients.

Cautions and Contraindications

This formula should be used with extreme caution in weak or pregnant patients. If severe diarrhea occurs, cold rice porridge should be taken. In cases with weakness, this formula should be taken, in turn, with another that strengthens the Spleen and augments the qi: one purges while the other tonifies.

It is not advisable to prepare this formula as a decoction. Experience and animal tests show that side effects increase when the herbs are boiled together rather than taken as a powder with a Jujubae Fructus *(dà zǎo)* decoction. By preparing the main herbs in this formula with vinegar before use, it is possible to reduce the potential side effects.

Commentary

This is a very strong formula that should be used only when absolutely necessary. If this pattern appears with a more superficial condition, the superficial condition must be resolved first using formulas like Cinnamon Twig Decoction *(guì zhī tāng)* or Minor Bupleurum Decoction *(xiǎo chái hú tāng)*. In relatively mild cases with an exterior condition, Minor Blue-green Dragon Decoction *(xiao qing long tang)* may be used to treat both. *Essential Teachings of [Zhu] Dan-Xi* recommends that Ten-Jujube Decoction *(shí zǎo tāng)* be prepared in pill form so that it is easier to take.

Glycyrrhizae Radix *(gān cǎo)* is often used to moderate the toxicity of other ingredients. However, it is not used here because it is traditionally believed to increase the toxicity of the particular herbs in this formula.

There are several reasons why it is advisable to take this formula, as recommended in the source text, "at daybreak" (i.e. between 3-5 A.M.) Suspended, thin mucus denotes a yin condition that needs to be moved in the direction of yang. The early morning, when yin is naturally transforming into yang, is the easiest time to do so. It is also the time when, according to *Discussion of Cold Damage,* pathologies of the lesser yang and terminal yin channels tend to resolve.

Suspended, thin mucus accumulates below the ribs, a region closely associated with the function of the Gallbladder and Liver, whose rising qi is in the ascendancy at daybreak. From this perspective, too, the early moning indicates the most favorable time for treatment.

Comparison

➤ Vs. Yu's ACHIEVEMENT POWDER (*Yǔ gōng sǎn*); *see* PAGE 94

Biomedical Indications

With the appropriate presentation, this formula may be used to treat a wide variety of biomedically-defined disorders including pleural and pericaridal effusions, pneumonia, cirrhosis with ascites, and nephritis, as well as increased gastric acidity, schizophremia, and epidemic hemorrhagic fever.

Alternate names

Three-Star Powder (*sān xīng sǎn*) in *Master Fu's Formulas for Reviving Infants*; Jujube Decoction (*dà zǎo tāng*) in *Cold Damage Revelations*

Associated Formula

控涎丹

Control Mucus Special Pill

kòng xián dān

SOURCE　*Discussion of Illnesses, Patterns, and Formulas Related to the Unification of the Three Etiologies* (1174)

Kansui Radix (*gān suì*)

Knoxiae Radix (*hóng dà jǐ*)

Sinapis Semen (*bái jiè zǐ*)

Grind equal amounts of each herb into powder and form into small pills. Take in 1-3g doses at bedtime with warm water. Dispels phlegm and expels thin mucus. For phlegm lurking above and below the diaphragm that obstructs the qi mechanism, characterized by sudden, excruciating pain in the thorax, neck, and lower back, a tightening sensation in the sinews and bones that evolves into a burning, piercing pain, a sticky, greasy tongue coating, and a wiry, slippery pulse. There may also be cold and painful extremities, unrelenting and severe headache, lethargy with a desire to sleep, a loss of desire for food and drink, coughing up of thick, sticky sputum, and a rattling sound in the throat at night or excessive salivation. While both this and the principal formula treat obstruction of the interior by fluids, this formula focuses on the thin mucus and phlegm in the chest and diaphragm with associated widespread pain, whereas the principal formula focuses on thin mucus in the chest and hypochondria with pain in these areas, abdominal distention, and edema. The word 'mucus' in the formula's name refers to heavy fluids in general, or to phlegm and thin mucus in particular.

甘遂半夏湯

Kansui and Pinellia Decoction

gān suì bàn xià tāng

SOURCE　*Essentials from the Golden Cabinet* (c. 220)

Kansui Radix (*gān suì*) 3g
Pinelliae Rhizoma praeparatum (*zhì bàn xià*) 5g
Paeoniae Radix (*sháo yào*) 5g
Glycyrrhizae Radix (*gān cǎo*) 3g

Decoction. The ingredients are decocted in 200ml of water until 50ml remain. One then adds 50ml of honey to the strained liquid, rapidly brings this mixture to a boil once or twice, and then administers it in a single dose. Drives out water, dispels phlegm, disperses knotting, eliminates fullness, relaxes hypertonicity, and stops pain. For the treatment of lingering thin mucus (留飲 *liú yǐn*) patterns characterized by fullness and focal distension of the chest and abdomen, hardness in the epigastrium, abdominal pain, diarrhea, a pale tongue with a white, slippery coating, and a deep or hidden pulse. There may also be nausea and vomiting, the back may feel cold, and the patient may be thirsty without wanting to drink.

When the transportation and transformation of fluid metabolism slows, the movement of water stops; it will then accumulate and can congeal into thin mucus, leading to edematous swelling and distention. The initial approach would normally be to restore transportation and transformation through warming, tonification, and the facilitation of urination. When, however, the thin mucus has accumulated deep within the body and the yang qi is unable to circulate, the pathogen can gather into a hard, excessive clump that resists more gentle treatment. This is lingering mucus in the interior, confirmed by the pulse, which is hidden and deep.

There are different lingering thin mucus patterns. The pattern treated by this formula relates to a severe accumulation of fluids in the interior that seeks an exit route via the bowels. The formula follows this natural momentum by forcefully driving out the fluids with the help of the toxic Kansui Radix (*gān suì*).

舟車丸（舟车丸）

Vessel and Vehicle Pill

zhōu chē wán

Because this formula is an extremely harsh and powerful purgative, the stool functions as a 'vessel and vehicle' for the removal of accumulation from the body.

Source　*Formulas from Benevolent Sages Compiled during the Taiping Era* (992)

Kansui Radix (*gān suì*) 30g
vinegar Genkwa Flos (*cù yuán huā*) 30g
vinegar Euphorbiae pekinensis Radix (*cù dà jǐ*) 30g
Pharbitidis Semen (*qiān niú zǐ*) 120g
Rhei Radix et Rhizoma (*dà huáng*) 60g
Citri reticulatae viride Pericarpium (*qīng pí*) 15g
Citri reticulatae Pericarpium (*chén pí*) 15g
Arecae Semen (*bīng láng*) 15g
Aucklandiae Radix (*mù xiāng*) 15g
Calomelas (*qīng fěn*) 3g

Method of Preparation　Grind the ingredients into powder and form into pills with water. Take in 3-6g doses with warm water on an empty stomach in the early morning. If the condition improves and the patient remains strong, it may be taken again (usually with a reduced dosage) 1-2 days later. Otherwise, the formula should not be taken more than once. This is the reason that present formulations contain Calomelas (qīng fěn), although it is generally regarded as an obsolete substance due to its toxicity.

Actions Promotes the movement of qi and harshly drives out water and heat accumulation

Indications

Ascites and distention in a robust patient accompanied by thirst, labored breathing, hard abdomen, constipation, scanty urine, and a submerged, rapid, and forceful pulse.

This is water and heat accumulation in the interior obstructing the qi mechanism. The constraint caused by the obstruction to the flow of qi by water or dampness produces heat. The water and heat accumulate and clog the entire abdomen, obstructing the qi in the Stomach and Intestines. This causes edema and ascites, and impedes the excretion of urine and stool. The resulting turbidity, lacking an outlet for drainage, produces further clogging and severe stagnation of qi. This, in turn, prevents the proper dissemination of fluids, leading to more distention, thirst, labored breathing, and a hard abdomen. The pulse reflects the accumulation of fluids and heat in the interior, and no deficiency of normal qi.

Analysis of Formula

This is a severe, acute condition in a person of otherwise robust health. To reduce the ascites and distention, the accumulation of water and heat must be harshly purged and driven out of the body. The chief ingredients, Kansui Radix (gān suì), Genkwa Flos (yuán huā), and Euphorbiae pekinensis Radix (jīng dà jǐ), are harsh expellants that purge water from the chest and abdomen. The deputies, Pharbitidis Semen (qiān niú zǐ) and Rhei Radix et Rhizoma (dà huáng), purge heat from the Intestines, expel water accumulation, and interact synergistically with the chief ingredients. Pharbitidis Semen (qiān niú zǐ) also drains water through the urine.

The assistant ingredients work indirectly to restore the proper flow of qi, thereby supporting the chief and deputy ingredients, whose actions are more direct. Citri reticulatae viride Pericarpium (qīng pí) spreads the Liver qi and breaks up clumping in the abdomen. Citri reticulatae Pericarpium (chén pí) promotes movement of the Lung and Spleen qi, helping to smooth the flow of qi in the thoracic and diaphragmatic regions. Arecae Semen (bīng láng) directs the qi downward, promotes urination, and breaks up clumping in the abdomen. Aucklandiae Radix (mù xiāng) unblocks the flow of qi in the three burners and guides out stagnation. Calomelas (qīng fěn) expels water, unblocks the bowels, and reinforces the actions of the chief and deputy ingredients.

Cautions and Contraindications

This formula is contraindicated during pregnancy and in persons who are weak or debilitated. Traditional texts discourage the use of Glycyrrhizae Radix (gān cǎo) with this formula as it is incompatible with some of its ingredients. Because the formula contains some extremely toxic substances, the dosage and duration of administration must be carefully regulated. After the acute condition has resolved, formulas that regulate and tonify the Spleen and Kidney should be prescribed to promote full recovery.

Commentary

The combination of harsh purgatives and strong, qi-moving ingredients makes this an extremely powerful formula that should be prescribed only in cases of emergency for persons of otherwise robust health. The Ming-dynasty physician Wang Ken-Tang did much to popularize the use of this formula in his influential work, *Indispensable Tools for Pattern Treatment*. Wang argued that because this formula was even stronger than Ten-Jujube Decoction (shí zǎo tāng), it was most suitable for those with a very robust constitution.

There has been controversy about the role of herbs that promote movement of qi in this formula. As some of the antecedent formulas lacked herbs such as Citri reticulatae Pericarpium (chén pí) and Arecae Semen (bīng láng), the Qing-dynasty physician Zhang Lu considered the use of these herbs as "superfluous adornments" unnecessary for driving water out of the body in the context of harsh purgation. Modern textbooks, including *Formulas* edited by Li Fei, on the other hand, argue that the physiology of qi and water are intimately connected and thus herbs that move qi and break up stagnation are essential in this formula.

Yet another opinion is that of Fei Bo-Xiong, from the late Qing. He considered the use of such strong purgation without the simultaneous use of Jujubae Fructus (dà zǎo) to be a serious mistake, and possibly fatal. This reflects a current within Chinese medicine that views with suspicion any deviations from the treatment strategies laid out by Zhang Zhong-Jing. Although the emergence of this view was influenced by many nonclinical factors, it deserves to be carefully reflected upon.

Biomedical Indications

With the appropriate presentation, this formula may be used to treat a variety of biomedically-defined disorders including ascites from cirrhosis and other causes, schistosomiasis, and uremia.

Alternate names

Divine Protection Vessel and Vehicle Pill (shén yòu zhōu chē wán) in *Liu He-Jian's Formulas*; Clean the Bowel Pill (jìng fǔ wán) in *Golden Mirror of the Medical Tradition*; Divine Protection Pill (shén yòu wán) in *Necessities for Women's Diseases*

禹功散

Yu's Achievement Powder

Yǔ gōng sǎn

The Great Yu was the last legendary leader of China's prehistoric tribal confederation. He is famous for having tamed the great floods of the Yellow River, a job in which his father had failed and that took him and his workers 13 years to accomplish. His success came to be known as 'Yu's achievement' (禹功 *Yǔ gōng*). This formula drives out edema that floods the body, an achievement likened to that of the Great Yu.

Source   *Confucians' Duties to Their Parents* (1228)

Pharbitidis Semen (*qiān niú zǐ*) 120g
dry-fried Foeniculi Fructus (*chǎo huí xiāng*). 30g

Method of Preparation   Grind the herbs into a fine powder and take 3-6g after mixing it with fresh ginger juice. At present, the usual dosage is 3g taken two to three times per day with fresh ginger juice or water.

Actions   Expels water, unblocks the bowels, moves the qi, and reduces edema

Indications

Generalized floating edema, abdominal distention, wheezing and fullness, constipation, urinary difficulty, and a submerged and forceful pulse. There may also be swelling and distention of the scrotum accompanied by a feeling of heaviness and pain, dampness, sweating, and reduced urination.

This is yang edema caused by water dampness invading the body and obstructing the qi dynamic. Water dampness collecting in the muscles and skin manifests as floating edema of the entire body. Water and qi accummulating in the interior and obstructing the qi dynamic leads to inhibited urination, constipation, wheezing, and fullness of the abdomen. As water dampness enters the blood vessels, it causes the pulse to become submerged. The forcefulness of the pulse reflects the constrained normal qi.

The same disease dynamic can also manifest as a water bulging disorder (水疝 *shuǐ shàn*). Here water dampness, which by its nature is a yin pathogen, accumulates in the lower burner, causing scrotal swelling and distention. Heaviness and pain indicate that the movement of qi has become obstructed. Functionally, this obstruction leads to reduced urination. Accumulated water dampness may seep to the outside instead, causing the scrotal region to become moist. This is referred to as 'damp sweating' (濕汗 *shī hàn*).

Analysis of Formula

Although yang water and water bulging are two distinct disorders in Chinese medicine, their underlying disease dynamic is the same. For this reason, they can be resolved by applying the same strategy of driving out water and moving the qi.

This formula uses cold and bitter Pharbitidis Semen (*qiān niú zǐ*) as the chief herb. Its nature is to direct downward. It excels at reducing edema by promoting urination and driving out water by means of purgation. The deputy is Foeniculi Fructus (*xiǎo huí xiāng*), which moves qi and stops pain. Its warmth moderates the cold nature of the chief herb, while its acrid nature aids restoration of the normal qi dynamic. Thus it considerably strengthens the power of the formula to drive out water. The assistant in the formula is Zingiberis Rhizoma recens (*shēng jiāng*), whose fresh juice is mixed with the powder before administration. This herb opens the interstices and pores to facilitate the movement of qi and the driving out of water dampness. Although the formula combines just three substances, their synergism is well thought out to achieve a powerful effect.

Cautions and Contraindications

This is a formula for excess disorders. Because of its purgative effects, it should be used with caution during pregnancy and in elderly or debilitated patients.

Commentary

Although this formula drives out water by purgation to treat excess disorders, it is milder in action than Ten-Jujube Decoction (*shí zǎo tāng*) or Vessel and Vehicle Pill (*zhōu chē wán*). The modern physician Qin Bo-Wei thus referred to it as a formula for 'draining out water' (瀉水 *xiè shuǐ*). Another well-known modern physician, Ran Xue-Feng, observes in *Annotated Fine Formulas from Generations of Famous Physicians*: "Compared to Ten-Jujube Decoction (*shí zǎo tāng*) and Vessel and Vehicle Pill (*zhōu chē wán*), this formula is smooth. It [acts] immediately without being harsh, it is moderate without being slack. People say it should not be used lightly. I say its correct [composition] permits it to be used frequently."

The formula's indication for yang edema stems from *Essential Teachings of [Zhu] Dan-Xi*, and that for bulging disorder from *Medical Mirror of Past and Present*. The source text, however, conceived of it as a gynecological formula indicated for abdominal and back pain after birth that is accompanied by white discharge, or the discharge of a white fatty substance caused by 'corrupted blood' (敗血 *bài xuè*) and 'noxious substances' (惡物 *è wù*). The famous modern Shanghai gynecology expert Shen Zhong-Li thus integrates this formula into his treatment of fibroids and ovarian cysts when there is a significant amount of water dampness and phlegm. Foeniculi Fructus (*xiǎo huí xiāng*) is considered by many classical and modern physicians to be an herb that enters the Conception and Penetrating vessels, supporting this formula's usage in treating gynecological disorders.

Comparison

➤ Vs. Ten-Jujube Decoction (*shí zǎo tāng*)

Both of these formulas drive out pathogenic water. The present formula focuses on driving out water and moving the qi, facilitating urination as well as purging water via the bowels. It is thus particularly indicated when water dampness obstructs the qi dynamic, reflected in a submerged and forceful pulse, or where water and qi clump in the lower burner manifesting in a water-bulging disorder. Ten-Jujube Decoction (*shí zǎo tāng*) relies on powerful toxic substances. For this reason, it combines strong purgation with tonification of the body's normal qi. It is specific for suspended thin mucus clogging up the chest and hypochondriac regions, as reflected in a submerged but wiry pulse.

Biomedical Indications

With the appropriate presentation, this formula may be used to treat a wide variety of biomedically-defined disorders such as cirrhosis with ascites, nephritis with edema, and hydrocele.

Modification

• Add Aucklandiae Radix (*mù xiāng*) to increase its ability to move the qi and stop pain. This addition comes from the modern physician Qin Bo-Wei.

Associated Formula

導水丸 (导水丸)

Guide Out Water Pill

dǎo shuǐ wán

SOURCE *Formulas from the Discussion Illuminating the Yellow Emperor's Basic Questions* (1172)

Pharbitidis Semen (*qiān niú zǐ*) 120g
Talcum (*huá shí*) 120g
Rhei Radix et Rhizoma (*dà huáng*) 60g
Scutellariae Radix (*huáng qín*) 60g

Grind the herbs into a fine powder and make into pills with water; 6-12g constitute one dose. Drains heat and drives out water. For generalized floating edema with constipation and reduced urination, thirst, dark urine, and a rapid pulse. Also for damp-heat backache and pains throughout the body caused by spreading of phlegm-dampness. Like the principal formula, Guide Out Water Pill (*dǎo shuǐ wán*) employs Pharbitidis Semen (*qiān niú zǐ*) as its chief herb and treats edema with constipation and reduced urination. However, due to the additions of Talcum (*huá shí*) and Rhei Radix et Rhizoma (*dà huáng*), its diuretic and purgative properties are distinctly stronger, while Scutellariae Radix (*huáng qín*) accentuates its ability to drain heat. For this reason, the formula is indicated for treating edema accompanied by damp-heat. Yu's Achievement Powder (*Yǔ gōng sǎn*), by contrast, is able to move qi in addition to driving out water. For this reason, it is indicated for yang edema accompanied by qi stagnation, accumulation, and pain.

己椒藶黃丸 (己椒苈黄丸)

Stephania, Zanthoxylum, Tingli Seed, and Rhubarb Pill

jǐ jiāo lì huáng wán

Source *Essentials from the Golden Cabinet* (c. 220)

Stephaniae tetrandrae Radix (*hàn fáng jǐ*) 30g
Zanthoxyli Semen (*jiāo mù*) 30g
Lepidii/ Descurainiae Semen (*tíng lì zǐ*) 30g
Rhei Radix et Rhizoma (*dà huáng*) 30g

Method of Preparation Form into pills with honey and take one pill (3-9g each) before meals three times daily.

Actions Drives out water, scours out thin mucus, moves the qi, and reduces distention

Indications

Abdominal distention, borborygmus, dryness of the mouth and tongue, constipation, reduced urination, a yellow, greasy tongue coating, and a wiry and slippery or a submerged, full, and slightly rapid pulse.

This is accumulation of water in the Stomach and Intestines with qi stagnation. Impediment of the qi dynamic by water causes abdominal distention and borborygmus. Stagnation also leads to yang qi constraint and development of heat within the Intestines, which manifests as constipation, a yellow, greasy tongue coating, and a wiry and slippery or a submerged, full, and slightly rapid pulse. Because the fluids are no longer dispersed, the mouth and tongue become dry, while impediment of qi transformation in the Bladder leads to reduced urination.

Analysis of Formula

The intention of this formula is to remove the root of the disorder by purging and driving out water, and to resolve the manifestations by moving qi and reducing fullness. The chief herb is bitter, cooling, and acrid Stephaniae tetrandrae Radix (*hàn fáng jǐ*), which expels pathogenic water via the urine. It is assisted by Zanthoxyli Semen (*jiāo mù*), an herb with a very similar nature and range of indications. Acting together, these two herbs strongly promote urination and thereby remove obstruction from the qi dynamic.

The remaining two herbs in the formula form another synergistic pairing, which drives out water and qi accumulation from the Intestines. Bitter, acrid, and strongly cooling Lepidii/ Descurainiae Semen (*tíng lì zǐ*) focuses on the Lungs, which are the upper source of water. If Lung qi flows smoothly, the waterways will be unimpeded. Lepidii/ Descurainiae Semen (*tíng lì zǐ*) drains Lung qi by forcefully breaking up stagnation and promoting urination. The Lungs are further related by way of an exterior/interior relationship to the Large Intestine. When the Lung qi directs downward, clearing and clarifying, passage through the bowels is unimpeded. Bitter and cooling Rhei Radix et Rhizoma *(dà huáng)* directs the qi downward and flushes accumulations from the Stomach and Intestines.

The four main herbs in the formula all direct qi downward to drive out water. To protect the Stomach qi, honey is added as a fifth substance in the preparation of the pills. Its sweet flavor moderates harshness, even as its moistening nature assists bowel movement.

Cautions and Contraindications

This formula is contraindicated in cases where the accumulation of fluids in the interior of the body is accompanied by Spleen deficiency. Like all purging formulas, it should only be used short term.

Commentary

The main characteristic of this formula is its strategy of eliminating different portions of pathogenic fluids via the urine and bowels, as explained by Cheng Lin in *True Explanation of the Essentials of the Golden Cabinet*:

> This is water qi in the Small Intestine. Stephaniae tetrandrae Radix *(hàn fáng jǐ)* and Zanthoxyli Semen *(jiāo mù)* guide out fluids at the front because [their] clear [portion] must be cleared via the urine. Rhei Radix et Rhizoma *(dà huáng)* and Lepidii/ Descurainiae Semen *(tíng lì zǐ)* push out fluids at the rear, because [their] turbid [portion] must be purged via the bowels. By separating [the clear from the turbid] and eliminating them at the front and the back, distention and fullness are diminished and water fluids move [normally once more]. The Spleen qi revolves and body fluids are generated.

This method of separation is a very important treatment principle in Chinese medicine that comports with the division of body fluids into clearer and more turbid portions, and with the different methods used in Chinese medicine to drain dampness via the urine and guide out phlegm via the bowels.

Note: The reader is referred to the discussion in *Chinese Herbal Medicine: Materia Medica* of herb identification related to *fáng jǐ* (Stephaniae/Cocculi/etc. Radix). At present, Stephaniae tetrandrae Radix *(hàn fáng jǐ)* is the herb that is used for *fáng jǐ*.

Biomedical Indications

With the appropriate presentation, this formula may be used to treat a wide variety of biomedically-defined disorders including pleural effusions, acute bronchial asthma, edema from cardiopulmonary disease, ascites, pyloric obstruction, rheumatic heart disease, and functional gastrointestinal disorders.

Alternate names

Zanthoxylum Pill *(jiāo mù wán)* in *Important Formulas Worth a Thousand Gold Pieces*; Stephania Pill *(fáng jǐ wán)* in *Comprehensive Recording of Sagely Beneficence*; Stephania, Zanthoxylum, and Tingli Seed Pill *(fáng jǐ jiāo lì wán)* in *Indispensable Tools for Pattern Treatment*

Modification

• For thirst indicating more severe heat in the Intestines, add 15g of Natrii Sulfas *(máng xiāo)*. (source text)

疏鑿飲子 (疏凿饮子)
Dredging and Cutting Drink
shū záo yǐn zi

Source *Formulas to Aid the Living* (1253)

Like Yu's Achievement Powder, this formula refers to the Great Yu, who controlled the devastating floods of the Yellow River. His father, Gun, had previously failed in this task by constructing huge dikes and banks. Yu changed tactics and decided to prevent the floods by dredging the river itself and by digging canals and trenches that diverted flood waters into the sea. Legend has it that this effort involved cutting a pathway through Mount Longmen, which was then obstructing the flow of the Yellow River. Later, the early 4th-century poet Guo Pu celebrated Yu's achievement with a memorable line: "Just like the [three] gorges of Badong, Xia [i.e., the Great Yu] later dredged [the rivers] and cut [a channel through the mountain]." Because this formula opens a pathway that guides pathogenic fluids from the body, it employs the same strategy by which the Great Yu succeeded in taming the floods.

Alismatis Rhizoma *(zé xiè)* 12g
Phaseoli Semen *(chì xiǎo dòu)* 15g
Phytolaccae Radix *(shāng lù)* 6g
Notopterygii Rhizoma seu Radix *(qiāng huó)* 9g
Arecae Pericarpium *(dà fù pí)* 15g
Zanthoxyli Semen *(jiāo mù)* 9g
Akebiae Caulis *(mù tōng)* .12g
Gentianae macrophyllae Radix *(qín jiāo)* 9g
Arecae Semen *(bīng láng)* .9g
Poriae Cutis *(fú líng pí)* 30g

The source text advises to take equal amounts of all the ingredients and make a paste of the herbs, then decoct 12g with 5 slices of Zingiberis Rhizoma recens *(shēng jiāng)* in half a cup of water until the liquid has been reduced by 70 percent. At present, the formula is prepared as a decoction, generally with the dosages noted above.

Actions Purges, drives out water, dredges wind, and discharges the exterior

Indications

Generalized edema, wheezing, dyspnea, restlessness and irritability, thirst, constipation, and urinary obstruction.

This is yang edema (陽水 *yáng shuǐ*) flooding both the interior and exterior and causing qi stagnation. This disorder is also referred to as a severe form of water qi (水氣 *shuǐ qì*). Water and dampness clogging the exterior and flooding the skin and muscles manifests as generalized floating edema accompanied by a subjective sensation of heaviness throughout the body. Water disturbing the Lungs causes its qi to rebel upward, which results in wheezing and dyspnea. Water clogging the interior obstructs the qi dynamic in the Triple Burner, preventing the Lung qi from directing downward and the passage of qi in the bowels. This causes restlessness, irritability, constipation, and urinary obstruction. Qi stagnation interferes with the diffusion of physiological fluids and produces thirst.

Analysis of Formula

This formula draws on all three of the basic strategies for the treatment of edema set forth in *Basic Questions* (Chapter 14): sweating, urination, and purgation. This is necessary because water has flooded the entire body and obstructed the regular ascending and descending functions of qi. In such a case, sweating opens the pores to treat edema in the exterior, while diuresis and purgation eliminate water from the interior.

The chief herb in the formula is bitter, cold, and toxic Phytolaccae Radix (*shāng lù*). It strongly moves the qi downward, opening both the urinary passages and the bowels to drive out water. Its action is comparable to that of Knoxiae Radix/Euphorbiae pekinensis Radix (*dà jǐ*) and Kansui Radix (*gān suì*) in both nature and effects. Five diuretic herbs serve as deputies: Poriae Cutis (*fú líng pí*), Akebiae Caulis (*mù tōng*), Zanthoxyli Semen (*jiāo mù*), Phaseoli Semen (*chì xiǎo dòu*), and Alismatis Rhizoma (*zé xiè*). Among these, Poriae Cutis (*fú líng pí*) and Alismatis Rhizoma (*zé xiè*) focus on promoting urination and dispeling dampness via the Bladder. Akebiae Caulis (*mù tōng*) and Phaseoli Semen (*chì xiǎo dòu*) are potent diuretics that drain pathogens from the Small Intestine. Phaseoli Semen (*chì xiǎo dòu*) is specific for pathogens that have acquired form (i.e., visible edema rather than mere dampness), while Akebiae Caulis (*mù tōng*) also invigorates the blood. Given concerns regarding the potential nephrotoxic side effects of the variations of *mù tōng* (Akebiae/Clematidis/etc. Caulis) found in the marketplace, it is advisable to substitute another herb for this herb. Tetrapanacis Medulla (*tōng cǎo*) or Plantaginis Semen (*chē qián zǐ*) may be used in the present case. Zanthoxyli Semen (*jiāo mù*) is indicated for abdominal distention in addition to its diuretic effects. Furthermore, both Poriae Cutis (*fú líng pí*) and Phaseoli Semen (*chì xiǎo dòu*) build up the Spleen. This prevents damage to the body's normal qi and supports the qi dynamic. Acting in combination, the chief and deputy herbs thus guide out water from the interior via the bowels.

Two groups of assistants support their action. Notopterygii Rhizoma seu Radix (*qiāng huó*), Gentianae macrophyllae Radix (*qín jiāo*), and Zingiberis Rhizoma recens (*shēng jiāng*) dredge the channels and exterior, open the pores and interstices, and promote sweating. This drains the water clogging the skin and muscles and facilitates the qi dynamic. Arecae Semen (*bīng láng*) and Arecae Pericarpium (*dà fù pí*) regulate the qi by moving it downward. Their use is indicated because water and dampness are yin pathogens that readily obstruct the qi dynamic. Qi stagnation, in turn, facilitates the generation of dampness and edema. Removing such stagnation restores the physiological movement of qi and helps in dispelling pathogenic water and diffusing physiological body fluids.

Cautions and Contraindications

The formula is only indicated for yang (i.e., excess) edema. Edema due to deficiency of the Spleen or Kidneys must be treated with appropriate warming and tonifying formulas. Use of the formula during pregnancy and in the absence of clear signs of excess and damp-heat is not advised.

Commentary

The special status of this formula in the history of Chinese medicine lies in its combination of diverse strategies for the treatment of edema that had previously been used separately. However, the formula does more than simply combine herbs that promote sweating, urination, and bowel movement. It utilizes the close relationship between qi and water intrinsic to the physiological qi dynamic to remove pathogenic water by means of strategies that differ according to the body region in which it is located. The qi in the skin and muscles tends to move outward. Thus, it is easiest to dispel water and dampness from this area by opening the pores and interstices and by promoting sweating. The qi in the interior moves downward, propelled by the downward directing of the bowels. Thus, it is easiest to drive out water from the interior via the urine and bowels. This is equivalent to the dredging and cutting strategy first used by the Great Yu, who exploited the water's own momentum in order to control it.

Comparison

➤ Vs. Minor Bluegreen Dragon Decoction (*xiǎo qīng lóng tāng*), True Warrior Decoction (*zhēn wǔ tāng*), Maidservant from Yue's Decoction (*yuè bì tāng*), and Five-Ingredient Powder with Poria (*wǔ líng sǎn*)

These are all formulas that are used to treat edema in both the exterior and the interior. The *Golden Mirror of the Medical Tradition* provides us with a useful comparison of these formulas:

Minor Bluegreen Dragon Decoction (*xiǎo qīng lóng tāng*), True Warrior Decoction (*zhēn wǔ tāng*), Maidservant from Yue's Decoction (*yuè bì tāng*), Five-Ingredient Powder with Poria (*wǔ líng sǎn*), and Dredging and Cutting Drink (*shū záo yǐn zi*) are five decoctions that all treat patterns characterized by the simultaneous presence of edema in the exterior and interior. Minor Bluegreen Dragon Decoction (*xiǎo qīng lóng tāng*) treats excess cold in the exterior and interior accompanied by edema. True Warrior Decoction (zhēn wǔ tāng) treats deficiency cold in the interior accompanied by edema. Both patterns are characterized by a lack of distention in the interior and a lack of [visible edematous] swelling in the exterior. Therefore, the first [formula] uses herbs like Ephedrae Herba (má huáng) and Cinnamomi Ramulus (guì zhī) to disperse the cold and move the water. The second uses herbs like Zingiberis Rhizoma recens (shēng jiāng) and Aconiti Radix lateralis praeparata (zhì fù zǐ) to warm the cold and control the water.

Maidservant from Yue's Decoction (yuè bì tāng) treats excess heat in the exterior and interior accompanied by edema. Five-Ingredient Powder with Poria (wǔ líng sǎn) treats deficiency heat in the exterior and interior accompanied by edema. Therefore, the first [formula] uses Ephedrae Herba (má huáng) and Gypsum fibrosum (shí gāo) to disperse water from the skin, clear heat from the muscles, and reduce swelling. The second uses Cinnamomi Ramulus (guì zhī), Poria (fú líng), Atractylodis macrocephalae Rhizoma (bái zhú), and Alismatis Rhizoma (zé xiè) to resolve the muscles and exterior heat, promote [movement] of water that has collected, and stop vomiting.

Dredging and Cutting Drink (shū záo yǐn zi) treats excess in both exterior and interior that is not characterized [by the predominance of either] heat or cold, but by an overwhelming excess of water dampness. [Such a pattern manifests with] generalized edema, wheezing, distention, and constipation.

Therefore, the formula uses Phytolaccae Radix (shāng lù) as chief, [an herb that is] specific for moving all kinds of water. It is assisted by Notopterygii Rhizoma seu Radix (qiāng huó), Gentianae macrophyllae Radix (qín jiāo), Arecae Pericarpium (dà fù pí), Poriae Cutis (fú líng pí), and Zingiberis Rhizomatis Cortex (shēng jiāng pí), which move the water in the exterior and disperse it via the skin. This is assisted by Arecae Semen (bīng láng), Phaseoli Semen (chì xiǎo dòu), Zanthoxyli Semen (jiāo mù), Alismatis Rhizoma (zé xiè), and Akebiae Caulis (mù tōng), which move the water in the interior and expel it via the urine and bowels. By separately reducing [edema] above and below, in the interior and exterior, according to its intrinsic momentum, [the formula] realizes the intention of the magical Yu, who dredged the rivers and cut canals [in order to control the floods].

Biomedical Indications

With the appropriate presentation, this formula may be used to treat a variety of biomedically-defined disorders including nephritis with edema and increased intracranial pressure.

Alternate name

Dredging and Cutting Powder (shū záo sǎn) in *Restoration of Life from the Groves of Medicine*

Comparative Tables of Principal Formulas

■ FORMULAS THAT PURGE HEAT ACCUMULATION

Common symptoms: constipation, fever, abdominal pain that increases upon pressure, dry tongue coating, submerged, excessive pulse; discontinue once diarrhea has been induced

Formula Name	Diagnosis	Indications	Remarks
Major Order the Qi Decoction (dà chéng qì tāng)	Yang brightness organ disorder with desiccated stool in the Intestines	Focal distention, fullness, dryness, hardness, a dry, yellow or dry, black tongue coating with prickles, and a submerged, excessive pulse	Vigorously purges heat accumulation.
Major Decoction [for Pathogens] Stuck in the Chest (dà xiàn xiōng tāng)	Clumping of heat and fluids in the chest and epigastrium	Hardness, fullness, and pain from the epigastrium to the lower abdomen that becomes unbearable with even the slightest pressure, a very dry tongue coating, and a submerged, tight, and forceful pulse	There may also be shortness of breath and irritability.

■ FORMULAS THAT WARM & PURGE

Common symptoms: constipation, abdominal pain, white tongue coating, submerged, tight pulse

Formula Name	Diagnosis	Indications	Remarks
Rhubarb and Aconite Accessory Root Decoction (dà huáng fù zǐ tāng)	Cold accumulation in the interior	Hypochondriac pain, chills, low-grade fever, cold hands and feet, a white, greasy tongue coating, and a submerged, tight, and wiry pulse	May also have low-grade fever.
Warm the Spleen Decoction (wēn pí tāng)	Cold accumulation in the interior with Spleen yang deficiency	Constipation or chronic red-and-white dysenteric disorders associated with abdominal pain, cold extremities, a white tongue coating, and a submerged, wiry pulse	Focuses on warming and tonifying Spleen yang and purging cold accumulation.

cont. ↘

Formula Name	Diagnosis	Indications	Remarks
Three-Substance Pill Prepared for Emergencies (sān wù bèi jí wán)	Sudden, severe cold accumulation	Sudden, severe epigastric and abdominal pain and distention, cyanotic complexion, a bluish-purple tongue, and a submerged, tight pulse	When severe, there may also be loss of consciousness.
Pinellia and Sulphur Pill (bàn liú wán)	Declining fire at the gate of vitality, with cold and turbid yin congealing and accumulating internally	Habitual constipation or chronic diarrhea, copious clear urine, cold extremities, abdominal pain, heavy or cold sensation in the lower back, a pale tongue with a white coating, and a submerged, slow pulse	This pattern is often found in the elderly.

■ FORMULAS THAT MOISTEN THE INTESTINES AND UNBLOCK THE BOWELS

Common symptoms: constipation

Formula Name	Diagnosis	Indications	Remarks
Five-Seed Pill (wǔ rén wán)	Desiccated Intestines	Dry stools that are difficult to pass, dry tongue, and a thin, rough pulse	For relatively mild problems.
Moisten the Intestines Pill from Master Shen's Book (rùn cháng wán)	Desiccated Intestines	Lusterless skin and nails, dry mouth and unquenchable thirst, a dry tongue, and a thin pulse	For very significant blood and yin deficiency.
Hemp Seed Pill (má zǐ rén wán)	Heat-dryness blocking the movement of fluids in the Spleen (Spleen bind)	Hard stool that is difficult to expel, normal to frequent urination, a dry, yellow tongue coating, and a submerged, rapid or floating, choppy pulse	Focuses on moistening dryness in the Intestines, draining heat, and moving qi.
Benefit the River [Flow] Decoction (jì chuān jiān)	Kidney deficiency constipation	Clear and copious urine, lower back pain, and a cold sensation in the back	Also for constipation due to Liver blood problems or essence depletion.

■ FORMULAS THAT SIMULTANEOUSLY ATTACK AND TONIFY

Common symptoms: constipation

Formula Name	Diagnosis	Indications	Remarks
Yellow Dragon Decoction (huáng lóng tāng)	Heat excess in the interior with qi and blood deficiency	Green, watery, and foul-smelling diarrhea, abdominal pain that increases upon pressure, fever, thirst, shortness of breath, lethargy, delirious speech, a dry, yellow or black tongue coating, and a deficient pulse	Also for constipation or firm, painful abdominal distention; when severe, there may be impaired consciousness.
Increase the Fluids and Order the Qi Decoction (zēng yè chéng qì tāng)	Deficiency of yin fluids with accumulation of dry stools in the Intestines	Dry stools that cannot be expelled even with a purging formula, distention and fullness of the epigastrium and abdomen, dry mouth and lips, a dry tongue with a thin, yellow or burnt yellow coating, and a rapid, thin pulse	Also used to treat various patterns of yang brightness excess with deficiency of yin fluids, such as toothache and skin diseases.

■ FORMULAS THAT DRIVE OUT EXCESS WATER

Common symptoms: constipation

Formula Name	Diagnosis	Indications	Remarks
Ten-Jujube Decoction (*shí zǎo tāng*)	Suspended, thin mucus clogging up the chest and hypochondriac regions	Cough with pain in the chest and hypochondria, hard focal distention in the epigastrium, dry heaves, shortness of breath, headache, vertigo, a white, slippery tongue coating, and a submerged, wiry pulse	Pain may extend to the back. Also used for edema due to obstruction from accumulation of thin mucus.
Vessel and Vehicle Pill (*zhōu chē wán*)	Water and heat accumulation in the interior obstructing the qi mechanism	Ascites and distention in a robust patient accompanied by thirst, labored breathing, a hard abdomen, constipation, scanty urine, and a submerged, rapid, and forceful pulse	Prescribed only in cases of emergency for those of otherwise robust health.
Yu's Achievement Powder (*yǔ gōng sǎn*)	Yang edema caused by water dampness invading the body and obstructing the qi dynamic	Generalized floating edema, abdominal distention, wheezing and fullness, constipation, inhibited urination, and a submerged and forceful pulse	May also be swelling and distention of the scrotum with heaviness, pain, dampness, and sweating.
Stephania, Zanthoxylum, Tingli Seed, and Rhubarb Pill (*jǐ jiāo lì huáng wán*)	Accumulation of water in the Stomach and Intestines with qi stagnation	Abdominal distention, borborygmus, dry mouth, constipation, reduced urination, a yellow, greasy tongue coating, and a wiry and slippery or submerged, full, and slightly rapid pulse	Should only be used short term.
Dredging and Cutting Drink (*shū záo yǐn zi*)	Yang edema flooding both the interior and exterior causing qi stagnation	Generalized edema, wheezing, dyspnea, restlessness and irritability, thirst, constipation, and urinary obstruction	Also known as a severe form of water qi.

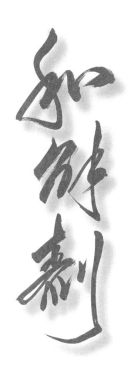

Chapter 3 Contents

Formulas that Harmonize

Formulas that Harmonize

A MONG THE EIGHT methods of treatment, the formulas in this chapter belong to the harmonizing method (和法 *hé fǎ*). In its widest sense, harmonization refers to the regulation of yin and yang within the body and thus to the goal of all treatment in Chinese medicine. The term, used in this way, occurs several times in the *Inner Classic,* and in ancient Chinese medicine was used interchangeably with the term for treating or curing (治 *zhì*). A somewhat similar usage can be found in *Discussion of Cold Damage* and *Essentials from the Golden Cabinet,* the late-Han dynasty texts from which the majority of formulas in this chapter are drawn. Their author, Zhang Zhong-Jing, describes the action of two formulas—Minor Order the Qi Decoction *(xiǎo chéng qì tāng)* and Cinnamon Twig Decoction *(guì zhī tāng)*—as harmonious (和 *hé*), which he contrasts to the action of stronger diaphoretic and purging formulas. Here, harmonious probably refers to relatively gentle treatment in general, rather than to any particular method. The use of the term 'harmonizing method' to refer to the strategies utilized in formulas such as Minor Bupleurum Decoction *(xiǎo chái hú tāng)* did not occur until 1156 with the publication of *Discussion Illuminating the Principles of Cold Damage.* In this book, Cheng Wu-Ji narrowed the concept of harmonization to mean a method of treatment appropriate for lesser yang-warp disorders:

> When there is a cold damage pathogen in the exterior, one must seep it from the body as sweat. When the pathogen is located in the interior, one must flush and scour it out as diarrhea. When it is neither in the exterior nor the interior but half outside and half inside, inducing sweating is not appropriate, nor do vomiting or purgation provide an answer. In this case, it is appropriate to resolve [the condition] by harmonization. Minor Bupleurum Decoction *(xiǎo chái hú tāng)* is the formula that harmonizes the exterior and the interior.

Many later commentators, including Zhang Jie-Bin and Cheng Guo-Peng, reminded their readers that the original meaning of harmonization was far broader and that it could be achieved by methods as diverse as tonification and purgation, or moistening dryness and drying dampness. By then, however, Cheng Wu-Ji's definition of harmonization was so firmly established that it could not be reversed. Instead, physicians expanded the scope of formulas included in the harmonization category. Besides formulas to treat lesser yang-warp disorders, it gradually came to include formulas that treat disharmonies between the Liver and Spleen, Gallbladder and Stomach, and Stomach and Intestines, as well as formulas that are indicated for malarial disorders.

The present content of this category was defined during the 1950s and 1960s in the People's Republic of China by physicians engaged in the systematization of traditional medicine. Pu Fu-Zhou, the most senior physician at the Academy of Chinese Medicine during this time, provided a concise definition:

> [Definition of] the harmonizing method: [Refers to] harmonizing in a narrow sense. Harmonization carries the meaning of

moderate use of dredging and resolving [strategies]. It brings balance to complex [conditions that present with] symptom pictures of interior-exterior, excess-deficiency, and cold-heat, as well as conditions of overabundance and debility that exist in the yin and yang organs, yin and yang, and qi and blood. (*Therapeutic Experiences of Pu Fu-Zhou*)

Harmonizing formulas should not be used in treating exterior disorders, as this will cause the disorder to advance to a deeper level. It is also important to remember that the presence of alternating fever and chills is not necessarily indicative of a lesser yang-warp disorder. This symptom may also appear in cases of terminal yin-warp disorders, severe organ deficiency, or deficiency of both qi and blood. The inappropriate use of harmonizing formulas in such cases will aggravate these problems.

For complex historical reasons, contemporary Chinese medicine in East Asia and the West associates psychosomatic disorders with conditions of the Liver or Gallbladder, or with Liver-Spleen disharmony. Disease due to emotional problems or to the stresses involved in coping with the rigors of modern life are therefore often treated with formulas selected from this category. While this disease-based approach may be successful in some cases, Chinese medical tradition suggests that it is better to differentiate patterns and apply treatment based on the symptoms and constitution exhibited by the individual patient.

Section 1

FORMULAS THAT HARMONIZE LESSER YANG-WARP DISORDERS

The lesser yang warp is generally considered to lie between the exterior greater yang and the interior yang brightness warps of the six warps of disease. The in-between nature of this warp (characterized as half-exterior, half-interior) means halfway between the exterior and the interior, and does not refer to concurrent exterior-interior conditions where the pathogenic influence is lodged in both the exterior and the interior. (For formulas that treat this type of pattern, see Chapter 7.) The dispersing and draining methods utilized in treating greater yang and yang brightness-warp disorders respectively cannot be used in treating lesser yang-warp disorders.

Identifying the type of fever will help to differentiate the warp: simultaneous fever and chills usually indicates a greater yang-warp disorder; fever without chills usually indicates a yang brightness-warp disorder; alternating fever and chills usually indicates a lesser yang-warp disorder. The Gallblad-

der (which corresponds to the leg lesser yang channel) is the organ most closely associated with this warp. A dry throat, bitter taste in the mouth, and sensation of fullness in the hypochondria are symptoms that occur along the course of the leg lesser yang channel. The typical pulse is wiry and forceful, indicating obstruction of the qi rising upward in the lesser yang.

Formulas that treat other externally-contracted conditions with similar signs and symptoms (e.g., heat in the Gallbladder and Triple Burner), although not regarded as purely lesser yang-warp disorders, are also included in this section. Given the wide-ranging functions of the Gallbladder and Triple Burner in organizing the distribution of yang qi and fluids, it is difficult to define the problems for which these formulas are indicated in terms of a single, tightly-defined pattern.

The core ingredients in these formulas consist of a pairing of Scutellariae Radix (*huáng qín*) with either Bupleuri Radix (*chái hú*) or Artemisiae annuae Herba (*qīng hāo*). These pairings are effective at reaching pathogens that are lodged in this half-exterior, half-interior aspect. Other herbs are added depending on which of the other aspects is affected by the pathogen. For example, for exterior pathogens, Zingiberis Rhizoma recens (*shēng jiāng*) might be added; to clear heat in the interior, add Coptidis Rhizoma (*huáng lián*); for phlegm, add Pinelliae Rhizoma praeparatum (*zhì bàn xià*) and Citri reticulatae Pericarpium (*chén pí*); and for significant qi stagnation, add Magnoliae officinalis Cortex (*hòu pò*) and Aurantii Fructus (*zhǐ ké*). Similarly, various types of interior deficiency often accompany these disorders. For qi deficiency, add Ginseng Radix (*rén shēn*), Atractylodis macrocephalae Rhizoma (*bái zhú*), or Jujubae Fructus (*dà zǎo*); for blood deficiency, Angelicae sinensis Radix (*dāng guī*) and Paeoniae Radix alba (*bái sháo*) are often prescribed.

小柴胡湯 (小柴胡汤)

Minor Bupleurum Decoction

xiǎo chái hú tāng

Source   *Discussion of Cold Damage* (c. 220)

Bupleuri Radix (*chái hú*) 24g
Scutellariae Radix (*huáng qín*) 9g
Pinelliae Rhizoma praeparatum (*zhì bàn xià*) 24g
Zingiberis Rhizoma recens (*shēng jiāng*) 9g
Ginseng Radix (*rén shēn*) 9g
Glycyrrhizae Radix praeparata (*zhì gān cǎo*) 9g
Jujubae Fructus (*dà zǎo*) . . . . 12 pieces

Method of Preparation   The source text advises to decoct the above ingredients in approximately 12 cups of water until 6 cups remain. The ingredients are removed and the strained decoction is further decocted until 3 cups remain. This is taken warm in three equal doses over the course of a day. At present, it is most often prepared as a decoction in the usual manner. Codonopsis Radix *(dǎng shēn)* is commonly substituted for Ginseng Radix *(rén shēn)* at 2-3 times its dosage. Most practitioners also reduce the dosage of Bupleuri Radix *(chái hú)* and Pinelliae Rhizoma praeparatum *(zhì bàn xià)* to 12g, Glycyrrhizae Radix praeparata *(zhì gān cǎo)* to 6g, and Jujubae Fructus *(dà zǎo)* to 4 pieces.

Actions   Harmonizes and releases lesser yang-warp disorders

Indications

Alternating fever and chills, dry throat, bitter taste in the mouth, dizziness, irritability, sensation of fullness in the chest and hypochondria (often experienced as difficulty in taking deep breaths), heartburn, nausea and vomiting, being downcast with no desire to eat, a thin, white tongue coating, and a wiry pulse. There may also be palpitations, coughing, or urinary dysfunction.

This is a cold pathogen constraining the lesser yang warp and impeding its ability to direct the clear upward and the turbid downward. The lesser yang defines the spaces in between the interior and exterior of the body. Its function is to direct the protective yang qi produced by the gate of vitality and the clear fluids upward and outward, and the turbid fluids downward from the upper to the lower burner. When a cold pathogen that has penetrated the exterior constrains the protective aspect, yang heat accumulates in the interior. The ensuing struggle between the protective yang and the pathogenic cold is reflected most clearly in the symptom of alternating chills and fever. When the pathogenic qi prevails, failure of the yang qi to warm the exterior causes chills. At more or less regular intervals, the constrained yang qi discharges to the exterior, which is experienced as fever by the patient. However, because this discharge is disorderly, it fails to dislodge the pathogen. Constrained heat rising upward in the interior also causes a bitter taste in the mouth, dry throat, and dizziness.

Other symptoms are associated with the Gallbladder, the organ that corresponds to the lesser yang. Qi constraint along the course of the Gallbladder channel may manifest as fullness of the chest and hypochondria or stiffness of the neck. Emotionally, such constraint is reflected in being downcast and laconic. If constrained Gallbladder qi attacks the Stomach, it causes heartburn, nausea, vomiting, and reduced appetite. If it attacks the Lungs, it causes coughing. If it blocks the distribution of fluids in the Triple Burner, it inhibits urination and causes an accumulation of phlegm fluids below the Heart that can lead to palpitations. The wiry pulse also indicates constraint, phlegm, and the involvement of the Gallbladder. The pulse is sometimes thin, which signifies a disorder that is in between the greater yang warp (where the pulse would be floating) and the yang brightness warp (where the pulse would be overflowing).

The source text also notes that this formula is indicated for heat entering the blood chamber (熱入血室 *rè rù xuè shì*). This is a presentation characterized by alternating fever and chills, dry throat, discomfort in the hypochondria, as well as agitation of the spirit that may develop into delirious speech. It is caused by the contraction of cold after childbirth or during menstruation.

During menstruation or following childbirth, women suffer from a deficiency of blood. Should they suffer invasion by a wind-cold pathogen, the pathogen can exploit this weakness to penetrate the blood chamber where it binds the blood. The blood and the blood chamber are closely associated with the Liver. Binding of the blood by pathogenic qi inhibits the Liver's function of dredging and discharging, leading to qi constraint with heat. This is reflected in alternating fever and chills, dry throat, and discomfort in the hypochondria. Heat rising upward through the terminal yin to harrass the Heart causes agitation of the spirit that may develop into delirious speech in more serious cases.

Analysis of Formula

This formula is designed to resolve the constraint located at the level of the lesser yang warp, or halfway between the exterior and interior, by means of a harmonizing strategy. The chief herb is Bupleuri Radix *(chái hú)*, the most important herb for venting pathogens in lesser yang-warp disorders in the Chinese materia medica. Combined with the deputy, Scutellariae Radix *(huáng qín)*, which drains heat from the Liver and Gallbladder (the interior aspect of the lesser yang warp), it vents the pathogenic influence and thereby releases lesser yang-warp disorders. Bupleuri Radix *(chái hú)* also spreads the Liver qi with an ascending, cooling action (contrary to most cooling herbs, which cause things to descend). This combination thereby clears the heat without causing it to sink deeper into the body.

One of the assistants, Pinelliae Rhizoma praeparatum *(zhì bàn xià)*, warms and transforms phlegm and turbidity in the middle burner. When combined with another assistant, Zingiberis Rhizoma recens *(shēng jiāng)*, it harmonizes the middle burner, directs rebellious qi downward, and stops nausea and vomiting. The remaining assistants, Ginseng Radix *(rén shēn)*, Glycyrrhizae Radix praeparata *(zhì gān cǎo)*, and Jujubae Fructus *(dà zǎo)*, support the normal qi and thereby prevent the pathogenic influence from penetrating to the interior. Glycyrrhizae Radix praeparata *(zhì gān cǎo)* and Jujubae Fructus *(dà zǎo)* also moderate the acrid, dry properties of Pinelliae Rhizoma praeparatum *(zhì bàn xià)* and Zingiberis Rhizoma recens *(shēng jiāng)*. The combination of Zingiberis Rhizoma recens *(shēng jiāng)* and Jujubae Fructus *(dà zǎo)* mildly regulates the nutritive and protective qi, and assists Bupleuri Radix *(chái hú)* in releasing the half-exterior aspects of this condition.

Cautions and Contraindications

This formula promotes the spreading out of yang qi, which can cause headache, dizziness, and bleeding of the gums if taken long term. These side effects can be reduced or eliminated if the formula is prepared according to the directions in the source text. For the same reason, unless considerably modified, it is contraindicated in patients with excess above and deficiency below, Liver fire, or bleeding of the gums. Use with caution in cases of ascendant Liver yang, hypertension, or vomiting of blood due to yin deficiency. Patients with relatively weak normal qi may experience fever and chills while taking this formula because the pathogenic influence is vented from the lesser yang warp via the greater yang.

Commentary

According to *Discussion of Cold Damage*, the common methods of treating externally-contracted diseases are inducing sweating (to release the exterior) and purging or vomiting (to expel interior accumulations). However, neither of these approaches is appropriate for treating a lesser yang disorder. The pathogenic influence is lodged too deeply in the interior to be released by sweating, which would only injure the fluids and the normal qi. Yet the pathogen has not penetrated deep enough to justify purging, which would injure the yin and could lead to palpitations with anxiety. Because the symptom of chest fullness is due to qi constraint rather than pathogenic accumulation, inducing vomiting is also inappropriate. This would merely injure the yang of the chest and could lead to palpitations. The preferred method, which unblocks the qi dynamic to clear heat constraint, vents pathogens from the lesser yang, and harmonizes fluid metabolism; it is known as harmonization, or literally 'harmonizing resolution' (和解 *hé jiě*).

Bupleuri Radix (chái hú) and Harmonizing Resolution

A passage in *Rectification of the Meaning of Materia Medica* explains the action of the chief herb in this formula, Bupleuri Radix (*chái hú*), and its role in the process of harmonizing resolution:

> Bupleuri Radix (*chái hú*) has a bitter flavor and therefore specifically focuses on pathogenic heat ... It grows in the early spring, its qi is fragrant, and its character light and clear. With both a light qi and flavor and an ascending, discharging nature constitutionally received in the spring, it is thus completely different, however, in both character and function from other bitter, cooling, draining, and downward-directing herbs. ... When pathogenic qi gradually enters into the interior and is no longer located merely at the muscle layer and surface [of the body] from which all other exterior-dispersing herbs can no longer vent it, only Bupleuri Radix (*chái hú*) with its clear and light qi and aromatic fragrance is able to dredge and drain it, guiding and lifting the pathogenic qi outward to be resolved via the exterior. This is why Bupleuri Radix (*chái hú*) is [included

among the herbs that] resolve the exterior, even if its action is different from other herbs that focus on resolving the exterior.

Wide Range of Application

Located in between the exterior and the interior and responsible for regulating the distribution of qi throughout the body, the lesser yang is referred to in Chapter 6 of *Basic Questions* as functioning like a 'pivot' (樞 *shū*). When the pivot becomes stuck, the qi dynamic breaks down. This gives Minor Bupleurum Decoction (*xiǎo chái hú tāng*) an extremely wide range of possible indications. The formula is mentioned over twenty times in *Discussion of Cold Damage* and *Essentials from the Golden Cabinet*. Paragraph 101 of *Discussion of Cold Damage* observes that "For cold damage or wind attack, when there is a [Minor] Bupleurum [Decoction (*xiǎo*) *chái hú* (*tāng*)] presentation, if there is only one sign, then that is it. It is not necessary that they all be present [to make the diagnosis]."

This statement sparked considerable discussion among commentators. Some interpreted it literally to mean that the presence of just one of the signs or symptoms listed in the source text warranted the use of Minor Bupleurum Decoction (*xiǎo chái hú tāng*). Others, however, read it as referring to the presence of just the chief signs (主症 *zhǔ zhèng*) like alternating chills and fever, fullness of the chest and hypochondria, downcast demeanor with lack of appetite, or irritability and nausea.

The late-Qing-dynasty physician Tang Zong-Hai prescribed this formula for a wide variety of problems. In *Discussion of Blood Patterns*, Tang's interpretation of its efficacy focuses on the relationship between the Gallbladder and Triple Burner within the lesser yang warp. In his discussion of pathophysiology, Tang's description provides one of the clearest expositions of Minor Bupleurum Decoction (*xiǎo chái hú tāng*) and its associated pattern:

> This is an invigorating formula that spreads out the exterior and harmonizes the interior, that lifts the clear upward and directs the turbid downward. The exterior of the human body [in this context refers to] the pivotal dynamic of the interstices and pores and the nutritive and protective [aspects]. The interior of the human body [refers to] the substantial supervisory function [exerted by] the Triple Burner on the yin and yang organs. In the interior, the lesser yang governs the Triple Burner, in the exterior it governs the interstices and pores. If we are discussing the nature of the lesser yang, we [mean] the qi of the ministerial fire with its root in the Gallbladder. If we are discussing its function, we [mean] the qi of clear yang that resides in the Stomach. The formula uses Ginseng Radix (*rén shēn*), Jujubae Fructus (*dà zǎo*), and Glycyrrhizae Radix (*gān cǎo*) to develop the patient's Stomach [qi]. It uses [the combination of] Scutellariae Radix (*huáng qín*) and Pinelliae Rhizoma praeparatum (*zhì bàn xià*) to direct turbid fire downward, and [the combination of] Bupleuri Radix (*chái hú*) and Zingiberis Rhizoma recens (*shēng jiāng*) to lift up the clear yang. Thus harmonizing and facilitating the patient's qi [dynamic], how would the interstices and Triple Burner not also be regulated?

Where the qi of the greater yang sinks into the anterior aspect of the chest from where it has no way out, one can also use this formula to clear the interior and harmonize the middle, raising and spreading the qi so that it does not clump but releases any exterior condition. Where fire constrains the Lung channel, inhibiting urination and the bowels, one uses it to disperse and unblock the upper burner. When the body fluids no longer clump, [urine and bowels] spontaneously [properly] move in the lower burner. One also uses it for fire from constraint in the Liver channel in order to guide Liver qi to spread upward so that wood is no longer constrained. Because [the formula] also contains substances that clear and direct downward, any remaining fire will definitely also be eliminated.

Historical Controversies

Given the wide range of possible indications for this formula, it is not surprising that commentators have differed on a number of diagnostic issues. The first concerns the nature of the alternating fever and chills for which this formula is prescribed. The traditional view is that, by contrast to malarial disorders, the alternation between fever and chills seen in lesser yang patterns has no set periodicity. However, this is not specifically stated in the source text. Furthermore, the literature contains many case records that document the successful use of Minor Bupleurum Decoction (*xiǎo chái hú tāng*) in cases of malaria.

Physicians also disagree about the precise meaning of "heat entering the blood chamber." Cheng Wu-Ji argued that blood chamber refers to the Penetrating vessel. Ke Qin thought that it was the Liver, while Zhang Jie-Bin believed it to be the Womb. Because the source text clearly links the onset of this disorder to blood loss during menstruation or birth, that is, from the Womb, most modern writers follow Zhang Jie-Bin's interpretation. The Womb is linked to the terminal yin, which in turn enjoys an interior/exterior relationship with the lesser yang. Using Minor Bupleurum Decoction (*xiǎo chái hú tāng*) can thus create an exit route for pathogenic heat from an organ that does not have its own link to the exterior.

Dosage of Bupleuri Radix (chái hú)

A third important point of historical debate concerns the function and dosage of the chief herb Bupleuri Radix (*chái hú*). From the Jin-Yuan period onward, physicians linked the ability of Bupleuri Radix (*chái hú*) to dredge Liver and Gallbladder qi and resolve the exterior to its capacity to lift up the yang qi. This is an elegant way of tying all of the many possible applications of this herb to one explanatory model. However, lifting up the yang qi is another way of saying that Bupleuri Radix (*chái hú*) stimulates the body's transformation of essence (water) into qi (fire). Some physicians thus became worried about the potential side effects of using Bupleuri Radix (*chái hú*). They argued that Bupleuri Radix (*chái hú*) and other uplifting herbs like Puerariae Radix (*gé gēn*) "plunder the yin" (劫陰 *jié yīn*) and should thus be used only

with extreme circumspection.

Owing to diverse cultural and social factors, these ideas became very influential among physicians and patients in southern China from the 16th century onward. These perceptions are an important reason for the large discrepancy between the dosage of Bupleuri Radix (*chái hú*) prescribed in the source text and the much lower dosage used by most modern practitioners. The latter believe that while the herb is quite safe for most patients, it should be used with caution in those with yin deficiency.

Other physicians, however, reject the entire explanatory framework on which these concerns are based. They point out that before Jin and Yuan dynasty physicians began describing this herb as lifting up the yang, it had been primarily used to open up obstructions. According to the *Divine Husbandman's Classic of the Materia Medica*, "Bupleuri Radix (*chái hú*) … governs clumping of qi in the Heart [i.e., the epigastrium], abdomen, bowels and Stomach, accumulation of food and drink, [as well as] fever and chills [caused by] pathogenic qi. It pushes out the old for the new to arrive." In pre-Song manuals like *Important Formulas Worth a Thousand Gold Pieces* or *Arcane Essentials from the Imperial Library*, Bupleuri Radix (*chái hú*) was thus used in accordance with quite different parameters than in later texts, namely, to dispel stasis in cases of mobile abdominal masses or menstrual irregularity, including amenorrhea; to resolve fever, including the fever of malaria and of consumptive disorders; and to drain downward by opening the digestive pathways.

When cultural shifts during the Qing dynasty stimulated a critical reexamination of Song-Jin-Yuan medicine, such older views gained new currency. Writers such as the 20th-century physician Zhang Ci-Gong, whose *Discussing Medicinal Substances* influenced generations of students in modern China, now completely rejected the proposition that Bupleuri Radix (*chái hú*) lifted up the qi. He argued that it must be used in a large dosage and is only appropriate for opening obstructions. His disciple, Zhu Liang-Chun, one of contemporary China's most influential clinicians who is renowned for his understanding of materia medica, tried to forge a compromise. In *Collected Experiences of Zhu Liang-Chun in Using Medicines*, Zhu argued that, depending on the dosage, Bupleuri Radix (*chái hú*) either lifts up the qi or unblocks by draining downward. For the former, useful in cases of qi constraint due to internal Liver disharmonies, Zhu recommends a dosage of 3-10g. For the latter, appropriate where constraint is caused by external pathogens, he recommends a dosage of 20-30g. Zhu also argued that the key sign for the use of Bupleuri Radix (*chái hú*) is a white and often relatively dirty and greasy tongue coating. This reflects the accumulation of phlegm fluids that is the invariable consequence of qi and fluid constraint, for which Bupleuri Radix (*chái hú*) is specifically indicated.

Use in the Modern Clinic

Over the centuries, physicians have extended the range of disorders for which Minor Bupleurum Decoction (*xiǎo chái hú tāng*) is indicated even further. Its use in modern practice can be grouped into six broad categories:

1. Febrile disorders with alternating fever and chills

2. Digestive disorders that present with signs of stagnation or clumping in the Liver and Gallbladder channels, or where loss of the Stomach's downward-directing function is accompanied by a wiry pulse

3. Gynecological disorders that match the presentations of heat entering the blood chamber where signs of blood stasis are accompanied by alternating chills and heat flushes

4. Urogenital disorders where signs of heat or inflammation are accompanied by qi stagnation

5. Miscellaneous disorders with a clear relationship to the lesser yang channels or related patterns, such as inflamed lymph glands in the neck or armpits, thyroid enlargement, hypertension, or palpitations

6. Nervous system and emotional disorders with a lesser yang presentation including insomnia, anxiety, headache, and nerve pain.

The case history literature also lists many instances where Minor Bupleurum Decoction (*xiǎo chái hú tāng*) is used to treat so-called 'strange disorders' (怪病 *guài bìng*). These are disorders that manifest with unusual symptoms or with presentations that are difficult to match with common patterns or disorders. The successful use of this formula in treating such disorders can be traced to the pivotal physiological function of the lesser yang warp, which is confirmed by the small number of signs and symptoms needed to diagnose a Minor Bupleurum Decoction pattern (*xiǎo chái hú tāng zhèng*).

The astute use of Minor Bupleurum Decoction (*xiǎo chái hú tāng*), furthermore, can play an important role in constitutional treatment. Here it is used to maintain physical, mental, and emotional equilibrium in those with a lesser yang temperament, as outlined by the late-Qing-dynasty physician Fei Boxiong:

> If I possess strong defenses, I do not need to engage in battles. Still, I may have a tendency toward feeling aggrieved. [In such cases] I can also use Bupleuri Radix (*chái hú*) to disperse pathogens from the lesser yang and Pinelliae Rhizoma praeparatum (*zhì bàn xià*) to eliminate phlegm and move the qi in order to transform rebelliousness. This is comparable to [a city] that is safe and secure yet from time to time allows the cavalry out to [excercise their horses] in a gallop, riding out without any distinct objective and returning without having seized anything. How could [any pathogen] not melt away like ice? (*Discussion of Medical Formulas*)

This suggests that for a constitutionally strong patient who holds grievances or stores emotions inside, it may be beneficial to occasionally give Minor Bupleurum Decoction (*xiǎo chái hú tāng*) as a way of exorcizing the emotional buildup and preventing the consequences of repressed emotions.

To tailor the use of this formula more specifically to its many possible indications, physicians devised many new formulas through judicious additions and substractions. Only the most famous of these are listed below. Minor Bupleurum Decoction (*xiǎo chái hú tāng*) is also often paired with other classical formulas. Typical examples include the combination with Cinnamon Twig Decoction (*guì zhī tāng*) to treat a joint disorder of the greater and lesser yang warps; with Minor Decoction [for Pathogens] Stuck in the Chest (*xiǎo xiàn xiōng tāng*) to treat cough with sticky phlegm and pain in the flanks; with Pinellia and Magnolia Bark Decoction (*bàn xià hòu pò tāng*) to treat qi stagnation in the chest, throat, and flanks often due to emotional factors; and with Five-Ingredient Powder with Poria (*wǔ líng sǎn*) to treat lesser yang disorders with pronounced urinary difficulty or edema.

Another commonly used strategy is to adjust the relative dosage of herbs within the formula to match specific presentations. If alternating fever and chills are the key presenting problem, the dosage of Bupleuri Radix (*chái hú*) should be two or three times that of Scutellariae Radix (*huáng qín*). If signs of internal heat like dryness of the throat and a bitter taste predominate, the dosage of Scutellariae Radix (*huáng qín*) may be increased until it matches that of Bupleuri Radix (*chái hú*). If nausea and abdominal fullness predominate, the dosage of Pinelliae Rhizoma praeparatum (*zhì bàn xià*) should be increased accordingly.

Comparisons

➢ Vs. Sweet Wormwood and Scutellaria Decoction to Clear the Gallbladder (*hāo qín qīng dǎn tāng*); *see* PAGE 112

➢ Vs. Frigid Extremities Powder (*sì nì sǎn*); *see* PAGE 119

➢ Vs. Major Bupleurum Decoction (*dà chái hú tāng*); *see* PAGE 288

➢ Vs. Cyperus and Inula Decoction (*xiāng fù xuán fù huā tāng*); *see* PAGE 790

Biomedical Indications

With the appropriate presentation, this formula may be used to treat a wide variety of biomedically-defined disorders. These can be divided into the following groups:

• Those manifesting with chest and hypochondriac pain including hepatitis, chronic cholecystitis, chronic gastritis, peptic ulcer disease, acute pancreatitis, pneumonia, and pleurisy

- Acute febrile illness such as upper respiratory tract infections, tonsilitis, conjunctivitis, malaria, typhoid fever of unknown origin, perimenstrual fevers, and postpartum fevers
- Those marked by periodicity such as bronchial asthma, epilepsy, angina pectoris, allergic rhinitis, and premenstrual syndrome
- Those affecting the pathways of the lesser yang channels such as migraine, intercostal neuralgia, periaural eczema, parotiditis, suppurative otitis media, and mastitis.

....

Alternate names

Bupleurum Deoction (*chái hú tāng*) in *Essentials from the Golden Cabinet;* Yellow Dragon Decoction (*huáng lóng tāng*) in *Important Formulas Worth a Thousand Gold Pieces;* Three Prohibitions Decoction (*sān jìn tāng*) in *Hard-Won Knowledge;* Ginseng Decoction (*rén shēn tāng*) in *Effective Formulas from Generations of Physicians);* Harmonizing and Resolving Powder (*hé jiě sǎn*) in *Six Texts on Cold Damage*

....

Modifications

- For irritability in the chest without nausea, remove Pinelliae Rhizoma praeparatum *(zhì bàn xià)* and Ginseng Radix *(rén shēn)* and add Trichosanthis Semen *(guā lóu rén)*. (source text)
- For pronunced thirst, remove Pinelliae Rhizoma praeparatum *(zhì bàn xià)* and add Trichosanthis Radix *(tiān huā fěn)*. (source text)
- For abdominal pain, remove Scutellariae Radix *(huáng qín)* and add Paeoniae Radix alba *(bái sháo)*. (source text)
- For hard focal distention and firmness below the ribs, remove Jujubae Fructus *(dà zǎo)* and add Ostreae Concha *(mǔ lì)*. (source text)
- For palpitations in the epigastric area with inhibited urination, remove Scutellariae Radix *(huáng qín)* and add Poria *(fú líng)*. (source text)
- For cases with no thirst and slight fever in the exterior, remove Ginseng Radix *(rén shēn)* and add Cinnamomi Ramulus *(guì zhī)*. (source text)
- For cough, remove Ginseng Radix *(rén shēn)*, Jujubae Fructus *(dà zǎo)*, and Zingiberis Rhizoma recens *(shēng jiāng)*, and add Schisandrae Fructus *(wǔ wèi zǐ)* and Zingiberis Rhizoma *(gān jiāng)*. (source text)
- For heat entering the blood chamber, add herbs like Persicae Semen *(táo rén)*, Carthami Flos *(hóng huā)*, and Moutan Cortex *(mǔ dān pí)*.
- For rough, scanty, dark, and painful urination, add Lysimachiae Herba *(jīn qián cǎo)* and Hedyotis diffusae Herba *(bái huā shé shé cǎo)*.
- For fever, aversion to wind, headache, a stifling sensation in the chest, constipation, loss of appetite, dark urine, irritability, thirst, a yellow tongue coating, and a tight pulse, add Cannabis Semen *(huǒ má rén)* and Aurantii Fructus immaturus *(zhǐ shí)*.
- For fever, coughing of yellow sputum, and chest pain, add Platycodi Radix *(jié gěng)*, Trichosanthis Fructus *(guā lóu)*, and Fritillariae cirrhosae Bulbus *(chuān bèi mǔ)*.
- For malarial disorders, add Artemisiae annuae Herba *(qīng hāo)* and Dichroae Radix *(cháng shān)*.
- For vertigo, add Chrysanthemi Flos *(jú huā)*, Uncariae Ramulus cum Uncis *(gōu téng)*, and Cassiae Semen *(jué míng zǐ)*.
- For coughs that are more severe around midnight, alternating fever and chills, and a bitter taste in the mouth, add Zingiberis Rhizoma *(gān jiāng)*, Asari Radix et Rhizoma *(xì xīn)*, and Schisandrae Fructus *(wǔ wèi zǐ)*. This application was pioneered by the Qing-dynasty physician Chen Nian-Zu, who also used it to treat coughs that did not respond to other treatment.
- For urinary tract infection with chills, fever, and urgent, frequent urination, combine with Six-Ingredient Pill with Rehmannia *(liù wèi dì huáng wán)*. This was developed by the 20th-century physician Yue Mei-Zhong.

Associated Formulas

柴胡桂枝湯 (柴胡桂枝汤)

Bupleurum and Cinnamon Twig Decoction

chái hú guì zhī tāng

SOURCE *Discussion of Cold Damage* (c. 220)

Cinnamomi Ramulus *(guì zhī)*	4.5g
Scutellariae Radix *(huáng qín)*	4.5g
Ginseng Radix *(rén shēn)*	4.5g
Glycyrrhizae Radix *(gān cǎo)*	3g
Pinelliae Rhizoma praeparatum *(zhì bàn xià)*	6-9g
Paeoniae Radix *(sháo yào)*	4.5g
Bupleuri Radix *(chái hú)*	12g
Zingiberis Rhizoma recens *(shēng jiāng)*	4.5g
Jujubae Fructus *(dà zǎo)*	6 pieces

At present, Paeoniae Radix alba *(bái sháo)* is the form of Paeoniae Radix *(sháo yào)* that is commonly used. Releases the muscle layer and exterior and harmonizes and releases lesser yang-warp disorders. The original indication is for lesser yang-warp disorders where the exterior has not been completely released, and joint pain with a 'crackling' sensation due to wind in the joints. It is thus frequently used for joint pain accompanied by lesser yang signs and symptoms as well as for fever accompanied by chills and aversion to wind. If fever is predominant, the dosage of Bupleuri Radix *(chái hú)* may be increased to as much as 30g. If chills are predominant, it should be decreased. If fever is accompanied by pronounced thirst, Gypsum fibrosum *(shí gāo)* may also be added. A mild sweat following ingestion of the formula is desirable.

The range of applications has since been expanded to treat a wide variety of conditions due to Liver qi constraint or Liver-Stomach disharmony against a background of Spleen qi deficiency and phlegm-dampness. These include allergic disorders such as rhinitis, urticaria, or skin rashes triggered by exposure to cold as well as chronic inflammatory conditions that match the core presentation. Modern Japanese physicians use the formula for treating hot flushes, sleep disorders (specifically for waking during sleep and sleep that does not refresh), tension headaches, and migraines specifically if there is a strong emotional element in the etiology. The formula may also be used for epigastric pain due to Liver and Spleen disharmony; in this case, it is advised to increase the dosage of Paeoniae Radix alba (bái sháo) by 2-3 times.

Comparison

➤ Vs. Bupleurum, Cinnamon Twig, and Ginger Decoction (chái hú guì zhī gān jiāng tāng); see page 141

柴胡加芒硝湯 (柴胡加芒硝汤)

Bupleurum Decoction plus Mirabilite

chái hú jiā máng xiāo tāng

Source Discussion of Cold Damage (c. 220)

Bupleuri Radix (chái hú) 8g
Scutellariae Radix (huáng qín) 3g
Ginseng Radix (rén shēn) 3g
Glycyrrhizae Radix praeparata (zhì gān cǎo) 3g
Zingiberis Rhizoma recens (shēng jiāng) 3g
Pinelliae Rhizoma praeparatum (zhì bàn xià) 3g
Jujubae Fructus (dà zǎo) .4 pieces
Natrii Sulfas (máng xiāo) 6g

Harmonizes and releases the lesser yang, softens hardness, and drains downward. For constipation and fullness in the chest and hypochondria with vomiting and alternating fever and chills (fever more pronounced in the afternoon). Often caused by inappropriate purging that injures the Stomach yin.

Comparison

➤ Vs. Major Bupleurum Decoction (dà chái hú tāng); see page 288

柴胡枳桔湯 (柴胡枳桔汤)

Bupleurum, Bitter Orange, and Platycodon Decoction

chái hú zhǐ jié tāng

Source Comprehensive Medicine According to Master Zhang (1695)

Bupleuri Radix (chái hú) 3-4.5g
Aurantii Fructus (zhǐ ké) 4.5g
ginger-fried Pinelliae Rhizoma praeparatum
    (jiāng bàn xià) 4.5g
Zingiberis Rhizoma recens (shēng jiāng) 3g
Platycodi Radix (jié gěng) 3g
Scutellariae Radix (huáng qín) 4.5g

Citri reticulatae Pericarpium (chén pí) 3-4.5g
Tea [picked before early May] (gǔ yǔ chá) 3g

Harmonizes and releases the lesser yang and promotes the smooth flow of qi in the chest and diaphragm. For alternating fever and chills, headache in the lateral aspect of the forehead, diminished hearing, vertigo, fullness and pain in the chest and hypochondria, a white tongue coating, a wiry, slippery pulse on the right, and a wiry, floating, and large pulse on the left.

柴胡四物湯 (柴胡四物汤)

Bupleurum and Four-Substance Decoction

chái hú sì wù tāng

Source Collection of Writings on the Mechanisms of Illness, Suitability of Qi, and the Safeguarding of Life as Discussed in Basic Questions (1186)

Bupleuri Radix (chái hú) 24g
Scutellariae Radix (huáng qín) 9g
Pinelliae Rhizoma praeparatum (zhì bàn xià) 9g
Glycyrrhizae Radix praeparata (zhì gān cǎo) 9g
Ginseng Radix (rén shēn) 9g
Paeoniae Radix alba (bái sháo) 45g
Rehmanniae Radix praeparata (shú dì huáng). 45g
Angelicae sinensis Radix (dāng guī) 45g
Chuanxiong Rhizoma (chuān xiōng) 45g

The source text advises to grind the herbs into powder and take as a draft in 9-12g doses. At present, it is prepared as a decoction with a proportionate reduction in dosage. For externally-contracted pathogenic influences that penetrate to the terminal yin warp, characterized by pain extending from the chest to the back and alternating fever and chills, with the symptoms often becoming worse at night. There may also be a pale tongue with dark-purple spots, and a wiry, thin pulse, which are signs of both blood deficiency and stasis. Also used for chronic consumptive disorders with alternating (slight) fever and chills, and colds contracted during menstruation.

柴平湯 (柴平汤)

Bupleurum and Calm the Stomach Decoction

chái píng tāng

Source Enumeration of Formulas Omitted from the Inner Classic (Song dynasty)

Bupleuri Radix (chái hú) 6g
Scutellariae Radix (huáng qín) 4.5g
Pinelliae Rhizoma praeparatum (zhì bàn xià) 3g
Glycyrrhizae Radix (gān cǎo) 1.5g
Ginseng Radix (rén shēn) 3g
Citri reticulatae Pericarpium (chén pí) 1.5g
Atractylodis Rhizoma (cāng zhú) 4.5g
Magnoliae officinalis Cortex (hòu pò) 3g

Harmonizes and releases the lesser yang, expels dampness, and harmonizes the Stomach. For malarial disorders due to dampness with alternating fever and chills (chills predominant), generalized body aches, a sensation of heaviness in the limbs, loss of appetite, and a soggy pulse.

柴胡清燥湯（柴胡清燥汤）

Bupleurum Decoction to Clear Dryness

chái hú qīng zào tāng

SOURCE *Discussion of Warm Epidemics* (1642)

Bupleuri Radix (*chái hú*). 6-12g
Scutellariae Radix (*huáng qín*). 4.5-9g
Glycyrrhizae Radix praeparata (*zhì gān cǎo*). 3-6g
Zingiberis Rhizoma recens (*shēng jiāng*). . . . . .2-4 slices
Jujubae Fructus (*dà zǎo*). 4-6 pieces
Citri reticulatae Pericarpium (*chén pí*). 6-9g
Trichosanthis Radix (*tiān huā fěn*). 9-12g
Anemarrhenae Rhizoma (*zhī mǔ*). 9-12g

The source text does not specify dosage. Harmonizes and releases the lesser yang, clears heat, and generates fluids. For heat entering the membrane source that has been improperly treated, causing incomplete clearing of heat and injury to the fluids.

加減小柴胡湯（加减小柴胡汤）

Modified Minor Bupleurum Decoction

jiā jiǎn xiǎo chái hú tāng

SOURCE *Six Texts on Cold Damage* (1445)

Turtle-blood Bupleuri Radix (*biē xuè bàn chái hú*)
wine-fried Scutellariae Radix (*jiǔ chǎo huáng qín*)
Rehmanniae Radix (*shēng dì huáng*)
Bubali Cornu (*shuǐ niú jiǎo*)
Moutan Cortex (*mǔ dān pí*)
Persicae Semen (*táo rén*)
Pinelliae Rhizoma praeparatum (*zhì bàn xià*)
Crataegi Fructus (*shān zhā*)
Glycyrrhizae Radix praeparata (*zhì gān cǎo*)
Zingiberis Rhizoma recens (*shēng jiāng*)

The source text does not specify dosage. Note that the original text calls for Rhinocerotis Cornu (*xī jiǎo*), which is no longer used, primarily due to the endangered species status of the rhinoceros. For heat entering the blood chamber causing clumping of blood, fever and chills with set periodicity, as in consumption. This formula was prescribed by Ye Tian-Shi for heat entering the blood chamber causing clumping of blood. He distinguished its use from that of the principal formula, where signs of qi deficiency should be present.

Note: Bupleuri Radix (*chái hú*) is treated with turtle blood to focus its effects deeper in the body and also to prevent it from depleting the yin.

蒿芩清膽湯（蒿芩清胆汤）

Sweet Wormwood and Scutellaria Decoction to Clear the Gallbladder

hāo qín qīng dǎn tāng

Source *Revised Popular Guide to the Discussion of Cold Damage* (Qing dynasty)

Artemisiae annuae Herba (*qīng hāo*). 4.5-6g
Scutellariae Radix (*huáng qín*). 4.5-9g
Bambusae Caulis in taeniam (*zhú rú*). 9g
Aurantii Fructus (*zhǐ ké*). 4.5g
Citri reticulatae Pericarpium (*chén pí*). 4.5g
Pinelliae Rhizoma praeparatum (*zhì bàn xià*). 4.5g
Poria rubra (*chì fú líng*). .9g
Jasper Powder (*bì yù sǎn*). 9g

Method of Preparation Decoction. The last ingredient is a powder composed of 6 parts Talcum (*huá shí*), 1 part Glycyrrhizae Radix (*gān cǎo*), and 1 part Indigo naturalis (*qīng dài*). It should be placed in a cheesecloth bag and cooked with the other ingredients. (This formula is discussed in Chapter 5.)

Actions Clears Gallbladder heat, harmonizes the Stomach qi, and transforms phlegm

Indications

Mild chills alternating with pronounced fever, a bitter taste in the mouth, a stifling sensation in the chest, spitting up bitter or sour fluids (or vomiting yellow, brackish fluids, or, in severe cases, dry heaves), thirst with or without a desire to drink, distention and pain in the chest and hypochondria, a red tongue with a thick, greasy coating that is usually white (but can be yellow or a combination of the two), and a pulse that is rapid while being slippery on the right and wiry on the left.

This is damp-heat and turbid phlegm in the lesser yang channels constraining the protective and nutritive qi. The alternating fever and chills (fever more intense) reflect the battle between the normal and pathogenic qi. The bitter taste in the mouth, stifling sensation in the chest, and distention and pain in the chest and abdomen are due to constraint in the lesser yang with inability of the clear yang to ascend. Gallbladder heat attacking the Stomach scorches the fluids and generates phlegm, leading to nausea and spitting up of sour or bitter fluids. Bile entering the Stomach causes vomiting of a yellow, brackish fluid or dry heaves. The presence of heat is also reflected in the red tongue body. The mixed tongue coating and pulse indicate Gallbladder and Stomach disharmony. Turbid phlegm in the Stomach causes a white, thick, greasy coating that turns white and yellow, and then just yellow as the heat becomes more severe. If the Stomach qi is strongly affected, the middle pulse on the right will be slippery, or the general character of the pulse will be soggy. A wiry pulse indicates Liver and Gallbladder disharmony.

Analysis of Formula

The chief ingredients, Artemisiae annuae Herba (*qīng hāo*) and Scutellariae Radix (*huáng qín*), drain damp-heat from the Liver and Gallbladder. Artemisiae annuae Herba (*qīng hāo*) also vents the exterior aspect of the lesser yang. The deputy, Bambusae Caulis in taeniam (*zhú rú*), drains heat from the Gallbladder and Stomach and stops the vomiting. The other deputies, Aurantii Fructus (*zhǐ ké*), Pinelliae Rhizoma praeparatum (*zhì bàn xià*), and Citri reticulatae Pericarpium *(chén pí)*, assist Bambusae Caulis in taeniam *(zhú rú)* in draining Gallbladder and Stomach heat, directing rebellious qi downward, harmonizing the Stomach, and transforming phlegm. The assistant ingredients, Poria rubra *(chì fú líng)*, Glycyrrhizae Radix *(gān cǎo)*, Talcum *(huá shí)*, and Indigo naturalis *(qīng dài)*, drain damp-heat through the urine to open constraint in the Triple Burner.

Cautions and Contraindications

This formula clears heat and transforms dampness. It is contraindicated in cases of phlegm-dampness due to yang deficiency.

Commentary

This is a combination of three formulas: Minor Bupleurum Decoction *(xiǎo chái hú tāng)*, which clears heat constraint from the lesser yang; Warm Gallbladder Decoction *(wēn dǎn tāng)*, which clears heat, expels phlegm, and regulates the Gallbladder and Stomach (see Chapter 17); and Jasper Powder *(bì yù sǎn)*, which clears heat, resolves toxicity, and expels dampness (see Chapter 5). Artemisiae annuae Herba *(qīng hāo)* is added to vent the exterior aspect.

The use of Artemisiae annuae Herba *(qīng hāo)* as the chief ingredient gives this formula a milder dispersing action than Minor Bupleurum Decoction *(xiǎo chái hú tāng)*, whose chief ingredient is Bupleuri Radix *(chái hú)*. Artemisiae annuae Herba *(qīng hāo)* is the colder of the two, while its aromatic nature makes it a specific herb for transforming damp-heat constraint in the lesser yang. The original formula uses only the tips of the fresh plant to focus its action on venting pathogenic heat to the exterior.

The author of this formula is the Qing-dynasty physician Yu Gen-Chu from Zhejiang province in southern China. Yu based his approach to the treatment of seasonal disorders on cold damage therapeutics, but integrated new approaches to the treatment of damp-warmth disorders that were then formulated in nearby Jiangsu. These focused particularly on the functions of the Triple Burner in order to eliminate pathogenic dampness from the body. This is reflected in the present formula, which contains Jasper Powder *(bì yù sǎn)*, an important formula in warm pathogen therapeutics.

In fact, it is its function of treating damp-heat or phlegm-heat in the Triple Burner that has allowed later generations of physicians to extend the indication of the formula beyond the narrow domain of seasonal disorders. Sweet Wormwood and Scutellaria Decoction to Clear the Gallbladder *(hāo qín qīng dǎn tāng)* can clear such pathogens from the course of the lesser yang channels when they cause symptoms like tinnitus, deafness, dizziness, jaundice, hemorrhoids, or urinary obstruction. It is equally effective in treating systemic manifestations of damp-heat such as night sweats, palpitations, or sleep dysfunctions.

Comparison

➢ Vs. Minor Bupleurum Decoction *(xiǎo chái hú tāng)*

Both formulas treat lesser yang patterns characterized by alternating chills and fever, discomfort in the hypochondria, nausea, and a bitter taste in the mouth. In Minor Bupleurum Decoction *(xiǎo chái hú tāng)* presentations, these symptoms arise from invasion of a wind-cold pathogen that primarily constrains the ascending of clear yang. In Sweet Wormwood and Scutellaria Decoction to Clear the Gallbladder *(hāo qín qīng dǎn tāng)* presentations, the constraint is due to a damp-warm pathogen that primarily constrains the downward-directing of turbid yin. This implies that in the former pattern, the chills will be relatively more pronounced, the pulse wiry, and the tongue normal with a dirty or greasy white coating. In the latter pattern, the chills are relatively mild. The pulse will be wiry in the left middle position only; on the right, it will be slippery and rapid. The tongue coating is also greasy and white, but the body will often be red.

Because the primary obstruction in both cases is in the lesser yang, both formulas treat dry retching as well as vomiting. However, cold damages the transportive and transformative functions of the middle burner, causing phlegm fluids to accumulate in the Stomach and epigastric area even as the throat becomes dry and urination is inhibited. Patients with a Minor Bupleurum Decoction *(xiǎo chái hú tāng)* presentation will thus vomit acidic fluids or expectorate white or clear sputum. Dampness, on the other hand, obstructs the flow of nutritive qi while heat injures the fluids. This generates thick, sticky phlegm in the Stomach. Patients with a Sweet Wormwood and Scutellaria Decoction to Clear the Gallbladder *(hāo qín qīng dǎn tāng)* presentation thus vomit sour bile and expectorate sticky, viscous, and yellowish phlegm.

Other Comparisons

This formula contains strong herbs for regulating the flow, transforming turbid dampness, and clearing heat. In these respects, it is similar to Bupleurum, Bitter Orange, and Platycodon Decoction *(chái hú zhǐ jié tāng)*, discussed above, but that formula is best for venting the half-exterior aspect of the lesser yang. It resembles Sweet Dew Special Pill to Eliminate Toxin *(gān lù xiāo dú dān)*, discussed in Chapter 16, in its treatment of damp-heat leading to qi-related disorders, but it focuses more on venting the pathogenic influence.

Biomedical Indications

With the appropriate presentation, this formula may be used to treat a wide variety of biomedically-defined disorders. Most commonly, this includes acute infections such as cholecystitis, icteric hepatitis, pyelonephritis, malaria, typhoid, pelvic inflammatory disease, pneumonia, and leptospirosis as well as reflux gastritis, aural vertigo, hypertension, and coronary artery disease.

Modifications

- For a thick, greasy tongue coating and fullness in the chest and diaphragm, add Magnoliae officinalis Cortex *(hòu pò)* and Pogostemonis/Agastaches Herba *(huò xiāng)*.

- For a strong fever, a soft and rapid pulse, and a yellow tongue coating, add Lonicerae Flos *(jīn yín huā)*, Forsythiae Fructus *(lián qiáo)*, and Isatidis Folium *(dà qīng yè)*.

- For severe vomiting, add Haematitum *(dài zhě shí)*.

- For acute jaundice with severe dampness, add Artemisiae scopariae Herba *(yīn chén)*, Gardeniae Fructus *(zhī zǐ)*, Curcumae Radix *(yù jīn)*, and Rhei Radix et Rhizoma *(dà huáng)*.

- For heat-predominant conditions with little dampness, remove Pinelliae Rhizoma praeparatum *(zhì bàn xià)*.

- For night sweats due to damp-heat in the Liver and Gallbladder, add Mori Folium *(sāng yè)*, Moutan Cortex *(mǔ dān pí)*, and Ostreae Concha *(mǔ lì)*.

- For tinnitus and diminished hearing due to damp-heat obstructing the lesser yang channel, add Acori tatarinowii Rhizoma *(shí chāng pǔ)*, Chrysanthemi Flos *(jú huā)*, Uncariae Ramulus cum Uncis *(gōu téng)*, and Alismatis Rhizoma *(zé xiè)*.

- For palpitations with anxiety and insomnia due to phlegm-heat, add Succinum *(hǔ pò)*, Coptidis Rhizoma *(huáng lián)*, and Alismatis Rhizoma *(zé xiè)*.

- For phlegm-heat in the Lungs, add Houttuyniae Herba *(yú xīng cǎo)*, Phragmitis Rhizoma *(lú gēn)*, and Benincasae Semen *(dōng guā zǐ)*.

柴胡加龍骨牡蠣湯 (柴胡加龙骨牡蛎汤)

Bupleurum plus Dragon Bone and Oyster Shell Decoction

chái hú jiā lóng gǔ mǔ lì tāng

Source   *Discussion of Cold Damage* (c. 220)

Bupleuri Radix *(chái hú)* 12g
Scutellariae Radix *(huáng qín)* 3g
Pinelliae Rhizoma praeparatum *(zhì bàn xià)* 6-9g
Ginseng Radix *(rén shēn)* 4.5g
Zingiberis Rhizoma recens *(shēng jiāng)* 4.5g
Cinnamomi Ramulus *(guì zhī)* 4.5g
Poria *(fú líng)* 4.5g
Fossilia Ossis Mastodi *(lóng gǔ)* 4.5g
Ostreae Concha *(mǔ lì)* 4.5g
Rhei Radix et Rhizoma *(dà huáng)* . . . . . (add just before end) 6g
Jujubae Fructus *(dà zǎo)* . . . . 6 pieces
Minium *(qiān dān)* 4.5g

Method of Preparation   Decoction. Take while still warm. In modern formulations, Haematitum *(dài zhě shí)* or Ferri Frusta *(shēng tiě luò)* is usually substituted for the toxic Minium

(qiān dān) and its dosage is often reduced to 1g. At present, Codonopsis Radix *(dǎng shēn)* or Pseudostellariae Radix *(tài zǐ shēn)* is usually substituted for Ginseng Radix *(rén shēn)* at 2-3 times its dosage.

Actions   Unblocks the three yang warps, and sedates and calms the spirit

Indications

Fullness in the chest, irritability with occasional attacks of fright palpitations, urinary difficulty, constipation, delirious speech, inability to rotate the trunk, a sensation of extreme heaviness throughout the body, a red tongue with a slippery coating, and a wiry, rapid pulse.

This condition is due to problems in all three of the yang channels. In the source text, this is attributed to the premature application of purgatives, which were used before the disease entered the yang brightness warp. The externally-contracted pathogenic influence takes advantage of the weakness caused by the purgatives and invades the interior, where it obstructs the qi dynamic to cause a complicated pattern characterized by excess as well as deficiency with symptoms in all three burners and in all yang organs. Difficulty in rotating the trunk and the wiry pulse indicate that constraint in the lesser yang channel is the fulcrum around which this pattern turns. This suggests that the original pattern was, in fact, a lesser yang pattern that was mistaken for a yang brightness pattern because it had persisted for a long period of time, or that the lesser yang is the pathway by which the pathogen is entering the interior. Fullness in the chest and irritability with occasional attacks of fright palpitations are due to the constraint of yang qi in the lesser yang flaring upward to attack the Heart. The red tongue and rapid pulse also reflect the presence of this heat. Clumping of heat and stools in the Intestines causes constipation, while heat in the yang brightness warp leads to the characteristic symptom of delirious speech. At the level of the Triple Burner and Bladder, which regulate the movement and transformation of fluids, constraint is reflected in urinary difficulty. Meanwhile, the improper treatment that gave rise to this disorder leaves a remnant of the pathogenic influence in the channels, a relatively superficial level of the body. At the same time, the yang qi is confined to the interior and cannot spread to the exterior. This causes a feeling of extreme heaviness throughout the body.

Analysis of Formula

Although this is a complicated pattern, the main problem is one of constraint. This is treated by unblocking the qi dynamic in order to disperse and drain pathogenic qi, while simultaneously supporting the middle burner as the fulcrum of this dynamic. The chief ingredients are those that address constraint in the three yang channels and their respective yang organs. Cinnamomi Ramulus *(guì zhī)* is a greater yang herb that is used here primarily to resolve the problems in the superficial levels and to promote the flow of yang qi in order to relieve the sensation of heaviness in the body. Bupleuri Radix *(chái hú)* and Scutellariae Radix *(huáng qín)* resolve lesser yang disorders, and release constraint at this level. The delirious speech and yang brightness-warp symptoms are addressed by Rhei Radix et Rhizoma *(dà huáng)*, which flushes clumping of heat and stools from the Intestines.

Among the assistant ingredients, Fossilia Ossis Mastodi *(lóng gǔ)*, Ostreae Concha *(mǔ lì)*, and Minium *(qiān dān)* are mineral substances that weigh down and calm the floating spirit. Ginseng Radix *(rén shēn)* and Poria *(fú líng)* strengthen the qi of the middle burner, and ensure that it is not further damaged by the treatment. Together, they also have a mild calming effect. The latter herb increases and promotes urination. Pinelliae Rhizoma praeparatum *(zhì bàn xià)* causes the qi to descend and works with Poria *(fú líng)* to transform disturbances of the fluids and to open up the diaphragm. It also assists Bupleuri Radix *(chái hú)* and Scutellariae Radix *(huáng qín)* in resolving the lesser yang-warp aspects of this disorder. The envoys, Zingiberis Rhizoma recens *(shēng jiāng)* and Jujubae Fructus *(dà zǎo)*, work together to regulate the relationship between the protective qi in the exterior and the nutritive qi in the interior. This helps focus the actions of the other ingredients on these critical aspects of the body.

Contraindications

Although this formula contains a small number of tonifying herbs, its focus is clearly on treating excess. It must not be used for conditions of deficiency. If prescribed inappropriately, symptoms such as anxiety, insomnia, irritability, or hypertension for which the formula may have been chosen will invariably get worse. In these cases, it is important to switch to a different formula immediately.

Commentary

This is a complex formula designed to treat a complex pattern. It incorporates hot and cold substances, purgatives and tonics, and has wide application. It is not surprising, therefore, that many different interpretations of the pattern and the formula itself have been expressed through the years. A commonly-held view of the mechanism of this disorder is that it began as a lesser yang-warp condition that was improperly purged, and that lesser yang (Liver and Gallbladder) dysfunction is at the core of the disorder. Some go so far as to characterize it as an interior lesser yang-warp disorder. This understanding is based partly on the fact that this formula is a variation of Minor Bupleurum Decoction *(xiǎo chái hú tāng)*, the quintessential formula for lesser yang-warp disorders, and partly on the presentation itself.

Yet the very complexity of the formula has made it problematic for generations of commentators. Some writers, such as the 17th-century physician Wang Hu, had such a hard time dealing with the complex nature of the formula and its combination of seemingly mutually contradictory medicinals, that they dared not use it. Others, like the 20th-century physician Lu Yuan-Lei, recognized the issues but learned to believe in its efficacy:

> Although this formula is a mixture [of different types of medicinals] and there are those who are inclined to suspect that it should not be used, if one institutes treatment based on the presentation [for which it is traditionally indicated], there are many for whom it is effective. As for the ingenuity with which the classic formulas are put together, honestly, today's knowledge is unable to completely understand it.

A practical understanding of these issues can be gained by attending carefully to the original indications as well as to the formula's composition. The source text attributes the pattern to the inappropriate use of purgatives in the treatment of a patient who has suffered from a cold damage disorder for 8 or 9 days. This implies that a basically deficient patient (whether due to inappropriate purgation or preexisting constitutional factors) presents with strong excess-type symptoms. This is reflected in the use of warm, tonifying herbs such as Ginseng Radix *(rén shēn)*, Cinnamomi Ramulus *(guì zhī)*, Poria *(fú líng)*, Jujubae Fructus *(dà zǎo)*, and Zingiberis Rhizoma recens *(shēng jiāng)*, which are combined with powerful draining and heat-clearing substances. The cardinal symptoms are those of a lesser yang-warp disorder, because the lesser yang is frequently understood to be the pivot at which disorders change from a yang to a yin pattern and vice versa. These include fullness in the chest accompanied by irritability, fright palpitations, or emotional instability and changing moods.

The definition of fright palpitations as a disorder caused by reaction to something in the environment (an unexpected sound, a frightening experience, etc.) may be read as an overreaction to stimulation that reflects the pathology outlined above, that is, a more fundamental deficiency that is conjoined to a strong excess-type manifestation. This can manifest in many different ways but is typical of all the conditions outlined above: hot flushes, irritability, vivid dreams, dizziness, etc. The advantage of this formula can be found in its ability to regulate (control) the excessive reaction, even as it tonifies the normal qi. Moreover, not only does it clear heat and settle the emotions, it also promotes fluid metabolism. This is important because fluid retention is a typical aspect of many depressive conditions or those where elation alternates with depression. Nie Hui-Min, a contemporary specialist in classical formulas, finds this formula particularly useful for depression because it addresses a very common yet intricate pathological dynamic in this disease by its complex set of functions: dredging the Liver, resolving constraint, harmonizing the lesser yang pivot, unblocking and opening up the three burners, draining heat to calm the spirit, and calming to regulate the spirit.

Over the centuries, the scope of this formula has been greatly expanded because of a realization that it can be effectively used in treating any disorder due to fright or to phlegm in the Liver-Gallbladder system. At present, it is used for a wide variety of internally-generated disorders that do not result from an acute, externally-contracted disease. In contemporary China, it is widely used in the treatment of epilepsy. The famous contemporary physician Zhao Xi-Wu recommends it for treating attacks of irregular heartbeat that occur at rest, reserving Prepared Licorice Decoction (*zhì gān cǎo tāng*) for the treatment of attacks brought on by activity. In both China and Japan, it is widely used to treat psychosomatic disorders in patients with a strong constitution, often instead of, or in combination with, biomedical tranquilizers. According to Wang Qi in *Explanation of the Discussion of Cold Damage,* "both within China and abroad, [this formula] is widely used to treat epilepsy, hypertension, hyperthyroidism, dizziness, alopecia, insomnia, and Meniere's disease."

When the severe aspects of this condition have been resolved, it is best to continue treatment with formulas such as Licorice, Wheat, and Jujube Decoction (*gān mài dà zǎo tāng*).

Comparisons

➤ Vs. Other Bupleurum-Based Formulas

This formula is similar to other harmonizing formulas that utilize Bupleuri Radix (*chái hú*) as the chief ingredient, where distention of the chest and flanks and a bitter taste constitute key points in the diagnosis. Like these formulas, it can be used to treat disorders characterized by lesser yang-type symptoms such as headache, tinnitus, or constraint, and for conditions characterized by loss of normal cognitive functions involving speech, memory, concentration, or sensation. However, compared to formulas such as Minor and Major Bupleurum Decoction (*xiǎo dà chái hú tāng*), Bupleurum and Cinnamon Twig Decoction (*chái hú guì zhī tāng*), or Bupleurum, Cinnamon Twig, and Ginger Decoction (*chái hú guì jiāng tāng*), these symptoms will typically be much more pronounced where this formula is indicated.

➤ Vs. Cinnamon Twig Decoction plus Dragon Bone and Oyster Shell (*guì zhī jiā lóng gǔ mǔ lì tāng*)

Both formulas treat disorders characterized by such key symptoms as insomnia, fright palpitations, and heightened sensitivity to external stimuli. However, Cinnamon Twig Decoction plus Dragon Bone and Oyster Shell (*guì zhī jiā lóng gǔ mǔ lì tāng*), discussed in Chapter 9, is indicated for patterns characterized by deficiency cold and loss of essence characterized by such symptoms as excessive sweating, palpitations, and tension in the lower abdomen. This formula, by

contrast, treats patterns characterized by excess heat and fluid retention with such symptoms such as restlessness, irritability, and impaired consciousness.

Biomedical Indications

With the appropriate presentation, this formula may be used to treat a wide variety of biomedically-defined disorders. Most commonly, this would include neuropsychiatric problems such as neurosis, depression, general anxiety disorder, schizophrenia, Parkinson's disease, and epilepsy. It has also been used for hypertension, first or second degree A-V block, supraventricular tachycardia, hyperthyroidism, Ménière's disease, spasm of the sternocleidomastoid muscle, gastritis, menopausal syndrome, erectile dysfunction, and postconcussion syndrome.

Alternate name

Bupleurum, Dragon Bone, and Oyster Shell Decoction (*chái hú lóng gǔ mǔ lì tāng*) in *General Discussion of the Disease of Cold Damage*

Modifications

- For nightmares, vertigo, fever, and other symptoms of vigorous Liver fire, add Gentianae Radix (*lóng dǎn cǎo*) and Prunellae Spica (*xià kū cǎo*).
- For cases with regular bowel movements, remove Rhei Radix et Rhizoma (*dà huáng*).
- For more pronounced phlegm symptoms, add Acori tatarinowii Rhizoma (*shí chāng pǔ*) and Polygalae Radix (*yuǎn zhì*).
- For constipation and manic behavior, remove Ginseng Radix (*rén shēn*) and increase the dosage of Rhei Radix et Rhizoma (*dà huáng*).
- For severe irritability and difficult sleep, add Succinum (*hǔ pò*), Ziziphi spinosae Semen (*suān zǎo rén*), and Polygoni multiflori Caulis (*yè jiāo téng*).
- For periodic spasms of the hands and feet with lightheadedness, dry mouth, dry stools, a greasy and yellow tongue coating, and a submerged and forceless pulse, substitute Pseudostellariae Radix (*tài zǐ shēn*) for Ginseng Radix (*rén shēn*) and add a large dose of Salviae miltiorrhizae Radix (*dān shēn*).
- For seizures, increase the dosage of Bupleuri Radix (*chái hú*) and add a large dose of Salviae miltiorrhizae Radix (*dān shēn*).
- For vertigo and headache after trauma to the head (postconcussion syndrome), replace Rhei Radix et Rhizoma (*dà huáng*) with wine-treated Rhei Radix et Rhizoma (*jiǔ zhì dà huáng*) and add Ligustici Rhizoma (*gǎo běn*) and Chrysanthemi Flos (*jú huā*).

- For stabbing pains in the chest, dark stools, and a dark purple tongue indicating qi and blood stasis, add Carthami Flos (hóng huā), Persicae Semen (táo rén), Paeoniae Radix rubra (chì sháo), Cyperi Rhizoma (xiāng fù), and Citri reticulatae viride Pericarpium (qīng pí).

- For bouts of severe anger, a red complexion, and red eyes indicating Liver fire, remove Cinnamomi Ramulus (guì zhī), Ginseng Radix (rén shēn), Zingiberis Rhizoma recens (shēng jiāng), and Jujubae Fructus (dà zǎo), and add Gentianae Radix (lóng dǎn cǎo), Gardeniae Fructus (zhī zǐ), Plantaginis Semen (chē qián zǐ), Alismatis Rhizoma (zé xiè), Akebiae Caulis (mù tōng), and Rehmanniae Radix (shēng dì huáng).

- For seizures or epilepsy characterized by phlegm with dizziness, disorientation, constipation, and a thick, greasy tongue coating, remove Cinnamomi Ramulus (guì zhī), Ginseng Radix (rén shēn), and Zingiberis Rhizoma recens (shēng jiāng), and add Chloriti Lapis/Micae Lapis aureus (méng shí), Aquilariae Lignum resinatum (chén xiāng), Ferri Frusta (shēng tiě luò), and Acori tatarinowii Rhizoma (shí chāng pú).

Section 2

FORMULAS THAT REGULATE AND HARMONIZE THE LIVER AND SPLEEN

The formulas in this section are used when there is an imbalance between the functions of the Liver and Spleen, which may result from either of two processes. When the Liver qi (which is normally spread smoothly throughout the body) is constrained, it can move transversely and violate the Spleen and Stomach. Conversely, when the Spleen qi is deficient, its transportive function is diminished, which in turn constrains the spreading of Liver qi. The most common symptoms of this disharmony are a stifling sensation in the chest, hypochondriac pain, epigastric and abdominal distention and pain, reduced appetite, diarrhea, and in severe cases, alternating chills and fever.

The qi-moving aspect of these formulas is generally not as strong as that of the formulas found in Chapter 12, but they also address the blood deficiency aspect of Liver disharmony. It is important to remember that these formulas are not intended primarily for conditions of deficiency; if they are used under those circumstances, the patient will become fatigued.

The crucial pairings in these formulas are herbs that dredge the Liver and regulate qi, such as Bupleuri Radix (chái hú), Aurantii Fructus (zhǐ ké), and Citri reticulatae Pericar-

pium (chén pí), with those that strengthen the Spleen, such as Atractylodis macrocephalae Rhizoma (bái zhú) and Poria (fú líng).

四逆散
Frigid Extremities Powder
sì nì sǎn

This formula is used in treating frigid extremities due to yang qi constrained in the interior, hence the name.

Source   *Discussion of Cold Damage* (c. 220)

Bupleuri Radix *(chái hú)* 9-12g
dry-fried Aurantii Fructus immaturus *(chǎo zhǐ shí)* 9-12g
Paeoniae Radix alba *(bái sháo)* 12-24g
Glycyrrhizae Radix praeparata *(zhì gān cǎo)* 6-9g

Method of Preparation   The source text advises to grind equal amounts of the herbs into powder and take in 6-9g doses three times a day. At present, it is usually taken as a decoction with the dosage indicated above.

Actions   Vents pathogenic qi, releases constraint, spreads the Liver qi, and regulates the Spleen

Indications

Cold fingers and toes while the body and head are warm. This may be accompanied by a sensation of irritability and fullness in the chest and epigastrium, cough, urinary difficulty, abdominal pain and severe diarrhea, a red tongue with a yellow coating, and a wiry pulse.

This is yang- or hot-type inversion (陽厥 *yáng jué*) due to internal constraint of yang qi that thereby fails to reach the extremities, causing cold fingers and toes (in contrast to devastated yang, where the entire limb is cold) and a warm body. The tongue signs reflect the presence of heat in the interior. The wiry pulse and sensation of irritability and fullness in the chest and abdomen reflect interior constraint. This type of 'frigid extremities' must be distinguished from similar presentations caused by excess heat or cold, as discussed in the COMMENTARY below.

Later generations of physicians expanded the use of this formula to the treatment of Liver-Spleen disharmony, characterized by hypochondriac pain and distention (sometimes with epigastric or abdominal pain and fullness) and a wiry, forceful pulse. This may be accompanied by a multitude of other digestive signs and symptoms including vomiting, constipation, diarrhea, lack of appetite, and a bitter taste in the mouth.

Analysis of Formula

Because the condition for which this formula is indicated is due to constraint and stagnation of the qi mechanism, its primary focus is to regulate the qi by venting heat and releasing constraint. Bupleuri Radix *(chái hú)* performs both of these functions well and is therefore the chief herb. Through its action on the lesser yang, it facilitates both the ascent of clear yang and the descent of turbid yin, as explained in *Explanation of the Classic of Materia Medica*: "Bupleuri Radix *(chái hú)* is clear and light, ascending and spreading out the Gallbladder qi. When the Gallbladder qi thrusts outward, the other twelve organs follow its dissipating transformation. Thus it is able to disperse any [kind of] clumped qi in the epigastrium, abdomen, Stomach, and Intestines."

The deputy is Aurantii Fructus immaturus *(zhǐ shí)*, which drains stagnation, breaks up stagnant qi, and reduces accumulation in the middle burner to facilitate the transportive and transformative functions of the Spleen and Stomach. Its bitterness directs downward to complement the chief herb's focus on dredging the lesser yang. This results in a stronger qi-regulating function and thereby the smooth dispersion of heat due to constraint.

The assistant is Paeoniae Radix alba *(bái sháo)*, which nourishes the Liver and preserves the yin. This herb holds things in; this is in contrast to the chief herb, which disperses. This combination is very effective in disseminating the Liver qi without injuring the Liver yin. The combination of the assistant with the envoy, Glycyrrhizae Radix praeparata *(zhì gān cǎo)*, moderates acute or colicky pain. The envoy also harmonizes the various actions of the other herbs in the formula and strengthens the Spleen to curb the Liver.

The entire formula is a primary exemplar of combining a small number of herbs in a way that leads to multilayered synergisms that can achieve profound effects: dispersing while also being astringing, dispersing yet nourishing, facilitating both ascent and descent, moving yang while moderating yin, dredging wood while assisting earth, and treating both the qi and blood. Frigid Extremities Powder *(sì nì sǎn)* vents pathogenic heat without injuring the normal qi so that moderate warmth can extend to all four extremities.

Cautions and Contraindications

This formula treats pain and distention in the hypochondria, epigastrium, and abdomen by unblocking the qi dynamic. It should not be used for yin deficiency with Liver constraint, which can present with similar symptoms.

Commentary

In the source text, the use of this formula is confined to the treatment of frigid extremities due to lesser yin-warp disharmony with a wide range of secondary signs and symptoms (see MODIFICATIONS below). This presentation often occurs in children.

This type of frigid extremities must be distinguished from both yin- or cold-type inversion and from severe heat inversion (熱深厥 *rè shēn jué*). Yin- or cold-type inversion

is characterized by exuberant yin preventing the diffusion of weak yang to the exterior. In this pattern, the entire area distal to the elbow and knee, or even the entire limb, may be cold. There will usually be other symptoms like generalized aversion to cold, desire to lie down, fatigue, abdominal pain, vomiting, diarrhea, a white tongue coating, and a weak pulse. This pattern is typically treated by Frigid Extremities Decoction *(sì nì tāng)*, discussed in Chapter 6. Severe heat inversion with frigid extremities, on the other hand, is due to exuberant heat in the interior constraining the diffusion of yang qi to the exterior. Here, ice-cold hands and feet (false cold) will be accompanied by symptoms of true heat like thirst, fever, burning heat in the Stomach and abdomen, irritability, restlessness, reduced dark urine, and constipation. Such patterns are typically treated with formulas such as White Tiger Decoction *(bái hǔ tāng)*, discussed in Chapter 4, or one of the Order the Qi Decoctions *(chéng qì tāng)*, discussed in Chapter 2.

Cold extremities due to yang-type inversion, for which this formula is indicated, can be differentiated from those patterns by the sensation of cold occurring only at the very tips of the extremities. This presentation was clearly described by the Ming-dynasty physician Li Zhong-Zi:

> While it is said that this pattern is called 'frigid extremities,' the extremities will not be extremely cold, the fingertips [may even be] slightly warm [to the touch], and the pulse is not submerged and faint. This is a pattern where the yin contains the yang and 'frigid extremities' results from the qi being unable to disseminate and flow freely.

In order to distinguish it more clearly from severe heat inversion, some texts refer to this as qi inversion (氣厥 *qì jué*) rather than yang-type inversion.

Several other patterns characterized by cold extremities are listed in *Discussion of Cold Damage*. Tangkuei Decoction for Frigid Extremities *(dāng guī sì nì tāng)* and its variations (see Chapter 6) treat conditions characterized by blood deficiency in which the patient feels cold (chills) and the entire hands and feet (not just the tips) are cold. Cinnamon Twig and Aconite Accessory Root Decoction *(guì zhī fù zǐ tāng)*, described in Chapter 1, treats dispersion of yang characterized by cold extremities and sweating that cannot be controlled, while Evodia Decoction *(wú zhū yú tāng)* and its variations (see Chapter 6) treat yin excess trapping yang, where cold extremities are accompanied by signs of phlegm or thin mucus in the Liver channel. Many other conditions not discussed in *Discussion of Cold Damage*, including qi stagnation and qi deficiency patterns, may also present with cold extremities. Great care should accordingly be taken to analyze the precise disease dynamic before formulating a treatment strategy.

It is also important to differentiate the use of the term 厥 *jué* as used in this context from that of other possible readings. As used in the *Inner Classic*, the term originally referred to a variety of conditions with sudden or temporary loss of consciousness that we render as 'collapse.' This was subsequently expanded to include certain conditions with symptoms of cold hands and feet that we render as 'inversion.' Similarly, the term 'frigid extremities' (四逆 *sì nì*, short for 四肢逆冷 *sì zhī nì lěng*), which literally means 'four rebellions,' narrowly means ice-cold limbs. In a wider sense, it encompasses different types of cold extremities, including the type for which this formula is indicated.

Discussion of Cold Damage lists Frigid Extremities Powder *(sì nì sǎn)* and its presentation in the chapter on lesser yin-warp disorders. This chapter also discusses the Frigid Extremities Decoction *(sì nì tāng)* presentation (see Chapter 6). It is in this context that the former is referred to as yang- or hot-type inversion and the latter as yin- or cold-type inversion. Because the precise relationship of Frigid Extremities Powder *(sì nì sǎn)* to the lesser yin warp is not easily deduced from the formula's composition, the exact nature of the pathology for which it is indicated became a topic of fierce debate among later commentators on *Discussion of Cold Damage*. Some writers, such as Shen Ming-Zong and Zhang Lu, note that the source text does not specify whether the condition is due to heat or cold. In addition, most of the modified formulas listed in the source text contain warming herbs, which would be inappropriate for a condition whose underlying pathology was associated with heat. Hence, they argue that the pathodynamic involved here must encompass the Spleen's control of the limbs, as suggested in a passage from Chapter 5 of *Basic Questions*: "The clear yang firms up the four limbs." They conclude that this condition arises in a person with a deficient Spleen who contracts a pathogenic influence that enters the lesser yin. This constrains the yang qi and prevents it from reaching the extremities. The constrained yang qi then generates heat. However, since there are no strong heat symptoms, the most appropriate strategy is to focus on regulating and harmonizing the movement of qi.

Among other commentators, the Qing-dynasty writer You Yi interprets the formula to be intended for eliminating pathogens from the half-exterior, half-interior by way of simultaneous venting and draining. The modern physician Lu Yuan-Lei likewise thinks of it as a lesser yang-warp formula. Lu's contemporary, Cheng Men-Xue, argues that the formula should have been listed for treating terminal yin-warp disorders because of its ability to regulate the Liver qi. The 18th-century editors of *Golden Mirror of the Medical Tradition* define it as acting on both the lesser yang and terminal yin. A later Qing-dynasty physician, Tang Zong-Hai, thinks that the formula achieves its effects by harmonizing the function of the pores and interstices.

Contemporary physicians, like the modern formula expert Chen Chao-Zu in his influential *Treatment Strategies and Formulas in Chinese Medicine*, attempt to resolve the tension between these many competing views by anchoring the presentation treated by Frigid Extremities Powder *(sì nì sǎn)* in biomedical pathophysiology. Chen defines the action of the formula as relaxing spasms of the smooth muscles. The Liver's relationship to the muscles explains the composition of the formula. The wide distribution of smooth muscle in the body explains its ability to treat problems in all organ systems of the body.

Traditional concepts offer at least as valid a resolution of these differences. In classical texts such as the *Inner Classic*, the lesser yang can include the Liver as well as Gallbladder and Triple Burner. From this perspective, the formula can be understood as breaking up obstructions of the qi dynamic comprising such varied manifestations as accumulation, focal distention, pain, phlegm, and harbored food that hinder the dispersion of ministerial fire from the interior to the exterior via this extended lesser yang system. In the exterior, this leads to a lack of warmth, while internally, it can cause the build-up of heat from constraint while depriving the muscles and sinews of physiologic fluids. Accordingly, one does not warm but vents the heat by means of Bupleuri Radix *(chái hú)* and breaks up stagnation with Aurantii Fructus immaturus *(zhǐ shí)*. In addition, the fluids must be nourished in order to moderate pain, which is achieved by softening the Liver with Paeoniae Radix alba *(bái sháo)* and Glycyrrhizae Radix *(gān cǎo)*.

Frigid Extremities Powder *(sì nì sǎn)* is thus useful in treating a disease dynamic that combines signs of excessive tension with both heat/dryness and cold/dampness. Examples include smelly, pain-free diarrhea; constipation with hard, pellet-like stools alternating with diarrhea; one-sided sinusitis or rhinitis with yellow mucus due to heat in the Gallbladder; and all kinds of inflammatory disorders in the abdomen (inflammation implying heat) that are also accompanied by pain and obstruction such as pancreatitis, gastritis, colitis, obstructed ovarian ducts, or calculi in both the biliary or urinary systems. Erectile dysfunction in men is another well-documented indication in modern clinical practice that is easily explained by the failure of ministerial fire to penetrate to the penis. Frigid Extremities Powder *(sì nì sǎn)* is also frequently used in the treatment of emotional distress marked by tension that is directed inward. It can also be used as an adjunct in the treatment of melancholia, sadness, or depression in the course of chronic illness resulting from internal constraint of ministerial fire.

Given the important role of Aurantii Fructus immaturus *(zhǐ shí)* in this formula, it is important to note that commentators disagree as to the precise identity of this herb. In the 11th century, Shen Kuo pointed out in *Dream Creek Essays* that the differentiation between the two herbs Aurantii Fructus immaturus *(zhǐ shí)* and Aurantii Fructus *(zhǐ ké)* was only introduced in the 5th century, three centuries after the writing of *Discussion of Cold Damage*. Previously, both herbs were known as Aurantii Fructus immaturus (*zhǐ shí*). Which of the two should be used in a modern prescription thus depends on the precise action one wishes to achieve. If one intends to focus on promoting the flow of qi in the exterior, Aurantii Fructus (*zhǐ ké*) with its action centered on the Lungs and Stomach may be more appropriate. If, on the other hand, one wishes to break up stagnant qi in the interior, Aurantii Fructus immaturus (*zhǐ shí*) with its downward-directing action focused on the lower body is the better choice.

Comparisons

➤ Vs. Minor Bupleurum Decoction (*xiǎo chái hú tāng*)

Both formulas dredge the lesser yang and vent pathogens to the exterior. They differ with respect to the kind of constraint they resolve. Minor Bupleurum Decoction (*xiǎo chái hú tāng*) focuses on venting a cold pathogen that obstructs the lesser yang. Hence, alternating fever and chills are a primary symptom, and the dosage of Bupleuri Radix (*chái hú*) is four times as large. Frigid Extremities Powder (*sì nì sǎn*) focuses on breaking up qi and fluid stagnation that prevents ministerial fire in the interior from diffusing outward. Hence, the main symptom is cold fingers and toes and the dosage of Bupleuri Radix (*chái hú*) is reduced accordingly.

The modern physician Cheng Men-Xue lists three additional symptoms as characteristic of Frigid Extremities Powder (*sì nì sǎn*) presentations:

1. A pulse that is submerged, thin, and tight indicating the constraint of yang qi in the interior. In a Minor Bupleurum Decoction (*xiǎo chái hú tāng*) presentation, the pulse is typically wiry.

2. Constipation with hard stools or severe diarrhea, reflecting stagnation of qi and fluids in the Intestines due to yang transformation failure. In a Minor Bupleurum Decoction (*xiǎo chái hú tāng*) presentation, these symptoms are absent.

3. Absence of sweating or sweating only from the head, also reflecting stagnation of fluids in the interior. In a Minor Bupleurum Decoction (*xiǎo chái hú tāng*) presentation, sweating may come and go in conjunction with the alternating fever and chills that characterize the presentation.

➤ Vs. Bupleurum Powder to Dredge the Liver (*chái hú shū gān sǎn*); *see* PAGE 513

➤ Vs. Linking Decoction (*yī guàn jiān*); *see* PAGE 382

➤ Vs. Rambling Powder (*xiāo yáo sǎn*); *see* PAGE 123

➤ Vs. Tangkuei and Peony Powder (*dāng guī sháo yào sǎn*); *see* PAGE 589.

➤ Vs. Tangkuei Decoction for Frigid Extremities (*dāng guī sì nì tāng*); *see* PAGE 254

Biomedical Indications

With the appropriate presentation, this formula may be used to treat a wide variety of biomedically-defined disorders. These can be divided into the following groups:

- Those marked by spasmodic abdominal pain such as cholecystitis, cholelithiasis, gastritis, gastric ptosis, peptic ulcers, allergic colitis, appendicitis, adhesive intestinal obstruction, pancreatitis, urinary tract stones, and dysmenorrhea

- Those that can be seen as related to emotional stress such as premenstrual syndrome, impotence, coronary artery disease, stress incontinence, enuresis, and perimenopausal syndrome

- Those marked by unsmooth excretions or secretions such as rhinitis, acute mastitis, blocked fallopian tubes, or encapsualted periappendical abscesses.

This formula has also been used in the treatment of intercostal neuralgia, neurogenic headache, trigeminal neuralgia, epilepsy, autonomic dystonia, hepatitis, allergic rhinitis, and epidemic hemorrhagic fever.

Modifications

- For cough, add Schisandrae Fructus (*wǔ wèi zǐ*) and Zingiberis Rhizoma (*gān jiāng*). (source text)

- For palpitations, add Cinnamomi Ramulus (*guì zhī*). (source text)

- For urinary difficulty, add Poria (*fú líng*). (source text)

- For abdominal pain, add Aconiti Radix lateralis praeparata (*zhì fù zǐ*). (source text)

- For epigastric pain with acid reflux, add Left Metal Pill (*zuo jin wan*).

- For blood deficiency with hypochondriac pain and irregular menstruation, remove Aurantii Fructus immaturus (*zhǐ shí*) and add Atractylodis macrocephalae Rhizoma (*bái zhú*), Poria (*fú líng*), and Angelicae sinensis Radix (*dāng guī*).

- For food stagnation with abdominal pain, add Crataegi Fructus (*shān zhā*), Hordei Fructus germinatus (*mài yá*), and Gigeriae galli Endothelium corneum (*jī nèi jīn*).

- For pinpoint fixed pain due to blood stasis, add Typhae Pollen (*pú huáng*), Trogopterori Faeces (*wǔ líng zhī*), and Salviae miltiorrhizae Radix (*dān shēn*).

- For painful menstruation, add Angelicae sinensis Radix (*dāng guī*), Linderae Radix (*wū yào*), Cyperi Rhizoma (*xiāng fù*), and Corydalis Rhizoma (*yán hú suǒ*).

- For damp-heat leukorrhea with lower abdominal pain and soreness of the lower back, combine with Two-Marvel Powder (*èr miào sǎn*).

- For breast abscess, add Citri reticulatae viride Pericarpium (qīng pí).
- For biliary tract disorders, add Artemisiae scopariae Herba (yīn chén), Salviae miltiorrhizae Radix (dān shēn), Curcumae Radix (yù jīn), Paeoniae Radix rubra (chì sháo), and Lysimachiae Herba (jīn qián cǎo).
- For intercostal neuralgia, add Trichosanthis Pericarpium (guā lóu pí), Allii macrostemi Bulbus (xiè bái), and Curcumae Radix (yù jīn).
- For roundworms, add Mume Fructus (wū méi) and Meliae Cortex (kǔ liàn gēn pí).
- For intestinal obstruction, add Rhei Radix et Rhizoma (dà huáng).
- For phlegm-heat obstruction manifesting with insomnia, irritability, and a tendency to become angry, combine with Minor Decoction [for Pathogens] Stuck in the Chest (xiǎo xiàn xiōng tāng).
- For distention after eating, belching, and reduced appetite, combine with Calm the Stomach Powder (píng wèi sǎn).
- For acute icteric hepatitis, combine with Virgate Wormwood Decoction (yīn chén hāo tāng).
- For red face, marked irritability, and insomnia, combine with a small dose of Coptis Decoction to Resolve Toxicity (huáng lián jiě dú tāng).

Associated Formulas

丹黃四逆散

Moutan and Phellodendron Powder for Frigid Extremities

dān huáng sì nì sǎn

Source   *New Explanations of Medical Formulas* (1980)

Bupleuri Radix (*chái hú*)	12g
Paeoniae Radix alba (*bái sháo*)	30-75g
Aurantii Fructus immaturus (*zhǐ shí*)	12g
Glycyrrhizae Radix (*gān cǎo*)	12g
Moutan Cortex (*mǔ dān pí*)	12g
Phellodendri Cortex (*huáng bǎi*)	12g

The dosage of Paeoniae Radix alba (*bái sháo*) depends on the severity of the abdominal pain. Clears heat, spreads the Liver qi, invigorates the blood, and relieves spasmodic pain. For early-stage appendicitis with right lower quadrant pain (along the Liver channel), fever, cold hands and feet, and signs and symptoms similar to those for which the principal formula is indicated.

枳實芍藥散 (枳实芍药散)

Unripe Bitter Orange and Peony Powder

zhǐ shí sháo yaò sǎn

Source   *Essentials from the Golden Cabinet* (c. 220)

charred Aurantii Fructus immaturus (*zhǐ shí tàn*)
Paeoniae Radix alba (*bái sháo*)

The source text advises to grind equal amounts of both herbs into a powder and to take seven 7 spoonfuls with wheat porridge. Moves the qi, harmonizes the blood, and moderates acute abdominal pain. For abdominal pain after childbirth with irritability and fullness such that one cannot lie down. Also treats pus-filled abscesses. While the main symptoms of this presentation indicate excess, its occurrence after childbirth suggests an underlying deficiency. Hence, the formula combines the breaking up of stagnation in the abdomen with nourishing blood, and dispersing with astringent activity. Taking the powder together with wheat porridge further augments the qi and harmonizes the Stomach. Whereas Frigid Extremities Powder (*sì nì sǎn*) is guided into the lesser yang by the inclusion of Bupleuri Radix (*chái hú*), this formula focuses on the Spleen and Stomach.

Some commentators interpret the action of this formula differently. The source text specifies that Aurantii Fructus immaturus (*zhǐ shí*) is to be fried until black. This is a common method of preparation for guiding herbs into the blood. If one also substitutes Paeoniae Radix rubra (*chì sháo*) for Paeoniae Radix alba (*bái sháo*), the formula can be used to move blood stasis from the lower abdomen and uterus. Here the formula moves both the qi and the blood and is milder than formulas containing Rhei Radix et Rhizoma (*dà huáng*) and various animal medicinals that break up and expel dead blood.

逍遙散 (逍遥散)

Rambling Powder

xiāo yáo sǎn

The characters 逍遥 (*xiāo yáo*) that give this formula its name may be translated as free and unfettered. They also refer to the title of the first chapter of *Zhuang Zi*, "Rambling Without a Destination," which includes many stories about soaring above a restricted world view. This formula similarly releases constraint and encourages the free-flow of Liver qi, allowing for open-mindedness and a free or rambling spirit.

Source   *Formulary of the Pharmacy Service for Benefiting the People in the Taiping Era* (1107)

Bupleuri Radix (*chái hú*)	30g (9g)
dry-fried Angelicae sinensis Radix (*chǎo dāng guī*)	30g (9g)
Paeoniae Radix alba (*bái sháo*)	30g (9g)
Atractylodis macrocephalae Rhizoma (*bái zhú*)	30g (9g)
Poria (*fú líng*)	30g (9g)
Glycyrrhizae Radix praeparata (*zhì gān cǎo*)	15g (4.5g)

Method of Preparation   Grind the ingredients into a powder and take as a draft in 6-9g doses with 6g of baked Zingiberis Rhizoma recens (*wēi jiāng*) and 3g of Menthae haplocalycis Herba (*bò hé*). This formula may also be prepared as a decoction with the dosage indicated in parentheses.

Actions   Spreads the Liver qi, strengthens the Spleen, and nourishes the blood

Indications

Hypochondriac pain (usually spasmodic), headache, vertigo, a bitter taste in the mouth, dry mouth and throat, fatigue, reduced appetite, pale-red tongue, and a wiry, deficient pulse.

There may also be alternating fever and chills and irregular menstruation or distended breasts.

The Liver governs dredging and discharging. According to its natural disposition, it favors smooth, unimpeded out-thrusting and resists being curbed and constrained. The Liver also stores blood and is yin in character. This dual nature is expressed in the Chinese saying, "The Liver is yin with respect to its essence and yang with respect to its function" (肝體陰用陽 *gān tǐ yīn yòng yáng*). When a person is unable to freely express their emotions, the Liver qi becomes constrained. Constraint leads to fire and hyperactivity of Liver yang, which damages the Liver blood. Conversely, blood deficiency implies qi excess or an inability of the Liver blood to regulate the smooth movement of Liver qi. When the Liver's dredging and discharging function is impeded, excess Liver/wood overcontrols Spleen/earth. This occurs even more readily when the Spleen is already deficient. Deficiency of the Spleen, whose function it is to transform nutrients into blood and qi, often leads to blood deficiency. Given these multiple pathophysiological relationships, the presentation treated by this formula is one of Liver constraint with blood deficiency and a frail Spleen.

Liver qi constraint is reflected in pain along the Liver channel, especially in the hypochondria. In women, this can manifest as distended breasts. In some patients, constraint of the Liver may affect its related channel, the Gallbladder, and lead to lesser yang-warp signs and symptoms such as alternating fever and chills and a bitter taste in the mouth. Liver constraint and blood deficiency cause headache, vertigo, and a dry mouth and throat. Fatigue and reduced appetite are symptoms of Spleen deficiency. The tongue and pulse signs reflect the constrained Liver qi and blood deficiency.

Analysis of Formula

Although the focus of this formula is on spreading the Liver qi to relieve the Liver constraint, nourishing herbs must also be included to treat a pattern that includes a deficiency of qi and blood. The chief herb, Bupleuri Radix (*chái hú*), spreads the Liver qi and relieves constraint. It also functions as an envoy that guides the entire formula into the Liver. Bitter and cooling as well as out-thrusting, Bupleuri Radix (*chái hú*) is particularly suitable for constraint that has transformed into heat. The deputies, Angelicae sinensis Radix (*dāng guī*) and Paeoniae Radix alba (*bái sháo*), work together to nourish the blood, strengthening the Liver so that it may discharge its functions more smoothly. These herbs also ensure that the acrid nature of the chief and envoys does not damage the Liver yin. Angelicae sinensis Radix (*dāng guī*) affects the qi of the blood, making it an important herb in the treatment of Liver constraint and blood deficiency. Paeoniae Radix alba (*bái sháo*) nourishes the yin while curbing the Liver yang and alleviating pain.

Essentials from the Golden Cabinet observes, "When one sees a Liver disorder, one knows that the Liver will transmit it to the Spleen. Therefore, one should first treat the Spleen." Two of the assistant herbs, Atractylodis macrocephalae Rhizoma (*bái zhú*) and Poria (*fú líng*), strengthen the Spleen. This curbs the tendency of wood (Liver) to invade earth (Spleen). In addition, augmenting the Spleen's transportive and transformative functions supports the treatment of any underlying blood deficiency. The other assistant, Glycyrrhizae Radix praeparata (*zhì gān cǎo*), tonifies the Spleen and, when combined with Paeoniae Radix alba (*bái sháo*), moderates the spasms that are an important aspect of this formula's indication. Baked Zingiberis Rhizoma recens (*wēi jiāng*), an envoy, harmonizes the Stomach and prevents the development of rebellious qi. The other envoy, Menthae haplocalycis Herba (*bò hé*), when used in small doses, enhances the chief herb's ability to relieve Liver constraint and to disperse the heat associated with that constraint.

Cautions and Contraindications

The chief herb in this formula dredges the Liver and vents heat. The formula is thus unsuitable for treating purely deficient disorders. Furthermore, while the formula is effective for treating psychoemotional disorders that manifest as Liver qi constraint, it does not address causes that go beyond a physiological disposition to express problems in this particular way.

Commentary

This is a variation of Frigid Extremities Powder (*sì nì sǎn*), which is widely used in internal medicine and in the treatment of women's disorders. It may be used for any condition with Liver constraint, blood deficiency, and Spleen deficiency characterized by hypochondriac pain, fatigue, reduced appetite, pale-red tongue, and a wiry, deficient pulse.

The wide range of applications for this formula is attributed by many physicians to the fact that its composition realizes the three basic treatment principles for Liver disorders listed in Chapter 22 of *Basic Questions*:

1. "When the Liver suffers from tension, quickly take sweet [flavors] to relax it."

2. "When the Liver requires dispersion, quickly take acrid flavors to disperse it."

3. "Use acrid [flavors] to tonify it and sour [flavors] to drain it."

From a physiological point of view, the specific characteristic of Rambling Powder (*xiāo yáo sǎn*) is its simultaneous treatment of excess and deficiency in both the Liver and Spleen. The modern physician Qin Bo-Wei succinctly analyzed the reasoning behind this strategy:

When the Liver and Spleen are both deficient, wood cannot dredge earth. If the Liver is unable to dredge and drain to facilitate an orderly [qi dynamic], if the Spleen is unable to strengthen the transportive functions and generate transformation, the manifestations of constraint take shape. … For this [type of disorder] one cannot simply write out formulas that dredge the Liver. (*Medical Lecture Notes of [Qin] Qian Zhai*)

Not surprisingly, some commentators, like the contemporary physician and formula expert Wang Mian-Zhi, thus argue that if constraint arises from Liver deficiency, then Angelicae sinensis Radix *(dāng guī)* and Paeoniae Radix alba *(bái sháo)* rather than Bupleuri Radix *(chái hú)* should be regarded as the formula's chief herbs. Furthermore, the manifestations of Liver constraint are seen as closely intertwined with emotional problems. Linking the Liver's governance of blood to the essential nature of female physiology, physicians throughout the history of Chinese medicine have maintained that women are specifically prone to this type of disorder. The discussion of the formula in *Discussion of Medical Formulas* by the late-Qing-dynasty physician Fei Bo-Xiong, an expert in the treatment of emotional disorders, is typical:

> Rambling Powder *(xiāo yáo sǎn)* employs the strategies of thrusting out Liver wood and disseminating Gallbladder qi within [the more fundamental approach] of regulating nutritive [qi] and supporting earth. It is an especially good formula for resolving constraint. The Liver is the strongest of the five yin organs. Among the seasons, it corresponds to the spring, among the five phases, to wood. It embodies the dynamic of development and growth. Whenever this [dynamic] is constrained, a person tends to become angry and tense and unable to return [to a state of tranquility]. When fire flourishes, it overcontrols metal, when wood flourishes, it overcontrols earth. Because it affects other organs, it is appropriate to put [this situation] in order. … If one adds the two herbs Salviae miltiorrhizae Radix *(dān shēn)* and Cyperi Rhizoma *(xiāng fù)* in order to regulate the menses [the effects of this formula] will be even more marvelous. This is because women are far more prone to constraint.

Despite such gender-based analysis, in contemporary practice, Rambling Powder *(xiāo yáo sǎn)* can be assumed to be as useful in the treatment of men as it is in the treatment of women. (See also the COMMENTARY in the entry for Escape Restraint Pill *(yuè jū wán)* in Chapter 12.) The manner in which the potential indications of this formula have been extended in modern China reflect this insight.

The famous 20th-century physician Yue Mei-Zhong recommended Augmented Rambling Powder *(jia wei xiao yao san)* with Prunellae Spica *(xià kū cǎo)*, Taxilli Herba *(sāng jì shēng)*, and Ligustri lucidi Fructus *(nǔ zhēn zǐ)* for treating hypertension. A modification of this formula based on Augmented Rambling Powder *(jiā wèi xiāo yáo sǎn)* with Chrysanthemi Flos *(jú huā)*, Lycii Fructus *(gǒu qǐ zǐ)*, and Acori tatarinowii Rhizoma *(shí chāng pǔ)* was devised by Wei Wen-Gui to treat various ophthalmological disorders including glaucoma, optic nerve atrophy, acute retrobulbar neuritis,

cortical blindness, and central retinitis.

Another important indication for its use in contemporary practice is the formula's ability to vent pathogens that invade the body against a background of deficiency. The 17th-century *Comprehensive Medicine According to Master Zhang* states that Rambling Powder *(xiāo yáo sǎn)* is effective for spontaneous sweating arising from Liver deficiency. This type of pathology implies a disharmony between nutritive and protective qi, a pathology that frequently underpins allergies, recurrent infections, and the inability to vent lingering pathogens. The modern physician Zhang Yao-Qing from Shanghai suggests that in blood deficient patients where a pathogen remains in the exterior, Menthae haplocalycis Herba *(bò hé)* and Zingiberis Rhizoma recens *(shēng jiāng)* should be made the chief herbs through an appropriate adjustment in dosage. If the pathogen penetrates into the lesser yang, the dosage of Bupleuri Radix *(chái hú)* may also be increased. Where blood deficiency is accompanied by internal heat, Menthae haplocalycis Herba *(bò hé)* and Glycyrrhizae Radix *(gān cǎo)* become the chief ingredients.

The very wide range of potential applications of this formula was already noted in the source text, which recommends it for such disorders as blood deficiency with fatigue, heat in the five centers, painful extremities and trunk, dizziness and heaviness of the head, palpitations, red cheeks, dry mouth and throat, fever, night sweats, reduced appetite, increased desire to sleep, contention between the blood and heat with irregular menstruation, periumbilical and abdominal pain, and malarial alternating fever and chills. The same text also recommends it for treating "virgin girls with weak blood and yin deficiency, disharmony of the nutritive and protective qi, phlegmy cough, tidal fever, and wasting of the limbs that slowly progresses to a steaming bone condition."

The many heat symptoms in these original indications suggest that the formula may be most useful for treating patterns characterized by significant constraint of yang qi, that is, the ministerial fire that is often understood to be under the Liver's control. Such constraint is enabled by deficiency of blood, which naturally leads to yang excess. This explains the use of Bupleuri Radix *(chái hú)* as the chief herb. Furthermore, prior to the Ming dynasty, the herbs Bupleuri Radix *(chái hú)* and Stellariae Radix *(yín chái hú)* were generally indistinguishable. Wang Mian-Zhi suggests that, in cases characterized by strong deficiency fire due to blood deficiency, Stellariae Radix *(yín chái hú)* may be the more appropriate choice.

Many different explanations for the formula's name can be found in the literature, besides that outlined above. Wang Zi-Jie, a teacher of Ye Tian-Shi, notes in *Selected Annotations to Ancient Formulas from the Garden of Crimson Snow*:

> According to the [1st-century dictionary] *Elucidations of the Signs and Explications of the Graphs*, the characters 逍遙 *(xiāo*

yáo) are interchangeable with [their homonyms] 消 (to reduce) and 搖 (to shake). The commentary to the [first chapter of] *Zhuang Zi*, "Rambling Without a Destination," states: 'When the sun rises it reduces the ice. Even though it is consumed, its essential nature is not exhausted. When a boat moves it shakes the water. Even though it is moved, its inner nature is not damaged.' Transferred to the domain of medicine [it implies that this formula] even as it reduces and disperses qi constraint and shakes and moves blood constraint, it never damages the normal qi.

Comparisons

➤ Vs. FRIGID EXTREMITIES POWDER *(sì nì sǎn)*

Both formulas treat Liver qi constraint that involves Liver-Spleen disharmony. Their presentations therefore share symptoms such as pain and distention in the hypochondria, alternating fever and chills, headache, dizziness, dryness of the mouth and throat, menstrual irregularity, and breast distention. However, Frigid Extremities Powder *(sì nì sǎn)* treats a purely excessive disorder where ministerial fire is constrained in the interior by clumping of qi and fluids. This is expressed in frigid extremities, diarrhea or constipation, and excess-type abdominal pain. Rambling Powder *(xiāo yáo sǎn)*, on the other hand, treats a disorder of mixed excess and deficiency where Liver qi constraint and blood and qi deficiency mutually generate and amplify each other. Qi deficiency symptoms like fatigue and reduced appetite, and blood deficiency symptoms like menstrual irregularity, pale tongue, and thin pulse, thus typically accompany the symptoms of excess outlined above.

➤ Vs. ESCAPE RESTRAINT PILL *(yuè jū wán)*

Both formulas treat Liver qi constraint and are frequently used to treat patterns characterized by a strong emotional component in both symptomatology and etiology. However, while Escape Restraint Pill *(yuè jū wán)* moves both the qi and the blood and is thus indicated solely for patterns of excess, Rambling Powder *(xiāo yáo sǎn)* tonifies the Spleen and Liver qi and blood and opens constraint and is thus indicated for mixed patterns of deficiency and excess. A second important difference is the type of constraint that is the primary focus of both formulas. Rambling Powder *(xiāo yáo sǎn)* contains bitter and cooling Bupleuri Radix *(chái hú)* as its chief herb. It is thus most suitable for patterns where constraint has transformed into heat, or, put another way, for constraint of yang qi or ministerial fire. Headache, vertigo, a bitter taste in the mouth, dry mouth and throat, or alternating fever and chills—all of which are due to fire from constraint—are thus core symptoms. Escape Restraint Pill *(yuè jū wán)*, on the other hand, contains Cyperi Rhizoma *(xiāng fù)* as the main herb for resolving Liver qi constraint. Acrid and warming in nature, it dredges stagnation of the more solid aspects of qi from the Liver channel. Hence, it is said to move the blood within the qi. Accordingly, key symptoms that would indicate the use of that formula include distention and pain, suggesting a more substantive type of stagnation that may extend from the qi to the fluids and even the blood.

➤ Vs. AUGMENTED LINDERA DECOCTION *(jiā wèi wū yào tāng)*; *see* PAGE 536

➤ Vs. LINKING DECOCTION *(yī guàn jiān)*; *see* PAGE 382

➤ Vs. TANGKUEI AND PEONY POWDER *(dāng guī sháo yào sǎn)*; *see* PAGE 589.

Biomedical Indications

With the appropriate presentation, this formula may be used to treat a wide variety of biomedically-defined disorders. These can be divided into the following groups:

• Those affecting the digestive system such as hepatitis, cholecystitis, peptic ulcers, gastric neurosis, cirrhosis, and chronic gastritis

• Women's disorders such as premenstrual syndrome fibrocystic breast disease, perimenopausal syndrome, pelvic inflammatory disease, and uterine fibroids.

The formula has also been used for goiter, schizophrenia, depression, optical neuritis, cataracts, and diabetes.

Alternate name

Rambling Decoction *(xiāo yáo tāng)* in *Comprehensive Recording of Sagely Beneficence*

Modifications

• For more severe hypochondriac pain with distention, remove Atractylodis macrocephalae Rhizoma *(bái zhú)* and add Cyperi Rhizoma *(xiāng fù)*.

• For intense, fixed pain due to blood stasis, add Moutan Cortex *(mǔ dān pí)*, Curcumae Radix *(yù jīn)*, and Sparganii Rhizoma *(sān léng)*.

• For vaginal discharge, add Lonicerae Flos *(jīn yín huā)* and *guàn zhòng* (Dryopteridis/Cyrtomii/etc. Rhizoma).

• For pain over the liver with fatigue and reduced appetite, remove baked Zingiberis Rhizoma recens *(wēi jiāng)* and Menthae haplocalycis Herba *(bò hé)* and add Cyperi Rhizoma *(xiāng fù)*, Citri sarcodactylis Fructus *(fó shǒu)*, Salviae miltiorrhizae Radix *(dān shēn)*, and Codonopsis Radix *(dǎng shēn)*.

• For enlarged liver and spleen, add Sepiae Endoconcha *(hǎi piāo xiāo)*, Trionycis Carapax *(biē jiǎ)*, and Ostreae Concha *(mǔ lì)*.

• For fibrocystic breasts, remove Glycyrrhizae Radix praeparata *(zhì gān cǎo)* and add Vaccariae Semen *(wáng bù liú xíng)*, Spatholobi Caulis *(jī xuè téng)*, Salviae miltiorrhizae Radix *(dān shēn)*, and Cyperi Rhizoma *(xiāng fù)*.

Variation

黑逍遙散 （黑逍遙散）

Black Rambling Powder

hēi xiāo yáo sǎn

SOURCE *Writings Taking Personal Responsibility for the Medical Tradition* (Qing dynasty)

For the same presentation as the principal formula, but with more severe blood deficiency characterized by premenstrual cramps, pain in the shoulders or shoulder blades, various types of discharge, excessive menstrual bleeding, and a wiry, deficient or wiry, rapid pulse, add Rehmanniae Radix praeparata *(shú dì huáng)*.

Associated Formulas

加味逍遙散 （加味逍遥散）

Augmented Rambling Powder

jiā wèi xiāo yáo sǎn

SOURCE *Summary of Internal Medicine* (Ming dynasty)

Angelicae sinensis Radix *(dāng guī)* 3g
Paeoniae Radix *(sháo yào)* 3g
Poria *(fú líng)* 3g
dry-fried Atractylodis macrocephalae Rhizoma *(chǎo bái zhú)* . . . 3g
Bupleuri Radix *(chái hú)* 3g
Moutan Cortex *(mǔ dān pí)* 1.5g
dry-fried Gardeniae Fructus *(chǎo zhī zǐ)* 1.5g
Glycyrrhizae Radix praeparata *(zhì gān cǎo)* 1.5g

Decoction. Take with a small amount of Zingiberis Rhizoma recens *(shēng jiāng)* and Menthae haplocalycis Herba *(bò hé)*. Spreads the Liver qi, strengthens the Spleen, nourishes the blood, and clears heat. For Liver constraint with Spleen deficiency that transforms into heat characterized by irritability, short temper with possible tidal fever and sweating, red eyes, dry mouth, palpitations, lower abdominal pressure, difficult, painful urination, and increased menstrual flow or uterine bleeding. In clinical practice, the heat treated by this formula is experienced as a subjective feeling of heat by the patient rather than as outright fever. When it becomes visible, it will manifest particularly in the upper half of the body, leading to facial flushing or flushing of the ear lobes. Children may present with mouth ulcers or swelling and distention of the breasts and nipples. In external medicine, the formula is used for treating itching or ulcers due to the heat of deficiency.

This variation is preferred to Rambling Powder *(xiāo yáo sǎn)* in contemporary Kampo medicine, where it is one of the main formulas for treating women's disorders ranging from infertility and menstrual problems to menopausal syndrome. Fire from Liver constraint readily damages the blood and leads to stagnation, especially if the blood is already deficient. This type of stagnation is relatively mild and often manifests symptomatically rather than with the more typical changes on the tongue commonly perceived to be indicative of blood stasis. Such symptoms may include painful menstruation, hard and painful breasts prior to menstruation, or tenderness of the lower abdomen on palpation. In such cases, one should add blood-moving herbs such as Rubiae Radix *(qiàn cǎo gēn)*, Carthami Flos *(hóng huā)*, and Persicae Semen *(táo rén)*. Add

Plantaginis Semen *(chē qián zǐ)* to focus the formula on the treatment of difficult, painful urination. At least ten other formulas by the same name, but with different additions or omissions, can be found in various historical sources.

Comparison

➢ Vs. MELIA TOOSENDAN POWDER *(jīn líng zǐ sǎn)*; *see* PAGE 524

➢ Vs. GENTIAN DECOCTION TO DRAIN THE LIVER *(lóng dǎn xiè gān tāng)*; *see* PAGE 200

抑肝散

Restrain the Liver Powder

yì gān sǎn

SOURCE *Synopsis for Protecting Infants* (1555)

dry-fried Atractylodis macrocephalae Rhizoma *(chǎo bái zhú)* . . . 3g
Poria *(fú líng)* 3g
Angelicae sinensis Radix *(dāng guī)* 3g
Chuanxiong Rhizoma *(chuān xiōng)* 2.4g
Uncariae Ramulus cum Uncis *(gōu téng)* 3g
Bupleuri Radix *(chái hú)* 1.5g
Glycyrrhizae Radix *(gān cǎo)* 1.5g

Taken as a draft, usually with the addition of 3g of Citri reticulatae Pericarpium *(chén pí)* and 4.5g of Pinelliae Rhizoma praeparatum *(zhì bàn xià)*. Calms the Liver and regulates the Liver blood and qi. Originally used in treating children for the heat of deficiency in the Liver channel with spasms, feverishness and bruxism, palpitations with anxiety, fever and chills, or spitting of sputum and saliva, abdominal distention, reduced appetite, and restless sleep due to the Liver (wood) overcontrolling the Spleen (earth). Its use has subsequently been expanded to cover a wide variety of chronic disorders of mixed deficiency and excess characterized by spasmodic movement including seizure disorders, hysteria, and night terrors. It can also be used to soothe frequent displays of temper or temper tantrums, irritability, impatience, aggressiveness, and insomnia.

In contemporary Japan, this formula is commonly used not only in the treatment of children, but also for Liver yang patterns in adults, specifically the elderly. Citri reticulatae Pericarpium *(chén pí)* 3g, and Pinelliae Rhizoma praeparatum *(zhì bàn xià)* 5g, are frequently added to produce a formula known as Restrain the Liver Powder with Tangerine Peel and Pinellia (抑肝散加陳皮半夏 *yì gān sǎn jiā chén pí bàn xià*). This is based on the experience that patients with Liver qi and blood deficiency often also present with phlegm. The reason for this is that the Liver plays a major role in dredging the channels, which promotes the free flow of qi and blood. When this is inhibited, the circulation of fluids is impeded, resulting in the production of phlegm even though, overall, the qi and blood are deficient. Compared to Rambling Powder *(xiāo yáo sǎn)*, this formula focuses more strongly on patterns characterized by the presence of wind and phlegm, as evidenced in such symptoms as tics, tremors, cramps, spasms, and headaches. Compared to Augmented Rambling Powder *(jiā wèi xiāo yáo sǎn)*, this formula is less able to clear heat from constraint, but better able to extinguish wind and transform phlegm.

疏肝理脾湯（疏肝理脾汤）

Dredge the Liver and Regulate the Spleen Decoction

shū gān lǐ pí tāng

SOURCE *New Explanations of Medical Formulas* (1980)

Bupleuri Radix (*chái hú*) 12g
Atractylodis macrocephalae Rhizoma (*bái zhú*) 12g
Cyperi Rhizoma (*xiāng fù*) 9g
Codonopsis Radix (*dǎng shēn*) 15g
Alismatis Rhizoma (*zé xiè*) 9g
Polygoni multiflori Radix (*hé shǒu wū*) 12g
Salviae miltiorrhizae Radix (*dān shēn*) 12g
Notoginseng Radix (*sān qī*) . . . . [powdered] 3g

Dredges the Liver qi, regulates the Spleen, and nourishes and invigorates the blood. For severe Liver qi constraint with clumping and Spleen deficiency leading to blood deficiency and blood stasis characterized by intense hypochondriac pain, irritability, insomnia, fatigue, a stifling sensation in the epigastrium, reduced appetite, and loose stools. Commonly used for chronic hepatitis and early stages of cirrhosis.

清肝達鬱湯（清肝达郁汤）

Clear the Liver and Thrust out Constraint Decoction

qīng gān dá yù tāng

SOURCE *Revised Popular Guide to the Discussion of Cold Damage* (Qing dynasty)

Gardeniae Fructus (*zhī zǐ*) 9g
Paeoniae Radix alba (*bái sháo*) 3g
Angelicae sinensis Radix (*dāng guī*) 3g
Bupleuri Radix (*chái hú*) 1.2g
Moutan Cortex (*mǔ dān pí*) 6g
Glycyrrhizae Radix praeparata (*zhì gān cǎo*) 1.8g
Citri reticulatae Exocarpium album (*jú bái*) 3g
Menthae haplocalycis Herba (*bò hé*) 1.2g
Chrysanthemi Flos (*jú huā*) 4.5g
Citri reticulatae Folium (*jú yè*) . . . . 5 leaves

Decoction. Clears the Liver, discharges fire, dredges constraint, and disseminates qi. For Liver constraint with chest fullness, pain in the hypochondria, abdominal fullness and pain, and a sensation of wanting to discharge the bowels without actually needing to, or the bowels not properly emptying after having had a bowel movement. This is a variation of Augmented Rambling Powder (*jiā wèi xiāo yáo sǎn*) that treats constrained Liver qi transforming into fire, which then overcontrols metal and leads to the bowel symptoms described above.

痛瀉要方（痛泻要方）

Important Formula for Painful Diarrhea

tòng xiè yào fāng

Source *Essential Teachings of [Zhu] Dan-Xi* (1481)

While the source text lists this formula, it does not specify a name. The first time the formula is given a name is in *Correct Transmission of Medicine* where it is called Important Formula for Discharging Pain (痛泄要方 *tòng xiè yào fāng*). The name was changed to Important Formula for Painful Diarrhea (痛瀉要方 *tòng xiè yào fāng*) in *Investigations of Medical Formulas*.

dry-fried Atractylodis macrocephalae Rhizoma
   (*chǎo bái zhú*) 90g (9-12g)
dry-fried Paeoniae Radix alba (*chǎo bái sháo* 60g (6-24g)
dry-fried Citri reticulatae Pericarpium (*chǎo chén pí*) 45g (4.5-9g)
Saposhnikoviae Radix (*fáng fēng*) 30-60g (3-6g)

Method of Preparation Grind the ingredients into powder and take in powder or pill form. May also be prepared as a decoction with the dosages indicated in parentheses.

Actions Tonifies the Spleen, softens the Liver, expels dampness, and stops diarrhea

Indications

Recurrent problems of borborygmus, abdominal pain, diarrhea with pain (which starts with the urge to defecate and subsides after completion), a thin, white tongue coating, and a wiry, moderate or wiry, thin pulse.

This is painful diarrhea due to Spleen deficiency with an overcontrolling Liver. Because of the mutual relationship between the Liver and Spleen, the presence of either Spleen deficiency or an overcontrolling Liver can lead to the development of the other. Unless properly treated, this close relationship also makes it easy for the condition to become recurrent. Diarrhea, which indicates a collapse of the Spleen qi, is caused by the Spleen's inability to transport nutrients upward; the resulting turbidity thereupon descends. The pain is caused by the transverse rebellion of Liver qi. The combination of the descent of the turbidity and the transverse rebellion of Liver qi leads to borborygmus (regarded as a form of wind in the abdomen). Pain before defecation with relief upon evacuation indicates constraint. A wiry pulse, which is either thin or moderate, reflects Liver constraint and Spleen deficiency. The tongue coating is unremarkable because the internally-generated dampness is directed downward and therefore does not affect the tongue. This type of tongue rules out damp excess and turbidity accumulating in the Intestines as the cause of the painful diarrhea.

Analysis of Formula

Atractylodis macrocephalae Rhizoma (*bái zhú*) strengthens the Spleen and dries dampness. In cases where a deficient Spleen interacts with an overcontrolling Liver, using this herb to nurture the Spleen (earth) will have the effect of controlling the Liver (wood). Paeoniae Radix alba (*bái sháo*) softens the overactive Liver and alleviates pain. The combination of these two herbs works very well to control wood and nurture the earth, thereby stopping the pain and diarrhea associated with this condition. As such, they are both regarded as chief herbs, although the first is sometimes given prominence. The deputy, Citri reticulatae Pericarpium (*chén pí*), is aromatic. It harmonizes the functions of the middle burner and transforms dampness. It also helps Atractylodis macrocephalae Rhizoma (*bái zhú*) strengthen the Spleen and eliminate dampness. Saposhnikoviae Radix (*fáng fēng*) serves as both an assistant and envoy. It enters the Liver and Spleen channels and helps relieve the overcontrol of the Spleen by the Liver, while focusing the actions of all the herbs on these two organs.

Cautions and Contraindications

This formula is not indicated in cases of diarrhea due to food damage. While this can also be accompanied by abdominal pain, the pain will usually disappear after the bowels have been evacuated and the food stagnation dispersed. Other differentiating symptoms are the presence of undigested food in the stools and particularly smelly stools. Borborygmus, if present, is frequently followed by the discharge of gas, which also is foul-smelling.

Commentary

According to the famous 20th-century physician Qin Bo-Wei, the pathogenesis of this disorder is that the deficient Spleen condition with abdominal distention usually occurs first. This causes the Liver to overcontrol the Spleen, with symptoms of abdominal pain and later diarrhea. The diarrhea is marked by a few distinguishing characteristics: it is relatively meager in volume; the patient feels more comfortable after each bowel movement; and the problem is recurrent. Qin noted that the pulse is usually wiry, thin, and transposed. By 'transposed' he meant that the right (Spleen) pulse is stronger than the left (Liver) pulse, which is a common, if paradoxical, sign of the Liver overcontrolling the Spleen. Regardless of which of the two organs is more affected, this condition often recurs during times of stress and Liver constraint.

There has been some discussion regarding why Saposhnikoviae Radix (*fáng fēng*) is used in this formula instead of Bupleuri Radix (*chái hú*), which is more commonly associated with treating Liver constraint. Four reasons are cited:

1. Saposhnikoviae Radix (*fáng fēng*) enters the Liver where its acrid flavor disperses constraint.

2. It enters the Spleen and Stomach and is frequently used as an envoy to guide other herbs into these organs. According to Li Dong-Yuan, "If one wants to tonify the Spleen and Stomach, [other herbs] will not move there unless guided by Saposhnikoviae Radix (*fáng fēng*)."

3. Its acrid and bitter flavors overcome dampness, while its nature is to ascend. By facilitating the ascent of clear qi, Saposhnikoviae Radix (*fáng fēng*) thus stops diarrhea.

4. Saposhnikoviae Radix (*fáng fēng*) tracks down and expels wind from the interior of the body, especially from the Intestines. This function is useful if the diarrhea is due to an external pathogen. Symptomatically, it treats borborygmus, which is also considered a type of wind.

In line with the emphasis on the treatment of wind suggested by the use of Saposhnikoviae Radix (*fáng fēng*), in the contemporary book *Collected Medical Writings of Li Ke-Shao*, that physician argues that this formula is most suitable for treating spasmic diarrhea, reflected in a wiry pulse:

> Irrespective of whether it is an acute or chronic disorder, and even when it is a case of daybreak diarrhea [which normally indicates Kidney deficiency], the only important [diagnostic] marker is the wiry pulse, or the spasmodic abdominal pain that accompanies [the diarrhea], or other symptoms that clearly indicate that the Liver qi is too strong.

Another well-known modern physician, Jiao Shu-De, notes in *Ten Lectures on Experiences with Formulas* that he uses this formula for daybreak diarrhea when there are signs of Liver constraint such as a slightly wiry pulse or aggravation of the symptoms upon getting angry. In these cases, he combines it with Four-Miracle Pill (*sì shén wán*) or Aconite Accessory Root Pill to Regulate the Middle (*fù zǐ lǐ zhōng wán*).

The contemporary physician and formula specialist Chen Chao-Zu goes so far as to suggest that the inclusion of Saposhnikoviae Radix (*fáng fēng*) in this formula is due to the fact that penetration by an external pathogen into the interior is the primary cause of the diarrhea treated by this formula:

> One must know that the cause of this presentation is externally-contracted wind-cold. It follows the lesser yang Triple Burner inward to the Intestinal passages where it lodges in the folds of the Small Intestine. Lingering for a long time without being expelled, it causes spasms that manifest as painful diarrhea. (*Treatment Strategies and Formulas in Chinese Medicine*)

These varied interpretations indicate the usefulness of this formula in treating chronic diarrhea and in treating diarrhea in deficient patients or the elderly. The contemporary physician Wang Mian-Zhi from Beijing recommends the addition of Cimicifugae Rhizoma (*shēng má*) in these cases, to assist the Spleen in raising the clear yang. For the same reason, namely, the as-yet-weak digestive system of infants and young children, he recommends it for use in pediatrics. Here, one often sees diarrhea that is yellow and watery but unaccompanied by heat symptoms. This is thought to indicate wind in Chinese medicine and so is amenable to treatment by this formula. Where cold accompanies the presentation, Wang recommends the addition of Zingiberis Rhizoma recens (*shēng jiāng*) or Zingiberis Rhizoma praeparatum (*páo jiāng*) to warm the middle.

Comparison

➢ Vs. Ginseng, Poria, and White Atractylodes Powder (*shēn líng bái zhú sǎn*); *see* page 316

Biomedical Indications

With the appropriate presentation, this formula may be used to treat a variety of biomedically-defined digestive disorders including various forms of colitis and indigestion in children.

Alternate names

White Atractylodes and Peony Powder (*baí zhú sháo yào sǎn*) in *Systematic Great Compendium of Medicine Past and Present*; White Atractylodes and Saposhnikovia Decoction (*baí zhú fáng fēng tāng*) in *Master Ye's Patterns and Treatments in Women's Diseases*; Saposhnikovia and Peony Decoction (*fáng fēng sháo yào tāng*) in *Essentials for Those Who Do Not Know Medicine*

Modifications

- For chronic diarrhea, add Cimicifugae Rhizoma (*shēng má*).

- For watery diarrhea, add Plantaginis Semen (*chē qián zǐ*), Poria (*fú líng*), and Zingiberis Rhizoma (*gān jiāng*).

- For porridge-like diarrhea, add Atractylodis Rhizoma (*cāng zhú*).

- For blood and pus in the stool, add Pulsatillae Radix (*bái tóu wēng*) and Scutellariae Radix (*huáng qín*).

- For diarrhea in children due to indigestion, add Crataegi Fructus (*shān zhā*).

- For tenesmus, add Arecae Semen (*bīng láng*) and Aucklandiae Radix (*mù xiāng*).

- For severe abdominal pain, double the dosage of Paeoniae Radix alba (*bái sháo*) and add Citri reticulatae viride Pericarpium (*qīng pí*) and Cyperi Rhizoma (*xiāng fù*).

- For urinary difficulty, add Talcum (*huá shí*).

- For severe qi deficiency, add Codonopsis Radix (*dǎng shēn*) and Glycyrrhizae Radix (*gān cǎo*).

- For diarrhea due to hypothyroid condition, substitute Puerariae Radix (*gé gēn*) for Saposhnikoviae Radix (*fáng fēng*), double the dosage of Paeoniae Radix alba (*bái sháo*), and add Ostreae Concha (*mǔ lì*) and Prunellae Spica (*xià kū cǎo*).

Section 3

FORMULAS THAT HARMONIZE THE STOMACH AND INTESTINES

The formulas in this section are used in treating conditions in which pathogenic influences have invaded the Stomach and Intestines leading to clumping and stagnation with simultaneous excess and deficiency. The ascending and descending functions of these organs are thereby disrupted, manifesting in symptoms of fullness and focal distention in the epigastrium, nausea, vomiting, abdominal pain and distention, borborygmus, and diarrhea. Obstruction of the yang qi leads to transformation failure in the middle burner with the simultaneous presence of dampness, phlegm, and heat. These conditions are traditionally described as mutual clumping of cold and heat. Because of their complexity, they must be treated with formulas that harmonize the various conflicting processes. For this purpose, these formulas usually combine acrid, warm herbs like Zingiberis Rhizoma (*gān jiāng*), Zingiberis Rhizoma recens (*shēng jiāng*), Pinelliae Rhizoma praeparatum (*zhì bàn xià*), and Cinnamomi Ramulus (*guì zhī*) that tonify deficiency and cause the clear yang to ascend with bitter, cold herbs like Coptidis Rhizoma (*huáng lián*) and Scutellariae Radix (*huáng qín*) that direct accumulation and turbidity downward.

半夏瀉心湯（半夏泻心汤）

Pinellia Decoction to Drain the Epigastrium

bàn xià xiè xīn tāng

Although the literal translation of this formula's name is Pinellia Drains the Heart Decoction, the word 'Heart' in this context refers to the area below the heart organ—the epigastrium—and not the heart organ itself. This formula eliminates focal distention and fullness in the epigastrium.

Source *Discussion of Cold Damage* (c. 220)

Pinelliae Rhizoma praeparatum (*zhì bàn xià*) 9-12g
Zingiberis Rhizoma (*gān jiāng*) 9g
Scutellariae Radix (*huáng qín*) 9g
Coptidis Rhizoma (*huáng lián*) 3g
Ginseng Radix (*rén shēn*) 9g
Jujubae Fructus (*dà zǎo*) . . . . 12 pieces
Glycyrrhizae Radix praeparata (*zhì gān cǎo*) 9g

Method of Preparation The source text advises to decoct the above ingredients in approximately 10 cups of water until 6 cups remain. The ingredients are removed, and the strained decoction is again decocted until 3 cups remain. This is taken warm in three equal doses over the course of a day. At present, it is generally prepared as a decoction. The dosage of Pinelliae Rhizoma praeparatum (*zhì bàn xià*) is usually increased by 3g and that of Glycyrrhizae Radix praeparata (*zhì gān cǎo*) is reduced by the same amount. Only four pieces of Jujubae Fructus (*dà zǎo*) are used. These adjustments are made to prevent middle burner distention. See the detailed discussion under Cinnamon Twig Decoction (*guì zhī tāng*) in Chapter 1.

Actions Harmonizes the Stomach, directs rebellious qi downward, disperses clumping, and eliminates focal distention

Indications

Epigastric focal distention, fullness, and tightness with very slight or no pain, dry heaves or frank vomiting, borborygmus with diarrhea, reduced appetite, a thin, yellow, and greasy tongue coating that may be red at the tip, and a wiry, rapid pulse.

The source texts attributes the presentation treated by this formula to improper purging of an exterior or half-exterior, half-interior condition in a patient with underlying Spleen and Stomach deficiency. The presence of a cold pathogen in the lesser yang leads to yang qi constraint with accumulation of phlegm fluids. Inappropriate purgation further damages the yang qi in the middle burner without expelling the pathogen. The result is a complex pathology known as 'clumping together of cold and heat' (寒熱互結 hán rè hù jié). Modern texts also speak of 'mixing of cold and heat' (寒熱錯雜 hán rè cuò zá). These terms describe a process where excess fluids accumulating in the Stomach and epigastrium clump with heat from constraint. Such clumping disrupts the qi dynamic of an already weakened middle burner, preventing the Spleen from raising the clear yang, and interfering with the Stomach's function of directing the turbid yin downward.

The main manifestation of this pathology is known as 'focal distention' (痞 pǐ). This refers to a focused, localized sensation of discomfort, blockage, and distention centered on the epigastrium. While the patient experiences a subjective sensation of fullness, the epigastrium itself is soft and palpation will reveal no masses or areas of hardness. There is only slight pain or no pain at all. Other key symptoms include dry heaves or vomiting above and diarrhea below. The simultaneous presence of excess and deficiency also causes a conflict between the different parts of the Intestines, which is manifested as borborygmus. The disruption of the digestive function leads to reduced appetite. The rising of the turbid yin and clumping of heat and fluids in the middle burner is also reflected in the yellow, greasy tongue coating and red tip of the tongue. The thin, greasy quality of the coating reflects the presence of congealed fluids, while the red tip reflects heat constrained in the epigastrium. The wiry, rapid pulse reflects internal clumping and heat.

This condition is not always caused by improper purging. It can arise whenever the ascending and downward-directing functions of the Spleen and Stomach are disturbed by the presence of dampness or phlegm constraining the middle burner yang. In all of these cases, clumping leading to focal distention in the epigastrium and the other symptoms described above will ensue.

Analysis of Formula

The primary goal of this formula is to drain the clumping that obstructs the qi dynamic in the epigastrium. This is supported by strategies that harmonize the middle burner. The chief herb is bitter, cold, and downward-draining Coptidis Rhizoma (huáng lián). As noted by Zhang Shan-Lei in Rectification of the Meaning of Materia Medica, this herb is specific for draining "constraint steaming of dampness and heat," the precise pathology at the heart of the present problem. Coptidis Rhizoma (huáng lián) also focuses on the epigastrium, making it an even more specific choice as the chief ingredient.

The chief is supported by three deputies. The first, bitter and cold Scutellariae Radix (huáng qín), is similar in action to Coptidis Rhizoma (huáng lián), strengthening its ability to dry, drain, and direct downward. As noted by the Song writer Su Song in Illustrated Classic of the Materia Medica, Scutellariae Radix (huáng qín) is used in all of Zhang Zhong-Jing's formulas to drain clumping from the epigastrium. The second deputy is acrid and warm Pinelliae Rhizoma praeparatum (zhì bàn xià). It enters the Stomach channel and disperses clumping, stops vomiting, and eliminates focal distention. The third deputy is acrid and very warm Zingiberis Rhizoma (gān jiāng), which enters the Spleen and Stomach. Assisting in the transformation of thin mucus while restoring yang qi to the middle burner, it treats both the root and branch of this pattern.

The assistants, Ginseng Radix (rén shēn) and Jujubae Fructus (dà zǎo), benefit the middle burner qi and prevent the dispersing actions of the chief and deputy herbs from injuring the normal qi. In this manner, they work with the chief herb to stop the vomiting. The envoy, Glycyrrhizae Radix praeparata (zhì gān cǎo), helps the assistant herbs tonify the middle qi and harmonizes the actions of the other ingredients. Because of the presence of the chief and deputy herbs, the assistant and envoy herbs are able to tonify without increasing the stagnation in the middle burner or aggravating the focal distention.

Cautions and Contraindications

This formula is indicated for focal distention caused by clumping of constrained heat and fluids in the epigastrium. Where such distention is due to qi stagnation or harbored food, this formula will not be effective.

Commentary

This is a variation of Minor Bupleurum Decoction (xiao chai hu tang) in which Bupleuri Radix (chái hú) and Zingiberis Rhizoma recens (shēng jiāng) have been replaced by Coptidis Rhizoma (huáng lián) and Zingiberis Rhizoma (gān jiāng). In Essentials from the Golden Cabinet, this formula is recommended for vomiting, borborygmus, and focal distention of the epigastrium. Later physicians prescribed it for treating Spleen and Stomach deficiency in patients that develop cold-heat complex due to an externally-contracted pathogenic influence.

In clinical practice, the use of this formula is suggested by the three cardinal symptoms of focal distention, vomiting, and diarrhea, especially if they occur together with a tongue that is red at the tip and has a thin, greasy, yellowish coating or a rapid, wiry pulse. As is common with relatively modern applications of Zhang Zhong-Jing formulas, not all of the three cardinal symptoms need be present for a diagnosis to be made. Several texts in various classical formula currents, for example, prescribe the formula in the treatment of dysenteric disorders alone. In *Categorized Collected Formulas*, the great 19th-century Japanese writer Yoshimasu Tōdō recommended the formula for the treatment of conditions where the ingestion of food or drink is followed shortly thereafter by borborygmus and diarrhea (without focal distention and vomiting). His contemporary, Asada Sohaku, stated that it treats hiccup and vomiting (without diarrhea or focal distention).

In Chinese, the term 'focal distention' describes not only a symptom, but also the disease dynamic treated by this formula. If it is written without the disease classifier, the character 否 *pǐ* refers to hexagram 12 of the *Classic of Changes* (䷋). This hexagram depicts an unfavorable situation where the communication between heaven and earth is obstructed and is often translated as 'standstill.' Its consequences in the medical domain are explained by Wu Kun:

> Because the middle [burner] qi is damaged and has been seized by a pathogen, it cannot cause the clear to ascend and direct the turbid downward. This obstruction in the middle is the same as heaven not connecting [with earth in hexagram 12] causing obstruction. *(Investigations of Medical Formulas)*

Several classical and contemporary writers argue that the descriptive term 'mutual clumping of cold and heat' in the traditional literature misrepresents this disease dynamic. The critique by the modern physician Jiang Jian-Guo, outlined in *Resolving Uncertainties about the [Discussion] of Cold Damage,* is representative of this current of thought. Jiang notes that heat and cold are opposites that can no more clump together than ice and fire. The term clumping, furthermore, is conventionally used to describe processes where physiological substances like body fluids or stool mix with a pathogen to cause obstruction. Neither heat nor cold are material substances, and hence they cannot clump together. In Jiang's opinion, Coptidis Rhizoma *(huáng lián)* and Scutellariae Radix *(huáng qín)* are therefore not utilized because they are cold, nor are Zingiberis Rhizoma *(gān jiāng)* and Pinelliae Rhizoma praeparatum *(zhì bàn xià)* chosen primarily because they are warm. Rather, bitter herbs are essential to direct downward while acrid herbs provide the physiological momentum necessary for completely draining obstruction from the epigastrium without further damaging the normal qi. In this view, Jiang is following in the footsteps of earli-er physicians who had similar views, chief among them Fei Bo-Xiong. In accordance with these arguments, in this text, Coptidis Rhizoma *(huáng lián)* has been designated the chief herb in this formula.

There is an opposing current that is exemplified by the Ming dynasty scholar-physician Ke Qin. Ke thought that because focal distention is essentially an obstruction to directing downward, Pinelliae Rhizoma praeparatum *(zhì bàn xià)* should be considered the chief herb. This view has been taken up by the majority of textbooks in contemporary China. It does not explain, however, why Coptidis Rhizoma *(huáng lián)* and Scutellariae Radix *(huáng qín)* are included in all five of the Drain the Epigastrium Decoctions *(xiè xīn tāng)* listed in *Discussion of Cold Damage,* while only this one carries Pinelliae Rhizoma praeparatum *(zhì bàn xià)* in its title. In *Collected Writings on Renewal of the Discussion of Cold Damage,* even Ke Qin admits that "To drain the epigastrium one must utilize Coptidis Rhizoma *(huáng lián)* and Scutellariae Radix *(huáng qín)*." Given this, the inclusion of Pinelliae Rhizoma praeparatum *(zhì bàn xià)* in the name of this formula likely represents an attempt to differentiate it from other Drain the Epigastrium Decoctions *(xiè xīn tāng),* rather than an effort to designate the chief herb.

For some modern uses, this issue will be moot. When there is relatively more heat, the chief ingredients are considered to be Coptidis Rhizoma *(huáng lián)* and Scutellariae Radix *(huáng qín);* when there is relatively more cold, the dosage of Zingiberis Rhizoma *(gān jiāng)* is increased; and when turbidity is the main issue, the dosage of Pinelliae Rhizoma praeparatum *(zhì bàn xià)* is increased.

Once the manner in which this formula opens the qi dynamic (and here specifically, the Stomach's downward-directing action) has been understood, the range of conditions for which this formula is effective widens. Besides the more obvious digestive problems, these include severe insomnia due to the failure of Stomach qi to descend, globus hystericus, mouth ulcers, chronic fatigue, as well as neck and shoulder stiffness.

Comparisons

➤ Vs. Minor Decoction [for Pathogens] Stuck in the Chest *(xiǎo xiàn xiōng tāng)* and Major Decoction [for Pathogens] Stuck in the Chest *(dà xiàn xiōng tāng)*

An epigastrium that is soft to the touch is of particular diagnostic significance in choosing this formula over the other two primary formulas from *Discussion of Cold Damage* that treat sinking of pathogenic influences due to inappropriate purging. Minor Decoction [for Pathogens] Stuck in the Chest *(xiǎo xiàn xiōng tāng)* is indicated for focal distention (with or without masses) in the chest and epigastrium that is painful to the touch. Major Decoction [for Pathogens] Stuck in the Chest (dà xiàn xiōng tāng) is indicated for a deeper, more severe condition in which the entire abdomen is hard, distended, and so painful that it cannot bear to be touched.

➢ Vs. Coptis Decoction (huáng lián tāng); see page 132

➢ Vs. Unripe Bitter Orange Pill to Reduce Focal Distention (zhǐ shí xiāo pǐ wán); see page 840

Biomedical Indications

With the appropriate presentation, this formula may be used to treat a variety of biomedically-defined disorders, primarily those affecting the digestive system such as gastritis, peptic ulcers, gastroesophageal reflux disease, chronic cholecystitis, colitis, and hepatitis. It has also been used for hyperthyroidism, chronic asthma, conjunctivitis, apthous ulcers, coronary artery disease, insomnia, amenorrhea, and morning sickness.

Alternate name

Drain the Epigastrium Decoction (xiè xīn tāng) in *Important Formulas Worth a Thousand Gold Pieces*

Modification

• For damp-heat aggregating in the middle burner with vomiting and focal distention, remove Ginseng Radix (rén shēn), Zingiberis Rhizoma (gān jiāng), Jujubae Fructus (dà zǎo), and Glycyrrhizae Radix praeparata (zhì gān cǎo) and add Aurantii Fructus immaturus (zhǐ shí) and Zingiberis Rhizoma recens (shēng jiāng).

Variation

甘草瀉心湯 （甘草泻心汤）

Licorice Decoction to Drain the Epigastrium

gān cǎo xiè xīn tāng

Source   *Discussion of Cold Damage* (c. 220)

For more severe Stomach qi deficiency characterized by undigested food in the stools and irritability, increase the dosage of Glycyrrhizae Radix praeparata (zhì gān cǎo) to 12g.

Chapter 3 of *Essentials from the Golden Cabinet* prescribes this formula for the treatment of 狐惑 hú huò (literally 'fox delusion') disorder, a condition characterized by erosions in the throat accompanied by fatigue and restlessness, and an aversion even to the smell of food. The effectiveness of the formula in treating this condition underlines the fact that the various Drain the Epigastrium Decoctions (xiè xīn tāng) do *not* treat Stomach organ disorders, but focus on opening the qi dynamic in order to facilitate the ascent of the clear and descent of the turbid. In contemporary practice, the formula is thus used for a variety of disorders involving the oral mucosa including gingivitis, stomatitis, and mouth ulcers as well as Behcet's disease, which in many ways resembles hú huò disorder.

This formula is used at present, particularly in Japan, for sleep disorders including difficulty in falling asleep, frequent waking, unrefreshing sleep, dream-disturbed sleep, talking in one's sleep, and somnambulism. This usage is based on the description of the formula's indication for the hú huò disorder in *Essentials from the Golden Cabinet*: "Hú huò disorder manifests like cold damage. The patient is silent and desires to sleep [but] the eyes cannot be closed [and when] they get up they are restless."

Ginseng Radix (rén shēn) is omitted in the source text's version of this formula but included in other classical texts, among them *Essentials from the Golden Cabinet, Thousand Ducat Formulas,* and *Arcane Essentials from the Imperial Library*. This implies that the formula can be modified to fit more precisely the presenting pattern. If deficiency is pronounced, Ginseng Radix (rén shēn) may be added; if excess is pronounced, it can be omitted. In cases of more severe cold, one may add Aconiti Radix lateralis praeparata (zhì fù zǐ), whereas Rhei Radix et Rhizoma (dà huáng) can be used for a stronger heat-draining effect.

A good example of such adjustment is a variation composed by the Qing-dynasty physician Wu Ju-Tong. Wu added Armeniacae Semen (xìng rén) and Aurantii Fructus immaturus (zhǐ shí) and removed Ginseng Radix (rén shēn), Zingiberis Rhizoma (gān jiāng), Jujubae Fructus (dà zǎo), and Glycyrrhizae Radix (gān cǎo) to treat yang brightness summerheat dampness characterized by lack of appetite, constipation, accumulation of turbidity and phlegm, and focal distention. Besides exemplifying the formula's wide scope of variation, this is one of the many examples indicating how closely cold damage and warm pathogen therapeutics are intertwined.

Associated Formulas

生薑瀉心湯 （生姜泻心汤）

Fresh Ginger Decoction to Drain the Epigastrium

shēng jiāng xiè xīn tāng

Source   *Discussion of Cold Damage* (c. 220)

Zingiberis Rhizoma recens (shēng jiāng) 12g
Zingiberis Rhizoma (gān jiāng) 3g
Pinelliae Rhizoma praeparatum (zhì bàn xià) 9g
Scutellariae Radix (huáng qín) 9g
Coptidis Rhizoma (huáng lián) 3g
Ginseng Radix (rén shēn) 9g
Glycyrrhizae Radix praeparata (zhì gān cǎo) 9g
Jujubae Fructus (dà zǎo) . . . . 12 pieces

Harmonizes the Stomach, reduces focal distention, disperses clumping, and expels water. For clumping of water and heat or Stomach deficiency with food stagnation and suspended thin mucus (懸飲 xuán yǐn) lingering internally, characterized by firm epigastric focal distention, dry heaves with a foul odor, the sound of fluids in the hypochondria, very loud borborygmus, and diarrhea. This formula adds a large dose of Zingiberis Rhizoma recens (shēng jiāng) because of its stronger action in dispersing water and opening phlegm. Note that at present, it is most common to use only four pieces of Jujubae Fructus (dà zǎo).

Comparison

➢ Vs. Inula and Haematite Decoction (xuán fù dài zhě tāng); see page 544

人參瀉心湯（人参泻心汤）

Ginseng Decoction to Drain the Epigastrium

rén shēn xiè xīn tāng

SOURCE *Systematic Differentiation of Warm Pathogen Diseases* (1798)

Ginseng Radix (*rén shēn*) 6g

Zingiberis Rhizoma (*gān jiāng*) .6g

Paeoniae Radix alba (*bái sháo*) 6g

Coptidis Rhizoma (*huáng lián*) 4.5g

Scutellariae Radix (*huáng qín*) 4.5g

Aurantii Fructus immaturus (*zhǐ shí*) 3g

Decoction. The source text advised to decoct the herbs in 5 cups of water until 3 cups remain. The decoction is strained and taken warm in two doses. The dregs are then decocted a second time in 1 cup of water. Unblocks the qi dynamic with acrid herbs, directs downward using bitter herbs, protects the yin, and assists the yang. For damp-heat in the upper burner that has not been cleared and has sunk into the interior due to deficiency. This causes veiling of consciousness, a slippery tongue coating, and a relaxed pulse.

黃連湯（黄连汤）

Coptis Decoction

huáng lián tāng

Source   *Discussion of Cold Damage* (c. 220)

Coptidis Rhizoma (*huáng lián*) 9g

Glycyrrhizae Radix praeparata (*zhì gān cǎo*) 9g

Zingiberis Rhizoma (*gān jiāng*) .9g

Cinnamomi Ramulus (*guì zhī*) 9g

Ginseng Radix (*rén shēn*) 6g

Pinelliae Rhizoma praeparatum (*zhì bàn xià*) 9g

Jujubae Fructus (*dà zǎo*) . . . . 10 pieces

Method of Preparation   The source text advises to decoct the above ingredients in approximately 10 cups of water until 6 cups remain. The ingredients are removed. The patient takes five doses of 1 cup each of the strained decoction warm, 3 cups during the day and 2 cups at night. At present, it is generally prepared as a decoction in the usual manner, most commonly with only four pieces of Jujubae Fructus (*dà zǎo*).

Actions   Regulates cold and heat, harmonizes the Stomach, and directs rebellious qi downward

Indications

Stifling sensation and irritability in the chest, nausea with an urge to vomit, abdominal pain, a white, greasy tongue coating, and a wiry pulse. There may also be fever and slight chills along with borborygmus and diarrhea.

This is heat above and cold below caused by the transmission of an external cold pathogen into the middle burner, impeding its ability to regulate ascending and descending. If fire in the upper burner cannot descend, it accumulates in the chest and causes a stifling sensation and irritability. Nausea with an urge to vomit is due to rebellious Stomach qi. Cold damaging the middle burner causes qi to stagnate, experienced as pain, and the Spleen to lose its transformative function, which results in diarrhea. Constraint of the qi dynamic with disharmony between the nutritive and protective qi manifests as fever and slight chills. These symptoms are not as pronounced as those of a greater yang pattern because the constraint does not involve the exterior. The white greasy tongue coating and the wiry pulse reflect the presence of a cold pathogen in the middle burner.

Analysis of Formula

This is a variation of Minor Bupleurum Decoction (*xiǎo chái hú tāng*) in which Scutellariae Radix (*huáng qín*) and Zingiberis Rhizoma recens (*shēng jiāng*) have been replaced with Cinnamomi Ramulus (*guì zhī*) and Zingiberis Rhizoma (*gān jiāng*). It can also be thought of as a variation of Pinellia Decoction to Drain the Epigastrium (*bàn xià xiè xīn tāng*), where Cinnamomi Ramulus (*guì zhī*) is substituted for Scutellariae Radix (*huáng qín*).

The chief ingredient is bitter, cold Coptidis Rhizoma (*huáng lián*), which drains the heat of excess from the chest and harmonizes the Stomach. The acrid, warm, and dispersing herbs Zingiberis Rhizoma (*gān jiāng*) and Cinnamomi Ramulus (*guì zhī*), which expel cold from the lower body to stop pain, serve as deputies. While Zingiberis Rhizoma (*gān jiāng*) excels at warming the Spleen and Stomach, Cinnamomi Ramulus (*guì zhī*) enters the nutritive qi to remove stagnation and harmonize its interaction with the protective yang. Another deputy, acrid and warm Pinelliae Rhizoma praeparatum (*zhì bàn xià*), harmonizes the Stomach by directing rebellious qi downward to stop nausea and vomiting. It also expands the chest and disperses clumping to reduce focal distention. This combination of bitter, downward-draining and acrid, yang-warming herbs effectively unblocks the qi dynamic, treating both the root and branch of this pattern.

The assistant herbs are Ginseng Radix (*rén shēn*), Jujubae Fructus (*dà zǎo*), and Glycyrrhizae Radix praeparata (*zhì gān cǎo*). They augment the qi and strengthen the Spleen, assisting the middle burner in maintaining its normal functions. Serving as the envoy, Glycyrrhizae Radix praeparata (*zhì gān cǎo*) has the additional task of harmonizing the opposing flavors and actions unfolded by the various herbs in this formula.

Cautions and Contraindications

This formula is indicated for nausea, vomiting, and abdominal pain in a presentation characterized by heat above and cold below. Where such symptoms are due to qi stagnation or harbored food, this formula will not be effective.

Commentary

This formula was first identified in paragraph 173 of *Discussion of Cold Damage*. The text defines an unspecified "pathogenic qi in the Stomach" to be the cause of the presentation. This provided later commentators with much room for interpretation. In his *Comprehensive Medicine According to Master Zhang*, the Qing-dynasty physician Zhang Lu utilized the concept of 'mutual clumping of cold and heat,' familiar from discussions of Pinellia Decoction to Drain the Epigastrium *(bàn xià xiè xīn tāng)*, to explain the disease dynamic of this pattern: "If heat and cold within the Stomach are not harmonious, focal distention and fullness in the Heart [ensues]."

Another perspective was offered by Yu Chang, Wang Zi-Jie, Zhang Nan, and the editors of *Golden Mirror of the Medical Tradition*, all of whom discussed this formula in relation to the treatment of plugged and rejecting disorder (關格 *guān gé*). Rejection (格 *gé*) is first described in *Divine Pivot*, Chapter 17: "If the yang qi is extremely exuberant, the yin qi cannot flourish. This is called rejection." *Discussion of Cold Damage* says that rejection manifests with a large, floating distal pulse, rebellious qi, and vomiting. This follows a similar discussion in *Basic Questions*, Chapter 9, where rejection of the yang qi is diagnosed when the carotid artery pulse at ST-9 (人迎 *rén yíng*) is four times as large as the radial artery pulse at LU-9 (寸口 *cùn kǒu*). The *Encyclopedia of Chinese Medicine* defines rejection as a condition where a cold pathogen in the chest prevents the Stomach qi from descending to connect with the yin. Besides nausea and incessant vomiting, rejection is characterized by cold extremities.

Linking this formula to the pathology of rejection disorders helps us understand why Zhang Zhong-Jing included Cinnamomi Ramulus *(guì zhī)* in this formula. For Cinnamomi Ramulus *(guì zhī)* is neither a primary herb for treating abdominal pain nor for treating rebellious qi due to cold. It does, however, tonify the yang of the chest and warm the nutritive qi in the vessels and middle burner. In a person with a weak and cold middle burner, the nutritive qi tends to be insufficient and is therefore easily obstructed by cold. Because nutritive qi is classified as yin, its obstruction causes a relative excess of protective yang. This excess accumulates in the chest, causing turbidity. Normally, the qi dynamic would seek to direct such turbidity downward. Here, however, this excess is rejected by the middle burner that is too cold and static to accept it. Hence, it rebels upward and causes vomiting.

The 18th-century writer Wang Zi-Jie explains the function of Cinnamomi Ramulus *(guì zhī)* in *Selected Annotations to Ancient Formulas from the Garden of Crimson Snow*: "Rejection manifests with vomiting and rebelliousness. Therefore, one introduces Cinnamomi Ramulus *(guì zhī)* to harmonize the Stomach and open the yang so that the yin qi can gradually vent upward from the middle burner." Unlike Pinellia Decoction to Drain the Epigastrium *(bàn xià xiè xīn tāng)*, which primarily drains downward, Coptidis Decoction *(huáng lián tāng)* thus regulates both ascending and downward-directing to facilitate the reconnection of yin and yang. This is explained by Fei Bo-Xiong in *Discussion of Medical Formulas*: "This [formula] changes the strategy of draining the epigastrium with Coptidis Rhizoma *(huáng lián)* and Zingiberis Rhizoma *(gān jiāng)* into one of raising the yang and directing the yin downward. The joint use of cooling and warming herbs to perform both dispersing and tonification makes this the perfection of the harmonizing method."

In clinical practice, typical features of 'heat above' include irritability and restlessness, palpitations, or upward-rushing qi with such symptoms as vomiting or dizziness. 'Cold below' manifests as abdominal pain or diarrhea. This can be reflected in a tongue that has a darkish body but a white and greasy coating, or a coating that is white and thick at the root and thin and yellow toward the front. Likewise, while the abdomen will tend to feel cold on palpation, the patient herself may experience sensations of heat in the chest or epigastrium.

Comparison

➢ Vs. Pinellia Decoction to Drain the Epigastrium *(bàn xià xiè xīn tāng)*

Both formulas combine acrid, warming and bitter, downward-directing herbs to harmonize the Stomach and Intestines, and both treat presentations characterized by vomiting and rebellious qi, diarrhea, and focal distention. Pinellia Decoction to Drain the Epigastrium *(bàn xià xiè xīn tāng)* is the more bitter of the two formulas. It is specific for focal distention, indicating clumping of fluids and qi in the epigastrium and upper burner. In Coptidis Decoction *(huáng lián tāng)*, Cinnamomi Ramulus *(guì zhī)* is substituted for Scutellariae Radix *(huáng qín)*. This makes the formula less effective in draining clumping, but better at warming the circulation of nutritive qi in the middle and upper burners. Combining ascending with downward-directing, Coptidis Decoction *(huáng lián tāng)* harmonizes problems of the nutritive and protective qi characterized by symptoms of heat above and cold below.

➢ Vs. Mume Pill *(wū méi wán)*; *see* page 851

Biomedical Indications

With the appropriate presentation, this formula may be used to treat a variety of biomedically-defined disorders, primarily those affecting the digestive system such as gastritis, hyper-acidic stomach, allergic colitis, and cholecystitis.

Modifications

- For sour vomiting, add Evodiae Fructus (*wú zhū yú*).
- For more pronounced diarrhea, add Poria (*fú líng*).

Associated Formula

乾薑黃連黃芩人參湯（干姜黄连黄芩人参汤）

Ginger, Coptis, Scutellaria, and Ginseng Decoction

gān jiāng huáng lián huáng qín rén shēn tāng

SOURCE   *Discussion of Cold Damage* (c. 220)

Zingiberis Rhizoma (*gān jiāng*) 9g
Scutellariae Radix (*huáng qín*) 9g
Coptidis Rhizoma (*huáng lián*) 9g
Ginseng Radix (*rén shēn*) 9g

Decoction. At present, the dosage of Coptidis Rhizoma (*huáng lián*) is commonly 3-6g and Codonopsis Radix (*dǎng shēn*) is substituted for Ginseng Radix (*rén shēn*). Unblocks the qi dynamic with acrid herbs and directs downward with bitter herbs, while regulating and tonifying the Spleen and Stomach. The source text traces its etiology to mistakenly purging a person with long-standing cold-type diarrhea who then contracts a cold damage disorder. This exacerbates the cold below, which 'rejects' the heat above (i.e., prevents it from moving downward as it should), leading to a disorder known as cold rejection (寒格 *hán gé*). The main manifestations are an increase in the diarrhea accompanied by vomiting, sometimes immediately after eating. In *Modern Explanation of Discussion of Cold Damage*, Lu Yuan-Lei explains the pathophysiology:

> All [cases] where eating in the morning is followed by vomiting at night [can be] blamed on Stomach cold. Vomiting immediately after eating [on the other hand, can be] blamed on Stomach heat. This is [a case] of Stomach heat, hence one uses Scutellariae Radix (*huáng qín*) and Coptidis Rhizoma (*huáng lián*). In the pattern [defining] this formula, even though the Stomach is hot, the Intestines are cold. Accordingly, it combines Scutellariae Radix (*huáng qín*) and Coptidis Rhizoma (*huáng lián*) with Zingiberis Rhizoma (*gān jiāng*) to treat heat above and cold below.

Use of this formula must be differentiated from that of Rhubarb and Licorice Decoction (*dà huáng gān cǎo tāng*), discussed in Chapter 2. While both formulas are indicated for vomiting due to heat (i.e., vomiting soon after eating), the latter formula treats patterns due to pure heat (i.e., heat in both the Stomach and Intestines). Often, therefore, vomiting will be accompanied by constipation. This formula, on the other hand, treats heat above and cold below. Although the textbook presentation of this pattern includes vomiting and diarrhea, this need not necessarily be the case in practice. As Ke Qin explains in *Further Appendices to the Discussion of Cold Damage*, "All those patients suffering from vomiting brought on by heat who do not benefit from [formulas based on] Aucklandiae Radix (*mù xiāng*), Amomi Fructus (*shā rén*), Citri reticulatae Pericarpium (*chén pí*), and Pinelliae Rhizoma praeparatum (*zhì bàn xià*) will feel at ease after taking this formula."

Section 4

. . . .

FORMULAS THAT TREAT MALARIAL DISORDERS AND VENT PATHOGENS FROM THE MEMBRANE SOURCE

Formulas for treating malarial disorders are included in this chapter because their main manifestation—chills followed by fever—resembles that of lesser yang-warp disorders. This section also includes formulas that vent pathogens from the membrane source (膜原 *mó yuán*), a body region implicated in the etiology of epidemic disorders that many physicians closely associate with the lesser yang.

Chinese medical doctrine holds that malarial disorders can be caused by a range of pathogens. These include wind, cold, heat, summerheat, and dampness, as well as various miasmatic qi and malarial toxins. If phlegm-dampness obstructs the qi dynamic, it is difficult for the body to vent these pathogens. They then lurk in the interior, typically in the greater yin or the membrane source, for long periods of time. The unsuccessful efforts of the protective qi to vent these pathogens is what produces the typical malaria attack. Hence the saying, "Without dampness, phlegm cannot form; without phlegm, malaria cannot form." All formulas in this section thus dispel phlegm-dampness and promote the proper movement of qi in addition to checking malarial pathogens.

Formulas that vent pathogens from the membrane source are not used solely to treat malarial disorders, but represent a very specific approach for dealing with epidemic infectious disorders that is closely related to the emergence of the warm pathogen disorder current in Chinese medicine. In contemporary practice, these formulas are frequently used to treat low-grade fevers or fevers of nonspecific etiology.

The core ingredients include Bupleuri Radix (*chái hú*) and Artemisiae annuae Herba (*qīng hāo*), which figure prominently in the formulas discussed above to help harmonize and vent lesser yang disorders. There are also herbs that are used primarily against malarial disorders such as Dichroae Radix (*cháng shān*) and Tsaoko Fructus (*cǎo guǒ*). As noted above, malarial disorders are commonly tied up with dampness and phlegm, which inhibit their treatment. For this reason, these formulas often contain herbs that dry dampness and transform phlegm such as Magnoliae officinalis Cortex (*hòu pò*), Pinelliae Rhizoma praeparatum (*zhì bàn xià*), Atractylodis Rhizoma (*cāng zhú*), and Poria (*fú líng*). Similarly, herbs that have a salutory effect on the qi dynamic, such as Arecae Semen (*bīng láng*), Citri reticulatae viride Pericarpium (*qīng pí*), Citri reticulatae Pericarpium (*chén pí*), and Aurantii Fructus (*zhǐ ké*), are frequently used in these formulas to facilitate the ascending/descending and dissemination of qi.

截瘧七寶飲（截疟七宝饮）

Seven-Treasure Drink to Check Malarial Disorders

jié nuè qī bǎo yǐn

Source   *Formulary of the Pharmacy Service for Benefiting the People in the Taiping Era* (1107)

Dichroae Radix *(cháng shān)* 3g
ginger Magnoliae officinalis Cortex *(jiāng hòu pò)* 1.5g
Citri reticulatae viride Pericarpium *(qīng pí)* 1.5g
Citri reticulatae Pericarpium *(chén pí)* 1.5g
Glycyrrhizae Radix praeparata *(zhì gān cǎo)* 1.5g
Arecae Semen *(bīng láng)* 1.5g
Tsaoko Fructus *(cǎo guǒ)* 1.5g

Method of Preparation   The source text advises to coarsely grind equal amounts of the herbs, which are then to be taken in 15g doses as a draft, prepared in a bowl of water with a tablespoon of wine. The dregs are discarded and the draft is left standing for a day. It is then heated up again before taking it warm. At present, the formula is prepared as a decoction, using the dosages above, with a small amount of wine, and is taken two hours before the onset of an attack (if the attacks are regular).

Actions   Dries dampness, expels phlegm, regulates the qi, and checks malarial disorders

Indications

Intense, unremitting attacks of alternating fever and chills, abdominal distention, a greasy, white tongue coating, and a wiry, slippery, floating, and large pulse at the distal position.

This is a phlegm-dampness malarial disorder. It arises when a malarial pathogen is contracted by a person with preexisting phlegm-dampness. The malarial pathogen lingers in the greater yin where it obstructs the ascending and downward-directing functions of the Spleen and Stomach. This aggravates the preexisting tendency toward production of phlegm and dampness. The Spleen and Stomach functions of ascending and downward-directing are closely intertwined with the movement and circulation of the nutritive and protective qi. When a malarial pathogen lurks in the nutritive qi (associated with the greater yin), the protective yang is drawn away from the exterior to battle the pathogen, resulting in chills. The ability of the protective qi to vent the pathogen to the surface is inhibited by the phlegm-dampness. As the protective qi rises toward the exterior, it causes high fever and sweating, but the pathogen is not completely expelled. This causes the process to recur at regular intervals.

The other symptoms reflect the presence of phlegm-dampness. These include a white, greasy tongue coating and a slippery pulse. Abdominal distention reflects constraint of the qi dynamic in the middle burner. The large, floating pulse indicates that normal qi is still strong and not yet exhausted by the battle with the pathogenic qi.

The source text indicates that the formula can also be used to treat excess-type malarial disorders that are not due to dampness and phlegm.

Analysis of Formula

Effective treatment of this condition requires venting the malarial pathogen and expelling the dampness and phlegm that is obstructing the qi dynamic. The formula thus combines herbs that are specific for checking malarial disorders with those that transform dampness and expel phlegm.

Bitter, acrid, cold, and toxic Dichroae Radix *(cháng shān)* combines all these actions and is therefore the chief herb. It is specific for checking malarial disorders but also expels phlegm and dredges and unblocks accumulated clumping in the interior. The two deputies, Arecae Semen *(bīng láng)* and Tsaoko Fructus *(cǎo guǒ)*, serve the function of opening the qi dynamic. This combination has a long history in the treatment of malarial disorders. Arecae Semen *(bīng láng)* promotes the descent of qi and thereby urination. Tsaoko Fructus *(cǎo guǒ)* is acrid and warming to strongly dry dampness. It also arouses the Spleen yang and facilitates the venting of lurking malarial pathogens to the exterior.

Three qi-moving herbs support the function of the deputies. The acrid, warming, and aromatic Magnoliae officinalis Cortex *(hòu pò)* transforms dampness. Bitter and warming Citri reticulatae viride Pericarpium *(qīng pí)* breaks up qi stagnation. Acrid and warming Citri reticulatae Pericarpium *(chén pí)* regulates the Spleen and moves the qi. Glycyrrhizae Radix praeparata *(zhì gān cǎo)* functions as the envoy that harmonizes the action of the entire formula while tonifying the Spleen and Stomach.

The wine that is added to the water before boiling the powder (or herbs) has the dual function of accelerating the action of the entire formula in venting the pathogen toward the exterior and of counteracting the toxicity of the chief herb. As *Delving into the Description of the Materia Medica* observes, "Used raw, [Dichroae Radix *(cháng shān)*] makes people vomit violently. Soak it in wine overnight, then steam thoroughly or dry-fry. If prepared properly, there will be no vomiting, and the malarial disorder will be more easily cured."

Cautions and Contraindications

Dichroae Radix *(cháng shān)*, the chief herb in this formula, is toxic in doses of 15-75g. Care should be taken not to exceed the safe dose. Preparation of the formula according to the instructions provided will help reduce side effects. This formula is not indicated for deficient or chronic conditions.

Commentary

This formula is suitable for all malarial disorders that are of an excessive nature. It is specific, however, to those where dampness and phlegm are obvious etiological factors. This formula influenced the approach to all subsequent treatment of malarial disorders, and the herbal combinations used here were taken up by later physicians in the treatment of other epidemic infectious diseases. The most influential of these was the Ming-dynasty physician Wu You-Ke, whose Reach the Source Drink (*dá yuán yǐn*) is discussed below.

Biomedical Indications

With the appropriate presentation, this formula may be used to treat malaria and similar biomedically-defined disorders.

Alternate names

Seven-Treasure Drink (*qī bǎo yǐn*) in *Formulary of the Pharmacy Service for Benefiting the People in the Taiping Era*; Seven-Treasure Powder (*qī bǎo sǎn*) in *Yang Family Formulas*; Seven-Treasure Decoction (*qī bǎo tāng*) in *Simple Book of Formulas*; Seven-Substance Decoction (*qī wù tāng*) in *Discussion of Formulas from Straight Directions from [Yang] Ren-Zhai*

Modifications

- For malarial attacks that occur with increasing frequency or do not respond to treatment, indicating that the pathogen has moved from the qi to the blood level, add herbs that invigorate the blood and expel stasis like Trogopterori Faeces (*wǔ líng zhī*) and Persicae Semen (*táo rén*).

- For strong chills, add Cinnamomi Ramulus (*guì zhī*).

- For nausea and vomiting, add Pinelliae Rhizoma praeparatum (*zhì bàn xià*) and Zingiberis Rhizoma recens (*shēng jiāng*).

Associated Formula

常山飲（常山饮）

Dichroa Drink

cháng shān yǐn

Source   *Formulary of the Pharmacy Service for Benefiting the People in the Taiping Era* (1107)

Anemarrhenae Rhizoma (*zhī mǔ*) 1000g
Dichroae Radix (*cháng shān*) 1000g
Tsaoko Fructus (*cǎo guǒ*) 1000g
Glycyrrhizae Radix praeparata (*zhì gān cǎo*) 1000g
Alpiniae officinarum Rhizoma (*gāo liáng jiāng*) 600g
Mume Fructus (*wū méi*) 500g

The source texts advises to grind the herbs into powder and prepare a draft by decocting 9g in 1 cup of water with 5 slices of Zingiberis Rhizoma recens (*shēng jiāng*) and 1 piece of Jujubae Fructus (*dà zǎo*) until one-third has evaporated. Checks malaria and treats phlegm by warming the yang and draining heat. Like the principal formula, Dichroa Drink (*cháng shān yǐn*) checks malaria by combining Dichroae Radix (*cháng shān*) and Tsaoko Fructus (*cǎo guǒ*). However, it focuses on harmonizing the yin and yang rather than moving qi stagnation and expelling phlegm. It utilizes Anemarrhenae Rhizoma

(*zhī mǔ*) to drain heat from the yang brightness and Mume Fructus (*wū méi*) to generate fluids, while Alpiniae officinarum Rhizoma (*gāo liáng jiāng*) and Glycyrrhizae Radix praeparata (*zhì gān cǎo*) warm the greater yin and tonify the qi. The Qing-dynasty physician Fei Bo-Xiong recommended this formula for malaria that did not respond to other treatments.

清脾湯（清脾汤）

Clear the Spleen Decoction

qīng pí tāng

Source   *Formulas to Aid the Living* (1253)

Citri reticulatae viride Pericarpium (*qīng pí*) 4.5-6g
ginger Magnoliae officinalis Cortex (*jiāng hòu pò*) 9-12g
Atractylodis macrocephalae Rhizoma (*bái zhú*) 9-12g
Tsaoko Fructus (*cǎo guǒ*) 6-9g
Bupleuri Radix (*chái hú*) 9-12g
Poria (*fú líng*) 9-12g
Pinelliae Rhizoma praeparatum (*zhì bàn xià*) 9-12g
Scutellariae Radix (*huáng qín*) 9-12g
Glycyrrhizae Radix praeparata (*zhì gān cǎo*) 1.5-3g

Method of Preparation   The source text advises to grind equal amounts of the herbs into a coarse mixture, prepare 12g of the mixture as a decoction, and take with 5 pieces of Zingiberis Rhizoma recens (*shēng jiāng*). At present, it is prepared as a decoction with a small amount of wine and is taken 2-3 times, beginning three hours before the onset of an attack (if the attacks are regular).

Actions   Harmonizes and resolves, clears heat, dries dampness, transforms phlegm, moves the qi, and improves the Spleen's transportive function

Indications

Alternating fever and chills (fever predominant) or fever without chills, focal distention, loss of appetite, a bitter taste in the mouth, irritability, thirst, dark urine, constipation, a yellow, greasy tongue coating, and a rapid, wiry pulse.

This is pure heat malaria (癉瘧 *dān nuè*) or warm malaria (溫瘧 *wēn nuè*) due to constraint arising from phlegm-dampness trapping heat. This accounts for the more severe heat signs of this type of malaria. During an attack, the fever is distinctly more pronounced than the chills, which may even be completely absent. Phlegm-dampness causes the pathogen to linger in the greater yin. Obstruction of the Spleen's transportive function manifests as focal distention and constipation. Constraint affects the lesser yang as well because it is the pathway for both qi and fluids. Yang qi constraint transforming into heat within the lesser yang manifests as irritability, a bitter taste, and dark urine. The physiological fluids are damaged, causing thirst. The yellow, greasy tongue coating and the rapid, wiry pulse indicate that the constraint caused by phlegm-dampness is generating heat.

Analysis of Formula

This is a variation of Minor Bupleurum Decoction *(xiǎo chái hú tāng)*, modified to treat pure heat malaria. The chief herbs are Bupleuri Radix *(chái hú)* and Scutellariae Radix *(huáng qín)*, a long-established combination for resolving the lesser yang, venting pathogens, and clearing heat. *Treasury of Words on the Materia Medica* observes that "Bupleuri Radix *(chái hú)* is the best [herb] for clearing the muscles and reducing fever. However, without Scutellariae Radix *(huáng qín)*, it can neither cool the muscles nor thrust out the exterior." Tsaoko Fructus *(cǎo guǒ)* and Pinelliae Rhizoma praeparatum *(zhì bàn xià)* are utilized as deputies to dry the dampness and transform the phlegm, opening the qi dynamic to facilitate the venting of the pathogen.

There are two groups of assistants. The first, Citri reticulatae viride Pericarpium *(qīng pí)* and Magnoliae officinalis Cortex *(hòu pò)*, moves the qi to expel the fullness and dry the dampness in accordance with the principles that "When the qi is transformed, dampness will also be transformed" and "When [the movement of] qi is smooth, phlegm will be eliminated." The second group of assistants, Atractylodis macrocephalae Rhizoma *(bái zhú)* and Poria *(fú líng)*, strengthens the Spleen, augments the qi, and dispels dampness. Not only do these herbs remove the cause of dampness, they also help to eliminate any excess fluid from the body. Glycyrrhizae Radix praeparata *(zhì gān cǎo)* serves as the envoy, harmonizing the formula and moderating its harshness. As a whole, the formula thus strengthens the normal qi while dispelling the pathogenic. It focuses on the Spleen but effectively vents pathogens from the lesser yang and the muscles.

Cautions and Contraindications

This formula is contraindicated for malarial disorders without phlegm-dampness.

Commentary

Although the formula professes to 'clear' the Spleen, the term is used here with a slightly different than usual meaning. The Ming-dynasty writer Wu Kun explained: "[Clearing here] does not mean clearing [in order to cool]. Rather, by attacking and eliminating the pathogen, the entire Spleen system is cleared." *(Investigations of Medical Formulas)*

Other commentators, including Zhang Lu and Wang Zi-Jie, argued that clearing refers to the lesser yang, which is obstructed by phlegm-dampness. Yet another current, represented by Wang Xu-Gao and He Lian-Chen, maintained that the formula checks malaria by flushing lurking pathogens from the membrane source, assuming that they have become stuck there by the presence of phlegm-dampness.

The most comprehensive explanation of this formula's action is perhaps provided by Ke Qin, quoted in the *Golden Mirror of the Medical Tradition*. Ke argued that the formula eliminates phlegm-dampness from the Spleen by focusing on moving the Stomach yang. The heat that dominates in pure heat malaria is, in fact, generated by obstruction of these yang functions by phlegm-dampness. The strategy devised by Yan Yong-He, the author of this formula, to deal with this problem was to separate the yin and yang pathogens, eliminating phlegm-dampness accumulation by facilitating downward-directing, and clearing heat constraint by venting it outward via the lesser yang.

Because this formula checks malaria while supporting the normal qi, it is commonly used to treat malarial disorders during pregnancy.

Comparison

➤ Vs. White Tiger plus Cinnamon Twig Decoction *(bái hǔ jiā guì zhī tāng)*

Both formulas can be used to treat pure heat or warm malaria characterized by little or no chills and a high fever that is accompanied by joint pain, thirst, nausea, and vomiting. White Tiger plus Cinnamon Twig Decoction *(bái hǔ jiā guì zhī tāng)* focuses on clearing heat from the yang brightness and facilitating the circulation of the nutritive qi. It is indicated for cases with very high fever, thirst, and distress. Clear the Spleen Decoction *(qīng pí tāng)* is used when phlegm-dampness traps lurking heat, indicated by signs of fullness in the membrane source (the epigastrium and hypochondria) and a bitter taste in the mouth.

Biomedical Indications

With the appropriate presentation, this formula may be used to treat malaria and similar biomedically-defined disorders.

....

Alternate names

Clear the Spleen Drink *(qīng pí yǐn zi)* in *Synopsis for Protecting Infants*; Clear the Spleen Drink *(qīng pí yǐn)* in *Comprehensive Outline on Benefiting Yin*; Nine-Ingredient Clear the Spleen Decoction *(jiǔ wèi qīng pí tāng)* in *New Discussion of Epidemic Diarrheal Diseases*

....

Modifications

- To strengthen the antipathogenic action of the formula, add Dichroae Radix *(cháng shān)* and Arecae Semen *(bīng láng)*.

- For severe fever, add Gypsum fibrosum *(shí gāo)*.

- For cases with pronounced phlegm-dampness, add Citri reticulatae Pericarpium *(chén pí)* and Atractylodis Rhizoma *(cāng zhú)*.

- For patients with a weak constitution and qi deficiency, add Ginseng Radix *(rén shēn)*.

達原飲 （达原饮）

Reach the Source Drink

dá yuán yǐn

The name of this formula is a play on two different meanings of the word 'source.' The chief herbs reach the level of the membrane source from which they expel the pathogenic qi that is regarded as the source of the epidemic disorders treated by this formula.

Source   *Discussion of Warm Epidemics* (1642)

Tsaoko Fructus (*cǎo guǒ*) 1.5g
Magnoliae officinalis Cortex (*hòu pò*) 3g
Arecae Semen (*bīng láng*) 6g
Scutellariae Radix (*huáng qín*) 3g
Anemarrhenae Rhizoma (*zhī mǔ*) 3g
Paeoniae Radix alba (*bái sháo*) 3g
Glycyrrhizae Radix (*gān cǎo*) 1.5g

Method of Preparation   Decoction. The source text recommends taking the decoction warm in the afternoon.

Actions   Opens the membrane source by thrusting out pathogens, clears away filth, and transforms turbidity

Indications

Alternating fever and chills (both strong) occurring 1-3 times a day at irregular intervals, a stifling sensation in the chest, nausea or vomiting, headache, irritability, and scanty, turbid, yellow urine. The tongue has deep-red edges and a thick, foul, and pasty coating. The pulse is wiry and rapid, and neither floating nor submerged.

This is foul turbidity entering the body via the nose and mouth to lodge in the membrane source (膜原 *mó yuán*). The membrane source is closely associated with the Triple Burner and its dual function of circulating yang qi and body fluids. Foul turbidity generates dampness, which compresses the yang qi in the interior. The ensuing battle between the strong pathogenic influence and the strong normal qi is expressed in intense fever and chills that appear at irregular intervals. Constraint of the qi dynamic by turbid dampness is also expressed in a stifling sensation in the chest, nausea, vomiting, and headache. Irritability, scanty, turbid, and yellow urine, and a rapid, wiry pulse reflect damp-heat from constraint. The pulse is neither floating nor submerged, reflecting the location of the pathogen in the membrance source, or the half-interior, half exterior. The tongue, with its dark-red edges and thick, foul, pasty coating in the center, precisely mirrors the nature of the pathology of turbid yin constraining yang.

Analysis of Formula

Appropriate treatment requires an appreciation of the complexity of this condition. The sweating method cannot be utilized because the pathogenic influences are not lodged in the exterior. Purgatives cannot be used because there is no clumping in the Stomach. The proper method of treatment is to transform the turbidity at the level of the membrane source, clear the heat, regulate the qi, and transform the dampness.

The three chief herbs in the formula effectively address this complex pattern. Tsaoko Fructus (*cǎo guǒ*) is an aromatic herb that transforms turbidity and thereby stops the vomiting and vents the pathogenic influences lurking in the half-exterior, half-interior level. Magnoliae officinalis Cortex (*hòu pò*), also an aromatic herb, transforms turbidity, expels dampness, and regulates the qi. Arecae Semen (*bīng láng*) disperses dampness and reduces stagnation by facilitating the flow of qi, thereby hastening the elimination of the pathogenic influences from the interior. The strong, acrid, and aromatic properties of these herbs enable them to reach and open up the membrane source, which is constrained by turbidity. Wu You-Ke, the author of this formula, sums this up in *Discussion of Warm Epidemics*: "Joining in a common effort, these three herbs directly reach the lair [where the pathogen hides] to rout the pathogenic qi, which thereupon quickly leaves the membrane source. This is what is meant by reaching the source."

The remaining four herbs in the formula deal with the secondary consequences of heat constraint, but do not actively contribute to the expulsion of the pathogenic qi. Scutellariae Radix (*huáng qín*), a deputy herb, clears heat and dries dampness. It is particularly useful for treating damp-heat in the Stomach and Gallbladder. Anemarrhenae Rhizoma (*zhī mǔ*), another deputy, clears heat, nourishes the yin, and prevents heat from injuring the yin and fluids. Paeoniae Radix alba (*bái sháo*), the third deputy, prevents the acrid, drying properties of the other herbs from damaging the yin and blood. The envoy, Glycyrrhizae Radix (*gān cǎo*), harmonizes the actions of the herbs in the formula.

Cautions and Contraindications

This formula is unsuitable for treating damp-warmth disorders where the manifestations of heat are stronger than those of dampness, or for lurking heat and constrained dampness. Furthermore, its use must be discontinued once the obstruction of the qi dynamic has been opened and the pathogen discharged. Such cases will often transmute into a heat pattern, as the yang qi that was previously pressed toward the interior now forcefully moves toward the outside. Repeated and inappropriate administration of this formula will cause ministerial fire to flare upward, stirring internal Liver wind with spasms and convulsions.

Commentary

The membrane source (膜原 *mó yuán*) is an anatomical structure first mentioned in Chapter 39 of *Basic Questions*, where it denotes an undefined entity located somewhere above the Stomach and Intestines. Later commentators took this as referring to a space in the region of the diaphragm. The concept is also connected with the 'vitals' (膏肓 *gāo huāng*), an area traditionally associated with difficult to cure disorders. From the 16th century onward, the membrane source became a concept of great importance to physicians associated with the warm pathogen disorder current, who viewed is as part of the half-exterior, half-interior aspect of the body. The famous Suzhou physician Xue Sheng-Bai observed: "The membrane source connects with the muscles and flesh in the exterior and with the yin and yang organs in the interior. It is the gate of the Triple Burner. In fact, it is the entire body's half-exterior, half-interior." (*Systematic Differentiation of Damp-Heat Disorders*)

At present, some conjecture that the anatomical substrate of the membrane source is the greater omentum, while others take it to be the pleura and peritoneum, or the membranes covering all the internal organs.

This formula was composed by the Ming-dynasty physician Wu You-Ke specifically for the treatment of epidemic disorders. Wu believed that such epidemics were caused by special types of pestilential qi (癘氣 *lì qì*) that differed from ordinary seasonal pathogens in the way they enter the body and where they reside once they have done so. Whereas seasonal pathogens enter through the pores and then penetrate to the channels and organs, epidemic qi enters through the mouth and nose to hide in the membrane source, where ordinary treatment strategies cannot reach it. In his main work, *Discussion of Warm Epidemics*, Wu You-Ke explained this disease dynamic:

> The pathogen enters through the nose and mouth. The place where it lodges is neither in the yin and yang organs of the inner aspect [of the body] nor in the channels of the outer aspect. It resides along both sides of the spine. [This space] is not far from the outer aspect and is next to the Stomach. It is on the boundary of the inner and outer aspects, half outer and half inner. According to the acupuncture classics, it is traversed by the membrane source.

Wu also identified an entirely new class of pathogens called heteropathic qi (雜氣 *zá qì*) that was responsible for epidemic disorders. Unlike seasonal pathogenic qi, heteropathic qi possesses distinctive characteristics that, once they had entered a person, cause the same kind of disorder irrespective of constitution, season, or other contextual factors. This, Wu argued, necessitated an entirely new approach to the treatment of these disorders. Rather than treating disorders based on pattern differentiation and taking into account the interplay of pathogenic and normal qi, the heteropathic qi had simply to be dislodged from its hiding place in the membrane source.

Many historians view Wu You-Ke's new doctrine as prefiguring Western ideas about specific pathogens by several

centuries. In Ming and Qing China, however, they did not lead to the development of a new medicine but were instead assimilated into traditional concepts of disease causation and dynamics. The modern textbook interpretation of Reach the Source Drink (*dá yuán yǐn*) as expelling damp-warmth pathogens from the middle burner is the product of this assimilative process. The early 20th-century physician Zhang Xi-Chun observed the potential dangers of this process and recommended that it only be used for early-stage epidemic disorders, which he considered to be contagious and spread by bacteria, and not for warm pathogen disorders, which he considered to be either contractions of seasonal warm qi or simply of externally-contracted cold that lurks in the membrane source for some time and transforms into heat to stir at an opportune moment.

In contemporary practice, venting of pathogens from the membrane source is defined by the combined use of the herbs Arecae Semen (*bīng láng*), Tsaoko Fructus (*cǎo guǒ*), and Magnoliae officinalis Cortex (*hòu pò*). Many physicians also view the development of a powdery coating on the tongue that looks like rice flour or curdled tofu to be the cardinal sign for the use of this formula. The coating is thought to reflect the trapping in the interior of strong yang protective qi by foul turbidity. The yang qi is unable to break through the constraint caused by the pathological dampness, hence the coating does not necessarily change in color from white to yellow. However, the strong heat in the interior consumes the fluids within this dampness, causing it to become dryish. It is important to note, however, that the source text itself does not specify this type of tongue coating.

Other key symptoms of the strong internal heat are headaches and fever. However, because the membrane source connects to all other parts of the body, the heat can break through anywhere. This accounts for the multitude of other symptoms associated with a Reach the Source Drink (*dá yuán yǐn*) presentation in the clinic. Zhou Xue-Hai's summary shows how far the definition of the disorder had changed by the late Qing:

> When a pathogen enters the membrane source there will often be a faint unease throughout the body. [This may manifest as] constant dizziness, constant sweating, constant fear of heat or cold, sudden shortness of breath, inability to carry out one's work, weakness of the four extremities, heat in the soles and palms, dark and rough urination, constant diarrhea or constipation, inability to digest, increased thirst, little appetite, a thick, greasy tongue coating, inability to sleep at night, or diverse and confused dreams. The manner in which [the disorder finally] discharges depends on the degree of toxicity of the pathogen and the strength or weakness of the normal qi. Cold transformation manifests in a warm [pathogen disorder] due to yang exuberance. Wind transformation manifests as diarrhea due to yin exuberance. [Summer-]heat transformation manifests as a malarial disorder where [the disorder] discharges through the exterior. Dampness transformation manifests as coughing

where [the disorder] discharges through the interior. It can also discharge in the form of painful obstruction with a sensation as if the body was filled with countless peach and plum pits that does not improve. It can also discharge [in the form of] faint/deep rashes (隱疹 *yǐn zhěn*) limited to one extremity or one location. These can emit year after year at distinctive periods in time without there [appearing to be] a permanent cure. (*Random Notes while Reading about Medicine*)

Many contemporary physicians prefer to use Bupleurum Drink to Reach the Source (*chái hú dá yuán yǐn*), discussed below, which they believe is more suitable for treating non-epidemic disorders.

Comparison

➢ Vs. Bupleurum Drink to Reach the Source (*chái hú dá yuán yǐn*)

Both of these formulas treat malarial disorders due to obstruction of the membrane source by foul turbidity. Reach the Source Drink (*dá yuán yǐn*) focuses on forcefully expelling foul turbidity. It is indicated where both the pathogenic qi and constitution are strong. This is reflected in more pronounced heat signs such as a rapid pulse and a yellow, greasy tongue coating. Bupleurum Drink to Reach the Source (*chái hú dá yuán yǐn*) focuses on phlegm-dampness obstructing the qi dynamic. This is reflected in focal distention and a white, coarse tongue coating that looks like rice flour or curdled cheese.

Biomedical Indications

With the appropriate presentation, this formula may be used to treat malaria, influenza, and similar biomedically-defined disorders.

Modifications

- For pain in the hypochondria, diminished hearing, and a bitter taste in the mouth, add Bupleuri Radix (*chái hú*). (source text)

- For back and neck pain, add Notopterygii Rhizoma seu Radix (*qiāng huó*). (source text)

- For pain in the orbital and frontal areas with dry nasal passages and insomnia, add Puerariae Radix (*gé gēn*). (source text)

- For fever and chills (chills predominant), marked distention, a sensation of heaviness in the limbs, and an extremely thick tongue coating (indicating the predominance of dampness), remove Paeoniae Radix alba (*bái sháo*) and Anemarrhenae Rhizoma (*zhī mǔ*) and add Eupatorii Herba (*pèi lán*) and Artemisiae scopariae Herba (*yīn chén*).

- For conditions that worsen in the afternoon and evening (indicating the predominance of heat), remove Arecae Semen (*bīng láng*) and add Gardeniae Fructus (*zhī zǐ*) and Cynanchi atrati Radix (*bái wēi*).

Associated Formulas

加減達原飲 （加減达原饮）

Modified Reach the Source Drink

jiā jiǎn dá yuán yǐn

Source   *Warp and Woof of Warm Heat Diseases* (1852)

Bupleuri Radix (*chái hú*)	4.5g
Magnoliae officinalis Cortex (*hòu pò*)	3g
Arecae Semen (*bīng láng*)	12g
Tsaoko Fructus (*cǎo guǒ*)	3g
Pogostemonis/Agastaches Herba (*huò xiāng*)	6g
Atractylodis Rhizoma (*cāng zhú*)	6g
Pinelliae Rhizoma praeparatum (*zhì bàn xià*)	6g
Acori tatarinowii Rhizoma (*shí chāng pǔ*)	1.8g
Six-to-One Powder (*liù yī sǎn*) (wrapped in cheese cloth)	1.5g

Prepare as a decoction. Opens damp constraint, vents the membrane source, and aromatically transforms foulness. For damp-heat obstructing the membrane source characterized by alternating fever and chills, lack of appetite, inability to differentiate flavors, and a white, greasy tongue coating. This is a modification of Reach the Source Drink (*dá yuán yǐn*) and Calm the Stomach Powder (*píng wèi sǎn*), originally authored by Xue Sheng-Bai and later modified by Wang Shi-Xiong. It is suitable for treating damp-warmth patterns characterized by alternating cold and heat where the symptoms of dampness are more pronounced than those of heat.

雷氏宣透膜原法

Lei's Method for Disseminating and Venting [Dampness and Heat from] the Membrane Source

Léi shì xuān tòu mó yuán fǎ

Source   *Discussion of Seasonal Diseases* (1882)

Magnoliae officinalis Cortex (*hòu pò*)	3g
Arecae Semen (*bīng láng*)	4.5g
Tsaoko Fructus (*cǎo guǒ*)	2.4g
Scutellariae Radix (*huáng qín*)	3g
Glycyrrhizae Radix (*gān cǎo*)	1.5g
Pogostemonis/Agastaches Folium (*huò xiāng yè*)	3g
Pinelliae Rhizoma praeparatum (*zhì bàn xià*)	6g
Zingiberis Rhizoma recens (*shēng jiāng*)	3 pieces

Decoction. Dispels and disperses turbid dampness from the membrane source. For turbid dampness obstructing the membrane source in a patient with a weak middle burner. Constraint of the membrane source by turbid dampness in a patient whose yang qi is weak does not generate as much heat as in the patient treated by the original formula. This is reflected in a tongue covered with a thick, white, powdery coating but no red edges. Other heat symptoms such as dark urine, restlessness, and high fever will also be less pronounced. Thus, the present formula replaces herbs that drain heat and nourish the yin with those that assist qi transformation in the middle burner. The resulting formula is considerably more warm and drying than the original. That being the case, even more care must be taken to stop using it once the pathological obstruction has been resolved and the fire begins to discharge through the Triple Burner.

柴胡達原飲 （柴胡达原饮）

Bupleurum Drink to Reach the Source

chái hú dá yuán yǐn

SOURCE *Revised Popular Guide to the Discussion of Cold Damage* (Qing dynasty)

Bupleuri Radix (chái hú) 4.5g
Magnoliae officinalis Cortex (hòu pò) 4.5
Aurantii Fructus (zhǐ ké) 4.5
Citri reticulatae viride Pericarpium (qīng pí) 4.5g
Glycyrrhizae Radix praeparata (zhì gān cǎo) 2.1g
Scutellariae Radix (huáng qín) 4.5g
Platycodi Radix (jié gěng) 3g
Tsaoko Fructus (cǎo guǒ) 1.8g
Arecae Semen (bīng láng) 6g
Nelumbinis Folium (hé yè) 9-15g

Transforms phlegm and dampness, vents disorders at the level of the membrane source. For phlegm-dampness obstructing the membrane source characterized by focal distention and fullness in the chest and epigastrium, irritability, dizziness or vertigo, a pasty sensation in the mouth, cough with sputum that is difficult to expectorate, intermittent fever and chills, a thick, white tongue coating that looks powdery and coarse like rice flour, and a wiry, slippery pulse. This condition is similar to that for which the principal formula is indicated, but with the addition of lesser yang signs and symptoms. To deal with these symptoms, Yu Gen-Chu, the author of the formula, added herbs like Bupleuri Radix (chái hú), Platycodi Radix (jié gěng), and Nelumbinis Folium (hé yè) that facilitate the rise of clear qi. Combined with downward-directing herbs like Magnoliae officinalis Cortex (hòu pò), Arecae Semen (bīng láng), and Citri reticulatae viride Pericarpium (qīng pí), the entire formula focuses more on opening the qi dynamic rather than on removing pathogenic or pestilential qi. For this reason, the early modern physician He Lian-Chen described it as "more nimble in its action" when compared to Wu You-Ke's original formula. Accordingly, it has become the formula of choice for many contemporary physicians when treating patterns associated with obstruction of the membrane source.

Comparison

➤ VS. REACH THE SOURCE DRINK (dá yuán yǐn);
　 see PAGE 139

柴胡桂薑湯 （柴胡桂姜汤）

Bupleurum, Cinnamon Twig, and Ginger Decoction

chái hú guì jiāng tāng

Source *Essentials from the Golden Cabinet* (c. 220)

Bupleuri Radix (chái hú) 24g
Cinnamomi Ramulus (guì zhī) 9g
Zingiberis Rhizoma (gān jiāng) 6g
Trichosanthis Radix (tiān huā fěn) 12g
Scutellariae Radix (huáng qín) 9g
Ostreae Concha (mǔ lì) 9g
Glycyrrhizae Radix praeparata (zhì gān cǎo) 9g

Method of Preparation Decoction. The method of preparation is the same as that for Minor Bupleurum Decoction (xiǎo chái hú tāng).

Actions Harmonizes and releases the lesser yang, disperses clumping, warms the interior, and dispels cold

Indications

Malarial disorders with pronounced chills and only light fever, or chills without fever. The extremities are cold and the patient is averse to wind. Other symptoms include headache, pain in the hypochondria, and thirst. The tongue has a white, slippery coating, and the pulse is wiry and tight on the left or wiry and slow on the right.

This is normal malaria (正瘧 zhēng nüè) caused by a lurking summerheat pathogen that hides deep in the yin aspect of the lesser yang and is stirred by a newly-contracted wind-cold disorder in late autumn. The wind-cold in the exterior pushes the protective yang qi into the interior where it encounters the lurking summerheat pathogen. Because the force of this pathogen (whose disposition is to vent toward the exterior) is relatively weak compared with the pathogen in the surface (whose disposition is to move toward the interior), chills are more pronounced than fever. The additional symptoms are those of constrained protective qi and fluids within the lesser yang.

Paragraph 147 of *Discussion of Cold Damage* lists a formula under the name of Bupleurum, Cinnamon Twig, and Ginger Decoction (chái hú guì zhī gān jiāng tāng) that is virtually identical to the present formula, except that the dosage of Ostreae Concha (mǔ lì) and Glycyrrhizae Radix praeparata (zhì gān cǎo) has been reduced from 9g to 6g each. This formula is indicated for alternating fever and chills, a sensation of fullness with clumping in the chest and hypochondria, irritability in the chest, urinary difficulty, thirst, and sweating from the head. This is generally interpreted to be a lesser yang disorder that is accompanied by fluids clumping in the interior.

A cold pathogen constraining the yang qi in the lesser yang Gallbladder channel will readily disrupt the circulation of fluids governed by the Triple Burner. In this case, fluids and constrained heat clump in the interior in the region of the hypochondria and diaphragm. This manifests as a sensation of fullness in the chest and hypochondria. As the qi dynamic of the lesser yang Triple Burner loses its regularity, the body is no longer irrigated, causing thirst above and urinary difficulty below. Heat constraint in the lesser yang Gallbladder, meanwhile, manifests in alternating chills and fever. Because the clumped water and heat cannot move downward, it rises upward to exit from the head as sweat. It also moves against the Heart, causing irritability. Although other lesser yang symptoms (e.g., wiry pulse, dizziness, bitter taste) are not specifically listed in the source text, they can also be present.

Analysis of Formula

This is a variation of Bupleurum and Cinnamon Twig Decoction (*chái hú guì zhī tāng*). The chief herbs are Cinnamomi Ramulus (*guì zhī*) and Bupleuri Radix (*chái hú*), which dredge constraint of protective qi in the exterior. The former disperses newly-contracted wind-cold, while the latter vents the lesser yang. Two deputies, Scutellariae Radix (*huáng qín*) and Ostreae Concha (*mǔ lì*), assist this action by focusing on the lurking heat in the interior. Scutellariae Radix (*huáng qín*) drains heat from the lesser yang, while Ostreae Concha (*mǔ lì*) is generally thought to work together with Cinnamomi Ramulus (*guì zhī*). Ostreae Concha (*mǔ lì*) has a long history in the treatment of malarial disorders, for which it is specifically indicated in *Divine Husbandman's Classic of the Materia Medica*. While its cooling action is of undoubted importance, its ability to soften and thereby remove constraint is equally useful. The modern text *One Hundred Supremely Effective Medicinals* thus recommends it for expelling pathogens from the greater yang, lesser yang, and terminal yin channels.

Two assistants, Trichosanthis Radix (*tiān huā fěn*) and Zingiberis Rhizoma (*gān jiāng*), support the function of the middle burner as the fulcrum of the qi dynamic. Trichosanthis Radix (*tiān huā fěn*) enriches the fluids of the Stomach, which have been damaged by heat constraint. Zingiberis Rhizoma (*gān jiāng*) warms the yang qi of the Spleen, enabling it to transform accumulated fluids. Glycyrrhizae Radix praeparata (*zhì gān cǎo*) functions as the envoy to harmonize the opposing flavors and qualities of the herbs in the formula, enabling them to disperse the pathogens that are at the root of this disorder while replenishing the body's own true qi.

The effectiveness of this formula in treating a lesser yang disorder accompanied by fluids clumping in the interior is based on the same synergistic effects.

Cautions and Contraindications

This formula treats a pattern of mixed excess and deficiency. It should not be prescribed for patterns of pure excess or deficiency.

Commentary

Most classical and modern commentators view this formula as part of the wider category of Bupleuri Radix (*chái hú*) formulas. As such, the clinical presentation of any condition for which it may be used must include the signs and symptoms, such as fullness and distention of the flanks and chest, or alternating fever and chills, that are typical of these formulas. Based on a doctrine first put forward by the Kampo physician Odai Yōdō, modern Chinese experts in cold damage therapeutics such as Liu Du-Zhou also argue that, provided such signs are present, the additional symptom of soft stools or diarrhea is the key indicator for use of this formula. They base this argument on two observations. First, the use of Zingib-

eris Rhizoma (*gān jiāng*) invariably indicates the presence of diarrhea in Zhang Zhong-Jing's therapeutic system. Second, according to paragraph 147 of *Discussion of Cold Damage*, the formula is used for a pattern that occurs in patients that have first been treated by inducing sweating and then by purgation. This is understood to mean that the yang in the interior has become deficient, leading to soft stools.

In the case histories published by Liu Du-Zhou and others, diarrhea or soft stools are often accompanied by reduced urination. This indicates that the condition cannot be one of simple yang deficiency (where urination would usually be increased), but that it must also involve damage to the yin fluids. An even more comprehensive interpretation of the formula's function thus focuses on the physiological interpenetration of the yang qi, with its protective function, and the yang fluids, which moisten as they move from the interior of the body to the exterior by way of the lesser yang. If this movement is constrained, water and fire lose their smooth interpenetration. Clumping together, they deprive the middle burner of both yang qi and yin fluids, even though neither is quantitatively deficient. In addition to diarrhea accompanied by reduced urination, this manifests in apparently contradictory symptoms like simultaneous fatigue and restlessness; depression accompanied by irritability or insomnia; or pallor with easy flushing of the head and neck.

At present, this formula is frequently prescribed for psychoemotional disorders, although its ability to harmonize the yin and yang and to disperse pathogens while strengthening the normal qi gives it a far wider range of possible applications. Contemporary Chinese internal medicine physicians thus use it to treat Liver and Gallbladder heat that occurs concurrently with Spleen and Stomach cold. Gynecologists think of it as a formula that can be used to readjust the harmonious interplay of qi, blood, and water that is so crucial to female physiology. Yet others exploit the ability of Ostreae Concha (*mǔ lì*) to disperse knotting and soften hardness and use this formula for the treatment of acne, scrofula, fibroadenoma of the breasts, or early stage cirrhosis.

Comparison

> Vs. Bupleurum and Cinnamon Twig Decoction (*chái hú guì zhī tāng*)

Both formulas treat conditions where a lesser yang-warp disorder is accompanied by an inability of the yang qi to properly control the circulation of fluids. Hence, both formulas manifest with symptoms of fever and chills as well as fluid accumulation. However, in a Bupleurum and Cinnamon Twig Decoction (*chái hú guì zhī tāng*) presentation, the dispersion of protective yang and fluids is constrained in the greater yang through cold in the exterior. This causes joint pain, fever, and slight chills. Furthermore, the yang qi that is unable to penetrate to the surface invades the Stomach, causing slight nausea. In a Bupleurum, Cinnamon Twig, and Ginger Decoction *(chái hú guì zhī gān jiāng tāng)* presentation, the dispersion of protective yang and fluids is constrained in the lesser yang Gallbladder and Triple Burner. This causes alternating fever and chills, clumping of heat and fluids in the body regions controlled by the lesser yang, thirst, and inhibited urination. The Stomach is not affected, however, hence there is no nausea.

➤ Vs. FIVE-ACCUMULATION POWDER *(wǔ jī sǎn)*; *see* PAGE 298

Biomedical Indications

With the appropriate presentation, this formula may be used to treat a variety of biomedically-defined disorders. These can be divided into the following groups:

- Acute infectious diseases such as the common cold, malaria, hepatitis, meningitis, pulmonary tuberculosis, pneumonia, and urinary tract infection
- Digestive problems such as bacillary dysentery, allergic colitis, chronic hepatitis, cholecystitis, postcholecystectomy diarrhea, gastritis, and peptic ulcers
- Those marked by nodularity such as scrofula, fibrocystic breast disease, and cirrhosis.

This formula has also been used for perimenopausal syndrome, postpartum fever, leukorrhea, erectile dysfunction, sinus tachycardia, gastric ptosis, insomnia, Ménière's disese, and diabetes.

Modifications

- For the early stages of malaria, add Dichroae Radix *(cháng shān)*.
- For dry coughs from damage to the fluids, add Asparagi Radix *(tiān mén dōng)* and Polygonati odorati Rhizoma *(yù zhú)*.
- For vertigo, add Alismatis Rhizoma *(zé xiè)* and Atractylodis macrocephalae Rhizoma *(bái zhú)*.
- For thirst with edema, take with Five-Ingredient Powder with Poria *(wǔ líng sǎn)*.
- For biliary system complaints, add Corydalis Rhizoma *(yán hú suǒ)*, Cyperi Rhizoma *(xiāng fù)*, and Toosendan Fructus *(chuān liàn zǐ)*.

Comparative Tables of Principal Formulas

■ FORMULAS THAT HARMONIZE LESSER YANG-WARP DISORDERS

Common symptoms: sensation of fullness in the chest and hypochondria, wiry pulse

Formula Name	Diagnosis	Indications	Remarks
Minor Bupleurum Decocotion *(xiǎo chái hú tāng)*	Lesser yang-warp disorder	Alternating fever and chills, dry throat, bitter taste, irritability, fullness in the chest and hypochondria, nausea and vomiting, being downcast with no desire to eat, a thin, white tongue coating, and a wiry pulse	Also indicated for a wide range of disorders including heat entering the blood chamber.
Sweet Wormwood and Scutellaria Decoction to Clear the Gallbladder *(hāo qín qīng dǎn tāng)*	Damp-heat and turbid phlegm in the lesser yang channels constraining the protective and nutritive qi	Mild chills alternating with pronounced fever, bitter taste, spitting up bitter or sour fluids, thirst, distention and pain in the chest and hypochondria, a red tongue with a thick, greasy white, and/or yellow coating, and a rapid pulse that is slippery on the right and wiry on the left	Also treats lesser yang channel damp-heat symptoms such as tinnitus or urinary obstruction and systemic damp-heat manifestations like night sweats.
Bupleurum plus Dragon Bone and Oyster Shell Decoction *(chái hú jiā lóng gǔ mǔ lì tāng)*	Problems in all three of the yang channels	Fullness in the chest, irritability, palpitations, urinary difficulty, constipation, delirious speech, sensation of heaviness, a red tongue with a slippery coating, and a wiry, rapid pulse	A pattern characterized by excess as well as deficiency with symptoms in all three burners and in all yang organs.

■ FORMULAS THAT REGULATE AND HARMONIZE THE LIVER AND SPLEEN

Common symptoms: hypochondriac or abdominal pain, wiry pulse

Formula Name	Diagnosis	Indications	Remarks
Frigid Extremities Powder (*sì nì sǎn*)	Yang- or hot-type inversion due to internal constraint of yang qi	Cold fingers and toes with a warm head and body, a sensation of irritability and fullness in the chest and epigastrium, cough, urinary difficulty, abdominal pain and severe diarrhea, a red tongue with a yellow coating, and a wiry pulse	Also used to treat various digestive problems due to Liver-Spleen disharmony.
Rambling Powder (*xiāo yáo sǎn*)	Liver constraint with blood deficiency and a frail Spleen	Hypochondriac pain, headache, vertigo, a bitter taste in the mouth, dry mouth and throat, fatigue, reduced appetite, a pale-red tongue, and a wiry, deficient pulse	Commonly used in internal medicine and in the treatment of women's disorders.
Important Formula for Painful Diarrhea (*tòng xiè yào fāng*)	Painful diarrhea due to Spleen deficiency with an overcontrolling Liver	Recurrent problems of borborygmus, abdominal pain, diarrhea with pain (which starts with the urge to defecate and subsides after completion), a thin, white tongue coating, and a wiry, moderate or wiry, thin pulse	Especially useful in treating chronic diarrhea, and diarrhea in deficient patients or the elderly.

■ FORMULAS THAT HARMONIZE THE STOMACH AND INTESTINES

Common symptoms: abdominal pain and distention, nausea or vomiting, borborygmus, diarrhea

Formula Name	Diagnosis	Indications	Remarks
Pinellia Decoction to Drain the Epigastrium (*bàn xià xiè xīn tāng*)	Clumping of constrained heat and fluids in the epigastrium	Epigastric focal distention, fullness and tightness with very slight or no pain, dry heaves or vomiting, borborygmus with diarrhea, reduced appetite, a thin, yellow, and greasy tongue coating that may be red at the tip, and a wiry, rapid pulse	This pattern is referred to as clumping together of cold and heat.
Coptis Decoction (*huáng lián tāng*)	Heat above and cold below due to an external cold pathogen transmitted into the middle burner	Stifling sensation and irritability in the chest, nausea, abdominal pain, a white, greasy tongue coating, and a wiry pulse. There may also be fever and slight chills along with borborygmus and diarrhea.	Focuses on regulating ascending and downward-directing to facilitate the reconnection of yin and yang.

■ FORMULAS THAT TREAT MALARIAL DISORDERS AND VENT PATHOGENS FROM THE MEMBRANE SOURCE

Common symptoms: alternating fever and chills, greasy tongue coating, wiry pulse

Formula Name	Diagnosis	Indications	Remarks
Seven-Treasure Drink to Check Malarial Disorders (*jié nuè qī bǎo yǐn*)	Phlegm-dampness malarial disorder	Intense, unremitting attacks of alternating fever and chills, abdominal distention, a greasy, white tongue coating, and a wiry, slippery, floating, and large pulse at the distal position	Also used to treat excess-type malarial disorders not due to dampness and phlegm.
Clear the Spleen Decoction (*qīng pí tāng*)	Pure heat malaria or warm malaria	Alternating fever and chills (fever predominant) or fever without chills, focal distention, loss of appetite, a bitter taste in the mouth, thirst, constipation, a yellow, greasy tongue coating, and a rapid, wiry pulse	Focuses on the Spleen but effectively vents pathogens from the lesser yang and muscles. Commonly used to treat malarial disorders during pregnancy.

cont. ↘

Formula Name	Diagnosis	Indications	Remarks
Reach the Source Drink (*dá yuán yǐn*)	Epidemic malarial disorder	Alternating fever and chills (both strong) occurring 1-3 times a day at irregular intervals, nausea or vomiting, headache, irritability, scanty and turbid urine, a tongue with deep-red edges and a thick, foul, and pasty coating, and a wiry, rapid pulse	Focuses on releasing pathogens by transforming turbidity in the membrane source; also used to treat influenza.
Bupleurum, Cinnamon Twig, and Ginger Decoction (*chái hú guì jiāng tāng*)	Normal malaria caused by an external cold pathogen encountering an internal lurking summerheat pathogen	Pronounced chills and only light fever or no fever, cold extremities, aversion to wind, headache, pain in the hypochondria, thirst, a white, slippery tongue coating, and a pulse that is either wiry and tight on the left or wiry and slow on the right	Also treats lesser yang disorders accompanied by clumping of fluids in the interior, or Liver-Gallbladder heat with Spleen-Stomach cold.

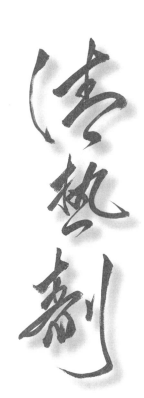

清熱劑

Chapter 4 Contents

Formulas that Clear Heat

Formulas that Clear Heat

4

THE TREATMENT STRATEGIES represented by the formulas in this chapter were first mentioned in the following passages from *Basic Questions:* "Cool what is hot" and "Use cold [substances] for hot causes" (Chapter 74); "Use clearing to treat warmth" and "Use cold [substances] to treat heat" (Chapter 70). The same idea is echoed in the *Divine Husbandman's Classic of the Materia Medica:* "Use cold medicines to treat heat." Among the eight methods of treatment, the formulas in this chapter utilize the clearing method (清法 *qīng fǎ*).

In its broadest sense, 'clearing heat' implies a process of purification and transformation that restores coolness and freshness to the body. The term is used to distinguish this strategy from others that address heat. The most important of these are purging, which treats the accumulation or clumping of heat in the interior (Chapter 3), and the venting of heat carried out by formulas that release the exterior and dispel wind-heat (Chapter 1). Heat-clearing formulas are used for all those problems where heat is present in the interior but where there are no signs of internal clumping that would imply a mixing of heat with body substances like fluids, phlegm, or stagnant food. Many modern textbooks thus refer to the former as 'heat without form' (無形之熱 *wú xíng zhī rè*) and to the latter as 'heat with form' (有形之熱 *yǒu xíng zhī rè*).

In a more narrow sense, clearing heat can be differentiated from 'draining fire' (泄火 *xiè huǒ*). Clearing removes the heat from the qi or blood levels without impeding their movement and transformation. To this end, one utilizes substances that are both acrid and cold like Mori Folium (*sāng yè*), Gypsum fibrosum (*shí gāo*), Bubali Cornu (*shuǐ niú jiǎo*), and Moutan Cortex (*mǔ dān pí*), or that unblock the pathways of qi in the Triple Burner like Gardeniae Fructus (*zhī zǐ*) or Lophatheri Herba (*dàn zhú yè*). By contrast, draining fire directs the fire downward and removes it from the body via the urine and bowels with herbs like Scutellariae Radix (*huáng qín*), Coptidis Rhizoma (*huáng lián*), Phellodendri Cortex (*huáng bǎi*), or Gentianae Radix (*lóng dǎn cǎo*). These herbs are very drying and readily damage the fluids. Their severe coldness can also damage the qi dynamic. For this reason, one should avoid using them too soon or in excessive amounts. Depending on the context, draining may be viewed as a mild form of purging, whereas clearing represents a venting of heat from deeper levels of the body.

The formulas in this chapter are grouped according to six major strategies. The first two, clearing heat in the qi level and clearing the nutritive and blood levels, are intimately associated with the theories of externally-contracted disease set forth in *Discussion of Cold Damage* and later by physicians associated with the warm pathogen disease current. Formulas that resolve toxicity are used for suppurative disorders or other conditions that present with the traditional manifestations of toxin with heat at the qi level. Formulas that clear heat from both the qi and blood levels combine strategies and formulas from the previous three groups to treat serious epidemic disorders that manifest with macular rashes or bleeding. The fifth strategy focuses on clearing heat from particular organs, which usually has a more localized presentation than is the case with other heat disorders. The sixth strategy is clearing heat from deficiency. This occurs when the blood or yin is severely depleted and is also called 'deficiency fire.'

Many other treatment strategies and formulas that rely on heat-clearing herbs to achieve their effect can be found in other chapters of this book. They include formulas that clear heat and open the orifices (Chapter 11), clear heat and extinguish internal wind (Chapter 14), clear heat and transform phlegm (Chapter 17), clear heat and stop bleeding (Chapter 13), clear damp-heat (Chapter 16), and release exterior-interior excess (Chapter 7).

In traditional Chinese medicine, the words 'warmth,' 'heat,' and 'fire' are often used interchangeably. The difference among them is one of degree and manifestation. Warmth is less intense than heat, while fire is more intense. Warmth and heat are terms that are more often applied to external pathogens, while fire is used to designate heat within specific organs. Fire is also used to describe conditions with grossly visible manifestations of heat such as bleeding, flushed face, and red eyes, even when the systemic level of heat is not particularly severe.

Before prescribing heat-clearing formulas, it is important to ascertain that there is no heat in the exterior and no clumping of heat in the interior. Should there be, one must clear the heat from the exterior or purge it, or use one of these strategies in conjunction with that of clearing heat. It is also important to clearly distinguish whether the condition is deficient or excessive in nature, and to identify the location (level and organ) of the disorder. Failure to do so will bring minimal results at best and may lead to complications.

Most of the herbs in these formulas are cold in nature. Cold substances readily injure the yang qi and produce cold. To avoid these side effects, it is important to include ingredients that protect the functions of the Stomach.

Most of these formulas are designed for treating relatively acute disorders. Their use should be discontinued once the heat has been successfully treated. It is also important to take the patient's overall condition or constitution into account. For example, great care must be exercised in treating a patient with long-standing yang deficiency who contracts a warm-heat pathogen disease. In this case, the cold ingredients in the formula must be used with utmost caution in order to prevent further injury to the yang. It is also essential to avoid mistaking the presence of false heat in patients with interior cold as a sign of excess heat. In that case, warming the interior will lead the floating fire back to its source.

If the use of heat-clearing formulas does not bring the desired effect, this is most likely due to deficiency of true yin. As described by Wang Bing, the Tang-dynasty editor of the *Inner Classic*: "Where [the use of] cold [herbs and formulas] does not [produce] cold, this is due to a lack of water." In such cases, enriching the yin and fortifying the water will clear the heat and reduce the fever.

Some patients with vigorous, blazing heat will vomit up orally-administered heat-clearing formulas. Should this occur, the addition of a small amount of ginger juice, or simply letting the decoction cool before taking it, will usually alleviate the problem.

Section 1

. . . .

FORMULAS THAT CLEAR QI-LEVEL HEAT

In Ye Tian-Shi's four-level system of differentiation (protective, qi, nutritive, and blood), qi-level disorders are marked by high fever, profuse sweating, irritability, thirst, and a flooding, large, and rapid pulse. This same presentation occurs in the yang brightness-warp channel disorder of the six-warp system of differentiation. Another type of qi-level disorder occurs when heat is not cleared during the recovery stage of a febrile disease, resulting in injury to both the qi and the yin. Manifestations include irritability, fever, sweating, and a sensation of constraint in the chest. Note that the presentation in both of these disorders includes thirst and irritability. The presence or absence of thirst often provides a clue for distinguishing this type of pattern from those lodged in either a deeper or more superficial level of the body.

The core ingredients in these formulas are those that clear heat and drain fire such as Gypsum fibrosum (*shí gāo*), Lophatheri Herba (*dàn zhú yè*), and Gardeniae Fructus (*zhī zǐ*).

Given the importance of the Stomach qi in these disorders, herbs that nourish the Stomach and harmonize the middle burner, such as Glycyrrhizae Radix (*gān cǎo*) and Nonglutinous rice (*jīng mǐ*), are often added.

Heat in the qi level often leads to high fevers and profuse sweating, which can damage the fluids. For this reason, it is common to add herbs that moisten and generate fluids such as Ginseng Radix (*rén shēn*), Ophiopogonis Radix (*mài mén dōng*), and Anemarrhenae Rhizoma (*zhī mǔ*).

When heat is constrained in the chest and diaphragm, it is helpful to include dispersing herbs such as Sojae Semen praeparatum (*dàn dòu chǐ*).

白虎湯（白虎汤）
White Tiger Decoction
bái hǔ tāng

The name of this formula is probably derived from Chinese mythology where the white tiger is the metal spirit of the west that appears in the autumn and heralds the end of summer's heat. It is used here as a metaphor for the heat-clearing action of the formula.

Source *Discussion of Cold Damage* (c. 220)

Gypsum fibrosum *(shí gāo)*. 48g (30-90g)
Anemarrhenae Rhizoma *(zhī mǔ)* 18g (9-15g)
Glycyrrhizae Radix praeparata *(zhì gān cǎo)* 6g (3-6g)
Nonglutinous rice *(jīng mǐ)*. 9-15g

Method of Preparation Decoction. Cook until the rice is done, then strain and ingest the liquid. The present day range of dosages are given in parentheses.

Actions Clears qi-level heat, drains Stomach fire, generates fluids, and alleviates thirst

Indications

High fever with profuse sweating and an aversion to heat, a red face, severe thirst and irritability, and a flooding, forceful or slippery, rapid pulse. May also include headache, toothache, or bleeding of the gums and nose.

This is blazing heat in the yang brightness-channel warp of the six warps of disease or the qi level of the four levels of disease. The yang brightness channels contain an abundance of qi and blood. A strong pathogenic influence attacking the yang brightness channels produces a presentation that is characterized by the 'four greats' (四大 *sì dà):* a great (high) fever, great thirst, great (profuse) sweating, and a great (flooding and big) pulse. Because the yang brightness channels traverse the head and face, severe heat in these channels causes headache and facial flushing. As the heat enters the interior, the simultaneous fever and chills that are the hallmark of exterior disorders evolve into the high fever that is characteristic of interior heat.

Although this is regarded as an interior disorder, it remains in the relatively superficial level of the channels. Thus, the heat primarily affects the superficial and upper aspects of the body. It forces out the fluids in the form of profuse sweating and dries the fluids in the Stomach, the upper yang brightness organ. This leads to severe thirst, irritability, and a dry mouth and tongue. The flooding pulse reflects the presence of a strong pathogenic influence in the channels and the equally strong reaction to it. The tongue may be red with either a dry white or a yellow coating; there may be heavy, labored breathing, and in severe cases, delirious speech, all of which are manifestations of interior heat.

Stomach fire can cause problems along the upper course of the Stomach (yang brightness) channel in the form of headache, toothache, and bleeding of the gums. This condition is similar to blazing heat at the same level of the body.

Analysis of Formula

This is a paradigmatic formula for the strategy of clearing heat with acrid, cold, and sweet substances, as opposed to draining it with bitter and cold herbs. This is the strategy

of choice where excess heat causes or occurs together with damage to the body fluids. Ke Qin, one of the foremost commentators of the cold damage current, explains:

> Conditions where earth is dry and fire scorches cannot be treated by [herbs with a] bitter, cold flavor. The *[Inner] Classic* states, sweetness first enters into the Spleen. It also states, use sweet [flavors] to drain it. … From this one knows that sweet, cold substances make the best formulas for draining Stomach fire and generating body fluids.

Gypsum fibrosum *(shí gāo)* is the chief ingredient in this formula. Its acrid, sweet, and extremely cold properties allow this single substance to achieve three different objectives: clear heat from the interior; vent pathogenic heat to the exterior and release heat constraint from the muscle layer and skin; and moisten and enrich the yin to support the generation of body fluids. The deputy, Anemarrhenae Rhizoma *(zhī mǔ),* is bitter, cold, and moistening. It assists Gypsum fibrosum *(shí gāo)* in clearing heat from the Lungs and Stomach to alleviate irritability, moistens dryness, and enriches the yin. The assistant and envoy ingredients, Glycyrrhizae Radix praeparata *(zhì gān cǎo)* and Nonglutinous rice *(jīng mǐ),* benefit the Stomach and protect the fluids. They also prevent the extremely cold properties of the other ingredients from injuring the middle burner.

Although the formula contains only four substances, their mutual interaction and support is elegantly designed. This allows the formula to clear severe heat from the interior without damaging the qi dynamic, and to support the generation of body fluids without inhibiting the venting of pathogenic heat.

Cautions and Contraindications

Systematic Differentiation of Warm Pathogen Diseases lists four primary contraindications for the use of this formula:

1. *A pulse that is floating, wiry, and thin.* Fever with a floating and wiry pulse indicates that the pathogen is located predominantly in the exterior, from which it must be dispersed. A thin, floating, or deficient pulse accompanied by fever, sweating, and an aversion to wind, on the other hand, indicates yin fire due to Spleen and Stomach deficiency that must be treated with sweet and warm herbs.

2. *A submerged pulse.* If this pulse is strong, it indicates that the pathogen has already moved into the yang organs and must be purged. If the submerged pulse is thin and weak, it reflects yang deficiency with false heat. The appropriate treatment strategy here is to augment the yang.

3. *The absence of thirst.* This can occur in the course of a damp-warmth disorder, where fever is due to obstruction of the yang qi by dampness. It also occurs when a warm pathogen disorder transforms from the qi into the nutritive level. In the former case, inappropriate use of White

Tiger Decoction (*bái hǔ tāng*) would further obstruct the yang qi, while in the latter case, it would prevent a venting of pathogenic heat from the nutritive into the qi level.

4. *The absence of sweating.* Within the context of feverish disorders, this will most likely occur either when the body fluids have been exhausted or where the exterior is obstructed by wind-cold. In the first case, one should enrich the yin, and in the second, release the exterior through sweating.

Zhang Xi-Chun argued that only the first two of Wu Ju-Tong's four points constitute absolute contraindications. In his personal experience, only about 20 percent of all cases for which White Tiger Decoction (*bái hǔ tāng*) is indicated present with both sweating and thirst. In all other cases, there will still be some obstruction in the exterior, causing a lack of sweating, or the fluids will not yet have been damaged so that the patient is not thirsty. Zhang Xi-Chun's experience resonates with Cheng Guo-Peng's analysis of the formula and is an important pointer in clinical practice.

Careful follow-up is advised in any case. Use of this formula should immediately stop if signs of headache, stiffness of the neck, icy-cold limbs, subjective sensations of cold, or impairment of mental faculties occur.

Commentary

This is Zhang Zhong-Jing's flagship formula for treating yang brightness channel-warp disorders where heat is 'without form' (無形 *wú xíng*). Most often, this is contrasted with yang brightness organ-warp disorders where heat acquires form with the appearance of constipation and abdominal pain.

Pathodynamics

Some commentators, however, offer a more complex view in which White Tiger Decoction (*bái hǔ tāng*) is indicated for an intermediate stage of yang brightness disorder due to its ability to clear heat from the interior and simultaneously vent it toward the exterior. A clear exposition of this argument is made by Cheng Guo-Peng in *Awakening of the Mind in Medical Studies:*

> A yang brightness channel disorder [manifests with] eye pain, a dry nose, and rinsing [the mouth] without a desire to swallow. There are not yet [any signs of] constipation, delirious speech, irritability, or thirst. This indicates an exterior condition where the interior is still in harmony. One therefore uses Kudzu Decoction (*gé gēn tāng*) to disperse [the pathogen from the exterior]. If the pathogen has already entered into the yang organs, fever transforms into tidal fever and there are symptoms such as delirious speech, irritability, thirst, constipation, and abdominal distention. This indicates that pathogenic qi has clumped and accumulated [in the interior]. One therefore uses [one of the] Order the Qi Decoctions (*chéng qì tāng*) to purge it. If a yang brightness channel disorder is just beginning to be transmitted to the yang organs, this manifests with symptoms

like steaming heat and spontaneous sweating, irritability, thirst, and delirious speech but not [yet] constipation or abdominal distention. It indicates that the heat pathogen has dispersed and flooded [throughout the body] but not yet clumped and become solid. One therefore uses White Tiger Decoction (*bái hǔ tāng*) to clear [heat from] the middle [burner] and thrust it out from the exterior, to harmonize and release it. These are the three methods for treating yang brightness. If [a physician] is not clear about [where the pathogen is located in relation to] channel and yang organ, treatment based on differentiation of patterns will be wrong. [Such a physician] deceives people like a petty thief.

Cheng's analysis is of great clinical value because it provides a deeper understanding of yang brightness disorders. Compared to the more conventional division into channel and organ-warp disorders, it has at least three distinct advantages:

1. It provides a clear definition of the pathological process at the heart of all White Tiger Decoction (*bái hǔ tāng*) presentations, namely, yang brightness-warp heat dispersing throughout the Triple Burner. The term Triple Burner here signifies that pathogenic fire is visible throughout the entire body rather than being localized in any single organ. It also suggests its method of resolution: through a treatment strategy that is focused neither on diaphoresis via the exterior nor on purgation via the interior. This is echoed in a passage from *Explaining [Zhang Zhong-Jing's] 113 Strategies* by the Qing-dynasty physician Wen Meng-Xiang: "In fact, this formula drains Triple Burner fire in order to treat the yang brightness [warp]."

2. It resolves the debate regarding the composition and usage of White Tiger Decoction (*bái hǔ tāng*) that has been offered by various physicians over the centuries by demonstrating that the chief herb in this formula must be Gypsum fibrosum (*shí gāo*) and not Anemarrhenae Rhizoma (*zhī mǔ*), as proposed by Cheng Wu-Ji and Xu Long, two influential commentators associated with the cold damage current. Gypsum fibrosum (*shí gāo*) is the only substance that addresses all aspects of the heat treated by this formula because it clears heat throughout the Triple Burner, as explained in *Miscellaneous Records of the Materia Medica:* "[Gypsum fibrosum (*shí gāo*) is good] at getting rid of headaches and generalized fever, strong heat throughout the three burners, [as well as] heat in the skin. It releases [heat from] the muscles by promoting sweating and it stops wasting thirst, irritability, and rebellious [qi]."

3. This view also helps us to understand why Chinese physicians were able to extend the application of this formula beyond its original indication. Most influential is Wu Ju-Tong's use of White Tiger Decoction (*bái hǔ tāng*) in *Systematic Differentiation of Warm Pathogen Diseases*, where he defines it as the formula of choice for the treatment of greater yin (i.e., Lung) qi-level disorders that present with the 'four greats.' Although the location of the disease here

is different, its dynamic remains the same. The physiology of both the Stomach and Lungs is closely tied up with that of the yang fluids, such that dryness is associated with the Lungs in five phase theory and with the yang brightness among the six channels. Thus, any damage to the yang fluids combined with pronounced yang qi excess produces the typical White Tiger Decoction (*bái hǔ tāng*) signs and symptoms. In fact, clinical experience bears out that the formula can be prescribed for any case that presents with severe heat in the qi level where the fluids are injured but there is no interior clumping, irrespective of the cause or manifestation. For example, sometimes in yang brightness channel disorders there is an absence of sweating because the heat is slightly constrained, or there may be profuse sweating with sensitivity to cold in the upper back. This formula is appropriate in both cases.

Issues Relating to Ingredients

Some physicians are overly cautious in prescribing this formula and therefore use it only rarely. This is because of the belief that the very cold nature of Gypsum fibrosum (*shí gāo*) is quite harmful to the yang qi. For this reason, Dendrobii Herba (*shí hú*) is sometimes substituted. However, if the diagnosis is accurate, this formula can be used without causing any unpleasant side effects. In fact, most physicians argue that unless Gypsum fibrosum (*shí gāo*) is prescribed in large doses, it does not achieve its intended effect. The early modern physician Zhang Xi-Chun, for instance, recommended a daily dosage of 120-240g and cited several case records within the archives of Chinese medicine that exceed this dosage by a large amount. Modern Chinese textbooks are slightly more conservative and recommend a daily dosage of between 30-120g. A normal course of treatment is 2-4 doses of the formula; in some cases, only one dose is needed. If treatment is ineffective after 6-7 doses, the practitioner must carefully reevaluate the situation. Side effects of an overdose of Gypsum fibrosum (*shí gāo*) include icy-cold limbs, labored and difficult breathing, and a rapid pulse.

This formula is frequently modified. For example, many modern-day practitioners do not use Nonglutinous rice (*jīng mǐ*), considering it to be both unnecessary and inadvisable to tonify the Stomach qi in conditions of heat excess. Zhang Xi-Chun replaced it with Dioscoreae Rhizoma (*shān yào*) because of its ability to supplement both the qi and yin. Also, unprepared Glycyrrhizae Radix (*gān cǎo*) is often used for its ability to generate fluids and thereby quench thirst.

In warm pathogen therapeutics, specifically in the treatment of epidemic disorders where strong heat is dispersed throughout the Triple Burner, White Tiger Decoction (*bái hǔ tāng*) is invariably used as the basis for the composition of larger formulas aimed at resolving toxicity or cooling heat from the blood as well as clearing qi-aspect heat.

Comparisons

➤ Vs. Ephedra, Apricot Kernel, Gypsum, and Licorice Decoction (*má xìng shí gān tāng*)

Both formulas clear qi-level heat from the interior. Frequently, such patterns occur in the course of cold damage disorders when cold transforms into heat. According to the early modern physician Cao Ying-Fu in *Records of Experiences with Classic Formulas*, Ephedra, Apricot Kernel, Gypsum, and Licorice Decoction (*má xìng shí gān tāng*) patterns occur when Ephedra Decoction (*má huáng tāng*) patterns transform into heat, that is, when a strong cold pathogen continues to bind the yang qi in the exterior. By contrast, White Tiger Decoction (*bái hǔ tāng*) patterns occur when Cinnamon Twig Decoction (*guì zhī tāng*) patterns transform into heat, that is, when the nutritive yin is unable to control the protective yang, a pattern that occurs more readily when wind is the primary pathogen within a wind-cold configuration.

➤ Vs. Coptis Decoction to Resolve Toxicity (*huáng lián jiě dú tāng*)

Both formulas treat pathogenic heat that disperses throughout the Triple Burner. They differ in that White Tiger Decoction (*bái hǔ tāng*) focuses entirely on the qi aspect, whereas Coptis Decoction to Resolve Toxicity (*huáng lián jiě dú tāng*) is able to drain fire that has already entered into the blood aspect. Thus, whereas the former treats patterns characterized by strong fever, sweating, and thirst, the latter treats patterns characterized by symptoms such as insomnia, irritability, and flushing (indicating heat disturbing the Pericardium), or nosebleeds, vomiting of blood, carbuncles, boils, or petechiae (indicating heat harassing the blood or congealing to produce toxic swellings).

➤ Vs. Five-Ingredient Powder with Poria (*wǔ líng sǎn*); see page 728

➤ Vs. Drain the White Powder (*xiè bái sǎn*); see page 187

➤ Vs. Tangkuei Decoction to Tonify the Blood (*dāng guī bǔ xuè tāng*); see page 340

Biomedical Indications

With the appropriate presentation, this formula may be used to treat a wide variety of biomedically-defined disorders. These can be divided into the following groups:

• The stage of acute infections marked by maximal fevers including influenza, scarlet fever, typhoid fever, encephalitis B, meningitis, lobar pneumonia, and hemorrhagic fever. It is also used for the somewhat similar increased metabolic state of hyperthyroidism and certain fevers related to cancers.

- Swollen, congested, and hemorrhagic skin and mucous membrane diseases including measles, dermatitis, recalcitrant allergic dermatitis, periodontitis, and acute stomatitis.
- It has also been used for sunstroke, diabetes, gastritis, psychiatric diseases, and unrelenting seepage after burns.

Modifications

- For concurrent wind-cold in the exterior, add Allii fistulosi Bulbus (cōng bái), Sojae Semen praeparatum (dàn dòu chǐ), and Asari Radix et Rhizoma (xì xīn).
- For red, swollen eyes and excruciating headache, add Coptidis Rhizoma (huáng lián) and Scutellariae Radix (huáng qín).
- For pain and swelling of the gums, headache, nosebleed, a dry mouth, thirst, and constipation due to Lung heat and Stomach fire, add Rhei Radix et Rhizoma (dà huáng).
- For wasting and thirsting disorder, or heat that severely injures the fluids resulting in thirst, irritability, and insatiable hunger, add Trichosanthis Radix (tiān huā fěn), Phragmitis Rhizoma (lú gēn), and Ophiopogonis Radix (mài mén dōng).
- For the subcutaneous blotches (petechiae), irritability and restlessness, disorientation, and insomnia associated with febrile disease and heat toxin, combine with Coptis Decoction to Resolve Toxicity (huáng lián jiě dú tāng).

Variations

白虎加人參湯 （白虎加人参汤）

White Tiger plus Ginseng Decoction
bái hǔ jiā rén shēn tāng

SOURCE *Discussion of Cold Damage* (c. 220)

For injury to the qi and fluids resulting from a summerheat disorder, or from sweating, vomiting, or purgation, or from exhaustion of qi in the course of a yang brightness disorder, add Ginseng Radix (rén shēn). Panacis quinquefolii Radix (xī yáng shēn) is often substituted for Ginseng Radix (rén shēn).

The pattern for which this formula is indicated manifests with the 'four greats' noted above (high fever, great thirst, profuse sweating, and big pulse). However, in addition, the pulse will be forceless, or there may be generalized weakness, or the person may feel a slight aversion to cold in their back, or the thirst will be unquenchable. All of these signs and symptoms indicate that the qi has been damaged. This readily occurs in the course of summerheat disorders and the invasion of strong heat pathogens.

Based on his extensive clinical experience, the early modern physician Zhang Xi-Chun argued that this formula can treat damage to the true yin in the course of acute febrile disorders where yin-enriching formulas that rely on herbs like Rehmanniae Radix (shēng dì huáng) or Scrophulariae Radix (xuán shēn) are ineffective. At present, thirst is taken as one of the cardinal symptoms indicating use of this formula rather than the principal formula. For this rea-

son, diabetes mellitus with Stomach fire is an important disorder for which White Tiger plus Ginseng Decoction (bái hǔ jiā rén shēn tāng) is indicated in contemporary practice.

Comparisons

➤ Vs. JADE SPRING PILL (yù quán wán); see PAGE 377

➤ Vs. CLEAR SUMMERHEAT AND AUGMENT THE QI DECOCTION FROM *Clarifying Doubts* (qīng shǔ yì qì tāng); see PAGE 244

白虎加桂枝湯 （白虎加桂枝汤）

White Tiger plus Cinnamon Twig Decoction
bái hǔ jiā guì zhī tāng

SOURCE *Essentials from the Golden Cabinet* (c. 220)

For wind-damp-heat painful obstruction characterized by high fever, sweating, irritability, thirst, pain and swelling of the joints, a white tongue coating, and a wiry, rapid pulse, add Cinnamomi Ramulus (guì zhī). Also used for warm malarial disorders with intense internal heat and mild external cold characterized by high fever, mild chills, aching joints, occasional vomiting, and a wiry, rapid pulse. The addition of warm and acrid Cinnamomi Ramulus (guì zhī) unblocks the channels and collaterals in the exterior, which in this pattern are obstructed by wind-dampness or wind-cold and prevent discharge of heat constraint from the interior. The pathogenesis of this pattern is cogently explained by Tang Zong-Hai in *Discussion of Blood Patterns*: "A body that is only hot and not [at all cold] indicates a normal White Tiger Decoction (bái hǔ tāng) pattern. One adds Cinnamomi Ramulus (guì zhī) if, in addition, the pattern [is characterized] by pain and irritability in the bones and joints. This is due to lurking cold in the sinews and joints. Hence, one employs Cinnamomi Ramulus (guì zhī) to drive it out."

In practice, this formula is frequently further modified to enhance its effects. For instance, to focus on malarial disorders, one might add Artemisiae annuae Herba (qīng hāo) and Dichroae Radix (cháng shān); for wind-type pain in the joints, add Lonicerae Caulis (rěn dōng téng); for damp-type pain and heaviness, add Atractylodis Rhizoma (cāng zhú); and for petechiae, add Scrophulariae Radix (xuán shēn) and Moutan Cortex (mǔ dān pí).

Comparisons

➤ Vs. CINNAMON TWIG, PEONY, AND ANEMARRHENA DECOCTION (guì zhī sháo yào zhī mǔ tāng); see PAGE 761

➤ Vs. CLEAR THE SPLEEN DECOCTION (qīng pí tāng); see PAGE 136

白虎加蒼朮湯 （白虎加苍术汤）

White Tiger plus Atractylodes Decoction
bái hǔ jiā cāng zhú tāng

SOURCE *Book to Safeguard Life Arranged According to Pattern* (1108)

For damp-warm-heat pathogen disease or damp painful obstruction that has transformed into heat characterized by fever, epigastric distention, profuse sweating, a generalized sensation of heaviness, cold feet, and a red, greasy tongue, add Atractylodis Rhizoma *(cāng zhú)*. This formula also treats wind-damp-heat painful obstruction with joint pain and generalized fever. Compared to White Tiger plus Cinnamon Twig Decoction *(bái hǔ jiā guì zhī tāng)*, which focuses on wind-predominant painful obstruction where pain comes and goes or moves around the body, this formula focuses on damp-predominant painful obstruction with swollen joints that are red and inflamed or hot to the touch.

Comparison

➤ Cinnamon Twig, Peony, and Anemarrhena Decoction *(guì zhī sháo yào zhī mǔ tāng)*; *see* page 761

羚犀白虎湯（羚犀白虎汤）
White Tiger with Antelope and Rhinoceros Horn Decoction
líng xī bái hǔ tāng

Source *Warp and Woof of Warm-Heat Pathogen Diseases* (1852)

For febrile diseases characterized by high fever, irritability, thirst, impaired consciousness, and convulsions due to injury to the qi and blood, add Saigae tataricae Cornu *(líng yáng jiǎo)* and Bubali Cornu *(shuǐ niú jiǎo)*.

白虎承氣湯（白虎承气汤）
White Tiger and Order the Qi Decoction
bái hǔ chéng qì tāng

Source *Revised Popular Guide to the Discussion of Cold Damage* (Qing dynasty)

For high fever, profuse sweating, irritability, thirst (with large consumption of fluids), constipation (with clumping of dry stool in the intestines), dark, scanty, and painful urination, and in severe cases, delirious speech or manic behavior, add Rhei Radix et Rhizoma *(dà huáng)* and Natrii Sulfas *(máng xiāo)*. This is a concurrent yang brightness channel- and organ-warp disorder.

Associated Formulas

柴胡白虎湯（柴胡白虎汤）
Bupleurum White Tiger Decoction
chái hú bái hǔ tāng

Source *Revised Popular Guide to the Discussion of Cold Damage* (Qing dynasty)

Bupleuri Radix *(chái hú)* 3g
Gypsum fibrosum *(shí gāo)* 24g
Trichosanthis Radix *(tiān huā fěn)* 9g
Scutellariae Radix *(huáng qín)* 4.5g
Anemarrhenae Rhizoma *(zhī mǔ)* 12g
Nonglutinous rice *(jīng mǐ)* 9g
Glycyrrhizae Radix *(gān cǎo)* 2.4g
Nelumbinis Folium recens *(xiān hé yè)* . . . 1 leaf

Harmonizes the lesser yang and clears yang brightness-warp heat. For severe fever that alternates with mild chills, sweating, irritability, thirst, and a wiry, forceful, and rapid pulse. This is a concurrent yang brightness- and lesser yang-warp disorder that is more commonly seen when the condition is near resolution (on the way out) than during its early stages (on the way in).

鎮逆白虎湯（镇逆白虎汤）
White Tiger Decoction to Suppress Rebellion
zhèn nì bái hǔ tāng

Source *Essays on Medicine Esteeming the Chinese and Respecting the Western* (1918-1934)

Gypsum fibrosum *(shí gāo)* 90g
Anemarrhenae Rhizoma *(zhī mǔ)* 45g
Pinelliae Rhizoma praeparatum *(zhì bàn xià)* . . . 24g
Bambusae Caulis in taeniam *(zhú rú)* . . . 18g

Decoction. Cook in 5 cups of water until reduced to 3 cups. Take 1 cup warm. Should not be taken again if the condition improves significantly within two hours. If the condition does not improve, take another cup (warm), and yet another two hours later, if necessary. Clears Stomach heat and regulates the Stomach qi. For cold damage or warm-heat pathogen diseases with heat entering the Stomach causing rebellious Stomach qi characterized by fever, thirst, other yang brightness-warp symptoms, and a feeling of fullness and stifling oppression in the epigastrium.

竹葉石膏湯（竹叶石膏汤）
Lophatherum and Gypsum Decoction
zhú yè shí gāo tāng

Source *Discussion of Cold Damage* (c. 220)

Lophatheri Herba *(dàn zhú yè)* 6-12g
Gypsum fibrosum *(shí gāo)* 30g
Ginseng Radix *(rén shēn)* 6g
Ophiopogonis Radix *(mài mén dōng)* . . . 9-18g
Pinelliae Rhizoma praeparatum *(zhì bàn xià)* . . . 9g
Glycyrrhizae Radix praeparata *(zhì gān cǎo)* . . . 3-6g
Nonglutinous rice *(jīng mǐ)* 12-15g

Method of Preparation Decoction. The liquid that is drained from the cooked rice is ingested.

Actions Clears heat, generates fluids, augments the qi, and harmonizes the Stomach

Note: The source text calls for Bambusae Folium (竹葉 *zhú yè*) and not Lophatheri Herba *(dàn zhú yè)*. This substitution can be traced back to the late 16th-century work *Comprehensive Outline of the Materia Medica* by Li Shi-Zhen and continues to the present. Nowadays, most sources say that Lophatheri Herba *(dàn zhú yè)* has a greater diuretic action than Bambusae Folium *(zhú yè)*, which is better for heat in the upper burner causing cough, irritability, and thirst.

Indications

Lingering fever (from a febrile disease) accompanied by vomiting, irritability, thirst, parched mouth, lips, and throat, choking cough, stifling sensation in the chest, red tongue with little coating, and a deficient, rapid pulse. Some patients experience restlessness and insomnia.

This is qi-level heat lingering in the Lungs and Stomach where it injures the qi and fluids. It usually occurs during the recovery stage or in the aftermath of a febrile disease. The more pronounced symptoms of heat have subsided, but a low-grade fever with sweating remains. The heat has disturbed the spirit, resulting in irritability and insomnia. Thirst, a very dry mouth and lips, and a red, dry tongue with little or no coating reflect injury to the yin and fluids. The stifling sensation in the chest is due to heat obstructing the flow of qi. Nausea, vomiting, and a choking cough indicate disharmony of qi flow in the Stomach and Lungs. The pulse is also indicative of heat and depleted fluids.

Overall, this is a mixed pattern of excess and deficiency where lingering pathogenic heat has damaged the qi and fluids, and where the disordered qi dynamic contributes to the body's inability to expel the pathogen.

Analysis of Formula

In *Discussion of Warm-Heat Pathogen [Disorders]*, one of the foundational texts of the warm pathogen disorder current, Ye Tian-Shi likened the problem treated by this formula to a situation where "one fears that although the stove no longer smokes, there is still fire within the ashes." Although the patient presents with clear signs that the qi and body fluids have been damaged, one must be careful not to feed this fire again. The appropriate strategy is to focus on clearing heat and only secondarily on tonifying the qi and fluids.

The chief ingredient is Gypsum fibrosum (*shí gāo*). Its cold nature clears lurking heat from the Lungs and Stomach. Its acrid flavor vents pathogenic heat to the exterior and helps to order the qi dynamic. Its sweetness generates fluids and stops thirst. Each of these three functions is supported by the three deputies. The first, Lophatheri Herba (*dàn zhú yè*), is sweet, bland, cold and enters into the Heart, Lung, and Stomach channels. It clears lingering heat through the urine but also vents it from the upper burner. The other two herbs, Ginseng Radix (*rén shēn*) and Ophiopogonis Radix (*mài mén dōng*), complement each other to moisten the Lungs and nourish the yin, benefit the Stomach and generate fluids, and clear heat from the Heart and eliminate irritability.

The assistant, Pinelliae Rhizoma praeparatum (*zhì bàn xià*), directs rebellious qi downward and thereby stops the vomiting. It is a warm and acrid substance and may therefore appear to be inappropriate in this formula. However, in concert with the heat-clearing and fluid-generating ingredients, it invigorates the Spleen qi and reduces the cloying, stag-

nating properties of Ophiopogonis Radix (*mài mén dōng*). The envoys, Glycyrrhizae Radix praeparata (*zhì gān cǎo*) and Nonglutinous rice (*jīng mǐ*), serve two functions. They assist Ginseng Radix (*rén shēn*) in tonifying the qi, and they harmonize the middle burner and nourish the Stomach, thereby protecting the Stomach against injury from Gypsum fibrosum (*shí gāo*). The formula's ability to simultaneously clear the remnants of heat and tonify the deficiency of qi is due to the combined actions of Gypsum fibrosum (*shí gāo*) and Ginseng Radix (*rén shēn*).

Cautions and Contraindications

This formula is not appropriate for febrile diseases where both the normal and pathogenic qi are abundant, when the fever remains high, or when the qi and yin have not yet been injured.

Commentary

When treating a patient who has had a febrile disease, it is very important to ascertain whether the pathogenic influence has in fact been cleared from the body. Lingering of the pathogenic influence in the qi level is a very common problem for which this formula is quite useful.

Formula Development

Regarded as a variation of White Tiger Decoction (*bái hǔ tāng*), this is an excellent example of how a relatively slight modification can change the entire focus of a formula. *Golden Mirror of the Medical Tradition* states that this "changes an extremely cold formula into a clearing and tonifying one." In *Continuing Discussing Cold Damage*, Zhang Lu argues that the substitution of Anemarrhenae Rhizoma (*zhī mǔ*) with Lophatheri Herba (*dàn zhú yè*), Ophiopogonis Radix (*mài mén dōng*), and Pinelliae Rhizoma (*bàn xià*) changes the indication of the original formula from one that treats a lurking warm pathogen to one that treats lurking heat.

By removing Lophatheri Herba (*dàn zhú yè*) and Gypsum fibrosum (*shí gāo*) from the formula and increasing the dosage of Ophiopogonis Radix (*mài mén dōng*), one obtains Ophiopogonis Decoction (*mài mén dōng tāng*), discussed in Chapter 15. This is a formula for treating dryness in the Lungs and Stomach without lingering heat. In spite of their different indications, all three formulas share a common emphasis on venting and clearing lingering heat from the qi level with acrid and cold herbs, even though in each case the yin is already damaged. Zhang Xi-Chun is the physician who best explained the reasoning behind this strategy. Relying too early on cold and sweet herbs like Rehmanniae Radix (*shēng dì huáng*), Scrophulariae Radix (*xuán shēn*), Asparagi Radix (*tiān mén dōng*), or Ophiopogonis Radix (*mài mén dōng*), which are aimed at replenishing fluids, obstructs the qi dynamic. This traps pathogenic heat and encourages rather than prevents the development of consumptive disorders.

Usage

Originally, the formula was prescribed only for the sequelae of cold damage disorders, but its scope was expanded significantly by later generations of physicians. *Straight Direction from Ren-Zhai*, for instance, prescribes it for "fever from lurking summerheat blazing in both the exterior and interior [characterized] by irritability and great thirst." *Prescriptions of Universal Benefit* recommends it for "being struck by summerheat with thirst, irritability, vomiting, rebellious qi, and a rapid pulse." Summerheat is thus another major indication. This type of pathogen readily injures the qi and fluids and may lead to a condition characterized by high fever, profuse sweating, extreme fatigue, severe thirst, a red and dry tongue, and a rapid pulse that is also deficient or thin.

Use of the formula is not limited, however, to feverish disorders and their sequelae. It can be used whenever there is evidence of excess heat in the Stomach that is accompanied by injury to the qi and yin. *Fine Formulas of Wonderful Efficacy* states that it treats "children who are deficient, severely emaciated, and have sparse qi, where the qi rebels causing a desire to vomit, and the four extremities are restless and the body hot." Ye Tian-Shi, in *Master Ye's Patterns and Treatments in Women's Diseases,* indicates its use for "irritability and thirst in pregnancy due to excess fire in the stomach channel." Dermatology experts prescribe the formula to treat prickly heat, and modern physicians use it for postoperative fever, nausea and vomiting, or for yang brightness-channel disorders such as mouth ulcers, toothache, and chronic gastritis.

Comparisons

➤ Vs. Other Formulas for Summerheat with Damage to the Qi and Yin

This formula is effective for treating fever from summerheat with damage to the qi and yin, but its use must be differentiated from that of other formulas for similar problems. Unlike White Tiger plus Ginseng Decoction *(bái hǔ jiā rén shēn tāng),* which treats cases with strong heat and damage to the qi, this formula treats cases where the qi and yin are both damaged. Unlike Generate the Pulse Powder *(shēng mài sǎn),* which focuses solely on augmenting the qi and generating fluids, Lophatherum and Gypsum Decoction *(zhú yè shí gāo tāng)* actively clears and vents pathogenic heat. Unlike Li Dong-Yuan's Tonify Spleen-Stomach, Drain Yin Fire, and Raise Yang Decoction *(bǔ pí wèi xiè yīn huǒ shēng yáng tāng),* which attends to the qi dynamic by draining damp-heat and raising the yang, the present formula focuses on generating fluids in cases where the yin is already damaged.

➤ Vs. Clear Summerheat and Augment the Qi Decoction *(qīng shǔ yì qì tāng); see* PAGE 244

➤ Vs. Lily Bulb and Rehmannia Decoction *(bǎi hé dì huáng tāng); see* PAGE 222

➤ Vs. Warm Gallbladder Decoction *(wēn dǎn tāng); see* PAGE 788

Biomedical Indications

With the appropriate presentation, this formula may be used to treat a variety of biomedically-defined disorders. These can be divided into the following groups:

• The recovery stage of infections such as pneumonia, encephalitis B, meningitis, measles, influenza, hemorrhagic fever, and scarlet fever
• Fevers from postsurgical infections or in response to chemotherapy or radiation therapy for cancer
• It has also been used for stomatitis, systemic lupus erythematosus, diabetes, and nervous exhaustion.

Modifications

• For insufficient Stomach qi and yin with only mild or no signs of Stomach heat, remove Gypsum fibrosum *(shí gāo).*
• For deficient Stomach yin with oral ulcerations and a red, dry tongue, add Trichosanthis Radix *(tiān huā fěn)* and Dendrobii Herba *(shí hú).*
• For intense, blazing Stomach fire with persistent hunger, add Trichosanthis Radix *(tiān huā fěn)* and Anemarrhenae Rhizoma *(zhī mǔ).*
• For vomiting or hiccups, add Phragmitis Rhizoma *(lú gēn).*
• For cough and wheezing, add Armeniacae Semen *(xìng rén).*
• For profuse sputum, add Fritillariae Bulbus *(bèi mǔ)* and Citri reticulatae Pericarpium *(chén pí).*
• For yin deficiency leading to yang deficiency with symptoms of abandonment, such as severe dyspnea or sweating, add Aconiti Radix lateralis praeparata *(zhì fù zǐ).*

Alternate names

Ginseng and Bamboo Leaf Decoction *(rén shēn zhú yè tāng)* in *Discussion of Illnesses, Patterns, and Formulas Related to the Unification of the Three Etiologies*; Gypsum and Bamboo Leaf Decoction *(shí gāo zhú yè tāng)* in *Simple Book of Formulas*

Associated Formula

加減竹葉石膏湯 (加减竹叶石膏汤)

Modified Lophatherum and Gypsum Decoction
jiā jiǎn zhú yè shí gāo tāng

SOURCE *Formula Based on the Experience of Ding Gan-Ren* (1927)

Lophatheri Herba *(dàn zhú yè)* . . . . .30 pieces
Mori Folium *(sāng yè)* 4.5g
Mori Cortex *(sāng bái pí)* 4.5g
Lonicerae Flos *(jīn yín huā)* 9g
Phragmitis Rhizoma *(lú gēn)* .30g
Gypsum fibrosum *(shí gāo)* 18g

Armeniacae Semen (xìng rén). 9g
Forsythiae Fructus (lián qiáo). 9g
white radish juice (bái luó bo zhì). 30g
Glycyrrhizae Radix (gān cǎo) 1.8g
Fritillariae thunbergii Bulbus (zhè bèi mǔ) 9g
Benincasae Semen (dōng guā rén) 12g

This is a special formula for treating the sequelae of measles and scarlet fever from a physician who made his name treating these conditions in the early 20th century. It is indicated for when the illness appears to be resolved but the fever does not subside. Additional signs and symptoms include fever, thirst, a painful throat, and coughing with copious sputum. Compared to the original formula, the qi and fluids are not damaged. Instead, heat lingering in the Lungs and Stomach is retained by phlegm. For this reason, Ophiopogonis Radix (mài mén dōng) and Ginseng Radix (rén shēn) are removed and replaced with herbs that strengthen the formula's capacity to clear heat in the exterior—Mori Folium (sāng yè), Lonicerae Flos (jīn yín huā) and Forsythiae Fructus (lián qiáo)—and drain it from the Lungs via the urine—Mori Cortex (sāng bái pí). Four other assistants are added to transform the phlegm-heat, namely Armeniacae Semen (xìng rén), Benincasae Semen (dōng guā rén), Fritillariae thunbergii Bulbus (zhè bèi mǔ), and white radish juice.

梔子豉湯 (栀子豉汤)

Gardenia and Prepared Soybean Decoction

zhī zǐ chǐ tāng

Source *Discussion of Cold Damage* (c. 220)

Gardeniae Fructus (zhī zǐ). 9g
Sojae Semen praeparatum (dàn dòu chǐ) 6-9g

Method of Preparation The source text advises to first put the Gardeniae Fructus (zhī zǐ) in about 4 cups of water and cook it down to 2½ cups; the other ingredient is then added and the decocting is continued until 1½ cups remain. At present, it is usually taken as a decoction with both ingredients cooked the same amount of time. If this formula induces vomiting, administration should be stopped.

Actions Clears heat and alleviates restlessness and irritability

Indications

Fever, irritability, insomnia with tossing and turning in bed, a stifling sensation in the chest with a soft epigastrium, hunger without a desire to eat, a slightly yellow tongue coating, and a slightly rapid pulse, or a strong, floating pulse at the distal position.

This is qi-level heat lingering in the superficial aspects of the yang brightness warp (the muscles and chest). Heat constrained in the qi level leads to fever. Heat constrained in the chest causes irritability and insomnia. In the source text, this condition is described as one of 'deficiency irritability' (虛 煩 xū fán). The term 'deficiency' here does not refer to depletion of the body's normal qi but to the fact that even though

constraint has caused heat to accumulate in the chest and epigastrium, both areas remain soft and pliable to the touch. Any feeling of obstruction is entirely subjective with no objective evidence of palpable lumps or distention. Thus, the condition is also said to be one of 'formless accumulation.' If the heat constraint is mild, it causes insomnia characterized by tossing and turning before falling asleep. If it is more severe, there will also be very restless sleep and the person will experience a stifling sensation in the chest. Heat in the Stomach increases the appetite, but because the qi dynamic is constrained, there is no desire to eat. The slightly yellow tongue coating and vigorous pulse at the distal position also indicate qi-level or superficial yang brightness-warp heat.

Analysis of Formula

The irritability and other symptoms of this disorder are due to constrained heat. When the heat is released, the irritability will disappear. The chief herb is Gardeniae Fructus (zhī zǐ). It is a bitter and cold herb that excels at clearing constrained heat from the Triple Burner, Heart, Stomach, and Liver by directing it downward and eliminating it via the urine. Zhu Dan-Xi observed that it "drains Triple Burner fire, cools epigastric heat, treats sensations of heat and pain in the cardiac region, dissipates pent-up heat, and mobilizes clumped qi." After noting that it is an essential herb for the treatment of heat in the chest, he explained that it has "a tremendous ability to drain fire downward and out through the urine, as by nature it winds its way downward." The deputy, Sojae Semen praeparatum (dàn dòu chǐ), supports the chief herb by dispersing what remains of the heat via the body's exterior. Compared to the chief herb, its cooling action is rather weak. Instead, its ability to disseminate constrained heat is derived from its power to dredge, vent, and spread. As *Treasury of Words on the Materia Medica* notes, "This is a superior medicinal for venting constraint."

As a seed, the soybean is considered heavy and thus able to reach the interior of the body. The flavor of the prepared herb, however, is acrid and sweet and its nature is accordingly to rise upward. Thus, Sojae Semen praeparatum (dàn dòu chǐ) is the substance of choice for many physicians (particularly those influenced by the doctrines of the warm pathogen disease current) who want to vent exterior heat that has become constrained in the interior of the body. To this end, they combine it with other herbs that direct its action to a specific area. In the present case, Gardeniae Fructus (zhī zǐ) focuses it on the qi level and chest, from which it vents heat from constraint.

Although the formula only contains two herbs, they develop multiple complementary synergies that succeed in the difficult task of eliminating a volatile pathogen. In Chinese texts, these synergies are expressed symbolically via complementary yin-yang associations. Gardeniae Fructus (zhī zǐ) is red and therefore related to the Heart while Sojae Semen praeparatum *(dàn dòu chǐ)* is black and associated with the Kidneys. The Heart is located above, from which Gardeniae Fructus *(zhī zǐ)* directs heat downward by way of its bitterness, while the Kidneys are located below, from which Sojae Semen praeparatum *(dàn dòu chǐ)* vents heat upward. These synergies also extend to the mode of preparation. Gardeniae Fructus *(zhī zǐ)* is decocted longer because it drains heat downward while Sojae Semen praeparatum *(dàn dòu chǐ)* is added at the end in order to maximize its acrid and light venting characteristics.

Cautions and Contraindications

Use with caution in patients with long-lasting Spleen deficiency and loose stools.

Commentary

The source text recommends this formula for the stifling and burning sensation in the chest and epigastrium, irritability, insomnia, and weakness that follow in the aftermath of treating a disease by sweating, vomiting, or purging. These symptoms are regarded as the consequence of relatively severe, lingering heat. *Readings from the Discussion of Cold Damage* cogently describes this process:

> Pathogenic influences in the exterior require sweating, in the epigastrium, vomiting, and in the abdomen, purging. In this case, after [inducing] sweating, vomiting, or purging, the pathogenic influence with form has been eliminated, but some left-over heat lingers in the areas of the chest and diaphragm. This causes the patient to suffer irritability of the Heart and insomnia. In a rather severe case, the heat and irritability increase, with more severe irritability and constraint in the Heart that is indescribable, and there will be a sense of unease whether lying down or being up. This is called anguish and vexation (懊憹 *ào nāo).*

This formula and its variations (see below) are all used to treat irritability due to lingering heat. They are usually indicated in the aftermath of a febrile disease or during a relapse. However, during the early Qing dynasty, Ke Qin, a well-known commentator on the *Discussion of Cold Damage*, noted that the formula had a far wider spectrum of indications: "It is able to dispel pathogenic qi, but it is also able to assist [in cases of treatment] mistakes. This is because it harmonizes the Stomach by unblocking the upper burner and directing the fluids downward." A little later, the scholar-physician Ye Tian-Shi took up this suggestion and prescribed the formula for a wide range of conditions. His influential *Case Records as a Guide to Clinical Practice* contains 37 cases in which Gardenia and Prepared Soybean Decoction *(zhī zǐ chǐ tāng)* is the main formula. Besides externally-contracted disorders like spring warmth, summerheat-dampness, and autumn dryness, cases of dizziness, focal distention, Heart pain, vomiting of blood, and coughing up of blood are also included.

Gardeniae Fructus *(zhī zǐ)* is undoubtedly the main herb for resolving such heat constraint because Zhang Zhong-Jing combines it with a range of different herbs such as Magnoliae officinalis Cortex *(hòu pò)*, Aurantii Fructus immaturus *(zhǐ shí)*, Phellodendri Cortex *(huáng bǎi)*, Zingiberis Rhizoma *(gān jiāng)*, or Rhei Radix et Rhizoma *(dà huáng)*, depending on the precise manifestations. Irritability and a stifling sensation in the chest are the cardinal symptoms in the clinic that distinguish the present formula from its VARIATIONS, listed below. These formulas may be combined, or the present formula may be used together with Bupleuri Radix *(chái hú)*, Pinelliae Rhizoma praeparatum *(zhì bàn xià)*, or Coptidis Rhizoma *(huáng lián)* based formulas, all of which address heat constraint in the area of the diaphragm and epigastrium.

Usage

In contemporary clinical practice, this formula thus has an extremely wide scope of application. Constraint may manifest with symptoms such as an inability to sit still, lie down quietly or relax, irritability, a tendency to flare into bouts of anger, difficulty in concentrating or staying focused, feelings of gloom, and depressive moods. Heat is experienced subjectively as an aversion to heat or as a hot or burning sensation, especially in the chest, while externally it manifests in symptoms such as red eyes, bad breath, increased hunger, dark urine, a red tongue, and a yellowish tongue coating.

Vomiting

The source texts notes that "[if administering the decoction] causes vomiting, it should not be taken again." Influential commentators like Cheng Wu-Ji, Fang You-Zhi, Wang Zi-Jie, and Ke Qin have taken this to mean that vomiting is a desired effect. They argue that because the pathogenic heat is located above the diaphragm, vomiting is the appropriate treatment strategy. However others, like Wang Hu, Wang Po, and Chen Yuan-Xi, think that this view is mistaken because the heat constraint has not acquired form and that there is accordingly no substance to vomit out. This is also the view expressed in contemporary textbooks. Nonetheless, some patients do vomit after taking this formula, and many do feel better having done so. When this occurs, as *Discussion of Cold Damage* points out, the patient should stop taking the herbs.

Comparisons

> Vs. DRAIN THE EPIGASTRIUM DECOCTION *(xiè xīn tāng)* AND MINOR DECOCTION [FOR PATHOGENS] STUCK IN THE CHEST *(xiǎo xiàn xiōng tāng)*

There are a few other formulas by Zhang Zhong-Jing that address accumulation in the chest characterized by fever, irritability, and varying degrees of chest discomfort. Drain the Epigastrium Decoction *(xiè xīn tāng),* discussed later in this chapter, is indicated when there is firm focal distention. Minor Decoction [for Pathogens] Stuck in the Chest (xiǎo xiàn xiōng tāng), discussed in Chapter 17, is indicated when there are tender and hard areas in the epigastrium.

➤ Vs. Warm Gallbladder Decoction (wēn dǎn tāng); see PAGE 788

Biomedical Indications

With the appropriate presentation, this formula may be used to treat a wide variety of biomedically-defined disorders. These can be divided into the following groups:

- Those related to disorders of the nervous system including insomnia, night terrors, neuroses, autonomic dystonia, various psychiatric disorders, and the neurological side effects of xanthine bronchodilators
- Upper gastrointestinal disorders including esophagitis, esophageal strictures, peptic ulcers, acute gastritis, and bile reflux gastritis
- Hemorrhages from the upper part of the body including upper GI bleeds, nosebleeds, and bronchiectasis
- A variety of inflammatory and infectious conditions including viral myocarditis, cholecystitis, icteric jaundice, bronchitis, pneumonia, pulmonary tuberculosis, prostatitis, cystitis, tonsillitis, periodontitis, glossitis, otitis media, and conjunctivitis
- The formula has also been used to treat hypertension and coronary artery disease.

Alternate names

Gardenia and Prepared Soybean Decoction (zhī zǐ xiāng chǐ tāng) in *General Discussion of the Disease of Cold Damage*; Prepared Soybean and Gardenia Decoction (xiāng chǐ zhī zǐ tāng) in *General Discussion of the Disease of Cold Damage*; Gardenia Decoction (zhī zǐ tāng) in *Comprehensive Recording of Sagely Beneficence*; Modified Gardenia Decoction (jiā jiǎn zhī zǐ tāng) in *Yun Qi-Zi's Notes on Pulse in Verse with Formulas*; Gardenia and Prepared Soybean Decoction (zhī zǐ dòu chǐ tāng) in *Indispensable Tools for Pattern Treatment*; Gardenia and Prepared Soybean Decoction (zhì chǐ tāng) in *Achieving Longevity by Guarding the Source*

Modifications

- For externally-contracted heat with lingering exterior symptoms, add Arctii Fructus (niú bàng zǐ) and Menthae haplocalycis Herba (bò hé).
- For more severe heat constraint and qi stagnation, add Curcumae Radix (yù jīn), Trichosanthis Fructus (guā lóu), and Aurantii Fructus (zhǐ ké).
- For a bitter taste in the mouth, yellow tongue coating, and other symptoms of severe interior heat, add Scutellariae Radix (huáng qín) and Forsythiae Fructus (lián qiáo).
- For nausea, vomiting, a greasy tongue coating, and other symptoms of dampness, add Pinelliae Rhizoma praepara-

tum (zhì bàn xià) and Bambusae Caulis in taeniam (zhú rú).
- For pain due to heat from constraint, combine with Toosendan Powder (jīn líng zǐ sǎn).

Variations

梔子甘草豉湯 (栀子甘草豉汤)
Gardenia, Licorice, and Prepared Soybean Decoction
zhī zǐ gān cǎo chǐ tāng

SOURCE　*Discussion of Cold Damage* (c. 220)

For shortness of breath, add Glycyrrhizae Radix (gān cǎo).

_____

梔子生薑豉湯 (栀子生姜豉汤)
Gardenia, Fresh Ginger, and Prepared Soybean Decoction
zhī zǐ shēng jiāng chǐ tāng

SOURCE　*Discussion of Cold Damage* (c. 220)

For vomiting, add Zingiberis Rhizoma recens (shēng jiāng).

_____

枳實梔子豉湯 (枳实栀子豉汤)
Bitter Orange, Gardenia, and Prepared Soybean Decoction
zhǐ shí zhī zǐ chǐ tāng

SOURCE　*Discussion of Cold Damage* (c. 220)

For fever and epigastric distention associated with a recurrence of disease due to overexertion or improper diet during convalescence, add Aurantii Fructus immaturus (zhǐ shí).

Associated Formulas

梔子乾薑湯 (栀子干姜汤)
Gardenia and Ginger Decoction
zhī zǐ gān jiāng tāng

SOURCE　*Discussion of Cold Damage* (c. 220)

Gardeniae Fructus (zhī zǐ) 9g

Clears heat and harmonizes the middle burner. For fever, slight irritability, abdominal pain, borborygmus, and diarrhea due to improper treatment by purging. This pattern may also occur in constitutionally yang-deficient patients who contract a warm pathogen at the qi level. In such cases, heat harasses the upper burner even as cold congeals in the middle.

_____

梔子厚樸湯 (栀子厚朴汤)
Gardenia and Magnolia Bark Decoction
zhī zǐ hòu pò tāng

SOURCE　*Discussion of Cold Damage* (c. 220)

Gardeniae Fructus (zhī zǐ) 9-12g
Magnoliae officinalis Cortex (hòu pò) 12g
Aurantii Fructus immaturus (zhǐ shí) 6-9g

Clears heat, alleviates irritability, and reduces fullness and distention. For irritability and abdominal distention after purging. This formula may be used to treat heat constraint as described above where abdominal distention due to qi stagnation is the key clinical sign. Stools will not necessarily be hard, but the patient may have a sensation of incomplete emptying. Other common symptoms are nausea, fullness, and belching.

栀子大黃湯 (栀子大黄汤)

Gardenia and Rhubarb Decoction

zhī zǐ dà huáng tāng

SOURCE   *Essentials from the Golden Cabinet* (c. 220)

Gardeniae Fructus (*zhī zǐ*)	9-12g
Sojae Semen praeparatum (*dàn dòu chǐ*)	9-12g
Aurantii Fructus immaturus (*zhǐ shí*)	6-9g
Rhei Radix et Rhizoma (*dà huáng*)	3g

Clears heat, alleviates irritability, unblocks the bowels, and reduces accumulation. For jaundice with distress and irritability sometimes accompanied by fever and generalized pain. Also for relapse of fever and constipation associated with a recurrence of disease due to improper diet during convalescence. The source text attributes the occurrence of jaundice in this pattern to the excessive consumption of alcohol, though later authors have not limited its use to this cause alone.

栀子芩葛湯 (栀子芩葛汤)

Gardenia, Scutellaria, and Kudzu Decoction

zhī zǐ qín gé tāng

SOURCE   *Unwilting Formulas* (Qing Dynasty)

Gardeniae Fructus (*zhī zǐ*)	9g
Sojae Semen praeparatum (*dàn dòu chǐ*)	9g
Puerariae Radix (*gé gēn*)	4.5g
Scutellariae Radix (*huáng qín*)	3g
Coptidis Rhizoma (*huáng lián*)	0.9g
Moutan Cortex (*mǔ dān pí*)	3g
Platycodi Radix (*jié gěng*)	3g
Glycyrrhizae Radix (*gān cǎo*)	1.5g

Clears heat from the exterior and interior of the yang brightness channel. For a warm pathogen heat disorder that is characterized by fever, aversion to wind, light sweating that does not resolve the problem, thirst, a painful throat, and a slightly red tongue with a thin, white, dry coating.

Section 2

FORMULAS THAT CLEAR NUTRITIVE-LEVEL HEAT AND COOL THE BLOOD

The nutritive (營 *yíng*) and blood (血 *xuè*) levels are the deepest of the four levels of disease. When heat enters the nutritive level, it causes fever that worsens at night, irritability, and insomnia. Sometimes there is delirious speech, and

there may also be faint, indistinct rashes. When heat enters the blood level, distinct rashes or hemorrhage appears. This is often accompanied by manic behavior and a reddish-purple tongue with prickles. Proper treatment of nutritive- and blood-level disorders requires more than simply clearing the nutritive level and cooling the blood. Since most of these disorders begin in the qi level, and also because the qi level is the main exit route through which a pathogen needs to be vented from the nutritive and blood levels, the formulas should also include herbs that clear heat from the qi level such as Lonicerae Flos (*jīn yín huā*), Forsythiae Fructus (*lián qiáo*), and Lophatheri Herba (*dàn zhú yè*). For a more detailed discussion of this issue, see the COMMENTARY under Clear the Nutritive Level Decoction (*qīng yíng tāng*) that follows below. Furthermore, the heat in these cases not only causes bleeding, but may also scorch the blood, which can lead to blood stasis. For this reason, ingredients that invigorate the blood, such as Moutan Cortex (*mǔ dān pí*) and Paeoniae Radix rubra (*chì sháo*), are often added.

清營湯 (清营汤)

Clear the Nutritive-Level Decoction

qīng yíng tāng

Source   *Systematic Differentiation of Warm Pathogen Diseases* (1798)

[Bubali Cornu (*shuǐ niú jiǎo*)	30-120g]
Scrophulariae Radix (*xuán shēn*)	9g
Rehmanniae Radix (*shēng dì huáng*)	15g
Ophiopogonis Radix (*mài mén dōng*)	9g
Lonicerae Flos (*jīn yín huā*)	9g
Forsythiae Fructus (*lián qiáo*)	6g
Coptidis Rhizoma (*huáng lián*)	4.5g
Lophatheri Herba (*dàn zhú yè*)	3g
Salviae miltiorrhizae Radix (*dān shēn*)	6g

Method of Preparation   Decoction. Bubali Cornu (*shuǐ niú jiǎo*) is in the form of powder or shavings and should be cooked separately for 15-20 minutes before adding the other ingredients. The original text calls for 9g of Rhinocerotis Cornu (*xī jiǎo*), which is taken in powdered form followed by the strained decoction. This is no longer done, primarily due to the endangered species status of the rhinoceros.

Actions   Clears the nutritive level, relieves fire toxin, drains heat, and nourishes the yin

Indications

High fever that worsens at night, severe irritability and restlessness, a scarlet, dry tongue, and a thin, rapid pulse. Some patients are thirsty, some delirious, and some exhibit faint and indistinct erythema and purpura.

This is heat entering the nutritive level. When a strong pathogenic influence enters the nutritive level there will be a high fever; because the yin (associated with night) is affected, the fever worsens at night. Heat also scorches the Heart and disturbs the spirit, causing irritability, restlessness, and in extreme cases, delirious speech. The presence or absence of thirst is an indication of whether heat remains in the qi level or has moved to the nutritive level. Thirst results from a 'plundering' of the Stomach fluids. Its presence indicates that heat remains in the qi level. Once the heat has almost completely moved to the nutritive level, the thirst will disappear. This is because the heat within the nutritive aspect 'steams' what remains of the fluids upward so that the patient does not feel thirsty even as their fluids continue to be exhausted. A yellow tongue coating may also be found in patients where heat lingers in the qi level. The faint, indistinct rashes indicate that heat is on the verge of entering the blood level. The scarlet, dry tongue and the thin, rapid pulse are important signs of heat in the nutritive level.

Analysis of Formula

The chief ingredient, bitter, salty, and cold Bubali Cornu *(shuǐ niú jiǎo),* clears heat from the nutritive level and the Heart, resolves toxicity, and calms the spirit. It is cold but does not cause obstruction, which makes it a useful substance for treating conditions with heat that has plunged into the interior. It also cools the blood and breaks up stasis. The deputies are Scrophulariae Radix *(xuán shēn),* which enriches the yin, directs fire downward, and resolves toxicity, Rehmanniae Radix *(shēng dì huáng),* which cools the blood and enriches the yin, and Ophiopogonis Radix *(mài mén dōng),* which clears heat, nourishes the yin, and generates fluids. These three ingredients, which comprise the formula Increase the Fluids Decoction *(zēng yè tāng),* discussed in Chapter 15, enhance the actions of the chief ingredient.

These ingredients reflect the core strategy for treating heat entering the nutritive level, as first outlined in *Basic Questions* (Chapter 74): "For hot pathogenic influences in the interior, treat with salty, cold [substances] with the assistance of bitter, sweet [substances]." By clearing heat and resolving toxicity, they directly focus on the root of the pathology, but they also enrich the yin and generate fluids and thereby push heat back into the qi aspect from which it can then be eliminated from the body. This important principle is explained by Ye Tian-Shi, from whose case records the formula is derived, in his *Warp and Woof of Warm-Heat Pathogen Diseases:* "Disturbances from [heat] entering the nutritive level can be [treated] by venting the heat through the qi [level]." This is the purpose of the assistants in the formula.

The assistants Lonicerae Flos *(jīn yín huā)* and Forsythiae Fructus *(lián qiáo)* clear heat and resolve toxicity. They are fragrant, aromatic, light, and excel at dissipating pathogenic heat. They are included to vent pathogenic heat toward the outside. This includes both the heat that remains in the qi level and that which is pushed there from the nutritive level

by the action of the deputy herbs. The third assistant, Lophatheri Herba *(dàn zhú yè),* is light and has a similar action. It also works together with the fourth assistant, cold and bitter Coptidis Rhizoma *(huáng lián),* to clear and drain heat from the Heart. The remaining assistant, Salviae miltiorrhizae Radix *(dān shēn),* prevents blood stasis, which can occur for two reasons: damage to the fluids due to heat entering into the blood, and the cooling action of the cold herbs in the formula, which slows down blood flow. This is why Ye Tian-Shi advised, "If one uses cooling herbs in heat disorders, one must assist them with substances that invigorate the blood, thereby avoiding anxieties about creating lurking ice." Some commentators consider Salviae miltiorrhizae Radix *(dān shēn)* to be the guiding herb in this formula that focuses the action of all the ingredients on the Heart.

Cautions and Contraindications

The source text cautions that this formula is contraindicated in cases with a white and slippery tongue coating, which is an indication of dampness. If used in cases with dampness, it will prolong the condition.

Commentary

Heat usually enters the nutritive level via the qi level. In the initial stages of a nutritive-level disorder in particular, some pathogenic heat usually remains in the qi aspect. The extent of this heat can be read from the level of a patient's thirst and the coating of the tongue. The greater the thirst and the thicker the tongue coating, the more qi-level heat remains. The more scarlet and dry the tongue body becomes, the deeper the heat has entered into the nutritive level. Some modern commentators therefore think of this formula as treating a mixed qi- and nutritive-level disorder. However, if this were the case, the balance between deputies and assistants in the formula would have to be different. It is more useful to think of the assistants as clearing both the heat that remains in the qi level and that which is pushed there again from the nutritive level by the chief and deputy herbs.

Why heat must be turned back into the qi level (轉氣 *zhuǎn qì)* before it can be vented from the body is also easy to understand. At the nutritive and blood levels, pathogenic heat is mixed up with the body's own substance. The only way to clear it from these levels directly is by way of bleeding. This is why rashes begin to appear when heat enters the nutritive level and why they turn into more severe bleeding as it sinks deeper into the blood level. To prevent these potentially fatal situations, it is essential to turn the heat back into the qi level as quickly as possible, from which it can be vented via the skin or drained via the bowels and urine.

In practice, a physician will adjust the dosage and number of assistants in the formula according to the degree of qi-level heat that is present. If qi-level heat is more prominent, the dosage of those herbs that treat this heat should be increased. Where there is no thirst, Coptidis Rhizoma (*huáng lián*) should be removed from the formula because the side effects of its dry, yin-damaging nature now exceed the benefits of its heat-draining properties.

Not all cases of heat entering the nutritive level are acute in nature. Sometimes, especially when the normal qi is strong, it will take longer for the heat to reach this level. But once it does, it will linger there.

Comparison

➤ Rhinoceros Horn and Rehmannia Decoction (*xī jiǎo dì huáng tāng*); see page 166

Biomedical Indications

With the appropriate presentation, this formula may be used to treat a variety of biomedically-defined disorders, primarily infectious, including encephalitis B, meningitis, typhoid, septicemia, and thrombocytopenic purpura.

Modifications

* For severe depletion of the yin and fluids, add Glehniae/ Adenophorae Radix (*shā shēn*) and Lycii Fructus (*gǒu qǐ zǐ*).
* For severe qi-level fire, add Gypsum fibrosum (*shí gāo*).
* For tremors and spasms, add Uncariae Ramulus cum Uncis (*gōu téng*), Saigae tataricae Cornu (*líng yáng jiǎo*), and Pheretima (*dì lóng*).
* For heat sinking into the Pericardium with high fever, convulsive spasms, and impaired consciousness, begin the treatment with Calm the Palace Pill with Cattle Gallstone (*ān gōng niú huáng wán*). Once these symptoms have subsided, use the principal formula.

Associated Formula

犀地透營湯 （犀地透营汤）

Rhinoceros Horn and Rhemannia Decoction for Venting the Nutritive Level

xī dì tòu yíng tāng

Source *Selected Formulas for Warm-Heat Pathogen Diseases* (c. 1900)

[Bubali Cornu (*shuǐ niú jiǎo*) . . . . 30-120g]
Rehmanniae Radix recens (*xiān dì huáng*) 12g
Sojae Semen praeparatum (*dàn dòu chǐ*) 6g
Moutan Cortex (*mǔ dān pí*) 6g
Forsythiae Fructus (*lián qiáo*) 9g
Gardeniae Fructus (*zhī zǐ*) 6g
Phragmitis Rhizoma (*lú gēn*) 60g
Junci Medulla (*dēng xīn cǎo*) .1.5g

Decoction. The source text specifies 2.4g of Rhinocerotis Cornu (*xī jiǎo*) and advises to first decoct Phragmitis Rhizoma (*lú gēn*) and

Junci Medulla (*dēng xīn cǎo*) and to use the strained liquid for decocting the other ingredients. For wind-warmth sinking into the interior leading to early-stage nutritive-level disorders, where the pathogen is located in between the protective and nutritive levels. Such disorders manifest with burning fever that is not accompanied by sweating, physical and mental irritability, restlessness that worsens at night, and transient periods of delirious speech. The patient is described as keeping both eyes either permanently open or closed, and, in severe cases, as having blood-shot eyes. The tongue has a white coating at the front, but is crimson at the root, or has a thin white coating on a red body. The pulse is rapid in the left distal position, and submerged and rapid (as if trapped) at the right distal position. In severe cases, the extremities may be cold. He Lian-Chen, the author of this formula, composed it to vent heat in the early stages of a nutritive-level disorder via the protective qi. Compared to the main formula, it contains no bitter, cold herbs that drain heat. Instead, it focuses on unblocking the qi dynamic in the upper burner and the exterior in order to vent wind-heat.

清宮湯 （清宫汤）
Clear the Palace Decoction

qīng gōng tāng

Source *Systematic Differentiation of Warm Pathogen Diseases* (1798)

Scrophulariae Radix (*xuán shēn*) 9g
Nelumbinis Plumula (*lián zǐ xīn*) 1.5g
Lophatheri Herba (*dàn zhú yè*) 6g
Forsythiae Fructus (*lián qiáo*) .6g
[Bubali Cornu (*shuǐ niú jiǎo*) . . . . 15-30g]
Ophiopogonis Radix (*mài mén dōng*) 9g

Method of Preparation Decoction. The source text specifies that 6g of Rhinocerotis Cornu (*xī jiǎo*) be shaved or powdered before being added to the decoction. To direct all of the main herbs directly into the Heart, Wu Ju-Tong, the author of the formula, specified that one should use their 'heart' (心 *xīn*), that is, the central portion of the herb. He appended an explanation to *Systematic Differentiation of Warm Pathogen Diseases*: "To use the heart of all [the substances in this formula is advised] because the heart signifies endless and unceasing production. Furthermore, the heart [of these substances] enters the Heart [of the patient]. They are substances that can clear foul-turbidity and that are suitable for tonifying the endless and unceasing production of qi within the Heart. Therefore, they can rescue life from the haziness [into which it has fallen]."

Actions Clears heat in the Heart and nourishes the yin fluids

Indications

Fever, impaired consciousness, disordered speech, and a crimson tongue without coating.

This is an externally-contracted warm pathogen disorder where excessive sweating has damaged the yin fluids of the Heart. This causes sinking of pathogenic heat into the Pericardium, which manifests as impaired consciousness. The crimson tongue reflects the pathogenic heat, and the lack of tongue coating reflects the damage to the yin fluids. Any accompanying symptoms will be those of heat at the nutritive level.

Analysis of Formula

The formula uses salty, cold, bitter, and sweet substances to clear and dissipate pathogenic heat from the Pericardium. Its chief herbs are Scrophulariae Radix *(xuán shēn)* and Bubali Cornu *(shuǐ niú jiǎo)*, both of which are black—associated with yin, water, and tranquility—and therefore able to control and calm the Heart—associated with yang, fire, and activity. Scrophulariae Radix *(xuán shēn)* is bitter in taste and moist in nature, and is especially suited for clearing Heart fire by means of tonifying its yin fluids. Bubali Cornu *(shuǐ niú jiǎo)* is salty, resolves toxicity, and focuses on clearing exuberant fire from the Heart.

Ophiopogonis Radix *(mài mén dōng)*, whose function here is to unblock the collateral vessels of the Heart, serves as deputy. This role is based on Wu Ju-Tong's analysis of a passage in *Divine Husbandman's Classic of the Materia Medica* where it says that Ophiopogonis Radix *(mài mén dōng)* "governs clumping of qi in the Heart and abdomen, damage to the center, and damage [due] to fullness [after eating], cutting off of the Stomach, vessels, and collaterals."

The two assistants are Forsythiae Fructus *(lián qiào)* and Lophatheri Herba *(dàn zhú yè)*, both of which clear heat from the qi level of the upper burner. Their function in this formula follows Ye Tian-Shi's treatment principle that pathogenic heat entering the nutritive level should be vented via the qi level. Forsythiae Fructus *(lián qiào)* resolves toxicity and dissipates clumps, while Lophatheri Herba *(dàn zhú yè)* enters into the Heart where its unblocks its orifices by draining heat via the urine and venting it via the exterior. The envoy in the formula is bitter and cold Nelumbinis Plumula *(lián zǐ xīn)*, which guides excessive Heart fire downward into the Kidneys and Kidney fire upward into the Heart to reestablish the normal physiological connection between water and fire in the body.

Cautions and Contraindications

In regard to this formula, the source text states, "Do not give it to those with a white, slippery tongue [coating]." This is because the formula could lead to the retention of any pathogenic dampness that is present.

Commentary

According to the *Classic of Difficulties* (Chapter 32), the Lungs are associated with the qi and protective qi, while the Heart is associated with the blood and nutritive qi. This passage later became the basis for Ye Tian-Shi's four-level system of differentiation in the diagnosis and treatment of warm pathogen heat disorders. A newly-contracted heat pathogen usually enters the body at the protective level of the upper burner, that is, the Lungs. From there it penetrates into the qi level, either within the Lungs, or the Stomach and Intestines. Only from there does it enter into the nutritive level. This type of disease development is known as a normal transmission (順傳 *shùn chuán*) and is treated with Clear the Nutritive Decoction *(qīng yíng tāng)*. However, under some circumstances, a very strong heat pathogen can penetrate directly from the protective level and the Lungs into the nutritive Level and the Pericardium. This is called an abnormal or rebellious transmission (逆傳 *nì chuán*) because it produces the serious pattern of heat sinking into the Pericardium. The present formula is indicated for this type of pathology.

As a nutritive-level disorder, the basic composition of the formula follows that outlined for Clear the Nutritive Decoction *(qīng yíng tāng)*. However, because the pathogenic heat has entered the nutritive level via the protective level, only very light herbs are needed to vent heat to the exterior. Furthermore, because the pathogenic heat remains completely within the upper burner, the formula avoids herbs such as Coptidis Rhizoma *(huáng lián)* or Rehmanniae Radix *(shēng dì huáng)* that might guide it downward into the middle burner. Instead, it focuses entirely on the Heart and its dynamic yin-yang relationship with the Kidneys. This principle is reflected in the choice of both the chief and envoy herbs, and is a prime example of the process of the thinking underpinning the composition of a formula in Chinese medicine.

Particularly noteworthy, too, is the choice of Ophiopogonis Radix *(mài mén dōng)* to open the collaterals of the Heart. Most physicians would select an herb that invigorates the blood and opens up areas of stasis. However, in a context where a very forceful yang pathogen has severely damaged the yin fluids of the Heart, the use of acrid, moving herbs could further aggravate the momentum of this pathology. An herb like Salviae miltiorrhizae Radix *(dān shēn)*, on the other hand, could easily pull the pathology deeper into the blood level. For this reason, Wu Ju-Tong selected a substance that opens the collaterals entirely by way of moistening and clearing.

The treatment strategy embodied in this formula, that is, simultaneous clearing of heat in both the protective and nutritive aspects, can be a very useful tool in the treatment of many internal medicine disorders. The formula may be combined with Clear the Nutritive Decoction *(qīng yíng tāng)* if the pathology requires.

Note that there are unrelated modern formulas with the same Chinese name in which 宮 *gōng* refers to the uterus (子宮 *zǐ gōng*). These would be translated as Clear the Uterus Decoction.

Biomedical Indications

With the appropriate presentation, this formula may be used to treat a variety of biomedically-defined disorders including meningitis, encephalitis B, septicemia, and leukemic crisis.

Modifications

- For pronounced phlegm-heat, add 5 spoonful each of Bambusae Succus (*zhú lì*) and pear juice. (source text)
- For hacking [cough] with phlegm that does not clear, add 4.5g of Trichosanthis Pericarpium (*guā lóu pí*). (source text)
- For gradual impairment of consciousness, add 9g of Lonicerae Flos (*jīn yín huā*), 6g of Nelumbinis Folium (*hé yè*), and 3g of Acori tatarinowii Rhizoma (*shí chāng pǔ*). (source text)

犀角地黃湯（犀角地黄汤）

Rhinoceros Horn and Rehmannia Decoction

xī jiǎo dì huáng tāng

Source　*Important Formulas Worth a Thousand Gold Pieces* (650)

[Bubali Cornu (*shuǐ niú jiǎo*) . . . . 30-120g]
Rehmanniae Radix (*shēng dì huáng*) 24g
Paeoniae Radix (*sháo yào*) 9g
Moutan Cortex (*mǔ dān pí*) 6g

Method of Preparation　The source text advises to use 3g of Rhinocerotis Cornu (*xī jiǎo*) and to coarsely grind and decoct the ingredients for a long period of time. At present, it is usually prepared as a decoction without grinding the ingredients, but increasing the dosage by 20-30 percent. Paeoniae Radix rubra (*chì sháo*) is the form of Paeoniae Radix (*sháo yào*) most commonly used. Bubali Cornu (*shuǐ niú jiǎo*) is powdered or shaved and should be cooked separately for 15-20 minutes before adding the other ingredients. Rehmanniae Radix recens (*xiān dì huáng*), with a three-fold increase in dosage, is preferred whenever possible over the dried form of the herb.

Actions　Clears heat, resolves fire toxicity, cools the blood, nourishes the yin, dispels blood stasis, and stops bleeding

Indications

Fever, various types of bleeding (including vomiting of blood, nosebleed, blood in the stool or urine, and rashes), black and tarry stools, abdominal distention and fullness, thirst with an inability to swallow, a scarlet tongue with prickles, and a thin, rapid pulse. Some patients become delirious.

This is heat entering the blood level, the deepest of the four levels of disease. When heat enters this level, it causes the blood to move recklessly and leave its normal pathways. In the upper part of the body, this manifests as nosebleed and

vomiting of blood; in the lower part, as blood in the urine and stool. Leakage into the skin results in maculopapular or other types of rash. When the heat is severe, the combination of bleeding and stasis will cause the rashes to turn purple. Blood forced into the Intestines by heat accumulates and stagnates. This leads to black and tarry stools together with distention and fullness in the abdomen. Heat generally causes thirst. However, a type of thirst peculiar to this condition arises when heat enters the deep (yin) levels of the body where it causes a bubbling and upward-boiling of the fluids. This results in a type of thirst in which the patient may wish to rinse his mouth with water, but has no desire to swallow it. A scarlet tongue body with prickles is a classic sign of heat in the blood level. Heat disturbing the Heart causes delirious speech.

Analysis of Formula

The basic strategy for treating pathogenic heat entering the blood level is outlined by Ye Tian-Shi in *Warp and Woof of Warm-Heat Pathogen Diseases*: "As soon as [a heat pathogen] enters into the blood it threatens to [simultaneously] consume and stir up the blood. One must [respond] directly by cooling and dispersing the blood [at the same time]." This is what the present formula achieves.

Bitter, salty, and cold Bubali Cornu (*shuǐ niú jiǎo*) is the chief herb in the formula. It clears Heart fire and resolves fire toxicity. It is cold but does not hinder the movement of blood, and is thus ideally suited to treat heat at the blood level. Injury to the yin fluids from severe heat and loss of blood requires that the yin be nourished. This is achieved by the deputy, Rehmanniae Radix (*shēng dì huáng*), which cools the blood, stops bleeding, nourishes the yin fluids, and clears heat. Two assistants focus on draining heat and enlivening blood to treat and prevent the blood stasis that may be caused by the severe heat or as a side effect of the cold ingredients in this formula. Paeoniae Radix rubra (*chì sháo*) cools and moves the blood, but also actively drains the heat pathogen. Moutan Cortex (*mǔ dān pí*) is bitter and slightly acrid. It drains heat to cool the blood and stops bleeding by dispersing static blood.

Cautions and Contraindications

Contraindicated in cases of bleeding due to yang deficiency or Spleen and Stomach deficiency

Commentary

In the source text, the use of this formula is limited to the treatment of externally-contracted disorders that have not been properly released by sweating and have therefore penetrated to the interior and affected the blood, causing nosebleed or vomiting of blood. In the Qing dynasty, this formula was representative of the treatment strategies to be used at the blood level in Ye Tian-Shi's four-level differentiation of warm pathogen heat disorders. It is now used for all types of bleeding accompanied by fever and a purple tongue. It is also widely used in gynecology, pediatrics, dermatology, and ophthalmology for problems due to both heat and blood stasis.

As early as the Ming dynasty, Zhang Jie-Bin suggested that the formula was able to promote sweating in order to vent pathogenic heat to the outside. He therefore suggested that one could substitute Cimicifugae Rhizoma (*shēng má*) for Rhinocerotis Cornu (*xī jiǎo*). This view was fiercely criticized by the Qing dynasty scholar-physician Fei Bo-Xiong, who argued that the use of an herb like Cimicifugae Rhizoma (*shēng má*), which is regarded as ascending in nature, was likely to aggravate bleeding in the upper body.

Zhang Lu, another Qing-dynasty physician, suggested adding Scutellariae Radix (*huáng qín*) and Rhei Radix et Rhizoma (*dà huáng*) to the formula if there are signs of interior excess, that is, if heat caused blood to congeal in the abdomen leading to a sensation of fullness that is palpable. If, on the other hand, the patient has only a subjective sensation of fullness accompanied by a slow pulse, he took this to indicate that there was no more yang in the blood and therefore added Cinnamomi Cortex (*ròu guì*). Wu Ju-Tong followed Zhang Lu's suggestions as far as heat accumulation was concerned, but listed internal yang deficiency as a contraindication of this formula. No consensus has yet emerged as to which of these diverse opinions is correct. Physicians must therefore exercise their own judgment in practice.

Comparison

➢ Vs. Clear the Nutritive-Level Decoction (*qīng yíng tāng*)

Both formulas contain Bubali Cornu (*shuǐ niú jiǎo*) and Rehmanniae Radix (*shēng dì huáng*) as chief and deputy ingredients. This indicates that nutritive- and blood-level disorders share a core pathology, that is, pathogenic heat that is damaging the fluids within the blood. At the nutritive level, the penetration of heat is still relatively superficial or recent and has not yet begun to stir the blood. This is reflected on the level of symptomatology in fever that worsens at night, disorders of consciousness or speech that come and go, a crimson tongue, and relatively indistinct rashes. To prevent the heat from moving deeper, one actively encourages it to turn back toward the qi level. This is why Clear the Nutritive-Level Decoction (*qīng yíng tāng*) focuses more strongly on enriching the yin fluids and why, in spite of its name, it contains several assistants that clear heat at the qi level.

As the heat penetrates more deeply, it increasingly consumes the yin fluids and begins to stir the blood into reckless movement. This is reflected in symptoms like bleeding and loss of consciousness, and in signs like a crimson tongue with prickles and an increasingly rapid pulse. To deal with this cri-

sis, the assistants in Rhinoceros Horn and Rehmannia Decoction (*xī jiǎo dì huáng tāng*) focus entirely on the blood. This is because the dangers arising from bleeding, blood stasis, and also potentially wind are now so acute that they demand our complete attention. Only when the heat has become less severe (i.e., when a blood-level disorder once again reverts to a nutritive-level disorder) does venting of the heat to the qi level once again become a possibility.

Biomedical Indications

With the appropriate presentation, this formula may be used to treat a variety of biomedically-defined disorders such as severe hepatitis, hepatic coma, disseminated intravascular coagulation, uremia, allergic purpura, leukemic crisis, as well as a variety of acute hemorrhages.

Alternate Names

Rehmannia Decoction (*dì huáng tāng*) in *General Discussion of the Disease of Cold Damage*; Resolve Toxin Decoction (*jiě dú tāng*) in *Comprehensive and Subtle Discussion on Children's Health*; Resolve Toxin Powder (*jiě dú sǎn*) in *Yang Family Formulas*. **Note:** The earliest extant reference to this formula appears in *Prescriptions with Short Articles* under the name Paeonia and Rhemannia Decoction (*sháo yào dì huáng tāng*).

Modifications

- For manic behavior, add Scutellariae Radix (*huáng qín*) and Rhei Radix et Rhizoma (*dà huáng*). (source text)

- For vomiting of blood, add Platycladi Cacumen (*cè bǎi yè*) and Imperatae Rhizoma (*bái máo gēn*).

- For blood in the stool, add Sanguisorbae Radix (*dì yú*) and Sophorae Flos immaturus (*huái mǐ*).

- For blood in the urine, add Imperatae Rhizoma (*bái máo gēn*) and Cirsii Herba (*xiǎo jì*).

- For severe injury to the yin and blood, substitute Paeoniae Radix alba (*bái sháo*) for Paeoniae Radix rubra (*chì sháo*).

- For a bad temper due to constraint, add Bupleuri Radix (*chái hú*), Scutellariae Radix (*huáng qín*), and Gardeniae Fructus (*zhī zǐ*).

- For rashes, add Arnebiae/Lithospermi Radix (*zǐ cǎo*) and Indigo naturalis (*qīng dài*).

- For severe bleeding, add powdered Notoginseng Radix (*sān qī*).

- For bleeding due to simultaneous reckless movement of hot blood and the inability of deficient qi to control the blood, add Astragali Radix (*huáng qí*) and Ginseng Radix (*rén shēn*).

- For high fever and impaired consciousness, combine with Calm the Palace Pill with Cattle Gallstone (*ān gōng niú huáng wán*).

Associated Formula

神犀丹

Magical Rhinoceros Special Pill

shén xī dān

SOURCE *Warp and Woof of Warm-Heat Pathogen Diseases* (1852)

Note: This is based on a prescription by Ye Tian-Shi.

[Bubali Cornu *(shuǐ niú jiǎo)*	450g]
Rehmanniae Radix *(shēng dì huáng)*	450g
Lonicerae Flos *(jīn yín huā)*	450g
Forsythiae Fructus *(lián qiáo)*	300g
Isatidis/Baphicacanthis Radix *(bǎn lán gēn)*	270g
Scutellariae Radix *(huáng qín)*	180g
Acori tatarinowii Rhizoma *(shí chāng pǔ)*	180g
Sojae Semen praeparatum *(dàn dòu chǐ)*	240g
Trichosanthis Radix *(tiān huā fěn)*	120g
Scrophulariae Radix *(xuán shēn)*	210g
Arnebiae/Lithospermi Radix *(zǐ cǎo)*	120g

Grind ingredients into powder mixed with Rehmannia juice and form into pills. Take 9g with cool water twice a day. Note that the source text uses 180g of Rhinocerotis Cornu *(xī jiǎo)*. Clears heat, opens up the orifices, cools the blood, and resolves fire toxicity. For warm-heat pathogen diseases, epidemic summerheat, and poxes characterized by severe heat toxin, delirious speech, deep-purple rashes, redness of the eyes, irritability, and a scarlet tongue (sometimes with a black coating). In contrast to the principal formula, which primarily cools and invigorates the blood, this formula focuses on resolving toxicity and opening the orifices.

Comparison

➢ Vs. Transform Maculae Decoction *(huà bān tāng)*; *see* PAGE 182

Section 3

....

FORMULAS THAT CLEAR HEAT AND RESOLVE TOXICITY

The formulas in this section are used in treating heat toxin with vigorous heat in the three burners characterized by fever, irritability, incoherent speech, nausea or vomiting, nosebleed, rashes, or various types of sores. Toxin is generally distinguished from heat by the presence of pustular lesions such as sores, or by the general 'sickness' of the patient. These formulas focus on heat toxin in the middle and upper burners, which may develop from constrained pathogenic influences generating heat, the accumulation of heat in the chest and diaphragm, or wind-heat epidemic toxin attacking the head or face. In addition, formulas that treat toxic sores characterized by localized redness, swelling, pain, and malaise are included.

The word 'toxin' (毒 *dú*) can mean different things depending on the context. It may refer to the cause of a disease, the pathological mechanism of a disease, or the toxicity of a substance, and is sometimes used interchangeably with the term for 'pathogenic influence' (邪 *xié*). In this chapter, toxin refers to the etiology or clinical presentation, not the toxicity of a substance. Chinese medicine also differentiates between yin and yang toxins, a distinction that dates back to Chapter 3 of *Essentials from the Golden Cabinet*. In general, yin toxin refers to toxicity accompanied by signs of cold, such as a pale or white complexion, white pus, or fatigue. Yang toxin refers to toxicity that manifests purely as heat. The formulas in this section address yang toxin.

The core ingredients in these formulas are those that clear heat and resolve toxicity, such as Coptidis Rhizoma *(huáng lián)*, Scutellariae Radix *(huáng qín)*, Phellodendri Cortex *(huáng bǎi)*, Lonicerae Flos *(jīn yín huā)*, Forsythiae Fructus *(lián qiáo)*, Isatidis/Baphicacanthis Radix *(bǎn lán gēn)*, and Taraxaci Herba *(pú gōng yīng)*. As heat toxicity is often constrained and clumped in the upper or superficial parts of the body, herbs that disperse wind and raise upward are often added, such as Menthae haplocalycis Herba *(bò hé)*, Arctii Fructus *(niú bàng zǐ)*, Bombyx batryticatus *(bái jiāng cán)*, and Saposhnikoviae Radix *(fáng fēng)*. When heat toxicity clumps in the middle burner, it can lead to constipation. Medicinals such as Rhei Radix et Rhizoma *(dà huáng)* and Natrii Sulfas *(máng xiāo)* are then used to drain out heat and unblock the bowels. Heat toxicity can clog up and collect, leading to local swelling and firmness, such as abscesses or boils. To treat these conditions, it is helpful to include herbs that transform phlegm and disperse clumping, such as Fritillariae Bulbus *(bèi mǔ)*, Citri reticulatae Pericarpium *(chén pí)*, and Bombyx batryticatus *(bái jiāng cán)*. These abscesses and other swellings can be extremely painful. Herbs that invigorate the blood and stop pain will then be necessary, such as Angelicae sinensis radicis Cauda *(dāng guī wěi)*, Olibanum *(rǔ xiāng)*, and Myrrha *(mò yào)*.

黄連解毒湯（黄连解毒汤）

Coptis Decoction to Resolve Toxicity

huáng lián jiě dú tāng

Source *Arcane Essentials from the Imperial Library* (752)

Coptidis Rhizoma *(huáng lián)*	9g
Scutellariae Radix *(huáng qín)*	6g
Phellodendri Cortex *(huáng bǎi)*	6g
Gardeniae Fructus *(zhī zǐ)*	6-12g

Method of Preparation Decoction. At present, the dosage of Coptidis Rhizoma *(huáng lián)* is generally one-half to one-third the amount specified. Some Japanese sources advise to take the decoction cool in order to enhance its cooling effects.

Actions Drains fire and resolves toxicity

Indications

High fever, irritability, a dry mouth and throat, incoherent speech, insomnia, dark urine, a red tongue with a yellow coating, and a rapid, forceful pulse. Also for nosebleed or vomiting of blood due to heat excess; carbuncles, deep-rooted boils, and other toxic swellings; and dysenteric disorders or jaundice due to damp-heat.

This is severe obstruction of the three burners by fire toxin (also known as 'heat toxin'), which pervades both the interior and exterior. Toxin can develop when an external pathogenic influence is transformed by constraint or from the accumulation of internally-generated heat. The fire toxin that ensues is present throughout the three burners and disturbs the spirit. This manifests as high fever, irritability, and in severe cases, incoherent speech and insomnia. The searing heat injures the fluids and dries the mouth and throat. Severe heat may also induce reckless movement of blood (especially in the upper part of the body), which causes nosebleeds or vomiting of blood. Injury to the blood vessels can result in leakage to the skin and the formation of purpura or rashes. Heat obstructing the muscle layer produces carbuncles, boils, and other types of suppurative swellings. The red tongue with a yellow coating and the fast, forceful pulse reflect the presence of fire toxin. In some cases, fire toxin from constraint may cause damp-heat dysenteric disorders or jaundice.

Analysis of Formula

Effective treatment of this condition requires that the heat (or fire) is drained from the entire body. Because the Heart corresponds to the fire phase, a substance that effectively drains fire from the Heart can cause an abatement of fire in all the other organs. Coptidis Rhizoma (huáng lián), the chief herb in this formula, does just this. It is also very useful in draining fire from the middle burner, a region of the body that, if not attended to, can give rise to many complications. The deputy, Scutellariae Radix (huáng qín), clears heat from the upper burner. Phellodendri Cortex (huáng bǎi), one of the assistants, clears heat from the lower burner. The other assistant, Gardeniae Fructus (zhī zǐ), drains heat from the three burners through the urine. This herb is particularly helpful in relieving irritability. Once the fire is effectively drained, the toxin will disappear.

Cautions and Contraindications

Because it is very bitter and cold, this formula should only be prescribed in cases of excess for patients of robust constitution. Since it can easily injure the yin, it should not be taken long term. If prescribed for conditions of heat in the nutritive or blood levels, it can readily injure the yin.

Commentary

This formula is suitable for all types of fire toxin obstructing the three burners. Such patterns are typically characterized by symptoms such as high fever, irritability, a dry mouth and throat, a red tongue with a yellow coating, and a rapid, strong pulse. Most commentators agree that the herbs that comprise the formula have been selected to drain heat and resolve toxicity from different sections of the Triple Burner. However, it is equally possible to think of their combination as a simple additive synergy where substances with the same basic action potentiate their individual effects. This perspective was first suggested by the Ming dynasty scholar-physician Zhang Jie-Bin:

> There is yin and yang fire, and heat [disorders] can be divided [according to whether they occur] above or below. According to the ancient formularies, Coptidis Rhizoma (huáng lián) clears the Heart, Scutellariae Radix (huáng qín) clears the Lungs, Dendrobii Herba (shí hú) and Paeoniae Radix (sháo yào) clear the Spleen, Gentianae Radix (lóng dǎn cǎo) clears the Liver, and Phellodendri Cortex (huáng bǎi) clears the Kidneys. Present usage generally adheres to this method. It is also a method of sticking [to custom without adapting to changing circumstance]. Generally, cold and cooling substances are all able to drain fire [irrespective of its location]. How could one claim that they cool here but do not cool there?

The contemporary formula expert Wang Mian-Zhi makes an interesting point regarding the emphasis on this formula's ability to resolve toxicity. He argues that this originally applied to its use in treating the effects of alcohol abuse. Alcohol is an acrid, dispersing, and strongly heating substance the effects of which are felt all over the body, that is, throughout the entire Triple Burner. In particular, although excess heat is itself a qi-aspect phenomenon, the effects of alcohol are focused on the blood. From this perspective, the present formula is particularly suitable for draining qi-aspect heat that stirs the blood, unlike White Tiger Decoction (bái hǔ tāng), which clears yang brightness heat that has spread throughout the Triple Burner. Furthermore, the aftereffects of alcohol consumption—insomnia, flushes, irritability, focal distention—provide useful clinical markers for using the formula in clinical practice.

Comparisons

➤ Vs. Major Order the Qi Decoction (dà chéng qì tāng)

Arcane Essentials from the Imperial Library differentiates the use of these formulas:

> The presence of dry stool in the Stomach causes a patient [to suffer from] delirious speech. Regular heat exuberance also causes a patient [to suffer from] delirious speech. In cases of constipation with delirious speech, it is appropriate to take Order the Qi Decoction (dà chéng qì tāng). [If the bowels are] open, [or even more if there is] dysentery with delirious speech, it is appropriate to take Four Substance Decoction with Coptis for Eliminating Heat (sì wèi huáng lián chú rè tāng) [another name for this formula].

In both cases, heat is located primarily in the yang brightness system but leads to different manifestations as it develops according to a different momentum. In the first case, heat enters into the bowels where it dries up the fluids and causes interior clumping with constipation. In the second case, it disperses throughout the three yang channels in the exterior and the Triple Burner in the interior. This is possible because the yang brightness is the 'sea of qi and blood' and the 'sea of the twelve channels.' Another perspective, suggested by the contemporary physician Ding Xue-Ping, is to attribute Order the Qi Decoction (*dà chéng qì tāng*) patterns to dry-heat and Coptis Decoction to Resolve Toxicity (*huáng lián jiě dú tāng*) patterns to damp-heat.

In clinical practice, yang toxin patterns are sometimes accompanied by constipation. In these cases, one can follow the clinical experience of the Qing-dynsaty physician Fei Bo-Xiong, who advised replacing Scutellariae Radix (*huáng qín*) with Rhei Radix et Rhizoma (*dà huáng*) in order to unblock the bowels and guide heat downward.

➢ Vs. WHITE TIGER DECOCTION (*bái hǔ tāng*); *see* PAGE 153

➢ Vs. DRAIN THE EPIGASTRIUM DECOCTION (*xiè xīn tāng*); *see* PAGE 172

Biomedical Indications

With the appropriate presentation, this formula may be used to treat a variety of biomedically-defined disorders, primarily infections such as septicemia, pyemia, dysentery, acute gastroenteritis, acute hepatitis, acute cholecystitis, pneumonia, urinary tract infections, stomatitis, periodontitis, meningitis, and encephalitis B. It is also used for insomnia, hypertension, and the sequelae of stroke.

Alternate names

Resolve Toxin Decoction (*jiě dú tāng*) in *Collection of Writings on the Mechanism of Disease, Suitability of Qi, and the Safeguarding of Life as Discussed in Basic Questions*; Fire Preparation Decoction (*huǒ jì tāng*) in *Pulse Causes, Patterns, and Treatments*; Coptis and Phellodendron Decoction (*huáng lián huáng bǎi tāng*) in *General Discussion of the Disease of Cold Damage*; Already Saved Resolve Toxin Decoction (*jì jì jiě dú tāng*) in *Lu Ban's Classic on Cultivating the Moon*; Three-Yellow Decoction to Resolve Toxicity (*sān huáng jiě dú tāng*) in *Awakening of the Mind in Medical Studies*; Three-Yellow Decoction (*sān huáng tāng*) in *Collection of Versatility*. **Note:** The origin of this formula is attributed to the Western Han dynasty physician Chun-Yu Yi, one of the earliest known physicians in the history of Chinese medicine. Its composition is first listed in *Emergency Prescriptions to Keep Up One's Sleeve*, but it has no name in that text.

Modifications

- For constipation, add Rhei Radix et Rhizoma (*dà huáng*).
- For jaundice due to obstruction from heat, add Artemisiae scopariae Herba (*yīn chén*) and Rhei Radix et Rhizoma (*dà huáng*).

- For dysenteric disorders with blood and mucus in the stool and tenesmus, add Aucklandiae Radix (*mù xiāng*), Arecae Semen (*bīng láng*), and Fraxini Cortex (*qín pí*).
- For damp-heat in the lower burner with urinary frequency, urgency, and discomfort, add Akebiae Caulis (*mù tōng*), Alismatis Rhizoma (*zé xiè*), and Plantaginis Semen (*chē qián zǐ*).
- For nosebleed, vomiting of blood, or erythema and purpura, add Rehmanniae Radix (*shēng dì huáng*), Moutan Cortex (*mǔ dān pí*), and Scrophulariae Radix (*xuán shēn*), or combine with Rhinoceros Horn and Rehmannia Decoction (*xī jiǎo dì huáng tāng*).
- For purulent lesions such as deep-rooted boils, combine with Five-Ingredient Decoction to Eliminate Toxin (*wǔ wèi xiāo dú yǐn*).

Associated Formulas

三黃石膏湯 （三黄石膏汤）

Three-Yellow and Gypsum Decoction from *Indispensable Tools for Pattern Treatment*

sān huáng shí gāo tāng

SOURCE *Indispensable Tools for Pattern Treatment* (1602)

Coptidis Rhizoma (*huáng lián*) 6g
Phellodendri Cortex (*huáng bǎi*) 3g
Scutellariae Radix (*huáng qín*) 4.5g
Gypsum fibrosum (*shí gāo*). 9g
Gardeniae Fructus (*zhī zǐ*) 3g
Scrophulariae Radix (*xuán shēn*) 3g
Anemarrhenae Rhizoma (*zhī mǔ*) 4.5g
Glycyrrhizae Radix (*gān cǎo*) 2.1g

Prepare as a decoction. Clears and drains heat from all three burners. This is one of a number of formulas by the same name and is a combination of the main formula and White Tiger Decoction (*bái hǔ tāng*). It is indicated for summerheat damage that manifests with severe fever due to heat and toxin spreading throughout the Triple Burner.

大黃連柏湯 （大黄连柏汤）

Rhubarb, Coptis, and Phellodendron Decoction

dà huáng lián bǎi tāng

SOURCE *Collected Medical Writings of Jiang Chun-Hua* (contemporary)

Rhei Radix et Rhizoma (*dà huáng*) . . . .(9g)
Coptidis Rhizoma (*huáng lián*) . . . .(6g)
Phellodendri Cortex (*huáng bǎi*) . . . .(6g)

Prepare as a decoction. The source text does not specify dosage. Drains heat and stops bleeding. For cough with bleeding that occurs in the course of rheumatic heart disease and is accompanied by a red complexion, a flooding, large pulse, and constipation. The pattern is caused by blood constrained within the Lungs. Rhei Radix et Rhizoma (*dà huáng*) is used as the chief herb to drain fire, stop bleeding, and guide the blood downward, which has the effect of easing blood constraint within the Lungs. The formula's author, Jiang Chun-Hua, was a leading figure in the movement to integrate Western and Chinese medicine in Maoist China, and this formula is representative of that approach.

瀉肝湯 （泻肝汤）

Drain the Liver Decoction

xiè gān tāng

SOURCE *Selections from the Clinical Experience of Guan You-Bo* (2006)

Artemisiae scopariae Herba (*yīn chén hāo*) 60g
Coptidis Rhizoma (*huáng lián*) 10g
Scutellariae Radix (*huáng qín*) 15g
Moutan Cortex (*mǔ dān pí*) 15g
Phellodendri Cortex (*huáng bǎi*) 15g
Rhei Radix et Rhizoma (*dà huáng*) . . . . (fried in alcohol) 10g
Gardeniae Fructus (*zhī zǐ*) 15g
Paeoniae Radix rubra (*chì sháo*) 15g
Lonicerae Flos (*jīn yín huā*) 30g
Taraxaci Herba (*pú gōng yīng*) 15g
Violae Herba (*zǐ huā dì dīng*) 15g
Chrysanthemi indici Flos (*yě jú huā*) 15g
Isatidis Radix (*bǎn lán gēn*) 30g
Paridis Rhizoma (*chóng lóu*)* 15g
Aurantii Fructus immaturus (*zhǐ shí*) 10g
Trichosanthis Fructus (*guā lóu*) 10g
Pinelliae Rhizoma (*bàn xià*) 10g

Prepare as a decoction and divide into four portions, which are taken in the course of one day. The source text stipulates that each dose should be taken with half a Greatest Treasure Special Pill (*zhì bǎo dān*). Drains heat and resolves toxicity, clears the liver, and cools the blood. For early stage hepatic coma with the patient drifting in and out of consciousness, yang-type jaundice, red eyes and complexion, pain in both flanks, abdominal distention, heavy breathing, foul breath, thirst, constipation, a red tongue with a yellow coating, and a wiry slippery pulse. This is another example of integrated Chinese and Western medicine in contemporary China. The formula combines Coptis Decoction to Resolve Toxicity (*huáng lián jiē dú tāng*) with Virgate Wormwood Decoction (*yīn chén hāo tāng*), Five-Ingredient Drink to Eliminate Toxin (*wǔ wèi xiāo dú yǐn*), and Minor Decoction [for Pathogens] Stuck in the Chest (*xiǎo xiàn xiōng tāng*). The author advises to take the formula for up to half a month or until the symptoms have improved by at least 50 percent. After that, the treatment strategy should change from attacking to tonifying.

黃連上清丸 （黄连上清丸）

Coptis Pill to Clear the Upper [Burner]

huáng lián shàng qīng wán

SOURCE *Nationwide Collection of TCM Patent Formulas* (1962)

---

*The source text calls for 草河車 *cǎo hé chē* ('herbal river vehicle'). This usually refers to the herb that is now conventionally called Paridis Rhizoma (*chóng lóu*), but could also be the herb known as Bistortae Rhizoma (*quán shēn*).

Coptidis Rhizoma (*huáng lián*) 240g
Scutellariae Radix (*huáng qín*) 240g
Phellodendri Cortex (*huáng bǎi*) 240g
Gardeniae Fructus (*zhī zǐ*) 240g
Rhei Radix et Rhizoma (*dà huáng*) 360g
Forsythiae Fructus (*lián qiáo*) 180g
Curcumae longae Rhizoma (*jiāng huáng*) 180g
Scrophulariae Radix (*xuán shēn*) 120g
Menthae haplocalycis Herba (*bò hé*) 120g
Angelicae sinensis radicis Cauda (*dāng guī wěi*) 120g
Puerariae Radix (*gé gēn*) 60g
Chuanxiong Rhizoma (*chuān xiōng*) 60g
Platycodi Radix (*jié gěng*) 60g
Trichosanthis Radix (*tiān huā fěn*) 60g

The ingredients are ground and formed into honey pills. The dosage is 9g/dose taken with green tea. Clears heat and resolves toxicity, drains fire, and unblocks the bowels. For acute red eyes, sore throat, mouth or tongue sores, dark, rough urination, and restlessness and heat in the heart and diaphragm. This formula is more balanced than the principal formula in that Puerariae Radix (*gé gēn*) and Trichosanthis Radix (*tiān huā fěn*) engender fluids and offset the fluid-damaging effects of the internal heat pathogen and the bitter herbs in the formula. Nonetheless, its bitter and cold herbs dictate that this formula be taken for only a short time.

In addition to the symptoms listed above, the formula is frequently applied to the treatment of toxic swellings in the upper body, sties, and conjunctivitis. It is also used to treat both internal and external acute ear infections.

Comparison

➢ Vs. SCHIZONEPETA AND FORSYTHIA DECOCTION (*jīng jiè lián qiáo tāng*); see PAGE 46

牛黃上清丸

Cattle Gallstone Pill to Clear the Upper [Burner]

niú huáng shàng qīng wán

SOURCE *Nationwide Collection of TCM Patent Formulas* (1962)

Coptidis Rhizoma (*huáng lián*) 24g
Scutellariae Radix (*huáng qín*) 75g
Phellodendri Cortex (*huáng bǎi*) 15g
Gardeniae Fructus (*zhī zǐ*) 75g
Bovis Calculus (*niú huáng*) 3g
Borneolum (*bīng piàn*) 15g
Rhei Radix et Rhizoma (*dà huáng*) 120g
Forsythiae Fructus (*lián qiáo*) 75g
Gypsum fibrosum (*shí gāo*) 120g
Chrysanthemi Flos (*jú huā*) 60g
Saposhnikoviae Radix (*fáng fēng*) 24g
Schizonepetae Herba (*jīng jiè*) 24g
Angelicae dahuricae Radix (*bái zhǐ*) 24g
Chuanxiong Rhizoma (*chuān xiōng*) 24g
Platycodi Radix (*jié gěng*) 24g
Glycyrrhizae Radix (*gān cǎo*) 15g
Menthae haplocalycis Herba (*bò hé*) 15g
Paeoniae Radix rubra (*chì sháo*) 24g
Angelicae sinensis Radix (*dāng guī*) 75g
Nelumbinis Plumula (*lián zǐ xīn*) 60g
Realgar (*xióng huáng*) 24g

Disperses wind-heat and drains and resolves fire toxicity. For head-ache, redness of the eyes, pain and swelling of the throat and gums, and ulcerations of the mouth and tongue due to fire.

清上防風湯 （清上防风汤）

Clear the Upper [Burner] Decoction with Saposhnikovia

qīng shàng fáng fēng tāng

SOURCE *Restoration of Health from the Myriad Diseases* (1587)

Saposhnikoviae Radix *(fáng fēng)*	3g
Forsythiae Fructus *(lián qiáo)*	2.2g
Platycodi Radix *(jié gěng)*	2.2g
Angelicae dahuricae Radix *(bái zhǐ)*	2.2g
Scutellariae Radix *(huáng qín)*	2g
Chuanxiong Rhizoma *(chuān xiōng)*	2g
Schizonepetae Herba *(jīng jiè)*	1.5g
Gardeniae Fructus *(zhī zǐ)*	1.5g
Coptidis Rhizoma *(huáng lián)*	1.5g
Menthae haplocalycis Herba *(bò hé)*	1.5g
Aurantii Fructus *(zhǐ ké)*	0.6g
Glycyrrhizae Radix *(gān cǎo)*	0.6g

The herbs are coarsely ground and then decocted. Modern practitioners generally increase the amount of all the ingredients. Clears heat, resolves toxicity, and dispels dampness and wind. This formula treats upper burner fire that presents with a wide variety of head and neck problems including headache, sores, pimples, or boils on the face or neck, infantile fetal heat, red and swollen eyes, red face and neck, and drinker's nose. It is also applied to acute eczema of the face and neck.

This formula can be seen as a modification of Coptis Decoction to Resolve Toxicity *(huáng lián jiě dú tāng)*, focusing the effects on the upper body while adding herbs that disperse wind, expel pus, and reduce accumulation.

Note that the source text suggests adding Bambusae Succus *(zhú lì)* to increase effectiveness. Because this liquid is usually not available in the West, one may consider substituting Bambusae Concretio silicea *(tiān zhú huáng)*.

Comparison

➢ Vs. SCHIZONEPETA AND FORSYTHIA DECOCTION *(jīng jiè lián qiáo tāng); see* PAGE 46

清涼飲子 （清涼饮子）

Clearing and Cooling Drink

qīng liáng yǐn zi

SOURCE *Symptom, Cause, Pulse, and Treatment* (Ming dynasty)

Scutellariae Radix *(huáng qín)*	6g
Coptidis Rhizoma *(huáng lián)*	6g
Gardeniae Fructus *(zhī zǐ)*	6g
Menthae haplocalycis Herba *(bò hé)*	4.5g
Moutan Cortex *(mǔ dān pí)*	4.5g
Angelicae sinensis Radix *(dāng guī)*	4.5g
Paeoniae Radix alba *(bái sháo)*	4.5g
Glycyrrhizae Radix *(gān cǎo)*	3g

Decoction. The source text does not list dosage, and these have been added based on contemporary usage. Clears fire and enriches the yin to treat excess fire from dryness in the upper burner leading to symptoms such as thirst, irritability, bleeding, and swelling. This is one of a number of similar formulas by the same name but with slightly different ingredients. It is used in contemporary practice to treat patterns of mixed excess and deficiency, such as herpes and stomatitis, manifesting with erosions and sores in the mouth.

瀉心湯 （泻心汤）

Drain the Epigastrium Decoction

xiè xīn tāng

The literal translation of this formula's name is Drain the Heart Decoction. In traditional Chinese medicine, the epigastrium is called the 'opening of the Heart' (心口 *xīn kǒu*).

Source *Essentials from the Golden Cabinet* (c. 220)

Rhei Radix et Rhizoma *(dà huáng)*	6g
Coptidis Rhizoma *(huáng lián)*	3g
Scutellariae Radix *(huáng qín)*	3g

Method of Preparation Decoction. Often at present the dosage of Coptidis Rhizoma *(huáng lián)* and Scutellariae Radix *(huáng qín)* is increased to 9g.

Actions Drains fire, resolves toxicity, and dries dampness

Indications

Fever, irritability and restlessness, flushed face, red eyes, dark urine, constipation, a greasy, yellow tongue coating, and in severe cases, delirious speech. Also for epigastric focal distention, jaundice, diarrhea and dysenteric disorders; or vomiting of blood or nosebleed; or red and swollen eyes and ears; or ulcerations of the tongue and mouth; or abscesses.

This is damp-heat excess with interior clumping. Fever, irritability, and restlessness, flushed face, red eyes, dark urine, constipation, a greasy, yellow tongue coating, epigastric focal distention, jaundice, diarrhea, and dysenteric disorders are manifestations of damp-heat excess and interior clumping. Vomiting of blood and nosebleed are caused by the reckless movement of hot blood. Red and swollen eyes and ears, ulcerations of the mouth and tongue, and abscesses are associated with fire toxin.

Analysis of Formula

This is one of the strongest heat-draining formulas in Chinese medicine. It focuses entirely on directing the qi downward in order to drain excess heat and fire from the body. Accordingly, in this formula Rhei Radix et Rhizoma *(dà huáng)*, the chief herb, is used more for its action in draining fire than for purging. However, this presentation does include signs of clumping; if accompanied by diarrhea or dysenteric disorders, purging will drain the heat and break up the clumping. In addition, this herb enters the blood level and is useful in the treatment of bleeding, especially in the upper part of the body. The deputies, Scutellariae Radix (huáng qín) and Coptidis Rhizoma (huáng lián), drain heat from the upper and middle burners. Together, the herbs in this formula drain heat from the three burners, primarily through the stool.

Cautions and Contraindications

Contraindicated in those with Spleen deficiency cold.

Commentary

Composition

There has been some controversy about the composition of this formula. In the extant edition of *Discussion of Cold Damage*, it lists only the two ingredients Rhei Radix et Rhizoma (dà huáng) and Coptidis Rhizoma (huáng lián), which are also prepared in a somewhat different manner (see below). This has led to two distinctly different views. The first is associated with Lin Yi, the official in charge of the Song state-sponsored editing of the medical classics. Lin interpreted the formula to include Scutellariae Radix (huáng qín). This interpretation is supported by the fact that the paired formula in that text, Aconite Accessory Root Decoction to Drain the Epigastrium (fù zǐ xiè xīn tāng), contains Scutellariae Radix (huáng qín). Furthermore, most, but not all, practitioners believe that the addition of Scutellariae Radix (huáng qín) improves the effectiveness of the formula in clearing heat and reducing focal distention.

A second view is to think of these as two different formulas, depending on whether Scutellariae Radix (huáng qín) is included. This interpretation is based on the different mode of preparation for the formula stipulated in paragraph 154 of *Discussion of Cold Damage*, which says to steep the ingredients in water that is just beginning to boil, press out the dregs, and then take warm. This turns the entire formula into an infusion rather than a decoction and fundamentally changes its action. We call this second formula Rhubarb and Coptis Infusion to Drain the Epigastrium (dà huáng huáng lián xiè xīn tāng) and discuss its properties and indications under VARIATIONS below.

Key Indicators

The main focus of the present formula is to direct fire downward and to drain excess heat. As such, it has four main areas of application, all of which must be accompanied by signs of excess fire such as dark urination, constipation, a bitter taste, a yellow tongue coating, and a rapid pulse:

1. Bleeding, especially from the upper body due to excess heat stirring the blood

2. Excess fire flaring throughout the body giving rise to conditions characterized by inflammation, particularly in the upper body and throughout the digestive system. Examples include mouth ulcers, gum disease, red and inflamed eyes, pain and ulceration of the throat, hemorrhoids, and early stage dysenteric disorders.

3. 'Unsettled Heart qi' (心氣不定 xīn qì bù dìng) due to excess fire harassing the spirit. The term is derived from Sun Si-Miao who substituted it for the term 'insufficient Heart qi' (心氣不足 xīn qì bù zú) in the source text. Although the flaring up of Heart fire may give rise to insufficiency of both qi and yin, Sun Si-Miao's analysis is widely considered to more accurately describe the presenting signs and symptoms. These include irritability, restlessness, and a sensation of oppression in the chest. Contemporary physicians also include manifestations of psychotic disorders and cardiovascular disease such as hypertension.

4. Jaundice due to damp-heat excess with focal distention, a greasy, yellow tongue coating, and a rapid, wiry pulse

Comparison

➢ Vs. COPTIS DECOCTION TO RESOLVE TOXICITY (huáng lián jiě dú tāng)

The focus of Coptis Decoction to Resolve Toxicity (huáng lián jiě dú tāng), which contains Gardeniae Fructus (zhī zǐ), is on draining heat from the three burners. Drain the Epigastrium Decoction (xiè xīn tāng), on the other hand, which contains Rhei Radix et Rhizoma (dà huáng), has purgative and heat-draining actions that are used to guide excess fire downward. This is known in Chinese medicine as 'employing draining as a substitute for clearing' (以瀉代清 yǐ xiè dài qīng). For this reason, the formula can be used in treating any condition of excess fire, particularly in the upper body, the Heart, and the Stomach and Intestines.

Biomedical Indications

With the appropriate presentation, this formula can be used to treat a wide variety of biomedically-defined disorders. These can be divided into the following groups:

- Infectious, purulent inflammations, especially those involving the head and neck such as carbuncles, furuncles, tonsilitis, and conjunctivitis

- Hemorrhages, including those from the optical fundus, lungs, stomach, colon, uterus, and brain, as well as hemorrhoids

- Cerebrovascular diseases including hypertension, atherosclerosis, and stroke

This formula has also been used for insomnia, schizophrenia, hypercholesterolemia, pleurisy, bacillary dysentery, cystitis, pelvic inflammatory disease, hepatolenticular degeneration, and trigeminal neuralgia.

Modifications

- For trigeminal neuralgia, add Scorpio (*quán xiē*), Scolopendra (*wú gōng*), and Cicadae Periostracum (*chán tuì*).
- For both yang brightness and terminal yin headache, add Frigid Extremities Powder (*sì nì sǎn*).

Variations

大黃黃連瀉心湯 （大黄黄连泻心汤）

Rhubarb and Coptis Infusion to Drain the Epigastrium

dà huáng huáng lián xiè xīn tāng

SOURCE　*Discussion of Cold Damage* (c. 220)

Rhei Radix et Rhizoma (*dà huáng*) 12g
Coptidis Rhizoma (*huáng lián*) 6g

METHOD OF PREPARATION　Infusion. The source text stipulates to steep the ingredients in 2 cups of water that is just starting to boil, press out the dregs, and then take warm in two doses. Drains fire, resolves toxicity, and dries dampness to treat hot focal distention. In the source text, this is defined as epigastric distention that is soft when pressed and accompanied by a floating pulse in the middle position. Hot focal distention occurs when heat pathogen without form collects in the epigastrium. The floating pulse here indicates the presence of heat. Because it is only felt in the middle position, it refers to heat in the middle burner that is causing blockage and focal distention. It is inappropriate to purge unless the heat has knotted with the dregs of digestion. However, from the pulse, it is clear that the pathogen is already in the interior. Combining two bitter, cooling, downward-draining herbs prepared as an infusion represents an elegant solution to this problem. It allows for the downward-draining of excess heat from the Stomach and thereby the resolution of focal distention without the use of purgation. As explained by Qian Huang: "With regard to [the epigastrium] being soft when pressed, it is just that it is formless pathogenic heat. Although the heat has no form, still it cannot be gotten rid of unless it is drained by bitter, cold [substances]; therefore this formula masters it."

Although the indications of this formula are similar to those of the principal formula, its effects are less harsh, and it thus has an even wider spectrum of application. For instance, it is used to treat all kinds of inflammatory conditions in the head, upper body, and throughout the digestive tract. Like the principal formula, it treats bleeding from the upper body orifices as well as heat excess harassing the spirit, hypertension, and heat excess skin disorders.

Use of this formula should be distinguished from others that drain focal distention from the epigastrium, particularly the various Pinellia Decoction to Drain the Epigastrium (*bàn xià xiè xīn tāng*) formulas. The presentations for which those formulas are indicated can easily be distinguished by the presence of cold/water excess in addition to heat/fire. This is reflected in such signs and symptoms as a greasy tongue coating, slippery pulse, cold-type diarrhea or borborygmus, and watery sputum.

附子瀉心湯 （附子泻心汤）

Aconite Accessory Root Infusion to Drain the Epigastrium

fù zǐ xiè xīn tāng

SOURCE　*Discussion of Cold Damage* (c. 220)

For focal distention due to damp-heat, vomiting, and diarrhea with sweating, aversion to cold, cold extremities, a submerged, thin pulse, and other signs of yang deficiency, add 3g of Aconiti Radix lateralis praeparata (*zhì fù zǐ*).

This can also be prepared as an infusion with all the ingredients except Aconiti Radix lateralis praeparata (*zhì fù zǐ*). This is steeped in 2 cups of water that is just starting to boil, the dregs are then pressed out, and the resulting liquid combined with decocted Aconiti Radix lateralis praeparata (*zhì fù zǐ*) and taken warm in two doses.

Associated Formula

內疏黃連湯 （内疏黄连汤）

Internal Dispersing Decoction with Coptis

nèi shū huáng lián tāng

SOURCE　*Collection of Writings on the Mechanism of Illness, Suitability of Qi, and the Safeguarding of Life as Discussed in Basic Questions* (1186)

Coptidis Rhizoma (*huáng lián*) 9g
Scutellariae Radix (*huáng qín*) 9g
Gardeniae Fructus (*zhī zǐ*) 9g
Forsythiae Fructus (*lián qiáo*) 9g
Menthae haplocalycis Herba (*bò hé*) 6g
Platycodi Radix (*jié gěng*) 6g
Glycyrrhizae Radix (*gān cǎo*) 6g
Angelicae sinensis Radix (*dāng guī*) 9g
Paeoniae Radix alba (*bái sháo*) 9g
Aucklandiae Radix (*mù xiāng*) 6g
Arecae Semen (*bīng láng*) 6g
Rhei Radix et Rhizoma (*dà huáng*) 6g

Clears heat and resolves toxicity, reduces swelling, and alleviates pain. For abscesses due to interior heat characterized by swelling with no change in skin color, fever, irritability, dry heaves, thirst, reduced urination, constipation, and a submerged, excessive pulse.

普濟消毒飲 （普济消毒饮）

Universal Benefit Drink to Eliminate Toxin

pǔ jì xiāo dú yǐn

This formula, devised during a period of widespread epidemics in China, was considered by its author to be a well-tested formula that could save many lives, hence the name.

Source　*Dong-Yuan's Tried and Tested Formulas* (1202)

Scutellariae Radix (*huáng qín*) 15g
Coptidis Rhizoma (*huáng lián*) 15g
Ginseng Radix (*rén shēn*) 9g
Arctii Fructus (*niú bàng zǐ*) 3g
Forsythiae Fructus (*lián qiáo*) 3g
Menthae haplocalycis Herba (*bò hé*) 3g
dry-fried Bombyx batryticatus (*chǎo jiāng cán*) 2g
Scrophulariae Radix (*xuán shēn*) 6g
Lasiosphaera/Calvatia (*mǎ bó*) 3g
Isatidis/Baphicacanthis Radix (*bǎn lán gēn*) 3g

Platycodi Radix (*jié gěng*) 6g
Glycyrrhizae Radix (*gān cǎo*) 6g
Citri reticulatae Exocarpium rubrum (*jú hóng*) 6g
Bupleuri Radix (*chái hú*) 6g
Cimicifugae Rhizoma (*shēng má*) 2g

Method of Preparation   The source text advises to grind the ingredients into powder and take half as a draft and the other half in the form of pills made with honey that are slowly dissolved in the mouth. At present, it is generally prepared as a decoction with Ginseng Radix (*rén shēn*) either reduced to a dosage of 3g or deleted.

Actions   Clears heat, eliminates fire toxin, and disperses wind-heat

Indications

Strong fever and chills, redness, swelling, and burning pain of the head and face, inability to open the eyes, dysfunction of the throat, dryness and thirst, a red tongue with a powdery-white or yellow coating, and a floating, rapid, and forceful pulse.

This is acute, massive febrile disorder of the head (大頭瘟 *dà toú wēn*), also known as massive epidemic disorder of the head (大頭天行 *dà toú tiān xíng*), due to a seasonal epidemic toxin associated with wind-heat and damp-phlegm. It is most commonly seen in children and is usually contracted during the winter or spring. It is characterized by a sudden onset and severe fire toxin. It is the severity and rapaciousness of the effects on the body of the underlying pathogenic influences that account for the use of the word 'toxin.'

The head is the meeting place of the body's yang qi and is the first area to be attacked by seasonal toxin. Here it festers and causes the redness, swelling, burning pain, and tenderness that characterize this disorder. In severe cases, the swelling may include the entire upper body. This condition reflects the battle raging between the powerful pathogenic influences and a robust host; the fever and chills are therefore both strong. The 'battleground' is the upper burner (the dwelling of the Lungs, Heart, and throat), hence the dysfunction of the throat. The severe heat also causes thirst, dryness, redness of the tongue and its powdery-white coating, and a floating, rapid pulse. If less severe, the tongue coating will be yellow.

Analysis of Formula

This condition requires two strategies: resolving the fire toxicity (the primary treatment principle that deals with the branch) and dispersing wind-heat (the secondary principle that deals with the root). A relatively large dose of the chief herbs, Coptidis Rhizoma (*huáng lián*) and Scutellariae Radix (*huáng qín*), is used to clear and drain the toxic heat from the upper burner. The use of wine serves to direct the actions of these herbs upward. There are two groups of deputies. Acrid and cool Arctii Fructus (*niú bàng zi*), Forsythiae Fructus

(*lián qiáo*), and Menthae haplocalycis Herba (*bò hé*), along with acrid and neutral Bombyx batryticatus (*bái jiāng cán*), disperse wind-heat from the upper burner, head, and face. Scrophulariae Radix (*xuán shēn*), Lasiosphaera/Calvatia (*mǎ bó*), Isatidis/Baphicacanthis Radix (*bǎn lán gēn*), Platycodi Radix (*jié gěng*), and Glycyrrhizae Radix (*gān cǎo*) clear heat from the throat and relieve the toxic fire there.

Citri reticulatae Exocarpium rubrum (*jú hóng*), the assistant, regulates the qi to ensure the free flow of blood and qi and thereby prevent the pathogenic influences from accumulating. This helps to reduce toxic swelling. Bupleuri Radix (*chái hú*) and Cimicifugae Rhizoma (*shēng má*) serve as envoys by raising the yang, dispersing wind-heat, and conducting the other ingredients to the head. They are also effective in dispersing stagnation due to fire.

Cautions and Contraindications

Because most of the herbs in this formula are bitter or acrid and have dispersing properties, it should be used with caution in treating those with yin deficiency.

Commentary

Although early observations of this disorder were recorded in the *Yellow Emperor's Inner Classic,* the understanding of its etiology and pathogenesis became more sophisticated during the Jin and Yuan dynasties, and perhaps was even better understood by the warm pathogen disease current of the Qing dynasty. Therefore, the Chinese medical literature discusses the disorder under a range of different names. Most writers, however, agree that Li Dong-Yuan's formula constitutes the treatment of choice. This consensus is reflected in a passage from Wu Ju-Tong's *Systematic Differentiation of Warm Pathogen Diseases:* "Treatment strategies [for this disorder] cannot go beyond Li Dong-Yuan's Universal Benefit Drink to Eliminate Toxin (*pǔ jì xiāo dú yǐn*)."

Nevertheless, Wu Ju-Tong felt entitled to make major adjustments to the use of the formula in the clinic. Noting that the inherent momentum of the disorder involved the excessive accumulation of heat toxin in the upper body and head, he suggested removing Bupleuri Radix (*chái hú*) and Cimicifugae Rhizoma (*shēng má*) and replacing them with Lonicerae Flos (*jīn yín huā*) and Schizonepetae Herba (*jīng jiè*). He argued that the addition of these light substances ensured that the formula would focus on the upper burner and head with little risk of guiding even more qi to this area. Such reasoning reflects a fundamental difference in style between Li Dong-Yuan's emphasis on supporting the body's normal qi and Wu Ju-Tong's adherence to the principles of the warm pathogen disease current, with its emphasis on the use of 'light substances to eliminate serious [disorders].' If the latter approach tries to prevent newly-contracted pathogens from moving deeper into the body, the Jin-Yuan medicine that Li

Dong-Yuan represents concentrates, instead, on supporting the body's resistance. These concerns not only underpin his use of Cimicifugae Rhizoma (*shēng má*) and Bupleuri Radix (*chái hú*), which are intended to facilitate the ascent of yang qi, but also explain the inclusion of a tonifying herb like Ginseng Radix (*rén shēn*) in a formula intended to resolve toxicity and clear heat.

The contemporary consensus is to include Ginseng Radix (*rén shēn*) only if the patient's consitution or presentation demands it. No such consensus exists regarding the use of Cimicifugae Rhizoma (*shēng má*) and Bupleuri Radix (*chái hú*). Those advocating inclusion refer to the well-established treatment strategy of discharging heat from constraint. They also point out the synergistic effects that arise from the combination with Coptidis Rhizoma (*huáng lián*) and Scutellariae Radix (*huáng qín*). Because these herbs drain fire downward, their matching balances out any excessive ascending or downward-directing effect that each pairing might cause on its own.

Proponents of the warm pathogen disease therapeutics, such as the Qing-dynasty physician Ye Lin, replied that such rationalizations cannot make up for Li Dong-Yuan's basic mistake. His own compromise was to omit Coptidis Rhizoma (*huáng lián*) and Cimicifugae Rhizoma (*shēng má*), but retain Scutellariae Radix (*huáng qín*) and Bupleuri Radix (*chái hú*). This argument, in turn, is based on Ye's own understanding of warm pathogen disorders as arising from lurking pathogens (伏邪 *fú xié*). According to the doctrines laid out in *Supplemental Critical Annotations to the Systematic Discussion of Warm Pathogen Diseases*, these lurking pathogens usually vent through the lesser yang and therefore justify the use of Bupleuri Radix (*chái hú*) and Scutellariae Radix (*huáng qín*).

Comparisons

➢ Vs. Sweet Dew Special Pill to Eliminate Toxin (*gān lù xiāo dú dān*); *see* page 704

➢ Vs. Immortals' Formula for Sustaining Life (*xiān fāng huó mìng yǐn*); *see* page 862

➢ Vs. Clear the Heart and Enable the Diaphragm Decoction (*qīng xīn lì gé tāng*); *see* page 887

Biomedical Indications

With the appropriate presentation, this formula may be used to treat a variety of biomedically-defined disorders, primarily acute infections including furuncles and carbuncles (especially affecting the head), parotiditis, tonsillitis, lymphadenditis, upper respiratory tract infections (primarily in children), hemorrhagic conjunctivitis, acute icteric hepatitis, infectious mononucleosis accompanied by hepatomegaly, and viral myocarditis.

Alternate names

The authorship of this formula is attributed to Li Dong-Yuan in 1202. It is first listed in a text by his student Luo Tian-Yi under the slightly different name 普濟消毒飲子 *pǔ jì xiāo dú yǐn zi*. Its modern name derives from a formula with the same indication but a slightly different composition listed in *Exemplars for Applying the Principles of External Medicine*, written during the Ming era. Wang Ang used the present name in his discussion of the formula in *Medical Formulas Collected and Analyzed*. Owing to the enormous influence of this work, it became the standard name in almost all later formularies, with the exception of *Discussion of Warm Epidemics*, which lists it as Universal Benefit Powder to Eliminate Toxin (*pǔ jì xiāo dú sǎn*).

Modifications

- For constipation, add Rhei Radix et Rhizoma (*dà huáng*). (source text)

- For more obvious exterior symptoms with less severe internal heat, reduce the dosage of Scutellariae Radix (*huáng qín*) and Coptidis Rhizoma (*huáng lián*) and add Schizonepetae Herba (*jīng jiè*), Saposhnikoviae Radix (*fáng fēng*), Menthae haplocalycis Herba (*bò hé*), and Mori Folium (*sāng yè*).

- When the exterior symptoms have disappeared and the internal heat is severe, remove Bupleuri Radix (*chái hú*) and Menthae haplocalycis Herba (*bò hé*) and add Lonicerae Flos (*jīn yín huā*) and Indigo naturalis (*qīng dài*).

- For internal heat with constipation, add Rhei Radix et Rhizoma (*dà huáng*), Aurantii Fructus immaturus (*zhǐ shí*), and Natrii Sulfas siccatus (*xuán míng fěn*).

- For hard, stubborn, localized swelling, add Moutan Cortex (*mǔ dān pí*), Paeoniae Radix rubra (*chì sháo*), Fritillariae thunbergii Bulbus (*zhè bèi mǔ*), Prunellae Spica (*xià kū cǎo*), and Luffae Fructus Retinervus (*sī guā luò*).

- For concurrent orchitis, add Meliae Cortex (*kǔ liàn gēn pí*) and Gentianae Radix (*lóng dǎn cǎo*).

Associated Formula

大頭瘟湯（大头瘟汤）

Massive Febrile Disorder of the Head Decoction
dà tóu wēn tāng

Source *Medical Collectanea of Kong Bo-Hua* (1988)

Gypsum fibrosum (*shí gāo*)	9g
Taraxaci Herba (*pú gōng yīng*)	12g
Forsythiae Fructus (*lián qiáo*)	9g
Menthae haplocalycis Herba (*bò hé*)	4.5g
Persicae Semen (*táo rén*)	9g
Armeniacae Semen (*xìng rén*)	9g
Lonicerae Flos (*jīn yín huā*)	15g
Gentianae Radix (*lóng dǎn cǎo*)	9g
Mori Folium (*sāng yè*)	9g
Phragmitis Rhizoma recens (*xiān lú gēn*)	30g
Bombyx batryticatus (*jiāng cán*)	9g
Nelumbinis Plumula (*lián zǐ xīn*)	6g
Anemarrhenae Rhizoma (*zhī mǔ*)	6g

Phellodendri Cortex (*huáng bǎi*) 6g
Talcum (*huá shí*) 12g
Cyathulae Radix (*chuān niú xī*) 9g
Trichosanthis Fructus (*quán guā lóu*) 24g
Nelumbinis Folium (*hé yè*) . . . . .1 leaf
Gardeniae Fructus (*zhī zǐ*) 9g
Lycii Cortex (*dì gǔ pí*) 9g
Nelumbinis Nodus rhizomatis (*ǒu jié*) 30g
Natrii Sulfas (*máng xiāo*) 4.5g
Plum Blossom Dotted Tongue Special Pill *
    (*méi huā diǎn shé dān*) . . . . 4 pills

Decoction. Clears heat, drains fire, dissipates clumps, and resolves toxicity. Indicated for massive febrile disorder of the head with severe swelling of the face and neck, chills and fevers, thirst, a white greasy tongue coating, and a wiry, slippery, and rapid pulse. The condition arises from obstruction of the upper burner by the pathogens wind, dampness, and heat. This formula was composed by Kong Bo-Hua, one of the Four Great Master Physicians (四大明醫 *sì dà míng yī*) of Beijing during the middle part of the 20th century, and unlike the original formula, reflects his personal emphasis on warm pathogen therapeutics.

涼膈散 （涼膈散）
Cool the Diaphragm Powder

liáng gé sǎn

This formula cools the diaphragm by clearing heat from the upper burner and draining heat from the middle burner. (The upper and middle burners straddle the diaphragm.)

Source   *Formulary of the Pharmacy Service for Benefiting the People in the Taiping Era* (1107)

Rhei Radix et Rhizoma (*dà huáng*) 600g (9g)
Natrii Sulfas (*máng xiāo*) 600g (9g)
Glycyrrhizae Radix (*gān cǎo*) .600g (9g)
Scutellariae Radix (*huáng qín*) 300g (4.5g)
Gardeniae Fructus (*zhī zǐ*) 300g (4.5g)
Forsythiae Fructus (*lián qiáo*) 1,200g (18g)
Menthae haplocalycis Herba (*bò hé*) 300g (4.5g)

Method of Preparation   Grind the ingredients into a powder and take 6-12g as a draft 2-3 times a day with a small amount of honey and 3g of Lophatheri Herba (*dàn zhú yè*). May also be prepared as a decoction using the dosages in parentheses above.

Actions   Drains fire and unblocks the bowels by clearing the upper burner and draining the middle burner

Indications

Sensation of heat and irritability in the chest and abdomen, delirious speech (in severe cases), thirst, flushed face and red lips, mouth and tongue sores, sore throat, swollen tongue, red eyes, nosebleed, constipation, dark, scanty urine, red tongue

body or edges with a dry, yellow, or white coating, and a rapid, possibly slippery pulse.

This pattern is one of formed or accumulated heat in the middle burner, and unformed or blazing heat in the upper burner. Heat in the chest and diaphragmatic regions produces a sensation of heat and irritability which, in severe cases, may evolve into delirious speech. Heat in the Stomach and Intestines injures the fluids and prevents them from rising to the mouth, which causes thirst. Dryness due to heat clumping in the yang organs interrupts the smooth flow of qi and causes constipation and dark, scanty urine. Heart fire blazing upward produces a flushed face, red lips, mouth and tongue sores, sore throat, and a swollen tongue. Heat in the Lungs, Heart, Spleen, and Liver manifests in signs of inflammation in their corresponding sensory organs (the nose, tongue, mouth, and eyes, respectively). A tongue with red edges and a white coating indicates that the heat is lodged primarily in the upper burner; redness covering the entire body of the tongue and a yellow coating indicates that heat is firmly established in both the upper and middle burners. A dry coating reflects the presence of dryness. A rapid pulse indicates heat, while a slippery pulse indicates clumping due to the accumulation of heat and dryness in the interior.

Analysis of Formula

In this pattern there is both unformed heat above and formed accumulation below, which requires a strategy of simultaneously clearing the heat and reducing the accumulation. The use of only one strategy will not alleviate the condition.

The large dose of Forsythiae Fructus (*lián qiáo*) indicates that it serves as the formula's chief herb, clearing heat and resolving toxicity. It enters the Heart channel to disperse pathogenic heat, eliminates all types of heat from the upper burner, and is a specific herb for treating sores. Two pair of deputies focus the action of the formula on the upper and middle burners. Scutellariae Radix (*huáng qín*) drains lurking heat from the Lungs and clears constrained heat from the diaphragm. Gardeniae Fructus (*zhī zǐ*) clears heat from all three burners through the urine and guides fire out from below. The second pair, Rhei Radix et Rhizoma (*dà huáng*) and Natrii Sulfas (*máng xiāo*), opens the bowels to flush heat from the middle burner.

Menthae haplocalycis Herba (*bò hé*) and Lophatheri Herba (*dàn zhú yè*) are light in nature. They serve as assistants that calm irritability and alleviate the attendant head and throat symptoms by dredging the protective qi and venting heat from the exterior. Glycyrrhizae Radix (*gān cǎo*) and the small amount of honey act as envoys that moderate and harmonize the fierce action of Rhei Radix et Rhizoma (*dà huáng*) and Natrii Sulfas (*máng xiāo*), protecting the Stomach and preventing the abdominal pain that sometimes accompanies the use of purgatives.

---

* Plum Blossom Dotted Tongue Special Pill (梅花點舌丹 *méi huā diǎn shé dān*) is a formula originally found in *Complete Compendium of Patterns and Treatments in External Medicine*. Because many of the ingredients in this formula have heavy metal toxicity or come from endangered species, it is presently considered obsolete and should not be added to this formula.

Overall, this formula can be interpreted as a variation of Regulate the Stomach and Order the Qi Decoction *(tiǎo wèi chéng qì tāng)* to which herbs that dredge the protective qi and clear heat from the upper burner have been added. This allows it to drain accumulation of heat from the upper and middle burners simultaneously, a strategy first discussed in Chapter 74 of *Basic Questions:* "Internal hot pathogenic influences should be treated with salty, cold [substances] assisted by [those that are] bitter and sweet."

Cautions and Contraindications

The use of this formula can readily injure the Spleen and Stomach qi. The dosage of Rhei Radix et Rhizoma *(dà huáng)* and Natrii Sulfas *(máng xiāo)* should therefore be reduced or omitted altogether once the constipation has been alleviated, or with the appearance of mild abdominal pain, pus in the stool, and fatigue. This formula is appropriate only for conditions of heat excess in the upper and middle burners, and is contraindicated during pregnancy and for patients who are very weak.

Commentary

Almost all commentators agree that the formula clears and drains heat from the upper and middle burners. Their views regarding the relative importance of each herb in the formula vary depending on which of the two actions they consider to be primary. A minority even extends the formula's action to all three burners. The mid-19th century scholar-physician Fei Bo-Xiong, for instance, argued that the combination of Rhei Radix et Rhizoma *(dà huáng)* and Natrii Sulfas *(máng xiāo)* also drains heat from the lower burner. Ding Xue-Ping, a contemporary physician from Shanghai, provides another divergent commentary in *Modern Explanations of Ancient Formulas:*

> This [formula] represents a joint strategy of dredging wind with acrid and cooling [substances], draining fire with bitter and cold [substances], and thrusting out [pathogens] via purgation with salty and bitter [substances. Its authors thereby] established the correct way [to treat] pathogenic fire that collects and clumps in the exterior, the interior, and the Triple Burner [simultaneously].

In *Convenient Reader of Established Formulas,* the late-Qing dynasty physician Zhang Bing-Cheng focused on describing the disease dynamic that leads to this pattern:

> All the various manifestations of this pattern outlined above are due to pathogenic fire in the upper and middle burners that is accompanied by clumped matter in the Stomach [made up of] harbored food or stools. Fire that has scattered, irrespective of whether it is [now] located in the interior or exterior, can be cured by clearing and dispersing. However, if [such fire] is accompanied by formed matter that has clumped and not been dispersed, one cannot completely recover from such an illness unless this clumping is [also] eliminated.

This explanation helps us understand the views of the late 17th-century physician Zhang Lu who thought that this formula works best for problems caused by a seasonal warm pathogen disorder. The source text also indicates its use "for any type of wind clogging [the qi dynamic]" (一切風壅 *yī qiè fēng yōng*). Wind-heat pathogens quickly penetrate into the body and can thus remain in the exterior (upper burner, Lungs), even as they are already entering into the interior (middle burner, Stomach). The Triple Burner, represented in the formula's name by the diaphragm, connects the exterior and interior, and must of necessity be involved in any such process.

This is comparable to a combined disorder of all three yang aspects in a cold damage disorder, which also necessitates a complex treatment strategy that hinges on the lesser yang. The difference is that in a warm pathogen disorder, heat in the exterior must be vented by means of light, acrid, and cooling herbs, whereas in a cold damage disorder, it is dispersed by means of acrid, warming herbs.

The scope of this formula's application has been extended to the treatment of childhood convulsions, macular rashes, and various types of pox where the heat evolves into such intense fire that it produces extremely dark, collapsed sores. Some practitioners use it for any type of skin disorder associated with the accumulation of heat in the upper and middle burners.

Comparisons

➤ Vs. Major Order the Qi Decoction *(dà chéng qì tāng)*

Both formulas flush fire from the middle burner by draining downward. A useful differentiation of their application is provided in *Comprehensive Medicine According to Master Zhang:*

> When Rhei Radix et Rhizoma *(dà huáng)* and Natrii Sulfas *(máng xiāo)* are combined with the [herbs] that weigh downward, Magnoliae officinalis Cortex *(hòu pò)* and Aurantii Fructus immaturus *(zhǐ shí)*, then lower burner heat is ordered by them and smoothly drains downward. When they are combined with the light ascending herbs Scutellariae Radix *(huáng qín)*, Gardeniae Fructus *(zhī zǐ)*, Forsythiae Fructus *(lián qiáo)*, and Menthae haplocalycis Herba *(bò hé)*, then upper burner heat is curbed and cleared downward.

➤ Vs. Saposhnikovia Powder that Sagely Unblocks *(fáng fēng tōng shèng sǎn)*

Both formulas treat the upper and middle burners and resolve the exterior while draining heat from the interior. Saposhnikovia Powder that Sagely Unblocks *(fáng fēng tōng shèng sǎn),* a modification of the present formula, is stronger at discharging and dispersing wind from the exterior. To compensate for this dispersing action, it also includes herbs that tonify the qi and blood. The present formula focuses on venting heat from constraint in the exterior. It is not indicated for patterns with wind in the exterior.

➤ Vs. Clear the Heart and Enable the Diaphragm Decoction *(qīng xīn lì gé tāng); see* page 887.

Biomedical Indications

With the appropriate presentation, this formula may be used to treat a variety of biomedically-defined disorders, primarily infections such as pharyngitis, stomatitis, tonsillitis, biliary tract infections, acute icteric hepatitis, conjunctivitis, lobar pneumonia, and multiple furuncles, as well as epilepsy and chronic renal failure.

....

Alternate names

Forsythia Drink *(lián qiáo yǐn zi)* in *Formulas from the Discussion Illuminating the Yellow Emperor's Basic Questions;* Forsythia Powder to Eliminate Toxin *(lián qiáo xiāo dú sǎn)* in *Essential Teachings on External Medicine*

....

Modifications

- For severe thirst, add Trichosanthis Radix *(tiān huā fěn)*.
- For severe mouth sores indicating excess Heart fire, add Coptidis Rhizoma *(huáng lián)* and Lycii Cortex *(dì gǔ pí)*.
- For childhood convulsions, add Uncariae Ramulus cum Uncis *(gōu téng)* and Saigae tataricae Cornu *(líng yáng jiǎo)*.
- For swollen and painful throat, strong fever, irritability, thirst, and no constipation, remove Rhei Radix et Rhizoma *(dà huáng)* and Natrii Sulfas *(máng xiāo)* and add Gypsum fibrosum *(shí gāo)*, Platycodi Radix *(jié gěng)*, Sophorae tonkinensis Radix *(shān dòu gēn)*, and Isatidis/Baphicacanthis Radix *(bǎn lán gēn)*.
- For nosebleed or vomiting of blood that does not stop, add Imperatae Rhizoma *(bái máo gēn)* and Nelumbinis Nodus rhizomatis *(ǒu jié)*.
- For jaundice, add Artemisiae scopariae Herba *(yīn chén)* and Curcumae Radix *(yù jīn)*.
- For yin deficiency, add Rehmanniae Radix *(shēng dì huáng)*, Scrophulariae Radix *(xuán shēn)*, and Ophiopogonis Radix *(mài mén dōng)*.
- For qi stagnation with distention and pain in the chest, add Bupleuri Radix *(chái hú)* and Toosendan Fructus *(chuān liàn zǐ)*.

Associated Formulas

加減涼膈散 （加减凉膈散）

Modified Cool the Diaphragm Powder

jiā jiǎn liáng gé sǎn

Source   *Golden Mirror of the Medical Tradition* (1742)

Menthae haplocalycis Herba *(bò hé)*
Gardeniae Fructus *(zhī zǐ)*
Scrophulariae Radix *(xuán shēn)*
Forsythiae Fructus *(lián qiáo)*
Glycyrrhizae Radix *(gān cǎo)*
Platycodi Radix *(jié gěng)*
Ophiopogonis Radix *(mài mén dōng)*
Arctii Fructus *(niú bàng zǐ)*
Scutellariae Radix *(huáng qín)*

The source text advises to grind equal amounts of the herbs into a powder and to decoct with water to take as a draft. Dredges wind, drains heat, and enriches the yin. For rashes that have already surfaced accompanied by loss of voice. This is wind-heat in the exterior with heat damaging the yin fluids. From a warm pathogen disorder perspective, it corresponds to a combined protective- and nutritive-level disorder. This formula is also indicated for skin disorders.

———————

清心涼膈散 （清心凉膈散）

Clear the Heart and Cool the Diaphragm Powder

qīng xīn liáng gé sǎn

Source   *Warp and Woof of Warm-Heat Pathogen Diseases* (1852)

Forsythiae Fructus *(lián qiáo)*	120g
Scutellariae Radix *(huáng qín)*	30g
Menthae haplocalycis Herba *(bò hé)*	30g
Gardeniae Fructus *(zhī zǐ)*	30g
Gypsum fibrosum *(shí gāo)*	60g
Platycodi Radix *(jié gěng)*	30g
Glycyrrhizae Radix *(gān cǎo)*	30g

Grind the ingredients into a coarse powder and take as a draft in 9g doses. Cools the diaphragm and drains heat. For heat toxin collecting in the qi level of the upper burner characterized by unremitting fever, thirst, irritability, red, swollen and macerated throat, and a red tongue with a yellow coating. Because heat has not clumped in the middle burner, the use of purgatives is not required. Instead, the formula focuses on venting heat from the exterior and clearing heat from the interior.

———————

人參瀉肺湯 （人参泻肺汤）

Ginseng Decoction to Drain the Lungs

rén shēn xiè fèi tāng

Source   *Golden Mirror of the Medical Tradition* (1742)

Ginseng Radix *(rén shēn)*	9g
Scutellariae Radix *(huáng qín)*	9g
Gardeniae Fructus *(zhī zǐ)*	9g
Aurantii Fructus *(zhǐ ké)*	6g
Menthae haplocalycis Herba *(bò hé)*	4.5g
Forsythiae Fructus *(lián qiáo)*	9g
Armeniacae Semen *(xìng rén)*	9g
Mori Cortex *(sāng bái pí)*	9g
Platycodi Radix *(jié gěng)*	9g
Natrii Sulfas *(máng xiāo)*	4.5g
Rhei Radix et Rhizoma *(dà huáng)*	(add near end) 4.5g
Glycyrrhizae Radix *(gān cǎo)*	3g

The source text says to take equal amounts of the ingredients; the dosages listed above reflect those in most contemporary texts. Clears heat, drains the Lungs, eliminates phlegm, and regulates the qi. For accumulation of heat in the Lungs that manifests as wheezing, distention, and fullness in the chest and diaphragm with copious sticky phlegm and inhibited stools.

Heat in the diaphragm and chest ascends to scorch the fluids and gives rise to phlegm-heat in the Lungs. Heat that descends into the region below the diaphragm can damage the yin and fluids there and result in heat accumulation in the Stomach and Intestines in the form of inhibited stools. This formula treats excess phlegm-heat accumulation in the chest and diaphragm. Because there is an inherent danger of damaging the normal qi when treating an excess pathogen, Ginseng Radix (*rén shēn*) is added to mitigate the damage caused by the pathogen itself and that brought about by the acrid and bitter herbs used to drain the Lungs. It also includes the moistening herbs Armeniacae Semen (*xìng rén*) and Mori Cortex (*sāng bái pí*) to prevent damage to the Lung yin and fluids by the heat pathogen and the formula's bitter, drying herbs.

This somewhat balanced approach allows what would otherwise be a severe formula to be given to patients whose state of qi and fluids might not tolerate a less conservative method. Nonetheless, for children, the elderly, and those with weak qi, one should reduce or eliminate Rhei Radix et Rhizoma (*dà huáng*) and Natrii Sulfas (*máng xiāo*). If constipation is a factor for these patients, substituting a large dose of Trichosanthis Fructus (*guā lóu*) for the harsh draining herbs may also be useful. The pattern treated by Ginseng Decoction to Drain the Lungs (*rén shēn xiè fèi tāng*) is one that often results from a wind-cold or wind-heat pathogen that sinks into the Lungs and diaphragm and transforms to phlegm-heat accumulation. In Western medicine, this often corresponds to bronchitis, pneumonia, tonsillitis, or pulmonary tuberculosis.

Section 4

FORMULAS THAT SIMULTANEOUSLY CLEAR HEAT FROM THE QI AND BLOOD LEVELS

When heat toxin enters the body in the course of an epidemic disorder, it can flood the entire body and produce patterns in which heat flares in both the qi and blood levels at the same time. Clinical manifestations include qi-level symptoms such as high fever, irritability, and thirst, accompanied by bleeding from the upper orifices and bleeding into the skin caused by chaotic movement of the blood, as well as by impaired consciousness and delirious speech due to heat toxin sinking into the interior. The treatment strategy for such complex disorders is to combine formulas that deal with the individual aspects of the pathology into new and larger formulas that can effectively address these serious and sometimes life-threatening conditions. This requires formulas that combine sub-

stances that clear qi-level heat, such as Gypsum fibrosum (*shí gāo*) and Anemarrhenae Rhizoma (*zhī mǔ*), those that clear the nutritive and cool the blood, such as Bubali Cornu (*shuǐ niú jiǎo*) and Rehmanniae Radix (*shēng dì huáng*), and those that clear heat and resolve toxicity, such as Coptidis Rhizoma (*huáng lián*) and Scutellariae Radix (*huáng qín*).

清瘟敗毒飲 (清瘟败毒饮)
Clear Epidemics and Overcome Toxicity Drink
qīng wēn bài dú yǐn

Source *Achievements Regarding Epidemic Rashes* (1794)

	Dose:	small	medium	large
Gypsum fibrosum (*shí gāo*)		24-36g	60-120g	180-240g
Rehmanniae Radix (*shēng dì huáng*)		6-12g	9-15g	18-30g
Coptidis Rhizoma (*huáng lián*)		3-4.5g	6-12g	12-18g
[Bubali Cornu (*shuǐ niú jiǎo*)				30-120g]
Gardeniae Fructus (*zhī zǐ*)				3-18g
Platycodi Radix (*jié gěng*)				1.5-12g
Scutellariae Radix (*huáng qín*)				1.5-12g
Anemarrhenae Rhizoma (*zhī mǔ*)				3-18g
Paeoniae Radix rubra (*chì sháo*)				3-18g
Scrophulariae Radix (*xuán shēn*)				3-18g
Forsythiae Fructus (*lián qiào*)				3-18g
Lophatheri Herba (*dàn zhú yè*)				1.5-12g
Glycyrrhizae Radix (*gān cǎo*)				1.5-12g
Moutan Cortex (*mǔ dān pí*)				3-18g

Note: The source text only lists dosage for the first four substances, specifying a small, medium, and large dose for each. It specifies 6-12g, 9-15g, or 18-24g of Rhinocerotis Cornu (*xī jiǎo*), which is no longer used due to the endangered status of the rhinoceros. The dosages for the last ten ingredients listed here are based on modern Chinese textbooks. They should likewise be adjusted in accordance with whether one chooses a small, medium, or large dose of the chief herbs. Physicians should use the pulse as indicator for determining the appropriate dosage: a submerged, thin, and rapid pulse (reflecting a more severe condition) requires a large dose; a floating, large, and rapid pulse (reflecting a less severe condition) requires a small dose; and a pulse in between these two extremes requires a medium dose.

Method of Preparation Cook Gypsum fibrosum (*shí gāo*) and Bubali Cornu (*shuǐ niú jiǎo*) first for 15-20 minutes.

Actions Clears heat, resolves toxicity, cools the blood, and drains fire

Indications

Intense fever, strong thirst, dry heaves, severe and stabbing headache, extreme irritability, and in severe cases, delirious speech, rashes, and nosebleed. The tongue is dark red, the lips are dark and scorched, and the pulse is either rapid, submerged, and thin or rapid, floating, and large.

This is an epidemic toxin warm pathogen disorder that manifests with severe fire in the qi and blood levels. Intense fever and strong thirst are signs of vigorous heat in the qi level. Severe, stabbing headache is due to fire toxin rising to the head. When fire enters the blood level, it disturbs the Heart and Liver, which causes extreme irritability; in severe cases, it causes incoherent or delirious speech. Fire at this level also incites the reckless movement of blood, which manifests in rashes, vomiting of blood, or nosebleed. A dark-red tongue with dark, scorched lips are signs of intense fire toxin in the qi and blood levels.

A submerged, thin, and rapid pulse occurs when intense fire toxin constrains the pulse. A submerged and rapid pulse that is not thin indicates that the fire toxin is less strong and the constraint less severe. A floating, large, and rapid pulse is a sign that there is no constraint at all and that the fire toxin is only light and superficial. If the fire toxin is not relieved, the pulse will become thin.

Analysis of Formula

This is a combination of three formulas discussed in earlier sections of this chapter, plus some additions. They are White Tiger Decoction (*bái hǔ tāng*), Rhinoceros Horn and Rehmannia Decoction (*xī jiǎo dì huáng tāng*), and Coptis Decoction to Resolve Toxicity (*huáng lián jiě dú tāng*). Among these, the functions of White Tiger Decoction (*bái hǔ tāng*) and its chief herb Gypsum fibrosum (*shí gāo*) are most important. Yu Lin, the formula's author, explains: "This is a very cold formula [intended] for resolving toxicity. Therefore, it uses a large dose of Gypsum fibrosum (*shí gāo*). By first calming the most extreme [manifestations of the disorder], that is, clearing the fire from all twelve channels, everything else will quiet down by itself."

In terms of individual ingredients, one group, composed of Gypsum fibrosum (*shí gāo*), Anemarrhenae Rhizoma (*zhī mǔ*), Glycyrrhizae Radix (*gān cǎo*), and Lophatheri Herba (*dàn zhú yè*), clears heat from the qi level. Another group, Bubali Cornu (*shuǐ niú jiǎo*), Rehmanniae Radix (*shēng dì huáng*), Moutan Cortex (*mǔ dān pí*), Paeoniae Radix rubra (*chì sháo*), and Scrophulariae Radix (*xuán shēn*), clears heat from the blood level. A third group, Coptidis Rhizoma (*huáng lián*), Scutellariae Radix (*huáng qín*), and Gardeniae Fructus (*zhī zǐ*), opens the Triple Burner by draining heat and toxic fire. Forsythiae Fructus (*lián qiáo*), when combined with Scrophulariae Radix (*xuán shēn*), resolves toxicity and disperses fire roaming throughout the body. Platycodi Radix (*jié gěng*) and Lophatheri Herba (*dàn zhú yè*) have an ascending action that conducts the actions of the other ingredients upward.

Cautions and Contraindications

Contraindicated in cases with yang deficiency or weakness of the Spleen and Stomach.

Commentary

Yu Lin's analysis and treatment of 'heat epidemics' (熱疫 *rè yì*) is highly original and based on a meticulous differentiation of their signs and symptoms, particularly of maculae and papules. He defined heat epidemic disorders primarily on the basis of rashes: "Black heat epidemic [disorders] are not cold damage disorders. Cold damage disorders do not manifest with maculae and papules." He also listed four symptoms that are shared by both disorders and that might lead to a misdiagnosis: headache, sweating, vomiting, and diarrhea. Unlike headaches due to lesser yang or yang brightness disorders, heat epidemic headaches are severe, stabbing, and feel as if the head is split. The head feels heavy and cannot be lifted. Unlike yang brightness channel disorders where sweating occurs over the entire body, sweating in heat epidemic disorders is limited to the head and upper body. The vomiting of heat epidemic disorders is not accompanied by flank pain or discomfort, as it would be in lesser yang disorders. Diarrhea is not accompanied by abdominal fullness, as in lesser yin disorders, but is characterized, instead, by constant evacuations that have a foul smell.

A special case is that of the 'stifled epidemic' (悶疫 *mēn yì*) disorder. This is a sudden, strong invasion of a turbid heat toxin that completely obstructs the qi dynamic in the interior such that exterior manifestations resemble those of abandonment of yang: a very pale complexion, icy-cold extremities, and cold sweats with big drops of fluid. The presence of heat in the interior is betrayed, however, by impaired consciousness, gripping abdominal pain, an unrelieved desire to vomit or defecate, splitting headache, and shaking of the head, all of which are due to heat toxins bottling-up the yang qi in the interior and the battle between the true and the pathogenic qi.

Dosage of Gypsum fibrosum (shí gāo)

Yu Lin stated that Gypsum fibrosum (*shí gāo*) alone is insufficient to treat such disorders. At the same time, it is the only substance capable of clearing heat from everywhere within the body. If qi-level heat is cleared, it is much easier to treat heat at other levels. Due to the strong nature of the heat pathogen, Yu advocated the use of a very large dosage of Gypsum fibrosum (*shí gāo*). This has caused much controversy among later physicians. The Qing-dynasty physician Zhuang Zhi-Ting, cited in *Warp and Woof of Warm-Heat Pathogen Diseases*, argued that a dosage of 15-90g was sufficient. The modern physician Jiao Shu-De, however, contends that doses of as much as 150-180g are frequently necessary. Wang Shi-Xiong, Yu Lin's great admirer, argued that there was no single, one-size-fits-all dosage, but that it was the nature of the particular disorder that determined the extent of medical intervention. Severe heat requires a severe response, and thus there was nothing wrong with Yu Lin's advocacy of using a very large dosage of heat-clearing herbs.

Comparison

➢ Vs. Transform Maculae Decoction (*huà bān tāng*); *see* PAGE 182

Biomedical Indications

With the appropriate presentation, this formula may be used to treat a variety of biomedically-defined disorders, primarily infections, including meningitis, encephalitis B, measles encephalitis, septicemia, pyemia, and epidemic hemorrhagic fever.

Modifications

- For constipation, add Rhei Radix et Rhizoma (*dà huáng*) and Natrii Sulfas (*máng xiāo*).
- For very high fever, add Isatidis Folium (*dà qīng yè*) and Isatidis/Baphicacanthis Radix (*bǎn lán gēn*).
- For a swollen face, add Violae Herba (*zǐ huā dì dīng*) and Rhei Radix et Rhizoma (*dà huáng*).
- For swollen parotid glands, add Indigo naturalis (*qīng dài*) and Lonicerae Flos (*jīn yín huā*).
- For soreness in the joints and a lower back that feels bruised, add Phellodendri Cortex (*huáng bǎi*) and Akebiae Caulis (*mù tōng*).
- For dark-purple rashes, add Arnebiae/Lithospermi Radix (*zǐ cǎo*), Carthami Flos (*hóng huā*), Persicae Semen (*táo rén*), and Angelicae sinensis Radix (*dāng guī*).
- For tremors caused by heat injuring the sinews, remove Platycodi Radix (*jié gěng*) and add Chrysanthemi Flos (*jú huā*) and Gentianae Radix (*lóng dǎn cǎo*).

化斑湯（化斑汤）
Transform Maculae Decoction
huà bān tāng

Source *Systematic Differentiation of Warm Pathogen Diseases* (1798)

Gypsum fibrosum (*shí gāo*)..30g
Anemarrhenae Rhizoma (*zhī mǔ*)........................12g
Glycyrrhizae Radix (*gān cǎo*)................................9g
Scrophulariae Radix (*xuán shēn*)..........................9g
[Bubali Cornu (*shuǐ niú jiǎo*)....................30-120g]
Nonglutinous rice (*jīng mǐ*)..........................9-15g

Method of Preparation Decoction. The source text specifies 6g of Rhinocerotis Cornu (*xī jiǎo*) in powdered form to be taken with the strained decoction. The other herbs are boiled with 8 cups of water until 3 cups remain, which are taken in three doses throughout the day. The dregs are cooked once more with less water and then taken as a single dose at night. The dosage of the individual herbs is adjusted according to the relative severity of qi- or blood-level symptoms.

Actions Clears qi-level heat and cools the blood

Indications

For warm pathogen heat disorders with heat entering the qi and blood levels. Heat sinking into the blood level causes fever that worsens at night, a dark-red macular rash, and a rapid pulse. However, the qi-level signs and symptoms, like thirst and a yellow tongue coating, do not subside, which indicates that the yang brightness qi level heat remains strong. This implies a very strong pathogen and a strong constitution.

Analysis of Formula

This formula can be regarded as a variation of White Tiger Decoction (*bái hǔ tāng*). The chief herb is Gypsum fibrosum (*shí gāo*), which clears the intense heat in the qi level that is the root cause of this presentation. Bubali Cornu (*shuǐ niú jiǎo*) and Scrophulariae Radix (*xuán shēn*) are the deputies. They resolve toxicity and clear heat in the blood, and nourish the yin fluids, thereby helping to vent the pathogen back to the qi level. Anemarrhenae Rhizoma (*zhī mǔ*) serves as an assistant to drain qi-level heat. Glycyrrhizae Radix (*gān cǎo*) and Nonglutinous rice (*jīng mǐ*) supplement the middle burner qi and harmonize the actions of the other ingredients.

Cautions and Contraindications

Contraindicated in cases with yang deficiency or weakness of the Spleen and Stomach.

Commentary

This formula is primarily used to treat macular rashes that result from heat in the qi and blood levels. Many physicians advise to add herbs that invigorate the blood and transform stasis, such as Moutan Cortex (*mǔ dān pí*), Paeoniae Radix rubra (*chì sháo*), and Rehmanniae Radix (*shēng dì huáng*), to increase its effectiveness. This is because blood-level heat readily leads to blood stasis, which engenders more heat and, in a vicious cycle, causes more bleeding. In addition, the cold nature of this formula itself can easily cause the blood to congeal and stagnate.

A total of nineteen different formulas named Transform Maculae Decoction (*huà bān tāng*) are listed in the *Encyclopedia of Chinese Medical Formulas*. Although they all address the same symptom, their individual constituents are quite different. A comparison of their composition and specific indications nevertheless allows us to make some useful generalizations regarding the treatment of maculopapular rashes with Chinese medicine. In terms of the disease dynamic addressed by these formulas, one can distinguish three main scenarios: (1) wind-heat constraining the flow of yang qi in the exterior such that the Lungs lose their ability to disseminate and direct downward, which in turn causes heat toxin to accumulate in the exterior from which it fails to be vented to the outside; (2) the more serious case of heat toxin sinking into the qi and blood levels in the course of a warm pathogen disorder, discussed above; and (3) late-stage rashes associated with a deficient pulse, which indicates qi and yin deficiency and the inability of the body to completely eliminate the pathogenic qi.

In terms of formula composition, one can also distinguish three main groups: (1) formulas that focus on venting pathogenic heat constraint from the skin and muscle layer with herbs like Arctii Fructus (*niú bàng zǐ*), Forsythiae Fructus (*lián qiáo*), Bupleuri Radix (*chái hú*), Cimicifugae Rhizoma (*shēng má*), Schizonepetae Herba (*jīng jiè*), Saposhnikoviae Radix (*fáng fēng*), and Scutellariae Radix (*huáng qín*); (2) formulas that focus on clearing heat and resolving toxicity from the qi and blood levels with herbs like Gypsum fibrosum (*shí gāo*), Anemarrhenae Rhizoma (*zhī mǔ*), Scrophulariae Radix (*xuán shēn*), Bubali Cornu (*shuǐ niú jiǎo*), Moutan Cortex (*mǔ dān pí*), and Rehmanniae Radix (*shēng dì huáng*); (3) formulas that treat late-stage rashes by combining herbs that augment the qi and nourish the yin, such as Ginseng Radix (*rén shēn*), Glycyrrhizae Radix (*gān cǎo*), and Scrophulariae Radix (*xuán shēn*), with those that clear heat, such as Gypsum fibrosum (*shí gāo*) and Anemarrhenae Rhizoma (*zhī mǔ*). Besides their relevance for treating warm pathogen disorders, these principles have important implications for the treatment of skin diseases in everyday clinical practice.

Comparisons

➢ Vs. Clear Epidemics and Overcome Toxicity Drink (*qīng wēn bài dú yǐn*) and Magical Rhinoceros Special Pill (*shén xī dān*)

All these formulas clear heat and resolve toxicity from both the qi and blood levels. They all are used in the treatment of macular and papular rashes. Clear Epidemics and Overcome Toxicity Drink (*qīng wēn bài dú yǐn*) focuses first on clearing heat from the yang brightness with a large dose of Gypsum fibrosum (*shí gāo*) as the chief substance. This is indicated where heat toxins flood the entire body or become constrained in the interior with symptoms of yang desertion on the outside. Magical Rhinoceros Special Pill (*shén xī dān*) uses the combination of Bubali Cornu (*shuǐ niú jiǎo*) and Acori tatarinowii Rhizoma (*shí chāng pú*) as chief herbs in order to clear heat from the Heart and open the orifices. Only secondarily does it focus on macular rashes. Transform Maculae Decoction (*huà bān tāng*) combines Gypsum fibrosum (*shí gāo*), Scrophulariae Radix (*xuán shēn*), and Bubali Cornu (*shuǐ niú jiǎo*) to focus equally on clearing heat from the qi and blood levels. Its main focus is on treating maculae that result from heat in the yang brightness and blood levels, rather than on relieving toxic heat constraint.

Associated Formula

人參化斑湯 （人参化斑汤）

Ginseng Transform Maculae Decoction

rén shēn huà bān tāng

Source　*Indispensable Tools for Pattern Treatment* (1602)

Ginseng Radix (*rén shēn*)	4.5g
Gypsum fibrosum (*shí gāo*)	9g
Polygonati odorati Rhizoma(*yù zhú*)	4.5g
Anemarrhenae Rhizoma (*zhī mǔ*)	4.5g
Glycyrrhizae Radix (*gān cǎo*)	1.5g
old stored rice (*chén cāng mǐ*)	9g

Decoction. Panacis quinquefolii Radix (*xī yáng shēn*) is nowadays regularly substituted for Ginseng Radix (*rén shēn*). For lurking pathogen disorders with heat flaring in both the qi and blood levels where, in spite of sweating or the emergence of macular rashes, the fever does not subside.

Another formula by the same name is listed in *Achieving Longevity by Guarding the Source*. This is also a variation of White Tiger Decoction (*bái hǔ tāng*) and contains the following ingredients: Ginseng Radix (*rén shēn*) 9g, Gypsum fibrosum (*shí gāo*) 30g, Anemarrhenae Rhizoma (*zhī mǔ*) 7.5g, Arnebiae/Lithospermi Radix (*zǐ cǎo*) 9g, Poria (*fú líng*) 9g, Angelicae sinensis Radix (*dāng guī*) 9g, and Glycyrrhizae Radix (*gān cǎo*) 9g. This formula clears heat, directs fire downward, and cools both the qi and blood. It is used for severe qi-level heat extending to the blood level with macular rashes and a sensation of insects crawling under the skin.

Section 5

FORMULAS THAT CLEAR HEAT FROM THE ORGANS

When heat excess develops in an organ, it will manifest in signs and symptoms that are characteristic of the pathology of that organ and its associated channel. While this type of disorder often occurs in the broader context of an externally-contracted disease, it is said to be at the organ level because its manifestations are clearly those of a particular organ. Just as often, however, these disorders can arise from internal causes. In treating such disorders, the choice of formula is based upon the organ affected, and the extent of its involvement.

- Heat or fire in the Lungs is primarily treated by herbs that clear the Lungs and drain out heat, such as Mori Cortex (*sāng bái pí*) and Scutellariae Radix (*huáng qín*). Lung heat can be very closely related to qi-level heat, and when this occurs, qi-level herbs that clear heat and resolve toxicity, such as Lonicerae Flos (*jīn yín huā*) and Forsythiae Fructus (*lián qiáo*), may be utilized. If there is lurking fire, herbs that clear this type of heat, such as Lycii Cortex (*dì gǔ pí*), are used.

- Heat or fire in the Spleen and Stomach are treated with herbs such as Gypsum fibrosum (*shí gāo*), Anemarrhenae Rhizoma (*zhī mǔ*), and Coptidis Rhizoma (*huáng lián*) that clear heat and fire from these organs. Heat in these organs often occurs in conjunction with constraint that leads to rebellion, and thus herbs that disperse or release constraint, such as Saposhnikoviae Radix (*fáng fēng*), Pogostemonis/Agastaches Herba (*huò xiāng*), or Cimicifugae Rhizoma (*shēng má*), are often added. In addition, heat in the Stomach can become quite intense, which readily affects the blood and yin, and thus herbs that cool the blood and nourish the yin, such as Rehmanniae Radix (*shēng dì huáng*), Rehmanniae Radix praeparata (*shú dì huáng*), and Ophiopogonis Radix (*mài mén dōng*), are often added.

- For overabundant heat in the Heart channel, the core ingredients are those that clear the Heart and drain fire, such as Lophatheri Herba (*dàn zhú yè*), Coptidis Rhizoma (*huáng lián*), and Gardeniae Fructus (*zhī zǐ*). Becuse the Heart has an interior-exterior relationship with the Small Intestine, heat affecting the Heart can be conducted out via the urine with such herbs as Akebiae Caulis (*mù tōng*) and Plantaginis Semen (*chē qián zǐ*). Additionally, heat in the Heart often ends up affecting the blood and readily injures the fluids, and thus herbs such as Rehmanniae Radix (*shēng dì huáng*) and Ophiopogonis Radix (*mài mén dōng*) are often used.

- Excess heat in the Liver and Gallbladder is primarily treated with herbs that clear the Liver and drain fire, such as Gentianae Radix (*lóng dǎn cǎo*), Gardeniae Fructus (*zhī zǐ*), and Prunellae Spica (*xià kū cǎo*). Liver and Gallbladder heat are often accompanied by dampness pouring downward, and thus herbs that clear heat and resolve dampness, such as Akebiae Caulis (*mù tōng*), Alismatis Rhizoma (*zé xiè*), and Plantaginis Semen (*chē qián zǐ*), are often used in these formulas. When Liver heat is due to constraint, one should add herbs that, when combined with heat-clearing herbs, can disperse heat from constraint; two examples are Notopterygii Rhizoma seu Radix (*qiāng huó*) and Saposhnikoviae Radix (*fáng fēng*). Not only does excessive Liver heat readily consume and damage the yin and blood, but the herbs used to treat it are often very drying. For this reason, formulas for excess Liver heat often include herbs that moisten the yin and blood, such as Angelicae sinensis Radix (*dāng guī*) and Rehmanniae Radix (*shēng dì huáng*).

- For heat in the Intestines, the primary herbs are those that clear the Intestines and resolve toxicity, such as Coptidis Rhizoma (*huáng lián*), Scutellariae Radix (*huáng qín*), Phellodendri Cortex (*huáng bǎi*), and Pulsatillae Radix (*bái tóu wēng*). This type of heat has a tendency to disrupt the functions of the qi and blood leading to dysenteric disorders and tenesmus, and hence herbs that promote the proper movement and regulate the qi and blood, such as Angelicae sinensis Radix (*dāng guī*), Paeoniae Radix (*sháo yào*), Aucklandiae Radix (*mù xiāng*), and Arecae Semen (*bīng láng*), are often added.

麻杏石甘湯（麻杏石甘汤）

Ephedra, Apricot Kernel, Gypsum, and Licorice Decoction

má xìng shí gān tāng

Source *Discussion of Cold Damage* (c. 220)

Ephedrae Herba (*má huáng*)........................12g
Gypsum fibrosum (*shí gāo*).........................24
Armeniacae Semen (*xìng rén*)........... 50 pieces (18g)
Glycyrrhizae Radix praeparata (*zhì gān cǎo*)..............6g

Method of Preparation The source text advises to cook Ephedrae Herba (*má huáng*) for a short time before adding the other ingredients. At present, this is not done, and the dosage of all ingredients is reduced by 30-50 percent.

Actions Facilitates the flow of Lung qi, clears heat, and calms wheezing by directing rebellious qi downward

Indications

Fever with or without sweating, thirst, wheezing, coughing, labored breathing, nasal flaring and pain, a thin tongue coating that can either be white or yellow, and a rapid pulse that can be floating or slippery.

This is heat lodged in the Lungs where it obstructs the flow of qi. It may be caused either by externally-contracted wind-heat or by wind-cold that has transformed into heat. The fever, thirst, yellow tongue coating, and rapid pulse are all indicative of heat. Wheezing, coughing, and labored breathing reflect obstruction of the Lung qi. When heat clogs the Lungs, they lose their ability to disseminate and direct downward. Upward rebellion of Lung qi leads specifically to wheezing, while internal steaming of the heat forces the fluids outward in the form of sweat. Note, however, that in more severe cases, the heat will deplete the fluids and there will be little or no sweating. The pulse and tongue will change according to how deeply the pathogen has entered the body: if there are still some lingering elements of an exterior condition, the pulse will be floating and the tongue coating may be white. Once the pathogen has moved completely from the exterior to the Lungs, the classic presentation for this formula will appear, with a yellow tongue coating and a slippery, rapid pulse.

Analysis of Formula

In order to treat heat lodged in the Lungs where it obstructs its normal functions, this formula employs a strategy of clearing the heat and directing the qi downward. One of the chief ingredients, Ephedrae Herba (má huáng), facilitates the circulation of Lung qi and thereby controls the wheezing. Its use is an example of the adage from the *Inner Classic*, "For fire [due to] constraint, discharge it" (火鬱發之 huǒ yù fā zhī). As a warm herb, it must be balanced by the other chief ingredient, Gypsum fibrosum (shí gāo), which drains heat from the Lungs and controls the diaphoretic action of Ephedrae Herba (má huáng). The dosage of these two ingredients must be adjusted according to the condition. For severe Lung heat (with relatively profuse sweating), the dosage of Ephedrae Herba (má huáng) is reduced and that of Gypsum fibrosum (shí gāo) is increased. If the condition has not completely left the exterior, the dosage of Ephedrae Herba (má huáng) is increased and that of Gypsum fibrosum (shí gāo) is reduced. Gypsum also clears heat from the Stomach (to relieve the thirst) and muscles (to relieve the fever and spontaneous sweating). The deputy, Armeniacae Semen (xìng rén), assists Ephedrae Herba (má huáng) in facilitating the flow of Lung qi. Together, these two herbs make a powerful combination for stopping wheezing by directing the rebellious Lung qi downward. Glycyrrhizae Radix praeparata (zhì gān cǎo), the envoy, moistens the Lungs, stops coughing, and harmonizes the actions of the other ingredients.

Cautions and Contraindications

Contraindicated for wheezing due to cold and in cases where the pathogenic influence lingers due to deficiency of the normal qi.

Commentary

This formula is a variation of Ephedra Decoction (ma huang tang), with Gypsum fibrosum (shí gāo) substituted for Cinnamomi Ramulus (guì zhī). It is a good example of how the substitution of just one ingredient can significantly alter the actions of a formula.

In paragraph 63 of *Discussion of Cold Damage*, this formula is prescribed for greater yang-stage disorders after sweating when Cinnamon Twig Decoction (guì zhī tāng) is inappropriate, if there is sweating and wheezing without intense heat. This requires some explanation as the formula can be used for patients with significant fevers.

Commentators such as You Yi have explained the last phrase to mean that there is no significant heat in the *exterior* because it has entered the Lung. Similarly, the contemporary physician Nie Hui-Min in *Nie's Study of Cold Damage* notes that this also means that the patient does not experience the *interior* heat of a *yang brightness* disorder with irritability and thirst. She notes that this is a way to differentiate this presentation from that of wheezing due to yang brightness heat upwardly disturbing the Lungs. Later generations of practitioners have used the formula in the treatment of cough with viscous and difficult-to-expectorate sputum, labored

breathing, a red tongue, and a rapid pulse, irrespective of the color of the tongue coating or the presence of fever or sweating. Others, however, such as the modern expert on classical formulas Huang Huang in *One-Hundred Classic Formulas*, consider sweating (indicating that the Lungs have lost their control over the opening and closing of the pores) to be a key symptom, but argue that this may be either a cold or hot sweat. Based on his analysis of both the presentation and the ingredients of this formula, the modern formula expert Chen Chao-Zu emphasizes that it is properly used when the fluids are somewhat stopped up and form thin mucus, but that it should not be used if the fluids are actually damaged.

This formula is used for a wide variety of Lung disorders. For example, it may be used in treating children with frequent and poorly controlled urination (the main complaint) accompanied by coughing and wheezing. This is an example of focusing treatment on the upper burner for disorders of the lower burner. It can also be used in treating allergic asthma or allergic rhinitis, both of which are conditions without fever and thus strong heat.

Comparisons

➤ Vs. Cinnamon Twig Decoction plus Magnolia Bark and Apricot Kernel (guì zhī jiā hòu pò xìng zǐ tāng)

Both formulas treat patterns characterized by wheezing and sweating. However, in a Cinnamon Twig Decoction plus Magnolia Bark and Apricot Kernel (guì zhī jiā hòu pò xìng zǐ tāng) presentation, these symptoms will be accompanied by an aversion to wind or drafts, and by subjective sensations of up-rushing qi. Furthermore, there will be none of the heat signs that are characteristic of an Ephedra, Apricot Kernel, Gypsum, and Licorice Decoction (má xìng shí gān tāng) presentation, such as a dry mouth, thirst, or flushing.

➤ Vs. Minor Bluegreen Dragon Decoction (xiǎo qīng lóng tāng)

Both formulas treat wheezing and coughing with sputum that may be white in color. However, a Minor Bluegreen Dragon Decoction (xiǎo qīng lóng tāng) presentation is characterized by aversion to cold, while an Ephedra, Apricot Kernel, Gypsum, and Licorice Decoction (má xìng shí gān tāng) presentation is defined by the presence of heat.

➤ Vs. White Tiger Decoction (bái hǔ tāng); *see* page 153

➤ Vs. Drain the White Powder (xiè bái sǎn); *see* page 187

Biomedical Indications

With the appropriate presentation, this formula may be used to treat a variety of biomedically-defined disorders, primarily infections, including upper respiratory tract infection, lobar pneumonia, bronchial pneumonia, bronchial asthma, pneumonitis from measles, bronchiolitis, pertussis, diphtheria, keratitis, and conjunctivitis.

Alternate names

This formula is often referred to by its full Chinese name with the herbs in a slightly different order: Ephedra, Apricot Kernel, Licorice, and Gypsum Decoction (*má huáng xìng rén gān cǎo shí gāo tāng*). Other names in historical sources include Ephedra and Apricot Kernel Decoction (*má huáng xìng rén tāng*) in *Formulas of Universal Benefit*; Ephedra, Apricot Kernel, Licorice, and Gypsum Decoction (*má huáng xìng zǐ cǎo gāo tāng*) in *Red Water and Dark Pearls*; Ephedra, Apricot Kernel, Licorice, and Gypsum Decoction (*má xìng gān shí tāng*) in *Comprehensive Medicine According to Master Zhang*; Four-Substance Licorice Decoction (*sì wù gān cǎo tāng*) in *Extension of the Important Formulas Worth a Thousand Gold Pieces*; and Ephedra, Apricot Kernel, Gypsum, and Licorice Decoction (*má xìng shí gān tāng*) in *Golden Mirror of the Medical Tradition*.

Modifications

- For severe heat, add Lonicerae Flos (*jīn yín huā*), Forsythiae Fructus (*lián qiáo*), Scutellariae Radix (*huáng qín*), and Houttuyniae Herba (*yú xīng cǎo*).

- For stubborn asthma, add Pinelliae Rhizoma praeparatum (*zhì bàn xià*), Trichosanthis Fructus (*guā lóu*), Citri reticulatae Pericarpium (*chén pí*), Aurantii Fructus immaturus (*zhǐ shí*), and Zingiberis Rhizoma recens (*shēng jiāng*).

- For wheezing and coughing with copious sputum, add Perillae Fructus (*zǐ sū zǐ*) and Lepidii/ Descurainiae Semen (*tíng lì zǐ*).

- For chills and no sweating, add Schizonepetae Herba (*jīng jiè*), Menthae haplocalycis Herba (*bò hé*), and Sojae Semen praeparatum (*dàn dòu chǐ*).

- For sinusitis, add Pheretima (*dì lóng*).

Associated Formulas

越婢湯 (越婢汤)

Maidservant from Yue's Decoction

Yuè bì tāng

SOURCE   *Essentials from the Golden Cabinet* (c. 220)

Ephedrae Herba (*má huáng*) 18g
Gypsum fibrosum (*shí gāo*) 24g
Zingiberis Rhizoma recens (*shēng jiāng*) 9g
Glycyrrhizae Radix (*gān cǎo*) 6g
Jujubae Fructus (*dà zǎo*) . . . . 15 pieces

Decoction. The source text advises to cook Ephedrae Herba (*má huáng*) for a short time before adding the other ingredients. At present, this is not done, and the dosage of all ingredients is reduced by one- to two-thirds. Induces sweating, disseminates the Lung qi, and moves water. For wind edema with aversion to drafts, generalized edema that begins in the face, slight fever, slight but continuous sweating, and a floating pulse. Since this is an acute condition and edema is the primary symptom, the dosage of Ephedrae Herba (*má huáng*) is larger than in the principal formula. Because of its ability to

treat a complex condition in a gentle manner (i.e., as a mild diaphoretic), this formula was named after the maidservants of southern China (*Yuè*) who were traditionally known to possess qualities of consideration and gentleness.

Comparisons

➤ Vs. DREDGING AND CUTTING DRINK
(*shū záo yǐn zi*); see PAGE 96

越婢加朮湯 (越婢朮湯)

Maidservant from Yue's Decoction plus Atractylodes

Yuè bì jiā zhú tāng

SOURCE   *Essentials from the Golden Cabinet* (c. 220)

Ephedrae Herba (*má huáng*) 18g
Gypsum fibrosum (*shí gāo*) 48g
Zingiberis Rhizoma recens (*shēng jiāng*) 9g
Glycyrrhizae Radix (*gān cǎo*) 6g
Atractylodis macrocephalae Rhizoma (*bái zhú*) 12g
Jujubae Fructus (*dà zǎo*) . . . . 15 pieces

Decoction. The source text advises to cook Ephedrae Herba (*má huáng*) for a short time before adding the other ingredients. At present, this is not done, and the dosage of all ingredients is reduced by one- to two-thirds. Induces sweating, disseminates the Lung qi, and moves water. For wind edema with edematous orbits, generalized edema, sore and heavy limbs, reduced urination, fever and chills, and a floating and slippery or submerged pulse. This formula is indicated for a more severe disorder than that for which Maidservant from Yue's Decoction (*Yuè bì tāng*) would be indicated.

越婢加半夏湯 (越婢半夏湯)

Maidservant from Yue's Decoction plus Pinellia

Yuè bì jiā bàn xià tāng

SOURCE   *Essentials from the Golden Cabinet* (c. 220)

Ephedrae Herba (*má huáng*) 18g
Gypsum fibrosum (*shí gāo*) 48g
Zingiberis Rhizoma recens (*shēng jiāng*) 9g
Glycyrrhizae Radix (*gān cǎo*) 6g
Pinelliae Rhizoma praeparatum (*zhì bàn xià*) 12g
Jujubae Fructus (*dà zǎo*) . . . . 15 pieces

Decoction. The source text advises to cook Ephedrae Herba (*má huáng*) for a short time before adding the other ingredients. At present, this is not done, and the dosage of all ingredients is reduced by one- to two-thirds. Disseminates the Lung qi, calms wheezing, dispels thin mucus, and clears heat. For wheezing with a productive cough where the sputum can be either yellowish or white, a dry mouth with a desire to drink, and sense of fullness in the chest and diaphragmatic area, and facial edema such that the eyes appear as if they were popping out of their sockets. Other symptoms are chills without sweating, mild to moderate feverishness, a red tongue with a yellow coating that may be greasy, and a pulse that is floating, large, and slippery or slippery and rapid. Often these patients have headaches, the sound of sputum in the throat, are nervous and anxious, and use the auxiliary muscles of respiration to breath; and some only have a dry mouth, but no thirst.

This is a condition known as Lung distention (肺胀 *fèi zhàng*) from chronic collection of heat and thin mucus internally with a superimposed externally-contracted wind condition.

五虎湯 (五虎汤)

Five-Tiger Decoction

wǔ hǔ tāng

SOURCE   *Collected Treatises of [Zhang] Jing-Yue* (1624)

Ephedrae Herba (*má huáng*) 2.1g
Gypsum fibrosum (*shí gāo*) 4.5g
Armeniacae Semen (*xìng rén*) 3g
Glycyrrhizae Radix (*gān cǎo*) 1.2g
Zingiberis Rhizoma recens (*shēng jiāng*) . . . . 3 slices
Jujubae Fructus (*dà zǎo*) . . . . 1 piece
Fine green tea (*xì chá*) 2.4g

Clears heat from the Lungs, disseminates the Lung qi, and stops coughing and wheezing. For labored breathing with heaving of the chest, a sensation of fullness in the chest, wheezing, and nasal flaring. This is due to wind-cold invading the body at BL-13 (*fèi shū*), after which it transforms into heat and obstructs the Lung channel. In contrast to the principal formula, this focuses more superficially on the Lung channel.

瀉白散 (泻白散)

Drain the White Powder

xiè bái sǎn

This formula is also called Drain the Lungs Powder (瀉肺散 *xiè fèi sǎn*), which suggests its action in draining heat from the Lungs. White may refer to the Lungs' correspondence to the metal phase and the color white.

Source   *Craft of Medicinal Treatment for Childhood Disease Patterns* (1119)

dry-fried Mori Cortex (*chǎo sāng bái pí*) 30g
Lycii Cortex (*dì gǔ pí*) 30g
Glycyrrhizae Radix praeparata (*zhì gān cǎo*) 3g
Nonglutinous rice (*jīng mǐ*) 15-30g

Method of Preparation   The source text advises to grind the herbs into a powder, cook with the rice, and take before meals. At present, it is usually taken as a decoction with the dosage reduced by two-thirds.

Actions   Drains heat from the Lungs and calms wheezing

Indications

Coughing, wheezing, and fever with skin that feels hot to the touch, all of which worsen in the late afternoon. There is also a dry mouth, little or difficult-to-expectorate sputum, a thin, rapid pulse, and a red tongue with a yellow coating.

This is lurking fire due to constrained heat in the Lungs. This heat causes the Lung qi to rebel, which manifests as coughing and wheezing. The Lungs govern the skin; lurking heat in the Lungs causes the skin to feel hot to the touch with light pressure. This so-called 'steaming' heat is thought to emanate from the skin itself. It should not be confused with the hot skin associated with a yang brightness-warp disorder, which originates in the flesh and feels hot at all levels of pressure. Constrained heat also injures the yin of the Lungs. For this reason, the coughing, wheezing, and fever all worsen in the afternoon when the Lung qi is at its nadir (the most yin time for the Lungs). This should be distinguished from conditions of Kidney yin deficiency where there is fever *only* in the afternoon. The dry mouth, thin and rapid pulse, and red tongue with a yellow coating are all indicative of heat.

Analysis of Formula

In order to treat constraint caused by lurking fire in the Lungs, the formula uses a strategy of clearing heat and draining fire, assisted by calming wheezing to address the symptoms. The chief herb, dry-fried Mori Cortex (*chǎo sāng bái pí*), drains constrained heat from the Lungs and thereby stops the coughing and wheezing. It combines a moistening nature with an acrid flavor, allowing it to drain heat without damaging the Lungs, which is regarded as the 'tender organ.' This is particularly suitable in a formula directed specifically at children. It is assisted by the deputy, Lycii Cortex (*dì gǔ pí*), which is sweet, bland, and bitter. It enters the Kidneys to clear heat from deficiency and into the Lungs to drain lurking fire. *Essentials of the Materia Medica* argues that it is able to vent heat pathogens from the Lungs that are retained following an external invasion and float to the surface from time to time as tidal fevers.

Both the chief and deputy consist of root bark (cortex), which in Chinese is called 'skin' (皮 *pí*). In the human body, the health of the Lungs is reflected in the skin. Traditionally, therefore, the peel or bark of plants was considered especially useful for treating the Lungs. If there is more heat from constraint than from deficiency, the dosage of the chief herb is increased; if there is more heat from deficiency, the dosage of the deputy is increased.

The assistants, Glycyrrhizae Radix praeparata (*zhì gān cǎo*) and Nonglutinous rice (*jīng mǐ*), protect the Stomach from the cold properties of the other herbs. In terms of the mother-child method, they also help the mother (i.e., earth, which corresponds to the Spleen and Stomach) nurture the child (i.e., metal, which corresponds to the Lungs).

Cautions and Contraindications

This formula is often modified to protect the Spleen from injury by the cold-natured herbs in the formula. It is contraindicated for coughing and wheezing due to wind-cold, wind-heat, or damp-phlegm.

Commentary

The source text refers to the disorder treated by this formula as 'Lung overabundance in children' (小兒肺盛 *xiǎo ér fèi shèng*). Not until the Ming and Qing eras did physicians define the nature of this overabundance as 'Lung fire' and provide a detailed analysis of the disease dynamic and etiology. With an overabundance of heat, the clearing and clarifying function of the Lungs is impaired and the qi rebels upward, producing a high, clear-sounding cough with little sputum. The heat itself is thought to arise from the oscillation between excess and deficiency that reflects the immaturely developed yin and yang in children. This pattern must therefore be distinguished from both external excess, where pathogenic heat constrains the diffusion of Lung qi, and internal deficiency, where an objective lack of fluids and essences is insufficient to moisten and cool the Lungs. For this reason, the formula focuses on draining heat without employing excessively cooling or bitter substances such as Gypsum fibrosum (*shí gāo*) or Scutellariae Radix (*huáng qín*) that would damage the qi dynamic; and it tonifies the qi and yin indirectly by strengthening earth and clearing deficiency heat rather than relying on sweet, moistening herbs such as Ophiopogonis Radix (*mài mén dōng*) or Asparagi Radix (*tiān mén dōng*) that would increase stagnation. The famous Qing-dynasty physician Fei Bo-Xiong concisely summed up this strategy: "Clearing Lung fire and supplementing the Spleen and Stomach—this is the method of caring for the mother [in order to treat the child]. If one were to add [bitter, cold herbs that damage the earth like] Coptidis Rhizoma (*huáng lián*), one would let go of the guiding [principles] laid down within the formula's composition."

Usage in Exterior Conditions

Physicians have long argued whether this formula can be used when a pathogenic factor is present in the exterior. *Symptom, Cause, Pulse, and Treatment* and the *Golden Mirror of the Medical Tradition* prescribe modifications of this formula to treat patterns where exterior wind-cold is tying the protective qi in the exterior. *Systematic Differentiation of Warm Pathogen Diseases*, on the other hand, contains a famous essay entitled "On Why Drain the White Powder (*xiè bái sǎn*) Cannot Be Used Rashly" in which its author, Wu Ju-Tong, explains:

> Throughout the ages the commentators on this formula only discuss its merits but do not [appear to] know about its drawbacks. … This formula is excellent for treating cough, ascending qi, and fever from deficiency in the wake of feverish disorders or pox in children, if no external pathogen remains but the true original [qi] is unable to return to its source [in the gate of vitality]. However, if one uses Mori Cortex (*sāng bái pí*) and Lycii Cortex (*dì gǔ pí*) where wind-cold or wind-warmth truly are in overabundance, or if one adds either of these herbs to other formulas [in the treatment of such disorders], it is like pouring oil into a soup. They will plug [the exterior and produce] clumping, so that [the disorder] cannot be resolved.

The early modern physician Zhang Shan-Lei forcefully repeated this warning, stating that unless there exist clear indications, use of this formula without significant modification is best avoided until all external pathogens have been cleared.

Comparisons

➤ Vs. WHITE TIGER DECOCTION (*bāi hú tāng*)

The basic organization of these two formulas is very similar. Sweet herbs to tonify earth are combined with substances that clear heat from the Lungs. Although White Tiger Decoction (*bāi hú tāng*) was originally used to treat yang brightness disorders, proponents of the warm pathogen disorder current broadened its scope to include the treatment of greater yin qi-level heat in the Lungs. It treats the overabundance of heat with some damage to the yang fluids. This pathology is effectively controlled by the chief ingredient Gypsum fibrosum (*shí gāo*), which clears heat in the interior and vents it to the outside. By contrast, Drain the White Powder (*xiè bái sǎn*) is indicated for Lung fire occurring against a background of yin deficiency. The pathology here is one of accumulation, which its chief herb Mori Cortex (*sāng bái pí*) effectively drains via the urine.

➤ Vs. EPHEDRA, APRICOT KERNEL, GYPSUM, AND LICORICE DECOCTION (*má xìng shí gān tāng*)

Both of these formulas treat wheezing and coughing due to heat constraining the diffusion and downward-directing of the Lung qi. However, Ephedra, Apricot Kernel, Gypsum, and Licorice Decoction (*má xìng shí gān tāng*) treats patterns characterized by heat excess arising either from the contraction of a cold pathogen that has transformed into heat or from excess internal heat. In both cases, the heat is pronounced, and the patient will most likely possess a strong constitution. Drain the White Powder (*xiè bái sǎn*), on the other hand, is indicated for Lung fire from constraint against a background of yin deficiency. This was originally thought to arise from the delicate balance between yin and yang in children, which readily allows the yang to escape the control of yin without either being objectively excessive or deficient. Symptomatically, Drain the White Powder (*xiè bái sǎn*) presentations are often characterized by a sensation of steaming heat in the afternoons and by skin that is warm to the touch but dry. Ephedra, Apricot Kernel, Gypsum, and Licorice Decoction (*má xìng shí gān tāng*) presentations will typically have light sweating and signs of excess heat, such as fever and thirst.

➤ Vs. ARREST WHEEZING DECOCTION (*dìng chuǎn tāng*); *see* PAGE 541

Biomedical Indications

With the appropriate presentation, this formula may be used to treat a variety of biomedically-defined disorders, primarily infections, including the early stages of measles, pneumonia, bronchitis, pertussis, conjunctivitis, herpes simplex, and urticaria.

Alternate names

Drain the Lungs Powder (*xiè fèi sǎn*) in *Craft of Medicines and Patterns for Children*; Drain the Lungs Decoction (*xiè fèi tāng*) in *Indispensable Tools for Pattern Treatment*

Modifications

- For mild phlegm, and to further protect the Spleen and Stomach, substitute Poria (*fú líng*) for Nonglutinous rice (*jīng mǐ*).
- For severe heat, add Scutellariae Radix (*huáng qín*) and Anemarrhenae Rhizoma (*zhī mǔ*).
- For obstruction due to phlegm, add Lepidii/ Descurainiae Semen (*tíng lì zǐ*) and Cynanchi stauntonii Rhizoma (*bái qián*).
- For cough due to dryness, add Trichosanthis Pericarpium (*guā lóu pí*), Armeniacae Semen (*xìng rén*), Fritillariae cirrhosae Bulbus (*chuān bèi mǔ*), and Glehniae/Adenophorae Radix (*shā shēn*).
- For heat from deficiency with afternoon fevers, add Artemisiae annuae Herba (*qīng hāo*), Trionycis Carapax (*biē jiǎ*), and Stellariae Radix (*yín chái hú*).

Variation

瀉白散 (泻白散)

Drain the White Powder from *Wondrous Lantern*

xiè bái sǎn

SOURCE   *Wondrous Lantern for Peering into the Origin and Development of Miscellaneous Diseases* (1773)

Add Ginseng Radix (*rén shēn*), Poria (*fú líng*), Anemarrhenae Rhizoma (*zhī mǔ*), and Scutellariae Radix (*huáng qín*) for coughing and wheezing due to heat from Lung qi deficiency.

Associated Formulas

瀉白散 (泻白散)

Drain the White Powder from *Indispensable Tools for Pattern Treatment*

xiè bái sǎn

SOURCE   *Indispensable Tools for Pattern Treatment* (1602)

Mori Cortex (*sāng bái pí*) 6g
Lycii Cortex (*dì gǔ pí*) 3g
Glycyrrhizae Radix praeparata (*zhì gān cǎo*) 3g
Fritillariae thunbergii Bulbus (*zhè bèi mǔ*) 3g
Platycodi Radix (*jié gěng*) 3g
Trichosanthis Semen (*guā lóu rén*) 4.5g
Zingiberis Rhizoma recens (*shēng jiāng*) . . . . .3 pieces

Drains heat from the Lungs, transforms phlegm and pus, and stops

coughing. For early-stage Lung abscess with coughing of dark-green or blood-streaked sputum that worsens in the morning.

桑丹瀉白湯 (桑丹泻白汤)

Mulberry Leaf and Moutan Decoction to Drain the White

sāng dān xiè bái tāng

SOURCE   *Revised Popular Guide to the Discussion of Cold Damage* (Qing dynasty)

Mori Cortex (*sāng bái pí*) 12g
Mori Folium (*sāng yè*) 9g
Lycii Cortex (*dì gǔ pí*) 15g
Moutan Cortex (*mǔ dān pí*) 4.5g
Bambusae Caulis in taeniam (*zhú rú*) 6g
Fritillariae cirrhosae Bulbus (*chuān bèi mǔ*) 9g
Nonglutinous rice (*jīng mǐ*) 9g
Glycyrrhizae Radix praeparata (*zhì gān cǎo*) 1.8g
Jujubae Fructus (*dà zǎo*) . . . . .2 pieces

Clears the Liver, drains and protects the Lungs. For Liver fire scorching the Lungs characterized by coughing that causes pain in the chest and flanks, an inability to rotate or bend the trunk, and in severe cases, coughing of blood or blood-streaked sputum.

葶藶大棗瀉肺湯 (葶苈大枣泻肺汤)

Lepidium/Descurainia and Jujube Decoction to Drain the Lungs

tíng lì dà zǎo xiè fèi tāng

SOURCE   *Essentials from the Golden Cabinet* (c. 220)

Lepidii/ Descurainiae Semen (*tíng lì zǐ*) 9-12g
Jujubae Fructus (*dà zǎo*) . . . . .12 pieces

The source text advises to cook Jujubae Fructus (*dà zǎo*) in 3 cups of water until 2 cups remain. This herb is discarded, and Lepidii/ Descurainiae Semen (*tíng lì zǐ*), which has been stewed and then pounded into a pill the size of a bullet, is added. This is cooked until only 1 cup of liquid remains. At present, it is typically prepared as a regular decoction with usually only 4 Jujubae Fructus (*dà zǎo*). Drains the Lungs, moves the fluids, drives out phlegm, and calms wheezing. For Lung abscess with phlegm in the chest characterized by coughing, wheezing, and a sense of fullness and distention in the chest. In the source text, the presentation includes superficial edema of the entire body (including the face and ears), nasal congestion with a clear discharge, and a loss of taste and smell. This formula focuses on draining phlegm and fluids from the Lungs.

辛夷清肺飲 (辛夷清肺饮)

Magnolia Flower Drink to Clear the Lungs

xīn yí qīng fèi yǐn

Source   *Orthodox Lineage of External Medicine* (1617)

Magnoliae Flos (*xīn yí*) 2.5g
Scutellariae Radix (*huáng qín*) 3g

Gardeniae Fructus (*zhī zǐ*). 3g
Ophiopogonis Radix (*mài mén dōng*) 3g
Lilii Bulbus (*bǎi hé*) 3g
Gypsum fibrosum (*shí gāo*) 3g
Glycyrrhizae Radix (*gān cǎo*) .1.5g
Eriobotryae Folium (*pí pá yè*) . . . . (remove hairs) 3g
Anemarrhenae Rhizoma (*zhī mǔ*) 3g
Cimicifugae Rhizoma (*shēng má*). 1g

Method of Preparation Use 2 cups boiled down to 0.8 cup, taken after meals.

Actions Disseminates Lung qi, clears heat, and unblocks the orifices (specifically the nose)

Indications

Nasal polyps, nasal congestion, atrophic rhinitis, sinusitis, and allergic rhinitis.

This formula treats the failure of the Lungs to disseminate the qi along with accumulation of Lung heat when these result in nasal congestion or nasal polyps. The patient will often present with a rapid pulse and a red tongue with a white or yellow coating.

Analysis of Formula

Magnoliae Flos (*xīn yí*), which disperses wind and unblocks the nose, serves as the chief herb in the formula. Scutellariae Radix (*huáng qín*), Gardeniae Fructus (*zhī zǐ*), Anemarrhenae Rhizoma (*zhī mǔ*), and Gypsum fibrosum (*shí gāo*) clear heat and resolve toxicity. Ophiopogonis Radix (*mài mén dōng*) works with Lilii Bulbus (*bǎi hé*) to enrich the yin and moisten the Lungs so as to offset damage to the Lung yin caused by the drying herbs in the formula and the stagnant heat inherent in this disorder. These herbs serve as deputies by addressing the heat congestion that is at the heart of this pattern.

The assistant herbs concentrate on assisting the chief ingredient in unblocking the nose by diffusing the Lung qi and directing it downward. Eriobotryae Folium (*pí pá yè*) clarifies and descends, thus directing the Lung qi downward and helping the Lung disseminate the qi. Cimicifugae Rhizoma (*shēng má*) raises the clear yang and clears heat and resolves toxicity. This combination of Eriobotryae Folium (*pí pá yè*) and Cimicifugae Rhizoma (*shēng má*) regulates the flow of qi in the upper body so that the turbid qi descends and the clear qi rises.

Glycyrrhizae Radix (*gān cǎo*) serves as envoy by harmonizing the formula, clearing heat, and resolving toxicity. In sum, the formula clears the heat from constrained stagnation, disseminates the Lung qi, and unblocks the nose.

Commentary

This formula is derived from the section on the treatment of nasal piles (鼻痔 *bì zhì*) in *Orthodox Lineage of External Medicine*. Here 'piles' refers to growths in the nose equivalent to what Western medicine calls nasal polyps. According to the text, nasal piles form because the "Lung qi is not clear [leading to] constrained stagnation of wind and dampness."

This is a concise way of saying that, because the Lung qi is not flowing freely to the nose, wind and dampness are not properly dispelled and dispersed and thus stagnate in the nose. If this is allowed to continue, the pile grows larger and larger until it completely blocks the nasal passage. *Golden Mirror of the Medical Tradition* cites the same formula for the treatment of this disorder and adds that, over time, the pile will turn purple and hard.

The source text says that when this formula is combined with the local application of a powder called Sal Ammoniac Powder (*náo shā sǎn*)* the nasal pile will gradually shrink. Due to the toxicity of two of the ingredients in this powder, Realgar (*xióng huáng*) and Calomelas (*qīng fěn*), it cannot be used in the modern Western clinic. This may explain why the main use of Magnolia Flower Drink to Clear the Lungs (*xīn yí qīng fèi yǐn*) at present is in the treatment of other outcomes of the failure of the Lung qi to disseminate and the ensuing stagnation of wind, dampness, and heat: mostly chronic rhinitis, nasal congestion, sinusitis, and allergic rhinitis. While surgery is the treatment of choice for most nasal polyps, this formula can be used postoperatively to prevent recurrence.

Because this formula disseminates the Lung qi and clears heat, with the addition of cough-relieving agents, it is also suitable for the treatment of Lung-heat cough with yellow phlegm. This is particularly true if the Lung-heat pattern includes nasal congestion. It should be noted, however, that Magnolia Flower Drink to Clear the Lungs (*xīn yí qīng fèi yǐn*) has little capacity to release pathogens from the body's exterior, so it would be inappropriate if the Lung heat is part of a respiratory disorder that includes signs such as aversion to wind and cold and a floating pulse. Also, despite the inclusion of such yin-tonifying agents as Ophiopogonis Radix (*mài mén dōng*) and Anemarrhenae Rhizoma (*zhī mǔ*), the formula is nevertheless drying and should therefore be used with caution in patients who exhibit signs of yin or fluid deficiency.

Biomedical Indications

With the appropriate presentation, this formula may be used to treat a variety of biomedically-defined disorders including nasal polyps, sinusitis, rhinitis, atrophic rhinitis or allergic rhinitis. With modifications, it can also treat chronic cough or bronchitis.

. . . .

Alternate name

Magnolia Flower Drink to Clear the Lungs (*xīn yí qīng fèi yǐn*) in *Golden Mirror of the Medical Tradition*

---

* Also from *Orthodox Lineage of External Medicine*, this formula contains Sal Ammoniac (*náo shā*) 3g, Calomelas (*qīng fěn*) 1g, Borneolum (*bīng piàn*) 0.2g, and Realgar (*xióng huáng*) 1g.

Modifications

- *Golden Mirror of the Medical Tradition* suggests adding Notopterygii Rhizoma seu Radix *(qiāng huó)*, Forsythiae Fructus *(lián qiáo)*, and Menthae haplocalycis Herba *(bò hé)*. This increases the formula's ability to dispel dampness, disseminate the Lung qi, and unblock the nose.

- For chronic rhinitis, add Paeoniae Radix rubra *(chì sháo)* and Puerariae Radix *(gé gēn)*.

- For Lung-heat cough, add Peucedani Radix *(qián hú)*, Benincasae Semen *(dōng guā zǐ)*, and Mori Cortex *(sāng bái pí)*.

瀉黃散（泻黄散）
Drain the Yellow Powder
xiè huáng sǎn

This formula is also called Drain the Spleen Powder *(xiè pí sǎn)*, which refers to its action in draining fire from the Spleen and Stomach. Yellow refers to the Spleen and Stomach's correspondence to the earth phase and to the color yellow.

Source   *Craft of Medicinal Treatment for Childhood Disease Patterns* (1119)

Gypsum fibrosum *(shí gāo)* 15g
Gardeniae Fructus *(zhī zǐ)* 3g
dry-fried Saposhnikoviae Radix *(chǎo fáng fēng)* 120g
Pogostemonis/Agastaches Folium *(huò xiāng yè)* 21g
Glycyrrhizae Radix *(gān cǎo)* 90g

Method of Preparation   The source text advises to grind the ingredients into a powder, toast lightly with honey and wine, and take as a draft in 3-6g doses. At present, it is prepared as a decoction with a reduction in dosage.

Actions   Clears lurking fire from the Spleen and Stomach

Indications

Mouth ulcers, bad breath, thirst, frequent hunger, dry mouth and lips, a red tongue, and a rapid pulse. Also for tongue thrusting in children.

This is lurking fire in the Spleen. The Spleen 'opens' through the mouth, thus Spleen fire is manifested in oral symptoms. Heat readily transfers from the Spleen to the Stomach (its paired organ), which leads to thirst and frequent hunger. Heat in the Spleen can also cause the tongue to become hot, dry, and red. A red tongue and a rapid pulse are signs of heat. The tongue is regarded as the 'sprout' of the Heart. Why then is tongue thrusting regarded as a sign of Spleen dysfunction? A branch of the Spleen channel reaches the root of the tongue and spreads through its underside. When heat disrupts the function of the channel, it stimulates the tongue and causes it to thrust outward. Heat in the Spleen may also cause the tongue to become hot and dry. It may then thrust out of the mouth in an effort to cool and moisten itself.

Analysis of Formula

This formula employs a strategy of clearing and dispersing to drain lurking fire from the Spleen and Stomach. Gypsum fibrosum *(shí gāo)*, one of the chief ingredients, is acrid and cooling and is one of the principal herbs for clearing heat from the middle burner. Gardeniae Fructus *(zhī zǐ)*, the other chief ingredient, drains heat from all three burners through the urine and enters the Heart to relieve irritability. Although these are the chief ingredients, their dosage is relatively small. This is to prevent their cooling and descending actions from further constraining or bottling-up the lurking fire. The large dosage of Saposhnikoviae Radix *(fáng fēng)*, one of the deputies, disperses the lurking Spleen fire in accordance with the principle of treating constrained fire by dispersal. If the condition is treated simply as a case of Stomach fire to be cleared and drained, and the dispersing action of this herb is omitted, there will be no improvement. Saposhnikoviae Radix *(fáng fēng)* also supports the physiological ascending function of the Spleen yang. Acting in concert, these three ingredients thus drain fire without injuring the Spleen and Stomach yang, and disperse constraint without fanning pathological fire.

The second deputy, Pogostemonis/Agastaches Folium *(huò xiāng yè)*, aromatically revives the Spleen. Working together with Saposhnikoviae Radix *(fáng fēng)*, it restores the qi mechanisms of the Spleen and Stomach and assists in dispersing the lurking fire. Glycyrrhizae Radix *(gān cǎo)*, honey, and the wine serve as assistants and envoys. Together they regulate the middle burner, drain fire, and harmonize the actions of the other ingredients in the formula.

Cautions and Contraindications

Contraindicated in cases with Stomach yin deficiency and tongue thrusting due to congenital qi deficiency.

Commentary

The composition of this formula provides an insight to the proper treatment of lurking heat (fire). Cold substances that drain heat from the middle burner play a very small role. What is needed are substances that gently clear and disperse, as recommended by the Qing-dynasty physician Wang Xu-Gao: "It is appropriate to drain lurking fire in the Spleen and Stomach very gently, unlike fire from excess that [needs] to be drained urgently." This is another example of flexibly applying the adage from the *Inner Classic*, "For fire from constraint, discharge it" (火鬱發之 *huǒ yù fā zhī*).

Nevertheless, the role of Saposhnikoviae Radix *(fáng fēng)* in the formula has been disputed. The early modern physician Zhang Shan-Lei, in particular, considered its inclusion, especially in such a high dosage, to be a mistake. He argued that it fans rather than disperses fire and should therefore be omitted. To settle this question, researchers at the Nanjing College of Chinese Medicine examined the functions of Saposhnikoviae Radix (*fáng fēng*) by means of animal experiments. They found that while the herb does not have any anti-inflammatory action when used on its own, such an effect can be produced by combining it with the other herbs in the formula. They also found that an 80 percent reduction in the dosage of Saposhnikoviae Radix (*fáng fēng*) did not markedly influence this action. For mouth ulcers or tongue thrusting, the dosage of Saposhnikoviae Radix (*fáng fēng*) is therefore often reduced today and other herbs that clear heat are added.

The large dosage of Glycyrrhizae Radix (*gān cǎo*) has likewise given rise to discussion, as its warming and cloying nature can be thought to inhibit the discharging effect of Saposhnikoviae Radix (*fáng fēng*). However, used in its unprepared form it actually drains fire, as elaborated in *Transforming the Significance of Medicinal Substances*: "Used unprepared, it is cooling and drains fire: it primarily disperses pathogens in the exterior, reduces swollen sores, eases sore throats, resolves the toxicity of all herbs, eliminates accumulated fire in the Stomach, and dispels urinary tract pain—this is the power of sweet coolness eliminating heat." This is its usage here.

This formula is also used in treating yellowing of the sclera due to Spleen heat.

Comparison

➤ Vs. Clear the Stomach Powder (*qīng wèi sǎn*)

Both formulas treat excess fire in the Spleen and Stomach manifesting with symptoms in the face and mouth. Clear the Stomach Powder (*qīng wèi sǎn*) focuses on resolving toxicity and clearing fire caused by damp-heat in the Stomach that penetrates into the blood. For this reason, the formula combines bitter, cold Coptidis Rhizoma (*huáng lián*) with herbs that cool the blood, while Cimicifugae Rhizoma (*shēng má*) guides the formula to the collaterals of the Stomach in the gums. The present formula focuses on draining lurking heat in the Spleen and Stomach that constrains their yang qi. Therefore, it pairs cold substances that clear the qi with warm and acrid herbs that facilitate the qi dynamic of the middle burner, but avoids bitter and cold herbs like Coptidis Rhizoma (*huáng lián*). This reasoning is summarized by Wang Xu-Gao, who makes a further useful comparison:

> Why [does the author of this formula] not use Coptidis Rhizoma (*huáng lián*) for lurking heat in the Spleen? Wu He-Gao says this is because he fears its drying action. This is not the case. It is because he fears its hindering [of the qi dynamic that would further trap the lurking heat]. White Tiger Decoction (*bái hǔ tāng*) treats flaring fire of the Lungs and Stomach that manifests with strong fever, irritability, thirst, and sweating. This formula treats constrained and steaming fire of the Stomach and Spleen that manifests with heat in the muscles and flesh, irritability, and thirst but no sweating. Therefore, it adds Saposhnikoviae Radix (*fáng fēng*) and Herba Agastaches seu

Pogostemi (*huò xiāng*), grasping the meaning [of the principle] that one should disperse fire from constraint.

Biomedical Indications

With the appropriate presentation, this formula may be used to treat a variety of biomedically-defined disorders including apthous ulcers and oral thrush.

Alternate names

Drain the Spleen Powder (*xiè pí sǎn*) in *Craft of Medicines and Patterns for Children*; Drain the Yellow Decoction (*xiè huáng tāng*) in *Mastery of Pox and Rashes*

Modifications

• For severe heat, add Coptidis Rhizoma (*huáng lián*).
• For irritability and restlessness, add Poria rubra (*chì fú líng*) and Junci Medulla (*dēng xīn cǎo*).

清胃散
Clear the Stomach Powder
qīng wèi sǎn

Source *Secrets from the Orchid Chamber* (1336)

Coptidis Rhizoma (*huáng lián*) 1.8g (3-6g)
Cimicifugae Rhizoma (*shēng má*) 3g (3-6g)
Moutan Cortex (*mǔ dān pí*) 1.5g (6-9g)
Rehmanniae Radix (*shēng dì huáng*) 0.9g (6-12g)
Angelicae sinensis radicis Corpus (*dāng guī shēn*) . .0.9g (6-12g)

Method of Preparation The source text advises to grind the ingredients into powder, prepare as a draft, and take cool. It also states that if administration does not improve the symptoms, the dosage of Coptidis Rhizoma (*huáng lián*) is to be increased by one-third. In any case, the dosage should be increased in the summer. At present, the formula is usually prepared as a decoction with the dosages specified in parentheses.

Actions Drains Stomach fire, cools the blood, and nourishes the yin

Indications

Toothache (especially when the pain extends into the head), facial swelling, fever, bad breath, a dry mouth, a red tongue with little coating, and a slippery, large, and rapid pulse. Also indicated for bleeding and sores of the gums, and for a swollen, painful tongue, lips, or jaw. The painful areas respond favorably to cold, and worsen with heat.

This is heat accumulation in the Stomach. The yang brightness Stomach channel, which contains an abundance of qi and blood, is a common place for conditions of excess to develop. This channel, and the yang brightness Large Intestine channel, supply the mouth and teeth. The accumulation of heat blocks the flow of qi in the channel and gives rise to rebellious fire, which causes toothache and headache. Fire also causes the flesh to fester, which manifests as sores and swelling in the mouth and bad breath. Bleeding of the gums is caused by fire that has injured the blood vessels. The sensitivity to changes in temperature, the red tongue with little coating, and the slippery, large, and rapid pulse are all signs of heat in the Stomach.

Analysis of Formula

The chief herb, Coptidis Rhizoma *(huáng lián),* attacks the Stomach fire and drains the accumulation of heat. When heat accumulates in the middle burner, the pure products of digestion are unable to rise and the turbid products are unable to descend. The deputy, Cimicifugae Rhizoma *(shēng má),* raises and disperses the heat and resolves toxicity. *Discussion of Medicinal Properties* lists it as a specific herb for toothache, ulcers, and festering sores in the mouth. Its synergy with Coptidis Rhizoma *(huáng lián)* ensures that draining of fire does not harm the qi dynamic, and that the ascent of yang does not further fan the rising fire. Cimicifugae Rhizoma *(shēng má)* also serves as the envoy, which directs the focus of the formula to the face and mouth. The remaining ingredients are regarded as assistants. Moutan Cortex *(mǔ dān pí)* and Rehmanniae Radix *(shēng dì huáng)* cool the blood and nourish the yin. Angelicae sinensis Radix *(dāng guī)* reduces swelling and alleviates pain by harmonizing the blood.

Cautions and Contraindications

Contraindicated in cases with toothache due to wind-cold, or tooth and gum problems due to Kidney deficiency.

Commentary

The source text notes that the cause of this disorder is the improper use of hot, tonic herbs. At present, the accumulation of heat in the Stomach is usually attributed to overconsumption of rich or fried foods, or (paradoxically) of cold foods, which constrains the yang qi and causes its transformation into fire.

This is a very effective formula in the treatment of toothache, swollen gums, and bleeding of the gums due to Stomach fire; it can be modified for treating many types of oral problems. While all commentators agree on these indications, they differ in their perspectives on the chief herb and, by implication, the precise disease dynamic that this formula treats. Modern textbooks generally follow the Qing-dynasty scholar Wang Ang in defining Coptidis Rhizoma *(huáng lián)* to be the chief herb. They give two apparently compelling reasons. First, Coptidis Rhizoma *(huáng lián)* is the herb with the closest affinity to the Stomach, which is the root of the disorder. Second, the source text itself emphasizes the role of Coptidis Rhizoma *(huáng lián)* as the chief herb by providing detailed instructions regarding adjustment of its dosage.

Other physicians have expressed divergent views. The late-Qing dynasty physician Tang Zong-Hai, for instance, emphasized the importance of Cimicifugae Rhizoma *(shēng má)* as representing the dispersing method by which the formula eliminates heat in accordance with the principle that fire from constraint should be discharged. His contemporary, Luo Mei, pointed to the absence in the list of indications of signs or symptoms that are usually associated with yang brightness channel disorders. For this reason, he considered the root of the disorder to be heat in the blood and accordingly designated Rehmanniae Radix *(shēng dì huáng)* as the chief herb.

Read together, these different perspectives lead to a deeper understanding of the disease process treated by this formula. As Ye Tian-Shi noted, "The gums are the collaterals of the Stomach." The collaterals pertain to blood, while signs and symptoms of the disorder imply the presence of fire toxin. Such toxin readily enters the blood in the Stomach via food, drink, or, as the source text notes, the improper use of medication. If blood is deficient, it will readily generate wind, which in turn leads fire toxin upward into the collaterals where it manifests as toothache and a progressive ulceration of the gums. To address all aspects of this pathology, the formula combines herbs that drain damp-heat from the Stomach, nourish and cool the blood, and disperse constraint and relieve toxic heat within the collaterals.

Comparisons

➤ Vs. Drain the Yellow Powder *(xiè huáng sǎn);* *see* page 191

➤ Vs. Jade Woman Decoction *(yù nǚ jiān),* Reed Decoction *(wěi jīng tāng); see* page 194

Biomedical Indications

With the appropriate presentation, this formula may be used to treat a variety of biomedically-defined disorders, primarily infections affecting the head, including stomatitis, periodontitis, glossitis, and trigeminal neuralgia.

Alternate names

Clear the Stomach Decoction *(qīng wèi tāng)* in *Complete Book on the Experience of Sores;* Disperse the Stomach Decoction *(xiāo wèi tāng)* in *Essentials for Those Who Do Not Know Medicine*

Modifications

• For strong thirst with a desire for cold beverages, remove Angelicae sinensis Radix *(dāng guī)* and add Scrophulariae Radix *(xuán shēn)* and Trichosanthis Radix *(tiān huā fěn).*

• For heat in the Large Intestine with constipation, add Rhei Radix et Rhizoma *(dà huáng).*

Associated Formula

清胃湯（清胃汤）

Clear the Stomach Decoction

qīng wèi tāng

SOURCE   *Golden Mirror of the Medical Tradition* (1742)

Gypsum fibrosum (*shí gāo*) 12g
Scutellariae Radix (*huáng qín*) 3g
Rehmanniae Radix (*shēng dì huáng*) 3g
Coptidis Rhizoma (*huáng lián*) 3g
Cimicifugae Rhizoma (*shēng má*) 3g
Moutan Cortex (*mǔ dān pí*) 4.5g

Clears fire from the Stomach and cools the blood. For bleeding gums and bad breath due to vigorous Stomach fire. In contrast to the principal formula, this focuses more on clearing vigorous Stomach heat.

玉女煎

Jade Woman Decoction

yù nǚ jiān

The origin of this name is unclear, but there are three theories. The first is that it refers to Gypsum fibrosum (*shí gāo*), an important ingredient of the formula, which, like jade, is cold and yin in nature. The second theory is that the name refers to the handmaiden of the Bodhisattva Guanyin, also known as the Jade Woman. Guanyin relieves the sorrows and cools the passions of the world, just like the yin-nourishing, fire-draining actions of this formula. The third theory is based on the ancient texts of alchemy, which refer to the Kidneys as the Jade Woman. This formula likewise treats problems associated with the Kidney yin.

Source   *Collected Treatises of [Zhang] Jing-yue* (1624)

Gypsum fibrosum (*shí gāo*) 6-15g
Rehmanniae Radix praeparata (*shú dì huáng*) 9-30g
Anemarrhenae Rhizoma (*zhī mǔ*) 4.56g
Ophiopogonis Radix (*mài mén dōng*) 6g
Achyranthis bidentatae Radix (*niú xī*) 4.5g

Method of Preparation   Decoction. At present, the dosage of Gypsum fibrosum (*shí gāo*) is usually 15-30g. Take either warm or cool.

Actions   Drains heat from the Stomach and nourishes the yin

Indications

Toothache, loose teeth, bleeding gums, frontal headache, irritability and fever, thirst with a desire to drink cold beverages, a dry, red tongue with a yellow coating, and a floating, slippery, deficient, and large pulse.

This is Kidney yin deficiency with vigorous Stomach fire. The teeth are associated with the Kidneys and are situated along the yang brightness channel. Heat in the Stomach may therefore cause toothache, while Kidney deficiency may cause the teeth to loosen. Bleeding gums result when heat injures the channels that supply the teeth. Stomach heat will travel through the channel and cause headache (usually frontal). The red tongue with a yellow coating and the floating, slippery, and large pulse are signs of Stomach heat. Irritability, fever, and thirst are also symptoms of heat. The dry tongue and deficient pulse are indicative of Kidney yin deficiency.

Analysis of Formula

Gypsum fibrosum (*shí gāo*) clears fire from the Stomach and thereby relieves the fever, irritability, and thirst. It is an important substance for treating toothache due to Stomach fire. Rehmanniae Radix praeparata (*shú dì huáng*) nourishes Kidney water insufficiency, which enables water to restrain fire. These are the chief ingredients in the formula. Anemarrhenae Rhizoma (*zhī mǔ*), one of the deputies, helps Gypsum fibrosum (*shí gāo*) clear heat from the Stomach and also nourishes the yin. Ophiopogonis Radix (*mài mén dōng*), the other deputy, is very effective in moistening the Stomach, generating fluids, and alleviating irritability. It nourishes the yin primarily in the middle and upper burners, and thus complements the action of Rehmanniae Radix praeparata (*shú dì huáng*), which nourishes the Kidney yin. Achyranthis bidentatae Radix (*niú xī*) serves as the envoy. It conducts the heat downward by guiding blood downward and thereby stops the 'overflow' of blood into the oral cavity.

Cautions and Contraindications

According to the source text, this formula is contraindicated in those with diarrhea.

Commentary

Zhang Jie-Bin, the author of this formula, defines its indications as "exhaustion of water and exuberance of fire with all six pulses floating, flooding, and large. This is insufficiency of the lesser yin and surplus of the yang brightness with manifestations such as irritability, feverishness, thirst, headache, toothache, and bleeding."

This pattern, where fire excess and yin deficiency are equally pronounced, clearly belongs in the domain of the miscellaneous diseases of internal medicine. The formula itself, however, is related to White Tiger Decoction (*bái hǔ tāng*), which is closely associated with the treatment of conditions arising from externally-contracted pathogens. With this in mind, the Qing-dynasty physician Wu Ju-Tong expanded the range of application of the formula to the treatment of warm pathogen disorders. *Systematic Differentiation of Warm Pathogen Diseases* contains two variations. The first substitutes Rehmanniae Radix (*shēng dì huáng*) for Rehmanniae Radix praeparata (*shú dì huáng*) and Scrophulariae Radix (*xuán shēn*) for Achyranthis bidentatae Radix (*niú xī*) to treat "greater yin warm pathogen disorders with fire blazing in both qi and blood [levels]." The other is listed under VARIATION below.

Controversy Surrounding Gypsum fibrosum (shí gāo)

Another Qing-dynasty physician, Chen Nian-Zu, severely criticized Zhang Jie-Bin for using Gypsum fibrosum *(shí gāo)*—which clears and disperses fire from excess—to treat fire associated with deficiency. Wang Shi-Xiong came to Zhang's defense by pointing out that Ye Tian-Shi's case records showed that the great Suzhou physician modified the formula to treat wasting and thirsting disorder from deficiency. Use of the formula for this indication remains popular today.

The early modern physician Tang Zong-Hai also joined the fray with an essay in *Discussion of Blood Patterns*. In his typically self-confident manner, he claimed that all previous writers had misunderstood the true dynamic underpinning the formula's efficacy:

> One can see that the general management of the blood is located in the gestational chamber and that the Womb and Penetrating vessel above pertain to the yang brightness. In a normal person, the juices that are transformed into blood in the yang brightness middle palace follow the Penetrating vessel and are transported down to the gestational chamber. In people who vomit blood, Womb fire stirs the qi to rebel, which joins above with the yang brightness and blood follows seeping [into the Stomach]. Incessant coughing is frequently [a sign] that the yang [qi] of the Penetrating [vessel] joins above with the yang brightness to produce all kinds of presentations [involving] hyperactivity and rebelliousness. The formula uses Gypsum fibrosum *(shí gāo)* and Anemarrhenae Rhizoma *(zhī mǔ)* to clear the heat of the yang brightness; Achyranthis bidentatae Radix *(niú xī)* to turn back the upward-rebelling qi; and Rehmanniae Radix praeparata *(shú dì huáng)* to enrich the yin of the Womb in order to normalize the dryness of the yang brightness. When the [rebellious] qi of the Penetrating vessel is extinguished, all symptoms of hyperactivity and rebelliousness are cured. When Zhang Jie-Bin composed this formula he was not clear about this. Chen Nian-Zu further belittled it, while Wang Shi-Xiong took it to treat a pattern of toothache caused by yin deficiency and Stomach fire. None of these [physicians] understood the connection between this formula and the Penetrating vessel, even though this is its true marvel. Ophiopogonis Decoction *(mài mén dōng tāng)* is a formula for treating rebelliousness of the Penetrating vessel by directing phlegm downward. The present formula treats rebelliousness of the Penetrating vessel by directing fire downward.

Comparisons

➤ Vs. CLEAR THE STOMACH POWDER *(qīng wèi sǎn)*

Both of these formulas treat toothache and gum problems from Stomach fire. However, Clear the Stomach Powder *(qīng wèi sǎn)* treats blazing fire caused by damp-heat and toxin. It uses Coptidis Rhizoma *(huáng lián)* as the chief herb to treat the root and follows the inherent momentum of the disorder by using Cimicifugae Rhizoma *(shēng má)* to vent heat to the exterior. By contrast, the principal formula treats yin deficiency with vigorous fire. This requires a strategy that directs the

fire downward, rather than dispersing it. For this reason, it utilizes Achyranthis bidentatae Radix *(niú xī)*, which causes fire to descend.

➤ Vs. ANEMARRHENA, PHELLODENDRON, AND REHMANNIA PILL *(zhī bǎi dì huáng wán)*

Jade Woman Decoction *(yù nǚ jiān)* nourishes the yin and drains fire excess from the Stomach. This contrasts with Anemarrhena, Phellodendron, and Rehmannia Pill *(zhī bǎi dì huáng wán)*, which nourishes the Kidney yin and drains excess fire from the gate of vitality.

Biomedical Indications

With the appropriate presentation, this formula may be used to treat a wide variety of biomedically-defined disorders including stomatitis, glossitis, periodontitis, diabetes, trigeminal neuralgia, and viral myocarditis.

Modifications

- For abundant heat in the qi level, add Gardeniae Fructus *(zhī zǐ)* and Lycii Cortex *(dì gǔ pí)*.

- For abundant heat in the blood level with more severe bleeding, replace Rehmanniae Radix praeparata *(shú dì huáng)* with Rehmanniae Radix *(shēng dì huáng)* and add Scrophulariae Radix *(xuán shēn)*.

- For severe yin deficiency with mild fire in the Stomach, add Ligustri lucidi Fructus *(nǚ zhēn zǐ)* and Ecliptae Herba *(mò hàn lián)*.

- Where toothache is the main symptom, replace Rehmanniae Radix praeparata *(shú dì huáng)* with Rehmanniae Radix *(shēng dì huáng)* and add Asari Radix et Rhizoma *(xì xīn)*.

- Where bleeding is the primary symptom, double the dosage of Gypsum fibrosum *(shí gāo)* and Achyranthis bidentatae Radix *(niú xī)* and add Imperatae Rhizoma *(bái máo gēn)* and Moutan Cortex *(mǔ dān pí)*.

- For a dark-purple tongue with no coating, add Glehniae/Adenophorae Radix *(shā shēn)* and Dendrobii Herba *(shí hú)*.

- For profuse sweating and severe thirst, add Schisandrae Fructus *(wǔ wèi zǐ)*.

Variation

竹葉玉女煎（竹叶玉女煎）

Lophatherum Jade Woman Decoction

zhú yè yù nǚ jiān

SOURCE *Systematic Differentiation of Warm Pathogen Diseases* (1798)

Wu Ju-Tong substituted Rehmanniae Radix *(shēng dì huáng)* for

Rehmanniae Radix praeparata (*shú dì huáng*) and added Lophatheri Herba (*dàn zhú yè*) for "warm pathogen disorders in women that occur at the onset of menstruation [and are characterized by] a rapid pulse, tinnitus, dry retching, irritability, thirst. ... If severe and not resolved after ten or more days, the pathogen sinks [into the blood] and causes tetany."

Associated Formula

新加玉女煎

Newly Augmented Jade Woman Decoction

xīn jiā yù nǚ jiān

SOURCE   *Revised Popular Guide to the Discussion of Cold Damage* (Qing dynasty)

Gypsum fibrosum (*shí gāo*)	15-30g
Rehmanniae Radix praeparata (*shú dì huáng*)	9-30g
Anemarrhenae Rhizoma (*zhī mǔ*)	3-6g
Ophiopogonis Radix (*mài mén dōng*)	6-9g
Achyranthis bidentatae Radix (*niú xī*)	3-6g
Fluoritum (*zǐ shí yīng*)	12g
Magnetitum (*cí shí*)	12g
Cynanchi atrati Radix (*bái wēi*)	12g
Haliotidis Concha (*shí jué míng*)	15g
salt-fried Pinelliae Rhizoma (*yán chǎo bàn xià*)	3g

Clears heat, extinguishes wind, and directs rebellious qi downward. For Liver and Gallbladder fire transforming into wind and causing the qi of the Penetrating vessel to rebel and flush upward to the Heart, with symptoms of cough, hiccup, or collapse all due to upward-flushing of qi. This is an example of another physician sharing Tang Zong-Hai's interpretation of the formula's action and expanding its range of application accordingly.

導赤散 （导赤散）

Guide Out the Red Powder

dǎo chì sǎn

This formula conducts heat out of the Heart channel through the Small Intestine. The color red corresponds to the Heart and Small Intestine channels.

Source   *Craft of Medicinal Treatment for Childhood Disease Patterns* (1119)

Rehmanniae Radix (*shēng dì huáng*)	3-6g
Akebiae Caulis (*mù tōng*)	3-6g
Lophatheri Herba (*dàn zhú yè*)	3-6g
Glycyrrhizae Radix tenuis (*gān cǎo shāo*)	3-6g

Method of Preparation   The source text advises to grind equal amounts of Rehmanniae Radix (*shēng dì huáng*), Akebiae Caulis (*mù tōng*), and Glycyrrhizae Radix tenuis (*gān cǎo shāo*) into a powder and take 9g as a draft after meals with a small amount of Lophatheri Herba (*dàn zhú yè*). At present, it is usually prepared as a decoction and the dosage of Rehmanniae Radix (*shēng dì huáng*) is increased to 12-15g.

Actions   Clears the Heart and promotes urination

Indications

Irritability with a sensation of heat in the chest, thirst with a desire to drink cold beverages, a red face, possibly sores around the mouth, a red tongue, and a rapid pulse. Also used for dark, scanty, rough, and painful urination, or even clearly visible blood in the urine.

The original indication for this formula is 'Heart heat' (心熱 *xīn rè*). Because the Heart is located in the chest and controls the spirit, the presence of heat in the Heart channel disturbs the spirit and causes irritability and a sensation of heat in the chest. The Heart channel has an internal pathway that travels up the esophagus and into the throat and mouth. Heat in this channel causes thirst with a desire for cold beverages and redness in the face. When heat travels up the Heart channel to the mouth, sores develop in the mouth and tongue, the 'sprout' of the Heart. When heat transfers to the Small Intestine channel (linked to the Heart channel in an interior-exterior relationship), the secretion of body fluids is disrupted and painful urinary dribbling ensues. The red tongue and rapid pulse are signs of heat. When the heat transferred into the Small Intestine channel is severe, the collaterals become scorched and leak blood into the urine.

Analysis of Formula

This formula guides out excess Heart fire via the Small Intestine. Accordingly, the chief herb in this formula is bitter and cold Akebiae Caulis (*mù tōng*). It clears heat from the Heart channel above, and clears heat and promotes urination within the Small Intestine channel below. It thus addresses both aspects of the pattern. The deputy, Rehmanniae Radix (*shēng dì huáng*), enters the Heart to cool the blood. It also enters the Kidneys to nourish the yin and generate fluids (strengthening the Kidney water), which controls the fire in the Heart. Its pairing with Akebiae Caulis (*mù tōng*) promotes urination without damaging the yin and tonifies the fluids without retaining the pathogenic qi. Lophatheri Herba (*dàn zhú yè*), the assistant, is used to alleviate irritability by clearing heat from the Heart. Glycyrrhizae Radix tenuis (*gān cǎo shāo*) serves as the envoy by treating painful urinary dribbling, in addition to resolving toxicity and harmonizing the actions of the other herbs in the formula. The tips are used because they are believed to focus the action of the herb on the urinary passageways.

Cautions and Contraindications

Use with caution in cases of Spleen and Stomach deficiency.

Commentary

The source text prescribes this formula for children with a pattern of heat in the Heart. According to its author, the famous Song-dynasty pediatrician Qian Yi, this pattern can be diagnosed "by examining [how a child] sleeps. There is warm breath in the [open] mouth and they may sleep face down with bouts of teeth grinding. All of these indicate Heart heat."

There has been considerable debate over whether this pattern denotes heat from excess or deficiency. The proponents of heat from excess argue that the presence of Akebiae Caulis (*mù tōng*) and Lophatheri Herba (*dàn zhú yè*), which leach out fluids, can also injure the yin. They would not have been included had the formula been intended for treating heat from deficiency. On the other side, the proponents of heat from deficiency argue that the absence of Coptidis Rhizoma (*huáng lián*), which treats heat excess in the Heart channel, would certainly have been included had the formula been intended for treating heat from excess.

A close look at the source text reveals that both of these views are incomplete. *Craft of Medicinal Treatment for Childhood Disease Patterns* contains a description of 'Heart qi excess' (心氣實 *xīn qì shí*) that lists a desire to sleep face up (*xǐ yǎng wò* 喜仰臥) as one of its signs. This pattern is treated with Drain the Epigastrium Decoction (*xiè xīn tāng*), a formula containing Coptidis Rhizoma (*huáng lián*) as its chief herb. Clearly, therefore, the pattern of Heart fire is not *simply* one of Heart excess. In another passage, Qian Yi notes that "Dark red [eyes imply] Heart heat. This is governed by Guide Out the Red Powder (*dǎo chì sǎn*). Pale red eyes [imply] Heart deficiency heat (心虛熱 *xīn xū rè*). This is governed by Rehmannia and Rhinoceros Powder (*shéng xī sǎn*)." The latter formula contains Rehmanniae Radix (*shēng dì huáng*) but not Akebiae Caulis (*mù tōng*). Clearly, therefore, Heart heat is not synonymous with heat from deficiency.

It follows that Qian Yi's disease category 'Heart heat' refers to a unique pattern that corresponds to an instability that *Golden Mirror of the Medical Tradition* defines as "water deficiency with fire that is not excessive" (水虛火不實 *shuǐ xū huǒ bù shí*). This description attempts to capture a pathology that reflects the immature development of the qi dynamic in children. Because the yin and yang are still unstable and ungrounded, the qi in children readily moves this way and then that, becoming hot or cold, excessive or deficient, without either aberration from the norm indicating a substantial underlying excess or deficiency. The present formula responds by guiding out fire excess without damaging the yin, and by generating yin fluids without retaining the pathogenic heat.

Usage

Over time, the original indication of this formula was expanded by successive generations of physicians. The 11th-century *Formulary of the Pharmacy Service for Benefiting the People in the Taiping Era*, for instance, lists its indications as internal heat in the Heart channel in both children and adults with irritability, a stifling sensation in the chest, and confusion, as well as urinary problems due to heat transferred from

the Heart to the Small Intestine. The 18th-century *Golden Mirror of the Medical Tradition* prescribes it for mouth ulcers and sores, pain in the throat, acute wheezing due to Heart heat punishing the Lungs, and urinary problems during pregnancy. The early modern physician Zhang Shan-Lei added Scutellariae Radix (*huáng qín*) to the formula and prescribed it for clearing heat from the Lungs.

Modifications

Since it was first published, the formula has been repeatedly modified. The medical literature therefore contains many formulas by the same name but with different ingredients. Additions to the original formula can be organized into three main groups:

1. Herbs that clear the Heart and drain fire, such as Bubali Cornu (*shuǐ niú jiǎo*), Forsythiae Fructus (*lián qiáo*), Gardeniae Fructus (*zhī zǐ*), and Scutellariae Radix (*huáng qín*)
2. Herbs that clear heat and promote urination, such as Plantaginis Semen (*chē qián zǐ*), Junci Medulla (*dēng xīn cǎo*), Imperatae Rhizoma (*bái máo gēn*), and Poria (*fú líng*)
3. Herbs that nourish the yin and augment the qi, such as Ophiopogonis Radix (*mài mén dōng*) and Ginseng Radix (*rén shēn*)

Comparisons

➤ Vs. Eight-Herb Powder for Rectification (*bā zhèng sǎn*); see PAGE 715

➤ Vs. Clear the Heart Drink with Lotus Seed (*qīng xīn lián zǐ yǐn*); see PAGE 198

Biomedical Indications

With the appropriate presentation, this formula may be used to treat a variety of biomedically-defined disorders including stomatitis, oral thrush, night terrors, pyelonephritis, cystitis, and urinary tract stones.

Alternate name

Guide Out the Red Decoction (*dǎo chì tāng*) in *Complete Book of Patterns and Treatments in External Medicine*

Modifications

- For yin deficiency, add Dendrobii Herba (*shí hú*) and Anemarrhenae Rhizoma (*zhī mǔ*).
- For blood in the urine, add Ecliptae Herba (*mò hàn lián*) and Imperatae Rhizoma (*bái máo gēn*).
- For ulcerated sores around the mouth, combine with Five-Ingredient Powder with Poria (*wǔ líng sǎn*).

Variations

瀉心導赤湯（泻心导赤汤）

Drain the Epigastrium and Guide Out the Red Decoction

xiè xīn dǎo chì tāng

Source   *Golden Mirror of the Medical Tradition* (1742)

Add Coptidis Rhizoma (*huáng lián*) and Junci Medulla (*dēng xīn cǎo*) and remove Lophatheri Herba (*dàn zhú yè*) for more severe symptoms, including tongue thrusting in children.

加減導赤瀉心湯（加减导赤泻心汤）

Modified Guide Out the Red and Drain the Epigastrium Decoction

jiā jiǎn dǎo chì xiè xīn tāng

Source   *Selected Formulas for Warm-Heat Pathogen Diseases* (c. 1900)

Coptidis Rhizoma (*huáng lián*) 3g
Gardeniae Fructus (*zhī zǐ*) 3g
[Bubali Cornu (*shuǐ niú jiǎo*) . . . . 12-15g]
Panacis quinquefolii Radix (*xī yáng shēn*) 3g
Scutellariae Radix (*huáng qín*) 3g
Augment the Primal Powder (*yì yuán sǎn*) 9g
Rehmanniae Radix (*shēng dì huáng*) 15g
Poriae Sclerotium pararadicis (*fú shén*) 6g
Nelumbinis Plumula (*lián zǐ xīn*) . . . . 30 pieces
Junci Medulla (*dēng xīn cǎo*) 1.5g

Decoction. The source text says to grind 1.5g of Rhinocerotis Cornu (*xī jiǎo*) into a powder and take with the decoction. Augment the Primal Powder (*yì yuán sǎn*) is wrapped in cloth and decocted together with the other ingredients. Treats wind-warmth that has transformed into fire and entered the Heart channel by way of adverse transmission. This can manifest as impaired consciousness without speech and the appearance of being drunk, speaking one or two sentences during sleep, red eyes, burnt lips, thirst with no desire to drink, eating only when offered food but no epigastric focal obstruction, fullness or constipation (that would account for the disinterest in food), reduced urination, blood in the urine, a dry, red tongue with a crimson tip, and a pulse that is thin and rapid on the left but not large and flooding on the right. These signs and symptoms indicate that although there is extreme heat in the blood level of the Heart, the spirit qi of the Heart organ itself is deficient.

This is an example of how the original formula can be used in the treatment of warm pathogen disorders. The inspiration for this application comes from Ye Tian-Shi, who added Coptidis Rhizoma (*huáng lián*) and Rhinocerotis Cornu (*xī jiǎo*) to Guide Out the Red Powder (*dǎo chì sǎn*) in order to treat heat entering the nutritive and blood levels in the course of wind-warmth disorders. He Lian-Chen further modified the formula to treat a situation where the Heart spirit had become deficient, manifesting in such signs as a disinclination to speak and lack of appetite.

清心蓮子飲（清心莲子饮）

Clear the Heart Drink with Lotus Seed

qīng xīn lián zǐ yǐn

Source   *Formulary of the Pharmacy Service for Benefiting the People in the Taiping Era* (1107)

Scutellariae Radix (*huáng qín*) 10g
Ophiopogonis Radix (*mài mén dōng*) 10g
Lycii Cortex (*dì gǔ pí*) 10g
Plantaginis Semen (*chē qián zǐ*) 10g
Glycyrrhizae Radix praeparata (*zhì gān cǎo*) 10g
Nelumbinis Semen (*lián zǐ*) 15g
Poria (*fú líng*) 15g
honey-fried Astragali Radix (*mì zhì huáng qí*) 15g
Ginseng Radix (*rén shēn*) 15g

Method of Preparation   Grind all of the ingredients into a powder and prepare as a draft by cooking 10g with 1½ cups of water until 80 percent of the water has evaporated. Remove the dregs and mix the draft with cold water before drinking. Take on an empty stomach.

Actions   Clears the Heart, augments the qi and yin, and stops turbid painful urinary dribbling

Indications

Seminal emission, turbid painful urinary dribbling, profuse uterine bleeding, and vaginal discharges. All of these symptoms are aggravated by overexertion. There may also be signs of kidney yin deficiency with a dry mouth and tongue, irritability, and fevers.

This is flourishing Heart fire against a background of qi and yin deficiency, where the Heart and Kidneys have lost their communication and damp-heat pours downward. If the Heart fire moves chaotically, it consumes the Heart yin such that the Heart fire is no longer directed downward to connect with the Kidneys below, while the Kidney water cannot support the Heart above. Exhaustion of water accompanied by chaotic movement of fire stirs the essence chamber and leads to seminal emissions. Damp-heat pouring downward collects in the Bladder, which loses its qi transformative function. The water passages become blocked and turbid painful urinary dribbling results. Heart fire and damp-heat harm the Conception and Penetrating vessels, which manifests as uterine bleeding and vaginal discharge. As heat becomes exuberant in the interior, the Heart spirit finds it difficult to be calm and the patient becomes irritable and feverish. Kidney yin deficiency with lack of fluids and deficiency fire flaring upward causes dryness of the mouth and tongue. Flourishing fire damages both the qi and yin, which further aggravates the stagnation of dampness and flaring of deficiency fire, leading to further consumption of qi and yin. This leads to a chronic condition where all symptoms are aggravated by overexertion.

Analysis of Formula

This is a pattern of mixed excess and deficiency that requires a complex treatment strategy: the clearing of Heart fire, augmentation of qi and yin, draining of damp-heat, and the stopping of leakage. Nelumbinis Semen (*lián zǐ*), which accomplishes all of these tasks, is the chief herb in the formula. Lycii Cortex (*dì gǔ pí*) and Scutellariae Radix (*huáng qín*) strengthen the power of the chief herb to clear heat and are therefore regarded as the deputies. Three groups of assistants address different aspects of the disease dynamic. Poria (*fú líng*) and Plantaginis Semen (*chē qián zǐ*) promote urination and separate heat from dampness. Ginseng Radix (*rén shēn*) and Astragali Radix (*huáng qí*) augment the qi and strengthen the body's transformative potential. Ophiopogonis Radix (*mài mén dōng*) clears the heat and tranquillizes the Heart by nourishing the yin. Glycyrrhizae Radix (*gān cǎo*) is the envoy and harmonizes the many different actions of the formula.

Overall, this formula focuses on clearing Heart fire, but this intention is strongly supported by the secondary functions of augmenting the qi and nourishing the yin, and of clearing and draining damp-heat. Once the pathogenic obstructions to the qi dynamic are removed, the Heart and Kidneys will connect once more, and the residual deficiencies can be resolved.

Commentary

The source text places considerable emphasis on the constitutional, emotional, and lifestyle issues that give rise to the disorders that are treated by this formula. These include excessive mental activity, anxieties, worry, depression, sexual overindulgence, overeating, and consumption of too much alcohol, as well as debility following in the aftermath of an illness. When, as the Ming-dynasty physician Wu Kun noted in *Investigations of Medical Formulas*, "a weak constitution is unable to cope with overexertion," these factors generate heat by way of constraint and deficiency as the qi dynamic becomes increasingly unable to keep yin and yang, fire and water connected to each other. It is therefore inappropriate to focus on draining fire with bitter and cold herbs that would further weaken the qi dynamic and especially the Heart. Instead, the formula strengthens the Heart's ability to direct fire downward while also clearing deficiency heat and dispelling damp-heat. This is what Wang Fu in *Collectanea of Investigations from the Realm of Medicine* refers to as "stopping the harm done by fire without [directly] treating fire." In this manner, as the source text points out, "it clears the Heart and nourishes the spirit, contains the essence and tonifies the deficiency, enriches and moistens the Stomach and Intestines. [In short] it regulates and smoothes [the interaction] of qi and blood."

Many physicians have interpreted this formula as treating more than just the Heart. Wu Kun saw it as focusing on over-exertion and as clearing heat from the yin and yang organs. Wang Ang also interpreted it as clearing heat from the five yin organs. The early modern writer Li Chou-Ren went even further in summing up the action of the formula in *Outline of Medical Formulas*: "Although its name [refers] to clearing the Heart, in reality it is a formula that clears the Lungs and Kidneys, that secures and binds." In clinical practice, therefore, the formula can be used to treat patterns of mixed excess and deficiency with overabundance of heat above and dampness and insecurity below.

Comparison

> Vs. Guide Out the Red Powder (*dǎo chì sǎn*)

In Chinese medicine it is said that, regarding the Heart, "blood is the essence, fire its function." Both of these formulas address an excess of the functional aspect of Heart activity by clearing the heat, tonifying the yin, and promoting urination. The principal formula strongly tonifies the Heart qi's ability to direct physiological fire downward, while Guide Out the Red Powder (*dǎo chì sǎn*) focuses on guiding out pathological fire via the Small Intestine. In practice, therefore, Guide Out the Red Powder (*dǎo chì sǎn*) is the formula of choice whenever the manifestations of fire in the Heart or Small Intestine channels are the dominant signs and symptoms of a mixed excess/deficiency disorder. The principal formula, on the other hand, is more suitable for treating chronic conditions with more severe symptoms of deficiency, where fire is also likely to be present in other organs besides the Heart. Neither formula is indicated for treating strong fire in the qi level with no signs of deficiency.

Biomedical Indications

With the appropriate presentation, this formula may be used to treat a variety of biomedically-defined disorders, primarily infections, including chronic nephritis, chronic prostatitis, chyluria, and myocarditis. It has also been used to treat nervous exhaustion and dysfunctional uterine bleeding.

Alternate name

Lotus Seed Drink to Clear the Heart (*lián zǐ qīng xīn yǐn*) in *Medical Formulas Collected and Analyzed*

Modifications

- For seminal emissions as the main symptom, add calcified Ostreae Concha (*mǔ lì*) and Fossilia Ossis Mastodi (*lóng gǔ*).
- For turbid painful urinary dribbling as the main symptom, add Dioscoreae hypoglaucae Rhizoma (*bì xiè*) and Acori tatarinowii Rhizoma (*shí chāng pú*).
- For uterine bleeding as the main symptom, add Ailanthi Cortex (*chūn pí*) and carbonized Schizonepetae Herba (*jīng jiè*).

- For overweight patients with turbid urination or blood in the urine and irritability due to pathogenic qi in the Heart, remove Lycii Cortex *(dì gǔ pí)* and Astragali Radix *(huáng qí)* and add Alpiniae oxyphyllae Fructus *(yì zhì rén)*, Polygalae Radix *(yuǎn zhì)*, Acori tatarinowii Rhizoma *(shí chāng pǔ)*, Atractylodis macrocephalae Rhizoma *(bái zhú)*, and Alismatis Rhizoma *(zé xiè)*. (Straight Direction from Ren-Zhai)

- For heat in the qi level with irritability, thirst, turbid urine, blood in the urine, painful urinary dribbling, or yin deficiency with fire flourishing, a bitter taste in the mouth, a dry throat, and slight fever, remove Nelumbinis Semen *(lián zǐ)*, Astragali Radix *(huáng qí)*, Poria *(fú líng)*, and Glycyrrhizae Radix *(gān cǎo)* and add Bupleuri Radix *(chái hú)*. (Assorted Works from Enlightened Physicians)

龍膽瀉肝湯 (龙胆泻肝汤)
Gentian Decoction to Drain the Liver
lóng dǎn xiè gān tāng

Source *Medical Formulas Collected and Analyzed* (1682)

Gentianae Radix *(lóng dǎn cǎo)* 3-9g
dry-fried Scutellariae Radix *(chǎo huáng qín)* 6-12g
Gardeniae Fructus *(zhī zǐ)* 6-12g
Akebiae Caulis *(mù tōng)* 3-6g
Plantaginis Semen *(chē qián zǐ)* 9-15g
Alismatis Rhizoma *(zé xiè)* 6-12g
Bupleuri Radix *(chái hú)* 3-9g
Rehmanniae Radix *(shēng dì huáng)* 9-15g
wine-washed Angelicae sinensis Radix *(jiǔ xǐ dāng guī)* 3-12g
Glycyrrhizae Radix *(gān cǎo)* 3-6g

Method of Preparation Decoction. No dosages are given in the source text and those provided here reflect current opinion. Gentianae Radix *(lóng dǎn cǎo)*, Gardeniae Fructus *(zhī zǐ)*, and Rehmanniae Radix *(shēng dì huáng)* are usually fried in wine to produce draining with dispersion.

Actions Drains fire excess from the Liver and Gallbladder, and clears and drains damp-heat from the lower burner

Indications

Pain in the hypochondria, headache, dizziness, red and sore eyes, hearing loss, swelling in the ears, a bitter taste in the mouth, irritability, short temper, a wiry, rapid, and forceful pulse, and a red tongue with a yellow coating. Also for difficult and painful urination with a sensation of heat in the urethra, swollen and pruritic external genitalia, or foul-smelling leukorrhea. In women, the menstrual cycle will be shortened and the menstrual blood will be reddish-purple in color.

This is heat excess in the Liver and/or Gallbladder channels. The Liver channel traverses the hypochondria and the external genitalia, and its corresponding sensory organ is the eyes. The Gallbladder channel (paired with the Liver channel in an exterior-interior relationship) begins at the outer canthus of the eye and crosses the lateral aspect (including the frontal and occipital areas) of the head. When heat excess enters these channels, it becomes constrained and cannot drain out. This leads to fire blazing upward to the head where it manifests with the symptoms described above.

A wiry, rapid, and forceful pulse and a red tongue with a yellow coating are signs of heat excess in the Liver channel. The Gallbladder and Triple Burner are both lesser yang channels. A disturbance in one of the lesser yang channels usually affects the other. When the Triple Burner channel is affected, water metabolism is disturbed and internal dampness is generated. A damp or humid climate can also induce dampness in the body. In both cases, damp-heat in the lower burner causes foul-smelling leukorrhea and other disorders of the external genitalia.

Analysis of Formula

To treat excess fire or damp-heat in the Liver and Gallbladder, this formula clears the fire and drains the damp-heat via the lower burner. The very cold and bitter nature of Gentianae Radix *(lóng dǎn cǎo)* makes it extremely effective in draining heat excess from the Liver and Gallbladder and eliminating damp-heat from the lower burner. Because these are the two primary functions of the formula, this ingredient serves as the chief herb. Two of the deputies, Scutellariae Radix *(huáng qín)* and Gardeniae Fructus *(zhī zǐ)*, assist the chief herb in draining the fire and eliminating the dampness. The other deputy, Bupleuri Radix *(chái hú)*, disperses heat due to constrained Liver and Gallbladder qi. Bupleuri Radix *(chái hú)* and Scutellariae Radix *(huáng qín)* comprise the classic combination for clearing lesser yang-channel heat. Bupleuri Radix *(chái hú)* also focuses the actions of the other herbs on the Liver and Gallbladder channels.

The assistant ingredients, Akebiae Caulis *(mù tōng)*, Plantaginis Semen *(chē qián zǐ)*, and Alismatis Rhizoma *(zé xiè)*, drain heat from the upper burner and eliminate damp-heat from the lower burner by promoting urination. This provides a pathway to drain Liver fire. Because the Liver stores the blood, heat in the Liver channel can readily injure the yin and blood. This situation is not helped by the bitter, drying herbs in the formula. Two assistants are therefore added to protect the yin and blood: Rehmanniae Radix *(shēng dì huáng)*, which supplements the yin, and Angelicae sinensis Radix *(dāng guī)*, which nourishes the blood without causing stasis. Similarly, because the cold and bitter nature of some of the ingredients readily injures the Stomach, Glycyrrhizae Radix *(gān cǎo)* is used as an envoy to harmonize the middle burner and regulate the actions of the other herbs in the formula.

Cautions and Contraindications

This formula can harm the Spleen. It should therefore not be taken long term or in large doses, nor in cases with Spleen deficiency or injury to the fluids.

Commentary

This formula can be used in treating a wide variety of complaints. There are three criteria for diagnosing heat in the Liver channel, the condition for which this formula is indicated: (1) a wiry, rapid pulse; (2) a red tongue or red dots along the sides of the tongue; and (3) dark urine or urinary difficulty.

All commentators agree that because 'the Liver carries ministerial fire within,' disruption of the flow of Liver qi in a person with a strong constitution produces Liver fire. There is less agreement, however, as to why such fire should so often manifest in the form of damp-heat. In the modern text *Elaboration of Medical Formulas*, Fu Yan-Kui and colleagues point to the relevance of the close relationship among the Liver, Gallbladder, and Triple Burner. Blazing heat in the Liver and Gallbladder channels obstructs water metabolism in the Triple Burner such that water is no longer properly excreted, and the accumulation of heat and water combine to form damp-heat. A contrary view is advanced in *Convenient Reader of Established Formulas*, whose author, Zhang Bing-Chen, thinks that dampness must already be constitutionally present or enter into the body from the outside. Both perspectives are clinically useful, but the fact that Liver function is responsible for both 'dispersing and draining' (疏瀉 *shū xiè*), and the presence of dampness and edema in many Liver pathologies irrespective of constitution or context, strongly favors the first view.

The herbs in this formula cool heat without causing stasis, dispel pathogenic qi, and cause it to descend without injuring the normal qi. It is an excellent formula for treating the symptoms and underlying mechanisms associated with Liver and Gallbladder heat excess that can be adjusted to fit the myriad manifestations of this pathology in clinical practice. Indeed, *Encyclopedia of Chinese Medical Formulas* lists 25 formulas with the same name but slightly different ingredients, a few of which are discussed below.

Comparisons

➤ Vs. Augmented Rambling Powder
   (*jiā wèi xiāo yáo sǎn*)

Augmented Rambling Powder (*jiā wèi xiāo yáo sǎn*) is indicated for a condition that lacks the full force of heat excess. Furthermore, while the present formula treats Liver and Gallbladder damp-heat, any dampness present in patterns treated by Augmented Rambling Powder (*jiā wèi xiāo yáo sǎn*) has its root in Spleen deficiency.

➤ Vs. Tangkuei, Gentian, and Aloe Pill (*dāng guī lóng huì wán*); *see* page 204

➤ Vs. Left Metal Pill (*zuǒ jīn wán*); *see* page 206

Biomedical Indications

With the appropriate presentation, this formula may be used to treat a variety of biomedically-defined disorders. These can be divided into the following groups:

- Infections such as furuncles, purulent otitis media, rhinitis, acute viral hepatitis, acute cholecystitis, acute pyelonephritis, acute cystitis, vulvitis, orchitis, and pelvic inflammatory disease
- Skin diseases such as herpes zoster, eczema, and drug rash
- Eye diseases such as acute conjunctivitis, optical fundal hemorrhage and hemorrhagic glaucoma
- Endocrine diseases such as hyperthyroidism, Cushing's syndrome, adrenal cortex hyperplasia, and polycystic ovary disease

It has also been used to treat migraine, hypertension, uterine prolapse, and polycythemia vera.

Alternate name

Drain the Liver Decoction (*xiè gān tāng*) in *Therapeutic Discernment through Pattern Classification*

Modifications

- For more severe signs of fire flaring and less dampness, remove Akebiae Caulis (*mù tōng*) and Plantaginis Semen (*chē qián zǐ*) and add Coptidis Rhizoma (*huáng lián*).
- For pronounced signs of dampness with less fire, remove Scutellariae Radix (*huáng qín*) and Rehmanniae Radix (*shēng dì huáng*) and add Talcum (*huá shí*) and Coicis Semen (*yì yǐ rén*).
- For pale-red leukorrhea and a wiry, rapid pulse, add Paeoniae Radix rubra (*chì sháo*) and Nelumbinis Stamen (*lián xū*).
- For ulcerations on the external genitalia in both men and women, or sores and abscesses, remove Bupleuri Radix (*chái hú*) and add Forsythiae Fructus (*lián qiáo*), Coptidis Rhizoma (*huáng lián*), and Rhei Radix et Rhizoma (*dà huáng*).
- For severe headache and painful, red eyes, add Chrysanthemi Flos (*jú huā*) and Mori Folium (*sāng yè*).
- For coughing up blood due to Liver fire injuring the Lungs (the fire of wood attacking metal), add Moutan Cortex (*mǔ dān pí*) and Platycladi Cacumen (*cè bǎi yè*).
- For tremors, add Uncariae Ramulus cum Uncis (*gōu téng*) and Fritillariae cirrhosae Bulbus (*chuān bèi mǔ*).

Associated Formulas

龍膽瀉肝湯 (龙胆泻肝汤)

Gentian Decoction to Drain the Liver from *Precious Mirror*

lóng dǎn xiè gān tāng

SOURCE *Precious Mirror of Health* (Yuan dynasty)

Scutellariae Radix *(huáng qín)*	2.1g
Bupleuri Radix *(chái hú)*	3g
Glycyrrhizae Radix *(gān cǎo)*	1.5g
Ginseng Radix *(rén shēn)*	1.5g
Ophiopogonis Radix *(mài mén dōng)*	1.5g
Asparagi Radix *(tiān mén dōng)*	1.5g
Coptidis Rhizoma *(huáng lián)*	1.5g
Anemarrhenae Rhizoma *(zhī mǔ)*	1.5g
Gentianae Radix *(lóng dǎn cǎo)*	1.5g
Gardeniae Fructus *(zhī zǐ)*	1.5g
Schisandrae Fructus *(wǔ wèi zǐ)*	10 pieces

The source text advises to grind the herbs into a powder and prepare as a draft by boiling with water, which is to be taken apart from meals. It can also be prepared as a decoction with a corresponding increase in the dosage of the individual ingredients. Clears the Liver, drains fire, enriches the yin, and generates fluids. For upward overflow of bile due to anger or overabundance of heat characterized by a bitter taste in the mouth, and Gallbladder pure heat (膽純熱 *dǎn chún rè*), which are periods of feverishness alternating with a sensation of normal temperature.

Compared to the original formula, which incorporates the three herbs that comprise Guide Out the Red Powder *(dǎo chì sǎn)*, this formula replaces the dampness-draining herbs with Generate the Pulse Powder *(shēng mài sǎn)*, Coptidis Rhizoma *(huáng lián)*, and Asparagi Radix *(tiān mén dōng)*. It is therefore indicated for heat without dampness that is injuring the fluids in the upper burner, or, in five-phase terminology, wood rebelling against metal.

A variation of this formula, found in *Symptom, Cause, Pulse, and Treatment*, substitutes Forsythiae Fructus *(lián qiáo)* for Schisandrae Fructus *(wǔ wèi zǐ)* for an even greater focus on clearing heat and resolving toxicity. In *Pattern Differentiation and Treatment for Women's Disorders [from the] Zhulin [Monastery]*, the monks of the Zhulin Monastery in Zhejiang, famous for their gynecological expertise, use a variation of this formula that removes Ophiopogonis Radix *(mài mén dōng)* to treat violent anger harming the Liver and stirring its fire that manifests as prolonged lochia.

清膽瀉火湯 (清胆泻火汤)

Clear the Gallbladder and Drain Fire Decoction

qīng dǎn xiè huǒ tāng

SOURCE *Integrated Chinese and Western Medical Treatment of the Acute Abdomen* (1973)

Bupleuri Radix *(chái hú)*	15g
Scutellariae Radix *(huáng qín)*	15g
Pinelliae Rhizoma praeparatum *(zhì bàn xià)*	9g
Artemisiae scopariae Herba *(yīn chén)*	30g
Gardeniae Fructus *(zhī zǐ)*	9g
Gentianae Radix *(lóng dǎn cǎo)*	9g
Curcumae Radix *(yù jīn)*	9g
Aucklandiae Radix *(mù xiāng)*	9g
Rhei Radix et Rhizoma *(dà huáng)* [add near end]	9g
Natrii Sulfas *(máng xiāo)* [dissolve in strained decoction]	9g

Spreads Liver qi, unblocks the interior, and resolves dampness. For unremitting pain in the hypochondria, a bitter taste in the mouth, dry mouth, alternating fever and chills, abdominal distention, a red or dark-red tongue with a yellow, dry coating, and a wiry, slippery, and rapid or a flooding, rapid pulse. This formula is designed to treat the fire excess type of acute cholecystitis.

瀉青丸 (泻青丸)

Drain the Green Pill

xiè qīng wán

Source *Craft of Medicinal Treatment for Childhood Disease Patterns* (1119)

Angelicae sinensis Radix *(dāng guī)*	30g
Gentianae Radix *(lóng dǎn cǎo)*	30g
Chuanxiong Rhizoma *(chuān xiōng)*	30g
Gardeniae Fructus *(zhī zǐ)*	30g
Rhei Radix et Rhizoma *(dà huáng)*	30g
Notopterygii Rhizoma seu Radix *(qiāng huó)*	30g
dry-fried Saposhnikoviae Radix *(chǎo fáng fēng)*	30g

Method of Preparation The source text advises to grind equal amounts of the herbs into a powder, add honey, and form into pills the size of a chicken head. One-half to one pill is dissolved in a decoction made from a small amount of Lophatheri Herba *(dàn zhú yè)* to which brown granulated sugar is added. At present, it is usually made into 6g pills with water and taken twice a day with warm water, or dissolved into the aforementioned decoction.

Actions Clears the Liver and drains fire

Indications

Red, sore, and swollen eyes, restlessness and irritability, dark urine, constipation, and a flooding, excessive pulse. Tremors or convulsions may also be present.

This is constrained fire in the Liver channel. The Liver 'opens' through the eyes, which become red and swollen when Liver fire flares upward. When fire is constrained in the interior, it deranges the Heart spirit, leading to restlessness, irritability, a propensity toward anger, insomnia, and restless sleep. The constrained heat also dries up the body fluids, leading to constipation and dark urine. The Liver governs the sinews. Fire from heat constraint causes the sinews to tighten up, which manifests as acute childhood fright wind with twitches or even convulsions. The flooding, excessive pulse reflects the overabundance of heat in the interior.

Analysis of Formula

Constrained fire in the Liver channel requires a strategy of clearing heat and draining fire. Bitter and cold Gentianae Radix *(lóng dǎn cǎo)* is the chief herb because it enters into the Liver channel and drains its fire. It is assisted by two deputies, Rhei Radix et Rhizoma *(dà huáng)* and Gardeniae Fructus *(zhī zǐ)*, which guide the Liver fire downward to eliminate it via the bowels and urinary tract. When fire becomes constrained and clumps in the Liver channel, the Liver loses its ability to thrust out the body's qi. *Basic Questions* (Chapter 22) advises: "To disperse the Liver, immediately take acrid [substances]." Thus, the formula uses two so-called 'wind herbs,' Notopterygii Rhizoma seu Radix *(qiāng huó)* and Saposhnikoviae Radix *(fáng fēng)*, as assistants. Such herbs resonate with the wood phase and have the ability to empower the out-thrusting and ascending nature of Liver qi. In the present context, they are used for 'treating fire constraint by discharging it.'

Another group of assistants, Angelicae sinensis Radix *(dāng guī)* and Chuanxiong Rhizoma *(chuān xiōng)*, nourish and move the Liver blood, preventing fire from damaging the yin. This is necessary because the Liver is 'yin in essence' and tends toward 'hardness.' Unless the Liver blood is strong and soft, the Liver qi cannot be controlled. Lophatheri Herba *(dàn zhú yè)* is the fifth assistant in this formula. It clears Heart fire and dispels restlessness and irritability by guiding heat out via the urine. The honey used to make the pills, and the sugar dissolved in the decoction, are envoys that relax the Liver and harmonize the formula with their sweetness.

Cautions and Contraindications

Contraindicated in those with a weak and deficient Spleen and Stomach.

Commentary

The original indication for this formula was childhood fright wind manifesting with Liver heat, muscle twitches, and a flooding, excessive pulse. Later physicians expanded the indication to the broader set of symptoms listed above and modified the formula accordingly. In view of the many cold herbs that it contains, the formula is generally understood to focus on clearing heat and draining fire. However, the primary pathogenic qi associated with the Liver is wind, not fire, and this, according to many well-known commentators, is the actual root of the pathology for which the formula works best.

According to *Golden Mirror of the Medical Tradition*:

> The Liver governs wind. Wind can engender fire. [However] treating the Liver does not [automatically] equate to treating wind. [And precisely because] it does not do so [the formula] utilizes Notopterygii Rhizoma seu Radix *(qiāng huó)* and Saposhnikoviae Radix *(fáng fēng)* to disperse Liver wind. Dispersing in this manner the fire of the Liver, it treats the root of the fire [with which this pattern manifests on the outside].

The famous modern scholar-physician Qin Bo-Wei likewise emphasized the formula's treatment of wind pathogens: "[It]

has the function of tracking down wind and dispersing fire, but [unlike Gentian Decoction to Drain the Liver *(lóng dǎn xiè gān tāng)* or Tangkuei, Gentian, and Aloe Pill *(dāng guī lóng huì wán)*] does not focus on unblocking the bowels or promoting urination [in order to drain fire]."

That Notopterygii Rhizoma seu Radix *(qiāng huó)* and Saposhnikoviae Radix *(fáng fēng)* were included in this formula to track down wind had already been noted by the 18th-century writer Wang Ang. Even earlier, the Ming-dynasty physician Wu Kun concluded his discussion of the formula in *Investigations of Medical Formulas* with this analysis: "It separates and reduces (分消 *fēn xiāo*) wind [from] heat above and below. This is how it drains [the Liver]."

The comments of these physicians illustrate how the understanding of a disease process informs the understanding of a formula's composition. This is wind engendering fire, where wind is perceived to be a pathological disposition that disorders and thereby constrains the Liver's function of dispersing and draining. This is a very different concept from that of internal wind, where deficiency of Liver yin or blood engenders wind and fire. For this reason, the wind here is not treated by enriching the yin and nourishing the blood, but by tracking it down and separating it from the fire that it engenders so that both can be eliminated by different means: the wind via the skin and the fire via the bowels and urine.

Comparison

➤ Vs. Tangkuei, Gentian, and Aloe Pill *(dāng guī lóng huì wán)*; see PAGE 204

Biomedical Indications

With the appropriate presentation, this formula may be used to treat a variety of biomedically-defined disorders including vascular headaches, hypertensive headaches, herpes zoster, insomnia, and panophthalmitis.

....

Alternate names

Cool the Liver Pill *(liáng gān wán)* in *Effective Formulas from Generations of Physicians*; Drain the Liver Pill *(xiè gān wán)* in *Formulas of Universal Benefit*

....

Associated Formulas

柴胡清肝湯 （柴胡清肝汤）

Bupleurum Decoction to Clear the Liver

chái hú qīng gān tāng

SOURCE   *Golden Mirror of the Medical Tradition* (1742)

Bupleuri Radix *(chái hú)*	4.5g
Rehmanniae Radix *(shēng dì huáng)*	4.5g
Angelicae sinensis Radix *(dāng guī)*	6g

Paeoniae Radix rubra (*chì sháo*) 4.5
Chuanxiong Rhizoma (*chuān xiōng*) 3g
Forsythiae Fructus (*lián qiáo*) 6g
Arctii Fructus (*niú bàng zǐ*) 4.5g
Scutellariae Radix (*huáng qín*) 3g
Gardeniae Fructus (*zhī zǐ*) 4.5g
Trichosanthis Radix (*tiān huā fěn*) 3g
Saposhnikoviae Radix (*fáng fēng*) 3g
Glycyrrhizae Radix (*gān cǎo*) 3g

Drains fire, resolves toxicity, spreads the Liver qi, and strengthens the Spleen. For early-stage sores along the lesser yang channel on the head. Also for clumping of fire toxin characterized by severe headache, flushed cheeks, bad breath, tinnitus, hearing loss, irritability, insomnia, coughing of viscous, thick sputum, dark urine, a red tongue, and a wiry, rapid pulse.

洗肝明目散
Wash the Liver to Clear the Eyes Powder
xǐ gān míng mù sǎn

SOURCE *Restoration of Health from the Myriad Diseases* (1587)

Angelicae sinensis radicis Cauda (*dāng guī wěi*) . . . .(8g)
Chuanxiong Rhizoma (*chuān xiōng*) . . . .(6g)
Paeoniae Radix rubra (*chì sháo*) . . . .(8g)
Rehmanniae Radix (*shēng dì huáng*) . . . .(8g)
Coptidis Rhizoma (*huáng lián*) . . . .(4g)
Scutellariae Radix (*huáng qín*) . . . .(8g)
Gardeniae Fructus (*zhī zǐ*) . . . .(8g)
Gypsum fibrosum (*shí gāo*) . . . .[cook first] (15g)
Forsythiae Fructus (*lián qiáo*) . . . .(8g)
Saposhnikoviae Radix (*fáng fēng*) . . . .(8g)
Schizonepetae Herba (*jīng jiè*) . . . .(8g)
Menthae haplocalycis Herba (*bò hé*) . . . . . .[add at end] (6g)
Notopterygii Rhizoma seu Radix (*qiāng huó*) . . . .(6g)
Viticis Fructus (*màn jīng zǐ*) . . . .(10g)
Chrysanthemi Flos (*jú huā*) . . . .(8g)
Tribuli Fructus (*cì jí lí*) . . . .(8g)
Cassiae Semen (*jué míng zǐ*) . . . .(8g)
Platycodi Radix (*jié gěng*) . . . .(6g)
Glycyrrhizae Radix (*gān cǎo*) . . . .(6g)

The source text instructs to grind equal amounts of the above ingredients to a coarse powder and then decoct. To be taken after meals. The dosage is not specified but 20-30g is typical for this type of decoction in the source text. The dosage and cooking details in parentheses are the editors' suggestions for a standard decoction. This formula dispels wind, clears heat, releases pathogens from the exterior, alleviates swelling and pain, and clears the eyes. It is used for acute wind-heat patterns that manifest as redness and swelling in and around the eyes with a rapid and floating pulse. This may present as conjunctivitis and conjunctivitis-like disorders, styes, orbital herpes infections, iritis, or scleritis. The pulse is rapid and floating. The Lung, Liver, and Stomach channels are most commonly involved in acute eye disorders, and this formula includes herbs to address all three.

洗肝散
Liver-Washing Powder
xǐ gān sǎn

SOURCE *Formulary of the Pharmacy Service for Benefiting the People in the Taiping Era* (1107)

Angelicae sinensis Radix (*dāng guī*) 60g (6-8g)
Menthae haplocalycis Herba (*bò hé*) . . . . . . .60g (6-8g—add at end)
Notopterygii Rhizoma seu Radix (*qiāng huó*) 60g (6-8g)
Saposhnikoviae Radix (*fáng fēng*) 60g (6-10g)
Gardeniae Fructus (*zhī zǐ*) 60g (6-10g)
Rhei Radix et Rhizoma (*dà huáng*) . . . . . . .60g (4-8g—add at end)
Glycyrrhizae Radix praeparata (*zhì gān cǎo*) 60g (4-8g)
Chuanxiong Rhizoma (*chuān xiōng*) 60g (4-8g)

Grind the above ingredients into a fine powder and take 6g each time washed down with cool water after meals. The amounts in parentheses are the editors' suggestions for a typical decoction. Dredges wind, disperses heat, clears the Liver, and drains fire. For red, swollen, and painful eyes that result from an ascendant attack of wind-heat. Accompanying symptoms can be excess tearing, astringent eyes, eye screens, clouded vision, constipation, dark, rough urination, and a strong, wiry pulse.

This formula lacks the eye-specific herbs in Wash the Liver to Clear the Eyes Powder (*xǐ gān míng mù sǎn*) as well as Rhei Radix et Rhizoma (*dà huáng*) to drain fire from the body through the stool. This allows it to focus more on clearing and dispersing ascendant, internal heat and drain it from the body. On the other hand, Wash the Liver to Clear the Eyes Powder (*xǐ gān míng mù sǎn*) contains many agents to dredge wind-heat from the exterior and disseminate Lung qi as well as several substances that work directly on the eyes. In this way, it is more effective at treating exterior wind-heat and dealing aggressively with the main eye symptoms of the pattern.

當歸龍薈丸 （当归龙荟丸）
Tangkuei, Gentian, and Aloe Pill
dāng guī lóng huì wán

Source *Formulas from the Discussion Illuminating the Yellow Emperor's Basic Questions* (1172)

Angelicae sinensis Radix (*dāng guī*) 30g
Gentianae Radix (*lóng dǎn cǎo*) 30g
Gardeniae Fructus (*zhī zǐ*) 30g
Coptidis Rhizoma (*huáng lián*) 30g
Phellodendri Cortex (*huáng bǎi*) 30g
Scutellariae Radix (*huáng qín*) 30g
Aloe (*lú huì*) 15g
Indigo naturalis (*qīng dài*) 15g
Rhei Radix et Rhizoma (*dà huáng*) 15g
Aucklandiae Radix (*mù xiāng*) 4.5g
Moschus (*shè xiāng*) 1.5g

Method of Preparation The source text advises to grind the herbs into a powder and form into pills the size of an aduki bean with honey. For children, the size is that of a hemp seed. Twenty pills per day are taken with a decoction made from Zingiberis Rhizoma recens (*shēng jiāng*). At present, the herbs are ground and mixed with water to form pills. Six grams are taken twice a day with water. The source text also forbids patients to take any substance that might induce fever, but specifically allows for the simultaneous use of Saposhnikovia Powder that Sagely Unblocks (*fáng fēng tōng shèng sǎn*).

Actions　Drains Liver and Gallbladder fire excess

Indications

Headache, vertigo, restlessness, delirious speech, mania, and fright wind in children. Often there is also constipation and dark, rough urination, or blockage of the throat with difficulty swallowing.

This is Liver and Gallbladder fire excess. Excessive excitation of the five emotions readily stirs the ministerial fire, causing upward-flushing. Because the Liver controls the ascent of qi and carries the ministerial fire inside, this upward-flushing tends to manifest as Liver and Gallbladder fire. The fire readily enters other channels and organs, too, as they take their direction from the Gallbladder. Liver and Gallbladder fire causes headache and vertigo. Fire entering the Heart manifests as restlessness, delirious speech, and mania. Fire in the Spleen and Intestines leads to constipation. Fire in the Triple Burner causes rough urination, while Lung fire causes blockage of the throat.

Analysis of Formula

The original name of the formula, Dragon Brain Pill (*lóng nǎo wǎn*), reflects the fact that bitter and very cold Gentianae Radix (*lóng dǎn cǎo*) is the chief herb. In the materia medica section of his *Collected Treatises of [Zhang] Jing-yue*, Zhang Jie-Bin notes that by itself, Gentianae Radix (*lóng dǎn cǎo*) undoubtedly enters the terminal yin and lesser yang. "But it [also] has a strong capacity to drain fire, and depending on where it is guided by the assistants and envoys [in a formula], it controls any fire." The second most important herb is the deputy Angelicae sinensis Radix (*dāng guī*), which softens the Liver by tonifying its blood. This is important because only a soft Liver (i.e., one whose blood is strong and mobile) can ensure the harmonious dispersing and draining of qi. In the present formula, even though it is warm, Angelicae sinensis Radix (*dāng guī*) addresses the secondary consequences of Liver fire and moderates the drying action of the other ingredients.

The various assistants are mostly cold and drain fire from different organs. Phragmitis Rhizoma (*lú huì*) and Indigo naturalis (*qīng dài*) drain the Liver; Coptidis Rhizoma (*huáng lián*) drains the Heart; Scutellariae Radix (*huáng qín*) drains the Lungs; Rhei Radix et Rhizoma (*dà huáng*) drains the yang brightness and eliminates clumping; Gardeniae Fructus (*zhī zǐ*) drains the Triple Burner. There are no herbs to drain fire from the Kidneys because the Kidneys are perceived as the source of physiological ministerial fire, which should not

be drained unless absolutely necessary. Ensuring that heat is cleared from the Stomach and that the Intestines are moistened is thus used as an indirect strategy to prevent damage to the Kidney yin by fire.

Aucklandiae Radix (*mù xiāng*) and Moschus (*shè xiāng*) are acrid and warm. They ensure that the bitter nature of the formula does not lead to a breakdown of the qi dynamic; they add regulation of the qi to the draining of fire. Zingiberis Rhizoma recens (*shēng jiāng*) and honey are the envoys that harmonize the protective and nutritive qi and thereby smooth the action of the entire formula.

Cautions and Contraindications

If the fire excess in the Liver and Gallbladder has not yet resulted in clumping, the formula should only be used after careful deliberation. It is contraindicated in cases of Spleen deficiency.

Commentary

This is an extremly cold and draining formula that focuses on directing fire downward in order to control the qi. It can be perceived as a variation of Coptis Decoction to Resolve Toxicity (*huáng lián jiě dú tāng*) that has been adjusted to treat Liver and Gallbladder fire that has spread throughout the entire body. Employing its fierce action is appropriate only where the Liver and Gallbladder fire has already led to clumping, that is, where the heat pathogen is acquiring form.

Suprisingly, then, the source text states that "regularly taking [this formula] unblocks the blood, augments the qi, and regulates the smooth [interpenetration] of yin and yang so that the disorder will not recur." This was not meant to encourage careless usage, but to point out that completely draining strong fire from the body may take some time. This is an example of treating a chronic condition that requires a longer period of application.

Comparisons

➤ Vs. Gentian Decoction to Drain the Liver (*lóng dǎn xiè gān tāng*) and Drain the Green Pill (*xiè qīng wán*)

All three formulas drain Liver and Gallbladder fire excess. Drain the Green Pill (*xiè qīng wán*) is the mildest of the three formulas. As well as clearing Liver heat and draining fire, it relieves constraint and tracks down wind. It balances the downward-draining of pathogenic fire with ascending of Liver qi and blood, and dispersing wind without promoting urination or bowel movement. Gentian Decoction to Drain the Liver (*lóng dǎn xiè gān tāng*) drains Liver fire and dispels dampness but also tonifies the blood and yin fluids. By focusing on the promotion of water metabolism, it drains fire through the urine and unblocks the Triple Burner. Tangkuei, Gentian, and Aloe Pill (*dāng guī lóng huì wán*) is the coldest of the three formulas. It drains fire from the entire body and focuses on purging via the bowels. It is most useful in cases of Liver and Gallbladder fire with clumping.

Biomedical Indications

With the appropriate presentation, this formula may be used to treat a variety of biomedically-defined disorders including vertigo, tinnitus, hearing loss, pharyngitis, psychosis, and epilepsy.

Alternate name

In the source text, this formula is called Dragon Brain Pill (龍腦丸 *lóng nǎo wǎn*).

左金丸
Left Metal Pill

zuǒ jīn wán

The origin of this name is unclear. The commentaries cite its connection to the traditional concept of the anatomy of the abdomen in which the area corresponding to wood (Liver) is situated to the left and is controlled by metal (Lungs). An alternative explanation is that the formula drains fire to protect the Lungs, which are then able to better control the Liver.

Source　*Essential Teachings of [Zhu] Dan-Xi* (1481)

Coptidis Rhizoma *(huáng lián)* 180g (15-18g)
Evodiae Fructus *(wú zhū yú)* 15-30g (2-3g)

Method of Preparation　The source text advises to grind the herbs into a powder and form into pills with water. Take in 2-3g doses 2-3 times a day. At present, it is usually prepared as a decoction with the dosage specified in parentheses.

Actions　Clears Liver heat, directs rebellious qi downward, and stops vomiting

Indications

Hypochondriac pain, indeterminate gnawing hunger, epigastric focal distention, vomiting, acid reflux, belching, a bitter taste in the mouth, a dry mouth, a red tongue with a yellow coating, and a wiry, rapid pulse.

This is heat in the Liver channel causing disharmony between the Liver and Stomach with pain localized along the Liver channel. Indeterminate gnawing hunger, focal distention, vomiting, and acid reflux are due to Liver heat disturbing the Stomach qi. The red tongue with a yellow coating and the wiry, rapid pulse reflect the presence of heat in the Liver and Stomach.

Analysis of Formula

The mechanisms underlying the pathology addressed by this formula are described in *Basic Questions* (Chapter 74): "All that rebels and rushes upward is associated with fire" and

"Vomiting and acid reflux are associated with heat." Fire and heat refer to the same pathogen. By focusing on draining heat, the formula thus effectively treats all the manifestations of this pattern.

Bitter, cold Coptidis Rhizoma *(huáng lián)* has two functions. The first is to drain fire from the Heart and thereby from the Liver. This is an application of a treatment principle stated in Chapter 69 of *Classic of Difficulties*: "In cases of excess, drain the child." Here, Coptidis Rhizoma *(huáng lián)* drains heat from the Heart (fire), which is the 'child' of the Liver (wood) in the generative cycle of the five phases. As the heat is drained from the Liver, it no longer rebels horizontally to invade the Stomach. The second function is to clear Stomach fire. As fire in the Stomach is drained downward, qi naturally follows and acid reflux is quelled. In this manner, Coptidis Rhizoma *(huáng lián)* treats the root and branch of the disorder at the same time, and is regarded as the chief herb.

Hot, acrid Evodiae Fructus *(wú zhū yú)*, the deputy, promotes the movement of qi and releases constraint by dispersing the Liver. It is also very effective in directing rebellious Stomach qi downward. Like the chief herb, it thereby also 'kills two birds with one stone.' The hot nature of the deputy is moderated by the cold nature of the chief herb, whose dosage is six times that of the deputy. The acrid nature of the deputy, on the other hand, ensures that physiological fire is not drained by the bitter, cold, downward-moving nature of the chief herb.

Cautions and Contraindications

Contraindicated in cases with acid reflux due to Stomach cold from deficiency.

Commentary

Composed of only two herbs, which complement each other on multiple levels, this is a very effective formula that has been a favorite of physicians associated with many diverse currents. The late 19th-century scholar-physician Fei Bo-Xiong sums up the essence of this formula in *Discussion of Medical Formulas*:

> The ingeniousness of this formula is due entirely [to its combination] of bitter, downward-directing and acrid, opening [herbs]. It treats not only the manifestations [associated with Liver disharmonly like] flank pain, Liver distention, acid reflux, and bulging qi, but can also be used to treat sudden turmoil disorder due to seasonal pathogens, cramping, vomiting, and diarrhea. In each case, it has a miraculous effect.

Chen Nian-Zu, another noted Qing-dynasty physician, explains the reasoning underlying this combination more precisely:

> [Herbs with a] bitter flavor are able to guide fire downward. The idea here is [one of resonance, which implies that phenomena

with] the same qi can mutually assist each other. [Herbs with] an acrid flavor can open constraint and disperse clumping. The idea here is that pain stops when [the flow of qi and blood] is unblocked.

The famous modern physician Qin Bo-Wei, on the other hand, limited the use of the formula to a more narrowly defined range of disorders, which is in line with the disease orientation of contemporary Chinese medicine. Consider Qin's assessment of the formula in *Medical Lecture Notes of [Qin] Qian-Zhai*, widely regarded as his most mature and accomplished work:

> I think that [in the treatment of] Liver fire patterns one rarely uses warm herbs as antagonistic assistants (反佐 *fǎn zǔo*). Furthermore, Coptidis Rhizoma (*huáng lián*) and Evodiae Fructus (*wú zhū yú*) do not enter into the same channels, so it is also very difficult to explain [the indication of this formula from that perspective]. If one examines its effectiveness, then this is most pronounced for [the two symptoms of] acid reflux and gnawing hunger. Its most important functions are thus [focused] on the Stomach. The basic function of Coptidis Rhizoma (*huáng lián*) is to harmonize the Stomach with bitter downward-directing. Evodiae Fructus (*wú zhū yú*) also disperses Stomach qi that has become constrained and clumped. In its combination of acrid and bitter flavors [the formula thus] resembles the various Drain the Epigastrium Decoctions (*xiè xīn tāng*). Therefore, if one increases the dosage of Evodiae Fructus (*wú zhū yú*) for cases of acid reflux with phlegm-dampness and sticky sputum, its efficacy will be even more pronounced.

Comparisons

➤ Vs. Gentian Decoction to Drain the Liver
(lóng dǎn xiè gān tāng)

The differences between these two formulas is a reflection of the differences between their chief herbs. Gentianae Radix (*lóng dǎn cǎo*) is more effective than Coptidis Rhizoma (*huáng lián*) in draining fire from the Liver but is unable to harmonize the functions of the Stomach. In fact, if too much of the herb is prescribed, it can easily induce nausea and vomiting.

➤ Vs. Melia Toosendan Powder
(jīn líng zǐ sǎn); see PAGE 524

Biomedical Indications

With the appropriate presentation, this formula may be used to treat biomedically-defined disorders of the upper digestive tract including esophagitis, gastritis, gastroesophageal reflux, and peptic ulcers.

Alternate names

Restore the Command Pill (*huí lìng wán*) in *Essential Teachings of [Zhu] Dan-Xi*; Evodia and Coptis Pill (*yú lián wán*) in *Introduction to Medicine* and in *Medical Formulas Collected and Analyzed*; Assist Metal Pill (*zǔo jīn wán*) in *Comprehensive Medicine According to* Master Zhang; Two-Ingredient Left Metal Pill (*èr wèi zuǒ jīn wán*) in *Nationwide Collection of TCM Patent Formulas*

Modifications

- For severe distention, add Toosendan Fructus (*chuān liàn zǐ*).
- For pronounced acid reflux, add Sepiae Endoconcha (*hǎi piāo xiāo*) and Arcae Concha (*wǎ léng zǐ*).
- For patients with constrained Liver qi who lack vitality, combine with Frigid Extremities Powder (*sì nì sǎn*).

Associated Formulas

戊己丸

Fifth and Sixth Heavenly Stem Pill
wù jǐ wán

SOURCE *Formulary of the Pharmacy Service for Benefiting the People in the Taiping Era* (1107)

dry-fried Coptidis Rhizoma (*chǎo huáng lián*)
dry-fried Evodiae Fructus (*chǎo wú zhū yú*)
dry-fried Paeoniae Radix alba (*chǎo bái sháo*)

Equal amounts of each herb are ground into powder and formed into pills with flour. Spreads the Liver qi and harmonizes the Spleen. This formula uses equal amounts of Coptidis Rhizoma (*huáng lián*) and Evodiae Fructus (*wú zhū yú*). It thus focuses equally on bitter downward-directing and acrid opening. It also adds Paeoniae Radix alba (*bái sháo*), which enters the Liver and Spleen and treats abdominal pain. In contrast to the original formula that focuses on Liver/Stomach disharmonies, this formula is indicated for Liver/Spleen disharmony with epigastric pain, acid reflux, abdominal pain, and diarrhea. It is also used for hot dysenteric disorders.

香連丸 (香连丸)

Aucklandia and Coptis Pill
xiāng lián wán

SOURCE *Formulary of the Pharmacy Service for Benefiting the People in the Taiping Era* (1107)

Coptidis Rhizoma (*huáng lián*) 600g
Evodiae Fructus (*wú zhū yú*) 300g
Aucklandiae Radix (*mù xiāng*) 150g

Fry Coptidis Rhizoma (*huáng lián*) with Evodiae Fructus (*wú zhū yú*), then discard the latter herb. Grind Coptidis Rhizoma (*huáng lián*) and Aucklandiae Radix (*mù xiāng*) and form into pills with vinegar. Take 9-12g with food. Clears heat, transforms dampness, promotes the movement of qi, and relieves dysenteric disorders. For red-and-white dysenteric disorders with focal distention and a stifling sensation in the chest and diaphragm due to damp-heat. Compared to the original formula, which uses Coptidis Rhizoma (*huáng lián*) and Evodiae Fructus (*wú zhū yú*) together, this formula is colder and more drying, as Evodiae Fructus (*wú zhū yú*) is discarded. Aucklandiae Radix (*mù xiāng*) is specific for treating tenesmus and focuses the action of the main herb on the Large Intestine.

芍藥湯 (芍药汤)

Peony Decoction

sháo yào tāng

Source   *Collection of Writings on the Dynamics of Illness, Suitability of Qi, and the Safeguarding of Life as Discussed in Basic Questions* (1186)

Paeoniae Radix *(sháo yào)*	30g (15-20g)
Angelicae sinensis Radix *(dāng guī)*	15g (6-9g)
Glycyrrhizae Radix praeparata *(zhì gān cǎo)*	6g (4.5g)
Aucklandiae Radix *(mù xiāng)*	6g (4.5g)
Arecae Semen *(bīng láng)*	6g (4.5g)
Coptidis Rhizoma *(huáng lián)*	15g (6-9g)
Scutellariae Radix *(huáng qín)*	15g (9-12g)
Rhei Radix et Rhizoma *(dà huáng)*	9g (6-9g)
Cinnamomi Cortex *(ròu guì)*	7.5g (1.5-3g)

Method of Preparation   Grind the ingredients into a coarse powder and take warm in 15g doses as a draft after meals. Note that the original text specifices 'official cinnamon' (官桂 *guān guì*), which is derived from the thinner bark of 6-7-year-old trees. Modern texts substitute Cinnamomi Cortex *(ròu guì)* and also use Paeoniae Radix alba *(bái sháo)*. At present, it is usually prepared as a decoction with the dosage specified in parentheses.

Actions   Regulates and harmonizes the qi and blood, clears heat, dries dampness, and resolves toxicity

Indications

Abdominal pain, tenesmus, difficulty with defecation, diarrhea with pus and blood (equal amounts), a burning sensation around the anus, dark, scanty urine, a greasy, slightly yellow tongue coating, and a rapid pulse.

This is dysenteric disorder due to damp-heat lodged in the Intestines where it causes the qi and blood to stagnate. This condition is frequently associated with food poisoning or the contraction of an epidemic toxin. Stagnation obstructs the flow of qi in the Intestines, producing abdominal pain and tenesmus. The damp-heat scorches the collaterals of the Intestines, which causes blood in the stool. The struggle between the normal qi and blood and the damp-heat brews in the Intestines and generates pus, which is expelled through the stool. Damp-heat in the lower burner causes scanty, dark urine and a burning sensation around the anus. The presence of damp-heat is also reflected in the greasy, slightly yellow tongue coating.

Analysis of Formula

The primary emphasis of this formula is to clear heat, dry dampness, and regulate the qi and blood in order to guide out the cause of the disorder. The chief herbs used for this purpose are bitter and very cooling Coptidis Rhizoma *(huáng lián)* and Scutellariae Radix *(huáng qín),* which resolve heat toxicity in the Intestines by clearing heat and drying dampness. A third bitter and cooling herb, Rhei Radix et Rhizoma *(dà huáng),* serves as the deputy to drain heat toxins through the stool. It also combines with the qi-moving herbs in the formula "to promote flow for disorders of flow" (不通則通 *bù tōng zé tōng*). Paeoniae Radix *(sháo yào),* used in a large dose to move the blood, expel the pus, relax urgency, and stop the pain, and Angelicae sinensis Radix *(dāng guī),* which tonifies, warms, and moves the blood, constitute a second group of deputies. Together, they regulate the nutritive qi and blood, following the adage that "by moving the blood, pus in the stools is naturally healed." When combined with Glycyrrhizae Radix *(gān cǎo),* Paeoniae Radix *(sháo yào)* also moderates the spasms and relieves abdominal pain.

Even though the formula treats a pattern of damp-heat, it uses a small amount of the strongly warming herb Cinnamomi Cortex *(ròu guì)* as an assistant. This herb enters the blood level and assists the blood-harmonizing herbs in moving the blood. It also acts as an opposing assistant, which means that it prevents the cold, bitter properties of the other herbs from either injuring the yang or constraining the pathogenic influences in the interior, and thereby transforming into smoldering damp-heat. The combination of Cinnamomi Cortex *(ròu guì)* with Rhei Radix et Rhizoma *(dà huáng)* is particularly adroit. While these two herbs work synergistically to invigorate the blood, the latter restrains the former from increasing the fire in the body. Two other assistants, Aucklandiae Radix *(mù xiāng)* and Arecae Semen *(bīng láng),* promote the movement of qi and help eliminate stagnation. They complement the actions of Paeoniae Radix *(sháo yào)* and Angelicae sinensis Radix *(dāng guī),* whose focus is to regulate the blood. Arecae Semen *(bīng láng)* also assists Rhei Radix et Rhizoma *(dà huáng)* in guiding out stagnation. Finally, Glycyrrhizae Radix *(gān cǎo)* serves as envoy. It harmonizes the functions of the Stomach and protects its qi from the harsh actions of the other herbs.

Cautions and Contraindications

This formula should not be used during the early stages of this disorder where there are also exterior symptoms, nor should it be used for chronic dysenteric disorders due to cold from deficiency.

Commentary

The source text explains the rationale of this formula: "When the stool contains pus and blood, the bleeding will stop when the qi moves; when the blood is moving normally, the pus in the stool will resolve by itself; when the qi is regulated, the tenesmus will disappear by itself." The emphasis given to the regulation of qi and blood in this passage has led to debates regarding the nature of the chief herbs in this formula. In *Discussion of Famous Physicians' Formulas Past and Present*, Luo Mei argued that such regulation was achieved via the combination of Paeoniae Radix *(sháo yào)* and Glycyrrhizae Radix *(gān cǎo)*. Hence, they should be regarded as the chief herbs.

Wang Ang, writing in *Medical Formulas Collected and Analyzed*, held that Paeoniae Radix (*sháo yào*) alone was the chief herb because it regulates the nutritive and protective qi.

The modern writer Chen Chao-Zu, in *Treatment Strategies and Formulas in Chinese Medicine*, puts forth a different view, that is, the chief herbs are Coptidis Rhizoma (*huáng lián*) and Scutellariae Radix (*huáng qín*). On the one hand, these two herbs directly treat the damp-heat that is at the root of this disorder. Additionally, historically, Peony Decoction (*sháo yào tāng*) can be viewed as a combination of Peony Decoction (*sháo yào tāng*), Drain the Epigastrium Decoction (*xiè xīn tāng*), and Aucklandia and Coptis Pill (*xiāng lián wán*). Bitter, cooling herbs are the chief ingredients in all of these formulas, and thus of the new combined formula as well.

Comparisons

➢ Vs. Pulsatilla Decoction (*bái tóu wēng tāng*)

The formula discussed here is used primarily for dysenteric disorders caused by damp-heat, while Pulsatilla Decoction (*bái tóu wēng tāng*) is used for dysenteric disorders caused by heat toxin scalding the Stomach and Intestines. One of the distinguishing characteristics of a damp-heat dysenteric disorder is the roughly equal amounts of blood and pus. Where the cause is heat toxin, however, the heat is much more pronounced, and there is thus more blood than pus in the stool.

➢ Vs. Pulsatilla Decoction (*bái tóu wēng tāng*); *see* PAGE 208

Biomedical Indications

With the appropriate presentation, this formula may be used to treat a variety of biomedically-defined disorders involving inflammation of the lower digestive tract including bacillary or amebic dysentery, acute enteritis, and ulcerative colitis.

Alternate names

Scutellaria and Peony Decoction (*huáng qín sháo yào tāng*) in *Displays of Enlightened Physicians*; White Peony Decoction (*bái sháo yào tāng*) in *A Physician's Teachings from the Heart*; Tangkuei and Peony Decoction (*dāng guī sháo yào tāng*) in *Golden Mirror of the Medical Tradition*

Modifications

• For a thick tongue coating and a slippery pulse (indicating food stagnation), remove Glycyrrhizae Radix (*gān cǎo*) and add Crataegi Fructus (*shān zhā*) and Massa medicata fermentata (*shén qū*).
• For heat that has injured the fluids with a dry tongue coating, remove Cinnamomi Cortex (*ròu guì*).
• For severe heat toxin, add Lonicerae Flos (*jīn yín huā*) and Pulsatillae Radix (*bái tóu wēng*).

• For severe bleeding, add Moutan Cortex (*mǔ dān pí*) and Sanguisorbae Radix (*dì yú*).
• For damp-heat toxin, add Sanguisorbae Radix (*dì yú*) and Sophorae Flos (*huái huā*).
• For white pus, add Zingiberis Rhizoma (*gān jiāng*).
• For more severe signs of dampness, add Atractylodis Rhizoma (*cāng zhú*), Poria (*fú líng*), and Amomi Fructus (*shā rén*).

黃芩湯（黄芩汤）

Scutellaria Decoction

huáng qín tāng

Source *Discussion of Cold Damage* (c. 220)

Scutellariae Radix (*huáng qín*) 9g
Radix Paeoniae (*sháo yào*) 9g
Glycyrrhizae Radix praeparata (*zhì gān cǎo*) 3g
Jujubae Fructus (*dà zǎo*) . . . . 4 pieces

Method of Preparation Decoction. The source text advises to take one portion during the day and another at night. Paeoniae Radix alba (*bái sháo*) is the type of Paeoniae Radix (*sháo yào*) that is generally used.

Actions Clears heat, alleviates dysenteric disorders, harmonizes the middle burner, and stops pain

Indications

Fever, a bitter taste in the mouth, abdominal pain, diarrhea, a red tongue with yellow coating, and a rapid or flooding pulse.

This is diarrhea or dysenteric disorder caused by heat constraint in the lesser yang that forces its way into the Stomach and Intestines. The disease dynamic is explained in *Discussion of Cold Damage* (paragraph 172): "For a combination disease of the greater and lesser yang with spontaneous diarrhea, give Scutellaria Decoction. If there is vomiting, Scutellaria plus Pinellia and Fresh Ginger Decoction masters it."

An external pathogen obstructing the protective qi within the greater yang manifests as fever. If it sinks deeper into the lesser yang, the constraint of ministerial fire causes a bitter taste in the mouth. The lesser yang occupies a half-exterior, half-interior position in between the greater yang and yang brightness. Because the nature of yang qi is to ascend, heat constraint in the lesser yang warp is usually discharged outward. If that route is blocked, the heat can force its way into the yang brightness to disturb the function of the Stomach and Intestines and cause vomiting or diarrhea. Because this is hot diarrhea, the stool will be sticky, foul-smelling, and may be accompanied by anal irritation and burning. Obstruction of the qi dynamic causes abdominal pain and, if severe, tenesmus. On the tongue, the heat will manifest in a yellow coating. Heat also causes the pulse to become rapid and flooding.

Analysis of Formula

Although the main manifestation treated by this formula appears to be heat in the Stomach and Intestines, its root is constraint in the lesser and greater yang channels. This must be dispersed if the manifestations are to be resolved. Using acrid and hot herbs to discharge the greater yang is inappropriate because this would increase the fire in the lesser yang and thereby aggravate the symptoms. Therefore, the formula focuses on clearing the heat and augmenting the yin. When the heat is cleared, the diarrhea will abate. When the yin is strong, the protective qi will expel the pathogen from the exterior by itself. *Medical Formulas Collected and Analyzed* explains this intention: "Why does the formula not use herbs for two channels if this is a combination disease of [the greater and lesser yang] channels? It is because this combination disease is accompanied by spontaneous diarrhea. This implies that the yang pathogen is moving into the interior. Therefore, [the formula] emphasizes [clearing heat from] the interior."

The formula's chief herb is bitter and cold Scutellariae Radix *(huáng qín)*. It drains heat from the lesser yang and yang brightness, resolves toxicity, and stops dysentery and diarrhea. Radix Paeoniae *(sháo yào)* serves as the deputy. Its coldness assists in draining heat from the middle burner, while its sourness astringes and contains the yin. Together with Glycyrrhizae Radix praeparata *(zhì gān cǎo)*, it also forms a synergistic pairing that is specific for abdominal cramping and pain. Glycyrrhizae Radix praeparata *(zhì gān cǎo)* resolves toxicity and, in conjunction with Jujubae Fructus *(dà zǎo)*, harmonizes the middle burner, augments the qi, and enriches the yin. Both herbs thus serve as assistants and envoys in this formula.

Cautions and Contraindications

This formula is not indicated for the initial stages of dysenteric or feverish disorders with pronounced exterior symptoms. It is contraindicated for dysenteric disorders due to cold or deficiency.

Commentary

The Qing dynasty *Medical Formulas Collected and Analyzed* praises this formula as "the ancestral formula on which generations [of physicians have based] the treatment of dysenteric disorders." The distinction between diarrhea and dysenteric disorders was not yet well established when the source text was written. Although most commentators consider it to treat dysenteric disorders, it can also be used for diarrhea from heat. Key indicators for the use of this formula in the clinic are thus symptoms such as abdominal cramping or tenesmus, a burning sensation at the anus, and a flooding pulse, which may or may not be accompanied by pus and blood in the stools.

This formula is generally regarded as a variation of Cinnamon Twig Decoction *(guì zhī tāng)*, with Scutellariae Radix *(huáng qín)* replacing Cinnamomi Ramulus *(guì zhī)* and Zingiberis Rhizoma recens *(shēng jiāng)*. This simple substitution changes a warm, dispersing formula into one that clears heat from the interior while staying true to its intention of strengthening the nutritive yin in order to augment the protective yang. Qing-dynasty physicians from the Suzhou region thus extended the use of this formula to the treatment of warm pathogen disorders where pathogenic heat had accumulated within the interior but the body's qi was unable to expel them. The early 17th-century physician Zhang Lu was one of the first to outline this strategy: "Scutellaria Decoction *(huáng qín tāng)* basically treats spring and summer warm pathogen heat where fever develops from within [i.e., without marked exterior symptoms like chills at the onset]."

Half a century later, Ye Tian-Shi extended this rationale to the treatment of lurking pathogens. In *Differentiating Lurking Pathogens and Externally-Contracted Diseases during Three Seasons,* he explained that "Cold that attacks the body in winter lurks in the Kidneys, transforms into heat, and manifests in the Gallbladder in the spring. The treatment for this situation is to take Scutellaria Decoction *(huáng qín tāng)* as the main formula to clear heat with bitter and cold herbs." Ye Tian-Shi's approach was based on a discussion in the *Inner Classic,* which postulates a deficiency of essence (or yin) to be the precondition for this kind of disorder. This makes his use of a formula derived from Cinnamon Twig Decoction *(guì zhī tāng)*, which harmonizes the nutritive yin to empower the function of the protective yang, both sensible and highly imaginative.

In the late 19th century, Liu Bao-Yi, another physician from the same general area, pushed Ye Tian-Shi's strategy even further. In *Encountering the Sources of Warm-Heat Pathogen Diseases,* Liu formulated a mature doctrine of lurking pathogen disorders that uses Scutellaria Decoction *(huáng qín tāng)*, to which Sojae Semen praeparatum *(dàn dòu chǐ)* and Scrophulariae Radix *(xuán shēn)* have been added, as the core formula for treating these disorders. Liu explained:

> In my humble opinion, there is nothing better than using Scutellaria Decoction *(huáng qín tāng)* plus Scrophulariae Radix *(xuán shēn)* and Sojae Semen praeparatum *(dàn dòu chǐ)*. It is the most appropriate method by far, with little need for alteration. This is because Scutellaria Decoction *(huáng qín tāng)* is specially designed to drain and cool internal heat. Scrophulariae Radix *(xuán shēn)* tonifies the Kidney yin. Sojae Semen praeparatum *(dàn dòu chǐ)* is made from black soybeans, which themselves enter the Kidney channel, and is prepared by steaming in a pent-up container—just like the pathogen itself before it begins to emerge. Because its nature and flavor are harmonious and neutral, without the drawback of strong diaphoresis or damage to the yin, it is just right for assisting the expression.

Liu Bao-Yi's reinterpretation is an example of how Chinese medicine developed historically before its encounter with the

West, and became, in turn, the foundation for an entirely new approach to the treatment of seasonal or feverish disorders.

Biomedical Indications

With the appropriate presentation, this formula may be used to treat a variety of biomedically-defined disorders, primarily those involving inflammation of the lower bowel such as amebic and bacillary dysentery, acute colitis, as well as pelvic inflammatory disease.

Modifications

- For upward rebellion of Stomach qi with retching and vomiting, add Pinelliae Rhizoma (*bàn xià*) and Zingiberis Rhizoma recens (*shēng jiāng*).

- For pronounced abdominal pain and tenesmus, add Aucklandiae Radix (*mù xiāng*) and Arecae Semen (*bīng láng*).

- For pus and blood in the stools, add Sanguisorbae Radix (*dì yú*) and Crataegi Fructus (*shān zhā*). Both herbs should be charred in order to increase their ability to stop the bleeding.

白頭翁湯 (白头翁汤)

Pulsatilla Decoction

bái tóu wēng tāng

Source   *Discussion of Cold Damage* (c. 220)

Pulsatillae Radix (*bái tóu wēng*) 6g (12-18g)
Coptidis Rhizoma (*huáng lián*) 9g (6-9g)
Phellodendri Cortex (*huáng bǎi*) 9g (9-12g)
Fraxini Cortex (*qín pí*) 9g (9-12g)

Method of Preparation   Decoction. The most commonly-used dosages at present are given in parentheses..

Actions   Clears heat, resolves toxicity, cools the blood, and alleviates dysenteric disorders

Indications

Abdominal pain, tenesmus, a burning sensation around the anus, diarrhea containing more blood than pus, thirst, a red tongue with a yellow coating, and a wiry, rapid pulse.

This is a hot dysenteric disorder due to heat toxin searing the Stomach and Intestines. This causes tenesmus, a burning sensation around the anus, blood and pus in the stools, a red tongue with a yellow coating, and a wiry, rapid pulse. The presence of damp-heat is reflected in the consistency of the stools and especially by the presence of pus.

Analysis of Formula

Pulsatillae Radix (*bái tóu wēng*) is the principal herb in the materia medica for treating dysenteric disorders. It serves as the chief herb in this formula because of its ability to clear damp-heat and resolve fire toxicity from the Large Intestine,

especially in the blood level. Bitter, cold Coptidis Rhizoma (*huáng lián*) clears damp-heat, especially from the Stomach and Intestines. Phellodendri Cortex (*huáng bǎi*) clears damp-heat from the lower burner. These two deputies assist the chief herb in clearing damp-heat and thereby relieve the dysenteric diarrhea. Cold, bitter, and astringent Fraxini Cortex (*qín pí*) serves as the assistant by restraining the diarrhea and enhancing the actions of the other herbs.

Cautions and Contraindications

Because this formula contains herbs that are bitter and cold in nature, it can readily injure the Spleen yang. It should therefore not be used long term, and is contraindicated in cases with Spleen yang deficiency.

Commentary

The source text recommends this formula for treating terminal yin-warp dysenteric disorders due to heat. This is regarded as a very serious condition where damp-heat or toxin penetrates into the blood level. The basic structure of the formula therefore emulates Coptis Decoction to Resolve Toxicity (*huáng lián jiě dú tāng*) to effectively deal with this pathology. However, whereas that formula extends its action to the entire body via the Triple Burner, the present formula focuses more specifically on the lower burner. As in the pattern treated by Scutellaria Decoction (*huáng qín tāng*), the Intestines, however, are merely the conduit through which the body attempts to eliminate damp-heat and toxins, whereas the root of the disorder lies in the terminal yin. This is reflected in the thirst and wiry pulse, key signs used in *Discussion of Cold Damage* to flag the presence of pathogens at this level.

In fact, dysenteric disorders can occur as a result of pathologies in each of the six warps, and with the exception of the greater yin warp, all of these involve thirst as a symptom. At the lesser yin warp, bowel movements will be clear and watery, permitting easy differentiation. Dysenteric disorders affecting the yang warps will also be of a hot type but can be differentiated on the basis of accompanying signs and symptoms.

For combined greater yang and yang brightness disorders, these include exterior symptoms like chills and fevers, or the acute onset of diarrhea shortly after such symptoms have abated. In combined greater yang and lesser yang patterns, thirst will be accompanied by a bitter taste in the mouth. In yang brightness-organ patterns, thirst will be accompanied by sweating, abdominal fullness, and signs of interior clumping.

The chief and assistant herbs in this formula combine to clear heat from the terminal yin. *Divine Husbandman's Classic of the Materia Medica,* which probably closely reflects the knowledge on which Zhang Zhong-Jing himself could draw, lists Pulsatillae Radix (*bái tóu wēng*) as a remedy for malarial disorders and abdominal masses. Later physicians deduced from its appearance—the plant apparently does not move in windy conditions but does move by itself when the weather is calm—an affinity to Liver disorders. Wu Ju-Tong, for instance, notes that it has the power of venting toxic heat pathogens from the lower burner blood level (i.e., terminal yin) upward and outward. This action follows the physiological direction of Liver qi, restoring its natural flow and assisting in removing stagnation from the Intestines. Meanwhile, the astringent properties of Fraxini Cortex (*qín pí*), the other herb in the formula that enteris the terminal yin, serve to retain the yin essences without which the Liver yin and blood lose their ability to control and harmonize the yang.

Usage

The use of this formula has been expanded to the treatment of other conditions due to heat toxin or damp-heat in the lower burner such as painful or bloody urinary dysfunction. Many of the materia medica books of the Ming and Qing periods note that the assistant herb, Fraxini Cortex (*qín pí*), is beneficial to the eyes. For example, in *Hidden Aspects of the Materia Medica*, the 16th-century writer Chen Jia-Mo noted that it is a specific herb for ophthalmology. For this reason, some modern practitioners use the formula in treating acute eye disorders due to damp-heat.

Comparisons

➢ Vs. Peony Decoction (*sháo yào tāng*) and Kudzu, Scutellaria, and Coptis Decoction (*gé gēn huáng qín huáng lián tāng*)

All of these formulas treat damp-heat dysenteric disorders. Peony Decoction (*sháo yào tāng*) has less heat-clearing and toxicity-resolving actions, but it does have ingredients that promote the movement of qi. It is therefore used for conditions with less heat and toxicity (less blood in the stool) and more qi stagnation (abdominal pain and tenesmus).

Kudzu, Scutellaria, and Coptis Decoction (*gé gēn huáng qín huáng lián tāng*) also treats hot dysenteric disorders and, like the present formula, relies on Coptidis Rhizoma (*huáng lián*). However, the pathogen treated by that formula is located in the qi level and still present in the upper burner. Accordingly, the formula uses Puerariae Radix (*gé gēn*) as chief herb in order to vent the pathogen from the exterior.

The present formula, by contrast, clears pathogens from the blood aspect in the lower burner and uses Pulsatillae Radix (*bái tóu wēng*) as the chief herb for this purpose. Key clinical markers suggesting its use include thirst, indicating heat, and blood in the stools, indicating that the heat has penetrated to the blood level.

➢ Vs. Peony Decoction (*sháo yào tāng*); *see* PAGE 208

Biomedical Indications

With the appropriate presentation, this formula may be used to treat a variety of biomedically-defined disorders, primarily bowel diseases such as amebic and bacillary dysentery and inflammatory bowel diseases. It has also been used for conjunctivitis, pelvic inflammatory disease, gonorrheal urethritis, hemorrhoids, and hysterical tremors.

Modifications

* For concurrent signs of an exterior condition such as chills and fever, add Puerariae Radix (*gé gēn*), Scutellariae Radix (*huáng qín*), Lonicerae Flos (*jīn yín huā*), and Forsythiae Fructus (*lián qiáo*).
* For severe tenesmus, add Aucklandiae Radix (*mù xiāng*), Paeoniae Radix alba (*bái sháo*), and Arecae Semen (*bīng láng*).
* For urinary frequency, urgency, and pain, add Akebiae Caulis (*mù tōng*), Imperatae Rhizoma (*bái máo gēn*), and Lysimachiae Herba (*jīn qián cǎo*).
* For hot, swollen, and painful eyes, add Chrysanthemi Flos (*jú huā*), Moutan Cortex (*mǔ dān pí*), and Carthami Flos (*hóng huā*).
* For amebic dysentery, add Granati Pericarpium (*shí liú pí*).
* For bacillary dysentery, add Fraxini Cortex (*qín pí*), Sanguisorbae Radix (*dì yú*), Agrimoniae Herba (*xiān hè cǎo*), and Aucklandiae Radix (*mù xiāng*).

Associated Formulas

白頭翁加甘草阿膠湯 （白头翁加甘草阿胶汤）

Pulsatilla Decoction plus Licorice and Ass-Hide Gelatin

bái tóu wēng jiā gān cǎo ē jiāo tāng

SOURCE *Essentials from the Golden Cabinet* (c. 220)

Pulsatillae Radix (*bái tóu wēng*) 6g
Glycyrrhizae Radix (*gān cǎo*) 6g
Asini Corii Colla (*ē jiāo*) . . . . 6g [add to strained decoction]
Fraxini Cortex (*qín pí*) 9g
Coptidis Rhizoma (*huáng lián*) 9g
Phellodendri Cortex (*huáng bǎi*) 9g

At present, the dosage of Pulsatillae Radix (*bái tóu wēng*) is usually increased 2-3 fold. Clears heat, resolves toxicity, nourishes the blood, and enriches the yin. For hot dysenteric disorders in cases with blood or yin deficiency. The source text recommends this formula for postpartum patients.

加味白頭翁湯 （加味白头翁汤）

Augmented Pulsatilla Decoction

jiā wèi bái tóu wēng tāng

SOURCE *Systematic Differentiation of Warm Pathogen Diseases* (1798)

Pulsatillae Radix (*bái tóu wēng*) 9g
Paeoniae Radix alba (*bái sháo*) 6g
Scutellariae Radix (*huáng qín*) 9g
Fraxini Cortex (*qín pí*) 6g
Coptidis Rhizoma (*huáng lián*) 6g
Phellodendri Cortex (*huáng bǎi*) 6g

Clears heat, resolves dampness, and alleviates dysenteric disorders. For damp-warm-heat pathogen diseases leading to hot dysenteric disorders characterized by tenesmus, diarrhea, and abdominal pain. The source text notes that the appropriate use of this formula depends on the pulse type, which should be big on the right and small on the left. This is interpreted to mean that the pathogenic influence enters through the upper and middle burners (reflected in the right, or more yang pulse) but becomes lodged in the lower burner (reflected in the left, or more yin pulse).

Section 6

. . . .

FORMULAS THAT CLEAR
HEAT FROM DEFICIENCY

Heat from deficiency can occur for many reasons. When it arises during the final stage of a warm-heat pathogen disease as the heat has depleted the yin or settled into the deep yin aspects of the body, it is characterized by fever at night that cools by morning. Chronic injury to the Liver and Kidneys from heat may present with similar symptoms, including tidal fever, steaming bone disorder, or a chronic, unremitting, low-grade fever.

The formulas used in treating this type of disorder consist of herbs that clear heat from deficiency and enrich the yin. When heat is cleared, yin can recover. When yin and yang are in harmony, the internal organs resume their normal function. This is different from the focus on tonifying deficiency and organ-based disharmonies that characterizes the formulas for yin deficiency, discussed in Chapter 8. What distinguishes the various formulas in this section from each other is the momentum (勢 *shì*) of the heat in each particular case, which leads to very characteristic presentations, as described below.

The core ingredients for clearing heat from deficiency are Artemisiae annuae Herba (*qīng hāo*), Lycii Cortex (*dì gǔ pí*), Gentianae macrophyllae Radix (*qín jiāo*), Stellariae Radix (*yín chái hú*), and Picrorhizae Rhizoma (*hú huáng lián*). Cloying, yin-enriching herbs are usually not used in these cases, as they could impede the clearing of the heat. Instead, substances such as Rehmanniae Radix (*shēng dì huáng*), Trionycis Carapax (*biē jiǎ*), and Anemarrhenae Rhizoma (*zhī mǔ*) that both enrich the yin and clear heat are used.

青蒿鱉甲湯（青蒿鳖甲汤）

Sweet Wormwood and Soft-Shelled Turtle Shell Decoction [Version 1]

qīng hāo biē jiǎ tāng

Source *Systematic Differentiation of Warm Pathogen Diseases* (1798)

Trionycis Carapax (*biē jiǎ*) 15g
Artemisiae annuae Herba (*qīng hāo*) . . . . [add near end] 6g
Rehmanniae Radix (*shēng dì huáng*) 12g
Anemarrhenae Rhizoma (*zhī mǔ*) 6g
Moutan Cortex (*mǔ dān pí*) 9g

Method of Preparation Decoction. The source text directs to decoct from 5 cups to 3 cups and take in two doses over the course of a day. Artemisiae annuae Herba (*qīng hāo*) should not be exposed to high temperatures for prolonged periods since this may destroy its active properties. For this reason, it is added to the preparation at the end.

Actions Nourishes the yin and vents heat

Indications

Night fever and morning coolness with no sweating as the fever recedes, emaciation with no loss of appetite, a red tongue with little coating, and a fine, rapid pulse.

This is heat lurking in the yin aspects of the body. It usually occurs during the later stages of a warm-heat pathogen disease when the heat has depleted the yin and fluids. Night fevers that recede in the morning indicate heat lurking in the yin aspects of the body. Because the yin and fluids are depleted, the body is unable to generate sweat, which would normally occur as a fever recedes. The fact that the patient does not lose their appetite indicates that the problem is not in the qi level, and that the digestive system is relatively unaffected. Nevertheless, injury to the yin and blood causes a general loss of nourishment and thus emaciation. The red tongue with little coating, and the fine, rapid pulse reflect injury to the yin.

Analysis of Formula

Once a heat pathogen has settled in the body it is unwise to nourish the yin since the cloying nature of the herbs used for this purpose will only serve to trap the heat inside. Nor should bitter, cold herbs that drain fire be prescribed, since their drying nature will cause further injury to the yin. The only proper course is to simultaneously nourish the yin and vent the heat pathogen. Salty, cold Trionycis Carapax (*biē jiǎ*) directly enters the yin to enrich the yin and reduce the fever from deficiency. Unlike other more cloying, yin-enriching herbs, this substance is able to enter the collaterals, track down pathogens, and actively clear heat from the deepest yin aspect of the body. It is coupled with the aromatic and acrid Artemisiae annuae Herba (*qīng hāo*), which vents the heat and expels it from the body. This very effective combination of substances, one of which focuses on the yin and the other on the yang, is the chief ingredient in the formula. Its action is summed up by Wu Ju-Tong in *Systematic Differentiation of Warm Pathogen Diseases*: "This formula ingeniously first enters [into the interior] and then issues [from the exterior]. Artemisiae annuae Herba *(qīng hāo)*, which is unable to enter into the yin aspect directly, is able to do so under the guidance of Trionycis Carapax *(biē jiǎ)*. Trionycis Carapax *(biē jiǎ)*, which by itself is unable to issue through the yang aspect, is able to do so under the guidance of Artemisiae annuae Herba *(qīng hāo)*."

The deputies, Rehmanniae Radix *(shēng dì huáng)* and Anemarrhenae Rhizoma *(zhī mǔ)*, assist Trionycis Carapax *(biē jiǎ)* in nourishing the yin and clearing heat from deficiency. The assistant, Moutan Cortex *(mǔ dān pí)*, drains heat from the yin and assists Artemisiae annuae Herba *(qīng hāo)* in venting and dispersing the heat. Together, the five substances that comprise this formula combine to nourish, clear, and vent, dealing with both the root and branch of this pattern.

Cautions and Contraindications

Contraindicated in the early stages of a warm-heat pathogen disease, when the pathogenic influence is still in the qi level, and also in cases with spasms or convulsions.

Commentary

Commentators provide different explanations of the disease dynamic that underlies the key symptom treated by this formula: night fever and morning coolness with an absence of sweating as the fever recedes. One theory is that when the body's protective qi, which circulates in the exterior during the day, enters the yin aspect of the body at night, it combines with the lurking heat already present there. This causes night fever. As the protective qi rises into the yang aspect again in the early morning, the fever recedes. Another theory is that nighttime fever is a manifestation of the battle between the body and the pathogenic qi. If the yin is deficient, this engagement can only take place at night when the yin is sufficiently strong.

The apparent contradiction between these views is best resolved by attending to how different physicians have used this formula in practice. Although it was originally intended to treat injury to the yin from a febrile disease, the formula has effectively been used in treating fever of various etiologies provided that the presentation is primarily one of yin deficiency with lurking heat. The famous modern physician Qin Bo-Wei used this formula for treating tidal fevers with Liver yin deficiency characterized by afternoon fever, fatigue, sweating, emaciation, and a thin, weak, and rapid pulse. In Qin's view, Trionycis Carapax *(biē jiǎ)* enters the Liver to enrich the yin, Moutan Cortex *(mǔ dān pí)* cools the Liver

blood, and Artemisiae annuae Herba *(qīng hāo)* vents heat from the lesser yang channel, which shares an exterior-interior relationship with the Liver channel.

If one analyzes the similarities between these different uses, one perceives a single mode of action at their core. The formula's combination of chief herbs clears heat due to constraint from the deepest parts of the body. Constraint at this level only occurs if the yin itself is so severely damaged that it can no longer moisten movement within the collaterals. As constraint implies a blockage that leads to heat, this symptom will present most obviously when yang within yin is strongest, that is, from the late afternoon to the early morning. As the protective qi retreats from the interior of the body, the symptoms of constraint diminish. But not being tied to sufficient yin, the body's yang qi also cannot fulfil its warming functions appropriately, explaining both the lack of sweating and the morning coolness.

This kind of disorder is different from an imbalance between yin and yang rooted in the Kidneys, which will present less with signs and symptoms of constraint (i.e., problems of movement) and more with symptoms indicating that fire and water are losing their connection (i.e., problems of holding). This is why Qin Bo-Wei explicitly spoke of a Liver rather than a Kidney disorder. In clinical practice, the thinking outlined here can be extended to disorders involving the extraordinary vessels.

Comparisons

➤ Vs. GREAT TONIFY THE YIN PILL *(dà bǔ yīn wán)*

The principal formula focuses more on the problems associated with externally-contracted disorders with remnants of heat, while Great Tonify the Yin Pill *(dà bǔ yīn wán)* addresses yin deficiency with exuberant fire in the Kidneys. Sweet Wormwood and Soft-Shelled Turtle Shell Decoction Version 1 *(qīng hāo biē jiǎ tāng)* treats yin deficiency with fire constraint in the Liver and the collaterals.

➤ Vs. COOL THE BONES POWDER *(qīng gǔ sǎn)*; *see* PAGE 215

➤ Vs. LARGE GENTIAN AND SOFT-SHELLED TURTLE SHELL POWDER *(qín jiāo biē jiǎ sǎn)*; *see* PAGE 218

Biomedical Indications

With the appropriate presentation, this formula may be used to treat a variety of biomedically-defined disorders such as low-grade fevers during the recovery phase of infectious diseases, fever of unknown origin, chronic pyelonephritis, and pulmonary or renal tuberculosis.

Alternate names

Sweet Wormwood and Soft-Shelled Turtle Shell Decoction *(qīng hāo biē jiǎ jiān)* in *Treatment Methods for Damp-Warm Seasonal Epidemics*

Modifications

- For Lung consumption, add Glehniae/Adenophorae Radix (shā shēn) and Ecliptae Herba (mò hàn lián).
- For pronounced coughing and wheezing, add Mori Cortex (sāng bái pí) and Asteris Radix (zǐ wǎn).
- For summertime night fever and morning coolness in children, add Cynanchi atrati Radix (bái wēi) and Nelumbinis Caulis (lián gěng).
- For blazing fire from deficiency, add Cynanchi atrati Radix (bái wēi) and Lycii Cortex (dì gǔ pí).
- For heat in the five centers, yellow urine, and a red tongue with a yellow coating, add Imperatae Rhizoma (bái máo gēn).
- For fevers of unknown origin due to yin deficiency, add Lycii Cortex (dì gǔ pí) and Cynanchi atrati Radix (bái wēi).

Associated Formulas

青蒿鱉甲湯 (青蒿鳖甲汤)

Sweet Wormwood and Soft-Shelled Turtle Shell Decoction [Version 2]

qīng hāo biē jiǎ tāng

SOURCE *Systematic Differentiation of Warm Pathogen Diseases* (1798)

Trionycis Carapax (biē jiǎ)	15g
Artemisiae annuae Herba (qīng hāo)	[add near end] 9g
Trichosanthis Radix (tiān huā fěn)	6g
Anemarrhenae Rhizoma (zhī mǔ)	6g
Mori Folium (sāng yè)	6g
Moutan Cortex (mǔ dān pí)	9g

Decoction. Clears heat and nourishes yin. For lesser yang patterns with relatively strong fever characterized by a wiry pulse on the left, night fevers with morning coolness, and thirst following sweating. This is one of two formulas by the same name occuring in the source text, which for convenience we have labelled Sweet Wormwood and Soft-Shelled Turtle Shell (Version 2). The lesser yang occupies a position half way between the exterior and the interior. In warm pathogen feverish disorders, the yin is readily damaged and pathogens in the lesser yang can then penetrate deep into the yin aspect of the body. This formula seeks to prevent such deterioration before it occurs.

Compared to the formula by the same name discussed in the main section (Version 1), this formula focuses more strongly on clearing heat from the yang aspects of the body. Compared to Minor Bupleurum Decoction (xiǎo chái hú tāng), which addresses a similar situation occurring in the course of cold damage disorders, this formula focuses more strongly on nourishing the yin in order to prevent the sinking of heat pathogens into the interior.

人參黃耆散 (人参黄芪散)

Ginseng and Astragalus Powder

rén shēn huáng qí sǎn

SOURCE *Precious Mirror of Health* (Yuan dynasty)

Ginseng Radix (rén shēn)	30g
Gentianae macrophyllae Radix (qín jiāo)	60g
Poria (fú líng)	60g
Anemarrhenae Rhizoma (zhī mǔ)	75g
Mori Cortex (sāng bái pí)	45g
Platycodi Radix (jié gěng)	30g
Asteris Radix (zǐ wǎn)	45g
Bupleuri Radix (chái hú)	75g
Astragali Radix (huáng qí)	105g
Lycii Cortex (dì gǔ pí)	60g
Rehmanniae Radix (shēng dì huáng)	60g
Pinelliae Rhizoma praeparatum (zhì bàn xià)	45g
Paeoniae Radix rubra (chì sháo)	45g
Asparagi Radix (tiān mén dōng)	90g
prepared Trionycis Carapax (zhì biē jiǎ)	90g
Glycyrrhizae Radix praeparata (zhì gān cǎo)	45g

Grind the ingredients into a powder and take in 9g doses twice a day as a draft on an empty stomach. May also be prepared as a decoction by reducing the dosage of the ingredients by approximately 90 percent. Enriches the yin, clears heat, augments the qi, strengthens the Spleen, stops coughing, and transforms phlegm. For deficiency consumption (虛癆 xū láo) characterized by lethargy, generalized weakness, coughing, scanty sputum, a dry throat, spontaneous sweating, reduced appetite, afternoon fever, a pale tongue with a dark-red tip, and a deficient, rapid pulse.

In contrast to the principal formula, this one focuses on treating yin, blood, and qi deficiency with lurking heat leading to steaming bone disorder and deficiency consumption that affects the Lungs and Spleen.

清骨散

Cool the Bones Powder

qīng gǔ sǎn

Source *Indispensable Tools for Pattern Treatment* (1602)

Stellariae Radix (yín chái hú)	4.5g
Anemarrhenae Rhizoma (zhī mǔ)	3g
Picrorhizae Rhizoma (hú huáng lián)	3g
Lycii Cortex (dì gǔ pí)	3g
Artemisiae annuae Herba (qīng hāo)	3g
Gentianae macrophyllae Radix (qín jiāo)	3g
vinegar-fried Trionycis Carapax (cù chǎo biē jiǎ)	3g
Glycyrrhizae Radix (gān cǎo)	1.5g

Method of Preparation The source text advises to take as a draft between meals. At present, it is usually prepared as a decoction with a doubling of the dosages.

Actions Clears heat from deficiency and alleviates steaming bone disorder

Indications

Afternoon tidal fever or unremitting, chronic low-grade fever, a sensation of heat in the bones but with flesh that is not warm to the touch, irritability, insomnia, emaciation, lethargy, red lips, dark-red cheeks, night sweats, thirst, a dry throat, a red tongue with little coating, and a thin, rapid pulse.

This is steaming bone disorder due to Liver and Kidney yin deficiency. Yin deficiency gives rise to fire, which disturbs the internal harmony of the body. The primary manifestations include afternoon tidal fever or unremitting, chronic low-grade fever. The Kidneys, which store the true yin and are associated with the bones, are affected by this condition. When fire from yin deficiency occurs at this level, the patient often experiences a subjective sensation of heat deep in the body (at the level of the bones), while the flesh itself is not necessarily warm to the touch. It is therefore called steaming bone disorder. The same process may also disturb the spirit and cause irritability and insomnia.

Long-term deficiency at the nutritive level, when further injured by blazing fire, leads to emaciation and lethargy. The deficient yin cannot control the yang, which allows the fire from deficiency to blaze upward where it manifests as red lips and dark-red cheeks. The deficient yin is unable to contain the fluids during the night (yin). It is at this time that the blazing fire from deficiency forces the fluids out of the body in the form of sweat. Yin deficiency also prevents the upper parts of the body from receiving moisture, giving rise to thirst and a dry throat. The red tongue with little coating and the thin, rapid pulse are classic signs of heat from yin deficiency.

Analysis of Formula

In this particular condition, although the yin must be nourished to ensure any lasting benefit, the primary focus should be on clearing the heat from deficiency. The substances that perform this function are different from the bitter, cold substances that clear heat from excess, as the latter would injure the yin. The distinction of this formula is that it utilizes most of the major substances that specifically clear heat from deficiency.

The chief ingredient, sweet and slightly cold Stellariae Radix *(yín chái hú)*, reduces the fever from deficiency without any of the draining tendencies that could further injure the yin. There are three deputies: Anemarrhenae Rhizoma *(zhī mǔ)*, which enriches the yin and clears heat from Kidney deficiency; Picrorhizae Rhizoma *(hú huáng lián)*, which clears heat from the blood level; and Lycii Cortex *(dì gǔ pí)*, which clears lingering heat from the Lungs above and heat from deficiency from the Liver and Kidneys below. These are the principal substances for clearing heat from deficiency and are especially useful in alleviating steaming bone disorder with sweating.

These herbs are supported by three assistants. The first is Artemisiae annuae Herba *(qīng hāo)*, which drains fire without injuring the qi or blood, and conducts heat at the level of the bones outward to the level of the muscles and the exterior. The second is Gentianae macrophyllae Radix *(qín jiāo)*, which clears heat from deficiency, especially from the Liver and Gallbladder. These two herbs vent heat externally, which

makes them a particularly useful combination for treating steaming bone disorder without sweating. The third assistant, salty and cold prepared Trionycis Carapax *(zhì biē jiǎ)*, enriches the yin, anchors the errant yang, and conducts the actions of the other herbs into the yin (deep) levels of the body. The formula's broad application is due to the combined actions of the chief, deputy, and assistant ingredients. The envoy, Glycyrrhizae Radix *(gān cǎo)*, harmonizes the actions of the other herbs and protects the Spleen and Stomach.

Commentary

The pattern for which this formula is indicated belongs to the class of deficiency consumption (虚勞 *xū láo*) disorders. This type of disorder is first mentioned in *Essentials from the Golden Cabinet*, written during the late Han. By the Song dynasty, the term had subsumed a large range of problems that included yin, yang, qi, and blood deficiencies as well as damage and harm to the yin and yang organs from both internal and external causes. Later generations of physicians tried to cull this profligacy by introducing a terminological differentiation between deficiency damage (虚損 *xū sǔn*), that is, disorders due to internal causes, and consumption sickness (癆瘵 *láo zhài*), which are disorders due to external pathogens. The present formula treats a particular manifestation of consumption sickness known as 'steaming bone disorder.' It presents with relatively severe heat from deficiency and is characterized by tidal fevers, emaciation, night sweats, a red tongue with little coating, and a rapid pulse.

The dynamic of such 'steaming' is succinctly analyzed in *Convenient Reader of Established Formulas* by the Qing dynasty physician Zhang Bing-Cheng:

> In terms of the disorder of steaming bones, the muscles and skin are not hot to the touch while there is a subjective sensation of heat within the bones that tends to issue from continuous steaming. Each night the five centers are irritable and hot. This arises from water being exhausted [so that] fire blazes because pathogenic heat lurks within the yin and blood. When [such a condition] persists, the more that yin is exhausted, the more that fire becomes overabundant. The more that fire becomes overabundant, the more that yin is exhausted. The [particular] momentum of this torment is that it continues until the yin is entirely spent. … Now, because the disorder begins with heat lurking within the yin, if one does not eliminate this heat, but vainly nourishes the yin, one does not get rid of the root of the disorder and will gain no benefit.

Comparison

> ➢ Vs. Sweet Wormwood and Soft-Shelled Turtle Shell Decoction Version 1 *(qīng hāo biē jiǎ tāng)*

Both formulas treat yin deficiency with heat and fever. However, Cool the Bones Powder *(qīng gǔ sǎn)* treats a process whereby heat lurking in the yin or blood 'steams' the yin to the outside, thereby progressively exhausting it. This momentum manifests in a fever from yin deficiency that appears to arise from within the bones and is accompanied by sweating as well as emanciation and other signs of heat from deficiency. Sweet Wormwood and Soft-Shelled Turtle Shell Decoction Version 1 (qīng hāo biē jiǎ tāng), on the other hand, treats a process whereby heat stagnates within the deep collaterals. This leads to night fevers and morning chills due to the diurnal movement of the body's yang qi, which at times aggravates and at times reduces the manifestations of constraint.

Biomedical Indications

With the appropriate presentation, this formula may be used to treat a variety of biomedically-defined disorders, primarily tuberculosis, but also postwound fevers.

Modifications

- For blood deficiency, add Angelicae sinensis Radix (dāng guī), Paeoniae Radix alba (bái sháo), and Rehmanniae Radix (shēng dì huáng). (source text)
- For coughing, add Asini Corii Colla (ē jiāo), Ophiopogonis Radix (mài mén dōng), and Schisandrae Fructus (wǔ wèi zǐ). (source text)
- For lack of appetite and soft stools indicating Spleen deficiency, remove bitter Picrorhizae Rhizoma (hú huáng lián), Gentianae macrophyllae Radix (qín jiāo), and Anemarrhenae Rhizoma (zhī mǔ) and add Lablab Semen album (biǎn dòu) and Dioscoreae Rhizoma (shān yào).
- For a pale and wan complexion, low voice, and shallow breathing, add Astragali Radix (huáng qí) and Codonopsis Radix (dǎng shēn).
- For more pronounced yin deficiency and less severe tidal fever, substitute Rehmanniae Radix (shēng dì huáng) for Picrorhizae Rhizoma (hú huáng lián) or use Great Tonify the Yin Pill (dà bǔ yīn wán).

Associated Formulas

清經散 （清经散）

Clear the Menses Powder

qīng jīng sǎn

SOURCE   *Fu Qing-Zhu's Women's Disorders* (17th century)

Moutan Cortex (mǔ dān pí) 6g
Paeoniae Radix alba (bái sháo) 6g
Rehmanniae Radix praeparata (shú dì huáng) 6g
Lycii Cortex (dì gǔ pí) 15g
Artemisiae annuae Herba (qīng hāo) 6g
Poria (fú líng) 3g
Phellodendri Cortex (huáng bǎi) 1.5g

Grind the ingredients into powder and take as a draft. May also be prepared as a decoction. Clears heat and cools the blood. For heat from deficiency leading to early periods with profuse, thick, and dark-red or purplish-red flow, irritability and a stifling sensation in

the epigastrium and abdomen, a red face, dry mouth, yellow urine, constipation, red tongue with a yellow coating, and a slippery, rapid pulse. This formula eliminates heat to prevent further injury to the yin and blood. When the blood becomes tranquil, the periods will resume their regular cycle.

地骨皮飲 （地骨皮饮）

Lycium Root Bark Drink

dì gǔ pí yǐn

SOURCE   *Shen's Book for Revering Life* (1773)

Lycii Cortex (dì gǔ pí) 60g
Bupleuri Radix (chái hú) 60g
Anemarrhenae Rhizoma (zhī mǔ) 7.5g
Glycyrrhizae Radix praeparata (zhì gān cǎo) 7.5g
Trionycis Carapax (biē jiǎ) 7.5g
Scutellariae Radix (huáng qín) 7.5g
Ginseng Radix (rén shēn) 7.5g
Poria rubra (chì fú líng) 15g

Grind the ingredients into a powder and take 6g as a draft with one piece of Zingiberis Rhizoma recens (shēng jiāng) and one piece of Mume Fructus (wūméi). Clears heat and nourishes the yin. For steaming bone disorder in children characterized by irritability in the diaphragm and palpitations. Also used for the later stages of cold damage disorders when the fever has not yet completely resolved.

秦艽鱉甲散 （秦艽鳖甲散）

Large Gentian and Soft-Shelled Turtle Shell Powder

qín jiāo biē jiǎ sǎn

Source   *Precious Mirror of Health* (Yuan dynasty)

Bupleuri Radix (chái hú) 30g
prepared Trionycis Carapax (zhì biē jiǎ) 30g
Lycii Cortex (dì gǔ pí) 30g
Gentianae macrophyllae Radix (qín jiāo) 15g
Angelicae sinensis Radix (dāng guī) 15g
Anemarrhenae Rhizoma (zhī mǔ) 15g

Method of Preparation   Grind the ingredients into a coarse powder and take in 15g doses with five leaves of Artemisiae annuae Herba (qīng hāo) and one piece of Mume Fructus (wū méi). At present, it is usually prepared as a decoction with a slight reduction in dosage.

Actions   Enriches the yin, nourishes the blood, clears heat, and alleviates steaming bone disorder

Indications

Night sweats, emaciation, red lips and cheeks, afternoon fevers, coughing with sticky yellow sputum or blood-streaked sputum, heat in the five centers, steaming bone fever, exhaustion, a faint, rapid pulse, and a red tongue with little coating.

This is wind consumption (風癆 *fēng láo*), a condition attributed to improper or unsuccessful treatment of an externally-contracted wind disorder in a patient with underlying yin deficiency. If yin is already deficient, improper treatment allows a wind pathogen to invade the interior of the body where it stirs up the body's yang qi and generates heat. Yin is unable to control wind-heat in the interior, which, due to its nature, moves toward the outside, taking with it the body's fluids. This pathology is most pronounced at night, when yin should be strong, causing night sweats. During the day, the same excess manifests in the form of steaming bone fever, red lips and cheeks, afternoon fevers, and heat in the five centers. As the yin becomes increasingly exhausted, the patient loses weight and becomes tired. Wind and fire mutually engender each other, scorching the Lungs to produce a dry cough with sticky sputum and, as the heat enters the blood, blood-streaked sputum. Heat and damage to the yin fluids are also reflected in the faint, rapid pulse and the red tongue that loses its coating.

Analysis of Formula

Treating a pattern where a deficiency of yin is aggravated by the invasion of a wind pathogen into the interior of the body requires a combined strategy of attack and tonification. Thus, the formula clears heat while enriching the yin and dispels wind while supporting the normal qi. This overall strategy is reflected in the synergistic pairing of Gentianae macrophyllae Radix (*qín jiāo*) and Trionycis Carapax (*biē jiǎ*), which are the chief substances in this formula. Acrid and bitter Gentianae macrophyllae Radix (*qín jiāo*) "treats wind, no matter whether it is old or new" (*Miscellaneous Writings of Famous Physicians*). It enters into the vessels as well as the collaterals and opens up areas of clumps in the interior and exterior. Trionycis Carapax (*biē jiǎ*) also enters the collaterals and bones to nourish the yin while focusing the action of Gentianae macrophyllae Radix (*qín jiāo*) on the interior.

Two other synergistic pairings support the actions of the chief herbs. Bupleuri Radix (*chái hú*) and Lycii Cortex (*dì gǔ pí*) serve as deputies to clear heat from deficiency and open the qi dynamic. The former "eliminates deficiency consumption irritability and heat by releasing and dispersing heat in the muscle layer" (*Origins of Medicine*). The latter is able to clear heat from within the bones and to drain fire from the Lungs. Anemarrhenae Rhizoma (*zhī mǔ*), which drains heat and enriches the yin, combines with Angelicae sinensis Radix (*dāng guī*), which nourishes and harmonizes the blood, in the role of assistants.

A small amount of Artemisiae annuae Herba (*qīng hāo*) is added to the formula in order to strengthen its ability to vent pathogenic heat. Sour and astringent Mume Fructus (*wū méi*), finally, has the dual task of reducing sweating and coughing while compensating for the actions of the acrid and

dispersing herbs in the formula. In this manner, the formula succeeds in getting rid of wind while nourishing the blood, addressing the cause while also preventing any relapse.

Cautions and Contraindications

Use of this formula is not indicated in cases of wind obstructing the exterior. It is contraindicated where the yin fluids are seriously exhausted, because the many acrid constituents in the formula may further aggravate such a condition.

Commentary

This formula was specifically composed to treat wind consumption (風癆 *fēng láo*), also known as Liver consumption (肝癆 *gān láo*). *Appendices to the Golden Cabinet* provides a useful definition:

> The disorder of wind consumption has steaming fever in the bones and muscles, alternating chills and fever, phlegm cough, night sweats, a yellow and emaciated [body], brittle hair, and foul breath. It may lead to childhood nutritional impairment with diarrhea. It comes about from a wind pathogen being stranded and stuck in the channels and collaterals [causing] constraint and stasis. This disorder frequently is associated with the Liver. It is therefore also called Liver consumption.

Other commentators, including Wu Kun and Xu Da-Chun, enlarge on this description and provide a clear account of the pathology that leads to its characteristic symptomatology. If the Liver blood is deficient, wind will readily invade into the interior of the body. Here the pathogen constrains the ministerial fire carried by the Liver. Ministerial fire then turns into pathological fire, leading to a process whereby two yang pathogens produce and reinforce each other to increase their destructive potential. Because this pathology centers on the Liver, the blood, and the vessels and collaterals, one may also see stiffness of the sinews, spasms of the extremities, pain and sensations of irritability in the joints, and weakness of the back and knees.

This analysis explains why the formula utilizes so many herbs that enter the Liver and dispel wind and heat from the channels and collaterals. The Qing-dynasty work *Collectanea of Investigations from the Realm of Medicine* by Wang Fu provides a vivid analogy:

> If a soup boils, one removes the lid [to let the steam] rise upward. Here yang is unable to be drawn out, becomes constrained, and thus heats internally. Gentianae macrophyllae Radix (*qín jiāo*), Bupleuri Radix (*chái hú*), Artemisiae annuae Herba (*qīng hāo*), and Mume Fructus (*wū méi*) act together to lift the lid [off this constraint to let the wind-heat] rise upward. How could the fire not be extinguished? The ministerial fire is a person's root of generation. [In treatment] one can [follow its] upward rising in order to expel [any excess]. One cannot restrain it to extinguish [wind and fire]. Why is the water not augmented? Enriching the yin has its [ability] to generate water, and when the fire is dispersed, the water will be able to enrich itself.

Comparison

➤ Vs. Sweet Wormwood and Soft-Shelled Turtle Shell Decoction Version 1 (*qīng hāo biē jiǎ tāng*)

Both formulas clear heat from deficiency, both focus on the Liver, and both treat fire arising from constraint due to the invasion of an external pathogen. However, Sweet Wormwood and Soft-Shelled Turtle Shell Decoction Version 1 (*qīng hāo biē jiǎ tāng*) focuses on lurking heat, whereas the present formula treats wind that has penetrated into the interior. For this reason, Sweet Wormwood and Soft-Shelled Turtle Shell Decoction Version 1 (*qīng hāo biē jiǎ tāng*) focuses on nourishing the fluids, which are more easily exhausted by heat. In fact, absence of sweating is one of the key indicators for the use of that formula. It also includes substances that vent heat. By comparison, the wind-dispersing characteristics of the present formula are much more pronounced. It also nourishes the blood rather than the fluids in order to harmonize the vessels and collaterals.

Biomedical Indications

With the appropriate presentation, this formula may be used to treat a variety of biomedically-defined disorders, primarily tuberculosis and fevers of unknown origin.

....

Alternate name

Large Gentian and Soft-Shelled Turtle Shell Decoction (*qín jiāo biē jiǎ yīn*) in *Six Texts on the Precis of Medicine*

....

Modifications

- For exhaustion of the yin fluids, add Rehmanniae Radix (*shēng dì huáng*).
- For pronounced sweating, add Astragali Radix (*huáng qí*).
- For pronounced coughing, add Fritillariae cirrhosae Bulbus (*chuān bèi mǔ*) and Trichosanthis Fructus (*guā lóu*).

當歸六黃湯 (当归六黄汤)
Tangkuei and Six-Yellow Decoction

dāng guī liù huáng tāng

The name of this formula is derived from its constituent herbs, which, except for Tangkuei, all include the word yellow in their names.

Source   *Secrets from the Orchid Chamber* (1336)

Angelicae sinensis Radix (*dāng guī*) 6-9g
Rehmanniae Radix (*shēng dì huáng*) 9-15g
Rehmanniae Radix praeparata (*shú dì huáng*) 9-15g
Coptidis Rhizoma (*huáng lián*) 3-6g
Scutellariae Radix (*huáng qín*) 6-12g
Phellodendri Cortex (*huáng bǎi*) 6-12g
Astragali Radix (*huáng qí*) 12-24g

Method of Preparation   The source text recommends grinding into a powder equal amounts of all the above ingredients, except for a double dosage of Astragali Radix (*huáng qí*), and taking 15g as a draft before meals. At present, it is more commonly taken as a decoction with the dosages indicated above.

Actions   Enriches the yin, drains fire, stabilizes the exterior, and stops sweating

Indications

Fever, night sweats, red face, dry mouth and parched lips, irritability, dry stools, dark and scanty urine, a red, dry tongue, and a rapid pulse.

This is night sweats due to raging fire in the interior with deficiency of blood and yin. The Heart is yang in that it is situated in the upper part of the trunk and is associated with fire. The Kidneys are yin in that they are situated in the lower part of the trunk and are associated with water. Normally, there is a give-and-take between these organs such that one regulates the other. In this disorder, however, there is an insufficiency of yin (water) which renders it incapable of properly controlling yang (fire), while raging fire above consumes water below.

During sleep, protective yang enters the nutritive yin; when the yin itself is deficient, it is unable to restrain the yang. This leads to instability of the exterior, especially at night. The unrestrained yang and the internal fire push the fluids out of the body in the form of sweat, which the deficient yin is unable to restrain. Fever and night sweats ensue. When the patient awakes, the protective yang leaves the nutritive yin and returns to the exterior so that the sweating stops. Ascending fire causes a red face, dry mouth, and parched lips. Because sweat is the fluid of the Heart, prolonged sweating injures the Heart yin, which manifests as irritability. Dry stools, dark and scanty urine, a red and dry tongue, and a rapid pulse are all characteristic of fire from deficiency.

Analysis of Formula

This formula enriches the yin and drains excess fire, but also stabilizes the exterior in order to control sweating. The chief herbs are Angelicae sinensis Radix (*dāng guī*), Rehmanniae Radix (*shēng dì huáng*), and Rehmanniae Radix praeparata (*shú dì huáng*). The first nourishes the blood and increases the fluids, which are then able to lubricate the Intestines and moisten the dry stools. The other two herbs enrich and nourish the yin fluids, blood, and essence. Sweet, bitter, and cooling Rehmanniae Radix (*shēng dì huáng*) is also particularly useful in treating heat from deficiency. Together, these herbs nourish water, which enables it to control the fire. One of the deputies, Coptidis Rhizoma (*huáng lián*), drains fire from the Heart. In concert with the other deputies, Scutellariae Radix (*huáng qín*) and Phellodendri Cortex (*huáng bǎi*), it relieves irritability and drains fire to remove the cause of damage to the yin. When the fire is drained, internal agitation will subside; and when the yin is fortified, the external draining of sweat will cease.

The severe, prolonged sweating injures the yang and destabilizes the protective qi in the exterior. To address this aspect of the disorder, a large dose of the assistant herb, Astragali Radix *(huáng qí),* is used to augment the qi and stabilize the exterior. This prevents excessive sweating from causing further injury to the yin and yang. It also protects the Stomach qi from the actions of the other herbs. In concert with Angelicae sinensis Radix *(dāng guī)* and Rehmanniae Radix praeparata *(shú dì huáng),* it makes a powerful combination for nourishing the qi and blood. When the qi and blood flourish, the interstices and pores tighten, and it is more difficult for sweat to improperly escape.

Cautions and Contraindications

This formula should be used with caution and in modified form, if at all, in cases with Spleen and Stomach deficiency.

Commentary

While the source text recommends this as "a sagely formula for the treatment of night sweats," it does not elaborate in any detail on the cause of the disease dynamic that it addresses. This was supplied by the Ming-dynasty physician Wu Kun in *Investigations of Medical Formulas:* "Yin deficiency with fire that causes people [to suffer from] night sweats is governed by this formula." By and large, this interpretation was accepted by later commentators and contemporary textbooks. In using this formula, it is important to understand, however, that while the formula nourishes the blood and enriches the yin, its bitter, cooling ingredients drain excess fire from the body. This implies that the formula does not treat sweating due to heat from deficiency but is for deficiency accompanied by excess fire. This dynamic is succinctly explained by the well-known Qing-dynasty author Xu Da-Chun in *Six Texts on the Precis of Medicine:* "When blood and qi are both exhausted, and fire disturbs the three burners, nutritive yin loses its defenses. How could there be no night sweats?"

In his analysis, Xu Da-Chun not only shows why the formula utilizes three bitter, cooling herbs (one associated with each of the three burners), but also resolves another question that has plagued commentators: How can one justify the use of the rather large dosage of Astragali Radix *(huáng qí),* a warming tonic that augments the functions of qi in the exterior, in a formula that treats yin deficiency? An answer can be deduced from other formulas composed by Li Dong-Yuan that also combine Astragali Radix *(huáng qí)* and Angelicae sinensis Radix *(dāng guī)* to treat conditions of deficiency in the exterior accompanied by internal heat, such as Tangkuei Decoction to Tonify the Blood *(dāng guī bǔ xuè tāng),*

discussed in Chapter 8. As shown there, Li Dong-Yuan uses Astragali Radix *(huáng qí)* to augment the qi in the exterior so that it can hold and direct the floating yang downward. This function is best understood by imagining Astragali Radix *(huáng qí)* not as an herb that raises the qi, but as one that tonifies the Lung qi and gathering qi, both of which direct the qi downward. The Lungs are also a check on the function of the Liver (as metal constrains wood), the organ associated with controlling the movement of yang qi throughout the three burners. Using Astragali Radix *(huáng qí)* to strengthen the Lungs is thus a useful adjunct to checking fire in the three burners by means of bitter, cooling herbs. An analysis of this process is provided by Ji Chu-Zhong, as recorded in *Discussion of Famous Physicians' Formulas Past and Present:*

> [Although] sweat fundamentally is the yin fluid [associated with] the Heart, its exiting and entering are related to the Liver and Lungs. The opening and closing of the nutritive level is managed by the Liver. The opening and closing of the protective level is managed by the Lungs. Given that both the nutritive and the protective have their own [kinds of] deficiency, they have their own [kinds of] sweating. The responsibility for yang deficiency sweating lies with the protective, that for yin deficiency sweating with the nutritive, and so they must mutually reinforce each other. If the protective qi is not secured in the exterior, this can arise from yin qi not [properly] storing. If nutritive qi is not being conserved in the center, this arises from yang qi not being [sufficiently] dense. Hence, there are two strategies for treating night sweats. In one, insufficient Liver blood leads to wood not generating fire such that the Heart also becomes deficient. Sour Jujube Decoction *(suān zǎo rén tāng)* [discussed in Chapter 10] tonifies the Liver, which will then tonify the Heart. In the other, [night sweats] are due to a surplus of Liver qi leading to wood insulting metal so that the Lungs also become deficient. Tangkuei and Six-Yellow Decoction *(dāng guī liù huáng tāng)* treats the Liver in order to treat the Lungs.

Some commentators, such as the modern physician Zhang Nian-Shun, go even further and argue that the formula was intended for night sweats associated with deficient protective qi coupled with vigorous fire that has injured the yin. Besides night sweats, this presentation includes fever, a red face, irritability, dark-yellow or red urine, a red tongue with a coating, and a flooding, rapid pulse. In this interpretation, because the deficiency of the protective qi is primary, Astragali Radix *(huáng qí)* is regarded as the chief herb, and because the deficiency of yin is due to vigorous fire, the heat-clearing herbs are regarded as deputies and the yin tonics as assistants.

Given that the actions of this formula in nourishing the yin and blood while draining fire from the three burners are rather strong, it is best used in cases where the middle qi has not been injured. It can be utilized in treating many types of disorders with night sweats including Lung consumption, steaming bone disorder, the aftermath of a severe febrile disease, and chronic nosebleeds.

Comparisons

➢ Vs. Tangkuei Decoction to Tonify the Blood (*dāng guī bǔ xuè tāng*); *see* page 340

➢ Vs. Oyster Shell Powder (*mǔ lì sǎn*); *see* page 422

Biomedical Indications

With the appropriate presentation, this formula may be used to treat a variety of biomedically-defined disorders including tuberculosis, diabetes, hyperthyroidism, perimenopausal syndrome, and nervous exhaustion.

Alternate name

Six Yellow Decoction (*liù huáng tāng*) in *Writings for Posterity of [Zhou] Shen-Zhai*

Modifications

• For especially severe sweating, add Ephedrae Radix (*má huáng gēn*) and Tritici Fructus levis (*fú xiǎo mài*).

• For yin deficiency without fire, remove Coptidis Rhizoma (*huáng lián*), Scutellariae Radix (*huáng qín*), and Phellodendri Cortex (*huáng bǎi*), and add Scrophulariae Radix (*xuán shēn*) and Ophiopogonis Radix (*mài mén dōng*).

• For tidal fever, dry mouth, a strong pulse at the rear position, and other signs of Kidney fire, add Testudinis Plastrum (*guī bǎn*) and Anemarrhenae Rhizoma (*zhī mǔ*)

百合地黃湯 (百合地黄汤)
Lily Bulb and Rehmannia Decoction

bǎi hé dì huáng tāng

Source   *Essentials from the Golden Cabinet* (c. 220)

Lilii Bulbus (*bǎi hé*) . . . . 7 bulbs (15-30g)
Rehmanniae Radix recens
   (*xiān dì huáng*) . . . . 1 cup of fresh juice (15-30g)

Method of Preparation   Decoction. The source text advises to wash the bulbs of Lilii Bulbus (*bǎi hé*), soak them overnight until white bubbles come out, and then discard the water before decocting them in 2 cups of spring water. When half the liquid has evaporated, discard the dregs and add 1 cup of juice from Rehmanniae Radix (*shēng dì huáng*). Decoct down until there are 1½ cups and take warm in divided doses. Once the disease has been affected, do not administer again. Usually after taking it, the stool is like lacquer.

At present, the formula is taken as a regular decoction with the dosage specified in parentheses, substituting Rehmanniae Radix (*shēng dì huáng*) for Rehmanniae Radix recens (*xiān dì huáng*). Tap water is used.

Actions   Moistens the Lungs, enriches the fluids, clears heat, and cools the blood

Indications

Mental disorientation, irritability, insomnia, palpitations, and other transient cognitive, sensory, and motor dysfunctions. These occur in the wake of an externally-contracted disorder and are accompanied by dark urine, a bitter taste in the mouth, and a slightly rapid pulse in a patient who has an otherwise normal appearance. The pulse is slightly rapid or weak and rapid, and the tongue will tend to have little coating.

This is the common manifestation of lily disorder (百合症 *bǎi hé zhèng*), first described in Chapter 3 of *Essentials from the Golden Cabinet*. The disorder is generally attributed to pathogenic heat entering the Lungs and penetrating into the nutritive or blood aspect. Because the nutritive and blood house the spirits or psychic aspects (五神 *wǔ shén*), heat at this level of the body will cause the spirits to become agitated and behave erratically. The dark urine and the bitter taste in the mouth point to the presence of pathogenic heat as the causative factor. However, because this heat has already damaged the yin and the qi, the pulse is either slightly rapid or weak and rapid, rather than forceful or flooding.

Analysis of Formula

To clear pathogenic heat from the body, this formula focuses on clearing heat via the urine and stools while simultaneously venting it from the nutritive and blood aspects by means of enriching the yin. The chief herb is sweet, slightly bitter, and cooling Lilii Bulbus (*bǎi hé*). Although modern materia medica list it as a tonifying herb, its classical usage is more complex, as explained by Zhang Shan-Lei in the following passage from *Rectification of the Meaning of Materia Medica*:

> Lilii Bulbus (*bǎi hé*) is sweet and cold, and is also a bitter, slippery, and moistening substance. Although the *Classic of the Materia Medica* calls it sweet and neutral, its main indications, ancient and modern, suggest that its nature is to clear heat, drain, and direct downward. When the *Classic of the Materia Medica* and *Miscellaneous Records* state that it 'governs pathogenic qi' and 'governs chills and fevers,' they are referring to a heat pathogen that has collected. [As to its treatment of the other symptoms] they are all due to its slippery, moistening ability to open up areas of clumping, and its unblocking, facilitating, draining, and guiding out actions. *Classic of the Materia Medica* also says that it tonifies the middle and augments the qi, and when texts like *Materia Medica of Ri Hua-Zi* state that it also quiets the spirit and strengthens the resolve, this refers to elimination of pathogenic heat and recovery of normal qi—it does not mean that sweet, cold substances tonify the qi.

The deputy herb is sweet and cooling Rehmanniae Radix (*shēng dì huáng*), or Rehmanniae Radix recens (*xiān dì huáng*) in the original formulation. It cools the heat in the blood, which disturbs the spirits, and enriches the yin fluids thereby venting heat from the nutritive and blood levels back toward the qi level from which it can be eliminated via the urine and bowels by the heat-clearing actions of Lilii Bulbus (*bǎi hé*). Together, this combination effectively eliminates pathogenic heat from the blood and nutritive levels without damaging the fluids through drying, or impeding the flow of qi through bitterness.

The spring water that the source text prescribes for the preparation of this decoction is described in the materia medica as being sweet and balanced and as possessing the therapeutic actions of resolving heat and harmonizing the middle burner. Used together with the main ingredients, it facilitates the downward-directing of heat to be cleared via the urine.

Cautions and Contraindications

This formula is not indicated for patterns presenting with excess fire in the Lungs and Heart, nor for patterns where yin deficiency is the main pathology.

Commentary

Originally this formula was designed to treat lily disorder (百合症 *bǎi hé zhèng*). Note that the word for lily in Chinese, 百合 *(bǎi hé)*, literally means one-hundred meetings. The manifestations of lily disorder (百合症 *bǎi hé zhèng*), for which this formula provides the basic method of treatment, were first described in Chapter 3 of *Essentials from the Golden Cabinet*.

> The hundred vessels all gather into one, [hence] each can lead to lily disorder. [Its presentation is as follows: The patient] desires food, yet does not want to eat; they are downcast and laconic; they want to lie down but are unable to lie down; they want to walk but are unable to walk. When they want to eat and drink, sometimes food can seem appetizing, but other times it stinks even before they smell it. They may feel cold yet have no chills; or they feel hot but have no fever. They have a bitter taste in the mouth and their urine is dark. The various medicines are ineffective and when they take medicine, there is intense vomiting and diarrhea. They are as if possessed. The physical appearance is normal, but the the pulse is faint and rapid.*

Over the centuries, comentators have struggled in various ways to explain the first part of this passage, which defines the disorder as rooted in pathophysiological changes arising from the one-hundred vessels, and to relate this to the manifestations described and the composition of the formula, with its focus on clearing heat and enriching fluids. Wei Li-Zhi in *The Original Meaning of Formulas Discussed in Essentials from the Golden Cabinet,* for instance, interprets the name of the disorder simply as pointing to the chief herb, Lilii Bulbus *(bǎi hé),* that is used to treat it. This is reflected in how we have rendered the disorder into English. Many other commentators, however, feel that the term 百 *bǎi* also, or even mainly, refers to the 'hundred vessels' (百脉 *bǎi mài*). The Qing-dynasty author You Yi, for instance, argues in *Personal Standards for the Essentials from the Golden Cabinet*: "The hundred vessels gather into one. When they divide, they be-

come the one-hundred vessels. When they join together, they become one gathering. Hence, if they become ill, there is nowhere in the body where the disease does not manifest."

Many commentators make a further connection between the first line of the source text and a passage in the *Inner Classic* that states that "the one-hundred vessels face the Lungs" (百脉朝肺 *bǎi mài cháo fèi*), although again this does not lead them to the same conclusions. Most contemporary textbooks, for example, explain the pathophysiology of this disorder as one of damage to Heart and Lung yin in the wake of febrile illness or caused by an emotional disorder where the lingering heat or fire from constraint have not been discharged. This analysis dates back to Qing-dynasty texts like *Golden Mirror of the Medical Orthodoxy* or *Rectification of the Meaning of the Golden Cabinet*, whose author, Zhang Shan-Lei, explains:

> This pattern is a result of a pathogenic influence interacting with the nutritive level of the Heart and the protective level of the Lungs. The Heart governs the hundred vessels, the Lungs govern the transformation of qi throughout the body. ... The reason that Lilii Bulbus *(bǎi hé)* is chosen in the treatment method ... is that the qi of Lilii Bulbus *(bǎi hé)* is extremely clearing, and enters the Lungs; its flavor is slightly bitter and enters the Heart; so it is most capable of clearing the upper burner, and thus serves as the chief.

There is also some controversy about a remark in the source text concerning when use of the formula should be stopped. Most commentators, including those who wrote *Golden Mirror of the Medical Tradition*, take the phrase in the source text 中病勿更服 *zhòng bìng wù gēng fú* as meaning "once [the formula] has gotten to the disease, do not give it again." They point out the fact that Rehmanniae Radix *(shēng dì huáng)*, if used long term, particularly when not required, can lead to dark, "lacquer-like" stools. Others, including Li Ke-Guang, a modern authority on *Essentials from the Golden Cabinet,* take the opposite view, stating that the phrase means "once [the formula] has gotten to the disease, do not change [the formula] administered."

This formula is just one of a range of formulas for the treatment of lily disorder listed in the source text. All are based on Lilii Bulbus *(bǎi hé)*, which is combined with heat-clearing substances such as Anemarrhenae Rhizoma *(zhī mǔ)* and Talcum *(huá shí)*, or heavy settlers like Haematitum *(dài zhě shí)*. The core pathology in all of these cases is that outlined above, but there is some difference as to the degree to which the presence of heat has damaged the yin and disordered the qi. Such differences arise from constitutional factors as well as from various kinds of inappropriate treatment explicitly referred to in the source text. For more detail on these formulas, see the VARIATIONS listed below.

Comparisons

➤ Vs. Licorice, Wheat, and Jujube Decoction
  (gān mài dà zǎo tāng)

---

* Note that this can also be read as "mildly rapid."

Both of these formulas are used in contemporary China to treat emotional and nervous system disorders characterized by symptoms such as insomnia, disorientation, confusion, or emotional instability. Licorice, Wheat, and Jujube Decoction (*gān mài dà zǎo tāng*), discussed in Chapter 10, treats restless organ disorder, a problem where the protective yang is no longer anchored by deficient nutritive yin and therefore begins to float away. For this reason, Licorice, Wheat, and Jujube Decoction (*gān mài dà zǎo tāng*) focuses on supplementing nutritive yin and holding on to floating yang. Lily disorder, on the other hand, is due to pathogenic heat that constrains the qi dynamic of the upper burner. For this reason, the various Bulbus Lily formulas focus on clearing qi from the Heart and Triple Burner via the urine as well as on nourishing yin.

➤ Vs. Lophatherum and Gypsum Decoction
   (*zhú yè shí gāo tāng*)

Both this formula and Lophatherum and Gypsum Decoction (*zhú yè shí gāo tāng*) can treat late-stage feverish disorders where an external pathogen has been resolved but some pathogenic heat remains in the body to cause symptoms such as irritability, restlessness, insomnia, and disorientation. However, Lophatherum and Gypsum Decoction (*zhú yè shí gāo tāng*) treats patterns where the pathogenic heat is located primarily in the Stomach and yang brightness warp and phlegm is present. The various Bulbus Lily formulas, on the other hand, focus on heat in the Triple Burner and Heart that is resolved via promoting urination. Thus, in clinical practice, this formula is useful in treating a wide variety of disorders manifesting with confusion and disorientation in both emotional and organic disease.

Biomedical Indications

With the appropriate presentation, this formula may be used to treat a variety of biomedically-defined disorders including the late stages of acute febrile diseases, perimenopausal syndrome, neuroses, autonomic dystonia, sleep walking, and hysteria. The formula, as well as some of its variations, have also been used to treat confusion associated with uremia, hepatic coma, and diabetes.

Modifications

- For damage to the fluids in the wake of a high fever causing insomnia, a dry throat, and irritability from heat without form, add Pseudostellariae Radix (*tài zǐ shēn*), Ziziphi spinosae Semen (*suān zǎo rén*), Ostreae Concha (*mǔ lì*), Polygoni multiflori Caulis (*yè jiāo téng*), and Talcum (*huá shí*) to promote clearing of heat via the urine and to calm the spirits.
- For hyperactive Heart fire and yin deficiency, combine with Bupleurum plus Dragon Bone and Oyster Shell Decoction (*chái hú jiā lóng gǔ mǔ lì tāng*) in order to nourish the blood and tonify deficiency.

- For Lung dryness and heat with cough, add Ophiopogonis Radix (*mài mén dōng*), Glehniae/Adenophorae Radix (*shā shēn*), Fritillariae Bulbus (*bèi mǔ*), and Glycyrrhizae Radix (*gān cǎo*).
- For lily disorder complicated by plum-pit qi, combine with Pinellia and Magnolia Bark Decoction (*bàn xià hòu pò tāng*).

Variations

百合知母湯 （百合知母汤）
Lily Bulb and Anemarrhena Decoction
bǎi hé zhī mǔ tāng
SOURCE   *Essentials from the Golden Cabinet* (c. 220)

Replace Rehmanniae Radix (*shēng dì huáng*) with Anemarrhenae Rhizoma (*zhī mǔ*) when the symptoms of heat have been mistaken for signs of a greater yang disorder, and the patient was improperly treated with the sweating method, which exhausts the yang fluids to produce dryness and exacerbates heat from constraint. This formula is particularly useful for treating lily disorder with pronounced symptoms involving the upper burner such as insomnia, dizziness, or heat clogging the Lungs with cough and restlessness.

――――――

滑石代赭湯 （滑石代赭汤）
Talcum and Hematite Decoction
huá shí dài zhě tāng
SOURCE   *Essentials from the Golden Cabinet* (c. 220)

Replace Rehmanniae Radix (*shēng dì huáng*) with Talcum (*huá shí*) and Haematitum (*dài zhě shí*) when the symptoms of heat have been mistaken for signs of a yang brightness disorder, and the patient was thus improperly purged. This damages the Stomach qi and causes it to rebel upward, leading to symptoms such as occasional retching or vomiting, while the heat remaining in the body leads to dry throat, thirst, and rough urination with dark urine. Compared to the principal formula, this variation focuses more strongly on directing the qi downward and on dispelling heat from the Triple Burner.

――――――

百合雞子黃湯 （百合鸡子黄汤）
Lily Bulb and Egg Yolk Decoction
bǎi hé jī zi huáng tāng
SOURCE   *Essentials from the Golden Cabinet* (c. 220)

Replace Rehmanniae Radix (*shēng dì huáng*) with egg yolk (*jī zi huáng*) when the symptoms related to appetite have been mistaken for phlegm lodged in the Stomach, and the patient was thus improperly induced to vomit. This damages the Spleen and Stomach yin and also adversely affects the downward-directing functions of the Lungs and Stomach, which manifests as increased irritability and restlessness, palpitations, and a feeling as if one were about to die accompanied by a rapid pulse. Compared to the principal formula, this more strongly nourishes the yin and essence, and focuses particularly on the middle burner and the Heart.

百合滑石散

Lily Bulb and Talcum Powder

bǎi hé huá shí sǎn

Source   *Essentials from the Golden Cabinet* (c. 220)

Replace Rehmanniae Radix (*shēng dì huáng*) with Talcum (*huá shí*)

when the problem is accompanied by a fever. This is attributed to strong constraint in the Triple Burner. The formula is taken as a powder to aid in its ability to disperse heat from constraint. Compared to the principal formula, this variation is stronger at clearing and directing heat downward. It is not indicated for long-term use because it can readily damage the yin fluids and must therefore be discontinued as soon as the fever begins to abate.

Comparative Tables of Principal Formulas

■ FORMULAS THAT CLEAR QI-LEVEL HEAT

Common symptoms: fever, irritability, thirst, red tongue, rapid pulse

Formula Name	Diagnosis	Indications	Remarks
White Tiger Decoction (*bái hǔ tāng*)	Blazing heat in the yang brightness channel warp	High fever, profuse sweating, aversion to heat, severe thirst, irritability, a red tongue with either a dry white or a yellow coating, and a flooding, forceful, or slippery and rapid pulse	Also treats headache, toothache, or bleeding of the gums and nose.
Lophatherum and Gypsum Decoction (*zhú yè shí gāo tāng*)	Qi-level heat lingering in the Lungs and Stomach	Lingering fever accompanied by vomiting, irritability, thirst, parched mouth, stifling sensation in the chest, a red tongue with little coating, and a deficient, rapid pulse	Primarily focuses on clearing heat and only secondarily on tonifying the qi and fluids; often occurs in the aftermath of a febrile disease.
Gardenia and Prepared Soybean Decoction (*zhì zǐ chǐ tāng*)	Qi-level heat lingering in the superficial aspects of the yang brightness warp (the muscles and chest)	Fever, irritability, insomnia with tossing and turning in bed, a stifling sensation in the chest with a soft epigastrium, hunger with no desire to eat, slightly yellow tongue coating, and a slightly rapid pulse, or a strong, floating pulse at the distal position	Focuses on eliminating constrained heat by simultaneously venting it outward and directing it downward.

■ FORMULAS THAT CLEAR HEAT FROM THE NUTRITIVE LEVEL AND COOL THE BLOOD

Common symptoms: fever (that worsens at night), irritability, a dry, scarlet tongue, a thin, rapid pulse

Formula Name	Diagnosis	Indications	Remarks
Clear the Nutritive-Level Decoction (*qīng yíng tāng*)	Heat entering the nutritive level	High fever that worsens at night, severe irritability and restlessness, a scarlet, dry tongue, and a thin, rapid pulse	Depending on the level of penetration, some patients may be thirsty, delirious, or exhibit faint and indistinct erythema and purpura.
Clear the Palace Decoction (*qīng gōng tāng*)	Externally-contracted warm pathogen disorder with damage to the yin fluids of the Heart	Fever, impaired consciousness, disordered speech, and a crimson tongue without coating	This is a serious pattern of pathogenic heat sinking into the Pericardium.
Rhinoceros Horn and Rehmannia Decoction (*xī jiǎo dì huáng tāng*)	Heat entering the blood level	Fever, various types of bleeding (including vomiting of blood, nosebleed, blood in the stool or urine, and rashes), black and tarry stools, abdominal distention and fullness, thirst with an inability to swallow, a scarlet tongue with prickles, and a thin, rapid pulse	Some patients become delirious. Widely used in gynecology, pediatrics, dermatology and ophthalmology for problems due to both heat and blood stasis.

■ FORMULAS THAT CLEAR HEAT AND RESOLVE TOXICITY

Common symptoms: fever, dryness/thirst, dark urine, rapid pulse, red tongue, redness and swellings of some type

Formula Name	Diagnosis	Indications	Remarks
Coptis Decoction to Resolve Toxicity *(huáng lián jiě dú tāng)*	Severe obstruction of the three burners by fire toxin	High fever, irritability, a dry mouth and throat, incoherent speech, insomnia, dark urine, a red tongue with a yellow coating, and a rapid, forceful pulse	Also for nosebleed due to heat excess, toxic swellings, and dysenteric disorders or jaundice due to damp-heat. Focuses on draining heat.
Drain the Epigastrium Decoction *(xiè xīn tāng)*	Damp-heat excess with interior clumping	Fever, irritability, restlessness, flushed face, red eyes, dark urine, constipation, a greasy, yellow tongue coating, and in severe cases, delirious speech	Also for epigastric focal distention, jaundice, dysenteric disorders, nosebleed, ulcerations or abscesses. Focuses on draining heat from the three burners, primarily through the stool.
Universal Benefit Drink to Eliminate Toxin *(pǔ jì xiāo dú yǐn)*	Epidemic toxin associated with wind-heat and damp-phlegm	Strong fever and chills, redness, swelling, and burning pain of the head and face, dysfunction of the throat, dryness and thirst, a red tongue with a powdery-white or yellow coating, and a floating, rapid, and forceful pulse	This is acute, massive febrile disorder of the head; focuses on relieving the toxic fire and dispersing wind-heat.
Cool the Diaphragm Powder *(liáng gé sǎn)*	Unformed blazing heat in the upper burner and formed accumulation in the middle burner	Sensation of heat and irritability in the chest and abdomen, thirst, flushed face, mouth/tongue sores, sore throat, nosebleed, constipation, scanty urine, red tongue body or edges with a dry and yellow or white coating, and a rapid, possibly slippery pulse	Also for various skin disorders and childhood convulsions. Focuses on clearing heat and reducing accumulation.

■ FORMULAS THAT SIMULTANEOUSLY CLEAR HEAT FROM THE QI AND BLOOD LEVELS

Common symptoms: high fever, thirst, red tongue with yellow coating, rapid pulse; both formulas can be used for carbuncles or other toxic swellings

Formula Name	Diagnosis	Indications	Remarks
Clear Epidemics and Overcome Toxicity Drink *(qīng wēn bài dú yǐn)*	Severe fire in the qi and blood levels	Intense fever, strong thirst, dry heaves, severe and stabbing headache, extreme irritability, scorched lips, a dark-red tongue, and a rapid pulse that is either submerged and thin or floating and large	Severe cases may present with delirious speech, rashes, and nosebleed.
Transform Maculae Decoction *(huà bān tāng)*	Heat entering into the qi and blood levels	Fever that worsens at night, a dark-red macular rash, thirst, yellow tongue coating, and a rapid pulse	Treats maculae that result from heat in the yang brightness and blood levels.

■ FORMULAS THAT CLEAR HEAT FROM THE ORGANS

Common indications for heat in the Lungs: fever, cough and wheezing, sinus pain or nasal congestion, red tongue with a yellow coating, and a rapid pulse

Formula Name	Diagnosis	Indications	Remarks
Ephedra, Apricot Kernel, Gypsum, and Licorice Decoction (*má xìng shí gān tāng*)	Heat lodged in the Lungs	Fever with or without sweating, thirst, wheezing, coughing, labored breathing, nasal flaring and pain, a thin and white or yellow tongue coating, and a rapid pulse that can be floating or slippery	Focuses on clearing heat and directing qi downward. Especially useful in children.
Drain the White Powder (*xiè bái sǎn*)	Lurking fire due to constrained heat in the Lungs	Coughing, wheezing, fever, and skin that feels hot to the touch (all of which worsen in the late afternoon), dry mouth, little or difficult-to-expectorate sputum, a red tongue with a yellow coating, and a thin, rapid pulse	Commonly used to treat children.
Magnolia Flower Drink to Clear the Lungs (*xīn yí qīng fèi yǐn*)	Stagnant heat in the Lungs	Nasal congestion or polyps with a red, coated tongue and a rapid pulse	Treats a wide range of nasal disorders.

Common indications for heat in the Spleen and Stomach: oral lesions or bleeding, dry mouth, red tongue

Formula Name	Diagnosis	Indications	Remarks
Drain the Yellow Powder (*xiè huáng sǎn*)	Lurking fire in the Spleen	Mouth ulcers, bad breath, thirst, frequent hunger, dry mouth and lips, a red tongue, and a rapid pulse	Also treats tongue thrusting in children, and yellowing of the sclera due to Spleen heat.
Clear the Stomach Powder (*qīng wèi sǎn*)	Heat accumulation in the Stomach	Toothache (especially when the pain extends into the head), facial swelling, fever, bad breath, dry mouth, a red tongue with little coating, and a slippery, large, and rapid pulse	Also treats bleeding/sores of the gums, and swollen, painful tongue, lips, or jaw. Areas of pain respond favorably to cold, and worsen with heat.
Jade Woman Decoction (*yù nǚ jiān*)	Kidney yin deficiency with vigorous Stomach fire	Toothache, loose teeth, bleeding gums, frontal headache, irritability, fever, thirst for cold beverages, a dry, red tongue with a yellow coating, and a floating, slippery, deficient, and large pulse	For wasting and thirsting disorder from deficiency.

Common indications for heat in the Heart: irritability, scanty/painful urination, red tongue, rapid pulse

Formula Name	Diagnosis	Indications	Remarks
Guide Out the Red Powder (*dǎo chì sǎn*)	Heat in the Heart and Small Intestine channels	Irritability with a sensation of heat in the chest, thirst with a desire to drink cold beverages, red face, possibly sores around the mouth, a red tongue, and a rapid pulse	Also used for dark, scanty, rough, and painful urination, or even clearly visible blood in the urine.
Clear the Heart Drink with Lotus Seed (*qīng xīn lián zǐ yǐn*)	Flourishing Heart fire with qi and yin deficiency	Seminal emission, turbid painful urinary dribbling, profuse uterine bleeding, and vaginal discharges (all of which are aggravated by overexertion)	There may also be signs of kidney yin deficiency with a dry mouth and tongue, irritability, and fever. Mixed excess and deficiency pattern.

Common indications for heat in the Liver: hypochondriac pain, bitter taste, dark urine, red tongue with a yellow coating, a wiry, rapid pulse

Formula Name	Diagnosis	Indications	Remarks
Gentian Decoction to Drain the Liver *(lóng dǎn xiè gān tāng)*	Heat excess in the Liver and/or Gallbladder channels	Pain in the hypochondria, headache, dizziness, red and sore eyes, hearing loss, swelling in the ears, bitter taste, irritability, short temper, a wiry, rapid, and forceful pulse, and a red tongue with a yellow coating	Also for difficult, painful urination with a sensation of heat in the urethra, swollen and pruritic external genitalia, or foul-smelling leukorrhea.
Drain the Green Pill *(xiè qīng wán)*	Constrained fire in the Liver channel	Red, sore, and swollen eyes, restlessness and irritability, dark urine, constipation, and a flooding, excessive pulse	Tremors or convulsions may also be present. Relatively strong formula for clearing heat and draining fire.
Tangkuei, Gentian, and Aloe Pill *(dāng guī lóng huì wán)*	Liver and Gallbladder fire excess	Headache, vertigo, restlessness, delirious speech, mania, and fright wind in children; often there is also constipation and dark, rough urination, or blockage of the throat with difficulty swallowing	Extremely cold and draining formula that focuses on directing fire downward in order to control the qi.
Left Metal Pill *(zuǒ jīn wán)*	Liver and Stomach disharmony from heat in the Liver channel	Hypochondriac pain, indeterminate gnawing hunger, epigastric focal distention, vomiting, acid reflux, bitter taste, dry mouth, a red tongue with a yellow coating, and a wiry, rapid pulse	Focuses on draining Liver heat and clearing Stomach fire.

Common indications for heat in the Intestines: abdominal pain, tenesmus, diarrhea with blood and/or pus, burning sensation around the anus, red tongue with a yellow coating, rapid pulse

Formula Name	Diagnosis	Indications	Remarks
Peony Decoction *(sháo yào tāng)*	Dysenteric disorder due to damp-heat lodged in the Intestines	Abdominal pain, tenesmus, difficulty with defecation, diarrhea with pus and blood (equal amounts), a burning sensation around the anus, dark, scanty urine, a greasy, slightly yellow tongue coating, and a rapid pulse	Combined focus on clearing damp-heat and regulating the qi.
Scutellaria Decoction *(huáng qín tāng)*	Dysenteric disorder due to heat constraint in the lesser yang moving into the Stomach and Intestines	Fever, a bitter taste in the mouth, abdominal pain, diarrhea, red tongue with yellow coating, and rapid or flooding pulse	Also for spontaneous diarrhea resulting from a combined disease of the greater and lesser yang warps.
Pulsatilla Decoction *(bái tóu wēng tāng)*	Hot dysenteric disorder due to heat toxin searing the Stomach and Intestines	Abdominal pain, tenesmus, burning sensation around the anus, diarrhea containing more blood than pus, thirst, red tongue with a yellow coating, and a wiry, rapid pulse	For terminal yin-warp dysenteric disorders due to heat. Also treats painful or bloody urinary disfunction and acute eye disorders.

■ FORMULAS THAT CLEAR HEAT FROM DEFICIENCY

Common symptoms: emaciation, night or afternoon fever, red tongue with little coating, a thin, rapid pulse

Formula Name	Diagnosis	Indications	Remarks
Sweet Wormwood and Soft-Shelled Turtle Shell Decoction (Version 1) (*qīng hào biē jiǎ tāng*)	Heat lurking in the yin aspects of the body	Night fever and morning coolness with no sweating as the fever recedes, emaciation with no loss of appetite, a red tongue with little coating, and a fine, rapid pulse	Often occurs in the aftermath of a febrile disease.
Cool the Bones Powder (*qīng gǔ sǎn*)	Steaming bone disorder due to Liver and Kidney yin deficiency	Afternoon tidal fever or unremitting, chronic low-grade fever, sensation of heat in the bones but with flesh that is not warm to the touch, irritability, insomnia, emaciation, lethargy, dark-red cheeks, night sweats, thirst, a dry throat, a red tongue with little coating, and a thin, rapid pulse	Focuses on clearing heat rather than tonifying the yin.
Large Gentian and Soft-Shelled Turtle Shell Powder (*qín jiāo biē jiǎ sǎn*)	Pathogenic wind penetrating the interior with preexisting yin deficiency	Night sweats, emaciation, red lips and cheeks, afternoon fever, coughing with sticky yellow sputum or blood-streaked sputum, heat in the five centers, steaming bone fever, exhaustion, a red tongue with little coating, and a faint, rapid pulse	This is wind consumption, also known as Liver consumption.
Tangkuei and Six-Yellow Decoction (*dāng guī liù huáng tāng*)	Raging fire in the interior with deficiency of blood and yin	Fever, night sweats, red face, dry mouth and parched lips, irritability, dry stools, dark and scanty urine, a red, dry tongue, and a rapid pulse	Specifically for night sweats that may accompany various disorders including Lung consumption, steaming bone disorder, the aftermath of a severe febrile disease, and chronic nosebleeds.
Lily Bulb and Rehmannia Decoction (*bǎi hé dì huáng tāng*)	Pathogenic heat entering the Lungs and penetrating into the nutritive or blood aspect	Mental disorientation, irritability, insomnia, palpitations, dark urine, a bitter taste in the mouth, a tongue with little coating, and a slightly rapid pulse in a patient with an otherwise normal appearance	Specifically for lily disorder.

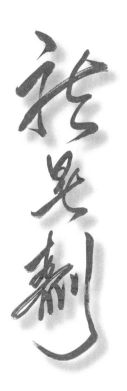

Chapter 5 Contents

Formulas that Dispel Summerheat

....

Formulas that Dispel Summerheat

THE FORMULAS IN this chapter dispel summerheat (暑 shǔ). Although summerheat is especially prevalent in late summer, like other seasonal pathogens it may also appear before or after its associated season. The 19th-century writer Wang Shi-Xiong defines summerheat as a pathogen that is entirely yang in nature and posseses no yin. Its effects on the body are dispersing, activating, and ascending. By inducing high fever and profuse sweating (the interstices and pores stay open more in the summer), summerheat injures the fluids, causing thirst and irritability. Because qi follows the fluids, their loss leads to qi deficiency with fatigue, shortness of breath, and even collapse.

Because the summer season is often accompanied by an increase in humidity, summerheat is generally accompanied by dampness. This, in fact, is one of the key features of summerheat damage that distinguishes it from warm-heat pathogen disorders. The latter occur closer in time to the spring and are more often accompanied by wind. *Basic Questions,* Chapter 31, notes: "With respect to cold damage that manifests as warm disorders, those of the early summer are warm pathogen diseases, those of the late summer are summerheat diseases. Summerheat exits via sweating. Therefore, [sweating should not be] impeded."

During hot spells, the increased consumption of cold beverages and exposure to drafts (attempts to 'cool off') are also conducive to the invasion of cold, either through the exterior or directly to the Spleen and Stomach. This can trap summerheat inside and prevent it from being vented to the outside. Effective treatment of summerheat disorders therefore requires that attention be given not only to cooling, but also to measures that reestablish the normal qi dynamic. These may include dispersal with acrid, warming or acrid, cooling herbs, augmenting the qi with warming and drying herbs, and generating fluids with sweet and cooling herbs.

Because dampness often accompanies summerheat, most of these formulas contain herbs that dry dampness or promote urination. If relieving summerheat is the primary strategy, the dosage of herbs that resolve dampness should be relatively low to avoid further injury to the fluids; if drying dampness is the primary focus, the dosage of herbs that relieve summerheat should not be too high since the cold, sweet nature of such herbs can generate more dampness.

Historically, summerheat disorders were long treated as a subcategory of cold damage disorders with formulas such as White Tiger Decoction *(bái hǔ tāng)* and its variants, discussed in Chapter 4. The first specialized formulas for the treatment of summerheat damage date to the Song dynasty. During the ensuing Jin-Yuan period, physicians like Zhang Yuan-Su and Li Dong-Yuan discussed summerheat damage in relation to its effect on the qi dynamic. By the early Qing, formulas for the treatment of summerheat damage were sufficiently recognized that Wang Ang, in *Medical Formulas Collected and Analyzed,* included a special section devoted just to them.

Between the 16th and 19th centuries, physicians associated with the warm pathogen disorder current in Chinese medicine developed entirely new approaches to the treatment of summerheat disorders. These drew on the work of the early 17th-century physician Zhang He-Teng, whose *Complete Treatise on Summerheat Damage* was the first specialist textbook on the subject. Zhang's ideas had little impact during his own lifetime but exerted great influence on the thinking of later physicians like Ye Tian-Shi, who observed in *Case Records as a Guide to Clinical Practice*: "Zhang [He-Teng] says that during the early stages of summerheat disorders one utilizes acrid, cooling [herbs. If the disorder] progresses, one uses sweet, cooling [herbs]. Furthermore, one also uses sour, discharging and sour, astringing [herbs]." Warm pathogen disorder therapeutics thus focused to a much greater extent than before on styles of treatment that ensured the healthy physiological functioning of the body fluids.

The five categories of formulas in this chapter represent a summary of these various strategies. A number of other formulas are regularly used in the treatment of summerheat disorders, but for historical reasons are included in other formula categories. They include White Tiger Decoction (*bái hǔ tāng*) and White Tiger plus Ginseng Decoction (*bái hǔ jiā rén shēn tāng*) (Chapter 4), Generate the Pulse Powder (*shēng mài sǎn*) (Chapter 8), and Sweet Dew Special Pill to Eliminate Toxin (*gān lù xiāo dú dān*) (Chapter 16).

Section 1

....

FORMULAS THAT DISPEL SUMMERHEAT AND CLEAR HEAT

The formulas in this section are indicated for relatively mild and superficial disorders characterized primarily by high fever, body heat, irritability, restlessness, sweating, thirst, and other heat symptoms. For this reason, they rely primarily on light, acrid or aromatic, cooling herbs such as Lonicerae Flos (*jīn yín huā*), Nelumbinis Folium (*hé yè*), and Lablab Flos (*biǎn dòu huā*). Summerheat readily damages the Heart and is often associated with dampnes. Thus, *Assorted Works from Enlightened Physicians* advises: "The best strategy for treating summerheat disorders is to clear the Heart and facilitate urination." Accordingly, herbs like Lophatheri Herba (*dàn zhú yè*) and Talcum (*huá shí*) are usually included in these formulas. More severe summerheat damage requires the use of more strongly cooling formulas such as the various modifications of White Tiger Decoctions (*bái hǔ tāng*), discussed in Chapter 4.

清絡飲（清络饮）
Clear the Collaterals Drink

qīng luò yǐn

The source text notes that this formula clears a lingering pathogen from the collaterals of the Lungs. The decoction may be drunk as a tea during the summer to prevent injury from summerheat.

Source *Systematic Differentiation of Warm Pathogen Diseases* (1798)

Lonicerae Flos recens (*xiān jīn yín huā*)..................6g
Lablab Flos recens(*xiān biǎn dòu huā*)..................6g
Citrulli Exocarpium (*xī guā*)..................6g
Luffae Fructus Retinervus (*sī guā luò*)..................6g
Nelumbinis Folium recens (*xiān hé yè*)..................6g
Lophatheri Herba (*dàn zhú yè*)..................6g

Method of Preparation Decoction. The source text advises to decoct the herbs in 2 cups of water until 1 cup remains. Two doses are taken per day.

Actions Resolves summerheat and clears the Lungs

Indications

Fever, mild thirst, unclear head and vision with lightheadedness and slight distention of the head, and a pink tongue with a thin, white coating.

This is mild summerheat injuring the qi level of the Lung channel or a summerheat-warmth pathogen that has not been fully released by sweating. The fever, mild thirst, and normal tongue reflect a mild, relatively superficial condition. The slight presence of dampness is reflected in the head symptoms. The location of these symptoms in the head, the most yang aspect of the body, is further evidence that the condition is confined to the superficial levels of the body.

Analysis of Formula

Cool, aromatic Lonicerae Flos recens (*xiān jīn yín huā*), one of the chief herbs, relieves summerheat. It "clears wind, fire, dampness, and heat from the collaterals and resolves pestilential, filthy turbid pathogens" (*Jottings from Repeated Celebration Hall*). The other chief herb, Nelumbinis Folium recens (*xiān hé yè*), clears and cools summerheat, facilitates the ascent of clear yang, and is an important herb for treating head symptoms like dizziness, headache, and muzziness due to turbid dampness obstructing the sensory orifices. It also stops thirst, generates yang fluids, and stops vomiting, diarrhea, and other symptoms associated with dampness obstructing the middle burner. Entering the Lung, the chief herbs combine to vent pathogenic qi from its collaterals to the exterior.

The chief herbs are assisted by two deputies that serve complementary functions. Aromatic Lablab Flos recens (*xiān biǎn dòu huā*) clears and disperses summerheat while strengthening the Spleen and harmonizing the Stomach. Citrulli Exocarpium *(xī guā)* is sweet and cooling, and thus better at relieving summerheat, stopping thirst, and generating fluids. The assistants are Luffae Fructus Retinervus *(sī guā luò)*, which specifically clears and vents the collaterals of the Lung, and Lophatheri Herba *(dàn zhú yè)*, which clears the Heart and promotes the smooth functioning of the water pathways. The latter herb also prevents summerheat from entering the Heart, and opens the way for the pathogenic influence to exit the Lung, the upper source of the water pathways.

Commentary

Fresh, aromatic herbs are used to relieve summerheat and eliminate the accompanying dampness. Not only is this because fresh herbs are more aromatic than the dried variety, but in China, such herbs are usually fresh during the summer season. Only small quantities of these herbs are used to gently relieve the summerheat, dispel the heat, and resolve the slight dampness in this mild, superficial condition. This action is reinforced by using flowers, leaves, and peels. All of the herbs thus resonate with the Lung, the body's most tender yin organ, while their floating nature naturally vents lingering pathogens toward the exterior. This is what Wu Ju-Tong, the author of the formula, meant when he wrote, in *Systematic Differentiation of Warm Pathogen Diseases*, "One treats the upper burner like a feather. Unless one's [touch] is light, one cannot grasp it."

Because the same dosage is used for all herbs, commentators disagree about which is the chief herb. Lonicerae Flos recens *(xiān jīn yín huā)* and Nelumbinis Folium recens *(xiān hé yè)* appear to be the two herbs that most closely match Wu Ju-Tong's stated intention of venting heat without form from the qi level in the upper burner. This intention—and its potential uses—are poetically described by the modern physician Ruan Xue-Feng in the following passage from *Annotated Fine Formulas from Generations of Famous Physicians*:

> If one examines this formula's [ability] to clear with cooling and aromatic [herbs], it appears to resemble Mulberry Leaf and Chrysanthemum Drink *(sāng jú yǐn)* yet does not disperse the exterior; it appears to resemble White Tiger Decoction *(bái hǔ tāng)* yet does not congeal [with] heavy [herbs]; it appears to resemble Six-to-One Powder *(liù yī sǎn)* yet does not clear [heat] through discharging. If [someone with] a summerheat pattern has already sweated, it is unnecessary to again vent the deficient exterior. If summerheat symptoms have already diminished, it is unnecessary to again clear the interior with very cold [herbs]. As the remnants of the pathogen have not yet been completely cleared up, one should not thicken the constraint by [premature] moistening and irrigating. Light, nimble, clearing, and aromatic [herbs] are sufficient to extinguish any flaring of the remaining cinders and calm any gleaming of the [pathogenic] qi. Dispersing [the pathogen] without dispersing [herbs], clearing [heat] without clearing [herbs], discharging [dampness] without discharging [herbs], the foul turbidity is naturally calmed and luxuriance naturally returns.

This kind of analysis provides us with deepened understanding. Not only for summerheat disorders, not only for the collaterals of the Lung, but for all kinds of heat patterns that move toward resolution [and] yet heat spreads to the collaterals from which it has not been cleared, one can adopt variations [of this strategy].

Biomedical Indications

With the appropriate presentation, this formula may be used to treat a variety of biomedically-defined disorders including hyperthermia, heat stroke, and rheumatic fever.

Modifications

- For a nonproductive cough with a clear, high pitch, add Glycyrrhizae Radix *(gān cǎo)*, Platycodi Radix *(jié gěng)*, Ophiopogonis Radix *(mài mén dōng)*, and Armeniacae Semen *(xìng rén)*.
- For summerheat in the exterior and dampness in the interior reflected in fever and chills with a lack of thirst and vomiting of blood, add Armeniacae Semen *(xìng rén)*, Talcum *(huá shí)*, and Coicis Semen *(yì yǐ rén)*.

Associated Formulas

五葉蘆根湯（五叶芦根汤）

Reed Decoction with Five Leaves

wǔ yè lú gēn tāng

SOURCE   *Writings on Damp-Heat Pathogen Diseases* (1852)

Pogostemonis/Agastaches Folium *(huò xiāng yè)* 6g
Menthae haplocalycis Herba *(bò hé)* 1.8g
Benincasae Semen *(dōng guā zǐ)* 15g
Eupatorii Folium *(pèi lán yè)* 4.5g
Eriobotryae Folium *(pí pá yè)* 15g
Phragmitis Rhizoma *(lú gēn)* 30g

Decoction. Disseminates upper burner yang qi and scours out summerheat with light, clearing, aromatic, and bland herbs. For mild damp-heat patterns characterized by fever, sweating, a slight stifling sensation in the chest and upper abdomen, hunger without a desire to eat, a bland taste, slight thirst but without an actual desire to drink, soft stools, hot urine, a mixed white and yellow tongue coating that is thin and sticky, and a pulse that is soggy on the right and slightly rapid on the left. This is damp-heat obstructing the clear yang in the upper burner, inhibiting the Lung's function of clarifying by directing downward. Like the main formula, Reed Decoction with Five Leaves *(wǔ yè lú gēn tāng)* relies on light herbs to disseminate the yang qi of the upper burner. However, because the dampness in this pattern is more pronounced, it also utilizes a treatment principle, first formulated by Ye Tian-Shi, that one should dispel dampness from below the heat. This is the function of Benincasae Semen *(dōng guā zǐ)* and Phragmitis Rhizoma *(lú gēn)*.

薷杏湯 （薷杏汤）

Mosla and Apricot Kernel Decoction

rú xìng tāng

Source *Selected Formulas for Warm-Heat Pathogen Diseases* (c. 1900)

Moslae Herba *(xiāng rú)* 2.4g
Armeniacae Semen *(xìng rén)* 4.5g
Forsythiae Fructus *(lián qiáo)* 4.5g
Augment the Primal Powder
  (yì yuán sǎn) . . . . [wrapped in a fresh lotus leaf] 9g
fresh Lophatheri Herba *(xiān dàn zhú yè)* . . . . 30 leaves
Luffae Folium *(sī guā yè)* 9g
Citrulli Praeparatio *(xī guā shuāng)* 30g
Lonicerae Flos *(jīn yín huā)* 60g

Decoction. Clears the upper burner while disseminating and facilitating the Lung qi to expel summerheat. For summerheat entering through the nose, attacking the protective qi, and accosting the Lungs characterized by a distended feeling in the head, a dirty complexion, fever without sweating, a burnt sensation in the body, dry mouth and teeth, incomplete and irregular bowel movements, yellow and reduced urination, a thin, dry, white tongue coating, and a pulse that is rapid and floating on the right but feels deficient if stronger pressure is applied.

This formula was composed by the early modern physician He Lian-Chen based on case records by Ye Tian-Shi. Compared to the main formula, it treats a pattern characterized by more severe heat obstructing the dissemination of Lung qi. As a result, the pores become obstructed, leading to severe heat just below the surface and rapid damage to the yang fluids. Although this is a potentially serious condition, it can be addressed with a small number of light herbs that open the surface to cause a light sweat. This strategy is known as 'light herbs being able to remove excess' (輕可去實 *qīng kě qù shí*). Compared with the principal formula, the chief herbs Moslae Herba *(xiāng rú)* and Armeniacae Semen *(xìng rén)* focus directly on the Lung qi and not merely on the collaterals of the Lung. Compared with Newly Augmented Mosla Drink *(xīn jiā xiāng rú yǐn)*, on the other hand, this formula is more light and nimble.

Note: Luffae Folium *(sī guā yè)* is bitter and slightly cold. It is used to clear heat and resolve toxicity, stop bleeding, and dispel summerheat. It is used for a wide variety of sores, bites, and burns, and for bleeding from trauma, as well as summerheat with irritability and thirst. At present, the normal dosage is 6-15g (15-60g when used fresh).

Section 2

FORMULAS THAT DISPEL SUMMERHEAT AND RESOLVE THE EXTERIOR

Attempts to 'cool off' during the heat of the summer, be it with the help of cold drinks, air conditioning, or cold showers, can easily lead to the contraction of wind-cold or wind-dampness. If the pathogen fetters the exterior, the diffusion of yang is constrained. If the damage is to the middle burner, the Spleen and Stomach lose their harmonious function. The clear yang no longer ascends while heat is trapped inside. Such pathologies require the use of acrid, warming herbs like Moslae Herba *(xiāng rú)* or Pogostemonis/Agastaches Herba *(huò xiāng)* that dispel summerheat and resolve the exterior. Depending on the nature of the accompanying signs and symptoms, these are combined with bitter herbs that dry interior dampness and strengthen the Spleen's transformative functions, such as Magnoliae officinalis Cortex *(hòu pò)*, Lablab Semen album *(biǎn dòu)*, and Coptidis Rhizoma *(huáng lián)*; or with acrid, cooling herbs that disperse qi constraint in the upper burner, such as Forsythiae Fructus *(lián qiáo)* or Lonicerae Flos *(jīn yín huā)*.

香薷散

Mosla Powder

xiāng rú sǎn

Source *Formulary of the Pharmacy Service for Benefiting the People in the Taiping Era* (1107)

Moslae Herba *(xiāng rú)* 480g (9-12g)
dry-fried Lablab Semen album *(chǎo biǎn dòu)* 240g (6-9g)
ginger Magnoliae officinalis Cortex *(jiāng hòu pò)* . . .240g (6-9g)

Method of Preparation Grind into a coarse powder and take 9g as a draft. Traditionally, a small amount of wine (equal to about one-tenth of the liquid in the draft) is added and the mixture is taken cold. May also be prepared as a decoction with the dosage indicated in parentheses.

Actions Releases the exterior, scatters cold, transforms dampness, and harmonizes the middle burner

Indications

Chills with skin that is warm to the touch, an absence of sweating, a sensation of heaviness in the head, headache, abdominal pain, vomiting, diarrhea, a stifling sensation in the chest, fatigued extremities, a white, greasy tongue coating, and a floating pulse.

This is exterior cold with interior dampness contracted in the summer. During the summer, the exterior may be affected by exposure to sudden cool breezes, and the interior may be injured by overconsumption of cold food or beverages. The combination of exterior cold and interior dampness causes a heavy, painful sensation in the head. The hot weather and interior dampness join in constraining the yang qi, leading to chills along with a warm, almost burning sensation in the skin. The cold and dampness condense in the abdomen, causing abdominal pain. They also attack the Spleen, which disrupts the ascending and descending of the qi dynamic, causing nausea and vomiting or diarrhea. Qi dysfunction and dampness produce a stifling sensation in the chest. The Spleen, which governs the extremities, cannot support them when it is encumbered by cold and dampness. This loss of support causes fatigue in the extremities. The white, greasy tongue coating reflects the presence of cold and dampness, while the floating pulse reflects an exterior condition.

Analysis of Formula

This condition requires simultaneous treatment of the exterior and interior. The chief herb, Moslae Herba *(xiāng rú)*, a warm, acrid, and aromatic substance, attacks the major aspects of this condition. It releases the exterior, harmonizes the ascending and descending functions of the Spleen, and disperses stagnant fluids by dispelling cold and dampness from the middle burner. The deputy, Lablab Semen album *(biǎn dòu)*, assists the chief herb by ameliorating the effects of summertime dampness on the Spleen. It also strengthens the Spleen, primarily by causing the turbid fluids and products of food transformation to descend, and the clear to ascend. The assistant, Magnoliae officinalis Cortex *(hòu pò)*, expels dampness and disperses fullness.

Cautions and Contraindications

The use of this formula in those with summerheat, other than yin summerheat, will severely injure the fluids and qi, increase heat in the body, and significantly aggravate the condition.

Commentary

This formula was originally designed for Spleen and Stomach disharmony due to both internal and external pathogens. These combine to cause a breakdown of the qi dynamic characterized by qi constraint, accumulation of dampness, and failure of the clear qi to ascend. According to Li Shi-Zhen, its indication was later extended to the treatment of summerheat disorders, and he was concerned that it would be used without the proper differentiation among various types of summerheat.

According to Zhang Jie-Bin, summerheat disorders can be differentiated into yin and yang types. Yin summerheat is caused by contraction of cold during the summer and is therefore a cold damage disorder. Should this occur, the cold would constrain the expansive dynamic of yang qi either in the exterior or in the middle burner, the fulcrum of the qi dynamic. This can happen very easily in the summer because the pores and interstices are open, and the upward and outward dynamic of qi leaves the interior relatively deficient. If exterior obstruction is predominant, a warm, dispersing, aromatic opening is indicated. If ingestion of cold food or drink has damaged the qi dynamic, warming of the center is most

important. Yang summerheat, on the other hand, is caused by the invasion of heat or damp-heat and therefore belongs to the category of warm pathogen disorders. It should be treated by clearing the heat, expelling the dampness, and supplementing the qi and fluids.

It follows that Mosla Powder *(xiāng rú sǎn)* is indicated for only the yin or cold type of summerheat. This is reflected in the warm, acrid nature of its constituent herbs. In fact, the chief herb in this formula, Moslae Herba *(xiāng rú)*, was characterized by Li Shi-Zhen as the summer equivalent of Ephedrae Herba *(má huáng)* because of its ability to stimulate sweating and release exterior cold. He also cautioned that to improperly use it in the treatment of yang summerheat would be harmful.

Given its original indication, this formula may be considered appropriate for any patient with a presentation of exterior cold and interior dampness, regardless of the season. It is especially useful in those patients with vomiting and diarrhea because of its action on the middle burner. However, its strongly aromatic nature can cause vomiting (particularly when taken warm) in patients with turbid dampness in the interior. For this reason, the draft or decoction should be allowed to cool before ingestion.

Comparisons

➤ Vs. Newly Augmented Mosla Drink *(xīn jiā xiāng rú yǐn)*; see page 238

➤ Vs. Patchouli/Agastache Powder to Rectify the Qi *(huò xiāng zhèng qì sǎn)*; see page 693

➤ Vs. Harmonize the Six Decoction *(liù hé tāng)*; see page 696

Biomedical Indications

With the appropriate presentation, this formula may be used to treat a variety of biomedically-defined disorders including acute gastroenteritis, bacillary dysentery, encephalitis B, enteric cholera, and acute tonsilitis.

....

Alternate Names

Mosla Decoction *(xiāng rú tāng)* in *Comprehensive Recording of Sagely Beneficence*; Mosla Drink *(xiāng rú yǐn)* in *Discussion of Formulas from Straight Directions from [Yang] Ren-Zhai*; Three-Substance Mosla Drink *(sān wù xiāng rú yǐn)* in *Medical Formulas Collected and Analyzed*

....

Modifications

• For a stronger exterior presentation, add Artemisiae annuae Herba *(qīng hāo)*.

• For severe cold with nasal obstruction, combine with Scallion and Prepared Soybean Decoction *(cōng chǐ tāng)*.

Variations

四味香薷飲 (四味香薷饮)

Four-Ingredient Drink with Mosla

sì wèi xiāng rú yǐn

SOURCE *Book to Safeguard Life Arranged According to Pattern* (1108)

Add ginger juice-fried Coptidis Rhizoma (*jiāng zhī huáng lián*) for interior dampness transformed into heat characterized by thirst and irritability.

五物香薷飲 (五物香薷饮)

Five-Substance Drink with Mosla

wǔ wù xiāng rú yǐn

SOURCE *Medical Formulas Collected and Analyzed* (1682)

Add Poria (*fú líng*) and Glycyrrhizae Radix (*gān cǎo*) for severe dampness in the interior characterized by abdominal distention and diarrhea.

六味香薷飲 (六味香薷饮)

Six-Ingredient Drink with Mosla

liù wèi xiāng rú yǐn

SOURCE *Medical Formulas Collected and Analyzed* (1682)

Add Chaenomelis Fructus (*mù guā*) to the previous formula if there is also stiffness in the calves.

Associated Formula

黃連香薷飲 (黄连香薷饮)

Coptis and Mosla Drink

huáng lián xiāng rú yǐn

SOURCE *Handed-Down Rare and Treasured Formulas* (Song dynasty)

Coptidis Rhizoma (*huáng lián*) 9g
Magnoliae officinalis Cortex (*hòu pò*) 9g
Olibanum (*rǔ xiāng*) 6g

The source text advises to mix Magnoliae officinalis Cortex (*hòu pò*) with 12g of Zingiberis Rhizomatis Succus (*jiāng zhī*), pestle into a paste, and fry until the color changes to purple. This is ground into a coarse powder with the remaining ingredients. Decoct 9g of this powder with 1 cup of water and 1 cup of wine until 1 cup remains. Let the sediment settle and drink the decoction cold twice a day. At present, it is prepared as a decoction to which Zingiberis Rhizoma recens (*shēng jiāng*) is added.

Resolves the exterior and disperses cold, dispels summerheat, and eliminates irritability. For consumption of cold food and drink that injures the Spleen and Stomach leading to sudden turmoil disorder with spasmodic diarrhea and vomiting, a squeezing pain in the central abdomen, cold sweats over the entire body, frigid extremities, restlessness, thirst, and an inability to settle down.

Compared to the original formula, Coptidis and Mosla Drink (*huáng lián xiāng rú yǐn*) combines equal amounts of cooling and warming herbs. This makes it suitable for patterns characterized by severe damp-heat in the interior with such symptoms as thirst, restlessness, and agitation. In contemporary practice, this condition may be caused by the cold wind from air conditioning systems attacking the exterior, trapping summerheat dampness in the interior. This formula is often effective for patterns characterized by a strong constitution, fever without chills, headache, uncomfortable limbs, focal distention, and nausea.

. . . .

Alternate names

The original name of this formula was Matchless Mosla Powder (*wú bǐ xiāng rú sǎn* 無比香薷散). It is listed as Mosla Powder (*xiāng rú sǎn* 香薷散) in *Book to Safeguard Life Arranged According to Pattern*, but later came to be known by its present name to differentiate it from other formulas of the same name.

十味香薷飲 (十味香薷饮)

Ten-Ingredient Drink with Mosla

shí wèi xiāng rú yǐn

SOURCE *Restoration of Health from the Myriad Diseases* (1587)

Moslae Herba (*xiāng rú*) 30g (9g)
prepared Astragali Radix (*zhì huáng qí*) 15g (6g)
Ginseng Radix (*rén shēn*) 15g (6g)
Atractylodis macrocephalae Rhizoma (*bái zhú*) 15g (6g)
Citri reticulatae Pericarpium (*chén pí*) 15g (6g)
Poria (*fú líng*) 15g (6g)
Chaenomelis Fructus (*mù guā*) 15g (6g)
ginger-fried Magnoliae officinalis Cortex (*jiāng chǎo hòu pò*) 15g (6g)
dry-fried Lablab Semen album (*chǎo biǎn dòu*) 15g (9g)
Glycyrrhizae Radix praeparata (*zhì gān cǎo*) 15g (6g)

Grind into a coarse powder and take as a draft. May also be prepared as a decoction, commonly with the dosages given in parentheses above. Releases exterior cold, transforms interior dampness, augments the qi, and strengthens the Spleen. For externally-contracted damp-cold characterized by mild fever and chills and relatively profuse sweating. The source text prescribes it for conditions contracted during the summertime. Compared to the original formula, Ten-Ingredient Drink with Mosla (*shí wèi xiāng rú yǐn*) treats excess and deficiency in equal measure. It is suitable for patients with preexisting Spleen deficiency and dampness who then contract a summerheat disorder. In this respect, the present formula is similar to Li Dong-Yuan's Clear Summerheat and Augment the Qi Decoction (*qīng shǔ yì qì tāng*), discussed later in this chapter. However, that formula focuses on summerheat dampness that has injured the qi and fluids. For this reason, it combines herbs that augment the qi and transform dampness with those that generate fluids. It does not treat patterns where a pathogen is also obstructing the exterior. Ten-Ingredient Drink with Mosla (*shí wèi xiāng rú yǐn*) focuses specifically on such a pattern, resolving the exterior as well as dispelling dampness from the interior. Furthermore, it is indicated for conditions marked by dampness where the body fluids themselves have not been damaged.

新加香薷飲（新加香薷饮）

Newly Augmented Mosla Drink

xīn jiā xiāng rú yǐn

Source   *Systematic Differentiation of Warm Pathogen Diseases* (1798)

Moslae Herba (*xiāng rú*) 6g
Lablab Flos recens (*xiān biǎn dòu huā*) 9g
Lablab Semen album (*biǎn dòu*). .9g
Magnoliae officinalis Cortex (*hòu pò*) 6g
Lonicerae Flos (*jīn yín huā*). 9g
Forsythiae Fructus (*lián qiáo*). .6g

Method of Preparation   Decoction. The source text advises to decoct the herbs with 5 cups of water until 2 cups remain. Take 1 cup to induce sweating and then another cup if sweating does not occur. The process is repeated if this still fails to induce sweating.

Actions   Dispels summerheat, releases the exterior, clears heat, and transforms dampness

Indications

Fever and chills without sweating, headache, thirst, flushed face, a stifling sensation in the chest, a heavy and aching body, dark and rough urination, a red tongue with a white, greasy tongue coating, a flooding pulse on the right and a small pulse on the left.

This is severe, early-stage summerheat in the Lung greater yin with superimposed contraction of cold fettering the exterior. It commonly occurs in the summer due to the gradual accumulation of damp-heat that is trapped by newly-contracted cold or wind-cold. When cold fetters the protective yang in the exterior the pores become blocked. This manifests as chills without sweating and headache. Constrained summerheat in the greater yin causes fever, a flushed face, and thirst. The simultaneous presence of dampness is reflected in a heavy and aching body. Damp-heat causes the Lungs and Triple Burner to lose their ability to direct fluids downward, which manifests as a stifling sensation in the chest and dark, rough urination. A red tongue with a white, greasy coating represents heat being constrained by cold and dampness. A flooding pulse indicates the presence of heat in the interior, while a short pulse on the left reflects the constraint of protective yang that cannot ascend toward the exterior via the lesser and greater yang.

Analysis of Formula

This is a variation of Coptidis and Mosla Decoction (*huáng lián xiāng rú yǐn*), also known as Mosla Drink (*xiāng rú yǐn*), in which Coptidis Rhizoma (*huáng lián*) has been replaced with Lonicerae Flos (*jīn yín huā*) and Forsythiae Fructus (*lián qiáo*). In this pattern, interior heat is located predominantly in the Lung greater yin (the upper burner). A bitter,

downward-draining herb like Coptidis Rhizoma (*huáng lián*) could easily cause the pathogen to move deeper into the body. To avoid this, the formula uses only light, cooling, and acrid herbs that thrust out the pathogen from the exterior.

The chief herb is acrid, warm, and aromatic Moslae Herba (*xiāng rú*). It enters the Lung collaterals to disperse the constraint of the protective yang. It also facilitates urination to aid in the resolution of dampness. Three deputies combine to clear summerheat. The first, Lablab Flos recens (*xiān biǎn dòu huā*), is aromatic and slightly cold. It disperses pathogens and resolves summerheat without damaging the fluids. If Lablab Flos recens (*xiān biǎn dòu huā*) is unavailable, the source text suggests the use of Lablab Testa recens (*xiān biǎn dòu yī*). Forsythiae Fructus (*lián qiáo*) and Lonicerae Flos (*jīn yín huā*) are both light, acrid, and cooling and vent wind-heat and foul turbidity through the exterior. Magnoliae officinalis Cortex (*hòu pò*) is added as an assistant, mindful of the adage that "Without warmth, dampness cannot be transformed." Moreover, its acrid, warming nature balances the acrid, cooling nature of the deputies.

Cautions and Contraindications

This formula is intended to induce sweating. It should not be used when fever is accompanied by sweating and must be discontinued once sweating occurs. For best effects, the decoction should be taken cold. Long-term use is not advised.

Commentary

This formula is another example of how physicians associated with the warm pathogen current in Chinese medicine adjusted established formulas to serve a new understanding of pathology. One of the most important innovations of the warm pathogen disorder current is the importance accorded to the Lung greater yin at the onset of externally-contracted disorders. Previously, damp-heat disorders, including summerheat, had been approached primarily through a focus on the functions of the Spleen and Stomach. Physicians such as Ye Tian-Shi, Xue Sheng-Bai, and Wu Ju-Tong argued that as long as pathogens had not yet entered the middle burner (absence of digestive symptoms), treating the middle burner could actually prolong the course of the illness by causing a pathogen to fall inward.

These physicians developed a style of treatment that relied on acrid and light herbs to thrust out pathogens that were obstructing the Lung greater yin. As Wu Ju-Tong noted in *Systematic Differentiation of Warm Pathogen Diseases*, "The position of the Lungs is the highest [in the body]. Herbs that are too heavy go past the place where the disorder is [actually] located."

The presentation for which Newly Augmented Mosla Drink (*xīn jiā xiāng rú yǐn*) is indicated mimics that of a cold damage disorder in its combination of chills, fever, body aches, and absence of sweating. Thus, some commentators, like the Qing-dynasty physician Zhang Bing-Cheng in *Convenient Reader of Established Formulas,* referred to this pattern as summerheat-wind. This description also draws our attention to factors like air conditioning that can be a major cause of this pattern in contemporary practice.

Comparison

➢ Vs. Mosla Powder *(xiāng rú sǎn)*

Both formulas treat summerheat disorders where cold constrains the diffusion of protective yang. Mosla Powder *(xiāng rú sǎn)* calls for a much larger dose of the chief herb Moslae Herba *(xiāng rú)* and uses wine to further augment the warming and dispersing properties of the formula. It strengthens the middle burner and is suitable for cases where cold has damaged the greater yin Spleen. Newly Augmented Mosla Drink *(xīn jiā xiāng rú yǐn)* utilizes a smaller dose of Moslae Herba *(xiāng rú)* and adds acrid, cooling herbs as deputies. It focuses on thrusting pathogens out from the greater yin Lung and is indicated for conditions characterized by more severe heat signs such as irritability, restlessness, and a flushed face.

Biomedical Indications

With the appropriate presentation, this formula may be used to treat a variety of biomedically-defined disorders including the common cold, influenza, acute gastroenteritis, and bacillary dysentery.

Modifications

- For more severe fever, add Artemisiae annuae Herba *(qīng hāo)* and Talcum *(huá shí)*.
- For heat flaring in the interior, add Rhei Radix et Rhizoma *(dà huáng)*.
- For more pronounced dampness, add Pogostemonis/ Agastaches Herba *(huò xiāng)* and Poria *(fú líng)*.

Section 3

FORMULAS THAT DISPEL SUMMERHEAT AND FACILITATE THE RESOLUTION OF DAMPNESS

Dampness frequently accompanies summerheat. When it is a significant factor, the patient will present with such symptoms as focal distention, a stifling sensation in the chest, muscle aches, heaviness of the body, nausea, diarrhea, and reduced urination. In these cases, treatment strategies that facilitate the resolution of dampness must accompany the dispelling of summerheat. Because dampness obstructs the

qi transformation of the Triple Burner, herbs that clear heat, facilitate urination, and do not damage the yin, such as Talcum *(huá shí)*, Gypsum fibrosum *(shí gāo)*, and Glauberitum *(hán shuǐ shí)*, are of primary importance. They may be combined with other herbs that facilitate the resolution of dampness, such as Alismatis Rhizoma *(zé xiè)* and Poria *(fú líng)*; with sweet herbs that relax, harmonize, and clear heat, such as Glycyrrhizae Radix *(gān cǎo)*; or with herbs that warm the yang to facilitate qi transformation, like Cinnamomi Ramulus *(guì zhī)*.

六一散

Six-to-One Powder

liù yī sǎn

This name is said to be derived from the ratio of the two ingredients in the formula.

Source *Formulas from the Discussion Illuminating the Yellow Emperor's Basic Questions* (1172)

Talcum *(huá shí)*
Glycyrrhizae Radix *(gān cǎo)*

Method of Preparation Grind six parts Talcum *(huá shí)* and one part Glycyrrhizae Radix *(gān cǎo)* into a powder and take 9-18g with warm water, or prepare as a decoction by placing the ingredients in a cheese cloth bag. The source text advises to use Glycyrrhizae Radix praeparata *(zhì gān cǎo)*.

Actions Clears summerheat, resolves dampness, and augments the qi

Indications

Fever, sweating, thirst, irritability, urinary difficulty, diarrhea, nausea, vomiting, a thin, yellow, and greasy tongue coating, and a soggy, rapid pulse. The formula also treats a range of other presentations including painful urinary dribbling and stony painful urinary dribbling due to damp-heat in the Bladder, and damp-heat skin disorders like papules, sores, and prickly heat.

Summerheat is a yang pathogenic influence whose nature is to ascend, disperse, and damage the yin fluids, which leads to fever and thirst. Associated with fire among the five phases, it readily disturbs the Heart and thereby gives rise to irritability. The combination of summerheat injuring the qi and dampness obstructing the interior gives rise to damp-heat, which disrupts the movement of qi and fluids within the Triple Burnner. The clear no longer ascends and the turbid no longer descends. When this impedes the middle burner, it manifests as nausea, vomiting, or diarrhea. If it impinges on the functioning of the Bladder, various types of painful urinary dribbling may present. If damp-heat accumulates in the skin and flesh, damp-heat skin disorders may result. The tongue signs reflect relatively mild summerheat-dampness, as does the soggy (damp) and rapid (summerheat) pulse.

Analysis of Formula

The proper treatment of summerheat requires an outlet. If accompanied by dampness, summerheat can be relieved by promoting urination. The chief ingredient, cold, bland Talcum (huá shí), clears summerheat and facilitates the resolution of dampness. Its nature is heavy, and it therefore directs downward. It is also slippery and able to facilitate passage through the apertures, be they the pores of the skin above or the urinary orifices below. Thus, Li Shi-Zhen considered Talcum (huá shí) to be an herb for clearing pathogenic heat from the entire Triple Burner, one whose actions were not limited to promoting urination. The deputy, Glycyrrhizae Radix (gān cǎo), harmonizes the middle and has a mild ability to clear heat and resolve toxicity. This combination not only promotes urination, but also generates fluids, thereby enabling the formula to perform its tasks without injuring the qi or fluids.

Cautions and Contraindications

Because this formula may injure the qi and fluids, use with caution when treating weak, elderly, or yin-deficient patients. Contraindicated in cases with copious, clear urine or in summerheat without dampness.

Commentary

This formula treats a yang-type summerheat disorder in Zhang Jie-Bin's two-fold classification scheme. Its author is Liu Wan-Su, one of the four great masters of the Jin-Yuan period, widely known for his focus on heat and fire pathogens. Liu Wan-Su recommended the formula for a wide range of conditions characterized by heat in the interior, matching the equally wide-ranging influence of Talcum (huá shí) on the Triple Burner.

> [This formula] treats body fever, vomiting, dysentery, diarrhea, Intestinal lumps with red and white dysentery, urinary blockage, and painful urinary dysfunction. It promotes urination but is particularly [useful] for stony painful urinary dribbling. … It [also] dissipates qi accumulation, unblocks the nine orifices and six yang organs, generates body fluids, removes stoppage and clumping, eliminates built-up water, stops thirst, eases the middle, eliminates irritability, heat, palpitations, abdominal distention, pain, and stifling [sensations]. It tonifies and augments the five yin organs and greatly nourishes the qi of Spleen and Kidneys. … In the interior, [it treats] internal damage [leading to] impotence. It calms the ethereal soul and settles the corporeal soul, [tonifies] all deficiency, and treats convulsions, fright palpitations, and forgetfulness. It stops irritability, fullness, shortness of breath, and coughing due to damage of the yin organs. [It helps where] food is not descending, pain in the muscles and flesh, mouth ulcers, and tooth decay. It brightens the ears and eyes, strengthens the sinews and bones, unblocks the blood vessels, harmonizes the blood and qi, reduces fluids and foodstuffs, safeguards the primal true [qi], [increases] endurance at work, labor, hunger and thirst, and dissipates heat by opening up the middle in all cases of external pathogen damage. Prolonged administration strengthens the resolve, lightens the body, preserves one's looks, and promotes longevity. Finally, it resolves summerheat stroke, cold damage, and epidemic [disorders], consumptive harm due to hunger, overeating, or any of the seven emotions, and fever left over after epidemic disorders or sweating. [It treats] recurrent consumption and resolves twice-contracted cold damage. It is able to dissipate and unblock clumps and stagnation throughout the body, and once the qi is harmonious, [the disease] will be cured.

As this lengthy passage shows, Liu Wan-Su attributed the formula's effectiveness to its ability to unblock clumping and stagnation, that is, to restore the normal physiological dissemination of qi and fluids throughout the entire body. This action centers on the physiology of the Triple Burner, which guides fluids downward from the Lungs above to the Bladder below. This intention is underlined by the deeper meaning of the formula's diverse names, outlined by the modern historian Zhao Cun-Yi in *Study of the Formula Names of Ancient Formulas in Chinese Medicine*:

> The name [of this formula] is 'six [to] one' not 'one [to] six.' [As in imperial China one wrote from top to bottom, this means that] the trigram of heaven 乾 [qián, which carries the number 1] stands below that for earth 坤 [kūn, which carries the number 6]. [Restoring] communication between yin and yang, the name [embodies the functioning of] the supreme Dao. Another name is Heaven Water Powder (天水散 tiān shuǐ sǎn). Heaven corresponds to the first [trigram] and generates water, which takes shape on earth, the sixth [trigram]. This has the meaning of [connecting] yin and yang. It is also called Augment the Primal Powder (益元散 yì yuán sǎn). By dispelling accumulated heat from the middle [burner] it benefits the qi that is primal to everything. Another name is Magical White Powder (神白散 shén baí sǎn) because the color [of the powder] is white and its [effects] are magical.

Earlier writers, such as the Ming-dynasty physician and teacher of Ye Tian-Shi, Wang Zi-Jie, had pointed out in *Selected Annotations to Ancient Formulas from the Garden of Crimson Snow* that the term 'white' refers to qi and the Lungs. Therefore, the formula

> empowers the clarifying, downward-directing of metal, so that its effects in treating summerheat-dampness pathogens damaging the upper burner are rapid. In the lower burner, its power to clear the waterways, flush heat, and leach dampness is also unmatched by other medicines.

To enhance its effectiveness in treating damp-heat pathologies constraining the Triple Burner, Liu Wan-Su also recommended that Six-to-One Powder (liù yī sǎn) be combined with other herbs to direct it toward specific areas of the body or focus it on specific pathodynamics. The formula is thus rarely used by itself and usually forms part of a larger prescription.

Zhang Xi-Chun, author of *Essays on Medicine Esteeming the Chinese and Respecting the Western*, provides a good example of how such adjustments are made in practice. Zhang noted that this formula is especially suited for use in southern China, a very humid region where summerheat commonly combines with dampness. In northern China, where the climate is much drier, summerheat more often combines with dryness. In his own practice in Liaoning and Tianjin, Zhang Xi-Chun thus halved the dosage of Talcum *(huá shí)* and replaced it with an equal amount of Gypsum fibrosum *(shí gāo)*.

Note that as a fine powder this formula can be applied externally to treat damp-heat rashes.

Comparison

➤ Vs. Cinnamon and Poria Sweet Dew Drink *(guì líng gān lù yǐn)*; see page 242

Biomedical Indications

With the appropriate presentation, this formula may be used to treat a variety of biomedically-defined disorders including stomach flu, gastroenteritis, heat stroke, cystitis, urethritis, and urinary tract stones.

Alternate names

Heaven's Water Pill *(tiān shuǐ sǎn)* in *Direct Investigation of Cold Damage*; Grand White Powder *(tài bái sǎn)* in *Direct Investigation of Cold Damage*; Divine White Powder *(shén bái sǎn)* in *Confucians' Duties to Their Parents*; Double Releasing Powder *(shuāng jiě sǎn)* in *Multitude of Marvellous Formulas for Sustaining Life*; Lubricate the Fetus Powder *(huá tāi sǎn)* in *Discussion on Supplemental Formulas Omitted from the Inner Classic*

Modifications

• For severe summerheat, add Citrulli Praeparatio *(xī guā shuāng)* and Lophatheri Herba *(dàn zhú yè)*.

• For severe thirst with a red tongue, add Ophiopogonis Radix *(mài mén dōng)*, Glehniae/Adenophorae Radix *(shā shēn)*, Dendrobii Herba *(shí hú)*, and Anemarrhenae Rhizoma *(zhī mǔ)*.

• For injury to the qi and fluids, add Panacis quinquefolii Radix *(xī yáng shēn)*.

• For stony painful urinary dysfunction, add Lysimachiae Herba *(jīn qián cǎo)*, Gigeriae galli Endothelium corneum *(jī nèi jīn)*, and Lygodii Spora *(hǎi jīn shā)*.

• For bloody painful urinary dysfunction, add Imperatae Rhizoma *(bái máo gēn)* and Cirsii Herba *(xiǎo jì)*.

• For cystitis or urethritis, add Phellodendri Cortex *(huáng bǎi)*.

• For dysenteric disorders with pus and blood during the summer caused by cold food or drink, add charred Gardeniae Fructus *(shān zhī zǐ tàn)* and Zingiberis Rhizoma *(gān jiāng)*.

Variations

雞蘇散 （鸡苏散）

Peppermint Powder

jī sū sǎn

Source *Formulas from the Discussion Illuminating the Yellow Emperor's Basic Questions* (1172)

Add one-third of one part Menthae haplocalycis Herba *(bò hé)* for concurrent exterior conditions with chills and an aversion to drafts, headache with a sensation of distention in the head, and cough.

———

益元散

Augment the Primal Powder

yì yuán sǎn

Source *Fine Formulas of Wonderful Efficacy* (1470)

The source text states to add one-third of one part Cinnabaris *(zhū shā)*, grind into a fine powder, and take 6g with warm water or a decoction prepared with Junci Medulla *(dēng xīn cǎo)*. For palpitations with anxiety, insomnia, or dream-disturbed sleep. This formula is also known as Cinnabaris Augment the Primal Powder *(chén shā yì yuán sǎn)*. Compared to the basic formula, this variation focuses more strongly on clearing heat from the Heart and calming the spirit.

Note: Due to its mercury content, Cinnabaris *(zhū shā)* is an obsolete substance and should not be used. A possible replacement is to add two parts Succinum *(hǔ pò)*. This formula is also indicated for stony painful urinary dribbling.

———

碧玉散

Jasper Powder

bì yù sǎn

Source *Formulas from the Discussion Illuminating the Yellow Emperor's Basic Questions* (1172)

Add one-third of one part Indigo naturalis *(qīng dài)* for summerheat with concurrent heat constraint in the Liver and Gallbladder manifesting with red eyes, sore throat and/or mouth and tongue sores.

Associated Formula

雷氏清涼滌暑法 （雷氏清涼滌暑法）

Master Lei's Method for Clearing, Cooling, and Scouring Out Summerheat

Léi shì qīng liáng dí shǔ fǎ

Source *Discussion of Seasonal Disorders* (1882)

Talcum *(huá shí)*	9g
Glycyrrhizae Radix *(gān cǎo)*	2.4g
Artemisiae annuae Herba *(qīng hāo)*	4.5g
Lablab Semen album *(bái biǎn dòu)*	3g
Forsythiae Fructus *(lián qiáo)*	9g
Poria *(fú líng)*	9g
Tetrapanacis Medulla *(tōng cǎo)*	3g

Decoct with one slice of Citrulli Exocarpium *(xī guā)*. For more severe manifestations of summerheat damage than those treated by the principal formula. Also for the treatment of summerheat diarrhea and lurking summerheat. Compared to the principal formula, Master Lei's Method for Clearing, Cooling, and Scouring Out Summerheat *(Léi shì qīng liǎng dí shǔ fǎ)* focuses more strongly on guiding out summerheat via the urine and on clearing heat from the Heart.

桂苓甘露飲 (桂苓甘露饮)
Cinnamon and Poria Sweet Dew Drink
guì líng gān lù yǐn

Like many formula names, Cinnamon and Poria Sweet Dew Drink at once evokes diverse references. It is first a reflection of the various components that make up this formula, namely Five-Ingredient Powder with Poria *(wǔ líng sǎn)*, in which cinnamon and poria are the main herbs, and Sweet Dew Powder *(gān lù sǎn)*. 'Cinnamon and poria' is also a reference to a special way of preparing poria that was common in imperial China and explained in the COMMENTARY below. Finally, the name suggests the formula's strategy for clearing summerheat and facilitating the resolution of dampness: "Overall, [it's action] resembles early autumn [when] the sweet dew descends to dispel the qi of summerheat." *(Selected Annotations to Ancient Formulas from the Garden of Crimson Snow)*

Source   *Formulas from the Discussion Illuminating the Yellow Emperor's Basic Questions* (1172)

Talcum *(huá shí)* 120g
Glycyrrhizae Radix praeparata *(zhì gān cǎo)* 60g
Gypsum fibrosum *(shí gāo)* 60g
Glauberitum *(hán shuǐ shí)* 60g
Cinnamomi Cortex *(ròu guì)* 15g
Polyporus *(zhū líng)* 15g
Poria *(fú líng)* 30g
Alismatis Rhizoma *(zé xiè)* 30g
Atractylodis macrocephalae Rhizoma *(bái zhú)* 15g

Method of Preparation   Grind the ingredients into a powder and take 9g with water. Taking the powder with a decoction prepared with Zingiberis Rhizoma recens *(shēng jiāng)* is said to enhance its effectiveness. Note that the source text calls for 'official cinnamon' (官桂 *guān guì*), which is a form of Cinnamomi Cortex *(ròu guì)* taken from the thinner bark of trees that are between 6- and 7-years old and which has less oil than the more commonly-used herb. The formula is generally prepared as a decoction with a proportionate reduction in the dosage of each ingredient.

Actions   Expels summerheat, clears heat, transforms the qi, and promotes the resolution of dampness

Indications

Fever, headache, irritability, thirst, urinary difficulty with reduced urine, or, in severe cases, sudden turmoil disorder (simultaneous vomiting and diarrhea) with abdominal fullness, pain, or stifling sensation during the summer.

This is summerheat with internal stagnation of water and dampness. Summerheat causes fever and headache. It injures the qi and fluids, which causes irritability and thirst. Internally, dampness leads to stagnation and the obstruction of the qi dynamic, which causes urinary difficulty with reduced output of urine. When summerheat-dampness is severe, injury to the Spleen and Stomach may occur; this disrupts their ascending and descending functions, and can lead to sudden turmoil disorder.

This formula is also used to treat vomiting, diarrhea, and fright wind in children caused by summerheat.

Analysis of Formula

The chief ingredient in this formula is Talcum *(huá shí)*. Sweet, cooling, and slippery, it unblocks stagnation, promotes passage through all the orifices, clears and resolves summerheat, and harmonizes the Stomach. It focuses on the central disease dynamic of this pattern as well as on both of the pathogens, summerheat and dampness. Two other minerals, Gypsum fibrosum *(shí gāo)* and Glauberitum *(hán shuǐ shí)*, serve as deputies. Both are acrid and cooling and strengthen the heat-clearing action of the formula. Together, the three minerals in the formula also develop a downward-directing action that promotes unblocking of the Triple Burner. Unlike bitter, cooling herbs, the sweet and salty flavor of these minerals does not dry the fluids or constrain the qi.

The various assistants in the formula focus on promoting the resolution of dampness. Polyporus *(zhū líng)*, Poria *(fú líng)*, and Alismatis Rhizoma *(zé xiè)* promote urination and expel dampness. Atractylodis macrocephalae Rhizoma *(bái zhú)* strengthens the Spleen. Together, these four ingredients restore the ascending and descending functions of the qi mechanism, transform the Bladder qi, and alleviate sudden turmoil disorder. Cinnamomi Cortex *(ròu guì)* assists in the transformation of qi in the lower burner. Its warming and drying nature also counterbalances the very cooling nature of the chief and deputies. Glycyrrhizae Radix *(gān cǎo)* functions as the envoy that harmonizes the diverse actions of the formula. Together with Talcum *(huá shí)*, it aids in the clearing of heat, and together with Poria *(fú líng)* and Atractylodis macrocephalae Rhizoma *(bái zhú)*, it strengthens the Spleen.

The balanced dynamic of the formula permits it to clear heat and promote proper water metabolism, and to expel pathogenic heat and water, without damaging the normal qi.

Cautions and Contraindications

This formula is indicated for treating summerheat damage presentations characterized by overwhelming heat and dampness, or heat that is more pronounced than dampness. It is not indicated for relatively mild presentations or for patterns where dampness is more pronounced than heat.

Commentary

This is a combination of Five-Ingredient Powder with Poria (*wǔ líng sǎn*) from *Discussion of Cold Damage* (discussed in Chapter 16), Six-to-One Powder (*liù yī sǎn*) by Liu Wan-Su (discussed above in this chapter), and Sweet Dew Powder (*gān lù sǎn*) by the famous Song-dynasty pediatrician Qian Yi. *Sweet Dew Powder* (*gān lù sǎn*), first listed as *Jade Dew Powder* (*yù lù sǎn*) in *Craft of Medicines and Patterns for Children*, is composed of Gypsum fibrosum (*shí gāo*), Glauberitum (*hán shuǐ shí*), and Glycyrrhizae Radix (*gān cǎo*). It is indicated for "exuberant heat generating wind with a tendency to fright twitching." This influence explains the special indication of the present formula in the treatment of summerheat disorders in children. At present, the formula is generally prescribed for a somewhat more severe condition of summerheat (located at a slightly deeper level) than the heat for which Six-to-One Powder (*liù yī sǎn*) is indicated.

In *The Refined in Medicine Remembered*, the late-Qing physician Fei Bo-Xiong observed that the use of this formula is indicated "when the underside of the tongue [looks] rough while the upper side appears as if there were chewed grains of rice on top." This reflects damage to the fluids in the interior (the underside or yin part of the tongue) with dampness obstructing the Triple Burner (the upper or more yang part of the tongue).

Comparison

➢ Vs. Six-to-One Powder (*liù yī sǎn*)

Both of these formulas contain Talcum (*huá shí*) and Glycyrrhizae Radix (*gān cǎo*) to unblock the constraint of summerheat and dampness. Comparing the two, the action of Six-to-One Powder (*liù yī sǎn*) is relatively mild. It is indicated for a milder disease dynamic in which dampness predominates and is focused on the Triple Burner and Bladder. Cinnamon and Poria Sweet Dew Drink (*guì líng gān lù yǐn*), on the other hand, is a large formula indicated for more severe presentations where both heat and dampness are pronounced. In addition to the Triple Burner, it focuses on the Stomach and Intestines.

Alternate names

Cinnamon, Poria, and White Atractylodes (*guì líng bái zhú sǎn*) in *Formulas from the Discussion Illuminating the Yellow Emperor's Basic Questions*; Cinnamon and Poria Sweet Dew Drink ((*guì líng gān lù yǐn*) in *Direct Investigation of Cold Damage*

Biomedical Indications

With the appropriate presentation, this formula may be used to treat a variety of biomedically-defined disorders including acute gastroenteritis, cholera, and heat stroke.

Associated Formulas

桂苓甘露飲 (桂苓甘露饮)

Cinnamon and Poria Sweet Dew Drink from *Confucians' Duties*

guì líng gān lù yǐn

SOURCE   *Confucians' Duties to their Parents* (1228)

Cinnamomi Cortex (*ròu guì*)	15g
Ginseng Radix (*rén shēn*)	15g
Pogostemonis/Agastaches Herba (*huò xiāng*)	15g
Poria (*fú líng*)	30g
Atractylodis macrocephalae Rhizoma (*bái zhú*)	30g
Glycyrrhizae Radix (*gān cǎo*)	30g
Puerariae Radix (*gé gēn*)	30g
Alismatis Rhizoma (*zé xiè*)	30g
Gypsum fibrosum (*shí gāo*)	30g
Glauberitum (*hán shuǐ shí*)	30g
Talcum (*huá shí*)	60g
Aucklandiae Radix (*mù xiāng*)	0.3g

The source text advises to grind the herbs into a powder and to take 9g with water or in a decoction prepared with Zingiberis Rhizoma recens (*shēng jiāng*). For lurking summerheat disorders that manifest with irritability, thirst, drinking that is followed by vomiting, and incessant watery diarrhea. Compared to the main formula, this one treats summerheat damage with more severe Spleen deficiency. Yu Chang sums up this difference in *Precepts for Physicians*:

> Liu Wan-Su's Cinnamon and Poria Sweet Dew Drink (*guì líng gān lù yǐn*) uses Five Poria Powder with Gypsum fibrosum (*shí gāo*). The intention is to generate yang fluids and augment Stomach deficiency. Zhang Ze-He's Cinnamon and Poria Sweet Dew Drink (*guì líng gān lù yǐn*) uses Ginseng Radix (*rén shēn*), Puerariae Radix (*gé gēn*), Glycyrrhizae Radix (*gān cǎo*), Pogostemonis/Agastaches Herba (*huò xiāng*), and Aucklandiae Radix (*mù xiāng*) to augment deficiency of the middle burner. It also eliminates turbidity.

三石湯 (三石汤)

Three Minerals Decoction

sān shí tāng

SOURCE   *Systematic Differentiation of Warm Pathogen Diseases* (1798)

Talcum (*huá shí*)	9g
Gypsum fibrosum (*shí gāo*)	15g
Glauberitum (*hán shuǐ shí*)	9g
Armeniacae Semen (*xìng rén*)	9g
Bambusae Caulis in taeniam (*zhú rú*)	6g
Lonicerae Flos (*jīn yín huā*)	9g
Succus Faecalis Aureus (*jīn zhī*)	one wine glass
Tetrapanacis Medulla (*tōng cǎo*)	6g

The source text advises to decoct the herbs with 5 cups of water until 2 cups remain. This is divided into two portions and consumed warm. Clears heat with acrid and cooling herbs and transforms turbidity with aromatic herbs. For qi-aspect summerheat and warm pathogen disorders with heat flooding the Triple Burner characterized by fever, a red face, focal distention, a stifling sensation in the chest, a fresh red tongue with a thin, yellow, slippery coating. The formula opens the qi dynamic by facilitating passage through the orifices, acting on the Lungs and Stomach to reduce heat and guide out turbidity. Compared to the principal formula, Three Minerals Decoction (*sān shí tāng*) is less potent in its ability to dispel dampness but stronger in clearing summerheat. Physicians in contemporary China also use the formula for treating phlegm-heat in contexts where they are concerned about damaging the fluids with acrid, drying herbs.

Note: Succus Faecalis Aureus (金汁 *jīn zhī*) is made by putting loose human stool in a clay pot and sealing it. It is then buried for three years and consumed. This substance is the clear water in the clay pot. It strongly clears heat and resolves toxicity. At present, it is not used; instead, either Isatidis Folium (*dà qīng yè*) or Coptidis Rhizoma (*huáng lián*) is substituted.

Section 4

FORMULAS THAT DISPEL SUMMERHEAT AND AUGMENT THE QI

As a yang pathogen, summerheat can readily damage the qi. This leads to symptoms such as fatigue and a deficient pulse that accompany the primary manifestation of heat. Such presentations require the use of treatment strategies that augment the qi in order to dispel summerheat. Formulas used for this purpose include herbs like Ginseng Radix (*rén shēn*), Pseudostellariae Radix (*tài zǐ shēn*), or Panacis quinquefolii Radix (*xī yáng shēn*) that tonify the qi and generate fluids. These are combined with other herbs that augment the qi and strengthen the Spleen and Stomach, such as Atractylodis macrocephalae Rhizoma (*bái zhú*) and Astragali Radix (*huáng qí*); with bitter, cooling herbs like Anemarrhenae Rhizoma (*zhī mǔ*) and Coptidis Rhizoma (*huáng lián*) that drain heat from the interior; and with herbs like Lophatheri Herba (*dàn zhú yè*) and Alismatis Rhizoma (*zé xiè*) that facilitate the resolution of dampness. Where damage to the qi is attributable to excessive sweating, qi deficiency will be accompanied by damage to the fluids. For these patterns, formulas like Generate the Pulse Powder (*shēng mài sǎn*) that tonify both the qi and yin should be used.

清暑益氣湯 (清暑益气汤)

Clear Summerheat and Augment the Qi Decoction

qīng shǔ yì qì tāng

Source   *Warp and Woof of Warm-Febrile Diseases* (1852)

Panacis quinquefolii Radix (*xī yáng shēn*) 4.5-6g
Citrulli Exocarpium (*xī guā*) 24-30g
Nelumbinis Caulis (*lián gěng*) 12-15g
Dendrobii Herba (*shí hú*) 12-15g
Ophiopogonis Radix (*mài mén dōng*) 6-9g
Lophatheri Herba (*dàn zhú yè*) 4.5-6g
Anemarrhenae Rhizoma (*zhī mǔ*) 4.5-6g
Coptidis Rhizoma (*huáng lián*) 2-3g
Glycyrrhizae Radix (*gān cǎo*) 2-3g
Nonglutinous rice (*jīng mǐ*) 12-15g

Method of Preparation   Decoction. The source text does not specify dosages.

Actions   Clears summerheat, augments the qi, nourishes the yin, and generates fluids

Indications

Fever, profuse sweating, irritability, thirst, scanty and dark urine, fatigued limbs, shortness of breath, apathy, and a deficient, rapid pulse.

This is summerheat injuring the qi and fluids. When summerheat penetrates to the interior there is fever, irritability, and a rapid pulse. The heat 'steaming' internally forces open the interstices and pores and causes profuse sweating. Summerheat, a yang pathogenic influence, readily injures the fluids, which is compounded by profuse sweating. This results in thirst with a desire to drink and dark, scanty urine. Qi attaches to the sweat as it leaves the body, causing qi deficiency with fatigued limbs, shortness of breath, apathy, and a deficient pulse.

Analysis of Formula

One of the chief herbs in this formula is Panacis quinquefolii Radix (*xī yáng shēn*), which augments the qi, generates fluids, nourishes the yin, and clears heat. In this it is aided by Dendrobii Herba (*shí hú*) and Ophiopogonis Radix (*mài mén dōng*), which nourish the yin of the Lungs and Stomach. The other chief herb, Citrulli Exocarpium (*xī guā*), is an important substance for clearing heat and releasing summerheat. It is aided by Nelumbinis Caulis (*lián gěng*), which has similar functions. The assistants include Lophatheri Herba (*dàn zhú yè*) and Anemarrhenae Rhizoma (*zhī mǔ*), which clear heat and resolve irritability and thirst. The bitter, cold Coptidis Rhizoma (*huáng lián*) is especially effective in quelling fire. Here it is used to assist in clearing heat and expelling summerheat. The other assistants, Glycyrrhizae Radix (*gān cǎo*) and Nonglutinous rice (*jīng mǐ*), augment the qi and nourish the Stomach. Not only do these ingredients assist in treating the underlying condition, they also prevent the cloying nature of the yin-nourishing herbs and the cold nature of the heat-clearing herbs from upsetting the Stomach.

Cautions and Contraindications

Because of the large number of cloying, yin-nourishing herbs, this formula should not be used without considerable modification in cases of summerheat-dampness. It is also inappropriate for conditions in which the pathogenic influence has already been resolved.

Commentary

From a five-phase perspective, fire controls metal. Summerheat is an excess of fire that damages metal, injuring both the qi and fluids. For this reason, physicians associated with the warm pathogen disorder current in Chinese medicine assign an important role to the Lungs in the onset of both windwarmth and summerheat disorders. The Lungs generate fluids by directing qi downward. Water follows this movement to stream into the Kidneys, which is why the Lungs are called the 'upper source of water.' If Lung qi is insufficient, it cannot direct this downward movement and fluids are lost through sweating. Hence, even though this formula focuses on clearing heat and augmenting the qi, its ultimate purpose is to conserve the fluids. In this, as discussed in the COMPARISON section below, it resembles formulas like White Tiger plus Ginseng Decoction (bái hǔ jiā rén shēn tāng) and Lophatherum and Gypsum Decoction (zhú yè shí gāo tāng).

This formula was composed by Wang Shi-Xiong, who included it in a commentary on Xue Sheng-Bai's *Writings on Damp-Heat Pathogen Diseases*. Xue Sheng-Bai had suggested using Li Dong-Yuan's Clear Summerheat and Augment the Qi Decoction (qīng shǔ yì qì tāng), listed below, to treat "damp-heat patterns [where] damp-heat has damaged the qi [as reflected in] fatigued limbs, diminished vitality, generalized fever, shallow breathing, Heart irritability, yellow urine, thirst, sweating, and a deficient pulse." Wang Shi-Xiong voiced his reply in *Warp and Woof of Warm-Heat Pathogen Diseases*: "The pulse and pattern all indicate that this [condition] should be treated by clearing summerheat and augmenting the qi. Although Li Dong-Yuan's formula defines itself as clearing summerheat, it does not really do this." To distinguish Wang Shi-Xiong's formula from that of Li Dong-Yuan, it is also known as Wang's Decoction to Clear Summerheat and Augment the Qi (Wáng shì qīng shǔ yì qì tāng).

Comparisons

➢ Vs. White Tiger plus Ginseng Decoction (bái hǔ jiā rén shēn tāng)

Both of these formulas treat heat excess with sweating and a deficient pulse. White Tiger plus Ginseng Decoction (bái hǔ jiā rén shēn tāng) is indicated for patterns characterized by pathogenic heat collecting in the qi aspect. The momentum of this heat is to discharge outward, thereby depleting the qi. Clear Summerheat and Augment the Qi Decoction (qīng shǔ yì qì tāng) treats summerheat collecting in the qi aspect. Summerheat connects with the Heart. The effect of this heat is to obstruct and dry out, causing irritability, yellow urine, and a dry mouth. Hence, this formula replaces Gypsum fibrosum

(shí gāo) with Coptidis Rhizoma (huáng lián) to remove the obstruction caused by the heat.

➢ Vs. Lophatherum and Gypsum Decoction (zhú yè shí gāo tāng)

Clear Summerheat and Augment the Qi Decoction (qīng shǔ yì qì tāng) is widely regarded as a modification of Lophatherum and Gypsum Decoction (zhú yè shí gāo tāng), which also can be used to treat summerheat damage. However, the latter formula is better suited for lingering heat in the Stomach that has not been completely cleared. Thus, its presentation includes symptoms like nausea and rebellious qi. Clear Summerheat and Augment the Qi Decoction (qīng shǔ yì qì tāng) focuses on the Lungs. Its presentation therefore includes symptoms like sweating and shortness of breath.

➢ Vs. Generate the Pulse Powder (shēng mài sǎn); see PAGE 330

Biomedical Indications

With the appropriate presentation, this formula may be used to treat a variety of biomedically-defined disorders including hyperthermia, heat stroke, fever of uknown origin, pneumonia, and during convalescence from an acute infectious disease.

Alternate name

Master Wang's Clear Summerheat and Augment the Qi Decoction (wáng shì qīng shǔ yì qì tāng) in *Handouts on Chinese Medical Formulas*

Modifications

• For mild summerheat with severe injury to the fluids, remove Coptidis Rhizoma (huáng lián).

• For a greasy, white tongue coating, remove Anemarrhenae Rhizoma (zhī mǔ) and Ophiopogonis Radix (mài mén dōng) and add Poria (fú líng).

• For unremitting fever in children during the summer, qi deficiency, and insufficient fluids, remove Coptidis Rhizoma (huáng lián) and Anemarrhenae Rhizoma (zhī mǔ) and add Cynanchi atrati Radix (bái wēi) and Lycii Cortex (dì gǔ pí).

Associated Formulas

清暑益氣湯 （清暑益气汤）

Clear Summerheat and Augment the Qi Decoction from *Clarifying Doubts*

qīng shǔ yì qì tāng

SOURCE *Clarifying Doubts about Damage from Internal and External Causes* (1247)

Astragali Radix (huáng qí) .4.5g (9-12g)

Ginseng Radix (*rén shēn*) 1.5g (3-4.5g)
Atractylodis Rhizoma (*cāng zhú*) 4.5g (6-9g)
Atractylodis macrocephalae Rhizoma (*bái zhú*) 1.5g (4.5-6g)
Ophiopogonis Radix (*mài mén dōng*) 0.9g (9-12g)
Schisandrae Fructus (*wǔ wèi zǐ*) 2g (3-6g)
Puerariae Radix (*gé gēn*) 0.9g (6-9g)
Citri reticulatae Pericarpium (*chén pí*) 1.5g (3-6g)
Citri reticulatae viride Pericarpium (*qīng pí*) 0.9g (3-6g)
Angelicae sinensis radicis Corpus (*dāng guī shēn*) 0.9g (6-9g)
Cimicifugae Rhizoma (*shēng má*) 3g (3-6g)
Alismatis Rhizoma (*zé xiè*) 1.5g (6-9g)
wine-fried Phellodendri Cortex (*jiǔ chǎo huáng bǎi*) . .0.6-0.9g (6-9g)
dry-fried Massa medicata fermentata (*chǎo shén qū*) . . . 1.5g (6-9g)
Glycyrrhizae Radix praeparata (*zhì gān cǎo*) 0.9g (2-3g)

Panacis quinquefolii Radix (*xī yáng shēn*) is often substituted for Ginseng Radix (*rén shēn*). The modern dosage (in parentheses) is larger than the dosage recommended in the source text. Clears summerheat, augments the qi, strengthens the Spleen, and dries dampness. For one with qi deficiency who contracts summerheat-dampness characterized by fever, headache, thirst, spontaneous sweating, fatigued limbs, loss of appetite, a sensation of fullness in the chest and a heavy body, loose stools, dark, scanty urine, a greasy tongue coating, and a deficient pulse.

The source text prescribes this formula for "for one who has over time exhausted their Spleen and Stomach by irregular eating or exhaustion, is assailed by the heat of summertime, and becomes ill." To treat this condition, Li Dong-Yuan modified Tonify the Middle to Augment the Qi Decoction (*bǔ zhōng yì qì tāng*), adding herbs that transform and leach out dampness, move the qi, and generate fluids to create what he called "a clearing and drying prescription." The source text also lists a number of variations:

> For severe discharge of sweat [leading to] fluid abandonment that must be urgently stopped, add Schisandrae Fructus (*wǔ wèi zǐ*), dry-fried Phellodendri Cortex (*chǎo huáng bǎi*), and Anemarrhenae Rhizoma (*zhī mǔ*). These [herbs] restrain and gather in. For damp-heat encroaching on the Kidneys and Liver with abnormal walking, atrophied and weak legs, and both feet askew, when [the patient] has already been attacked by an atrophy pathogen, add wine-washed Phellodendri Cortex (*jiǔ huáng bǎi*) and Anemarrhenae Rhizoma (*zhī mǔ*) to let the force of qi gush out through both feet. If the bowel movements are bound up and stagnant, occuring just every second or third day and causing loss of appetite, there is heat lurking within the blood so that it does not get moistened. Add Angelicae sinensis radicis Caput (*dāng guī tóu*), Rehmanniae Radix (*shēng dì huáng*), ground Persicae Semen (*táo rén ní*), and ground Cannabis Semen (*huǒ má rén ní*) to moisten it.

Through the centuries, physicians, among them the 17th-century writer Wang Shi-Jie and the contemporary scholar Qiu Pei-Ran, have recommended Li Dong-Yuan's formula for obese or deficient patients (indicating Spleen deficiency) who contract a summerheat pathogen. Not everyone, however, shared this view. The 19th-century scholar-physician Fei Bo-Xiong is representative of the doubters. Fei observed that this formula

> is extremely complex in terms of its constituents. It contains tonifying herbs to tonify and eliminating herbs to eliminate, ascending herbs to ascend, and downward-draining herbs to drain. But how do they know where it is appropriate to go? The main focus of treatment is to direct downward because chest fullness and gasping for breath are listed [as symptoms]. Therefore, Astragali Radix (*huáng qí*) and Cimicifugae Rhizoma (*shēng má*) would be contraindicated.

In my opinion, it is sufficient to clear the Heart, nourish the Stomach, strengthen the Spleen, and promote the resolution of dampness. Why make such a big effort for such a trifling matter? It is my sincere conviction that because of formulas such as this, Dong-Yuan does not deserve the flattery [he is so often accorded].

雷氏清涼滌暑湯（雷氏清凉涤暑汤）
Master Lei's Decoction to Clear, Cool, and Remove Summerheat
Léi shì qīng liáng dí shǔ tāng

SOURCE *Discussion of Seasonal Diseases* (1882)

Talcum (*huá shí*) 9g
Glycyrrhizae Radix (*gān cǎo*) 2.4g
Artemisiae annuae Herba (*qīng hāo*) 4.5g
Lablab Semen album (*biǎn dòu*) 3g
Forsythiae Fructus (*lián qiáo*) 9g
Poria (*fú líng*) 9g
Tetrapanacis Medulla (*tōng cǎo*) 3g
Citrulli Praeparatio (*xī guā shuāng*) . . . . 1 piece

Relieves summerheat and leaches out dampness. For externally-contracted summerheat and dampness in the upper burner characterized by fever and chills, sweating, light-headedness, coughing, and a thin, slightly greasy tongue coating.

Section 5

. . . .

FORMULAS THAT DISPEL SUMMERHEAT AND PRESERVE THE BODY FLUIDS

Summerheat has a yang, rising, and dispersing nature. It causes sweating and readily damages the body fluids. In the early stages of summerheat disorders, one guards the yin by focusing on the yang. The key strategies are to clear heat to stop sweating and resolve constraint within the Triple Burner by facilitating the resolution of dampness. Herbs like Ophiopogonis Radix (*mài mén dōng*) or Panacis quinquefolii Radix (*xī yáng shēn*) that generate fluids may be added to these formulas as assistants. The use of sour, astringent herbs is avoided, however, as this may prevent the effective discharge of pathogenic heat. Only when damage to the body fluids becomes a dominant aspect of a presentation—reflected in such manifestations as wasting and thirsting disorder, a cracked tongue, or a thin pulse—does it become necessary to shift strategies. The formulas in this section utilize sour, astringent herbs like Mume Fructus (*wū méi*) and Chaenomelis Fructus (*mù guā*) to astringe the fluids and prevent the loss of yin essence. They combine these sour herbs with bitter, cold herbs that drain heat from the interior and sweet, cold herbs that enrich the yin and generate fluids.

吳氏連梅湯 (吴氏连梅汤)

Master Wu's Coptis and Mume Decoction

Wú shì lián méi tāng

Source   *Systematic Differentiation of Warm Pathogen Diseases* (1798)

Coptidis Rhizoma (*huáng lián*) 6g
Mume Fructus (*wū méi*) 9g
Ophiopogonis Radix (*mài mén dōng*) 9g
Rehmanniae Radix (*shēng dì huáng*) 9g
Asini Corii Colla (*ē jiāo*) 6g

Method of Preparation   Decoction. The source text advises to decoct the herbs in 5 cups of water until 2 cups remain and then administer in two doses. The source text advises to take Purple Snow Special Pill (*zǐ xuě dān*) before taking this formula if clouding of consciousness is severe.

Actions   Drains heat, preserves fluids, and transforms yin

Indications

Wasting and thirsting, heat in the Heart, irritability and restlessness, paralysis and clouding of consciousness, a dry, cracked tongue, and a submerged and thin pulse.

This is pathogenic summerheat entering into the lesser yin and terminal yin warps. Summerheat first enters into the chest and the Heart, causing irritability and restlessness. The Heart and Kidneys are associated with the lesser yin warp. If summerheat persists, it damages the body fluids that are governed by the Kidneys. This manifests as waisting and thirsting. If summerheat damages the body fluids in the terminal yin, it stirs wind in the muscles and sinews, which are governed by the Liver; this causes paralysis. If wind enters the Pericardium, it clouds the consciousness. The tongue and pulse signs here are manifestations of the damage to the yin and fluids.

Analysis of Formula

The formula combines bitter, cold herbs to drain heat from the Heart with sour and sweet herbs to transform the yin. The chief herb is bitter and cold Coptidis Rhizoma (*huáng lián*). It enters the Heart to drain pathogenic summerheat, removing the root cause of this pathology. The deputy is sour, astringent, and warm Mume Fructus (*wū méi*). It enters the Stomach to generate yang fluids and stop the thirst, and is a specific herb for treating wasting and thirsting. The combination of Coptidis Rhizoma (*huáng lián*) and Mume Fructus (*wū méi*) is a well-established synergistic pairing in the Chinese materia medica, as in Mume Pill (*wū méi wán*). It allows Coptidis Rhizoma (*huáng lián*) to drain the heat without injuring the normal qi, while preventing the restraining action of Mume Fructus (*wū méi*) from improperly retaining the pathogenic heat within the body. The bitterness of Coptidis

Rhizoma (*huáng lián*), furthermore, focuses the sourness of Mume Fructus (*wū méi*) on the yin aspect of the fluids that were damaged within the lesser yin.

Three assistants aid the generation of body fluids. Sweet, cooling Ophiopogonis Radix (*mài mén dōng*) and Rehmanniae Radix (*shēng dì huáng*) tonify the water to stop the thirst and extinguish the wind. Their sweetness is restrained by the sourness of Mume Fructus (*wū méi*) and guided toward transformation into yin. Asini Corii Colla (*ē jiāo*) tonifies the blood and increases the yin fluids, softening the Liver to extinguish the wind and assisting the Kidneys to govern the water. Asini Corii Colla (*ē jiāo*), black in color and sinking in nature, also serves as an envoy that guides the formula into the interior and the lesser yin and terminal yin warps.

If there is severe clouding of consciousness, Purple Snow Special Pill (*zǐ xuě dān*) is administered first to open the orifices. Wu Ju-Tong, the formula's author, describes the purpose of this strategy as first creating an opening through which the pathogen can be eliminated from the body, after which Mume Fructus (*wū méi*) and Coptidis Rhizoma (*huáng lián*) can enter.

Cautions and Contraindications

This formula is contraindicated for summerheat damage without severe loss of fluids. The presence of thirst, irritability, and restlessness are not indications unless they are accompanied by a submerged and thin pulse, a dry, cracked tongue, or other signs of wasting.

Commentary

Using sour, astringent herbs is normally contraindicated in situations where a pathogen remains in the body. This formula circumvents this difficulty through its judicious combination of sour and bitter herbs, which drain pathogenic heat, and sour and sweet herbs, which transform the yin to soften the Liver. The astringent action of Mume Fructus (*wū méi*) is thus guided toward restraining the fluids for the purpose of harmonizing the physiological movement of qi, without which the pathogens cannot be eliminated nor the symptoms of wasting and thirsting or paralysis brought under control.

Modern physicians have extended the use of this formula to treat diabetes.

Biomedical Indications

With the appropriate presentation, this formula may be used to treat a variety of biomedically-defined disorders including paroxysmal supraventricular tachycardia and diabetes.

Associated Formula

人參烏梅湯 (人参乌梅汤)

Ginseng and Mume Decoction
rén shēn wū méi tāng

SOURCE *Systematic Differentiation of Warm Pathogen Diseases* (1798)

Ginseng Radix *(rén shēn)* 4.5g
Mume Fructus *(wū méi)* . . . . flesh 0.9g
Chaenomelis Fructus *(mù guā)* 2.4g
Dioscoreae Rhizoma *(shān yào)* 9g
Nelumbinis Semen *(lián zǐ)* 3g

Decoction. In contemporary practice, Ginseng Radix *(rén shēn)* is often replaced with Panacis quinquefolii Radix *(xī yáng shēn)*. Generates fluids, tonifies qi, and eliminates pathogenic summerheat. For the late stages of a summerheat disorder with damage to both the qi and yin due to excessive sweating. The formula combines sweet and sour herbs to transform the yin and stop spasms, and slightly bitter and sour herbs to drain the pathogenic heat. This follows a strategy first outlined by the Ming-dynasty writer Zhang He-Teng: "to continue treating [the late stages of summerheat] by means of sour draining and sour retaining [herbs]."

Comparative Tables of Principal Formulas

■ FORMULAS THAT DISPEL SUMMERHEAT AND CLEAR HEAT

Formula Name	Diagnosis	Indications	Remarks
Clear the Collaterals Drink *(qīng luò yǐn)*	Mild summerheat injuring the qi level of the Lung channel	Fever, mild thirst, unclear head and vision with light-headedness and slight distention of the head, a pink tongue with a thin, white coating	Also for a summerheat-warmth pathogen that has not been fully released by sweating.

■ FORMULAS THAT DISPEL SUMMERHEAT AND RESOLVE THE EXTERIOR

Common symptoms: chills, headache, stifling sensation in the chest, white, greasy tongue coating

Formula Name	Diagnosis	Indications	Remarks
Mosla Powder *(xiāng rú sǎn)*	Exterior cold with interior dampness contracted in the summer	Chills with skin that is warm to the touch, absence of sweating, sensation of heaviness in the head, headache, abdominal pain, vomiting, diarrhea, stifling sensation in the chest, fatigued limbs, a white, greasy tongue coating, and a floating pulse	Also for any presentation of exterior cold and interior dampness, regardless of the season, especially when accompanied by vomiting and diarrhea.
Newly Augmented Mosla Drink *(xīn jiā xiāng rú yǐn)*	Severe, early-stage summerheat in the Lung greater yin with superimposed contraction of cold fettering the exterior	Fever and chills without sweating, headache, thirst, flushed face, stifling sensation in the chest, heavy and aching body, dark and rough urination, a red tongue with a white, greasy coating, and a flooding pulse on the right and a small pulse on the left	For more severe heat signs.

■ FORMULAS THAT DISPEL SUMMERHEAT AND FACILITATE THE RESOLUTION OF DAMPNESS

Common symptoms: fever, irritability, thirst, vomiting, diarrhea, urinary difficulty

Formula Name	Diagnosis	Indications	Remarks
Six-to-One Powder *(liù yī sǎn)*	Summerheat with dampness in the interior	Fever, sweating, thirst, irritability, urinary difficulty, diarrhea, nausea, vomiting, a thin, yellow, and greasy tongue coating, and a soggy, rapid pulse	Also for painful urinary dysfunction and damp-heat skin disorders.
Cinnamon and Poria Sweet Dew Drink *(guì líng gān lù yǐn)*	Summerheat with internal stagnation of water and dampness	Fever, headache, irritability, thirst, urinary difficulty with reduced urine, or in severe cases, sudden turmoil disorder with abdominal fullness, pain, or stifling sensation	Also for vomiting, diarrhea, and fright wind in children caused by summerheat.

■ FORMULAS THAT DISPEL SUMMERHEAT AND AUGMENT THE QI

Formula Name	Diagnosis	Indications	Remarks
Clear Summerheat and Augment the Qi Decoction *(qīng shǔ yì qì tāng)*	Summerheat injuring the qi and fluids	Fever, profuse sweating, irritability, thirst, scanty and dark urine, fatigued limbs, shortness of breath, apathy, and a deficient, rapid pulse	Focuses on replenishing the fluids while clearing heat and augmenting the qi.

■ FORMULAS THAT DISPEL SUMMERHEAT AND PRESERVE THE BODY FLUIDS

Formula Name	Diagnosis	Indications	Remarks
Master Wu's Coptis and Mume Decoction *(Wú shì lián méi tāng)*	Summerheat entering into the lesser yin and terminal yin warps	Wasting and thirsting, heat in the Heart, irritability and restlessness, paralysis, clouding of consciousness, a dry, cracked tongue, and a submerged, thin pulse	Also used by modern physicians to treat diabetes.

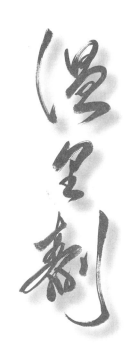

Chapter 6 Contents

Formulas that Warm Interior Cold

Formulas that Warm Interior Cold

6

THE FORMULAS IN this chapter contain as their chief ingredients herbs that are warming and heating. Such herbs dispel cold from the interior of the body by assisting the yang, and unblock the channels and collaterals by dispersing cold. Among the eight methods of treatment, they belong to the warming method (溫法 *wēn fǎ*), which applies the simple dictum from Chapter 74 of *Basic Questions):* "Use heat in treating cold." Cold in the interior may be externally-contracted, or it may be internally-generated from yang or qi deficiency. Externally-contracted cold can directly invade the interior, or it can first attack the exterior, and then, if not properly treated, penetrate to deeper levels of the body. The excessive or improper use of cooling herbs and medicinals, and the consumption of cooling food and beverages, can also lead to interior cold.

Historically, the warming method has been accorded great significance in the treatment of disease by Chinese medicine. Twenty-eight percent of all herbs discussed in the *Divine Husbandman's Classic of the Materia Medica,* for instance, have significant warming or heating properties. These herbs continue to form the foundation of interior warming formulas today. *Discussion of Cold Damage* and *Essentials from the Golden Cabinet* likewise focus to a significant extent on supporting and harmonizing the body's yang qi with the help of warming and heating formulas. Formulas recorded by Zhang Zhong-Jing in these two texts make up most of the content of this chapter. Warming formulas are

of particular significance in the treatment of disorders associated with the three yin warps and of many yin organ patterns.

The second most important influence on the development of treatment strategies that warm the interior was the appearance of the warm tonification current (溫補學派 *wēn bǔ xué pài)* during the Ming dynasty. New doctrines regarding the functions of the gate of vitality led physicians like Xue Ji, Zhang Jie-Bin, and Zhao Xian-Ke to reemphasize the life-enhancing functions of the yang qi as the foundation of all vital processes. Responding to critics who advocated tonification of the yin, Zhang Jie-Bin replied: "Zhu Dan-Xi says 'Excess of qi leads to fire.' On reading this, I reply, 'Insufficiency of qi leads to cold.'" The proponents of warm tonification did not devise any radically new treatment strategies, however, but mainly focused on reconfiguring Zhang Zhong-Jing's original formulas through addition and substraction. Thus, since the Han, only a small number of new formulas that warm the interior were integrated into popular formularies. These include Wang Wei-De's Balmy Yang Decoction (*yáng hé tāng),* discussed in Chapter 21, and Wang Qing-Ren's Restore and Revive the Yang Decoction (*huí yáng jiù jí tāng),* discussed in section 3 below.

Different types of warming formulas are prescribed for treating cold in different levels of the body, and they are so arranged in this chapter. For relatively superficial disorders, formulas that warm the channels and disperse cold are used (section 1). Cold has a tendency to invade the middle burner, and when it does so, formulas that warm the middle and dispel cold should be prescribed (section 2). The most severe conditions associated with cold are those that devastate the yang. These can be life-threatening and require the use of formulas that rescue the devastated yang (section 3).

The formulas in this chapter are not the only ones for treating conditions associated with cold. Formulas that treat cold in the exterior are discussed in Chapter 1, and those that warm and transform phlegm-cold are discussed in Chapter 17. Formulas that tonify the yang (Chapter 8) are also used for treating cold disorders. However, there is a very basic difference between formulas that primarily warm and those that primarily tonify the yang. The former, which are the subject of this chapter, focus on mobilizing the yang qi in order to dispel cold. This includes supporting the transformational processes in the upper and middle burners that depend on the supply of yang qi. By contrast, formulas that tonify the yang focus on strengthening the transformational processes that produce the yang qi in the lower burner and the gate of vitality.

The formulas in this chapter contain substances of a heating and drying nature. They must therefore be used with caution in patients with yin deficiency or blood loss, and should never be used in cases with true heat and false cold, which is characterized by cold extremities, aversion to wind, a dry mouth and thirst, constipation, and a red tongue, among other markers.

The dosage of the chief ingredients in these formulas, particularly Aconiti Radix lateralis praeparata *(zhì fù zǐ)* and Zingiberis Rhizoma *(gān jiāng)*, must be adjusted to suit the season, climate, and constitution of the individual patient. If the dosage is too small, it will have no therapeutic effect; if it is too large, it may cause such side effects as a dry mouth, a burning sensation in the tongue, palpitations, and manic behavior.

Patients with pronounced or long-standing internal cold, particularly with cold in the middle burner, may have difficulty ingesting warming formulas. In severe cases, vomiting may be induced by even small amounts of a decoction or pill. In such cases, it is often necessary to include a small dose of a cooling herb such as Coptidis Rhizoma *(huáng lián)* in the formulation of a prescription, or to take the decoction cold in order to facilitate its assimilation This is an example of the strategy known as 'employing cooling [to treat conditions] caused by cold.' The effectiveness of this strategy may seem odd but is easily explained. Very severe cold pushes what heat remains to the surface of the body, including that from the digestive tract. A small amount of cooling will reduce this surface heat to allow penetration of the heating herbs into the interior.

Section 1

FORMULAS THAT WARM THE CHANNELS AND DISPERSE COLD

The formulas in this section treat cold pathogens congealing in the channels and collaterals where they obstruct the flow of qi and blood. This gives rise to cold inversion, cold-type obstruction patterns, and yin sores. It occurs more readily in patients with preexisting blood and nutritive qi deficiency, where the body's yang lacks substance to which it might attach itself. The formulas scatter cold with the help of herbs like Cinnamomi Ramulus *(guì zhī)*, Asari Radix et Rhizoma *(xì xīn)*, Ephedrae Herba *(má huáng)*, and Zingiberis Rhizoma recens *(shēng jiāng)*. To address any underlying deficiency, they combine these with herbs like Angelicae sinensis Radix *(dāng guī)*, Paeoniae Radix *(sháo yào)*, Astragali Radix *(huáng qí)*, or Cervi Cornu pantotrichum *(lù róng)* that tonify the qi and blood.

當歸四逆湯 (当归四逆汤)
Tangkuei Decoction for Frigid Extremities
dāng guī sì nì tāng

The term that we translate as frigid extremities (四逆 *sì nì*) literally means 'four rebellions' or 'four contraries.' In this condition, the limbs are cold, and instead of being normally extended, they 'rebel' or behave in a contrary manner by flexing and drawing inward toward the body in order to keep warm.

Source   *Discussion of Cold Damage* (c. 220)

Angelicae sinensis Radix *(dāng guī)* 9g
Paeoniae Radix *(sháo yào)* 9g
Cinnamomi Ramulus *(guì zhī)* 9g
Asari Radix et Rhizoma *(xì xīn)* 6g
Glycyrrhizae Radix praeparata *(zhì gān cǎo)* 6g
Jujubae Fructus *(dà zǎo)* . . . . 25 pieces
Akebiae Caulis *(mù tōng)* 6g

Method of Preparation   Decoction. The source text advises to take three times a day. At present, Paeoniae Radix alba *(bái sháo)* is the type of Paeoniae Radix *(sháo yào)* most commonly used (see the discussion under Cinnamon Twig Decoction *(guì zhī tāng)* in Chapter 1), and the dosage of Jujubae Fructus *(dà zǎo)* is reduced to 4-5 pieces. While the source text lists 通草 *tōng cǎo* as one of the ingredients, studies in the history of the Chinese materia medica (known as 本草學 *běn cǎo xué*) have shown that at least since the 10th century, the plant that was earlier known as 通草 *tōng cǎo* was then called Akebiae Caulis (木通 *mù* *tōng)*. For that reason, and the corollary clinical considerations, Akebiae Caulis *(mù tōng)* is what is used in this formula.

Actions   Warms the channels, disperses cold, nourishes the blood, and unblocks the blood vessels

Indications

Long-standing cold hands and feet that are both cold to the touch and feel very cold to the patient, a pale tongue with a white coating, and a submerged, thin pulse or one that is so thin that it is almost imperceptible

The extremities are rooted in the yang. The hands and feet become cold when they are deprived of the warmth and nourishment of the yang qi. However, the yang qi also needs something to which it can attach itself in order to be carried to the extremities. Because the pattern for which this formula is indicated is characterized by cold hands (up to the wrists) and feet (up to the ankles), a thin pulse that is almost imperceptible (due to blood deficiency and the congealing effects of cold) but no other indications of yang deficiency or ascendant yin, it is regarded as being due to cold in the channels in a patient with underlying blood deficiency. Such reasoning is based on a passage from Chapter 39 of *Basic Questions*: "When cold qi enters into the channels and slows down [their flow, the blood merely] trickles and does not move [properly]." The pale tongue is further evidence of blood deficiency, while the thin, white coating is indicative of cold.

Analysis of Formula

This formula is representative of a treatment strategy that simultaneously nourishes the blood and unblocks the vessels. It is comprised of two groups of herbs that address these complementary goals. The chief ingredient of the first group, Angelicae sinensis Radix *(dāng guī)*, is acrid, sweet, and warming. It tonifies and invigorates the blood to eliminate cold. Its blood-tonifying action is strengthened by the deputy ingredient, Paeoniae Radix *(sháo yào)*. The chief ingredient of the second group, Cinnamomi Ramulus *(guì zhī)*, warms the channels and disperses cold from the nutritive qi. When combined with its deputy, Asari Radix et Rhizoma *(xì xīn)*, it disperses both internal and external cold. The combination of Cinnamomi Ramulus *(guì zhī)* and Paeoniae Radix *(sháo yào)* harmonizes the protective and nutritive qi, thereby helping to eliminate cold from the more superficial levels of the body. The assistant herbs, Glycyrrhizae Radix praeparata *(zhì gān cǎo)* and Jujubae Fructus *(dà zǎo)*, augment the qi and strengthen the Spleen. They assist the first group in tonifying the blood and the second group in facilitating the flow of qi. The envoy, Akebiae Caulis *(mù tōng)*, facilitates the flow in the channels and vessels and also drains the static heat that may accumulate even in these conditions as the qi is fettered by cold. This strengthens the actions of the other ingredients and focuses their effects on the channels.

Cautions and Contraindications

This formula should be used with caution during the spring and summer seasons, or in warm climates, since it readily injures the fluids. It is contraindicated in patients with fire from yin deficiency.

Commentary

Treatment of Frigid Extremities

This formula is regarded as a variation of Cinnamon Twig Decoction *(guì zhī tāng)*. The source text notes that it is indicated for cold injuring the terminal yin with "extremely cold hands and feet and a pulse that is thin almost to the point of being imperceptible." In *Discussion of Medical Formulas*, the Qing-dynasty scholar-physician Fei Bo-Xiong explained the connection between the formula and its indication:

> The terminal yin is the channel [responsible] for storing the blood. Therefore, Tangkuei Decoction for Frigid Extremities *(dāng guī sì nì tāng)* focuses on harmonizing the nutritive [qi]. It includes Cinnamomi Ramulus *(guì zhī)* and Asari Radix et Rhizoma *(xì xīn)* to harmonize the protective qi. When the nutritive and protective qi are harmonized, frigidity of the extremities resolves by itself. In spite of the presence of cold [as the main pathogen], the formula does not employ Aconiti Radix lateralis praeparata *(zhì fù zǐ)* or Zingiberis Rhizoma *(gān jiāng)* out of fear that their excessively drying [nature] may cut off yin and consume the blood.

Some commentators, however, found it difficult to accept that frigid extremities from cold deficiency might be treated without the use of the warming and dispersing herbs Aconiti Radix lateralis praeparata *(zhì fù zǐ)* and Zingiberis Rhizoma *(gān jiāng)*. The most influential representative of this current, the Qing-dynasty physician Ke Qin, advanced a critique in *Collected Writings on Renewal of the Discussion of Cold Damage* that demonstrates that even the formulas of sages like Zhang Zhong-Jing were not beyond the reproach of classically-oriented physicians:

> The pattern [discussed] in this section [of *Discussion of Cold Damage*] is an interior [pattern]. One should use Frigid Extremities Decoction *(sì nì tāng)* as the foundation and add Angelicae sinensis Radix *(dāng guī)*. Poria Frigid Extremities Decoction *(fú líng sì nì tāng)* is an example [of when this type of modification is permitted]. Using [a variation of] Cinnamon Twig Decoction *(guì zhī tāng)* to attack the exterior [when the illness is in the interior] is wrong.

Nevertheless, most commentators agree with Fei Bo-Xiong's interpretation. They view the formula as an example of the versatility of Cinnamon Twig Decoction *(guì zhī tāng)* in treating conditions arising from cold entering the nutritive qi (see Chapter 1). Astragalus and Cinnamon Twig Five-Substance Decoction *(huáng qí guì zhī wǔ wù tāng)*, discussed below, Cinnamon Twig plus Aconite Accessory Root Decoction *(guì zhī jiā fù zǐ tāng)*, discussed in Chapter 1, and Cinnamon Twig, Peony, and Anemarrhena Decoction (guì zhī sháo yào zhī mǔ tāng), discussed in Chapter 16, are other examples. Because the nutritive qi circulates within the vessels, obstruction to its flow frequently manifests as painful obstruction patterns in the extremities. The role of Cinnamomi Ramulus (guì zhī) in all of these formulas is to lead the yang into the yin, the protective into the nutritive, and to facilitate its dispersion and resolve stagnation.

The type of frigid extremities disorder for which this formula is indicated—deficient blood and nutritive qi fettered by cold—must be distinguished from other possible manifestations of this disorder, as discussed below in the COMPARISON section.

Dosage of Jujubae Fructus (dà zǎo)

This formula's focus on the nutritive qi—that aspect of the body's qi that is produced in the middle burner, fills the vessels, and forms the basis for the production of blood—also helps explain the large dosage of Jujubae Fructus (dà zǎo) included in the original formula. According to Li Shi-Zhen, Jujubae Fructus (dà zǎo) is an herb for the "Spleen channel blood level." *Seeking Accuracy in the Materia Medica* further explains that it "is sweet so that it tonifies the middle, warm so that it augments the qi. When the Spleen and Stomach are tonified, the twelve channels are naturally unblocked." Nevertheless, ever since the Jin-Yuan epoch, physicians have reduced the dosage of this herb in this and many other formulas due to concerns about its cloying nature. Practitioners should exercise their own judgment in weighing priorities.

Expanded Usage

The use of this formula has been expanded over the centuries to encompass a variety of conditions due to cold invading the channels with underlying blood deficiency. Common manifestations include headache (including migraines), pain in the joints, irregular menstruation, abdominal pain and cold, pain in the lower back and legs, and chest pain. In all the cases, the symptoms tend to be precipitated or aggravated by exposure to cold, including cold food or drink. Moreover, based on Japanese precedents, the modern physician Huang Huang in *One-Hundred Classic Formulas* extended its use to patterns where the key symptoms of cold extremities and faint pulse are accompanied by signs of disordered body fluids. This might include increased sweating, particularly of the feet, vaginal discharge, increased salivation, or changes in urination. The thinking behind this usage is that cold also inhibits the normal dissemination of body fluids. In this formula, the issue is addressed by including the herbs Akebiae Caulis (mù tōng) and Asari Radix et Rhizoma (xì xīn), which, besides unblocking the vessels and dispersing cold, also facilitate water metabolism and promote urination.

Comparison

> ➤ Vs. OTHER FORMULAS THAT TREAT COLD HANDS AND FEET AS A PRIMARY SYMPTOM

Discussion of Cold Damage prescribes the present formula for a pattern known as "inversion [characterized by] cold" (厥寒 jué hán). Typically, this is a more long-standing condition seen in patients who are generally averse to cold, but where the hands and feet feel colder to the patient than the rest of the body, and where the cold affects the entire hand and foot instead of just the fingers and toes. The nails and lips tend to be purple, and the general complexion will be pale. The presence of pain is another important clinical marker.

This must be distinguished from yin- or cold-type inversion disorder due to interior cold from deficiency. This is referred to in the source text as "inversion [characterized by] frigidity" (厥冷 jué lěng) and is treated with Frigid Extremities Decoction (sì nì tāng), which is discussed later in this chapter. In this pattern, the entire limb—and not just the hands and feet—are cold. In addition, the patient will also experience lethargy, an increased desire to sleep, watery diarrhea, and a submerged pulse.

The third pattern is cold extremities due to constrained qi, for which Frigid Extremities Powder (sì nì sǎn), discussed in Chapter 3, is indicated. This pattern is known as yang- or hot-type inversion. Generally, only the tips of the hands and feet will be cold, the nails and lips are of normal color, the pulse is wiry rather than thin, and there are usually some heat signs visible elsewhere in the body. These may include subjective sensations of heat, irritability, insomnia, constipation, dark urine, and a red tongue with a yellow coating. There is often an emotional component to the disorder. In special cases where intense heat leads to cold extremities, formulas that clear interior heat, such as White Tiger Decoction (bái hǔ tāng) (see Chapter 4) or Major Order the Qi Decoction (dà chéng qì tāng) (see Chapter 2), are required.

Biomedical Indications

With the appropriate presentation, this formula may be used to treat a wide variety of biomedically-defined disorders, primarily those involving narrowing or occlusive problems with the peripheral circulation, such as vascular headaches, Raynaud's disease, thromboangiitis obliterans, frostbite, impotence, varicocele, and scleroderma. It has also been used for other vascular problems such as Takayasu's arteritis, basilar artery insufficiency, and coronary artery insufficiency.

It has also been used to treat painful conditions with cold extremities such as hypertensive headache, traumatic headache, gingivitis, trigeminal neuralgia, lower back sprains, sciatica, periarthritis of the shoulders, peptic ulcer, cholecystitis, pelvic inflammatory disease, and pain from cancers.

The presentation for this formula can also be seen in such diverse diseases as Meniere's disease, idiopathic purpura, chronic urticaria, prostatitis, perimenstural edema, tenosynovitis, postoperative adhesions, as well as the early stages of upper respiratory tract infections.

Modifications

- For persistent, mild headache, vertigo, and tinnitus, add Angelicae dahuricae Radix *(bái zhǐ)* and Saposhnikoviae Radix *(fáng fēng)*.

- For vague epigastric pain that responds well to the application of heat or pressure, and spitting of clear fluids, add Evodiae Fructus *(wú zhū yú)*, Citri sarcodactylis Fructus *(fó shǒu)*, and Codonopsis Radix *(dǎng shēn)*.

- For cold and pain in the lower abdomen during menstruation (which is scanty), add Leonuri Herba *(yì mǔ cǎo)* and Cyperi Rhizoma *(xiāng fù)*.

- For bulging disorders due to cold, add Linderae Radix *(wū yào)*, Foeniculi Fructus *(xiǎo huí xiāng)*, and Alpiniae officinarum Rhizoma *(gāo liáng jiāng)*.

- For chronic, resistant sciatica, add Aconiti Radix lateralis praeparata *(zhì fù zǐ)*, Rhei Radix et Rhizoma *(dà huáng)*, Dipsaci Radix *(xù duàn)*, and Cibotii Rhizoma *(gǒu jǐ)*.

Variation

當歸四逆加吳茱萸生薑湯
（当归四逆加吴茱萸生姜汤）

Tangkuei Decoction for Frigid Extremities plus Evodia and Fresh Ginger

dāng guī sì nì jiā wú zhū yú shēng jiāng tāng

SOURCE *Discussion of Cold Damage* (c. 220)

For a similar presentation with chronic cold in the middle burner or in the Conception and Penetrating vessels characterized by loose stools, nausea and vomiting, abdominal pain, and an extremely thin pulse, add Evodiae Fructus *(wú zhū yú)* and Zingiberis Rhizoma recens *(shēng jiāng)*. These two herbs enter into the terminal yin and yang brightness to disperse chronic stagnation and prolonged cold. The source text advises to decoct the herbs with 6 cups each of water and weak rice wine (清酒 *qīng jiǔ*) until about half the liquid has evaporated. The strained decoction is then divided into five portions and taken warm. The wine used for boiling the herbs further strengthens the cold-dispersing properties of the formula. It is indicated when a Tangkuei Decoction for Frigid Extremities *(dāng guī sì nì tāng)* pattern is complicated by chronic stagnation and cold. Japanese texts therefore advise that it be used as a prophylactic for chillblains and frostbite that may be taken throughout late autumn and winter. Such a pattern is still less severe than the condition for which Frigid Extremities Decoction *(sì nì tāng)* is indicated.

黃耆桂枝五物湯（黄芪桂枝五物汤）

Astragalus and Cinnamon Twig Five-Substance Decoction

huáng qí guì zhī wǔ wù tāng

Source *Essentials from the Golden Cabinet* (c. 220)

Astragali Radix *(huáng qí)*	9g
Paeoniae Radix *(sháo yào)*	9g
Cinnamomi Ramulus *(guì zhī)*	9g
Zingiberis Rhizoma recens *(shēng jiāng)*	18g
Jujubae Fructus *(dà zǎo)*	12 pieces

Method of Preparation   Decoction. The source text advises to take three times a day. At present the dosage of Astragali Radix *(huáng qí)* and Zingiberis Rhizoma recens *(shēng jiāng)* is usually 12g.

Actions   Augments the qi, warms and harmonizes the channels, and unblocks painful obstruction

Indications

Relatively superficial numbness without pain, paresthesias and numbness of the skin and flesh, and a faint, choppy, and tight pulse

This is painful obstruction of the blood. A passage in Chapter 72 of *Basic Questions* states: "If the normal qi is stored in the interior, pathogens cannot attack." When protective and nutritive qi are both deficient, wind-cold invading the superficial layers of the body lodges in the blood vessels and obstructs the movement of qi and blood. Failing to nourish and moisten the skin, it thickens and becomes insensitive. This is experienced as superficial numbness. Stagnation of the blood vessels caused by pathogenic wind-cold is reflected in a faint, choppy, and tight pulse.

Analysis of Formula

This formula utilizes a strategy of warming the channels and tonifying deficiency in order to overcome peripheral obstructions to the movement of blood. As its name indicates, Astragali Radix *(huáng qí)* and Cinnamomi Ramulus *(guì zhī)* jointly serve as the chief herbs. Sweet and warming, Astragali Radix *(huáng qí)* strongly tonifies the original qi, helping the normal qi to expel pathogenic qi while simultaneously firming up the skin and exterior. Its usage embodies a treatment strategy first outlined in Chapter 4 of *Divine Pivot*: "When yin and yang, form and qi are both insufficient, do not take care of it with needles, but regulate by means of sweet herbs." Cinnamomi Ramulus *(guì zhī)* warms the nutritive qi in the channels and unblocks the yang. Astragali Radix *(huáng qí)* increases the ability of Cinnamomi Ramulus *(guì zhī)* to augment the qi and stimulate the protective yang. Cinnamomi Ramulus *(guì zhī)* increases the capacity of Astragali Radix *(huáng qí)* to firm up the exterior without retaining pathogenic qi. In combination, the two chief herbs synergistically augment the qi, warm the yang, harmonize the blood, and unblock the channels.

Paeoniae Radix (sháo yào), which nourishes the blood, harmonizes the nutritive qi, and unblocks painful obstruction, functions as the deputy. In combination with Cinnamomi Ramulus (guì zhī), it harmonizes the nutritive and protective qi. In combination with Astragali Radix (huáng qí), it firms up the exterior and nourishes the yin. Because the pathogen is located in the skin, the formula uses a large dose of Zingiberis Rhizoma recens (shēng jiāng) as an assistant. Acrid and warming, it opens the interstices and pores, disperses wind-cold from the exterior, and, together with Cinnamomi Ramulus (guì zhī), warms and moves the blood vessels. Jujubae Fructus (dà zǎo) serves as envoy, regulating the formula by means of its sweetness and assisting Cinnamomi Ramulus (guì zhī), Zingiberis Rhizoma recens (shēng jiāng), and Paeoniae Radix (sháo yào) in regulating the nutritive and protective qi.

This formula can thus be regarded as a variation of Cinnamon Twig Decoction (guì zhī tāng), in which Glycyrrhizae Radix praeparata (zhì gān cǎo) has been replaced by Astragali Radix (huáng qí) and the dosage of Zingiberis Rhizoma recens (shēng jiāng) has been increased. Glycyrrhizae Radix (gān cǎo) is used in many of Zhang Zhong-Jing's formulas to facilitate the flow of blood by relaxing the vessels. Astragali Radix (huáng qí), on the other hand, which strongly acts on the upper burner, stimulates and supports the pulsating rhythm of the gathering qi and thereby assists movement in the vessels. In this manner, the formula not only expels wind-cold, but also facilitates movement in the vessels to cure painful obstruction of the blood.

Commentary

Essentials of the Golden Cabinet defines painful obstruction of the blood, the pattern for which this formula is indicated, as "joint feebleness of yin and yang." Most commentators interpret the reference to yin and yang in this context as referring to the protective and nutritive qi. Elaborating on the source text, *Discussion of the Origins of the Symptoms of Disease* provides the following explanation:

> Painful obstruction of the blood arises from a pathogen entering into the yin vessels of a deficient body. Blood is yin. The pathogen enters into the blood [causing] painful obstruction. Hence, it is called painful obstruction of the blood. Its manifestation in the body is as if being blown upon by a light wind. It arises in overly emotional people (憂樂之人 *yōu lè zhī rén*)* with weak bones and overabundant flesh who, because of sweating due to fatiguing work, have frequent tremors when lying down, so their skin and interstices are open and can be

invaded by wind pathogens. On examining the pulse, [one finds] it to be faint and weak at the distal pulse position, and slightly tight in the middle position. In painful obstruction of the blood, it is appropriate to draw the yang qi up [by using] needles. Through harmonizing the blood vessels and eliminating tightness [from the pulse, the condition] is cured.

Symptomatically, numbness and parasthesia are the most distinctive features of painful obstruction of the blood. More severe cases may manifest with aching of the entire body, a manifestation that the source text defines as "resembling wind painful obstruction." Painful obstruction of the blood must also be distinguished from wind-stroke in the channels. Both are caused by the invasion of wind and characterized by numbness. However, in wind-stroke patterns the wind invades more deeply, obstructing the vessels and collaterals and denying nourishment to the sinews and blood vessels. This results in functional impairment such as paralysis and hemiplegia. Astragalus and Cinnamon Twig Five-Substance Decoction (huáng qí guì zhī wǔ wù tāng) is therefore inappropriate to treat the acute stages of wind-stroke when more strongly dispersing formulas are required. *Discussion of Seasonal Diseases* does, however, recommend it for treating the sequelae of wind-stroke: "This formula treats disability from wind, hemiplegia, weakness of the hands and feet, and inability to walk. [In these cases, the formula] shows its power [only] if it is used for a long time."

Most modern texts translate the term 不仁 *bù rén* as 'insensitivity' or 'numbness.' As in many other instances, however, the original Chinese meaning is more comprehensive and includes pain and itching. For example, in *Personal Standards for the Essentials from the Golden Cabinet*, the Qing dynasty physician Long Zai-Jing states that 不仁 *bù rén* refers to "stubborn painful obstruction of the entire body [that is characterized] by pain, itching, and insensitivity." In clinical practice, the formula can thus be used to treat various types of neuralgia and even abdominal or chest pain, provided that the pulse is submerged, feeble, and forceless, and the tongue is pale and puffy.

Biomedical Indications

With the appropriate presentation, this formula may be used to treat a wide variety of biomedically-defined disorders. One group deals with numbness and loss of sensitivity such as polyneuritis, diabetic neuropathy, scleroderma, dermatomyositis, Bell's palsy, common peroneal neuropathy, Raynaud's disease, Takayasu's arteritis, and thromboangiitis obliterans. This formula has also been used in the treatment of related dermatological disorders including ulcers of the lower extremities, bedsores, urticaria, and idipathic thrombocytopenic purpura.

A second group consists of disorders marked by pain, weakness, tightness, or spasms of the extremities such as sci-

---

*Note that in *Essentials of the Golden Cabinet* (Chapter 6), the term used here is "the venerated and honored" (夫尊榮人 *fū zūn róng rén*), that is, those who normally do not perform physical labor.

atica, cervical disc disease, rheumatoid arthritis, periarthritis of the shoulder, focal seizures, sequelae of stroke, restless leg syndrome, and facial tics.

The formula has been used for a wide variety of other problems as well, including postpartum conditions, urinary retention, chronic prostatitis, nephritis, obesity, pneumonia, and coronary artery disease.

Alternate names

Astragalus Decoction (*huáng qí tāng*) in *Comprehensive Recording of Sagely Beneficence*; Astragalus Five-Substance Decoction (*huáng qí wǔ wù tāng*) in *Illnesses, Patterns, and Formulas Related to the Unification of the Three Etiologies*; Cinnamon Twig Five-Substance Decoction (*guì zhī wǔ wù tāng*) in *Complete Collection of Red Water and Dark Pearls*; Five-Substance Decoction (*wǔ wù tāng*) in *Precious Mirror of Oriental Medicine*

Modifications

- For more pronounced qi deficiency, increase the dosage of Astragali Radix (*huáng qí*) and add Codonopsis Radix (*dǎng shēn*).
- For blood deficiency, add Angelicae sinensis Radix (*dāng guī*) and Spatholobi Caulis (*jī xuè téng*).
- For yang deficiency with frigid extremities, add Aconiti Radix lateralis praeparata (*zhì fù zǐ*).
- For spasms of the sinews, numbness, and painful obstruction, add Chaenomelis Fructus (*mù guā*) and Zaocys (*wū shāo shé*).
- For dispersing a more severe wind pathogen, add Saposhnikoviae Radix (*fáng fēng*) and *fáng jǐ* (Stephaniae/Cocculi/etc. Radix).
- For blood stasis, add Carthami Flos (*hóng huā*) and Persicae Semen (*táo rén*).

Section 2

FORMULAS THAT WARM THE MIDDLE AND DISPEL COLD

The formulas in this section are used to treat cold from deficiency in the middle burner. The Spleen and Stomach control the transformation and transportation of food and nutrients, and play a pivotal role in regulating the ascending and descending functions of the qi. When the yang qi of these organs is weak and the patient suffers an invasion of external cold, the qi dynamic is disrupted causing epigastric and abdominal distention and pain, fatigue, cold extremities, a white, slippery tongue coating, and a submerged pulse that is either slow or thin. Sometimes there is also acid reflux, nau-

sea and vomiting, abdominal pain with diarrhea, reduced appetite, or reduced thirst.

The chief herbs in formulas used to treat these disorders are warming and acrid or heating and acrid in nature. The most important of these is Zingiberis Rhizoma (*gān jiāng*), whose color resembles that of earth. Other frequently used herbs are Caryophylli Flos (*dīng xiāng*), Alpiniae officinarum Rhizoma (*gāo liáng jiāng*), Cinnamomi Ramulus (*guì zhī*), Zingiberis Rhizoma recens (*shēng jiāng*), Zanthoxyli Pericarpium (*huā jiāo*), and Evodiae Fructus (*wú zhū yú*). Depending on the pattern treated, they may be combined with herbs that strengthen the Spleen and augment the qi, such as Astragali Radix (*huáng qí*), Ginseng Radix (*rén shēn*), or Atractylodis macrocephalae Rhizoma (*bái zhú*); or with herbs that nourish the blood and enrich the yin, such as Angelicae sinensis Radix (*dāng guī*), Paeoniae Radix alba (*bái sháo*), or Rehmanniae Radix praeparata (*shú dì huáng*).

理中丸

Regulate the Middle Pill

lǐ zhōng wán

This formula regulates the yang qi of the Spleen and Stomach, which occupy the middle burner, hence the name. In some contexts, the formula is used as a decoction. Accordingly, it is also known as Regulate the Middle Decoction (*lǐ zhōng tāng*).

Source *Discussion of Cold Damage* (c. 220)

Zingiberis Rhizoma (*gān jiāng*)	9g
Ginseng Radix (*rén shēn*)	9g
Atractylodis macrocephalae Rhizoma (*bái zhú*)	9g
Glycyrrhizae Radix praeparata (*zhì gān cǎo*)	9g

Method of Preparation Grind the ingredients into a powder and form into pills with honey. The source text advises to take three times a day and twice at night with warm water. At present, it is taken 2-3 times a day in 9g doses. It may also be prepared as a decoction. The pill form is often taken with warm rice porridge. Except in acute cases, at present, Codonopsis Radix (*dǎng shēn*) is generally substituted for Ginseng Radix (*rén shēn*) at 2-3 times its dosage.

Actions Warms the middle burner and strengthens the Spleen and Stomach

Indications

This formula is used to treat a number of different patterns, the most important of which is middle burner cold from deficiency, also known as middle burner yang deficiency, characterized by diarrhea with watery stools, nausea and vomiting, no particular thirst, loss of appetite, abdominal pain, a pale tongue with a white coating, and a submerged, thin pulse.

A second important pattern is bleeding due to middle burner yang deficiency, including nose bleeds, vomiting of blood, excessive menstrual bleeding, bleeding from the rectum, and various types of internal bleeding. In all cases, the blood is pale and the bleeding is accompanied by cold extremities, a wan complexion, pale tongue, frail pulse, and other symptoms indicating middle burner cold.

Other presentations include chronic childhood convulsions (驚風 *jīng fēng*) characterized by emaciation, cold hands and feet, vomiting, and diarrhea; spitting of frothy saliva during the recovery stage of an illness; sudden turmoil disorder with cold marked by an absence of thirst; and chest painful obstruction characterized by rigid focal distention in the heart region, a sense of fullness in the chest, and pain in the hypochondria that shoots toward the heart.

When the Spleen yang is deficient, the clear yang cannot ascend, which causes diarrhea with watery stools. When the Stomach loses its ability to make the turbid yin descend, nausea and vomiting ensue. The loss of appetite is indicative of Spleen deficiency. When cold invades the abdomen, it causes contraction, and thus pain. This process is reflected in the saying, "When the yang is deficient, the yin ascends." The absence of thirst is indicative of cold. Cold from deficiency is also reflected in the pale tongue with a white coating and the submerged, thin pulse.

The Spleen governs the blood, and the power of qi contains the blood. Cold invading the middle burner or insufficiency of Spleen yang impairs these functions. If the Spleen qi lacks the power to contain the blood, bleeding may occur throughout the body. This disease dynamic is aptly summarized by Tang Zong-Hai in *Discussion of Blood Patterns*: "When the classics state that the Spleen governs the blood, [they mean that] the movement of blood above and below depends entirely on the Spleen. If the Spleen yang is deficient, it is unable to govern the blood."

Chronic childhood convulsions (驚風 *jīng fēng*) are attributed to disharmony of the protective and nutritive qi due to insufficient development of middle burner yang. This is manifested in such symptoms as emaciation, cold hands and feet, vomiting, and diarrhea. Spitting of frothy saliva in the recovery stage of an illness indicates damage to the Spleen yang, which is unable to contain the yang fluids.

Sudden turmoil disorder can be caused by an external cold pathogen that directly attacks the middle burner, especially where the Spleen and Stomach are deficient due to irregular eating and a poor diet. Damage to the middle burner yang qi results in insufficient separation of the clear and turbid, as well as a disorder in the ascending and descending actions of the qi dynamic, which manifests in vomiting and diarrhea.

Chest obstruction is characterized by exuberance of yin and deficiency of yang. The cold of deficiency in the middle burner slows down the movement of qi, causing the yin fluids and blood to stagnate in the chest. Yin occupying the position of yang manifests as rigid focal distention in the heart region, a sense of fullness in the chest, and pain in the hypochondria that shoots toward the heart.

Analysis of Formula

This formula treats deficiency cold of the middle burner. Without warming and heating herbs, the cold cannot be dispelled, but without tonification, what is deficient cannot be augmented. For this reason, the formula employs a combined strategy of warming the interior to dispel the cold and tonifying the qi of the Spleen and Stomach.

The chief herb, Zingiberis Rhizoma *(gān jiāng)*, warms the Spleen and Stomach yang and eliminates interior cold, the primary function of this formula. The yang and the qi are intimately related. The deputy herb, Ginseng Radix *(rén shēn)*, strongly tonifies the source qi; this reinforces the yang and rectifies the ascending and descending functions of the middle burner. When the Spleen is deficient, its ability to transform and transport is impaired, which leads to internal stagnation of water and dampness. The assistant herb, Atractylodis macrocephalae Rhizoma *(bái zhú)*, not only aids the deputy herb in tonifying the Spleen and Stomach, but also strengthens the Spleen and dries dampness. This combination of herbs—one warming, one tonifying, and one drying—is quite effective in warming and improving the functions of the middle burner. The envoy, Glycyrrhizae Radix praeparata *(zhì gān cǎo)*, augments the qi of the middle burner and harmonizes the actions of the other herbs in the formula.

Cautions and Contraindications

Because this formula contains ingredients that warm and dry, it should not be used for externally-contracted disorders with fever or yin deficiency. For sudden turmoil disorder, its use should be discontinued once the vomiting and diarrhea have stopped.

Commentary

The reliance of the digestive functions of the middle burner on the yang qi supplied by the gate of vitality makes it particularly vulnerable to damage from cold. The reliance of other organ systems on postnatal essences, in turn, implies that impairment of the transportive and transformative functions of the middle burner will be felt throughout the body. In *Clear Explanations to the Discussion of Cold Damage and Later Systematic Differentiations,* the early Qing-dynasty physician Cheng Ying-Mao explains this pathology:

> The movement of yang begins with warmth. [When the Spleen] receives the warm qi, it transports the food essences. The food qi ascends and the qi of the middle [burner] is supported. Hence, the name [of this formula refers to] regulating the middle. In fact, its power to regulate the middle is bestowed by the yang of the middle burner. If Stomach yang is deficient, the qi of the middle burner is plundered, the chest center [no longer carries out its] disseminating functions, and the six yang organs lose their powers of sprinkling and ripening. It is like re-

moving firewood from under the cauldron. Clear food diarrhea below, loss of taste above, deprivation of the five yin organs, and all other manifestations result from this.

Cheng Ying-Mao's analysis deserves some attention because, unlike contemporary textbooks, it focuses on the functions of the middle burner yang (indicated by reference to the Stomach as a yang organ) rather than on the Spleen. The original use of this formula in *Discussion of Cold Damage*, where it is listed as treating greater yin disorders, corroborates this view. Greater yin disorders imply a deficiency in the functions of the middle burner yang, as opposed to the yang excess disorders grouped under the yang brightness category. In Chinese medicine, this is summed up in the saying, "Excess means the yang brightness, deficiency the greater yin." In *Formulas in Verse from the Scholar's Studio in Two Volumes*, the modern scholar-physician Cheng Men-Xue explains this relationship:

> The greater yin and yang brightness, a yin and a yang organ, Spleen and Stomach as fellow officials, these two are integrated with each other … [The fact that] patterns listed under the heading of greater yin disorders [include] vomiting and inability to get food down [indicate that these] are not simply Spleen but also Stomach disorders. One should [therefore] differentiate according to the maxim, 'Because heat [patterns] are yang, they are subordinated to the yang brightness and the Stomach yang organ. Because cold [patterns] are yin, they are subordinated to the greater yin and the Spleen yin organ. However, if the Spleen is cold, the Stomach is also cold. Therefore, greater yin [disorders] include vomiting and the inability to get food down. When the Stomach is hot, the Spleen is also hot. Therefore, yang brightness [disorders] include the Spleen bind pattern.' [In all these cases, one does not view the Spleen and Stomach separately, but] merely differentiates according to what is primary or secondary.

Cheng also provides a useful differentiation of the similarities and differences of greater yin and yang brightness disorders:

> [When] the greater yin stores cold, there is clear, thin diarrhea below, not all of the food is transformed, and the urine is clear and increased. This is very different from foul-smelling heat-type diarrhea with a yellow or red color and the consistency of soup, tenesmus, and the hot, dark, and reduced urination [associated with yang brightness disorders]. In greater yin disorders, the abdomen is soft on palpation, whereas in yang brightness disorders, it is hard. Abdominal distention in yang brightness disorders is unrelieved, whereas in greater yin disorders there are periods of aggravation and amelioration. Although there are commonalities, there are also clear differences [allowing us] to differentiate excess and deficiency.

Key Indicators

In clinical practice, therefore, the following signs and symptoms are key clinical markers for use of this formula:

- Abdominal distention or pain in patients with a soft and lax abdomen that is not relieved by belching or the passing of wind

- Pain that is mild and chronic rather than acute and relieved by warmth or warming foods
- Abnormal stools that tend to be soft and loose but can also be hard if untransformed fluids are directly eliminated via the bladder.

Since its first listing in *Discussion of Cold Damage*, subsequent generations of physicians have used Regulate the Middle Pill (*lǐ zhōng wán*) as the foundation for a large number of new formulas that extend its range. These include pox and rashes (based on its ability to treat the root of deficiency wind), blood stasis-type abdominal pain (which develops against a background of cold and blood deficiency), and lower back pain (caused by blood deficiency due to middle burner cold). Depending on the type of disorder treated, the formula is prescribed as a pill (more suitable for patterns characterized by mild symptoms like spitting of thin saliva) or as a decoction (indicated for patterns that are more acute, such as sudden turmoil disorder or bleeding).

Controversy Surrounding the Chief Ingredient

Physicians have argued over the nature of the chief herb in this formula. The Song dynasty commentator Cheng Wu-Ji contended that it was Ginseng Radix (*rén shēn*) because of its ability to tonify the middle burner. Others, like the modern physician Cai Lu-Xin, argue that the chief herb is Zingiberis Rhizoma (*gān jiāng*) because of its ability to warm and support the yang. In practice, most physicians adopt a flexible approach that focuses on the interaction between the various ingredients of the formula, adjusting their relative dosage according to the presenting symptoms.

Comparisons

➤ Vs. Magnolia Bark Decoction for Warming the Middle (*hòu pò wēn zhōng tāng*)

Both of these formulas treat diarrhea due to cold in the middle burner. Magnolia Bark Decoction for Warming the Middle (*hòu pò wēn zhōng tāng*) strongly dries dampness and promotes movement of the qi but does not tonify. It is used for invasion of damp-cold into the middle burner marked by epigastric and abdominal distention and fullness, and a white, slippery tongue coating. By contrast, Regulate the Middle Pill (*lǐ zhōng wán*) is used for cold from deficiency or invasion of cold without dampness. In this presentation, distention and fullness are absent, but there is nausea and vomiting, and the pulse is submerged and thin.

➤ Vs. Four-Gentlemen Decoction (*sì jūn zǐ tāng*)

Both formulas treat patterns characterized by deficiency of the middle burner with symptoms such as reduced appetite, fatigue, and abdominal distention. However, Four-Gentlemen Decoction (*sì jūn zǐ tāng*) focuses on qi deficiency leading to impaired movement and transformation. In practice, therefore, this formula is often modified by including herbs that move the qi or promote water metabolism in order to deal with increased dampness and qi stagnation due to qi deficiency. Regulate the Middle Pill *(lǐ zhōng wán)*, on the other hand, focuses on yang deficiency leading to symptoms such as abdominal distention and pain, increased urination, and aversion to cold.

➤ Vs. Frigid Extremities Decoction *(sì nì tāng)*; see PAGE 277

➤ Vs. Licorice, Ginger, Poria and White Atractylodes Decoction *(gān cǎo gān jiāng fù líng bái zhú tāng)*; see PAGE 743

➤ Vs. Mume Pill *(wū méi wán)*; see PAGE 851

Biomedical Indications

With the appropriate presentation, this formula can be used to treat a wide variety of biomedically-defined disorders. One group deals with abdominal pain and diarrhea and includes gastroenteritis (particularly in children), peptic ulcers, functional digestive problems, irritable bowel syndrome, chronic dysentery, and ulcerative colitis. Another group deals with fluid and mucous issues, including allergic rhinitis, benign prostatic hypertrophy, gastritis from biliary reflux, chronic bronchitis, vaginitis, and pelvic inflammatory disease. It has also been used for exudative eczema and dermatitis, and for an assortment of problems marked by bleeding, including bronchiectasis, upper GI bleeds, allergic purpura, idiopathic thrombocytopenic purpura, and functional uterine bleeding. Finally, it has been a foundation prescription for some types of chest pain, including those from coronary artery disease.

Alternate names

Four-Fold Smoothing Regulate the Middle Pill *(sì shùn lǐ zhōng wán)* in *Important Formulas Worth a Thousand Gold Pieces for any Emergency*; White Atractylodes Pill *(bái zhú wán)* in *Comprehensive Recording of Sagely Beneficence*; Regulate the Middle Pill *(tiáo zhōng wán)* in *Craft of Medicines and Patterns for Children*; Major Regulate the Middle Pill *(dà lǐ zhōng wán)* in *Effective Formulas from Generations of Physicians*; Smooth Flavor Pill *(shùn wèi wán)* in *Formulas of Universal Benefit*; Ginseng Regulate the Middle Pill *(rén shēn lǐ zhōng wán)* in *Essential Dynamics of Pestilential Sores*; Ginseng Decoction *(rén shēn tāng)* in *Essentials from the Golden Cabinet*; Treat the Middle Decoction *(zhì zhōng tāng)* in *Important Formulas Worth a Thousand Gold Pieces*; Ginseng Decoction to Regulate the Middle *(rén shēn lǐ zhōng tāng)* in *Fine Formulas for Women*

Modifications

• For severe vomiting, add Zingiberis Rhizoma recens *(shēng jiāng)*.
• For bleeding due to yang deficiency, substitute Zingiberis Rhizoma praeparatum *(páo jiāng)* for Zingiberis Rhizoma *(gān jiāng)* and add Astragali Radix *(huáng qí)*, Angelicae

sinensis Radix *(dāng guī)*, and Asini Corii Colla *(ē jiāo)*.
• For palpitations, add Poria *(fú líng)*.
• For 'butterflies' above the navel indicating Kidney deficiency with water qi encroaching upward, remove Atractylodis macrocephalae Rhizoma *(bái zhú)* and add Cinnamomi Ramulus *(guì zhī)* to direct the rebellious qi downward.
• For vomiting of thin fluids, increase the dosage of Atractylodis macrocephalae Rhizoma *(bái zhú)*.
• For more severe signs of cold marked by cold extremities, add Aconiti Radix lateralis praeparata *(zhì fù zǐ)* and Cinnamomi Cortex *(ròu guì)*.
• For incessant coughing, add Pinelliae Rhizoma praeparatum *(zhì bàn xià)*, Citri reticulatae Pericarpium *(chén pí)*, Asari Radix et Rhizoma *(xì xīn)*, and Schisandrae Fructus *(wǔ wèi zǐ)*.
• For cold-type jaundice, add Artemisiae scopariae Herba *(yīn chén)*.
• For yang deficiency bleeding, add Astragali Radix *(huáng qí)*, Angelicae sinensis Radix *(dāng guī)*, and Asini Corii Colla *(ē jiāo)*.
• For wheezing, fullness, edema, and reduced urination, combine with Five-Ingredient Powder with Poria *(wǔ líng sǎn)*.

Variations

連理湯 (连理汤)
Regulating Decoction with Coptis
lián lǐ tāng

SOURCE *Symptom, Cause, Pulse, and Treatment* (Ming dynasty)

For the same presentation as the principal formula with vomiting of sour fluids, thirst, reduced urination, and mouth ulcers, add Coptidis Rhizoma *(huáng lián)*. This is chronic constraint due to cold bottling up the fluids, which accumulate and gradually transform into damp-heat.

丁萸理中湯 (丁萸理中汤)
Clove and Evodia Decoction to Regulate the Middle
dīng yú lǐ zhōng tāng

SOURCE *Golden Mirror of the Medical Tradition* (1742)

For Stomach cold in children characterized by vomiting that is neither sour nor foul-smelling (especially vomiting in the evening what was eaten in the morning), undigested particles of food in the stool, cold extremities, and a pale complexion and lips, add Caryophylli Flos *(dīng xiāng)* and Evodiae Fructus *(wú zhū yú)*.

桂附理中湯 (桂附理中汤)
Cinnamon and Prepared Aconite Accessory Root Decoction to Regulate the Middle
guì fù lǐ zhōng tāng

SOURCE *Traditional Chinese Internal Medicine* (1970s)

For severe cold from deficiency of the Spleen, Stomach, and Kidneys characterized by diarrhea with undigested food or daybreak diarrhea, aversion to cold, cold extremities, back pain, reduced appetite, a pale tongue with a white coating, and a submerged, slow, and deficient pulse, add Cinnamomi Cortex (*ròu guì*) and Aconiti Radix lateralis praeparata (*zhì fù zǐ*).

Associated Formulas

治中丸

Treat the Middle Pill

zhì zhōng wán

SOURCE   *Simple Formulas for Health* (1905)

Ginseng Radix (*rén shēn*) 60g
Zingiberis Rhizoma (*gān jiāng*) 60g
Atractylodis macrocephalae Rhizoma (*bái zhú*) 60g
Glycyrrhizae Radix praeparata (*zhì gān cǎo*) 60g
Citri reticulatae Pericarpium (*chén pí*) 60g

For sudden turmoil disorder characterized by epigastric and abdominal pain, a desire to vomit without actually vomiting, and a desire to defecate without actually doing so. One variation of the formula uses Citri reticulatae Semen (*jú hé*) instead of Citri reticulatae Pericarpium (*chén pí*).

———————

附子理中丸

Aconite Accessory Root Pill to Regulate the Middle

fù zǐ lǐ zhōng wán

SOURCE   *Formulary of the Pharmacy Service for Benefiting the People in the Taiping Era* (1148)

Aconiti Radix lateralis praeparata (*zhì fù zǐ*) 90g
Zingiberis Rhizoma praeparatum (*páo jiāng*) 90g
Ginseng Radix (*rén shēn*) 90g
Atractylodis macrocephalae Rhizoma (*bái zhú*) 90g
Glycyrrhizae Radix praeparata (*zhì gān cǎo*) 90g

Grind the ingredients into a fine powder and form into 3g pills with honey. Make a draft of one pill, and take warm on an empty stomach. Warms the yang, dispels cold, augments the qi, and strengthens the Spleen. For more severe internal cold than that for which the principal formula is indicated, with abdominal and epigastric pain, vomiting and diarrhea, inability to keep food down, a cold body with very cold extremities, mild sweating, and a faint pulse. Also very effective for chronic or recurrent oral ulcers due to cold from deficiency of the Spleen and Stomach. At present, this is more popular than the principal formula.

———————

枳實理中丸 (枳实理中丸)

Unripe Bitter Orange Pill to Regulate the Middle

zhǐ shí lǐ zhōng wán

SOURCE   *Formulary of the Pharmacy Service for Benefiting the People in the Taiping Era* (1148)

Aurantii Fructus immaturus (*zhǐ shí*) 30g
Zingiberis Rhizoma (*gān jiāng*) 60g
Ginseng Radix (*rén shēn*) 60g

Atractylodis macrocephalae Rhizoma (*bái zhú*) 60g
Poria (*fú líng*) 60g
Glycyrrhizae Radix praeparata (*zhì gān cǎo*) 60g

Grind the ingredients into powder and form into yolk-sized (3-6g) pills with honey. Take with hot water. Strengthens the Spleen, warms the middle, and dissipates clumps. For cold from deficiency of the Spleen and Stomach with clumping characterized by abdominal fullness, distention, and pain.

吳茱萸湯 (吴茱萸汤)

Evodia Decoction

wú zhū yú tāng

Source   *Discussion of Cold Damage* (c. 220)

Evodiae Fructus (*wú zhū yú*) 9-12g
Zingiberis Rhizoma recens (*shēng jiāng*) 18g
Ginseng Radix (*rén shēn*) 9g
Jujubae Fructus (*dà zǎo*) . . . . 12 pieces

Method of Preparation   Decoction. At present, Codonopsis Radix (*dǎng shēn*) is often substituted for Ginseng Radix (*rén shēn*) with 2-3 times the dosage. Most practitioners use a slightly lower dosage than specified here, and only 4 pieces of Jujubae Fructus (*dà zǎo*). The dosage is reduced to prevent distention in the middle burner.

Actions   Warms and tonifies the Liver and Stomach, directs rebellious qi downward, and stops vomiting

Indications

In the source text the formula is prescribed for three different patterns:

- Yang brightness-warp pattern characterized by vomiting immediately after eating, indeterminate gnawing hunger, and acid reflux with or without epigastric pain
- Terminal yin-warp pattern characterized by dry heaves or spitting of clear fluids with a vertex headache
- Lesser yin-warp pattern characterized by vomiting and diarrhea with cold hands and feet, and agitation so severe that the patient wants to die.

In all cases, the tongue is not red, but has a white, slippery coating and the pulse is thin and slow or thin and wiry.

In terms of its disease dynamic, the first pattern is one of Stomach deficiency cold, where cold in the Stomach causes stagnation and pain. Stagnation leads to upward rebellion of Stomach qi, manifesting as vomiting. When the Stomach is deficient, it is unable to accept food. This causes vomiting immediately after eating. Indeterminate gnawing hunger is commonly interpreted as a sign of phlegm that irritates the Stomach qi. In the present context, this phlegm is due to fluid accumulation caused by deficiency of the Stomach yang.

The second presentation is thought to be due to Stomach and Liver deficiency cold. Cold in the Liver inhibits its ability to cause the clear to ascend, while Stomach cold inhibits its ability to direct the turbid downward. This results in the accumulation of turbid fluids manifesting as headache at the vertex (the end point of the foot terminal yin Liver channel) as well as dry heaves or spitting of clear fluids.

The third presentation is due to cold attacking the middle burner. In this pattern, the movement of Stomach qi is misdirected while the yang qi produced in the gate of vitality is neither spread to the limbs, resulting in cold hands and feet, nor to the middle burner, resulting in diarrhea. The combination of headache, vomiting, diarrhea, and cold hands and feet is so unbearable that the patient feels as if they want to die.

To summarize, although there are different manifestations of this disorder, they all share a common primary symptom (vomiting) and mechanism (Stomach deficiency cold). There is no heat present because the tongue is not red, nor is the pulse rapid. The white, slippery tongue coating and the thin and slow or thin and wiry pulse reflect the cold from deficiency and the disruption of the ascending and descending functions of the middle burner.

Analysis of Formula

To treat patterns characterized by rebelliousness due to cold in the Liver and Stomach, this formula employs a combined strategy of warming and tonifying the interior while directing rebellious qi downward in order to stop the vomiting. The chief ingredient, acrid, hot Evodiae Fructus (wú zhū yú), enters the Liver, Stomach, and Spleen. It warms the middle, disperses cold, promotes the movement of qi, and directs rebellious qi downward. It thereby addresses all the major pathological processes at the root of the various presentations treated by this formula. Because vomiting is such an important symptom in each, it must be addressed directly. The rather large dose of the deputy herb, Zingiberis Rhizoma recens (shēng jiāng), helps the chief herb accomplish this task by warming the Stomach and directing its qi downward. While Zingiberis Rhizoma recens (shēng jiāng) excels at dispersing clear fluids from the Stomach, Evodiae Fructus (wú zhū yú) treats acid reflux due to Liver cold accosting the Stomach; in addition, its bitterness directs the Stomach qi downward. Together, the two herbs combine to treat all aspects of vomiting due to cold-phlegm.

In order to treat deficiency cold, one must not only warm, but also tonify. The assistant ingredient, Ginseng Radix (rén shēn), serves this function by strengthening the middle burner. It also promotes the generation of fluids and calms the spirit (severe vomiting damages the Spleen and Stomach, injures the fluids, and disturbs the spirit). The envoy, sweet Jujubae Fructus (dà zǎo), moderates the acrid, drying properties of the chief and deputy ingredients, and supports the qi-tonifying action of the assistant ingredient.

Cautions and Contraindications

For particularly severe vomiting, the decoction will be easier to keep down if taken cool. Rarely, patients may experience a transitory sensation of discomfort in the chest, dizziness, and a worsening of the headache after taking the decoction. These symptoms will disappear once the formula begins to take effect (within 30 minutes). The patient should rest after taking the decoction to minimize these side effects. This formula is contraindicated in cases with vomiting or acid reflux due to heat.

Commentary

This is a very useful formula for treating a wide range of conditions with vomiting due to Stomach or Liver disharmony. Clinically, the term 'vomiting' should be taken in a very wide sense of the word to include such symptoms as excessive flow of thin and frothy saliva. The mechanism underlying this disorder was first mentioned in Chapter 39 of Basic Questions: "When cold [pathogenic] qi resides in the Intestines and Stomach, it strongly rebels upward to depart. This leads to pain and vomiting." Here, as in all classical sources, the problem to be treated is understood as a process characterized by a distinctive dynamic that reflects not only pathological change, but also the body's own attempt at self-healing. Only by understanding this dynamic can the formula be effectively utilized. After all, vomiting and diarrhea due to deficiency cold in the middle or lower burner are also treated by a number of other formulas, including Regulate the Middle Pill (lǐ zhōng wán) and Frigid Extremities Decoction (sì nì tāng). In Elaborating on the Subtleties of Cold Damage, the early modern physician Cao Ying-Fu clearly differentiates between the different dynamics:

> A lesser yin disorder where [the diffusion of yang qi to] the exterior is cut off and which is not [complicated by] additional patterns is characterized by vomiting and diarrhea, and abnormal coldness of the extremities. That the [appropriate] formulas to treat this [pattern] are Regulate the Middle Pill (lǐ zhōng wán) and Frigid Extremities Decoction (sì nì tāng) is undisputed. The reason for the abnormally cold extremities [in this case] is the weak and frail yang qi of the middle cavity caused by vomiting above and diarrhea below, which is unable to spread out to the extremities. In attending to the same [constellation of] diarrhea, vomiting, and abnormally cold extremities, but accompanied by irritability and restlessness [that make] one wish to die, one must [however] not rashly prescribe either Regulate the Middle Pill (lǐ zhōng wán) or Frigid Extremities Decoction (sì nì tāng). If the yang qi of the middle burner is deficient [the connection between] above and below is obstructed and does not afford free passage. Floating yang harasses the upper [burner] causing pathological irritability and restlessness. If the middle cavity is obstructed, heating herbs like Zingiberis Rhizoma (gān jiāng) and Aconiti Radix lateralis praeparata (zhì fù zǐ) are unable to spread out to the lower [burner]. Instead, they [would] reinforce the floating heat above the obstruction,

aggravating the vomiting. Therefore, it is only appropriate to moderate and regulate [such a pathology].

[Evodia Decoction (*wú zhū yú tāng*)] utilizes the middle and lower burner warming herb Evodiae Fructus (*wú zhū yú*) in order to direct the vomiting and rebelliousness downward. The remaining herbs, Ginseng Radix (*rén shēn*), Zingiberis Rhizoma recens (*shēng jiāng*), and Jujubae Fructus (*dà zǎo*), are all used to increase the Stomach juices and assist the Spleen yang. As the middle burner qi is gradually harmonized, the body fluids are unblocked and regulated, ascending and flowing downward into the four extremities, while the vomiting, irritability, and restlessness should stop. If [the presence of pathological] water qi is slight, the diarrhea below will follow suit and also stop. However, if the vomiting, irritability, and restlessness have stopped but the diarrhea persists, one can then prescribe Regulate the Middle Pill (*lǐ zhōng wán*) or Frigid Extremities Decoction (*sì nì tāng*) to improve any remaining [problems]. [If treated in this manner] there is no pattern that will not be cured. This can be verified by experience independent of my words.

Cao Ying-Fu's analysis focuses on the deficiency aspect of the pathology treated by this formula. In *Selected Annotations to Ancient Formulas from the Garden of Crimson Snow,* the Qing-dynasty physician Wang Zi-Jie explains why the formula is directed at the Liver and terminal yin channel in order to open the obstruction in the middle burner.

Evodia Decoction (*wú zhū yú tāng*) is a medicinal for the terminal yin and yang brightness [warps]. [As it states in Chapter 74 of *Basic Questions*], 'The terminal yin is the [warp] where the two yin reach their utmost limit.' Hence, all yang [and therefore] the generation of qi are centered on it. Accordingly, when [Zhang] Zhong-Jing treated the terminal yin, he emphasized to protect the generation of qi. If the generation of qi is completely exhausted, the turbid yin rises upward to interfere with the [function of the] yang brightness, [leading to] spitting up of frothy sputum and a desire to vomit what one has eaten. Restlessness and irritability [that make one] wish to die show that the yang of the lesser yin also [is affected]. Accordingly, he employs Evodiae Fructus (*wú zhū yú*), which enters directly into the terminal yin, in order to enlist its severely constrained yang [qi], while Ginseng Radix (*rén shēn*) arouses the joint virtues of thunder (震 *zhèn*) and earth (坤 *kūn*) [the trigrams associated with the wood and earth phases, respectively] to protect the generation of qi. Zingiberis Rhizoma recens (*shēng jiāng*) and Jujubae Fructus (*dà zǎo*), meanwhile, are used to regulate the nutritive and protective [aspects]. In this manner, Ginseng Radix (*rén shēn*) and Evodiae Fructus (*wú zhū yú*) contain the frothy sputum, stop the vomiting, and calm the vexation by ordering and disseminating the middle and lower burners, but without [directly] treating the Lungs and Heart.

Other Indications

Besides vomiting, headache is the second most important indication for Evodia Decoction (*wú zhū yú tāng*). In contemporary practice, the distinctive type of migraine headache for which it is often prescribed presents as follows: A typical attack will be accompanied by muscular tightness

of the neck, nausea, vomiting, excessive salivation, and cold extremities. Although the patient feels tired, weak, and cold, bouts of vomiting (which mark attempts by the body to unblock the middle burner) may be accompanied by facial flushing, irritability, and restlessness, indicating the floating upward of yang. Unlike patterns where obstruction of the middle burner by phlegm is a major factor, the vomiting here does not significantly ameliorate the attacks. In fact, it may further exacerbate them by depleting the already deficient qi and yang. Although the decoction is bitter and strong-tasting, it is usually well tolerated by those for whom it is indicated. During an attack, it should be taken in small sips.

This formula is also used to treat epigastric and abdominal pain due to deficiency cold. This practice is traced back to *Comprehensive Recording of Sage-like Benefit*, where a formula named Ginseng Decoction (*rén shēn tāng*) with the same composition as Evodia Decoction (*wú zhū yú tāng*) is indicated for 'Heart pain.' Here, as elsewhere, the term 'Heart' stands for the epigastrium, the region below the heart.

Comparison

➢ Vs. Clove and Persimmon Calyx Decoction (*dīng xiāng shì dì tāng*); *see* PAGE 548

Biomedical Indications

With the appropriate presentation, this formula may be used to treat a variety of biomedically-defined disorders, which can be divided into the following groups:

- Those associated with vomiting of clear fluids such as chronic gastritis, acute gastroenteritis, cholecystitis, morning sickness, pyloric spasm, and recalitrant perimenopausal vomiting

- Those associated with excruciating headaches including neurogenic headache, migraine headache, headaches from increased intracranial pressures, hypertension, trigeminal neuralgia, and Ménière's disease

- Eye disorders that involve pain accompanied by nausea and vomiting including eye fatigue, corneal ulcers, conjunctivitis, acute congestive glaucoma, and recalcitrant hordeolum

- Digestive disorders marked by abdominal pain and diarrhea such as gastritis, peptic ulcers, chronic hepatitis, chronic cholecystitis, bacillary dysentery, and ulcerative colitis.

It has also been used for a variety of miscellaneous problems including chronic nephritis, renal failure, infertility, Kehsan's syndrome, urticaria, and thrombocytopenic purpura.

Alternate names

Evodia Decoction (*zhū yú tāng*) in *Essentials from the Golden Cabinet*; Evodia and Ginseng Decoction (*zhū yú rén shēn tāng*) in *Discussion of Illnesses, Patterns, and Formulas Related to the*

Unification of the Three Etiologies; Three-Ingredient Evodia Decoction (*sān wèi zhū yú tāng*) in *Introduction to Medicine*; Ginseng and Evodia Decoction (*shēn yú tāng*) in *Introduction to Medicine*; Four Miracle Decoction (*sì shén jiān*) in *Collection Picked by Immortals*; Evodia Decoction (*wú zhū tāng*) in *Accounts of Formulas and Symptoms*

Modifications

- For severe vomiting or morning sickness, add Pinelliae Rhizoma praeparatum (*zhì bàn xià*) and Amomi Fructus (*shā rén*).

- For severe headache, add Chuanxiong Rhizoma (*chuān xiōng*) and Angelicae sinensis Radix (*dāng guī*).

- For severe cold, add Zanthoxyli Pericarpium (*huā jiāo*) and Zingiberis Rhizoma (*gān jiāng*).

- For severe epigastric pain, add Salviae miltiorrhizae Radix (*dān shēn*) and Aucklandiae Radix (*mù xiāng*).

- For palpitations and insomnia, add Angelicae sinensis Radix (*dāng guī*) and Poria (*fú líng*).

- For bulging disorders due to cold, add Aconiti Radix lateralis praeparata (*zhì fù zǐ*)

- For acid reflux, add Arcae Concha (*wǎ léng zǐ*) and Sepiae Endoconcha (*hǎi piāo xiāo*).

Associated Formulas

吳茱萸湯（吴茱萸汤）

Evodia Decoction from *Comprehensive Recording*

wú zhū yú tāng

SOURCE   *Comprehensive Recording of Sagely Beneficence from the Zhenghe Era* (1117)

Evodiae Fructus (*wú zhū yú*)	60g
Cinnamomi Cortex (*ròu guì*)	60g
Magnoliae officinalis Cortex (*hòu pò*), prepared in ginger juice	60g
Zingiberis Rhizoma praeparatum (*páo jiāng*)	60g
Zanthoxyli Pericarpium (*huā jiāo*), prepared	15g
Citri reticulatae Pericarpium (*chén pí*)	15g
Atractylodis macrocephalae Rhizoma (*bái zhú*)	15g

Grind the herbs into a powder, and use 9g to prepare as a draft by boiling in one large cup of water with 3 slices of Zingiberis Rhizoma recens (*shēng jiāng*) until one-fifth has evaporated. The source text advises to discard the dregs and drink the draft on an empty stomach. Warms the middle burner, disperses cold, and transforms dampness. Treats cold qi generating turbidity, which in turn leads to distention. In contrast to the principal formula, this variation is more dispersing. Treating both the root and the branch, it is indicated where cold leads to visible symptoms of stagnation.

延年半夏湯（延年半夏汤）

Pinellia Decoction to Extend Life

yán nián bàn xià tāng

SOURCE   *Arcane Essentials from the Imperial Library* (752)

Ginseng Radix (*rén shēn*)	2g
Aurantii Fructus immaturus (*zhǐ shí*)	1g
Evodiae Fructus (*wú zhū yú*)	1g
Pinelliae Rhizoma praeparatum (*zhì bàn xià*)	5g
Zingiberis Rhizoma (*gān jiāng*)	2g
Trionycis Carapax (*biē jiǎ*)	3g
Platycodi Radix (*jié gěng*)	3g
Arecae Semen (*bīng láng*)	3g
Peucedani Radix (*qián hú*)	3g

Decoction. Although this formula is first listed in a Tang dynasty Chinese source text, it is more frequently used at present in Kampo medicine, and the dosages given are those indicated in contemporary Japanese sources. The formula is specific for internal cold leading to stagnation of fluids, generating phlegm and blocking the descent of qi. This manifests as pain in the chest, shoulder stiffness, abdominal distention and pain, and a tendency toward constipation. These symptoms will be accompanied by signs of cold in the interior such as cold feet, an aversion to cold, facial pallor, fatigue, and headaches accompanied by heavy headedness indicating that the clear yang is failing to ascend. The formula is thought to be particularly effective for left-sided symptoms, that is, stiffness and pain in the left shoulder and back, pain in the left breast or the left hypochondrium, and tension of the left rectus abdominus muscle. It is therefore used in the treatment of chronic pancreatitis, intercostal neuralgia, and digestive disorders, often with a psychosomatic component.

小建中湯（小建中汤）

Minor Construct the Middle Decoction

xiǎo jiàn zhōng tāng

This formula 'constructs' (strengthens) the Spleen and Stomach, the organ systems of the middle burner. Because the middle burner serves as the foundation for the physiological functioning of all other organ systems, 'constructing the middle' extends to a harmonization of yin and yang in general. Compared to Major Construct the Middle Decoction (*dà jiàn zhōng tāng*), the tonifying and warming properties of this formula are relatively mild, hence its 'minor' appellation.

Source   *Discussion of Cold Damage* (c. 220)

Maltosum (*yí táng*)	18-30g
Cinnamomi Ramulus (*guì zhī*)	9g
Paeoniae Radix (*sháo yào*)	18g
Glycyrrhizae Radix praeparata (*zhì gān cǎo*)	6g
Zingiberis Rhizoma recens (*shēng jiāng*)	9g
Jujubae Fructus (*dà zǎo*)	12 pieces

Method of Preparation   Add Maltosum (*yí táng*) to the strained decoction. If this substance is not available, substitute honey. Do *not*, however, substitute cane sugar as its sweet and cold nature will cause further injury to the Spleen. At present, Paeoniae Radix alba (*bái sháo*) is the form of Paeoniae Radix (*sháo yào*) used, and only 3-5 pieces of Jujubae Fructus (*dà zǎo*) are prescribed.

Actions   Warms and tonifies the middle burner and moderates the spasmodic abdominal pain

Indications

Intermittent, spasmodic abdominal pain that responds favorably to local application of warmth and pressure, a lusterless complexion, reduced appetite, a pale tongue with a white coating, and a thin, wiry, and moderate pulse. There may also be low-grade fever, palpitations, irritability, cold and sore extremities with nonspecific discomfort, and a dry mouth and throat.

The various patterns treated by this formula are all due to consumptive deficiency (虛勞 *xū láo*). The term 'consumptive deficiency' here refers to middle burner deficiency cold (brought on by overwork, improper eating habits, poor diet, etc.) leading to insufficiency of transportation and transformation. When the abdomen is deprived of the warmth of the yang qi, the result is intermittent, spasmodic abdominal pain that responds favorably to local application of warmth and pressure. A lusterless complexion, reduced appetite, and pale tongue with a white coating indicate cold from deficiency of the middle burner. The pulse is of particular interest. The combination of deficiency cold and the body's reaction to the pain caused by it results in a thin, wiry, and moderate pulse.

The middle burner is the source of the transformation and transportation of nutrients in the body. When it is weakened, the yin and yang both suffer, leading to dissipation of both qi and blood. Lack of regulation between the nutritive and protective qi ensues because the protective yang is no longer controlled by the nutritive yin. This can manifest as low-grade fever combined with cold, soreness, and general discomfort in the extremities. The lack of proper transportation combined with cold from deficiency leads to the seemingly paradoxical signs of a pale tongue with a dry throat. Note that if the patient is thirsty, there will be a desire for hot beverages. The inadequate supply of nutritive qi to the Heart, combined with the insufficiency of protective yang, causes palpitations, irritability, and a complexion that lacks luster.

Analysis of Formula

Proper treatment of this condition requires strengthening the middle qi and regulating the yin and yang. The chief ingredient, Maltosum (*yí táng*), is distilled from grains such as rice, wheat, or barley, all of which are associated with sweetness and earth. For this reason, *Records of Thoughtful Differentiation of Materia Medica* describes it as the "quintessence of a quintessence." Containing the very essence of earth makes it ideally suited to tonifying the middle burner in a condition characterized by contradictory signs of heat and cold, constraint and deficiency. It tonifies both the qi and blood, generates fluids, alleviates thirst, and moderates spasmodic abdominal pain. It is complemented by the deputies, Cinnamomi Ramulus (*guì zhī*), which warms the middle burner and disperses cold, and Paeoniae Radix alba (*bái sháo*), whose sweet and sour taste benefits the yin. As in Cinnamon

Twig Decoction (*guì zhī tāng*), this combination harmonizes the nutritive and protective qi, one warming, the other cooling, one dispersing, the other astringing. When combined with Maltosum (*yí táng*), their balanced opposition enhances the balancing and moderating actions of the chief herb. This function is further augmented by the relative dosage of the two deputies: in Cinnamon Twig Decoction (*guì zhī tāng*) they are equal, while here the dosage of Paeoniae Radix alba (*bái sháo*) is doubled.

The protective qi is yang in nature; its tonification requires acrid, warming herbs. The nutritive qi is yin; its tonification requires sweet herbs. The assistants, Zingiberis Rhizoma recens (*shēng jiāng*) and Jujubae Fructus (*dà zǎo*), combine these functions while also strengthening the middle burner. The envoy, Glycyrrhizae Radix praeparata (*zhì gān cǎo*), works with the deputies to stop spasmodic abdominal pain. It also harmonizes the functions of the middle burner and of the formula in general.

Overall, this formula emphasizes the use of sweet and warming herbs to tonify the cold of deficiency but balances these with acrid and sour herbs to harmonize the protective and nutritive qi. It thus synthesizes two of the most fundamental strategies of Chinese medicine: the combination of acrid and sweet herbs to facilitate the transformation into yang, and sour and sweet herbs to facilitate the transformation into yin.

Cautions and Contraindications

Contraindicated for heat from yin deficiency. It should not be used without modification in patients with vomiting or roundworms because these conditions are often aggravated by sweet substances. It must also be modified in cases with abdominal distention.

Commentary

This is a popular formula that can be used for a variety of consumptive disorders with yang deficiency. It is the primary formula for treating abdominal pain due to cold from deficiency, characterized by abdominal pain that responds favorably to warmth and accompanied by cold, sore extremities. There should be no signs of heat, such as constipation or yellow urine. It may also be used in treating jaundice and dysenteric disorders due to cold from deficiency. A second major area of application is pediatrics where it is used to treat a wide range of disorders associated with cold from deficiency. In Japan, it is especially popular for treating enuresis but is also used for sleeping disorders, headaches, allergies, recurrent infections, cramping, and abdominal pain. Important clinical markers for both types of problems include:

- A generally weak and debilitated disposition associated with the loss of essence such that the patient looks pale, is easily exhausted, has low resistance to stress of various kinds, feels cold but sweats easily, has a weak back and knees or a variety of aches and pains, and anxiety

- Superficial tension of the rectus abdomini muscles, especially in the upper abdomen, in a person with a bloated but weak abdomen, and with no pain on palpation; in children, especially, the peristaltic movement of the bowels may become visible

- A tendency to hyperexcitability that can manifest in muscular cramping or tension, pains that come and go or move about, irritability, nervousness, palpitations, excessive dreaming, nosebleeds, and similar symptoms

- A pale and tender tongue with various types of coating, from thinnish white and yellow to a more thick white, depending on the nature and degree of constraint accompanying the fundamental deficiency.

The ingredients of this formula are the same as those in Cinnamon Twig Decoction plus Peony (*guì zhī jiā sháo yào tāng*) with the addition of Maltosum (*yí táng*). This illustrates how the therapeutic focus of a formula may be changed by altering the dosage of the ingredients and their ratio to one another. Depending upon their view of the underlying mechanism, various commentators have designated Maltosum (*yí táng*), Paeoniae Radix alba (*bái sháo*), or Cinnamomi Ramulus (*guì zhī*) as the chief ingredient in the formula.

Issues Surrounding Paeoniae Radix (*sháo yào*)

As with Cinnamon Twig Decoction (*guì zhī tāng*) and its many variations, the source text does not specify which kind of Paeoniae Radix (*sháo yào*) should be used, as there was no such differentiation during Han times. Most commentators, however, agree on the use of Paeoniae Radix alba (*bái sháo*), citing three main reasons. First, it tonifies the blood and enriches the yin, both of which are lacking due to deficiency cold in the middle burner. Second, it harmonizes the interior and moderates the spasmodic abdominal pain that is the key symptom of one of the patterns of consumptive deficiency. Third, it softens the Liver and thereby stops the pain, providing another perspective from which the action of this formula may be viewed, namely, as Liver qi (wind-like in nature) invading a weak earth. However, where deficiency cold causes signs of blood stasis, or where constipation is a symptom, the use of Paeoniae Radix rubra (*chì sháo*) should be considered.

In *Investigations of Medical Formulas*, the Ming-dynasty physician Wu Kun suggested substituting Cinnamomi Cortex (*ròu guì*), which he considered to be better at warming the interior, for Cinnamomi Ramulus (*guì zhī*). This suggestion was taken up by Fei Bo-Xiong in *Discussion of Medical Formulas*. Fei argued that Cinnamomi Cortex (*ròu guì*) has the ability to counteract (literally 'kill' 殺 *shā*) wood, thus assisting Paeoniae Radix alba (*bái sháo*) in restraining the Liver qi.

Following the experience of these physicians, one may use Cinnamomi Ramulus (*guì zhī*) where exterior symptoms like cold limbs and fever predominate, and Cinnamomi Cortex (*ròu guì*) where interior symptoms like abdominal pain are predominant in the presentation.

Comparisons

➢ Vs. Cinnamon Twig Decoction (*guì zhī tāng*)

Both formulas harmonize the nutritive and protective qi and can be used to treat symptoms such as fever with aversion to wind and cold. They also can be used to treat greater yin disorders that involve the Spleen. However, Cinnamon Twig Decoction (*guì zhī tāng*), which contains Cinnamomi Ramulus (*guì zhī*) as its chief herb, focuses on releasing the muscle layer. It is indicated where wind-cold invades from the exterior and obstructs the circulation of nutritive qi, in cases where such invasion is accompanied by signs of middle burner deficiency such as diarrhea. The pulse will be relaxed and floating. It can also be used where the protective yang is unable to move the nutritive yin, resulting in disharmony between the two. Minor Construct the Middle Decoction (*xiǎo jiàn zhōng tāng*), on the other hand, treats deficiency in the interior characterized by a substantive insufficiency of both yin and yang, which no longer interpenetrate each other. This leads to symptoms of wind (spasmodic pain) in the interior. In these cases, the pulse will be submerged, thin, and wiry.

➢ Vs. Tonify the Middle to Augment the Qi Decoction (*bǔ zhōng yì qì tāng*)

Both formulas can be used to treat conditions with heat. Minor Construct the Middle Decoction (*xiǎo jiàn zhōng tāng*) is used when the condition is due to a lack of regulation between the yin and yang. This usage illustrates the method of treating fever with sweet, warming substances. The characteristic low-grade fever (precipitated and aggravated by overexertion) is often accompanied by cool extremities and a desire to drink hot beverages. This distinguishes it from the heat due to yin deficiency, in which the palms are always warm and there is a desire to drink cool beverages. Some commentators view it as the inspiration behind Li Dong-Yuan's composition of Tonify the Middle to Augment the Qi Decoction (*bǔ zhōng yì qì tāng*), discussed in Chapter 8, which also relies on sweet, warming herbs to treat fever. However, whereas the present formula focuses on deficiency cold, Tonify the Middle to Augment the Qi Decoction (*bǔ zhōng yì qì tāng*) focuses on constraint from qi deficiency.

➢ Vs. Major Construct the Middle Decoction (*dà jiàn zhōng tāng*); see page 269

Biomedical Indications

With the appropriate presentation, this formula may be used

to treat a variety of biomedically-defined disorders. One group includes those with paroxysmal spasmodic pain, such as chronic gastritis, peptic ulcers, inflammatory bowel disease, autonomic dystonia, chronic hepatitis, cholelithiasis, chronic nephritis, benign prostatic hypertrophy, and migraines. It is also used for problems marked by palpitations and dizziness, such as anemia, hypoglycemia, and hyptension. It has also been used for an assortment of miscellaneous disorders, including fever of unknown origin, enuresis, idiopathic thrombocytopenic purpura, hemolytic jaundice, and leukemia.

Alternate names

Peony Decoction (*sháo yào tāng*) in *Records of Proven Formulas Past and Present*; Cinnamon Bark Decoction (*guì xīn tāng*) in *Comprehensive Recording of Sagely Beneficence*; Construct the Middle Decoction (*jiàn zhōng tāng*) in *Clarification of the Theory of Cold Damage*; Cinnamon Twig and Peony Decoction (*guì zhī sháo yào tāng*) in *Thorough Understanding of Cold Damage with Charts and Songs to Safeguard Life*

Modifications

- For more severe cold, substitute Cinnamomi Cortex (*ròu guì*) for Cinnamomi Ramulus (*guì zhī*).

- For relapse due to consumption of raw or cold food, increase the dosage of Cinnamomi Ramulus (*guì zhī*) and add Linderae Radix (*wū yào*).

- For concurrent qi stagnation, add Aucklandiae Radix (*mù xiāng*) and Gigeriae galli Endothelium corneum (*jī nèi jīn*).

- For diarrhea, add Atractylodis macrocephalae Rhizoma (*bái zhú*).

- For roundworms, reduce the dosage of Maltosum (*yí táng*) and Paeoniae Radix alba (*bái sháo*) and add Mume Fructus (*wū méi*).

- For abdominal fullness or nausea after taking this formula, add Citri reticulatae Pericarpium (*chén pí*) and Amomi Fructus (*shā rén*) to moderate the cloying nature of the sweet herbs.

Variations

黄耆建中湯 (黄芪建中汤)

Astragalus Decoction to Construct the Middle

huáng qí jiàn zhōng tāng

SOURCE *Essentials from the Golden Cabinet* (c. 220)

For more severe qi deficiency characterized by spontaneous sweating, shortness of breath, occasional fevers, and a thin, faint, frail pulse, add 9g Astragali Radix (*huáng qí*) to the principal (source) formula. The source text prescribes it for "spasmodic abdominal pain" and "all (kinds of) insufficiency." In contrast to the principal formula, it also tonifies the qi of both Spleen and Lungs. In *Gathering of Songs for Golden Cabinet Formulas*, Chen Yuan-Xi noted that "it

thus excels at tonifying deficiency and plugging the pores, firming up the interstices, and unblocking the collaterals." In clinical practice, it is used to treat abdominal pain from deficiency cold associated with gastritis, peptic or duodenal ulcers, or colitis. It is also a popular formula in the treatment of allergies and in pediatrics.

This formula is often further modified to fit particular presentations. For shortness of breath and chest fullness due to thin mucus, one can increase the dosage of Zingiberis Rhizoma recens (*shēng jiāng*). For abdominal fullness, one can remove the cloying sweetness of Jujubae Fructus (*dà zǎo*) and substitute 4.5g of Poria (*fú líng*). For Lung deficiency where the Lungs' clearing and clarifying function is impaired, one can add Pinelliae Rhizoma praeparatum (*zhì bàn xià*).

歸耆建中湯 (归芪建中汤)

Tangkuei and Astragalus Decoction to Construct the Middle

guī qí jiàn zhōng tāng

SOURCE Experiential formula composed by Hanaoka Seshū (1760-1835)

This is Minor Construct the Middle Decoction (*xiǎo jiàn zhōng tāng*) with the addition of Angelicae sinensis Radix (*dāng guī*) and Astragali Radix (*huáng qí*). It tonifies the qi and blood, warms and strengthens the middle burner, and moderates spasmodic abdominal pain. This formula, like the principal formula, treats abdominal pain, but here the patient has both qi and blood deficiency. The addition of Astragali Radix (*huáng qí*) increases the formula's ability to tonify the qi, and adds the functions of engendering flesh and outthrusting pus. For this reason, it is often used to treat suppurating sores and skin ulcers associated with chronic qi deficiency. In Japan, this thinking has led to its use in the treatment of chronic deficiency-type middle ear infections. Because it also contains Angelicae sinensis Radix (*dāng guī*) to tonify blood, the formula is often suited to blood deficiency patterns that occur after giving birth, significant illness, or surgery.

Comparison

➤ Vs. POWDER TO SUPPORT THE INTERIOR WORTH A THOUSAND GOLD PIECES (*qiān jīn nèi tuō sǎn*); *see* PAGE 874

Associated Formulas

內補當歸建中湯 (内补当归建中汤)

Internally Tonifying Tangkuei Decoction to Construct the Middle

nèi bǔ dāng guī jiàn zhōng tāng

SOURCE *Important Formulas Worth a Thousand Gold Pieces for any Emergency* (7th century)

Angelicae sinensis Radix (*dāng guī*)	12g
Paeoniae Radix (*sháo yào*)	18g
Glycyrrhizae Radix (*gān cǎo*)	6g
Zingiberis Rhizoma recens (*shēng jiāng*)	18g
Cinnamomi Cortex (*ròu guì*)	9g
Jujubae Fructus (*dà zǎo*)	10 pieces

Decoction. For cases with severe deficiency, dissolve 18g of Malto-sum (yí táng) into the strained decoction. Warms the middle burner, tonifies deficiency, relaxes hypertonicity, and stops pain. For post-partum emaciation and weakness with persistent, tight abdominal pain, shortness of breath, reduced appetite, dry lips and mouth, a wan complexion, and reduced breast milk. The addition of the blood-tonifying herb Angelicae sinensis Radix (dāng guī) to the principal formula focuses its action more strongly on nourishing the blood, which is lacking during the postpartum period.

In clinical practice, this formula, too, is often further modified to fit particular presentations. Astragali Radix (huáng qí) can be added to enhance the Spleen's ability to produce blood, making it Tangkuei and Astragalus Decoction to Construct the Middle (guī qí jiàn zhōng tāng), discussed above. In cases of more severe blood loss or inces-sant postpartum bleeding, the source text advises to add 18g of Reh-manniae Radix praeparata (shú dì huáng) and 6g of Asini Corii Colla (ē jiāo) to nourish the blood and enrich the yin.

安中散

Calm the Middle Powder

ān zhōng sǎn

SOURCE *Formulary of the Pharmacy Service for Benefiting the People in the Taiping Era* (1148)

Cinnamomi Cortex (ròu guì) 150g
Corydalis Rhizoma (yán hú suǒ) 150g
calcined Ostreae Concha (duàn mǔ lì) . . . . [cook first] 120g
Foeniculi Fructus (xiǎo huí xiāng) 150g
Zingiberis Rhizoma praeparatum (páo jiāng) 150g
Alpiniae officinarum Rhizoma (gāo liáng jiāng) 150g
Glycyrrhizae Radix (gān cǎo) 300g

The source text recommends grinding the ingredients to a fine pow-der and taking 6g with warm wine. At present, it is usually taken as a decoction with a marked reduction in dosage. Note that most modern formulations substitute Amomi Fructus (shā rén) for Zin-giberis Rhizoma praeparatum (páo jiāng) and Cinnamomi Ramulus (guì zhī) for Cinnamomi Cortex (ròu guì). Warms and strengthens the middle burner, regulates the qi, and invigorates the blood. For spasmodic epigastric pain due to cold from deficiency of the Spleen and Stomach with qi stagnation and blood stasis, often accompanied by nausea and vomiting or spitting up of sour liquids, a feeling of fullness and distention in the chest and abdomen, and sharp pains. The pains occur when the stomach is empty. The patient will present with a moist tongue with a white coating, and a large, frail pulse. The patient is commonly thin, has poor general muscle tone, a flabby ab-domen, and experiences palpitations that feel as if they are located in the periumbilical area. Most modern formulations add 4-5g of Poria (fú líng) to strengthen the formula's ability to treat palpitations.

大建中湯（大建中汤）

Major Construct the Middle Decoction

dà jiàn zhōng tāng

This formula constructs (strengthens) the middle qi. The appel-lation 'major' indicates that the formula is relatively strong.

SOURCE *Essentials from the Golden Cabinet* (c. 220)

Zanthoxyli Pericarpium (huā jiāo) 3-9g
Zingiberis Rhizoma (gān jiāng) 12g
Ginseng Radix (rén shēn) 6g
Maltosum (yí táng) 18-30g

Method of Preparation   Add Maltosum (yí táng) to the strained decoction. If this substance is not available, substitute honey. Do *not*, however, use cane sugar as a substitute. Its sweet and cold nature will cause further injury to the Spleen. At present, Codonopsis Radix (dǎng shēn) is usually substituted for Ginseng Radix (rén shēn) at 2-3 times its dosage, the lower dosage of Zanthoxyli Pericarpium (huā jiāo) is used, and the dosage of the other two ingredients is reduced by one-half. The source text advises to eat rice porridge after taking the formula, which toni-fies the Spleen and Stomach. This advice is based on the maxim in Chapter 22 of *Basic Questions*: "Effective medicine attacks the pathogenic influences, and the five grains are used for nourish-ment."

Actions   Warms and tonifies middle burner deficiency, directs rebellious qi downward, and alleviates pain

Indications

Excruciating epigastric and abdominal pain such that the pa-tient cannot tolerate being touched, a strong sensation of cold in the epigastrium, vomiting to the point of being unable to eat, a white, slippery tongue coating, and a thin and tight or slow and wiry (or, especially in severe cases, hidden) pulse. There may also be borborygmus.

This is weakness and deficiency of the middle burner yang (the root) and yin or cold that is ascendant in the inte-rior (the manifestation). This combination of deficiency and excess is reflected in the distinctive characteristics of the pain and cold in the abdomen. Vigorous cold in the interior leads to an upsurge of cold qi, which produces a strong sensation of cold in the epigastrium. The Stomach qi follows the upsurge of cold qi, causing vomiting and an inability to keep food down. The tongue coating reflects the presence of vigorous cold in the interior. A thin pulse is indicative of yang deficien-cy, and a tight pulse reflects cold in the interior. If the cold is more severe, the pulse will be slow (indicating cold) and wiry (pain). In especially severe cases when the pain is intolerable, the pulse will be hidden. If the cold causes the fluids to con-gest, borborygmus will ensue.

Analysis of Formula

This formula combines warming dispersion with warming tonification to address both the root and branch. The chief ingredient, very hot and acrid Zanthoxyli Pericarpium (huā jiāo), stimulates the yang of the middle burner and dispels cold, thereby alleviating the pain. This herb also warms the gate of vitality, extending its action from the mobilization of yang at its root all the way up to the upper burner. The deputy, Zingiberis Rhizoma (gān jiāng), reinforces the chief ingredient and also quiets the upsurge of cold qi. Without this upsurge, the Stomach qi would not rebel upward and the vomiting would thus cease. The assistant ingredients, Ginseng Radix *(rén shēn)* and Maltosum *(yí táng)*, tonify and strengthen the middle qi, which ameliorates the painful abdominal spasms. Maltosum *(yí táng)* is also regarded by some commentators as counteracting the excessively acrid and drying actions of the chief herb, which might otherwise readily injure the normal qi.

Cautions and Contraindications

This formula is contraindicated in cases with internal clumping, damp-heat, or yin and blood deficiency.

Commentary

This is an important formula for treating severe abdominal pain or colic. The onset of symptoms can often be traced to eating or drinking something cold, especially in patients with preexisting yang deficiency of the middle burner.

Treatment Strategy

Because the presenting symptoms of pain and cold are so severe, most commentators think that warming dispersion is the core strategy of this formula. In *Annotated Fine Formulas from Generations of Famous Physicians*, the modern physician Ran Xue-Feng provides a poetic explanation of how this strategy relates to the name of the formula:

> [In my efforts] to grasp how this formula constructs the middle [I was led] to the saying that when a disorder [extends from] above to below, one treats the middle. If one tonified the middle, the deficiency would not be reversed. If one only eased the middle, the qi [dynamic] would not be unblocked. Hence, only by borrowing the strong acridity and strong warming of Zanthoxyli Pericarpium *(huā jiāo)* and Zingiberis Rhizoma *(gān jiāng)* is [the yang qi] aroused and the middle burner qi constructed after it has been vanquished. … When the sun comes out, the small fires [in people's homes] are extinguished. Human beings take the postnatal grain qi as their root. When the yang of the middle burner returns, the yang of the upper and lower burners also returns. When the qi of the middle burner is calm, can there be anything [within the body] that lacks foundation? [As to the formula] being called 'major,' this is because it does not [directly] stop pain, yet the pain stops; it does not warm the lower burner, yet eliminates its [excess] yin; it does not warm the upper burner, yet disseminates the upper burner yang. The formula's subtlety stems from [the combination of] all of these [functions].

Ran Xue-Feng's view represents the modern consensus. A different view, however, is represented in the writing of the late Qing-dynasty physician Mo Wen-Quan. According to this view, strengthening the middle qi is the formula's primary function, and Maltosum *(yí táng)* is its chief herb. Writing in *Speaking of Studying the Classic*, Mo explained:

> [This formula takes] Maltosum *(yí táng)* as its chief, Zingiberis Rhizoma *(gān jiāng)* as the deputy, and Ginseng Radix *(rén shēn)* and Zanthoxyli Pericarpium *(huā jiāo)* as assistants. As the major acrid and sweet dispersing formula, it [represents] the strategy of toppling [the pathogenic cold] by means of warmth. The reason its name is 'construct the middle' likewise is due to its inclusion of Maltosum *(yí táng)* [which is also the chief herb in] Minor Construct the Middle Decoction *(xiǎo jiàn zhōng tāng)*—[in both cases, it is] the same name and the same meaning.

Although ultimately this dispute cannot be resolved, it is worth pointing out that both sides agree about the formula's ability to strongly stimulate the yang qi of the middle burner. This not only requires herbs that strongly warm, but others that nourish the nutritive qi of the middle burner. Without the latter, the yang qi would have nothing to which it might attach, and this could aggravate the uncontrolled upward rushing of qi. It is for this reason, too, that the formula does not contain the strongly warming Aconiti Radix lateralis praeparata *(zhì fù zǐ)*, but only herbs whose primary action is centered on the middle burner.

Controversy Surrounding the Original Indication

Another dispute concerns an ambiguous passage in *Essentials of the Golden Cabinet's* descripion of the symptomatology associated with this formula: "The cold in the abdomen rushes upward causing the skin to rise up, resembling something that has head and feet." Commentators like the Qing-dynasty scholar Wang Ang, writing in *Medical Formulas Collected and Analyzed*, interpreted this to be a description of the upsurging qi that is such a significant aspect of the pattern. However, in *Personal Standards for the Essentials from the Golden Cabinet*, the Qing-dynasty writer You Yi argued instead that it referred to 'worms' (蟲物 *chóng wù*) agitated by the cold in the abdomen. Zanthoxyli Pericarpium *(huā jiāo)* has long been used as an herb that kills worms and is included by Zhang Zhong-Jing in formulas like Mume Pill *(wū méi wán)* that explicitly refer to worms in the description of patterns they treat. The case history literature also includes cases where this formula is used to treat roundworm infestation. The antiparasitic action of the formula, therefore, deserves further investigation.

Usage

In contemporary Japan, Major Construct the Middle Decoction *(dà jiàn zhōng tāng)* has become an important formula for preventing postoperative ileus and is routinely prescribed in hospital settings. A related usage is that of treating morphine-induced constipation in cancer patients.

Comparison

➤ Vs. Minor Construct the Middle Decoction
 (xiǎo jiàn zhōng tāng)

Both formulas warm the middle burner and tonify deficiency, and both treat pain due to cold against a background of deficiency. In the pattern for which Major Construct the Middle Decoction (dà jiàn zhōng tāng) is indicated, the middle burner cold is severe and primary. This is a very acute presentation characterized by severe pain, a strong sensation of cold in the abdomen, and upsurging of qi with nausea and vomiting. Minor Construct the Middle Decoction (xiǎo jiàn zhōng tāng), on the other hand, focuses on deficiency of both the yin and yang and disharmony between the nutritive and protective qi. While Minor Construct the Middle Decoction (xiǎo jiàn zhōng tāng) patterns also include abdominal pain, it is a milder form characterized by periods of remission. Furthermore, in addition to symptoms of deficiency cold, there will also be apparently contradictory symptoms like thirst, dry mouth, fever, or irritability.

Biomedical Indications

With the appropriate presentation, this formula may be used to treat a wide variety of biomedically-defined disorders such as chronic gastritis, gastric ulcer, duodenal ulcer, chronic pancreatitis, chronic cholecystitis, urinary calculi, intestinal spasms, and uncomplicated intestinal obstruction. It is commonly used in Japan for postoperative ileus or cases of severe constipation.

Alternate name

Three-Substance Major Construct the Middle Decoction (sān wù dà jiàn zhōng tāng) in Comprehensive Medicine According to Master Zhang

Modifications

- For roundworms, reduce the dosage of Maltosum (yí táng) and add Mume Fructus (wū méi), Arecae Semen (bīng láng), and Quisqualis Fructus (shǐ jūn zǐ).
- To strengthen the pain-relieving actions of the formula, add Salviae miltiorrhizae Radix (dān shēn), Corydalis Rhizoma (yán hú suǒ), and Aucklandiae Radix (mù xiāng).
- For nausea, add Pinelliae Rhizoma praeparatum (zhì bàn xià) and Zingiberis Rhizoma recens (shēng jiāng).
- For numb hands and feet, add Cinnamomi Ramulus (guì zhī).

Associated Formula

附子粳米湯 (附子粳米汤)

Aconite Accessory Root and Glutinous Rice Decoction

fù zǐ jīng mǐ tāng

SOURCE   *Essentials from the Golden Cabinet* (c. 220)

Aconiti Radix lateralis praeparata (zhì fù zǐ) 15g
Pinelliae Rhizoma praeparatum (zhì bàn xià) 65g
Glycyrrhizae Radix (gān cǎo) 15g
Jujubae Fructus (dà zǎo) 30g
Nonglutinous rice (jīng mǐ) 80g

Decoction. The source text recommends that the ingredients be boiled in 8 cups of water until the rice is cooked, then discard the dregs and drink the liquid in three doses over the course of a day. Warms the middle burner and stops pain and vomiting. For cold qi in the abdomen characterized by borborygmus, sharp pain, rebelliousness and fullness in chest and flanks, nausea, vomiting, and a pale tongue with a greasy, white coating. Frigid extremities may be present. In comparison to the principal formula, Aconite Accessory Root and Glutinous Rice Decoction (fù zǐ jīng mǐ tāng) focuses more specifically on the Stomach in cases where cold pathogenic qi has invaded, resulting in the accumulation of yin fluids and impairment of the Stomach's downward-directing function. Thus, its tonifying action is milder, while its ability to regulate the qi and transform fluids—both through the drying action of Pinelliae Rhizoma praeparatum (zhì bàn xià) in the Stomach and the warming action of Aconiti Radix lateralis praeparata (zhì fù zǐ) that centers on the lesser yin Kidneys—is more pronounced. Once the turbid yin is directed downward and the fluids are transformed, the stagnation will be resolved and the pain and vomiting will cease.

甘草乾薑湯 (甘草干姜汤)

Licorice and Ginger Decoction

gān cǎo gān jiāng tāng

Source   *Essentials from the Golden Cabinet* (c. 220)

Glycyrrhizae Radix praeparata (zhì gān cǎo) 12g
Zingiberis Rhizoma praeparatum (páo jiāng) 6g

Method of Preparation   Decoction

Actions   Warms the Lungs and strengthens the Stomach

Indications

Cold extremities, absence of thirst, a dry throat, excessive salivation with spitting up of clear fluids, absence of coughing, irritability, dizziness, frequent urination, a pale, moist tongue without a coating, and a pulse that is either frail or submerged and slow.

This is deficiency cold Lung atrophy. The term 'Lung atrophy' (肺痿 fèi wěi) implies a decline in the Lung's ability to govern the qi. Here this is due to cold in the Lungs, which impedes its dissemination and control of the fluids. This manifests in a number of ways in different parts of the body. In the mouth, it appears as excessive salivation and spitting up of clear fluids. The absence of thirst is important because it distinguishes this pattern from Lung atrophy due to heat. The failure of the Lungs to disseminate the fluids is likewise responsible for the paradoxical dryness of the throat, indicating a generalized lack of irrigation throughout the body. Instead, the fluids seep directly into the Bladder from which they are voided through increased urination. There is no coughing because the Lung qi, although weak, is not obstructed. Because cold prevents the clear yang from rising upward, there is dizziness, irritability, and coldness of the limbs. The pale and moist tongue without a coating, and the pulse that is either frail or submerged and slow, reflect the presence of deficiency cold.

Analysis of Formula

The Lungs are a tender organ that is easily damaged by dryness and excessively acrid medicines. Internal cold, however, must be dispelled with acrid and heating herbs that are by their nature drying. To overcome this difficulty, the formula employs an indirect strategy that focuses as much on the middle as on the upper burner, and on the mother in order to treat the child. The first ingredient, Zingiberis Rhizoma *(gān jiāng)*, warms the Lungs and disperses cold. It is used here primarily to restore the yang of the chest. However, its acrid, hot nature can readily deplete the source qi. To ameliorate this effect, the form used is Zingiberis Rhizoma praeparatum *(páo jiāng)*, as blast-frying reduces it acrid and dispersing characteristics. The second herb, Glycyrrhizae Radix praeparata *(zhì gān cǎo),* is added to tonify the qi. Together these herbs warm and strengthen the Stomach, which in turn helps to resolve the disorder in the Lungs (through the generative cycle of the five phases). This is called 'nurturing the earth (Stomach) to generate the metal (Lungs).' The combination of sweet and acrid herbs warms the yang and augments the qi in a balanced manner.

Commentary

The disease category Lung atrophy was first described and analyzed in Chapter 7 of *Essentials from the Golden Cabinet,* where it is further subdivided into two distinctive patterns. The first, deficiency cold, is treated by the present formula. The second, deficiency heat, is treated by Ophiopogonis Decoction *(mài mén dōng tāng),* discussed in Chapter 15. The defining symptom in both patterns is excessive salivation. The key symptoms that distinguish the patterns from each other is the abscence of coughing and thirst in case of deficiency cold and the presence of these symptoms in case of deficiency heat. This is because in the latter, the fluids are actually damaged (manifesting as thirst), which, in turn, causes a relative excess of yang where the qi rebels upward (manifesting as coughing).

A pattern of deficiency cold Lung atrophy must be further differentiated from the various patterns of wasting and thirsting disorder, with which it shares the symptom of frequent urination. This can be done by attending to fluid intake. In deficiency cold Lung atrophy, the patient is not thirsty. Wasting and thirsting disorder patterns, on the other hand, are characterized by a desire for drink, with the patient "urinating twice for each time they drink."

The source text also states that, "If drinking of [Licorice and Ginger] Decoction *(gān cǎo gān jiāng tāng)* causes thirst, it is [then a pattern] that belongs to [the category of] wasting and thristing disorder." While contemporary Chinese text-books frequently dismiss this sentence as irrelevant, a passage in Chapter 37 of *Basic Questions* also connects Lung cold to wasting and thirsting disorder: "When the Heart shifts cold to the Lungs, the Lungs waste. [In cases of] Lung wasting one urinates twice for each time one drinks. [The patient] dies because there is no treatment [for this kind of disorder]." In clinical practice, where wasting and thirsting disorder not infrequently presents with qi or yang deficiency patterns, this passage can thus be of crucial significance in pointing us toward the right diagnosis.

This formula is the foundation for two other important scripts, Regulate the Middle Pill *(li zhong wan)* and Frigid Extremities Decoction *(sì nì tāng),* which is discussed later in this chapter. Some authorities recommend the use of Zingiberis Rhizoma praeparatum *(páo jiāng)* all the time; others use Zingiberis Rhizoma *(gān jiāng)* unless there is bleeding.

Usage

Over the centuries, the use of this formula has been expanded to include abdominal pain due to Spleen and Stomach deficiency, and bleeding due to Spleen yang deficiency. While it usually serves as a component in a larger formula, it can be quite effective by itself in the treatment of bleeding (especially spitting up blood and bleeding from the nose) due to Spleen yang deficiency. This effect is due to the synergy between the channel-warming function of Zingiberis Rhizoma praeparatum *(páo jiāng),* a primary herb for bleeding due to cold, and the Spleen-tonifying action of Glycyrrhizae Radix *(gān cǎo),* which helps reassert its governance of blood.

Comparison

➢ Vs. Ephedra Decoction *(má huáng tāng)*

Both of these formulas treat patterns of Lung cold. However, Ephedra Decoction *(má huáng tāng)* patterns are conditions of excess where cold has invaded from outside, obstructing the diffusion of protective yang and fluids in the exterior. This manifests as fever and chills, a hacking cough without much sputum, no sweating, and usually reduced urination. By contrast, Licorice and Ginger Decoction *(gān cǎo gān jiāng tāng)* patterns are conditions of mixed excess and deficiency where deficiency of yang is unable to vanquish yin, giving rise to contradictory symptoms like excessive saliva without cough, urinary frequency, and a dry throat without thirst, irritability, and frigid extremities.

Biomedical Indications

With the appropriate presentation, this formula may be used to treat a wide variety of biomedically-defined disorders. One group involves clear secretions and excretions, including enuresis, excessive drooling, allergic rhinitis, and hayfever. Another involves bleeding, such as recurrent epistaxis or dysfunctional uterine bleeding. It has also been used for peptic ulcer, chronic gastritis, and emphysema.

Modifications

- For incontinence of urine, add Alpiniae oxyphyllae Fructus (*yì zhì rén*) and Linderae Radix (*wū yào*).
- For epigastric and abdominal pain due to cold from deficiency of the Spleen and Stomach, add Alpiniae officinarum Rhizoma (*gāo liáng jiāng*) and Cinnamomi Cortex (*ròu guì*).
- For nosebleeds, blood in the stool, or vomiting of blood due to cold from deficiency, use Zingiberis Rhizoma praeparatum (*páo jiāng*) instead of raw Zingiberis Rhizoma (*gān jiāng*).

Associated Formula

生薑甘草湯 （生姜甘草汤）

Fresh Ginger and Licorice Decoction

shēng jiāng gān cǎo tāng

SOURCE *Important Formulas Worth a Thousand Gold Pieces* (7th century)

Zingiberis Rhizoma recens (*shēng jiāng*) 15g
Glycyrrhizae Radix (*gān cǎo*) 12g
Ginseng Radix (*rén shēn*) 9g
Jujubae Fructus (*dà zǎo*) . . . . .12 pieces

Warms the Stomach and Lungs and augments the qi. For Lung atrophy with coughing, spitting of clear fluids, dry mouth, and thirst. Because this condition is more one of qi deficiency than of yang deficiency, there is coughing and thirst.

白朮附子湯 （白术附子汤）

White Atractylodes and Aconite Accessory Root Decoction

bái zhú fù zǐ tāng

Source   *Essentials of the Golden Cabinet* (c. 220)

Atractylodis macrocephalae Rhizoma (*bái zhú*) 12g
Aconiti Radix lateralis praeparata (*zhì fù zǐ*) 9g
Zingiberis Rhizoma recens (*shēng jiāng*) 9g
Glycyrrhizae Radix praeparata (*zhì gān cǎo*) 6g
Jujubae Fructus (*dà zǎo*) . . . . .12 pieces

Method of Preparation   Decoction. The source text advises to boil the ingredients in the equivalent of 600ml of water until one-third has evaporated. The strained liquid is then taken in three doses. After the first dose, the pain, for which the decoction is prescribed, should begin to abate. After three doses, it should be gone. If, after taking the decoction, the patient feels as if they are 'veiled' (如冒狀 *rú mào zhuàng*), this is not an adverse sign, but an indication that the chief herbs have not yet achieved their intended result.

Actions   Warms the channels, disperses cold, builds up the middle burner, and promotes the resolution of dampness

Indications

Pain throughout the body characterized by an inability to rotate the body, hard stools, normal urination, and a floating, thin, and moderate pulse. There is no thirst or nausea.

This is a wind-cold-dampness obstruction pattern due to yang deficiency with dampness being predominant. This is reflected in the symptomatology, where stiffness and lack of movement predominate over pain. Dampness is associated with Spleen earth, although in the pattern here the Spleen itself is not the root of the disorder. This can be deduced from the fact that there is neither nausea nor diarrhea. Rather, deficiency of yang rooted in the lesser yin Kidneys fails to provide the warmth necessary for transportation. As a consequence, an excess of dampness within the Spleen (the yin aspect of the middle burner) impedes the movement of fluids in the Stomach and Intestines (the yang aspect of the middle burner) resulting in dry stools accompanied by an abscence of thirst. This disease dynamic is also reflected in the pulse. It is superficial because the pathogen is predominantly in the exterior. It is thin because there is insufficient yang to move the physiological body fluids. It is moderate because of the accumulation of dampness in the channels and collaterals.

Analysis of Formula

This is a variation of Cinnamon Twig plus Aconite Accessory Root Decoction (*guì zhī jiā fù zǐ tāng*) in which Atractylodis macrocephalae Rhizoma (*bái zhú*) has been substituted for Cinnamomi Ramulus (*guì zhī*). Aconiti Radix lateralis praeparata (*zhì fù zǐ*) is the chief herb because it is strongly warming and dispersing, mobilizing the yang qi at the gate of vitality to spread throughout the entire body, reaching the exterior, the middle burner, and the Intestines. Warming, sweet, and bitter, Atractylodis macrocephalae Rhizoma (*bái zhú*) dries dampness and augments the qi. In combination with the acrid and warming Aconiti Radix lateralis praeparata (*zhì fù zǐ*), this action is focused on the muscles and flesh in the exterior. Although the more acrid Atractylodis Rhizoma (*cāng zhú*) might seem to be a more obvious choice here, Atractylodis macrocephalae Rhizoma (*bái zhú*) is preferred because it stops sweating and thus counterbalances the dispersing action of the chief herb. Sweating is contraindicated in the present case because there is already dryness in the Intestines.

The combination of Jujubae Fructus (*dà zǎo*), Glycyrrhizae Radix (*gān cǎo*), and Zingiberis Rhizoma recens (*shēng jiāng*) is familiar from many other formulas, including Cinnamon Twig Decoction (*guì zhī tāng*). Together, they harmonize the nutritive and protective qi, assist the qi transformation of the middle burner, and smooth the diverse actions of the formula into a single whole. The formula adjusts the yin and yang of the Spleen and Stomach (and thereby the flesh), reducing excessive dampness without injuring the fluids, and promoting the movement of yang without dispersing the qi.

Cautions and Contraindications

This is a heating and tonifying formula. It must not be used in cases of hard stools caused by heat or yin deficiency.

Commentary

This formula is an example of a strategy known as 'augmenting fire to generate earth.' Although it is generally used in the treatment of painful obstruction patterns where dampness predominates, an important secondary indication is the treatment of headache and dizziness due to internal wind from yang deficiency. In *Precepts for Physicians*, the Ming dynasty physician-scholar Yu Chang provided a clear analysis of the disease dynamic that leads to such patterns:

> According [to established practice] this formula treats patients who are deficient in Kidney qi. When external wind enters the Kidneys, it resembles a bird in a cave. Yin wind is dull but stops at neither day nor night. As the wind avails itself of the turbid yin qi within the Kidneys, it rebels and attacks the top. The person will suffer from heaviness in the head and dizziness, which are extremely difficult to endure. Because the Stomach qi is also deficient and unable to discrminate the flavors, the formula completely avoids the use of wind herbs [whose acrid nature would deplete the qi]. Instead, it uses Aconiti Radix lateralis praeparata (*zhì fù zi*) to warm the water yin organ and Atractylodis macrocephalae Rhizoma (*bái zhú*) and Glycyrrhizae Radix (*gān cǎo*) to warm the earth yin organ. If water and earth are both warm, the turbid yin qi will always hurry downward and the symptoms of heavy-headedness, dizziness, and lack of interest in food will disappear.

Other indications for which this formula has been used include wind-stroke, and constipation and diarrhea due to generalized yang and qi deficiency in children. In fact, although the source text explicitly mentions hard stools in the list of symptoms associated with this pattern, it is not accepted by contemporary practitioners as a necessary condition for prescribing the formula. This is because the presence of cold in the middle burner can also give rise to loose stools.

Comparison

➤ Vs. Cinnamon Twig plus Aconite Accessory Root Decoction (*guì zhī jiā fù zi tāng*) & Licorice and Aconite Accessory Root Decoction (*gān cǎo fù zi tāng*)

All three formulas treat wind-dampness painful obstruction that occurs against a background of yang deficiency. Cinnamon Twig and Aconite Accessory Root Decoction (*guì zhī fù zi tāng*) patterns are characterized by body pain, inability to rotate the body, and a floating, deficient, and rough pulse. This formula focuses particularly on expelling wind and pathogens that are primarily located in the exterior. Atracty-

lodes Macrocephalae and Aconite Accessory Root Decoction (*bái zhú fù zi tāng*) patterns present in a similar manner, but with hard stools and a floating, thin, and moderate pulse. This formula focuses particularly on transforming dampness and on the muscles and flesh. Licorice and Aconite Accessory Root Decoction (*gān cǎo fù zi tāng*) patterns are characterized by even more severe or deep-seated pain, inability to flex or extend the joints, sweating, shortness of breath, and urinary difficulty. This formula focuses on the joints and on moderating and expelling wind-dampness.

Biomedical Indications

With the appropriate presentation, this formula may be used to treat a variety of biomedically-defined disorders such as degenerative joint disease and arthropathy, post-stroke debility, and pediatric diarrhea.

Modifications

- For wind-dampness painful obstruction with numbness and loss of movement in the joints, add Mori Ramulus (*sāng zhī*) and Spatholobi Caulis (*jī xuè téng*).

- For more severe internal dampness indicated by a thick, white, and greasy tongue coating, substitute Atractylodis Rhizoma (*cāng zhú*) for Atractylodis macrocephalae Rhizoma (*bái zhú*) and add Coicis Semen (*yì yǐ rén*).

- For sweating due to qi deficiency, add Codonopsis Radix (*dǎng shēn*).

Associated Formulas

白朮附子湯 (白术附子汤)

Atractylodes Macrocephalae and Aconite Accessory Root Decoction from *Arcane Essentials*

bái zhú fù zi tāng

Source *Arcane Essentials from the Imperial Library* (752)

Atractylodis macrocephalae Rhizoma (*bái zhú*) 9g
Aconiti Radix lateralis praeparata (*zhì fù zi*) 6g
Glycyrrhizae Radix praeparata (*zhì gān cǎo*) 6g
Cinnamomi Cortex (*ròu guì*) 12g

Decoction. The source text advises to drink the decoction in three portions over the course of a day. Warms the channels, disperses cold, strengthens the middle burner, and promotes the resolution of dampness. For yang deficiency wind characterized by dizziness and heavy-headedness, or wind-dampness painful obstruction with pain in the bones and joints that can be neither flexed nor extended. In acute cases, the pain will be very severe and accompanied by sweating, shortness of breath, urinary difficulty, an aversion to wind so strong that the patient is unwilling to uncover, and slight edema. Compared to the principal formula, this variation focuses more strongly on augmenting the yang at the gate of vitality.

Note: In the source text, this formula is attributed to *Easily [Applicable] Effective and Essential Dynamics* (近效機要 *Jìn xiào jī yào*), which is no longer extant.

茵陳附子乾薑湯（茵陈附子干姜汤）

Virigate Wormwood, Aconite Accessory Root, and Ginger Decoction

yīn chén fù zǐ gān jiāng tāng

SOURCE　*Precious Mirror of Health* (Yuan dynasty)

Aconiti Radix lateralis praeparata (*zhì fù zǐ*) 6g
Zingiberis Rhizoma praeparatum (*páo jiāng*) 6g
Artemisiae scopariae Herba (*yīn chén*) 3.6g
Atractylodis macrocephalae Rhizoma (*bái zhú*) 1.2g
Alpiniae katsumadai Semen (*cǎo dòu kòu*) 3g
Poria (*fú líng*) 0.9g
Aurantii Fructus immaturus (*zhǐ shí*). 1.5g
Pinelliae Rhizoma praeparatum (*zhì bàn xià*) 1.5g
Alismatis Rhizoma (*zé xiè*) 1.5g
Citri reticulatae Pericarpium (*chén pí*). 0.9g

Decoction. The source text advises to decoct the above ingredients with five slices of Zingiberis Rhizoma recens (*shēng jiāng*) in 1½ cups of water until 1 cup remains, discard the dregs, and drink the strained liquid cold. Warms the middle, disperses cold, dries dampness, and unblocks the qi dynamic. For cold-dampness yin-type jaundice caused by the over-prescribing of cooling medicinals characterized by cold extremities, skin that is cold to the touch, hard focal distention in the epigastrium, dry eyes that do not want to open, diarrhea, fatigue, and a desire to lie down. Compared to damp-heat or yang-type jaundice, yin-type jaundice is dark in color and lacks shine. For more detail, see the discussion under Virgate Wormwood Decoction (*yīn chén hāo tāng*) in Chapter 16.

Section 3

FORMULAS THAT RESCUE DEVASTATED YANG

The formulas in this section are used to treat debilitated yang and exuberant yin with cold in both the exterior and interior. In extreme cases, this may lead to exuberant yin repelling yang, or upcast yang. Such patterns are characterized by cold extremities, aversion to cold, fatigue, a desire to lie down and curl up, clear, watery diarrhea, and a submerged, faint, and almost imperceptible pulse. In severe cases, the patient will break into a strong sweat that seems to pour out like water. Only formulas that contain substances with strong warming properties, such as Aconiti Radix lateralis praeparata (*zhì fù zǐ*), Cinnamomi Cortex (*ròu guì*), Zingiberis Rhizoma (*gān jiāng*), Psoraleae Fructus (*bǔ gǔ zhī*), and Trigonelle Semen (*hú lú bā*), are able to rescue the yang in such cases. Among these, Aconiti Radix lateralis praeparata (*zhì fù zǐ*) is the most important herb because it is strongly warming, acrid, drying, and enters all twelve channels.

Depending on the context, these chief herbs are combined with four different types of deputies and assistants. In cases of severe debility of the fire at the gate of vitality, or sudden abandonment of yang, one should add herbs that tonify the qi, such as Ginseng Radix (*rén shēn*), Glycyrrhizae Radix (*gān cǎo*), or Atractylodis macrocephalae Rhizoma (*bái zhú*), because the force generated by acrid herbs alone is too light to secure abandonment. Where the yin and yang separate or fail to interpenetrate due to exuberance of yin cold in the interior, one should add herbs that unblock the yang and open the orifices, such as Allii fistulosi Bulbus (*cōng bái*) or Moschus (*shè xiāng*). In order to prevent yang abandonment, one can also add astringent herbs like Schisandrae Fructus (*wǔ wèi zǐ*), Myristicae Semen (*ròu dòu kòu*), or Halloysitum rubrum (*chì shí zhī*). Where accumulation of yin cold leads to qi stagnation, one can add a small amount of qi-moving herbs like Citri reticulatae Pericarpium (*chén pí*), Aucklandiae Radix (*mù xiāng*), or Toosendan Fructus (*chuān liàn zǐ*) to promote the dispersion of cold and facilitate the revival of yang.

四逆湯（四逆汤）

Frigid Extremities Decoction

sì nì tāng

This formula treats disorders in which the extremities become frigid due to devastated yang. Its name literally means the 'four rebellions' (四逆 *sì nì*). Some commentators think that this refers to the fact that the extremities curl up from the cold rather than extend properly. Another view is that the yang qi disobeys its charge of warming the four extremities, which are sometimes described as 'the root of all yang' in the body due to the fact that all twelve primary channels begin or end in the arms and legs.

Source　*Discussion of Cold Damage* (c. 220)

Aconiti Radix lateralis (*fù zǐ*) . . . . 1 piece (6-9g)
Zingiberis Rhizoma (*gān jiāng*). 4.5g
Glycyrrhizae Radix praeparata (*zhì gān cǎo*) 6g

Method of Preparation　Prepare as a decoction and take warm. At present, the less toxic Aconiti Radix lateralis praeparata (*zhì fù zǐ*) is almost always substituted for Aconiti Radix lateralis (*fù zǐ*) and the dosage of Zingiberis Rhizoma (*gān jiāng*) is often doubled. Cook Aconiti Radix lateralis praeparata (*zhì fù zǐ*) for 30 minutes to one hour before adding the other ingredients. (The larger the dosage, the longer it should be cooked.)

Actions　Rescues devastated yang, warms the middle burner, and stops diarrhea.

Indications

Extremely cold extremities, aversion to cold, curling up when lying down, lethargy with a constant desire to sleep, vomiting, diarrhea with undigested food particles, abdominal pain and cold, lack of thirst, a pale tongue with a white, slippery coating, and a submerged and thin or faint pulse.

This is a cold inversion pattern most typically associated with a lesser yin disorder. Cold is a yin pathogenic influence that readily injures the yang qi. The fire at the gate of vitality, which is the foundation of the body's yang qi, is responsible for transmitting warmth to all the organs. When cold invades the interior and injures this fire, its warming function is inhibited, which is manifested in various signs of deficiency and cold. The most typical of these are extreme cold in the extremities, aversion to cold, curling up when lying down, and lethargy with a constant desire to sleep.

The Spleen and Stomach, which transform food and fluids into refined essence, depend on the fire at the gate of vitality to carry out their respective functions. When it is deficient, the middle burner is reduced to a 'cauldron without a fire underneath;' thus it cannot digest, assimilate, transform, or transport the essence of food and fluids. As a result, the clear yang cannot ascend, nor can the turbid yin properly descend. Vomiting, diarrhea with undigested food particles, and an absence of thirst ensue. Because cold contracts, congeals, and stagnates, congealed cold and qi stagnation causes pain and cold in the abdomen.

The yang qi also nourishes the spirit. When the yang qi is sufficient, the spirit will be vigorous, but when the spirit is deprived of nourishment, it will weaken, which manifests as lethargy and a desire to sleep. A pale tongue with a white, slippery coating and a submerged or faint and thin pulse are also indicative of yang deficiency with internal cold. The wording of the source text makes clear that the pulse here is thin not because the yin or blood is deficient, but because it is primarily faint, implying that there is insufficient yang to move the pulse, which therefore becomes thin. This interpretation follows a passage in Chapter 39 of *Basic Questions*: "The cold qi enters into the channels and slows down [their flow]. They trickle but do not move. [If cold] lodges outside of the blood vessels, the blood will be lacking. If it lodges within the blood vessels, the qi is obstructed."

Analysis of Formula

The basic strategy for treating severe cold that has entered deeply into the interior is outlined in Chapter 74 of *Basic Questions*: "Cold pernicious qi in the interior is treated with sweet, heating [herbs] assisted by bitter, acrid [herbs]" and, "If a cold pernicious qi is victorious, it can be levelled by means of acrid, heating [herbs]."

When the yang is debilitated and the yin flourishes, as reflected in a faint pulse and frigid extremities, one must use a strongly heating and acrid herb to break through the yin and revive the yang. Aconiti Radix lateralis praeparata *(zhì fù zǐ)* serves this purpose and is therefore designated as the chief herb in the formula. It is especially effective in warming and stimulating the fire at the gate of vitality so that it disseminates throughout the body and reaches the extremities. In

Discourse on Tracing Back to the Source of [the Discussion] of Cold Damage, Qian Huang notes:

> Acrid and heating Aconiti Radix lateralis praeparata *(zhì fù zǐ)* goes directly to the lower burner to strongly tonify the true yang at the gate of vitality. Therefore, it is able to treat cold pathogens that rebel upward from the lower burner, assisting the ascent of the clear yang, which rises to the four extremities. As the yang returns, the qi warms, and the four limbs no longer suffer from inversion frigidity.

The deputy, Zingiberis Rhizoma *(gān jiāng)*, warms the middle burner and eliminates cold, which strengthens the Spleen's functions of transforming and transporting food and fluids. The chief and deputy ingredients work synergistically: the deputy assists the chief in strengthening the fire at the gate of vitality, while the chief assists the deputy in strengthening the yang of the middle burner. These herbs are used together in order to realize the full potential of each. In fact, it is traditionally said that Aconiti Radix lateralis praeparata *(zhì fù zǐ)* is not hot if it is used apart from Zingiberis Rhizoma *(gān jiāng)*. The field of action of these two herbs is also complementary. The chief ingredient warms the entire body by traveling through all of the twelve channels, while the focus of the deputy ingredient is primarily on the Spleen, Stomach, and Lungs.

The assistant herb, Glycyrrhizae Radix praeparata *(zhì gān cǎo)*, augments the qi, strengthens the Spleen, reduces the toxicity of the chief ingredient, and moderates the drying properties of the chief and deputy ingredients. Being sweet, it also provides a substratum to which the acrid and heating qi of the chief and deputy herbs can attach in order to achieve their intended functions without merely dissipating. This function is so important to the overall effectiveness of the formula that some physicians even consider Glycyrrhizae Radix *(gān cǎo)* to be the chief herb (see COMMENTARY below).

Cautions and Contraindications

This formula is contraindicated in cases with true heat and false cold characterized by cold extremities, thirst with a desire to drink cool beverages, dark urine, and a red tongue with a yellow coating.

Commentary

The significance of this formula lies in its ability to strengthen the yang of both the gate of vitality and the middle burner. Furthermore, it is formulated in such a way as to warm and strengthen the yang without injuring the yin. This is important here because the formula's indications include vomiting or diarrhea, both of which can injure the yin. The moderating and qi-augmenting qualities of Glycyrrhizae Radix *(gān cǎo)* make an important contribution to the efficacy of this formula. In fact, it is listed first in the source text, and its dosage is as large or larger than that of the other ingredients.

Both Cheng Wu-Ji, the famous Song-dynasty commentator on the *Discussion of Cold Damage*, and the editors of the *Golden Mirror of the Medical Tradition* therefore considered Glycyrrhizae Radix (*gān cǎo*) to be the chief herb. The modern Shanghai physician Cheng Men-Xue admonished his students "not to think lightly" of it because it lacked the apparent power of the heating herbs.

The importance of this formula is demonstrated by the fact that it is mentioned twelve times in *Discussion of Cold Damage*. The scope of its use is succinctly summed up by the Qing-dynasty physician Wang Zi-Jie in *Selected Annotations to Ancient Formulas from the Garden of Crimson Snow*:

> [This formula] can be used in patterns of all three yin warps as well as one [i.e., the greater] yang warp [provided they] are characterized by inversion [as the key symptom]. One employs it in lesser yin [disorders] in order to rescue the yang of the primal sea [i.e., the Kidneys]. In greater yin [disorders], one uses it to warm cold within the yin organ [i.e., the Spleen]. Terminal yin [disorders characterized by] lack of warmth and inversion where devastation of yang is threatening cannot be helped without this [formula]. Finally, one also uses it in greater yang [disorders] where inappropriate sweating has devastated the yang.

Key Indicators

Wang Zi-Jie emphasizes that frigid extremities is the chief indicator for this formula. According to the Qing-dynasty physician Fei Bo-Xiong, the arms must be cold up to (or beyond) the elbows and the legs up to (or beyond) the knees to warrant use of Frigid Extremities Decoction (*sì nì tāng*). This type of disorder is called 'inversion rebellion' (厥逆 *jué nì*) or 'frigid extremities' (四逆 *sì nì*). Classical texts describe three types of inversion (厥 *jué*) disorders: emotional problems accompanied by a sensation of qi rushing upward from the abdomen to the chest; sudden fainting; and extreme cold in the extremities. This formula is indicated only for the last type of disorder. Furthermore, while the character 逆 *nì* often refers to a contrary flow of qi, as in rebellious qi, the term 四逆 *sì nì* or 'four rebellions' refers to the symptom of frigid extremities, which here is due to yang qi deficiency and internal cold.

The second most important symptom, according to Fei Bo-Xiong, is the pulse, which must be submerged and thin and faint. The modern physician Cheng Men-Xue concurs. In *Formulas in Verse from the Scholar's Studio in Two Volumes*, he advises: "Whenever one sees a pulse that is faint and thin [in a patient who is also] lethargic with a constant desire to sleep, this is the manifestation of deficiency cold. You should be decisive in [selecting this formula] without hesitation so that later you do not regret having wasted an opportunity [for successful treatment]." Note that the pulse here appears to be thin because it is so weak. This is different from the pulse associated with Tangkuei Decoction for Frigid Extremities (*dāng guī sì nì tāng*) patterns, discussed above, which can be

so thin as to become almost imperceptible. The root in the first case is devasted yang unable to invigorate the blood, while in the second, it is deficient blood invaded by cold.

Usage

The onset of these symptoms can be very acute and use of the formula is documented for conditions like shock, myocardial infarction, and severe blood loss. As often, however, the formula is used for less severe disorders. The late 19th-century physician Zheng Shou-Quan, for instance, observed that cases of exhausted yang are relatively rare, and that treatment in such cases is often unsuccessful in any event. Although he considered this formula to be effective, he recommended that it be used when the yang was merely deficient and not yet exhausted.

This formula may also be used in treating conditions with true cold and false heat. This is a fairly frequent occurrence in clinical practice when exuberant yin in the interior forces yang to float to the surface. Besides classical symptoms like flushing, a dry throat, or a yellow tongue coating, one may also observe severely high blood pressure or a raised heart beat. Modern clinicians also use it for disorders such as chronic inflammatory conditions with a yang-deficient presentation. When the false heat signs include a flushed face and irritability, the decoction should be taken cool.

Aconiti Radix lateralis (fù zǐ)

There has been much debate among commentators regarding both the type of Aconiti Radix lateralis (*fù zǐ*) to be used and its dosage. Traditionally-minded physicians like Cheng Men-Xue point out that in *Discussions of Cold Damage*, Zhang Zhong-Jing uses untreated Aconiti Radix lateralis (*fù zǐ*) to treat serious and acute disorders but that its toxicity is moderated both by the use of Zingiberis Rhizoma (*gān jiāng*) and Glycyrrhizae Radix (*gān cǎo*), as well as by extended boiling. For this reason, Cheng Men-Xue recommends that it also be used untreated in this formula. However, according to Chinese laws governing poisons, the unprepared herb is not available at all except through a very small number of herb preparation factories, and then only by special prescription. This means that at present, the unprepared herb is no longer used, except in some topical preparations. Physicians in contemporary China consider 6-10g to be the standard dosage for Aconiti Radix lateralis praeparata (*zhì fù zǐ*) in this formula, but may increase it up to 150g for very acute cases.

Comparisons

➢ Vs. True Warrior Decoction (*zhēn wǔ tāng*)

Both formulas treat patterns characterized by debilitated yang and exuberant yin. The patterns differ in the nature of the yin excess and, by implication, their disease dynamic. True Warrior Decoction *(zhēn wǔ tāng)* warms the yang and promotes water metabolism to treat water collecting in the interior. The excess of water (which quells fire) is as important here as the deficiency of yang. By contrast, Frigid Extremities Decoction *(sì nì tāng)* revives the yang and stems rebelliousness in cases where the yang is too debilitated to move and transform the yin. As a result, there are frigid extremities, watery diarrhea, and a floating upward of the yang.

➤ Vs. Regulate the Middle Pill *(lǐ zhōng wán)*

Both formulas treat diarrhea due to cold from deficiency. In *Discussion of Cold Damage* the diarrhea treated by Regulate the Middle Pill *(lǐ zhōng wán)* is referred to as 'spontaneous diarrhea' (自利 *zì lì*). This is interpreted to mean diarrhea that comes and goes in relation to factors such as food intake, climate, or physical and mental exhaustion. It implies that diarrhea occurs when the yang and qi of the middle burner become deficient relative to the task they have to carry out. In a Frigid Extremities Decoction *(sì nì tāng)* pattern, on the other hand, the diarrhea is incessant. This is because the yang of the middle burner has been cut off from its source in the gate of vitality. This is also reflected in the fact that the extremities in a Regulate the Middle Pill *(lǐ zhōng wán)* pattern may be warm, whereas in a Frigid Extremities Decoction *(sì nì tāng)* pattern, they must be cold.

➤ Vs. Tangkuei Decoction for Frigid Extremities *(dāng guī sì nì tāng)*; *see* page 254

➤ Vs. Ginseng and Aconite Accessory Root Decoction *(shēn fù tāng)*; *see* page 280

➤ Vs. Mume Pill *(wū méi wán)*; *see* page 851

Biomedical Indications

With the appropriate presentation, this formula may be used to treat a wide variety of biomedically-defined disorders. One group involves circulatory problems such as acute cardiac insufficiency, cerebrovascular insufficiency, and shock from a variety of causes. Another involves severe digestive dysfunction such as acute gastroenteritis, chronic colitis, and cirrhosis. It has also been used for such disorders as hypopituitarism, hypothyroidism, adrenal insufficiency, functional uterine bleeding, chronic prostatitis, recurrent aphthous ulcers, and intractable arthritis.

Modifications

- For intractable arthritis due to wind-dampness, add Cinnamomi Cortex *(ròu guì)* and Atractylodis macrocephalae Rhizoma *(bái zhú)*.
- For edema or leukorrhea due to cold from deficiency of the Spleen and Kidneys, add Codonopsis Radix *(dǎng shēn)* Poria *(fú líng)* and Alismatis Rhizoma *(zé xiè)*.

Variation

四逆加人參湯 (四逆加人参汤)

Frigid Extremities Decoction plus Ginseng

sì nì jiā rén shēn tāng

Source   *Discussion of Cold Damage* (c. 220)

If the diarrhea ceases but the extremities remain cold (indicating severe injury to the yin and blood, which harms the source qi), add Ginseng Radix *(rén shēn)*. In contrast to the principal formula, this focuses more on nourishing the yin (fluids) and qi aspects of this type of inversion. When the qi returns, blood will be generated again. In clinical practice, this formula is also used to treat Frigid Extremities Decoction *(sì nì tāng)* patterns characterized by severe breathlessness.

Associated Formulas

通脈四逆湯 (通脉四逆汤)

Unblock the Pulse Decoction for Frigid Extremities

tōng mài sì nì tāng

Source   *Discussion of Cold Damage* (c. 220)

Glycyrrhizae Radix praeparata *(zhì gān cǎo)* 6g
Aconiti Radix lateralis *(shēng fù zǐ)* . . . . 1 big piece (12-24g)
Zingiberis Rhizoma *(gān jiāng)* 9-12g

Decoction. At present, the less toxic Aconiti Radix lateralis praeparata *(zhì fù zǐ)* is always substituted for Aconiti Radix lateralis *(shēng fù zǐ)*. Even in its prepared form, it should be cooked for 30 minutes to one hour before adding the other ingredients (the larger the dosage, the longer it should be cooked). Restores the yang and unblocks the pulse. For lesser yin disorders with true cold in the interior and false heat in the exterior characterized by diarrhea with undigested food particles, cold extremities, a faint or hidden pulse that is almost imperceptible, but no aversion to cold. The patient may have a flushed face, the diarrhea may cease, or the pulse may be imperceptible. In this pattern, the yin in the interior is so strong that it rejects the yang, which thereupon floats to the exterior. The pathologocial nature of this outward movement of yang manifests in symptoms like dry retching and pain in the throat. Another way of viewing this problem is as a lesser yin stage with relatively severe yang deficiency of the Heart. This is a more serious condition than that for which the principal formula is used; thus, the dosage of Aconiti Radix lateralis praeparata *(zhì fù zǐ)* is increased.

白通湯 (白通汤)

White Penetrating Decoction

bái tōng tāng

Source   *Discussion of Cold Damage* (c. 220)

Allii fistulosi Bulbus *(cōng bái)* . . . . 4 pieces
Zingiberis Rhizoma *(gān jiāng)* 3g
Aconiti Radix lateralis *(shēng fù zǐ)* . . . . 1 piece (9-15g)

Decoction. At present, the less toxic Aconiti Radix lateralis praeparata *(zhì fù zǐ)* is substituted for Aconiti Radix lateralis *(shēng fù zǐ)* and the dosage of Zingiberis Rhizoma *(gān jiāng)* increased by at least half. Cook Aconiti Radix lateralis praeparata *(zhì fù zǐ)* for 30 minutes to one hour before adding the other ingredients (the larger the dosage, the longer it should be cooked). Unblocks the yang and breaks up accumulations of yin. This is a lesser yin disorder characterized by diarrhea, lassitude, cold extremities, flushed face, and a faint pulse. The symptoms of this pattern indicate that yin is increasing and accumulating in the lower part of the body, forcing the weakened yang to the upper part of the body. In order to prevent yang desertion, the formula employs Allii fistulosi Bulbus *(cōng bái)*, which is specific for unblocking the vessels, as manifested in the symptom of facial flushing.

Comparison

➤ Vs. Restore and Revive the Yang Decoction *(huí yáng jiù jí tāng)*; see page 279

回陽救急湯 (回阳救急汤)
Restore and Revive the Yang Decoction

huí yáng jiù jí tāng

Source   *Six Texts on Cold Damage* (1445)

Aconiti Radix lateralis praeparata *(zhì fù zǐ)*. 9g
Zingiberis Rhizoma *(gān jiāng)*. 4.5g
Cinnamomi Cortex *(ròu guì)*. 3g
Ginseng Radix *(rén shēn)*. 6g
dry-fried Atractylodis macrocephalae Rhizoma *(chǎo bái zhú)* .9g
Poria *(fú líng)*. 9g
Citri reticulatae Pericarpium *(chén pí)*. 6g
Glycyrrhizae Radix praeparata *(zhì gān cǎo)* 4.5g
Schisandrae Fructus *(wǔ wèi zǐ)*. 3g
Pinelliae Rhizoma praeparatum *(zhì bàn xià)*. 9g

Method of Preparation   Decoction. Cook with 3 pieces of Zingiberis Rhizoma recens *(shēng jiāng)*. The source text does not specify the dosage. Take 0.1g of Moschus *(shè xiāng)* followed by the strained decoction.

Actions   Restores and revives the yang, augments the qi, and revives the pulse

Indications

Chills, a propensity to curl up when lying down, cold extremities, vomiting, diarrhea, abdominal pain, lethargy with a constant desire to sleep, a pale tongue with a white coating, and a submerged, faint, or (in severe cases) imperceptible pulse. There may also be severe chills or cyanosis of the fingernails and lips. This is an extremely dangerous type of abandoned disorder.

This is pathogenic cold directly attacking all three yin warps in a patient with weak, exhausted true yang. Cold is a yin pathogen that readily injures the yang qi. If a person with a yang deficient constitution is exposed to cold, the protective yang is too weak to repel the pathogen. The cold therefore directly enters into the three yin warps, leading to exhaustion of true yang. Loss of the yang qi's warmth manifests as chills,

cold extremities, and a propensity to curl up when lying down. As the true yang becomes exhausted, it can no longer warm the middle burner, which loses its ability to transport and transform. The clear yang no longer ascends, and the turbid yin no longer descends, manifesting in vomiting and diarrhea. Yin cold in the interior causes the qi to contract and the fluids to congeal, leading to abdominal pain. If the spirit fails to be stimulated by the yang qi of the minsterial fire, a person becomes lethargic with an increasing desire to sleep. Because cold congeals the blood, the nails and lips become cyanotic, the chills become increasingly severe, the pulse slows down and becomes submerged and forceless, and, in extreme cases, may even be imperceptible.

Analysis of Formula

To treat a condition where cold has attacked all three yin warps and the yang is exhausted, one must restore and revive the yang, stem rebelliousness, augment the qi, and generate the pulse. To this end, the formula employs three strongly acrid and heating chief herbs: Aconiti Radix lateralis praeparata *(zhì fù zǐ)*, Zingiberis Rhizoma *(gān jiāng)*, and Cinnamomi Cortex *(ròu guì)*. Because the qi is very weak, the dispersing action of these herbs could lead to abandoned yang if they were used on their own. For this reason, the formula adds Six-Gentlemen Decoction *(liù jūn zǐ tāng)*, discussed in Chapter 8, as a deputy. Together, its four herbs—Ginseng Radix *(rén shēn)*, Atractylodis macrocephalae Rhizoma *(bái zhú)*, Poria *(fú líng)*, and Glycyrrhizae Radix praeparata *(zhì gān cǎo)*—augment the Spleen and Stomach. Strengthening the middle burner serves to regulate the dispersal of yang without hindering its restoration.

Sour and astringent Schisandrae Fructus *(wǔ wèi zǐ)* serves as an assistant to prevent dispersal of the true yang, while in combination with Ginseng Radix *(rén shēn)*, it acts to generate the pulse. A relatively small dosage ensures that its astringency does not impede the dispersing action of the chief herbs. A very small amount of Moschus *(shè xiāng)*, which is acrid and aromatic, is used as a second assistant because its scurrying nature excels at unblocking the vessels. The two assistants, one acrid and the other sour, one scurrying and the other astringent, offer a complementary dynamic that promotes the dispersal of yang to generate the pulse. Zingiberis Rhizoma recens *(shēng jiāng)* and Glycyrrhizae Radix praeparata *(zhì gān cǎo)*, an ingredient of Six-Gentlemen Decoction *(liù jūn zǐ tāng)*, function as envoys that harmonize the formula and balance the slightly toxic nature of Aconiti Radix lateralis praeparata *(zhì fù zǐ)*.

Cautions and Contraindications

This is a very strong heating and dispersing formula. It should not be used long term or with too high a dosage. As soon as warmth returns to the limbs, its use should be discontinued.

Commentary

Cold directly attacking the three yin warps is a relatively acute condition that requires urgent attention. According to Tao Hua, the author of this formula, it can be distinguished from cold that has penetrated into the interior via the yang warps by the complete absence of fever or headache at the onset of the disorder. In addition to the obvious middle burner symptoms, the pulse is of central importance in identifying this pattern. If the weak and therefore thin pulse associated with Frigid Extremities Decoction (*sì nì tāng*) indicates that there is insufficient yang to move the yin, the submerged, slow, weak, and (at times) imperceptible pulse associated with this pattern signifies yang deficiency coupled with a deficiency of nutritive qi. The nutritive qi is produced in the middle burner and fills the vessels. Without it, the protective yang has nothing with which to attach itself. If it is lost in a situation where there is also no yang, the pulse becomes imperceptible.

The formula therefore addresses a pattern where both protective yang and nutritive yin are deficient. In *Revised Popular Guide to the Discussion of Cold Damage*, He Xiu-Shan is cited as calling it "the most beneficial formula for augmenting the qi and generating the pulse." In the same text, He Lian-Chen stipulates that it could also be used for damage to the original yang caused by using excessively cooling and draining formulas when treating a warm pathogen disorder. In *Discussion of Medical Formulas*, Fei Bo-Xiong explains how it achieves these effects by comparing it with the purely heating Frigid Extremities Decoction (*sì nì tāng*):

> This formula can be used to treat moderate patterns of middle burner cold. If its [name] refers to 'meeting urgent needs' (救急 *jiù jí*), this indicates the combination of Zingiberis Rhizoma (*gān jiāng*) and Aconiti Radix lateralis praeparata (*zhì fù zǐ*) with Six-Gentlemen Decoction (*liù jūn zǐ tāng*) and Schisandrae Fructus (*wǔ wèi zǐ*). This [combination] moderates any excessiveness in the nature of Zingiberis Rhizoma (*gān jiāng*) and Aconiti Radix lateralis praeparata (*zhì fù zǐ*). This differs [significantly] from the [manner in which] Frigid Extremities Decoction (*sì nì tāng*) removes one obstacle after another.

Comparisons

➤ Vs. Generate the Pulse Powder (*shēng mài sǎn*)

The earliest formula for generating the pulse (生脉 *shēng mài*) when it becomes imperciptible is Sun Si-Miao's Generate the Pulse Powder (*shēng mài sǎn*), discussed in Chapter 8. That formula treats a condition where the pulse disappears due to concurrent deficiency of qi and body fluids. By contrast, the present formula contains two of the three herbs used in Generate the Pulse Powder (*shēng mài sǎn*), namely, Ginseng Radix (*rén shēn*) and Schisandrae Fructus (*wǔ wèi zǐ*). By combining these two with strongly heating and unblocking herbs, it creates a new formula that treats an imperceptible pulse caused by excess cold and deficient nutritive qi.

➤ Vs. White Penetrating Decoction (*bái tōng tāng*)

White Penetrating Decoction (*bái tōng tāng*) also unblocks the vessels but treats a pattern characterized by a strong and tight pulse. Because the fluids are not deficient, this formula simply uses acrid and heating herbs that scatter cold to remove the yin excess

Biomedical Indications

With the appropriate presentation, this formula may be used to treat a variety of biomedically-defined disorders including myocardial infarction, cardiogenic shock, acute gastroenteritis, food posioning, and hypotension.

Alternate names

Restore and Revive the Yang Decoction (*huí yáng jí jiù tāng*) in *Achieving Longevity by Guarding the Source*; Restore the Yang and Return the Root Decoction (*huí yáng fǎn běn tāng*) in *Medical Formulas from Straight Directions in Haojing*

Modifications

* For spitting of thin sputum or abdominal pain due to cold, add salt-fried Evodiae Fructus (*wú zhū yú*).
* For incessant diarrhea, add Astragali Radix (*huáng qí*) and Cimicifugae Rhizoma (*shēng má*).
* For incessant vomiting, add freshly-pressed Zingiberis Rhizomatis Succus (*jiāng zhī*).

Variation

回陽救急湯 (回阳救急汤)

Restore and Revive the Yang Decoction from *Revised Popular Guide*

huí yáng jiù jí tāng

Source *Revised Popular Guide to the Discussion of Cold Damage* (Qing dynasty)

Add 9g of cinnabar Ophiopogonis Radix (*zhū mài dōng*) to the original formula. When combined with Ginseng Radix (*rén shēn*) and Schisandrae Fructus (*wǔ wèi zǐ*), this makes Generate the Pulse Powder (*shēng mài sǎn*), discussed in Chapter 8, which increases the qi-augmenting potential of the entire formula. However, because Ophiopogonis Radix (*mài mén dōng*) is cold in nature, it must be used with caution so as not to impede the recovery of the yang.

參附湯 (参附汤)

Ginseng and Aconite Accessory Root Decoction

shēn fù tāng

Source *Classified Compilation of Medical Prescriptions* (1445)

Ginseng Radix (*rén shēn*) 15g (9g)
Aconiti Radix lateralis praeparata (*zhì fù zǐ*) 30g (15g)

Method of Preparation   Decoction. The dosage commonly used at present is indicated in parentheses. The source text advises to decoct in water in which Zingiberis Rhizoma recens (*shēng jiāng*) and Jujubae Fructus (*dà zǎo*) have been boiled. Ginseng Radix (*rén shēn*) may be separately prepared by cooking in a double boiler and adding the resulting liquid to a strained decoction of Aconiti Radix lateralis praeparata (*zhì fù zǐ*). Ginseng Radix (*rén shēn*) must be used because Codonopsis Radix (*dǎng shēn*) cannot adequately tonify the source qi in this condition.

Actions   Restores the yang, strongly tonifies the source qi, and rescues the qi from collapse due to devastated yang

Indications

Cold extremities, sweating, weak breathing and shortness of breath, dizziness, an extremely pale complexion, a pale tongue, and a faint pulse that is almost imperceptible

This is severe deficiency of the source qi with sudden collapse of the yang qi. The function of the yang qi is to warm the body and promote the physiological activity of the entire organism. Its source is the gate of vitality in the lower burner and its strength is an expression of the prenatal constitution. As the most yang aspect of the qi dynamic, it must attach itself to more substantive elements, such as the nutritive qi, body fluids, or blood, in order to carry out its functions. If this happens, the interpenetration of yin and yang ensures the smooth functioning of the qi dynamic. On the other hand, if the yang qi collapses, all physiological processes begin to break down and the movement of any other type of qi ceases. In sudden collapse, the processes that are most visibly affected are at the more yang aspects of the qi dynamic associated with the Heart and Lungs. If the yang qi is unable to support the pulse, this manifests as cold extremities and a faint, almost imperceptible, pulse. If it is unable to stabilize the superficial levels of the body, this leads to sweating and a drainage of the yin and fluids. Weak breathing and shortness of breath, dizziness, pale complexion, and a pale tongue indicate yang deficiency leading to Lung qi deficiency.

Analysis of Formula

To restore the exhausted yang and rescue the qi from collapse, very warm and strongly tonifying herbs must be used. The chief ingredient, sweet and warm Ginseng Radix (*rén shēn*), strongly tonifies the source qi within the Heart and Lungs, augmenting the qi and enriching the fluids. The deputy, Aconiti Radix lateralis praeparata (*zhì fù zǐ*), warms and tonifies the true yang at the gate of vitality. Together with the main herb, it assists the Spleen earth at the center of all transformation in the body. In this manner, it unfolds a rapid supportive action into the entire qi dynamic, even though it is composed of just two herbs. It is therefore suitable for conditions of acute collapse of the yang qi.

Cautions and Contraindications

This is a very strong tonic designed for the treatment of acute conditions. It should not be administered long term. Once the yang qi has been restored and the acute stage has passed, the pattern of disharmony should be reevaluated and the formula modified accordingly. Extended use generates fire, which injures the yin and consumes the blood.

Commentary

When the yang qi suddenly collapses, the functions of ascending, descending, entering, and leaving come to a halt, which presents a life-threatening condition. The powerful tonifying action of this formula makes it suitable for emergencies. Hospitals of traditional medicine in China prepare the formula as a solution and administer it intravenously.

One way of explaining its rapid life-saving efficacy is its dual tonification of pre- and postnatal yang and qi. The *Golden Mirror of the Medical Tradition* takes this approach:

> No [herb] excels at tonifying the postnatal qi like Ginseng Radix (*rén shēn*). No herb is as good at tonifying the prenatal qi as Aconiti Radix lateralis praeparata (*zhì fù zǐ*). This is [the principle] on which Ginseng and Aconite Accessory Root Decoction (*shēn fù tāng*) is established. Mutually accentuating, if used appropriately, these two herbs are able to transform qi in a flash as if out of thin air, and to generate yang in an instant within the gate of vitality. This formula possesses the most spirit-like agility.

Another explanation is provided by the early modern physician Tang Zong-Hai in *Discussion of Blood Patterns*. Tang emphasizes the formula's action on the lower and upper burners:

> A person's original qi originates in the Kidneys and emerges through the Lungs. If the Lung yin cannot exert its governance of rhythm, the Kidney yang will be unable to return to its source, leading to a pattern [characterized by] wheezing and abandonment. One uses Aconiti Radix lateralis praeparata (*zhì fù zǐ*), which enters into the Kidneys, to tonify the root of yang qi. One uses Ginseng Radix (*rén shēn*), which enters into the Lungs, to assist the governance of qi emission. The two herbs mutually assist each other to strongly tonify the yang qi. Qi is the yang of water and water is the yin of qi. Ginseng Radix (*rén shēn*) tonifies the yin of qi, while Aconiti Radix lateralis praeparata (*zhì fù zǐ*) tonifies the yang of water. If one understands this, one understands everything about the strategy for tonifying the qi.

Comparison

> ➤ Vs. Frigid Extremities Decoction (*sì nì tāng*)

Both formulas treat patterns characterized by yang debilitation and an overabundance of yin with frigid extremities and a weak pulse. Frigid Extremities Decoction (*sì nì tāng*) focuses on conditions where the yang is debilitated but has not abandoned the organism. Thus, it uses strongly warming, acrid herbs to disperse the cold and restore the yang. Ginseng and Aconite Accessory Root Decoction (*shēn fù tāng*), on the other hand, treats patterns characterized by qi abandonment with symptoms like wheezing, sweating, and a very faint pulse. Thus, it balances the dispersion of cold with the tonification of qi and fluids in order to secure the qi and yang.

Biomedical Indications

With the appropriate presentation, this formula may be used to treat a variety of biomedically-defined disorders including cardiac failure, myocardial infarction, cardiogenic shock, postpartum hemorrhage, uterine bleeding, and other causes of hypovolemic shock.

Alternate names

Aconite Accessory Root and Ginseng Decoction (*fù shēn tāng*) in *Systematic Great Compendium of Medicine Past and Present*; Turn Around Inversion Decoction to Make Childbirth Safe (*zhuǎn jué ān chǎn tāng*) in *Master Ye's Patterns and Treatments in Women's Diseases*

Modification

- For shock or cardiac failure, add Fossilia Ossis Mastodi (*lóng gǔ*), Ostreae Concha (*mǔ lì*), Paeoniae Radix alba (*bái sháo*), and Glycyrrhizae Radix praeparata (*zhì gān cǎo*).

Associated Formula

獨參湯 （独参汤）

Unaccompanied Ginseng Decoction

dú shēn tāng

SOURCE   *Miraculous Book of Ten Remedies* (1348)

Ginseng Radix (*rén shēn*) 60g

Prepare as a decoction with 5 pieces of Jujubae Fructus (*dà zǎo*). At present, no more than half the specified dosage is used. Tonifies the source qi and stabilizes collapse. For acute, severe blood loss or heart failure characterized by an extremely pale complexion, lethargic state, cold extremities, excessive sweating, weak breathing, and a faint or thin pulse that is almost imperceptible. This is called 'qi collapse following the [loss of] blood.' In contrast to the principal formula, which is used for chronic deficient yang patterns that have reached a critical stage, the emphasis of this formula is on strengthening the exhausted qi associated with acute, severe blood loss.

Comparative Tables of Principal Formulas

■ FORMULAS THAT WARM THE CHANNELS AND DISPERSE COLD

Common symptoms: relatively superficial cold in patients with blood deficiency

Formula Name	Diagnosis	Indications	Remarks
Tangkuei Decoction for Frigid Extremities (*dāng guī sì nì tāng*)	Cold in the channels with underlying blood deficiency	Long-standing cold hands and feet that are both cold to the touch and feel very cold to the patient, a pale tongue with a white coating, and a submerged, thin pulse or one that is thin and almost imperceptible	Also used to treat irregular menstruation and various types of pain that are aggravated by exposure to cold.
Astragalus and Cinnamon Twig Five-Substance Decoction (*huáng qí guì zhī wǔ wù tāng*)	Painful obstruction of the blood	Relatively superficial numbness without pain, paresthesias and numbness of the skin and flesh, and a faint, choppy, and tight pulse	Focuses on expelling wind-cold from the superficial layers of the body and moving the vessels.

■ FORMULAS THAT WARM THE MIDDLE AND DISPEL COLD

Common symptoms: abdominal pain, pale tongue with a white coating, thin pulse

Formula Name	Diagnosis	Indications	Remarks
Regulate the Middle Pill (*lǐ zhōng wán*)	Middle burner cold from deficiency	Diarrhea with watery stool, nausea and vomiting, no particular thirst, loss of appetite, abdominal pain, a pale tongue with a white coating, and a submerged, thin pulse	Also for greater yin disorders, and middle burner yang deficiency patterns such as chronic bleeding, chronic childhood convulsions, and painful obstruction of the chest.

cont. ↘

Formula Name	Diagnosis	Indications	Remarks
Evodia Decoction (*wú zhū yú tāng*)	Stomach deficiency cold with Liver involvement	Vomiting from either yang brightness or lesser yin-warp disorders, and terminal yin-warp headache, a tongue that is not red, but has a white, slippery coating, and a thin pulse that is either slow or wiry	For a wide range of conditions with vomiting due to Stomach or Liver disharmony.
Minor Construct the Middle Decoction (*xiǎo jiàn zhōng tāng*)	Middle burner deficiency cold with insufficiency of transportation and transformation	Intermittent, spasmodic abdominal pain that responds favorably to local application of warmth and pressure, lusterless complexion, reduced appetite, a pale tongue with a white coating, and a thin, wiry, and moderate pulse	There may also be low-grade fever, palpitations, irritability, cold and sore extremities, and a dry mouth and throat.
Major Construct the Middle Decoction (*dà jiàn zhōng tāng*)	Middle burner yang deficiency with internal ascendence of cold	Excruciating epigastric and abdominal pain, strong sensation of cold in the epigastrium, severe vomiting, a white, slippery tongue coating, and a thin and tight or slow and wiry pulse	Also used for postoperative ileus.
Licorice and Ginger Decoction (*gān cǎo gān jiāng tāng*)	Deficiency cold Lung atrophy	Cold extremities, absence of thirst or coughing, dry throat, spitting up of clear fluids, irritability, dizziness, frequent urination, a pale, moist tongue without coating, and a frail or submerged and slow pulse	Also for abdominal pain due to Spleen and Stomach deficiency, and bleeding due to Spleen yang deficiency.
White Atractylodes and Aconite Accessory Root Decoction (*baí zhú fù zǐ tāng*)	Wind-cold-dampness obstruction due to yang deficiency	Pain throughout the body characterized by an inability to rotate the body, hard stools, normal urination, lack of thirst or nausea, and a floating, thin, and moderate pulse	Also used for headaches and dizziness, wind-stroke, constipation, and diarrhea.

■ FORMULAS THAT RESCUE DEVASTATED YANG

Common symptoms: emergencies with cold extremities, lethargy, pale tongue, faint pulse

Formula Name	Diagnosis	Indications	Remarks
Frigid Extremities Decoction (*sì nì tāng*)	Cold inversion typically associated with a lesser yin-warp pattern	Extremely cold extremities, lethargy with a constant desire to sleep, vomiting, diarrhea with undigested food, abdominal pain and cold, lack of thirst, a pale tongue with a white, slippery coating, and a submerged, thin or submerged, faint pulse	Strengthens the yang of both the gate of vitality and the middle burner without injuring the yin.
Restore and Revive the Yang Decoction (*huí yáng jiù jí tāng*)	Pathogenic cold directly attacking all three yin warps with exhausted yang	Chills, cold extremities, vomiting, diarrhea, abdominal pain, lethargy with a constant desire to sleep, a pale tongue with a white coating, and a submerged, faint, or imperceptible pulse	There may also be severe chills or cyanosis of the fingernails and lips. This is an extremely dangerous type of abandoned disorder.
Ginseng and Aconite Accessory Root Decoction (*shēn fù tāng*)	Severe deficiency of the source qi with sudden collapse of the yang qi	Cold extremities, sweating, weak breathing and shortness of breath, dizziness, an extremely pale complexion, a pale tongue, and a faint pulse that is almost imperceptible	For patterns characterized by qi abandonment.

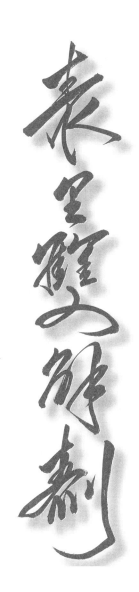

Chapter 7 Contents

Formulas that Release Exterior-Interior Excess

Formulas that Release Exterior-Interior Excess

IN EXTERNALLY-CONTRACTED diseases there is often a stage where the pathogenic influence remains lodged in the exterior even though it has already penetrated into the interior. Similar problems may occur if a person with an interior disorder contracts a new pathogen, which then obstructs the exterior. In each case, the patient will present with a combined exterior-interior disorder.

There are three basic treatment strategies for dealing with such problems: resolve the exterior first and then treat the interior, dispel the pathogen from the interior first and then treat the exterior, or simultaneously treat the interior and exterior. The formulas in this chapter utilize the third approach. This is most appropriate when the pathogens in the exterior and interior are both relatively strong. In clinical practice, these are often relatively acute disorders where both the exterior and interior require urgent attention. If the exterior is released without treating the interior, the condition will worsen; if the interior is treated without releasing the exterior, the pathogenic influences cannot be completely eliminated from the body. A similar scenario applies where exterior excess is combined with interior deficiency, as discussed in Chapter 1.

Although the core strategies used in the formulas discussed here—sweating, warming, cooling, and purging—were already known to the authors of the *Inner Classic,* it was Zhang Zhong-Jing at the end of the Han dynasty who first composed specific formulas to treat exterior-interior excess patterns: Major Bupleurum Decoction *(dà chái hú tāng)*

for combined yang brightness and lesser yang disorders; Seven-Substance Decoction with Magnolia Bark *(hòu pò qī wù tāng)* for combined yang brightness and greater yang disorders; Kudzu, Scutellaria, and Coptis Decoction *(gé gēn huáng qín huáng lián tāng)* for yang brightness disorders with heat pathogens in both the exterior and interior; and Cinnamon Twig and Ginseng Decoction *(guì zhī rén shēn tāng)* for cold in the interior complicated by wind-cold in the greater yang. These formulas continue to be widely used today. They also became the models for all later formulas in this section.

Besides Zhang Zhong-Jing, the second most influential physician to focus on the joint treatment of internal and external excess disorders was Liu Wan-Su, one of the four masters of the Jin-Yuan period (1115-1368). His clinical strategies focused on the elimination of fire from the body and he invented a method known as 'double releasing' (雙解 *shuāng jiě),* exemplified by Saposhnikovia Powder that Sagely Unblocks *(fáng fēng tōng shèng sǎn)* and its variations. This method aims at releasing wind-cold from the exterior by means of sweating, while simultaneously draining internal heat via the stool and urine.

In contemporary Chinese medicine, external disorders are generally divided into heat- and cold-type disorders, while interior disorders are divided into deficiency and excess as well as heat and cold disorders. Accordingly, formulas in this chapter can be divided according to whether heat or cold in the exterior combines with heat or cold excess in the interior.

Accurate diagnosis is imperative for successful use of these formulas. The practitioner must identify which pathogenic influence is involved, its location (interior or exterior), and the extent of its development (level or warp) before the appropriate formula can be selected and modified to match the precise pattern. Once a formula's composition and its indication have been understood, however, its use can be expanded beyond its original indication to problems facing every clinician in contemporary practice.

Section 1

....

FORMULAS THAT RELEASE THE EXTERIOR AND PURGE THE INTERIOR

The formulas in this group are indicated for patterns characterized by the presence of an externally-contracted pathogen in the exterior while excess accumulation obstructs the interior. The term 'interior' here does not generally refer to the organs as opposed to the channels, but more often to the bowels associated with the yang brightness as opposed to the greater and lesser yang warps, or the exterior of the yang brightness warp itself. This is because heat excess in the interior is typically a manifestation of a yang brightness pattern.

The patterns treated by formulas in this section are characterized by fever and chills that are accompanied by abdominal fullness, constipation, and a red tongue with a yellow coating. Formulas that treat these disorders combine herbs that release the exterior, such as Cinnamomi Ramulus (*guì zhī*), Ephedrae Herba (*má huáng*), Bupleuri Radix (*chái hú*), Menthae haplocalycis Herba (*bò hé*), Schizonepetae Herba (*jīng jiè*), and Saposhnikoviae Radix (*fáng fēng*), with herbs that purge accumulation from the interior, such as Rhei Radix et Rhizoma (*dà huáng*) and Natrii Sulfas (*máng xiāo*).

大柴胡湯 (大柴胡汤)
Major Bupleurum Decoction
dà chái hú tāng

Source   *Discussion of Cold Damage* (c. 220)

Bupleuri Radix (*chái hú*)..............................24g
Scutellariae Radix (*huáng qín*)........................9g
prepared Aurantii Fructus immaturus (*zhì zhǐ shí*)....6-9g
Rhei Radix et Rhizoma (*dà huáng*).....................6g
Paeoniae Radix (*sháo yào*)............................9g
Pinelliae Rhizoma praeparatum (*zhì bàn xià*).........24g
Zingiberis Rhizoma recens (*shēng jiāng*).............15g
Jujubae Fructus (*dà zǎo*)........................12 pieces

Method of Preparation   The source text advises to decoct the above ingredients in approximately 12 cups of water until 6 cups remain. The ingredients are removed, and the strained decoction is further decocted until 3 cups remain. This is taken warm in three equal doses over the course of a day. At present, it is generally prepared as a decoction in the usual manner. The above dosages are based on the source text; at present, most practitioners use 12-15g of Bupleuri Radix (*chái hú*) and Pinelliae Rhizoma praeparatum (*zhì bàn xià*), 6-9g of Zingiberis Rhizoma recens (*shēng jiāng*), and 4 pieces of Jujubae Fructus (*dà zǎo*). Paeoniae Radix alba (*bái sháo*) is the most common form of Paeoniae Radix (*sháo yào*) that is currently used.

Actions   Harmonizes and releases the lesser yang, and drains internal clumping due to heat

Indications

Alternating fever and chills, fullness in the chest and hypochondria (with or without pain), a bitter taste in the mouth, nausea, continuous vomiting, hard focal distention or fullness and pain in the epigastrium, burning diarrhea or no bowel movements, melancholy, slight irritability, a yellow tongue coating, and a wiry, forceful pulse.

This is a concurrent lesser yang and yang brightness-warp disorder. The alternating fever and chills, sensation of fullness in the chest and hypochondria, bitter taste in the mouth, and wiry pulse are indicative of a lesser yang-warp disorder. The sensation of firm masses or distention and pain in the epigastrium, absence of bowel movements or hot, burning diarrhea, yellow coating on the tongue, and forceful pulse are indicative of a yang brightness organ-warp disorder. It is not uncommon to find a flooding or excessive pulse. The yang brightness signs indicate that the pathogen has moved deeper into the body. Compared to a purely lesser yang condition, the heat and constraint are thus more severe. This explains the symptoms of uncontrolled vomiting, melancholy, and increased irritability.

This formula can also be used for commingled heat with diarrhea (協熱下利 *xié rè xià lì*). This is a pattern, first outlined in *Discussion of Cold Damage*, where diarrhea is accompanied by heat. The term 'heat' in this context may denote fever, that is, an objective rise in body temperature accessible to the physician by means of palpation, as well as mere subjective sensations experienced by the patient but not accessible to the physician. In both cases, neither the pulse nor the tongue reflects the presence of heat, which differentiates this pattern from excess heat yang brightness patterns.

Analysis of Formula

Because it focuses on a combined lesser yang and yang brightness disorder this formula combines a strategy of harmonization with one of downward draining. Harmonization vents the pathogen in the exterior via the lesser yang, while downward draining expels the heat knotting in the interior.

Although normally purging heat from the interior would be contraindicated in lesser yang disorders, it is permitted here due to the simultaneous occurrence of a yang brightness interior excess pattern.

This formula has two chief herbs. Bupleuri Radix *(chái hú)* dredges the lesser yang and releases the exterior. Rhei Radix et Rhizoma *(dà huáng)* enters the yang brightness to drain heat and open the bowels. These functions are amplified by two deputies. The first, bitter and cold Scutellariae Radix *(huáng qín)*, combines with Bupleuri Radix *(chái hú)* to clear heat from the lesser yang but also assists Rhei Radix et Rhizoma *(dà huáng)* in draining heat from the bowels. The second, Aurantii Fructus immaturus *(zhǐ shí)*, is a strong regulator of qi movement that breaks up qi stagnation and reduces focal distention and fullness in the chest and abdomen. When combined with Bupleuri Radix *(chái hú)*, its ability to facilitate the flow of qi is greatly strengthened. When combined with Rhei Radix et Rhizoma *(dà huáng)*, it breaks up clumping in the bowels.

One of the assistants, Paeoniae Radix *(sháo yào)*, relaxes urgency and stops pain. In concert with Aurantii Fructus immaturus *(zhǐ shí)* and Rhei Radix et Rhizoma *(dà huáng)*, it treats the pain from excess in the abdomen. The other assistant, Pinelliae Rhizoma praeparatum *(zhì bàn xià)*, harmonizes the middle burner and directs the rebellious Stomach qi downward. When combined with one of the envoys, Zingiberis Rhizoma recens *(shēng jiāng)*, it effectively stops the vomiting. The other envoy, Jujubae Fructus *(dà zǎo)*, strengthens the ability of Paeoniae Radix *(sháo yào)* to soften the Liver and reduce abdominal spasms. This combination also protects the yin from injury by pathogenic heat and from the harsh draining properties of Rhei Radix et Rhizoma *(dà huáng)* and Aurantii Fructus immaturus *(zhǐ shí)*. The combination of Zingiberis Rhizoma recens *(shēng jiāng)* and Jujubae Fructus *(dà zǎo)* mildly regulates the nutritive and protective qi, and assists in the release of the pathogenic influence.

Commentary

This is the first formula in the history of Chinese medicine to focus on simultaneously venting heat from the exterior and draining it from the interior. It is therefore the model on which all the other formulas in this section are based.

Used for concurrent lesser yang and yang brightness organ disorders, this formula is based on two formulas that separately treat each of these single-warp conditions: Minor Bupleurum Decoction *(xiǎo chái hú tāng)* for the lesser yang, and Major Order the Qi Decoction *(dà chéng qì tāng)* for the yang brightness. Ginseng Radix *(rén shēn)* and Glycyrrhizae Radix praeparata *(zhì gān cǎo)* are omitted to prevent the tonifying and cloying properties of these herbs from obstructing the flow, which would aggravate the problems of vomiting and defecation. Since the abdominal pain is more

severe than the distention, Magnoliae officinalis Cortex *(hòu pò)* and Natrii Sulfas *(máng xiāo)* are omitted, and Paeoniae Radix *(sháo yào)* is added. Depending on which type of Paeoniae Radix *(sháo yào)* is chosen, one can achieve a different effect. Paeoniae Radix alba *(bái sháo)* helps relax urgency by tonifying the fluids. Paeoniae Radix rubra *(chì sháo)* will focus more strongly on cooling the blood and unblocking stasis. Although purging is generally inappropriate for lesser yang-warp disorders, concurrent lesser yang and yang brightness organ-warp disorders require the use of purgatives to attack the interior aspect of the problem.

Rhei Radix et Rhizoma (dà huáng)

Although this formula is found in both *Discussion of Cold Damage* and *Essentials from the Golden Cabinet,* only the latter lists Rhei Radix et Rhizoma *(dà huáng)* as an ingredient. Later commentators therefore argued over whether inclusion of this herb in the formula is essential. There are three different views. The first, represented by the Song text *Three Works on the Discussion of Cold Damage* by Xu Shu-Wei, held that Rhei Radix et Rhizoma *(dà huáng)* is essential: "Rhei Radix et Rhizoma *(dà huáng)* is an essential herb in [treating] cold damage. Its omission from Major Bupleurum Decoction *(dà chái hú tāng)* must [have been] an error."

The opposite view was expressed by the Ming-dynasty commentator Ke Qin. In *Collected Writings on Renewal of the Discussion of Cold Damage,* Ke argued that in this disorder the pathogen is just beginning to enter the Stomach organ, obstructing its opening but not yet its central portion. This is reflected in the symptoms of hard focal distention in the epigastric region and diarrhea. These symptoms indicate that the passages of the bowels are still open, hence the use of Rhei Radix et Rhizoma *(dà huáng)* is not yet necessary.

Finally, in *Essays on Medicine Esteeming the Chinese and Respecting the Western,* the early modern physician Zhang Xi-Chun attempted to reconcile these opposing views:

> Later generations [of physicians following Zhang Zhong-Jing] feared the fierceness of Rhei Radix et Rhizoma *(dà huáng)* and tended to replace it with Aurantii Fructus immaturus *(zhǐ shí)*. They [argued] that if a formula did not work, one could then still add Rhei Radix et Rhizoma *(dà huáng)* without, however, removing Aurantii Fructus immaturus *(zhǐ shí)*. This is the origin of [the dispute over] why, on one occasion [in Zhang Zhong-Jing's works,] the formula Major Bupleurum Decoction *(dà chái hú tāng)* contains Rhei Radix et Rhizoma *(dà huáng)*, and on another it does not.

Most modern textbooks include Rhei Radix et Rhizoma *(dà huáng)*, arguing that it is essential to flush clumping heat from the Intestines. One should also note that, in relation to the other herbs in the formula, the dosage of Rhei Radix et Rhizoma *(dà huáng)* is actually very low. Hence, as the modern physician He Lian-Chen commented: "In addition to harmonizing [the middle] and resolving [the exterior, the formula] only gently purges." Most prepared products of this formula contain Rhei Radix et Rhizoma (dà huáng).

Usage

Major Bupleurum Decoction (dà chái hú tāng) may be used to treat either diarrhea (due to accumulation of heat in the Intestines) or constipation. It may also be used for Liver and Gallbladder fire causing headache, tinnitus, diminished hearing and vision, red eyes, manic behavior, or palpitations with anxiety if the presentation also includes epigastric fullness and pain, a bitter taste in the mouth, a red tongue with yellow coating, and a fast, wiry pulse. Another important modern usage is wheezing caused by inability of the qi to descend due to the obstruction of the epigastric area and flanks.

This is also an important formula for treating fevers, and not just those presenting with alternating heat and cold. More important is the presence of such markers as tension and fullness in the flanks and epigastrium aggravated by pressure, and a rather acute and accelerated disease process. Note that it may be necessary to press quite deeply in those who are overweight before the characteristic abdominal signs are elicited, while they will be felt more superficially in those who are thin.

Comparisons

➤ Vs. Minor Bupleurum Decoction (xiǎo chái hú tāng)

Both of these formulas treat lesser yang-warp disorders. However, a Major Bupleurum Decoction (dà xiǎo chái hú tāng) presentation is characterized by more severe vomiting (rather than occasional vomiting or just nausea) caused by stronger heat. Thus, the formula contains a much larger dosage (24g vs. 9g) of Zingiberis Rhizoma recens (shēng jiāng). Symptomatically, Zingiberis Rhizoma recens (shēng jiāng) stops nausea and vomiting while functionally, it assists Bupleuri Radix (chái hú) in venting the pathogen to the exterior. A Major Bupleurum Decoction (dà chái hú tāng) presentation must also have symptoms of heat in the yang brightness organ with clumping, such as abdominal fullness, focal distention, and pain.

Because Minor Bupleurum Decoction (xiǎo chái hú tāng) contains herbs that harmonize and tonify the Spleen and Stomach, it can be used when heat has already been purged from the interior but some heat still remains in the exterior. In these cases, the formula not only effectively vents any lingering pathogen but also strengthens the qi of the middle burner that has been weakened by the prior purgation.

➤ Vs. Bupleurum Decoction plus Mirabilite (chái hú jiā máng xiāo tāng)

Relative to this formula, Major Bupleurum Decoction (dà xiǎo

chái hú tāng) focuses on disorders of excess with hard focal distention of the epigastrium and an absence of injury to the Stomach qi. The fever will tend to be constant and rise in the afternoon. By contrast, Bupleurum Decoction plus Mirabilite (chái hú jiā máng xiāo tāng) is indicated for constipation and fullness in the chest and hypochondria with alternating fever and chills that are more pronounced in the afternoon.

➤ Vs. Major Order the Qi Decoction (dà chéng qì tāng); see page 66

Biomedical Indications

With the appropriate presentation, this formula may be used to treat a variety of biomedically-defined disorders. One group involves the upper digestive system and includes cholecystitis, cholelithiasis, pancreatitis, and peptic ulcers as well as viral hepatitis, enteric fever, and scarlet fever. In these cases, the formula is usually given in high doses as a decoction in order to produce a rapid effect. The other group involves metabolic and autonomic disruptions such as diabetes, hypertension, hyperlipidemia, fatty liver, and obesity. In these cases, the formula is usually given in lower doses over longer periods of time, often in the form of concentrated powders.

Modifications

- For marked chest and epigastric pain and distention, add Aucklandiae Radix (mù xiāng), Curcumae Radix (yù jīn), and Artemisiae scopariae Herba (yīn chén).
- For severe abdominal pain, add Corydalis Rhizoma (yán hú suǒ), Linderae Radix (wū yào), and Cyperi Rhizoma (xiāng fù).
- For severe nausea and vomiting, add Bambusae Caulis in taeniam (zhú rú), Inulae Flos (xuán fù huā), and Coptidis Rhizoma (huáng lián).
- For uncontrolled, continuous vomiting, add Coptidis Rhizoma (huáng lián) and Evodiae Fructus (wú zhū yú).
- For manic behavior due to Liver Fire, add Indigo naturalis (qīng dài), Gardeniae Fructus (zhī zǐ), Moutan Cortex (mǔ dān pí), and Natrii Sulfas (máng xiāo).
- For acute jaundice, add Gardeniae Fructus (zhī zǐ) and Phellodendri Cortex (huáng bǎi).
- For marked chills, add Ephedrae Herba (má huáng), Forsythiae Fructus (lián qiáo), and Phaseoli Semen (chì xiǎo dòu).
- For acute cholecystitis, add Lonicerae Flos (jīn yín huā), Forsythiae Fructus (lián qiáo), Taraxaci Herba (pú gōng yīng), and Violae Herba (zǐ huā dì dīng).
- For gallstones, add Lysimachiae Herba (jīn qián cǎo), Pyrrosiae Folium (shí wěi), and Lygodii Spora (hǎi jīn shā).
- For pancreatitis, combine with Pinellia Decoction to Drain the Epigastrium (bàn xià xiè xīn tāng).

- For intercostal neuralgia, combine with Minor Decoction [for Pathogens] Stuck in the Chest (*xiǎo xiàn xiōng tāng*).

Associated Formulas

厚朴七物湯 （厚朴七物汤）

Seven-Substance Decoction with Magnolia Bark

hòu pò qī wù tāng

SOURCE *Essentials from the Golden Cabinet* (c. 220)

Magnoliae officinalis Cortex (*hòu pò*) 24g
Glycyrrhizae Radix (*gān cǎo*) 9g
Rhei Radix et Rhizoma (*dà huáng*) 9g
Aurantii Fructus immaturus (*zhǐ shí*) 9g
Cinnamomi Ramulus (*guì zhī*) 6g
Zingiberis Rhizoma recens (*shēng jiāng*) 15g
Jujubae Fructus (*dà zǎo*) . . . . 12 pieces

Dosage is based on the source text. At present, 15g of Magnoliae officinalis Cortex (*hòu pò*), 6g of Glycyrrhizae Radix (*gān cǎo*), 12g of Zingiberis Rhizoma recens (*shēng jiāng*), and 4 pieces of Jujubae Fructus (*dà zǎo*) are used. Releases the muscles and the exterior, promotes the movement of qi, and unblocks the bowels. For externally-contracted disorders where the exterior is not yet released, but excess has already developed in the interior. Such a condition develops due to improper treatment or failure to treat an external condition. Manifestations include symptoms of interior excess such as a sensation of fullness in the abdomen and no bowel movements, accompanied by signs that a pathogen remains in the exterior such as fever and a floating, rapid pulse.

In contrast to the principal formula, this is indicated for concurrent greater yang and yang brightness-warp disorders, focusing on the interior aspect. It can thus be viewed as a combination of Cinnamon Twig Decoction (*guì zhī tāng*) and Minor Order the Qi Decoction (*xiǎo chéng qì tāng*). Paeoniae Radix (*sháo yào*) is omitted from the formula because there is no abdominal pain in this pattern.

加味大柴胡湯 （加味大柴胡汤）

Augmented Major Bupleurum Decoction

jiā wèi dà chái hú tāng

SOURCE *Revised and Expanded Discussion of Warm-Heat Pathogen Diseases* (1907)

Bupleuri Radix (*chái hú*) 4.5g
Scutellariae Radix (*huáng qín*) 9g
Paeoniae Radix alba (*bái sháo*) 9g
Pinelliae Rhizoma praeparatum (*zhì bàn xià*) 9g
Aurantii Fructus immaturus (*zhǐ shí*) 4.5g
Rhei Radix et Rhizoma (*dà huáng*) 9g
Jujubae Fructus (*dà zǎo*) . . . . 3 pieces
Zingiberis Rhizoma recens (*shēng jiāng*) . . . . 3 slices
Persicae Semen (*táo rén*) 12g
Paeoniae Radix rubra (*chì sháo*) 6g

Decoction. This formula is specific for cold damage disorders in women occurring with menstruation where the pathogen enters into the lesser yang channel that traverses the ear. The battle between the normal and pathogenic qi causes clumping and obstruction, which manifests in a loss of hearing. These symptoms may be accompanied by fullness and pain in the back, hypochondria, and lower abdomen.

清胰湯 （清胰汤）

Clear the Pancreas Decoction

qīng yí tāng

SOURCE *Integrated Chinese and Western Medical Treatment of the Acute Abdomen* (1973)

Bupleuri Radix (*chái hú*) 15g
Scutellariae Radix (*huáng qín*) 9g
Picrorhizae Rhizoma (*hú huáng lián*) 9g
Paeoniae Radix alba (*bái sháo*) 15g
Aucklandiae Radix (*mù xiāng*) . . . . [add near end] 9g
Corydalis Rhizoma (*yán hú suǒ*) 9g
Rhei Radix et Rhizoma (*dà huáng*) . . . . [add near end] 15g
Natrii Sulfas (*máng xiāo*) . . . . [add to strained decoction] 9g

Clears and drains heat excess, spreads the Liver qi, promotes the movement of qi, and alleviates pain. For stabbing, diffuse pain in the epigastrium that extends to the back, loss of appetite, alternating fever and chills, pain in the abdomen, and constipation. This presentation most commonly occurs during acute pancreatitis. Although there are many formulas by this name in modern China (all of which are used to treat acute pancreatitis), this is the best known. It was composed by physicians at the Nankai Hospital in Tianjin, who have also formulated a range of formulas based on Major Bupleurum Decoction (*dà chái hú tāng*) to treat cholecystitis. These can be found in the source text.

The physicians at the Nankai Hospital also suggest a number of modifications to adjust the formula more precisely to the pattern:

- For severe dampness with jaundice, add Artemisiae scopariae Herba (*yīn chén*), Gardeniae Fructus (*zhī zǐ*), and Gentianae Radix (*lóng dǎn cǎo*).

- For severe vomiting, add Pinelliae Rhizoma praeparatum (*zhì bàn xià*) and Haematitum (*dài zhě shí*).

- For severe pain, add Toosendan Fructus (*chuān liàn zǐ*) and increase the dosage of Corydalis Rhizoma (*yán hú suǒ*).

- For food accumulation, add Raphani Semen (*lái fú zǐ*), Massa medicata fermentata (*shén qū*), Hordei Fructus germinatus (*mài yá*), and Crataegi Fructus (*shān zhā*).

- For fullness of the chest, add Magnoliae officinalis Cortex (*hòu pò*) and Aurantii Fructus immaturus (*zhǐ shí*).

- For back pain, add Trichosanthis Fructus (*quán guā lóu*), Allii macrostemi Bulbus (*xiè bái*), Saposhnikoviae Radix (*fáng fēng*), and Gentianae macrophyllae Radix (*qín jiāo*).

- For tapeworms in the bile duct, add Arecae Semen (*bīng láng*), Quisqualis Fructus (*shǐ jūn zǐ*), and Meliae Cortex (*kǔ liàn gēn pí*).

- For patients with a deficient constitution and interior cold, remove Rhei Radix et Rhizoma (*dà huáng*) and Natrii Sulfas (*máng xiāo*) and add Aconiti Radix lateralis praeparata (*zhì fù zǐ*) and Zingiberis Rhizoma (*gān jiāng*).

防風通聖散 (防风通圣散)

Saposhnikovia Powder that Sagely Unblocks

fáng fēng tōng shèng sǎn

This formula induces sweating without injuring the exterior, and purges without injuring the interior. Its ability to unblock is sage-like in its subtlety, hence the name.

Source   *Formulas from the Discussion Illuminating the Yellow Emperor's Basic Questions* (1172)

Saposhnikoviae Radix (*fáng fēng*) 15g
Ephedrae Herba (*má huáng*) 15g
Rhei Radix et Rhizoma (*dà huáng*) 15g
Natrii Sulfas (*máng xiāo*) 15g
Schizonepetae Herba (*jīng jiè*) 15g
Menthae haplocalycis Herba (*bò hé*) 15g
Gardeniae Fructus (*zhī zǐ*) 15g
Talcum (*huá shí*) 90g
Gypsum fibrosum (*shí gāo*) 30g
Forsythiae Fructus (*lián qiáo*) 15g
Scutellariae Radix (*huáng qín*) 30g
Platycodi Radix (*jié gěng*) 30g
Chuanxiong Rhizoma (*chuān xiōng*) 15g
Angelicae sinensis Radix (*dāng guī*) 15g
Paeoniae Radix alba (*bái sháo*) .15g
Atractylodis macrocephalae Rhizoma (*bái zhú*) 15g
Glycyrrhizae Radix (*gān cǎo*) 60g

Method of Preparation   Grind into powder and take 6-9g as a draft with three pieces of Zingiberis Rhizoma recens (*shēng jiāng*). May also be prepared as a decoction with a proportionate reduction in dosage.

Actions   Disperses wind, releases the exterior, drains heat, and unblocks the bowels

Indications

Strong fever and chills, light-headedness, dizziness, red and sore eyes, difficulty in swallowing, nasal congestion with thick and sticky nasal discharge and saliva, a bitter taste in the mouth, dry mouth, focal distention with a stifling sensation in the chest and diaphragm, constipation, dark, rough urination, a yellow, greasy tongue coating, and a flooding, rapid or wiry, slippery pulse.

This is heat excess in both the exterior and interior, either from wind-heat invading a person with preexisting internal accumulation of heat or from an invasion of wind-heat that causes the heat to lodge simultaneously in both the exterior and interior. The strong fever and chills are signs of exterior wind-heat. Because it tends to attack the upper parts of the body, wind-heat causes dizziness and red, sore eyes. It also attacks the Lungs and causes difficulty in swallowing and nasal congestion with thick and sticky nasal discharge and saliva. Interior heat, accumulating primarily in the Lungs and Stomach, is reflected in the bitter taste in the mouth, dry mouth,

focal distention with a stifling sensation in the chest and diaphragm, constipation, dark, rough urination, greasy, yellow tongue coating, and flooding, rapid or wiry, slippery pulse.

Analysis of Formula

To treat heat excess in both the exterior and interior, this formula utilizes a combined strategy of dispersing wind-heat from the exterior and draining heat from the interior via both the urine and stool. Two of the chief herbs, Saposhnikoviae Radix (*fáng fēng*) and Ephedrae Herba (*má huáng*), disperse wind and release the exterior by inducing sweating. Although quite hot in nature (moderated by the other herbs), Ephedrae Herba (*má huáng*) has strong exterior-releasing properties. The other chief herbs, wine-washed Rhei Radix et Rhizoma (*jiǔ dà huáng*) and Natrii Sulfas (*máng xiāo*), a powerful combination, expel heat through the stool. Treating Rhei Radix et Rhizoma (*dà huáng*) in wine strengthens its effect on the circulation while mitigating its purgative properties. This is important because too strong of a purgative will cause the exterior disorder to penetrate more deeply into the body. Among the deputies, Schizonepetae Herba (*jīng jiè*) and Menthae haplocalycis Herba (*bò hé*) assist Saposhnikoviae Radix (*fáng fēng*) and Ephedrae Herba (*má huáng*) in releasing the exterior, while Gardeniae Fructus (*zhī zǐ*) and Talcum (*huá shí*) drain heat through the urine. Because heat has settled primarily in the Lungs and Stomach, the other deputies, Gypsum fibrosum (*shí gāo*), Forsythiae Fructus (*lián qiáo*), Scutellariae Radix (*huáng qín*), and Platycodi Radix (*jié gěng*), are added to clear heat from these organs. The ascending nature of Platycodi Radix (*jié gěng*) complements the descending nature of the purgatives in their separate actions of expelling heat. Such combinations are frequently used in treating complex exterior and interior disorders.

Among the assistant herbs, Chuanxiong Rhizoma (*chuān xiōng*), Angelicae sinensis Radix (*dāng guī*), and Paeoniae Radix alba (*bái sháo*) harmonize the blood, which helps to disperse wind. Because wind-dispersing and heat-clearing ingredients can injure the Spleen, Atractylodis macrocephalae Rhizoma (*bái zhú*), the other assistant, is added to strengthen this organ. Glycyrrhizae Radix (*gān cǎo*), an envoy, indirectly protects the Spleen by harmonizing the actions of the other ingredients. In concert with Platycodi Radix (*jié gěng*), it also improves the functioning of the throat to alleviate difficulty in swallowing. The other envoy, Zingiberis Rhizoma recens (*shēng jiāng*), strengthens the Stomach to prevent the ingredients from causing stomach upset.

Commentary

This formula, which some physicians regard as a variation of Cool the Diaphragm Powder (*liáng gé sǎn*), is used for excess heat in both the exterior and interior. It is representative of the strategy of 'double releasing' (雙解 *shuāng jiě*), that is, releasing the exterior while clearing, draining, or purging heat from the interior, which was devised by Liu Wan-Su, one of the great masters of the Jin-Yuan period. Liu argued that "all six [pathogenic] qi can transform into fire" and that special attention should therefore be paid to eliminating it from the body. These ideas later became focal points for the development of warm pathogen therapeutics during the Ming and Qing epochs. Liu Wan-Su thus opened the way for an important transformation in Chinese medicine, as he himself noted:

> The double-releasing [strategy] that I have constructed in the acrid, cold Sagely Unblocking formula does not follow the model of [Zhang] Zhong-Jing with [reliance on] exterior-releasing herbs like Cinnamomi Ramulus *(guì zhī)* and Ephedrae Herba *(má huáng)*. It is not that I am showing off, as it contains the [correct] principles.

The use of acrid, warm herbs like Ephedrae Herba *(má huáng)*, Saposhnikoviae Radix *(fáng fēng)*, and Schizonepetae Herba *(jīng jiè)* to treat wind-heat in the exterior nevertheless distinguishes this formula from the treatment strategies developed later by physicians like Ye Tian-Shi and Wu Ju-Tong. Although their use is moderated by the inclusion of herbs that tonify the blood, in contemporary clinical practice, it would be foolish to ignore the subsequent developments in Chinese medicine that occurred during the centuries that followed. Thus, where aversion to cold is not very pronounced, some modern textbooks, such as *Formulas* edited by Li Fei, suggest that Ephedrae Herba *(má huáng)* be removed from the prescription.

From the perspective of the six warps of disease, this formula treats a disorder that simultaneously affects the greater yang (exterior), yang brightness (interior heat), and lesser yin (focal distention with a stifling sensation in the chest and diaphragm). The source text recommends the formula for all wind-heat disorders with constipation, dark, rough urination, facial sores, and red, sore eyes, since such conditions can progress to internally-generated wind with stiff tongue or clenched jaw.

Usage

The indications for this formula today are not limited to those discussed above, but may also include some types of carbuncles, skin rashes, manic behavior, Intestinal wind, and heat rash. Many modern practitioners use the formula to treat obesity with exterior-interior heat. Modern Japanese physicians also prescribe it for constitutional treatment of metabolic disorders in patients with a strong constitution, excess heat, and constipation. Some recommend that it be taken by these patients twice a year for one to two months in the spring and autumn as a kind of cleanser in order to prevent the accumulation of heat excess.

Comparison

➢ Vs. Cool the Diaphragm Powder *(liáng gé sǎn)*; *see* PAGE 177

Biomedical Indications

With the appropriate presentation, this formula may be used to treat a wide range of biomedically-defined disorders that affect a variety of systems, such as the common cold, hypertension, migraine, obesity, habitual constipation, hemorrhoids, facial boils, and acute conjunctivitis.

Alternate name

Sagely Unblocking Powder *(tōng shèng sǎn)* in *Teachings on the Manifestion and Root of Cold Damage, Categorized and Gathered*

Modifications

• For cases without strong chills, remove Ephedrae Herba *(má huáng)*.

• For cases without strong fever, remove Gypsum fibrosum *(shí gāo)*.

• For cough and sputum, add Pinelliae Rhizoma praeparatum *(zhì bàn xià)* fried in ginger juice.

Variation

雙解通聖散 (双解通圣散)

Double Releasing Powder that Sagely Unblocks

shuāng jiě tōng shèng sǎn

SOURCE *Golden Mirror of the Medical Tradition* (1742)

Remove Rhei Radix et Rhizoma *(dà huáng)* and Natrii Sulfas *(máng xiāo)* for cases without constipation.

Associated Formula

祛風至寶丹 (祛风至宝丹)

Greatest Treasure Special Pill to Dispel Wind

qū fēng zhì bǎo dān

SOURCE *Wondrous Lantern for Peering into the Origin and Development of Miscellaneous Diseases* (1773)

Talcum *(huá shí)*	45g
Chuanxiong Rhizoma *(chuān xiōng)*	37.5g
Angelicae sinensis Radix *(dāng guī)*	37.5g
Glycyrrhizae Radix *(gān cǎo)*	30g
Paeoniae Radix alba *(bái sháo)*	21g
Saposhnikoviae Radix *(fáng fēng)*	21g
Atractylodis macrocephalae Rhizoma *(bái zhú)*	19.5g
Gypsum fibrosum *(shí gāo)*	15g
Scutellariae Radix *(huáng qín)*	15g
Platycodi Radix *(jié gěng)*	15g
Rehmanniae Radix praeparata *(shú dì huáng)*	15g
Gastrodiae Rhizoma *(tiān má)*	15g
Ginseng Radix *(rén shēn)*	15g

Notopterygii Rhizoma seu Radix (qiāng huó) 15g
Angelicae pubescentis Radix (dú huó) 15g
Gardeniae Fructus (zhī zǐ) 9g
Forsythiae Fructus (lián qiáo) 7.5g
Schizonepetae Herba (jīng jiè) 15g
Menthae haplocalycis Herba (bò hé) 15g
Ephedrae Herba (má huáng) 15g
Rhei Radix et Rhizoma (dà huáng) 15g
Natrii Sulfas (máng xiāo) 15g
Coptidis Rhizoma (huáng lián) 15g
Phellodendri Cortex (huáng bǎi) 15g
Asari Radix et Rhizoma (xì xīn) 15g
Scorpio (quán xiē) 15g

Grind the ingredients into powder and form into pills with honey. Take 1-2 pills (approximately 6g each) once a day with tea or warm wine. Dispels wind, clears heat, and unblocks the bowels. Treats organ-type wind-stroke characterized by facial asymmetry, paraplegia or hemiplegia, impaired consciousness, or sudden loss of consciousness with strong heat symptoms. While the principal formula is indicated for invasion of wind-heat with accumulation of heat in the interior, this formula is prescribed for wind-stroke with internally-generated wind and heat.

Section 2

FORMULAS THAT RELEASE THE EXTERIOR AND CLEAR THE INTERIOR

The formulas in this section are indicated for patterns characterized by pathogens in the exterior with simultaneous blazing heat in the interior. Such patterns are characterized by chills and fever occurring together with irritability and restlessness, thirst, dysenteric disorders due to heat, wheezing, and a rapid pulse. Because heat in the interior has not yet clumped, it is treated by clearing and draining rather than by purging. The formulas in this group thus combine herbs like Ephedrae Herba (má huáng), Sojae Semen praeparatum (dàn dòu chǐ), and Puerariae Radix (gé gēn) with Gypsum fibrosum (shí gāo), Coptidis Rhizoma (huáng lián), or Scutellariae Radix (huáng qín).

葛根黃芩黃連湯（葛根黄芩黄连汤）
Kudzu, Scutellaria, and Coptis Decoction
gé gēn huáng qín huáng lián tāng

Source   *Discussion of Cold Damage* (c. 220)

Puerariae Radix (gé gēn) 15-24g
Scutellariae Radix (huáng qín) 9g
Coptidis Rhizoma (huáng lián) 6g
Glycyrrhizae Radix praeparata (zhì gān cǎo) 6g

Method of Preparation   Decoction. The source text advises to cook Puerariae Radix (gé gēn) first, a practice which is not commonly followed at present. According to the Qing-dynasty author Ke Qin, the intention of this mode of preparation is to emphasize the formula's focus on the exterior rather than the interior.

Actions   Releases the exterior and drains heat

Indications

Fever, sweating, thirst, dysenteric diarrhea characterized by especially foul-smelling stools and a burning sensation around the anus, a sensation of irritability and heat in the chest and epigastrium, possible wheezing, a red tongue with yellow coating, and a rapid pulse.

In this pattern, the exterior has not been completely released, but the interior is already ablaze with heat. As noted in the source text, this can be caused by improper treatment of an exterior disorder with purgatives. Purging drives the pathogenic influence into the yang brightness warp where it gives rise to dysenteric diarrhea with heat, characterized by especially foul-smelling stools and a burning sensation around the anus. There is also a sensation of irritability and heat in the chest. The presence of interior heat is reflected in the fever, thirst, the red tongue with a yellow coating, and the rapid pulse. As the condition progresses inward from the exterior, it causes 'steaming' of the muscle layer that manifests as sweat. When fire in the interior attacks the Lungs, wheezing results.

Analysis of Formula

To address the pathodynamic at the root of this pattern, one must resolve the exterior by dispersing constraint from the muscle layer, while also draining heat from the Stomach and Intestines. Puerariae Radix (gé gēn), used in a relatively large dosage, acts as the chief herb. It releases the exterior, clears heat, and treats dysenteric diarrhea by raising the clear yang of the Spleen and Stomach. It is a specific herb for patterns where a cold pathogen in the exterior is transforming into heat, as explained in Zhou Yan's *Records of Thoughtful Differentiation of Materia Medica*: "When the greater yang stage is about to become the yang brightness stage of an exterior disease, Puerariae Radix (gé gēn) is essential." Yet the text goes on to say that "If the Stomach yin is pouring downward, Puerariae Radix (gé gēn) can also lift the yin qi in order to alleviate diarrhea." This makes it ideally suited for the present condition.

The deputy, Coptidis Rhizoma (huáng lián), drains heat (especially yang brightness-warp heat) while its bitterness dries dampness in the Stomach and Intestines, thereby stopping the diarrhea. The assistant, Scutellariae Radix (huáng qín), is also bitter and cold. It is helpful for treating problems in the relatively superficial levels of the body where it is used to drain heat from the Lungs and to stop wheezing (if present). It also enters into the Intestines and is frequently prescribed in the treatment of dysenteric disorders due to damp-heat. Glycyrrhizae Radix praeparata *(zhì gān cǎo)* harmonizes the actions of the other herbs and protects the middle burner from further injury.

Cautions and Contraindications

Contraindicated for dysenteric disorders without fever and a submerged, slow pulse.

Commentary

Although this formula treats both the interior and exterior, its primary focus is on draining interior heat. Referring to this condition, *Medical Formulas Collected and Analyzed* notes that "The pathogenic influence being driven into the interior is seven-tenths [of the condition]; its lingering in the exterior is three-tenths." *Discussion of Cold Damage* (paragraph 34) observes that this condition is due to improperly treating a greater yang disorder by purging when it should have been treated with the exterior-releasing Cinnamon Twig Decoction *(guì zhī tāng)*. For this reason, the ensuing pattern can be regarded as a simultaneous greater yang and yang brightness disorder.

The early modern scholar-physician Yun Tie-Qiao went even further and argued that the formula only drains interior heat. His view was that if a pathogen was still left in the exterior, one should only use Cinnamon Twig Decoction *(guì zhī tāng)* or Kudzu Decoction *(gé gēn tāng)*. Contemporary teaching manuals like *Explicating the Discussion of Cold Damage* have followed Yun's lead. They hold that the function of the herb Puerariae Radix *(gé gēn)* is to clear heat and raise the yang and that once the heat has been drained from the interior, the sweating and wheezing will stop, too.

Cheng Men-Xue, a famous modern physician and former head of the Shanghai College of Chinese Medicine, offered yet another innovative interpretation. He argued that the formula treats dysentery caused by a lurking pathogen, which, according to Chinese medical doctrine, collects and develops most often in the yang brightness warp. The bitter, cold herbs in the formula drain this lurking heat toxin. Chinese medical doctrine also holds that lurking pathogens trigger a disorder only when the invasion of a new pathogen arouses the body's antipathogenic qi into action. In Cheng Men-Xue's opinion, Puerariae Radix *(gé gēn)* is included in the formula to release this new pathogen from the muscle layer and discharge heat constraint.

Usage

Irrespective of the prior treatment history, the use of this formula has been expanded to include any early-stage dy-

senteric disorder characterized by fever, foul-smelling stools, a burning sensation in the anus, a red tongue with a yellow coating, and a rapid pulse. This condition is identified as lower burner damp-heat with lingering exterior symptoms. A variation of the formula Patchouli/Agastache Powder to Rectify the Qi *(huò xiāng zhèng qì sǎn)* can be used if the heat is not severe.

The use of Kudzu, Scutellaria, and Coptis Decoction *(gé gēn huáng qín huáng lián tāng)* was further expanded during the late Qing dynasty by Lu Mao-Xiu to cover yang brightness warm pathogen disorders and, in particular, the occurrence of sand papules (痧疹 *shā zhěn*). In *Medical Texts from Bettering the World Studio,* Lu argued that this formula was "the essential method for treating sand papules" because of its ability to simultaneously resolve the exterior and drain heat from the interior without overemphasizing either aspect.

In contemporary clinical practice, the formula is also used for conditions characterized by subjective sensations of heat such as periomenopausal hot flushes or hypertension. Another usage is prolapse of the anus where the uplifting properties of Puerariae Radix *(gé gēn)* are exploited to help the qi in the greater yin to ascend. In contrast to Tonify the Middle to Augment the Qi Decoction *(bǔ zhōng yì qì tāng)*, which is used for deficiency conditions, Kudzu, Scutellaria, and Coptis Decoction *(gé gēn huáng qín huáng lián tāng)* is appropriate where prolapse occurs as a result of heat excess diarrhea.

Comparision

➤ Vs. Other Commonly-Used Formulas for Acute Dysenteric Disorders

Kudzu, Scutellaria, and Coptis Decoction *(gé gēn huáng qín huáng lián tāng)* treats dysenteric disorders due to damp-heat in the yang brightness qi aspect. A pathogen in the exterior may or may not be present. Heat is more severe than dampness, hence there must be thirst, anal burning, fever, a rapid pulse or other pronounced heat signs. Another commonly-used formula for dysenteric disorders is Pulsatilla Decoction *(bái tóu wēng tāng)*, which is used for interior patterns with blood and pus in the stool and no chest or abdominal symptoms. Here the heat is located in the terminal yin blood aspect, complicated by damp-heat in the Large Intestine. Under the proper circumstances, that formula can be combined with the principal formula.

The application of these formulas should be differentiated from that of Scutellaria Decoction *(huáng qín tāng)*, which treats dysentery that occurs in the course of a simultaneous greater yang and lesser yang disorder. This is characterized by more severe abdominal pain. Peony Decoction *(sháo yào tāng)* also treats dysentery with abdominal pain and stools that contain both blood and a white discharge of pus or phlegm. Its distinguishing feature is that it drains damp-heat while simultaneously regulating qi and blood, that is, there will already be signs of blood deficiency.

➤ Vs. Cinnamon Twig and Ginseng Decoction
(guì zhī rén shēn tāng); see PAGE 300

➤ Vs. Kudzu Decoction (gé gēn tāng); see PAGE 20

➤ Vs. Pulsatilla Decoction (bái tóu wēng tāng);
see PAGE 211

Biomedical Indications

With the appropriate presentation, this formula may be used to treat a variety of biomedically-defined disorders. One group is comprised of diseases that affect the digestive tract including stomach flu, acute enteritis, bacillary dysentery, enteric fever, and toxic gastroenteritis. Another group is comprised of other types of acute infections such as pneumonia, encephalitis B, and measles. A third involves vascular disorders such as coronary artery disease, hypertension, and cerebrovascular disease. There are also miscellaneous disorders that are treated by this formula including cervical spine disease, perimenopausal syndrome, rectal prolapse, stroke, eczema, and diabetes.

Alternate names

Kudzu Decoction (gé gēn tāng) in Divinely Ingenious Surefire Formulas; Coptis and Kudzu Decoction (huáng lián gé gēn tāng) in Formulas of Universal Benefit; Kudzu, Coptis, and Scutellaria Decoction (gé gēn huáng lián huáng qín tāng) in Formula Appearances from the Inner Platform of the Golden Mirror; Kudzu and Scutellaria Decoction (gé gēn huáng qín tāng) in Complete Compendium of Cold Damage.

Modifications

• For abdominal pain, add Aucklandiae Radix (mù xiāng) and Paeoniae Radix alba (bái sháo).

• For tenesmus, add Aucklandiae Radix (mù xiāng) and Arecae Semen (bīng láng).

• For high fever and stools containing blood or pus, add Pulsatillae Radix (bái tóu wēng) and Fraxini Cortex (qín pí).

• For more prominent exterior signs and symptoms, add Chrysanthemi Flos (jú huā).

• For pronounced wheezing, add Mori Cortex (sāng bái pí).

• For pronounced dampness indicated by a greasy tongue coating and a slippery pulse, add Lonicerae Flos (jīn yín huā) and Plantaginis Semen (chē qián zǐ).

• For nausea and vomiting, add Pinelliae Rhizoma (bàn xià) and Bambusae Caulis in taeniam (zhú rú).

• For concurrent food stagnation, add Crataegi Fructus (shān zhā) and Massa medicata fermentata (shén qū).

石膏湯 (石膏汤)
Gypsum Decoction
shí gāo tāng

Source   *Arcane Essentials from the Imperial Library (752)*

Gypsum fibrosum (shí gāo) 6g
Ephedrae Herba (má huáng) .9g
Sojae Semen praeparatum (dàn dòu chǐ) 9g
Coptidis Rhizoma (huáng lián) 6g
Scutellariae Radix (huáng qín) 6g
Phellodendri Cortex (huáng bǎi) 6g
Gardeniae Fructus (zhī zǐ) .6-9g

Method of Preparation   Decoction. The aim of the formula is to induce mild sweating. At present, the usual dosage of Gypsum fibrosum (shí gāo) is 15-30g.

Actions   Clears heat, resolves toxicity, and releases the exterior

Indications

Strong fever and chills without sweating, headache, a generalized sensation of heaviness and tightness, red face and eyes, dry nasal passages, thirst, irritability and insomnia (leading in severe cases to delirium), possible nosebleeds, coughing up blood or skin blotches, and a rapid, slippery or rapid, flooding pulse.

This is cold damage in which heat blazes in the interior while the exterior condition still lingers. The fever and chills, absence of sweating, headache, and sensation of heaviness and tightness reflect severe greater yang-warp cold damage. The strength of the fever, red face and eyes, dry nasal passages, thirst, irritability, insomnia, delirious speech, and rapid pulse reflect blazing heat in the interior. The presence of bleeding or skin blotches indicates that the heat has caused reckless movement of hot blood.

Analysis of Formula

Although this formula is designed for conditions of excess in both the exterior and interior, its focus is on clearing the particularly severe interior heat. The chief ingredient, cold-natured Gypsum fibrosum (shí gāo), clears heat and eliminates irritability. One of the deputies, strong and warm Ephedrae Herba (má huáng), releases the exterior by inducing sweating. Another deputy, Sojae Semen praeparatum (dàn dòu chǐ), also releases the exterior and relieves irritability. The four assistants, Coptidis Rhizoma (huáng lián), Scutellariae Radix (huáng qín), Phellodendri Cortex (huáng bǎi), and Gardeniae Fructus (zhī zǐ), are all very bitter and very cold herbs that excel at draining heat and resolving toxicity in the interior. Together with Gypsum fibrosum (shí gāo), these five herbs clear and drain interior heat from all three burners.

Cautions and Contraindications

The effect of this formula is very drying. It must not be used where the absence of sweating is due to deficiency of yin fluids in patients with significant deficiency.

Commentary

According to *Golden Mirror of the Medical Tradition*, this formula combines the treatment strategies of Major Bluegreen Dragon Decoction *(dà qīng lóng tāng)*, discussed in Chapter 1, and Coptis Decoction to Resolve Toxicity *(huáng lián jiě dú tāng)*, discussed in Chapter 4. This suggests that the condition it treats often arises in the course of an unresolved greater yang pattern causing severe internal heat to accumulate and transform into toxin that spreads throughout the Triple Burner and thus the entire body. The ensuing pathodynamic is reflected in a very specific constellation of signs and symptoms: strong internal heat, a rapid, flooding pulse at all six positions, but the absence of sweating. This implies that heat constraint in the exterior is still very severe, justifying the use of Ephedrae Herba *(má huáng)*.

Comparison

➤ Vs. Major Bluegreen Dragon Decoction *(dà qīng lóng tāng)*

The presentations for both of these formulas include similar symptoms due to heat in the interior and yang constraint in the exterior. However, the heat treated by the principal formula is not only more severe, but has spread throughout all three burners. By contrast, Major Bluegreen Dragon Decoction *(dà qīng lóng tāng)* focuses on patterns with stronger yang qi constraint in the exterior but less blazing heat in the interior, or heat that has not yet transformed into toxin. Later generations of physicians developed a number of new formulas based on Gypsum Decoction *(shí gāo tāng)*, some of which are listed below.

Biomedical Indications

With the appropriate presentation, this formula may be used to treat a variety of biomedically-defined disorders, primarily infectious, including tonsillitis, pertussis, measles, and pneumonia.

Alternate name

Three-Yellow and Gypsum Decoction *(sān huáng shí gāo tāng)* in *General Discussion of the Disease of Cold Damage*

Variation

石膏湯 (石膏汤)

Gypsum Decoction from *Six Texts*

shí gāo tāng

SOURCE *Six Texts on Cold Damage* (1445)

Add Zingiberis Rhizoma recens *(shēng jiāng)*, Jujubae Fructus *(dà zǎo)*, and green tea for heat in all three burners with generalized pain.

Associated Formulas

雙解加蔥豉湯 (双解加葱豉汤)

Double Releasing Decoction with Spring Onions and Prepared Soybeans

shuāng jiě jiā cōng chǐ tāng

SOURCE *Comprehensive Medicine According to Master Zhang* (1695)

Schizonepetae Herba *(jīng jiè)*	3g
Menthae haplocalycis Herba *(bò hé)*	8g
Allii fistulosi Bulbus *(cōng bái)*	2 stalks
Sojae Semen praeparatum *(dàn dòu chǐ)*	4.5g
dry-fried Gardeniae Fructus *(jiāo zhī zǐ)*	4.5g
Forsythiae Fructus *(lián qiáo)*	4.5g
Platycodi Radix *(jié gěng)*	2.4g
Glycyrrhizae Radix *(gān cǎo)*	1.5g
Gypsum fibrosum *(shí gāo)*	6g
Talcum *(huá shí)*	9g
Chuanxiong Rhizoma *(chuān xiōng)*	1.5g
Angelicae sinensis Radix *(dāng guī)*	2.4g
Paeoniae Radix rubra *(chì sháo)*	3g
Scutellariae Radix *(huáng qín)*	3g

Decoction. Unblocks the Triple Burner, releases the exterior, and clears heat from the interior. For warm pathogen heat disorders characterized by aversion to wind and heat, high fever, and a superficial and tight pulse. This is a modification of the principal formula and is intended for clearing heat that has spread throughout the Triple Burner but has not yet produced clumping. Hence, it can be vented outward through the exterior via sweating and discharged downward via the urine. The early modern physician He Lian-Chen notes: "The meaning of 'double releasing' (雙解 *shuāng jiě*) really is to promote sweating and facilitate urination. Liu He-Jian [i.e., Liu Wan-Su] excelled in treating fire. This formula [which is based on his ideas] truly advanced the strategies for obtaining results in treating warm pathogen heat disorders." (*Collected Select Formulas for Warm Heat Pathogen Disease*)

The contemporary physician Ding Xue-Ping argues that the efficacy of this formula is due to its understanding of warm pathogen disorders:

Our ancestors said, 'The yang brightness is the source for the formation of warm [pathogen disorders]. The Liver and Gallbladder are the marshes where warm [pathogen disorders] form.' For warm pathogen heat [disorders] or summerheat dampness [disorders] to develop, lurking pathogens collected but hidden away must be present. Because [it stirs up such lurking heat] the transmission and development of warm pathogen [disorders] is most rapid. Often, even though the pathogen at the protective level has not yet been released, qi level interior heat is already blazing. This is a so-called combined protective and qi [level disorder]. When Master Zhang [composed] this formula, he genuinely delivered the most subtle understanding of this disease dynamic. Allii fistulosi Bulbus *(cōng bái)* and Sojae Semen praeparatum *(dàn dòu chǐ)* are light and clearing to dissipate and vent. Schizonepetae Herba *(jīng jiè)* and Menthae haplocalycis Herba (bò hé) disperse wind-heat from the upper burner. Acrid and cooling, [these herbs] are used to discharge the pathogen from the protective level. Gypsum fibrosum (shí gāo), Platycodi Radix (jié gěng), and Astragali Radix (huáng qí) clear qi-level heat from the Stomach and Lungs. Gardeniae Fructus (zhī zǐ), Scutellariae Radix (huáng qín), Angelicae sinensis Radix (dāng guī), Paeoniae Radix rubra (chì sháo), and Chuanxiong Rhizoma (chuān xiōng) discharge constraint and lurking fire from the Liver and Gallbladder. Talcum (huá shí) and Glycyrrhizae Radix (gān cǎo) guide the heat to move downward.

六神通解散

Six-Miracle Powder to Unblock and Release

liù shén tōng jiě sǎn

SOURCE *Comprehensive Medicine According to Master Zhang* (1695)

Ephedrae Herba (má huáng)	15g
Gypsum fibrosum (shí gāo)	15g
Atractylodis Rhizoma (cāng zhú)	2.4g
Scutellariae Radix (huáng qín)	4.5g
Talcum (huá shí)	9g
Glycyrrhizae Radix (gān cǎo)	1.5g
Sojae Semen praeparatum (dàn dòu chǐ)	9g
Allii fistulosi Bulbus (cōng bái)	3 stalks

Clears heat and transforms dampness. This is damp-heat accumulating in the Triple Burner with wind-cold binding the exterior. Such a condition can easily occur during the summer months due to sudden exposure to cold, a situation that is becoming more prevalent due to the widespread use of air conditioning. The condition presents with headache, fever and chills without sweating, a bitter taste in the mouth, reduced urination or blood in the urine, a stifling sensation in the chest, fatigue, aching of the limbs, nausea, and a yellow, greasy tongue coating. The formula simultaneously disperses cold in the exterior, clears heat from the yang brightness channel and the upper burner, and drains dampness. Some physicians recommend replacing Ephedrae Herba (má huáng) with Moslae Herba (xiāng rú).

Section 3

....

FORMULAS THAT RELEASE THE EXTERIOR AND WARM THE INTERIOR

The formulas in this group are indicated for patterns characterized by the presence of a pathogen in the exterior with simultaneous excess cold in the interior. Such patterns are characterized by chills and fever, which are accompanied by cold and pain in the epigastrium or abdomen, diarrhea or dystenteric disorders, a white tongue coating, and a slow pulse. To treat these patterns, the formulas in this group combine exterior-releasing herbs like Cinnamomi Ramulus (guì zhī) and Ephedrae Herba (má huáng) with interior-warming herbs like Cinnamomi Cortex (ròu guì) and Zingiberis Rhizoma (gān jiāng).

五積散 (五积散)

Five-Accumulation Powder

wǔ jī sǎn

This formula treats disorders associated with the five types of accumulation: cold, dampness, qi, blood, and phlegm.

SOURCE *Secret Formulas to Manage Trauma and Reconnect Fractures Received from an Immortal* (c. 846)

Ephedrae Herba (má huáng)	180g (1.5-4.5g)
Angelicae dahuricae Radix (bái zhǐ)	90g (1.5-4.5g)
Zingiberis Rhizoma (gān jiāng)	120g (1.5-4.5g)
Cinnamomi Cortex (ròu guì)	90g (1.5-4.5g)
Atractylodis Rhizoma (cāng zhú)	600g (3-9g)
Magnoliae officinalis Cortex (hòu pò)	120g (1.5-4.5g)
Citri reticulatae Pericarpium (chén pí)	180g (3-9g)
Pinelliae Rhizoma praeparatum (zhì bàn xià)	90g (3-9g)
Poria (fú líng)	90g (3-9g)
Platycodi Radix (jié gěng)	600g (3-9g)
Aurantii Fructus (zhǐ ké)	180g (1.5-4.5g)
Angelicae sinensis Radix (dāng guī)	90g (1.5-4.5g)
Paeoniae Radix alba (bái sháo)	90g (1.5-4.5g)
Chuanxiong Rhizoma (chuān xiōng)	90g (1.5-4.5g)
Glycyrrhizae Radix (gān cǎo)	90g (1.5-4.5g)

Method of Preparation   Grind the ingredients into a coarse powder and set Cinnamomi Cortex (ròu guì) and Aurantii Fructus (zhǐ ké) aside. Fry the remaining ingredients over low heat until the powder changes color, and then allow it to cool. Add the powder made from the other two ingredients and take 9g as a draft with 3 pieces of Zingiberis Rhizoma recens (shēng jiāng). May also be prepared as a decoction with the dosages indicated in parentheses.

Actions   Releases the exterior, warms the interior, smoothes the flow of qi, transforms phlegm, invigorates the blood, and reduces accumulation

Indications

Fever and chills without sweating, headache, body aches, stiff neck and back, a sensation of fullness in the chest and abdomen, nausea and aversion to food, vomiting, abdominal pain and cold, diarrhea with borborygmus, a white and greasy tongue coating, and a pulse that can be submerged and wiry or floating and slow. In women, the disharmony between qi and blood may also manifest as cold-type epigastric and abdominal pain, or menstrual irregularity.

This is externally-contracted wind-cold with internal injury due to cold (usually caused by improper diet). Such a pattern is usually found in patients with interior cold who also contract wind-cold. The fever and chills without sweating, headache, body aches, and stiff neck and back reflect the presence of exterior wind-cold. Internal damage by cold, or harbored cold accumulation, impairs the Spleen's functions of moving and transformation, leading to phlegm obstruction, qi stagnation, and disharmony between qi and blood. When cold (which is contractile in nature) invades the exterior, it accelerates this process and leads to the five accumulations of cold, dampness, qi, blood, and phlegm. This is reflected in the sensation of fullness in the chest and abdomen, nausea and aversion to food, vomiting, abdominal pain, and diarrhea with borborygmus. The tongue will typically have a white, greasy coating. The pulse may be submerged and wiry, or floating and slow, depending on which aspect of the disease dynamic predominates. In women, interior cold with stagnation of qi or accumulation of phlegm and dampness can lead to menstrual irregularities and painful menstruation.

Analysis of Formula

This formula treats five types of accumulation (五積 *wǔ jī*)—cold, dampness, phlegm, qi, and blood—caused by a combination of wind-cold in the exterior and cold damaging the interior. Because cold is the primary pathogen, the formula focuses on promoting sweating to resolve the exterior and on warming the interior to dispel internal cold. These main strategies are supported by drying of dampness, transformation of phlegm, strengthening of the Spleen's transportive function, regulation of qi, and moving of blood.

Two of the chief herbs, Ephedrae Herba (*má huáng*) and Angelicae dahuricae Radix (*bái zhǐ*), release cold from the exterior; the other chief herbs, Zingiberis Rhizoma (*gān jiāng*) and Cinnamomi Cortex (*ròu guì*), warm the interior and expel cold. The synergistic action of these four herbs addresses cold in both the exterior and interior. The other herbs focus on the other four accumulations: Atractylodis Rhizoma (*cāng zhú*) and Magnoliae officinalis Cortex (*hòu pò*) dry dampness and eliminate its stagnation; Citri reticulatae Pericarpium (*chén pí*), Pinelliae Rhizoma praeparatum (*zhì bàn xià*), and Poria (*fú líng*) strengthen the Spleen and transform phlegm; Platycodi Radix (*jié gěng*), which causes the qi to ascend, and Aurantii Fructus (*zhǐ ké*), which causes it to descend, resolve qi stagnation and assist in the transformation of phlegm; and Angelicae sinensis Radix (*dāng guī*), Paeoniae Radix alba (*bái sháo*), and Chuanxiong Rhizoma (*chuān xiōng*) nourish and invigorate the blood. Glycyrrhizae Radix (*gān cǎo*) harmonizes the actions of the other herbs and strengthens the middle burner.

Cautions and Contraindications

This formula is contraindicated in cases with damp-heat or yin deficiency.

Commentary

The main strategies incorporated in this formula—releasing the exterior, warming the interior, smoothing the flow of qi,

and reducing accumulation—are of a dispersing nature and focus on the qi. The supporting strategies address dampness, phlegm, and blood. The ingredients for the supporting strategies are basically those that comprise Calm the Stomach Powder (*píng wèi sǎn*) (Chapter 16), Two-Aged [Herb] Decoction (*èr chén tāng*) (Chapter 17), and Four-Substance Decoction (*sì wù tāng*) (Chapter 8).

The complexity of this formula was not welcomed by all commentators. As the Ming-dynasty physician Yu Chang noted in *Precepts for Physicians*:

> Because this formula can treat many disorders, the unrefined practitioners are happy to use it. … Although with its separate [herbs for] the interior and exterior, it was composed for internal cold [compounded by an] externally-contracted [pathogen], it is not really [like one of Zhang] Zhong-Jing's formulas [which treat both] the interior and exterior [by combining] Ephedrae Herba (*má huáng*), Cinnamomi Ramulus (*guì zhī*), Zingiberis Rhizoma (*gān jiāng*), and Aconiti Radix lateralis praeparata (*zhì fù zǐ*).

Scholar-physicians like the Qing-dynasty writer Zhang Lu, writing in *Continuing Discussing Cold Damage*, therefore advised to use the formula only if it was adjusted to the precise disease dynamic:

> Such a complex compound formula should not simply be used inflexibly in its entirety. If there is no blood disorder, one does not need to use Chuanxiong Rhizoma (*chuān xiōng*) and Angelicae sinensis Radix (*dāng guī*). If [the patient] has no cough, why trouble with Aurantii Fructus (*zhǐ ké*) and Platycodi Radix (*jié gěng*)? If there are no headaches, why take Angelicae dahuricae Radix (*bái zhǐ*)? Or if [the patient] sweats, should Ephedrae Herba (*má huáng*) be given? One must add or subtract [herbs] according to a careful assessment of the foundation of the disorder. Doing so is what is known as the ingenious use of compound formulas.

According to *Formulary of the Pharmacy Service for Benefiting the People in the Taiping Era*, damp-cold is the primary pathological mechanism of this condition and Atractylodis Rhizoma (*cāng zhú*) is the chief herb, which is reflected in the size of its dosage. The different interpretation provided in the analysis section above is the modern view. Clinically, the difference between externally-contracted wind-cold with internal injury due to cold, and externally-contracted damp-cold, is usually insignificant. For example, the use of this formula has been expanded in recent times to include treatment of the acute exacerbations of bronchial asthma, which can be due to either of the above mechanisms.

Usage

At the present time, this formula is used primarily for treating the accumulation of food in the interior with externally-contracted wind-cold. It is also employed in gynecological practice to treat menstrual irregularity and painful menstruation due to cold congealing the vessels and collaterals. Another possible indication is cold in the lower body with heat in the upper body. In this case, obstruction of the qi dynamic by the five accumulations prevents yang qi from the exterior from returning into the interior. In clinical practice, one may see symptoms such as hot flushes or unusual warmth in the upper body that is not accompanied by sweating, even though the lower body is cold and the person prefers heat and warm food.

Herb Preparation

Besides the method of preparation outlined above, the literature provides several other methods that emphasize either the exterior-releasing or interior-warming properties of this formula. *Medical Formulas Collected and Analyzed* contains a formula known as Prepared Five Accumulation Powder (*shú liào wǔ jī sǎn*), which is prepared by frying all the ingredients except Aurantii Fructus (*zhǐ ké*), Cinnamomi Cortex (*ròu guì*), Angelicae dahuricae Radix (*bái zhǐ*), and Citri reticulatae Pericarpium (*chén pí*) before decocting. This increases the capacity of the formula for warming cold and dispersing pathogenic accumulations. *Simple Book of Formulas* contains a formula known as Unprepared Five Accumulation Powder (*shēng liào wǔ jī sǎn*), which is prepared by decocting all the ingredients without frying them. This increases the capacity of the formula for discharging wind and dispersing cold.

Comparison

> ➤ Vs. Bupleurum, Cinnamon Twig, and Ginger Decoction (*chái hú guì zhī gān jiāng tāng*)

Both this formula and Bupleurum, Cinnamon Twig, and Ginger Decoction (*chái hú guì zhī gān jiāng tāng*) treat interior cold complicated by wind-cold in the exterior. Five Accumulation Powder (*wǔ jī sǎn*) treats patterns where the newly-contracted wind-cold remains in the yang brightness warp, while the symptoms of internal cold-dampness are centered on the middle burner. Cold is more pronounced than dampness, with phlegm and blood stasis a secondary complication. Although there may be heat at the top, this is weak and will not be accompanied by sweating. By contrast, Bupleurum, Cinnamon Twig, and Ginger Decoction (*chái hú guì zhī gān jiāng tāng*) treats patterns where the pathogen has penetrated to the lesser yang warp, while internal cold-dampness is centered on the Triple Burner. This leads to thin mucus gathering in the interior with some signs of interior heat from constraint, such as sweating from the head.

Biomedical Indications

With the appropriate presentation, this formula may be used to treat a variety of biomedically-defined disorders including recurrent upper respiratory tract infections, bronchitis, gastritis, and sciatica.

Alternate names

Expedite Life Decoction (*cuī shēng tāng*) in *Easy and Simple Formulas*; Extraordinary Merit Five-Accumulation Powder (*yì gōng wǔ jī sǎn*) in *My Humble Complete Collection of Fine Formulas*; Cooked Grain Five-Accumulation Powder (*shú liào wǔ jī sǎn*) in *Medical Formulas Collected and Analyzed*; Hundred-Disease Worry-Free Powder (*bǎi bìng wú yōu sǎn*) and Regulate the Middle and Construct the Stomach Decoction (*tiáo zhōng jiàn wèi tāng*) in *Zheng Family Secret Formulas for Women's Diseases*

Modifications

- For more acute exterior cold, substitute Cinnamomi Ramulus (*guì zhī*) for Cinnamomi Cortex (*ròu guì*).
- For deficient exterior disorders with sweating, remove Ephedrae Herba (*má huáng*) and Atractylodis Rhizoma (*cāng zhú*).
- For qi deficiency with weakness, remove Aurantii Fructus (*zhǐ ké*) and Citri reticulatae Pericarpium (*chén pí*) and add Ginseng Radix (*rén shēn*) and Atractylodis macrocephalae Rhizoma (*bái zhú*).
- For severe cold with intense abdominal pain, add Evodiae Fructus (*wú zhū yú*).
- For irregular menstruation with epigastric and abdominal pain due to cold, remove Ephedrae Herba (*má huáng*) and Angelicae dahuricae Radix (*bái zhǐ*) and add Cyperi Rhizoma (*xiāng fù*), Corydalis Rhizoma (*yán hú suǒ*), and Artemisiae argyi Folium (*ài yè*).

桂枝人参湯（桂枝人参汤）

Cinnamon Twig and Ginseng Decoction

guì zhī rén shēn tāng

Source   *Discussion of Cold Damage* (c. 220)

Cinnamomi Ramulus (*guì zhī*) 12g
Glycyrrhizae Radix praeparata (*zhì gān cǎo*) 12g
Atractylodis macrocephalae Rhizoma (*bái zhú*) 9g
Ginseng Radix (*rén shēn*) 9g
Zingiberis Rhizoma (*gān jiāng*) 9g

Method of Preparation   Decoction. The source text advises to boil all of the herbs with the exception of Cinnamomi Ramulus (*guì zhī*) in 9 cups of water until 4 cups have evaporated. Cinnamomi Ramulus (*guì zhī*) is added and the herbs are then decocted until an additional 2 cups have evaporated. The dregs are removed and the decoction is divided into three doses. Two doses are taken warm during the day and the third at night

Actions   Releases the exterior, warms the interior, augments the qi, and eliminates focal distention

Indications

Mild exterior symptoms (fever, chills, headache, joint pains, etc.) accompanied by severe diarrhea and hard focal distention in the epigastrium.

This is a greater yang disorder that has not been released accompanied by cold obstructing the greater yin. In the source text, the etiology of this pattern is attributed to repeated inappropriate purging. This has damaged the Spleen and Stomach yang and caused the pathogen to fall inward where it blocks the qi dynamic of the middle burner. The result is a complex exterior-interior disorder. The mild greater yang-warp symptoms indicate that the pathogen still remains in the exterior. Cold obstructing the downward directing of the Stomach causes hard (i.e., palpable) focal distention in the epigastrium. The severe diarrhea reflects damage to the Spleen yang.

Analysis of Formula

The formula treats a pattern where cold is present in both the exterior and interior. This requires a combined strategy of resolving the exterior with acrid, warming herbs while simultaneously warming the interior and augmenting the qi. These strategies are reflected in the qualities of the two chief herbs. Acrid, warming Cinnamomi Ramulus (*guì zhī*) releases the exterior through its warming action on the greater yang warp, but also helps to direct turbid qi downward by means of its acrid fragrance. It is added to the formula after the other ingredients have been decocted to keep its actions separate from those of the other herbs and allow it to focus entirely on the exterior. Ginseng Radix (*rén shēn*) strongly tonifies the primal qi, assisting movement and transformation, and ascending and downward directing.

Acrid and heating Zingiberis Rhizoma (*gān jiāng*) serves as the deputy. It warms the middle burner, dispelling interior cold and boosting the Spleen and Stomach yang qi. If the Spleen's transportive and transformative functions fail, dampness will readily form. To address this problem, Atractylodis macrocephalae Rhizoma (*bái zhú*) is added as an assistant, strengthening the Spleen, drying dampness, and stopping diarrhea. Glycyrrhizae Radix praeparata (*zhì gān cǎo*) is sweet and balanced, entering the Spleen to harmonize the entire formula and assist Ginseng Radix (*rén shēn*) and Atractylodis macrocephalae Rhizoma (*bái zhú*) in strengthening the Spleen.

Cautions and Contraindications

This formula is strongly warming and drying. It is contraindicated for patterns with interior heat or yin deficiency.

Commentary

This formula can be regarded as a variation of Regulate the Middle Pill (*lǐ zhōng wán*), discussed in Chapter 6, with the dosage of Glycyrrhizae Radix praeparata (*zhì gān cǎo*) increased and Cinnamomi Ramulus (*guì zhī*) added to release the exterior. It is one of several formulas listed in *Discussion of Cold Damage* for treating 'commingled heat with diarrhea'

(協熱利下 *xié rè lì xià*). In these patterns, diarrhea is accompanied by heat. The term 'heat' in this context may denote fever, that is, an objective rise in body temperature accessible to the physician by means of palpation, as well as mere subjective sensations experienced by the patient but not accessible to the physician. Because neither the pulse nor tongue indicate the presence of heat, these types of diarrhea are not due to heat excess. In this particular pattern, the diarrhea is described as unstoppable. This is because the constraint of protective yang in the greater yang warp, which manifests as heat, disables diffusion of yang qi to the middle burner. Vice versa, interior cold blocks the protective yang from diffusing outward in order to dislodge wind-cold from the exterior.

Usage

Commentators have debated whether this formula might be used to treat interior cold patterns without wind-cold in the exterior. A narrow interpretation, focusing on the role of Cinnamomi Ramulus (*guì zhī*) in resolving exterior wind-cold, might suggest not. A more profound interpretation, however, is offered by the Qing-dynasty writer Chen Nian-Zu in *Summary Songs for Formulas from Changsha*. Chen's view deepens our understanding of the disease dynamic and opens new modes of application:

> The qi of the greater yang enters and exits the Heart and chest. In the present case, the yang qi governed by the greater yang has been mistakenly purged and has fallen downward. As a consequence, the turbid yin qi of cold water reversely occupies the position of yang, causing hard focal distention in the epigastrium. [This disease dynamic] can be referenced to the [discussion of] Licorice Decoction to Drain the Epigastrium (*gān cǎo xiè xīn tāng*) in section [158 of *Discussion of Cold Damage*], where it says: '[In this case] there is no clumping of heat, only Stomach deficiency. Guest qi rebels upward, causing hardness.'

Based on interpretations such as this, contemporary physicians in China and Japan use the formula to treat internal medicine disorders characterized by obstruction of the qi dynamic due to cold in the middle burner. Typically, these will present with symptoms of deficiency (e.g., diarrhea, fatigue after eating, cold extremities, increased urination) accompanied by symptoms of excess indicating clumping of cold and fluids (e.g., hard focal distention, bloating, abdominal pain relieved by warmth, nausea), up-rushing of yang (vomiting, hot flushes), and the inability of the turbid yin to descend (headaches, migraines, excessive salivation). In these cases, it is advisable to decoct Cinnamomi Ramulus (*guì zhī*) together with the other ingredients to direct its action to the interior where it will treat sensations of up-rushing, palpitations, and similar manifestations.

Another modern indication is chest painful obstruction occurring against a background of Spleen yang deficiency.

Excessive turbidity caused by the failure of Spleen transformation combined with deficiency of yang qi in the chest readily results in blockage of the blood vessels, particularly following exposure to cold or after eating. With the same intention, the formula can also be used to treat aches and pains in the muscles and joints, skin rashes, headaches, migraines, and pain in the throat. In all of these cases, the dosage of Cinnamomi Ramulus (guì zhī) may be increased to augment the formula's moving and unblocking actions.

Comparison

➤ Vs. Kudzu, Scutellaria, and Coptis Decoction (gé gēn huáng qín huáng lián tāng)

Both Cinnamon Twig and Ginseng Decoction (guì zhī rén shēn tāng) and Kudzu, Scutellaria, and Coptis Decoction (gé gēn huáng qín huáng lián tāng) treat commingled heat with diarrhea. A Kudzu, Scutellaria, and Coptis Decoction (gé gēn huáng qín huáng lián tāng) presentation is caused by a wind-cold pathogen in the yang brightness exterior that has already penetrated into the interior. Such patterns typically occur in patients with strong yang qi tending toward heat transformation. The diarrhea is therefore of the hot-type: it will have a foul odor and may be accompanied by burning of the anus. Pain is not a prominent feature or will disappear after passing of stools. By contrast, a Cinnamon Twig and Ginseng Decoction (guì zhī rén shēn tāng) presentation is caused by a wind-cold pathogen in the greater yang exterior that has also penetrated into the interior where it has damaged the middle burner yang. Such patterns typically occur in patients with weak yang qi tending toward cold transformation. The diarrhea is therefore of the cold type: it will be watery and have no odor. Any accompanying pain will improve with the application of warmth.

Biomedical Indications

With the appropriate presentation, this formula may be used to treat a variety of biomedically-defined disorders. One group is acute infectious gastrointestinal diseases, including the common cold with gastrointestinal symptoms and acute gastroenteritis. Another is long-term digestive dysfunctions such as chronic gastritis, peptic ulcer, functional indigestion, chronic cholecystitis, and chronic colitis. It has also been used for viral myocarditis and coronary heart disease.

Alternate name

Cinnamon Twig Decoction plus Ginseng (guì zhī jiā rén shēn tāng) in *Yun Qi-Zi's Collection for Safeguarding Life*

Modifications

- For more severe interior cold, add Aconiti Radix lateralis praeparata (zhì fù zǐ).
- For abdominal pain, add Paeoniae Radix alba (bái sháo).
- For incessant diarrhea that cannot be stopped, add Astragali Radix (huáng qí) and Cimicifugae Rhizoma (shēng má).

Comparative Tables of Principal Formulas

■ FORMULAS THAT RELEASE THE EXTERIOR AND PURGE THE INTERIOR

Common symptoms: fever and chills, epigastric distention, fullness in the chest and hypochondria, bitter taste, constipation, yellow tongue coating

Formula Name	Diagnosis	Indications	Remarks
Major Bupleurum Decoction (dà chái hú tāng)	Concurrent lesser yang and yang brightness-warp disorder	Alternating fever and chills, fullness in the chest and hypochondria, bitter taste, nausea, vomiting, epigastric distention or fullness and pain, burning diarrhea or no bowel movements, slight irritability, a yellow tongue coating, and a wiry, forceful pulse	For a wide range of symptoms accompanying obstruction of the epigastric area and flanks including headache, tinnitus, wheezing, and fevers.
Saposhnikovia Powder that Sagely Unblocks (fáng fēng tōng shèng sǎn)	Heat excess in both the exterior and interior	Strong fever and chills, dizziness, red and sore eyes, nasal congestion with thick discharge, bitter taste, dry mouth, focal distention, stifling sensation in the chest and diaphragm, constipation, dark, rough urination, a yellow, greasy tongue coating, and a flooding, rapid or wiry, slippery pulse	For a disorder which simultaneously affects the greater yang, yang brightness, and lesser yin warps.

■ FORMULAS THAT RELEASE THE EXTERIOR AND CLEAR THE INTERIOR

Common symptoms: fever, irritability, thirst, rapid pulse

Formula Name	Diagnosis	Indications	Remarks
Kudzu, Scutellaria, and Coptis Decoction (*gé gēn huáng qín huáng lián tāng*)	Incompletely resolved exterior with blazing interior heat	Fever, sweating, thirst, dysenteric diarrhea with especially foul-smelling stools, burning sensation around the anus, a sensation of irritability and heat in the chest and epigastrium, possible wheezing, a red tongue with yellow coating, and a rapid pulse	For simultaneous greater yang and yang brightness-warp disorders. Focuses on draining interior heat.
Gypsum Decoction (*shí gāo tāng*)	Exterior cold damage with blazing interior heat	Strong fever and chills without sweating, headache, thirst, irritability and insomnia, possible nosebleeds, coughing up blood or skin blotches, and a rapid, slippery or rapid, flooding pulse	Focuses on clearing severe interior heat.

■ FORMULAS THAT RELEASE THE EXTERIOR AND WARM THE INTERIOR

Common symptoms: chills and fever, cold and pain in the epigastrium or abdomen, diarrhea or dysenteric disorders, white tongue coating, slow pulse

Formula Name	Diagnosis	Indications	Remarks
Five-Accumulation Powder (*wǔ jī sǎn*)	Externally-contracted wind-cold with internal injury due to cold	Fever and chills without sweating, headache, body aches, a sensation of fullness in the chest and abdomen, nausea, vomiting, abdominal pain and cold, diarrhea, a white and greasy tongue coating, and a submerged, wiry or floating, slow pulse	Also for food accumulation with exterior wind-cold, painful or irregular menstruation due to cold, and cold in the lower body with heat in the upper body.
Cinnamon Twig and Ginseng Decoction (*guì zhī rén shēn tāng*)	Unresolved greater yang-warp disorder with cold obstructing the greater yin warp	Mild exterior symptoms (fever, chills, headache, joint pains, etc.) accompanied by severe diarrhea and hard focal distention in the epigastrium	For a complex pattern with cold in both the exterior and interior.

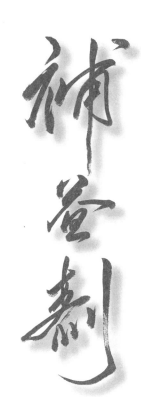

補遺劑

Chapter 8 Contents

Formulas that Tonify

Formulas that Tonify

THE FORMULAS IN this chapter are used in treating various forms of deficiency by tonifying, augmenting, nourishing, enriching, fortifying or supplementing the qi, blood, yin, or yang. Among the eight methods of treatment, the formulas here belong to the tonifying method (補法 *bǔ fǎ*). Early references to this method of treatment can be found in many passages of *Basic Questions*. For example, Chapter 20 admonishes "Tonify that which is deficient" while Chapter 74 advises "Augment those who [suffer from] harm, warm those who [suffer from] overexertion" and Chapter 5 notes that, "When the form (形 *xíng*) is insufficient, one warms by means of the qi [of herbs]; when the essence is insufficient, one tonifies by means of the flavor [of herbs]."

The *Classic of Difficulties* elaborated on these pragmatic instructions by tying the idea of tonification to the doctrine of the yin and yang organs: "When the Lungs are harmed, augment the qi. When the Heart is harmed, regulate the nutritive and protective [qi]. When the Spleen is harmed, regulate the diet and adjust [exposure] to heat and cold. When the Liver is harmed, relax the middle [burner]. When the Kidneys are harmed, augment the essence" (Chapter 19). The text also applied the five-phase doctrine as a model from which general treatment strategies could be deduced. The principle, "For deficiency, tonify the mother" (Chapter 75), continues to be applied in contemporary practice. This means that one should tonify the organ that corresponds to the phase that precedes that of the deficient organ in the cycle of mutual generation. For example, the Kidneys (water) are tonified for treating Liver (wood) deficiency, and the Spleen (earth) is tonified for treating Lung (metal) deficiency. This principle may be applied even when the situation does not adhere strictly to five-phase criteria. An example is that of tonifying the gate of vitality (the Kidney fire) rather than the Heart (fire phase) in treating deficiency of the Spleen (earth).

That tonification was an important concern to physicians early in the history of Chinese medicine can be discerned from an analysis of the herbs discussed in the *Divine Husbandman's Classic of the Materia Medica*. About 20 percent of these are what would today be classified as tonifying herbs. On the other hand, tonifying formulas are relatively rare in such early medical classics as *Discussion of Cold Damage* or *Essentials from the Golden Cabinet*. The majority of well-known formulas in use today were composed in the period from the Song to the Ming dynasties. The Song dynasty *Formulas from Benevolent Sages Compiled during the Taiping Era*, for instance, contains the classic formulas Four-Gentlemen Decoction *(sì jūn zǐ tāng)*, Four-Substance Decoction *(sì wù tāng)*, Ginseng, Poria, and White Atractylodes Powder *(shēn líng bái zhú sǎn)*, and All-Inclusive Great Tonifying Decoction *(shí quán dà bǔ tāng)*. During the same period, the pediatrican Qian Yi composed a number of formulas for tonifying deficiency of the five yin organs including the famous Six-Ingredient Pill with Rehmannia *(liù wèi dì huáng wán)*.

During the Jin-Yuan dynasties, Li Dong-Yuan emphasized the role of the Spleen and Stomach in formulas like Tonify the Middle to Augment the Qi Decoction *(bǔ zhōng yì qì tāng)*, for tonifying the qi, and Tangkuei Decoction to Tonify the Blood *(dāng guī bǔ xuè tāng)*, for tonifing the blood. Li's emphasis on tonification with sweet and warming herbs was continued during the Ming dynasty by physicians like Zhang Jie-Bin, who extended it to the tonification of Kidney yang and essence with formulas like Restore the Right [Kidney] Pill *(yòu guī wán)* and Restore the Left [Kidney] Drink *(zuǒ guī yǐn)*. Tonification of yin, on the other hand, was shaped most importantly by Zhu Dan-Xi, the last of the four great masters of the Jin-Yuan period. Formulas like Hidden Tiger Pill *(hǔ qián wán)* or Great Tonify the Yin Pill *(dà bǔ yīn wán)* focus on enriching Kidney essence while simultaneously directing fire downward. Under the influence of physicians belonging to the warm pathogen current, this approach was extended to the tonification of the Stomach, Lung, and Liver yin with an emphasis on generating fluids; Benefit the Stomach Decoction *(yì wèi tāng)* and Increase the Fluids Decoction *(zēng yè tāng)* (both discussed in Chapter 16) are well-known examples.

At present, tonifying formulas are used not only to treat illness, but also to increase resistance to disease, improve performance, and deal with the side effects of biomedical interventions such as chemotherapy or radiation therapy. Their undoubted benefit in these and other areas of contemporary practice should not distract us, however, from the fact that, like any other medical intervention, tonification must be used responsibly, and that, if used incorrectly and without regard to pattern differentiation, it can cause its own side effects.

Manifestations of deficiency are quite diverse and can arise in a wide variety of contexts. They may be due to constitutional factors, bad diet, overwork, emotional stress, trauma, illness, as well as the side effects of medical treatment. Patterns of deficiency patterns can be differentiated by aspect (yin, yang, qi, or blood) or a combination of aspects (yang and qi, yin and blood); by organ (Liver, Heart, Spleen, Lungs, Kidneys) or a combination of organs (Liver-Kidney, Spleen-Lungs); or by both aspect and organ (Lung qi deficiency, Kidney yang deficiency).

Because of the integral relationship between the qi and blood, tonifying one will have a salutary effect on the other. The adage "Qi is the commander of blood, and blood is the mother of qi" suggests that qi moves the blood and that blood nourishes the qi. This understanding of the relationship between qi and blood deficiency is reflected in a passage from *Discussion of the Spleen and Stomach*: "For blood deficiency, use Ginseng Radix *(rén shēn)* to tonify, because when the yang [qi] is exuberant, it will generate yin blood." Astragali Radix *(huáng qí)* is another commonly used herb in many blood-tonifying formulas because of its ability to augment the qi of the middle and upper burners.

A similar relationship exists between the yin and yang, illustrated in the following passage from *Collected Treatises of*

[Zhang] Jing-Yue: "To tonify the yang well, you must search for the yang within the yin.... To tonify the yin well, you must search for the yin within the yang." Many formulas that tonify the yang therefore contain ingredients which tonify the yin, and vice versa. Strategies for tonification are sometimes explained by the theory of the five phases.

Because these formulas are designed specifically for conditions of deficiency, it is essential that deficiency and excess be properly differentiated. Conditions due to severe excess sometimes resemble those from deficiency, manifesting in such symptoms as weight loss and reduced vitality. This is clearly analyzed in another passage from *Collected Treatises of [Zhang] Jing-Yue*:

> Extreme deficiency disorders [sometimes] turn into their opposite exhibiting an exuberant force, while strong excess disorders may conversely manifest with marked emaciation. One must not fail to differentiate these. Disorders arising from the seven emotions, over-eating, exhaustion, or damage due to [over-indulgence] in alcohol and sex, as well as those disorders occurring because of insufficient prenatal [endowment], all frequently manifest with patterns [including] body fever, constipation, upcast yang, distention, fullness, deficiency mania, or false macules. Although they resemble disorders characterized by surplus, their excess is due to insufficiency.

Remember also that chronic conditions are not necessarily due to deficiency, nor are all deficient conditions chronic. It is not uncommon for an externally-contracted disease to injure the qi, blood, yin, or yang. In such cases, one should combine ingredients that expel the pathogenic influence with those that tonify. Formulas that simultaneously tonify and treat excess are found in other chapters of the book (see particularly Chapters 1-3).

Tonifying formulas have very specific effects and indications. They should therefore not be used indiscriminately, like vitamins, just because it is assumed that "everyone can use a little tonification." This is not true. Side effects will often develop when tonics are prescribed for those who are not suffering from deficiency. These include fever, headache, rash, pimples, insomnia, irritability, and digestive upset.

The rich, cloying nature of tonifying herbs places a burden on the digestive system. It is therefore usually necessary to add ingredients that promote digestion and assimilation, such as those that strengthen the Spleen, harmonize the Stomach, and regulate the qi. It is also advisable to reduce the dosage of tonifying ingredients for patients with marked Spleen and Stomach qi deficiency. Furthermore, it is essential that the dosage be adjusted to the relative severity of the condition. Mild, chronic conditions require a smaller dosage than do acute, life-threatening conditions.

Tonifying formulas are generally cooked for a rather long period of time over a low flame and are taken on an empty stomach to realize their full effect. Of course, these rules do not apply in emergencies.

Section 1

FORMULAS THAT TONIFY THE QI

Formulas that tonify the qi are primarily used in treating conditions that involve the Spleen and Lungs. These organs produce the body's qi, which is derived from food absorbed by the Spleen and from air taken in by the Lungs. General symptoms of qi deficiency include lethargy and fatigue. An important hallmark of disorders associated with qi deficiency is that they are precipitated by activity and improve with rest.

The Spleen and Stomach, located in the middle burner, are the source for the production and transformation of qi and blood. If the Spleen is deficient, the qi will in turn be deficient. Similarly, for tonification of the qi of any organ to be effective, the Spleen must itself be tonified and strengthened. When the transportive function of the Spleen and Stomach is healthy, the normal qi will be abundant. The primary indications of Spleen qi deficiency include fatigue, shortness of breath (with little exertion), laconic speech, a shiny, pale complexion, reduced appetite, loose stools, and a weak pulse. When qi deficiency is accompanied by qi stagnation, acrid herbs that facilitate the Spleen's functions of assimilation and transportation, such as Citri reticulatae Pericarpium (*chén pí*), Aucklandiae Radix (*mù xiāng*), or Amomi Fructus (*shā rén*), are usually added to tonifying formulas.

The qi of the Spleen and Stomach is also known as the middle qi. In addition to controlling digestion, the middle qi has many other functions that are related to its pivotal role in the ascending and descending actions of the qi mechanism. When the qi of the middle burner is deficient, it will manifest above in symptoms of shortness of breath and laconic speech, and below in symptoms of prolapse, bleeding, and incontinence. Tonifying the middle qi will raise the sunken yang qi and thereby restore the qi mechanism. Herbs that facilitate the upward movement of qi in the body, such as Bupleuri Radix (*chái hú*), Cimicifugae Rhizoma (*shēng má*), or Saposhnikoviae Radix (*fáng fēng*), are commonly added to formulas that treat these patterns.

Lung qi deficiency manifests as chronic cough accompanied by generalized weakness, a low voice, and profuse sweating (the Lungs control the skin and the interstices and pores). Because the fluids may be injured by profuse sweating, these formulas also address the effects of injury to the yin and fluids by adding yin-tonifying herbs like Ophiopogonis Radix (*mài mén dōng*) or Glehniae/Adenophorae Radix (*shā shēn*), and astringent herbs like Schisandrae Fructus (*wǔ wèi zǐ*) or Mume Fructus (*wū méi*). Tonifying the qi and yin 'firms up' or consolidates the protective qi and thereby helps reduce sweating. This gives these formulas a stabilizing effect.

When the Spleen and Lungs lose control over water metabolism, leading to the accumulation of internal dampness, herbs that leach out dampness and facilitate water metabolism, such as Poria (*fú líng*) or Coicis Semen (*yì yǐ rén*), and those that transform phlegm, like Pinelliae Rhizoma praeparatum (*zhì bàn xià*), are added to qi-tonifying formulas. When qi deficiency leads to or is accompanied by blood deficiency, blood tonics like Paeoniae Radix alba (*bái sháo*), Angelicae sinensis Radix (*dāng guī*), and Lycii Fructus (*gǒu qǐ zǐ*) are added. Because qi deficiency implies an inability of the qi to move substances in the body, the dosage of these herbs should be kept low in order that their greasy nature not obstruct the qi dynamic.

For cases with deficiency of Heart qi (usually more complex, because of the Heart's close relationship to the blood), the reader is referred to those formulas which tonify the blood (this chapter) and calm the spirit (Chapter 13). For conditions with deficiency of the Kidney qi, including Kidney yang deficiency and unstable Kidney qi, consult the formulas that tonify the yang (this chapter) and stabilize and bind (Chapter 12).

四君子湯 (四君子汤)
Four-Gentlemen Decoction
sì jūn zǐ tāng

Traditionally in China, a 'gentleman' was a person whose virtue and achievements made him stand out from the common people. From the Confucian perspective, becoming a gentleman implies a process of self-cultivation through which one develops a rounded personality. The four herbs of which this formula is composed are balanced and harmonious, and therefore have the qualities of a gentleman, as explained by the Qing-dynasty writer Zhang Lu:

> For qi deficiency, one tonifies using sweet [herbs] like Ginseng Radix (*rén shēn*), Atractylodis macrocephalae Rhizoma (*bái zhú*), Poria (*fú líng*), and Glycyrrhizae Radix (*gān cǎo*). Sweet and warming, they augment the Stomach. They [thus] have the ability to strengthen the transportive [functions of the middle burner]. As they all have the virtue of being thoroughly harmonious, they are considered gentlemen.

Source *Formulary of the Pharmacy Service for Benefiting the People in the Taiping Era* (1107)

Ginseng Radix (*rén shēn*) .... (3-9g)
Atractylodis macrocephalae Rhizoma (*bái zhú*) .... (6-9g)
Poria (*fú líng*) .... (6-9g)
Glycyrrhizae Radix praeparata (*zhì gān cǎo*) .... (3-6g)

Method of Preparation The source text advises to grind equal amounts of the ingredients into a fine powder and take 6g as a draft, either with plain or lightly salted water. It need not be taken at any particular time. At present, it is usually prepared as a decoction with the dosage specified in parentheses, but with Codonopsis Radix (*dǎng shēn*) substituted for Ginseng Radix (*rén shēn*) at 2-3 times its dosage.

Actions Tonifies the qi and strengthens the Spleen

Indications

Pallid complexion, low and soft voice, reduced appetite, loose stools, and weakness in the limbs. The body of the tongue is pale, and the pulse is deficient and/or frail.

This is the classic presentation of Spleen qi deficiency, usually caused by improper eating habits, excessive deliberation, or overworking. When the Spleen qi is deficient, the transformation of food into blood and qi will be impaired. This manifests as a pallid complexion and a low, soft voice. Spleen deficiency also leads to a decline in that organ's transportive functions and thus a lack of transport through the Stomach. This manifests as reduced appetite and unformed stools. Because the Spleen governs the limbs, the patient will first experience weakness in the limbs. The pale tongue and deficient and/or frail pulse are typical signs of Spleen qi deficiency.

Analysis of Formula

When Spleen and Stomach qi deficiency is marked by weakness in transportation and transformation, the main treatment strategy is to tonify the qi and strengthen the Spleen. The chief herb in this formula is sweet, warm Ginseng Radix (rén shēn), a powerful tonic for the Spleen qi. In most modern formulations, however, Codonopsis Radix (dǎng shēn) is substituted both because it is well-suited for this pattern and is significantly less expensive. The deputy, bitter and warm Atractylodis macrocephalae Rhizoma (bái zhú), strengthens the Spleen and dries dampness. These two herbs work synergistically to improve the transportive and transformative functions of the Spleen, that is, the Spleen qi.

The assistant herb is Poria (fú líng), a sweet, bland substance that leaches out dampness. It also assists the chief and deputy herbs in strengthening the Spleen. The envoy, Glycyrrhizae Radix praeparata (zhì gān cǎo), warms and regulates the middle burner. The combination of these two herbs is instructive. Poria (fú líng) moderates the cloying nature of Glycyrrhizae Radix praeparata (zhì gān cǎo) to prevent abdominal distention, while the tonifying properties of Glycyrrhizae Radix praeparata (zhì gān cǎo) moderate the draining properties of the former ingredient.

Together, the herbs in this formula tonify the Spleen while also dispelling dampness and supporting transportation. They tonify the middle burner while also moving its qi and are warming without being excessively drying. In this way, they work harmoniously together as a simple but effective formula that lives up to its name.

Cautions and Contraindications

The long-term use of this formula may result in a dry mouth, thirst, and irritability. It should not be used without modification in patients with high fever, heat from deficiency, or a combination of irritability, thirst, and constipation.

Commentary

This is one of the basic formulas for tonifying the qi. Fei Bo-Xiong even referred to it as the "gold standard" (金科玉律 jīn kē yù lǜ) for all such formulas. Its distinguishing characteristic is its harmonious and moderate nature. Unlike many of the other qi-tonifying formulas, which are quite warm and drying, this one opens the qi dynamic without relying on acrid, qi-moving herbs. The original instructions for use of this formula, relying on a dosage that is far lower than is generally used nowadays, further underlines this moderate mode of action.

In some ways, this formula can be viewed as a modification of Regulate the Middle Pill (lǐ zhōng wán), with Poria (fú líng) substituted for Zingiberis Rhizoma (gān jiāng). This is an example of how the substitution of a single herb can change the basic nature of a formula, in this case from one that dispels cold from the middle burner to one that tonifies the Spleen. As is usually the case in contemporary practice, the precise mode of action of the formula is further modified by adjusting the nature of the individual ingredients to fit the presentation of the patient. As explained above under ANALYSIS OF FORMULA, Codonopsis Radix (dǎng shēn) is commonly substituted for Ginseng Radix (rén shēn). However, if the formula is used to treat deficiency of primal qi, this substitution is not recommended. If dampness is pronounced, unprepared Atractylodis macrocephalae Rhizoma (bái zhú) is used and is made the chief herb of the formula by increasing its dosage. If, on the other hand, there are signs of yin deficiency caused by the Spleen's inability to assimilate fluids and move them to the Lungs, it is advisable to fry Atractylodis macrocephalae Rhizoma (bái zhú) in honey in order to moderate its drying properties. Moreover, the original formula employs Glycyrrhizae Radix (gān cǎo) rather than Glycyrrhizae Radix praeparata (zhì gān cǎo), to underline the fact that it was being used not only as a harmonizing herb, but also for its tonifying and toxicity-resolving properties.

Clinically, the formula may be used in treating any disorder for which deficient Spleen qi is considered to be the root. The original indications summarize the essence of such patterns: deficiency of nutritive and protective qi, weakness of the yin and yang organs, distention and fullness of the epigastrium and abdomen, generalized lack of appetite, borborygmi, diarrhea, vomiting, and belching. Successive generations of physicians have modified the formula to expand its use. Some examples are discussed under VARIATIONS and ASSOCIATED FORMULAS below. Others include Tonify the Middle to Augment the Qi Decoction (bǔ zhōng yì qì tāng), discussed later in this section, and Restore the Spleen Decoction (guī pí tāng), discussed later in this chapter. At present, it is usually modified and augmented with other herbs in the clinic. Many contemporary practitioners base their treatment of childhood nutritional impairment on this formula.

Comparisons

➢ Vs. Ginseng, Poria, and White Atractylodes Powder *(shēn líng bái zhú sǎn)*; see page 315

➢ Vs. Tonify the Middle to Augment the Qi Decoction *(bǔ zhōng yì qì tāng)*; see page 321

➢ Vs. Regulate the Middle Pill *(lǐ zhōng wán)*; see page 259

Biomedical Indications

With the appropriate presentation, this formula may be used to treat a wide variety of biomedically-defined disorders. These can be organized into the following groups:

• Those primarily affecting the digestive system such as chronic gastritis, peptic ulcer, irritable bowel syndrome, chronic hepatitis, and to reduce the recovery time after gastric surgery

• Fever of unknown origin, recurrent nosebleeds, and sequelae of infections, especially in children

• Hemopoietic fuctions in anemia and neutropenia, as well as the basis for adjunctive therapy in conjunction with chemotherapy or radiation therapy for cancer patients.

In addition, this formula has been used for such problems as diabetes mellitus, periodic paralysis, coronary artery disease, uterine fibroids, and chronic bronchitis.

Alternate names

White Atractylodes Powder *(bái zhú sǎn)* in *Effective Medical Formulas Arranged by Category by Master Zhu*; Four-Sages Decoction *(sì shèng tāng)* in *Invoking Blessings for Healthy Children*; Ginseng Powder *(rén shēn sǎn)* in *Formulas of Universal Benefit*; Warm the Middle Decoction *(wēn zhōng tāng)* in *Complete Collection of Charts and Texts Past and Present*; Four-Gentlemen Decoction *(sì jūn tāng)* in *Effective Formulas from the Hall of Literature*

Modifications

• For indigestion, reduced appetite, abdominal distention, and weight loss, add Cyperi Rhizoma *(xiāng fù)* and Magnoliae officinalis Cortex *(hòu pò)*.

• For morning sickness, add Amomi Fructus *(shā rén)*, Citri reticulatae Pericarpium *(chén pí)*, and Magnoliae officinalis Cortex *(hòu pò)*.

• For edema during pregnancy, take with Five-Peel Drink *(wǔ pí yǐn)*.

• For periodic paralysis, add Astragali Radix *(huáng qí)*, Ophiopogonis Radix *(mài mén dōng)*, Angelicae dahuricae Radix *(bái zhǐ)*, and Saposhnikoviae Radix *(fáng fēng)*.

• For uterine fibroids, add Curcumae Rhizoma *(é zhú)*, Sparganii Rhizoma *(sān léng)*, and Achyranthis bidentatae Radix *(niú xī)*.

• For palpitations and insomnia, add Ziziphi spinosae Semen *(suān zǎo rén)*.

Associated Formulas

異功散 （异功散）

Extraordinary Merit Powder

yì gōng sǎn

Source *Craft of Medicinal Treatment for Childhood Disease Patterns* (1119)

Ginseng Radix *(rén shēn)* .... (3-9g)
Atractylodis macrocephalae Rhizoma *(bái zhú)* .... (6-9g)
Poria *(fú líng)* .... (6-9g)
Glycyrrhizae Radix praeparata *(zhì gān cǎo)* .... (3-6g)
Citri reticulatae Pericarpium *(chén pí)* .... (6-9g)

The source text advises to grind equal amounts of the ingredients into a fine powder and take as a draft with Zingiberis Rhizoma recens *(shēng jiāng)* and Jujubae Fructus *(dà zǎo)*. At present, it is usually prepared as a decoction with Codonopsis Radix *(dǎng shēn)* substituted for Ginseng Radix *(rén shēn)* at 2-3 times its dosage. Strengthens the Spleen, augments the qi, and harmonizes the Stomach. This formula treats Spleen deficiency leading to an irregular appetite accompanied by a stifling sensation in the chest and epigastrium, and sometimes nausea and vomiting. Compared to the principal formula, this variation focuses more strongly on moving the qi and harmonizing the Stomach. It is widely used in the treatment of digestive disorders in children.

六君子湯 （六君子汤）

Six-Gentlemen Decoction

liù jūn zǐ tāng

Source *Formulary of the Pharmacy Service for Benefiting the People in the Taiping Era* (1107)

Ginseng Radix *(rén shēn)* 3g
Atractylodis macrocephalae Rhizoma *(bái zhú)* 4.5g
Poria *(fú líng)* 3g
Glycyrrhizae Radix praeparata *(zhì gān cǎo)* 3g
Citri reticulatae Pericarpium *(chén pí)* 3g
Pinelliae Rhizoma praeparatum *(zhì bàn xià)* 4.5g

Strengthens the Spleen, transforms phlegm, and stops vomiting. For concurrent deficient Spleen qi and phlegm characterized by a loss of appetite, nausea or vomiting, focal distention and a stifling sensation in the chest and epigastrium, and often coughing of copious, thin, and white sputum. This formula combines the principal formula with Two-Aged [Herb] Decoction *(èr chén tāng)*. At present, Codonopsis Radix *(dǎng shēn)* is usually substituted for Ginseng Radix *(rén shēn)* at 2-3 times its dosage, and the dosage of the other herbs is commonly increased by 1.5-2 times. Compared to the principal formula, the dosage of Atractylodis macrocephalae Rhizoma *(bái zhú)* here is increased, and two drying herbs that direct the qi downward are added. In addition to tonifying the qi, this focuses the formula's action on removing obstruction to the middle burner by phlegm-dampness, characterized by rebellious qi of the Stomach and Lungs.

Although it is a variation of Four-Gentlemen Decoction *(sì jūn zǐ tāng)*, this formula has become a major formula in its own right, spawning a multitude of new formulas that take it, rather than Four-Gentlemen Decoction (*sì jūn zǐ tāng*), as their model. Some examples include:

- Adding Coptidis Rhizoma (*huáng lián*) makes Coptis Six-Gentlemen Decoction (*huáng lián liù jūn zǐ tāng*), used for indefinable epigastric discomfort. (*Comprehensive Medicine According to Master Zhang*)

- Adding Paeoniae Radix alba (*bái sháo*) and Bupleuri Radix (*chái hú*) gives Bupleurum and Peony Six-Gentlemen Decoction (*chái sháo liù jūn zǐ tāng*), used for Spleen-deficient abdominal pain, menstrual pain, diarrhea during menstruation, and chronic low-grade fevers. (*Formulary of the Pharmacy Service for Benefiting the People in the Taiping Era*)

- Adding Atractylodis Rhizoma (*cāng zhú*), Bupleuri Radix (*chái hú*), and Cimicifugae Rhizoma (*shēng má*) makes the modern formula Augmented Six-Gentlemen Decoction (*jiā wèi liù jūn zǐ tāng*), used for chronic vaginal discharges.

Comparisons

➤ Vs. Open the Spleen Pill (*qǐ pí wán*); see page 313

➤ Vs. Ginseng, Poria, and White Atractylodes Powder (*shēn líng bái zhú sǎn*); see page 315

香砂六君子湯 (香砂六君子汤)

Six-Gentlemen Decoction with Aucklandia and Amomum

xiāng shā liù jūn zǐ tāng

Source *Discussion of Famous Physicians' Formulas Past and Present* (1675)

Ginseng Radix (*rén shēn*) 3g
Atractylodis macrocephalae Rhizoma (*bái zhú*) 6g
Poria (*fú líng*) 6g
Glycyrrhizae Radix praeparata (*zhì gān cǎo*) 2.1g
Citri reticulatae Pericarpium (*chén pí*) 2.4g
Pinelliae Rhizoma praeparatum (*zhì bàn xià*) 3g
Amomi Fructus (*shā rén*) 2.4g
Aucklandiae Radix (*mù xiāng*) 2.1g
Zingiberis Rhizoma recens (*shēng jiāng*) 6g

Strengthens the Spleen, harmonizes the Stomach, regulates the qi, and alleviates pain. For Spleen and Stomach qi deficiency with damp-cold stagnating in the middle burner. Symptoms include reduced appetite with a feeling of surfeit after eating very little, belching, abdominal distention or pain, and sometimes vomiting and diarrhea. At present, Codonopsis Radix (*dǎng shēn*) is usually substituted for Ginseng Radix (*rén shēn*) at 2-3 times its dosage, and the dosage of the other herbs is commonly increased by 1.5-2 times.

This formula is regarded as a variation of Six-Gentlemen Decoction (*liù jūn zǐ tāng*). Compared to that formula, it is even more drying and moving, such that it regulates the qi as much as it tonifies it. Moreover, the literature lists a number of different formulas by the same name, but that replace Aucklandiae Radix (*mù xiāng*) with Pogostemonis/Agastaches Herba (*huò xiāng*) or Cyperi Rhizoma (*xiāng fù*). The formula should therefore be adjusted to fit the pattern.

香砂養胃湯 (香砂养胃汤)

Nourish the Stomach Decoction with Aucklandia and Amomum

xiāng shā yǎng wèi tāng

Source *Restoration of Health from the Myriad Diseases* (1587)

Ginseng Radix (*rén shēn*) 1.5g
Atractylodis macrocephalae Rhizoma (*bái zhú*) 3g
Poria (*fú líng*) 2.4g
Atractylodis Rhizoma (*cāng zhú*) 2.4g
ginger-juice fried Magnoliae officinalis Cortex
  (*jiāng zhī chǎo hòu pò*) 2.4g
Citri reticulatae Pericarpium (*chén pí*) 2.4g
dry-fried Cyperi Rhizoma (*chǎo xiāng fù*) 2.4g
Amomi Fructus rotundus (*bái dòu kòu*) 2.1g
Aucklandiae Radix (*mù xiāng*) 1.5g
Amomi Fructus (*shā rén*) 2.4g
Zingiberis Rhizoma recens (*shēng jiāng*) .3g
Glycyrrhizae Radix praeparata (*zhì gān cǎo*) 1.5-3g
Jujubae Fructus (*dà zǎo*) 1.5-3g

Strengthens and harmonizes the Spleen and Stomach and resolves dampness. For disharmony between the Spleen and Stomach together with dampness manifested as reduced appetite, a loss of taste, inability to eat more than a little at a time, bloating after eating, focal distention, an uncomfortable feeling in the epigastrium, and generalized weakness. At present, Codonopsis Radix (*dǎng shēn*) is usually substituted for Ginseng Radix (*rén shēn*) at 2-3 times its dosage.

六神散

Six-Miracle Powder from *Indispensable Tools for Pattern Treatment*

liù shén sǎn

Source *Indispensable Tools for Pattern Treatment* (1602)

Ginseng Radix (*rén shēn*) 15g
Atractylodis macrocephalae Rhizoma (*bái zhú*) 30g
Poria (*fú líng*) 30g
Glycyrrhizae Radix praeparata (*zhì gān cǎo*) 30g
Lablab Semen album (*biǎn dòu*) 30g
honey-prepared Astragali Radix (*zhì huáng qí*) 30g

Grind the ingredients into a powder and take as a draft in 6g doses with 1 piece of Zingiberis Rhizoma recens (*shēng jiāng*) and 1 piece of Jujubae Fructus (*dà zǎo*). At present, Codonopsis Radix (*dǎng shēn*) is usually substituted for Ginseng Radix (*rén shēn*) at 2-3 times its dosage. Augments the qi, tonifies the middle burner, and regulates the Stomach. For Spleen and Stomach deficiency leading to a lack of fluids. This internal deficiency with reduction in the intake of food and fluids leads to a form of heat from deficiency. Note that although there are at least five rather well-known formulas by this name, each serves a very different function from the other.

啓脾丸 (启脾丸)

Open the Spleen Pill

qǐ pí wán

SOURCE　*Restoration of Health from the Myriad Diseases* (1587)

Ginseng Radix (*rén shēn*)..............................37.5g (10g)
Atractylodis macrocephalae Rhizoma (*bái zhú*).........37.5g (10g)
Poria (*fú líng*)......................................37.5g (10g)
Dioscoreae Rhizoma (*shān yào*)........................37.5g (10g)
Nelumbinis Semen (*lián zǐ*)...........................37.5g (10g)
Crataegi Fructus (*shān zhā*)..............................19g (5g)
Citri reticulatae Pericarpium (*chén pí*)................19g (10g)
Alismatis Rhizoma (*zé xiè*)...............................19g (5g)
Glycyrrhizae Radix (*gān cǎo*).............................19g (5g)

The source text advises to grind the above ingredients into a powder, mix with refined honey, and form into very small pills (about the size of a sesame seed). The dosage is 23 pills, most likely taken 2-3 times a day on an empty stomach with rice porridge. If used as a decoction, the dosages in parentheses can be taken as a reference. Builds up the Spleen, transforms dampness, harmonizes the Stomach, and disperses food accumulation. Treats middle burner deficiency with food stagnation and dampness. Symptoms include no desire to eat or drink, diarrhea, abdominal pain, vomiting, belching that smells rotten or sour, a greasy or turbid tongue coating, and a weak, soggy pulse. These symptoms may be the result of simple stagnant food accumulation in children or adults with constitutional Spleen deficiency, or may be part of a childhood nutritional impairment pattern.

This formula was originally designed for children with childhood nutritional impairment and accumulations (疳積 *gān jī*) and thus simultaneously treats the root and branch of this problem. In these patients, simply treating the symptoms with a more dispersing formula like Preserve Harmony Pill (*bǎo hé wán*) runs the risk of further damaging the middle burner qi. Similarly, addressing only the root would likely be ineffective because the stagnation that characterizes the pattern has rendered the digestive system unable to process the tonifying herbs, which would likely worsen the situation. At present, while still popular in the pediatric clinic, Open the Spleen Pill (*qǐ pí wán*) is also used to treat digestive accumulation problems in deficient patients of all ages. This includes the formula's use in treating qi-deficiency types of obesity.

Comparisons

➤ VS. SIX-GENTLEMEN DECOCTION (*liù jūn zǐ tāng*)

Both formulas tonify and regulate the middle burner qi and transform dampness to treat deficient middle burner qi that gives rise to diarrhea, belching, and lack of appetite. However, Open the Spleen Pill is better at dispersing food stagnation and also treating diarrhea. Six-Gentlemen Decoction (*liù jūn zǐ tāng*), on the other hand, is better at transforming dampness and causing the Stomach qi to descend. For cases of accumulation diarrhea where dampness is less significant, Open the Spleen Pill (*qǐ pí wán*) is the preferred formula.

➤ VS. FAT BABY PILL FROM *Golden Mirror*
　　(*Jīn jiàn féi ér wán*)

Both formulas treat childhood nutritional impairment by dispersing accumulation and supplementing the middle burner. Fat Baby Pill

from *Golden Mirror (Jīn jiàn féi ér wán)* concentrates on dispersing food accumulation and clearing the heat that arises from accumulation of food and dampness in the digestive tract. In addition, it expels parasites. This inclusive approach makes the formula a good candidate for entrenched cases of childhood nutritional impairment, but renders it much less able than Open the Spleen Pill (*qǐ pí wán*) to supplement the middle. Open the Spleen Pill (*qǐ pí wán*), on the other hand, is far less able than Fat Baby Pill from *Golden Mirror (Jīn jiàn féi ér wán)* to disperse stagnation. It also contains no agents to clear heat or expel parasites. Open the Spleen Pill (*qǐ pí wán*) is best suited for mild, early cases of childhood nutritional impairment. When using Fat Baby Pill from *Golden Mirror (Jīn jiàn féi ér wán)* in patients who are significantly deficient, it is helpful to alternate it with doses of Open the Spleen Pill (*qǐ pí wán*) to ensure that the middle burner qi is not depleted by the bitter, dispersing nature of Fat Baby Pill from *Golden Mirror (Jīn jiàn féi ér wán)*.

Modifications

- For significant diarrhea, add Myristicae Semen (*ròu dòu kòu*).
- For cold abdominal pain, add Zingiberis Rhizoma (*gān jiāng*).
- To increase the formula's ability to disperse food accumulation, add Hordei Fructus germinatus (*mài yá*) and Massa medicata fermentata (*shén qū*).
- For childhood nutritional impairment, add Quisqualis Fructus (*shǐ jūn zǐ*).

固真湯 (固真汤)

Stabilize the True Decoction

gù zhēn tāng

SOURCE　*Indispensable Tools for Pattern Treatment* (1602)

Ginseng Radix (*rén shēn*)......................................7.5g
Aconiti Radix lateralis praeparata (*zhì fù zǐ*)................7.5g
Poria (*fú líng*)...7.5g
Atractylodis macrocephalae Rhizoma (*bái zhú*)..................7.5g
Dioscoreae Rhizoma (*shān yào*)...................................6g
Honey-prepared Astragali Radix (*mì zhì huáng qí*)................6g
Cinnamomi Cortex (*ròu guì*)......................................6g
Glycyrrhizae Radix (*gān cǎo*)....................................6g

The decoction is taken with 3 slices of Zingiberis Rhizoma recens (*shēng jiāng*) and 1 piece of Jujubae Fructus (*dà zǎo*). Warms and tonifies the Spleen and Kidneys, restores the yang, and dispels cold. For chronic Spleen wind from exhaustion of the true or yang qi. Manifestations include a lethargic and blunted affect or frank somnambulance, a pasty-white complexion, profuse sweating, rhythmic spasms of the hands and feet, clear, liquid diarrhea, a pale tongue with a thin, white coating, and a submerged, faint pulse. This condition most often occurs as the sequelae to a prolonged bout of vomiting and diarrhea.

保元湯 (保元汤)

Preserve the Primal Decoction

baǒ yuán tāng

SOURCE　*Collected Treatises of [Zhang] Jing-Yue* (1624)

Astragali Radix (*huáng qí*) 9g
Ginseng Radix (*rén shēn*) 3g
Glycyrrhizae Radix praeparata (*zhì gān cǎo*) 3g
Cinnamomi Cortex (*ròu guì*) 1.5-2.1g

Decocted with a handful of glutinous rice. Tonifies the qi and warms the yang. For deficiency and consumption with insufficient primal (source) qi. Manifestations include fatigue and lethargy, shortness of breath, and aversion to cold. May also be accompanied by pain, or vomiting and diarrhea. Recommended for consumption when the low-grade fever is thought to be due to qi deficiency and a floating, errant yang. If the formula is inappropriate, the condition will quickly worsen; if it is helpful, it may take a few months to show definite improvement. Originally used for smallpox with deficient qi characterized by a pox-like rash with recessed heads. Compared to the principal formula, this variation focuses purely on tonification without moving stagnation or draining dampness.

Note: This formula was first recorded in the *Mirror of the Heart of Universal Love,* which is no longer extant.

參苓白朮散 (参苓白术散)
Ginseng, Poria, and White Atractylodes Powder

shēn líng bái zhú sǎn

Source   *Formulary of the Pharmacy Service for Benefiting the People in the Taiping Era* (1107)

Ginseng Radix (*rén shēn*) 1000g
Atractylodis macrocephalae Rhizoma (*bái zhú*) 1000g
Poria (*fú líng*) 1000g
Glycyrrhizae Radix praeparata (*zhì gān cǎo*) 1000g
Dioscoreae Rhizoma (*shān yào*) 1000g
dry-fried Lablab Semen album (*chǎo biǎn dòu*) 750g
Nelumbinis Semen (*lián zǐ*) 500g
Coicis Semen (*yì yǐ rén*) 500g
Amomi Fructus (*shā rén*) 500g
dry-fried Platycodi Radix (*chǎo jié gěng*) 500g

Method of Preparation   The source text advises to grind the ingredients into a powder and take in 6g doses with warm water. At present, Codonopsis Radix (*dǎng shēn*) or Pseudostellariae Radix (*tài zǐ shēn*) is usually substituted for Ginseng Radix (*rén shēn*) at 2-2.5 times its dosage. Often prepared as a decoction with approximately one-hundredth the dosage specified above.

Actions   Augments the qi, strengthens the Spleen, leaches out dampness, and stops diarrhea

Indications

Loose stools or diarrhea, reduced appetite, weakness of the extremities, weight loss, distention and a stifling sensation in the chest and epigastrium, pallid and wan complexion, a pale tongue with a white coating, and a thin, moderate or deficient, moderate pulse. There may also be vomiting.

This is Spleen qi deficiency leading to internally-generated dampness. The Spleen is responsible for transforming and transporting food and nutrients, which it sends upward and to the extremities. When the Spleen qi is weakened, usually from improper eating habits or overworking, the fluids accumulate and transform into dampness. The primary signs of this process are loose stools or diarrhea and a white coating on the tongue. When the Spleen and Stomach qi are weakened, the individual cannot take in food, which manifests as reduced appetite. The loss of the Spleen's ability to transform and transport nutrients leads to weight loss, weakness of the extremities, and a pallid and wan complexion. The internally-generated dampness obstructs the qi mechanism in the middle burner, which manifests as distention and a stifling sensation in the chest and epigastrium. In some patients this can lead to rebellious Stomach qi, manifested as vomiting. The pale tongue body and the thin or deficient pulse reflect Spleen and Stomach qi deficiency, while the tongue coating and moderate pulse reflect dampness.

In other contexts, the same pathological process may also manifest as Lung and Spleen qi deficiency with accumulation of phlegm-dampness. The formula also treats this pattern, which is characterized by coughing up copious amounts of white sputum and a thin, slippery pulse, in addition to the symptoms outlined above. When phlegm-dampness accumulates in the middle burner, it often collects in the Lungs, the upper source of water metabolism, leading to coughing up of white phlegm. The pulse is thin because the physiological fluids are reduced, and slippery due to the presence of pathological phlegm-dampness.

Analysis of Formula

The primary focus of this formula is to tonify and strengthen the Spleen qi. The chief herbs are Ginseng Radix (*rén shēn*), Atractylodis macrocephalae Rhizoma (*bái zhú*), Poria (*fú líng*), and Glycyrrhizae Radix praeparata (*zhì gān cǎo*), which together comprise Four-Gentlemen Decoction (*sì jūn zǐ tāng*), discussed immediately above. The reader is referred there for a discussion of how these herbs interact in tonifying the Spleen qi.

The deputy herbs include Dioscoreae Rhizoma (*shān yào*), which tonifies the Spleen and supports the chief herbs; Coicis Semen (*yì yǐ rén*), which strengthens the Spleen and leaches out dampness; and Lablab Semen album (*biǎn dòu*) and Nelumbinis Semen (*lián zǐ*), which strengthen the Spleen and stop diarrhea. In relation to the chief herbs, the deputies support the functions of Atractylodis macrocephalae Rhizoma (*bái zhú*) and Poria (*fú líng*) in strengthening the Spleen and eliminating dampness, which are the most important aspects of this condition.

Amomi Fructus (*shā rén*) serves as the assistant herb. It transforms dampness and promotes the movement of qi. The latter action enables the formula to tonify without causing stagnation. The envoy, Platycodi Radix (*jié gěng*), unblocks the flow of Lung qi. Its functions are threefold: by disseminating the Lung qi, it helps spread nourishment throughout the body; its ascending nature helps treat the diarrhea; and it guides the actions of the other herbs into the Lungs. This last function prevents the development of Lung deficiency, which is a common sequela of Spleen deficiency.

Cautions and Contraindications

Use with caution, and then only after significant modification, in cases with concurrent heat from yin deficiency.

Commentary

This variation of Four-Gentlemen Decoction (*sì jūn zǐ tāng*) is used when diarrhea and vomiting are the main symptoms or for chronic cough with copious sputum due to Lung deficiency. This is known as 'cultivating the earth [Spleen] to generate metal [Lungs].' It achieves its effect by focusing on the ascending and downward-directing functions of the greater yin, tonifying the qi to raise the clear yang, and eliminating turbid yin by promoting the water metabolism.

The use of Platycodi Radix (*jié gěng*) in the formula is particularly important in this respect and has been hugely influential on subsequent generations of physicians. Its action is described in *Feng's Secret Records from the Brocade Purse*: "Platycodi Radix (*jié gěng*) enters the Lungs. It can ascend as well as direct [the qi] downward. Consequently, it connects the qi of heaven with the pathways of the earth so that one need not worry about obstruction." The same sentiments are echoed by Wang Ang in *Medical Formulas Collected and Analyzed*: "Platycodi Radix (*jié gěng*) is sweet and bitter, entering the Lungs. It is able to carry all herbs upward to float. It also can connect the qi of heaven with the pathways of the earth, allowing the qi to ascend and descend, augmenting as well as harmonizing [the qi dynamic]." Said to be "like a boat that can lift other herbs upward" so as to focus the action of the entire formula on the upper burner, Platycodi Radix (*jié gěng*) thus enhances the effectiveness of the formula in two important ways. First, it directs qi tonification toward the Lungs, where it more effectively moves the qi and thereby the fluids within the body. Second, by focusing the formula's action on the upper burner, it facilitates the ascent of the clear yang. When the clear yang rises, the turbid yin naturally descends. Were this focus lacking, the many dampness-draining herbs in the formula might readily further imbalance the functions of an already weakened middle burner. But in combination with Platycodi Radix (*jié gěng*), they guide out dampness without injuring the qi.

The formula's focus on preserving as well as augmenting the qi is underscored by the inclusion of Dioscoreae Rhizoma (*shān yào*) and Nelumbinis Semen (*lián zǐ*) as deputies. Dioscoreae Rhizoma (*shān yào*) not only tonifies the qi of the Spleen and Lungs, but also that of the Kidneys, enhancing their function of securing and holding. It is a major herb for

the treatment of diarrhea, urinary frequency, and spermatorrhea. Similarly, Nelumbinis Semen (*lián zǐ*) tonifies the Spleen and Kidneys to stop the diarrhea and stabilize the essence. Thus, even as it drains turbid dampness, the formula prevents the leaking of yin essences. For this reason, this formula is traditionally prescribed to treat diarrhea at the onset of menstrual flow, or leukorrhea (considered by many to indicate a leaking of essences) in relatively obese women with edema and other signs of Spleen deficiency with dampness. More recently, this usage has been expanded to the treatment of chronic proteinuria in patients with edema and signs of qi deficiency. Given its emphasis on the use of bland and neutral rather than acrid and warm herbs, some physicians go even further and view the formula as tonifying not just the Spleen qi, but also the Spleen yin. The contemporary physician Ding Xue-Ping explains:

> The Ming writer Hu Shen-Rou states in *Five Texts by [Hu] Shen-Rou*: '[Herbs with a] bland [flavor] nourish the Stomach qi, [those] that are slightly sweet nourish the Spleen yin. This is the secret of success in treating deficiency and consumption (癆 *láo*).' Whoever has not fully comprehended the secret to the successful recovery from deficiency and injury can arrive there [by way of these words]. The nature and taste of Ginseng Radix (*rén shēn*), Atractylodis macrocephalae Rhizoma (*bái zhú*), Poria (*fú líng*), and Glycyrrhizae Radix (*gān cǎo*) are balanced. Calmly and gently, they augment the qi to strengthen the Spleen. Lablab Semen album (*bái biǎn dòu*), Dioscoreae Rhizoma (*shān yào*), Nelumbinis Semen (*lián zǐ*), and Coicis Semen (*yì yǐ rén*) all have a sweet and bland flavor. They are excellent [herbs] for nourishing the Spleen yin. After any illness or after birth when the body is deficient and has not recovered [its former strength], or where the Spleen yin has been damaged by vomiting or diarrhea, administering [this formula] is always appropriate. [The composition of this formula] truly helps us comprehend the basic principle of deficiency, and is a guide to treating harm.

Comparisons

➤ Vs. FOUR-GENTLEMEN DECOCTION (*sì jūn zǐ tāng*)

Both formulas tonify the qi and strengthen the Spleen. The difference is that Four-Gentlemen Decoction (*sì jūn zǐ tāng*) focuses solely on those functions, while this formula also harmonizes the Stomach, leaches out dampness, and tonifies the Lungs. It is thus especially suited for the treatment of chronic diarrhea or other kinds of leakage due to Spleen deficiency and dampness.

➤ Vs. SIX-GENTLEMEN DECOCTION (*liù jūn zǐ tāng*)

Both formulas treat Spleen deficiency complicated by the presence of phlegm-dampness. Each can be said to embody the principle of 'cultivating the earth [Spleen] to generate metal [Lungs].' However, Six-Gentlemen Decoction (*liù jūn zǐ tāng*) contains Pinelliae Rhizoma praeparatum (*zhì bàn xià*) and Citri reticulatae Pericarpium (*chén pí*), both relatively acrid and drying herbs. It is thus better at drying dampness and transforming phlegm. This formula, on the other hand, contains bland and sweet herbs that promote water metabolism and secure the essence. It is thus better at treating chronic deficiency disorders characterized by loss of essence or damage to the yin.

➤ Vs. Important Formula for Painful Diarrhea (tòng xiè yào fāng)

Both are important formulas for treating diarrhea, but they can be differentiated in terms of their focus on excess versus deficiency. Important Formula for Painful Diarrhea (tòng xiè yào fāng) treats patterns where Liver wood excess overcomes Spleen earth. This is characterized by painful diarrhea, often triggered by stress. Ginseng, Poria, and White Atractylodes Powder (shēn líng bái zhú sǎn) treats patterns of deficiency where Spleen earth is encumbered by phlegm-dampness. Here, the stools will be soft or even contain phlegm, and the symptoms are aggravated by dietary irregularities or exhaustion.

➤ Vs. Four-Miracle Pill (sì shén wán); see PAGE 431.

➤ Vs. Harmonize the Six Decoction (liù hé tāng); see PAGE 696

Biomedical Indications

With the appropriate presentation, this formula may be used to treat a wide variety of biomedically-defined disorders including chronic gastritis and enteritis, gastrointestinal side effects of chemotherapy and radiation therapy, irritable bowel syndrome, chronic hepatitis, chronic bronchitis, chronic nephritis, various forms of anemia, diabetes mellitus, malabsorption syndromes, and malnutrition (especially in children).

Alternate names

White Atractylodes Powder to Regulate the Source (bái zhú tiáo yuán sǎn) in Complete Collection on Pox and Rashes; Ginseng and White Atractylodes Drink (shēn zhú yǐn) in Comprehensive Medicine According to Master Zhang; White Atractylodes Powder (bái zhú sǎn) in Nationwide Collection of TCM Patent Formulas

Modifications

- For coughing up copious, watery sputum with generalized weakness and a stifling sensation in the chest, add Citri reticulatae Pericarpium (chén pí), Pinelliae Rhizoma praeparatum (zhì bàn xià), and Armeniacae Semen (xìng rén).
- For interior cold with abdominal pain, add Zingiberis Rhizoma (gān jiāng) and Cinnamomi Cortex (ròu guì).
- For reduced appetite, add Crataegi Fructus (shān zhā), Massa medicata fermentata (shén qū), and Hordei Fructus germinatus (mài yá).

- For childhood nutritional impairment, remove Platycodi Radix (jié gěng) and add Gigeriae galli Endothelium corneum (jī nèi jīn).
- For a dusky-yellow color of the skin and eyes with lethargy, focal distention in the epigastrium, pain in the hypochondria, and nausea, add Frigid Extremities Powder (sì nì sǎn).
- For postpartum fever with spontaneous sweating, add Tangkuei Decoction to Tonify the Blood (dāng guī bǔ xuè tāng).
- For diabetes mellitus, add Astragali Radix (huáng qí), Schisandrae Fructus (wǔ wèi zǐ), and Gigeriae galli Endothelium corneum (jī nèi jīn).
- For chronic proteinuria accompanied by edema of the legs and signs of Spleen deficiency, add Astragali Radix (huáng qí).

Variation

參苓白朮散（参苓白术散）

Ginseng, Poria, and White Atractylodes Powder from *Medical Formulas Collected and Analyzed*

shēn líng bái zhú sǎn

Source   *Medical Formulas Collected and Analyzed* (1682)

Add Citri reticulatae Pericarpium (chén pí) to strengthen the formula's ability to benefit the Spleen and expel dampness.

Associated Formulas

七味白朮散

Seven-Ingredient Powder with White Atractylodes

qī wèi bái zhú sǎn

Source   *Craft of Medicinal Treatment for Childhood Disease Patterns* (1119)

Ginseng Radix (rén shēn) 7.5g
Atractylodis macrocephalae Rhizoma (bái zhú) 15g
Poria (fú líng) 15g
Glycyrrhizae Radix praeparata (zhì gān cǎo) 3g
Aucklandiae Radix (mù xiāng) 6g
Pogostemonis/Agastaches Folium (huò xiāng yè) 15g
Puerariae Radix (gé gēn) 15-30g

At present, Codonopsis Radix (dǎng shēn) is usually substituted for Ginseng Radix (rén shēn), at 2-3 times its dosage. Strengthens the Spleen and stops diarrhea. For persistent vomiting and diarrhea due to Spleen and Stomach deficiency. The long-term reduction in food intake leads to exhaustion of the essence and fluids with emaciation, which in turn leads to severe thirst, irritability, and in extreme cases, seizures. The author of this formula, Qian Yi, regarded it as particularly effective in treating this problem in children. The use of Puerariae Radix (gé gēn) is said to stimulate, or literally 'drum and dance' (鼓舞 gǔ wǔ), the Stomach qi upward to help stop the diarrhea. As much as 30g of this ingredient may be used if there is thirst.

保胎資生丸（保胎资生丸）

Protect the Fetus and Aid Life Pill

bǎo tāi zī shēng wán

SOURCE *Extensive Notes on Medicine from the First-Awakened Studio* (1613)

Ginseng Radix (*rén shēn*)..........................90g
Atractylodis macrocephalae Rhizoma (*bái zhú*)..........90
Poria (*fú líng*)..........................45g
Citri reticulatae Pericarpium (*chén pí*)..........60g
Crataegi Fructus (*shān zhā*)..........60g
Glycyrrhizae Radix praeparata (*zhì gān cǎo*)..........15g
dry-fried Dioscoreae Rhizoma (*chǎo shān yào*)..........45g
dry-fried Coptidis Rhizoma (*chǎo huáng lián*)..........9g
dry-fried Coicis Semen (*chǎo yì yǐ rén*)..........45g
dry-fried Lablab Semen album (*chǎo biǎn dòu*)..........45g
Amomi Fructus rotundus (*bái dòu kòu*)..........10.5g
Pogostemonis/Agastaches Folium (*huò xiāng yè*)..........15g
dry-fried Nelumbinis Semen (*chǎo lián ròu*)..........45g
dry-fried Alismatis Rhizoma (*chǎo zé xiè*)..........10.5g
Platycodi Radix (*jié gěng*)..........15g
dry-fried Euryales Semen (*chǎo qiàn shí*)..........45g
dry-fried Hordei Fructus germinatus (*chǎo mài yá*)..........30g

Form the ingredients into pills with honey and take in 6g doses. At present, Codonopsis Radix (*dǎng shēn*) or Pseudostellariae Radix (*tài zǐ shēn*) is usually substituted for Ginseng Radix (*rén shēn*) at 2-3 times its dosage. When taken as a decoction, dosages are reduced by approximately 90 percent. Augments the qi, strengthens the Spleen, harmonizes the Stomach, and calms a restless fetus. For morning sickness or threatened miscarriage in women with deficient Spleen qi together with qi stagnation. The source text notes that because the yang brightness channel nourishes the fetus, when it is weak (especially in the first trimester), the fetus is deprived of nourishment, which can lead to miscarriage. The use of this formula has been expanded to include deficiency of the Spleen and Stomach with concurrent damp-heat characterized by a reduced appetite, diarrhea, weakness, and weight loss.

補中益氣湯（补中益气汤）

Tonify the Middle to Augment the Qi Decoction

bǔ zhōng yì qì tāng

Source *Clarifying Doubts about Damage from Internal and External Causes* (1247)

The name of the formula indicates that tonification of the middle burner qi is placed at the service of augmenting the qi dynamic. More generally, as pointed out by Wang Zi-Jie in *Selected Annotations to Ancient Formulas from the Garden of Crimson Snow*:

[Analyzing the composition of] this formula, it turns out that its particular emphasis lies not in tonifying the Spleen and Liver … but that its significance lies in … raising and lifting the clear yang qi and promoting the revolving movement of the middle [burner]. Hence, it is not merely called 'tonify the middle' but [the author] additionally explained that it augments the qi.

Astragali Radix (*huáng qí*)..........3g (12-24g)
Ginseng Radix (*rén shēn*)..........0.9g (9-12g)
Atractylodis macrocephalae Rhizoma (*bái zhú*)..........0.9g (9-12g)
Glycyrrhizae Radix praeparata (*zhì gān cǎo*)..........1.5g (3-6g)
wine-washed Angelicae sinensis Radix (*jiǔ xǐ dāng guī*) 6g (6-12g)
Citri reticulatae Pericarpium (*chén pí*)..........0.9g (6-9g)
Cimicifugae Rhizoma (*shēng má*)..........0.9g (3-6g)
Bupleuri Radix (*chái hú*)..........0.9g (3-9g)

Method of Preparation The source text advises to coarsely grind the ingredients and prepare as a decoction by cooking 2 bowls of liquid down to 1 (if the patient is weak, use smaller bowls). Take the strained liquid warm between meals. At present, it is usually prepared as a decoction with the larger dosage specified in parentheses. Also, Codonopsis Radix (*dǎng shēn*) is usually substituted for Ginseng Radix (*rén shēn*) at 2-3 times its dosage.

Actions Tonifies the middle burner, augments the qi, raises the yang, and lifts what has sunken

Indications

This formula is used to treat three different patterns that may occur alone or in conjunction with each other.

The first is Spleen and Stomach deficiency with inability to raise the clear characterized by dizziness, unsteadiness, impaired or unclear vision, deafness, tinnitus, shortness of breath, laconic speech, a weak voice, a shiny, pale complexion, reduced intake of food, loose stools, a pale tongue, and a frail pulse.

The second is qi deficiency fever. Typically, this manifests as intermittent fever that worsens upon exertion, spontaneous sweating, aversion to cold, a thirst for warm beverages, a pale and swollen tongue, and a large but forceless pulse.

The third is sinking of the middle burner qi characterized by hemorrhoids, rectal or uterine prolapse, prolapse of the internal organs, chronic diarrhea or dysentery, irregular uterine bleeding, reduced intake of food, loose stools, a pale tongue, and a deficient and soft pulse.

The food assimilated by the Spleen and Stomach nourishes the various organs and structures of the body. Hence, they are referred to as "the root of the postnatal constitution, the source of generation and transformation of the nutritive and protective [qi], of qi and blood." Raising the clear essence of food and drink to the upper burner, while directing the turbid waste products downward to the lower burner, the Spleen and Stomach serve as the fulcrum for the entire qi dynamic. Thus, failure of the Spleen to raise the refined essences (the clear yang) means that the turbid yin cannot be directed downward. This leads to obstruction of the sensory orifices (related to the upper burner) causing such symptoms as dizziness, unsteadiness, impaired or unclear vision, deafness, and tinnitus. The laconic speech, weak voice, and shiny, pale complexion indicate that the Lung qi of the upper burner is not nourished by the essences from the middle burner.

Reduced intake of food, loose stools, a pale tongue, and a frail pulse identify this as a pattern of middle burner deficiency and distinguish it from patterns of excess that manifest with similar symptoms (such as obstruction of the sensory orifices by phlegm-dampness or static blood).

As the foundation of the postnatal constitution, the qi of the middle burner supports the circulation of all the qi throughout the body. This includes the upward and outward diffusion of protective yang from the gate of vitality in the lower burner as well as the circulation of gathering qi controlled by the Lungs in the upper burner. If production of qi in the middle burner fails, the upward movement of protective yang is constrained, resulting in intermittent fever that worsens whenever extra demands are placed on the body. Failure of the protective yang to circulate in the superficial levels of the body between the interstices and pores manifests as aversion to cold that can be alleviated by wearing more clothing. This distinguishes it from the aversion to cold due to externally-contracted disorders, which is not as easily alleviated. Spontaneous sweating and thirst for warm beverages indicate failure of the Lung qi to control the circulation of fluids. The pale and swollen tongue reflects the stagnation of fluids and the deficiency of qi that characterize this pattern. A large but forceless pulse (which appears to be flooding but disappears with pressure) indicates that the nutritive qi of the middle burner has lost its ability to fill and restrain the pulse.

Hemorrhoids, prolapse of the uterus, bowel, or other internal organs, chronic diarrhea, irregular uterine bleeding and similar symptoms indicate that the Spleen qi has lost its ability to hold things in place. This is known as 'sinking of the middle burner qi.' Typically, there will also be other symptoms of qi deficiency such as reduced intake of food, loose stools, a pale tongue, and a deficient and soft pulse.

Analysis of Formula

The chief herb, Astragali Radix (huáng qí), strongly augments the qi (particularly its superficial aspects) and raises the yang qi of the Spleen and Stomach. It thereby addresses the root of the patterns treated by this formula, while also preventing further loss of qi through leakage to the outside. This was emphasized by Li Dong-Yuan, the author of the formula: "In any deficiency of Spleen and Stomach the Lung qi is the first to be cut off [because it is the child of earth]. Therefore, I use Astragali Radix (huáng qí) in order to augment the skin and body hair and close the pores and interstices and not let spontaneous sweating [further] harm the primal qi." The deputy herbs, Ginseng Radix (rén shēn) (or Codonopsis Radix [dǎng shēn]), Atractylodis macrocephalae Rhizoma (bái zhú), and Glycyrrhizae Radix praeparata (zhì gān cǎo), are sweet and warm and tonify the qi of the middle burner. For a discussion of the interactions of these herbs, the reader is referred to Four-Gentlemen Decoction (sì jūn zǐ tāng) above.

There are two assistant herbs. The first is Angelicae sinensis Radix (dāng guī), which tonifies the qi in the blood. It works synergistically with the qi-tonifying herbs in this formula (especially the chief herb) to augment the qi by invigorating the blood. It also moistens and fills the blood, thereby preventing the warming and drying qi tonics from damaging the yin. The second assistant is Citri reticulatae Pericarpium (chén pí), which regulates the qi. Its use in this formula is twofold: it facilitates digestion of the tonifying herbs (which are quite rich and cloying) and thereby increases their effectiveness; and its qi-regulating properties contribute slightly to the qi-raising action of the formula. The envoys, Cimicifugae Rhizoma (shēng má) and Bupleuri Radix (chái hú), are generally believed to help raise the sunken yang qi, especially in conjunction with the chief herb. Their precise action, however, has been the subject of considerable debate, as described in the COMMENTARY below.

Cautions and Contraindications

This formula is contraindicated for fever due to heat from yin deficiency or for excess disorders caused by the contraction of external pathogens. It is also contraindicated for patterns rooted in deficiency of the lower base. This has been summed up in the Ming text *Discussion of Famous Physicians' Formulas Past and Present*:

> [The indications of this formula] refer to sinking of the clear yang. They do not refer to deficiency of the lower burner where the clear yang [is unable] to rise. If one raises [the qi] even more, when a person's proximal pulses are both deficient and faint, when kidney water is consumed, or when the fire at the gate of vitality is feeble, then this is like shaking a big tree by grasping it at its roots.

It should also be remembered that this formula is not indicated in all instances of prolapse, but only in those due to qi deficiency.

Commentary

This is the most famous formula composed by Li Dong-Yuan (also known as Li Gao), one of the four great masters of the Jin-Yuan era. Li Dong-Yuan is widely regarded as the founder of the 'tonify the earth current' (補土派 bǔ tǔ paì) in Chinese medicine, and Tonify the Middle to Augment the Qi Decoction (bǔ zhōng yì qì tāng) duly reflects the central importance its author attributed to the functions of the Spleen and Stomach. It has had a far-reaching influence on the development of Chinese medicine, with whole schools of practice based on this single formula. Yet the wider concerns and world views that distinguish Jin-Yuan medicine from previous periods in the history of Chinese medicine are just as important in understanding the principles of practice embodied in this formula's composition. These include a focus on the raising and downward-directing of qi in the body, and a concern with fire as both physiological function and pathological agent.

Not surprisingly given the popularity of this formula, there has been much discussion regarding its precise mode of action, its indications and contraindications. The ambivalent wording of the source text, always a factor in Chinese medical debates but particularly pronounced in the case of Li Dong-Yuan's writings, means that these discussions can never be truly closed. Thus, while there is no final word on this formula, here is our attempt to cut through the thicket of diverse opinions informed by a wide reading of these debates.

Treatment of Yin Fire

Because the first text in which this formula occurs is *Clarifying Doubts about Damage from Internal and External Causes*, it is, above all, a formula for the treatment of fevers that arise from a dysfunction of the yin and yang organs in the interior or yin aspect of the body, and not from the penetration of pathogenic cold into the exterior or yang aspect of the body. In the opinion of Ding Guang-Di, a modern expert on Jin-Yuan medicine, this is the true meaning of the term 'yin fire' (陰火 *yīn huǒ*). In Li Dong-Yuan's thinking, this usually involves deficiency of qi, specifically the failure of the middle burner to manage the qi. This function includes both the ascent of clear yang from the lower burner *and* the ability of qi at the surface to contain the qi and thereby help move it downward. Although it is the former function that has received most attention, the latter was also clearly important to Li Dong-Yuan, as becomes apparent when we examine the entire family of formulas he built around Astragali Radix (*huáng qí*).

The clear yang is normally distributed throughout the body via the lesser yang (which encompasses the Gallbladder, Triple Burner, and, in some readings, also the Liver), a system to which Li Dong-Yuan attributes as much importance as he does to the functions of the Spleen and Stomach. The yang qi, by its very nature, is hot. When it stagnates, symptoms of heat or fever arise. Being yang in nature, the tendency of such heat is to move outward and upward, leading to symptoms of apparent excess such as fever, dizziness, headache, tinnitus, or panting. These are exacerbated by deficiency of qi in the exterior, which fails to direct fire downward. Overall, therefore, the symptom picture may resemble that caused by the penetration of external pathogens. On closer inspection, however, it is found to be distinctly different.

First, many of the signs and symptoms among the indications for this formula have an on-again, off-again nature and are brought on by exertion. This is because the extent of injury to the qi in this condition does not always prevent the clear yang from rising. This is different from the on/off nature of symptoms in a lesser yang-stage disorder, which come and go irrespective of energy levels. It is also completely different from greater yang and yang brightness fevers, which never

abate, and from the false heat of yang deficiency, which is accompanied by signs of true cold.

Second, because they are signs of yin fire, yang symptoms such as fever, headache, dizziness, palpitations, tinnitus, and so on will tend to manifest in a yin manner: the palms of the hands and feet will tend to be hotter than the exterior surface; the pulse will be large but forceless; fever will be accompanied by sweating and an aversion to cold; headache is aggravated by exertion, and so on.

Third, although signs of yin fire may be the most obvious or troublesome to a patient, they are never more than manifestations.

Other Indications

Failure of the middle burner qi to facilitate raising the clear yang is the root of all patterns treated by this formula. Thus, it also can be used to treat patterns characterized by the sinking of middle burner qi, but without any obvious signs of yin fire. In clinical practice, such patterns may be subdivided into four groups:

- Failure of middle burner qi to assist the spreading of protective qi in the upper burner, leading to instability of the exterior characterized by aversion to cold, spontaneous sweating, and a proclivity toward catching colds or other infections

- Failure of middle burner qi to contain essences, manifesting as bleeding (particularly from the lower part of the body), diarrhea, urinary incontinence, premature ejaculation, etc.

- Failure of middle burner qi to facilitate uplifting, manifesting as abdominal bloating, constipation, urinary obstruction, or prolapse of internal organs

- Failure of middle burner qi to lift the yang that leads to turbid yin not being directed downward, which in turn leads to obstruction of the sensory orifices characterized by such symptoms as tinnitus, visual disturbances, or dizziness

All the symptoms tend to be chronic and are accompanied by signs of middle burner qi deficiency.

The strategy Li Dong-Yuan devised to deal with the problem of yin fire is widely known as 'eliminating heat with sweet and warming herbs' (甘溫除熱 *gān wēn chú rè*). The source text is somewhat more specific: "[To treat] disorders [characterized by] internal damage and insufficiency … one should use sweet and warming formulas. By tonifying the middle [burner of such patients], raising their yang, and draining fire with sweet and cooling [substances,] they will be cured." There has been considerable debate among later commentators about the extent to which this statement of intent is reflected in the composition of Tonify the Middle to Augment the Qi Decoction (*bǔ zhōng yì qì tāng*) and its many modifications and variants.

Debates over Composition and Mode of Action

In *Discussion of the Spleen and Stomach* by the same author, it is noted that Astragali Radix *(huáng qí)*, Ginseng Radix *(rén shēn)*, and Glycyrrhizae Radix *(gān cǎo)* "are sagely herbs for eliminating damp-heat and irritability heat." The source text for the formula states that Atractylodis macrocephalae Rhizoma *(bái zhú)* "eliminates heat from the Stomach and promotes blood in between the lower back and umbilicus." Based on these statements, some writers have imputed a direct heat-clearing action into these qi-tonifying herbs. However, given their warming nature, this view is rejected by the majority of commentators who regard the qi-tonifying herbs as addressing the root of the disorder while the heat and fever are eliminated by one or more of three other groups of herbs regularly deployed by Li Dong-Yuan: acrid herbs that raise the yang; moistening herbs that tonify the blood and yin; and bitter, cooling herbs that drain fire.

Acrid herbs that raise the yang are also known as 'wind herbs' (風藥 *fēng yaò*). In Tonify the Middle to Augment the Qi Decoction *(bǔ zhōng yì qì tāng)*, these are represented by Bupleuri Radix *(chái hú)* and Cimicifugae Rhizoma *(shēng má)*, both of which are also cooling and thus directly address the yin fire from constraint. In other formulas by Li Dong-Yuan that embody the same principles of composition, herbs such as Puerariae Radix *(gé gēn)*, Saposhnikoviae Radix *(fáng fēng)*, Angelicae pubescentis Radix *(dú huó)*, or Notopterygii Rhizoma seu Radix *(qiāng huó)* are used to achieve a similar effect. Acrid and warming in nature, these herbs open constraint and thereby facilitate the unhindered movement of the yang qi. Because it is in the nature of yang qi to move upward, one can assume that the primary function of these wind herbs is to unblock the qi dynamic rather than directly cause the qi to ascend.

Tonify the Middle to Augment the Qi Decoction *(bǔ zhōng yì qì tāng)* contains Angelicae sinensis Radix *(dāng guī)* to tonify the blood. In related formulas, Li Dong-Yuan uses similar herbs, such as Paeoniae Radix alba *(bái sháo)*, Ophiopogonis Radix *(mài mén dōng)*, Asparagi Radix *(tiān mén dōng)*, and Rehmanniae Radix *(shēng dì huáng)*. If the middle burner qi is insufficient, the production of blood and body fluids will be impeded. Heat, which consumes yin, and the loss of essences due to qi deficiency further aggravate this condition. Including moistening, yin-tonifying herbs as assistants effectively deals with this secondary disease dynamic. However, due to their cloying nature, their dosage should be kept to a minimum.

There are no bitter, cooling herbs in Tonify the Middle to Augment the Qi Decoction *(bǔ zhōng yì qì tāng)*. The source text states, however, that "a small [amount may] be added" (少加 *shǎo jiā*) if this seems to be indicated. Formulas like Tonify Spleen-Stomach, Drain Yin Fire, and Raise Yang Decoction *(bǔ pí wèi xiè yīn huǒ shēng yáng tāng)*, Raise the

Yang and Augment the Stomach Decoction *(shēng yáng yì wèi tāng)*, or Augment the Qi and Increase Acuity Decoction *(yì qì cōng míng tāng)*, discussed later in this chapter, contain these herbs as core ingredients. Unlike the acrid herbs that clear heat from constraint and facilitate the qi dynamic, bitter and cooling herbs drain excess and impede the ascent of yang. For this reason, their use is generally contraindicated in patterns where the sinking of qi is a root problem. Yet, because deficiency of the middle burner qi causes all kinds of transformative processes in the body to work less effectively, excess heat can arise as a secondary problem. This can manifest as damp-heat (particularly in the middle or lower burners, but also in the joints, muscles, and exterior of the body), as Heart fire (when the Heart qi is not sufficiently strong to guide fire downward), or as phlegm-heat (particularly in the Stomach, where it arises from undigested food). In these cases, the use of bitter, cooling herbs may become necessary to effectively deal with such secondary manifestations. They are not, however, essential ingredients of Tonify the Middle to Augment the Qi Decoction *(bǔ zhōng yì qì tāng)*.

Qi deficiency of the middle burner readily gives rise to dampness, which further aggravates the constraint that leads to yin fire. Thus many variations of Tonify the Middle to Augment the Qi Decoction *(bǔ zhōng yì qì tāng)* also contain herbs that aromatically transform and dry dampness, or that promote water metabolism and leach out dampness. Because many of these herbs direct the qi downward, they too should be used judiciously and added only if warranted by the presentation.

Influence of the Formula on the Development of Chinese Medicine

The influence of this formula on the development of Chinese medicine goes far beyond its clinical application, however. Zhu Dan-Xi considered Li Dong-Yuan to be the first physician to establish a framework for discussing disorders due to internal damage (i.e., deficiency disorders). His own concerns regarding the treatment of yin deficiency and yang excess are directly influenced by Li Dong-Yuan's doctrine of yin fire. During the Ming dynasty, physicians like Xue Ji, Li Zhong-Zi, Wang Ken-Tang, and Zhang Jie-Bin were guided by Li Dong-Yuan's emphasis on promoting the function of yang qi in their development of the current of warm tonification (溫補學派 *wēn bǔ xué paì*). Li Dong-Yuan directly influenced the development of the doctrines on the pathology and treatment of ancestral qi by the early 20th-century physician Zhang Xi-Chun. Such widespread influence naturally led to excesses, and the indiscriminate use of acrid and warming herbs by physicians claiming to be Li Dong-Yuan's acolytes was duly criticized by commentators like Ye Tian-Shi. Yet even he noted that "No one expounded on the Spleen and Stomach like Li Dong-Yuan."

Note that although the formula is widely considered to stem from *Discussion of the Spleen and Stomach*, it is also listed in a slightly earlier book by Li Dong-Yuan, *Clarifying Doubts about Damage from Internal and External Causes*. This title is now viewed as the source text.

Comparisons

➤ Vs. Four-Gentlemen Decoction *(sì jūn zǐ tāng)*

Both of these formulas treat deficiency of the middle burner manifesting with symptoms such as fatigue, pallor, lack of appetite, and diarrhea. The main difference is that Four-Gentlemen Decoction *(sì jūn zǐ tāng)* focuses primarily on tonifying the transportive and transformative functions of the Spleen and Stomach. Tonify the Middle to Augment the Qi Decoction *(bǔ zhōng yì qì tāng)*, on the other hand, focuses on the qi dynamic, augmenting the power of the qi to lift the yang and direct the turbid yin downward. It is thus better suited for treating patterns characterized by the downward sinking of qi, such as various types of prolapse, incontinence, or heavy menstruation; by heat from constraint, such as deficient fevers or chronic inflammatory conditions; or by failure of the qi and turbid yin to be directed downward, leading to such symptoms as headache, dizziness, and tinnitus.

These differences are crucially reflected in the pulse and complexion. Middle burner qi deficiency, for which Four-Gentlemen Decoction *(sì jūn zǐ tāng)* is indicated, is typically accompanied by a frail pulse and a pale and wan complexion. The pulse in patterns for which Tonify the Middle to Augment the Qi Decoction *(bǔ zhōng yì qì tāng)* is indicated is typically large and deficient, indicating the upward and outward movement of yang that cannot be contained by deficient qi. The complexion tends to be pale and shiny, again reflecting the combination of internal deficiency and external excess.

➤ Vs. Raise the Sunken Decoction *(shēng xiàn tāng)*

Both of these formulas are used to treat patterns of deficiency characterized by the downward sinking of qi. Tonify the Middle to Augment the Qi Decoction *(bǔ zhōng yì qì tāng)* focuses on the middle burner and enhances the Spleen's ability to contain essences by lifting the qi. It is thus used for prolapse, incontinence, and bleeding from the lower body. Raise the Sunken Decoction *(shēng xiàn tāng)*, on the other hand, focuses on the gathering qi of the upper burner. The function of the gathering qi is to invigorate and move. For this reason, this formula is indicated for patterns of severe qi deficiency characterized by loss of dynamic functions anywhere in the body, and particularly those relating to cardiovascular function. These include dyspnea, wheezing and panting, aversion to cold, or chills alternating with fever, palpitations, and signs of spirit disturbances ranging from lack of concentration to loss of consciousness.

Here, too, the pulse is an important sign in differentiating the two formulas. While the pulse in Tonify the Middle to Augment the Qi Decoction *(bǔ zhōng yì qì tāng)* presentations is typically large and deficient, particularly in the middle position, in patterns for which Raise the Sunken Decoction *(shēng xiàn tāng)* is indicated, it will be deep, slow, and weak, particularly in the proximal position, or characterized by severe irregularities that make it difficult to define a clear pattern.

➤ Vs. Restore the Spleen Decoction *(guī pí tāng)*; *see* PAGE 354

➤ Vs. Six-Ingredient Pill with Rehmannia *(liù wèi dì huáng wán); see* PAGE 367

➤ Vs. Minor Construct the Middle Decoction *(xiǎo jiàn zhōng tāng); see* PAGE 266

Biomedical Indications

With the appropriate presentation, this formula may be used to treat a wide variety of biomedically-defined disorders. These can be divided into the following groups:

- Those marked by signs of heat such as fever of unknown origin, chronic hepatitis, various types of arrhythmias, hypertension, chronic bronchitis, chronic rhinitis, apthous ulcers, chronic laryngitis, and the side effects of radiation treatments
- Those related to a slackening of muscles or other tissues such as uterine prolapse, prolapsed rectum, gastroptosis, hernias, stress incontinence, myasthenia gravis, primary hypotension, and constipation due to decreased peristalsis
- Those related to flow of turbid substances in the lower parts of the body, including dysfunctional uterine bleeding, leukorrhea, and chyluria.

This formula has also been used in the treatment of many other conditions such as postpartum problems (including urinary incontinence, lochioschesis, and insufficient lactation), recurrent miscarriages, infertility in both men and women, corneal ulcers, cerebral arteriosclerosis, Alzheimer's disease, pernicious anemia, paralytic strabismus leukopenia, chronic nephritis, the side effects of immunosuppressive treatment, and as a general adaptogen.

Alternate name

King of Medicine Decoction *(yī wáng tāng)* in *Rhymed Formula Mnemonics*

Modifications

- For abdominal pain, increase the dosage of Glycyrrhizae Radix praeparata *(zhì gān cǎo)* and add Paeoniae Radix alba *(bái sháo)*. (source text)

- For pronounced aversion to cold, add Cinnamomi Cortex (*ròu guì*). (source text)

- For pronounced headache, add Viticis Fructus (*màn jīng zǐ*). If it becomes severe, also add Chuanxiong Rhizoma (*chuān xiōng*). (source text)

- For headache at the vertex or pain inside the head, add Ligustici Rhizoma (*gǎo běn*). (source text)

- For severe pain, add Asari Radix et Rhizoma (*xì xīn*). (source text)

- For generalized pain or a sensation of heaviness in the body (both of which are due to dampness), take with Five-Ingredient Powder with Poria (*wǔ líng sǎn*) and remove Cinnamomi Ramulus (*guì zhī*). (source text)

- For diarrhea due to excessive deliberation, add Aucklandiae Radix (*mù xiāng*).

- For vertigo and headache, add Chuanxiong Rhizoma (*chuān xiōng*) and Pinelliae Rhizoma praeparatum (*zhì bàn xià*).

- For tinnitus and diminished hearing due to qi deficiency (with a relatively low pitch to the ringing), add Corni Fructus (*shān zhū yú*) and Alpiniae oxyphyllae Fructus (*yì zhì rén*).

- For diminished visual acuity or double vision, add Lycii Fructus (*gǒu qǐ zǐ*) and Chuanxiong Rhizoma (*chuān xiōng*).

- For recurrent miscarriage, add Eucommiae Cortex (*dù zhòng*) and Cuscutae Semen (*tù sī zǐ*).

- For leukorrhea, add Atractylodis Rhizoma (*cāng zhú*) and Phellodendri Cortex (*huáng bǎi*).

- For abdominal distention, add Aurantii Fructus immaturus (*zhǐ shí*), Magnoliae officinalis Cortex (*hòu pò*), Aucklandiae Radix (*mù xiāng*), and Amomi Fructus (*shā rén*).

- For bulging disorders, add Citri reticulatae Semen (*jú hé*), Foeniculi Fructus (*xiǎo huí xiāng*), and Litchi Semen (*lì zhī hé*).

- For constipation due to Spleen deficiency, add honey and sesame oil.

- For painful urinary difficulty in the elderly due to sunken yang qi, add Alismatis Rhizoma (*zé xiè*) and Akebiae Caulis (*mù tōng*).

- For premenstrual diarrhea, add Zingiberis Rhizoma praeparatum (*páo jiāng*) and Coptidis Rhizoma (*huáng lián*).

- For enuresis in children, add Mantidis Oötheca (*sāng piāo xiāo*) and Alpiniae oxyphyllae Fructus (*yì zhì rén*).

- For chronic rhinitis, add Xanthii Fructus (*cāng ěr zǐ*) and Magnoliae Flos (*xīn yí huā*).

- For corneal ulcers, add Eriocauli Flos (*gǔ jīng cǎo*), Cassiae Semen (*jué míng zǐ*), and Dioscoreae Rhizoma (*shān yào*).

Associated Formulas

加減補中益氣湯 （加减补中益气汤）
Modified Tonify the Middle to Augment the Qi Decoction
jiā jiǎn bǔ zhōng yì qì tāng

SOURCE *Discussion of the Spleen and Stomach* (13th century)

Astragali Radix (*huáng qí*) 9g
Ginseng Radix (*rén shēn*). 9g
Atractylodis macrocephalae Rhizoma (*bái zhú*). 6g
Glycyrrhizae Radix praeparata (*zhì gān cǎo*). 3g
Citri reticulatae Pericarpium (*chén pí*) 6g
Cimicifugae Rhizoma (*shēng má*) 3g
Bupleuri Radix (*chái hú*) 3g
Asini Corii Colla (*ē jiāo*)
  [dissolve in strained decoction]. 6g
Artemisiae argyi Folium (*ài yè*). 6g

Tonifies the qi, raises the yang, and calms the fetus. For constitutionally weak women in the fourth or fifth month of pregnancy who present with fatigue and lethargy, lower back pain, abdominal distention, excessive or insufficient movement of the fetus, spotting, and a slippery pulse without strength. At present, Codonopsis Radix (*dǎng shēn*) is usually substituted for Ginseng Radix (*rén shēn*) at 2-3 times its dosage.

調中益氣湯 （调中益气汤）
Regulate the Middle to Augment the Qi Decoction
tiáo zhōng yì qì tāng

SOURCE *Discussion of the Spleen and Stomach* (13th century)

Astragali Radix (*huáng qí*). 3g (12-20g)
Ginseng Radix (*rén shēn*). 1.5g (9-12g)
Atractylodis Rhizoma (*cāng zhú*). 1.5g (9-12g)
Glycyrrhizae Radix praeparata (*zhì gān cǎo*). . 1.5g (3-6g)
Aucklandiae Radix (*mù xiāng*). 0.3-0.6g (6-9g)
Citri reticulatae Pericarpium (*chén pí*) 0.6g (6-9g)
Cimicifugae Rhizoma (*shēng má*) 0.6g (3-6g)
Bupleuri Radix (*chái hú*) 0.6g (3-9g)

Leaches out dampness and strengthens the Spleen and Stomach. For a sensation of heaviness in the body, irritability, pain in the joints, difficulty in flexing and extending the joints, loss of appetite, either an inability to rest calmly or hypersomnia, a sensation of fullness in the chest, shortness of breath, a productive cough with sticky sputum, frequent, clear urination, either frequent diarrhea or constipation, and a flooding, moderate, and wiry pulse that is choppy when pressed hard. At present, the dosage specified in parentheses is usually prescribed, and Codonopsis Radix (*dǎng shēn*) is generally substituted for Ginseng Radix (*rén shēn*), at 2-3 times its dosage.

補脾胃瀉陰火升陽湯 （补脾胃泻阴火升阳汤）
Tonify Spleen-Stomach, Drain Yin Fire, and Raise Yang Decoction
bǔ pí wèi xiè yīn huǒ shēng yáng tāng

SOURCE *Discussion of the Spleen and Stomach* (13th century)

Bupleuri Radix (*chái hú*) 45g
Glycyrrhizae Radix praeparata (*zhì gān cǎo*). 30g

Astragali Radix (*huáng qí*) 30g
Atractylodis Rhizoma (*cāng zhú*) 30g
Notopterygii Rhizoma seu Radix (*qiāng huó*) 30g
Cimicifugae Rhizoma (*shēng má*) 24g
Ginseng Radix (*rén shēn*) 21g
Scutellariae Radix (*huáng qín*) 21g
Coptidis Rhizoma (*huáng lián*) . . . . 15g (fried in wine)

Grind the herbs into a fine powder and take 9g as a draft. The source text says to add a small amount of Gypsum fibrosum (*shí gāo*) if the formula is prescribed during the summer. Tonifies the Spleen, augments the qi, lifts the yang and drains fire. For fire constraint and fever due to overeating that has damaged the Stomach or exhaustion that has injured the Spleen. Compared to the principal formula, this variation focuses more strongly on unblocking constraint of the yang qi and directing excess fire downward rather than on tonifying the middle burner. The heat will be so strong that the skin feels burning hot to the touch. Li Dong-Yuan thought that this type of disorder occurs mainly in the spring, when the body's yang qi is strongly rising of its own accord. When the middle burner is weak, the qi loses its ability to manage this upward movement. This leads to constraint, which is resolved by the acrid, opening herbs, but also requires draining downward of excess fire by means of bitter, cooling herbs. This is different from the pattern treated by Tangkuei Decoction to Tonify the Blood (*dāng guī bǔ xuè tāng*), discussed below, which is also characterized by strong heat at the surface, but due to a sudden loss of blood. In that formula, Astragali Radix (*huáng qí*) is employed to strengthen the qi in the exterior so as to facilitate the downward-directing function.

益氣聰明湯 （益气聪明汤）

Augment the Qi and Increase Acuity Decoction

yì qì cōng míng tāng

SOURCE *Dong-Yuan's Tried and Tested Formulas* (1202)

Astragali Radix (*huáng qí*) 15g
Ginseng Radix (*rén shēn*) 15g
Glycyrrhizae Radix (*gān cǎo*) 15g
Cimicifugae Rhizoma (*shēng má*) 9g
Puerariae Radix (*gé gēn*) 9g
Viticis Fructus (*màn jīng zǐ*) 4.5g
Paeoniae Radix (*sháo yào*) 3g
wine-fried Phellodendri Cortex (*jiǔ chǎo huáng bǎi*) 3g

Grind the ingredients into a coarse powder and take 9g doses as a draft. The source text recommends that it be taken warm at bedtime and at daybreak. Strengthens and raises the middle burner qi and improves visual and aural acuity. For long-term deficiency of the middle burner qi that results in pterygium or other obstructive visual disorders, chronic visual disturbances, tinnitus, or hearing loss. At present, Codonopsis Radix (*dǎng shēn*) is usually substituted for Ginseng Radix (*rén shēn*) at 2-3 times its dosage. Most physicians follow *Medical Formulas Collected and Analyzed* in using Paeoniae Radix alba (*bái sháo*). The source text recommends frying Phellodendri Cortex (*huáng bǎi*) in alcohol. The ascending nature of the alcohol focuses the action of the herb on the head. The text also advises to remove this herb from the formula in patients with severe Spleen qi deficiency and to increase its dosage in patients with more severe heat signs or during the hot summer months.

舉元煎 （举元煎）

Lift the Source Decoction

jǔ yuán jiān

SOURCE *Collected Treatises of [Zhang] Jing-Yue* (1624)

honey-prepared Astragali Radix (*mì zhì huáng qí*) 9-15g
Ginseng Radix (*rén shēn*) 9-15g
Glycyrrhizae Radix praeparata (*zhì gān cǎo*) 3-6g
dry-fried Cimicifugae Rhizoma (*chǎo shēng má*) 1.5-2.1g
Atractylodis macrocephalae Rhizoma (*bái zhú*) 3-6g

Tonifies the qi in order to tonify the blood. For collapse due to qi deficiency leading to severe blood loss and devastated yang. Most commonly occurs in women with excessive menstruation or uterine bleeding. The blood is pale and watery and is accompanied by palpitations, shortness or breath, laconic speech, a sinking sensation in the lower abdomen, fatigue, a shiny, pale complexion, a pale tongue with a moist, thin coating, and a deficient, frail, and forceless pulse. The source text recommends adding Cinnamomi Cortex (*ròu guì*), Aconiti Radix lateralis praeparata (*zhì fù zǐ*), and Zingiberis Rhizoma (*gān jiāng*) for signs and symptoms of cold.

This is one of many formulas that demonstrate Li Dong-Yuan's influence on the medical style of Zhang Jie-Bin, and through him, on the development of the current of warming and tonification. What distinguishes this current from Li Dong-Yuan's medicine is its concern for supporting the yang qi at its source in the lower burner, rather than merely raising it by way of the middle burner.

升陷湯 （升陷汤）

Raise the Sunken Decoction

shēng xiàn tāng

SOURCE *Essays on Medicine Esteeming the Chinese and Respecting the Western* (1918-1934)

Astragali Radix (*huáng qí*) 18g
Anemarrhenae Rhizoma (*zhī mǔ*) 9g
Bupleuri Radix (*chái hú*) 4.5g
Platycodi Radix (*jié gěng*) 4.5g
Cimicifugae Rhizoma (*shēng má*) 3g

Augments the qi and raises what is sinking. For sinking of the gathering qi in the chest characterized by shortness of breath, difficult and rapid breathing, and a submerged, slow, and frail pulse. For severe qi deficiency, add Ginseng Radix (*rén shēn*) and Corni Fructus (*shān zhū yú*).

This formula was composed by the early modern physician Zhang Xi-Chun, who extended Li Dong-Yuan's approach to raising the gathering qi to the upper burner. Zhang Xi-Chun argued that the functions of gathering qi, which he called the 'great qi' (大氣 *dà qì*), had been underestimated by physicians throughout the history of Chinese medicine. These functions extended to vitalizing physiological activity throughout the body and all organ systems. Under normal conditions, the gathering qi accumulates in the chest, which is therefore known as the 'upper sea of qi' (上氣海 *shàng qì hǎi*). Chronic diarrhea, an overdose of herbs that break up stagnant qi, overly strenuous activity, major illness, and other factors that exhaust the qi or that direct it excessively downward may diminish the gathering qi in the chest. In these cases, it is essential not merely to tonify the qi, but also to lead it into the chest. This is accomplished by the inclusion of Platycodi Radix (*jié gěng*) in the present formula. Moreover, using Astragali Radix (*huáng qí*) as the only qi-tonifying herb ensures that tonification is entirely focused on the upper burner. Anemarrhenae Rhizoma (*zhī mǔ*) is added as an assistant to counteract the warming nature of Astragali Radix (*huáng qí*) that might otherwise dry the yin fluids of the upper burner.

This is one of Zhang Xi-Chun's most important formulas around which he developed an entirely new approach to treating chronic as well as acute, life-threatening disorders. Zhang Xi-Chun's ideas have exerted an important influence on the development of contemporary Chinese medical practice, and this formula has become important specifically in the treatment of cardiovascular disorders.

Comparisons

➢ Vs. Tonify the Middle to Augment the Qi Decoction (*bǔ zhōng yì qì tāng*); see page 321

➢ Vs. Generate the Pulse Powder (*shēng mài sǎn*); see page 330

升陽益胃湯 (升阳益胃汤)
Raise the Yang and Augment the Stomach Decoction
shēng yáng yì wèi tāng

This formula raises the body's yang qi by tonifying the yang ascending and transportive functions of the middle burner. The reference to the Stomach in the name of the formula refers to this focus on the yang functions of the middle burner. However, it does not imply that the formula only, or even primarily, tonifies the Stomach organ.

Source   *Clarifying Doubts about Injury from Internal and External Causes* (1247)

Astragali Radix (*huáng qí*) 60g
Pinelliae Rhizoma praeparatum (*zhì bàn xià*) 30g
Ginseng Radix (*rén shēn*) 30g
Glycyrrhizae Radix praeparata (*zhì gān cǎo*) 30g
Angelicae pubescentis Radix (*dú huó*) 15g
Saposhnikoviae Radix (*fáng fēng*) 15g
Paeoniae Radix alba (*bái sháo*) 15g
Notopterygii Rhizoma seu Radix (*qiāng huó*) 15g
Citri reticulatae Pericarpium (*chén pí*) 12g
Poria (*fú líng*) 12g
Bupleuri Radix (*chái hú*) 9g
Alismatis Rhizoma (*zé xiè*) 9g
Atractylodis macrocephalae Rhizoma (*bái zhú*) 9g
Coptidis Rhizoma (*huáng lián*) 3g

Method of Preparation   Grind the ingredients into a powder and take 9-15g as a draft with 5 slices of Zingiberis Rhizoma recens (*shēng jiāng*) and 2 pieces of Jujubae Fructus (*dà zǎo*). At present, when taken as a decoction, the dosages are roughly halved.

Actions   Strengthens the Spleen, augments the qi, raises the yang, and leaches out dampness

Indications

Loss of taste, reduced appetite, fullness and distention of the abdomen, irregular bowel movements, fatigue and lethargy, a sensation of heaviness in the body, pain in the joints, chills, aversion to wind, dizziness, tinnitus, reduced and dark urination, a shiny pale complexion, and a dry mouth and tongue.

This is Spleen and Stomach qi deficiency with damp-heat flowing down into the lower burner where it stagnates and obstructs the qi dynamic. The Spleen governs transportation and transformation. It likes dryness and abhors dampness. Its qi seeks to ascend. If the qi of the Spleen and Stomach is frail, the appetite will be reduced, one's sense of taste will diminish, and bowel movements will become irregular. When the clear yang fails to ascend, the upper orifices will be deprived of nourishment, leading to dizziness and tinnitus. Failure of earth to support metal manifests as Lung qi deficiency with chills, aversion to wind, and a shiny, pale complexion. As dampness accumulates as a result of the Spleen's inability to transform food, it obstructs the qi dynamic. Consequently, the abdomen feels distended and full, the body becomes heavy and the joints painful, and there is often a generalized feeling of fatigue and lethargy. When dampness flows downward into the lower burner, it constrains the movement of yang qi, leading to a buildup of damp-heat. This manifests as reduced and dark urination, and a dry mouth and tongue.

Analysis of Formula

This formula treats patterns characterized by Spleen and Stomach qi deficiency and the accumulation of damp-heat. It therefore employs a strategy of building up the middle burner qi in conjunction with eliminating dampness and clearing heat.

The chief herb is Astragali Radix (*huáng qí*), which tonifies both the Spleen and Lung qi to treat both the root and branch of this disorder. Because the Lungs are responsible for directing water downward into the Bladder, they play an important role in removing dampness from the body. Strengthening the Lung qi will thus not only stabilize the exterior, but also actively eliminate the pathogenic dampness. Ginseng Radix (*rén shēn*), Glycyrrhizae Radix praeparata (*zhì gān cǎo*), and Atractylodis macrocephalae Rhizoma (*bái zhú*) serve as deputies. Together with the three assistants, Poria (*fú líng*), Pinelliae Rhizoma praeparatum (*zhì bàn xià*), and Citri reticulatae Pericarpium (*chén pí*), they constitute the formula Six-Gentlemen Decoction (*liù jūn zǐ tāng*), discussed earlier in the chapter. This is a balanced formula that tonifies and regulates the functions of the middle burner by focusing on building Spleen qi, draining dampness, and opening the qi dynamic. This action is further supported by Alismatis Rhizoma (*zé xiè*), another assistant, which drains dampness and heat from the lower burner. This facilitates the ascent of clear yang, making Alismatis Rhizoma (*zé xiè*) an important herb in the treatment of dizziness and tinnitus caused by the accumulation of damp-heat in the lower burner.

The four herbs Angelicae pubescentis Radix (*dú huó*), Notopterygii Rhizoma seu Radix (*qiāng huó*), Saposhnikoviae Radix (*fáng fēng*), and Bupleuri Radix (*chái hú*) constitute a second group of assistants. Acrid and dispersing in nature, these so-called wind herbs facilitate the movement of yang qi in the body. Together with Astragali Radix (*huáng qí*), Ginseng Radix (*rén shēn*), and Atractylodis macrocephalae Rhizoma (*bái zhú*), they strengthen the ascending movement of the qi dynamic, allowing the qi to move from below to above without obstruction. Two other assistants, Coptidis Rhizoma (*huáng lián*) and Paeoniae Radix (*sháo yào*), balance the warming, drying, and dispersing nature of these wind herbs. Bitter and strongly cooling Coptidis Rhizoma (*huáng lián*) drains damp-heat, which builds up as a result of qi constraint. Paeoniae Radix (*sháo yào*) nourishes and cools the blood to remove heat from a deeper stratum of physiological function. Most physicians use Paeoniae Radix alba (*bái sháo*) because of its astringent nature, as explained by Wu Kun in *Investigations of Medical Formulas*: "When the ancients employed acrid, dispersing [herbs,] they would necessarily combine them with sour, astringent [herbs] to protect [the body] from the fierceness [of the former]. This [embodies] the [use of] controlling [measures by] military strategists."

Zingiberis Rhizoma recens (*shēng jiāng*) and Jujubae Fructus (*dà zǎo*) serve as envoys that regulate the protective and nutritive qi by gently supporting the transportive and transformative functions of the middle burner. Together with Glycyrrhizae Radix praeparata (*zhì gān cǎo*), they also moderate the diverse functions of the many different herbs in this formula.

Cautions and Contraindications

Although this formula treats damp-heat disorders, its focus is on tonifying the qi of the middle burner. It is therefore contraindicated in patterns characterized by dampness in the absence of deficiency of the middle burner. In fact, the source text specifically instructs to remove the draining herbs Poria (*fú líng*) and Alismatis Rhizoma (*zé xiè*) unless their inclusion is indicated by symptoms reflecting obstruction of the lower burner qi dynamic, such as painful urinary dribbling.

Commentary

This is another of Li Dong-Yuan's flagship formulas that embody his doctrine of strengthening the yang functions of the middle burner (ascending, transportation) in order to expel pathogenic qi from the body. This is explained by the Qing-dynasty physician Yu Chang in *Precepts for Physicians*:

[Regarding] ascending yang to augment the Stomach [it is like this]: When a person's yang qi is constrained within the Stomach earth [because] the Stomach is deficient and [therefore] unable to raise the yang qi, then, according to the *Inner Classic's* strategy of discharging fire from constraint, [one must] augment the Stomach in order to discharge the fire.

This is the same basic treatment strategy that informed the composition of Tonify the Middle to Augment the Qi Decoction (*bǔ zhōng yì qì tāng*), discussed above. However, whereas that formula focused primarily on raising the yang and discharging fire constraint, the present formula adds to this the downward-directing of turbid dampness and draining of excess heat. It is thus suited for treating more complex disorders where tonifying the qi (treating the root) is not sufficient because of the presence of relatively severe pathogenic qi. In the pattern for which this formula is indicated, the primary pathogen is dampness or damp-heat, which inhibits the qi dynamic of an already deficient middle burner. This constrains the yang qi produced in the gate of vitality, preventing it from acting as a source of transformation.

Some commentators, like the Qing dynasty physician Wang Zi-Jie, have interpreted the composition of the formula to be designed for treating disorders that occur in the aftermath of a damp-heat disorder that penetrates the body via the Lungs. At present, therefore, this formula is often used for problems in the upper burner (Lungs) that affect the lower burner and lead to problems like vaginal discharge.

The formula is also used to treat allergic disorders involving the skin, respiratory, and digestive systems. Its efficacy in treating such disorders can be explained as harmonizing disharmonies between the protective and nutritive qi that cause the body to overreact to certain stimuli. Unlike Cinnamon Twig Decoction (*guì zhī tāng*), which treats patterns distinguished by the simultaneous presence of heat and cold, this formula focuses on disorders characterized by the presence of dampness.

The efficacy of this formula can be increased by attending to diet and exercise, as the source text explains:

[Those patients] fond of eating should abstain from eating until satiated for a few days [while taking this decoction, because eating] might further damage the Stomach and reduce the power of the herbs. [Patients] whose Stomach qi does not afford transportation and uplifting should eat light or fine foods in order to assist the power of the herbs by augmenting their uplifting and floating qi and enriching the Stomach qi. One should be cautious with bland foods [as these] may damage the power of the herbs by assisting the draining and sinking [nature of] the pathogen. One can also engage in light exercise to facilitate the Stomach and the herb's ability to transport and uplift. One must be cautious [however] with strenuous exercise so as not to further damage the qi. It is best when the Spleen and Stomach are peaceful. When the Stomach qi has been somewhat strengthened, one may eat a little fruit to assist the power of the herbs.

Biomedical Indications

With the appropriate presentation, this formula may be used to treat a variety of biomedically-defined disorders including chronic inflammatory bowel disease, atrophic gastritis, chronic cholecystitis, chronic pelvic inflammatory disease, fever of unknown origin, periodontal disease, and urticaria.

Alternate name

Augment the Stomach Decoction (*yì wèi tāng*) in *Precious Mirror for Advancement of Medicine*

Modifications

- For diarrhea with perianal burning indicating the presence of damp-heat in the Large Intestine, add Scutellariae Radix (*huáng qín*).
- If body aches are not severe, remove Notopterygii Rhizoma seu Radix (*qiāng huó*) and Angelicae pubescentis Radix (*dú huó*).
- In patterns without dry mouth, remove Coptidis Rhizoma (*huáng lián*).
- If urination is normal, remove Poria (*fú líng*) and Alismatis Rhizoma (*zé xiè*).

Associated Formula

升陽散火湯 （升阳散火汤）

Raise the Yang and Disperse Fire Decoction

shēng yáng sàn huǒ tāng

Source   *Clarifying Doubts about Damage from Internal and External Causes* (1247)

Cimicifugae Rhizoma (*shēng má*) 15g
Puerariae Radix (*gé gēn*) 15g
Angelicae pubescentis Radix (*dú huó*) 15g
Notopterygii Rhizoma seu Radix (*qiāng huó*) 15g
Paeoniae Radix alba (*bái sháo*) 15g
Ginseng Radix (*rén shēn*) 15g
Saposhnikoviae Radix (*fáng fēng*) 7.5g
Bupleuri Radix (*chái hú*) 24g
Glycyrrhizae Radix (*gān cǎo*) 6g
Glycyrrhizae Radix praeparata (*zhì gān cǎo*) 9g

The source text advises to coarsely grind to the size of a hemp seed and take 15g of the resulting powder as a draft, cooking 2 cups of water down to one 1 cup of strained liquid. Take warm. Raises the yang, disperses fire, benefits the qi, and preserves the yin. For fire from constraint in the yang warps that consumes the qi and damages the fluids, manifesting as extremities that are both subjectively and objectively hot in very fatigued patients. This particular type of heat from constraint usually occurs in patients with underlying blood and Stomach deficiency who, often through eating too much cold food or other dietary issues, restrain the yang qi within the Spleen earth.

Note: In *Secrets from the Orchid Chamber*, this formula is known as Bupleurum and Cimicifuga Decoction (柴胡升麻湯 *chái hú shēng má tāng*).

玉屏風散 （玉屏风散）

Jade Windscreen Powder

yù píng fēng sǎn

In Chinese, the word 屏風 *píng fēng* denotes a screen used to protect the inside of a room against wind. It is also an alternate name for the herb Saposhnikoviae Radix (*fáng fēng*). The formula serves as a screen or barrier against the invasion of wind, using this herb for that purpose. According to the Qing-dynasty physician Ke Qin, it was considered as precious and valuable as jade, hence the name.

Source   *Researching Original Formulas* (1213)

honey-prepared Astragali Radix (*mì zhì huáng qí*) 60g
Atractylodis macrocephalae Rhizoma (*bái zhú*) 60g
Saposhnikoviae Radix (*fáng fēng*) 30g

Method of Preparation   The source text advises to grind the ingredients into a powder and take in 9g doses as a draft with one piece of Jujubae Fructus (*dà zǎo*). At present, it is usually taken twice daily in 6-9g doses with warm, boiled water. Two-to-six times the specified dosage of Astragali Radix (*huáng qí*) is often used. For relatively acute conditions, it can be prepared as a decoction with a proportionate reduction (about 75%) in the dosage of the herbs.

Actions   Augments the qi, stabilizes the exterior, and stops sweating

Indications

Aversion to drafts, spontaneous sweating, recurrent colds, a shiny, pale complexion, a pale tongue with a white coating, and a floating, deficient, and soft pulse.

This is deficiency of the exterior with weak and unstable protective qi. The Lungs govern the qi, skin, and body hair. By virtue of their control of the protective qi, they guard the exterior of the body and ward off pathogenic influences. Part of this mechanism is regulating the opening and closing of the interstices and pores. When the qi is weak and cannot stabilize the superficial aspects of the body, the interstices and pores will not properly close. Not only does this give rise to spontaneous sweating and aversion to drafts, it also increases one's susceptibility to invasion by external pathogenic influences, and thus to recurrent colds. The shiny, pale complexion and pale tongue reflect deficiency of qi, while the floating, deficient, and soft pulse reflects weakness in the superficial level of the body's energies.

Analysis of Formula

The chief herb, Astragali Radix (*huáng qí*), is an extremely powerful substance for strengthening the qi and stabilizing the exterior. It tonifies the superficial or exterior aspects of the Lungs and Spleen, and is well-suited to this pattern, as noted in *Seeking Accuracy in the Materia Medica*: "[It] enters the Lungs to tonify the qi, and it enters the exterior to firm up the protective [qi]. It is foremost among all herbs that tonify the qi."

The deputy, Atractylodis macrocephalae Rhizoma *(bái zhú),* strengthens the Spleen and augments the qi. It reinforces the actions of the chief herb and strengthens the metal (Lungs) by cultivating the earth (Spleen). Early pharmacopeias such as the *Divine Husbandman's Classic of the Materia Medica* claim that Atractylodis macrocephalae Rhizoma *(bái zhú)* "stops sweating." Sun Si-Miao's *Important Formulas Worth a Thousand Gold Pieces* contains a formula for "sweating that does not stop" consisting solely of this herb. Although this indication has fallen out of use, it is highly likely to have influenced the composition of the formula. The combination of chief and deputy generates qi by tonifying the Spleen, which is the source of qi and blood. The exterior is thereby stabilized, and sweat will no longer leak from the interstices and pores. This also prevents pathogenic influences from easily penetrating the outer defenses of the body.

Saposhnikoviae Radix *(fáng fēng),* the assistant, circulates in the exterior of the body where it expels wind, the major pathogenic influence at this level on which the others ride to invade the body. Regarded as "the moistening medicinal among the wind herbs," it is chosen here over other dispersing herbs because it does not damage the fluids and thereby further injure the Lungs, the "tender organ." In concert with the chief herb, it stabilizes the exterior without causing the pathogenic influences to linger, and expels pathogenic influences without harming the normal qi. This is an example of dispersing while tonifying.

Cautions and Contraindications

Although the formula disperses pathogenic wind-dampness, it is unsuitable for treating excess patterns. Its focus is on preventing pathogenic qi from entering the body, not on dispersing pathogenic qi from the body. Unless significantly modified, it is thus unsuited for releasing pathogenic qi from the exterior in patterns of excess, even where such excess occurs against a background of qi deficiency.

Commentary

At least 40 texts in the Chinese medical literature list formulas that consist of Astragali Radix *(huáng qí),* Atractylodis macrocephalae Rhizoma *(bái zhú),* and Saposhnikoviae Radix *(fáng fēng).* Not all of these formulas retain the original name, and the relative dosage of the constituent herbs also differs. In the present formula, the relative dosage is 2:2:1. By contrast, Jade Windscreen Powder *(yù píng fēng sǎn),* listed in *Essential Teachings of [Zhu] Dan-Xi,* uses a ratio of 1:1:1, while a formula by the name of Atractylodes and Saposhnikovia Decoction *(bái zhú fáng fēng tāng),* listed in *Precious Mirror of Oriental Medicine,* uses a ratio of 1:1:2.

Inherent in these differences in dosage are disagreements over the nature of the chief and deputy herbs in the formula. Most commentators agree that Astragali Radix *(huáng qí)* is the chief herb. Some physicians therefore massively increase its dosage to enhance the formula's effect in stabilizing the exterior. Others, like the Ming-dynasty writer Wang Ken-Tang in *Indispensable Tools for Pattern Treatment,* argue that Saposhnikoviae Radix *(fáng fēng)* should be designated the deputy because the strategy of simultaneously dispersing and stabilizing the exterior is more important than that of strengthening the qi. Accordingly, these commentators tend to increase the dosage of that herb.

Along with differences in relative dosage, there are very different opinions about usage. Some, such as Wang Ang in *Medical Formulas Collected and Analyzed,* held that, with appropriate modifications, this formula can be used to actively disperse pathogenic qi from the exterior:

> A decoction of equal amounts of the aforementioned three herbs is called Astragalus Decoction *(huáng qí tāng).* Zhang Yuan-Su used it as a substitute for Cinnamon Twig Decoction *(guì zhī tāng)* in treating fever with sweating in spring and summer [accompanied by] a feeble and frail pulse and aversion to wind-cold. If aversion to wind is severe, he added Cinnamomi Ramulus *(guì zhī).*

The opposing view, that this formula must not be used to treat acute exterior disorders, is represented by Fei Bo-Xiong in *Discussion of Medical Formulas:*

> The herbs [in this formula] secure the exterior and disperse wind. It is appropriate to use them to secure the exterior. To say, however, that with appropriate modifications [this formula] can be used to replace Ephedra Decoction *(má huáng tāng)* or Cinnamon Twig Decoction *(guì zhī tāng),* that is, [to treat patterns characterized by] exterior excess where the pathogen has no way out, is absolutely impermissible. Such ideas do people great harm and must not be followed.

In clinical practice, the dosage of tonifying and dispersing herbs can be adapted to match the relationship between the strength of the pathogen and the deficiency of qi. Furthermore, one can also adjust the relative dosage of Astragali Radix *(huáng qí)* and Atractylodis macrocephalae Rhizoma *(bái zhú)* depending on whether Spleen or Lung qi deficiency is more pronounced.

In contemporary practice, this formula is commonly taken to prevent colds, particularly in those who suffer from recurrent colds. Although it is effective in treating this problem, it may take time and require patience. Usually the formula must be administered for at least a month before any effect is demonstrated (i.e., less frequent and less severe colds). When taken to prevent colds, the formula is usually prepared as a powder, and when taken to treat colds, as a decoction.

Its ability to expel wind pathogens that keep entering the body because of qi deficiency also makes it a formula of choice for treating allergies that involve a response located at the qi level or that involve the Lung and Spleen functional systems (i.e., urticaria, asthma, rhinitis, hayfever, etc.), which occur against a background of qi deficiency.

Note that the source of this formula is identified in many Chinese formularies as *Essential Teachings of [Zhu] Dan-Xi*. However, the Ming work *Classified Compilation of Medical Prescriptions* states that the formula first appeared in the no longer extant *Researching Original Formulas* (究原方 *jiū yuán fāng*), which dates to 1213. For that reason, it is appropriate to consider the older text to be the original source.

Comparisons

➤ Vs. CINNAMON TWIG DECOCTION (*guì zhī tāng*)

Both formulas treat conditions known as exterior deficiency. Cinnamon Twig Decoction (*guì zhī tāng*) is designed for relatively acute conditions with fever and aversion to cold, where sweating does not resolve the problem. In such cases, although the exterior can be considered deficient, the pathogenic influence is strong. By contrast, Jade Windscreen Powder (*yù píng fēng sǎn*) is designed for ongoing, chronic problems marked by spontaneous sweating together with aversion to drafts and recurrent colds. In this case, the deficiency of the normal qi is not strong enough to prevent wind pathogens from reentering once they have been dispersed. Some physicians nevertheless think that both formulas can complement each other at different times in treating the same patient, or may even combine them in treating the same patient at the same time. Based on the this line of reasoning, Jade Windscreen Powder (*yù píng fēng sǎn*) is also used in special circumstances for acute attacks of wind-cold, that is, in cases where patients are so deficient that they are unable to tolerate even the weakest dispersing formula, yet still require some exterior-releasing action.

➤ Vs. TONIFY THE LUNGS DECOCTION (*bǔ fèi tāng*); *see* PAGE 331

➤ Vs. OYSTER SHELL POWDER (*mǔ lì sǎn*); *see* PAGE 421

Biomedical Indications

With the appropriate presentation, this formula may be used to treat a variety of biomedically-defined disorders including recurrent upper respiratory infections, glomerulonephritis, allergic rhinitis, chronic urticaria, and bronchial asthma.

Modifications

• For externally-contracted disorders with aversion to wind, sweating, and a moderate pulse, add Cinnamomi Ramulus (*guì zhī*).
• For persistent sweating, add Ostreae Concha (*mǔ lì*), Tritici Fructus levis (*fú xiǎo mài*), and Schisandrae Fructus (*wǔ wèi zǐ*).

• For chronic or allergic rhinitis with the appropriate presentation, add Magnoliae Flos (*xīn yí huā*), Xanthii Fructus (*cāng ěr zǐ*), and Angelicae dahuricae Radix (*bái zhǐ*).
• For bronchitis in children, add Dioscoreae Rhizoma (*shān yào*), Citri reticulatae Pericarpium (*chén pí*), and Jujubae Fructus (*dà zǎo*).
• For night sweats where qi deficiency in the exterior is a major factor in the loss of yin fluids, add Schisandrae Fructus (*wǔ wèi zǐ*), Tritici Fructus levis (*fú xiǎo mài*), and Paeoniae Radix alba (*bái sháo*).
• For hypotension, combine with Generate the Pulse Powder (*shēng mài sǎn*).
• For allergic rhinitis, combine with Xanthium Powder (*cāng ěr zǐ sǎn*).

生脈散 (生脉散)
Generate the Pulse Powder
shēng mài sǎn

A pulse without enough force (qi) or volume (fluids) is very weak. The name of this formula is derived from its effect in tonifying the qi and generating fluids and thereby restoring a normal pulse.

Source   *Expounding on the Origins of Medicine* (Yuan)

Ginseng Radix (*rén shēn*) 1.5g (9-15g)
Ophiopogonis Radix (*mài mén dōng*) 1.5g (9-12g)
Schisandrae Fructus (*wǔ wèi zǐ*) . . . . 7 seeds (3-6g)

Method of Preparation   Decoction. Generally taken three times a day. The source text recommends using running water in preparing the decoction, and notes that it does not matter when the formula is administered. At present, the dosage (in parentheses) is larger than that specified in the source text. If the condition is not critical or the qi deficiency is not pronounced, Codonopsis Radix (*dǎng shēn*) may be substituted for Ginseng Radix (*rén shēn*) at 2-3 times its dosage. In cases with pronounced yin deficiency or internal heat, Panacis quinquefolii Radix (*xī yáng shēn*) is often used as a substitute.

Actions   Augments the qi, generates fluids, preserves the yin, and stops excessive sweating

Indications

Chronic cough with sparse sputum that is difficult to expectorate, shortness of breath, spontaneous sweating, a dry mouth and tongue, a pale, red tongue with a dry, thin coating, and a deficient, rapid or deficient, thin pulse.

This is concurrent deficiency of qi and yin, primarily of the Lungs. Chronic cough not only injures the Lung qi, but is also a manifestation of injured Lung qi, as are shortness of breath and spontaneous sweating. Prolonged, profuse sweating injures the fluids and yin, which is manifested here in the sparse sputum that is difficult to expectorate, and the dry mouth and tongue. The pulse is deficient, which reflects deficient qi, and rapid or thin, which reflects deficient yin.

A similar pattern can develop over a relatively short period of time due to profuse sweating, as in summerheat-stroke or heat-stroke. The dynamic in such cases is that excessive sweating injures not just the fluids or yin, but also the qi, which attaches itself to the body fluids. When qi deficiency develops quickly, it almost always produces a tendency to curl up, as well as shortness of breath and laconic speech. The pulse in this pattern will be deficient and rapid, indicating the outward movement of qi due to pathogenic heat.

Analysis of Formula

The chief herb, Ginseng Radix *(rén shēn),* strongly tonifies the source qi and strengthens the qi that generates fluids and calms the spirit. When the source qi is strong, the Lung qi is replete and properly regulates the interstices and pores so that the fluids are no longer lost through the superficial levels of the body. The deputy herb is Ophiopogonis Radix *(mài mén dōng),* which nourishes the yin and moistens the Lungs. It also benefits the Stomach and generates fluids, and clears heat from the Heart to eliminate the irritability that may occur with this condition. The chief herb acts on the qi of the fluids, while the deputy herb acts directly on the fluids, a combination that gives the formula a very strong, fluid-generating effect. The assistant, Schisandrae Fructus *(wǔ wèi zǐ),* restrains the leakage of Lung qi (and sweat) and generates fluids in the Kidneys. By tonifying the Kidneys, it also checks the excessive ascent of qi. In concert with the deputy, it forms a powerful combination for generating fluids. Together with the chief herb, it enables the formula to rescue the injured qi and yin. This formula is simple yet well-balanced: the chief herb tonifies, the deputy clears, and the assistant restrains leakage.

Cautions and Contraindications

This formula should be used only with extreme caution in cases with high fever, or where the pathogenic influence has not been resolved or has yet to injure the fluids. If it is used in cases where the external pathogenic influence remains in the system, it will prolong the disease.

Commentary

The author of this formula, Zhang Yuan-Su, designed it "to tonify insufficiency of source or primal qi within the Lungs" due to "lurking heat in the Lungs with a pulse that threatens to be cut off." His disciple, Li Dong-Yuan, expanded on this indication by using the formula for the treatment of summerheat injuring the true or source qi. Later generations of physicians used these concepts to extend the usage of this formula in two different directions. The first, represented by members of the warm pathogen current, emphasized its ability to treat severe damage to the qi and body fluids in the course of externally-contracted heat disorders. *Systematic Differentiation of Warm Pathogen Diseases*, for instance, describes the disease dynamic treated by Generate the Pulse Powder *(shēng mài sǎn)* as one of "excessive dispersion and discharge of yang qi leading to interior deficiency with inability to manage containment" characterized by "severe sweating and a dispersed, large pulse."

A second group of physicians focused instead on the formula's ability to tonify the Lung qi and yin and thus strengthen the Lungs as the body's "upper source of water." Tang Zong-Hai's analysis in *Discussion of Blood Patterns* is representative of this view: "Combining sweet and sour [herbs] to transform [into] yin with [herbs that] clear and moisten Lung metal, this is the herald [of the later formula] Clear Dryness and Rescue the Lungs Decoction *(qīng zào jiù fèi tāng)."*

More recently, this formula has been widely used in the treatment of acute shock as well as various types of heart disease, including palpitations and coronary artery disease. For this reason, it is often administered intravenously in hospital settings. It is particularly useful in treating palpitations with a stifling sensation in the chest, shortness of breath, sweating, a dry mouth and thirst, poor sleep, a pale, red, and dry tongue, and a slow-irregular or consistently-irregular pulse. Combined with other formulas such as Tonify the Middle to Augment the Qi Decoction *(bǔ zhōng yì qì tāng),* it is used to treat dizziness and vertigo caused by low blood pressure, or with Drive Out Stasis from the Mansion of Blood Decoction *(xuè fǔ zhú yū tāng)* to treat arterial obstruction and occlusion, which also often manifests with dizziness and vertigo.

Other traditional indications include external medicine disorders where excessive discharge of pus or leakage from abscesses or sores has depleted the qi and body fluids, and it is used in pediatrics, where the frailty of qi and yin in children readily leads to their depletion upon invasion of external pathogens. Another modern indication is its use (with the modifications listed below) in the treatment of dark, scanty, and difficult urination caused or accompanied by excessive sweating, where the use of diuretics would be contraindicated.

When this formula is used for treating a critical condition, no substitution should be made for Ginseng Radix *(rén shēn).* It is interesting to note that under the entry for this herb in *Divine Husbandman's Classic of the Materia Medica*, it is said to "tonify the five yin organs, calm the essential spirit, steady the soul, and relieve palpitations with anxiety." All of these functions are drawn upon in this formula. However, for debility following a febrile disease or for cases with pronounced yin deficiency and internal heat, Panacis quinquefolii Radix *(xī yáng shēn),* which tonifies both the qi and the yin, is preferred.

Comparisons

➢ Vs. Clear Summerheat and Augment the Qi Decoction (qīng shǔ yì qì tāng)

Both formulas are indicated for the treatment of summer-heat-stroke with profuse sweating and damage to the qi and yang fluids. However, Clear Summerheat and Augment the Qi Decoction (qīng shǔ yì qì tāng) treats patterns characterized by the presence of strong pathogenic qi at the qi level in a person with weak normal qi. This is indicated by symptoms such as fever, Heart irritability, dark and scanty urination, and a red tongue with yellow coating. The present formula, on the other hand, treats patterns of deficiency without the presence of pathogenic qi but with damage to the yang fluids and the original qi. This is indicated by a dry cough with little phlegm that is difficult to expectorate.

➢ Vs. Raise the Sunken Decoction (shēng xiàn tāng)

Both formulas are used in contemporary practice to treat deficiency of qi in the upper burner that manifests as cardiovascular disorders. This is based on the idea that while the Heart governs the vessels and pulse (脈 mài), it is the Lung or gathering qi that provides the vessels with movement and the pulse with its rhythm. Raise the Sunken Decoction (shēng xiàn tāng) only treats the qi. It does not treat any specific organ, and it does not augment the fluids. The present formula tonifies the Lung qi and yin. Thus, it not only strengthens the Lung's ability to promote the pulse, but also fills the vessels with fluids.

➢ Vs. Other formulas for Acute Collapse

This is one of the few formulas that are used in treating acute collapse. Two others are Ginseng and Aconite Accessory Root Decoction (shēn fù tāng), which is used for sudden exhaustion of the yang qi, and Frigid Extremities Decoction (sì nì tāng), indicated for extremely weak yang qi with internal ascent of yin cold. (Both of these formulas are discussed in Chapter 6.) It is of the utmost importance that the diagnosis be very clear before any of these formulas are prescribed.

➢ Vs. Prepared Licorice Decoction (zhì gān cǎo tāng); see PAGE 358

➢ Vs. Restore and Revive the Yang Decoction (huí yáng jiù jí tāng); see PAGE 279

Biomedical Indications

This formula may be used to treat a wide variety of biomedically-defined disorders. These can be divided into the following groups:

• Those primarily involving the cardiovascular system such as coronary artery disease, acute myocardial infarction, myocarditis, heart arrhytmias, congestive heart disease, and various types of shock

• Those affecting the pulmonary system including chronic bronchitis, pulmonary tuberculosis, and cardiopulmonary disease.

It has also been used in treating such problems as the recovery phase of acute infections, sunstroke, senility, sclerema neonatorum, and neurasthenia-like disorders.

Alternate names

Generate the Pulse Decoction (shēng mài tāng) in *Essential Teachings of [Zhu] Dan-Xi*; Ginseng and Ophiopogon Powder (shēn mài sǎn) in *Eight Notes on Conforming to [the Rules of] Life*; Generate the Pulse Drink (shēng mài yǐn) in *Medical Records*; Ginseng Powder to Generate the Pulse (rén shēn shēng mài sǎn) in *Symptom, Cause, Pulse, and Treatment*; Settle the Lungs Decoction (dìng fèi tāng) in *Compendium of the Rules of Conduct for Physicians*; Ginseng and Ophiopogon Five-Ingredient Drink (shēn mài wǔ wèi yǐn) in *Essential Teachings on Pregnancy and Childbirth*

Modifications

• For profuse sweating with dark, scanty, and difficult urination, add Astragali Radix (huáng qí) and Angelicae sinensis Radix (dāng guī). It is important in this type of condition to avoid the use of herbs that leach out dampness.

• For severe coughing, add Farfarae Flos (kuǎn dōng huā) and Lilii Bulbus (bǎi hé).

• For irritability with relatively severe insomnia, add Ziziphi spinosae Semen (suān zǎo rén) and Albiziae Cortex (hé huān pí).

• For marked palpitations, add Cinnamomi Ramulus (guì zhī), Fossilia Ossis Mastodi (lóng gǔ), and Ostreae Concha (mǔ lì).

• For coronary artery disease, add Glycyrrhizae Radix praeparata (zhì gān cǎo), Salviae miltiorrhizae Radix (dān shēn), Carthami Flos (hóng huā), and Paeoniae Radix rubra (chì sháo).

Associated Formula

加減生脈散 （加減生脉散）

Modified Generate the Pulse Powder
jiā jiǎn shēng mài sǎn

SOURCE *Systematic Differentiation of Warm Pathogen Diseases* (1798)

Glehniae/Adenophorae Radix (shā shēn) 9g
Ophiopogonis Radix (mài mén dōng) 9g
Rehmanniae Radix (shēng dì huáng) 9g
Schisandrae Fructus (wǔ wèi zǐ) 3g
Moutan Cortex (mǔ dān pí) 6g

Clears heat from the blood level, generates fluids, and restrains leakage. For greater yin-stage disorders with smoldering summerheat. The pathogenic influence is in the blood level, and the exterior is deficient. Manifestations include thirst, profuse sweating, and a dark-red tongue.

補肺湯（补肺汤）

Tonify the Lungs Decoction

bǔ fèi tāng

Source *Everlasting Categorization of Inscribed Formulas* (1331)

Ginseng Radix *(rén shēn)* 9g
Astragali Radix *(huáng qí)* 24g
Rehmanniae Radix praeparata *(shú dì huáng)* 24g
Schisandrae Fructus *(wǔ wèi zǐ)* 6g
Asteris Radix *(zǐ wǎn)* 9g
Mori Cortex *(sāng bái pí)* 12g

Method of Preparation Decoction. At present, Codonopsis Radix *(dǎng shēn)* is often substituted for Ginseng Radix *(rén shēn)* at 2-3 times its dosage.

Actions Augments the qi and stabilizes the exterior

Indications

Shortness of breath, spontaneous sweating, occasional chills and feverishness, coughing, wheezing, a pale tongue, and a frail or deficient and large pulse.

This is Lung qi deficiency. The Lungs control the body's qi. When the Lung qi is weak and unstable, the individual is likely to experience shortness of breath, spontaneous sweating, and occasional chills or feverishness. The weakened qi's inability to stabilize the exterior of the body leads to recurrent colds with resulting cough. The wheezing in this case is primarily due to deficient Lung qi, but also involves the inability of the Kidneys to grasp the qi. The pale tongue, and the frail or deficient and large pulse, reflect the deficiency of qi.

Analysis of Formula

The chief herbs in this formula are Ginseng Radix *(rén shēn)* and Astragali Radix *(huáng qí),* which work synergistically to tonify the qi and fortify the protective qi. Two of the deputies act on the upper part of the body: Mori Cortex *(sāng bái pí)* causes the Lung qi to descend, and Asteris Radix *(zǐ wǎn)* moistens the Lungs and stops the coughing. The other deputy, Schisandrae Fructus *(wǔ wèi zǐ),* preserves the Lung qi and helps the Kidneys grasp the qi. In concert with the assistant ingredient, Rehmanniae Radix praeparata *(shú dì huáng),* which tonifies the essence, it tonifies the lower and basal aspects of the body.

Commentary

This can be seen as a variation of Generate the Pulse Powder *(shēng mài sǎn)* for which the main indication is chronic cough due to Lung deficiency. The cough may either be dry or productive. Although this may appear to be contradictory, both manifestations can result from the same underlying disease dynamic. The Lungs are the 'upper source of water.' Through their control of the skin and pores, they regulate the dispersion of body fluids to the exterior. Through their

downward direction of qi, they move the fluids into the lower burner and the Kidneys. If the Lung qi is too weak to fulfill these functions, water accumulates in the Lungs, which becomes visible as phlegm. The Kidneys, furthermore, are no longer nourished by the water they receive from the Lungs. As the Kidney yin declines, water is no longer steamed upward to moisten the Lungs, causing dryness. Such dryness further weakens the qi, both because the lack of yin control can lead to the leakage of qi as sweat, and because, without the movement-facilitating moisture afforded by the body fluids, the qi stagnates and over time diminishes.

The composition of this formula succeeds in addressing all of these problems. It tonifies the Lung qi with Ginseng Radix *(rén shēn)* and Astragali Radix *(huáng qí),* facilitates moistening, downward-directing, and the draining of excess pathological water through the urine with Mori Cortex *(sāng bái pí)* and Asteris Radix *(zǐ wǎn),* nourishes the Kidney yin with Rehmanniae Radix praeparata *(shú dì huáng),* and astringes the excessive upward and outward movement of qi and fluids with Schisandrae Fructus *(wǔ wèi zǐ).* This makes it an ideal formula for treating chronic cough in older patients or in those weakened by another illness or medical treatment.

This formula also is a good example of the use of Rehmanniae Radix praeparata *(shú dì huáng)* in the treatment of phlegm disorders. This topic is discussed in more detail in the COMMENTARY section of Six-Ingredient Pill with Rehmannia *(liù wèi dì huáng wán).*

Note that there are many other formulas with this name, over 15 of which are identified in *Thousand Ducat Formulas* alone. At present, this one is the most commonly used.

Comparison

➤ Vs. JADE WINDSCREEN POWDER *(yù píng fēng sǎn)*

Both formulas not only tonify the Lungs and qi, but also stabilize the exterior. However, while Jade Windscreen Powder *(yù píng fēng sǎn)* focuses primarily on relieving the spontaneous sweating and recurrent colds, this formula focuses on tonifying the Lungs to relieve the persistent coughing.

人參蛤蚧散（人参蛤蚧散）

Ginseng and Gecko Powder

rén shēn gé jiè sǎn

Source *Formulas of Broad Benefit* (1047)

Gecko *(gé jiè)* . . . . .1 pair
Ginseng Radix *(rén shēn)* 60g
Poria *(fú líng)* 60g
Mori Cortex *(sāng bái pí)* 60g
Armeniacae Semen *(xìng rén)* .180
Fritillariae cirrhosae Bulbus *(chuān bèi mǔ)* 60g

Anemarrhenae Rhizoma (*zhī mǔ*) .60g
Glycyrrhizae Radix praeparata (*zhì gān cǎo*) 150g

Method of Preparation   Grind the ingredients into a fine powder. The source text recommends that the powder be kept in a ceramic vessel and taken throughout the day like a tea. At present, it is usually taken in 3-6g doses with warm water twice a day (morning and evening) on an empty stomach.

Actions   Tonifies the qi, augments the Kidneys, stops coughing, and arrests wheezing

Indications

Chronic coughing and wheezing, thick, yellow sputum, coughing of pus and blood, a sensation of heat and irritability in the chest, facial edema, gradual emaciation, a purple tongue with either a thin and white or a greasy, thin, and yellow tongue coating, and a floating, deficient pulse, especially at the distal position.

This is Lung and Kidney qi deficiency with phlegm-heat collecting internally, which manifests externally as coughing and wheezing. Together, the Lungs and Kidneys govern the entering and exiting of qi. When these functions are impaired, deficient qi rebels upward causing coughing and wheezing. Because this is a condition of deficiency, the coughing lacks force, and the voice is weak. Exhalation is easier than inhalation, indicating failure of the Kidneys to accept qi and of the Lungs to move it downward. In conditions of excess, where coughing and wheezing are due to obstruction of the upper burner qi dynamic by external or internal pathogens, this is usually reversed. Together with their control over the qi, the Lungs and Kidneys also control water metabolism. Should this break down, body fluids accumulate in the form of phlegm and thin mucus. The constraint and stagnation which accompanies the accumulation of phlegm and thin mucus may, over time, transform into heat, which manifests as chronic coughing and wheezing, thick, yellow sputum, and a sensation of heat and irritability in the chest. Heat and chronic coughing injure the blood collaterals, which may appear as coughing of pus and blood or blood-streaked sputum. When the Lung qi has been injured in this manner, it is unable to regulate the water channels and facial edema ensues. Over time, this may progress to Lung atrophy and its associated symptom of gradual emaciation.

In cases of Lung qi deficiency with stagnation and retention of damp-phlegm, there is typically a purple tongue with either a thin and white or a greasy, thin, and yellow tongue coating. A floating and deficient pulse, especially at the distal position, is also indicative of Lung qi deficiency.

Analysis of Formula

This is a case in which both the root (Lung and Kidney qi deficiency) and branch (heat and phlegm) must be treated. The chief ingredient, Gecko (*gé jiè*), enters the Lung and

Kidney channels to tonify the Kidneys and thereby restore their ability to grasp the qi and thus arrest wheezing. It is salty and warming, and thus able to tonify the qi dynamic without inducing more heat. The other chief ingredient is Ginseng Radix (*rén shēn*), which strongly tonifies the source qi, increases the qi of the Lungs and Spleen, but also slightly moistens, and in this way complements the action of Gecko (*gé jiè*). Poria (*fú líng*), which benefits the Spleen by draining dampness, and Glycyrrhizae Radix praeparata (*zhì gān cǎo*), which harmonizes the actions of the other herbs and assists in tonifying the source qi, serve as deputies. Focusing on the treatment of Spleen earth, they treat problems of Lung metal and Kidney water via the generating and controlling relationships of the five phases.

Two sets of paired herbs serve as assistants. The first is the combination of Mori Cortex (*sāng bái pí*) and Armeniacae Semen (*xìng rén*), which regulates the Lung qi and directs rebellious qi downward. These two ingredients work especially well together when there is heat in the Lungs due to constraint. The second pair consists of Fritillariae cirrhosae Bulbus (*chuān bèi mǔ*), which clears heat, moistens the Lungs, releases constraint, and transforms phlegm, and Anemarrhenae Rhizoma (*zhī mǔ*), which serves the dual purpose of draining heat from the Lungs and Kidneys without damaging the yin. This pair comprises the formula Fritillaria and Anemarrhena Powder (*èr mǔ sǎn*), discussed in Chapter 17.

Overall, the herbs combine in this formula to tonify the qi without obstructing the qi dynamic, and clear heat and transform phlegm without damaging the qi. This makes it especially useful in the treatment of chronic patterns characterized by the simultaneous presence of both deficiency and excess.

Cautions and Contraindications

Contraindicated in cases with any evidence of an externally-contracted pathogenic influence.

Commentary

The harmonization of the Lungs and Kidneys that is the basis of this formula leads to the regulation of qi as well as water metabolism. Because the movement and transformation of qi and water within the body is so closely intertwined, whenever one is impaired, the other will also show symptoms and must be treated. Hence, as the contemporary physician Chen Chao-Zu reminds us, "In all Lung conditions, no matter whether acute or chronic, the [simultaneous] regulation of fluids and qi is the catch [around which treatment turns]."

The heat in this presentation is due to stasis, thus neither strongly warming herbs to boost the Kidney yang nor yin-enriching herbs to subdue the heat of deficiency are needed. Rather, this is a type of excess heat that results from the knotting of phlegm-fluids and yang qi within the upper burner.

This heat must be cleared in order to open the qi dynamic, but where it has taken on form it must also be drained. This is achieved by the combination of Fritillariae cirrhosae Bulbus (*chuān bèi mǔ*), Mori Cortex (*sāng bái pí*), Anemarrhenae Rhizoma (*zhī mǔ*), and Armeniacae Semen (*xìng rén*).

Biomedical Indications

With the appropriate presentation, this formula may be used to treat a wide variety of biomedically-defined disorders including chronic bronchitis, bronchial asthma, emphysema, bronchiectasis, pulmonary heart disease, and pulmonary tuberculosis.

Associated Formula

人參胡桃湯（人参胡桃汤）

Ginseng and Walnut Decoction

rén shēn hú táo tāng

Source *Formulas to Aid the Living* (1253)

Juglandis Semen (*hé táo rén*)	5 nuts
Ginseng Radix (*rén shēn*)	small piece (6-9g)
Zingiberis Rhizoma recens (*shēng jiāng*)	5 pieces

Tonifies the Lungs and Kidneys, arrests wheezing, and stops coughing. For deficiency of both the Lungs and Kidneys in which the inability of the Kidneys to grasp the qi and the deficiency of the Lung qi leads to rebellious qi of the Lungs. Manifestations include coughing, wheezing, fullness in the chest, and an inability to lie supine. Although both this and the principal formula are used in treating coughing and wheezing due to Lung qi deficiency, the principal formula is slightly cold and has a stronger effect. It is therefore used when there is marked heat and phlegm. By contrast, this formula is somewhat weaker and slightly warm, and is therefore better suited to milder patterns with some degree of cold.

Section 2

FORMULAS THAT TONIFY THE BLOOD

Disorders of the blood can be divided into three basic types: blood deficiency, blood stasis, and blood loss. (A fourth aspect is heat in the blood level.) Although each type has its own distinctive characteristics, they often blend into each other. Chronic blood deficiency commonly leads to blood stasis; blood stasis can lead to a reduction in the production and circulation of blood (known as 'bad blood preventing the generation of new blood'); and blood loss is one of the most common etiologies of blood deficiency.

The formulas in this section are used in treating conditions due to blood deficiency. The reader is referred to Chapter 2 for formulas that treat blood-level heat, Chapter 10 for formulas that transform blood stasis, and Chapter 11 for formulas that stop bleeding.

Common indications of blood deficiency include dizziness, vertigo, a pale and lusterless complexion, a pale tongue and lips, dry and cracked nails, palpitations, dry and itchy skin, insomnia, constipation, long menstrual cycles with scanty, pale flow, and a thin pulse. Clinically, a condition of blood deficiency is often encountered in women due to the loss of menstrual blood or in any patient who has lost blood or suffered from chronic malnutrition.

Formulas to tonify the blood focus particularly on the physiological functions of the Heart, Liver, and Spleen, which govern, store, and control the blood, respectively. Because of the integral relationship between the qi and blood, tonifying one will have a salutary effect on the other. The adage "Qi is the commander of blood, and blood is the mother of qi" suggests that qi moves the blood and that blood nourishes the qi. This understanding of the relationship between qi and blood deficiency is reflected in a passage from *Discussion of the Spleen and Stomach*: "For blood deficiency, use Ginseng Radix (*rén shēn*) to tonify, because when the yang [qi] is exuberant, it will generate yin blood." Astragali Radix (*huáng qí*) is another commonly used herb in many blood-tonifying formulas because of its ability to augment the qi of the middle and upper burners. Restore the Spleen Decoction (*guī pí tāng*) and Tangkuei Decoction to Tonify the Blood (*dāng guī bǔ xuè tāng*) are well-known examples. Herbs that invigorate the blood and transform stasis are also frequently added to blood-tonifying formulas for the reasons outlined above. These include Carthami Flos (*hóng huā*), Persicae Semen (*táo rén*), Salviae miltiorrhizae Radix (*dān shēn*), Chuanxiong Rhizoma (*chuān xiōng*), and Paeoniae Radix rubra (*chì sháo*).

四物湯（四物汤）

Four-Substance Decoction

sì wù tāng

Source *Secret Formulas to Manage Trauma and Reconnect Fractures Received from an Immortal* (c. 846)

The name of this formula refers to the four herbs of which it is comprised. However, as explained by Wang Zi-Jie in *Selected Annotations to Ancient Formulas from the Garden of Crimson Snow*, the emphasis is on the total effect achieved by these substances rather than on the individual ingredients: "[The term] substance [in the name] Four-Substance Decoction refers to similar things (類 *lèi*). [The formula is composed of] four similar substances that possess one nature and achieve one function. They move together without impeding each other."

Rehmanniae Radix praeparata (*shú dì huáng*)	(9-12g)
Paeoniae Radix alba (*bái sháo*)	(9-12g)
Angelicae sinensis Radix (*dāng guī*)	(9-12g)
Chuanxiong Rhizoma (*chuān xiōng*)	(3-6g)

Method of Preparation   The source text advises to coarsely grind equal amounts of the ingredients and take in 9g doses as a draft before meals. At present, it is usually prepared as a decoction with the dosage specified in parentheses.

Actions   Tonifies the blood and regulates the Liver

Indications

Dizziness, blurred vision, lusterless complexion and nails, generalized muscle tension, insomnia, palpitations, a thin body lacking strength, irregular menstruation with little flow or amenorrhea, periumbilical and lower abdominal pain, a pale tongue, and a thin and wiry or thin and choppy pulse. Also used for menorrhagia, hard abdominal masses with recurrent pain, restless fetus disorder, or lochioschesis with a firm and painful abdomen and sporadic fever and chills.

This is generalized blood deficiency and stagnation. From an organ perspective, this is associated primarily with the complex of functional systems that Chinese medicine refers to as the 'sea of blood,' that is, the Liver, Penetrating vessel, and Womb. When the Liver blood is deficient, it is unable to rise and nourish the head. This manifests as dizziness and a lusterless complexion. The Liver's ability to supply its associated sensory organ (eyes) and tissues (muscles and sinews) is also impaired, which leads to blurred vision or chronic eye strain and generalized muscle tension. As the blood becomes deficient, the muscles will diminish, and the body will become thin and lack strength. The health of the Liver is also reflected in the nails; when the Liver blood is deficient, the nails will become soft, dry, and lusterless (described as being 'wretched').

A normal menstrual cycle depends on the health of the Penetrating vessel, the Womb, and the Liver. When the sea of blood is empty, the menses are typically irregular with a scanty flow. There may even be amenorrhea. However, when the blood becomes disordered, menorrhagia may also occur. When the blood is deficient, it does not move well, and there is a tendency for blood stasis to develop. This commonly manifests as periumbilical and lower abdominal pain, often occurring at the onset of menstruation, which is due to stasis and insufficiency of blood in the Womb. This same process can also lead to hard abdominal masses with recurrent pain, restless fetus, or lochioschesis.

The blood houses the spirit and the Liver the ethereal soul. When the blood becomes deficient, the spirit and ethereal soul no longer have a place to which to return. As a result, one becomes restless, and sleep is disturbed. The Heart is also dependent on the Liver blood; when it is deficient, one may experience palpitations. The pale tongue reflects blood deficiency, as does the thin pulse. The wiry or choppy quality of the pulse, which almost always accompanies this condition, signals the stasis of blood and demonstrates the link between blood deficiency and stasis.

Analysis of Formula

This formula tonifies and regulates the blood. All of its ingredients enter the blood, but they are often divided into two groups based on their function. The first group consists of 'blood in the blood' herbs that are entirely yin in nature and only nourish the blood. The first of these, Rehmanniae Radix praeparata (shú dì huáng), has a very strong tonifying effect on the Liver and Kidneys and is said to nourish the yin of the blood. In *Collected Treatises of [Zhang] Jing-Yue*, the Ming-dynasty physician Zhang Jie-Bin, who so admired the functions of this herb that he was given the nickname "Rhemannia Zhang," explained that "it tonifies the true yin of the five yin organs, and therefore is most important for those organs that have much blood … no channel deficient in yin blood can be treated without Rehmanniae Radix praeparata (shú dì huáng)." Paeoniae Radix alba (bái sháo) tonifies the blood and preserves the yin. Its sour and astringent character helps to settle the muscle spasms caused by blood deficiency, and it is particularly well-suited to treat abdominal pain. In concert with Rehmanniae Radix praeparata (shú dì huáng), it provides a strong tonic for the blood. However, because these two herbs are rich, cloying, and astringent in nature, there is a risk that their use will lead to blood stasis. This is prevented by the second group of herbs, which treat the 'qi in the blood.'

Angelicae sinensis Radix (dāng guī) is warming and moistening, entering the Liver and Heart to tonify and invigorate the blood. Quoting once more from *Collected Treatises of [Zhang] Jing-Yue*, "It moves as it tonifies and it tonifies as it moves. It truly is the qi herb within the blood. It is also a sagely herb for the blood." It also moistens the Intestines and regulates the dynamic between the Liver (movement) and Kidneys (storage). Chuanxiong Rhizoma (chuān xiōng) primarily acts to invigorate the blood and promote the movement of qi. Above, it directs the blood to the head, relieving symptoms like headache, dizziness, and blurred vision, while below, it moves the sea of blood. Facilitating the flow of blood through the vessels and collaterals, it releases constraint, opens knotting, and alleviates pain. The combination of these herbs with the first group facilitates the production of blood. At the same time, the ability of Paeoniae Radix alba (bái sháo) to preserve the yin prevents the aromatic nature of these two herbs from injuring the yin.

Overall, the formula thus regulates the blood by providing both tonification and movement. If the blood-deficient aspect of the presentation is predominant, the dosage of the first group of herbs should be increased. Conversely, if blood stasis is predominant, the dosage of the second group should be increased. For this reason, the hierarchy of ingredients in this formula will change depending on the pattern treated, as outlined in the COMMENTARY below.

Cautions and Contraindications

This formula should not be used in treating acute, severe blood loss or other problems of blood deficiency characterized by severe weakness and labored breathing. Due to the cloying nature of its main ingredients, the formula is inappropriate for treating patterns characterized by an overabundance of dampness with abdominal fullness, poor appetite, and loose stools.

Commentary

It is widely accepted that this formula is a variation of Ass-Hide Gelatin and Mugwort Decoction (*jiāo ài tāng*) from *Essentials from the Golden Cabinet*, discussed in Chapter 13. Its first listing in the medical literature can be traced to a Tang-dynasty text on trauma, *Secret Formulas to Manage Trauma and Reconnect Fractures Received from an Immortal*, in which it was used it to treat trauma and static blood in the Intestines. Because the original formula focused on chronic uterine bleeding while the new intended usage was to move and generate the blood, Asini Corii Colla (*ē jiāo*), Artemisiae argyi Folium (*ài yè*), and Glycyrrhizae Radix (*gān cǎo*) were removed; Rehmanniae Radix (*shēng dì huáng*) was replaced by Rehmanniae Radix praeparata (*shú dì huáng*); and Paeoniae Radix alba (*bái sháo*) was clearly identified as the type of Paeoniae Radix (*sháo yào*) to be used. The use of this new formula in the treatment of gynecological disorders was first suggested in the Song-dynasty text *Formulary of the Pharmacy Service for Benefiting the People in the Taiping Era*, which said that this formula:

> Regulates and augments the nutritive and protective [qi], enriches and nourishes the qi and blood. It treats deficiency injury to the Conception and Penetrating vessels [characterized by] irregular menstruation, continuous abdominal pain, irregular uterine bleeding, mobile abdominal masses and hard lumps, or intermittent pain. It is suitable for pregnant women who are habitually cold with threatened miscarriage, restless fetus, and incessant bleeding. It is also [indicated] for deficiency following birth with wind and cold contending in the interior, retained lochia, knotting generating abdominal masses, hardness and pain in the lower abdomen, and occasional chills and fever.

Ever since, Four-Substance Decoction (*sì wù tāng*) has been used as a basic formula for tonifying the blood and regulating menstruation, for which it is very effective. It can be used (with appropriate modification) in treating almost any problem of menstruation or birth in which the nails are lusterless, the tongue is pale, and the pulse is thin. It has many derivatives, some of which are listed under VARIATIONS and ASSOCIATED FORMULAS below, and also Eight-Treasure Decoction (*bā zhēn tāng*), which is discussed in the following section.

Because the formula moves as well as tonifies, most commentators take Rehmanniae Radix praeparata (*shú dì huáng*)

and Angelicae sinensis Radix (*dāng guī*) to be the key herbs in the formula, and a majority consider Rehmanniae Radix praeparata (*shú dì huáng*) to be the chief herb. Others have different ideas about what herbs work best and use Rehmanniae Radix (*shēng dì huáng*) instead of Rehmanniae Radix praeparata (*shú dì huáng*) and Paeoniae Radix rubra (*chì sháo*) instead of Paeoniae Radix alba (*bái sháo*), retaining the original composition of Ass-Hide Gelatin and Mugwort Decoction (*jiāo ài tāng*).

Another common way to modify the formula consists of varying the relative dosage of the ingredients. As a general rule, the contemporary physician Pu Fu-Zhou recommends that "The dosage of Chuanxiong Rhizoma (*chuān xiōng*) should be low, on average about half that of Angelicae sinensis Radix (*dāng guī*); that of Rehmanniae Radix praeparata (*shú dì huáng*) should be twice that of Angelicae sinensis Radix (*dāng guī*)." Another influential modern physician, Qin Bo-Wei, advised that "For the purpose of nourishing blood, the dosage of Rehmanniae Radix praeparata (*shú dì huáng*) and Angelicae sinensis Radix (*dāng guī*) should be highest, followed by that of Paeoniae Radix alba (*bái sháo*). If one does not use Rehmanniae Radix praeparata (*shú dì huáng*), then the dosage of Paeoniae Radix alba (*bái sháo*) should generally exceed that of Angelicae sinensis Radix (*dāng guī*)."

Some practitioners recommend keeping modifications to a minimum, following the advice given by the Qing-dynasty physician Zhang Lu in *Discussing the Remainders of the [Discussion of] Cold Damage*:

> Four-Substance Decoction (*sì wù tāng*) is a special formula for [treating patterns] where the yin blood has become ill. It is, however, not a formula for regulating and tonifying the true yin. Hence, when a considerable number of formularies state that Four-Substance Decoction (*sì wù tāng*) tonifies the yin and this is [interpreted by] later generations [of physicians as licensing] the treatment of yin deficiency manifesting with heat, the up-flaring of fire with bleeding, and similar patterns, then this is ignorant [practice] whose harm continues to the present day. With regard to its specific usage in gynecology, [it is common practice] to casually add herbs [that treat] wind, food [stagnation], phlegm, or qi, so that today [use of] the original Four-Substance Decoction (*sì wù tāng*) has become all confused and disorderly. Among all of these later physicians who would like [their modifications] to become [accepted] standards, there are hardly any worth using.

To effectively regulate menstruation, which is the most important clinical usage of this formula, a small number of core modifications are thus generally sufficient:

- For heavy bleeding, reduce the dosage of Chuanxiong Rhizoma (*chuān xiōng*) and add Artemisiae argyi Folium (*ài yè*) and Asini Corii Colla (*ē jiāo*); or add qi tonics such as Ginseng Radix (*rén shēn*) or Astragali Radix (*huáng qí*).

- For painful menstruation, add Linderae Radix (*wū yào*), Cyperi Rhizoma (*xiāng fù*), and Citri reticulatae viride

Pericarpium (qīng pí) if qi stagnation is pronounced; or Corydalis Rhizoma (yán hú suǒ), Persicae Semen (táo rén), and Carthami Flos (hóng huā) if blood stasis is pronounced.

- For pronounced heat prior to menstruation, add herbs that clear and drain heat such as Moutan Cortex (mǔ dān pí), Lycii Cortex (dì gǔ pí), or Phellodendri Cortex (huáng bǎi).

Comparisons

> Vs. Tangkuei Decoction to Tonify the Blood (dāng guī bǔ xuè tāng) and Restore the Spleen Decoction (guī pí tāng)

All three formulas can be used to tonify the blood and treat heavy menstruation, or blood deficiency resulting from heavy menstruation. Both Tangkuei Decoction to Tonify the Blood (dāng guī bǔ xuè tāng) and Restore the Spleen Decoction (guī pí tāng) tonify the qi in order to tonify the blood. Another way to put this is that they improve the assimilation functions of the Spleen and Stomach in order to facilitate the production of blood. Because the Spleen manages blood by providing the qi that contains it, both of these formulas are also used to treat excessive bleeding: the former is used for acute blood loss, while the latter is better for chronic conditions accompanied by signs of Spleen deficiency. Both formulas combine Astragali Radix (huáng qí) and Angelicae sinensis Radix (dāng guī) in order to focus the qi on the production and containment of blood.

Four-Substance Decoction (sì wù tāng) focuses on the Liver and on the Governing and Conception vessels. It aims to tonify the blood in its role as an essence rather than the functions that produce and manage it, even if, as Wu Kun points out in Investigations of Medical Formulas, this also involves the digestive functions of the middle burner:

> Plants are not sentient. How can they then generate blood? When one says that the [herbs in this formula] generate blood, one means that Paeoniae Radix (sháo yào) and Rehmanniae Radix praeparata (shú dì huáng) are able to nourish the yin of the five yin organs, and that Chuanxiong Rhizoma (chuān xiōng) is able to regulate the qi within the nutritive [aspect]. When the five yin organs function harmoniously, they generate blood. If one says that the four substances [themselves] generate blood, then this is not so. The master says: When the blood is deficient, one can use this formula to regulate [the condition and production of blood]. However, in [cases of] excessive blood loss from either the upper or lower [body orifices] accompanied by the symptom of [labored] breathing, use of the four substances is forbidden.

In clinical practice, the patterns of blood deficiency for which Four-Substance Decoction (sì wù tāng) is indicated will thus invariably show signs of dryness because essence is lacking. The digestive function, on the other hand, is not impaired. By

contrast, Restore the Spleen Decoction (guī pí tāng) patterns are characterized by the presence of dampness that comes from Spleen deficiency. Tangkuei Decoction to Tonify the Blood (dāng guī bǔ xuè tāng) is differentiated from both formulas by its use in acute bleeding patterns.

> Vs. Arborvitae Seed Pill for Women's Diseases (nǚ kē bái zǐ rén wán); see PAGE 343

Biomedical Indications

With the appropriate presentation, this formula may be used to treat a wide variety of biomedically-defined disorders, primarily those related to obstetrics and gynecology such as irregular menstruation as primary dysmenorrhea, irregular menstruation, threatened miscarriage, postpartum weakness, and insufficient lactation. It has also been used for anemia of various etiologies, urticaria, plantar warts, allergic purpura, and neurogenic headache.

Alternate names

Rehmannia Decoction (dì suǐ tāng) in Comprehensive Recording of Sagely Beneficence; Major Chuanxiong Decoction (dà chuān xiōng tāng) in Ji-Feng's Formulas of Universal Benefit

Modifications

- For restless fetus disorder with continuous bleeding from the vagina, add Artemisiae argyi Folium (ài yè) and Asini Corii Colla (ē jiāo).
- For signs of heat, substitute Rehmanniae Radix (shēng dì huáng) for Rehmanniae Radix praeparata (shú dì huáng) and add Scutellariae Radix (huáng qín) and Moutan Cortex (mǔ dān pí).
- For a predominance of blood stasis, substitute Paeoniae Radix rubra (chì sháo) for Paeoniae Radix alba (bái sháo) and add Persicae Semen (táo rén) and Carthami Flos (hóng huā).
- For qi deficiency, add Ginseng Radix (rén shēn) and Astragali Radix (huáng qí).
- For blood deficiency with internal cold, add Cinnamomi Cortex (ròu guì) and Evodiae Fructus (wú zhū yú).
- For blood deficiency and cold in the Womb, add Artemisiae argyi Folium (ài yè) and Cyperi Rhizoma (xiāng fù).
- For a short menstrual cycle with steaming bone disorder in which the fever worsens early in the evening, add Lycii Cortex (dì gǔ pí) and Moutan Cortex (mǔ dān pí).
- For dry and itchy skin, add Saposhnikoviae Radix (fáng fēng) and Schizonepetae Herba (jīng jiè).
- For premenstrual vomiting and nosebleed due to excessive heat, add Coptidis Rhizoma (huáng lián), Scutellariae Radix (huáng qín), and Rhei Radix et Rhizoma (dà huáng).

Variant

桃紅四物湯 （桃红四物汤）

Four-Substance Decoction with Safflower and Peach Pit

táo hóng sì wù tāng

Source   *Supreme Commanders of the Medical Ramparts* (1291)

Add Persicae Semen (*táo rén*) and Carthami Flos (*hóng huā*) to tonify and invigorate the blood and regulate menstruation. For concurrent blood deficiency and blood stasis leading to a shortened menstrual cycle with copious bleeding of dark-purple, sticky blood, with or without clots. Also used when menstruation is accompanied by abdominal pain and distention due to the same mechanism.

Associated Formulas

聖愈湯 （圣愈汤）

Sage-Like Healing Decoction

shèng yù tāng

Source   *Secrets from the Orchid Chamber* (1336)

Rehmanniae Radix (*shēng dì huáng*) 9g
Rehmanniae Radix praeparata (*shú dì huáng*) 9g
Chuanxiong Rhizoma (*chuān xiōng*) 9g
Ginseng Radix (*rén shēn*) 9g
Angelicae sinensis Radix (*dāng guī*) 1.5g
Astragali Radix (*huáng qí*) 1.5g

Augments the qi, tonifies the blood, and preserves the blood. For qi and blood deficiency manifested as a constant ache in the lower abdomen that occurs either during or just after menstruation and responds favorably to pressure. The menstrual flow is scanty and pale. The patient has a pale complexion, is lethargic and withdrawn, and has a pale tongue with a thin coating, and a thin, frail pulse. The source text recommends this formula for treating sores that bleed profusely and cause irritability and insomnia. Note that at present, the dosage of the last two herbs is usually increased 8-10 fold. There are several other formulas by the same name.

―――――

溫清飲 （温清饮）

Warming and Clearing Drink

wēn qīng yǐn

Source   *Song Family Secret Texts on Women's Disorders* (1612)

Coptidis Rhizoma (*huáng lián*) 3g
Scutellariae Radix (*huáng qín*) 3g
Phellodendri Cortex (*huáng bǎi*) 3g
Gardeniae Fructus (*zhī zǐ*) 3g
Rehmanniae Radix praeparata (*shú dì huáng*) 3g
Chuanxiong Rhizoma (*chuān xiōng*) 3g
Angelicae sinensis Radix (*dāng guī*) 3g
Paeoniae Radix alba (*bái sháo*) 3g

Drains fire, resolves toxicity, tonifies the blood, and stops bleeding. For chronic, continuous, and excessive uterine bleeding due to heat accompanied by pale complexion, stabbing pain in the abdomen, and alternating fever and chills. This is a combination of Four-Substance Decoction (*sì wù tāng*) and Coptis Decoction to Resolve Toxicity (*huáng lián jiě dú tāng*), discussed in Chapter 4. The name refers to the formula's ability to warm the chills that often accompany blood deficiency (blood is the substratum that carries the warmth of yang qi around the body), while simultaneously clearing heat from the blood, which in this case is the cause of the blood deficiency (blood heat consumes yin blood). In clinical practice, this is reflected in symptoms like heat in the upper body while the lower body is cold, irritability and restlessness despite fatigue and exhaustion, a submerged but rapid pulse, and a dry tongue with a red tip and a thin white coating. At present, this formula is also commonly used for stubborn skin diseases such as eczema, dermatitis, and urticaria characterized by dry, itchy, and inflamed skin.

―――――

芩連四物湯 （芩连四物汤）

Four-Substance Decoction with Scutellaria and Coptis

qín lián sì wù tāng

Source   *Wondrous Lantern for Peering into the Origin and Development of Miscellaneous Diseases* (1773)

Scutellariae Radix (*huáng qín*) 3-6g
Coptidis Rhizoma (*huáng lián*) 3-6g
Ophiopogonis Radix (*mài mén dōng*) 9-12g
Chuanxiong Rhizoma (*chuān xiōng*) 3-6g
Angelicae sinensis Radix (*dāng guī*) 9-12g
Paeoniae Radix alba (*bái sháo*) 9-12g
Rehmanniae Radix (*shēng dì huáng*) 9-12g

Tonifies the blood and drains heat. For concurrent blood deficiency and excessive heat. This may manifest in one of several ways, including a short menstrual cycle with purple blood and a heavy flow, or a red, sticky vaginal discharge with tidal fever, a greenish hue to the complexion, dizziness, blurred vision, palpitations, insomnia, and irritability. Dosage is not specified in the source text.

Comparison

➢ Vs. Delayed Menstruation Drink (*guò qī yǐn*); see page 342

―――――

補肝湯 （补肝汤）

Tonify the Liver Decoction

bǔ gān tāng

Source   *Golden Mirror of the Medical Tradition* (1742)

Angelicae sinensis Radix (*dāng guī*) 9-12g
Chuanxiong Rhizoma (*chuān xiōng*) 6-9g
Paeoniae Radix alba (*bái sháo*) 9-15g
Rehmanniae Radix praeparata (*shú dì huáng*) 15-24g
Ziziphi spinosae Semen (*suān zǎo rén*) 6-9g
Chaenomelis Fructus (*mù guā*) 6-9g
Glycyrrhizae Radix praeparata (*zhì gān cǎo*) 3-6g

Tonifies and regulates the blood and nourishes the Liver yin. For Liver blood and yin deficiency leading to headache, dizziness, tinnitus, dry eyes, photophobia, blurred vision, irritability, bad temper, numbness, and muscle twitches. Additional signs include malar flush, a red and dry tongue, and a wiry, thin, and rapid pulse. Dosage is not specified in the source text.

玉燭散 （玉烛散）

Jade Candle Powder

yù zhú sǎn

SOURCE   *Confucians' Duties to Their Parents* (1228)

Angelicae sinensis Radix (*dāng guī*)
Chuanxiong Rhizoma (*chuān xiōng*)
Rehmanniae Radix praeparata (*shú dì huáng*)
Paeoniae Radix alba (*bái sháo*)
Rhei Radix et Rhizoma (*dà huáng*)
Natrii Sulfas (*máng xiāo*)
Glycyrrhizae Radix (*gān cǎo*)

Grind equal amounts of the ingredients into a powder and take 24g as a draft before meals. Tonifies and invigorates the blood and purges accumulation in the interior. For amenorrhea due to blood stasis and excessive heat. Also used for blood deficiency with interior heat manifesting as hard stools and constipation.

加味四物湯 （加味四物汤）

Augmented Four-Substance Decoction

jiā wèi sì wù tāng

SOURCE   *Fang's Orthodox Lineage of Pulse and Symptoms* (1749)

Angelicae sinensis Radix (*dāng guī*) 3g
Ophiopogonis Radix (*mài mén dōng*) 3g
Phellodendri Cortex (*huáng bǎi*) 3g
Atractylodis Rhizoma (*cāng zhú*) 3g
Rehmanniae Radix praeparata (*shú dì huáng*) 9g
Paeoniae Radix alba (*bái sháo*) 2.1g
Chuanxiong Rhizoma (*chuān xiōng*) 2.1g
Eucommiae Cortex (*dù zhòng*) 2.1g
Schisandrae Fructus (*wǔ wèi zǐ*) 1.5g
Ginseng Radix (*rén shēn*) 1.5g
Coptidis Rhizoma (*huáng lián*) 1.5g
Anemarrhenae Rhizoma (*zhī mǔ*) 0.9g
Achyranthis bidentatae Radix (*niú xī*) 0.9g

Tonifies the blood, dries dampness, and strengthens the limbs. For any type of atrophy disorder with weakness of the limbs and difficulty in moving.

當歸雞血藤湯 （当归鸡血藤汤）

Tangkuei and Spatholobus Decoction

dāng guī jī xuè téng tāng

SOURCE   *Traditional Chinese Traumatology* (c. 1960)

Angelicae sinensis Radix (*dāng guī*) 15g
Rehmanniae Radix praeparata (*shú dì huáng*) 15g
Longan Arillus (*lóng yǎn ròu*) .6g
Paeoniae Radix alba (*bái sháo*) 9g
Salviae miltiorrhizae Radix (*dān shēn*) 9g
Spatholobi Caulis (*jī xuè téng*) 15g

Tonifies the qi and blood. For qi and blood deficiency that develops after traumatic injury. Also for leukopenia or thrombocytopenia during radiation therapy or chemotherapy for tumors.

七物降下湯 （七物降下汤）

Seven-Substance Decoction for Directing Downward

qī wù jiàng xià tāng

SOURCE   *Practice of Syndrome Treatment in Kampo* (1963)

Uncariae Ramulus cum Uncis (*gōu téng*) 4g
Angelicae sinensis Radix (*dāng guī*) 3g
Chuanxiong Rhizoma (*chuān xiōng*) 3g
Paeoniae Radix alba (*bái sháo*) 3g
Rehmanniae Radix praeparata (*shú dì huáng*) 3g
Astragali Radix (*huáng qí*) 3g
Phellodendri Cortex (*huáng bǎi*) 2g

Tonifies and invigorates the blood, tonifies the qi, and extinguishes internal wind. For qi and blood deficiency accompanied by liver yang excess. This is a famous Kampo formula composed by the Japanese physician Otsuka Keisetsu for the treatment of hypertension. It is indicated for patterns characterized by headache, flushing, tension of the neck and shoulders, sensitivity to cold (especially in the lower body), tinnitus, urinary frequency, dry skin, and a tendency to become tired.

當歸補血湯 （当归补血汤）

Tangkuei Decoction to Tonify the Blood

dāng guī bǔ xuè tāng

Source   *Clarifying Doubts about Injury from Internal and External Causes* (1247)

Astragali Radix (*huáng qí*) 30g
wine-washed Angelicae sinensis Radix (*jiǔ xǐ dāng guī*) 6g

Method of Preparation   The source text advises to grind the herbs into a coarse powder and prepare as a decoction.

Actions   Tonifies the qi and generates blood

Indications

Hot sensation in the muscles, a red face, irritability, thirst with a desire to drink warm beverages, a pale tongue, and a flooding, large, and deficient pulse that is forceless when pressed hard. Also for fever and headache due to loss of blood.

This is a pattern of heat from deficiency characterized by blood deficiency and floating yang. Blood stores qi by providing a substance to which its dynamic can attach itself. When the blood is deficient, the yin is then unable to contain the yang, which floats to the superficial aspects of the body. This is explained by Tang Zong-Hai in *Discussion of Blood Patterns*: "When the blood is deficient, this [manifests with] fever and sweating. For when the blood does not match the qi, the qi becomes exuberant and discharges to the outside." Symptomatically, the classic signs of 'floating yang' include a hot sensation in the muscles, a red face, irritability, and thirst with a desire for warm beverages. The definitive (almost pathognomonic) sign is the flooding, large, and deficient pulse that reflects perfectly the weak yang qi dilating in an attempt to reach the superficial parts of the body. The pale tongue is indicative of blood deficiency. The same pathological mechanism underlies the fever that follows a severe loss of blood. In these cases, headache occurs because the process is relatively acute and therefore has some force behind it: when the yang floats to the head, it causes pain.

Analysis of Formula

In the pattern treated by this formula, blood deficiency is the root, but floating yang is the primary external manifestation or branch. Blood is difficult to generate, while qi easily disperses. Following the adage, "In acute conditions treat the branch," the formula thus focuses on preventing the qi from discharging. For this purpose, the formula employs a large dosage of Astragali Radix (*huáng qí*) as its chief herb. Astragali Radix (*huáng qí*) not only strongly tonifies the original qi of the Spleen, but also secures the exterior, as explained in *Rectification of the Meaning of Materia Medica:* "Its cortex reaches directly to the exterior skin and muscle, securing the protective yang and amply filling the exterior level. These are its specific strengths, so it is really marvelous for all disorders involving exterior deficiency." Turning this qi inward will, in turn, facilitate the production of blood, which is produced by the qi transformations of the middle burner. Furthermore, augmenting qi also supports movement and transformation, and thereby reinforces the generation of blood on a second level. A smaller dosage of Angelicae sinensis Radix (*dāng guī*) is utilized as a deputy to address the root cause. Among the blood-tonifying herbs, Angelicae sinensis Radix (*dāng guī*) in particular is used here for two reasons. First, it tonifies but also invigorates the blood, and therefore works better in generating new blood than do other, more cloying substances. In a related manner, it also replenishes the 'qi of the blood' and therefore works particularly well in conjunction with Astragali Radix (*huáng qí*), which indirectly tonifies the blood by tonifying the qi, as previously explained.

Cautions and Contraindications

Use with caution in cases with tidal fever from yin deficiency.

Commentary

Original and Later Indications

Like many other formulas composed by the Jin-dynasty physician Li Dong-Yuan, this formula treats a pattern characterized by the fever of deficiency as its main manifestation. On first glance, the symptoms (fever, irritability, thirst, a red face, and a flooding, large pulse) are similar to those of a White Tiger Decoction (*bái hǔ tāng*) pattern. However, the latter formula is used for treating a yang brightness pattern characterized by manifestations typical of excess: high fever with profuse sweating, strong thirst for cold beverages, and an ex-

cessive pulse. This formula, by contrast, is for a pattern of blood deficiency characterized by manifestations typical of deficiency: low-grade fever, slight sweating, a thirst for warm beverages, and a deficient pulse. Needless to say, prescribing one of these formulas when the other is indicated could have disastrous consequences.

In the literature, the pattern treated by this formula is commonly associated with consumptive fatigue (癆倦 *láo juàn*), a form of blood deficiency caused by injury to the source qi. This disorder was first described in *Basic Questions,* Chapter 62: "With what is called consumptive fatigue, the qi of the form is debilitated and meager. The qi from food does not ascend, and there is no movement in the upper burner; nor is the lower epigastrium open. The Stomach qi becomes hot [from constraint] and the heat sears the chest. Therefore, there is internal heat." This suggests that internal injury from consumptive fatigue depletes the source qi, which in turn causes the nutritive qi and blood to become deficient. Li Dong-Yuan attributed such deficiency to lack of food, poverty, and overwork, and proposed a strategy of sweet, warming tonification as key to treating the resulting patterns. The combination of Astragali Radix (*huáng qí*) and Angelicae sinensis Radix (*dāng guī*) reflects this approach and is found in many other of Li Dong-Yuan's formulas, most importantly Tonify the Middle to Augment the Qi Decoction (*bǔ zhōng yì qì tāng*). Taking up these ideas, later physicians incorporated the combination into many other important formulas, including Restore the Spleen Decoction (*guī pí tāng*), Tangkuei and Six-Yellow Decoction (*dāng guī liù huáng tāng*), and Tonify the Yang to Restore Five-Tenths Decoction (*bǔ yáng huán wǔ tāng*).

The range of indications for the present formula itself was also expanded over time. One of its major uses at present is for bleeding associated with deficient qi failing to control the blood. Another very common use is in the treatment of sores that do not heal for a long period of time after ulcerating, but continue to exude a thin, pale fluid. These are called 'yin-type ulcers' and are attributed to weakness of the protective qi and blood, which inhibits the normal healing process. In this case, the formula acts to support the protective qi, resolve toxicity, and generate flesh to heal the sore.

Debates about Action and Usage

That the formula treats blood deficiency but uses a qi-tonifying herb as its main ingredient has led to intense debates among commentators regarding the precise functions of Astragali Radix (*huáng qí*). Five distinct positions have emerged in these debates:

• The first, represented by Wu Kun in *Investigations of Medical Formulas,* holds that Astragali Radix (*huáng qí*) "tonifies the qi in order to tonify the blood," based on the view that the growth of yin depends in the last instance on the generative capacities of yang.

- The second view, represented by Wang Ang in *Medical Formulas Collected and Analyzed,* assumes that the formula treats deficiency of both the qi and blood and thus needs two different herbs to deal with these two problems.

- A third group of physicians, represented by Wang Fu in *Collectanea of Investigations from the Realm of Medicine,* holds that Astragali Radix (*huáng qí*) tonifies the Spleen and Stomach as the postnatal source of blood.

- A fourth position, represented by Zhang Bin-Cheng in *Convenient Reader of Established Formulas,* is that it is used as an emergency measure to secure floating yang.

- Finally, a fifth group of physicians, represented by Chen Nian-Zu in *Compendium of Songs on Modern Formulas,* argues that the fever treated by this formula is due to unresolved heat constrained at the level of the skin and hair. In the opinion of these physicians, Astragali Radix (*huáng qí*) is light and slightly warming so that it can enter this part of the body from which it clears heat by promoting sweating.

Although all five perspectives are validated by the indications for which this formula has been used, that of Zhang Bin-Cheng appears to come closest to the original indications. As outlined above, Li Dong-Yuan specifically composed this formula to treat a pattern resembling White Tiger Decoction (*bái hǔ tāng*), from which it is distinguished merely by the deficient pulse. If White Tiger Decoction (*bái hǔ tāng*) treats patterns where the outward dispersion of yang qi has become excessive, this implies that the present formula must treat patterns of deficiency characterized by the same pathodynamic. This justifies the large dosage of Astragali Radix (*huáng qí*) and its use as chief herb in the formula. Many commentators therefore suggest that the dosage of this herb be reduced considerably if the formula is used to treat blood deficiency without floating yang or combined qi and blood deficiency.

Comparisons

➤ Vs. White Tiger Decoction (*bái hǔ tāng*)

Both formulas treat feverishness, hot sensations in the muscles, flushing, irritability, restlessness, and other symptoms of heat through to the exterior. White Tiger Decoction (*bái hǔ tāng*) treats patterns of yang brightness excess, as reflected in thirst with a desire for cold drinks, profuse sweating, and a flooding, excessive pulse that is forceful when pressed. By contrast, Tangkuei Decoction to Tonify the Blood (*dāng guī bǔ xuè tāng*) treats patterns of deficiency where the qi in the exterior is too weak to contain the yang. This is reflected in thirst with a desire for warm drinks, sweating aggravated by exertion, and a large but deficient pulse that appears strong at the surface but is revealed as weak with pressure.

➤ Vs. Other formulas that Treat Heat due to Qi Deficiency

This is one of a number of different formulas that can be used to treat internal heat due to qi deficiency, where the use of bitter, cold, heat-draining or sweet, cooling, yin-nourishing herbs and formulas would be contraindicated. Tangkuei Decoction to Tonify the Blood (*dāng guī bǔ xuè tāng*) treats patterns characterized by blood deficiency failing to secure the yang, which then floats to the exterior. Rambling Powder (*xiāo yáo sǎn*) or Six-Gentlemen Decoction (*liù jūn zǐ tāng*) plus Bupleuri Radix (*chái hú*) can be used to treat patterns where the yang qi becomes constrained in the interior. Tonify the Middle to Augment the Qi Decoction (*bǔ zhōng yì qì tāng*) treats yang qi constraint due to failure of the clear qi to ascend. Tonify Spleen-Stomach, Drain Yin Fire, and Raise Yang Decoction (*bǔ pí wèi xiè yīn huǒ shēng yáng tāng*) treats patterns characterized by relatively severe constraint and fire excess due to inability of the qi to manage the ascent and descent of fire. Finally, Minor Construct the Middle Decoction (*xiǎo jiàn zhōng tāng*) treats patterns characterized by nutritive qi deficiency leading to a relative excess of protective qi.

➤ Vs. Tangkuei and Six-Yellow Decoction (*dāng guī liù huáng tāng*)

Both of these formulas treat flushing and feverishness and contain the synergistic combination of Astragali Radix (*huáng qí*) and Angelicae sinensis Radix (*dāng guī*). However, Tangkuei and Six-Yellow Decoction (*dāng guī liù huáng tāng*) focuses on enriching the yin and draining excess fire while the function of stabilizing the exterior in order to control sweating is secondary. It is therefore used to treat fever and night sweats accompanied by a dry mouth and parched lips, irritability, dry stools, dark and scanty urine, a red, dry tongue, and a rapid pulse. Tangkuei Decoction to Tonify the Blood (*dāng guī bǔ xuè tang*), on the other hand, focuses on tonifying deficient qi in the exterior. For this reason, it uses a very large dosage of Astragali Radix (*huáng qí*), but none of the bitter, cooling, or yin-tonifying herbs used in Tangkuei and Six-Yellow Decoction (*dāng guī liù huáng tāng*).

➤ Vs. Four-Substance Decoction (*sì wù tāng*);
see PAGE 336

➤ Vs. Eight-Treasure Decoction (*bā zhēn tāng*);
see PAGE 347

Biomedical Indications

With the appropriate presentation, this formula may be used to treat a wide variety of biomedically-defined disorders, particularly those affecting women such as perimenstrual and postpartum fevers, and dysfunctional uterine bleeding. It is also used for various types of anemia, thrombocytopenic purpura, leukopenia, and nonhealing sores and ulcers.

Alternate names

Astragalus and Tangkuei Decoction (*huáng qí dāng guī tāng*) in *Secrets from the Orchid Chamber*; Tonify the Blood Decoction (*bŭ xuè tāng*) in *Pulse Causes, Patterns, and Treatments*; Astragalus and Tangkuei Decoction (*qí guī tāng*) in *Writings for Posterity of [Zhou] Shen-Zhai*; Astragalus Decoction to Tonify the Blood (*huáng qí bŭ xuè tāng*) in *Essential Teachings on Fetuses and Childbirth*

....

Modifications

- For bleeding due to qi failing to secure the blood, add Agrimoniae Herba (*xiān hè cǎo*) and Crinis carbonisatus (*xuè yú tàn*).

- For ulcerated sores in which the toxin has not been completely discharged, add Lonicerae Flos (*jīn yín huā*) and Glycyrrhizae Radix (*gān cǎo*).

- For allergic purpura, add Bombyx batryticatus (*bái jiāng cán*) and Achyranthis bidentatae Radix (*niú xī*).

過期飲 （过期饮）
Delayed Menstruation Drink
guò qī yǐn

Source   *Indispensable Tools for Pattern Treatment* (1602)

Angelicae sinensis Radix (*dāng guī*) 6g
Paeoniae Radix alba (*bái sháo*) 6g
Rehmanniae Radix praeparata (*shú dì huáng*). 6g
Cyperi Rhizoma (*xiāng fù*) 6g
Chuanxiong Rhizoma (*chuān xiōng*) 3g
Carthami Flos (*hóng huā*) 2.1g
Persicae Semen (*táo rén*) 1.8g
Curcumae Rhizoma (*é zhú*) 1.5g
Akebiae Caulis (*mù tōng*) 1.5g
Glycyrrhizae Radix praeparata (*zhì gān cǎo*). 1.2g
Cinnamomi Cortex (*ròu guì*) 1.2g

Method of Preparation   The source text recommends cooking 2 cups down to 1 and drinking the decoction warm before meals.

Actions   Warms the menses, dispels blood stasis, and nourishes the blood

Indications

Overdue menses with scanty menstrual flow (often with blood clots) and pain and distention in the lower abdomen before and during menses. The pulse is submerged and strong.

The main causes of overdue menses are qi constraint, phlegm obstruction, blood cold, blood deficiency, and blood stasis. Delayed Menstruation Drink (*guò qī yǐn*) addresses the disorder when it stems from blood deficiency and blood stasis in patients who tend to be cold. As might be expected, these factors give rise to stagnant qi as well. This combination of factors inhibits the free flow of blood and menses, and causes pain and distention in the lower abdomen.

Analysis of Formula

Failure of blood to move smoothly is regarded as a condition of excess, while scanty menstrual flow is a sign of deficiency. Thus, the pattern to which this formula attends is considered to be one of excess within deficiency. The principle of treatment should be to promote movement through areas of stasis and constraint and to tonify what is insufficient.

The formula uses Rehmanniae Radix praeparata (*shú dì huáng*) to nourish and tonify the blood, replenish the essence, and tonify the body. Angelicae sinensis Radix (*dāng guī*) nourishes and invigorates the blood, warms the menses, and relieves pain. The combination of these two herbs tonifies insufficiency in the nutritive level and the blood. Because this is the primary source of the problem, these are considered the chief herbs. The deputies are Chuanxiong Rhizoma (*chuān xiōng*), Carthami Flos (*hóng huā*), Persicae Semen (*táo rén*), and Curcumae Rhizoma (*é zhú*), which invigorate the blood and move stasis. Two of the assistants are Akebiae Caulis (*mù tōng*), which promotes the flow of fluids, and Cyperi Rhizoma (*xiāng fù*), which supports the body's qi dynamic. These eight herbs work together to remedy qi constraint, blood stasis, and stagnant fluids. Of these three pathologies, the emphasis is on managing blood stasis without exacerbating the underlying deficiency. Similarly, the deficiency is tonified without exacerbating the stagnation of blood and qi. Since the patient for whom this formula is intended is inclined toward cold, Cinnamomi Cortex (*ròu guì*) is included as an assistant to warm the lower burner and thwart congealing and clumping from cold. Cramping pain in the lower abdomen accounts for the inclusion of the last two assisants, Glycyrrhizae Radix (*gān cǎo*) and Paeoniae Radix alba (*bái sháo*), to soften the Liver and moderate the pain. Cold contributes to the congealing of blood and intensifies blood stasis by causing the vessels to contract. Warm and acrid Cinnamomi Cortex (*ròu guì*) can disperse cold, and for this reason is combined with Glycyrrhizae Radix (*gān cǎo*) and Paeoniae Radix alba (*bái sháo*) as a remedy for cold abdominal pain. The formula nourishes the blood and moves stasis, dispels the cold (a function sometimes expressed as warming the menses), and relieves the pain. It moves and disperses without depleting the yin-blood, and nourishes the yin-blood without causing further stasis.

Cautions and Contraindications

This formula is inappropriate for those who do not present with blood deficiency and cold. Also, because it contains blood-moving agents, it should not be given to those who bleed heavily during menses or to those who may be pregnant.

Commentary

Wang Ken-Tang, the author of the source text, opens his discussion of menstrual timing with a quote from the Ming-dynasty physician Wang Zi-Heng: "when yang is in excess, the [menses] will arrive early, when yin is incomplete, [the menses] will be delayed." The implication of this statement is that yin-blood deficiency (incomplete yin) is a main cause of overdue menses. Wang goes on to say that this formula treats overdue menses and inhibited menstrual flow when these symptoms are due to blood deficiency and stagnant qi.

Wang recognized that there are many factors that can give rise to overdue menses and provided the following advice from Zhu Dan-Xi:

> For scanty menstrual flow that arrives late, [use] Chuanxiong Rhizoma (chuān xiōng), Angelicae sinensis Radix (dāng guī), Ginseng Radix (rén shēn), Atractylodis macrocephalae Rhizoma (bái zhú), and phlegm herbs. If the late-arriving menstrual flow is pale in color [and] phlegm is copious, [use] Two-Aged [Herb] Decoction (èr chén tāng) adding Chuanxiong Rhizoma (chuān xiōng) and Angelicae sinensis Radix (dāng guī). If the late-arriving menstrual flow is purple and has clots, [this is] blood heat. There will be pain. [Use] Four-Substance Decoction (sì wù tāng) modified with Cyperi Rhizoma (xiāng fù) and Coptidis Rhizoma (huáng lián).

Wang further cited the Ming-dynasty physician Xue Ji-Zhuan, who emphasized treating the blood deficiency that is the basis of this disorder:

> For late-arriving periods owing to Spleen channel blood deficiency, Ginseng Decoction to Nourish Luxuriance (rén shēn yǎng yíng tāng) is suitable. If the cause is scant Liver blood, Six-Flavor Pill with Rehmannia (liù wèi dì huáng wán) is appropriate. If the root is qi deficiency and weakness of blood, Eight-Treasure Decoction (bā zhēn tāng) is fitting.

Clinically, it is helpful to combine these formulas with Delayed Menstruation Drink (guò qī yǐn) when the stasis is mild. If, however, the stasis is severe, it is best to clear the stasis before tonifying.

Most modern practitioners consider the original dosages for this formula to be too small. One should therefore increase various ingredients according to the patient's presenting pattern. If blood deficiency is paramount, increase Angelicae sinensis Radix (dāng guī) and Rehmanniae Radix (shēng dì huáng). If stasis is dominant and deficiency is not extreme, increase the dosage of Carthami Flos (hóng huā), Persicae Semen (táo rén), and Chuanxiong Rhizoma (chuān xiōng).

Though originally intended for overdue menses, this formula is now also used for painful menstruation owing to blood deficiency and stasis of qi and blood. In this case, it is usually given for 4-5 days prior to the onset of the period and is continued through the first day of the period.

Comparison

➤ Vs. Four-Substance Decoction with Safflower and Peach Pit (táo hóng sì wù tāng)

Delayed Menstruation Drink (guò qī yǐn) can be seen as a warmer variation of Four-Substance Decoction with Safflower and Peach Pit (táo hóng sì wù tāng), which can also move the qi and fluids. It is thus well-suited for a woman with overdue menses together with fluid retention and qi stagnation (manifesting as discomfort in the lower abdomen and emotional distress). If, on the other hand, the main symptoms associated with overdue menses are heavily clotted blood, a purple tongue, and stabbing pain, Four-Substance Decoction with Safflower and Peach Pit (táo hóng sì wù tāng) may be a better choice.

Biomedical Indications

With the appropriate presentation, this formula may be used to treat a variety of biomedically-defined disorders, particularly those affecting women such as irregular menstruation and dysmenorrhea.

Modifications

- Where the cold is extreme and the lower abdominal pain is relieved by warmth, add Evodiae Fructus (wú zhū yú), Foeniculi Fructus (xiǎo huí xiāng), and Zingiberis Rhizoma (gān jiāng).
- For qi stagnation, add Linderae Radix (wū yào).
- If dampness is present or fluid retention is extreme, add Poria (fú líng) and Atractylodis Rhizoma (cāng zhú).
- For phlegm, add Poria (fú líng), Citri reticulatae Pericarpium (chén pí), and Pinelliae Rhizoma praeparatum (zhì bàn xià).

女科柏子仁丸
Arborvitae Seed Pills for Women's Disorders

nǚ kē bǎi zǐ rén wán

Source   *Fine Formulas for Women* (1237)

Rehmanniae Radix praeparata (shú dì huáng) 96g (15-30g)
Lycopi Herba (zé lán) 64g (12g)
Dipsaci Radix (xù duàn) 64g (12g)
Selaginellae tamariscinae Herba (juǎn bǎi) 16g (9g)
Achyranthis bidentatae Radix (niú xī) 16g (9g)
Platycladi Semen (bǎi zǐ rén) 16g (9g)

Method of Preparation   Grind the ingredients into a powder and form into small pills with the addition of honey. The source text prescribes 30 pills the size of the seeds of the Chinese parasol tree on an empty stomach. At present, it is often taken as a decoction. The dosages above are the suggestions of the editors.

Actions   Quiets the spirit, invigorates the blood, nourishes the blood, and unblocks the menses

Indications

Amenorrhea of gradual onset from long-term blood deficiency. Attendant symptoms include general disquietude, gradually worsening afternoon tidal fevers, emaciation, and achy and uncomfortable flesh and bones of the hands and feet. The formula also treats irregular menstruation or scanty menses from deficiency of yin and blood accompanied by blood stasis.

The source text puts the above symptoms in the context of "yin deficiency blood weakness [which allows] yang to roam and overwhelm. Scarce water cannot extinguish the abundance of fire [leaving] fire to accelerate its drying effect on water [thus resulting in] devastation of fluids." The author goes on to say that the treatment principle in such circumstances is to "nourish the blood and augment the yin. One should be cautious not to use toxic herbs to unblock." The text also mentions that, despite obvious heat signs, one should not use cool herbs such as Artemisiae annuae Herba *(qīng hāo)* in this situation because to do so would cause the blood to congeal, which would aggravate the disorder.

Analysis of Formula

The formula contains mild and moderate herbs to gently nourish and move the blood and nourish the Heart. The chief herb, Platycladi Semen *(bǎi zǐ rén)*, is a good example of the gentle and nourishing nature of this formula. *Comprehensive Outline of the Materia Medica* states that this herb:

> Nourishes Heart qi, moistens Kidney dryness, quiets the ethereal soul, and settles the corporeal soul. Its nature is balanced, and it is neither cold nor drying. Its flavor is sweet and tonifying, it is acrid and yet can moisten, its qi is clear and fragrant, and it can penetrate the Heart and Kidney and augment the Spleen and Stomach.

Rehmanniae Radix praeparata *(shú dì huáng)*, the deputy herb, enriches the Kidney yin and nourishes the blood, thus addressing the two main causes of the disorder. Achyranthis bidentatae Radix *(niú xī)* nourishes the Liver and Kidney, invigorates the blood, dispels stasis, and guides the blood downward. Dipsaci Radix *(xù duàn)* tonifies the Liver but can also break up blood stasis. Because the author of this formula wanted to avoid strong moving herbs for this pattern, the movement of the blood is promoted with herbs that tonify or nourish as they promote movement.

Lycopi Herba *(zé lán)* is a blood-moving agent that is acrid, bitter, fragrant, and drying. It is often contraindicated in cases of blood deficiency. In this formula, however, its drying nature is offset by the inclusion of a large dosage of Rehmanniae Radix praeparata *(shú dì huáng)*. The acrid, dispersing, and fragrant Spleen-arousing nature of Lycopi Herba *(zé lán)* also helps to obviate the stagnation that Rehmanniae Radix praeparata *(shú dì huáng)* might otherwise engender. Lycopi Herba *(zé lán)* unblocks the menses, invigorates the blood,

and dispels stasis. It joins with the more moderate Achyranthis bidentatae Radix *(niú xī)* and Dipsaci Radix *(xù duàn)* to move the blood and dispel stasis.

The last of the four assistants is Selaginellae tamariscinae Herba (卷柏 *juǎn bǎi)*, which has the English name of tamariskoid spikemoss. It is acrid and neutral, enters the Liver and Heart channels, and stops bleeding when charred, but otherwise invigorates the blood and unblocks the channels.

Commentary

In the early 20th-century gynecology text *Compendium of Secrets for Women's Diseases*, Chen Lian-Fang cites Arborvitae Seed Pill for Women's Disorders *(nǚ kē bái zǐ rén wán)* as one of the four formulas for the treatment of withered-blood amenorrhea (血枯經閉 *xuè kū jīng bì)*, which is one of the two main categories of amenorrhea, the other being blood obstruction (血隔 *xuè gé)*. The two can be distinguished by studying the history of the disorder and its attendant symptoms. In the same text, Zhang Jing-Yue notes:

> Liver disease withered-blood pattern and blood-obstruction pattern are similar, both displaying the symptom of amenorrhea. [However, in truth,] they are as different as ice and hot coals. Withering [signals] exhaustion, blood deficiency in the extreme. Obstruction [signals] blockage; the blood's foundation is not deficient [and there is evidence of] rebellion [from] qi [stagnation], cold, or accumulation.

The onset may be gradual in both patterns, but the presence of pain or other symptoms of rebellion and excess in the blood-obstruction type, and the attendant symptoms of blood and yin deficiency in the blood-withering type, are important markers for differentiation. Chen Lian-Fang suggests Arborvitae Seed Pill for Women's Disorders *(nǚ kē bái zǐ rén wán)* for withered-blood amenorrhea in patients who exhibit blood deficiency with fire from yin deficiency. The thinking here matches that of the formula's author, Chen Zi-Ming, who stated that the formula is for women who are "gradually losing weight, have irritating pain in the flesh and bones of the hands and feet, gradually worsening tidal fevers, and a faint and rapid pulse."

Although it treats patients with signs of deficiency fire, Arborvitae Seed Pill for Women's Disorders *(nǚ kē bái zǐ rén wán)* is a warm and nourishing formula. Its author warned against the use of cold herbs that would aggravate the stagnation and damage the yin and qi. Instead, he advised that withered-blood amenorrhea required the use of nourishing and gently moving agents, as the signs of heat will fall away naturally as their root cause is eradicated.

Comparison

➣ Vs. Four-Substance Decoction *(sì wù tāng)*

Both of these formulas treat menstrual irregularities owing to blood deficiency and blood stasis. The difference lies in their focus. While Four-Substance Decoction (sì wù tāng) is better suited for blood deficiency, it is less able than Arborvitae Seed Pill for Women's Disorders (nǔ kē bái zǐ rén wán) to move the blood and dispel stasis, nor can it treat the disturbance of the spirit that is part of the pattern that Arborvitae Seed Pill for Women's Disorders (nǔ kē bái zǐ rén wán) treats. For cases where blood deficiency is paramount and stasis secondary, the two formulas can be used together.

Biomedical Indications

With the appropriate presentation, this formula may be used to treat a variety of biomedically-defined disorders including amenorrhea and irregular menstruation.

Modifications

- For severe blood stasis, manifestIng in stabbing pain in the lower abdomen, purple tongue color, and clotted menstrual blood, add Verbenae Herba (mǎ biān cǎo), Persicae Semen (táo rén), Carthami Flos (hóng huā), and Spatholobi Caulis (jī xuè téng).

- If the patient suffers from Spleen-deficient digestive difficulties, replace Rehmanniae Radix praeparata (shú dì huáng) with Two-Solstice Pill (èr zhì wán).

- For blood-deficient headaches, add Angelicae sinensis Radix (dāng guī) and Chuanxiong Rhizoma (chuān xiōng).

- For insomnia, add Albiziae Cortex (hé huān pí) and Spatholobi Caulis (jī xuè téng).

- For amenorrhea due to a meager amount of blood, add Lycopi Herba (zé lán), Angelicae sinensis Radix (dāng guī), Glycyrrhizae Radix (gān cǎo), and Paeoniae Radix alba (bái sháo). In Golden Mirror of the Medical Tradition, the combination of these four herbs is called Lycopus Decoction (zé lán tāng).

芍藥甘草湯 (芍药甘草汤)
Peony and Licorice Decoction

sháo yào gān cǎo tāng

Source   Discussion of Cold Damage (c. 220)

Paeoniae Radix (sháo yào) 12g (30g-100g)
Glycyrrhizae Radix praeparata (zhì gān cǎo) 12g (10-30g)

Method of Preparation   Decoction. Paeoniae Radix alba (bái sháo) is the form of Radix Paeoniae that is generally used in this formula. At present, the dosage that is commonly used is specified in parentheses.

Actions   Nourishes the blood, augments the yin, moderates painful spasms, and alleviates pain

Indications

Irritability, slight chills, spasms of the calf muscles, and the absence of coating on the tongue. The formula also treats cramps in the hands, and abdominal pain that improves with pressure.

This formula was originally used for the first pattern described here, which was said to occur when the inappropriate use of sweating had injured the blood or yin. At present, it is used for any type of pain in the calves with blood deficiency or injury to the fluids. The irritability and lack of tongue coating are attributed to injury to the yin. The slight chills are due to weakness of the yang that follows injury to the yin, and may not always be present. The spasms, cramps, and abdominal pain are typically spasmodic, wind-like manifestations that are commonly associated with patterns of Liver blood deficiency or exuberant wood (Liver) overwhelming earth (Spleen). The fact that the pain improves with pressure indicates that it is neither due to heat (i.e., inflammatory in nature) nor to an organic lesion.

Analysis of Formula

The chief herb is Paeoniae Radix alba (bái sháo), which nourishes the blood and preserves the yin. It enters the Spleen, softens the Liver, and alleviates pain. It thereby addresses the primary aspects of this condition. The Liver is a hard, 'edgy' organ, and its qi has a tendency to rebel transversely. This herb is effective in moderating the wayward inclinations of the Liver qi, especially when it overacts on earth, and preserving the Liver yin; this is what is meant by 'softening of the Liver.' Glycyrrhizae Radix praeparata (zhì gān cǎo) augments the qi of the middle burner, especially that of the Spleen, and moderates urgency. Together, these herbs regulate the relationship between the Liver and Spleen and nourish the sinews and blood, which in turn stops the spasms and pain.

Commentary

This formula is very popular for treating a wide variety of pain syndromes associated with spasms and cramps. In Treatment Strategies and Formulas in Chinese Medicine, the contemporary physician Chen Chao-Zu identifies the following markers for use of this formula:

- Hypertonicity of the extremities characterized by difficult extension and flexion

- Pain in the head, body, or limbs due to arterial spasms, characterized by severe pulling pain

- Abdominal pain characterized by tightness and distention that responds favorably to pressure

- Hypertonicity of smooth muscle leading to symptoms such as wheezing, coughing, hiccup, vomiting, or diarrhea characterized by subjective sensations of severe discomfort.

The formula is also used to overcome aconite toxicity.

The strategy by which this formula addresses these problems is widely known as 'transforming yin with sweet and sour [herbs].' There are two very different interpretations of this adage in the literature. The first interprets 'transforming' to mean 'forming' and focuses on the yin-nourishing qualities of the formula. The second reads 'transforming yin' as implying a more dynamic action of opening obstruction by means of regulating the qi. Fei Bo-Xiong's analysis of the formula in *Discussion of Medical Formulas* is representative of the latter view:

> If there is no free flow, there will be pain. When the abdomen and middle [burner] are not harmonized, the qi rebels and there is turbid yin. In this case, one employs the method of transforming yin with sweet and sour herbs in order to naturally diminish rebellious qi. This is also the wisdom [implied in the notion of] softening [excessive] restraint.

An interpretation that reconciles the two views was offered by Chen Chao-Zu. Chen pointed out that the source text uses equal amounts of Glycyrrhizae Radix (*gān cǎo*) and Paeoniae Radix alba (*bái sháo*), implying that both sweet and sour flavors are equally important constituents of the formula. This accords with Chapter 22 of *Basic Questions*, which admonishes: "When the Liver suffers from tension, urgently take sweet [medicinals] in order to moderate it." The yin-nourishing action of sweet herbs, in other words, is a primary tool for moderating hypertonicity throughout the body, and sweet herbs like Glycyrrhizae Radix (*gān cǎo*), Jujubae Fructus (*dà zǎo*), and Maltosum (*yí táng*) are consistently used in classical formulas for this purpose. Rather than merely harmonizing the middle burner or the actions of the other herbs, sweet flavors thus actively control the yang. Softening and moderating in nature, they relax tension, restore free flow, and thereby alleviate pain.

Biomedical Indications

With the appropriate presentation, this formula may be used to treat a very wide variety of biomedically-defined disorders. These can be divided into the following groups:

- Pain and discomfort from spasms of skeletal muscles, ligaments, and related tissues including fibromyalgia, cramping calf muscles, vaginismus, priaprism, laryngeal spasm, poststroke contractures, periarthritis of the shoulder, acute lumbar strain, and spinal osteophytes

- Pain, often severe, from smooth muscle spasm such as biliary colic, renal colic, gastric spasm, intestinal adhesions, peptic ulcers, atrophic gastritis, bronchial asthma, pertussis, ulcerative colitis, end-stage hepatic carcinoma, and threatened miscarriage

- Bone and joint pain such as rheumatoid arthritis, heel pain, cervical spine syndrome, necrosis of the femoral head, and disc disease

- Neuralgia, including trigeminal neuralgia, intercostal neuralgia, postherpetic neuralgia, sciatica, and diabetic neuropathy

- Disorders marked by involuntary stimulation such as recalcitrant hiccups, restless leg syndrome, bruxism, facial tics, Parkinson's disease, essential tremor, atrial fibrillation, night terrors, and enuresis

- Bleeding disorders such as thrombocytopenic purpura, allergic purpura, upper GI bleeding, bronchiectasis, and recurrent nosebleeds

- Problems due to decreases in humoral functionality such as male and female infertility, hypotestosteronemia, impotence from increased prolactin levels, and myasthenia gravis.

In addition, this formula has also been used for treating hepatitis, diabetes, acute mastitis, bacillary dysentery, habitual constipation, anal fissures, and coronary artery disease.

Modifications

- For fixed pain that increases with pressure, substitute Paeoniae Radix rubra (*chì sháo*) for Paeoniae Radix alba (*bái sháo*).

- For a slow pulse and other signs of cold, add Zingiberis Rhizoma (*gān jiāng*).

- For a flooding pulse and other signs of heat, add Coptidis Rhizoma (*huáng lián*).

- To increase the efficacy of the formula in treating spasms of the calf muscles, add Achyranthis bidentatae Radix (*niú xī*) and Chaenomelis Fructus (*mù guā*).

- For abdominal pain, add Cyperi Rhizoma (*xiāng fù*).

- For wind rash, add Cicadae Periostracum (*chán tuì*), Jujubae Fructus (*dà zǎo*), and Kochiae Fructus (*dì fū zǐ*).

- For spasms of the extremities and stiff neck and back associated with encephalitis, after the fever has broken, add Scorpio (*quán xiē*) and Scolopendra (*wú gōng*).

Associated Formula

芍藥甘草附子湯 (芍药甘草附子汤)

Peony, Licorice, and Aconite Accessory Root Decoction
sháo yào gān cǎo fù zǐ tāng

SOURCE *Discussion of Cold Damage* (c. 220)

Paeoniae Radix (*sháo yào*) 9g
Glycyrrhizae Radix praeparata (*zhì gān cǎo*) 9g
Aconiti Radix lateralis praeparata (*zhì fù zǐ*) 3g

This formula supports the yang and benefits the yin. It is used for treating those with constitutional weakness in whom sweating was inappropriately induced and who thereafter develop chills and a slow, submerged pulse. Paeoniae Radix alba (*bái sháo*) is the variety of Radix Paeoniae most often used in this formula.

當歸生薑羊肉湯（当归生姜羊肉汤）

Mutton Stew with Tangkuei and Fresh Ginger

dāng guī shēng jiāng yáng ròu tāng

Source   *Essentials from the Golden Cabinet* (c. 220)

Angelicae sinensis Radix *(dāng guī)* 9g
Zingiberis Rhizoma recens *(shēng jiāng)* 15g
mutton *(yáng ròu)* 48g

Method of Preparation   Prepare as a stew by simmering in 8 cups of water until it is reduced to 3 cups of liquid.

Actions   Warms the interior, nourishes the blood, and alleviates pain

Indications

Postpartum abdominal pain, cold abdominal hernial pain, or spasmodic pain in the flanks. The pain responds favorably to pressure and warmth. The pulse is submerged, wiry, and forceless.

This is a pattern of interior deficiency with cold blood. In the postpartum period, the blood is often deficient because of loss of blood and essence during birth. If an external cold pathogenic influence takes advantage of this weakened condition and invades the body, it will lodge in the blood level and obstruct the dynamic of both qi and blood. Because deficiency is the primary etiology, the pain will respond favorably to pressure, and because it is a cold disorder, it will respond favorably to warmth. The pulse is submerged and wiry because of the pain from interior cold, and forceless because of the deficiency. This type of cold abdominal hernial pain and spasmodic flank pain may also occur in individuals with constitutional blood deficiency.

Analysis of Formula

The chief ingredient is mutton *(yáng ròu)*. Heating, sweet, and acrid in nature, mutton strongly tonifies the fire at the gate of vitality, nourishes the blood, and augments the qi. Angelicae sinensis Radix *(dāng guī)*, which tonifies without causing stagnation, and warms without drying, serves as deputy. It is also an excellent herb for generating blood, which is required in this condition. Acrid, warm Zingiberis Rhizoma recens *(shēng jiāng)* scatters the cold and serves as the assistant ingredient. It also facilitates digestion of the chief ingredient and thereby indirectly aids in tonification. Because it warms, it also assists the deputy in moving the blood. The combination of these three ingredients not only nourishes the blood, but also disperses the cold and thereby relieves the pain.

Commentary

This formula is an example of 'food as medicine.' It embodies the principle of 'unblocking [through] tonification' (通補

tōng bǔ), taken up by later physicians, with the use of such herbs as Cistanches Herba *(ròu cōng róng)* or Morindae officinalis Radix *(bā jǐ tiān)*. By this is meant the use of herbs with a thick flavor capable of tonifying the blood and essence, yet which are also warming and moving in nature so that they can unblock the pain from deficiency. It is important to note that when the formula is used in treating hernial pain, it should be taken after the acute stage has resolved. It will not help in acute conditions. Its use has been expanded to include dysmenorrhea, leukorrhea, lower back pain, and abdominal pain associated with cold from deficiency.

Biomedical Indications

With the appropriate presentation, this formula may be used to treat a variety of biomedically-defined disorders such as postpartum weakness, hernia, leukorrhea, male infertility, and thrombocytopenic purpura.

Modifications

- For severe cold, increase the dosage of Zingiberis Rhizoma recens *(shēng jiāng)* to 48 grams. (source text)
- For severe pain and vomiting, add 6g of Citri reticulatae Pericarpium *(chén pí)* and 3g of Atractylodis macrocephalae Rhizoma *(bái zhú)*. (source text)
- For severe pain, add a large amount (over 30g) of Paeoniae Radix alba *(bái sháo)*.
- For profuse, continuous sweating postpartum, add Astragali Radix *(huáng qí)*.
- For lochioschesis, add Cinnamomi Ramulus *(guì zhī)*.

Section 3

. . . .

FORMULAS THAT TONIFY THE QI AND BLOOD

八珍湯（八珍汤）

Eight-Treasure Decoction

bā zhēn tāng

This formula is composed of eight ingredients that are highly valued for their ability to tonify the qi and blood, hence the name.

Source   *Experiential Formulas from the Auspicious Bamboo Hall* (1326)

Ginseng Radix *(rén shēn)* 30g (6-9g)
Atractylodis macrocephalae Rhizoma *(bái zhú)* 30g (9-12g)
Poria *(fú líng)* 30g (12-15g)
Glycyrrhizae Radix praeparata *(zhì gān cǎo)* 30g (3-6g)
Rehmanniae Radix praeparata *(shú dì huáng)* 30g (15-18g)

Paeoniae Radix alba *(bái sháo)* 30g (12-15g)
Angelicae sinensis Radix *(dāng guī)* 30g (12-15g)
Chuanxiong Rhizoma *(chuān xiōng)* 30g (6-9g)

Method of Preparation The source text advises to grind the herbs into a coarse powder and prepare as a draft by boiling 9g of the powder in 200ml of water together with 5 slices of Zingiberis Rhizoma recens *(shēng jiāng)* and 1 piece of Jujubae Fructus *(dà zǎo)*. At present, it is usually prepared as a decoction with the dosage specified in parentheses. Codonopsis Radix *(dǎng shēn)* is usually substituted for Ginseng Radix *(rén shēn)* at 2-3 times its dosage.

Actions Tonifies and augments the qi and blood

Indications

Pallid or sallow complexion, palpitations with anxiety that may be continuous, reduced appetite, shortness of breath, laconic speech, extremities that are easily fatigued, lightheadedness and/or vertigo, a pale tongue with a white coating, and a pulse which is either thin and frail or large, deficient, and without strength.

This is concurrent deficiency of the qi and blood, most often due to imbalances caused by chronic disease or excessive loss of blood. The Lungs control the body's qi; when the qi is deficient, the Lung qi will also be deficient. This manifests as shortness of breath and laconic speech. A poor appetite is almost a pathognomonic sign of Spleen qi deficiency. In this case, the Spleen qi is too weak to transform and transport nutrients to the extremities. When this is combined with blood deficiency, the extremities are easily fatigued. Concurrent deficiency of the qi and blood also prevents nourishment (the clear yang and the blood) from reaching the head and Heart. This leads to palpitations (which may be continuous), lightheadedness and/or vertigo, and a pallid or sallow complexion. The complexion will be more pallid if the condition is primarily one of qi deficiency, and more sallow if blood deficiency predominates. The pale tongue with a white coating combines signs of blood and qi deficiency. If blood deficiency predominates, the pulse will be thin and frail, and if qi deficiency predominates, the pulse will be large, deficient, and without strength.

Analysis of Formula

To treat patterns caused by both qi and blood deficiency, this formula pays equal attention to both. All the chief herbs are warming in nature. Ginseng Radix *(rén shēn)* augments the qi, and Rehmanniae Radix praeparata *(shú dì huáng)* nourishes the blood. Two of the deputies, Atractylodis macrocephalae Rhizoma *(bái zhú)* and Poria *(fú líng)*, strengthen the Spleen and dry or leach-out dampness, thereby assisting Ginseng Radix *(rén shēn)* in strengthening the qi of the Spleen and Lungs. The other deputies, Paeoniae Radix alba *(bái sháo)* and Angelicae sinensis Radix *(dāng guī)*, nourish the blood and thereby reinforce the action of Rehmanniae Radix praeparata *(shú dì huáng)*.

One of the assistants, Chuanxiong Rhizoma *(chuān xiōng)*, invigorates the blood and promotes the movement of qi. The other, Glycyrrhizae Radix praeparata *(zhì gān cǎo)*, augments the qi and harmonizes the middle burner. The envoys are Zingiberis Rhizoma recens *(shēng jiāng)* and Jujubae Fructus *(dà zǎo)*, which regulate the absorptive function of the Stomach and Spleen. This is especially important because it allows the other herbs in the formula to be absorbed. The envoys also regulate the relationship between the protective and nutritive qi, which allows a patient suffering from deficiency to recover without developing other problems.

Commentary

This formula is a combination of Four-Gentlemen Decoction *(sì jūn zǐ tāng)* and Four-Substance Decoction *(sì wù tāng)*. The reader is referred to those formulas for a more complete discussion of the interaction among the ingredients. Because one of these formulas tonifies the qi and the other one the blood, most commentators interpret the combined formulas as simply additive. The one exception is the modern physician Zhang Shan-Lei, who views the formula as acting primarily on the middle burner, as discussed in this passage from *Annotated and Corrected Synopsis of Shen's Women's Disorders*:

> Based on the physiological function of the ingredients, one can say that Four-Gentlemen Decoction *(sì jūn zǐ tāng)* [consists of] qi herbs, which are able to support the Spleen yang. Four-Substance Decoction *(sì wù tāng)* [consists of] blood herbs, which are able to nourish the Spleen yin. The former relates to qi, the latter to blood. Hence, one can explain [this formula] as focusing on the Spleen and Stomach, and one need not just generalize about Four-Gentlemen Decoction *(sì jūn zǐ tāng)* tonifying qi and Four-Substance Decoction *(sì wù tāng)* tonifying blood.

If one examines the original indications of the formula, there is some justification for Zhang's focus on the middle burner. These are listed in the source texts as abdominal pain, complete disinterest in food, frailty of the yin and yang organs, diarrhea, hardness and pain in the lower abdomen, and periodic chills and fevers. Furthermore, although originally a women's formula, it has long been used to treat any pattern in both men and women where both the qi and blood are deficient. The presentation may include chills and fever, weight loss, abscesses that neither suppurate nor improve, and continuous spotting from uterine bleeding.

Comparisons

> ➤ Vs. Tangkuei Decoction to Tonify the Blood *(dāng guī bǔ xuè tāng)*

Both formulas can be used to tonify the qi and blood in the treatment of fevers, uterine bleeding, or nonhealing abscesses or sores. However, the primary action of Tangkuei Decoction to Tonify the Blood *(dāng guī bǔ xuè tāng)* is to secure the floating yang, whereas the present formula aims at nourishing the qi and blood more generally.

➤ Vs. All-Inclusive Great Tonifying Decoction (*shí quán dà bǔ tāng*); *see* PAGE 349

Alternate name

Eight-Substance Decoction (*bā wù tāng*) in *Correct Transmission of Medicine*

Biomedical Indications

With the appropriate presentation, this formula may be used to treat a wide variety of biomedically-defined disorders including various forms of anemia, chronic hepatitis, dysfunctional uterine bleeding, habitual miscarriage, nonhealing ulcers, and nervous exhaustion.

Modifications

- For insomnia, add Ziziphi spinosae Semen (*suān zǎo rén*) and Armeniacae Semen (*xìng rén*).

- For Stomach deficiency with reduced appetite, add Amomi Fructus (*shā rén*) and Massa medicata fermentata (*shén qū*).

- For galactorrhea from deficiency and weakness of the Stomach qi that causes it to become unstable, remove Chuanxiong Rhizoma (*chuān xiōng*) and add Astragali Radix (*huáng qí*), Schisandrae Fructus (*wǔ wèi zǐ*), and Euryales Semen (*qiàn shí*).

Associated Formula

八珍益母湯 （八珍益母汤）

Eight-Treasure Pill to Benefit Mothers

bā zhēn yì mǔ wán

SOURCE   *Collected Treatises of [Zhang] Jing-Yue* (1624)

Ginseng Radix (*rén shēn*) 30g
dry-fried Atractylodis macrocephalae Rhizoma
    (*chǎo bái zhú*) 30g
Poria (*fú líng*) 30g
Chuanxiong Rhizoma (*chuān xiōng*) 30g
Angelicae sinensis Radix (*dāng guī*) 60g
Rehmanniae Radix praeparata (*shú dì huáng*) 60g
Glycyrrhizae Radix praeparata (*zhì gān cǎo*) 15g
vinegar friend Paeoniae Radix alba (*cù chǎo bái sháo*) . . . 30g
Leonuri Herba (*yì mǔ cǎo*) 120g

Grind the ingredients into a fine powder and form into pills with honey. Take on an empty stomach with honey water or wine. Tonifies deficiency and invigorates the blood. For qi and blood deficiency with blood stasis leading to such problems as irregular menstruation and red-and-white vaginal discharge. Accompanying signs and symptoms include reduced appetite, weak extremities, soreness in the lower back, and abdominal distention. Also used for infertility and a restless fetus.

十全大補湯 （十全大补汤）

All-Inclusive Great Tonifying Decoction

shí quán dà bǔ tāng

This formula is composed of ten herbs that strongly tonify the qi and blood, extending its action to the entire body, hence the name.

Source   *Transmitted Trustworthy and Suitable Formulas* (1180)

Ginseng Radix (*rén shēn*) . . . . (6-9g)
Atractylodis macrocephalae Rhizoma (*bái zhú*) . . . . . . (9-12g)
Poria (*fú líng*) . . . . (12-15g)
Glycyrrhizae Radix praeparata (*zhì gān cǎo*) . . . . (3-6g)
Rehmanniae Radix praeparata (*shú dì huáng*) . . . . . . (15-18g)
Paeoniae Radix alba (*bái sháo*) . . . . (12-15g)
Angelicae sinensis Radix (*dāng guī*) . . . . (12-15g)
Chuanxiong Rhizoma (*chuān xiōng*) . . . . (6-9g)
Cinnamomi Cortex (*ròu guì*) . . . . (6-9g)
Astragali Radix (*huáng qí*) . . . . (15-18g)

Method of Preparation   The source text advises to coarsely grind equal amounts of the ingredients and take 6g as a draft with 3 pieces of Zingiberis Rhizoma recens (*shēng jiāng*) and 2 pieces of Jujubae Fructus (*dà zǎo*). At present, it is usually taken as a decoction with the dosage specified in parentheses. Codonopsis Radix (*dǎng shēn*) is usually substituted for Ginseng Radix (*rén shēn*) at 2-3 times its dosage.

Actions   Warms and tonifies the qi and blood

Indications

A wan complexion, fatigue, reduced appetite, dizziness, listlessness, dyspnea, palpitations, spontaneous sweating, night sweats, cold extremities, spermatorrhea, a pale tongue, and a thin and frail pulse. The formula is also used to treat sores that do not heal, irregular periods, or continuous spotting from uterine bleeding.

This is combined qi and blood deficiency, often seen in consumptive disorders. When the qi is deficient, the entire body loses its warmth and nourishment, leading to symptoms like fatigue, listlessness, dyspnea, spontaneous sweating, cold extremities, and a frail pulse. When the blood is deficient, the organs, channels, and collaterals are no longer moistened and nourished, leading to symptoms like a wan complexion, dizziness, palpitations, night sweats, a pale tongue, and a thin pulse. If the qi and blood fail to nourish the Penetrating and Conception vessels, the sea of blood becomes empty, leading to irregular periods and uterine bleeding in women, and to spermatorrhoea in men. If the muscle sinews, bones, and joints are not nourished, this leads to sores that do not heal.

Analysis of Formula

This formula is a combination of Four-Gentlemen Decoction (*sì jūn zǐ tāng*), the primary formula for tonifying the qi, and Four-Substance Decoction (*sì wù tāng*), the primary formula for tonifying the blood, to which Astragali Radix (*huáng qí*) and Cinnamomi Cortex (*ròu guì*) have been added. Sweet and warming Astragali Radix (*huáng qí*) is described in *Seeking Accuracy in the Materia Medica* as "the first among all of the qi-tonifying herbs." Entirely yang in nature, it powerfully stimulates the qi dynamic, raises the yang, and disperses the blood and essences throughout the entire body. Acrid and strongly warming Cinnamomi Cortex (*ròu guì*) tonifies the fire at the gate of vitality to assist the yang. Its warmth enters the blood to open the vessels and facilitate the movement of blood, and it stimulates the qi dynamic and transformation throughout the entire body, as described by Zhang Bin-Cheng in the early 20th-century work *Convenient Reader of Established Formulas*: "The tonifying properties of all herbs that receive the power of its warming nourishment are greatly increased. Therefore, their efficacy is also greatly increased. Not only yang deficiency, but also yin deficiency can be warmed, because without the yang, the yin cannot be generated." Overall, therefore, this formula can be said to stimulate, tonify, and gather the power of qi and yang in order to stimulate the production and transformation of blood.

Cautions and Contraindications

This is a strong tonifying formula. It must not be used for treating disorders of excess reflected in such symptoms as a thick tongue coating or a strong and forceful pulse.

Commentary

This is a very commonly used formula for qi and blood deficiency with a predominance of deficient qi tending toward cold. Regarding its action, the Qing-dynasty physician Wang Zi-Jie in *Selected Annotations to Ancient Formulas from the Garden of Crimson Snow* provides an analysis of the formula that extends beyond simple qi and blood tonification and that provides an alternative interpretation of its name:

> Adding Astragali Radix (*huáng qí*) and Cinnamomi Cortex (*ròu guì*) to Four-Gentlemen Decoction (*sì jūn zǐ tāng*) and Four-Substance Decoction (*sì wù tāng*) produces a complex strategy of hardening and softening. The Spleen is a soft organ, which is controlled by the hardening herbs in Four-Gentlemen Decoction (*sì jūn zǐ tāng*). Concerned that excessive hardening may harm its softness, one adds Astragali Radix (*huáng qí*) to support the softening qi. The Liver is a hard organ, which is controlled by the softening herbs in Four-Substance Decoction (*sì wù tāng*). Concerned that excessive softening may harm its hardness, one adds Cinnamomi Cortex (*ròu guì*) in order to shield its hardness. Attentive to every detail, this [new formula] can truly be referred to as all-inclusive. For only the tonification of Liver and Spleen can be called 'great,' as explained in Chapter 29 of *Basic Questions* 29: "The Spleen normally contacts the Stomach and is the essence or earth. Modeling itself on heaven and earth, the earth produces the myriad things.' Thus, it is the root of the postnatal life. Although the Liver is a male yin organ that occupies an inferior position, one has nevertheless to worry about its ability of using its excess to exploit any deficiency. Hence, one must include a strategy whereby harden-

ing and softening [herbs] mutually control each other in any [formula] that augments and tonifies. Harmonizing the Liver and constructing the Spleen, [this formula restores] the unceasing transformative [processes] of the middle palace, establishing it like heaven and earth as a place for the production of the myriad things. Therefore, it is called 'all-inclusive tonification.'

In contemporary practice, this formula is often used palliatively in the treatment of severe chronic and incurable disorders like cancer. It is also used to assist in the recovery from surgery, severe blood loss, or major illness. Some physicians advise to take it for up to two weeks before surgery to minimize the risk of complications and provide a basis for healing and recovery. Similarly, it is used to minimize the side effects of radiation therapy or chemotherapy, when it is also often prescribed up to a week before biomedical treatment begins.

Due to its composition, many physicians view this formula to be a variation of Eight-Treasure Decoction (*bā zhēn tāng*), discussed above. However, the text in which this formula was first listed was published in 1180, which is 146 years before the text in which Eight-Treasure Decoction (*bā zhēn tāng*) is discussed for the first time. Furthermore, a formula called Internally Tonifying Decoction with Astragalus (*nèi bǔ huáng qí tāng*), whose composition is very similar to that of All-Inclusive Great Tonifying Decoction (*shí quán dà bǔ tāng*), can be found in *Formulas Bequeathed by the Unorthodox Genius Liu Juan-Zi*, published in 499. Given the influence of this formulary, Internally Tonifying Decoction with Astragalus (*nèi bǔ huáng qí tāng*), listed under ASSOCIATED FORMULAS below, must thus be considered the true ancestor of the present formula.

Comparisons

➤ Vs. EIGHT-TREASURE DECOCTION (*bā zhēn tāng*)

Both fomulas tonify the qi and blood and are derived from the combination of Four-Gentlemen Decoction (*sì jūn zǐ tāng*) and Four-Substance Decoction (*sì wù tāng*). Although quite similar in composition, the present formula focuses more strongly on warming the yang and moving the qi and blood. It is thus preferred for patterns that include symptoms like cold extremities or weakness in the lower body. Eight-Treasure Decoction (*bā zhēn tāng*), on the other hand, can be used for patterns characterized by periodic chills and fevers.

➤ Vs. GINSENG DECOCTION TO NOURISH LUXURIANCE (*rén shēn yǎng róng tāng*); see PAGE 352

Biomedical Indications

With the appropriate presentation, this formula may be used to treat a wide variety of biomedically-defined disorders including various forms of anemia, nervous exhaustion, chronic urticaria, nonhealing ulcers, to improve postoperative recovery, and as adjunctive treatment to chemotherapy and radiation therapy.

Alternate names

Ten Tonic Decoction (shí bǔ tāng) in *Simple Book of Formulas*; All-Inclusive Drink (shí quán yǐn) in *Formulary of the Pharmacy Service for Benefiting the People in the Taiping Era*; Great Tonifying All-Inclusive Powder (dà bǔ shí quán sǎn) in *Supreme Commanders of the Medical Ramparts*; Thousand Gold Powder (qiān jīn sǎn) in *Essential Teachings of [Zhu] Dan-Xi*; All-Inclusive Great Tonifying Powder (shí quán dà bǔ sǎn) in *Indispensable Tools for Pattern Treatment*; Augmented Eight-Treasure Decoction (jiā wèi bā zhēn tāng) in *Master Luo's Distillation of Medical Knowedge*

Modifications

- For palpitations, add Schisandrae Fructus (wǔ wèi zǐ) and Ziziphi spinosae Semen (suān zǎo rén).

- For severe sweating, add Ostreae Concha (mǔ lì) and Fossilia Ossis Mastodi (lóng gǔ).

- For Lung and Heart yin deficiency in chronic conditions like bronchial carcinoma or tuberculosis, add Polygalae Radix (yuǎn zhì), Schisandrae Fructus (wǔ wèi zǐ), and Aurantii Fructus (zhǐ ké).

Associated Formulas

內補黃耆湯 (内补黄芪汤)

Internally Tonifying Decoction with Astragalus

nèi bǔ huáng qí tāng

Source   *Formulas Bequeathed by the Unorthodox Genius Liu Juan-Zi* (499)

dry-fried Astragali Radix (chǎo huáng qí)	3g (9-18g)
Ophiopogonis Radix (mài mén dōng)	3g (9-12g)
Rehmanniae Radix praeparata (shú dì huáng)	3g (9-12g)
Poria (fú líng)	3g (9-12g)
Ginseng Radix (rén shēn)	3g (6-9g)
Glycyrrhizae Radix praeparata (zhì gān cǎo)	4.5g (3-6g)
dry-fried Paeoniae Radix alba (chǎo bái sháo)	4.5g (6-12g)
dry-fried Polygalae Radix (chǎo yuǎn zhì)	4.5g (6-12g)
Chuanxiong Rhizoma (chuān xiōng)	4.5g (6-9g)
Cinnamomi Cortex (ròu guì)	4.5g (3-6g)
wine-washed Angelicae sinensis Radix (jiǔ xǐ dāng guī)	4.5g (6-12g)

Prepare as a decoction by boiling with 3 slices of Zingiberis Rhizoma recens (shēng jiāng) and 1 piece of Jujubae Fructus (dà zǎo). Augments and tonifies the qi and blood and promotes tissue growth. For qi and blood deficiency caused by discharging ulcers and sores, with symptoms of pain at the location of the sore, fatigue, laconic speech, spontaneous sweating, dry mouth, a pale tongue with thin coating, and a thin, frail pulse. Also used for fever and uterine bleeding. This is the formula from which All-Inclusive Great Tonifying Decoction (shí quán dà bǔ tāng) was derived. The pattern treated by this formula shows few signs of Spleen deficiency, but some yin deficiency. Hence, it uses Ophiopogonis Radix (mài mén dōng) instead of Atractylodis macrocephalae Rhizoma (bái zhú). It also uses Polygalae Radix (yuǎn zhì) to move the qi and settle the Heart and thereby treat the pain. In clinical practice, this formula is used more commonly in external medicine, whereas All-Inclusive Great Tonifying Decoction (shí quán dà bǔ tāng) is used more commonly in internal medicine and gynecology.

Comparison

➤ Vs. Ginseng Decoction to Nourish Luxuriance (rén shēn yǎng róng tāng); see PAGE 352

腸寧湯 (肠宁汤)

Intestinal Serenity Decoction

cháng níng tāng

Source   *Women's Diseases According to Fu Qing-Zhu* (1826)

Angelicae sinensis Radix (dāng guī)	30g
Rehmanniae Radix praeparata (shú dì huáng)	30g
Ginseng Radix (rén shēn)	9g
Ophiopogonis Radix (mài mén dōng)	9g
Asini Corii Colla (ē jiāo) [dissolve in strained decoction]	9g
Dioscoreae Rhizoma (shān yào)	9g
Dipsaci Radix (xù duàn)	6g
Cinnamomi Cortex (ròu guì) [powdered]	0.6g
Glycyrrhizae Radix (gān cǎo)	3g

Tonifies the blood, augments the qi, and alleviates pain. For postpartum abdominal pain that responds favorably to pressure. This type of pain is very common and is due to loss of blood with resulting qi and blood deficiency. Note that in this case, it is unnecessary to use herbs that are specifically for pain, as proper tonification will relieve the problem.

人參養榮湯 (人参养荣汤)

Ginseng Decoction to Nourish Luxuriance

rén shēn yǎng róng tāng

Source   *Discussion of Illnesses, Patterns, and Formulas Related to the Unification of the Three Etiologies* (1174)

The name of the formula in the source text simply reads Nourish Luxuriance Decoction (yǎng róng tāng). The present name appears for the first time in *Formulary of the Pharmacy Service for Benefiting the People in the Taiping Era*. Due to the enormous influence of this work, it has been maintained by later authors. See the COMMENTARY section for a detailed discussion of the formula's name and its translation into English.

Paeoniae Radix alba (bái sháo)	90g
Angelicae sinensis Radix (dāng guī)	30g
Citri reticulatae Pericarpium (chén pí)	30g
Astragali Radix (huáng qí)	30g
Cinnamomi Cortex (ròu guì)	30g
Ginseng Radix (rén shēn)	30g
Atractylodis macrocephalae Rhizoma (bái zhú)	30g
Glycyrrhizae Radix praeparata (zhì gān cǎo)	30g
Rehmanniae Radix praeparata (shú dì huáng)	22.5g
Schisandrae Fructus (wǔ wèi zǐ)	22.5g
Poria (fú líng)	22.5g
dry-fried Polygalae Radix (chǎo yuǎn zhì)	15g

Method of Preparation   The source texts advises to grind the ingredients into a powder and take 12g as a draft with 3 pieces of

Zingiberis Rhizoma recens (shēng jiāng) and 2 pieces of Jujubae Fructus (dà zǎo). At present, it is usually prepared as a decoction with an appropriate reduction in the dosage of the individual herbs. Codonopsis Radix (dǎng shēn) is usually substituted for Ginseng Radix (rén shēn) at 2-3 times its dosage.

Actions Augments the qi, tonifies the blood, nourishes the Heart, and calms the spirit

Indications

Palpitations, forgetfulness, restlessness at night, feverishness, reduced appetite, fatigue, cough, shortness of breath, dyspnea on exertion, weight loss, dry skin, and a dry mouth and throat. The formula is also used to treat chronic, nonhealing sores.

This is Heart and Spleen qi and blood deficiency due to accumulating damage from overexertion. When the Spleen qi becomes deficient and frail, one easily tires and loses one's appetite. As earth fails to nourish metal, the Lung qi also becomes deficient leading to shortness of breath, coughing, and dyspnea on exertion. Blood nourishes, moistens, and fills the entire body. Blood deficiency is thus reflected in weight loss and dry skin. The Heart spirit resides in the blood. When the blood becomes deficient, the spirit is no longer settled and loses its function to focus the body-person, which is manifested in symptoms like palpitations, forgetfulness, and restlessness at night. Insufficient yin blood loosing control over the yang qi causes feverishness and a dry mouth and throat. When the qi and blood are deficient, the body's ability to restore itself is impaired, tissue growth is retarded, and sores and wounds easily become chronic and fail to heal.

Analysis of Formula

This formula treats Spleen and Heart qi and blood deficiency characterized by symptoms of internal heat and dryness. For this purpose, it uses Paeoniae Radix alba (bái sháo) and Ginseng Radix (rén shēn) as the chief herbs. Sour and cooling Paeoniae Radix alba (bái sháo) enters the Spleen to nourish the blood and restrain the yang. Ginseng Radix (rén shēn) strongly augments the source qi, generates fluids and tonifies the Spleen, Lungs, and Heart. Together, these two herbs address the pathodynamic treated by this formula and harmonize all of the organs that are directly affected by it. Angelicae sinensis Radix (dāng guī) and Rehmanniae Radix praeparata (shú dì huáng) support Paeoniae Radix alba (bái sháo) in nourishing the blood. Astragali Radix (huáng qí), Atractylodis macrocephalae Rhizoma (bái zhú), Poria (fú líng), and Glycyrrhizae Radix praeparata (zhì gān cǎo) help Ginseng Radix (rén shēn) tonify the qi. Cinnamomi Cortex (ròu guì) warms the yang qi to stimulate all physiological activity. These seven herbs serve as deputies. Three assistants balance the tonifying properties of the chief and deputy herbs, by moving the qi and regulating the qi dynamic. Acrid and warming Citri reticulatae Pericarpium (chén pí) enters the Lungs and Spleen to move the qi and harmonize the Stomach, preventing the cloying characteristics of the tonifying herbs from obstructing the qi dynamic. Bitter, acrid, and warming Polygalae Radix (yuǎn zhì) regulates the Heart qi and establishes harmonious communication between the Heart and Kidneys to settle the spirit and calm palpitations. Sweet, sour, and warming Schisandrae Fructus (wǔ wèi zǐ) restrains the qi and prevents excessive sweating, ensuring that augmented qi is not dispersed to the outside but turned toward the inside and the blood. Zingiberis Rhizoma recens (shēng jiāng) and Jujubae Fructus (dà zǎo), which are added to the formula when decocting, serve as assistants by regulating the nutritive and protective qi and harmonizing the Spleen and Stomach. They ensure that this complex formula is properly assimilated, and blend its many ingredients into a harmonious whole.

Cautions and Contraindications

This formula is not indicated for qi and blood deficiency patterns accompanied by symptoms of pronounced cold.

Commentary

This formula is similar in composition to that of All-Inclusive Great Tonifying Decoction (shí quán dà bǔ tāng), discussed above, yet decisively different in its focus on the Spleen and Heart rather than on the Spleen and Liver. This is reflected in the formula's original name, Nourish Luxuriance Decoction (yǎng róng tāng). In the Chinese medical literature, the term 榮 róng is often used interchangeably with the term 營 yíng and therefore translated into English as 'nutritive' or 'constructive' qi. Both terms, furthermore, are often equated to the term 血 xuè or blood. In Discussion of Medical Formulas, the Qing-dynasty physician Fei Bo-Xiong attempted to tease out the subtle differences between these terms:

> To grasp the meaning of [the term] blood [one must understand two other terms]. The first is róng, which means luxuriance. Without blood, there is nothing to moisten the yin and yang organs, irrigate the channels and vessels, and nourish the hundred bones. All of this embodies the meaning [of blood as something] that enriches [and promotes] growth. The second [term] is yíng, which [conveys the image of] barracks and their enclosing walls. Without blood, there is nothing to fill the form, firm the interstices and pores, and secure the hundred vessels. All of this embodies the meaning [of blood as something] that guards [the body-person] from the inside.

This passage clarifies that while the terms xuè, róng, and yíng refer to the same thing, they imply different perspectives. If xuè refers to the overall entity, that is, blood as a thing, then róng and yíng are more dynamic, capturing two different aspects of what this thing does. Here, róng embodies the yin aspect of blood's dynamic: its ability to vitalize the body by means of its moistening and enriching nature. Yíng, on the other hand, refers to blood's active function of securing the body by providing it with substance: a yin place to which yang qi can attach itself. For that reason, the term *yíng* invariably invokes as its counterpart *wèi*, or protective yang, whereas *xuè* invokes qi.

The term *yíng*, furthermore, is generally associated in the medical literature with the Spleen and Heart, while *xuè* is more often associated with the Liver and other aspects of the sea of blood in the lower burner, that is, the Penetrating vessel and the Womb. This makes sense as the Liver and sea of blood store blood (emphasizing its substantive nature), whereas the Heart and Spleen exert functional control over the blood (producing it, governing it). The term *róng* lacks such definitive associations, but the pattern for which this formula is indicated clearly relates to the more functional aspects of the blood. Besides symptoms pointing to a loss of luxuriance (dryness, weight loss, and a diminished ability to promote tissue growth), symptoms indicating diminished functioning of both the Spleen and Heart (fatigue, lack of appetite, forgetfulness, restlessness, palpitations, and a general lack of focus) are most prominent.

A closer look at the chief herbs supports this analysis. Ginseng Radix (*rén shēn*) strengthens the qi of the Spleen and Heart; it tonifies but also generates fluids. While Paeoniae Radix alba (*bái sháo*) is primarily associated with the Liver in contemporary Chinese medical textbooks, in the premodern literature it was much more closely associated with the Spleen and the nutritive qi. In *Materia Medica of Ri Hua-Zi*, it is said to benefit the Spleen. In *Origins of Medicine*, written not too long after the source text for this formula, Zhang Yuan-Su lists the six functions of Paeoniae Radix alba (*bái sháo*) as follows: "First, it calms the Spleen channel; second, it treats abdominal pain; third, it restrains Stomach qi; fourth, it stops diarrhea and dysentery; fifth, it harmonizes the blood vessels; sixth, it secures the interstices and pores."

Based on this analysis, the pathodynamic treated by this formula—and thereby its distinctive characteristics vis-à-vis other formulas in this category—are cast into relief. Ginseng Decoction to Nourish Luxuriance (*rén shēn yǎng róng tāng*) does not primarily tonify blood as a substance, but as an essence that achieves distinctive effects: moistening and the promotion of growth. For that reason, it centers on the Spleen and Heart, refocusing the actions of the qi and yang that had become unsecured precisely because of this lack of luxuriance onto the production of blood once more.

Comparisons

➤ Vs. All-Inclusive Great Tonifying Decoction (*shí quán dà bǔ tāng*)

Both formulas treat qi and blood deficiency with similar compositions. However, in using Paeoniae Radix alba (*bái sháo*) as its main herb, Ginseng Decoction to Nourish Luxuriance (*rén shēn yǎng róng tāng*) is more cooling in nature, while

the inclusion of Polygalae Radix (*yuǎn zhì*) and Schisandrae Fructus (*wǔ wèi zǐ*) allows it to focus on the Heart, restraining and regulating its qi in order to control the yang and produce blood. All-Inclusive Great Tonifying Decoction (*shí quán dà bǔ tāng*), on the other hand, contains Chuanxiong Rhizoma (*chuān xiōng*), a warming Liver herb. It is thus more suited for treating blood deficiency accompanied by symptoms of cold in the treatment of gynecological disorders and for patterns characterized by symptoms of Liver blood deficiency.

➤ Vs. Tonifying Decoction with Astragalus (*nèi bǔ huáng qí tāng*)

These formulas resemble each other in both composition and indications, sharing nine of their key herbs. Ginseng Decoction to Nourish Luxuriance (*rén shēn yǎng róng tang*) focuses on the Spleen and qi with the addition of Atractylodis macrocephalae Rhizoma (*bái zhú*), Citri reticulatae Pericarpium (*chén pí*), and Schisandrae Fructus (*wǔ wèi zǐ*). Internally Tonifying Decoction with Astragalus (*nèi bǔ huáng qí tāng*) focuses more on the Liver and fluids with the use of Chuanxiong Rhizoma (*chuān xiōng*) and Ophiopogonis Radix (*mài mén dōng*), which help it promote healing in external medicine patterns.

➤ Vs. Restore the Spleen Decoction (*guī pí tāng*); *see* page 354

Biomedical Indications

With the appropriate presentation, this formula may be used to treat a wide variety of biomedically-defined disorders including various forms of anemia, nonhealing ulcers, and nervous exhaustion, and to treat debility after a severe illness.

Modifications

- For spermatorrhea, add Fossilia Ossis Mastodi (*lóng gǔ*).
- For coughing, add Asini Corii Colla (*ē jiāo*).
- When heat symptoms are not pronounced, reduce the dosage of Paeoniae Radix alba (*bái sháo*).

Associated Formula

香貝養榮湯（香贝养荣汤）

Cyperus and Fritillaria Decoction to Nourish Luxuriance
xiāng bèi yǎng róng tāng

SOURCE   *Golden Mirror of the Medical Tradition* (1742)

dry-fried Atractylodis macrocephalae Rhizoma
(*chǎo bái zhú*) 6g
Ginseng Radix (*rén shēn*) 3g
Poria (*fú líng*) 3g
Citri reticulatae Pericarpium (*chén pí*) 3g
Rehmanniae Radix praeparata (*shú dì huáng*) 3g
Chuanxiong Rhizoma (*chuān xiōng*) 3g

Angelicae sinensis Radix (dāng guī) 3g
Fritillariae Bulbus (bèi mǔ) 3g
Cyperi Rhizoma (xiāng fù) 3g
Paeoniae Radix alba (bái sháo) 3g
Platycodi Radix (jié gěng) 1.5g
Glycyrrhizae Radix (gān cǎo) 1.5g
Zingiberis Rhizoma recens (shēng jiāng) . . . . .3 slices
Jujubae Fructus (dà zǎo) . . . . .2 pieces

Tonifies the qi, nourishes the blood, regulates the qi, and transforms phlegm. For hard masses on the side of the neck, breasts, or axillae in patients with qi and blood deficiency.

歸脾湯 （归脾汤）
Restore the Spleen Decoction
guī pí tāng

The actions of this formula benefit the Spleen qi and thereby restore its control over the blood, hence the name. Zhang Shan-Lei explained its name in *Annotated and Corrected Synopsis of Shen's Women's Disorders*:

> The [reason this formula] is called Restore the Spleen [Decoction] and not Tonify Blood [Decoction] is that when the Spleen and Stomach receive the essences from food, the middle burner transforms them into a red [substance]. It is therefore the source of blood. Placing the essences under the charge of the Spleen is thus the intention of this formula's composition, even if it is not directly stated. In this, one sees its true brilliance.

Source   *Categorized Essentials for Normalizing the Structure* (1529)

Ginseng Radix (rén shēn) 3g (3-6g)
dry-fried Astragali Radix (chǎo huáng qí) 3g (9-12g)
Atractylodis macrocephalae Rhizoma (bái zhú) 3g (9-12g)
Poria (fú líng) 3g (9-12g)
dry-fried Ziziphi spinosae Semen (chǎo suān zǎo rén) . 3g (9-12g)
Longan Arillus (lóng yǎn ròu) 3g (6-9g)
Aucklandiae Radix (mù xiāng) 1.5g (3-6g)
Glycyrrhizae Radix praeparata (zhì gān cǎo) 0.9g (3-6g)
Angelicae sinensis Radix (dāng guī) 3g (6-9g)
processed Polygalae Radix (zhì yuǎn zhì) 3g (3-6g)

Method of Preparation   The source text advises to take as a decoction with Zingiberis Rhizoma recens (shēng jiāng) and Jujubae Fructus (dà zǎo). At present, it is usually prepared with the dosages specified in parentheses. Codonopsis Radix (dǎng shēn) is generally substituted for Ginseng Radix (rén shēn) at 2-3 times its dosage, and Poriae Sclerotium pararadicis (fú shén) is substituted for Poria (fú líng).

Actions   Augments the qi, tonifies the blood, strengthens the Spleen, and nourishes the Heart

Indications

Forgetfulness, palpitations (with or without anxiety), insomnia, dream-disturbed sleep, anxiety and phobia, feverishness,

withdrawal, reduced appetite, a pallid and wan complexion, a pale tongue with a thin, white coating, and a thin, frail pulse. Chronic bleeding syndromes may also be part of the presentation. Women may experience early periods with copious, pale blood or prolonged, almost continuous periods with little flow.

Excessive deliberation for a long period of time or obsessive behavior injures both the Spleen and Heart and leads to this disorder. The primary injury is to the Spleen, which is the organ that generates blood. When it is weak, the blood becomes deficient and is unable to nourish the Heart. The Heart stores the spirit and the Spleen stores the intention (意 yì). When they are insufficient, one loses the ability to concentrate and becomes forgetful. Spleen qi deficiency manifests as a reduction in appetite and withdrawal. When the Heart is deprived of nourishment, the patient may have palpitations, with or without anxiety. When this affects the spirit, the patient will present with anxiety and phobia, insomnia, and dream-disturbed sleep. Blood deficiency may give rise to the feverishness associated with heat from deficiency. The pallid and wan complexion, pale tongue with a thin, white coating, and the thin, frail pulse are all signs of qi and blood deficiency.

Another way of analyzing the etiology of this disorder is through the generation cycle of the five phases. In this cycle, the relationship between fire (Heart) and earth (Spleen) is one of mother and child. When the child is deficient, the mother will in turn become drained and deficient. Here, the Spleen deficiency brought on by excessive deliberation (or other causes) will lead to deficiency of the Heart. Because the relationship between these two organs is expressed primarily through the blood, it is the blood aspects of the organs that are primarily affected.

Analysis of Formula

The chief herbs in this formula focus on the Spleen. Ginseng Radix (rén shēn) and Astragali Radix (huáng qí) are very powerful substances for tonifying the Spleen qi. Atractylodis macrocephalae Rhizoma (bái zhú) strengthens the Spleen and dries dampness, while Glycyrrhizae Radix praeparata (zhì gān cǎo) tonifies the Spleen and augments the qi. Together, these four herbs have a strong tonifying effect on the Spleen, which enables it to generate blood.

The deputies 'root' the spirit by tonifying the blood and calming the spirit. Longan Arillus (lóng yǎn ròu) performs both of these functions, while Angelicae sinensis Radix (dāng guī) tonifies the blood and regulates the menses. The combination of Angelicae sinensis Radix (dāng guī) and Astragali Radix (huáng qí) is very effective in generating and tonifying the blood. Ziziphi spinosae Semen (suān zǎo rén) and Poriae Sclerotium pararadicis (fú shén) both serve to calm the spirit, while the latter ingredient also reinforces the Spleen-tonifying action of the chief herbs. The final deputy, processed Polygalae Radix (zhì yuǎn zhì), calms the spirit by facilitating the flow of qi in the Heart. It is especially effective when it is balanced by the astringent properties of Ziziphi spinosae Semen (suān zǎo rén).

The assistant herb, Aucklandiae Radix (mù xiāng), regulates the qi and revives the Spleen. It is especially effective when combined with Atractylodis macrocephalae Rhizoma (bái zhú). Its use also prevents indigestion due to the rich, cloying properties of the other herbs. Although it only functions as an assistant, in Discussion of Famous Physicians' Formulas Past and Present, Zhang Lu described its use as inspired: "This formula enriches and nourishes the Spleen and Heart by inciting the lesser fire [of qi transformation]. Its subtlety expresses itself in the use of Aucklandiae Radix (mù xiāng) to regulate and facilitate the qi [dynamic]." The envoys, Zingiberis Rhizoma recens (shēng jiāng) and Jujubae Fructus (dà zǎo), improve the appetite and regulate the nutritive and protective qi, thereby facilitating the actions of the other ingredients. They also assist the chief herbs in strengthening the Spleen.

Commentary

This formula is appropriate for treating any disorder due to qi and blood deficiency where Spleen deficiency constitutes the root and symptoms of Heart deficiency are secondary manifestations. In clinical practice, this encompasses three main manifestations: (1) restless Heart spirit; (2) qi and blood deficiency; and (3) the inability of the Spleen to control the blood. Psychoemotional symptoms are an important aspect of this formula's indications. Their relationship to blood deficiency is explained in Collected Treatises of [Zhang] Jing-Yue:

> In [cases of] blood deficiency there is nothing to nourish the Heart. If the Heart is deficient, the spirit has no abode. Therefore, [patients with such a condition] have manifestations of the ethereal and corporeal souls not being quiet, such as being easily startled, fearful, not wishing to leave a place, prone to unreasonable and rash thinking, unable to sleep until deep into the night, or suddenly falling asleep and waking again just as suddenly.

In Selected Annotations to Ancient Formulas from the Garden of Crimson Snow, Wang Zi-Jie provides an alternative explanation of the formula's name that relates it specifically to the treatment of such manifestations. Wang's interpretation is of interest also for its different approach to the formula's composition:

> Return to the Spleen [Decoction implies that this formula] regulates the four [spirits of the other] yin organs—the ethereal and corporeal souls, the spirit, and the resolve—so that they return to the Spleen. … Astragali Radix (huáng qí) is added [to the formula] because it moves directly to the Lungs to secure the corporeal soul. Ziziphi spinosae Semen (suān zǎo

rén) goes to the Heart to astringe the spirit. Angelicae sinensis Radix (dāng guī) enters the Liver where its fragrance delights the ethereal soul. Polygalae Radix (yuǎn zhì) enters the Kidneys where its acridity opens the resolve. Connecting and regulating [the movement of the spirits] above and below the diaphragm, the four yin organs are calmed and harmonized, so that the ethereal and corporeal souls, the spirit, and the resolve naturally return to the Spleen.

From a contemporary perspective, this formula can be viewed as a modified combination of Four-Gentlemen Decoction (sì jūn zǐ tāng) and Tangkuei Decoction to Tonify the Blood (dāng guī bǔ xuè tāng). It acquired this structure, however, only after several centuries of ongoing development and modification. A formula called Restore the Spleen Decoction (guī pí tāng) first appeared in Formulas to Aid the Living by the Song-dynasty scholar-physician Yan Yong-He. This formula, which did not yet include the herbs Angelicae sinensis Radix (dāng guī) and Polygalae Radix (yuǎn zhì), was recommended for the treatment of palpitations with anxiety and forgetfulness from long-term pensiveness injuring the Spleen and Heart. In the Yuan-dynasty text Effective Formulas from Generations of Physicians, its use was expanded to include bleeding disorders caused by Spleen qi deficiency. It was during the Ming dynasty that the court physician Xue Ji added those two herbs. Because of Xue Ji's enormous influence, this became the standard version of the formula accepted by later physicians. During the Qing dynasty, Gu Yang-Wu proposed to increase the blood-tonifying properties of the formula by adding Rehmanniae Radix praeparata (shú dì huáng) to Xue Ji's version. This new formula, popularized as Black Restore the Spleen Decoction (hēi guī pí tāng) in the ophthalmology text Guide to the Silver Seas, was quickly criticized by influential physicians like Fei Bo-Xiong as being too heavy, and therefore never achieved the popularity of Xue Ji's version.

Comparisons

➤ Vs. Tonify the Middle to Augment the Qi Decoction (bǔ zhōng yì qì tāng)

Both formulas strengthen the Spleen, but they have different applications. Restore the Spleen Decoction (guī pí tāng) is used for Spleen and Heart deficiency with palpitations, withdrawal, reduced appetite, and perhaps chronic bleeding. By contrast, Tonify the Middle to Augment the Qi Decoction (bǔ zhōng yì qì tāng) is used for Spleen and Stomach qi deficiency with shortness of breath, weight loss, withdrawal, and perhaps signs of ptosis or sinking. While it is true that, with modifications, they can be made to look quite similar, it is better to use the one that was designed for the primary dynamic of the disorder.

➤ Vs. Ginseng Decoction to Nourish Luxuriance (rén shēn yǎng róng tāng)

Both formulas tonify the blood by focusing on the functions of the Spleen and Heart qi in the production and regulation of blood. Their differences are cogently summed up by the 19th-century physician Tang Zong-Hai in *Discussion of Blood Patterns*:

> The Heart focuses on generating blood, the Spleen focuses on governing blood. Nourish Luxuriance Decoction (*yǎng róng tāng*) primarily treats the Heart, while Restore the Spleen Decoction (*guī pí tāng*) primarily treats the Spleen. Heart blood is generated in the Spleen, hence Nourish Luxuriance Decoction (*yǎng róng tāng*) tonifies the Spleen in order to augment the [functions of the] Heart. Spleen earth is generated by fire, hence Restore the Spleen Decoction (*guī pí tāng*) guides the Heart fire toward the generation of Spleen [earth]. More generally, making the Spleen qi abundant lets it contain the blood to [prevent it from] leaking.

➤ Vs. Prepared Licorice Decoction (*zhì gān cǎo tāng*); see PAGE 358.

➤ Vs. Stabilize Gushing Decoction (*gù chōng tāng*); see PAGE 444.

➤ Vs. Four-Substance Decoction (*sì wù tāng*); see PAGE 336

➤ Vs. Sour Jujube Decoction (*suān zǎo rén tāng*); see PAGE 465.

➤ Vs. Yellow Earth Decoction (*huáng tǔ tāng*); see PAGE 610

Biomedical Indications

With the appropriate presentation, this formula may be used to treat a wide variety of biomedically-defined disorders. These can be divided into the following groups:

- Those affecting the neurological system such as postconcussion syndrome, myasthenia gravis, and nervous exhaustion

- Those affecting the hematological system such as anemia (especially from chronic disease) and thrombocytopenic or allergic purpura

- Those affecting the cardiovascular system such as congestive heart disease and supraventricular tachycardia

- Gynecological problems such as cervicitis and dysfunctional uterine bleeding

- Digestive disorders such as peptic ulcers and nonspecific colitis

- Psychoemotional disorders such as depression, anxiety, the now outdated disorder neurasthenia that is still diagnosed in Asia, and disorders involving mood changes including

perimenopausal syndrome, insomnia, and treatment of addiction.

This formula has also been used in the treatment of hypertension, Ménière's disease, and diabetes.

....

Alternate names

Return the Spleen Powder (*guī pí sǎn*) in *Mirror of Medicine Past and Present*; Augmented Return the Spleen Decoction (*jiā wèi guī pí tāng*) in *Mirror of Medicine Past and Present*; Return the Spleen Drink (*guī pí yǐn*) in *True Transmission on Pox Studies*; Return the Spleen Decoction to Nourish the Nutritive (*guī pí yǎng yíng tāng*) in *Collected Know-How Gained through Practice and Study for the Treatment of Itchy Disorders*

....

Modifications

- For numbness in the upper extremities, add Notopterygii Rhizoma seu Radix (*qiāng huó*) and Chuanxiong Rhizoma (*chuān xiōng*).

- For numbness in the lower back and lower extremities, add Clematidis Radix (*wēi líng xiān*), Angelicae pubescentis Radix (*dú huó*), and Achyranthis bidentatae Radix (*niú xī*).

- For painful menstruation with clots in the blood, add Curcumae Radix (*yù jīn*) and Cyperi Rhizoma (*xiāng fù*).

- For very dark menstrual blood, add Carthami Flos (*hóng huā*), Moutan Cortex (*mǔ dān pí*), and Gardeniae Fructus (*zhī zǐ*).

- For menstruation that suddenly changes in volume and flows continuously, add Corni Fructus (*shān zhū yú*) and Schisandrae Fructus (*wǔ wèi zǐ*).

Associated Formula

固本止崩湯 （固本止崩汤）

Stabilize the Root and Stop Excessive Uterine Bleeding Decoction

gù běn zhǐ bēng tāng

SOURCE *Women's Diseases According to Fu Qing-Zhu* (1826)

Rehmanniae Radix praeparata (*shú dì huáng*) 30g
Atractylodis macrocephalae Rhizoma (*bái zhú*) 30g
Ginseng Radix (*rén shēn*) 9g
Astragali Radix (*huáng qí*) 9g
Angelicae sinensis Radix (*dāng guī*) 15g
Zingiberis Rhizoma praeparatum (*páo jiāng*) 6g

Tonifies the blood, augments the qi, and stops bleeding. For inability of the Spleen to control the blood leading to either sudden, severe uterine bleeding or persistent uterine bleeding with continuous spotting. The blood is pale and watery. Accompanying signs and symptoms include a shiny, pale complexion or slight facial edema, lightheadedness, fatigue, lack of warmth in the extremities, shortness of breath, a stifling sensation in the chest, loose stools, a pale and swollen tongue body with teeth marks, and a thin and frail or hollow pulse.

炙甘草湯 (炙甘草汤)
Prepared Licorice Decoction
zhì gān cǎo tāng

This formula is also known as Restore the Pulse Decoction (*fù mài tāng*). It was given this name because of its ability to revive the qi and blood and thus restore the pulse to healthful vigor. This name is used in some of the later modifications of the formula.

Source   *Discussion of Cold Damage* (c. 220)

Glycyrrhizae Radix praeparata *(zhì gān cǎo)* 12g
Ginseng Radix *(rén shēn)* 6g
Cinnamomi Ramulus *(guì zhī)* .9g
Rehmanniae Radix *(shēng dì huáng)* 48g
Ophiopogonis Radix *(mài mén dōng)* 9g
Asini Corii Colla *(ē jiāo)* . . . . . [dissolve in strained decoction] 6g
Cannabis Semen *(huǒ má rén)* . . . . [crush] 9g
Zingiberis Rhizoma recens *(shēng jiāng)* 9g
Jujubae Fructus *(dà zǎo)* . . . . 30 pieces

Method of Preparation   The source text advises to cook the ingredients in approximately 1 liter of liquid consisting of seven-fifteenths rice wine and eight-fifteenths water. At present, it is prepared as a decoction with 10ml of rice wine added at the end. Regardless of how it is prepared, the resulting liquid is divided into thirds and taken in three doses over the course of a day. At present, only half the dosage of Rehmanniae Radix *(shēng dì huáng)*, and only 5-10 pieces of Jujubae Fructus *(dà zǎo)*, are used. Codonopsis Radix *(dǎng shēn)* is usually substituted for Ginseng Radix *(rén shēn)* at 2-3 times its dosage.

Actions   Augments the qi, nourishes the blood, enriches the yin, and restores the pulse

Indications

The main pattern for which this formula is used presents with palpitations that may be accompanied by anxiety, irritability, insomnia, emaciation, shortness of breath, constipation, a dry mouth and throat, a pale, shiny tongue, and a pulse that is consistently irregular, slow-irregular, or thin, faint, and forceless.

This is another of the consumptive conditions with qi and blood deficiency. The Heart controls the pulse and is nourished by the qi and blood. When the Heart is undernourished, it loses its vitality, which manifests as palpitations accompanied by anxiety. The Heart blood provides the foundation for the activities of the spirit; when it is deficient, the spirit has no place to calmly reside. This leads to irritability and insomnia. Qi and blood deficiency also manifest as emaciation and shortness of breath. The blood and fluids are intimately related, such that deficiency of one usually leads to deficiency of the other. Insufficient fluids lead to constipation, a dry mouth and throat, and a lack of coating on the tongue. A pale tongue is a sign of qi and blood deficiency. When the qi is deficient and can only weakly push a pulse that is lacking

in blood, the pulse will either be irregular or thin, frail, and forceless.

A second pattern for which this formula is used presents with coughing of frothy sputum or coughing of blood-streaked sputum accompanied by emaciation, shortness of breath, irritability, insomnia, spontaneous sweating or night sweats, a dry throat and tongue, constipation, heat from deficiency, and a deficient, rapid pulse.

This is Lung atrophy due to consumption. When the Lung qi is deficient, it rebels upward leading to coughing, shortness of breath, spontaneous sweating, and a deficient pulse. Damage to the body fluids by long-standing consumption leads to dryness, manifesting in symptoms like dry throat and tongue, constipation, and frothy sputum (i.e., water that cannot be contained by the dry mucous membranes). Yin deficiency invariably leads to symptoms of yang excess such as irritability, insomnia, night sweats, heat from deficiency, and a rapid pulse.

Analysis of Formula

The chief ingredient, Glycyrrhizae Radix praeparata *(zhì gān cǎo)*, augments the qi of the middle burner. Used in a large dosage, it nourishes the Heart and, according to *Materia Medica of Ri Hua-Zi*, "quiets the ethereal soul and settles the corporeal soul." Rehmanniae Radix *(shēng dì huáng)*, also used with a rather large dosage, serves as deputy. Sweet and cooling, enriching and moistening, it restores the Heart yin and tonifies the blood. Together with Glycyrrhizae Radix praeparata *(zhì gān cǎo)*, it fills the vessels with qi and fluids, providing the basis for returning the pulse to its normal status.

There are seven assistants, which can be divided into three functional groups. Ginseng Radix *(rén shēn)* strongly tonifies the source qi and thus all of the organs. It also calms the spirit, which relieves the palpitations and anxiety, especially when combined with the chief ingredient. Jujubae Fructus *(dà zǎo)* benefits the Spleen and nourishes the Heart. The combination of these two herbs with Glycyrrhizae Radix praeparata *(zhì gān cǎo)* tonifies the qi of the Spleen and Stomach (the postnatal qi), which is the root of the Heart qi and the source of blood generation.

Asini Corii Colla *(ē jiāo)* effectively enriches the yin, tonifies the blood, and moistens dryness. Ophiopogonis Radix *(mài mén dōng)* moistens dryness in the Stomach and Lungs (upper burner), while Cannabis Semen *(huǒ má rén)* nourishes the yin and moistens the Intestines (lower burner). Together, these three herbs assist Rehmanniae Radix *(shēng dì huáng)* in enriching the yin, moistening dryness, and cooling heat from deficiency.

Cinnamomi Ramulus *(guì zhī)* unblocks the flow of Heart qi. Its combination with Ginseng Radix *(rén shēn)* strengthens this effect. This is an important aspect of the treatment of palpitations, and the herb is found in every formula devised by Zhang Zhong-Jing for treating this symptom. Zingiberis Rhizoma recens *(shēng jiāng)* is used to strengthen the Stomach and enable it to cope with the tonifying substances in the formula. In concert with Jujubae Fructus *(dà zǎo)*, it also regulates the relationship between the protective and nutritive qi. This function plays an important part in restoring vitality to individuals suffering from consumption, as it enables their systems to revive without developing other problems.

Wine serves as the envoy by helping the assistant ingredients keep things moving. Although this condition is due to an underlying deficiency, there is also an element of stagnation due to both cold and dryness. Both must be treated if the condition is to be dealt with effectively.

Cautions and Contraindications

This formula should not be used without modification in cases with heat from deficient yin or where there is severe diarrhea.

Commentary

This is the principal formula for the treatment of irregular pulses, of which there are two major types: slow-irregular, also known as knotted (結 *jié*), which is a slow pulse with an occasional dropped beat; and consistently-irregular or intermittent (代 *dài)*, in which beats are dropped at regular intervals. These pulses are attributed to deficient yang, which is unable to circulate the pulse qi, along with deficient yin, which is unable to nourish the Heart blood. A third type of irregular pulse, called rapid-irregular or hasty (促 *cù)*, is attributed to excessive heat with stagnation and cannot be treated with this formula.

Debates about the Formula's Composition

The composition of this formula is very complex, combining qi-, yin-, and blood-tonifying substances with herbs that move the yang qi. This complexity reflects the complex pathodynamic of the conditions for which it is indicated. These are often chronic in nature and require long-term treatment. The effects of this formula thus take time to develop and should not be judged unless it has been taken for at least 10 days.

Two main issues have drawn the interest of commentators regarding the composition of the original formula itself: identifying which of the ingredients is the chief herb and explaining the precise functions and interactions among the various ingredients. Some writers, like the Ming dynasty cold-damage expert Ke Qin, consider Rehmanniae Radix *(shēng dì huáng)* to be the chief herb:

> This [formula] is used for Heart deficiency [presenting with] a consistently irregular or slow-irregular pulse. Employing Rehmanniae Radix *(shēng dì huáng)* as chief and Ophiopogonis Radix *(mài mén dōng)* as assistant to forcefully tonify the true yin, it blazed a trail for later generations of scholars [by laying down a strategy] for enriching the yin.

Ke Qin's opinion, and that of others who think like him, including You Yi and Zhang Xi-Chun, is not merely based on the fact that Rehmanniae Radix *(shēng dì huáng)* is the ingredient with the highest dosage. These physicians believe that deficiency of yin fluids is at the root of the pattern treated by this formula and that only tonification of the fluids can treat the problem at its source. Other commentators, like Qian Huang, oppose this view with the simple observation that the name of the formula is Prepared Licorice Decoction *(zhì gān cǎo tāng)*, therefore the chief herb should be Glycyrrhizae Radix praeparata *(zhì gān cǎo)*. The dosage of this herb is much higher than one might expect were it used in its usual role as an assistant or envoy. However, if that is the case, which of its actions makes it so important?

A majority of commentators simply note that Glycyrrhizae Radix praeparata *(zhì gān cǎo)* tonifies the qi and the middle burner, but they do not explain why this makes it more important than any of the other qi tonics in the formula. A more plausible argument is presented by the contemporary physician Yue Mei-Zhong, who points out that the functions attributed to this herb have changed over time. Older pharmacopeias like *Miscellaneous Records of Famous Physicians*, for instance, defined Glycyrrhizae Radix *(gān cǎo)* as "unblocking the blood vessels and facilitating the force of qi."

Use of Cinnamomi Ramulus (guì zhī)

This question is related to the use of Cinnamomi Ramulus *(guì zhī)*. These two herbs, Cinnamomi Ramulus *(guì zhī)* and Glycyrrhizae Radix *(gān cǎo)*, are combined in a formula from *Discussion of Cold Damage*, Cinnamon Twig and Licorice Decoction *(guì zhī gān cǎo tāng)*, for the treatment of mild injury to the Heart yang from too much sweating that manifests as palpitations that respond favorably to pressure over the chest. This combination activates the Heart yang, according to the strategy of 'transforming the yang with acrid and sweet herbs.' Here, the large dosage of Glycyrrhizae Radix praeparata *(zhì gān cǎo)*, especially when combined with a similarly large dosage of Jujubae Fructus *(dà zǎo)*, provides a basis for the production of nutritive qi into which Cinnamomi Ramulus *(guì zhī)* then enters as a moving and mobilizing force. In the words of Yu Chang, writing in *Precepts for Physicians*:

> Because Cinnamomi Ramulus *(guì zhī)* is acrid and warming, it does not seem to be appropriate [for use in a condition characterized by yin deficiency]. But [those who think so] do not understand that Cinnamomi Ramulus *(guì zhī)* is able to unblock [the movement] of nutritive and protective [qi] to convey the body fluids. When the nutritive and protective [qi] are unblocked and the body fluids are conveyed, then the Lung qi transports and the turbid froth gradually moves downward. It is indeed a special herb. Therefore, one says that it treats the Heart by warming the yin fluids within it.

Later Usage

The use of this formula has been expanded over the centuries. In *Supplement to Important Formulas Worth a Thousand Gold Pieces*, the Tang-dynasty physician Sun Si-Miao recommended it for a variety of consumptive disorders. A little later, Wang Tao, in *Arcane Essentials from the Imperial Library*, suggested its use in the treatment of Lung atrophy, which has since become the second most important indication. It is one of the earliest yin-tonifying formulas in the Chinese medical literature, which, according to *Introduction to Medicine*, influenced the development of the entire field because "All enriching tonifying formulas are [in fact] modifications of this formula."

Physicians, most notably those associated with the warm pathogen disorder current, adapted it to many new uses. Ye Tian-Shi prescribed it in the treatment of generalized body numbness due to exhaustion of the protective and nutritive qi. Substituting cooling, restraining, or heavy sedating medicinals like Paeoniae Radix alba *(bái sháo)*, Ziziphi spinosae Semen *(suān zǎo rén)*, or Ostreae Concha *(mǔ lì)* for the acrid, warming ingredients in this formula, Ye devised treatments for internal wind arising in the course of warm pathogen disorders or from yin and blood deficiency. Wu Ju-Tong, likewise, modified it for treating conditions of yin deficiency, creating a number of formulas that have become classics in their own right (see ASSOCIATED FORMULAS below and Three-Shell Decoction to Restore the Pulse [*sān jiǎ fù mài tāng*] in Chapter 14).

Comparisons

➤ Vs. RESTORE THE SPLEEN DECOCTION *(guī pí tāng)*

While both formulas tonify the qi and blood and treat palpitations, Restore the Spleen Decoction *(guī pí tāng)* is stronger at tonifying the qi. It focuses on strengthening the Spleen and calming the spirit. It can be used to treat patterns of Spleen qi and Heart Blood deficiency, as well as bleeding attributed to inability of the Spleen to contain the blood. Prepared Licorice Decoction *(zhì gān cǎo tāng)*, on the other hand, is stronger at nourishing the blood and the yin fluids. In addition, it also opens the yang with acrid and warming herbs. Its action does not focus on the middle burner, but on harmonizing the nutritive and protective qi to restore the pulse.

➤ Vs. GENERATE THE PULSE POWDER *(shēng mài sǎn)*

Both formulas tonify the qi and yin, treat deficiency of both the Heart and the Lungs, and focus on the pulse. Both can also be used to treat chronic coughs. Prepared Licorice Decoction *(zhì gān cǎo tāng)* strongly tonifies both the qi and yin and focuses on the root of the coughing by fortifying the Lung's restraining action. Because it contains acrid and warming herbs, it is not suitable for treating patterns characterized by

internal heat. Generate the Pulse Powder *(shēng mài sǎn)*, on the other hand, combines tonifying with restraining herbs to treat both the root and branch. Although it contains Ginseng Radix *(rén shēn)*, even this warming herb is not drying and, in fact, generates fluids. It is therefore better at stopping coughs and can be used both to clear heat and tonify the qi and yin.

➤ Vs. EMPEROR OF HEAVEN'S SPECIAL PILL TO TONIFY THE HEART *(tiān wáng bǔ xīn dān)*

Both of these formulas tonify the yin and blood to treat patterns manifesting with palpitations, anxiety, insomnia, and dry stools. However, Emperor of Heaven's Special Pill to Tonify the Heart *(tiān wáng bǔ xīn dān)* focuses on tonifying the fluids as well as the blood in patterns where Heart yang flares upward due to deficiency. This causes the spirit to lose its anchoring in the blood, leading to insomnia, dream-disturbed sleep, anxiety, and restlessness as the main symptoms. The pulse will be thin and perhaps rapid. These problems are addressed by the inclusion of herbs that calm the spirit such as Ziziphi spinosae Semen *(suān zǎo rén)*, Platycladi Semen *(bǎi zǐ rén)*, and Polygalae Radix *(yuǎn zhì)*. Prepared Licorice Decoction *(zhì gān cǎo tāng)*, on the other hand, focuses on nourishing the blood and the yang functions of the Heart in addition to enriching the fluids. The main symptom is an irregular pulse. To address these issues, warming and qi-tonifying herbs like Ginseng Radix *(rén shēn)*, Glycyrrhizae Radix *(gān cǎo)*, and Cinnamomi Ramulus *(guì zhī)* are the key ingredients of that formula.

Biomedical Indications

With the appropriate presentation, this formula may be used to treat a variety of biomedically-defined disorders, primarily those centering around irregular heartbeats such as sick sinus syndrome, atrial flutter, atrial fibrillation, coronary artery disease, viral myocarditis, rheumatic heart disease, and hyperthyroidism. It has also been used for various types of anemia and upper GI bleeding secondary to cirrhosis.

Alternate names

Restore the Pulse Decoction *(fù mài tāng)* in *Discussion of Cold Damage*; Licorice Decoction *(gān cǎo tāng)* in *Formulas of Universal Benefit*

Modifications

- For Lung atrophy, reduce the dosage or remove Cinnamomi Ramulus *(guì zhī)* and Zingiberis Rhizoma recens *(shēng jiāng)*, remove the wine, and add Stemonae Radix *(bǎi bù)* and Gecko *(gé jiè)*.
- For chest pain and discomfort, add Salviae miltiorrhizae Radix *(dān shēn)* and Persicae Semen *(táo rén)*.
- For nosebleed from yin deficiency, increase the dosage of Rehmanniae Radix *(shēng dì huáng)* and Ophiopogonis

Radix *(mài mén dōng)* and add Scutellariae Radix *(huáng qín)* and Coptidis Rhizoma *(huáng lián)*.

• For insomnia, substitute Ziziphi spinosae Semen *(suān zǎo rén)* for Cannabis Semen *(huǒ má rén)*. One may also add Platycladi Semen *(bǎi zǐ rén)* or heavy, settling substances like Fossilia Dentis Mastodi *(lóng chǐ)* and Magnetitum *(cí shí)*.

Associated Formula

加減復脈湯 (加减复脉汤)

Modified Restore the Pulse Decoction

jiā jiǎn fù mài tāng

Source *Systematic Differentiation of Warm Pathogen Diseases* (1798)

Glycyrrhizae Radix praeparata *(zhì gān cǎo)* 18g
Rehmanniae Radix *(shēng dì huáng)* 18g
Paeoniae Radix alba *(bái sháo)* 18g
Ophiopogonis Radix *(mài mén dōng)* 15g
Asini Corii Colla *(ē jiāo)* . . . . [dissolve in strained decoction] 9g
Cannabis Semen *(huǒ má rén)* . . . .[crush] 9g

Nourishes the blood, preserves the yin, generates fluids, and moistens dryness. For yang brightness organ-warp disorders in which purging has eliminated the excessive heat but has also depleted the yin and fluids. This is characterized by fever, a red face, heat in the palms and soles (in severe cases the hands and feet become hot), a dry mouth and tongue, and a large, deficient pulse. The composition of this formula is based on the strategy of using 'sour and sweet (herbs) to transform (into) yin,' for which the combination of Paeoniae Radix alba *(bái sháo)* and Glycyrrhizae Radix *(gān cǎo)* is the exemplar (see discussion under Peony and Licorice Decoction [*sháo yào gān cǎo tang*] above). By means of this strategy, the formula controls the yang that is beginning to float away (reflected in the large, deficient pulse) without actually treating the yang itself. This is important in treating conditions such as this, where yang excess is purely a result of yin deficiency, because one wants to avoid moving any of the body's qi into the yang aspect.

泰山磐石散

Taishan Bedrock Powder

Tàishān pán shí sǎn

The original name of this formula was Great Mountain Bedrock Powder (太山磐石散 *tài shān pán shí sǎn*). The influential Ming-dynasty physician Zhang Jie-Bin changed 太 *tài*, meaning 'great,' to its homonym 泰 *tài*, referring to Taishan, one of China's four most important mountains and widely regarded as a symbol of stability. The formula secures the fetus by nourishing the Conception and Penetrating vessels, making them strong like Taishan and bedrock-firm.

Source *Systematic Great Compendium of Medicine Past and Present* (1556)

Ginseng Radix *(rén shēn)* 3g
Astragali Radix *(huáng qí)* 3g
Atractylodis macrocephalae Rhizoma *(bái zhú)* 1.5g

Glycyrrhizae Radix praeparata *(zhì gān cǎo)* 1.5g
Angelicae sinensis Radix *(dāng guī)* .3g
Chuanxiong Rhizoma *(chuān xiōng)* 2.4g
Paeoniae Radix alba *(bái sháo)* 2.4g
Rehmanniae Radix praeparata *(shú dì huáng)* 2.4g
Dipsaci Radix *(xù duàn)* 3g
Scutellariae Radix *(huáng qín)* 3g
Amomi Fructus *(shā rén)* 1.5g
Glutinous rice *(nuò mǐ)* . . . . 1 scoop

Method of Preparation Decoct with 300ml of water until one-fifth remains. The decoction is to be taken away from meals. At present, the dosage of most ingredients is usually increased slightly, except for Astragali Radix *(huáng qí)* and Rehmanniae Radix praeparata *(shú dì huáng)*, which are increased 4-5 fold. When used to prevent miscarriage, it is usually taken once or twice a week from the second to the fourth or fifth month of pregnancy.

Actions Augments the qi, strengthens the Spleen, nourishes the blood, and quiets the fetus

Indications

Restless fetus, threatened miscarriage, or habitual miscarriage. There will be a pale complexion, fatigue, a lack of appetite, a pale tongue with a slippery coating, and a slippery but forceless pulse.

This is qi and blood deficiency with lack of nourishment to the fetus. Qi and blood deficiency in women causes the sea of blood—a system that encompasses the Womb, Liver, and Conception and Penetrating vessels—to become malnourished. When the woman becomes pregnant, this system's role in supporting fetal growth and development is impaired. The fetus becomes restless and miscarriage is threatened, or may well be habitual. The pale complexion, fatigue, and lack of appetite indicate Spleen and Stomach deficiency, while the pale tongue is a manifestation of blood deficiency. The slippery but forceless pulse indicates a restless fetus pattern, where the body is unable to secure the fetus.

Analysis of Formula

This formula utilizes a strategy of augmenting the qi, strengthening the Spleen, and nourishing the blood in order to secure the fetus and prevent miscarriage. The chief herbs are Ginseng Radix *(rén shēn)*, which strongly tonifies the primal qi to secure the fetus, and Rehmanniae Radix praeparata *(shú dì huáng)*, which tonifies the blood and enriches the yin, to nourish the fetal origin. Together, these two herbs treat qi and blood deficiency in the Conception and Penetrating vessels, which is the precondition for healthy fetal development. Each of the three deputies utilizes a different strategy to quiet the fetus: Dipsaci Radix *(xù duàn)* tonifies the Kidneys, Scutellariae Radix *(huáng qín)* drains heat, and Atractylodis macrocephalae Rhizoma *(bái zhú)* tonifies the Spleen. These herbs are extensively used in formulas treating habitual or threatened miscarriage. Focusing on the branch rather than the root, they deal with the acute problem of threatened miscarriage.

Astragali Radix (huáng qí) assists Ginseng Radix (rén shēn) and Atractylodis macrocephalae Rhizoma (bái zhú) in tonifying the qi. Angelicae sinensis Radix (dāng guī), Paeoniae Radix alba (bái sháo), and Chuanxiong Rhizoma (chuān xiōng) assist Rehmanniae Radix praeparata (shú dì huáng) in tonifying and regulating the blood. Together, they serve as assistants, nourishing the Liver blood and ensuring that its qi is strong and ascending. This is important inasmuch as many Chinese medicine physicians consider the Liver to be the root of a woman's physiology. Amomi Fructus (shā rén) moves the qi, harmonizes the Stomach, quiets the fetus, stops nausea, and facilitates the digestion of the more cloying tonifying herbs. Glutinous rice also tonifies the Spleen and Stomach, and as a sweet substance, harmonizes the actions of the other ingredients. Facilitating digestion and tonifying the Penetrating vessel via the Stomach, these herbs serve as envoys.

Cautions and Contraindications

While taking this formula, women are advised to avoid alcohol as well as sour, spicy, and hot foods, and to regulate their emotions.

Commentary

This formula tonifies and nourishes all the physiological systems that Chinese medicine associates with fetal development and a healthy pregnancy: Liver, Kidneys, Spleen and Stomach, the Womb, and the Conception and Penetrating vessels. Its composition is based on Eight-Treasure Decoction (bā zhēn tāng), discussed above, by removing Poria (fú líng) from the original formula and adding Astragali Radix (huáng qí), Scutellariae Radix (huáng qín), Dipsaci Radix (xù duàn), Amomi Fructus (shā rén), and Glutinous rice (nuò mǐ). Poria (fú líng), which has a bland nature that moves the fluids and thereby the qi downward, is not generally appropriate in pregnancy unless there is, in fact, edema. Most of the added herbs, on the other hand, are commonly used to 'quiet the fetus' (安胎 ān tāi), that is, to prevent miscarriage. These substitutions thus transform a formula that tonifies the qi and blood into one with a very specific focus and narrow range of application.

In clinical practice, the formula is typically prescribed for several months, taking one bag of the decoction per week. If there is nausea and vomiting, the formula should be modified by adding herbs such as Bambusae Caulis in taeniam (zhú rú), Pinelliae Rhizoma praeparatum (zhì bàn xià), Zingiberis Rhizoma recens (shēng jiāng), Eriobotryae Folium (pí pá yè), and Coptidis Rhizoma (huáng lián). If there is severe depletion of fluids due to vomiting, herbs such as Ophiopogonis Radix (mài mén dōng) and Scrophulariae Radix (xuán shēn) may also be added.

Comparison

> ➤ Vs. Worry-Free Formula to Protect Birth (bǎo chǎn wú yōu fāng); see page 361

Biomedical Indications

With the appropriate presentation, this formula may be used to treat such biomedically-defined disorders as threatened miscarriage or recurrent miscarriage.

....

Alternate name

Calm the Fetus Powder (ān tāi tāng) in Effective Formulas from the Hall of Literature

....

Modifications

• For more severe heat, increase the dosage of Astragali Radix (huáng qí) and reduce that of Amomi Fructus (shā rén).

• For patients with a weak Stomach, increase the dosage of Amomi Fructus (shā rén) and reduce that of Scutellariae Radix (huáng qín).

• For nausea and vomiting, add Pinelliae Rhizoma praeparatum (zhì bàn xià), Zingiberis Rhizoma recens (shēng jiāng), Bambusae Caulis in taeniam (zhú rú), or Eriobotryae Folium (pí pá yè).

• For vomiting of yellow or greenish bile, add Coptidis Rhizoma (huáng lián).

• For more severe deficiency with soreness of the back and knees, add Eucommiae Cortex (dù zhòng) and Cuscutae Semen (tù sī zǐ).

• For insomnia and palpitations, add Ziziphi spinosae Semen (suān zǎo rén), Longan Arillus (lóng yǎn ròu), and Polygoni multiflori Caulis (yè jiāo téng).

• For threatened miscarriage with vaginal bleeding, add Asini Corii Colla (ē jiāo) and Artemisiae argyi Folium (ài yè).

保產無憂方（保产无忧方）
Worry-Free Formula to Protect Birth
bǎo chǎn wú yōu fāng

Source Fu Qing-Zhu's Women's Disorders (1826)

wine-washed Angelicae sinensis Radix (dāng guī) 4.5g
charred Schizonepetae Herba (jīng jiè) 2.4g
honey-prepared Astragali Radix (mì zhì huáng qí) 2.4g
Cuscutae Semen (tù sī zǐ) . . . . [wine-fried] 4.5g
ginger-fried Magnoliae officinalis Cortex (hòu pò) 2.1g
Notopterygii Rhizoma seu Radix (qiāng huó) 1.8g
Fritillariae cirrhosae Bulbus (chuān bèi mǔ) 6g
wine-fried Paeoniae Radix alba (bái sháo) 3.6g
Glycyrrhizae Radix (gān cǎo) 1.5g
Chuanxiong Rhizoma (chuān xiōng) 4.5g
vinegar-fried Artemisiae argyi Folium (ài yè) 6g
Zingiberis Rhizoma recens (shēng jiāng) . . . . 3 slices

Method of Preparation The source text suggests decocting the above ingredients and taking the liquid hot. Although not mentioned in the discussion of this formula, in a related formula in the same section, Fritillariae cirrhosae Bulbus *(chuān bèi mǔ)* is "added after the decoction is completely cooked." This is usually interpreted to mean that one should mix the powdered herb into the cooked decoction.

Actions Supplements the qi, nourishes the blood, regulates the qi, quiets the fetus, and expedites delivery

Indications

This formula has been used historically to treat deficiency of qi and blood that results in a restless fetus, tendency to miscarriage, malpositioned fetus, and difficult delivery. In addition, it is considered a prophylactic against miscarriage and difficult delivery.

While not explicitly stated in premodern texts, the implication is that this formula treats qi and blood deficiency that leaves the Penetrating and Conception vessels unsecured. This disharmony in the vessels most responsible for a smooth pregnancy and delivery can give rise to the symptoms listed above.

Analysis of Formula

Angelicae sinensis Radix *(dāng guī)*, Chuanxiong Rhizoma *(chuān xiōng),* and Paeoniae Radix alba *(bái sháo)* work together to nourish and harmonize the blood. Paeoniae Radix alba *(bái sháo)* is sour and astringent and is positioned to counter the pungent and dispersing tendency of Angelicae sinensis Radix *(dāng guī)* and Chuanxiong Rhizoma *(chuān xiōng),* while at the same time contributing to blood supplementation. Astragali Radix *(huáng qí)* and Glycyrrhizae Radix *(gān cǎo)* supplement the qi and support the fetus. These herbs address the root condition and, except for Glycyrrhizae Radix *(gān cǎo)*, comprise the chief herbs in the formula. Schizonepetae Herba *(jīng jiè)* and Notopterygii Rhizoma seu Radix *(qiāng huó)* lend an upward bearing to the formula and thus work with the qi-supplementing agents to support the fetus. *Essentials of the Materia Medica* states that Notopterygii Rhizoma seu Radix *(qiāng huó)* drains the Liver qi and tracks down Liver wind. *Thorough Investigations of the Materia Medica* points out that Schizonepetae Herba *(jīng jiè)* can clear heat and cool the blood by virtue of its ability to disperse stasis and clumps. These two ingredients disperse the stagnation of qi and blood and dispel internal wind. Because they address factors that can disrupt pregnancy that are not addressed by the chief herbs, they function as deputies. Aurantii Fructus *(zhǐ ké)* and Magnoliae officinalis Cortex *(hòu pò)* expand the chest and regulate the qi. Artemisiae argyi Folium *(ài yè)* warms the uterus, and Zingiberis Rhizoma recens *(shēng jiāng)* warms the middle and smooths the flow of qi. Zingiberis Rhizoma recens *(shēng jiāng)* supplements the Kidneys and secures the fetus while Fritillariae cirrhosae

Bulbus *(chuān bèi mǔ)* is cold and moistening and is traditionally known for its ability to move the fetus and provide for a smooth delivery. These herbs address issues that are not addressed by the chief and deputy herbs, and also help prevent the tonifying chief herbs from causing stagnation. They function as assistants in this formula. Glycyrrhizae Radix *(gān cǎo)* and Zingiberis Rhizoma recens *(shēng jiāng)* also harmonize and serve the role of envoy. All told, the formula works to supplement the blood and qi and secure the fetus without causing undue stagnation in the middle burner (Spleen-Liver).

Cautions and Contraindications

This formula is designed for women with qi and blood deficiency. It is not suitable for those who present with signs of fire from yin deficiency.

Commentary

This formula is first mentioned in the 13th-century text *Formulas to Aid the Living.* The modification presented here was composed by the famous Qing-dynasty gynecologist Fu Qing-Zhu. Only Carthami Flos *(hóng huā)* is removed from the original formula. To ensure the correct position of the fetus and a smooth delivery, the formula is traditionally given 3-5 times per month during the sixth and seventh months of pregnancy. Modern texts recommend 4-7 day courses beginning in the 28th week. Alternatively, after 3-5 packets of herbs, the situation can be reassessed and the herbs continued for up to 15 days until the fetus assumes a correct position.

During the sixth and seventh months when the goal of the formula is to ensure the correct position of the fetus and prepare the mother's body for the future birth, Fritillariae cirrhosae Bulbus *(chuān bèi mǔ)* may be removed from the formula as its primary role is to provide for a smooth delivery.

Once labor begins, the formula is prescribed as needed, and usually 2-4 doses is sufficient. At this time, especially if labor is prolonged, Ginseng Radix *(rén shēn)* is frequently added to the formula to supplement the mother's qi and give her more strength to endure the birthing process.

Comparison

➢ Vs. Taishan Bedrock Powder *(Tàishān pán shí sǎn)*

Both formulas treat habitual miscarriage and threatened abortion owing to deficiency of qi and blood. Taishan Bedrock Powder *(Tàishān pán shí sǎn)* addresses these symptoms when the qi and blood deficiency gives rise to substantial heat that disturbs the fetus and places the pregnancy at risk. Worry-Free Formula to Protect Birth *(bǎo chǎn wú yōu fāng),* on the other hand, only clears the heat by removing knotting and does not directly address the heat itself. This approach is fitting for more moderate heat in women who are slightly more deficient than those for whom Taishan Bedrock Powder *(Tàishān pán shí sǎn)* is appropriate. It has the added functions of treating inhibited urination during pregnancy, correcting fetal position in the sixth and seventh months of pregnancy, and of promoting a smooth delivery when administered during the birthing process itself. The difference between these formulas is indeed subtle and is revealed only by the degree of restlessness of the fetus and the intensity of other heat signs such as irritability, a red tongue tip, and a rapid pulse.

Biomedical Indications

With the appropriate presentation, this formula may be used to treat such biomedically-defined disorders as fetal malposition, difficult delivery, habitual miscarriage, threatened abortion, and inhibited urination during pregnancy.

Modifications

- For difficult delivery, add Carthami Flos *(hóng huā)*.
- For securing the fetus, add Eucommiae Cortex *(dù zhòng)* and Taxilli Herba *(sāng jì shēng)* and increase the dosage of Paeoniae Radix alba *(bái sháo)*.
- To aid the pelvic bones to part during delivery, add Testudinis Plastrum *(guī bǎn)*, Cyathulae Radix *(chuān niú xī)*, and Ginseng Radix *(rén shēn)*.
- For cases of deficiency, add Ginseng Radix *(rén shēn)*.

何人飲 (何人饮)
Fleeceflower Root and Ginseng Drink

hé rén yǐn

Source   *Collected Treatises of [Zhang] Jing-Yue* (1624)

Polygoni multiflori Radix *(hé shǒu wū)* 9-30g
Ginseng Radix *(rén shēn)* 9-15g
An-gelicae sinensis Radix *(dāng guī)* 6-9g
Citri reticulatae Pericarpium *(chén pí)* 6-9g
baked Zingiberis Rhizoma recens *(wēi jiāng)* 6-15g

Method of Preparation   Decoction. Sometimes prepared in a mixture of wine and water. At present, Codonopsis Radix *(dǎng shēn)* is usually substituted for Ginseng Radix *(rén shēn)* at 2-3 times its dosage. Take 2-3 hours before the onset of attacks.

Actions   Tonifies the blood and qi and treats malarial disorders

Indications

Chronic, unrelenting malarial disorders with a wan complexion, emaciation, a pale tongue, and a moderate, large, deficient pulse. The slightest amount of exertion will lead to an exacerbation of the intermittent fever and chills.

If prolonged and unrelenting, malarial disorders can profoundly affect the qi and blood. This is because such disorders are most closely associated with the Gallbladder channel, which over time and through its connection with the Liver,

will affect the blood. Liver and Gallbladder disorders have an adverse influence on the Spleen and Stomach (the transformational source of qi and blood), which leads to qi and blood deficiency. A wan complexion, emaciation, pale tongue, and large, deficient pulse are typical manifestations of qi and blood deficiency. As in most conditions of deficiency, slight exertion will aggravate the symptoms.

Analysis of Formula

The ingredients in this formula treat malarial disorder, nourish the blood (focusing on the Liver), and augment the qi (focusing on the Spleen). One of the chief herbs is Polygoni multiflori Radix *(hé shǒu wū)*, which tonifies the Liver and Kidneys, benefits the essence and blood, and is also said to have a mild effect on malarial disorders. It therefore acts upon all of the important aspects of this condition except for the Spleen qi. That aspect is addressed by the other chief herb, Ginseng Radix *(rén shēn)*, the most powerful of all qi tonics. The deputies are Angelicae sinensis Radix *(dāng guī)*, which assists Polygoni multiflori Radix *(hé shǒu wū)* in nourishing the Liver blood, and baked Zingiberis Rhizoma recens *(wēi jiāng)*, which warms the middle burner and strengthens the Stomach. This herb works synergistically with Ginseng Radix *(rén shēn)*. The assistant is Citri reticulatae Pericarpium *(chén pí)*, which regulates the qi of the middle burner and prevents the tonifying herbs from causing stagnation.

Cautions and Contraindications

Contraindicated during the early stages of a malarial disorder and in cases that have not yet become deficient.

Commentary

The first mention of the condition treated by this formula is found in Chapter 36 of *Basic Questions*: "When the pulse is moderate, large, and deficient in malarial disorders, medicinal substances should be used rather than needles." This is an important formula in the treatment of malarial disorders because if the ordinary type of antimalarial treatment is used, the patient will become even more depleted.

Some writers prescribe this formula for use in conditions where malaria is accompanied by dysenteric disorders or where improvement of dysenteric symptoms is followed by aggravation of malarial symptoms. This explains the use of herbs for warming, tonifying, and regulating the middle burner. They also suggest adjusting the dosage of these ingredients according to the actual presentation. For instance, if qi deficiency is pronounced, the dosage of Ginseng Radix *(rén shēn)* can be increased to 30g while that of Citri reticulatae Pericarpium *(chén pí)* should be reduced or the herb completely omitted from the formula. In cases with severe cold in the middle burner, the dosage of Zingiberis Rhizoma recens *(shēng jiāng)* might be increased to 15g.

Biomedical Indications

With the appropriate presentation, this formula may be used to treat the biomedically-defined disorder of chronic malaria.

Modifications

- For increased efficacy, add Artemisiae annuae Herba (*qīng hāo*), Astragali Radix (*huáng qí*), and Mume Fructus (*wū méi*).
- For severe qi deficiency, add Atractylodis macrocephalae Rhizoma (*bái zhú*) and Glycyrrhizae Radix praeparata (*zhì gān cǎo*).
- For focal distention or masses in the hypochondria, add Paeoniae Radix alba (*bái sháo*) and Trionycis Carapax (*biē jiǎ*).
- For thirst, a red tongue, and little or no tongue coating, add Trichosanthis Radix (*tiān huā fěn*), Ophiopogonis Radix (*mài mén dōng*), and Schisandrae Fructus (*wǔ wèi zǐ*).
- For fatigue, spontaneous sweating, and a pale complexion, add Astragali Radix (*huáng qí*) and Oryzae glutinosae Radix (*nuò dào gēn xū*).

地黃飲子 (地黄饮子)
Rehmannia Drink from *A Simple Book*

dì huáng yǐn zi

Source   *A Simple Book of Formulas* (1191)

Ginseng Radix (*rén shēn*)
prepared Astragali Radix (*zhì huáng qí*)
Glycyrrhizae Radix praeparata (*zhì gān cǎo*)
Rehmanniae Radix (*shēng dì huáng*)
Rehmanniae Radix praeparata (*shú dì huáng*)
Asparagi Radix (*tiān mén dōng*)
Ophiopogonis Radix (*mài mén dōng*)
Eriobotryae Folium (*pí pá yè*)
Dendrobii Herba (*shí hú*)
Alismatis Rhizoma (*zé xiè*)
Aurantii Fructus (*zhǐ ké*)

Method of Preparation   Grind equal amounts of the herbs into a coarse powder and decoct 9g as a draft.

Actions   Generates essence, tonifies the blood, nourishes the yin, and moistens dryness

Indications

Thirst, irritability and restlessness, a dry throat, flushed face, fatigue, and spontaneous sweating.

This is wasting and thirsting disorder due to heat collecting in the yang brightness warp where it has depleted the blood and damaged the qi. Thirst here is caused by heat collecting in the Stomach, depleting the fluids. This, is turn, leads to irritability (associated with the Heart) and restlessness (associated with the Kidneys), indicating that the heat has damaged the blood and essence. When the blood and essence are damaged, the ministerial fire is no longer controlled and flares upward, causing a dry throat. Facial flushing is due to heat in the yang brightness warp flaring upward. The heat also consumes the qi, leading to fatigue and spontaneous sweating.

Analysis of Formula

The pattern for which this formula is indicated is complex and requires simultaneous treatment of the root and branch. Many of the symptoms reflect damage to the qi, blood, and body fluids. This is treated by three groups of herbs. The first is comprised of Ginseng Radix (*rén shēn*), Astragali Radix (*huáng qí*), and Glycyrrhizae Radix praeparata (*zhì gān cǎo*). These herbs tonify the qi of the greater yin warp to assist with transformation and transportation. The second group, consisting of Rehmanniae Radix praeparata (*shú dì huáng*) and Rehmanniae Radix (*shēng dì huáng*), tonifies the blood and essence. The third group, comprised of Ophiopogonis Radix (*mài mén dōng*), Asparagi Radix (*tiān mén dōng*), and Dendrobii Herba (*shí hú*), focuses on generating fluids and nourishing the yin. The root of the disorder, however, is heat collecting in the yang brightness warp due to constraint of the body's qi dynamic. For this reason, the formula includes Eriobotryae Folium (*pí pá yè*), which directs the Stomach qi downward and clears heat, as well as Alismatis Rhizoma (*zé xiè*) and Aurantii Fructus (*zhǐ ké*). Together, these two herbs unblock the yang organs, draining heat from the Heart and Kidneys via the urine and from the Stomach and Intestines via the bowels.

Cautions and Contraindications

This is a tonifying and moistening formula. It must not be prescribed for wasting and thirsting disorder due to excess heat or yang deficiency.

Commentary

Wasting and thirsting disorder where thirst is the main symptom is traditionally classified as an upper burner pattern. Its root is usually Heart fire, but it can also be caused by heat collecting in the Stomach. In *Medical Formulas Collected and Analyzed*, the Qing-dynasty scholar Wang Ang explains the dynamics of this process:

> In all cases [of wasting and thirsting disorder,] fire is exuberant and water debilitated. The *Classic* states: 'Clumping of the two yang is called wasting.' The two yang [here] refers to the yang brightness. The hand yang brightness Large Intestine governs the yang fluids. A wasting disorder [manifesting] with yellow eyes and thirst is due to insufficiency of yang fluids. The foot yang brightness Stomach governs the blood. Heat [in the Stomach] causes digestion of food and [manifests] in becoming easily hungry. This is due to lurking heat within the blood with insufficiency of blood.

The most likely cause of this pattern is improper diet, including the excessive consumption of heating and cloying foods that generate heat and obstruct the qi dynamic. Shen Jin-Ao thus presents this formula along with Jade Spring Pill (*yù quán wán*), discussed below, for the treatment of wasting from internal heat constraint (消癉 *xiāo dàn*). He says the following about the formula:

> It generates essence, supplements the blood, nourishes dryness, and relieves thirst. Alismatis Rhizoma (*zé xiè*) and Aurantii Fructus (*zhǐ ké*) assist by guiding out from and dredging the two Intestines. This results in Heart fire descending; thus, the Small Intestine is cleared and free-flowing. Lung metal is moistened and the flow of the Large Intestine is smooth. Deep-seated heat is dispersed and thirst is spontaneously relieved.

Heat from constraint damages the qi and fluids but because the Stomach is the 'sea of blood,' it also readily penetrates into the blood, where over the long term, it leads to blood and essence deficiency. The 19th-century physician Fei Bo-Xiong emphasized this aspect in his interpretation of the formula:

> The subtlety of this formula lies in its augmenting the source of water in addition to clearing metal and moistening the Lungs. It furthermore includes Alismatis Rhizoma (*zé xiè*) and Aurantii Fructus (*zhǐ ké*) to drain constrained heat. When in this manner the thirst is stopped, irritability and restlessness are also eliminated.

The earliest reference to this formula, in *Simple Book of Formulas*, recommends it for wasting and thirsting from collected heat in the yang brightness. The pattern includes damage to the yin and qi with symptoms of thirst, vexing heat, lassitude of the spirit, and spontaneous sweating. Zhu Dan-Xi also lists the formula as Rehmannia Drink (*dì huáng yǐn zi*) in *Essential Teachings of [Zhu] Dan-Xi*. His version is identical, except for the omission of Aurantii Fructus (*zhǐ ké*). Zhu states that the formula is suited for treating wasting and thirsting disorder with irritability, dry throat, and red face. Note that there is another, more commonly-used formula called Rehmannia Drink from *Comprehensive Recording of Sagely Beneficence*. That formula is discussed later in this chapter among the formulas that tonify both the yin and the yang.

Comparison

➤ Vs. Jade Spring Pill (*yù quán wán*)

Both of these formulas tonify the yin and enrich the fluids and are used in practice for the treatment of wasting thirst. Rehmannia Drink from *A Simple Book (dì huáng yǐn zi)* contains more herbs that directly nourish the yin than does Jade Spring Pill (*yù quán wán*). In addition, it has a greater ability to guide fire downward and dispense it through the urine and stool. It relies on Aurantii Fructus (*zhǐ ké*) to promote free flow in the chest and Large Intestine, and on the down-ward-moving herbs Alismatis Rhizoma (*zé xiè*) and Eriobotryae Folium (*pí pá yè*) to move the qi and fire downward. The actions of these herbs, combined with those that nourish the yin and qi, make it a well-rounded formula in cases where Heart and Small Intestine heat are prominent in a setting of qi and yin deficiency. By contrast, Jade Spring Pill (*yù quán wán*) is better suited for tonifying the Spleen and Lungs, generating fluids, and adjusting the water pathways.

Biomedical Indications

With the appropriate presentation, this formula may be used to treat a variety of biomedically-defined disorders such as diabetes and hypoglycemia.

Section 4

....

FORMULAS THAT NOURISH AND TONIFY THE YIN

These formulas are used when the body fluids and essences are damaged such that yin becomes deficient and yang relatively excessive. This type of condition may occur for many reasons and usually affects two groups of organs. When the disorder is relatively superficial, with damage predominantly to the yang fluids, it is regarded as dryness of the Lungs and Stomach (see Chapter 15). Damage to the yin fluids or essences, which occurs more often in connection with chronic disorders, affects the Liver and Kidneys, which is the focus of the formulas here. The therapeutic strategies for these disorders focus on nourishing and enriching the Kidney and Liver yin and regulating the storage and transformation of fluids in the lower burner as a means of tonification.

The yin of the Kidneys and Liver serves as the basic reserve of yin for the entire body. In some texts, it is referred to as the 'true' or 'fundamental yin.' Many long-term problems associated with environment or lifestyle (e.g., excessive sexual activity, a hard-driven lifestyle, or a dry environment with insufficient fluid intake) will, over time, deplete the Kidney and Liver yin, thereby damaging the true yin. Common symptoms include soreness and weakness of the lower back and legs, lightheadedness, vertigo, tidal fever with malar flush, irritability, heat in the five centers, night sweats, insomnia, and spontaneous emissions. The tongue is usually red and thin with little or no coating. The pulse is rapid and thin. In clinical practice, such textbook presentations are often complicated, however, by concomitant signs of other problems such as yang or qi deficiency, water toxin, phlegm, or blood stasis. In such cases, care must be taken to properly assess root and branch, selecting and modifying treatment strategies and formulas accordingly.

The chief ingredients of the formulas in this section are for the most part nourishing in nature and therefore have rich, cloying characteristics. They include Asparagi Radix (*tiān mén dōng*), Dendrobii Herba (*shí hú*), Polygonati odorati Rhizoma (*yù zhú*), Rehmanniae Radix (*shēng dì huáng*), Rehmanniae Radix praeparata (*shú dì huáng*), Schisandrae Fructus (*wǔ wèi zǐ*), Trionycis Carapax (*biē jiǎ*), and Testudinis Plastrum (*guī bǎn*).

Herbs that tonify the blood, such as Angelicae sinensis Radix (*dāng guī*) and Paeoniae Radix alba (*bái sháo*), are also used. This makes sense, as blood is also an essence, and damage to one type of essence readily damages others. This is why herbs like Rehmanniae Radix praeparata (*shú dì huáng*) and Lycii Fructus (*gǒu qǐ zǐ*) can be used to tonify both substances.

Three other types of ingredients are combined with the chief herbs in the formulas discussed here:

- Substances that tonify the yang such as Cervi Cornus Colla (*lù jiǎo jiāo*), Eucommiae Cortex (*dù zhòng*), Cibotii Rhizoma (*gǒu jǐ*), and Cuscutae Semen (*tù sī zǐ*). Because the yin and yang have the same source, deficiency of one readily leads to deficiency of the other. Furthermore, tonifying the yang is a strategy for dynamically integrating yin tonification into the body's physiology, as explained by Zhang Jie-Bin in the *Classified Classic*: "Experts in tonifying the yang invariably assist the yang from within the yin. For when yang avails itself of the assistance of yin, generation and transformation are never exhausted."

- Because yin deficiency gives rise to yang excess, which usually manifests as heat, many formulas also include herbs that clear fire or drain heat such as Moutan Cortex (*mǔ dān pí*), Anemarrhenae Rhizoma (*zhī mǔ*), or Phellodendri Cortex (*huáng bǎi*).

- Finally, another common addition to these formulas are herbs like Poria (*fú líng*), Alismatis Rhizoma (*zé xiè*), Amomi Fructus (*shā rén*), or Citri reticulatae Pericarpium (*chén pí*) that promote the movement of fluids and qi. This is done to prevent the formulas from clogging the body's digestion and water metabolism. Even so, the formulas discussed here should be used with caution and appropriately modified in patients with weakness of the Spleen and Stomach. It is also important to remember that if an active pathogenic influence is still the main problem, the use of these formulas is contraindicated.

六味地黃丸（六味地黄丸）
Six-Ingredient Pill with Rehmannia
liù wèi dì huáng wán

Source *Craft of Medicinal Treatment for Childhood Disease Patterns* (1119)

Rehmanniae Radix praeparata (*shú dì huáng*)	240g
Corni Fructus (*shān zhū yú*)	120g
Dioscoreae Rhizoma (*shān yào*)	120g
Poria (*fú líng*)	90g
Moutan Cortex (*mǔ dān pí*)	90g
Alismatis Rhizoma (*zé xiè*)	90g

Method of Preparation Grind the ingredients into a powder and form into small pills with honey. Take in 9g doses three times a day. May also be prepared as a decoction with one-tenth the specified dosage.

Clinically, this formula is prepared as a decoction for treating relatively intense fire from deficiency, eye disorders, or weakened Spleen and Stomach function. The pill or concentrate forms are used for patients with edema, reduced urination, or for those with restricted fluid intake. For long-term constitutional treatment, pills are the preferred method of preparation.

Actions Enriches the yin and nourishes the Kidneys

Indications

Soreness and weakness in the lower back, lightheadedness, vertigo, tinnitus, diminished hearing, night sweats, spontaneous and nocturnal emissions, a red tongue with little coating, and a rapid, thin pulse. The patient may also present with a variety of other symptoms including hot palms and soles, a chronic dry and sore throat, toothache, or wasting and thirsting disorder.

This is the classic presentation of Kidney and Liver yin deficiency. The lower back is the abode of the Kidneys, which are also associated with the bones and are responsible for generating marrow (which gives the bones their resiliency and strength). When the Kidneys are weak, the marrow will become depleted, and there will be general weakness of the skeletal structure, which is focused in the area of the body most closely associated with the Kidneys, the lower back and legs. Kidney and Liver yin deficiency also mean that the essence (Kidneys) and blood (Liver) are not flourishing and are therefore unable to nourish the upper parts of the body, primarily the sensory orifices. The eyes are nourished by the Liver; lack of nourishment manifests as lightheadedness and vertigo. The ears are nourished by the Kidneys; lack of nourishment manifests as tinnitus and diminished hearing. When the yin is deficient, it cannot retain substances during the night, which is the time associated with yin. This leads to night sweats and nocturnal emissions. The deficient yin is also unable to preserve the essence, which is manifested in men as spontaneous emissions. Yin deficiency and internally-generated heat is reflected in the red color of the tongue and its less-than-normal moisture (little or no coating), and also in the pulse, which has little volume (thin) and is rapid.

Depending on the individual and the particular etiology of the Kidney and Liver yin deficiency, other problems may also occur. If the heat from deficiency is more severe, the patient may present with hot palms and soles, a flushed face, or a dry and sore throat. If the heat transforms into fire and ascends to the teeth (which are connected with the Kidneys), there may be toothache. And if the Kidney qi is also unstable, there may be wasting and thirsting disorder with copious urination.

Analysis of Formula

This formula focuses on tonifying the yin and thereby allowing it to flourish. When this is achieved, the other signs and symptoms will disappear.

This formula is an elegant combination of two groups of ingredients, each consisting of three herbs. The first group is comprised of the tonifying herbs. The chief herb, Rehmanniae Radix praeparata *(shú dì huáng),* strongly enriches the Kidney yin and essence. One of the deputies, Corni Fructus *(shān zhū yú),* nourishes the Liver and restrains the leakage of essence. It performs the latter function by inhibiting the improper dispersion and drainage through the Liver, thereby enabling the essence to build up in the Kidneys. For this to occur, a substance with the strong, essence-building properties of the chief herb is also required. The other deputy, Dioscoreae Rhizoma *(shān yào),* stabilizes the essence by tonifying the Spleen. To reinforce the essence and improve its function, the Spleen (the source of postnatal essence) must function properly.

The second group of ingredients has a predominantly draining action in the context of this formula. They are regarded as the assistants. Alismatis Rhizoma *(zé xiè)* clears and drains the overabundance of Kidney fire. It is used here to prevent the rich, cloying properties of the chief herb from congesting the mechanisms of the Kidneys, which will induce even more fire from deficiency. Moutan Cortex *(mǔ dān pí)* clears and drains Liver fire and is used here to counterbalance the warm properties of Corni Fructus *(shān zhū yú).* Poria *(fú líng)* is a bland herb that leaches out dampness from the Spleen. It is paired with Dioscoreae Rhizoma *(shān yào)* to strengthen the transportive functions of the Spleen. This prevents the formula from clogging up the digestive process and reinforces the Spleen's function of nourishing the body. Poria *(fú líng)* and Alismatis Rhizoma *(zé xiè)* work together to improve the metabolism of fluids and promote urination, thereby preventing a buildup of stagnant fluids.

Cautions and Contraindications

This formula has cloying properties and should be used with caution in cases with indigestion, diarrhea due to Spleen deficiency, or a white, greasy tongue coating.

Commentary

Original Indications and Main Usage

This formula is a variation of Kidney Qi Pill *(shèn qì wán),* discussed below. Its author, the famous Song-dynasty pedia-trician Qian Yi, removed the heating herbs Cinnamomi Ramulus *(guì zhī)* and Aconiti Radix lateralis praeparata *(zhì fù zǐ)* from that formula and substituted Rehmanniae Radix praeparata *(shú dì huáng)* for Rehmanniae Radix *(shēng dì huáng).* This created an entirely new formula with very different indications. In the source text, the indication was slow development in children reflected in the so-called 'five retardations' (五遲 *wǔ chí):* "Kidney timidity (腎怯 *shèn qiè)* with loss of voice, nonclosure of the anterior fontanel, insufficient spirit, excessive visibility of the whites of the eyes, and a shiny, pale complexion." It was not until the Ming dynasty, however, that Six-Ingredient Pill with Rehmannia *(liù wèi dì huáng wán)* came to be seen as the paradigmatic formula for the treatment of yin deficiency. The key person in this process was the famous court physician Xue Ji, who attributed to it the ability to "fortify water in order to control fire" and used it as one of his main formulas. Xue Ji's influence was channeled particularly through the proponents of warm tonification, a group of physicians that flourished during the Ming era who regarded the Kidneys as the most important organ in the body. Through their writing and teaching, these physicians established Six-Ingredient Pill with Rehmannia *(liù wèi dì huáng wán)* as one of the most widely used formulas in Chinese medicine, with many equally famous variations (see ASSOCIATED FORMULAS below).

Because the Kidneys house the true yin, problems of the type described above can influence all the other yin organs. For example, the Heart and Kidneys are both lesser yin organs, the former being relatively yang, as it is situated higher in the body. Kidney yin deficiency often results in a lack of control over the yang (Heart), with fire from deficiency blazing upward through the lesser yin channels. This manifests as a dry throat, pain in the tongue, night sweats, and insomnia. However, despite this interrelationship among the yin organs, not all disorders of yin deficiency can be treated with this formula. This was noted by the modern physician Qin Bo-Wei in *Medical Lecture Notes of [Qin] Qian-Zhai:*

> The most important indication of Six-Ingredient Pill with Rehmannia *(liù wèi dì huáng wán)* is Kidney yin deficiency due to harm from exhaustion leading to patterns [characterized by] emaciation and lower back pain. The literature also says that it treats insufficiency of the Liver and Kidneys or of all three [major] yin organs together, as well as listing spontaneous sweating, night sweats, overflowing of water that turns into phlegm, loss of semen, bloody stools, throat pain, toothache [and similar symptoms]. … It is able to treat all of these, but when all is said and done, one must clearly see the main cause, the main organ [involved], and the main pattern, and make modifications according to the specific nature of the disorder. If one mistakenly assumes that one can treat all yin deficiency patterns [in the same manner], and treat them all with Six-Ingredient Pill with Rehmannia *(liù wèi dì huáng wán),* one's success in the clinic will most definitely not be very high.

Debates about Composition and Usage: Deficiency, Fire, Phlegm, and Thin Mucus

The debates underlying Qin Bo-Wei's discussion relate to two different aspects of the formula's composition and usage. The first is its main focus of action. Whereas physicians like Qian Yi, Xue Ji, or Qin Bo-Wei clearly define this to be the Kidneys, others accorded it more comprehensive effects. In *Discussion of Medical Formulas*, for example, Fei Bo-Xiong states that "This formula does not merely treat deficiency of the Kidneys and Liver. It truly is a formula for treating all three [major] yin organs [i.e., the Kidneys, Liver, and Spleen]." Zhang Bing-Cheng, another late-Qing-dynasty writer, made an even bolder claim in *Convenient Reader of Established Formulas*, exending its effects even further to blood tonification: "This formula strongly tonifies the three organs Kidneys, Liver, and Spleen. [It is thereby indicated for] patterns characterized by insufficiency of true yin, and of exhaustion damage to the essence and blood."

A second topic of debate concerned the inclusion of the three so-called "draining" herbs in the formula, which may seem odd given its use for severe deficiency disorders. To answer this question, one must look at the indications for the formula from which it was derived, Kidney Qi Pill (*shèn qì wán*). These include wasting thirst, phlegm, and thin mucus, urinary difficulty from a shifted bladder (轉胞 *zhuàn bāo*), and other disorders of water transformation. Since the Kidneys govern the fluids of the entire body, and the Kidneys, Liver, and Spleen all play a major role in the transformation and regulation of fluid metabolism, this is not surprising. In the patterns treated by Kidney Qi Pill (*shèn qì wán*) these symptoms arise from deficiency of yang. Deficiency of yin, however, can cause the same problems. This is because the yin here is unable to control the yang, which floats to the upper burner and the body surface as heat from deficiency rather than contributing to fluid transformation in the lower and middle burners. In *Assorted Works from Enlightened Physicians*, Xue Ji, the main popularizer of this formula, revealed his clear understanding of this action when he stated:

> In those [suffering from] insufficiency of Kidney channel yin essence where the yang is not transformed and the fire of deficiency moves chaotically causing the previously outlined symptoms [of yin deficiency with flourishing fire as well as coughing of blood,] the use of Six-Ingredient Pill with Rehmannia (*liù wèi dì huáng wán*) is indicated to make the yin flourish so that it transforms the yang.

Thus, both the fire of deficiency and phlegm often present together in conditions of yin deficiency, constituting the pathophysiological equivalent of false heat and thin mucus that characterizes yang deficiency patterns. In both cases, fire and phlegm/thin mucus can be seen as internal pathogens that must be treated just as much as the deficiency that gave rise to them. This is clearly stated by Gong Ju-Zhong, an-

other Ming dynasty court physician, in *Understanding in an Instant,* one of of the key texts on phlegm-fire in Chinese medicine:

> The ancients composed Six-Ingredient Pill with Rehmannia (*liù wèi dì huáng wán*) in order to treat all kinds of phlegm-fire patterns. It is also said that one can take it irrespective of whether one is ill or not yet ill. [To understand this] one must deeply penetrate to the mysteries of disease. How then is this? … When the ancients used tonifying herbs, they always simultaneously drained the pathogenic [qi that is caused by deficiency]. When these pathogens are removed, the tonifying herbs become [even more] potent. [Being able to] open and close at the same time, this is truly miraculous. Later generations no longer understood this principle. Focusing solely on tonification will, over the long term, cause harm through unilateral dominance. Is the composition of Six-Ingredient Pill not divine?

Thus, the presence of phlegm or thin mucus is not a contraindication for this formula as long as the root cause is Kidney yin, rather than Spleen yang, deficiency. In clinical practice, loose stools, as well as difficulty in digesting this formula will be the key markers for making this differentiation.

Name of the Formula

Note that in Chinese medicine the term 味 *wèi*, which translates as 'flavor' or 'taste,' is often used to simply designate the ingredients of a formula, and that is reflected in our translation of this formula's name as Six-Ingredient Pill with Rhemannia. However, in the present case, some commentators, including Wang Zi-Jie, understand the name in a more specific way, based in part on a passage from Chapter 5 of *Basic Questions*: "When the essences are deficient, use the flavor [of herbs] to tonify them." This is generally interpreted as referring to the yin quality of a medicinal substance (i.e., its capacity to nourish and tonify), as opposed to its yang quality or qi (i.e., its capacity to move, disperse, ascend, etc.). From this perspective, for a formula like this one that is aimed at tonifying the Kidney essences, the term 味 *wèi* is used with this connotation in mind, making it 'Six Flavors Pill.' This formula is well-balanced, treating all the yin organs of the body, combining tonification with draining. To achieve this effect it makes use of all six flavors (bitter, sour, sweet, salty, acrid, and bland) making it both clinically effective, but also a model for the composition of a well-rounded formula.

Comparisons

> ➢ Vs. Tonify the Middle to Augment the Qi Decoction (*bǔ zhōng yì qì tāng*)

Comparing these two formulas will help illuminate the concept of ascending and descending functions in traditional Chinese medicine. This comparison was first made by the 18th-century physician You Yi. When the yang is deficient, the qi collapses. A combination of relatively 'light' herbs should therefore be used to strengthen and raise it. This is the thrust of Tonify the Middle to Augment the Qi Decoction (bǔ zhōng yì qì tāng). By contrast, when the yin is deficient, the qi rises but does not return downward. Thus, cloying, 'heavy' herbs such as Rehmanniae Radix praeparata (shú dì huáng) are combined with herbs that leach out fluids through the urine to encourage the qi to descend. This is the mechanism underlying Six-Ingredient Pill with Rehmannia (liù wèi dì huáng wán). Similarly, collapse of the qi is usually accompanied by some stagnation. To move the qi, Citri reticulatae Pericarpium (chén pí) is used in Tonify the Middle to Augment the Qi Decoction (bǔ zhōng yì qì tāng). By contrast, when the qi floats, there is usually heat. To clear this type of heat from yin deficiency, Moutan Cortex (mǔ dān pí) is used in Six-Ingredient Pill with Rehmannia (liù wèi dì huáng wán).

➤ Vs. Restore the Left [Kidney] Pill (zuǒ guī wán); see page 371

➤ Vs. Great Tonify the Yin Pill (dà bǔ yīn wán); see page 375

➤ Vs. Two-Solstice Pill (èr zhì wán); see page 384

Biomedical Indications

With the appropriate presentation, this formula may be used to treat a wide variety of biomedically-defined disorders. These can be divided into the following groups:

- Genitourinary disorders such as chronic nephritis, prostate diseases, chronic glomerulonephritis, urinary tract infection, renal tuberculosis
- Endocrine disorders such as diabetes mellitus, hyperthyroidism, and diabetes insipidus
- Cardiovascular disease such as hypertension, atherosclerosis, and coronary artery disease
- Women's disorders such as perimenopausal syndrome and dysfunctional uterine bleeding
- Ophthalmic diseases such as cataracts, glaucoma, central retinopathy, optic nerve atrophy, and optic neuritis.

This formula has also been used for neurasthenia, pulmonary tuberculosis, chronic hepatitis, cirrhosis, and failure to thrive.

Alternate names

Tonify the Kidneys Rehmannia Pill (bǔ shèn dì huáng wán) in *Effective Formulas*; Tonify the Liver and Kidneys Rehmannia Pill (bǔ gān shèn dì huáng wán) in *Fine Formulas of Wonderful Efficacy*; Six Ingredient Pill (liù wèi wán) in *Fine Formulas for Women*; Rehmannia Pill (dì huáng wán) in *Assorted Works from Enlightened Physicians*

Modifications

- For severe depletion of the fluids with heat signs, substitute Rehmanniae Radix (shēng dì huáng) for Rehmanniae Radix praeparata (shú dì huáng).

- For wasting and thirsting disorder, remove Alismatis Rhizoma (zé xiè) and add a large dosage (at least 30g when prepared as a decoction) of Trichosanthis Radix (tiān huā fěn).
- For Spleen deficiency, add Atractylodis macrocephalae Rhizoma (bái zhú), Amomi Fructus (shā rén), and Citri reticulatae Pericarpium (chén pí).
- For childhood nutritional impairment with abdominal distention and loose, watery stools, remove Rehmanniae Radix praeparata (shú dì huáng) and add Atractylodis macrocephalae Rhizoma (bái zhú), Gigeriae galli Endothelium corneum (jī nèi jīn), and Amomi Fructus (shā rén).
- For optic neuritis, optic nerve atrophy, or central retinitis, add Bupleuri Radix (chái hú), Angelicae sinensis Radix (dāng guī), and Schisandrae Fructus (wǔ wèi zǐ).
- For hypertension, add Mori Folium (sāng yè), Pheretima (dì lóng), and Achyranthis bidentatae Radix (niú xī).
- For chronic nephritis, add Leonuri Herba (yì mǔ cǎo), Trichosanthis Radix (tiān huā fěn), and Lophatheri Herba (dàn zhú yè).
- For irregualr menstruation, add Artemisiae argyi Folium (ài yè) and Cyperi Rhizoma (xiāng fù).

Variations

都氣丸（都气丸）

Capital Qi Pill

dū qì wán

Source *Symptom, Cause, Pulse, and Treatment* (1706)

For chronic wheezing disorders in those who are always short of breath and begin wheezing with little exertion, add Schisandrae Fructus (wǔ wèi zǐ). This formula is also used to treat premature ejaculation or spermatorrhea from Kidney deficiency. Schisandrae Fructus (wǔ wèi zǐ) tonifies and gently warms the Kidneys, while its sourness prevents its qi from ascending in an uncontrolled fashion, focusing it instead on Kidney qi transformation. This makes it a formula whose range of application is between that of Kidney Qi Pill (shèn qì wán) and Anemarrhena, Phellodendron, and Rehmannia Pill (zhī bǎi dì huáng wán).

───────────

杞菊地黃丸（杞菊地黄丸）

Lycium Fruit, Chrysanthemum, and Rehmannia Pill

qǐ jú dì huáng wán

Source *Complete Treatise on Measles* (Yuan Dynasty)

For dry eyes with diminished visual acuity, photophobia, tearing when exposed to drafts, or painful eyes, add Lycii Fructus (gǒu qǐ zǐ) and white Chrysanthemi Flos (jú huā). The use of this formula has been expanded to include all conditions of Kidney and Liver yin deficiency in which Liver deficiency is the predominant aspect.

知柏地黃丸（知柏地黄丸）

Anemarrhena, Phellodendron, and Rehmannia Pill

zhī bǎi dì huáng wán

Source   *Investigations of Medical Formulas* (1584)

For yin deficiency with vigorous fire, consumptive heat, or steam-ing bone disorder characterized by night sweats, a dry mouth and tongue, and a large pulse only in the rear position, add salt-fried Anemarrhenae Rhizoma *(yán chǎo zhī mǔ)* and salt-fried Phello-dendri Cortex *(yán chǎo huáng bǎi)*. Also for urinary difficulty and lower back pain from damp-heat in the lower burner in patients with underlying Kidney yin deficiency. When using this formula, it is important to remember that Anemarrhenae Rhizoma *(zhī mǔ)* and Phellodendri Cortex *(huáng bǎi)* are, in fact, bitter, cooling herbs that drain excess heat from the body. The pathodynamic is thus one of yin fire, a pathodynamic explained in detail in the COMMENTARY section to Great Tonify the Yin Pill *(dà bǔ yīn wán)*, discussed below. A key clinical marker is the flooding proxi-mal pulse on both wrists.

Comparisons

➤ Vs. GREAT TONIFY THE YIN PILL *(dà bǔ yīn wán)*; *see* PAGE 375

➤ Vs. JADE WOMAN DECOCTION *(yù nǚ jiān)*; *see* PAGE 194

八仙長壽丸（八仙长寿丸）

Eight-Immortal Pill for Longevity

bā xiān cháng shòu wán

Source   *Achieving Longevity by Guarding the Source* (1615)

For deficient yin consumptive disorders with cough, coughing of blood, tidal fevers, and night sweats, add Ophiopogonis Radix *(mài mén dōng)* and Schisandrae Fructus *(wǔ wèi zǐ)*. This formula is used for many different types of conditions due to yin deficiency of the Lungs and Kidneys. It is used in contemporary practice to treat yin deficiency in older patients characterized by generalized weak-ness and fatigue, a lusterless or wan complexion, lack of appetite, phlegm, coughing, frequent urination, impotence, and weakness in the lower body. Compared to Capital Qi Pill *(dū qì wán)*, this formula supports both the upper and lower sources of water trans-formation in the body.

加味六味地黃丸（加味六味地黄丸）

Augmented Six-Ingredient Pill with Rehmannia

jiā wèi liù wèi dì huáng wán

Source   *Golden Mirror of the Medical Tradition* (1742)

For children with slow mental development, a lusterless complex-ion, fatigue, lethargy, a pale tongue, and a forceless, submerged pulse, add Cervi Cornu pantotrichum *(lù róng)*, Acanthopanacis Cortex *(wǔ jiā pí)*, and Moschus *(shè xiāng)*. This formula is used for a wide range of developmental disorders.

耳聾左慈丸（耳聋左慈丸）

Pill for Deafness that is Kind to the Left [Kidney]

ěr lóng zuǒ cí wán

Source   *Discussion of Widespread Warm Epidemics* (1642)

For continuous, cicada-like tinnitus that worsens at night, hearing loss, irritability, insomnia, vertigo with blurry vision, and a thin and frail or thin and rapid pulse, add Magnetitum *(cí shí)*, Acori tatari-nowii Rhizoma *(shí chāng pǔ)*, and Schisandrae Fructus *(wǔ wèi zǐ)*. This formula is widely used for hearing loss due to old age.

Associated Formulas

當歸地黃飲（当归地黄饮）

Tangkuei and Rehmannia Decoction

dāng guī dì huáng yǐn

Source   *Collected Treatises of [Zhang] Jing-Yue* (1624)

Angelicae sinensis Radix *(dāng guī)* 6-9g
Rehmanniae Radix praeparata *(shú dì huáng)* 9-15g
Dioscoreae Rhizoma *(shān yào)* 6g
Eucommiae Cortex *(dù zhòng)* 6g
Achyranthis bidentatae Radix *(niú xī)* 4.5g
Corni Fructus *(shān zhū yú)* 3g
Glycyrrhizae Radix praeparata *(zhì gān cǎo)* 2.4g

Enriches the Kidney and Liver yin, nourishes the blood, and regu-lates the menstrual cycle. This is a very useful formula in treating Kidney and Liver yin deficiency in women. For pain and weakness in the lower back and legs, reduced menstrual flow, foot and heel pain, a pale, dry tongue, and a submerged, thin pulse. The patient may also experience lightheadedness and tinnitus.

八味地黃丸（八味地黄丸）

Eight-Ingredient Pill with Rehmannia

bā wèi dì huáng wán

Source   *Women's Diseases According to Fu Qing-Zhu* (1826)

Corni Fructus *(shān zhū yú)* 24g
Dioscoreae Rhizoma *(shān yào)* 24g
Moutan Cortex *(mǔ dān pí)* 24g
Poria *(fú líng)* 24g
Rehmanniae Radix praeparata *(shú dì huáng)* 24g
Alismatis Rhizoma *(zé xiè)* 15g
Schisandrae Fructus *(wǔ wèi zǐ)* 15g
honey-prepared Astragali Radix *(zhì huáng qí)* 30g

Grind the ingredients into a powder and form into pills with honey. Take before bedtime. Tonifies the yin, nourishes the blood, and stops excessive sweating. For postpartum continuous sweating from defi-ciency. *Note:* There are many formulas by this name, and in Japan it refers to Kidney Qi Pill *(shèn qì wán)*.

明目地黃丸（明目地黄丸）

Improve Vision Pill with Rehmannia

míng mù dì huáng wán

Source   *Scrutiny of the Priceless Jade Case* (1642)

Rehmanniae Radix praeparata (shú dì huáng) 120g
Rehmanniae Radix (shēng dì huáng) 60g
Dioscoreae Rhizoma (shān yào) 60g
Alismatis Rhizoma (zé xiè) 60g
Corni Fructus (shān zhū yú) 60g
Moutan Cortex (mǔ dān pí) 60g
Bupleuri Radix (chái hú) 60g
Poriae Sclerotium pararadicis (fú shén) 60g
Angelicae sinensis Radix (dāng guī) 60g
Schisandrae Fructus (wǔ wèi zǐ) 60g

Grind the ingredients into a powder and form into pills with honey. Take in 9g doses. Nourishes the Liver, enriches the Kidneys, and improves the vision. For blurry or diminished vision due to Liver and Kidney deficiency. This formula is more effective in nourishing the blood and treating eye disorders than Lycium Fruit, Chrysanthemum, and Rehmannia Pill (qǐ jú dì huáng wán), discussed above. The source text advises that patients taking this formula should abstain from eating turnips.

Comparison

➢ Vs. Preserve Vistas Pill (zhù jīng wán); see page 392

滋腎明目湯 (滋肾明目汤)
Enrich the Kidneys and Improve Vision Decoction
zī shèn míng mù tāng

Source   *Restoration of Health from the Myriad Diseases* (1587)

Angelicae sinensis Radix (dāng guī) 2parts (6g)
Chuanxiong Rhizoma (chuān xiōng) 2parts (6g)
Paeoniae Radix alba (bái sháo) .2parts (6g)
Rehmanniae Radix (shēng dì huáng) 2parts (6g)
Rehmanniae Radix praeparata (shú dì huáng) 2parts (6g)
Ginseng Radix (rén shēn) 1part (3g)
Platycodi Radix (jié gěng) 1part (3g)
Gardeniae Fructus (zhī zǐ) 1part (3g)
Coptidis Rhizoma (huáng lián) .1part (3g)
Angelicae dahuricae Radix (bái zhǐ) 1part (3g)
Viticis Fructus (màn jīng zǐ) 1part (3g)
Chrysanthemi Flos (jú huā) 1part (3g)
Glycyrrhizae Radix (gān cǎo) 1part (3g)

Grind the ingredients and cook with a pinch of tea and a coil of Junci Medulla (dēng xīn cǎo). Only relative dosages are given in the text; those shown above in parenthesis are the editors' suggestions. Enriches the yin, nourishes the blood, tonifies the qi, clears heat, resolves toxicity, and brightens the eyes. The indications in the source text are for eye pain in the presence of spirit consumption (瘰神 láo shén), Kidney deficiency, or scant blood. In addition, the formula addresses visual dizziness and, with modifications, wind-heat and red and swollen eyes in patients who are constitutionally yin-blood deficient.

This formula treats eye disorders in old or weak patients who display obvious signs of blood deficiency and heat. While several of the herbs in the formula are generally not recommended for patients with yin-blood deficiency, in this formula, the strong basis of blood-

supplementing herbs allows their use. At present, the formula is used in treating chronic nervous exhaustion, diminished visual acuity, easily-tired eyes, excessive tearing, itching, or pain in the eyes, and cataracts as well as for constitutionally weak patients who contract wind-heat eye disorders such as conjunctivitis or sties, or patients who suffer pain or swelling following surgery or other invasive procedures at or near the eyes.

Note: This formula is also known as Kidney Qi Eye-Brightening Decoction (shèn qì míng mù tāng).

左歸丸 (左归丸)
Restore the Left [Kidney] Pill
zuǒ guī wán

According to Chapter 36 of the *Classic of Difficulties*, the left Kidney is called the 'true Kidney,' while the right is called the 'gate of vitality.' Zhang Jie-Bin, the author of this formula, regarded the left Kidney as the source of the true or source yin. He noted that "to fortify the governance of water, one nurtures the source yin, [which is] the left Kidney." Hence the formula's name.

Source   *Collected Treatises of [Zhang] Jing-Yue* (1624)

Rehmanniae Radix praeparata (shú dì huáng) 240g
dry-fried Dioscoreae Rhizoma (chǎo shān yào) 120g
Lycii Fructus (gǒu qǐ zǐ) 120g
Corni Fructus (shān zhū yú) 120g
wine-prepared Cyathulae Radix (jiǔ chuān niú xī) 90g
Cuscutae Semen (tù sī zǐ) 120g
Cervi Cornus Colla (lù jiǎo jiāo) 120g
Testudinis Plastri Colla (guī bǎn jiāo) 120g

Method of Preparation   Grind the ingredients into a powder and form into pills with honey. Take in 15g doses twice a day with salted water.

Actions   Nourishes the yin, enriches the Kidneys, fills the essence, and augments the marrow

Indications

Lightheadedness, vertigo, tinnitus, soreness and weakness in the lower back and legs, spontaneous and nocturnal emissions, spontaneous and night sweats, dry mouth and throat, thirst, a red, shiny tongue, and a thin, rapid pulse.

When the true yin of the Kidneys is damaged, the essence and marrow will be depleted. Lightheadedness, veritigo, and tinnitus indicate that the yin has lost its ability to anchor the yang. Because the Kidneys reside in the lower back, there will also be soreness in this area. Yin deficiency always leads to some degree of internal fire, which causes the essence (housed in the Kidneys) to move recklessly. This leads to spontaneous emissions. The same process forces the fluids to dissipate externally in the form of sweat at night, which is the time of day associated with the yin. The depletion of fluids leads to internal dryness, evidenced in the dry mouth and throat, thirst with a desire to drink, and the peeled, shiny tongue. A thin, rapid pulse is a classic sign of yin deficiency.

Analysis of Formula

This formula strongly tonifies the true yin, employing chiefly sweet herbs to fortify water while avoiding all draining of yang or essence. The chief herb is Rehmanniae Radix praeparata (*shú dì huáng*). Zhang Jie-Bin described its actions thus:

> It is able to tonify the true yin of the five yin organs. … It is not possible to [treat] deficiency of yin blood in the twelve channels without Rehmanniae Radix praeparata (*shú dì huáng*). … [Likewise,] spirit dispersal due to yin deficiency cannot be gathered in sufficiently without [the ability of] Rehmanniae Radix praeparata (*shú dì huáng*) to conserve. When the yin is deficient and fire ascends, one cannot direct it downward sufficiently without the heaviness of Rehmanniae Radix praeparata (*shú dì huáng*). Restless movement [due to] yin deficiency cannot be sedated sufficiently without the stillness of Rehmanniae Radix praeparata (*shú dì huáng*). And hardness and tension due to yin deficiency cannot be relaxed sufficiently without the sweetness of Rehmanniae Radix praeparata (*shú dì huáng*).

Altogether there are five deputies. Corni Fructus (*shān zhū yú*) and Lycii Fructus (*gǒu qǐ zǐ*) nourish the Liver blood. Here they work synergistically with the chief herb. Dioscoreae Rhizoma (*shān yào*) benefits the yin and tonifies the Spleen as the source of the postnatal constitution. Two animal-based medicinals, Cervi Cornus Colla (*lù jiǎo jiāo*) and Testudinis Plastri Colla (*guī bǎn jiāo*), are added to push the action of the formula even further toward the tonification of essence. Testudinis Plastri Colla (*guī bǎn jiāo*) is sweet, salty, and cooling and thus able to sedate Liver yang as well as cool heat from deficiency. Cervi Cornus Colla (*lù jiǎo jiāo*) is sweet, salty, and slightly warming, entering the Governing vessel to tonify the essence and blood and mobilize the yang.

One of the assistants is Cyathulae Radix (*chuān niú xī*), which augments the Liver and Kidneys, strengthens the back and knees, and builds the sinews and bones. Due to its moving and draining character, Achyranthis bidentatae Radix (*niú xī*) is suggested as a substitute when the formula is used to treat spontaneous emissions. Cuscutae Semen (*tù sī zǐ*) tonifies the Kidney yin and yang and secures the essence, supporting the overall action of the formula in a balanced manner.

Cautions and Contraindications

Use with caution in cases with Spleen and Stomach deficiency, and then only with modifications. This formula should only be considered in patterns without any signs of excess heat such as a yellow tongue coating or a wiry and rapid pulse.

Commentary

This is one of the flagship formulas composed by Zhang Jie-Bin that reflects the emphasis on warm tonification prevalent among many physicians during the Ming dynasty. The core assumption of this approach is succinctly summarized in Zhang Jie-Bin's dictum, "Yang is not [ever really] excessive, but yin is often deficient." Unlike earlier physicians who often combined yin tonification with the draining of yang excess (assuming that such excess was a contributing factor in the exhaustion of yin), proponents of warm tonification emphasized pure tonification. For this purpose, Zhang Jie-Bin employed Six-Ingredient Pill with Rehmannia (*liù wèi dì huáng wán*) and Kidney Qi Pill (*shèn qì wán*) as his foundational formulas, but removed from them the "three draining [herbs]" Poria (*fú líng*), Alismatis Rhizoma (*zé xiè*), and Moutan Cortex (*mǔ dān pí*). Instead, he added herbs that further tonified the yin essence and blood and that gently stimulated and moved the yang. For example, Cuscutae Semen (*tù sī zǐ*) tonifies the Kidney qi. Cervi Cornus Colla (*lù jiǎo jiāo*) and Testudinis Plastri Colla (*guī bǎn jiāo*) enter the Governing and Conception vessels, which organize and control the movement of both the yin and yang in the body. This reflects the fundamental importance that Zhang Jie-Bin attached to the role of the yang qi as the motivating force in the body's physiology. Without yang assisting in the transformation of yin, physiological activity would cease, while the yin itself depends on the transformative potential of the yang for its own production. Thus, Zhang noted in his *Classified Classic*, "Experts in tonifying the yin invariably assist the yin by means of the yang. For when the yin avails itself of the ascending [power] of the yang, the fountainhead is never used up." This strategy had a tremendous influence on later generations of physicians and remains, to the present day, one of the core principles underlying strategies aimed at tonifying the Kidney yin.

Comparisons

➢ Vs. Six-Ingredient Pill with Rehmannia (*liù wèi dì huáng wán*)

Both formulas tonify the Kidneys and Liver. The difference is that while Six-Ingredient Pill with Rehmannia (*liù wèi dì huáng wán*) is a mixture of tonifying and draining herbs that are used to clear signs of fire from deficiency (vertigo, hot palms and soles, etc.), the ingredients in Restore the Left [Kidney] Pill (*zuǒ guī wán*) directly tonify and are used for treating relatively pure conditions of deficiency with little fire. Because of its more balanced formulation, Six-Ingredient Pill with Rehmannia (*liù wèi dì huáng wán*) is more suitable for long-term use, while use of Restore the Left [Kidney] Pill (*zuǒ guī wán*) should be restricted to short-term supplementation of severe deficiency.

➢ Vs. Tortoise Shell and Deer Antler Two-Immortal Syrup (*guī lù èr xiān jiāo*); *see* page 408

Biomedical Indications

With the appropriate presentation, this formula may be used to treat a wide variety of biomedically-defined disorders such as chronic bronchitis, chronic nephritis, and hypertension, especially in the elderly. It is also used for lumbar strain and infertility.

Modifications

- For spontaneous emissions, remove Cyathulae Radix (*chuān niú xī*).
- For patterns without heat signs, remove Testudinis Plastri Colla (*guī bǎn jiāo*).
- For deficiency of true yin with upflaring of fire, remove Lycii Fructus (*gǒu qǐ zǐ*) and Testudinis Plastri Colla (*guī bǎn jiāo*) and add Ligustri lucidi Fructus (*nǚ zhēn zǐ*) and Ophiopogonis Radix (*mài mén dōng*).
- For fire scorching the Lungs with a dry cough and little phlegm, add Lilii Bulbus (*bǎi hé*).
- For heat at night, add Lycii Cortex (*dì gǔ pí*).
- For urinary obstruction, add Poria (*fú líng*).
- For dry stools, remove Cuscutae Semen (*tù sī zǐ*) and add Cistanches Herba (*ròu cōng róng*).
- For qi deficiency, add Ginseng Radix (*rén shēn*).

Associated Formulas

左歸飲 （左归饮）

Restore the Left [Kidney] Drink

zuǒ guī yǐn

Source   *Collected Treatises of [Zhang] Jing-Yue (1624)*

Rehmanniae Radix praeparata (*shú dì huáng*) 6-60g
Dioscoreae Rhizoma (*shān yào*) 3-6g
Lycii Fructus (*gǒu qǐ zǐ*) 6g
Poria (*fú líng*) 4.5g
Corni Fructus (*shān zhū yú*) 3-6g
Glycyrrhizae Radix praeparata (*zhì gān cǎo*) 3g

Decoction. Depending on the desired strength of the treatment, the dosage of Rehmanniae Radix praeparata (*shú dì huáng*) is either at the lower or upper limit specified above. At present, the larger dosage is more commonly used.

Nourishes the yin and tonifies the Kidneys. For deficiency of the Kidneys (especially the marrow and essence) with lower back soreness, spontaneous emissions, night sweats, a dry mouth and throat, thirst with a desire to drink, a peeled, shiny tongue, and a thin, rapid pulse.

This is a milder version of the pill analyzed above. Its use as a drink rather than as a decoction (which implies that a shorter period of boiling is necessary) reflects its intended use as a mildly tonifying formula. The source text lists a number of possible modifications that widen its range of indications:

- For heat in the Lungs with irritability, add Ophiopogonis Radix (*mài mén dōng*).
- For blood stasis, add Moutan Cortex (*mǔ dān pí*).
- For heat in the Spleen with frequent hunger that cannot be satisfied, add Paeoniae Radix alba (*bái sháo*).

- For heat in the Kidneys with steaming bone disorder and profuse sweating, add Lycii Cortex (*dì gǔ pí*).

固陰煎 （固阴煎）

Stabilize the Yin Decoction

gù yīn jiān

Source   *Collected Treatises of [Zhang] Jing-Yue (1624)*

Ginseng Radix (*rén shēn*) 3-6g
Rehmanniae Radix praeparata (*shú dì huáng*) 9-15g
Dioscoreae Rhizoma (*shān yào*) 6g
Corni Fructus (*shān zhū yú*) 4.5g
Polygalae Radix (*yuǎn zhì*) 2.1g
Glycyrrhizae Radix praeparata (*zhì gān cǎo*) 3-6g
Schisandrae Fructus (*wǔ wèi zǐ*) 3-6g
Cuscutae Semen (*tù sī zǐ*) 6-9g

Enriches and tonifies the Kidneys and regulates the Penetrating and Conception vessels. For early or late menstrual periods that are scanty and light-colored due to Kidney deficiency. Accompanied by lightheadedness, tinnitus, lower back pain that can be severe, urinary frequency at night, soft stools, and a submerged, frail pulse. The patient may also experience distention and a sensation of prolapse in the lower abdomen.

大補元煎 （大补元煎）

Great Tonify the Primal Decoction

dà bǔ yuán jiān

Source   *Collected Treatises of [Zhang] Jing-Yue (1624)*

Ginseng Radix (*rén shēn*) 3-9g
Dioscoreae Rhizoma (*shān yào*) 6g
Rehmanniae Radix praeparata (*shú dì huáng*) 9-90g
Eucommiae Cortex (*dù zhòng*) 6g
Angelicae sinensis Radix (*dāng guī*) 6-9g
Corni Fructus (*shān zhū yú*) 3g
Lycii Fructus (*gǒu qǐ zǐ*) 6-9g
Glycyrrhizae Radix praeparata (*zhì gān cǎo*) 3-6g

Tonifies the yin and blood and benefits the yang and qi. The relative dosage of the herbs depends upon which aspect of the disorder predominates. Originally used for severe injury to the primal or source qi and blood in either men or women, it is now used primarily for uterine prolapse accompanied by soreness and weakness in the lower back, severe lower abdominal distention, urinary frequency that worsens at night, tinnitus, hearing loss, dizziness, a pale-red tongue, and a submerged, frail pulse.

大補陰丸 （大补阴丸）

Great Tonify the Yin Pill

dà bǔ yīn wán

The name of this formula in the source text is Great Tonifying Pill (*dà bǔ wán*). This name reflects both the composition of the pill, which focuses on the use of rich, tonifying substances, as well as its intention, namely, to tonify the true yin. To emphasize the latter function, in *Correct Transmission of Medicine* the name was changed to Great Tonify the Yin Pill (*dà bǔ yīn wán*).

Source   *Essential Teachings of [Zhu] Dan-Xi* (1481)

Rehmanniae Radix praeparata (*shú dì huáng*) 180g
crisp Testudinis Plastrum (*sū guī bǎn*) 180g
dry-fried Phellodendri Cortex (*chǎo huáng bǎi*) 120g
wine-fried Anemarrhenae Rhizoma (*jiǔ chǎo zhī mǔ*) 120g

Method of Preparation   Grind the ingredients into a powder, cook with the marrow from pigs' vertebrae, add honey, and form into pills. The normal dosage is 6-9g taken twice a day with salted water. May also be prepared as a decoction by reducing the dosage of each ingredient by a factor of 8-10. The marrow is usually omitted when prepared as a decoction.

Actions   Enriches the yin and directs fire downward

Indications

Steaming bone disorder with afternoon tidal fever, night sweats, spontaneous emissions, irritability, a sensation of heat and pain in the knees and legs that is sometimes accompanied by weakness, a red tongue with little coating, and a pulse that is rapid and forceful in the rear position. May also be accompanied by coughing of blood or constant hunger.

This is yin deficiency and flourishing fire, with both pathologies contributing equally to the pattern. Internally-generated heat against a background of yin deficiency leads to tidal fever (which appears as the yin becomes ascendant) and night sweats (a forcing out of the fluids during the yin phase of the daily cycle). The deficient yin is unable to restrain the essence, which moves recklessly and manifests as spontaneous emissions in men. When the rising fire disturbs the spirit, the patient will become irritable. Intense heat from deficiency in the Kidneys and Liver causes heat and pain (and sometimes weakness) in the knees and legs, which is the area of the body governed by those organs. A red tongue with little coating is a classic sign of yin deficiency with heat. A rapid, forceful pulse in the rear position is a manifestation of intense heat in the Kidneys. If the rising fire attacks the collaterals of the Lungs, the patient will cough blood; if it disturbs the Stomach, there will be constant hunger.

Analysis of Formula

A vicious cycle whereby exhausted yin is unable to control the up-flaring fire, while the fire continually scorches and thereby depletes the yin, can only be treated by a strategy known as 'cultivating the root and clearing the source' (培 其本,清其源 *péi qí běn, qīng qí yuán*). Cultivating the root refers to nourishing and enriching the yin essence; clearing the source refers to draining the flourishing fire that flares out of control. Both aspects of treatment are essential: if only the root is cultivated, it will be difficult to clear the fire, and if only the source is cleared, the disorder will recur with more intensity.

The ingredients that cultivate the root are Rehmanniae Radix praeparata (*shú dì huáng*), which is a very effective herb for enriching and tonifying the Liver and Kidneys, and Testudinis Plastrum (*guī bǎn*), which nourishes the yin and weighs down the floating yang fire. The use of these ingredients is a good example of enriching the water to control the fire. This effect is greatly amplified by the herbs that clear the source. These are Phellodendri Cortex (*huáng bǎi*), which quells Kidney fire, and Anemarrhenae Rhizoma (*zhī mǔ*), which clears heat, enriches the Lungs, and generates fluids. These herbs work synergistically, one of which focuses on the lower burner and the other on the upper burner. They are fried in order to moderate their bitter, cold properties. The ratio of yin-tonifying to fire-draining substances in this formula is 3:2, indicating that yin deficiency is regarded as the root and fire as the branch of this pattern. For this reason, Rehmanniae Radix praeparata (*shú dì huáng*) and Testudinis Plastrum (*guī bǎn*) are considered the chief herbs, while Phellodendri Cortex (*huáng bǎi*) and Anemarrhenae Rhizoma (*zhī mǔ*) function as deputies.

Cooking the ingredients in the marrow from the vertebrae of pigs serves two functions. One is to tonify the essence and marrow, and the other is to moderate the bitter, drying properties of Phellodendri Cortex (*huáng bǎi*), which otherwise could damage the yin. The latter function is also served by the use of honey. These two substances therefore serve as assistants and envoys in this formula.

Cautions and Contraindications

Use with caution in patients with poor appetite and loose stools. It is contraindicated in cases of fire from excess.

Commentary

Yin Fire

A characteristic aspect of Jin-Yuan-Ming medicine is its concern with fire. Physicians during this period thus devised many new strategies for cultivating physiological fire and eliminating pathological fire from the body. A second important change in medical thinking during this time was a shift in focus from external to internal causes of disease. This is reflected in the new concept of yin fire (陰火 *yīn huǒ*) used by physicians in the Jin-Yuan period to distinguish disorders where the origin of the pathological fire was perceived to lie within the body (yin) from those due to pathogens that penetrate the body from without (yang). The description of yin fire pathology was linked to newly emergent doctrines regarding the physiological activities of fire in the body, more specifically, the role of the fire at the gate of vitality. Increasingly, this fire came to be seen as supporting all physiological transformation and thus essential to life itself. Disease occurred when this fire became stagnant or raged out of control. Among the various masters of this period, Li Dong-Yuan is known for analyzing yin fire pathologies caused by middle burner qi deficiency, while Zhu Dan-Xi became famous for the treatment of yin fire arising in the context of yin deficiency. This formula is representative of Zhu's approach.

Actions of Great Tonify the Yin Pill (dà bǔ yīn wán)

In *Essential Teachings of [Zhu] Dan-Xi*, the actions of this formula are described as "directing yin fire downward, while tonifying Kidney water." In *Compendium of Songs on Modern Formulas*, the Qing-dynasty writer Chen Nian-Zu explained how the formula's composition achieves these objectives:

> Anemarrhenae Rhizoma (zhī mǔ) and Phellodendri Cortex (huáng bǎi) are cooling and can eliminate heat; they are bitter and can direct fire downward. Bitterness leads to dryness, hence [the formula] uses pig marrow to moisten and Rehmanniae Radix praeparata (shú dì huáng) to enrich. This is a common strategy for treating the fever of yin deficiency. Merely using cooling herbs to eliminate heat, however, does not constitute treatment [on the basis] of an exhaustive investigation of the root. Thus, the chief [ingredient] of the formula is Testudinis Plastrum (guī bǎn). [Its use embodies] the strategy of using shells to subdue the yang. Compared to Six-Ingredient Pill with Rehmannia (liù wèi dì huáng wán), the power of [Zhu] Dan-Xi's formula [to treat yin fire] is thus even more outstanding. Thus, if physicians like Li Shi-Cai [Li Zhong-Zi], Xue Li-Zhai, or Zhang Jie-Bin [merely] added bitter, cooling [substances to yin-tonifying formulas, but did not simultaneously subdue the yang, this shows] that they did not really understand the subtleties of [the relationship between] yin and yang in nature.

Here, Chen seeks to show that the formula addresses a pathological process whose momentum tends toward the separation of yin and yang. If yin is deficient, it loses its ability to control yang. This requires not only that the fire be quelled and the water tonified, but also that the upward-flaring yang be turned downward in order that it reconnect with the ever diminishing yin. For Chen, this is achieved by means of Testudinis Plastrum (guī bǎn), which nourishes the yin essence while simultaneously subduing the yang, and thereby becomes the fulcrum around which the entire formula turns.

However, Testudinis Plastrum (guī bǎn) is not included in all of Zhu Dan-Xi's formulas to treat the fire of deficiency. Thus, as Chen himself acknowledged earlier in the quoted passage, the downward-draining action of Phellodendri Cortex (huáng bǎi) and Anemarrhenae Rhizoma (zhī mǔ) has a similar effect on the aberrant yang. Bitterness is the flavor that resonates with fire and the Heart, and bitter herbs thus excel at guiding fire downward. Phellodendri Cortex (huáng bǎi), in particular, is consistently used by physicians for this purpose. In *Patterns and Treatment of Miscellaneous Disorders*, the Qing-dynasty physician Xu Da-Chun therefore praises Phellodendri Cortex (huáng bǎi) as "the primary substance for clearing blazing and overabundant lower burner ministe-

rial fire, thereby pacifying ministerial fire [overall] and giving the true yin some shade so that irritability, dryness, and thirst will not return."

In his writings, Zhu Dan-Xi implied that this action tonified the Kidneys. This statement was taken literally by some of his followers, setting up heated debates with those who held that bitter, cold herbs drain excess fire from the body. In *Origins of Medicine*, Li Dong-Yuan's teacher Zhang Yuan-Su, for instance, lists as one of the main actions of Phellodendri Cortex (huáng bǎi) the ability "[to] drain dragon fire from the Bladder." Dragon fire is another term for ministerial fire or the fire at the gate of vitality, that is, the body's yang qi, which emerges at the Bladder to be distributed throughout the body via the lesser yang.

The following passage from the late 18th-century *Materia Medica of Combinations* successfully resolves this tension by explaining how Phellodendri Cortex (huáng bǎi) "tonifies" the yin and then how it does not:

> [It] tonifies water through its ability to clear the yin-fire blazing upward from below: when the fire is cleared, water is fortified and condenses [as is normal]—this is tonifying without tonifying. Note that this pathogenic heat in the midst of yin is not originally the true fire at the gate of vitality, and so there is no harm in using bitter, cold herbs to expel it. When the true water of the Kidneys is insufficient so that the true fire floats deficiently upward, then Rehmanniae Radix (shēng dì huáng) and Rehmanniae Radix praeparata (shú dì huáng) must be used to enrich the Kidneys. When the water is sufficient, fire will naturally return to its place of containment. If Phellodendri Cortex (huáng bǎi) and Anemarrhenae Rhizoma (zhī mǔ) are mistakenly used, as the water becomes dried [by their bitterness], the fire will blaze even higher, and contrary to one's intention, the yang will become separated from the yin and fly away. This is irredeemable.

It follows that when the present formula is said to treat the fire of deficiency, it is best understood as yin deficiency accompanied by vigorous fire (vigorous to the extent that it can be drained from the body) and not merely as deficiency of yin invariably accompanied by a certain degree of floating yang. The excessive nature of the fire in this pattern can be found in the strong and flooding pulses in both rear positions as well as in the other symptoms denoting heat excess, such as coughing up of blood-tinged sputum, constant hunger, restlessness, and seminal emissions.

In contemporary practice the formula is used, for instance, to treat patterns of deficient yin and hyperactive yang associated with disorders such as hyperthyroidism or diabetes. The progressive nature of these disorders provides a good example of disease processes where excess fire can rapidly erode the yin while deficient yin essence becomes increasingly unable to contain the up-flaring yang, such that only a treatment focused simultaneously on both aspects of the disorder holds out the promise of success.

Comparisons

➤ Vs. Six-Ingredient Pill with Rehmannia *(liù wèi dì huáng wán)*

The indications of these two formulas overlap. Great Tonify the Yin Pill *(dà bǔ yīn wán)* has a stronger effect in treating yin deficiency with ascendant yang, especially in causing the fire from deficiency to descend. Six-Ingredient Pill with Rehmannia *(liù wèi dì huáng wán)* contains herbs that regulate the water metabolism. It focuses on the Kidneys, but also treats the Liver and Spleen. It can thus be used to treat yin deficiency that is accompanied by phlegm or other signs of water excess, while regulating the qi dynamic through the adjustment of organ functions. Great Tonify the Yin Pill *(dà bǔ yīn wán)*, on the other hand, seeks to conserve water by focusing primarily on quelling excess fire, as noted by the modern physician Ran Xue-Feng. In *Building Efficacious Formulas on the Eight Methods,* Ran observed that the herbs in this formula

> are used to rapidly pacify fire, rapidly restrain fire, rapidly subdue fire, and rapidly contain fire. Eliminating even a minute amount of fire means protecting an [equivalent] amount of yin fluids. And containing even a minute amount of yin fluids implies protecting an [equivalent] amount of primal qi.

➤ Vs. Anemarrhena, Phellodendron, and Rehmannia Pill *(zhī bái dì huáng wán)*

Both formulas treat patterns where yin deficiency is accompanied by vigorous fire manifesting with symptoms such as night sweats, a dry mouth and tongue, and a large pulse only in the rear position. Both formulas also use the combination of Anemarrhenae Rhizoma *(zhī mǔ)* and Phellodendri Cortex *(huáng bǎi)* to control hyperactive yang and drain excess fire, as well as Rehmanniae Radix praeparata *(shú dì huáng)* to tonify the Kidney yin. However, by using a heavy substance such as Testudinis Plastrum *(guī bǎn)*, Great Tonify the Yin Pill *(dà bǔ yīn wán)* is able to control the yang more successfully. By contrast, Anemarrhena, Phellodendron, and Rehmannia Pill *(zhī bái dì huáng wán)*, which is built on Six-Ingredient Pill with Rehmannia *(liù wèi dì huáng wán)*, focuses more strongly on supplementing the yin. Furthermore, as an animal substance, Testudinis Plastrum *(guī bǎn)* tonifies the essence and is frequently associated in the literature with deficiency of the Conception vessel. Six-Ingredient Pill with Rehmannia *(liù wèi dì huáng wán)*, on the other hand, regulates the water metabolism as well as tonifying the yin of the Kidneys, Liver, and Spleen.

➤ Vs. Hidden Tiger Pill *(hǔ qián wán)*; see pages 379

➤ Vs. Great Creation Pill *(dà zào wán)*; see pages 380

➤ Vs. Open the Gate Pill *(tōng guān wán)*; see pages 719

➤ Vs. Sweet Wormwood and Soft-Shelled Turtle Shell Decoction [Version 1] *(qīng hāo biē jiǎ tāng)*; *see* page 213

Biomedical Indications

With the appropriate presentation, this formula may be used to treat a wide variety of biomedically-defined disorders, including tuberculosis (of the lungs, kidneys, or bones), bronchiectasis, diabetes mellitus, hyperthyroid conditions, and nervous exhaustion.

Alternate name

Tonify the Yin Pill *(bǔ yīn wán)* in *Comprehensive Outline of the Materia Medica*

Modifications

- For severe night sweats, add Ostreae Concha *(mǔ lì)* and Tritici Fructus levis *(fú xiǎo mài)*.
- For coughing of blood, add Agrimoniae Herba *(xiān hè cǎo)* and Platycladi Cacumen *(cè bǎi yè)*.
- For sputum that is difficult to expectorate, add Stemonae Radix *(bǎi bù)* and Farfarae Flos *(kuǎn dōng huā)*.
- For severe, spontaneous emissions, add Euryales Semen *(qiàn shí)* and Rosae laevigatae Fructus *(jīn yīng zǐ)*.

玉泉丸
Jade Spring Pill
yù quán wán

The name of this formula refers to saliva, which is said to flow from the jade spring situated on the underside of the tongue. 'Jade spring' is a designation that brings to mind a cool, ever-flowing source of liquid.

Source   *Straight Direction from [Yang] Ren-Zhai (1264)*

Ophiopogonis Radix *(mài mén dōng)* . [remove the center] 37.5g
Ginseng Radix *(rén shēn)* 37.5g
Poria *(fú líng)* 37.5g
Astragali Radix *(huáng qí)*
. . . . [half honey-fried & half untreated] 37.5g
Mume Fructus *(wū méi)* . . . . [roasted] 37.5g
Glycyrrhizae Radix *(gān cǎo)* 37.5g
Trichosanthis Radix *(tiān huā fěn)* 56g
Puerariae Radix *(gé gēn)* 56g

Method of Preparation   Grind the ingredients into a powder and mix with refined honey to make honey pills. Each pill should be made the size of a bullet (or a large marble). Take one pill per dose with warm water. At present, this formula is usually taken as a prepared medicine.

Actions   Augments the qi, nourishes the yin, clears heat, and generates yang fluids

Indications

Treats wasting and thirsting disorder (消渴 *xiāo kě*), which overlaps with the disease of diabetes in modern biomedicine. The main symptoms include irritability with thirst, urinary frequency, dry mouth, increased appetite, and weight loss. The pulse is large and rapid, and the tongue is red and dry.

Analysis of Formula

In this formula, Ginseng Radix (*rén shēn*), Astragali Radix (*huáng qí*), and Poria (*fú líng*) augment the qi. The sweet and sour flavors of Glycyrrhizae Radix (*gān cǎo*) and Mume Fructus (*wū méi*) transform the yin. Ophiopogonis Radix (*mài mén dōng*) and Trichosanthis Radix (*tiān huā fěn*) clear heat, generate yang fluids, nourish the yin, and relieve irritability and thirst. Puerariae Radix (*gé gēn*) generates yang fluids and clears heat from the yang brightness channels. Thus, the heat is cleared, the qi augmented, the yin nourished, and the fluids generated to relieve thirst, mitigate irritability, and address the pattern's main symptoms.

This formula takes a unique approach to the treatment of yin deficiency. With Ophiopogonis Radix (*mài mén dōng*) as the only true yin-nourishing herb in the formula, this combination relies on the qi-supplementing agents Astragali Radix (*huáng qí*) and Ginseng Radix (*rén shēn*) to support the Spleen and Lung and thus help the body to transform and transport yin and fluids. In tandem with Poria (*fú líng*), these qi herbs not only supplement the middle, but also adjust the water pathways. These four herbs serve as the chief ingredients and treat the root of the disorder, leaving Puerariae Radix (*gé gēn*), Mume Fructus (*wū méi*), and Trichosanthis Radix (*tiān huā fěn*), the deputies, to address the manifestations of fluid depletion, such as thirst and a dry mouth.

Commentary

Zhu Dan-Xi paid particular attention to the discussion of wasting and thirsting disorder in which he mentions Jade Spring Pill (*yù quán wán*). Here is a condensed version of Zhu Dan-Xi's discussion of the subject from the Qing-dynasty text *Supplemented Collections on Patterns and Treatments*:

> [The *Inner Classic* states that] water's origin is the Kidneys, and its end point is the Lungs. True water has no limit. Where then does thirst come from? [When] people think only of alcohol or sexual activity or overdo spicy, hot [foods], or spoil their palates with sweet and fatty foods … [this] causes fire to flame upward and parch the yang fluids and leads to this disease.

Jade Spring Pill (*yù quán wán*) is listed in *Essential Teachings of [Zhu] Dan-Xi* especially for wasting and thirsting disorders that present with irritability, thirst, and dry mouth. This emphasis implies that the formula is best for upper wasting. Modern texts agree, and prescribe this formula for upper burner wasting and thirsting, especially in those cases where the symptoms stem from a lack of nourishment in the Heart and Lungs and heat flaming in the upper burner.

In *Wondrous Lantern for Peering into the Origin and Development of Miscellaneous Diseases*, Shen Jin-Ao identifies Jade Spring Pill (*yù quán wán*) as a treatment for a particular disorder called 'wasting from internal heat constraint' (消癉 *xiāo dàn*). He asserts that the cause of this disorder is yin deficiency of the Liver, Heart, and Kidney channels that, in turn, generates internal heat. This, he claims, is what the classics call 'heat-attack' (熱中 *rè zhòng*). Shen understood this disorder to stem from frailty of the five yin organs whose nutritive aspect was unable to flourish. The resulting yin deficiency and heat constraint combine to cause disquietude of the qi in these organs. Additionally, heat lingering in the nutritive aspect further damages the yin and fluids and wastes the flesh. Shen considered this disorder to be a constitutional weakness with which one is born, which therefore differs from the wasting and thirsting disorder brought on by intemperance in one's lifestyle.

The proper use of Jade Spring Pill (*yù quán wán*) requires careful consideration. It is appropriate for situations where the qi and yang fluids are exhausted or when the yin-fluid deficiency is due to the failure of the Spleen and Lungs to transport and transform fluids. If the yin is severely deficient and the Spleen and Lung qi is not exceptionally compromised, a formula that more directly nourishes the yin, such as Rehmannia Drink from *A Simple Book* (*dì huáng yǐn zi*), discussed above, is a better option. In modern China, Jade Spring Pill (*yù quán wán*) is mistakenly viewed by some lay people as a treatment for diabetes, irrespective of cause or stage of disease, in much the same way that Generating and Transforming Decoction (*shēng huà tāng*) is frequently used indiscriminately in postpartum women. For proper treatment of any disorder, the analysis of the cause, nature, and severity of the disorder, along with careful consideration of the constitution of the patient, should guide the treatment. Blanket treatment of a given disease by a single formula is often ineffective and, on occasion, even harmful.

Jade Spring Pill (*yù quán wán*) includes herbs to supplement deficiency of the qi and yin, clear heat, and generate fluids. It is best suited for diabetes-like disorders that present with deficiency. Note that a patient need not present with blood sugar levels out of the normal range to be classified as having either of the patterns discussed here. Early treatment, before the symptoms are extreme, will bring a much higher chance of success.

Note that the ingredients of the prepared medicines by this name can vary. Some versions of Jade Spring Pill (*yù quán wán*) add Dioscoreae Rhizoma (*shān yào*) and/or Glehniae/Adenophorae Radix (*shā shēn*).

Comparisons

➤ Vs. White Tiger plus Ginseng Decoction *(bái hǔ jiā rén shēn tāng)*

Both formulas nourish the yin, generate fluids, and clear heat. They are frequently assigned to treat upper wasting disorders. White Tiger plus Ginseng Decoction *(bái hǔ jiā rén shēn tāng)* from *Discussion of Cold Damage* was originally for patients who had been mistakenly given purging or diaphoretic formulas to treat cold damage presenting with great thirst, high fever, heavy sweating, and a large and flooding pulse. For upper wasting disorders, it is better able to clear heat than Jade Spring Pill *(yù quán wán)*, but is far less adept at tonification. By contrast, Jade Spring Pill *(yù quán wán)* is better able to tonify the Spleen and Lungs, generate fluids, and adjust the water pathways. If heat signs are extreme, one may well begin treatment with White Tiger plus Ginseng Decoction *(bái hǔ jiā rén shēn tāng)* and gradually switch to Jade Spring Pill *(yù quán wán)* as the heat signs mitigate.

➤ Vs. Rehmannia Drink from *A Simple Book (dì huáng yǐn zi)*, 364

Biomedical Indications

With the appropriate presentation, this formula may be used to treat a variety of biomedically-defined disorders such as diabetes and hyperglycemia.

Modifications

- If yin deficiency is prominent, add Rehmanniae Radix *(shēng dì huáng)*.

- For upper wasting with strong heat signs, add Anemarrhenae Rhizoma *(zhī mǔ)* and Gypsum fibrosum *(shí gāo)*.

- For dark urine, add Alismatis Rhizoma *(zé xiè)*.

- For internal heat constraint, add Paeoniae Radix alba *(bái sháo)* and Moutan Cortex *(mǔ dān pí)*.

虎潜丸 （虎潜丸）
Hidden Tiger Pill

hǔ qián wán

The tiger is a symbol of yin in Chinese mythology. The most common explanation of the formula's name is that by enriching the yin, it causes fire to descend, nourishes the essence, and strengthens the sinews and bones. Another name for the formula is thus Hidden Tiger Pill for Strengthening One's Steps *(jiàn bù hǔ qián wán)*. There are several other interpretations, however, which are linked, in turn, to different views regarding the formula's properties. These are discussed in the COMMENTARY section below.

Source *Teachings of [Zhu] Dan-xi* (1481)

wine-fried Phellodendri Cortex *(jiǔ chǎo huáng bǎi)* 240g
wine-fried Anemarrhenae Rhizoma *(jiǔ chǎo zhī mǔ)* 30g
Rehmanniae Radix praeparata *(shú dì huáng)* 60g
wine-fried Testudinis Plastrum *(jiǔ chǎo guī bǎn)* 120g
Paeoniae Radix alba *(bái sháo)* .60g
Tigris Os *(hǔ gǔ)* 60g
Cynomorii Herba *(suǒ yáng)* 45g
Zingiberis Rhizoma *(gān jiāng)* .15g
Citri reticulatae Pericarpium *(chén pí)* 60g

Method of Preparation The source text advises to grind the ingredients into a powder and form into pills with wine. Some texts advise to decoct the ingredients together with mutton. At present, it is usually made into 9g pills with honey. The normal dosage is one pill every morning and evening, taken with salted or warm water. May also be prepared as a decoction with an appropriate reduction in dosage.

Note that Tigris Os *(hǔ gǔ)* is generally not available since all tigers are protected species and trade in their body parts is prohibited. Some use the bones of other animals, particularly Canis Os *(gǒu gǔ)* or Felinis Os *(māo gǔ)*, especially the former. There are other substitutions as well, including Taraxaci Herba *(pú gōng yīng)* for its anti-inflammatory action, and Drynariae Rhizoma *(gǔ suì bǔ)* or Clematidis Radix *(wēi líng xiān)* plus Vespae Nidus *(lù fēng fáng)*, all of which affect the Governing vessel.

Actions Enriches the yin, directs fire downward, and strengthens the sinews and bones

Indications

Weakness of the lower back and knees, deterioration of the sinews and bones with general reduction in function, wasting of the muscles of the legs and feet, difficulty in walking, a red tongue with little coating, and a thin, frail pulse. The formula also treats dizziness, tinnitus, spontaneous emissions, and urinary incontinence.

This is atrophy disorder due to Liver and Kidney deficiency. There is heat from deficiency in these organs and also deficiency of their associated substances, blood and essence. This leads to a lack of nourishment in their associated tissues, the sinews and bones, which manifests as weakness and wasting. Because the Kidneys and Liver govern the lower back and knees, this type of deficiency results in weakness in those areas of the body. The weakness and wasting of the sinews and bones makes walking difficult. A red tongue with little coating is a classic sign of yin deficiency, and a thin, frail pulse reflects deficiency of the blood and essence. Dizziness, tinnitus, spontaneous emissions, and urinary incontinence are other signs of Liver and Kidney yin deficiency accompanied by up-flaring of fire.

Analysis of Formula

This formula serves two functions: it enriches the yin and directs the errant fire downward in order to treat the root cause of the disorder, and it strengthens the bones and sinews in order to treat the branch. To accomplish these ends, the formula utilizes three groups of ingredients: bitter, cooling herbs to drain and direct fire downward, sweet and salty substances that enrich the yin and nourish the blood, and acrid, warming herbs that tonify the yang and move the qi.

The synergistic combination of Phellodendri Cortex (*huáng bǎi*) and Testudinis Plastrum (*guī bǎn*) serves as the chief ingredients. The larger dosage of the first ingredient indicates that the primary thrust of the formula is to cause the fire to descend. Phellodendri Cortex (*huáng bǎi*) also plays an important role in the treatment of atrophy disorder by drying dampness in the bones and lower burner. Sweet, salty, and cooling Testudinis Plastrum (*guī bǎn*) enriches the yin and anchors the errant yang, augments the marrow, and fills the essence so as to tonify the Kidneys and strengthen the bones. Together, these two substances tonify the insufficiency of both the Liver and Kidneys, while simultaneously draining the ministerial fire that flares out of control. They are complemented in these tasks by the two deputies, Anemarrhenae Rhizoma (*zhī mǔ*), which drains fire and clears heat, and Rehmanniae Radix praeparata (*shú dì huáng*), which enriches the yin and tonifies the Kidneys. The reader is referred to Great Tonify the Yin Pill (*dà bǔ yīn wán*) above for a more thorough discussion of the interactions among these four herbs. Because malnourishment of the sinews is such an important aspect of this disorder, Paeoniae Radix alba (*bái sháo*) is added as a third deputy to nourish the sinews and tonify the blood.

The second group of ingredients, Tigris Os (*hǔ gǔ*) and Cynomorii Herba (*suǒ yáng*), acts as assistants to strengthen the sinews and bones. Tigris Os (*hǔ gǔ*), or tiger bone, helps the bones directly (an action derived, at least in part, on sympathetic magical reasoning), while the latter ingredient warms the yang and benefits the essence with a focus on the bones. This combination is a very strong one for treating weakness of the bones and sinews, and its effect is strengthened by the first group of ingredients.

The final two ingredients serve miscellaneous functions and are also regarded as assistants. Zingiberis Rhizoma (*gān jiāng*) moderates the bitter, cold properties of Phellodendri Cortex (*huáng bǎi*), assists the yin tonics in generating blood, and warms the middle burner. Citri reticulatae Pericarpium (*chén pí*) regulates the qi and the middle burner. The combination of these ingredients warms and tonifies the Spleen and Stomach, and thereby aids in the digestion and assimilation of the formula. This is particularly important when using a formula that nourishes the yin. Taking the pills with salted water, which serves as an envoy, guides the entire formula into the lower burner, particularly the Kidneys, and underlines the formula's yin-tonifying properties.

Cautions and Contraindications

Remember that atrophy disorder can occur for many reasons. If it is due to Spleen and Stomach deficiency or invasion of damp-heat, the use of this formula is contraindicated.

Commentary

The first discussion of the pattern treated by this formula is found in Chapter 44 ("On Atrophy") in *Basic Questions*:

> When the Liver qi is hot, the Gallbladder will drain, the mouth becomes bitter, and the sinews and membranes become dry. When the sinews and membranes are dry, there is a sensation of severe tightness in the sinews, which contract. This development is called atrophy of the sinews. ... When the Kidney qi is hot, the lower spine will not move, the bones will become desiccated, and the marrow will be depleted. This development is called atrophy of the bones.

To treat this pattern, Zhu Dan-Xi, the author of the formula, employed a variation of Great Tonify the Yin Pill (*dà bǔ yīn wán*), used for treating fire with yin deficiency, to which he added Tigris Os (*hǔ gǔ*) and other substances that assist the yang and move the qi. In this manner, the formula succeeds in nourishing the essence and blood and strengthening the bones and sinews, without further obstructing the channels and collaterals. Later generations of physicians expanded the tonifying properties of this formula by adding substances like Eucommiae Cortex (*dù zhòng*), Angelicae sinensis Radix (*dāng guī*), Achyranthis bidentatae Radix (*niú xī*), and mutton that nourish the blood and augment the Kidneys. Alternatively, herbs such as Ginseng Radix (*rén shēn*) and Astragali Radix (*huáng qí*) were added to tonify and strengthen the qi.

Physicians have interpreted the formula's name in four somewhat different ways. The prevailing view is that the tiger symbolizes yin and that 'hidden' refers to storing, thus underlining the formula's properties of tonifying yin essence. Zhang Lu elaborates on this view in his *Comprehensive Medicine According to Master Zhang*:

> The tiger's body is yin in nature. Therefore, [even though] it is indomitable and moves well, it prefers to hide. If yin substances follow their salty nature, they also remain hidden and do not move. By activating their vigorous power [by way of its warm and yang-moving substances], they bestow great benefit to the lower body.

Finally, in *Discussion of Medical Formulas*, the late Qing-dynasty physician Fei Bo-Xiong argued that the formula "extinguishes deficiency wind of the Liver and Kidneys. The [behavior of] wind follows the same principle as that of the tiger. Hiding, the tiger thus [implies] that wind is extinguished."

Although these views differ in their interpretation of the words 'tiger' and 'hidden,' they all arrive at the same end point: that in order to treat the wind-type manifestations that characterize this pattern (tightness of the sinews, dizziness), it is essential to enrich the yin and nourish the water.

Comparison

➤ Vs. Great Tonifying the Yin Pill *(dà bǔ yīn wán)*

Both formulas enrich the Kidneys and tonify the Liver, while also directing fire downward. Great Tonifying the Yin Pill *(dà bǔ yīn wán)* is intended for long-term use. For that reason, the formula is administered in pill form and is primarily used to enrich and tonify the blood and essence. Hidden Tiger Pill *(hǔ qián wán)* also moves the yang and is tonifying without being cloying. It is ideal for strengthening the sinews and bones in atrophy disorders of the lower body due to yin deficiency and uncontrolled ministerial fire.

Biomedical Indications

With the appropriate presentation, this formula may be used to treat a wide variety of biomedically-defined disorders including sequelae of polio and tuberculosis of the knee.

Alternate name

Fast-Paced Hidden Tiger Pill *(jiàn bù hǔ qián wán)* in *Collected Formulas from the Crane-Feeding Pavilion*

Modifications

• For more severe fire manifesting as steaming bone fever, remove Zingiberis Rhizoma *(gān jiāng)* and substitute Rehmanniae Radix *(shēng dì huáng)* for Rehmanniae Radix praeparata *(shú dì huáng)*.

• For patterns characterized by a pale yellowish complexion, palpitations, a pale tongue body, and a thin pulse, add Astragali Radix *(huáng qí)*, Codonopsis Radix *(dǎng shēn)*, and Angelicae sinensis Radix *(dāng guī)*.

• For chronic yin deficiency that is also harming the yang characterized by aversion to cold, impotence, clear and copious urine, and a pale tongue, remove Anemarrhenae Rhizoma *(zhī mǔ)* and Phellodendri Cortex *(huáng bǎi)* and add Cervi Cornus Colla *(lù jiǎo jiāo)*, Psoraleae Fructus *(bǔ gǔ zhī)*, Epimedii Herba *(yín yáng huò)*, Morindae officinalis Radix *(bā jǐ tiān)*, Aconiti Radix lateralis praeparata *(zhì fù zǐ)*, and Cinnamomi Cortex *(ròu guì)*.

Variation

虎潜丸 (虎潛丸)

Hidden Tiger Pill from *Medical Formulas Collected and Analyzed*

hǔ qián wán

Source   *Medical Formulas Collected and Analyzed* (1682)

For a more severe condition, add Angelicae sinensis Radix *(dāng guī)* and Achyranthis bidentatae Radix *(niú xī)*. Cook with mutton and wine and form into pills.

大造丸

Great Creation Pill

dà zào wán

The name of this formula is derived from its function of nourishing and enriching the root of the body to help a patient recover from emaciation, and from the use of a placenta, which is emblematic of creation. The word 'great' is a reference to the potent action of this formula in treating deficiency of essences, which is said to give patients a 'new lease on life' (再造 *zài zào*).

Source   *Essential Formulas to Support Longevity* (1534)

Hominis Placenta *(zǐ hé chē)* 0.9g
crispy Testudinis Plastrum Testudinis Plastrum *(sū guī bǎn)* . . 60g
Phellodendri Cortex *(huáng bǎi)* 45g
Eucommiae Cortex *(dù zhòng)* 45g
Achyranthis bidentatae Radix *(niú xī)* 36g
Ophiopogonis Radix *(mài mén dōng)* 36g
Asparagi Radix *(tiān mén dōng)* 36g
Rehmanniae Radix *(shēng dì huáng)* 150g
Ginseng Radix *(rén shēn)* 30g

Method of Preparation   Grind the ingredients into a powder and form into pills with honey. The normal dosage is 9-12g once each morning. The source text recommends that Rehmanniae Radix *(shēng dì huáng)* be boiled briefly with Amomi Fructus *(shā rén)* and Poria *(fú líng)*, after which the latter herbs are discarded. This method is used to help the body assimilate the formula but is rarely followed nowadays. At present, Testudinis Plastrum *(guī bǎn)* is first deep-fried so that it can be ground into a powder.

Note that owing to the perceived risks of contamination of Hominis Placenta *(zǐ hé chē)* by viruses such as those related to hepatitis and HIV, this item is not frequently used in the West. Further, many countries, including the United States, prohibit the importation of human body parts. Possible substitutes include herbs that are said to have a tonifying action with respect to the essence such as Polygoni multiflori Radix *(hé shǒu wū)*, Polygonati Rhizoma *(huáng jīng)*, Cuscutae Semen *(tù sī zǐ)*, and Taxilli Herba *(sāng jì shēng)*.

Actions   Tonifies the Kidneys, enriches the yin, drains heat, and anchors the yang

Indications

Steaming bone disorder, cough with sticky sputum that is difficult to expectorate, emaciation, tinnitus, dizziness, tidal fever, a dry mouth and parched throat, heat in the five centers, and night sweats.

The simultaneous appearance of cough and steaming bone disorder signifies that the root of this disorder is in the Kidneys and that its manifestations are in the Lungs. The Kidney yin is deficient and damaged and is therefore unable to control the yang, which becomes hyperactive and leads to steaming bone disorder. Fire also attacks the Lungs where it produces a cough with sticky sputum that is difficult to expectorate. Because the substance of the body is damaged and the qi is unable to circulate (due to damage to the Lungs), the patient becomes emaciated. If the uncontrolled yang disturbs the sensory orifices, the patient will experience such symptoms as tinnitus and dizziness. The tidal fever, dry mouth and parched throat, heat in the five centers, and night sweats are characteristic of severe yin deficiency.

Analysis of Formula

The primary focus of this formula is to nourish and enrich the yin, and secondarily to clear heat and anchor the uncontrolled yang. The chief ingredient is Hominis Placenta *(zǐ hé chē)*, a very strong tonic for the blood and essence. The deputy ingredients assist the chief ingredient in tonifying the Kidneys in general and the Kidney yin in particular. They are Rehmanniae Radix *(shēng dì huáng)*, Achyranthis bidentatae Radix *(niú xī)*, Eucommiae Cortex *(dù zhòng)*, and Testudinis Plastrum *(guī bǎn)*. The latter ingredient also anchors the yang and, in concert with the fire-draining Phellodendri Cortex *(huáng bǎi)*, is very effective in controlling the hyperactive yang. All of these ingredients treat the Kidneys.

The remaining herbs work on the Lungs and are regarded as assistants. Ginseng Radix *(rén shēn)*, in concert with Ophiopogonis Radix *(mài mén dōng)* and Asparagi Radix *(tiān mén dōng)*, is very effective in tonifying the Lung qi and benefiting the Lung yin. This combination is particularly useful in treating the cough and emaciation due to yin deficiency.

Commentary

This formula treats both the root and branch of this disorder and is therefore particularly effective in treating consumptive disorders with emaciation. The use of Hominis Placenta *(zǐ hé chē)* as chief herb implies that the pathology extends beyond damage to the yin fluids and reaches the essence. Besides coughing and tidal fever, emaciation is thus the key indication for this formula. More acute cases of coughing with tidal fever are lesser yang or greater yin phlegm-dampness patterns, for which this formula is inappropriate.

The inclusion of Ginseng Radix *(rén shēn)*, furthermore, suggests that the primal qi is also insufficient. Therefore, the formula is also suitable for problems that occur postpartum when a woman's essence and qi are depleted. If the formula is used to treat tuberculosis, it is best thought of as a complement to biomedical treatment.

Comparison

➤ Vs. Great Tonify the Yin Pill *(dà bǔ yīn wán)*

Both formulas treat yin deficiency with up-flaring of fire. Great Tonify the Yin Pill *(dà bǔ yīn wán)* has less enriching

actions and focuses on bringing down the fire from deficiency. By contrast, Great Creation Pill *(dà zào wán)* focuses more on tonifying as well as nourishing the Lungs. The location of the fire, too, is different in both cases. In patterns for which Great Tonify the Yin Pill *(dà bǔ yīn wán)* is indicated, the fire is located predominantly in the Kidney and Liver channels. In patterns for which Great Creation Pill *(dà zào wán)* is indicated, it flares upward to scorch the Lungs.

Biomedical Indications

With the appropriate presentation, this formula may be used to treat a wide variety of biomedically-defined disorders including exhaustion from a chronic disease, pulmonary tuberculosis, chronic obstructive pulmonary disease, various endocrine disorders, neurasthenia, and fever of unknown origin.

Modifications

- For more severe signs of heat, add Artemisiae annuae Herba *(qīng hāo)*, Anemarrhenae Rhizoma *(zhī mǔ)*, and Moutan Cortex *(mǔ dān pí)*.

- For more severe signs of yin deficiency and wasting, add Paeoniae Radix alba *(bái sháo)*, Scrophulariae Radix *(xuán shēn)*, and Schisandrae Fructus *(wǔ wèi zǐ)*.

Associated Formula

大造丸

Great Creation Pill from *Collected Treatises of [Zhang] Jing-Yue*

dà zào wán

Source   *Collected Treatises of [Zhang] Jing-Yue* (1624)

Hominis Placenta *(zǐ hé chē)* . . . . 1 whole placenta
Rehmanniae Radix *(shēng dì huáng)* 45g
Asparagi Radix *(tiān mén dōng)* 21g
Angelicae sinensis Radix *(dāng guī)* 21g
Lycii Fructus *(gǒu qǐ zǐ)* 21g
Achyranthis bidentatae Radix *(niú xī)* 21g
Schisandrae Fructus *(wǔ wèi zǐ)* 21g
Cistanches Herba *(ròu cōng róng)* 21g
Phellodendri Cortex *(huáng bǎi)* 21g
Cynomorii Herba *(suǒ yáng)* 21g
Eucommiae Cortex *(dù zhòng)* 30g

Enriches the yin and secures the yang. For yin deficiency and heat in the blood from deficiency and overwork characterized by loss of hearing and diminished visual acuity, premature graying of hair, and loss of memory. In contrast to the principal formula, this variation focuses less on clearing heat from the Lungs and more on moistening and nourishing the blood, and also on assisting the yang. It is thus indicated for patterns where deficiency of essence manifests with signs that the blood is no longer able to carry out its moistening, lubricating, and nourishing functions.

一貫煎 （一貫煎）

Linking Decoction

yī guàn jiān

The name of this formula is believed to refer to a passage from Chapter 4 of the *Analects*, where Confucius tells his disciple Zeng Zi, "My way consists of one [principle] that links everything." In the context of this formula and its composition, the name may be understood as a reference to the Liver, which is "yin in essence but manifests through its yang functions." The formula treats Liver qi constraint (a disorder of its yang functions) mainly through the use of enriching herbs (tonifying its yin nature). To this end, the formula combines enriching, moistening, and softening herbs that act on the yin with one that is bitter and cooling and acts on the yang. They are linked by their joint effect on Liver function.

Source *Continuation of Famous Physicians' Cases Organized by Categories* (1770)

Rehmanniae Radix (*shēng dì huáng*) 18-45g
Lycii Fructus (*gǒu qǐ zǐ*) 9-18g
Glehniae/Adenophorae Radix (*shā shēn*) 9g
Ophiopogonis Radix (*mài mén dōng*) 9g
Angelicae sinensis Radix (*dāng guī*) 9g
Toosendan Fructus (*chuān liàn zǐ*) 4.5g

Method of Preparation Decoction.

Actions Enriches the yin and spreads the Liver qi

Indications

Hypochondriac, epigastric, and chest pain, a dry and parched mouth and throat, acid reflux, a red and dry tongue, and a thin, frail or deficient, wiry pulse.

This is yin deficiency of the Liver and Kidneys with qi stagnation. The yin deficiency may be caused by fire from constraint, or it may be an independent, but concurrent condition. The Liver is "yin in essence but manifests through its yang functions." This means that while its ability to activate and control movement is the most visible external manifestation of its function, it depends entirely on its ability to store blood to carry out this function in a physiologically balanced manner. This is why here, the deficiency of yin inhibits the dispersing and dredging function of the Liver. The Liver channel traverses the hypochondria and chest. Insufficient Liver blood deprives the channel of its moisture and nourishment, which in turn causes qi stagnation and thereby pain in the chest and hypochondria. Many patients characterize this pain as being tight or 'dry,' as if things were being stretched tight on the inside, although this part of the history may be difficult to elicit.

Because the Liver spreads and controls the yang qi, stagnation of Liver qi often results in fire from constraint that rebels transversely and attacks the Stomach. Not only does this generate epigastric pain and distention, but also acid reflux. The lack of flow, together with yin deficiency, causes a dry and parched mouth and throat as well as a red and dry tongue. The pulse will vary depending on the relative intensity of the yin deficiency and constraint. When yin deficiency predominates, the pulse will be thin and frail, but when constraint is more significant, the pulse will be deficient and wiry.

Analysis of Formula

This formula combines the primary strategy of nourishing Liver yin with the secondary strategy of dispersing Liver qi and clearing heat in order to treat conditions due to Liver qi constraint occurring against a background of Liver yin and blood deficiency. The chief, Lycii Fructus (*gǒu qǐ zǐ*), softens the Liver by satisfying its needs, that is, by nourishing its blood and the yin of its mother organ, the Kidneys. It is widely regarded as a moistening herb, a function that implies the facilitation of movement. It enters the Lungs, and some writers, such as the modern physician Zhang Xi-Chun, believe that it also clears heat. In this way, it can facilitate the Lungs' function of regulating the qi. The deputy herb is Angelicae sinensis Radix (*dāng guī*), which also nourishes the blood, but with its acrid and warming nature, focuses the formula's action on moving the qi and blood rather than merely tonifying the yin. However, because deficiency is the root of the disorder, the three assistant herbs all tonify the yin. Sweet and cooling Rehmanniae Radix (*shēng dì huáng*) is used in a large dosage to enrich the fluids, soften the Liver, and clear heat from constraint. Glehniae/Adenophorae Radix (*shā shēn*) and Ophiopogonis Radix (*mài mén dōng*) enrich and nourish the yin fluids of the Stomach and Lungs. They treat the parched mouth and throat while indirectly helping to soften the Liver. From a five-phase perspective, or that of the qi dynamic, improving the downward-directing functions of the Lung and Stomach helps to counterbalance and control Liver excess.

The envoy is Toosendan Fructus (*chuān liàn zǐ*), which is used to disperse the constrained Liver qi and thereby directly attack the pain. Ordinarily, the bitter nature of this herb would tend to damage the yin. In this formula, however, this property is mitigated by the sweet, moistening nature of the other herbs in the formula. Conversely, the other herbs have a cloying tendency that can easily clog the digestive process and hinder the movement of qi. This tendency is moderated here by the presence of the envoy.

Cautions and Contraindications

This formula should *never* be used for pain and distention from dampness or phlegm, as this will severely aggravate the condition.

Commentary

Liver qi constraint generally requires the use of acrid, moving herbs in order to unblock stagnation and open the channels and collaterals. However, the movement of qi also depends on fluids to moisten and control it. Without water, the physiological yang qi turns into pathological fire; without lubrication, the acrid nature of the qi is no longer smoothed, and the qi stagnates, causing distention and pain.

This formula treats patterns where constraint is due to such a lack of cooling and lubrication. Its effectiveness can be attributed to its moistening on two different levels, both of which have a bearing on the smooth flow of qi. The chief and deputy, Lycii Fructus (*gǒu qǐ zǐ*) and Angelicae sinensis Radix (*dāng guī*), work on the level of Liver blood. Lycii Fructus (*gǒu qǐ zǐ*) also enriches the essence and thus supports the Liver through its mother organ, the Kidneys. This combination may be regarded as a variation of Four-Substance Decoction (*sì wù tāng*), adapted for the purpose of opening constraint by substituting the cloying, acrid, and astringent herbs with one that is both tonifying and lubricating. The assistants focus on the level of the fluids. Rehmanniae Radix (*shēng dì huáng*) enters the blood, where it clears heat and generates fluids. Ophiopogonis Radix (*mài mén dōng*) and Glehniae/Adenophorae Radix (*shā shēn*) generate fluids in the upper and middle burners. These three herbs constitute a variation of *Increase the Fluids Decoction (zēng yè tāng)*, discussed in Chapter 15, which has been adapted to facilitate movement rather than clear heat.

Overall, the formula succeeds in harmonizing Liver function by attending to all the relationships of generation and control encompassed within the five-phase model. Different sources describe the action and composition of this formula from various perspectives. For instance, Rehmanniae Radix (*shēng dì huáng*) is often defined as a chief herb.

The original indications of the formula focus on pain in the ribs and epigastrium, the areas controlled by the Liver and Stomach. Because it can be viewed as opening constraint due to dryness in a more general manner, however, its use has been expanded to include many other patterns thought to arise from the same pathology. A discussion of the formula by the modern physician Zhang Shan-Lei is often cited to support this usage. Writing in *Careful Deliberations on Wind Stroke*, Zhang observed: "This [formula] can be used to treat all kinds of disorders arising [within a context where] the blood is insufficient, the collaterals plugged up, and the Liver and Gallbladder are out of control. It has a particularly outstanding effect if there is no blocked phlegm or accumulation of thin mucus." Manifestations of such disorders include pain in other parts of the body, particularly those traversed by the Liver channel, such as menstrual pain and bulging disorders, chronic abdominal pain, amenorrhea, abdominal masses with Liver and Kidney yin deficiency, Lung consumption, and wasting and thirsting disorder. It has also been used in treating certain stages and the sequelae of warm pathogen disorders.

Comparisons

➤ Vs. Frigid Extremities Powder (*sì nì sǎn*) and Rambling Powder (*xiāo yáo sǎn*)

All of these formulas treat hypochondriac pain due to Liver constraint. There are, however, differences among them. The ability of Frigid Extremities Powder (*sì nì sǎn*) to relieve Liver constraint is relatively strong, and it is used for hypochondriac pain with cold extremities. Rambling Powder (*xiāo yáo sǎn*) is used more in cases of Liver constraint following emotional upset where there is disharmony between the Liver and Spleen manifested in fatigue, lethargy, reduced appetite, and a pale tongue. In the case of Linking Decoction (*yī guàn jiān*), it is the deficiency of Liver yin that leads to constraint, heat, and pain. The heat from constraint then attacks the Stomach, as described above. Thus, this script is formulated to enrich and nourish the Liver and Kidney yin in order to soften the Liver, while also dispersing the constrained Liver qi, reflected in the dry mouth and thin pulse.

Biomedical Indications

With the appropriate presentation, this formula may be used to treat a wide variety of biomedically-defined disorders such as chronic active hepatitis, cirrhosis, liver pain due to liver cancer, costochondritis, peptic ulcer, essential hypertension, hypertension during pregnancy, Addison's disease, thrombocytopenic purpura, pulmonary tuberculosis, diabetes mellitus, chronic orchitis, restless leg syndrome, and nervous exhaustion.

Modifications

- For headache, dizziness, blurred vision, or other signs of Liver wind, add Paeoniae Radix alba (*bái sháo*) and Scrophulariae Radix (*xuán shēn*).
- For constipation, add Trichosanthis Semen (*guā lóu rén*).
- For heat from deficiency, add Lycii Cortex (*dì gǔ pí*).
- For severe yin deficiency with a dry tongue, add Dendrobii Herba (*shí hú*).
- For firmness over the area of pain, add Trionycis Carapax (*biē jiǎ*).
- For severe abdominal pain, add Paeoniae Radix alba (*bái sháo*) and Glycyrrhizae Radix (*gān cǎo*).
- For a very dry and bitter mouth, add a small amount of Coptidis Rhizoma (*huáng lián*).
- For weakness in the lower extremities, add Achyranthis bidentatae Radix (*niú xī*) and Coicis Semen (*yì yǐ rén*).
- For hypertension with more severe Liver and Kidney deficiency, add Taxilli Herba (*sāng jì shēng*) and Eucommiae Cortex (*dù zhòng*).
- For hypertension with more Liver heat, add Prunellae Spica (*xià kū cǎo*) and Scutellariae Radix (*huáng qín*).

Associated Formula

滋水清肝飲 （滋水清肝饮）

Enrich Water and Clear the Liver Drink

zī shuǐ qīng gān yǐn

SOURCE *Externally-Contracted Patterns from Xitang (1725)*

Rehmanniae Radix praeparata (*shú dì huáng*) 15g
Corni Fructus (*shān zhū yú*) 12g
Dioscoreae Rhizoma (*shān yào*) 12g
Moutan Cortex (*mǔ dān pí*) 9g
Poria (*fú líng*) 9g
Alismatis Rhizoma (*zé xiè*) 6g
Bupleuri Radix (*chái hú*) 6g
Paeoniae Radix alba (*bái sháo*) 12g
Gardeniae Fructus (*zhī zǐ*) 9g
Ziziphi spinosae Semen (*suān zǎo rén*) 12g
Angelicae sinensis Radix (*dāng guī*) 9g

Decoction. The source text does not specify dosage; those above are suggested by the editors. Enriches the yin and clears the Liver. For Kidney yin deficiency and Liver constraint transforming into fire manifesting with indistinct burning pain in the flanks, irritability, bouts of anger, a dry mouth with a bitter taste, insomnia or dream-disturbed sleep, dry stools, or burning pain in the epigastric area, gnawing hunger, acid reflux, soreness and weakness of the back and knees, dizziness, headaches, early periods, a red tongue with little coating, and a wiry, thin, and rapid pulse. This is a combination of Six-Ingredient Pill with Rehmannia (*liù wèi dì huáng wán*) and Augmented Rambling Powder (*jiā wèi xiāo yáo sǎn*), discussed in Chapter 3. The indications of this formula match those of Linking Decoction (*yī guàn jiān*), discussed above. However, this formula focuses more on treating Kidney deficiency as the root of the disorder and on leading the qi and fire back to their source in the lower burner. Such uncontrolled yang, which is an important aspect of the pattern, is experienced by the patient as a feeling of fullness or swelling in the face and extremities that may or may not be visible. Linking Decoction (*yī guàn jiān*), on the other hand, focuses on generating fluids, moistening dryness, and checking Liver excess by supplementing the downward-directing functions of the Stomach and Lungs. Key signs here, therefore, are dryness of the mouth and tongue, as well as a thin and wiry pulse.

二至丸

Two-Solstice Pill

èr zhì wán

The two herbs that comprise this formula should be picked at the solstices, the ultimate yin and yang times of the year. The formula is also used to treat the Liver and Kidney yin, which is the ultimate source of nourishment for the entire body.

Source *Essential Formulas to Support Longevity (1534)*

Ligustri lucidi Fructus (*nǔ zhēn zǐ*)
Ecliptae Herba (*mò hàn lián*)

Method of Preparation The source text specifies that the first herb should be picked at the winter solstice, and the second at the summer solstice. Grind equal amounts of the ingredients into a powder and form into pills with honey. In some cases, a concentrate is made of the second herb, to which a powdered form of the first herb and honey are then added to form into pills. Originally taken before bedtime with wine; at present, it is taken in 9-15g doses 2-3 times a day. May also be prepared as a decoction.

Actions Tonifies and benefits the Liver and Kidneys

Indications

Weakness and soreness of the lower back and knees, or even weakness and atrophy of the lower extremities, dry and parched mouth and throat, dizziness and blurred vision, insomnia and dream-disturbed sleep, spontaneous emissions, premature graying or loss of hair, and a red, dry tongue.

This condition is due to deficiency of the Liver and Kidney yin. The Kidneys govern the bones and generate the marrow. When the Kidney yin is deficient, the yin and essence are unable to properly moisten and nurture the lower parts of the body; weakness and soreness of the lower back and knees ensue. In severe cases, this process can lead to weakness and atrophy of the lower extremities. The Kidney channel winds its way through the throat to reach the tongue. When the fluids are insufficient, the throat and mouth become parched, and the tongue becomes red and dry. The eyes are the adornment of the Liver. When the Liver yin is deficient, dizziness and blurred vision may occur. In addition to blood, the Liver also stores the ethereal soul. When the Liver yin is deficient, the ethereal soul has no place to reside at night, and the patient will complain of insomnia and dream-disturbed sleep. Deficiency of the Kidney and Liver yin also leaves no place for the essence to be stored, which often manifests as spontaneous emissions. Premature graying or loss of hair are another sign of Liver and Kidney deficiency.

Analysis of Formula

This formula is an elegant combination of two herbs. Ligustri lucidi Fructus (*nǔ zhēn zǐ*) is a sweet, bitter, and cool herb that enriches the Kidneys and nourishes the Liver. Ecliptae Herba (*mò hàn lián*) is a sweet, sour, and cold herb that nourishes the yin, benefits the essence, and cools the blood to stop bleeding. Together, they nourish the yin aspects of the Liver and Kidneys, without being cloying.

Cautions and Contraindications

The two herbs in this formula are cooling and should therefore be used with caution in patients with weak digestive systems.

Commentary

The original name of this formula was Ligustrum Special Pill (女貞丹 *nǔ zhēn dān*), which suggests the potent tonifying properties attributed to it and also suggests which of the two ingredients should be regarded as chief. The actions listed in the source text are "[the ability] to make [the hair black like that of a] crow, strengthen the back, knees, and insufficient yin." Its modern name stems from the Ming-dynasty physician Wang San-Cai, who emphasized that the two herbs should be harvested at the two solstices. His interpretation of the formula's actions is that it "clears the upper [burner] and tonifies the lower [burner]." This is a reference to the formula's ability to clear heat as well as tonify deficiency.

At present, this formula is widely used in China, both alone and as an additive to other formulas when the Liver and Kidney yin needs to be tonified. It is considered safe and relatively mild. Many physicians think that it must be prescribed long-term to achieve its effects. *New Compilation of Materia Medica* observes that if Ligustri lucidi Fructus (*nǔ zhēn zǐ*)

> is prescribed gently [i.e., long-term in a low dosage], it performs meritorious service. If it is used [to act] quickly, it has little effect. Therefore, if it is used quickly, it is virtually impossible to score a success. If it is used gently, it truly prolongs life into perpetuity. This, therefore, is its most appropriate use in people.

Comparison

➤ Vs. Six-Ingredient Pill with Rehmannia (*liù wèi dì huáng wán*)

Although these two formulas are quite similar in usage, Six-Ingredient Pill with Rehmannia (*liù wèi dì huáng wán*) is regarded as a slightly stronger formulation. Two-Solstice Pill (*èr zhì wán*) is preferred when chronic bleeding is part of the presentation and is considered by some to be superior in treating premature graying or loss of hair.

Biomedical Indications

With the appropriate presentation, this formula may be used to treat a variety of biomedically-defined disorders including insomnia, menorrhagia, and other forms of hemorrhage.

Modification

• For a slightly stronger effect, add Mori Fructus (*sāng shèn*).

Associated Formula

桑麻丸

Mulberry Leaf and Sesame Seed Pill

sāng má wán

SOURCE *Achieving Longevity by Guarding the Source* (1615)

Mori Folium (*sāng yè*) 500g
Sesami Semen nigrum (*hēi zhī má*) 120g

Make a concentrate from the second herb, add 500g of honey and a powdered form of the first herb. Form into 9g pills and take one pill

twice a day. For best results, take with salted water in the morning and wine in the evening. Enriches the Liver and Kidneys, clears the head and eyes, and expels wind-dampness. For yin deficiency with dried blood and wind-dampness characterized by dizziness, blurred vision, chronic cough, constipation with very dry stools, and dry, flaky skin accompanied by numbness and painful obstruction.

Compared with Two-Solstice Pill (*èr zhì wán*), which is stronger at tonifying the yin and cooling the blood, this formula focuses on nourishing the blood and moistening dryness. For that reason, the main formula is used when yin deficiency below is accompanied by heat above, with such symptoms as tinnitus, dizziness, and early graying of hair. By contrast, this associated formula is used when yin deficiency is accompanied by dryness and wind in the skin, channels, and collaterals.

百合固金湯 (百合固金汤)

Lily Bulb Decoction to Preserve the Metal

bǎi hé gù jīn tāng

This formula acts to preserve and stabilize the function of the Lungs, which is associated with the metal phase, and one of its chief herbs is lily bulb (*bǎi hé*), hence the name.

Source *Writings for Posterity of [Zhou] Shen-Zhai* (1573)

Lilii Bulbus (*bǎi hé*) 4.5g
Rehmanniae Radix (*shēng dì huáng*) 9g
Rehmanniae Radix praeparata (*shú dì huáng*) 9g
Ophiopogonis Radix (*mài mén dōng*) 4.5g
Scrophulariae Radix (*xuán shēn*) 2.4g
Fritillariae Bulbus (*bèi mǔ*) 4.5g
Platycodi Radix (*jié gěng*) 2.4g
Angelicae sinensis Radix (*dāng guī*) 9g
Paeoniae Radix alba (*bái sháo*) .3g
Glycyrrhizae Radix (*gān cǎo*) 3g

Method of Preparation Decoction. At present, most practitioners use 2-3 times the specified dosage, and some texts advise to increase the dosage of Lilii Bulbus (*bǎi hé*) to 24 grams. Fritillariae cirrhosae Bulbus (*chuān bèi mǔ*) is generally the species of Fritillariae used.

Actions Nourishes the yin, moistens the Lungs, transforms phlegm, and stops coughing

Indications

Coughing with blood-streaked sputum, wheezing, a dry and sore throat, hot palms and soles, night sweats, a red tongue with little coating, and a thin, rapid pulse.

This is internal dryness of the Lungs due to Lung and Kidney yin deficiency with heat from deficiency. The Lungs and Kidneys are known respectively as the upper and lower sources of water. In this pattern both are deficient, as reflected in the dry throat, dry tongue with little coating, and thin pulse. Deficiency of yin always implies an excess of yang. This manifests as heat from deficiency that rises from the Kidneys to cause a sore throat, 'steams' the delicate, uppermost organ (the Lungs), and interferes with the regulation of Lung qi, producing coughing and wheezing. Heat from deficiency also 'scorches' the collaterals of the Lungs, leading to blood-streaked sputum. The red tongue color and the rapid pulse are other classic signs of internal heat.

Analysis of Formula

The treatment strategy underpinning the composition of this formula is one of simultaneously generating metal and water in order to enrich the yin and control heat from deficiency. Lilii Bulbus *(bǎi hé)*, one of the chief herbs in the formula, moistens and nourishes dryness in the Lungs, and clears heat. Another of the chief herbs, Rehmanniae Radix *(shēng dì huáng)*, strongly enriches the yin and tonifies the Kidneys. It also performs the important function of cooling the blood to stop the bleeding. Rehmanniae Radix praeparata *(shú dì huáng)*, the third chief herb, is a very powerful tonic for the Liver and Kidney yin. In concert with Rehmanniae Radix *(shēng dì huáng)*, it is also especially helpful in treating fire due to yin deficiency. One of the deputies, Ophiopogonis Radix *(mài mén dōng)*, is an important herb for tonifying the yin, especially that of the upper burner. It also potentiates the actions of Lilii Bulbus *(bǎi hé)* on the Lungs and the yin-tonifying actions of the two other chief herbs. The other deputy, Scrophulariae Radix *(xuán shēn)*, helps the Kidney water ascend to the Lungs and is extremely useful in clearing fire from deficiency and treating steaming bone condition.

Fritillariae cirrhosae Bulbus *(chuān bèi mǔ)*, one of the assistants, moistens the Lungs, transforms phlegm, and stops coughing. Another assistant, Platycodi Radix *(jié gěng)*, facilitates the movement of Lung qi and stops coughing, especially when combined with Fritillariae cirrhosae Bulbus *(chuān bèi mǔ)*. The other assistant herbs, Angelicae sinensis Radix *(dāng guī)* and Paeoniae Radix alba *(bái sháo)*, nourish the blood to support the yin. In ancient materia medica, Angelicae sinensis Radix *(dāng guī)* was regarded as being useful in stopping coughs. Another way of viewing the actions of Paeoniae Radix alba *(bái sháo)* and Angelicae sinensis Radix *(dāng guī)* is that, by calming the Liver, they protect the Lungs from violation. The envoy, Glycyrrhizae Radix *(gān cǎo)*, harmonizes the actions of the other herbs and, in combination with Platycodi Radix *(jié gěng)*, improves the condition of the throat.

Cautions and Contraindications

Most of the herbs in this formula are of a sweet, cold, and cloying nature. For this reason, it should be used with caution or modified (using herbs that strengthen the Spleen and regulate the qi) in cases with Spleen deficiency or food stagnation. Failure to do so may result in indigestion or diarrhea. It should not be used for patients with exterior conditions.

Commentary

This formula was originally composed to treat consumptive disorders affecting the Lungs that are caused by underlying Kidney yin deficiency. In *Collectanea of Investigations from the Realm of Medicine*, the Qing-dynasty physician Wang Fu provides a detailed explanation of the strategy underlying its composition:

> [In Chapter 8 of *Basic Questions* it states that] the Lungs hold the office of prime minister and are the issuer of management and regulation. Its location close to the Heart makes it innately antagonistic to fire. If Lung metal clarifies and clears [fire] and the five yin organs are calm, [the Lung qi is] not restrained by its [natural] aversion to fire. [Hence, it is able to exercise its charge of] management and regulation in a spontaneous and unhurried manner. Qi is [then] governed and disorders [characterized] by dispersal and rebelliousness will not exist. When the Lungs become deficient [their charge of] management is no longer regulated, and they are incapable of generating qi. Qi rebels and the vessels become chaotic. In such [a situation,] it is appropriate to use sour [herbs and formulas] to restrain [the excess]. However, by their nature, the Lungs have much qi and little blood and are easily impaired by dryness. If a person's Kidney water is exhausted or impaired, the ministerial fire flares upward. Although metal generates water, this is insufficient to triumph over fire. This [is the cause] of Lung consumption. If sovereign fire becomes fearless [because it is] assisted by ministerial fire, [the two] combine, flaring upward and damaging the healthy Lungs. Contrary to the [normal physiological function outlined above, this is a situation] where Lung deficiency arises because of Kidney deficiency and Lung function is overexerted. … [In its composition, this formula thus] focuses on controlling fire so that it does not punish metal. Secondarily, it assists metal so that it can generate Kidney water below. This is why the intention [also expressed in the formula's name] is ultimately to preserve metal.

In practice, the formula is thus most suitable for treating cases of chronic cough or throat pain accompanied by blood loss: the former indicating yin deficiency, the latter, the uncontrolled upward movement of fire. Once these symptoms have abated, a different strategy should be selected, following the advice of Fei Bo-Xiong, another Qing-dynasty physician, in *Discussion of Medical Formulas*: "Li Shi-Zai said: 'After clearing metal one must urgently attend to the mother.' This understanding is outstanding. I [therefore] say: 'When the throat pain has been entirely alleviated, one should urgently nurture earth to generate metal.'"

Comparisons

➤ Vs. Tonify the Lungs Decoction with Ass-Hide Gelatin *(bǔ fèi ē jiāo tāng)*

While similar, Lily Bulb Decoction to Preserve the Metal *(bǎi hé gù jīn tāng)* possesses stronger yin-nourishing actions. Tonify the Lungs Decoction with Ass-Hide Gelatin *(bǔ fèi ē jiāo tāng)* focuses on clearing heat and stopping the bleeding.

➤ Vs. Clear Dryness and Rescue the Lungs
   Decoction *(qīng zào jiù fèi tāng)*

Both of these formulas moisten and nourish the Lung yin. However, Lily Bulb Decoction to Preserve the Metal *(bǎi hé gù jīn tāng)* only nourishes the Lung and Kidney yin and treats fire from deficiency. Throat pain is one of its main symptoms. Clear Dryness and Rescue the Lungs Decoction *(qīng zào jiù fèi tāng)*, which augments the qi and has a slight, exterior-releasing action, also addresses injury to the qi and yin. However, its main action is in clearing excess heat from the qi aspect.

➤ Vs. Fritillaria and Trichosanthes Fruit Powder
   (bèi mǔ guā lóu sǎn)

Both of these formulas treat Lung dryness with phlegm. However, Fritillaria and Trichosanthes Fruit Powder *(bèi mǔ guā lóu sǎn)* primarily transforms phlegm and is used when the phlegm is severe, the dryness is not intense, and the yin is not yet deficient. By contrast, Lily Bulb Decoction to Preserve the Metal *(bǎi hé gù jīn tāng)* focuses on moistening the Lungs and is used when the dryness is more severe than the phlegm and the yin is already deficient.

➤ Vs. Precious Jade Syrup *(qióng yù gāo)*; see page 391

Biomedical Indications

With the appropriate presentation, this formula may be used to treat a wide variety of biomedically-defined disorders such as chronic bronchitis, bronchiectasis, chronic pharyngitis, spontaneous pneumothorax, corpulmonale, silicosis, and pulmonary tuberculosis.

Modifications

- For copious sputum, add Trichosanthis Semen *(guā lóu rén)* and Mori Cortex *(sāng bái pí)*.
- For coughing up profuse blood, remove Platycodi Radix *(jié gěng)*, which has an ascending action, and add Imperatae Rhizoma *(bái máo gēn)* and Agrimoniae Herba *(xiān hè cǎo)*.
- For pronounced fever and dark-yellow sputum, add Anemarrhenae Rhizoma *(zhī mǔ)* and Houttuyniae Herba *(yú xīng cǎo)*.
- For lung cancer with yin deficiency, add Houttuyniae Herba *(yú xīng cǎo)*, Paeoniae Radix rubra *(chì sháo)*, Agkistrodon/Bungarus *(bái huā shé)*, and Scutellariae barbatae Herba *(bàn zhī lián)*.

Associated Formula

益氣清金湯 (益气清金汤)

Augment Qi and Clear the Metal Decoction

yì qì qīng jīn tāng

Source   *Golden Mirror of the Medical Tradition* (1742)

Platycodi Radix *(jié gěng)* 9g
Scutellariae Radix *(huáng qín)* 6g
Fritillariae thunbergii Bulbus *(zhè bèi mǔ)* 4.5g
Ophiopogonis Radix *(mài mén dōng)* 4.5g
dry-fried Arctii Fructus *(chǎo niú bàng zǐ)* 4.5g
Ginseng Radix *(rén shēn)* 3g
Poria *(fú líng)* 3g
Citri reticulatae Pericarpium *(chén pí)* 3g
Gardeniae Fructus *(zhī zǐ)* 3g
Menthae haplocalycis Herba *(bò hé)* 3g
Glycyrrhizae Radix *(gān cǎo)* 3g
Perillae Folium *(zǐ sū yè)* 1.5g
Lophatheri Herba *(dàn zhú yè)* . . . . 30 leaves

Decoction. Clears the Lungs, benefits the throat, transforms phlegm, and disperses clumps. For heat from constraint in the Lung channel as well as throat problems caused by harm to the qi from excessive speaking. This often manifests as a chronic inflammatory disorder or swelling in the throat that may or may not be painful. In contrast to the principal formula, Augment Qi and Clear the Metal Decoction *(yì qì qīng jīn tāng)* focuses on clearing the Lungs, resolving toxicity, benefitting the throat, and transforming phlegm to disperse clumps and reduce swellings. Although it also tonifies the qi and yin, these functions are secondary.

補肺阿膠湯 (补肺阿胶汤)

Tonify the Lungs Decoction with Ass-Hide Gelatin

bǔ fèi ē jiāo tāng

Source   *Craft of Medicinal Treatment for Childhood Disease Patterns* (1119)

Asini Corii Colla *(ē jiāo)* 45g (9g)
Aristolochiae Fructus *(mǎ dōu líng)* 15g (6g)
dry-fried Armeniacae Semen *(chǎo xìng rén)* 70 (6g)
dry-fried Arctii Fructus *(chǎo niú bàng zǐ)* 7.5g (3g)
dry-fried Glutinous rice *(chǎo nuò mǐ)* 30g (6g)
Glycyrrhizae Radix praeparata *(zhì gān cǎo)* 7.5g (3g)

Method of Preparation   The source text advises to dry-fry Asini Corii Colla *(ē jiāo)* with wheat bran, pound it and form into balls with glutinous rice flour, grind the other ingredients into a powder, and take as a draft in 3-6g doses. At present, it is prepared as a decoction with the dosages given above, and Asini Corii Colla *(ē jiāo)* dissolved in water and added to the strained decoction.

Actions   Nourishes the yin, tonifies the Lungs, controls coughing, and stops bleeding

Indications

Cough with wheezing, a dry and parched throat, scanty or blood-streaked sputum, a red tongue with little coating, and a floating, thin, and rapid pulse.

This is Lung yin deficiency with vigorous heat, which disrupts the flow of Lung qi and results in cough with wheezing. The dry throat and cough with scanty sputum is due to scorching of the fluids. Heat also scorches the collaterals of the Lungs, leading to blood-streaked sputum. The tongue signs reflect heat from yin deficiency. The floating, rapid pulse indicates heat in the Lungs, the most superficial of the yin organs. The tongue signs and the thin pulse also indicate that this is not an externally-contracted exterior disorder, which would show no change in the color of the tongue body (or only a red tip) and some coating would remain.

Analysis of Formula

This formula treats both the branch (heat) and the root (Lung yin deficiency) of the disorder. The chief ingredient, Asini Corii Colla *(ē jiāo)*, nourishes the yin and tonifies the Lungs, stops the bleeding, and nourishes the blood. The deputy ingredients treat the manifestations: Aristolochiae Fructus *(mǎ dōu líng)* clears heat and stops the coughing; Armeniacae Semen *(xìng rén)* directs the Lung qi downward and calms the wheezing; and Arctii Fructus *(niú bàng zǐ)* spreads the Lung qi and unblocks areas of congestion in the throat. The assistants, Nonglutinous rice *(jīng mǐ)* and Glycyrrhizae Radix praeparata *(zhì gān cǎo)*, tonify the Spleen and benefit the Lungs. This combination cultivates the earth (Spleen) to generate metal (Lungs) in order to tonify the Lungs and prevents the other herbs from disrupting the digestive process.

Cautions & Contraindications

This formula should not be used if there is Lung deficiency without heat, when there is any cold in the exterior, or when there in internal phlegm.

Commentary

The primary function of Asini Corii Colla *(ē jiāo)* is to tonify the blood and stop the bleeding. Any moistening effect that this substance has on the Lungs is secondary. The actions of the three deputy ingredients, which focus on clearing heat, directing Lung qi downward, and unblocking the throat, are also not directly tonifying with respect to either the Lung qi or yin. Many commentators thus think that the designation of this formula as one that 'tonifies the Lungs' is misleading. In fact, its original name, Ass-hide Gelatin Powder *(ē jiāo sǎn)*, draws attention to the chief herb rather than to the Lungs. In clinical practice, therefore, its primary indication is cough with blood-streaked sputum rather than yin deficiency with empty fire.

The use of Arctii Fructus *(niú bàng zǐ)* in the formula, and the presence of a floating pulse in the presentation, has led other commentators to identify this as a formula for treating externally-contracted disorders with Lung yin deficiency. Most clinicians do not share this extreme view.

Comparison

➤ Vs. Lily Bulb Decoction to Preserve the Metal *(bǎi hé gù jīn tāng)*; see page 385

➤ Vs. Nine-Immortal Powder *(jiǔ xiān sǎn)*; see page 424

Biomedical Indications

With the appropriate presentation, this formula may be used to treat a wide variety of biomedically-defined disorders such as chronic bronchitis, bronchiectasis, pulmonary tuberculosis, and chronic pharyngitis.

....

Alternate names

The formula was first listed under the name Ass-hide Gelatin Powder *(ē jiāo sǎn)* in the source text. It is likely that the name was later changed to differentiate this formula from others with the same name. It is also known as Tonify the Lungs Powder *(bǔ fèi sǎn)* in *Craft of Medicines and Patterns for Children*; Tonify the Lungs Powder with Ass-Hide Gelatin *(bǔ fèi ē jiāo sǎn)* in *Comprehensive Outline of the Materia Medica*; and Clear the Lungs Drink *(qīng fèi yǐn)* in *Complete Book on Treating Pox and Rashes*.

....

Modifications

- For blood-streaked sputum with severe heat signs due to Liver fire violating the Lungs, add Indigo naturalis *(qīng dài)* and Gardeniae Fructus *(zhī zǐ)*.

- For cough with very little phlegm that is difficult to cough up, add Trichosanthis Pericarpium *(guā lóu pí)* and Fritillariae cirrhosae Bulbus *(chuān bèi mǔ)*.

Associated Formula

月華丸（月华丸）

Moonlight Pill

yuè huá wán

Source *Awakening the Mind in Medical Studies* (1732)

Asparagi Radix *(tiān mén dōng)*	30g
Ophiopogonis Radix *(mài mén dōng)*	30g
Rehmanniae Radix *(shēng dì huáng)*	30g
Rehmanniae Radix praeparata *(shú dì huáng)*	30g
Dioscoreae Rhizoma *(shān yào)*	30g
Stemonae Radix *(bǎi bù)*	30g
Glehniae/Adenophorae Radix *(shā shēn)*	30g
Fritillariae cirrhosae Bulbus *(chuān bèi mǔ)*	30g
Asini Corii Colla *(ē jiāo)*	30g
Poria *(fú líng)*	15g
Lutrae Jecur *(tǎ gān)*	[otter liver] 15g
Notoginseng Radix *(sān qī)*	15g
white Chrysanthemi Flos *(bái jú huā)*	60g
Mori Folium *(sāng yè)*	60g

The source text advises to take 30g each of Mori Folium *(sāng yè)* and white Chrysanthemi Flos *(bái jú huā)*, which are cooked to a thickened consistency; the Asini Corii Colla *(ē jiāo)* is then melted in. This paste is then mixed with honey and the powder of the remaining herbs is used to make pills. Take one bullet-sized pill three times a day. At present, the ingredients are made into a paste with the addition of honey and formed into pills, which are taken in 15g doses three times a day. Enriches the yin, moistens the Lungs, controls coughing, and stops bleeding. For Lung and Kidney yin deficiency characterized by chronic cough or consumptive cough with tidal fever, heat in the five centers, emaciation, dry and nonproductive cough or cough with blood-streaked sputum, a dry mouth and throat, a sensation of fullness in the chest with reduced appetite, shortness of breath, laconic speech, difficult bowel movements, scanty urine, a red and dry tongue, and a thin and rapid pulse. In contrast to the principal formula, this has a stronger tonifying action on the yin of the Lungs and Kidneys, and is particularly useful in treating Lung consumption.

Note: Lutrae Jecur (獺肝 *tǎ gān*), or otter liver, is sweet, salty, neutral, and toxic, entering the Liver and Kidney channels. It nourishes the yin, eliminates heat, calms coughs, and stops bleeding. The normal dosage in decoctions is 3-6g. However, it is no longer used.

Comparison

➤ Vs. Decoction to Enrich Yin and Direct Fire Downward (*zī yīn jiàng huǒ tāng*); see PAGE 389

滋陰降火湯 (滋阴降火汤)
Decoction to Enrich Yin and Direct Fire Downward
zī yīn jiàng huǒ tāng

Source *Restoration of Health from the Myriad Diseases* (1587)

wine-washed Angelicae sinensis Radix (*jiǔ dāng guī*) 4g
wine-washed Paeoniae Radix alba (*jiǔ bái sháo*) 7g
ginger-juice fried Rehmanniae Radix praeparata
  (*jiāng zhì shú dì huáng*) 3g
Rehmanniae Radix (*shēng dì huáng*) 2.5g
center-removed Asparagi Radix (*tiān mén dōng*) 3g
center-removed Ophiopogonis Radix (*mài mén dōng*) 3g
honey-fried Citri reticulatae Pericarpium (*chén pí*) 2.5g
Atractylodis macrocephalae Rhizoma (*bái zhú*) 3g
Anemarrhenae Rhizoma (*zhī mǔ*) 2.5g
Phellodendri Cortex (*huáng bǎi*) 2.5g
Glycyrrhizae Radix praeparata (*zhì gān cǎo*) 1.5g
Zingiberis Rhizoma recens (*shēng jiāng*) . . . . 3 slices
Jujubae Fructus (*dà zǎo*) . . . . 1 piece

Method of Preparation   The source text suggests decocting the above ingredients and adding a small amount of Bambusae Succus (*zhú lì*), Infantis Urina (*tóng biàn*), and Zingiberis Rhizomatis Succus (*jiāng zhī*) before taking the decoction. At present, these items are omitted. The text also recommends that for best results, the formula be taken along with Six-Ingredient Pill with Rehmannia (*liù wèi dì huáng wán*).

Actions   Enrich the yin, nourish the blood, and direct fire downward

Indications

Fire from yin deficiency that gives rise to cough that may or may not be productive, wheezing, night sweats, dry mouth, fever, coughing of blood, wasting and thirsting, and steaming bones. The formula can also address the fire of deficiency scorching the throat with symptoms such as sore throat, throat sores, raspy voice, and dry throat.

Analysis of Formula

The various symptoms associated with this consumptive pattern all stem from yin deficiency with deficiency fire. The exhaustion of yin and blood that characterizes this pattern may be attributable to an undisciplined lifestyle or a constitutional deficiency. Alternatively, the cause may be a contagious consumptive disease. The treatment principle is to tonify the yin and blood while simultaneously tonifying the middle burner and draining the fire from deficiency.

This formula is built on the foundation of Four-Substance Decoction (*sì wù tāng*) supplemented with Atractylodis macrocephalae Rhizoma (*bái zhú*), Citri reticulatae Pericarpium (*chén pí*), Zingiberis Rhizoma recens (*shēng jiāng*), Glycyrrhizae Radix praeparata (*zhì gān cǎo*), and Jujubae Fructus (*dà zǎo*) to regulate the middle burner. This prevents the cloying, yin-nourishing herbs in the formula from overwhelming the digestive function of the Spleen-Stomach. Asparagi Radix (*tiān mén dōng*) and Ophiopogonis Radix (*mài mén dōng*) are included to further supplement the yin, relieve the cough, and moisten the Lungs. Phellodendri Cortex (*huáng bǎi*) and Anemarrhenae Rhizoma (*zhī mǔ*) drain the fire from deficiency.

Rehmanniae Radix (*shēng dì huáng*), Rehmanniae Radix praeparata (*shú dì huáng*), Ophiopogonis Radix (*mài mén dōng*), Asparagi Radix (*tiān mén dōng*), Angelicae sinensis Radix (*dāng guī*), and Paeoniae Radix alba (*bái sháo*) all nourish the yin and blood. They treat the root of the pattern for which this formula is designed and comprise the chief ingredients. Atractylodis macrocephalae Rhizoma (*bái zhú*), Citri reticulatae Pericarpium (*chén pí*), and Zingiberis Rhizoma recens (*shēng jiāng*) support the middle burner and serve as deputies. The assistants, Phellodendri Cortex (*huáng bǎi*) and Anemarrhenae Rhizoma (*zhī mǔ*), drain the fire of deficiency and thereby the manifestations of night sweats, cough, and fever. Glycyrrhizae Radix praeparata (*zhì gān cǎo*) harmonizes the formula and serves as the envoy.

This combination of herbs nourishes the yin and blood and drains the deficiency fire without compromising the middle burner. Thus, the symptoms of deficiency fire such as night sweats, cough, coughing of blood, steaming bones, dry mouth, fever, and thirst gradually recede.

Commentary

This formula treats consumptive disorder, in both its broad and narrow sense, as long as the fire from yin deficiency is the prominent characteristic of the pattern. In its narrow sense, consumptive disorder is known as 'consumptive disease' (癆瘵 *láo zhài*), and in its broader sense, 'deficiency consumption' (虛癆 *xū láo*). Deficiency consumption disorders are caused by overwork or over-indulgence. Overexertion can lead to the consumption of one's qi and essence.

The symptoms of this exhaustion-based consumptive disorder will differ depending on which aspect of the body has suffered consumption: yin, yang, qi, or blood. Yin-deficiency consumption presents with dry cough, dry throat, tidal fevers, night sweats, heat in the five centers, headache, visual dizziness, dry eyes, tinnitus, aching lower back, and weak legs. Qi consumption is marked by fatigue, lack of appetite, and flaccidity, while blood consumption manifests as insomnia, dizziness, scanty menses, and a pale complexion.

This formula addresses deficiency consumption that primarily displays signs of yin deficiency. Since the formula includes herbs to supplement the blood and qi, it can also treat the multiple deficiencies of qi, yin, and blood that frequently occur in this pattern.

According to *Formulas to Aid the Living,* the narrow meaning of consumptive disease is a "devastating contagious disease that can wipe out an entire household." This disorder, generally thought to be modern-day tuberculosis, occurs when a weakened normal qi is attacked by a type of contagious pest (蟲 *chóng*). Common symptoms of consumptive disease include fatigue, cough, spitting of blood, tidal fevers, night sweats, and gradual weight loss.

Note that some versions of this formula include Chuanxiong Rhizoma (*chuān xiōng*), but ours excludes it. This is probably due to the fact that many practitioners feel that the herb should be used with caution, if at all, in cases of heat from deficiency.

Comparison

➤ Vs. MOONLIGHT PILL (*yuè huá wán*)

Both formulas treat consumptive disease, and both tonify the yin and blood. Decoction to Enrich Yin and Direct Fire Downward (*zī yīn jiàng huǒ tāng*) is better able to drain fire from deficiency and supplement the middle. Moonlight Pill (*yuè huá wán*), on the other hand, can more effectively relieve cough and stanch bleeding but is less useful for symptoms such as steaming bones and night sweats.

Biomedical Indications

With the appropriate presentation, this formula may be used to treat a wide variety of biomedically-defined disorders including pulmonary tuberculosis, pneumonia, pleurisy, acute or chronic bronchitis, pharyngitis, laryngitis, renal tuberculosis, pyelitis, diabetes and perimenopausal syndrome.

Modifications

- For steaming bones and consumptive heat, add Lycii Cortex (*dì gǔ pí*) and either Stellariae Radix (*yín chái hú*) or Bupleuri Radix (*chái hú*). If the heat persists, add 1 gram of Zingiberis Rhizoma praeparatum (*páo jiāng*). (source text)
- For incessant night sweats with deficiency of qi and blood,

add Astragali Radix (*huáng qí*) and Ziziphi spinosae Semen (*suān zǎo rén*). (source text)
- For phlegm-fire cough with wheezing, add Mori Cortex (*sāng bái pí*), Asteris Radix (*zǐ wǎn*), Scutellariae Radix (*huáng qín*), and Bambusae Succus (*zhú lì*). (source text)
- For dry cough, sore throat, throat sores, and loss of voice, add Scutellariae Radix (*huáng qín*), Trichosanthis Semen (*guā lóu rén*), Fritillariae thunbergii Bulbus (*zhè bèi mǔ*), Schisandrae Fructus (*wǔ wèi zǐ*), Armeniacae Semen (*xìng rén*), Mori Cortex (*sāng bái pí*), Asteris Radix (*zǐ wǎn*), and Gardeniae Fructus (*zhī zǐ*). (source text)
- For nocturnal emissions, add Dioscoreae Rhizoma (*shān yào*), Ostreae Concha (*mǔ lì*), Eucommiae Cortex (*dù zhòng*), Psoraleae Fructus (*bǔ gǔ zhī*), and Achyranthis bidentatae Radix (*niú xī*). Remove Asparagi Radix (*tiān mén dōng*). (source text)
- For consumptive disease, add Stemonae Radix (*bǎi bù*) and Mori Cortex (*sāng bái pí*).
- If the qi is deficient, add Cordyceps (*dōng chóng xià cǎo*).
- With coughing of blood, add Asini Corii Colla (*ē jiāo*), Bletillae Rhizoma (*bái jí*), and Imperatae Rhizoma (*bái máo gēn*).
- For nonproductive cough, add Lilii Bulbus (*bǎi hé*).
- If the middle burner is compromised with lack of appetite and loose stools, reduce or remove Asparagi Radix (*tiān mén dōng*), Ophiopogonis Radix (*mài mén dōng*), and Rehmanniae Radix (*shēng dì huáng*) and add Codonopsis Radix (*dǎng shēn*), Coicis Semen (*yì yǐ rén*), Amomi Fructus (*shā rén*), and Nelumbinis Semen (*lián zǐ*). (source text)

瓊玉膏 (琼玉膏)
Precious Jade Syrup

qióng yù gāo

Source *Hong's Collection of Experiential Formulas* (1170)

The Chinese term 瓊玉 *qióng yù* refers to particularly beautiful and precious jade, and jade is related to fluids. According to *Discussion of Famous Physicians' Formulas Past and Present,* "[This formula] raises us from deep-seated illness, making it more precious than exquisite jade. Thus, it was given the name Precious Jade Syrup."

Ginseng Radix (*rén shēn*) 750g
Rehmanniae Radix (*shēng dì huáng*) 8kg
Poria (*fú líng*) 1.5kg
good quality honey (*bái mì*) 5kg

Method of Preparation Syrup. The modern way to prepare the syrup is to boil the herbs in water three times: the first time for 4 hours, the second time for 3 hours, and the third time for 2 hours. The strained liquid so obtained is then mixed together and allowed to settle. The clear liquid at the top is filtered off, while the denser liquid at the bottom is mixed with the honey by warming it over a low flame. The liquid is filtered once more to remove any froth before allowing it to cool down. The recommended dosage is 9-15g twice a day to be taken with warm water. Note that the source text calls for Korean ginseng.

Actions　Enriches the yin, moistens the Lungs, augments the qi, and tonifies the Spleen

Indications

Dry cough with little sputum accompanied by a dry throat or spitting of blood, muscle wasting, shortness of breath, weakness, a red tongue with little coating, and a thin, rapid pulse.

This is yin deficiency consumptive disorder, a chronic condition where the normal qi is progressively depleted until the yin of the Lungs and Kidneys is exhausted. When the Lungs lose their ability to moisten and the fluids are depleted, qi rebels upward, causing cough with little sputum. Yin deficiency leads to an up-flaring of empty fire, which dries the throat. Fire also damages the Lung collaterals, causing spitting of blood. Attributed to fire from deficiency, this manifests as sporadic coughing up of a few drops of blood rather than blood-streaked sputum or vomiting of blood. Chronic Lung deficiency drains earth (Spleen) because a child depletes its mother, leading to muscle wasting and loss of weight. More generalized signs of qi deficiency are weakness and shortness of breath. The tongue and pulse reflect the yin deficiency that is the root of this disorder.

Analysis of Formula

The chief herb in this formula is Rehmanniae Radix *(shēng dì huáng)*, which enriches the Kidney yin, clears heat, cools the blood, and directs empty fire downward to stop the bleeding. Good quality honey, described as 'whitish' in Chinese, serves as the deputy. Sweet and balanced in its action, it moistens the Lungs, stops coughing, enriches the Spleen, and augments the Stomach. According to *Transforming the Significance of Medicinal Substances*:

> Honey is the essence of all varieties of flowers gathered by the bees. Its sweet taste governs tonification, [hence] it enriches and nourishes the five yin organs. Its slippery nature governs facilitation [of movement, hence] it lubricates the Triple Burner. Where the Lungs are desiccated and the lobes retracted in physically weakened people who cough incessantly, it leads to the development of a dry Lung presentation. As there is neither cold nor heat [pathogens present,] medicines are seldom effective. [But few people] will not respond to using two morsels of old honey daily for about a month. The intention [of this strategy] is to moisten dryness.

Together, Rehmanniae Radix *(shēng dì huáng)* and honey tonify the yin of both metal and water, moisten dryness, and facilitate movement to stop coughing.

Ginseng Radix *(rén shēn)* and Poria *(fú líng)* serve as assistants to augment the qi and build up the Spleen. The inten-

tion is to build up earth in order to tonify metal. By improving the Spleen's transportive and transformative functions, these two herbs facilitate the assimilation of what is a very rich formula and reduce the risk that the cloying nature of the chief and deputy herbs will obstruct the qi dynamic.

The preparation of the formula as a syrup makes this a very mild-acting formula that must be taken long-term (i.e., for 1-2 months) to be effective.

Cautions and Contraindications

Although the formula contains herbs that tonify the middle burner and drain dampness, its main purpose is to enrich the yin. Thus, it should not be used where there are clear signs of deficiency of the middle burner such as soft stools or bloating after eating. The formula is strongly tonifying and is indicated for long-term use. If the patient contracts an external pathogen, its use should be discontinued until the pathogen has been cleared.

Commentary

This formula is one of the first medicinal syrups found in Chinese formularies. It has therefore exerted considerable influence on the practice of Chinese medicine, particularly in the Yangzi River delta. According to the source text, its original range of application was wider than that listed in contemporary textbooks:

> It fills the essence and tonifies the marrow [so that] blood transforms into sinews, the myriad spirits are all satisfied, the five yin organs are filled to the brim, the marrow is excessive and the blood full, white hair turns black, excessive aging is turned back toward youthfulness, and there are no nightmares or thoughts at night.

Later generations modified the formula in various ways. The Ming-dynasty text *Correct Transmission of Medicine*, for example, added Succinum *(hǔ pò)* and Aquilariae Lignum resinatum *(chén xiāng)* to facilitate the moving aspects of the formula, the first focusing on enlivening the blood and quieting the Heart, and the second on directing the qi downward into the Kidneys. *Selected Formulas to Support Longevity*, on the other hand, focused more on the tonification of essence and fluids by adding Ophiopogonis Radix *(mài mén dōng)*, Asparagi Radix *(tiān mén dōng)*, and Lycii Fructus *(gǒu qǐ zǐ)*. Meanwhile, the range of indications was gradually narrowed until, in *Golden Mirror of the Medical Tradition*, all that remained was "deficiency consumption and Lung atrophy."

As one of the first formulas to simultaneously tonify the Lung and Kidney yin in order to treat dryness, Precious Jade Syrup *(qióng yù gāo)* established a precedent that is reflected in many other formulas discussed in this chapter. At the same time, its use of Ginseng Radix *(rén shēn)* and Poria *(fú líng)* adhered to the strategy of building earth in order to tonify metal that was first employed in Ophiopogonis Decoction *(mài mén dōng tāng).* The inclusion of Poria *(fú líng)* has attracted particular attention from the commentators. The 19th-century physician Fei Bo-Xiong noted in *Discussion of Medical Formulas*:

> Ginseng Radix *(rén shēn)* and Rehmanniae Radix *(shēng dì huáng)* simultaneously tonify the qi and blood to mutually generate metal and water. [The author] furthermore adds Poria *(fú líng)* in order to settle the Heart and tonify the earth. As water ascends and fire directs downward, the coughing stops by itself.

In *Annotated Fine Formulas from Generations of Famous Physicians*, the modern physician Ruan Xue-Feng provides a somewhat different interpretation:

> The marvel [of this formula] lies in how Poria *(fú líng)* filters out [dampness] and promotes water metabolism through draining downward. [In this manner,] it promotes [the function of the] Bladder in order to unblock the yang organs. … Poria *(fú líng)* in this formula transforms the qi in order to unblock the yang in the lower burner.

Ruan Xue-Feng's commentary is important, not only in its explanation of a specific herb's usage, but because it points to the essential difference between those formulas that moisten dryness and those that tonify yin. While the intention of the latter is merely to add substance, the ultimate purpose of the former is always to facilitate movement. This is why formulas that tonify the yin generally focus on the Kidneys (concerned with storage of essence and fluids) while those that moisten focus on the Lungs (concerned with the movement of fluids and qi).

Another major impact of Precious Jade Syrup *(qióng yù gāo)* on the development of Chinese medicine was its role in popularizing the use of medicinal syrups. Used initially for the treatment of chronic deficiency disorders, syrups gradually developed into a popular instrument for strengthening a person's constitution, preventing illness, and promoting longevity. Up to the present day, patients in the Yangzi delta still visit their Chinese medicine physicians in late fall for the prescription of a tailor-made syrup. Composed of a mixture of tonifying and moving herbs, the syrup is then taken in the middle of winter to prevent illness during the following year.

Comparisons

➤ Vs. Ophiopogonis Decoction *(mài mén dōng tāng)* and Lily Bulb Decoction to Preserve the Metal *(bǎi hé gù jīn tāng).*

All of these formulas nourish the yin and moisten the Lungs to treat dry cough. Ophiopogonis Decoction *(mài mén dōng tāng)* focuses on treating Lung and Stomach yin in order to direct the qi and fire that have rebelled upward and accumulated in the Lungs downward again. The formula is thus indicated for coughing of frothy saliva or vomiting. Lily Bulb Decoction to Preserve the Metal *(bǎi hé gù jīn tāng)* focuses on tonifying the Kidney and Lung yin in order to clear the fire of deficiency from flaring upward. The formula is thus indicated for cough with blood-streaked phlegm. Precious Jade Syrup *(qióng yù gāo)* focuses on enriching desiccated Lungs and Kidneys accompanied by Spleen deficiency. It is indicated for a dry cough without any phlegm in weak and frail patients.

Biomedical Indications

With the appropriate presentation, this formula may be used to treat a variety of biomedically-defined disorders including diabetes, chronic cough, and pulmonary tuberculosis.

Alternate names

Immortal Precious Jade Syrup *(shén xiān qióng yù gāo)* recorded in *Essential Additions to Observations on Formulas Gathered*; Rehmannia Radix Syrup *(shēng di huáng gāo)* in *Straight Direction from [Yang] Ren-Zhai*; Precious Jade Gelatin *(qióng yù jiāo)* in *The Rectification of Deficiency and an Examination of its Origins*

Associated Formula

三才湯 （三才汤）

Three-Talents Decoction

sān caí tāng

Source *Medical Formulas Collected and Analyzed* (1682)

Asparagi Radix *(tiān mén dōng)*
Rehmanniae Radix praeparata *(shú dì huáng)*
Ginseng Radix *(rén shēn)*

Use equal amounts of the three herbs to make a decoction. Nourishes the yin, augments the qi, moistens the Lungs, and stops coughing. For consumptive coughing from Lung and Spleen deficiency. This is a variation of Three-Talents Pill *(sān caí wán)*, first listed in *Confucians' Duties to Their Parents*. Compared to Precious Jade Syrup *(qióng yù gāo)*, this formula contains Rehmanniae Radix praeparata *(shú dì huáng)* and is prepared as a decoction. This implies a stronger focus on the tonification of yin and blood and the expectation of a quicker effect. Both formulas treat weak and emaciated patients suffering from a dry cough. In clinical practice, one uses Three-Talents Decoction *(sān caí tāng)* for a simple cough, while Precious Jade Syrup *(qióng yù gāo)* is indicated where the cough is accompanied by occasional spitting of small amounts of blood.

駐景丸 （驻景丸）

Preserve Vistas Pill

zhù jǐng wán

The name of this formula is derived from its ability to preserve the vision, which enables the eyes to take in panoramic vistas.

Source *Indispensable Tools for Pattern Treatment* (1602)

Cuscutae Semen *(tù sī zǐ)* 150g
Rehmanniae Radix praeparata *(shú dì huáng)*. 120g
Plantaginis Semen *(chē qián zǐ)* 60g

Method of Preparation　Grind the ingredients into a powder and form into pills with honey. Take 6-12g before meals with a soup made from Poria *(fú líng)* and Acori tatarinowii Rhizoma *(shí chāng pǔ)*. May also be prepared as a decoction by reducing the dosage to about one-tenth of that specified above.

Actions　Tonifies and nourishes the Liver and Kidneys, enriches the yin, and improves the vision

Indications

Diminished visual acuity and blurred vision that worsens with exertion and improves with rest, soreness and weakness of the lower back and legs, and a thin, frail pulse.

This is diminished vision due to Liver and Kidney deficiency, with some dampness caused by a reduction in fluid metabolism. The Liver stores the blood and is associated with the eyes. Good vision requires that the eyes are nourished with blood. The Kidneys store the essence. Good vision also requires that the essence from all of the organs reaches the eyes. When the Liver and Kidneys are deficient, the eyes are deprived of the nourishment from blood, and the essence does not reach the eyes in full strength. This leads to diminished visual acuity in general, and blurred vision in particular. Dampness can also block the sensory organs and aggravate the symptoms. Symptoms that worsen with exertion and improve with rest are characteristic of deficiency. The soreness and weakness in the lower back, as well as the thin pulse, are indicative of Liver and Kidney deficiency, while the frail aspect of the pulse reflects a combination of deficiency and dampness.

Analysis of Formula

One of the chief herbs, Rehmanniae Radix praeparata *(shú dì huáng)*, enriches the yin and tonifies the Kidneys. It also nourishes the blood, especially of the Liver. In concert with the other chief herb, Cuscutae Semen *(tù sī zǐ)*, which tonifies the Liver and Kidneys, it has a powerful effect on the root cause of this disorder. When the Liver blood is ample, the eyes are nourished and the vision is acute; when the Kidney essence is sufficient, it rises to the eyes and keeps them clear. The deputy, Plantaginis Semen *(chē qián zǐ)*, improves visual acuity by promoting the proper metabolism of fluids and the draining of dampness.

The assistant herbs are aromatic Acori tatarinowii Rhizoma *(shí chāng pǔ)*, which transforms turbidity, and bland Poria *(fú líng)*, which leaches out dampness. These ingredients improve visual acuity by transforming and draining dampness, and also ensure that the rich, cloying nature of the chief herbs does not cause stagnation. This is an excellent example of using herbs with seemingly contradictory actions to produce a desired effect.

Commentary

This formula focuses on treating both excess and deficiency,

tonifying the Kidneys below and draining pathogenic water from above. It thereby responds to a pathological dynamic that is at the heart of many eye disorders, first described in Chapter 10 of *Divine Pivot*: "When the Kidneys are perturbed … the eyes blur and one cannot see clearly." In conjunction with the other symptoms listed in the passage, such as wheezing, restlessness, and gnawing hunger, it appears to describe a pattern where the qi is unable to return to the Kidneys in the lower burner and thus rebels upward. This qi, of course, is partly water, which should move to the lower burner to be transformed by the Bladder under the control of the Kidneys. Chapter 22 of *Basic Questions* attributes the same kind of eye disorder to Liver deficiency. Again, the Liver not only has the function of storing blood, but also of mobilizing the qi and fluids. Any impairment of Liver and Kidney function in the lower burner may thus be accompanied by water excess in the upper burner.

In practice, this impairment may be due to excess as well as deficiency. This formula is indicated only if other signs corroborate the diagnosis. Yang deficiency should be treated with formulas like True Warrior Decoction *(zhēn wǔ tāng)*, Poria, Cinnamon Twig, Atractylodes, and Licorice Decoction *(líng guì zhú gān tāng)*, or Five-Ingredient Powder with Poria *(wǔ líng sǎn)* with the addition of herbs like Plantaginis Herba *(chē qián cǎo)* that transform the qi and move water. Damp-heat disorders, on the other hand, should be treated with formulas like Sweet Wormwood and Scutellaria Decoction to Clear the Gallbladder *(hāo qín qīng dǎn tāng)*, Three-Seed Decoction *(sān rén tāng)*, or Gentian Decoction to Drain the Liver *(lóng dǎn xiè gān tāng)*.

Comparison

➢ Vs. Improve Vision Pill with Rehmannia *(míng mù dì huáng wán)*

Both formulas treat diminished visual acuity and blurred vision. Preserve Vistas Pill *(zhù jǐng wán)* is more effective in treating chronically poor vision due to deficiency of essence accompanied by dampness. It focuses more on the Kidneys, and contains a larger dosage of dampness-leaching herbs. By contrast, Improve Vision Pill with Rehmannia *(míng mù dì huáng wán)* is more effective in treating chronic visual disorders due primarily to blood deficiency, heat from deficiency, and associated Kidney problems.

Associated Formulas

駐景丸加減方 （驻景丸加减方）

Formula Modified from Preserve Vistas Pill

zhù jǐng wán jiā jiǎn fāng

SOURCE　*Methodology for Using the Six Warps in Ophthalmology* (1979)

Cuscutae Semen (*tù sī zǐ*)............................240g
Broussonetiae Fructus (*chǔ shí zǐ*)................240g
Lycii Fructus (*gǒu qǐ zǐ*).............................60g
Plantaginis Semen (*chē qián zǐ*)....................60g
Glauberitum (*hán shuǐ shí*)..........................90g
Schisandrae Fructus (*wǔ wèi zǐ*)....................60g
Leonuri Fructus (*chōng wèi zǐ*).....................180g
Notoginseng Radix (*sān qī*)...........................15g
Hominis Placenta (*zǐ hé chē*)...........................9g
Chaenomelis Fructus (*mù guā*)..........................6g

Grind the ingredients into a powder and make into pills with honey. Take 30g per day with warm water. Tonifies the blood and essence, regulates water metabolism, clears the Liver, and brightens the eyes. For impaired vision, especially for difficulty seeing in the distance, while close-up vision remains relatively unimpaired. This is a formula devised by Chen Da-Fu, an expert in the treatment of eye disorders from Chengdu.

This formula uses many seeds, which are thought to both embody the potential of essence and to direct the qi downward. Two herbs have been included for reasons related to the author's understanding of biomedical pathophysiology. Chaenomelis Fructus (*mù guā*), which is traditionally associated with relaxing the sinews, is thought to have a beneficial effect on the optic nerve, which is viewed as a kind of sinew. Notoginseng Radix (*sān qī*) moves the blood and transforms stasis, helping Plantaginis Semen (*chē qián zǐ*) move excess water toward the lower burner, as well as benefiting microcirculation in the eyes.

石斛夜光丸

Dendrobium Pill for Night Vision

shí hú yè guāng wán

SOURCE *Experiential Formulas from the Auspicious Bamboo Hall* (1326)

dry-fried Asparagi Radix (*chǎo tiān mén dōng*)..............30g
Ginseng Radix (*rén shēn*)............................30g
Poria (*fú líng*).....................................30g
prepared Ophiopogonis Radix (*zhì mài mén dōng*).........30g
Rehmanniae Radix praeparata (*shú dì huáng*)............30g
Cuscutae Semen (*tù sī zǐ*)..........................22.5g
white Chrysanthemi Flos (*bái jú huā*)...............22.5g
dry-fried Cassiae Semen (*chǎo jué míng zǐ*).........22.5g
dry-fried Armeniacae Semen (*chǎo xìng rén*).........22.5g
Dioscoreae Rhizoma (*shān yào*).......................30g
Lycii Fructus (*gǒu qǐ zǐ*)..........................22.5g
wine-prepared Achyranthis bidentatae Radix (*jiǔ niú xī*).........21g
dry-fried Schisandrae Fructus (*chǎo wǔ wèi zǐ*)........15g
dry-fried Astragali complanati Semen (*chǎo shā yuàn zǐ*).......15g
Dendrobii Herba (*shí hú*).........................22.5g
wine-prepared Cistanches Herba (*jiǔ cōng róng*)........15g
Chuanxiong Rhizoma (*chuān xiōng*)....................15g
Glycyrrhizae Radix praeparata (*zhì gān cǎo*).........15g
bran-fried Aurantii Fructus (*fū chǎo zhǐ ké*)........15g
Celosiae Semen (*qīng xiāng zǐ*)......................15g
Saposhnikoviae Radix (*fáng fēng*)....................15g
Coptidis Rhizoma (*huáng lián*).......................15g
[Bubali Cornu (*shuǐ niú jiǎo*).......................45g]
Saigae tataricae Cornu (*líng yáng jiǎo*).............15g

Grind the ingredients into a powder and form into 9g pills with honey. Take one pill in the morning and another in the evening with salted water. Note that the original text calls for 15g of Rhinocerotis Cornu (*xī jiǎo*), which is no longer done, primarily due to the endangered status of the rhinoceros. Extinguishes Liver wind, enriches the yin, and improves the vision. For visual disturbances due to insufficient Liver and Kidney yin leading to fire from deficiency and internal wind. This is characterized by enlarged pupils, blurred vision, photophobia, excessive tearing, lightheadedness, and vertigo. At present, it is used for various ophthalmological problems, especially cataracts, as well as appropriate cases of hypertension.

益胃湯 (益胃汤)

Benefit the Stomach Decoction

yì wèi tāng

Source *Systematic Differentiation of Warm Pathogen Diseases* (1798)

Glehniae/Adenophorae Radix (*shā shēn*)...............9g
Ophiopogonis Radix (*mài mén dōng*)..................15g
Rehmanniae Radix (*shēng dì huáng*).................15g
dry-fried Polygonati odorati Rhizoma (*chǎo yù zhú*).......4.5g
Saccharum cristallisatum (*bīng táng*)................3g

Method of Preparation Boil the ingredients in 5 cups of water until 2 cups remain. Divide into two portions and drink warm. The herbs are then decocted again with the same amount of water until 1 cup remains, which is taken as a third dose.

Actions Benefits the Stomach and generates fluids

Indications

A faint or indistinct pain or burning in the epigastric region, hunger but no desire to actually eat, a dry mouth and throat, constipation, retching, hiccup, a dry, red tongue with scanty coating, and a thin rapid pulse.

This is Stomach yin deficiency. The Stomach is in charge of receiving food and drink. It likes moisture and abhors dryness. Chronic Stomach disorders, fevers that scorch the yin fluids, habitual consumption of spicy, acrid foods, the overuse of laxatives, vomiting, or inappropriate purging can all harm the Stomach yin, deplete the fluids, and thereby generate internal heat. When the Stomach yin becomes insufficient, it fails to moisten the collaterals, causing a faint or indistinct pain or burning in the epigastric region. The heat, reflecting excessive yang, makes the patient feel hungry, but because this heat arises from deficiency, there is no desire to actually eat. Insufficient fluids in the Stomach can cause constipation characterized by dry stools. Alternatively, yin deficiency with yang excess harms the Stomach's downward-directing functions, causing retching and hiccup. The root of the disorder is reflected in the dry, red tongue with scanty coating, and the thin, rapid pulse.

Analysis of Formula

To treat Stomach yin deficiency, this formula benefits the Stomach and generates fluids. Its chief herbs are Rehmanniae Radix *(shēng dì huáng)* and Ophiopogonis Radix *(mài mén dōng)*, both of which are sweet, cooling, and moistening and thereby address both the root (yin deficiency) and the branch (internal heat). The deputies, Glehniae Radix *(běi shā shēn)* and Polygonati odorati Rhizoma *(yù zhú)*, have a similar action. Entering the Stomach channel, they also direct the action of the chief herbs more specifically to this organ. Saccharum cristallisatum *(bīng táng)* moistens the Lungs, benefits the Stomach, and, as a primarily sweet substance, moderates the actions of the other herbs. It is therefore considered to be both the assistant and the envoy in this formula. The combined actions of these five herbs nourishes the yin without being cloying, which would further obstruct the downward-directing function of the Stomach. The herbs clear heat without being excessively cooling or even drying, and thereby treat Stomach heat without damaging the yang qi.

Cautions and Contraindications

This formula is cooling, enriching, and moistening. It is inappropriate for patients with dampness obstructing the middle burner, which manifests as focal distention and a greasy tongue coating.

Commentary

This formula was composed by the Qing-dynasty writer Wu Ju-Tong to treat qi-level yang brightness-warp warm pathogen disorders where sweating occurs after the condition has been purged. Wu Ju-Tong interpreted such a pattern to mean that the Stomach yin had been injured, since after purgation has drained pathogenic heat from the body, the patient should normally recover. Thus, the sweating in this case does not indicate an attempt by the body to disperse a pathogen from the exterior, but is an uncontrolled upward movement of the yang qi that carries the fluids with it and leaks them to the outside. Because, in a warm pathogen disorder, heat quickly injures the body fluids, the emphasis in treatment thus should not be on directing the yang downward, nor on clearing the heat, but on nourishing the Stomach yin.

The combination of the two chief herbs in this formula—Ophiopogonis Radix *(mài mén dōng)* and Rehmanniae Radix *(shēng dì huáng)*—was commonly employed by Wu Ju-Tong for the purpose of restoring fluids that have been damaged by heat pathogens. Increase the Fluids Decoction *(zēng yè tāng)*, discussed in Chapter 15, can be regarded as the model for this usage. That formula, in turn, can be viewed as being derived from Prepared Licorice Decoction *(zhì gān cǎo tāng)*, discussed above, which was composed for the purpose of treating injury to both the qi and fluids in the course of a cold damage disorder. Wu Ju-Tong borrowed the two

sweet, cooling, and moistening ingredients from that formula and combined them with herbs such as Scrophulariae Radix *(xuán shēn)*, Trichosanthis Radix *(tiān huā fěn)*, and Polygonati odorati Rhizoma *(yù zhú)*. This is another example of the close relationship between the strategies for the treatment of cold damage and warm pathogen disorders.

Although the formula was originally composed for treating patterns that arise in the course of warm pathogen disorders, it is used at present to treat any pattern where Stomach yin deficiency is the root. Besides the symptoms listed above, such patterns may also manifest with dizziness, ulcerations in the oral cavity, picky eating in children, as well as dental problems.

Biomedical Indications

With the appropriate presentation, this formula may be used to treat a variety of biomedically-defined disorders including chronic gastritis and diabetes.

Modifications

- For yin deficiency with more pronounced internal heat or fever, add Scrophulariae Radix *(xuán shēn)* and Trichosanthis Radix *(tiān huā fěn)*.
- For conccurent qi deficiency, add Pseudostellariae Radix *(tài zǐ shēn)* and Dioscoreae Rhizoma *(shān yào)*.
- For gnawing hunger with no desire for food, add sweet and sour herbs like Mume Fructus *(wū méi)*, Chaenomelis Fructus *(mù guā)*, Paeoniae Radix alba *(bái sháo)*, and Glycyrrhizae Radix *(gān cǎo)*, as well as herbs that transform food stagnation and move the qi such as Setariae (Oryzae) Fructus germinatus *(gǔ yá)*, Hordei Fructus germinatus *(mài yá)*, Massa medicata fermentata *(shén qū)*, and Citri reticulatae Pericarpium *(chén pí)*.
- For faint or indistinct pain or burning in the epigastric region, add Paeoniae Radix alba *(bái sháo)* and Glycyrrhizae Radix *(gān cǎo)*.
- For retching or hiccup, add Bambusae Caulis in taeniam *(zhú rú)* and Eriobotryae Folium *(pí pá yè)*.
- For dry stools, add Angelicae sinensis Radix *(dāng guī)*, Paeoniae Radix alba *(bái sháo)*, Cannabis Semen *(huǒ má rén)*, Sesami Semen nigrum *(hēi zhī má)*, and Achyranthis bidentatae Radix *(niú xī)*.

Associated Formulas

甘露飲 (甘露饮)

Sweet Dew Drink

gān lù yǐn

SOURCE   *Formulary of the Pharmacy Service for Benefiting the People in the Taiping Era* (1107)

Rehmanniae Radix *(shēng dì huáng)* 9g
Rehmanniae Radix praeparata *(shú dì huáng)* 9g

Dendrobii Herba (*shí hú*) 9g
Asparagi Radix (*tiān mén dōng*) .12g
Ophiopogonis Radix (*mài mén dōng*) 12g
Scutellariae Radix (*huáng qín*) 9g
Artemisiae scopariae Herba (*yīn chén*) 9g
Aurantii Fructus (*zhǐ ké*) 9g
Eriobotryae Folium (*pí pá yè*) 24g
Glycyrrhizae Radix (*gān cǎo*) 6g

The source text advises to coarsely grind equal amounts of the ingredients and take in 6g doses as a draft. At present, it is usually prepared as a decoction with the dosage specified above. Nourishes the yin, clears heat, disseminates the Lung qi, and resolves dampness. This is residual heat in the yang brightness warp that arises in the course of a cold damage disorder and damages the yang fluids. The residual heat, often also involving a degree of dampness, is reflected in the swollen gums with or without pus, mouth ulcers, bad breath, sore throat, and the dry, red tongue with a yellow, greasy coating. All yang brightness-warp patterns are characterized by heat excess and damage to the yang fluids. The customary treatment strategy at this stage is to focus on clearing and draining pathogenic heat. This orders the qi dynamic and prevents further damage to the fluids. In this case, however, the dry tongue and sore throat in the absence of signs indicating knotting of heat in the interior suggests that dryness is predominant. For this reason, the formula focuses on generating fluids as the primary route for supporting the normal qi. The use of this formula has been expanded recently to include treatment of some eye disorders (the Stomach channel terminates near the eyes) as well as other conditions with yin deficiency and damp-heat.

Section 5

FORMULAS THAT WARM AND TONIFY THE YANG

The formulas in this section are used for treating patterns of yang deficiency by warming and tonifying the yang. In contemporary China, they are used above all for tonification of the Kidney yang. There are two reasons for this. First, for both historical and physiological reasons, formulas that tonify the yang of the Spleen and Heart are generally listed as formulas that warm the interior (discussed in Chapter 3). Second, contemporary Chinese medicine emphasizes an organ-centered perspective. In this view, the functions of the Kidneys include those of the gate of vitality, even though throughout history many physicians considered them to be different physiological and anatomical entities. These differences of opinion will be highlighted in some of the COMMENTARY sections of the formulas below.

The principal manifestation of the type of yang deficiency treated by the formulas in this section is systemic exhaustion, usually accompanied by a sensation of cold or aversion to cold. Because this type of cold is due to deficiency, that is, something that the body is lacking, simply wearing more clothing will often alleviate it. This is in contrast to the sensation of cold or chills associated with an exterior condition, which cannot be alleviated by putting on more clothing. Other common manifestations of yang deficiency include withdrawal into oneself, aversion to cold, cold extremities, soreness and weakness of the lower back and lower extremities, a pale tongue, and a submerged, frail pulse (particularly at the proximal position on the right). Accompanying signs and symptoms are manifold and include impotence, spermatorrhea, watery leukorrhea, enuresis, frequent and copious urination, wheezing, daybreak diarrhea, and wasting and thirsting disorder.

In these formulas, the interdependence of yin and yang is clearly seen. Ingredients that tonify the yang are generally combined with those that tonify the yin. Neither yang nor yin can exist and flourish independently of the other. In this respect, yin and yang are said to have a mutual root and should be tonified together so that yang may be generated from yin. Sometimes this is achieved by combining a yin-tonifying herb like Rehmanniae Radix praeparata (*shú dì huáng*) with one that mobilizes the yang, such as Aconiti Radix lateralis praeparata (*zhì fù zǐ*) or Cinnamomi Cortex (*ròu guì*). At other times, these functions are inherent to a greater or lesser extent within individual substances, such as Cervi Cornu pantotrichum (*lù róng*) (which is warming, but is itself the essence of an animal), Cistanches Herba (*ròu cōng róng*) (which is both moistening and yang-tonifying), or Cuscutae Semen (*tù sī zǐ*) (which tonifies both the yang and the yin).

Because the production of yang qi is intimately associated with the transformation of water, yang deficiency invariably is accompanied by fluid pathologies. For this reason, the formulas in this section tend to include herbs that promote the metabolism of water, drain dampness, or transform phlegm.

腎氣丸（肾气丸）

Kidney Qi Pill

shèn qì wán

In Chapter 5 of *Basic Questions*, it is noted that "the lesser [Kidney] fire generates qi." This formula combines herbs that nourish the yin with those that tonify the yang, not so much to tonify the Kidney fire itself, but as a means of generating Kidney qi. It is therefore named 'Kidney Qi Pill' rather than 'Kidney Yang Pill' (see COMMENTARY below).

Source   *Essentials from the Golden Cabinet* (c. 220)

Rehmanniae Radix (*shēng dì huáng*) 24g
Corni Fructus (*shān zhū yú*) 12g
Dioscoreae Rhizoma (*shān yào*) .12g
baked Aconiti Radix lateralis (*bāo fù zǐ*) 3g
Cinnamomi Ramulus (*guì zhī*) 3g
Alismatis Rhizoma (*zé xiè*) 9g
Poria (*fú líng*) 9g
Moutan Cortex (*mǔ dān pí*) 9g

Method of Preparation   Grind the ingredients into a powder and form into small pills with honey. Take 6-9g of the pills once or twice daily with warm water. Rehmanniae Radix praeparata *(shú dì huáng)* is often substituted for Rehmanniae Radix *(shēng dì huáng)*, and Cinnamomi Cortex *(ròu guì)* for Cinnamomi Ramulus *(guì zhī)*. At present, when prepared as pills, the dosage of the ingredients is increased by a factor of ten. May also be prepared as a decoction.

Actions   Warms and tonifies the Kidney yang

Indications

Lower back pain, weakness of the lower extremities, a cold sensation in the lower half of the body, tenseness in the lower abdomen, a pale, swollen tongue with a thin, white, and moist coating, and an empty or frail pulse that is submerged and faint at the proximal position. The patient may also be irritable to the point of experiencing difficulty lying down, and will breathe most comfortably while leaning against something. There is either urinary difficulty with edema, or excessive urination, sometimes to the point of incontinence.

This is the classic presentation of Kidney yang deficiency with insufficient fire at the gate of vitality. From an organ systems perspective, the Kidneys are the foundation of the pre-natal essence and store the essence. Essence transforms into qi, and the qi that arises from the transformation of Kidney essence is what is meant by the term 'Kidney qi.' Kidney qi is also known as 'Kidney yang' or 'source yang,' as it is the basis for the yang of the entire body and the source of motivating power underlying the body's functions of movement.

The Kidneys govern the bones and reside in the lower back, and the Kidney channel ascends from the foot and enters the spine to pass upward through the lower back. Kidney deficiency is therefore accompanied by lower back pain and weakness of the lower extremities. From the spine, a branch of the channel diverges and enters the abdomen. When the Kidney yang is deficient, it is unable to warm the lower burner, which causes a cold sensation in the lower half of the body and tenseness in the lower abdomen. Stagnation of water and fluids produces a pale, swollen tongue with a thin, white, and moist coating. Kidney yang deficiency generally manifests as an empty or frail pulse that is submerged and faint at the proximal (Kidney) position.

The yang qi of the Kidneys drives the functional transformation and movement of water in the body, directing the pure upward and the turbid downward. When the Kidney yang is insufficient, its ability to regulate the ascent and descent of water and fluids is impaired. Various symptoms of urinary difficulty may result. If the Kidneys are unable to transform qi and move water, there will be urinary difficulty and edema. The water and qi may also rebel upward, causing panting and irritability to the point that the patient will have difficulty lying down, and will lean against something for support. In those instances where the debilitated Kidney qi is unable to provide stability in the governance of water, the Bladder may lose its ability to restrain the water, manifesting as frequent and copious urination, or, in severe cases, incontinence.

Analysis of Formula

To treat Kidney yang deficiency this formula employs a strategy of tonifying the Kidneys in order to assist the yang. Following the adage coined by Wang Bing, the Tang commentator on the *Inner Classic*, "In order to benefit the source of fire, one must eliminate the yin that conceals it," the formula also uses as assistants herbs that promote the metabolism of water. Its chief herbs are acrid and strongly warming Aconiti Radix lateralis praeparata *(zhì fù zǐ)*, which tonifies the source fire, dispels cold, and eliminates dampness, and acrid, sweet, and warming Cinnamomi Ramulus *(guì zhī)*, which benefits the joints, warms the channels, and unblocks the vessels. Aconiti Radix lateralis praeparata *(zhì fù zǐ)* also strongly promotes movement and reaches down to the source to warm chronic cold, while Cinnamomi Ramulus *(guì zhī)* also promotes qi transformation in the Bladder. Together, these herb not only assist the yang and enhance the metabolism of water, but also promote the unhindered dispersion of yang throughout the body. The relatively small dosage of these ingredients suggests that they are intended only to slightly generate yang in order to strengthen the Kidney qi.

There are three deputies. The first, sweet and cooling Rehmanniae Radix *(shēng dì huáng)*, enriches the yin and generates fluids. Its large dosage relative to the other ingredients reflects the importance of tonifying the Kidneys and replenishing the yin, one of the principles underlying the composition of this formula. This principle was summed up by Zhang Jie-Bin in an oft-quoted passage from his *Classified Classic*: "Experts in tonifying the yang invariably assist the yang from within the yin. For when yang avails itself of the assistance of yin, generation and transformation are never exhausted." The other deputies are Corni Fructus *(shān zhū yú)* and Dioscoreae Rhizoma *(shān yào)*, which tonify the Liver and benefit the Spleen in order to tonify and reinforce the essence and blood. Sour and slightly warming Corni Fructus *(shān zhū yú)* tonifies the Liver and Kidneys, thereby helping to preserve the essential qi while nourishing the yin and reinforcing the blood. Strengthening the Kidney qi is beneficial to its role as repository of the body's yin and yang. It also ensures that nourishment will be supplied to the Liver, which derives its essence from the Kidneys. The supply of yin and essence to the Liver serves to facilitate the free and smooth operation of its spreading function. Sweet and bland Dioscoreae Rhizoma *(shān yào)* strengthens the Spleen, stabilizes the Kidneys, and nourishes the essence. It is effective in treating deficiency and various consumptive patterns.

The three assistants are Alismatis Rhizoma *(zé xiè)*, Poria *(fú líng)*, and Moutan Cortex *(mǔ dān pí)*. Their purpose is to regulate the three yin organs: the Kidneys, Liver, and Spleen. Alismatis Rhizoma *(zé xiè)* unblocks and regulates the water passageways, Poria *(fú líng)* strengthens the Spleen and drains dampness, and Moutan Cortex *(mǔ dān pí)* clears heat and quells Liver fire. These herbs work synergistically with Rehmanniae Radix *(shēng dì huáng)*, Corni Fructus *(shān zhū yú)*, and Dioscoreae Rhizoma *(shān yào)* to provide a draining action as an accompaniment to the primary strategy of tonification. Thus, Alismatis Rhizoma *(zé xiè)* and Poria *(fú líng)* unblock and regulate the water passageways, strengthen the Spleen, and drain dampness to enable Cinnamomi Ramulus *(guì zhī)* to warm the Bladder and promote urination by assisting in the transformation of that organ's qi. Moutan Cortex *(mǔ dān pí)* cools the blood, dispels blood stasis, and, in concert with Cinnamomi Ramulus *(guì zhī)*, helps move blood stasis. Together, these two herbs invigorate the blood and thereby facilitate its unimpeded flow to the Kidneys. This accelerates the recovery of that organ.

In summary, this elegantly-balanced formula nourishes without being cloying, warms without producing dryness, tonifies the deficiency of yin to promote the generation of qi, assists the frail yang in its transformation of water, and stimulates the yang to overcome this disorder by restoring the functional capacity of the Kidneys.

Cautions and Contraindications

Contraindicated in cases of yin deficiency with a dry mouth and throat and a red tongue with little coating.

Commentary

Original and Later Indications

This enormously influential formula was composed by the Han-dynasty physician Zhang Zhong-Jing to treat Kidney deficiency patterns across a wide spectrum of illnesses. One primary indication is phlegm and thin mucus, reflecting a disruption of water metabolism due to deficiency. It is also indicated for lower burner-type wasting and thirsting disorder with Kidney yang deficiency characterized by thirst and frequent and copious urination. When the Kidney yang is deficient, it is unable to 'steam' the fluids to the upper part of the body, which causes thirst. The frequent, copious urination is caused by the inability of the deficient Kidneys to stabilize the water and fluids, as well as restrain the Bladder. Zhang Zhong-Jing further prescribed it for treating leg qi disorder in which water and dampness pour into the legs and cause edema of such severity that it interferes with the ability to walk. In fact, the source text recommends it be used for leg qi that ascends and enters the lower abdomen where it causes numbness. Retention of water and dampness in the lower abdomen may lead to numbness. Kidney deficiency with inability to regulate the metabolism of water is also the basis for its indication in deficiency consumption disorders character-

ized by backache, hypertonicity of the lower abdomen, and urinary dysfunction.

Later generations of physicians extended its indications to include all kinds of Kidney and Spleen yang deficiency patterns as well as weak fire at the gate of vitality. It also served as the model for a range of new formulas, the most famous of which is Six-Ingredient Pill with Rehmannia *(liù wèi dì huáng wán)*. In that formula, the Song-dynasty pediatrician Qian Yi removed the two warming ingredients Aconiti Radix lateralis praeparata *(zhì fù zǐ)* and Cinnamomi Ramulus *(guì zhī)*, and substituted Rehmanniae Radix *(shēng dì huáng)* with Rehmanniae Radix praeparata *(shú dì huáng)* to produce a formula that tonifies the Liver and Kidney blood and yin. In other cases, physicians added ingredients to produce variants for the tonification of yang, some of which are listed below.

Another important aspect of the formula is its ability to lead the fire back to its source in the Kidneys. This aspect was highlighted by a modification made during the Tang dynasty that replaced Cinnamomi Ramulus *(guì zhī)* with Cinnamomi Cortex *(ròu guì)* in order to accentuate the warming and tonification of the lower burner that leads the fire back to its source in the Kidneys. The use of this modification is appropriate in treating waning fire at the gate of vitality with deficient yang floating upward characterized by a flushed face, wheezing, severe sweating, weakness and cold of the lower extremities, and a deficient, rootless pulse. This condition should be distinguished from the flushed face and Kidney symptoms associated with Kidney yin insufficiency with ascending fire from deficiency, for which this formula is generally contraindicated.

Debates about the Formula's Composition

The well-balanced design of this formula, which drains in the course of tonifying, has been the subject of much comment by later generations of physicians. Their discussion ranges across a number of different topics and helps to elucidate the formula's composition, function, and clinical usage. The first topic concerns the use of draining herbs in a formula intended to tonify the yang. The renowned Ming-dynasty physician, Li Shi-Zhen, offered this insight:

> Poria *(fú líng)* and Alismatis Rhizoma *(zé xiè)* are both aimed at draining the pathogenic qi from the Bladder. [When] the ancient physicians used tonifying herbs, they necessarily combined them with [herbs that] drain the pathogenic influences. When the pathogenic influences are removed, the tonics gain in strength.

The Qing-dynasty writer Wang Ang noted in his book *Medical Formulas Collected and Analyzed* that these herbs also serve another function: "This formula uses Alismatis Rhizoma *(zé xiè)* like an enemy whose purpose is to connect with and guide Aconiti Radix lateralis praeparata *(zhì fù zǐ)* and Cinnamomi Ramulus *(guì zhī)* into the Kidneys." In fact, most of the formulas in this section contain both draining and tonifying ingredients, the use of which can be traced back to this formula.

A second topic of debate concerns the identity of the chief ingredient. One group of commentators, represented by Wang Lü in his book *Discourse on Tracing Back to the Medical Classics*, considered the chief herb to be Rehmanniae Radix (shēng dì huáng) because its dosage is the largest of all the herbs and also because it enters into the Kidneys to enrich the yin fluids. This function is emphasized even more by those physicians who suggested substituting the warming and tonifying Rehmanniae Radix praeparata (shú dì huáng) for the colder and less Kidney-focused Rehmanniae Radix (shēng dì huáng). Another view is represented by Wang Yi-Luo in *Practical Established Formulas*, who argued that Aconiti Radix lateralis praeparata (zhì fù zǐ) and Cinnamomi Ramulus (guì zhī) should be considered the chief herbs. Although these are interior-warming and yang-moving rather than Kidney-tonifying herbs, they generate qi when combined with yin-tonifying substances, in accordance with Zhang Jie-Bin's dictum to "assist the yang from within the yin." Again, the substitution of Cinnamomi Cortex (ròu guì) for Cinnamomi Ramulus (guì zhī), standard in modern practice, was thought to underscore this function.

Debates about the Formula's Function

Regarding the overall action of the formula, some scholars maintain that it primarily tonifies the yin, others that it nourishes the Liver, and still others that it provides balanced, moderate tonification of the yin and yang. It is perceived as being both very warming and only slightly stimulating of the Kidney fire. Some view it as generating yang via the gate of vitality, others via the Kidneys. Rather than discussing these many opinions in detail, an understanding of the formula's actions and indications may best be reached by grasping the connection among three important aspects that may appear odd to the contemporary practitioner:

- The inclusion in the original formula of Rehmanniae Radix (shēng dì huáng), which enriches the fluids, rather than Rehmanniae Radix praeparata (shú dì huáng), which tonifies the Kidneys
- The use of Cinnamomi Ramulus (guì zhī), which unblocks and moves the yang, rather than Cinnamomi Cortex (ròu guì), which warms and tonifies the yang
- The emphasis on treating the Kidney qi rather than the Kidney yang, as emphasized in the literature.

Indeed, none of these things makes sense if the primary intention of the formula was simply to nourish the yin in order to generate yang. An explanation that is probably more congruent with Zhang Zhong-Jing's intentions emerges from examining the commonalities among the various disorders for

which the formula is prescribed in the source text: a disorder of water metabolism centered on the lower burner, leading to either the retention of excessive water in the body (associated with reduced urination, edema, and thin mucus) or its excessive loss (associated with increased urination and thirst). All of these imply a deficiency of physiological fluids combined with an excess of pathological fluids, which in this case results from insufficient Kidney qi.

The yin aspect of Kidney function is the storage of yin fluids, and its yang aspect may be summed up as regulating the physiology of these fluids via control of opening and closing (開闔 kāi hé). This function of opening and closing should be understood dynamically as also encompassing Bladder qi transformation, since the Bladder is the yang complement of the Kidneys. By regulating the amount of water in the body, the Kidney-Bladder system also regulates fire and yang. The more fluids that are kept in the body, the more yang that is needed to move them. If this yang qi is lacking, water and fire are no longer regulated, resulting in a chronic condition that affects all the fluids of the body, including blood. Accumulation of pathological fluids accompanied by deficiency of physiological fluids invariably leads to blood stasis. This becomes visible, for instance, in changes of pigmentation on the forehead, the cheeks, and around the eyes (but also in other areas of the body), and the lack of blood supply to the entire body that is characteristic of deficiency and overwork disorders for which this formula is indicated. This complex, interconnected pathophysiology is cogently summarized in *Annotated and Corrected Craft of Medicines and Patterns for Children* by the modern physician Zhang Shan-Lei:

> Master [Zhang] Zhong[-Jing]'s Eight-Ingredient [Pill = Kidney Qi Pill (shèn qì wán)] was in its entirety composed as a strategy for incomplete Kidney qi unable to activate the true yang with urinary difficulty. … As a general principle in the composition of this formula, therefore, not a single herb [has been included] without considering its [effect] on promoting water metabolism. The formula's name [in referring] to Kidney qi emphasizes the term 'qi.' The very low dosage of Aconiti Radix lateralis praeparata (zhì fù zǐ) and Cinnamomi Ramulus (guì zhī) does nothing more than utilize their warmth and radiance to whisper encouragement to the true yang within the Kidneys, facilitating unimpeded urinary passage.

Viewed from this perspective, the formula's combination of Cinnamomi Ramulus (guì zhī) and Alismatis Rhizoma (zé xiè) is a standard strategy for promoting water metabolism found in many other formulas by Zhang Zhong-Jing, including Five-Ingredient Powder with Poria (wǔ líng sǎn) and Poria, Cinnamon Twig, Atractylodes, and Licorice Decoction (líng guì zhú gān tāng). Similarly, the combination of Cinnamomi Ramulus (guì zhī), Poria (fú líng), and Moutan Cortex (mǔ dān pí) are used by Zhang to treat blood stasis resulting from retained fluids, for example, in Cinnamon Twig and Poria Pill (guì zhī fú líng wán).

Rehmanniae Radix (*shēng dì huáng*), likewise, is not used to tonify the Kidneys but to enrich the fluids. In *Divine Husbandman's Classic of the Materia Medica*, the book that most likely reflects the pharmacological knowledge from which Zhang Zhong-Jing would have drawn, this herb was said to drive out blood obstruction. In the same text, Corni Fructus (*shān zhū yú*) is reported to drive out damp-cold painful obstruction, reflecting an action related to water metabolism. As Zhang Xi-Chun argued in his early 20th-century work, *Essays on Medicine Esteeming the Chinese and Respecting the Western*, this formula was prepared as a pill to ensure that the moving properties of Rehmanniae Radix (*shēng dì huáng*) were not diminished by decocting it.

Given the above, the presentation for this formula will include signs such as a swollen, pale tongue with visible indentations (indicating an excess of retained fluids in the context of yang deficiency) accompanied by a submerged, fine, and frail pulse in the distal position (indicating Kidney deficiency with diminished physiological fluids as well as a tendency to blood stasis). If yang deficiency below is accompanied by floating yang above, the pulse may be flooding and large at the surface but frail below, or floating and large toward the distal positions but submerged, fine, and frail toward the proximal positions. In Japanese Kampo, hypertonicity of the rectus abdominis muscle in the lower abdomen accompanied by general weakness of the abdomen is considered to be another important marker for the use of this formula.

Comparisons

➤ Vs. True Warrior Decoction (*zhēn wǔ tāng*)

Both formulas are used for problems of fluid metabolism due to Kidney yang deficiency. However, True Warrior Decoction (*zhēn wǔ tāng*) focuses on lesser yin-warp disorders characterized by more severe flooding of the entire body by pathogenic fluids. There are more severe manifestations of yin excess, including abdominal pain that is aggravated by cold, deep aching and heaviness in the extremities, and a pale or dark, swollen tongue. Kidney Qi Pill (*shèn qì wán*), on the other hand, is for problems of fluid metabolism due to Kidney qi deficiency characterized by problems of opening and closing. Accordingly, the symptoms of deficiency and stagnation will be relatively more pronounced than those of yin excess.

➤ Vs. Restore the Right [Kidney] Pill (*yòu guī wán*); see PAGE 402

Biomedical Indications

With the appropriate presentation, this formula may be used to treat a wide variety of biomedically-defined disorders. These can be divided into the following groups:

- Endocrine disorders including diabetes mellitus, primary hyperaldosteronism, hypothyroidism, perimenopausal syndrome, and Addison's disease

- Urinary disorders including chronic glomerular, interstitial or diffuse nephritis, pyelonephritis, renal tuberculosis, renal stones, cystitis, chronic urethritis, benign prostatic hypertrophy, paralysis of the detrusor muscle, postpartum urinary retention, postsurgical urinary incontinence, and urinary retention from spinal cord injuries

- Disorders of the eyes, ears, nose, and throat including cataracts, glaucoma, vitreous opacity, keratitis, chronic rhinitis, chronic tonsillitis, Ménière's disease, neurogenic tinnitus, recurrent aphthous ulcers, and periodontal disease

- Genital disorders including erectile dysfunction, premature ejaculation, infertility (male and female), and dysmenorrhea

- Respiratory disease including emphysema, chronic bronchitis, and bronchial asthma.

This formula has also been used in the treatment of eczema, sciatica, ascites, rectal prolapse, cerebral hemorrhage, atherosclerosis, and hypertension.

Alternate names

Eight-Ingredient Kidney Qi Pill (*bā wèi shèn qì wán*) in *Essentials from the Golden Cabinet*; Rehmannia Pill (*dì huáng wán*) in *Formulas from Benevolent Sages Compiled during the Taiping Era*; Eight-Immortal Pill (*bā xiān wán*) in *Book on Nourishing the Elderly and Serving One's Parents*; Supplement the Kidney Pill with Eight Ingredients (*bǔ shèn bā wèi wán*) in *Comprehensive Recording of Sagely Beneficence*; Eight-Ingredient Pill (*bā wèi wán*) in *Suitable Formulas*; Eight-Ingredient Pill with Rehmannia (*bā wèi dì huáng wán*) in *Discussion of Formulas for Pediatric Pox and Rashes*; Aconite Accessory Root Pill with Eight Ingredients (*fù zǐ bā wèi wán*) in *Formulas Categorized by the Stratagems of Pattern Treatment*; Kidney Qi Pill from the *Golden Cabinet* (*Jīn guì shèn qì wán*) in *Complete Collection of Red Water and Dark Pearls*; Cinnamon and Aconite Accessory Root Pill with Eight Ingredients (*guì fù bā wèi wán*) in *Concise Medical Guidelines*; Cinnamon, Aconite Accessory Root, and Rehmannia Pill (*guì fù dì huáng wán*) in *Concise Medical Guidelines*; Aconite Accessory Root and Cinnamon Pill with Eight Ingredients (*fù guì bā wèi wán*) in *Discussion of Medical Formulas*; Cinnamon and Aconite Accessory Root Eight-Ingredients Pill with Rehmannia (*guì fù bā wèi dì huáng wán*) in *Essential Teachings on Pregnancy and Childbirth*

Modifications

- To strengthen the effect of warming and tonifying the Kidney yang, substitute Cinnamomi Cortex (*ròu guì*) for Cinnamomi Ramulus (*guì zhī*).

- For urination at night, add Schisandrae Fructus (*wǔ wèi zǐ*).

- For frequent, copious, and clear urination with emaciation, add Psoraleae Fructus (*bǔ gǔ zhī*) and Cervi Cornu pantotrichum (*lù róng*).

- For impotence, add Morindae officinalis Radix (*bā jǐ tiān*), Cistanches Herba (*ròu cōng róng*), Cynomorii Herba (*suǒ yáng*), and Lycii Fructus (*gǒu qǐ zǐ*).

- For painful urinary dribbling due to cold lodging in the lower burner characterized by frequent, scanty urination with continuous dripping, add Cervi Cornu pantotrichum (*lù róng*) and Aquilariae Lignum resinatum (*chén xiāng*).

- For incontinence or turbid urine after overuse of excessively bitter and cold herbs, remove Alismatis Rhizoma (*zé xiè*) and add Schisandrae Fructus (*wǔ wèi zǐ*).

- For edema of the lower extremities, combine with Five-Peel Drink (*wǔ pí yǐn*).

Associated Formulas

加味腎氣丸 （加味肾气丸）

Augmented Kidney Qi Pill

jiā wèi shèn qì wán

SOURCE *Formulas to Aid the Living* (1253)

Rehmanniae Radix praeparata (*shú dì huáng*) 15g
Corni Fructus (*shān zhū yú*) 30g
dry-fried Dioscoreae Rhizoma (*chǎo shān yào*) 30g
Alismatis Rhizoma (*zé xiè*) 30g
Poria (*fú líng*) 30g
Moutan Cortex (*mǔ dān pí*) 30g
Cinnamomi Cortex (*ròu guì*) 15g
baked Aconiti Radix lateralis (*bāo fù zǐ*) 15g
wine-prepared Cyathulae Radix (*jiǔ chuān niú xī*) 15g
Plantaginis Semen (*chē qián zǐ*) 30g

Grind the ingredients into a powder and form into pills with honey. Take on an empty stomach with rice water, which is said to tonify the Stomach. Warms the yang, tonifies the Kidneys, assists the qi in transforming water, promotes urination, and reduces edema. For Kidney deficiency with overflow of water, aversion to cold, cold extremities, scanty urination, edema of the legs, abdominal distention, soreness of the lower back, a pale, swollen, tooth-marked tongue with a white, slippery coating, and a submerged, wiry pulse. In contrast to the principal formula, the dosage of the interior-warming herbs Aconiti Radix lateralis praeparata (*zhì fù zǐ*) and Cinnamomi Cortex (*ròu guì*) has been significantly increased, while that of Rehmanniae Radix praeparata (*shú dì huáng*) has been decreased. Moreover, the addition of Cyathulae Radix (*chuān niú xī*) and Plantaginis Semen (*chē qián zǐ*) increases its downward-directing and diuretic functions. As a result, it has a stronger effect on water metabolism and is often used for edema due to Kidney yang deficiency. It is also suitable for directing floating fire from the gate of vitality downward to its source. This is known in Chinese medicine as 'leading the dragon back into the sea.' Note that the source text specifies "official cinnamon" (官桂 *guān guì*), which is taken from the thinner bark of 6- or 7-year-old trees. This is thought to be a relatively dry form of Cinnamomi Cortex (*ròu guì*) and is used to warm the middle and dry dampness. This formula is also referred to as Kidney Qi Pill from *Formulas to Aid the Living* (*jì shēng shèn qì wán*) in order to distinguish it more clearly from the principal formula.

十補丸 （十补丸）

Ten-Tonic Pill

shí bǔ wán

SOURCE *Formulas to Aid the Living* (1253)

baked Aconiti Radix lateralis (*bāo fù zǐ*) 60g (9g)
Schisandrae Fructus (*wǔ wèi zǐ*) 60g (9g)
Corni Fructus (*shān zhū yú*) 30g (9g)
dry-fried Dioscoreae Rhizoma (*chǎo shān yào*) 30g (9g)
Moutan Cortex (*mǔ dān pí*) 30g (9g)
Cervi Cornu pantotrichum (*lù róng*) 30g (3g)
Rehmanniae Radix praeparata (*shú dì huáng*) 30g (9g)
Cinnamomi Cortex (*ròu guì*) 3g
Poria (*fú líng*) 30g (6g)
Alismatis Rhizoma (*zé xiè*) 30g (6g)

Grind the ingredients into a fine powder and form into pills with honey. Take on an empty stomach with salted wine. Warms and tonifies the Kidney yang. For patterns of Kidney deficiency characterized by a dark complexion, cold and edematous lower extremities, tinnitus, hearing loss, emaciation, weakness of the legs and knees, urinary difficulty, and lower back pain. In contrast to the principal formula, this has a stronger effect on the essence and the qi-grasping function of the Kidneys.

———————

無比山藥丸 （无比山药丸）

Incomparable Dioscorea Pill

wú bǐ shān yào wán

SOURCE *Important Formulas Worth a Thousand Gold Pieces* (650)

Dioscoreae Rhizoma (*shān yào*) 60g
Cistanches Herba (*ròu cōng róng*) 120g
Schisandrae Fructus (*wǔ wèi zǐ*) 180g
Cuscutae Semen (*tù sī zǐ*) 90g
Eucommiae Cortex (*dù zhòng*) 90g
Achyranthis bidentatae Radix (*niú xī*) 30g
Alismatis Rhizoma (*zé xiè*) 30g
Rehmanniae Radix (*shēng dì huáng*) 30g
Corni Fructus (*shān zhū yú*) 30g
Poriae Sclerotium pararadicis (*fú shén*) 30g
Morindae officinalis Radix (*bā jǐ tiān*) 30g
Halloysitum rubrum (*chì shí zhī*) 30g

Grind the ingredients into a powder and form into pills with honey. The recommended dosage is 20-30 pills to be taken twice a day before meals with wine. Nourishes the yin, assists the yang, augments the qi, and firms the Kidneys. For Kidney deficiency depletion damage characterized by soreness or pain of the waist and back, dizziness, tinnitus, frequent and clear urination or dribbling that starts and stops, a pale tongue, and a submerged and frail pulse.

Unlike the principal formula, Incomparable Dioscorea Pill (*wú bǐ shān yào wán*) uses herbs that tonify the Kidney yang directly rather than taking the detour via tonifying the yin while also warming the fire at the gate of vitality. It thus focuses less on treating an imbalance of water and fire manifesting as a disorder of water metabolism and more on deficiency fatigue arising from a lack of essence and yang qi.

Note that the original name of this formula, 無比薯蕷丸 *wù bí shǔ yù wán,* used a different term for dioscorea.

右歸丸（右归丸）
Restore the Right [Kidney] Pill

yòu guī wán

The right Kidney is regarded by many in the Chinese medical tradition to be the seat of the gate of vitality, associated with the Kidney yang. This formula focuses on warming and tonifying the Kidney yang, thereby restoring function and potency to the right Kidney.

Source *Collected Treatises of [Zhang] Jing-Yue* (1624)

Aconiti Radix lateralis praeparata *(zhì fù zǐ)* 60-180g
Cinnamomi Cortex *(ròu guì)* 60-120g
Cervi Cornus Colla *(lù jiǎo jiāo)* 120g
Rehmanniae Radix praeparata *(shú dì huáng)* 240g
Corni Fructus *(shān zhū yú)* 90g
dry-fried Dioscoreae Rhizoma *(chǎo shān yào)* 120g
dry-fried Lycii Fructus *(chǎo gǒu qǐ zǐ)* 120g
Cuscutae Semen *(tù sī zǐ)* 120g
Eucommiae Cortex *(dù zhòng)* 120g
Angelicae sinensis Radix *(dāng guī)* 90g

Method of Preparation Grind the ingredients into a fine powder and form into pills with honey. Take 9-15g with warm water 2-3 times daily. May also be prepared as a decoction with an appropriate reduction in the dosage of the ingredients.

Actions Warms and tonifies the Kidney yang, replenishes the essence, and tonifies the blood

Indications

Exhaustion from long-term illness, aversion to cold, coolness of the extremities, impotence, spermatorrhea, and aching and weakness of the lower back and knees. There may also be infertility, loose stools (sometimes with undigested food particles), incontinence, and edema of the lower extremities.

This is Kidney yang deficiency with waning of the fire at the gate of vitality. The source text describes the condition as

> primal (source) yang deficiency and decline of the prenatal endowment such that the fire at the gate of vitality wanes. Because it is unable to generate earth, the Spleen and Stomach are cold and deficient. ... cold is in the lower burner and pathogenic water arises, leading to floating edema.

The root aspect of this condition, Kidney yang deficiency, causes such symptoms as aversion to cold, coolness of the extremities, impotence, spermatorrhea, aching and weakness of the lower back and knees, infertility, incontinence, and edema of the lower extremities. The secondary aspect, cold and deficiency of the middle burner, causes loose stools to the point of containing undigested food particles.

Analysis of Formula

The chief ingredients, Aconiti Radix lateralis praeparata *(zhì fù zǐ),* Cinnamomi Cortex *(ròu guì),* and Cervi Cornus Colla *(lù jiǎo jiāo),* warm and fortify the source yang. Cervi Cornus Colla *(lù jiǎo jiāo)* also has a certain 'flesh-and-blood' quality that replenishes the essence and tonifies the marrow. The deputies, Rehmanniae Radix praeparata *(shú dì huáng),* Corni Fructus *(shān zhū yú),* Dioscoreae Rhizoma *(shān yào),* Lycii Fructus *(gǒu qǐ zǐ),* Cuscutae Semen *(tù sī zǐ),* and Eucommiae Cortex *(dù zhòng),* nourish the yin to benefit the Kidneys, nourish the Liver, and tonify the Spleen. Specifically, sweet and warm Rehmanniae Radix praeparata *(shú dì huáng)* nourishes the yin and tonifies the Kidneys, especially the blood. Corni Fructus *(shān zhū yú)* and Dioscoreae Rhizoma *(shān yào)* tonify the Liver and benefit the Spleen in order to indirectly tonify and supplement the essence and blood. Lycii Fructus *(gǒu qǐ zǐ),* Cuscutae Semen *(tù sī zǐ),* and Eucommiae Cortex *(dù zhòng)* nourish and tonify the Liver and Kidneys; they are especially helpful in treating lower back pain and weakness. Angelicae sinensis Radix *(dāng guī)* is added to tonify the blood and nourish the Liver.

Cautions and Contraindications

Because this formula tonifies without draining, it is inappropriate when Kidney deficiency is accompanied by dampness or turbidity.

Commentary

This formula can be viewed as a variation of Kidney Qi Pill *(shèn qì wán).* The primary modifications are the increase in the dosage of the warming herbs that fortify the yang, omission of the three herbs that are predominantly draining in nature—Poria *(fú líng),* Alismatis Rhizoma *(zé xiè),* and Moutan Cortex *(mǔ dān pí)*—and the addition of ingredients that strengthen the tonifying action of the formula and increase both the yin and yang of the Kidneys—Cervi Cornus Colla *(lù jiǎo jiāo),* Cuscutae Semen *(tù sī zǐ),* Eucommiae Cortex *(dù zhòng),* and Lycii Fructus *(gǒu qǐ zǐ)).* Some physicians prefer to use Cervi Cornu pantotrichum *(lù róng)* in place of Cervi Cornus Colla *(lù jiǎo jiāo)* because of its superior ability to replenish essence.

This is one of the best formulas for treating Kidney yang deficiency with insufficiency of essence and blood. It is commonly used for waning of the fire at the gate of vitality, most often seen in the elderly and those suffering from chronic diseases. Although this disorder gives rise to symptoms in both the middle (Spleen) and lower burners (Kidneys), according to the source text, its etiology is invariably the insufficiency of source yang. This formula is designed to "increase the source of fire by firming up the source yang of the right [Kidney]." That is to say, it tonifies the 'yang within the yin' since the Kidneys themselves are associated with yin. For this reason, one should combine ingredients that nourish the yin and replenish the essence with ingredients that firm up and tonify the Kidney yang. This is the most commonly-used approach for firming up and tonifying the source yang.

Comparison

➤ Vs. KIDNEY QI PILL *(shèn qì wán)*

Both formulas warm and fortify the source yang and tonify the Kidneys. However, Restore the Right [Kidney] Pill *(yòu guī wán)* focuses on tonification without draining. In addition to Aconiti Radix lateralis praeparata *(zhì fù zǐ)* and Cinnamomi Cortex *(ròu guì)*, which secure and tonify the fire at the gate of vitality (or source yang), it primarily relies on Kidney tonics. These herbs are not only warming, but are also sweet in nature, supplying the body with essences that can nourish deficiency. For this reason, this formula is indicated for the treatment of chronic disorders characterized by weakness and exhaustion in addition to cold.

Kidney Qi Pill *(shèn qì wán)*, on the other hand, uses low dosages of Aconiti Radix lateralis praeparata *(zhì fù zǐ)* and Cinnamomi Ramulus *(guì zhī)* to "generate qi [with the help] of a little fire" (少火生氣 *shǎo huǒ shēng qì*), as well as herbs that promote water metabolism and move the yin. The qi referred to in this adage is the qi of the Kidneys and Bladder, the qi that facilitates the transformation of water in the lower burner. Accordingly, Kidney Qi Pill *(shèn qì wán)* is used to treat water excess due to Kidney yang deficiency.

Biomedical Indications

With the appropriate presentation, this formula may be used to treat a wide variety of biomedically-defined disorders such as nephrotic syndrome, osteoporosis, infertility (especially due to low sperm count), various forms of anemia, leukopenia, and asthma.

Modifications

- For waning of the yang and qi deficiency, add Ginseng Radix *(rén shēn)* in quantities of 60-90g, or as much as 150-180g, depending on the severity of the deficiency. The addition of this herb accelerates the effect of the formula. (source text)
- For yang deficiency with manifestations of spermatorrhea, turbid leukorrhea, and/or pasty stools, add wine-treated Psoraleae Fructus *(bǔ gǔ zhī)*. (source text)
- For incessant Kidney diarrhea, add Schisandrae Fructus *(wǔ wèi zǐ)* and Myristicae Semen *(ròu dòu kòu)*. (source text)

- For reduced appetite, poor digestion, nausea, and acid reflux due to cold and deficiency of the Spleen and Stomach, add Zingiberis Rhizoma *(gān jiāng)*. (source text)
- For incessant abdominal pain, add Evodiae Fructus *(wú zhū yú)*. (source text)
- For impotence, add Morindae officinalis Radix *(bā jǐ tiān)* and Cistanches Herba *(ròu cōng róng)*. (source text)

Associated Formulas

右歸飲（右归饮）

Restore the Right [Kidney] Drink

yòu guī yǐn

SOURCE   *Collected Treatises of [Zhang] Jing-Yue (1624)*

Rehmanniae Radix praeparata *(shú dì huáng)* 6-60g
dry-fried Dioscoreae Rhizoma *(chǎo shān yào)* 6g
Corni Fructus *(shān zhū yú)* 3g
Lycii Fructus *(gǒu qǐ zǐ)* 6g
Glycyrrhizae Radix praeparata *(zhì gān cǎo)* 3-6g
Eucommiae Cortex *(dù zhòng)* 6g
Cinnamomi Cortex *(ròu guì)* 3-6g
Aconiti Radix lateralis praeparata *(zhì fù zǐ)* 3-9g

Warms the Kidneys and replenishes the essence. For Kidney yang deficiency with feebleness and exhaustion, abdominal pain, sore lower back, cold extremities, and a thin pulse. Also for patterns of true cold and false heat in which the preponderance of yin causes a separation of the yang, which floats to the exterior; that is to say, the excessive yin causes the remaining yang to move to the superficial levels of the body. This formula is slightly weaker than the principal formula.

青娥丸

Young Maiden Pill

qīng é wán

SOURCE   *Formulary of the Pharmacy Service for Benefiting the People in the Taiping Era (1107)*

ginger-juice fried Eucommiae Cortex
   (jiāng zhī chǎo dù zhòng) 480g
wine-fried Psoraleae Fructus *(jiǔ chǎo bǔ gǔ zhī)* 240g
Juglandis Semen *(hé táo rén)* 150g

Grind the ingredients into a powder and form into pills with 120g of Allii sativi Bulbus *(dà suàn)* that has been crushed to a paste. May also be formed into pills with honey. Take in 3g doses on an empty stomach with warm wine. Tonifies the Kidneys, strengthens the lower back, and alleviates lower back pain. For severe lower back pain from Kidney yang deficiency with damage from wind-cold-dampness, or due to injury from trauma. The pain is continuous, and it is hard to stand up from a seated position, difficult to bend forward or backward, and impossible to rotate the trunk. The pain is accompanied by weakness of the legs and extreme exhaustion. There may also be dizziness, earache, dribbling urination, or vaginal discharge. All of these symptoms improve with bed rest. There is also a tense sensation in the lower abdomen, cold extremities, a pale and shiny complexion, pale tongue, and a submerged, thin pulse.

菟絲子丸（菟丝子丸）
Cuscuta Seed Pill

tù sī zǐ wán

Source *Formulas to Aid the Living* (1253)

Cuscutae Semen *(tù sī zǐ)* 60g
Cervi Cornu pantotrichum *(lù róng)* 30g
Cistanches Herba *(ròu cōng róng)* 60g
Dioscoreae Rhizoma *(shān yào)* 30g
Aconiti Radix lateralis praeparata *(zhì fù zǐ)* 30g
Linderae Radix *(wū yào)* 30g
Schisandrae Fructus *(wǔ wèi zǐ)* 30g
Mantidis Oötheca *(sāng piāo xiāo)* 30g
Alpiniae oxyphyllae Fructus *(yì zhì rén)* 30g
calcined Ostreae Concha *(duàn mǔ lì)* 60g
Gigeriae galli Endothelium corneum *(jī nèi jīn)* 15g

Method of Preparation Grind the ingredients into a powder and form into pills with wine. Take 3-9g with salted water 2-3 times daily before meals. May also be taken as a decoction with an appropriate reduction in dosage.

Actions Warms the Kidneys and prevents abnormal leakage

Indications

Exhaustion, aversion to cold, frail physique, dizziness, lower back pain, weakness of the lower extremities, frequent, scanty urination with continuous dripping, and a submerged, thin pulse that is especially frail at the proximal position.

This is Kidney qi deficiency with an inability to grasp the essence. The exhaustion is due to weakness of the essence and blood of the Kidneys, while the aversion to cold stems from insufficient warmth due to yang qi deficiency. The frail physique, dizziness, lower back pain, and weakness of the lower extremities is due to exhaustion of the source qi, which is unable to fill out the skin and flesh externally, or to distribute the qi and blood internally. When the Kidneys are deficient, the Bladder may lose its power to restrain, which results in frequent and scanty urination with continuous dripping.

Analysis of Formula

This formula combines strategies for tonifying the Kidney yang and essence with those that bind and grasp the Kidney qi. The chief ingredients, Cuscutae Semen *(tù sī zǐ)*, Cervi Cornu pantotrichum *(lù róng)*, Cistanches Herba *(ròu cōng róng)*, and Dioscoreae Rhizoma *(shān yào)*, work together to tonify the Kidneys. One of the deputies, Aconiti Radix lateralis praeparata *(zhì fù zǐ)*, warms the Kidney yang. Together with another deputy, Linderae Radix *(wū yào)*, it moves and dispels the cold qi from the Kidneys and Bladder. A third deputy, Schisandrae Fructus *(wǔ wèi zǐ)*, binds and grasps the Kidney qi. It is aided in this function by the astringent, assistant ingredients Mantidis Oötheca *(sāng piāo xiāo)*, Alpiniae oxyphyllae Fructus *(yì zhì rén)*, and calcined Ostreae Concha *(duàn mǔ lì)*. Gigeriae galli Endothelium corneum *(jī nèi jīn)*

is used for treating the urinary frequency and incontinence, and serves as the envoy in this formula.

Commentary

When the qi-grasping function of the Kidneys is weak, abnormal leakage of urine may result. Although this is but a manifestation of the underlying disorder, it is important that it be treated. To that end, this formula combines astringent ingredients with tonifying ingredients that work on the root cause of the disorder. This accelerates the healing process and helps to effect a long-term cure. If the absorbing and grasping function of the Kidneys is strong, the recovery from Kidney qi deficiency or injury will be faster and more complete since it ensures that the full potential of qi is rooted in the Kidneys.

This formula is named after Cuscutae Semen *(tù sī zǐ)*, which has a weaker yang-tonifying effect than Cervi Cornu pantotrichum *(lù róng)* and warms the gate of vitality less than Aconiti Radix lateralis praeparata *(zhì fù zǐ)*. However, *Miscellaneous Records [of Famous Physicians]* states that it treats "cold in the penis, leakage of semen, and excessive dribbling of urine." This is the main focus of the formula, as many of the formula's other ingredients also excel at constraining leakage.

Biomedical Indications

With the appropriate presentation, this formula may be used to treat a variety of biomedically-defined disorders such as urinary incontinence, seminal emissions, and premature ejaculation.

贊育丹（赞育丹）
Special Pill to Aid Fertility

zàn yù dān

Source *Collected Treatises of [Zhang] Jing-Yue* (1624)

Aconiti Radix lateralis praeparata *(zhì fù zǐ)* 60g
Cinnamomi Cortex *(ròu guì)* .60g
Cistanches Herba *(ròu cōng róng)* 120g
Morindae officinalis Radix *(bā jǐ tiān)* 120g
Epimedii Herba *(yín yáng huò)* 120g
Cnidii Fructus *(shé chuáng zǐ)* 60g
Allii tuberosi Semen *(jiǔ zǐ)* .120g
Curculiginis Rhizoma *(xiān máo)* 120g
Corni Fructus *(shān zhū yú)* 120g
Eucommiae Cortex *(dù zhòng)* 120g
Rehmanniae Radix praeparata *(shú dì huáng)* 240g
Angelicae sinensis Radix *(dāng guī)* 180g
Lycii Fructus *(gǒu qǐ zǐ)* 180g
Atractylodis macrocephalae Rhizoma *(bái zhú)* 240g

Method of Preparation Grind the ingredients into a powder and form into pills with honey. Take 3-9g twice a day. May also be prepared as a decoction with an appropriate reduction in the dosage of the ingredients.

Actions Warms and tonifies the lower base (Kidneys)

Indications

Impotence or infertility, listlessness and dispiritedness, aching and weakness of the lower back, a pale, shiny complexion, and a submerged, thin pulse.

This is impotence or infertility due to waning of the fire at the gate of vitality and cold and deficiency of the essential qi. Clinical experience has shown that these problems typically involve not only debilitation of the source yang, but also deficiency of the qi and blood. Thus, in addition to the primary symptom of impotence or infertility, most patients will also present with such symptoms as listlessness and dispiritedness, aching and weakness of the lower back, a pale, shiny complexion, and a submerged, thin pulse.

Analysis of Formula

The strategy underlying this formula is to tonify and warm the Kidneys in order to promote fertility. The chief ingredients tonify the Kidneys and strengthen the yang. These include Aconiti Radix lateralis praeparata (zhì fù zǐ), Cinnamomi Cortex (ròu guì), Cistanches Herba (ròu cōng róng), Morindae officinalis Radix (bā jǐ tiān), Epimedii Herba (yín yáng huò), Cnidii Fructus (shé chuáng zǐ), Allii tuberosi Semen (jiǔ zǐ), Curculiginis Rhizoma (xiān máo), Corni Fructus (shān zhū yú), and Eucommiae Cortex (dù zhòng). When all of these herbs are gathered together into one formula, the action of tonifying the Kidneys and promoting the yang becomes quite powerful.

The deputies, Rehmanniae Radix praeparata (shú dì huáng), Angelicae sinensis Radix (dāng guī), and Lycii Fructus (gǒu qǐ zǐ), are combined with the chief ingredients to tonify the yin and replenish the essence. The assistant, Atractylodis macrocephalae Rhizoma (bái zhú), is added for its ability to strengthen the Spleen and eliminate dampness. Not only does it strengthen the transportive function of the Spleen and Stomach, it also transforms and transports the essence to a slight extent, thereby assisting the formula in tonifying and replenishing the Kidney essence.

Commentary

When the fire at the gate of vitality is waning, the strategy should be strong tonification and warming of the Kidney yang. A large number of ingredients are incorporated for this purpose. However, in accordance with the principle that one should tonify the Kidney yin when tonifying the Kidney yang, three other ingredients are added for the specific purpose of nourishing and moistening the yin and blood. This ensures that the yin and yang remain in harmony and are rooted to each other at the source. The use of strong warming agents such as Aconiti Radix lateralis praeparata (zhì fù zǐ) and Cinnamomi Cortex (ròu guì) must be balanced in this manner to avoid injuring the Kidney yin. Otherwise, the unbalanced utilization of yang tonics and cold-dispelling herbs may injure the yin, resulting in manifestations of both Kidney yin and yang deficiency.

Although deficient fire at the gate of vitality is an important cause of impotence and infertility, patterns involving blood stasis, dampness obstructing the movement of qi in the lower burner, and toxins are also often seen. Although this formula contains some herbs that move the blood and promote water metabolism, these are insufficient in terms of both strength and dosage to be effective in treating such patterns.

Biomedical Indications

With the appropriate presentation, this formula may be used to treat a variety of biomedically-defined disorders such as infertility (both male and female) and erectile dysfunction.

Modifications

- To increase the efficacy of the formula in treating infertility, add Ginseng Radix (rén shēn) and Cervi Cornu pantotrichum (lù róng).
- To increase the efficacy of the formula in treating impotence, add Chuanxiong Rhizoma (chuān xiōng), Poria (fú líng), and Scolopendra (wú gōng) to move the blood, drain dampness, and unblock the collaterals.

Associated Formula

還少丹 （还少丹）

Rejuvenation Special Pill

huán shào dān

Source   *Hong's Collection of Experiential Formulas* (1170)

Rehmanniae Radix praeparata (shú dì huáng) 18 (9-12)
Dioscoreae Rhizoma (shān yào). 45 (9-15)
wine-soaked Achyranthis bidentatae Radix (niú xī) 45 (9-12)
Lycii Fructus (gǒu qǐ zǐ). 15 (9-12)
Corni Fructus (shān zhū yú) 30 (9-12)
Poria (fú líng) 30 (9-12)
wine-fried with ginger juice Eucommiae Cortex
   (dù zhòng) 30 (9-12)
Polygalae Radix (yuǎn zhì) 30 (6-9)
Schisandrae Fructus (wǔ wèi zǐ). 30 (6-9)
wine-steamed Broussonetiae Fructus (chǔ shí zǐ). 30 (6-9)
dry-fried Foeniculi Fructus (xiǎo huí xiāng) 30 (6-9)
wine-soaked Morindae officinalis Radix (bā jǐ tiān) 30 (9-12)
Cistanches Herba (ròu cōng róng) 30 (12-15)
Acori tatarinowii Rhizoma (shí chāng pǔ) 15 (6-9)

The source text recommends grinding the above herbs and mixing them with honey and steamed Jujubae Fructus (dà zǎo) to make pills. The normal dosage is 9g twice a day taken with warm salt water. At present, it is usually taken as a decoction with the dosages in parentheses, plus 2-3 pieces of Jujubae Fructus (dà zǎo). Tonifies the Spleen and Kidney and nourishes the Heart. Enriches the yin, nourishes the blood and yang, and augments the qi. For insufficiency of essence and blood from Kidney, Heart, and Spleen deficiency that manifests as fatigue, heavy and painful lower back pain, dream-disturbed sleep, general weakness, lack of interest in food or drink, fever, night sweats, seminal emissions or vaginal discharge, impotence, emaciation, loose teeth, and signs of premature aging. The pulse for this pattern is moderate and weak. One unique aspect of this formula is that it treats the Kidney, Spleen, and Heart. While it lacks the simple elegance of Six-Ingredient Pill with Rehmannia *(liù wèi dì huáng wán)*, it is still quite well-balanced and can address specific complaints relating to loss of essence, listless spirit, and abdominal cold. The well-known modern practitioner Jiao Shu-De recommends it, with the addition of Cuscutae Semen *(tù sī zǐ)* and Cervi Cornu pantotrichum *(lù róng)*, for impotence or reduced sex drive. It is also used for ophthalmological disorders with significant Kidney deficiency.

Section 6

FORMULAS THAT TONIFY BOTH THE YIN AND THE YANG

Yin essences depend for their generation on the transformative powers of the yang qi. The yang qi, in turn, is produced from and controlled by the yin essence. Over time, therefore, yin deficiency will invariably lead to yang deficiency and vice versa. This process may be slow and progressive (as in the course of a chronic illness), or relatively acute (as in the course of a feverish disorder). Alternatively, yin and yang deficiency may be the constitutional basis from which a disorder arises.

The formulas in this section treat these combined yin and yang deficiency disorders. For this reason, they typically combine herbs that tonify the yin, such as Trionycis Carapax *(biē jiǎ)*, Rehmanniae Radix praeparata *(shú dì huáng)*, Corni Fructus *(shān zhū yú)*, Lycii Fructus *(gǒu qǐ zǐ)*, or Ophiopogonis Radix *(mài mén dōng)*, with those that tonify the yang, such as Cervi Cornu pantotrichum *(lù róng)*, Morindae officinalis Radix *(bā jǐ tiān)*, Cistanches Herba *(ròu cōng róng)*, or Eucommiae Cortex *(dù zhòng)*. Other herbs are added as necessary, as outlined in preceding sections. In practice, one type of deficiency will tend to predominate, a fact that must be reflected in the selection and modification of appropriate formulas.

地黃飲子 (地黄饮子)
Rehmannia Drink
dì huáng yǐn zi

Source *Comprehensive Recording of Sagely Beneficence from the Zhenghe Era* (1117)

Rehmanniae Radix praeparata *(shú dì huáng)* 30g
dried fried Corni Fructus *(chǎo shān zhū yú)* 30g
wine-prepared Cistanches Herba *(jiǔ cōng róng)* 30g
Morindae officinalis Radix *(bā jǐ tiān)* 30g
baked Aconiti Radix lateralis *(bāo fù zǐ)* 30g
Cinnamomi Cortex *(ròu guì)* 30g
Dendrobii Herba *(shí hú)* .30g
Poria *(fú líng)* 30g
dry-fried Schisandrae Fructus *(chǎo wǔ wèi zǐ)* 30g
prepared Ophiopogonis Radix *(zhì mài mén dōng)* 15g
Acori tatarinowii Rhizoma *(shí chāng pú)* 15g
Polygalae Radix *(yuǎn zhì)* 15g

Method of Preparation The source text advises to grind equal amounts of the ingredients into a powder. A dose of 9-15g of the powder is then decocted with 3 slices of Zingiberis Rhizoma recens *(shēng jiāng)* and 2 pieces of Jujubae Fructus *(dà zǎo)* in a cup of water until about one-third of the liquid remains. The draft is taken warm before meals. At present, it is usually prepared as a decoction.

Actions Enriches the Kidney yin, tonifies the Kidney yang, opens the orifices, and transforms phlegm

Indications

Stiffness of the tongue with an inability to speak, disability or paralysis of the lower extremities, a dry mouth with an absence of thirst, a greasy, yellow tongue coating, and a submerged, slow, thin, and frail pulse.

This is mute paraplegia (喑痱 *yīn fèi*) due to deficiency and waning of the lower base (the Kidney yin and yang) together with an upward-flaring of deficient yang that takes the turbid phlegm with it. Above, deficient yang fire scorches the fluids of the throat, while turbid phlegm blocks the orifices.

Stiffness of the tongue and inability to speak is due to three processes. The Kidney channel nourishes the root of the tongue. When the lower base is deficient, the Kidneys are unable to send nourishment to the root of the tongue, leaving the voice without a 'root.' Upward-flaring of fire from deficiency accompanied by turbid phlegm blocks the orifices and closes the 'gate' of the voice. Finally, because the tongue is the 'sprout' of the Heart, when the Heart qi is consumed by the fire of deficiency, it is unable to reach the tongue. This leaves the voice without a 'ruler,' hence the inability to speak.

The Kidneys govern the bones. Deficiency and waning of the lower base weakens the sinews and bones, which leads to disability or paralysis of the lower extremities.

Analysis of Formula

In order to treat a pattern characterized by deficiency below and turbid phlegm flooding the upper body, this formula combines a core strategy of warming and tonifying the lower source with a secondary strategy of opening the orifices and transforming the phlegm. Two of the chief ingredients, Rehmanniae Radix praeparata *(shú dì huáng)* and Corni Fructus *(shān zhū yú)*, enrich and tonify the Kidneys, strengthen Kidney water, and augment the essence. The other chief ingredients, Cistanches Herba *(ròu cōng róng)* and

Morindae officinalis Radix (bā jǐ tiān), warm and tonify the Kidney yang without being excessively drying, while also fortifying the sinews and strengthening the bones. Together, these four herbs address the root of the disorder by tonifying the deficiency of the lower source in its various aspects. Two of the deputies, Aconiti Radix lateralis praeparata (zhì fù zǐ) and Cinnamomi Cortex (ròu guì), assist Cistanches Herba (ròu cōng róng) and Morindae officinalis Radix (bā jǐ tiān) in warming and nourishing the source yang. Cinnamomi Cortex (ròu guì) is especially effective in guiding the errant fire from deficiency back to its source in the gate of vitality. The other deputies, Dendrobii Herba (shí hú) and Ophiopogonis Radix (mài mén dōng), enrich the yin fluids and cool the fire from deficiency, while simultaneously moderating the drying actions of Aconiti Radix lateralis praeparata (zhì fù zǐ) and Cinnamomi Cortex (ròu guì). In combination with Rehmanniae Radix praeparata (shú dì huáng) and Corni Fructus (shān zhū yú), they tonify the postnatal constitution in order to nourish the prenatal essences. A fifth deputy, Schisandrae Fructus (wǔ wèi zǐ), combines in its astringent action with Corni Fructus (shān zhū yú) to aid Cinnamomi Cortex (ròu guì) in restraining the floating yang. Together, the five deputies assist the chief ingredients in enriching the yin and warming the yang, thereby regulating the functions of the lower burner.

Among the assistants, Acori tatarinowii Rhizoma (shí chāng pǔ), Polygalae Radix (yuǎn zhì), and Poria (fú líng) open the orifices, transform phlegm, and calm the spirit. Polygalae Radix (yuǎn zhì) is ascending in nature, directing the qi from the Kidneys to the Heart, while Acori tatarinowii Rhizoma (shí chāng pǔ) directs the qi from the Heart toward the Kidneys in the lower burner. With Poria (fú líng) assisting the functions of the Spleen and Stomach as the fulcrum of the qi dynamic, the three assistants facilitate communication between the Heart and the Kidneys to adjust the relationship between water and fire to effectively treat the manifestation of the disorder.

The envoys, Zingiberis Rhizoma recens (shēng jiāng) and Jujubae Fructus (dà zǎo), adjust and harmonize the nutritive and protective qi. In Formulas from the Discussion Illuminating the Yellow Emperor's Basic Questions, which some commentators list as the source text of this formula, Zhang Yuan-Su recommends adding a few leaves of Menthae haplocalycis Herba (bò hé) to the draft before boiling. This has the additional benefit of cooling the throat, though more importantly, the light nature of Menthae haplocalycis Herba (bò hé) focuses the power of the formula's action on the throat as the locus of the most important symptom.

Cautions and Contraindications

This formula is indicated for conditions of severe deficiency and is contraindicated for disorders of excess, such as ascendant Liver yang. Because it contains herbs that are very warm and dry in nature, it should not be taken long term. If it must be prescribed for as long as a few weeks, substitute Curculiginis Rhizoma (xiān máo) and Epimedii Herba (yín yáng huò) for Aconiti Radix lateralis praeparata (zhì fù zǐ) and Cinnamomi Cortex (ròu guì).

Commentary

This formula can be viewed as a combination of Kidney Qi Pill (shèn qì wán), analyzed above, and Settle the Emotions Pill (dìng zhì wán), discussed in Chapter 10. It is an important formula for treating the sequelae of wind-stroke, such as aphasia and disability or paralysis of the lower extremities. Wind-stroke is traditionally divided into 'true wind-stroke' (真中風 zhēn zhòng fēng) and 'quasi-wind-stroke' (類中風 lèi zhòng fēng). True wind-stroke is caused by an attack of pathogenic wind from the outside. Quasi-wind-stroke is an internal disorder caused by yin deficiency, yang deficiency, or both. If the Kidney yang is deficient, phlegm and dampness tend to develop. If the true yin is deficient, fire tends to develop. Yang deficiency more often leads to abandoned disorders or sudden collapse, while yin deficiency more often leads to patterns with vigorous fire. This formula is used in treating patterns of quasi-wind-stroke caused by Kidney deficiency. It contains a blend of ingredients that are not often found together: herbs that warm the Kidney yang, herbs that nourish the yin, herbs that open the orifices, and herbs that calm the spirit.

Because the source text merely defines Kidney deficiency as the root but does not identify a precise pathology, commentators have proposed a number of different mechanisms to explain both the disease dynamic and the action of this formula. Three theories can be distinguished:

- Kidney qi deficiency is the root cause. If the Kidney qi is too deficient to transform the fluids and anchor the qi, turbid yin will float upward to usurp the place of fire above, while the nutritive qi will fail to nourish the leg sinews and bones below. This theory can be traced back to Precepts for Physicians by Yu Chang.

- The focus of the pathogenesis of this disorder should be on the floating yang secondary to waning fire at the gate of vitality. Many commentators have taken this position, including Chen Nian-Zu in Compendium of Songs on Modern Formulas. This view is bolstered by the implied consumption of the yin fluids by fire due to the inclusion of the cooling, moistening herbs Ophiopogonis Radix (mài mén dōng) and Dendrobii Herba (shí hú).

- Deficiency of both Kidney yin and yang is responsible, according to the contemporary physician Zhang Shan-Lei in Careful Deliberations on Wind-Stroke. From this perspective, the flood of turbid yin above is secondary to the abandonment of yin and yang below.

Use of this formula is indicated if the pulse is submerged and weak or minute, and the tongue is pale and moist with a slippery, white coating. These signs help differentiate this pattern from Liver yang type wind-stroke, which will be accompanied by a pulse that is wiry or large, as well as a red tongue. The use of this formula has been expanded to include the treatment of Kidney deficiency without the associated problems with speech or paralysis, although there should always be signs of dryness accompanied by excess of turbid yin above. Such disorders include insomnia, edema, or dryness and itching of the skin. In order to focus the action of the herbs on the upper burner, it is important not to decoct the ingredients for too long, as indicated in the formula's name (a 'drink' rather than a 'decoction') and underscored time and again by various commentators.

Because mute paraplegia is referred to as wind paraplegia (風痱 *fēng fèi*) in other texts, this formula is listed in some classical and modern textbooks as a wind-dispelling formula. We have placed it here because there are no herbs in this formula that treat wind directly.

Comparison

➤ Vs. Tortoise Shell and Deer Antler Two-Immortal Syrup (*guī lù èr xiān jiāo*); *see* page 408

Biomedical Indications

With the appropriate presentation, this formula may be used to treat a variety of biomedically-defined disorders such as end-stage hypertension, cerebrovascular disease, the sequelae of stroke, transverse myelitis, amyotrophic lateral sclerosis, sequelae of cerebrovascular accident, Parkinson's disease, and secondary hypertension associated with chronic glomerulonephritis and pyelonephritis.

Modifications

• For disability of the lower extremities, and irritated, hot joints associated with Kidney yin deficiency, add Taxilli Herba (*sāng jì shēng*), Lycii Cortex (*dì gǔ pí*), and Trionycis Carapax (*biē jiǎ*).
• For severe Kidney yang deficiency with cold affecting the lower back and knees, add Epimedii Herba (*yín yáng huò*) and Curculiginis Rhizoma (*xiān máo*).
• For concurrent qi deficiency, add Astragali Radix (*huáng qí*) and Codonopsis Radix (*dǎng shēn*).
• For disability of the lower extremities without aphasia, remove Acori tatarinowii Rhizoma (*shí chāng pǔ*), Polygalae Radix (*yuǎn zhì*), and Menthae haplocalycis Herba (*bò hé*).
• For yin deficiency and vigorous phlegm-fire without yang deficiency, remove Cinnamomi Cortex (*ròu guì*) and Aconiti Radix lateralis praeparata (*zhì fù zǐ*) and add Fritillariae cirrhosae Bulbus (*chuān bèi mǔ*), Bambusae Succus (*zhú lì*), Arisaema cum Bile (*dǎn nán xīng*), and Bambusae Concretio silicea (*tiān zhú huáng*).

龜鹿二仙膠 （龟鹿二仙胶）
Tortoise Shell and Deer Antler Two-Immortal Syrup
guī lù èr xiān jiāo

In Chinese folklore, the tortoise and deer are regarded as animals that live a long life. They have thus become symbols of strength and longevity. This formula combines products derived from these two animals for the purpose of restoring vitality, thereby giving long life to those who take it; hence, the reference to the two immortals in the name.

Source *Concise Medicine* (1587)

Cervi Cornu (*lù jiǎo*) 5000g
Testudinis Plastrum (*guī bǎn*) 2500g
Lycii Fructus (*gǒu qǐ zǐ*) 900g
Ginseng Radix (*rén shēn*) 450g

Method of Preparation Prepared as a syrup. Take in 3-9g doses with wine or lightly salted, warm water.

Actions Nourishes and replenishes the yin, tonifies the essence, augments the qi, and tonifies and strengthens the yang

Indications

Emaciation, weakness, spermatorrhea, impotence, diminished visual acuity, aching and weakness of the lower back and knees, daybreak diarrhea, and a thin, frail pulse.

This is Kidney yin and yang deficiency accompanied by insufficiency of essence and blood in the Conception and Governing vessels. *Basic Questions*, Chapter 4, states that "Essence is the root of life." If essence is depleted, either because of constitutional weakness or by illness, or if it is wasted through overwork or a lifestyle focused on excess, symptoms of essence deficiency will become manifest, implicating particularly those organs and functions charged with the storage and maintenance of essence: the Kidneys and the eight extraordinary vessels. Impotence and infertility are the primary manifestations of essence depletion. If essence fails to nourish the blood, the person becomes emaciated. Liver blood and Kidney yin share the same source; hence, essence depletion will lead to diminished visual acuity above and aching and weakness of the lower back and knees below. Daybreak diarrhea is another classic sign of Kidney deficiency, reflecting that the Kidneys are failing in their function of guarding opening and closing. A thin, frail pulse reflects deficiency of essence, blood, and qi.

Analysis of Formula

This formula reaches beyond the qi and blood to the yin and yang, and still further to the essence and marrow, in order to replenish the deepest sources of energy in the body. For this purpose, it utilizes two chief ingredients that embody vitality and longevity on the symbolic level, while nourishing essence, blood, and qi through their medicinal functions. Cervi Cornus Colla *(lù jiǎo jiāo)* is sweet, salty, and warming and is thereby able to fortify the yang, augment the essence, and nourish the blood. It is complemented by Testudinis Plastri Colla *(guī bǎn jiāo)*, which is sweet and salty but slightly cooling, filling the essence, tonifying the marrow, enriching the yang and nourishing the blood. Made of 'flesh and blood,' these two substances powerfully tonify the essence, yin, and yang without leaning too much in either direction. Sweet, bitter, and warming Ginseng Radix *(rén shēn)* is the most important herb for tonifying the source qi. Combined with the two chief ingredients, it aids the transformation of essence into qi, and, conversely, of qi into essence. Sweet and balanced Lycii Fructus *(gǒu qǐ zǐ)* tonifies the Kidneys, augments the essence, and nourishes the Liver blood to brighten the eyes, addressing both the root and branch of the pattern treated by the formula.

This formula is prepared as a syrup, indicating that it is intended to be used long term. Taking it together with alcohol balances any stagnating properties that such a strongly tonifying formula may have on the qi dynamic.

Cautions and Contraindications

This formula is very cloying and is unsuitable for patients with Spleen and Stomach deficiency. It is warming in nature and therefore contraindicated in patients with fire from yin deficiency.

Commentary

This formula is an example of how the symbolic and practical meet in the formulation of treatment strategies in Chinese medicine. Its composition is based on the adage that essences need to be tonified with substances strong in flavor (i.e., those that nourish) rather than qi (i.e., those that are dynamic). Animal products, which contain flesh and blood, are thought to be more useful for nourishing the essences than plants, which are somewhat more removed from human physiology. The deer and the tortoise are also, of course, potent symbols in Chinese mythology, representing power and longevity, yang and yin. Cervi Cornu pantotrichum *(lù róng)* and Testudinis Plastrum *(guī bǎn)* are thought to enter into the eight extraordinary vessels, particularly the Governing and Conception vessels, regarded by many Chinese physicians to constitute one of the most fundamental levels of human physiology.

In its avoidance of draining herbs, this Ming-dynasty formula represents an approach to tonification that is substantially different from Zhang Zhong-Jing's emphasis on balancing tonification of the normal qi with draining of pathogens as well as paying attention to the movement of qi and blood. This style of treatment later formed the foundation of Ye Tian-Shi's

doctrine of tonification via the eight extraordinary vessels, which rejects the use of cloying substances like Rehmanniae Radix praeparata *(shú dì huáng)* or Glycyrrhizae Radix *(gān cǎo)* and focuses, instead, on animal products containing blood, a substance thought to be both tonifying and moving.

Use of this formula is thus most appropriate in cases of severe depletion due to prolonged illness or long-term general debility characterized by few, if any, signs of excess.

Comparisons

➢ Vs. Restore the Left [Kidney] Pill *(zuò guī wán)*

Both formulas contain the same core of animal products that can be used to fill the essence and augment the marrow in patterns characterized by deficiency of the true source. However, in Restore the Left [Kidney] Pill *(zuò guī wán)*, the chief herb is Rehmanniae Radix praeparata *(shú dì huáng)*, while in Tortoise Shell and Deer Antler Two-Immortal Syrup *(guī lù èr xiān jiāo)*, Cervi Cornus Colla *(lù jiǎo jiāo)* and Testudinis Plastri Colla *(guī bǎn jiāo)* are the chief ingredients and are prescribed with a much larger dosage. Ye Tian-Shi argued that cloying herbs such as Rehmanniae Radix praeparata *(shú dì huáng)* do not enter the extraordinary vessels. Hence, while this formula can be used to tonify essence and qi at the level of the Governing and Conception vessels, Restore the Left [Kidney] Pill *(zuò guī wán)* is more appropriate for treating Kidney deficiency patterns.

➢ Vs. Rehmannia Drink *(dì huáng yǐn zi)*

Both formulas treat simultaneous deficiency of yin and yang. However, Rehmannia Drink *(dì huáng yǐn zi)* treats patterns characterized by floating yang and turbid phlegm above with dryness at the level of the yin fluids. By contrast, Tortoise Shell and Deer Antler Two-Immortal Syrup *(guī lù èr xiān jiāo)* treats patterns characterized entirely by symptoms of deficiency with no signs of excess.

➢ Vs. Seven-Treasure Special Pill for Beautiful Whiskers *(qī bǎo měi rán dān)*; *see* page 409

Biomedical Indications

With the appropriate presentation, this formula may be used to treat a variety of biomedically-defined disorders including severe anemia, endocrine-related developmental disorders, reduced sexual function, and nervous exhaustion.

Alternate names

Tortoise Shell and Deer Antler Two-Immortal Syrup *(guī lù èr xiān gāo)* in *Dissecting the Secrets of Sustaining Life*; Two-Immortal Syrup *(èr xiān jiāo)* in *Wondrous Lantern for Peering into the Origin and Development of Miscellaneous Diseases*; Tortoise Shell and Deer Antler Two [-Ingredient] Syrup *(guī lù èr jiāo)* in *Nationwide Collection of TCM Patent Formulas*

七寶美髯丹 (七宝美髯丹)

Seven-Treasure Special Pill for Beautiful Whiskers

qī bǎo měi rán dān

This formula is used primarily for treating premature graying of the hair. Black whiskers were considered more beautiful than gray, and there are seven ingredients in the pill, hence the name.

Source *Comprehensive Outline of the Materia Medica* (1590)

Polygoni multiflori Radix (*hé shǒu wū*)
  [steam in black sesame seeds] 1000g
Poria (*fú líng*) 500g
Poria rubra (*chì fú líng*) 500g
Achyranthis bidentatae Radix (*niú xī*) 240g
wine-washed Angelicae sinensis Radix (*jiǔ xǐ dāng guī*) 240g
Lycii Fructus (*gǒu qǐ zǐ*) 240g
Cuscutae Semen (*tù sī zǐ*) 240g
Psoraleae Fructus (*bǔ gǔ zhī*)
  [dry-fry with black sesame seeds] 120g

Method of Preparation Grind the ingredients into a powder and form into 9g pills with honey. The normal dosage is one pill in the morning and evening taken with warm, salted water. Pots made from iron are specifically forbidden for use in the preparation of this decoction.

Actions Enriches the Kidney yin and nourishes the Liver blood

Indications

Premature graying of the hair or hair loss, loose teeth, spontaneous and nocturnal emissions, and soreness and weakness of the lower back and knees.

Healthy hair depends on the sufficiency of blood stored in the Liver. When the Liver blood is deficient, it is unable to rise and nourish the head; the hair then turns gray or falls out. The health of the Kidneys is expressed in the hair of the head, and graying or loss of hair is a sign of Kidney deficiency. The teeth depend on the sufficiency of bone matter, which is governed by the Kidneys. The Kidneys also generate marrow, which is thought to keep the teeth in place; if the Kidneys are deficient, the teeth will become loose and readily fall out. Nocturnal and spontaneous emissions are classic signs of Kidney yin deficiency, while soreness and weakness of the lower back and knees are signs of Liver and Kidney deficiency.

Analysis of Formula

The chief herb is Polygoni multiflori Radix (*hé shǒu wū*), used here in a relatively large dosage. Its bitterness enables it to strengthen the sinews and bones, and its astringent properties enable it to stabilize the essence and thus the Kidneys. Two of the deputies, Lycii Fructus (*gǒu qǐ zǐ*) and Cuscutae Semen (*tù sī zǐ*), nourish the Liver and Kidneys. In concert with the chief herb, they supplement and stabilize the essence and thereby help stop nocturnal and spontaneous emissions.

Achyranthis bidentatae Radix (*niú xī*), the other deputy, is used for its ability to strengthen the sinews and bones in general, and the lower back and knees in particular. Because of its effect on the Liver blood, Angelicae sinensis Radix (*dāng guī*) is added as an assistant ingredient to help the chief and deputy herbs nourish the hair.

All of the above herbs are yin in nature, but if the yin is without yang, it will be unable to transform the condition. The warm herb Psoraleae Fructus (*bǔ gǔ zhī*), which tonifies the yang, is therefore added as an 'opposing assistant' to find the yang in the yin. Similarly, if there is tonification without any draining, it is possible that the formula will inhibit the Bladder's function of draining turbidity. For this reason, Poria (*fú líng*) is added as another assistant to leach out any dampness or turbidity in the body. The use of black sesame seeds, Sesami Semen nigrum (*hēi zhī má*), in processing some of the herbs strengthens the yin-nourishing properties of the formula. It is regarded as the envoy ingredient.

Cautions and Contraindications

This formula is quite cloying in nature and should therefore be used with caution (if at all) in patients with Spleen deficiency.

Commentary

The composition of this formula is attributed to the Ming-dynasty Daoist and master physician Shao Ying-Jie (邵應節), who successfully prescribed the formula to Emperor Shizong (1522-1566). In *Essential Formulas to Support Longevity*, a famous Ming physician, Wu Min, provides a useful account of what to expect when prescribing this formula:

> After taking [this formula] for three to four days, urination increases or changes in color, indicating that miscellaneous diseases are being eliminated from the five organs. After two weeks, the lips turn red from the generation of fluids and one will not have to get up again at night [to urinate]. If one experiences slight abdominal pain, this is nothing to worry about as this is the disease being tracked down. After three weeks, the body feels light and comfortable and then the breasts become red and moist. After one month, one feels an acrid and sour [sensation] in the nose, indicating that all kinds of wind and [associated] disorders are leaving. After forty-nine days, [the formula has] tonified the blood and generated essence, drained the fire and benefited the water, strengthened the sinews and bones, and turned the hair black.

Owing to its balanced composition, combining tonification with draining, securing with moving, this formula is regarded as a model for treating problems associated with aging.

Comparison

➤ Vs. Tortoise Shell and Deer Antler Two-Immortal Syrup (*guī lù èr xiān jiāo*)

Both formulas tonify the yin and yang, promote vitality, and are used to prevent and treat disorders associated with aging. Tortoise Shell and Deer Antler Two-Immortal Syrup *(guī lù èr xiān jiāo)*, which contains two animal substances, is stronger at generating essence and blood. These substances also enter the Governing and Conception vessels, regulating the organization and flow of qi at a deep level. This function is further enhanced by the inclusion of Ginseng Radix *(rén shēn)*, which strongly tonifies the original qi. Seven-Treasure Special Pill for Beautiful Whiskers *(qī bǎo měi rán dān)* is relatively more warming and moving while also moistening and securing. Rather than treating the Governing and Conception vessels, it tonifies the Liver and Kidneys, not just promoting the generation of blood and essence, but also draining the pathogenic qi from the qi and blood by the inclusion of dampness-draining Poria *(fú líng)* and blood-moving Achyranthis bidentatae Radix *(niú xī)*.

Biomedical Indications

With the appropriate presentation, this formula may be used to treat a variety of biomedically-defined disorders including alopecia, premature graying of the hair, many types of dental problems, impotence, and infertility in males.

Alternate names

Seven-Gem Pill of Utmost Treasures *(qī zhēn zhì bǎo dān)* and Black Whiskers Pill to Strengthen Yang *(wū xū jiàn yáng dān)* in *Essential Formulas to Support Longevity*; Beautiful Whiskers Pill *(měi rán dān)* in *Precious Mirror for Advancement of Medicine*; Seven-Treasure Pill for Beautiful Whiskers *(qī bǎo měi rán wán)* in *Nationwide Collection of TCM Patent Formulas*; Flowery Knotweed Pill to Tonify and Augment *(hé shǒu bǔ yì wán)* in *Practical Manual of Prepared Chinese Medicine*

Modifications

- For pronounced backache and aversion to cold, add Morindae officinalis Radix *(bā jǐ tiān)*, Curculiginis Rhizoma *(xiān máo)*, and Epimedii Herba *(yín yáng huò)*.

- For a lusterless complexion and dizziness, add Rehmanniae Radix praeparata *(shú dì huáng)* and Paeoniae Radix alba *(bái sháo)*.

- For seminal emissions, add Astragali complanati Semen *(shā yuàn zǐ)*, Euryales Semen *(qiàn shí)*, calcined Ostreae Concha *(duàn mǔ lì)*, and calcined Fossilia Ossis Mastodi *(duàn lóng gǔ)*.

二仙湯 (二仙汤)

Two-Immortal Decoction

èr xiān tāng

The name of this formula is derived from the word 仙 *xiān*, which means immortal or celestial being. It appears in the names of the two chief ingredients, Curculiginis Rhizoma (仙茅 *xiān máo*) and Epimedii Herba (仙靈脾 *xiān líng pí*), more commonly known as 淫羊藿 *yín yáng huò*.

Source   *Clinical Handbook of Chinese Medical Formulas* (1950s)

Curculiginis Rhizoma *(xiān máo)* 6-15g
Epimedii Herba *(yín yáng huò)* 9-15g
Morindae officinalis Radix *(bā jǐ tiān)* 9g
Phellodendri Cortex *(huáng bǎi)* .4.5-9g
Anemarrhenae Rhizoma *(zhī mǔ)* 4.5-9g
Angelicae sinensis Radix *(dāng guī)* 9g

Method of Preparation   Decoction

Actions   Warms the Kidney yang, tonifies the Kidney essence, drains fire from the Kidneys, and regulates the Penetrating and Conception vessels

Indications

Symptoms of menopause including hypertension, menstrual irregularity, hot flushes, sweating, nervousness, fatigue, lassitude, depression, irritability, insomnia, palpitations, and urinary frequency. The formula may also be used for other chronic disorders which present with signs and symptoms of Kidney yang deficiency and flaring-up of fire at the gate of vitality.

This is deficiency of both the Kidney yin and yang accompanied by a flaring-up of fire at the gate of vitality. This is a complicated pattern of disharmony that can present with rather complex patterns of symptoms, such as those seen in menopause. In contemporary Chinese medicine, menopause can be associated with deficiency of the Penetrating and Conception vessels. Together with a decline of the Kidney qi, this produces such symptoms as menstrual disturbances or amenorrhea, hot flushes, sweating, and nervousness. From a combined Western and Chinese medical perspective, this process can also lead to hypertension. Waning of the Kidney yang is responsible for such symptoms as fatigue, lassitude, depression, and urinary frequency. Ascending fire at the gate of vitality presents with irritability, insomnia, and palpitations.

Analysis of Formula

The treatment strategy underlying the composition of this formula is to tonify the Kidney yin and yang as well as drain flaring fire at the gate of vitality. Curculiginis Rhizoma *(xiān máo)* and Epimedii Herba *(yín yáng huò)* are the chief herbs in this formula. Together with the deputy, Morindae officinalis Radix *(bā jǐ tiān)*, they warm the Kidney yang and tonify the Kidney essence. Epimedii Herba *(yín yáng huò)* also tonifies the yin and yang and harnesses the ascendant fire, which makes it an ideal ingredient for this particular pattern of disharmony. Two of the assistants, Phellodendri Cortex *(huáng bǎi)* and Anemarrhenae Rhizoma *(zhī mǔ)*, drain ascending fire at the gate of vitality. The other assistant, Angelicae sinensis Radix *(dāng guī)*, moistens and nourishes the blood and regulates the Penetrating and Conception vessels.

Commentary

This is a modern formula composed by the Shanghai physician Zhang Bo-Na during the 1950s to treat hypertension in menopausal women. It is an example of how traditional therapeutic strategies were employed at the time in the search for solutions to modern, often biomedically-defined, health care problems. The formula may also be effective in treating other types of hypertension, but further research is needed to determine whether it has any special properties in this regard. Its use has already been extended to other chronic disorders such as amenorrhea, schizophrenia occurring during menopause, nephritis, and pyelonephritis. With appropriate modifications, it is generally applicable to chronic disorders with manifestations of fire above and Kidney deficiency below.

The special feature of this formula is its combination of herbs that strengthen the yang with those that nourish the blood and others that drain fire. Although the number of ingredients is small, its design and underlying strategy are complex. The formula focuses on two particular aspects of the disharmony: deficiency of Kidney yang in the lower part of the body, and the flaring-up of fire at the gate of vitality, which manifests in the upper part of the body. Clinical presentations may include signs and symptoms that also occur in patterns characterized by Liver and Kidney yin deficiency with ascending fire. In those cases, there will be no signs of yang deficiency or coldness below.

The strategy of this formula is to warm the Kidney yang while quelling flaring fire at the gate of vitality. In addition to these seemingly contradictory but actually complementary actions, the formula also tonifies the essence and blood. Tonifying the blood counterbalances the action of the warming herbs to prevent further injury to the already deficient yin and essence, but is also, of course, a typical presentation of postmenopause. For example, Curculiginis Rhizoma *(xiān máo)* is often contraindicated in cases of yin deficiency with heat signs. However, its powerful effect on the Kidneys and yang can be used here because of the counterbalance provided by the cooling properties of Phellodendri Cortex *(huáng bǎi)* and Anemarrhenae Rhizoma *(zhī mǔ)*. In addition, its drying action is moderated by Anemarrhenae Rhizoma *(zhī mǔ)*, which nurtures the yin while draining fire, and Angelicae sinensis Radix *(dāng guī)*, which moistens the Intestines.

From a classical perspective, the symptoms of excess treated by this formula fall under the category of yin fire. The reader is referred to the COMMENTARY section under Great Tonify the Yin Pill *(dà bǔ yīn wán)* for a detailed discussion of this concept, particularly in relation to the use of the cooling, bitter herbs Phellodendri Cortex *(huáng bǎi)* and Anemarrhenae Rhizoma *(zhī mǔ)*.

Biomedical Indications

With the appropriate presentation, this formula may be used to treat a variety of biomedically-defined disorders such as perimenopausal syndrome, essential hypertension, chronic glomerulonephritis, chronic pyelonephritis, polycystic kidneys, renal vascular disease, hyperthyroidism, urinary tract infection, and hypofunction of the anterior pituitary.

Comparative Tables of Principal Formulas

■ FORMULAS THAT TONIFY THE QI

Common symptoms: weakness, shortness of breath, reduced appetite, pale tongue, deficient pulse

Formula Name	Diagnosis	Indications	Remarks
Four-Gentlemen Decoction *(sì jūn zǐ tāng)*	Spleen qi deficiency	Pallid complexion, low and soft voice, loose stools, weakness in the limbs, a pale tongue, and a deficient and/or frail pulse	A harmonious and moderate formula for tonifying the Spleen qi.
Ginseng, Poria, and White Atractylodes Powder *(shēn líng bái zhú sǎn)*	Spleen qi deficiency leading to internally-generated dampness	Loose stools or diarrhea, weakness of the extremities, distention and a stifling sensation in the chest and epigastrium with possible vomiting, pallid complexion, a pale tongue with a white coating, and a thin, moderate or deficient, moderate pulse	Also for chronic cough with copious sputum due to Lung and Spleen deficiency.
Tonify the Middle to Augment the Qi Decoction *(bǔ zhōng yì qì tāng)*	Deficiency of the Spleen and Stomach with inability to raise the clear yang	Dizziness, impaired vision, tinnitus, intermittent fever that worsens upon exertion, spontaneous sweating, aversion to cold, a thirst for warm beverages, shortness of breath, a shiny, pale complexion, loose stools, a pale, possibly swollen tongue, and a pulse that is frail or large but forceless	Also for fever from qi deficiency and various patterns resulting from sinking of the middle burner qi including prolapse, diarrhea, and bleeding disorders.

cont. ↘

Raise the Yang and Augment the Stomach Decoction (*shēng yáng yì wèi tāng*)	Spleen and Stomach qi deficiency with damp-heat in the lower burner	Loss of taste, abdominal fullness and distention, irregular bowel movements, fatigue, heaviness, pain in the joints, chills, aversion to wind, dizziness, reduced and dark urine, and a dry mouth and tongue	Focuses on building up middle burner qi in conjunction with eliminating dampness and clearing heat.
Jade Windscreen Powder (*yù píng fēng sǎn*)	Deficiency of the protective qi	Aversion to drafts, spontaneous sweating, recurrent colds, a shiny, pale complexion, a pale tongue with a white coating, and a floating, deficient, and soft pulse	Also for chronic colds, allergies, asthma, and urticaria.
Generate the Pulse Powder (*shēng mài sǎn*)	Simultaneous Lung qi and yin deficiency	Chronic cough with sparse sputum that is difficult to expectorate, shortness of breath, spontaneous sweating, dry mouth, a pale, red tongue with a dry, thin coating, and a deficient, rapid or deficient, thin pulse	Also for palpitations presenting alongside shortness of breath and a dry mouth, heat-stroke, acute shock, and various forms of heart disease.
Tonify the Lungs Decoction (*bǔ fèi tāng*)	Lung qi deficiency	Shortness of breath, spontaneous sweating, occasional chills and feverishness, coughing, wheezing, a pale tongue, and a frail or deficient and large pulse	For chronic cough due to Lung deficiency.
Ginseng and Gecko Powder (*rén shēn gé jiè sǎn*)	Lung and Kidney qi deficiency with phlegm-heat collecting internally	Chronic coughing and wheezing, thick, yellow sputum, coughing of pus and blood, a sensation of heat and irritability in the chest, facial edema, gradual emaciation, a purple tongue with a thin, white or thin, greasy, and yellow coating, and a floating, deficient pulse, especially at the distal position	This is a deficient condition and therefore the coughing lacks force and exhalation is easier than inhalation. May progress to Lung atrophy.

■ FORMULAS THAT TONIFY THE BLOOD

Common symptoms: menstrual disorders, irritability, pale tongue, thin, deficient, or submerged pulse

Formula Name	Diagnosis	Indications	Remarks
Four-Substance Decoction (*sì wù tāng*)	Generalized blood deficiency and stagnation	Dizziness, lusterless complexion and nails, muscle tension, insomnia, irregular menses with little flow, lower abdominal pain, a pale tongue, and a thin and wiry or thin and choppy pulse	Also for menorrhagia, hard abdominal masses with recurrent pain, and restless fetus disorder.
Tangkuei Decoction to Tonify the Blood (*dāng guī bǔ xuè tāng*)	Deficiency heat pattern from blood deficiency and floating yang	Hot sensation in the muscles, red face, irritability, thirst for warm beverages, a pale tongue, and a flooding, large, and deficient pulse that is forceless when pressed hard	Also for fever and headache due to loss of blood, bleeding disorders, and nonhealing, yin-type ulcers.
Delayed Menstruation Drink (*guò qī yǐn*)	Blood deficiency and stasis in patients who tend to be cold	Overdue menses, scanty menstrual flow (often with blood clots), pain and distention in the lower abdomen before and during the menses, and a submerged and strong pulse	Also for painful menses owing to blood deficiency and stasis of qi and blood.
Arborvitae Seed Pill for Women's Disorders (*nǔ kē bái zǐ rén wán*)	Gradual onset amenorrhea from blood deficiency	General disquietude, afternoon tidal fevers, emaciation, and achy and uncomfortable flesh and bones of the hands and feet	Also for irregular menstruation or scanty menses from deficiency of yin and blood accompanied by blood stasis.
Peony and Licorice Decoction (*sháo yào gān cǎo tāng*)	Blood deficiency or injury to the fluids	Irritability, slight chills, spasms of the calf muscles, and lack of coating on the tongue	For various pain syndromes associated with spasms and cramps (particularly the abdomen).

cont. ↘

Mutton Stew with Tangkuei and Fresh Ginger (*dāng guī shēng jiāng yáng ròu tāng*)	Interior deficiency with cold blood	Postpartum abdominal pain, cold abdominal hernial pain, or spasmodic pain in the flanks, all of which respond favorably to pressure and warmth, and a submerged, wiry, and forceless pulse	Also for dysmenorrhea, leukorrhea, lower back pain, and abdominal pain associated with cold from deficiency.

■ FORMULAS THAT TONIFY THE QI AND BLOOD

Common symptoms: loss of appetite, fatigue, pallid/wan complexion, emaciation, palpitations, pale tongue, forceless pulse

Formula Name	Diagnosis	Indications	Remarks
Eight-Treasure Decoction (*bā zhēn tāng*)	Qi and blood deficiency	Pallid or sallow complexion, palpitations, anxiety, reduced appetite, laconic speech, easily-fatigued extremities, light-headedness and/or vertigo, a pale tongue with a white coating, and a pulse that is either thin and frail or large, deficient, and without strength	Symptoms may also include chills and fever, weight loss, non-healing abscesses, and continuous spotting from uterine bleeding.
All-Inclusive Great Tonifying Decoction (*shí quán dà bǔ tāng*)	Qi and blood deficiency with a tendency toward internal cold	Wan complexion, fatigue, reduced appetite, dizziness, listlessness, palpitations, spontaneous or night sweating, cold extremities, spermatorrhea, a pale tongue, and a thin and frail pulse	Focuses on warming and tonifying. Also used to treat sores that do not heal, irregular periods, or continuous spotting from uterine bleeding.
Ginseng Decoction to Nourish Luxuriance (*rén shēn yǎng róng tāng*)	Heart and Spleen qi and blood deficiency with internal heat and dryness	Palpitations, forgetfulness, restlessness at night, feverishness, reduced appetite, fatigue, cough, dyspnea on exertion, weight loss, dry skin, and a dry mouth and throat	Also for chronic, nonhealing sores.
Restore the Spleen Decoction (*guī pí tāng*)	Spleen qi and Heart blood deficiency	Forgetfulness, palpitations, insomnia, dream-disturbed sleep, anxiety and phobia, feverishness, reduced appetite, pallid and wan complexion, early or prolonged menses, a pale tongue with a thin, white coating, and a thin, frail pulse	Also for chronic bleeding syndromes.
Prepared Licorice Decoction (*zhì gān cǎo tāng*)	Consumptive conditions with qi and blood deficiency	Palpitations with anxiety, irritability, insomnia, emaciation, shortness of breath, constipation, dry mouth and throat, a pale, shiny tongue, and a pulse that is consistently irregular, slow-irregular, or thin, faint, and forceless	Focuses on tonifying deficiency while addressing elements of stagnation due to cold and dryness. This is the principal formula for irregular pulses; also for Lung atrophy.
Taishan Bedrock Powder (*Tàishān pán shí sǎn*)	Qi and blood deficiency with lack of nourishment of the fetus	Restless fetus, threatened or habitual miscarriage, pale complexion, fatigue, lack of appetite, a pale tongue with a slippery coating, and a slippery but forceless pulse	Focuses on tonifying the qi and blood to prevent miscarriage.
Worry-Free Formula to Protect Birth (*bǎo chǎn wú yōu fāng*)	Qi and blood deficiency with unsecured Penetrating and Conception vessels	Restless fetus, tendency to miscarriage, malpositioned fetus, and difficult delivery	Also considered a prophylactic against miscarriage and difficult delivery.
Fleeceflower Root and Ginseng Drink (*hé rén yǐn*)	Malarial disorders with qi and blood deficiency	Chronic, unrelenting malarial disorders with a wan complexion, emaciation, intermittent fever and chills aggravated by slight exertion, a pale tongue, and a moderate, large, deficient pulse	Treats deficiency-type malarial disorders without further depleting the patient.

cont. ↘

Rehmannia Drink from *A Simple Book (dì huáng yǐn zi)*	Wasting and thirsting disorder due to heat in the yang brightness warp with depleted qi and blood	Thirst, irritability, restlessness, dry throat, flushed face, fatigue, and spontaneous sweating	Focuses on tonifying the qi, blood, and yin, while guiding out heat.

■ FORMULAS THAT NOURISH AND TONIFY THE YIN

Common symptoms: sore and weak lower back, dry mouth and throat, irritability of some type, red and dry tongue, thin and rapid pulse

Formula Name	Diagnosis	Indications	Remarks
Six-Ingredient Pill with Rehmannia *(liù wèi dì huáng wán)*	Kidney and Liver yin deficiency	Lower back soreness and weakness, light headedness, vertigo, tinnitus, diminished hearing, night sweats, spontaneous and nocturnal emissions, possibly hot palms and soles or chronic sore throat, a red tongue with little coating, and a rapid, thin pulse	The representative formula of this group, it is balanced between enriching the yin and treating fire from deficiency.
Restore the Left [Kidney] Pill *(zuǒ guī wán)*	Kidney yin deficiency with damage to the essence and marrow	Lightheadedness, tinnitus, lower back soreness, spontaneous emissions, night sweats, dry mouth and throat, thirst, a peeled, shiny tongue, and a thin, rapid pulse	Focuses on treating deficiency and therefore for patients with no signs of fire.
Great Tonify the Yin Pill *(dà bǔ yīn wán)*	Yin deficiency and flourishing fire	Afternoon tidal fever, night sweats, spontaneous emissions, irritability, a sensation of heat and pain in the knees and legs, a red tongue with little coating, and a pulse that is rapid and forceful in the rear position	Focuses on causing the fire from deficiency to descend and less on tonifying.
Jade Spring Pill *(yù quán wán)*	Wasting and thirsting disorder with exhausted qi and fluids	Irritability, thirst, urinary frequency, dry mouth, increased appetite, weight loss, a large and rapid pulse, and a red, dry tongue	Focuses on tonifying the Spleen and Lungs, generating fluids, and adjusting the water pathways.
Hidden Tiger Pill *(hǔ qián wán)*	Atrophy disorder due to Liver and Kidney deficiency	Weakness of the lower back and knees, deterioration of the sinews and bones, wasting of the legs and feet, difficulty walking, a red tongue with little coating, and a thin, frail pulse	Also for dizziness, tinnitus, spontaneous emissions, and urinary incontinence.
Great Creation Pill *(dà zào wán)*	Kidney and Lung yin deficiency	Cough with sticky sputum that is difficult to expectorate, emaciation, tinnitus, dizziness, tidal fever, dry mouth and throat, heat in the five centers, and night sweats	Especially useful for consumptive disorders with emaciation.
Linking Decoction *(yī guàn jiān)*	Liver and Kidney yin deficiency with qi stagnation	Hypochondriac, epigastric, and chest pain, dry and parched mouth and throat, acid reflux, a red and dry tongue, and a thin, frail or deficient, wiry pulse	Not for pain and distention from dampness or phlegm.
Two-Solstice Pill *(èr zhì wán)*	Liver and Kidney yin deficiency	Weakness and soreness of the lower back and knees, dry mouth and throat, dizziness, blurred vision, insomnia, spontaneous emissions, premature graying or loss of hair, and a red, dry tongue	Also for chronic bleeding problems.
Lily Bulb Decoction to Preserve the Metal *(bǎi hé gù jīn tāng)*	Lung and Kidney yin deficiency with heat from deficiency	Coughing with blood-streaked sputum, wheezing, a dry and sore throat, hot palms and soles, night sweats, a red tongue with little coating, and a thin, rapid pulse	This is internal dryness of the Lungs; this formula focuses on nourishing the yin.

cont. ↘

Tonify the Lungs Decoction with Ass-Hide Gelatin (bǔ fèi ē jiāo tāng)	Lung yin deficiency with vigorous heat	Cough with wheezing, dry and parched throat, scanty or blood-streaked sputum, a red tongue with little coating, and a floating, thin, and rapid pulse	Focuses on clearing heat and stopping bleeding.
Decoction to Enrich Yin and Direct Fire Downward (zī yīn jiàng huǒ tāng)	Yin deficiency with fire from deficiency	Cough that may or may not be productive, wheezing, night sweats, dry mouth, fever, coughing of blood, sore and dry throat, throat sores, and raspy voice	For consumptive disorders such as wasting and thirsting and steaming bones.
Precious Jade Syrup (qióng yù gāo)	Lung and Kidney yin deficiency consumptive disorder	Dry cough with little sputum, dry throat or spitting of blood, muscle wasting, shortness of breath, weakness, a red tongue with little coating, and a thin, rapid pulse	Tonifying formula for long-term use (not during external pathogenic invasion).
Preserve Vistas Pill (zhù jīng wán)	Liver and Kidney deficiency with some dampness	Diminished visual acuity and blurred vision that worsens with exertion and improves with rest, soreness and weakness of the lower back and legs, and a thin, frail pulse	Focuses on tonifying the Kidneys below and draining pathogenic water from above.
Benefit the Stomach Decoction (yì wèi tāng)	Stomach yin deficiency	Faint or indistinct pain or burning in the epigastric region, hunger but no desire to eat, dry mouth and throat, constipation, retching, a dry, red tongue with scanty coating, and a thin, rapid pulse	Also for dizziness, ulcerations in the oral cavity, picky eating in children, as well as dental problems.

■ FORMULAS THAT WARM AND TONIFY THE YANG

Common symptoms: fatigue, aversion to cold, lower back pain, weakness in lower extremities, pale and swollen tongue, thin and frail pulse (especially in the proximal position)

Formula Name	Diagnosis	Indications	Remarks
Kidney Qi Pill (shèn qì wán)	Kidney yang deficiency	Cold, pain, and weakness of the lower back and legs, tense lower abdomen, urinary disorders, a pale, swollen tongue with a thin, white, and moist coating, and an empty or frail pulse that is submerged and faint at the proximal position	Particularly useful when there are abnormalities in water metabolism. Also for leg qi and thin mucus.
Restore the Right [Kidney] Pill (yòu guī wán)	Kidney yang deficiency with waning of the fire at the gate of vitality	Exhaustion from long-term illness, aversion to cold, cold extremities, impotence, spermatorrhea, aching and weakness of the lower back and knees, and possibly infertility, loose stools, incontinence, or edema	Focuses on tonification and therefore not for patients with dampness or turbidity.
Cuscuta Seed Pill (tù sī zǐ wán)	Kidney qi deficiency with an inability to grasp the essence	Exhaustion, aversion to cold, frail physique, dizziness, lower back pain, weakness of the lower extremities, frequent, scanty urination with continuous dripping, and a submerged, thin pulse that is especially frail at the proximal position	Focuses on constraining leakage.
Special Pill to Aid Fertility (zàn yù dān)	Waning of the fire at the gate of vitality with cold and deficiency of the essential qi	Impotence or infertility, listlessness and dispiritedness, aching and weakness of the lower back, a pale, shiny complexion, and a submerged, thin pulse	Focuses on tonifying and warming the Kidneys to promote fertility.

■ FORMULAS THAT TONIFY BOTH THE YIN AND THE YANG

Common symptoms: soreness and weakness of the lower back and knees, sexual disorders, generalized debility or exhaustion, frail pulse

Formula Name	Diagnosis	Indications	Remarks
Rehmannia Drink (dì huáng yǐn zi)	Kidney yin and yang deficiency with upward-flaring of deficient yang and phlegm turbidity blocking the orifices	Mute paraplegia with stiffness of the tongue, inability to speak, disability or paralysis of the lower extremities, dry mouth with no thirst, a greasy, yellow tongue coating, and a submerged, slow, thin, and frail pulse	Also for other Kidney deficiency disorders including insomnia, edema, or dryness and itching of the skin.
Tortoise Shell and Deer Antler Two-Immortal Syrup (guī lù èr xiān jiāo)	Kidney yin and yang deficiency with insufficiency of essence and blood in the Conception and Governing vessels	Emaciation, weakness, spermatorrhea, impotence, diminished visual acuity, aching and weakness of the lower back and knees, daybreak diarrhea, and a thin, frail pulse	Most appropriate in cases of severe depletion.
Seven-Treasure Special Pill for Beautiful Whiskers (qī bǎo měi rán dān)	Deficiency of Liver blood and Kidney yin	Premature graying of the hair or hair loss, loose teeth, spontaneous and nocturnal emissions, and soreness and weakness of the lower back and knees	Used to prevent and treat disorders associated with aging.
Two-Immortal Decoction (èr xiān tāng)	Kidney yin and yang deficiency with flaring-up of fire at the gate of vitality	Symptoms of menopause including hypertension, menstrual irregularity, hot flushes, sweating, fatigue, depression, irritability, insomnia, palpitations, and urinary frequency	Also for other chronic disorders with symptoms of Kidney yang deficiency and flaring-up of fire at the gate of vitality.

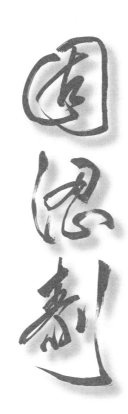

Chapter 9 Contents

Formulas that Stabilize and Bind

Formulas that Stabilize and Bind

9

I N CHINESE MEDICINE, the qi, blood, essence, and body fluids are regarded as treasures that nourish and sustain the human body. Under normal conditions, the body maintains physiologically appropriate levels of these substances by regulating production and discharge. Some leakage of substances (including sweat, sputum, blood, urine, stool, sperm, vaginal discharge) and qi is thus a normal aspect of healthy physiological function.

There are two common causes for the improper discharge or leakage of qi and substances from the body. First, they can be forced out by conditions of excess involving heat, for example, exterior wind-heat, phlegm-heat in the Lungs, hot blood, or damp-heat in the lower burner. Second, the deficiency or weakening of those processes that normally hold in the fluids and other substances causes instability. It is the latter problem that is addressed by the formulas in this chapter. The most common strategy underlying these formulas is to combine tonifying substances that strengthen these processes with astringent substances that stabilize or 'firm up' the physiological functions of holding and restraining and thereby prevent abnormal leakage and discharge.

Among the ten types of traditional formulas, those in this chapter are said to stabilize and bind (固澀 *gù sè*). This strategy was first mentioned in *Basic Questions* (Chapter 74): "For [problems of] dispersion, retain" and "Astringent [substances] can stabilize [cases of] abandonment." The term abandonment (脱 *tuō*) refers to a condition in which there is an external draining of the body's fundamental substances.

This is a serious condition that requires immediate and strong intervention. Generally, this is done by tonifying the primal qi by administering Ginseng Radix *(rén shēn)* as a stand-alone herb. If there are signs of cold indicating loss of yang qi, Ginseng Radix *(rén shēn)* is often combined with Aconiti Radix lateralis praeparata *(zhì fù zǐ)*. Other formulas for this condition are found in Chapter 6.

There are five major categories of formulas that stabilize and bind: those that stabilize the exterior and stop sweating; those that secure the Lungs and stop coughing; those that bind up the Intestines and secure abandoned conditions; those that secure the essence and stop enuresis; and those that secure irregular uterine bleeding and stop vaginal discharge.

It is important to bear in mind that while these formulas are designed for problems such as abandonment that are caused by exhaustion of the normal qi and essence, they primarily focus on the symptoms or branch. To effect a long-term cure, once the symptoms are resolved, one should continue treatment with formulas that address the root or underlying cause.

It is imperative that these formulas *not* be used in treating conditions of excess, such as profuse sweating from acute febrile disease (Chapter 4), spontaneous emissions due to fire from excess (Chapter 4), acute dysenteric disorders (Chapter 4), diarrhea from food stagnation (Chapter 18), or uterine bleeding from the reckless movement of hot blood (Chapter 13). If these formulas are used in cases with lingering, externally-contracted pathogenic influences, those influences will remain in the body for a long time.

Section 1

....

FORMULAS THAT STABILIZE THE EXTERIOR AND STOP SWEATING

Sweating is an important sign in Chinese medicine, providing information about the movement of yang qi and fluids toward the exterior of the body and in the exterior itself. Abnormal sweating can be due to a wide variety of pathologies and is treated with a large number of formulas found throughout many chapters of this book. The formulas in this section only treat sweating that does not involve either a condition of excess (of wind, heat, dampness) or pronounced deficiency (of qi, yin, or yang). This usually results from a disharmony between the nutritive and protective qi due to internal rather than external causes. It may manifest as spontaneous sweating or night sweats, and is frequently accompanied by symptoms such as a pallid complexion, shortness of breath, palpitations, a pale tongue, and a thin, deficient, or frail pulse. The treatment strategy here is to tonify the qi so as to stabilize or 'firm up' the protective qi, while enriching and unblocking constraint in the movement of the nutritive qi.

In clinical practice, deficiency of protective qi in the exterior invariably means that the body is having difficulty expelling pathogens or that it is easier for them to invade the exterior in the first place. Such deficiency, furthermore, is often complicated by deficiency of qi at deeper functional levels in the body. For this reason, formulas such as Jade Windscreen Powder *(yù píng fēng sǎn)*, discussed in Chapter 8, modified Cinnamon Twig Decoction *(guì zhī tāng)*, discussed in Chapter 1, and modified True Warrior Decoction *(zhēn wǔ tāng)*, discussed in Chapter 16, are also commonly used to stop this type of sweating.

The core ingredients of these formulas are those that directly stabilize the exterior and stop sweating, such as Ostreae Concha *(mǔ lì)* and Astragali Radix *(huáng qí)*. Because the exterior is stronger when the qi in general is stronger, herbs that strengthen the Spleen and augment the qi, such as Atractylodis macrocephalae Rhizoma *(bái zhú)*, are often added. When Heart heat is part of the clinical picture, sweet, cooling herbs that enter the Heart, such as Tritici Fructus *(xiǎo mài)*, are added. Often these patients harbor some slight wind in the exterior. Should that occur, one should add herbs that dispel wind from the exterior, such as Saposhnikoviae Radix *(fáng fēng)*.

牡蠣散 （牡蛎散）

Oyster Shell Powder

mǔ lì sǎn

Source *Formulary of the Pharmacy Service for Benefiting the People in the Taiping Era* (1107)

calcined Ostreae Concha *(duàn mǔ lì)* 30g (15-30g)
Astragali Radix *(huáng qí)* 30g (9-15g)
Ephedrae Radix *(má huáng gēn)* 30g (3-9g)
Tritici Fructus levis *(fú xiǎo mài)* 30g (15-30g)

Method of Preparation Grind the first three ingredients into a powder, add the fourth herb, and take 9g as a draft. The source text recommends that it be taken twice a day. May also be prepared as a decoction with the dosage indicated in parentheses.

Note: The source text specifies Tritici Fructus *(xiǎo mài)* instead of Tritici Fructus levis *(fú xiǎo mài)*. These are the ripe grains of wheat that do not float. They are sweet and slightly cold, and enter the Heart channel. They nourish the Heart qi and eliminate irritability. In contemporary practice, Tritici Fructus levis *(fú xiǎo mài)* is used because its floating nature focuses the action even more strongly on the surface of the body.

Actions Inhibits sweating and stabilizes the exterior

Indications

Spontaneous sweating that worsens at night, palpitations, easily startled, shortness of breath, irritability, general debility, lethargy, a pale-red tongue, and a thin, frail pulse.

Sweating that is neither due to exertion nor occurs at night is called 'spontaneous sweating' and is associated with deficient qi. Sweating that comes on with sleep and ends upon awakening is called 'night sweats,' literally 'thieving sweat' (盗 汗 *dào hàn)*. It is associated with deficient yin. The pattern for which this formula is indicated involves both spontaneous sweating due to unstable protective qi (associated with the Lungs) and night sweats due to constrained heat at the level of the nutritive qi (associated with the Heart).

Sweat is the fluid of the Heart. Prolonged sweating thus can reflect physiological disturbances at the level of Heart qi or yin and, in turn, can exacerbate such disorders. When deficient nutritive qi (yin) is unable to properly anchor the protective qi (yang), it begins to float, becomes more deficient, and aggravates the sweating until it becomes most pronounced at night. This type of sweating, a combination of spontaneous and night sweats, is a manifestation of both deficient qi and yin, albeit at the yin level of qi, rather than that of the essences. Injury to the Heart qi also manifests as palpitations, anxiety, being easily startled, shortness of breath, and general debility. The combination of irritability and lethargy is often a sign of deficient qi with concurrent heat from constraint. The pale-red tongue and thin, frail pulse are also characteristic of deficiency of both qi and constrained heat.

Analysis of Formula

This formula employs two strategies first outlined in *Basic Questions*—"Astringe what is dispersing" and "Tonify what is deficient"—to inhibit sweating and secure the exterior. The chief ingredient, salty and slightly cooling Ostreae Concha (*mǔ lì*), restrains the yin, anchors the floating yang, inhibits sweating, and relieves irritability. The deputy, Astragali Radix (*huáng qí*), strongly tonifies the Lung qi and is of particular benefit to the superficial protective qi. It strengthens the protective qi and stabilizes the exterior. The combination of these two ingredients, one of which benefits the nutritive level and the other the protective level, is especially effective in treating this condition. The deputy is also very helpful in treating the symptoms associated with deficient qi, including shortness of breath and general debility.

One of the assistants, Ephedrae Radix (*má huáng gēn*), assists the chief ingredient in augmenting the Heart qi, restraining sweat, and stabilizing the exterior. Its nature is to move to the exterior of the body, but its action is to direct the qi downward. It thereby complements the action of Ostreae Concha (*mǔ lì*), which anchors the yang, while focusing the tonifying actions of Astragali Radix (*huáng qí*) on the exterior. The other assistant is the sweet, salty, and slightly cooling Tritici Fructus levis (*fú xiǎo mài*). It mildly nourishes the Heart qi and clears heat from constraint by venting it to the surface, thereby removing one of the causes of sweating in this pattern. When this is accomplished, the normal qi will be restored, the sweating will cease, and the symptoms of Heart qi distress will abate.

Cautions and Contraindications

This formula is inappropriate for treating the profuse, oily sweat associated with exhaustion of the yin or yang.

Commentary

The composition and actions of this formula are very subtle and require some explanation. It is indicated for spontaneous sweating that worsens at night and has become chronic. Because Chinese medicine associates daytime with yang and nighttime with yin, night sweats are generally thought to reflect some degree of yin deficiency. Many textbooks thus define Heart yin deficiency to be one of the underlying causes of the pattern treated by this formula. The problem with this explanation is that none of the herbs in the formula tonifies yin at the level of the substances. They neither enrich the fluids nor do they nourish the blood. Yin deficiency, in this context, thus does not imply a structural deficiency of Heart fluids or blood, but rather constraint, that is, functional deficiency, at the level of the nutritive qi. Nutritive qi is the most solid type of qi. It only flows in the vessels and thus is inti-

mately associated with the Heart. Being relatively more solid, moist, and cool than protective qi, which is lighter, warmer, and also circulates outside of the vessels, the relationship between these two functions is readily captured in the relational framework of yin/yang discourse.

Once this is understood, the actions and indications of this formula are immediately apparent. It treats chronic deficiency at the qi level, involving both the protective and nutritive qi. When the nutritive qi is weak, the flow of qi in the vessels becomes constrained, generating heat. This heat manifests as restlessness and irritability, but also moves the fluids within the vessels toward the exterior. As the protective qi is also deficient, it is too weak to direct the fluids downward toward the interior again, hence they manifest as sweating. This dual deficiency is reflected in the combination of Astragali Radix (*huáng qí*) and Tritici Fructus levis (*fú xiǎo mài*). Astragali Radix (*huáng qí*) is sweet and warm, entering the middle burner to augment the qi and entering the exterior to stabilize the protective qi. Its mechanism of action is thus to strengthen and secure the protective yang in order to stop sweating. Tritici Fructus levis (*fú xiǎo mài*) is sweet and cooling, and enters the Heart channel to inhibit the Heart yang fluids. Because it is light in weight, it travels to the exterior to clear heat. Together, they support the qi in controlling the opening and closing of the pores, clearing heat from the pores and interstices, and securing the Heart fluids.

Because this is qi deficiency, sweating occurs throughout the day and will be aggravated by exertion. However, because constraint at the level of the nutritive qi is the root (indicated by the many Heart symptoms that make up this pattern), sweating worsens at night when the protective yang moves toward the interior. Aggravating constraint within the vessels, its relative lack at the exterior is now even less able to constrain the leakage of fluids. This is well captured by the Qing-dynasty commentator Fei Bo-Xiong, who, in his *Discussion of Medical Formulas,* summed up the action of this formula in a single sentence: "All [that needs to be said] about the strategy [embodied in this formula] is that it secures the exterior and clears irritability and thereby stops sweating." Key markers in diagnosis are symptoms that indicate constraint from deficiency at the level of the nutritive qi such as reduced appetite, dizziness, palpitations, and fatigue.

The literature lists at least sixty-nine formulas by this name, of which at least twelve stop sweating as their main function. This is by far the most common one.

Comparisons

➢ Vs. Jade Windscreen Powder (*yù píng fēng sǎn*)

Both of these formulas treat sweating from qi deficiency. However, Jade Windscreen Powder (*yù píng fēng sǎn*) is for deficiency of protective qi at the level of the Lungs with recurrent penetration of wind into the exterior. This is characterized by spontaneous sweating accompanied by aversion to wind or drafts, as well as recurrent infections or allergies. Oyster Shell Powder (mǔ lì sǎn), on the other hand, also treats deficiency of protective qi, but this is complicated here by constraint from deficiency at the level of the nutritive qi. Because the nutritive qi is associated with the Heart, there are symptoms of Heart qi deficiency such as anxiety and palpitations. Because of the presence of heat from constraint, there will be irritability and restlessness, and the sweating tends to worsen at night.

➤ Vs. Tangkuei and Six-Yellow Decoction (dāng guī liù huáng tāng)

Both of these formulas stabilize the exterior, stop sweating, and enrich the yin. Although this formula has a rather weak yin-enriching action and does not clear heat, it is nonetheless effective at restraining sweating. It is therefore commonly used for excessive sweating in weak patients, but should be avoided in treating night sweats due to raging fire from deficiency. The latter condition is precisely that for which Tangkuei and Six-Yellow Decoction (dāng guī liù huáng tāng) was designed.

Biomedical Indications

With the appropriate presentation, this formula may be used to treat a variety of biomedically-defined disorders including excessive sweating postpartum or post-surgery, autonomic dystonia, and pulmonary tuberculosis.

Alternate names

Wheat-Brew Decoction (mài jiān tāng) in *Correct Transmission of Medicine*; Wheat-Brew Powder (mài jiān sǎn) in *Precious Mirror of Health*; Oyster Shell Drink (mǔ lì yǐn) in *Essentials for Those Who Do Not Know Medicine*

Modifications

- To strengthen the formula, add Schisandrae Fructus (wǔ wèi zǐ).

- To increase tonification of the nutritive qi, add Atractylodis macrocephalae Rhizoma (bái zhú) and Ginseng Radix (rén shēn).

- To increase tonification of the yin fluids, add Paeoniae Radix alba (bái sháo) or Rehmanniae Radix (shēng dì huáng).

- For yang deficiency, add Atractylodis macrocephalae Rhizoma (bái zhú) and Aconiti Radix lateralis praeparata (zhì fù zǐ).

- For blood deficiency, add Polygoni multiflori Radix (hé shǒu wū) and Rehmanniae Radix praeparata (shú dì huáng).

- For pronounced yin deficiency, add Rehmanniae Radix (shēng dì huáng) and Paeoniae Radix alba (bái sháo).

- For insomnia, add Ziziphi spinosae Semen (suān zǎo rén) and Platycladi Semen (bǎi zǐ rén).

Associated Formulas

柏子仁丸
Arborvitae Seed Pill
bǎi zǐ rén wán

SOURCE　*Formulas of Universal Benefit from My Practice* (1132)

Platycladi Semen (bǎi zǐ rén)	60g
Pinelliae Rhizoma praeparatum (zhì bàn xià)	60g
Ostreae Concha (mǔ lì)	30g
Ginseng Radix (rén shēn)	30g
Ephedrae Radix (má huáng gēn)	30g
Atractylodis macrocephalae Rhizoma (bái zhú)	30g
Schisandrae Fructus (wǔ wèi zǐ)	30g
Tritici Fructus levis (fú xiǎo mài)	15g

Grind the herbs into a powder and make into small pills by mixing it with the flesh of Jujubae Fructus (dà zǎo). Take 30-50 pills twice a day on an empty stomach with rice broth. Tonifies the qi, nourishes the Heart, secures the exterior, and stops sweating. For sweating arising from Heart qi and yin deficiency characterized by night sweats and restless sleep. In contrast to the principal formula, this formula more strongly tonifies and regulates the Heart qi, while not focusing on the protective qi.

固表止汗湯 (固表止汗汤)
Stabilize the Exterior and Stop Sweating Decoction
gù biǎo zhǐ hàn tāng

SOURCE　*Case Histories of Huang Wen-Dong* (2001)

Astragali Radix (huáng qí)	10g
Atractylodis macrocephalae Rhizoma (bái zhú)	12g
Glycyrrhizae Radix praeparata (zhì gān cǎo)	4.5g
Ophiopogonis Radix (mài mén dōng)	9g
Schisandrae Fructus (wǔ wèi zǐ)	4.5g
Artemisiae annuae Herba (qīng hāo)	9g
Cynanchi atrati Radix (bái wēi)	9g
Ostreae Concha (mǔ lì)	30g
Fossilia Ossis Mastodi (lóng gǔ)	15g
Tritici Fructus levis (fú xiǎo mài)	30g
Oryzae glutinosae Radix (nuò dào gēn xū)	30g

Decoction. Augments the qi, secures the exterior, nourishes the Heart, and stops sweating. For sweating associated with tuberculosis that does not abate in spite of the use of antibiotic treatment. The sweating is associated with sensations of heat when lying down and will be chronic. Digestion is normal, the tongue pale, and the pulse thin and rapid. This is a combination of a number of different formulas including the principal formula, Jade Windscreen Powder (yù píng fēng sǎn), and Generate the Pulse Powder (shēng mài sǎn). It is stronger at both tonifying the qi and clearing heat from deficiency.

Section 2

FORMULAS THAT SECURE THE LUNGS AND STOP COUGHING

Chronic coughing leads to Lung deficiency by exhausting the qi and yin of that organ. In addition to a persistent, shallow cough, the patient will also present with spontaneous sweating and a deficient, rapid pulse. Treatment must be directed at both the branch and the root of the disorder: if the coughing (branch) continues, the Lungs will be unable to recover, and unless the qi and yin (root) are relatively healthy, there is no way to stop the coughing. To treat such a condition requires the use of balanced formulas that combine tonification of qi and yin with support for the Lungs' dynamic functions of dissemination, clearing, and downward directing, and that balance astringent herbs to secure the Lungs with moistening herbs to facilitate the movement of Lung qi.

The core ingredients of formulas that secure the Lungs are restraining herbs such as Schisandrae Fructus (*wǔ wèi zǐ*), Mume Fructus (*wū méi*), and Papaveris Pericarpium (*yīng sù ké*).

九仙散

Nine-Immortal Powder

jiǔ xiān sǎn

This formula contains nine ingredients and is said to be so effective that it must have been devised by immortals, hence the name.

Source *Precious Mirror of Health* (Yuan dynasty)

Ginseng Radix (*rén shēn*) 30g
honey-prepared Papaveris Pericarpium (*mì zhì yīng sù ké*) . .240g
Mume Fructus (*wū méi*) 30g
Schisandrae Fructus (*wǔ wèi zǐ*) 30g
Asini Corii Colla (*ē jiāo*) 30g
Farfarae Flos (*kuǎn dōng huā*) 30g
Fritillariae Bulbus (*bèi mǔ*) 15g
Platycodi Radix (*jié gěng*) 30g
Mori Cortex (*sāng bái pí*) 30g

Method of Preparation The source text advises to grind the ingredients into a powder and take warm as a draft with 2 pieces of Zingiberis Rhizoma recens (*shēng jiāng*) and 1 piece of Jujubae Fructus (*dà zǎo*). At present, it is often prepared as a decoction with an appropriate reduction in dosages. Fritillariae cirrhosae Bulbus (*chuān bèi mǔ*) is the form of Fritillariae Bulbus (*bèi mǔ*) that is generally used. Because Papaveris Pericarpium (*yīng sù ké*) is an obsolete substance, such medicinals as Chebulae Fructus (*hē zǐ*), Galla chinensis (*wǔ bèi zǐ*), or Ginkgo Semen (*bái guǒ*) may be substituted.

Actions Secures the Lungs, stops coughing, augments the qi, and nourishes the yin

Indications

Chronic, unremitting cough with wheezing, a shiny-white complexion, shortness of breath, spontaneous sweating, and a deficient, rapid pulse.

Chronic coughing will exhaust both the qi and yin of the Lungs, which in turn causes further coughing. The deficiency of Lung qi causes wheezing, a shiny-white complexion, shortness of breath, and a deficient pulse. The Lungs govern the skin and the exterior of the body; weak Lung qi opens up the interstices and pores and results in spontaneous sweating. Injury to the Lung yin is reflected in the nonproductive cough as well as the rapid pulse.

Analysis of Formula

To effectively treat this disorder, one must address both the chronic cough (branch) and the deficiency of Lung qi and yin (root). This is achieved by combining within one formula all four of the main strategies for treating cough: disseminating, clarifying, moistening, and securing the Lungs. The formula's chief ingredient, astringent and sour Papaveris Pericarpium (*yīng sù ké*), is most effective in restraining the Lungs and stopping coughing. Frying it in honey increases its moistening quality and helps it to transform phlegm. As this substance is illegal in most countries, other medicinals that secure the Lungs, such as Chebulae Fructus (*hē zǐ*), Galla chinensis (*wǔ bèi zǐ*), or Ginkgo Semen (*bái guǒ*) are substituted. Two deputies, Schisandrae Fructus (*wǔ wèi zǐ*) and Mume Fructus (*wū méi*), assist the chief ingredient in securing the Lungs and stopping the coughing. According to Li Shi-Zhen, author of *Comprehensive Outline of the Materia Medica*, Mume Fructus (*wū méi*) is also an herb that enhances the efficacy of Papaveris Pericarpium (*yīng sù ké*) by moderating its side effects. In addition, Schisandrae Fructus (*wǔ wèi zǐ*) also helps Ginseng Radix (*rén shēn*) augment the Lung qi.

Most of the remaining herbs function as assistants. These can be divided into two groups. The first is comprised of herbs that tonify the qi and yin. Asini Corii Colla (*ē jiāo*), which nourishes the Lung yin, also serves a minor astringent function. Ginseng Radix (*rén shēn*) is perhaps the most effective herb in the materia medica for tonifying and augmenting the qi; it supports the Lungs' function of dissemination. The second group of assistants is comprised of herbs that facilitate the Lungs' clarifying and downward-directing functions. Farfarae Flos (*kuǎn dōng huā*), Fritillariae Bulbus (*bèi mǔ*), and Mori Cortex (*sāng bái pí*) stop the coughing, transform phlegm, and direct the rebellious qi downward to calm the wheezing. Fritillariae Bulbus (*bèi mǔ*) and Mori Cortex (*sāng bái pí*) also combine to clear Lung heat, while Farfarae Flos (*kuǎn dōng huā*) is lubricating and moistening.

Platycodi Radix (*jié gěng*) focuses the actions of all the ingredients on the Lungs, while also disseminating the Lungs and transforming the phlegm. Hence, it serves as an envoy.

Zingiberis Rhizoma recens (shēng jiāng) and Jujubae Fructus (dà zǎo) regulate the interaction between the nutritive and protective qi, thereby reinforcing the general effect of the formula and enabling the Lungs to more quickly recover.

Cautions and Contraindications

This formula has rather strong Lung-restraining and antitussive effects. Without significant modification, it should not be used in cases with pronounced phlegm or where there is a concurrent exterior condition, even if the patient has suffered from long-term, unremitting cough and otherwise fits the presentation.

Commentary

This formula was composed by the imperial physician Wang Zi-Zhao (王子昭) and is noted in the source text as being extremely effective for any kind of cough. Its composition was influenced by the clientele that Wang treated at court, demanding both tonification and the need to avoid side effects. This explains the use of herbs that equally address the branch and the root.

Suppressing a cough with astringent herbs can be a useful tool because it counteracts the loss of qi and fluids that accompanies coughing, which itself is an attempt by the Lungs to overcome obstruction. However, this treatment strategy is only suitable for the later stages of cough, when the pathogen has already been eliminated. This point was made in *Essentials of Zhu Dan-Xi's Treatment Methods*: "Papaveris Pericarpium (yīng sù ké) is widely employed by those treating cough. [There is no reason, therefore, why] one should doubt [its usefulness]. Nevertheless, one must first eliminate the root of the disorder. It is an herb [to be used] only after [such treatment] has come to an end."

Comparison

➢ Vs. Tonify the Lungs Decoction with Ass-Hide Gelatin (bǔ fèi ē jiāo tāng)

Both of these formulas stop coughing and contain herbs that augment the Lungs and tonify the yin. However, Nine-Immortal Powder (jiǔ xiān sǎn) uses three astringent herbs as chief and deputies to focus on securing the Lungs to stop the cough. This action is balanced by the tonic herbs, making it a balanced formula for treating both the root and branch. It is indicated for chronic disorders characterized by both qi and yin deficiency and therefore accompanied by spontaneous sweating and a deficient, rapid pulse. Tonify the Lungs Decoction with Ass-Hide Gelatin (bǔ fèi ē jiāo tāng), on the other hand, uses Asini Corii Colla (ē jiāo) as the chief herb, reflecting a focus on enriching the yin to tonify the Lungs, while the deputies Aristolochiae Fructus (mǎ dōu líng) and Arctii Fructus (niú bàng zǐ) clear heat to support the Lungs' disseminating and downward-directing functions. This formula is indicated where yin deficiency is the clear root of the

coughing, as reflected in a dry throat, blood-streaked sputum, and floating, thin, and rapid pulse.

Biomedical Indications

With the appropriate presentation, this formula may be used to treat a variety of biomedically-defined disorders including chronic bronchitis, asthma, emphysema, silicosis, and pertussis.

Modifications

- For more severe yin deficiency with a red tongue without coating, add Glehniae/Adenophorae Radix (shā shēn) and Ophiopogonis Radix (mài mén dōng).

- For phlegm manifested as profuse sputum, remove honey-prepared Papaveris Pericarpium (mì zhì yīng sù ké) and Mume Fructus (wū méi) and add Trichosanthis Fructus (guā lóu) and Citri reticulatae Pericarpium (chén pí).

- For concurrent exterior cold, remove honey-prepared Papaveris Pericarpium (mì zhì yīng sù ké) and Mume Fructus (wū méi) and add Ephedrae Herba (má huáng) and Cinnamomi Ramulus (guì zhī).

- For concurrent exterior heat, remove honey-prepared Papaveris Pericarpium (mì zhì yīng sù ké) and Mume Fructus (wū méi) and add Mori Folium (sāng yè) and Chrysanthemi Flos (jú huā).

Section 3

. . . .

FORMULAS THAT BIND UP THE INTESTINES AND SECURE ABANDONED CONDITIONS

The formulas in this section are used for Spleen and Kidney cold from deficiency characterized by chronic, unremitting diarrhea or dysenteric disorders that, if severe, can lead to incontinence of stool. Accompanying signs and symptoms include lethargy, weakness, abdominal pain that responds favorably to warmth or pressure, reduced appetite, a pale tongue with a white coating, and a submerged, slow pulse.

Because these formulas consist primarily of warm, tonifying substances with astringent properties, qi-regulating herbs are added to prevent stagnation of the qi and its associated distention. And because chronic diarrhea causes the middle qi to sink, many of the formulas also contain substances that raise the qi, which helps stop the diarrhea.

These formulas are designed for long-term problems and should not be used for acute, excessive disorders, or those with remnants of damp-heat. If improperly prescribed, the pathogenic influences will linger in the body for a long time.

The core ingredients of these formulas are those that bind up the Intestines and stop diarrhea, particularly Myristicae Semen (*ròu dòu kòu*), Chebulae Fructus (*hē zǐ*), and Schisandrae Fructus (*wǔ wèi zǐ*). Because these problems usually have a component of interior cold, warming herbs such as Zingiberis Rhizoma (*gān jiāng*), Cinnamomi Cortex (*ròu guì*), and Evodiae Fructus (*wú zhū yú*) are often added. Similarly, the processes that lead to these conditions tax the Spleen qi, so herbs that strengthen it, such as Ginseng Radix (*rén shēn*) and Atractylodis macrocephalae Rhizoma (*bái zhú*), are also helpful. Diarrhea leads to loss of yin and blood, and herbs that enrich the yin and nourish the blood, such as Angelicae sinensis Radix (*dāng guī*) and Paeoniae Radix alba (*bái sháo*), are often added. Finally, because the digestive systems of such patients are not working properly, herbs such as Citri reticulatae Pericarpium (*chén pí*) and Caryophylli Flos (*dīng xiāng*) are used to regulate the qi and transform dampness.

真人養臟湯 (真人养脏汤)

True Man's Decoction to Nourish the Organs

zhēn rén yǎng zàng tāng

This formula nourishes the organs by warming the middle and restraining leakage from the Intestines. It is said to have been handed down by the Tang-dynasty hermit Lü Dong-Bin, one of the eight immortal hermits of Chinese legend, whose Daoist name was 'pure-yang' (純陽子 *chún yáng zi*). The formula was thus originally known as Pure-Yang True Man's Decoction to Nourish the Organs (*chún yáng zhēn rén yǎng zàng tāng*). It assumed its present name in *Straight Direction from [Yang] Ren-Zhai* and has been known as such ever since.

Source   *Formulary of the Pharmacy Service for Benefiting the People in the Taiping Era* (1107)

Ginseng Radix (*rén shēn*) 18g (3-6g)
dry-fried Atractylodis macrocephalae Rhizoma
    (*chǎo bái zhú*) 18g (9-12g)
Cinnamomi Cortex (*ròu guì*) 24g (3-4.5g)
roasted Myristicae Semen (*wēi ròu dòu kòu*) 15g (9-15g)
Chebulae Fructus (*hē zǐ*) 36g (6-15g)
honey-prepared Papaveris Pericarpium
    (*mì zhì yīng sù ké*) 108g (6-20g)
Paeoniae Radix alba (*bái sháo*) 48g (9-15g)
Angelicae sinensis Radix (*dāng guī*) 18g (6-12g)
Aucklandiae Radix (*mù xiāng*) 42g (6-9g)
Glycyrrhizae Radix praeparata (*zhì gān cǎo*) 24g (3-9g)

Method of Preparation   The source text advises to grind the ingredients into a coarse powder and take 6g as a draft before meals. At present, it is usually prepared as a decoction with the dosage indicated in parentheses. Codonopsis Radix (*dǎng shēn*) is generally substituted for Ginseng Radix (*rén shēn*) at 2-3 times its dosage.

Actions   Warms the middle, tonifies deficiency, restrains leakage from the Intestines, and stops diarrhea

Indications

Chronic diarrhea or dysenteric disorders with unremitting diarrhea to the point of incontinence, and, in severe cases, prolapsed rectum. The diarrhea may contain pus and blood, and there may also be tenesmus. Accompanying symptoms include mild, persistent abdominal pain that responds favorably to local pressure or warmth, lethargy, a wan complexion, reduced appetite, soreness of the lower back, lack of strength in the legs, a pale tongue with a white coating, and a slow, thin pulse.

This is chronic diarrhea or dysenteric disorder causing a leaking type of abandonment (滑脱 *huá tuō*), which indicates that the body is no longer able to contain the contents of the Intestines. In such cases, the Spleen qi has become deficient and the Intestines have lost their stability and capacity to absorb. This results in unremitting diarrhea to the point of incontinence. When severe, there may be sinking of the Spleen (or middle) qi, which manifests as prolapse of the rectum. Long-term diarrhea not only leads to deficiency of the Spleen qi and yang, but also invariably involves the Kidneys. This aggravates the diarrhea, which further injures the Spleen and Kidneys, which in turn worsens the diarrhea, and so on in a vicious circle.

When the Spleen and Kidneys are deficient and cold, there is fatigue and lethargy as well as mild, persistent abdominal pain that responds favorably to local pressure or warmth. When the Spleen is weak, the appetite declines, food intake is reduced, and the complexion becomes wan. Kidney yang deficiency is further expressed in the sore lower back and lack of strength in the legs. The pale tongue with a white coating and the slow, thin pulse are indicative of yang deficiency of the Spleen and Kidneys.

Analysis of Formula

The focus of this formula is on binding up the Intestines to secure abandoned conditions, while also warming the middle and tonifying deficiency. Such a dual strategy is necessary because, unless the loss of essence from the body is stopped, any attempt to nourish the organs will fail. To lead the body back to a state where it is able to contain the loss of essence via the bowels, however, also requires that the organs in charge of these functions—the Spleen, Stomach, and Intestines—be nourished. Following the principle, "In acute [disorders, first] treat the manifestations," the focus, however, is on securing abandonment with the help of an astringent strategy.

The chief herb, Papaveris Pericarpium praeparatum (*zhì yīng sù ké*), is an astringent that can be used to treat both cough and severe diarrhea or dysenteric disorders. Its pain-killing properties address the tenesmus that is part of the presentation. Two deputies, bitter, sour, neutral, and astringent Chebulae Fructus (*hē zǐ*) and acrid, warming, and astringent roasted Myristicae Semen (*wēi ròu dòu kòu*), support the actions of the chief herb while also warming the Spleen yang. There are five assistants. Ginseng Radix *(rén shēn)* and Atractylodis macrocephalae Rhizoma *(bái zhú)*, especially when combined, are very effective in strengthening the Spleen and augmenting the middle qi. Cinnamomi Cortex *(ròu guì)* warms the Kidney yang and Spleen to dispel cold, and helps the chief herb strengthen the Spleen. Chronic diarrhea depletes the fluids, which exhausts the yin and blood. Paeoniae Radix alba *(bái sháo)* and Angelicae sinensis Radix *(dāng guī)* tonify the yin and blood. Stronger yin-tonifying substances are too cloying and would overwhelm the capacity of the digestive system; in any event, they are unnecessary in the context of this disorder. Aucklandiae Radix *(mù xiāng)* serves as an envoy to revive the Spleen and regulate the qi, thereby helping with digestion and abdominal pain. This particular qi-regulating herb is chosen because of its specific ability to alleviate tenesmus. Although its use may appear to be contraindicated in a condition of excessive movement, it actually prevents the astringent, binding properties of the other herbs from causing stagnation. A second envoy, Glycyrrhizae Radix praeparata *(zhì gān cǎo)*, helps the chief herb tonify the middle burner, works with Paeoniae Radix alba *(bái sháo)* to alleviate abdominal pain, and harmonizes the actions of the other herbs.

Cautions and Contraindications

This formula should *never* be used in treating disorders of excess or when stagnation or damp-heat is present. Patients taking this formula should avoid alcohol, wheat, cold or raw foods, fish, and greasy foods.

Commentary

This formula is used for severe cases in which the diarrhea is incessant to the point of incontinence, the tongue is pale with a white coating, and the pulse is slow and thin. The source text notes that this formula is gentle enough to be used in treating acute diarrhea in the elderly, pregnant women, and children. Its effect in these cases should be immediate. It can be used to treat prolapse of the rectum where this is due to Spleen and Kidney yang deficiency. This pattern must be distinguished from that due to sinking of Spleen qi, for which Tonify the Middle to Augment the Qi Decoction *(bǔ zhōng yì qì tāng)*, discussed in Chapter 8, is indicated, and also from that due to dryness clumping the Intestines, which should be treated with a formula such as Hemp Seed Pill *(má zǐ rén wán)*, discussed in Chapter 2.

There is much disagreement about the order of importance of the different groups of herbs in this formula. Some commentators believe that the qi-tonifying herbs are most important because treating the root is more important in a chronic disorder like this than treating the branch. Whatever their disagreements regarding the relative importance of

the various herbs, most commentators agree that its complex structure is necessary, as explained in Fei Bo-Xiong's *Discussion of Medical Formulas*:

> This is another [example] of astringent [herbs] within [the context] of a warming strategy. Adding herbs to tonify both the qi and blood makes it most suitable for treating chronic disorders with deficiency of the normal [qi].

This formula was criticized in the writings of the classical formula current, such as *Compendium of Songs on Modern Formulas* by Fei's contemporary, Chen Nian-Zu:

> This [is an example] of a formula that collects herbs [from many different formulas] to treat a disorder beloved by market-stall physicians. I am the only one who opposes this [practice]. However, using a high dosage of Aucklandiae Radix *(mù xiāng)* [to make] an astringent [formula] not constraining is a view with which I can get along very well.

Note that Chen's reference to 'market-stall physicians' referred not to some local competitors, but rather to eminent scholar-physicians such as Zhang Jie-Bin, who held a different viewpoint. The classical formula approach to treating chronic dysenteric disorders would be to use an astringent formula such as Peach Blossom Decoction *(táo huā tāng)* to stop the diarrhea, followed by another formula to tonify the normal qi.

Comparisons

➢ Vs. Peach Blossom Decoction *(táo huā tāng); see* PAGE 428

➢ Vs. Four-Miracle Pill *(sì shén wán); see* PAGE 431

Biomedical Indications

With the appropriate presentation, this formula may be used to treat a variety of biomedically-defined disorders including chronic colitis, chronic diarrhea in children, ulcerative colitis, Crohn's disease, chronic dysentery, and recalcitrant diarrhea as a result of diabetes. It is also used for rectal prolapse accompanying any of these conditions.

Alternate names

Nourish the Organs Decoction *(yǎng zàng tāng)* in *Discussion of Formulas from Straight Directions from [Yang] Ren-Zhai*; True Man's Powder for Nourishing the Organs *(zhēn rén yǎng zàng sǎn)* in *Nationwide Collection of TCM Patent Formulas*; Nourish the Organs Powder *(yǎng zàng sǎn)* in *Nationwide Collection of TCM Patent Formulas*.

Modifications

• For diarrhea with undigested food particles, cold extremities, and a submerged, faint pulse, add Zingiberis Rhizoma *(gān jiāng)* and Aconiti Radix lateralis praeparata *(zhì fù zǐ)*.

- For prolapsed rectum, add Astragali Radix *(huáng qí)* and Cimicifugae Rhizoma *(shēng má)*.
- For severe abdominal pain, add Arecae Semen *(bīng láng)*.

桃花湯 (桃花汤)
Peach Blossom Decoction

táo huā tāng

The name of this formula is generally thought to be related to the chief ingredient, either because it is the color of peach blossoms, as suggested by Zhang Zhi-Cong, or because it is also known as peach blossom stone (桃花石 *táo huā shí*), as explained by Li Shi-Zhen. A very different derivation was suggested by Wang Zi-Jie: "Peach Blossom Decoction is not so named because of its color. It is used [to treat] yang deficiency of the Kidney organ. [Its effect] is like the warmth [of the spring] returning to a cold winter valley. Hence the name."

Source *Discussion of Cold Damage* (c. 220)

Halloysitum rubrum *(chì shí zhī)* 48g (30g)
Zingiberis Rhizoma *(gān jiāng)* 3g (9g)
Nonglutinous rice *(jīng mǐ)* 30g

Method of Preparation Decoction. In the source text, half of the Halloysitum rubrum *(chì shí zhī)* is decocted and the other half powdered and taken first, followed by the strained decoction. At present, it is usually taken in powdered form with the dosage indicated in parentheses.

Actions Warms the middle, dispels cold, binds up the bowels, and stops dysenteric disorders

Indications

Chronic dysenteric disorders with dark blood and pus in the stool, abdominal pain that responds favorably to local pressure or warmth, a pale tongue, and a pulse that is slow and frail or faint and thin.

The first stages of a dysenteric disorder are usually due to damp-heat, but over time the Spleen and Stomach are injured and the condition transforms into one of cold from deficiency and the loss of fluids. Deficiency of the middle burner (Spleen and Stomach) yang combined with weak fire in the lower burner prevents food from being digested, transformed, or transported, and inhibits the metabolism of water. This leads to internal obstruction of damp-cold, which disrupts the qi mechanism of the Large Intestine. The obstruction and disruption injure the collaterals of the Intestines, and dark blood and pus appear in the stool. The lack of bright color in the blood, the presence of pus, and the absence of a strong odor distinguishes this disorder from that caused by damp-heat. Abdominal pain that responds favorably to local pressure or warmth is a classic symptom of Spleen and Kidney yang deficiency. The pale tongue, and the pulse that is slow and frail or faint and thin, also reflect weakness of the Spleen and Kidney yang.

Analysis of Formula

This formula employs three strategies first outlined in *Basic Questions*—bind that which is dispersing, warm that which is cold, and tonify that which is deficient—in order to treat unremitting diarrhea or dysentery due to yang deficiency. The chief ingredient, warming and astringent Halloysitum rubrum *(chì shí zhī)*, binds up the Intestines and stabilizes the abandoned disorder. Due to its warming nature, it is particularly useful for treating blood and pus in the stool due to cold from deficiency. Half of the formula is taken as a powder so that the substance itself reaches the Intestines; this will increase its absorptive action. The deputy ingredient, Zingiberis Rhizoma *(gān jiāng)*, calms the middle burner and expels cold. Assisting the original yang, it revitalizes the Spleen's transportive and transformative functions so that it is able once more to contain essence. The contemporary physician Zhang Xi-Chun argues that because the formation of pus in the pattern treated by this formula is due to cold, Zingiberis Rhizoma *(gān jiāng)* has the additional functions of dispelling cold from the blood by means of its warmth and of opening stasis by means of its acridity, thereby effectively dealing with the root and branch of pus formation. The assistant, Nonglutinous rice *(jīng mǐ)*, nourishes the Stomach and harmonizes the middle burner. It helps the other ingredients improve the function of the Stomach and Intestines.

Cautions and Contraindications

This formula is astringent and warming in nature and therefore contraindicated for dysenteric disorders due to damp-heat. Such patterns are treated by formulas like Peony Decoction *(sháo yào tāng)*, Scutellaria Decoction *(huáng qín tāng)*, or Pulsatilla Decoction *(bái tóu wēng tāng)*, discussed in Chapter 4.

Commentary

While this formula warms the middle and binds up the Intestines, its tonifying action is minimal. Without significant modification, it is therefore used only in treating the branch, and not the root, of this disorder. After the diarrhea has stopped, other formulas should be used to treat the root. This is reflected in the source text, which states that its administration may be discontinued after just one dose, provided the diarrhea stops.

This formula was first mentioned in *Discussion of Cold Damage* (paragraph 306) where it is recommended for "lesser yin disorders with dysenteric diarrhea and pus and blood in the stools." The text goes on to mention a number of other symptoms that may be observed in this pattern. They include abdominal pain, urinary difficulty, incessant diarrhea, and blood in the stools. Some commentators think that the presence of symptoms that do not directly relate to the stools, that is, abdominal pain and urinary dysfunction, constitute key markers for successfully using the formula in clinical practice. This has allowed contemporary physicians to expand its use to patterns of cold from deficiency occurring in the context of disorders such as rectal abscesses, bowel cancer, hemorrhoids, or anal fistulae. The modern Shanghai physician Cheng Men-Xue (cited in *Contemporary Explanations of Ancient Formulas*) provides one of the clearest differentiations of these symptoms:

> When using Peach Blossom Decoction (*táo huā tāng*) to treat pus and blood in the stools, abdominal pain, and dysenteric diarrhea, the pain must be chronic with a slow pulse and a dark complexion or other distinctive manifestations of cold. The pus in these [cases] is leakage and loss of intestinal mucous lubricant with a jelly-like appearance like that of fish brain. The bleeding [is caused] by internal damage to the yin collaterals and has a pale black color, or it will be stagnant, dark, and not fresh. The abdominal pain is not due to stagnation, nor heat, but to the cold of deficiency damaging the Intestines, thus, it will respond very favorably to warmth and pressure. These [signs] are very different from the abdominal pain, pus, and bleeding [that accompany] heat-type dysenteric disorders.

Because dysenteric diarrhea is usually associated with damp-heat, Cheng's statement that this is a lesser yin disorder suggests that it is a relatively chronic problem involving deficient Kidney yang and loss of absorptive capacity in the lower burner. Historically, there has been disagreement about the etiology of this disorder. Some commentators believe that it results from a transfer of heat to the lesser yin channel, while others believe that it is due primarily to cold from deficiency in the lower burner. At present, both etiologies are accepted.

Comparisons

➤ Vs. Yellow Earth Decoction (*huáng tǔ tāng*)

Both of these formulas from *Essentials from the Golden Cabinet* can be used to treat blood in the stools associated with yang deficiency. They are very similar in terms of their composition in that each uses a mineral substance to bind up the Intestines and stop bleeding, Halloysitum rubrum (*chì shí zhī*) versus Terra flava usta (*zào xīn tǔ*); a warming, acrid herb to assist the original yang, Zingiberis Rhizoma (*gān jiāng*) versus Aconiti Radix lateralis praeparata (*zhì fù zǐ*); and a sweet herb to tonify the middle, Nonglutinous rice (*jīng mǐ*) versus Glycyrrhizae Radix (*gān cǎo*). However, whereas Peach Blossom Decoction (*táo huā tāng*) treats lesser yin patterns where the blood congeals due to excess cold, characterized by dark-colored blood and pus, Yellow Earth Decoction (*huáng tǔ tāng*) treats bleeding due to damp-heat penetrating into the blood aspect, characterized by fresh-looking blood. For this reason it also includes bitter, cold Scutellariae Radix (*huáng qín*) in order to drain damp-heat, as well as Rehmanniae Radix praeparata (*shú dì huáng*) and Asini Corii Colla (*ē jiāo*) to harmonize the blood.

➤ Vs. True Man's Decoction to Nourish the Organs (*zhēn rén yǎng zàng tāng*)

Both of these formulas warm and tonify the Spleen yang in order to treat unremitting diarrhea and dysentery, but they differ in their focus and composition. True Man's Decoction to Nourish the Organs (*zhēn rén yǎng zàng tāng*) uses a very large dose of Papaveris Pericarpium (*yīng sù ké*) as its chief ingredient and thus focuses primarily on stopping excessive bowel movements. Secondarily, it tonifies and warms the middle burner qi and also tonifies the blood. It is thus indicated primarily for Spleen qi and yang deficiency leading to severe diarrhea. Peach Blossom Decoction (*táo huā tāng*), on the other hand, focuses on warming and binding the Large Intestine, employing Halloysitum rubrum (*chì shí zhī*) to bind up the Intestines and stop the bleeding. Although the pattern it treats often results from yang deficiency of the middle burner, its focus is on treating the manifestation. Clinically, the use of this formula should be followed by one that treats the root once the acute symptoms have been relieved.

➤ Vs. Halt the Carts Pill (*zhù chē wán*); see PAGE 433

Biomedical Indications

With the appropriate presentation, this formula may be used to treat a variety of biomedically-defined disorders including ulcerative colitis, Crohn's disease, peptic ulcer, chronic dysentery, hemorrhoids, and dysfunctional uterine bleeding.

....

Alternate name

Three-Substance Peach Blossom Decoction (*sān wù táo huā tāng*) in *Restoration of Life from the Groves of Medicine*

....

Modifications

• For more severe abandoned disorders with incontinence of stool, add Codonopsis Radix (*dǎng shēn*) and roasted Myristicae Semen (*wēi ròu dòu kòu*).

• For more severe abdominal pain, add Paeoniae Radix alba (*bái sháo*) and Cinnamomi Ramulus (*guì zhī*).

• For icy-cold hands and feet and a submerged, faint pulse, add Aconiti Radix lateralis praeparata (*zhì fù zǐ*).

• For chronic Intestinal wind with bleeding, substitute Zingiberis Rhizoma praeparatum (*páo jiāng*) for Zingiberis Rhizoma (*gān jiāng*).

• For chronic leukorrhea from Spleen and Kidney deficiency, take with Four-Miracle Pill (*sì shén wán*).

• For chronic amebic dysentery, remove nonglutinous rice and add Dioscoreae Rhizoma (*shān yào*), Fossilia Ossis Mastodi (*lóng gǔ*), Ostreae Concha (*mǔ lì*), Sanguisorbae Radix (*dì yú*), and Fraxini Cortex (*qín pí*).

Associated Formula

赤石脂禹糧湯 (赤石脂禹余粮汤)

Halloysite and Limonitum Decoction

chì shí zhī yǔ yú liáng tāng

<small>SOURCE</small> *Discussion of Cold Damage* (c. 220)

Halloysitum rubrum (*chì shí zhī*) 30g (12g)
Limonitum (*yǔ yú liáng*) 30g (12g)

Grind the two herbs into a powder and decoct with 6 cups of water until 3 cups remain. Strain and take warm in three doses. The commonly-used dosages at present are in parentheses. Binds up the Intestines and stops diarrhea. For chronic diarrhea or dysenteric disorders causing a leaky, abandoned condition. These symptoms will often be accompanied by reduced urination or urinary dysfunction. The source text prescribes this formula to treat incessant diarrhea that does not respond to the use of formulas that leach out dampness, treat damp-heat, or warm the interior. According to the commentators, this suggests that the treatment must focus on the lower burner and on binding up the Intestines. In contrast to the principal formula, Halloysite and Limonitum Decoction (*chì shí zhī yǔ yú liáng tāng*) focuses only on binding up the Intestines and not on assisting the original yang. It is thus unsuitable for treating patterns characterized by the discharge of blood and pus, indicating stasis of blood due to cold.

四神丸

Four-Miracle Pill

sì shén wán

The four ingredients in this formula work so quickly that it appears to be a miracle, hence the name.

Source *Summary of Internal Medicine* (Ming dynasty)

Psoraleae Fructus (*bǔ gǔ zhī*) 120g
dry-fried Evodiae Fructus (*chǎo wú zhū yú*) 30g
Myristicae Semen (*ròu dòu kòu*) 60g
Schisandrae Fructus (*wǔ wèi zǐ*) 60g

Method of Preparation Grind the ingredients into a powder and decoct with 240g of Zingiberis Rhizoma recens (*shēng jiāng*) and 100 pieces of Jujubae Fructus (*dà zǎo*). When the latter are thoroughly cooked, remove them and Zingiberis Rhizoma recens (*shēng jiāng*) from the decoction. The remaining ingredients are formed into pills. Take 9-12g at bedtime with salted or boiled water. May also be prepared as a decoction with an appropriate reduction in the dosage of the ingredients.

Actions Warms and tonifies the Spleen and Kidneys, binds up the Intestines, and stops diarrhea

Indications

Diarrhea that occurs daily just before sunrise, lack of interest in food and inability to digest what is eaten, soreness of the lower back with cold limbs, fatigue and lethargy, a pale tongue with a thin, white coating, and a submerged, slow, and forceless pulse. There may also be abdominal pain.

This is daybreak diarrhea (五更瀉 *wǔ gēng xiè*), also called 'cock-crow diarrhea' because it occurs every day just before sunrise. This is the time of day when the yin is at its peak and the yang is starting to rise. Because this is the yang within the yin, diarrhea occurring at this time reflects a problem of yin transforming into yang, or yang rising out of the yin. Yang also refers to fire, and yin to water. If the fire at the gate of vitality (source yang) is weak, the yang will not properly rise and the yin will suddenly descend, causing diarrhea at this time.

As explained in more detail in the COMMENTARY below, the pathodynamic that leads to this manifestation involves the Kidneys' governance of opening and closing, the Spleen functions of transportation and transformation, and the Liver's ability to control the spreading of ministerial fire throughout the body. When the yang of the Spleen and Kidneys is deficient, there is a lack of interest in food, and because the deficient Spleen yang is unable to 'cook' or decompose food, what is eaten is not digested. Pain results from cold contracting the abdomen as a result of the Liver being unable to disseminate fire. The Spleen governs the limbs, and the lower back is the province of the Kidneys; yang deficiency of these organs leads to soreness of the lower back and cold limbs. When the yang is deficient, the spirit cannot become fully animated. This lack of animation is manifested in fatigue, lethargy, and a 'dispirited' demeanor. A pale tongue with a thin, white coating and a submerged, slow, and forceless pulse are characteristic of cold from deficiency.

Analysis of Formula

This formula treats patterns due to insufficient fire at the gate of vitality, which is unable to supply the Kidneys and Spleen with the warmth they require to carry out their transformative processes. To treat the ensuing diarrhea, this formula employs a dual strategy of warming and binding to deal with both the root and branch. The chief herb is acrid, bitter, and warm Psoraleae Fructus (*bǔ gǔ zhī*). It directly tonifies the gate of vitality and benefits earth (Spleen) by fortifying this aspect of fire. It also has an astringent nature that acts on the Kidneys to secure the primal yang, and on the Spleen to stop the diarrhea. According to *Commentary on the Divine Husbandman's Classic of Materia Medica*, it generates yang from within yin, thus making it an ideal herb for the treatment of daybreak diarrhea from yang deficiency. The deputy, Myristicae Semen (*ròu dòu kòu*), warms the Spleen and Kidneys and binds up the Intestines. It works synergistically with the chief herb by focusing its actions on the Intestines. It is often used to treat lack of appetite due to cold from deficiency.

One of the assistants, Evodiae Fructus (*wú zhū yú*), disperses cold in the middle burner (Spleen and Stomach) and thereby complements the action of the chief herb (which warms the source of the prenatal qi) by warming the source of the postnatal qi. Entering the Liver channel, it dredges Liver constraint, promoting the movement of qi and stopping pain, all of which are aspects of this pattern. The other assistant, Schisandrae Fructus (wŭ wèi zǐ), is a strong, warm, and astringent herb that strengthens the deputy's ability to bind up the Intestines. It also works synergistically with Evodiae Fructus (wú zhū yú), one herb being warm, acrid, drying, and strongly dispersing, the other sour, sweet, and astringent. The envoys, which are added to the decoction but removed before the pills are made, include Zingiberis Rhizoma recens (shēng jiāng), which disperses cold and activates the metabolism of water, and Jujubae Fructus (dà zǎo), which nourishes the Spleen and Stomach.

When the Spleen and Kidneys are warmed and the Large Intestine is stabilized, the transformation and transportation of foodstuffs will resume, and the diarrhea will stop.

Cautions and Contraindications

Without modification, this formula should not be used if there is accumulation or stagnation in the Stomach or Intestines. One should also avoid raw or cooling foods while taking this formula.

Commentary

This formula is very effective for daybreak diarrhea. It was devised by the Ming-dynasty physician Xue Ji, a strong proponent of warming and tonification who emphasized organ systems as core rubrics in pattern differentiation. Like many other physicians associated with this current of thought, Xue Ji focused particularly on the Spleen and Kidneys as the two organ systems whose physiological agencies he viewed as most closely intertwined with the functions of the original yang. Thus, the original indications of this formula were "deficiency and frailty of Spleen and Kidneys, soft stools, and disinterest in food, [and] also patterns [characterized] by diarrhea and abdominal pain." To treat this pattern, Xue combined two existing formulas from Xu Shu-Wei's 12th-century book, *Formulas of Universal Benefit from My Practice:* Two-Miracle Pill (èr shén wán), composed of Psoraleae Fructus (bǔ gǔ zhī) and Myristicae Semen (ròu dòu kòu), and Schisandra Pill (wǔ wèi zǐ sǎn), composed of Evodiae Fructus (wú zhū yú) and Schisandrae Fructus (wǔ wèi zǐ). The first of these formulas treated "deficiency and frailty of Spleen and Kidneys with total disinterest in food," the second "Kidney diarrhea," a term equated by some authors with daybreak diarrhea. It is via this association that the new formula came to be regarded as the exemplar for the treatment of this disorder.

Our brief genealogy of Four-Miracle Pill (sì shén wán) allows two important observations regarding the use of this formula in the clinic. First, its use is not limited in any strict sense to daybreak diarrhea, but extends more widely to patterns presenting with diarrhea, abdominal pain, and lack of appetite. All of these reflect deficiency of the fire at the gate of vitality that extends, in particular, to the Spleen and Kidneys. Secondly, inasmuch as the formula does treat daybreak diarrhea, its use of Evodiae Fructus (wú zhū yú) and Schisandrae Fructus (wǔ wèi zǐ) is of particular significance. The joint action of these herbs, which combine acrid and warming dispersion with sweet and sour restraining, is a classic strategy for tonifying the function of constrained Liver yang attributable to cold from deficiency. There is no particular reason why diarrhea due to Kidney and Spleen yang deficiency should only occur at daybreak. It is more likely that such deficiency will manifest with diarrhea that has no fixed pattern or that is aggravated by the intake of cold foods. An understanding of the Liver's role in the dissemination of ministerial fire is needed to fully grasp the disease dynamic that leads to daybreak diarrhea (i.e., diarrhea that only occurs at this time).

If the Kidney is in control of the storage and release (opening and closing) of the ministerial fire produced in the gate of vitality, the Liver is in charge of its dispersal throughout the three burners. If this dispersal is constrained by Liver deficiency, it will manifest in a manner typical of Liver wood pathology: suddenly, rebelliously, and at a moment that reflects the transformation of yin into yang corresponding to the terminal yin. All of these are present in daybreak diarrhea. In addition, the Chinese medical literature associates daybreak diarrhea with other Liver-related problems: food and alcohol accumulation, for instance, as well as Liver fire. Many commentators, too, have been explicit about the contribution of Liver constraint to the pattern treated by Four-Miracle Pill (sì shén wán). Ke Qin's discussion in *Golden Mirror of the Medical Tradition* is one of the most perceptive:

> Diarrhea is an abdominal disorder, and the abdomen is where all three yin meet. A loss of regulation in any one organ can lead to diarrhea. Therefore, Zhang Zhong-Jing devised formulas that master diarrhea from [disorders] of the three yin. … However, even if for one organ there are six different strategies, when all three organs connect with each other [in causing the problem], it would remain for a long time without ever being cured, such as the symptom of having diarrhea after the first watch [i.e., after 1 A.M.]. [The treatment methods] had not yet reached this [problem].
>
> Now, from the time the cock crows to daybreak, [although] the sky is dark, it is [the time] of yang within the yin. When the yang qi should arrive but does not, a deficient pathogen is able to remain without being expelled, causing diarrhea at dawn. This has four reasons: first, a deficient Spleen unable to control water; second, a deficient Kidney unable to move water; third, frail fire at the gate of vitality unable to generate earth; fourth, a lesser yang whose qi is too deficient to spread out. Acting as an assistant, the acridity and warmth of Evodiae Fructus (wú zhū yú) is used to expedite the propensity that the Liver wood has to disperse, thereby opening the way for water qi to propagate [allowing the body] to receive spring's generation.

Over the centuries, physicians developed the formula further by following three basic strategies:

- Add herbs to warm the Kidneys and augment fire, such as Aconiti Radix lateralis praeparata (zhì fù zǐ), Zingiberis Rhizoma praeparatum (páo jiāng), Piperis longi Fructus (bì bá), Sulfur (liú huáng), or Zanthoxyli Pericarpium (huā jiāo).
- Add herbs to warm the middle and disperse cold, such as Zingiberis Rhizoma (gān jiāng), Aucklandiae Radix (mù xiāng), or Foeniculi Fructus (xiǎo huí xiāng).
- Add herbs that warm the Kidneys and tonify the Spleen, such as Ginseng Radix (rén shēn), Atractylodis macrocephalae Rhizoma (bái zhú), Morindae officinalis Radix (bā jǐ tiān), and Poria (fú líng).

With these and similar additions, the formula's range of indications has been much expanded to treat loss of other essences, such as excessive urination or sweating, and other symptoms manifesting at daybreak, such as asthma, sweating, headache, low back pain, fever, cramps, and abdominal pain. The key, as always, is a correct understanding of the underlying pathodynamic. A pale tongue with a white coating, and a submerged, forceless pulse will be key markers in the clinic.

Comparisons

➢ Vs. True Man's Decoction to Nourish the Organs (zhēn rén yǎng zàng tāng)

Both of these formulas are warming and are used to treat chronic diarrhea associated with cold and deficiency of the Spleen and Kidneys. They differ in their focus on the middle and lower burner, respectively, and also in the relative weight placed on binding and warming properties. True Man's Decoction to Nourish the Organs (zhēn rén yǎng zàng tāng) focuses primarily on stopping excessive bowel movements. Secondarily, it tonifies and warms the middle burner qi and also tonifies the blood. It is therefore the formula of choice for uncontrollable bowel movements associated with deficiency, irrespective of when they occur. By contrast, Four-Miracle Pill (sì shén wán) is primarily a warming formula that augments the fire at the gate of vitality and its dissemination to the middle burner. Astringent herbs are used only as assistants. The formula is thus used primarily for early morning diarrhea, but also for other types of leakage due to insufficient fire at the gate of vitality.

➢ Vs. Ginseng, Poria, and White Atractylodes Powder (shēn líng bái zhú sǎn)

Both of these are important formulas for treating diarrhea, but they can be differentiated in terms of their focus on qi versus yang deficiency. Ginseng, Poria, and White Atractylodes Powder (shēn líng bái zhú sǎn) treats patterns of deficiency where Spleen earth is encumbered by phlegm-dampness. Here the stools will be soft or may even contain phlegm, and symptoms worsen in relation to dietary irregularities or

exhaustion. Systemic symptoms include fatigue, poor appetite, and weak muscles. By contrast, Four-Miracle Pill (sì shén wán) augments the fire at the gate of vitality in order to treat the diarrhea associated with Kidney and Spleen yang deficiency. Diarrhea in these cases is often watery and contains undigested food. The patient will be cold and tired.

Biomedical Indications

With the appropriate presentation, this formula may be used to treat a variety of biomedically-defined disorders including chronic colitis, chronic dysentery, irritable bowel syndrome, tuberculosis of the colon, allergic colitis, and lower back pain.

Alternate names

Chronic Diarrhea Pill (jiǔ xiè wán) and Old Paper Four-Miracle Pill (gù zhǐ sì shén wán) in Nationwide Collection of TCM Patent Formulas; Warm the Kidneys Pill to Check Diarrhea (wēn shèn zhǐ xiè wán) in Chinese Medical Formulas

Modifications

- For prolapsed rectum, add Astragali Radix (huáng qí), Codonopsis Radix (dǎng shēn), and Cimicifugae Rhizoma (shēng má).
- For uncontrolled diarrhea, add Papaveris Pericarpium (yīng sù ké) and Chebulae Fructus (hē zǐ).
- For more severe yang deficiency with backache and cold extremities, add Aconiti Radix lateralis praeparata (zhì fù zǐ) and Cinnamomi Cortex (ròu guì).
- For interior cold with abdominal pain and nausea, combine with Regulate the Middle Pill (lǐ zhōng wán).

Associated Formula

澹寮四神丸

Four-Miracle Pill from the Tranquil Hut

dàn liáo sì shén wán

SOURCE Indispensable Tools for Pattern Treatment (1602)

Psoraleae Fructus (bǔ gǔ zhī) 120g
Myristicae Semen (ròu dòu kòu) 60g
Foeniculi Fructus (xiǎo huí xiāng) 30g
Aucklandiae Radix (mù xiāng) 15g

The method of preparation is identical to that of the principal formula. Tonifies the Kidneys, reinforces the yang, regulates the Spleen qi, and stops diarrhea. For chronic diarrhea or daybreak diarrhea due to cold from deficiency of the Spleen and Kidneys with stagnation of the middle qi. In contrast to the principal formula, this is for conditions with more severe abdominal pain. In Discussion of Medical Formulas, the Qing-dynasty physician Fei Bo-Xiong succinctly explained its differences from the principal formula:

> The gate of vitality produces the fire used [in the course] of daily [activity]. It steams the Spleen and Stomach to transport and transform the food. For Kidney diarrhea, Two-Miracle Pill

(*èr shén wán*) is appropriate. In case of Spleen diarrhea with hyperactive wood controlling earth, Evodiae Fructus (*wú zhū yú*) is able to disperse the qi of the terminal yin. Therefore, it can be used to curb wood. If that is not the case, then there is nothing better than removing Schisandrae Fructus (*wǔ wèi zǐ*) and Evodiae Fructus (*wú zhū yú*) and replacing them with Foeniculi Fructus (*xiǎo huí xiāng*) and Aucklandiae Radix (*mù xiāng*).

駐車丸 (驻车丸)
Halt the Carts Pill
zhù chē wán

Within Mahāyāna Buddhism, the three types of Buddha correspond to different programs of skillful means (*upāya*) or expedient practices. Chapter 3 of the *Lotus Sutra* compares the three types of Buddha to three carts, namely, a goat cart, a deer cart, and an ox cart. Some authors in the history of Chinese medicine took up this idea and linked the three carts to the three burners when referring to the transformative movement of essence, qi, and spirit in the body. This formula treats dysenteric disorders due to problems in the qi dynamic, expressed in terms of the uncontrolled movement of the three carts, leading to leakage from the carts.

Source   *Arcane Essentials from the Imperial Library* (752)

Coptidis Rhizoma (*huáng lián*) .180g
Zingiberis Rhizoma (*gān jiāng*) .60g
Angelicae sinensis Radix (*dāng guī*) 90g
Asini Corii Colla (*ē jiāo*) 90g

Method of Preparation   Grind the herbs into a powder, mix with 3-year-old vinegar, and make into pills. Take 30 pills twice daily. At present, 6-9g of pills are taken 2-3 times daily with rice broth or warm water. Can also be prepared as a decoction with an appropriate reduction in the dosages of the individual ingredients.

Actions   Drains heat, dries dampness, nourishes the yin, and stops dysenteric disorders

Indications

Discharge of blood and pus from the bowels (blood and pus can be mixed up with each other) that comes and goes, tenesmus, continuous abdominal pain, irritability of the chest, a red tongue with little coating, and a thin, rapid pulse.

This is chronic or intermittent dysenteric disorder due to damp-heat that has not been eliminated and gradually damages both the yin and yang. Damp-heat that remains in the Intestines for a long period of time leads to stagnation of qi and stasis of blood. These various pathogens intermingle, causing the discharge of blood and pus from the bowels as well as tenesmus. Chronic or intermittent dysenteric disorders invariably damage the blood and yin, and, over the long term, the Spleen yang as well. The former manifests as irritability, a red tongue with little coating, and a thin and rapid pulse. The latter manifests as continuous abdominal pain due to failure of the yang to warm and move the Spleen qi.

Analysis of Formula

The pattern treated by this formula is one of excess complicated by deficiency, where the chronic retention of damp-heat has led to deficiency of the yang qi and yin blood. To treat this pattern, the formula combines four strategies from *Basic Questions*: cool what is hot, disperse what has clumped, restrain what has dispersed, and tonify what is deficient. Its chief herb is bitter and cooling Coptidis Rhizoma (*huáng lián*), which drains fire and dries dampness, making it a key herb in the treatment of dysenteric disorders. There are two deputies. The first is Asini Corii Colla (*ē jiāo*), which enriches the yin and nourishes the blood, and is described in *Comprehensive Outline of the Materia Medica* as treating "Intestinal wind and dysenteric diarrhea." The second is Angelicae sinensis Radix (*dāng guī*), which nourishes and harmonizes the blood, and, according to *Delving into the Description of the Materia Medica*, "stops hot dysenteric disorders and abdominal pain." Acting synergistically, the two deputies nourish the blood and support the normal qi, as well as prevent the bitter, drying Coptidis Rhizoma (*huáng lián*) from further damaging the yin. Acrid, warming Zingiberis Rhizoma (*gān jiāng*) serves as an assistant to warm the middle, expel dampness, and supports the normal qi. In combination with Coptidis Rhizoma (*huáng lián*), it forms a synergistic pair in which its bitterness directs the turbid qi downward, and its acridity raises the clear and also balances both excessive cooling and heating. Mature vinegar, added in the production of the pills, serves as an envoy and adds an astringent quality.

Cautions and Contraindications

This formula is contraindicated for the initial stages of a dysenteric disorder, where treatment should focus on eliminating the pathogenic qi. The source text advises to avoid pork, cold beverages, and greasy food while taking this formula.

Commentary

This formula can be viewed as a variation of Pinellia Decoction to Drain the Epigastrium (*bàn xià xiè xīn tāng*) or Mume Pill (*wū méi wán*), both of which combine acrid, warming Zingiberis Rhizoma (*gān jiāng*) with bitter, cooling Coptidis Rhizoma (*huáng lián*) to treat a variety of Intestinal patterns, including dysenteric disorders.

Over the centuries, different texts have published contradictory information about the type of dysenteric disorder for which this formula is indicated. These include cold (*Important Formulas Worth a Thousand Gold Pieces*), mixed cold and heat (*Arcane Essentials from the Imperial Library*), heat from deficiency (*Convenient Reader of Established Formulas*), and "all kinds of dysenteric disorders" (*Formulary of the Pharmacy Service for Benefiting the People in the Taiping Era*).

One elegant approach to this formula that focuses on the qi dynamic is described by Zhang Lu in *Extension of the*

Important Formulas Worth a Thousand Gold Pieces:

> The human body possesses [three] carts. Attaching to the spine in order to move, they are the transport systems of essence, qi, and spirit. The goat cart pertains to the qi aspect and should [by right] be located in the upper [burner]. However, because it manages qi transformation in the generation of essence, it is, on the contrary, located in the lower [burner]. The deer cart pertains to the Kidney aspect and should [by right] be located in the lower [burner]. However, because it manages fire transformation in the augmentation of qi, it is, on the contrary, located in the middle [burner]. The ox cart pertains to the Spleen aspect. It should [by right] be located in the middle [burner]. However, because it manages grain transformation to create spirit, it is, on the contrary, located in the upper [burner]. In a healthy person, all of these systems [function] normally. If a healthy person loses normal function due to diarrhea, dysenteric disorders, profuse bleeding, or abandoned disorders, very often this is due to excessive and hasty movement of the deer cart. [As the movement of the] goat cart becomes excessive, essence and blood are no longer stored. [As the movement of the] ox cart becomes excessive [too], but unable to follow the galloping deer cart, food [transformation] becomes depleted.

> Therefore, one uses Zingiberis Rhizoma (*gān jiāng*) to assist healthy transportation by the ox cart, Coptidis Rhizoma (*huáng lián*) to pull up the dangerously tilting deer cart, Asini Corii Colla (*ē jiāo*) to help the goat cart's rushing approach, and Angelicae sinensis Radix (*dāng guī*) to regulate the chaotic dispersal of qi and blood so as to return the essence, qi, and blood to their [normal] order and avoid a crisis due to profuse bleeding or abandonment. By means of Zingiberis Rhizoma (*gān jiāng*), one can achieve recovery from cold dysenteric disorder. By means of Coptidis Rhizoma (*huáng lián*), one can heal hot dysenteric disorders. By combining Zingiberis Rhizoma (*gān jiāng*) and Coptidis Rhizoma (*huáng lián*), one can resolve mixed hot and cold dysenteric disorders. Asini Corii Colla (*ē jiāo*) is able to enrich what Zingiberis Rhizoma (*gān jiāng*) dries. Angelicae sinensis Radix (*dāng guī*) can harmonize what Coptidis Rhizoma (*huáng lián*) cools. Not only is this a miraculous elixir for chronic dysenteric disorders, it is also a specific medicine for intermittent dysenteric disorders.

Comparison

➤ Vs. Peach Blossom Decoction (*táo huā tāng*)

Both formulas employ Zingiberis Rhizoma (*gān jiāng*) in the treatment of chronic dysenteric disorders. Because Peach Blossom Decoction (*táo huā tāng*) uses Halloysitum rubrum (*chì shí zhī*) as the chief ingredient, it is specific for patterns of cold from deficiency. By contrast, Halt the Carts Pill (*zhù chē wán*) uses Coptidis Rhizoma (*huáng lián*) as the chief herb to focus on regulating the qi dynamic, expelling the pathogenic qi, and supporting normal qi. It is specific for damp-heat patterns complicated by deficiency of blood and yang.

Biomedical Indications

With the appropriate presentation, this formula may be used to treat such biomedically-defined disorders as bacillary dysentery.

Alternate names

Minor Coptis Pill (*xiǎo lián wán*) in *Pediatrics: Categorized and Brought Together*; Minor Halt the Vehicles Pill (*xiǎo zhù chē wán*) in *Introduction to Medicine*

....

Modification

• For severe abdominal pain, add Paeoniae Radix alba (*bái sháo*) and Aucklandiae Radix (*mù xiāng*).

益黄散（益黄散）
Benefit the Yellow Powder
yì huáng sǎn

Yellow is the color associated with earth, and by extension, with the Spleen and Stomach. This formula builds up the middle burner and regulates its qi, hence the name.

Source   *Craft of Medicines and Patterns for Children* (1119)

Citri reticulatae Pericarpium (*chén pí*).................30g
Caryophylli Flos (*dīng xiāng*)........................6g
Citri reticulatae viride Pericarpium (*qīng pí*)..............15g
prepared Chebulae Fructus (*páo hē zǐ*)...............15g
Glycyrrhizae Radix praeparata (*zhì gān cǎo*)...........15g

Method of Preparation   The source text advises to grind the ingredients into a powder and take as a draft in 6-9g doses. At present, it is usually prepared as a decoction with an appropriate reduction in dosage.

Actions   Strengthens the Spleen, harmonizes the Stomach, regulates the qi, and stops diarrhea

Indications

This formula treats two patterns seen primarily in babies and young children. The first is Spleen and Stomach deficiency with qi stagnation characterized by abdominal pain and distention, vomiting, unremitting diarrhea, and no desire for food. The second is childhood nutritional impairment characterized by fatigue, a yellow complexion, a grossly bloated abdomen, and wasting of the rest of the body.

In the Foreword to the source text, Qian Yi, the most famous pediatrician in the history of Chinese medicine, stated:

> The organ systems [of babies and small children] are weak and frail. They readily become deficient or excessive, cold or hot. This is especially the case for the Spleen and Stomach, the organs at the fulcrum of the transformative process in the body. When their transportive or transformative functions are impaired, food and milk accumulate and stagnate in the interior, obstructing the qi dynamic. This manifests as abdominal pain, distention, and lack of appetite. When raising and downward-directing become disordered, vomiting and unremitting diarrhea ensue. If such problems become chronic, or if the Spleen and Stomach are constitutionally deficient, leading to fatigue, a yellow complexion, a grossly bloated abdomen, and wasting of the rest of the body, this is called childhood nutritional impairment.

Analysis of Formula

This formula treats a pattern of deficiency complicated by excess by combining several different treatment strategies outlined in *Basic Questions*: tonify what is deficient, disperse what has clumped, restrain what has dispersed, and warm what is cold. Its chief herb is Citri reticulatae Pericarpium (*chén pí*). It is acrid and thus disperses and regulates the qi; it is bitter and warming and thus dries dampness. According to Li Dong-Yuan, it is the primary herb for regulating the qi of the Spleen and Stomach, and such regulation must be the focus of any formula treating these organs.

There are three deputies. Bitter, acrid, and warming Citri reticulatae viride Pericarpium (*qīng pí*) regulates the qi and dredges the Liver to disperse food stagnation and drain excess Liver qi that has encroached on the Spleen. Sweet and warming Glycyrrhizae Radix praeparata (*zhì gān cǎo*) tonifies the middle burner and augments the qi. Sour, astringent, and restraining prepared Chebulae Fructus (*páo hē zǐ*) enters the Spleen and regulates the middle burner to stop diarrhea, warms the Stomach, and binds up the Intestines. This herb must be used blast-fried, baked, or dry-fried; otherwise, it enters the Lungs to direct the qi downward. It is also indicated for abdominal fullness and distention as well as food stagnation. Acrid and warming Caryophylli Flos (*dīng xiāng*) serves as the assistant, warming the middle burner to disperse the cold and directing rebellious qi downward to stop the vomiting.

Together, the three aromatic herbs Citri reticulatae Pericarpium (*chén pí*), Citri reticulatae viride Pericarpium (*qīng pí*), and Caryophylli Flos (*dīng xiāng*) delight the Spleen and strengthen the Stomach. Citri reticulatae Pericarpium (*chén pí*), Citri reticulatae viride Pericarpium (*qīng pí*), and prepared Chebulae Fructus (*páo hē zǐ*) work synergistically to regulate the qi and disperse stagnation, stopping both the diarrhea and vomiting. Glycyrrhizae Radix (*gān cǎo*) moderates spasmodic abdominal pain.

Cautions and Contraindications

This formula is warming and therefore contraindicated in patterns associated with hot dysenteric disorders.

Commentary

Qian Yi also called this formula Tonify the Spleen Powder (*bǔ pí sǎn*), yet it does not contain any tonifying herbs. It is listed as an astringent formula for the treatment of incessant diarrhea and vomiting, yet is composed primarily of acrid, warming, and qi-regulating herbs. These apparent contradictions are the key to understanding the formula's mode of action and the many patterns and disorders for which it can be used in the clinic. In the source text, these include not only the digestive problems listed under INDICATIONS, but also other problems that Qian associated with disordered Spleen

and Stomach function in children, such as dribbling of saliva, chronic fright, sores, cough, jaundice, edema, and night crying. Qian also used it to treat diverse patterns associated with wind damage, such as muscle twitches in the evening or at night, cold hands and feet, and diarrhea and vomiting. Later generations of physicians expanded this spectrum even further. Zhang Yuan-Su defined it as the representative formula for tonifying the Spleen, while Xu Da-Chun used it to treat abdominal pain and diarrhea in pregnancy where the pulse is tight.

Clearly, then, the term 'deficiency' here must not be read to mean depletion, but rather deficiency of function. In children, this is due to the immature development of their organ systems, which quickly respond to any internal or external stress with such deficient reactions. Where the Spleen and Stomach are concerned, this manifests as an inability to properly execute the functions of transportation and transformation, and of regulating raising and downward-directing. Treatment by means of tonifying the qi would merely aggravate such a condition. Instead, it is best addressed by a strategy that combines sweet harmonization with aromatic stimulation, acrid and warm moving, bitter drying, and sour securing.

Biomedical Indications

With the appropriate presentation, this formula may be used to treat a variety of biomedically-defined disorders such as pediatric gastroenteritis and epilepsy.

Alternate names

Tonify the Spleen Powder (*bǔ pí sǎn*) in *Craft of Medicines and Patterns for Children*; Augment the Yellow Decoction (*yì huáng tāng*) in *Fine Formulas from Experience*; Master Qian's Augment the Yellow Powder (*Qián shì yì huáng sǎn*) in *Investigations of Medical Formulas*; Augment the Spleen Powder (*yì pí sǎn*) in *Chinese Medical Formulas*

Modifications

- For more severe food stagnation, add Gigeriae galli Endothelium corneum (*jī nèi jīn*) and Hordei Fructus germinatus (*mài yá*).

- For more pronounced qi deficiency, add Ginseng Radix (*rén shēn*) and Atractylodis macrocephalae Rhizoma (*bái zhú*).

Section 4

FORMULAS THAT SECURE THE ESSENCE AND STOP ENURESIS

The formulas in this section are used for deficient Kidneys that have lost their ability to store, causing instability in the lower burner. This, in turn, can destabilize the gate of essence (leading to spermatorrhea of various types) and the Bladder (leading to loss of bladder control), or deprive the fetus of nourishment and stability (leading to restless fetus disorder or miscarriage). Accompanying signs and symptoms include weakness and soreness of the lower back, tinnitus, forgetfulness, a pale tongue with a white coating, and a pulse that is thin, frail, and weak. Important herbs to treat this type of instability include Fossilia Ossis Mastodi (lóng gǔ), Ostreae Concha (mǔ lì), Mantidis Oötheca (sāng piāo xiāo), Nelumbinis Stamen (lián xū), and Astragali complanati Semen (shā yuàn zǐ). Because of the close relationship among the Kidneys, Heart, and Spleen, formulas that secure the essence and stop enuresis also include herbs that calm the spirit and settle the emotions, such as Poriae Sclerotium pararadicis (fú shén) or Acori tatarinowii Rhizoma (shí chāng pú), herbs that tonify and augment the qi of the Spleen and Kidneys, such as Dioscoreae Rhizoma (shān yào), or herbs that warm and regulate the Kidney qi, such as Linderae Radix (wū yào).

金鎖固精丸 （金锁固精丸）

Metal Lock Pill to Stabilize the Essence

jīn suǒ gù jīng wán

This formula stabilizes the essence (i.e., restrains the loss of semen) as effectively as a metal lock closes a chest, hence the name.

Source   *Medical Formulas Collected and Analyzed* (1682)

dry-fried Astragali complanati Semen *(chǎo shā yuàn zǐ)* 60g
Euryales Semen *(qiàn shí)* 60g
Nelumbinis Stamen *(lián xū)* 60g
calcined Fossilia Ossis Mastodi *(duàn lóng gǔ)* 30g
calcined Ostreae Concha *(duàn mǔ lì)* 30g

Method of Preparation   Grind the ingredients into a powder and form into pills with approximately 60 g of powdered Nelumbinis Semen *(lián zǐ)*. Take in 9g doses on an empty stomach with salted water. May also be prepared as a decoction with a proportionate reduction in the dosage of the ingredients.

Actions   Stabilizes the Kidneys and binds up the semen

Indications

Chronic spermatorrhea, impotence, fatigue and weakness, sore and weak limbs, lower back pain, tinnitus, a pale tongue with a white coating, and a thin, frail pulse.

There are many possible causes of spermatorrhea, but it is most often associated with dysfunction of the Kidneys and Liver. The Kidneys store the essence (of which semen is a material manifestation) of all the organs, and the Liver governs the free-flowing or spreading functions of the body. The Liver (wood) depends on the Kidneys (water) for nourishment, and the gate of essence in the Kidneys requires a calm Liver to be stable. When the Kidneys are deficient, they cannot store the essence (or semen); accordingly, the gate of essence be-

comes destabilized, and spermatorrhea (usually chronic) results. Blazing fire at the gate of vitality (often associated with Kidney deficiency or Liver yang excess) disturbing the chamber of the essence, which leads to an intemperate spreading of essence, is the other main cause of spermatorrhea.

By and large, wet dreams are due to blazing fire, while spontaneous emissions (spermatorrhea that occurs without dreams) are caused by instability at the gate of essence. This formula is designed primarily for the latter problem, although it can be modified to treat the former. Kidney deficiency and shortage of essence leads to weakness of the qi, which manifests as fatigue, weakness, and sore and weak limbs. The lower back is the dwelling of the Kidneys; lower back pain is a classic symptom of Kidney deficiency. The sensory organ most closely associated with the Kidneys is the ears; Kidney deficiency manifests as tinnitus. The pale tongue with a white coating and the thin, frail pulse are also characteristic of Kidney deficiency.

Analysis of Formula

This formula employs two strategies first outlined in *Basic Questions*—tonify what is deficient, and restrain what is dispersed—to secure the leakage due to Kidney deficiency. The chief ingredient, Astragali complanati Semen *(shā yuàn zǐ)*, provides both of the fundamental actions of this formula: it tonifies the Kidneys and benefits the essence, and stops the leakage of semen by stabilizing the gate of essence. The deputy ingredients, Nelumbinis Semen *(lián zǐ)*, Nelumbinis Stamen *(lián xū)*, and Euryales Semen *(qiàn shí)*, are all aquatic plants, sweet and astringent in action, but moist by nature, that assist the chief ingredient in stabilizing the gate of essence and stopping the leakage of semen. Nelumbinis Stamen *(lián xū)* and Euryales Semen *(qiàn shí)* also tonify the postnatal constitution via the Spleen. From a five-phase perspective, a strong earth helps to control water, and thereby prevents the leakage of semen. Nelumbinis Semen *(lián zǐ)* and Nelumbinis Stamen *(lián xū)* also nourish the Heart to calm the spirit. A calm Heart guards against excessive stirring of the ministerial fire at the gate of vitality. The assistants, calcined Fossilia Ossis Mastodi *(duàn lóng gǔ)* and calcined Ostreae Concha *(duàn mǔ lì)*, are powerful restraining substances that bind the semen and prevent it from leaking. Heavy in nature, they also calm the Liver and subdue the yang, assisting in the prevention of spermatorrhea from yet another direction.

Cautions and Contraindications

The herbs in this formula are primarily astringent, restraining substances. The formula is contraindicated in cases of damp-heat in the lower burner and should be modified if used for spermatorrhea at night due to blazing fire from deficiency. In case of fever from externally-contracted pathogens, use of the formula should be discontinued to avoid retention of the pathogen. Acrid, spicy, and hot foods as well as sexual intercourse should be avoided while taking this formula.

Commentary

Although this is a Qing-dynasty formula, its author, Wang Ang, claims in the Foreword to *Medical Formulas Collected and Analyzed* that this is "a compilation of ancient formulas." Several formulas by this name can be found in older texts, albeit with different compositions. Wang Ang himself attributed the type of spermatorrhea treated by this formula to "fire flaring upward and water hastening downward, [in other words] Heart and Kidneys not communicating." Based on their interpretation of the actions of individual ingredients, later commentators extended the analysis of the underlying pathodynamic to include the Spleen and Liver. However, Wang's analysis is more consistent with the ingredients of the formula, which focus on the leg lesser yin, that is, the Kidneys.

Although this formula simultaneously tonifies the Kidneys (root) and stops the leakage of semen (branch), it is weighted toward the latter function. When spermatorrhea has ceased, one should therefore use Kidney tonics to finish the treatment. This formula is most often used for chronic spermatorrhea and for incontinence of urine, but it can also be used in treating any problem judged to be due to loss of essence. For example, some modern practitioners attribute the same etiology to myasthenia gravis and have used the formula, successfully in some cases, in the treatment of that disease. Other indications include diarrhea that occurs when walking or running, profuse uterine bleeding, as well as postpartum disorders associated with weak Kidneys unable to contain the essence, such as excessive sweating, diarrhea, and urinary incontinence.

Comparisons

➤ Vs. Mantis Egg-Case Powder (*sāng piāo xiāo sǎn*); see
   page 438

Biomedical Indications

With the appropriate presentation, this formula may be used to treat a variety of biomedically-defined disorders such as sexual dysfunction, chyluria, chronic prostatitis, spermatocystitis, postpartum incontinence, nervous exhaustion, diabetes, and myasthenia gravis.

Alternate name

Stabilize the Essence Pill (*gù jīng wán*) in *Applications of Chinese Medical Prescriptions*

Modifications

- For Kidney yang deficiency with frequent urination and a submerged, frail pulse, add Psoraleae Fructus (*bǔ gǔ zhī*) and Corni Fructus (*shān zhū yú*).

- For blazing fire from yin deficiency with wet dreams, irritability, insomnia, a dry, red tongue, and a thin, rapid pulse, add Testudinis Plastrum (*guī bǎn*) and Ligustri lucidi Fructus (*nǚ zhēn zǐ*).

- For constipation, add Cistanches Herba (*ròu cōng róng*) and Angelicae sinensis Radix (*dāng guī*).

- For diarrhea, add Psoraleae Fructus (*bǔ gǔ zhī*), Cuscutae Semen (*tù sī zǐ*), and Schisandrae Fructus (*wǔ wèi zǐ*).

- For impotence from Kidney yang deficiency, add Cynomorii Herba (*suǒ yáng*), Epimedii Herba (*yín yáng huò*), Morindae officinalis Radix (*bā jǐ tiān*), and Curculiginis Rhizoma (*xiān máo*).

- For deficiency of Kidney essence, add Rehmanniae Radix praeparata (*shú dì huáng*) and Hominis Placenta (*zǐ hé chē*).

- For hyperactive Liver yang, add Haliotidis Concha (*shí jué míng*), Haematitum (*dài zhě shí*), and Paeoniae Radix alba (*bái sháo*).

- For blazing Heart fire, add Coptidis Rhizoma (*huáng lián*) and Ophiopogonis Radix (*mài mén dōng*).

- For Spleen deficiency, add Codonopsis Radix (*dǎng shēn*), Atractylodis macrocephalae Rhizoma (*bái zhú*), and Dioscoreae Rhizoma (*shān yào*).

Associated Formula

水陸二仙丹 （水陆二仙丹）

Water and Earth Immortals Special Pill

shuǐ lù èr xiān dān

Source   *Materia Medica Arranged According to Pattern* (1108)

Euryales Semen (*qiàn shí*)
Rosae laevigatae Fructus (*jīn yīng zǐ*)

Grind equal amounts of the ingredients and form into pills with honey. Take 9-15g before meals with either salted water or warm wine. May also be prepared as a decoction. Tonifies the Kidneys and binds up the essence. For white, cloudy spermatorrhea or leukorrhea that is strictly from yang deficiency. This formula focuses almost entirely on the manifestation. It is often added to other formulas in treating patients with this condition. The name of the formula is derived from the fact that Euryales Semen (*qiàn shí*) grows in the water and Rosae laevigatae Fructus (*jīn yīng zǐ*) grows on land.

桑螵蛸散

Mantis Egg-Case Powder

sāng piāo xiāo sǎn

Source   *Extension of the Materia Medica* (1116)

Mantidis Oötheca (*sāng piāo xiāo*)	30g (9-12g)
Fossilia Ossis Mastodi (*lóng gǔ*)	30g (12-30g)
Ginseng Radix (*rén shēn*)	30g (9-12g)
Poriae Sclerotium pararadicis (*fú shén*)	30g (9-12g)

Polygalae Radix *(yuǎn zhì)* 30g (3-6g)

Acori tatarinowii Rhizoma *(shí chāng pǔ)* 30g (6-9g)

prepared Testudinis Plastrum *(zhì guī bǎn)* 30g (9-15g)

Angelicae sinensis Radix *(dāng guī)* 30g (6-9g)

Method of Preparation Grind the ingredients into a powder and take 6g at bedtime. In the source text, the powder is often taken with a decoction of Ginseng Radix *(rén shēn)*. At present, Codonopsis Radix *(dǎng shēn)* is usually substituted for Ginseng Radix *(rén shēn)* at 2-3 times its dosage. May also be prepared as a decoction with the dosage indicated in parentheses.

Actions Regulates and tonifies the Heart and Kidneys, stabilizes the essence, and stops leakage

Indications

Frequent urination (sometimes to the point of incontinence), urine the color of rice water (gray and cloudy), sometimes accompanied by spermatorrhea. Other signs and symptoms include disorientation, forgetfulness, a pale tongue with a white coating, and a thin, slow, and frail pulse.

Frequent urination to the point of incontinence and spermatorrhea may represent either a condition of excess (vigorous fire in the lower burner) or deficiency (most commonly, Kidney and Heart deficiency, or weakness of the Spleen and Kidney qi). The condition for which this formula is indicated is Kidney and Heart qi deficiency. Sometimes this disorder is referred to as the 'Bladder losing its restraint' (膀胱失約 *páng guāng shī yuē)*, as the Bladder depends on the Kidneys both to transform the qi that gives it power and to restrain it.

The etiology of this disorder is often related to problems in the relationship between the spirit (Heart) and will (Kidneys). When the Kidneys are deficient, they are unable to properly store, and frequent urination and spermatorrhea ensue. The incontinence is characterized by the patient being aware of the urge to urinate but is unable to suppress it. Gray, cloudy urine is another symptom that is peculiar to this condition and linked by some commentators to the Small Intestine (the yang complement of the Heart) failing in its function of separating the clear from the turbid. The deficiency of Heart qi causes disorientation and forgetfulness. The pale tongue with a white coating and the thin, slow, and frail pulse also reflect deficiency of both the Heart and Kidneys.

Analysis of Formula

This formula employs a strategy of treating both the root and branch, tonifying the Heart and Kidneys as well as stopping the leakage. The chief ingredient, sweet, salty, and neutral Mantidis Oötheca *(sāng piāo xiāo)*, tonifies the Kidneys and gate of vitality, stabilizes the essence, and stops leakage. It attacks both the root and branch of this disorder and is a specific medicinal for both enuresis in children and cloudy urine. The two deputies are sweet and astringent Fossilia Ossis Mastodi *(lóng gǔ)* and sweet and salty Testudinis Plastrum

(guī bǎn). The former helps the chief ingredient in binding up the essence, calms the spirit, and steadies the will. The latter enriches the yin, subdues the yang, and tonifies the Kidneys. As a synergistic pairing, the two deputies facilitate communication between Heart and Kidneys by augmenting the yin and directing the yang downward.

Among the assistants, Ginseng Radix *(rén shēn)* strongly tonifies the source qi. Strong source qi is a prerequisite for a healthy mind. It also tonifies the Heart. The other assistants, Poriae Sclerotium pararadicis *(fú shén)*, Polygalae Radix *(yuǎn zhì)*, and Acori tatarinowii Rhizoma *(shí chāng pǔ)*, calm the spirit and steady the will. The first facilitates communication between the Heart qi and the Kidneys; the second facilitates communication between the Kidney qi and the Heart; and the third opens up the sensory orifices of the Heart and spirit. This demonstrates the importance of the mental functions in the pathogenesis and treatment of this particular problem. Angelicae sinensis Radix *(dāng guī)* nourishes the blood and yin. Together with the other ingredients in this formula, it regulates and tonifies the qi and blood, which is essential for revitalization to occur.

Cautions and Contraindications

This formula is contraindicated for incontinence due to either vigorous fire in the lower burner or damp-heat. Patients with these disorders usually present with painful urination.

Commentary

This formula is based on two Tang-era formulas from *Important Formulas Worth a Thousand Gold Pieces* that were designed to treat problems from Heart qi deficiency and turbid phlegm clouding the Heart orifices. The new formula adds Angelicae sinensis Radix *(dāng guī)* and Mantidis Oötheca *(sāng piāo xiāo)*. In outlining its indications and principles of composition, the source text makes it clear that the main purpose of Mantidis Oötheca *(sāng piāo xiāo)* is to guide the focus of the action to the Kidneys, as it was designed to treat a pattern with Heart qi deficiency as its root and Kidney and Bladder losing their restraint as its branch. This was cogently expressed by the Qing-dynasty imperial physician, Wang Jiu-Feng: "Although the storage of essence is controlled by the Kidneys, its buildup and discharge are [determined] by the Heart."

Disorientation or forgetfulness, a pale tongue with a white coating, and a thin, slow, and frail pulse are thus the controlling symptoms in the pattern for which this formula is indicated. It can be used to treat frequent urination, inability to control urination in both children and the elderly, as well as bed-wetting, provided that these symptoms imply a lack of focus on the part of the Heart. It is also effective in treating spermatorrhea due to deficiency of the Heart and Kidneys that is associated with dreams or overactive fantasies. The source text attributes this disorder to excessive sexual activity, but the formula can also be used in treating similar symptoms from other causes, provided that the underlying pathodynamic is the same. In clinical practice, the main differential diagnosis will be patterns due to flaring fire or Kidney and Spleen deficiency. When the symptoms improve, this formula should be replaced with one that is more tonifying and regulating.

Comparisons

➤ Vs. Metal Lock Pill to Stabilize the Essence (*jīn suǒ gù jīng wán*)

Both formulas treat patterns characterized by urinary incontinence and spermatorrhea due to failure of communication between the Heart and Kidneys. Metal Lock Pill to Stabilize the Essence (*jīn suǒ gù jīng wán*) focuses on tonifying the Kidneys and securing the essence to treat patterns of Kidney deficiency. By contrast, Mantis Egg-Case Powder (*sāng piāo xiāo sǎn*) focuses on tonifying the Heart while securing the essence and stopping urination to treat patterns of Heart deficiency. In practice, the former is often associated with premature ejaculation or nocturnal emissions without dreams, the latter with heightened sexual arousal and nocturnal emissions with dreams.

➤ Vs. Restrict the Fountain Pill (*suō quán wán*); see PAGE 439

Biomedical Indications

With the appropriate presentation, this formula may be used to treat a wide variety of biomedically-defined disorders including pediatric enuresis, diabetes, neurosis, prolapsed uterus, and autonomic dystonia.

Modifications

• For palpitations and insomnia, add Schisandrae Fructus (*wǔ wèi zǐ*) and Ziziphi spinosae Semen (*suān zǎo rén*).

• For severe Kidney yang deficiency with a sensation of coldness, add Morindae officinalis Radix (*bā jǐ tiān*), Cinnamomi Cortex (*ròu guì*), and Aconiti Radix lateralis praeparata (*zhì fù zǐ*).

• For unremitting incontinence, combine with Restrict the Fountain Pill (*suō quán wán*).

• For severe spermatorrhea, combine with Water and Earth Immortals Special Pill (*shuǐ lù èr xiān dān*).

• For severe, long-term uterine prolapse with frequent urination and discharge from the uterus, add Astragali Radix (*huáng qí*), Cimicifugae Rhizoma (*shēng má*), and Bupleuri Radix (*chái hú*). This can both be taken orally and applied externally to the prolapsed uterus.

Associated Formula

茯菟丹

Poria and Cuscuta Special Pill

fú tù dān

Source   *Formulary of the Pharmacy Service for Benefiting the People in the Taiping Era* (1107)

Cuscutae Semen (*tù sī zǐ*)	150g
Schisandrae Fructus (*wǔ wèi zǐ*)	210g
Dioscoreae Rhizoma (*shān yào*)	60g
Nelumbinis Semen (*lián zǐ*)	60g
Poria (*fú líng*)	90g

Soak Cuscutae Semen (*tù sī zǐ*) in wine and decoct with the other ingredients to make a paste, which is then formed into pills. Take 9g twice a day. Stabilizes the Kidney qi, stops leakage, and strengthens the Spleen. For milky, turbid spermatorrhea accompanied by listlessness, a shiny, white complexion, reduced appetite, a pale tongue with a white coating, and a submerged, frail pulse. In contrast to the principal formula, which is for Heart and Kidney deficiency, this is indicated for deficiency of the Spleen and Kidney qi.

縮泉丸 (缩泉丸)

Restrict the Fountain Pill

suō quán wán

This formula treats increased urination to the point of incontinence caused by Bladder and Kidney deficiency. Its name is a reference to a passage from Chapter 17 of *Basic Questions*: "When water flows endlessly from the fountain, this is due to the Bladder's failure to store."

Source   *Formulas Kept by the Wei Family* (1227)

Alpiniae oxyphyllae Fructus (*yán chǎo yì zhì rén*)	(9-12g)
Linderae Radix (*wū yào*)	(6-12g)
dry-fried Dioscoreae Rhizoma (*chǎo shān yào*)	(9-15g)

Method of Preparation   Combine equal amounts of the first two herbs with a paste made from the third herb and form into pills. The normal dosage is 6g taken twice a day. Originally taken with salted wine or rice water; at present, it is usually taken with boiled water. May also be prepared as a decoction with the dosages indicated in parentheses.

Actions   Warms the Kidneys, dispels cold, shuts off urinary frequency, and stops leakage

Indications

Frequent, clear, and prolonged urination or enuresis accompanied by a pale tongue with a white coating and a submerged, frail pulse.

The Bladder stores and discharges urine, but its functions are almost totally dependent on the Kidneys. When the Kidney qi is deficient, it fails to transform the Bladder qi, and diminished Bladder function ensues. This condition is due to cold from deficiency of the Kidneys in which the Bladder loses its restraint, which manifests as frequent, clear, and prolonged urination or enuresis. The pale tongue with a white coating and the submerged, frail pulse are indicative of cold from deficiency of the Kidneys.

Analysis of Formula

To treat the symptom of increased urination, this formula focuses on tonifying the lower source and warming the Kidneys in order to disperse cold. The strategy is to tonify the qi dynamic of the lower burner in order to achieve a restraining effect. Alpiniae oxyphyllae Fructus *(yì zhì rén)* warms the Kidneys and helps them grasp the qi. (The term 'grasp the qi' refers here to control over urination—the qi of the Bladder—rather than to breathing.) It also warms the Spleen, which assists in governing the fluids by way of the control cycle of the five phases. Tonifying the postnatal qi, it also indirectly strengthens the prenatal qi. These functions, together with its direct action in stabilizing and binding up the urine, make it the chief herb in the formula. The deputy, Linderae Radix *(wū yào),* disperses cold (either excessive or deficient) in the lower burner and thereby helps transform the Bladder qi and restrain urination. It is particularly effective in dispersing the cold qi between the Kidneys and Bladder. The assistant herb, Dioscoreae Rhizoma *(shān yào),* strengthens the Spleen, tonifies the Kidneys, and binds up the essence. It thereby supports the actions of the chief herb.

Cautions and Contraindications

Spicy and other stimulating types of food should not be eaten while taking this formula.

Commentary

This is a warm (but not drying) formula that eliminates cold from deficiency in the lower parts of the body. When the Kidney qi is restored, it will reassert its control over the fluids. This includes not only urination, but other body fluids as well, all of which are subject to control by the Kidneys, as explained by Zhang Jie-Bin in *Appendices to the Classified Classic:* "The Kidneys govern water. They store the essence received from the five yang and six yin organs. Therefore, the five yin fluids are all regarded as being [types of] essence, and all essence is governed by the Kidneys." For this reason, later writers expanded the use of this formula to patterns characterized by excessive salivation, weeping of the breast, excessive nasal discharge, diarrhea, vaginal discharge, and profuse uterine bleeding. However, this simple formula is rather weak and therefore often inadequate by itself to resolve the problem. In practice, it is therefore often combined with other formulas suited to treating the underlying pathodynamic.

The genealogy of this formula is complex, and modern commentators cite a number of different source texts or list different ingredients. In the source text, it was known as Special Pill for Securing the True (固真丹 *gù zhēn dān).* About

200 years later in *Classified Compilation of Medical Prescriptions,* another formula appeared with the same indication but different ingredients, namely, Alpiniae oxyphyllae Fructus *(yì zhì rén),* Linderae Radix *(wū yào),* Zanthoxyli Pericarpium *(huā jiāo),* and Evodiae Fructus *(wú zhū yú).* This formula was called Restrict the Fountain Pill *(suō quán wán).* Over time, many authors applied this name to the warming formula from the Wei family.

Comparison

> Vs. Mantis Egg-Case Powder *(sāng piāo xiāo sǎn)*

Both formulas treat increased urination, urinary incontinence, and bedwetting as well as spermatorrhoea. However, Mantis Egg-Case Powder *(sāng piāo xiāo sǎn)* treats patterns due to failure of the Heart and Kidneys to communicate, where Heart qi deficiency is the root. This formula is indicated for symptoms such as forgetfulness, a pale tongue with a white coating, and a thin, slow, and frail pulse. The urine may be turbid due to failure of the Small Intestine to separate the clear from the turbid. Restrict the Fountain Pill *(suō quán wán),* on the other hand, treats patterns due to cold from deficiency of the Kidneys leading to the inability of the Kidneys to control the fluids. This manifests with symptoms of cold such as a pale tongue with a white coating, a submerged and frail pulse, and frequent, clear, and prolonged urination or enuresis.

Biomedical Indications

With the appropriate presentation, this formula may be used to treat a variety of biomedically-defined disorders such as stress incontinence and overactive bladder.

Modifications

- For a stronger effect, add Aconiti Radix lateralis praeparata *(zhì fù zǐ),* Rubi Fructus *(fù pén zǐ),* and Schisandrae Fructus *(wǔ wèi zǐ).*

- For Kidney yang deficiency, add herbs like Morindae officinalis Radix *(bā jǐ tiān),* Psoraleae Fructus *(bǔ gǔ zhī),* and Cuscutae Semen *(tù sī zǐ).*

- For enuresis associated with emotional instability, add Ziziphi spinosae Semen *(suān zǎo rén)* and Schisandrae Fructus *(wǔ wèi zǐ).*

桂枝加龍骨牡蠣湯
（桂枝加龙骨牡蛎汤）

Cinnamon Twig Decoction plus Dragon Bone and Oyster Shell
guì zhī jiā lóng gǔ mǔ lì tāng

Source *Essentials from the Golden Cabinet* (c. 220)

Cinnamomi Ramulus *(guì zhī)* 9g
Paeoniae Radix alba *(bái sháo)* 9g
Fossilia Ossis Mastodi *(lóng gǔ)* 9g
Ostreae Concha *(mǔ lì)* 9g
Zingiberis Rhizoma recens *(shēng jiāng)* 9g
Jujubae Fructus *(dà zǎo)* . . . . 12 pieces
Glycyrrhizae Radix *(gān cǎo)* 6g

Method of Preparation   Decoction. At present, the dosage of each of the mineral substances is 15-30g. (They need not be cooked first.) Also, only 4 pieces of Jujubae Fructus *(dà zǎo)* are used.

Actions   Restrains the essence, suppresses rebellion, and regulates and harmonizes the yin and yang

Indications

Spermatorrhea (in men) or dreaming of sexual intercourse (in women), lower abdominal contraction and pain, a cold sensation at the tip of the penis, occasionally watery diarrhea, dizziness, palpitations, insomnia and dream-disturbed sleep, loss of hair, and a hollow, slightly tight pulse.

This pattern is one of deficiency of both the yin and yang, neither of which are secured, leading to floating of deficient yang above and draining of yin essence below. As such, it is a consumptive disorder with the loss of essence as its basis, evidenced by the loss of semen or dreaming of sexual intercourse (the female equivalent of wet dreams). Its etiology is described in the source text as due to excessive sexual activity or loss of blood, though in practice, it can be due to any type of deficiency and overwork. The deficient yin is unable to contain and nourish the yang, which then floats upward. The deficient yang is unable to guard and attend to the yin, which in turn is discharged below. As the yang floats upward, it separates from the yin, manifesting as false yang above and relative yin excess (cold) below. Because this yin excess is due to deficiency, its manifestations are localized as lower abdominal contraction and pain and a cold sensation in the genitals, instead of more widespread pain and coldness. Occasionally, the patient will also have watery diarrhea. The floating yang manifests as dizziness, palpitations, insomnia, and dream-disturbed sleep. The depletion of the essence leads to blood and essence deficiency, which causes hair loss and aggravates the dizziness and palpitations. The hollow pulse reflects the floating yang, while the slight tightness reflects cold from deficiency.

Analysis of Formula

This formula employs a harmonizing strategy in order to restrain the essence and suppress rebellion. The chief ingredients are Cinnamomi Ramulus *(guì zhī)* and Paeoniae Radix alba *(bái sháo)*. The former warms the yang, and the latter restrains the yin. Warming the yang helps it attend to the yin; restraining the yin enables it to contain and nourish the yang. In the context of this formula, the ability of these ingredients

to regulate the nutritive and protective qi helps restore proper communication between the yin and yang above and below.

This process is encouraged by the deputies, Fossilia Ossis Mastodi *(lóng gǔ)*, which weighs down or anchors the yang so that it reunites with the yin, and Ostreae Concha *(mǔ lì)*, which is particularly effective in helping the yin restrain the yang. The deputies also weigh down the actions of the chief ingredients so that they work on a deeper level than they ordinarily would; that is, instead of merely regulating the nutritive and protective qi, they also regulate the yin and yang. The assistants, Zingiberis Rhizoma recens *(shēng jiāng)* and Jujubae Fructus *(dà zǎo)*, reinforce the regulating and nourishing actions of the chief ingredients. The envoy, Glycyrrhizae Radix *(gān cǎo)*, harmonizes the actions of the other ingredients in the formula.

Cautions and Contraindications

Although this is a harmonizing formula, the pattern treated is one of deficiency. This will be reflected in a floating or big but weak pulse. The formula is not indicated when the pulse is deep and thin but full, or superficial but forceful.

Commentary

This formula is a modification of Cinnamon Twig Decoction *(guì zhī tāng)*, discussed in Chapter 1. As with that formula, the focus here is on harmonizing the interpenetration of yin and yang, rather than on regulating the function of specific organ systems. Whereas in the pattern associated with Cinnamon Twig Decoction *(guì zhī tāng)*, the nutritive and protective qi become disordered due to cold from the outside obstructing the flow of the nutritive qi and thereby causing it to become deficient, here, deficiency arises from overwork or other types of exhaustion and is therefore more severe. As with that formula, however, the most obvious outward signs are those of 'deficiency excess' or false yang.

In contemporary practice, this pattern presents as generalized nervous excitability which, based on the individual's constitution and life history, will express itself in many different ways. Typical manifestations include vasomotor symptoms such as hot flushes, sweating, or palpitations associated with nervousness and anxiety; a generalized overreaction to external stimuli, such as being easily startled or oversensitive to noise; generalized muscle tension, usually in thin patients, palpable during abdominal diagnosis as tension of the rectus abdominis muscles, particularly of the lower abdomen; sleep disturbances such as difficulty falling or staying asleep, dream-disturbed sleep, nightmares, or nonrestorative sleep; and frequent urination associated with nervous excitability or neurotic symptoms involving the urogenital system. Some writers consider the formula to be most appropriate for treating yang deficiency compounded by qi and blood deficiency and internal damp-cold. Besides the symptoms discussed above, such patients will also present with cold extremities as well as pain and weakness of the lower back and lower extremities.

Comparisons

➤ Vs. Bupleurum plus Dragon Bone and Oyster Shell Decoction (*chái hú jiā lóng gǔ mǔ lì tāng*); see PAGE 115

Biomedical Indications

With the appropriate presentation, this formula may be used to treat a wide variety of biomedically-defined disorders, primarily those marked by palpitations or anxiety including ventricular tachycardia, myocarditis, functional premature beats, hyperthyroidism, hysteria, nervous exhaustion, and epilepsy. It is also used for disorders in children such as pneumonia, enuresis, and night terrors. It has been used for a variety of other problems such as male infertility, erectile dysfunction, benign prostatic hypertrophy, urticaria, bronchial asthma, chronic gastritis, and perimenopausal syndrome.

Modifications

• For severe loss of semen, add Rubi Fructus (*fù pén zǐ*) and Rosae laevigatae Fructus (*jīn yīng zǐ*).

• For reckless fire, add Phellodendri Cortex (*huáng bǎi*) and Anemarrhenae Rhizoma (*zhī mǔ*).

• For qi deficiency, add Astragali Radix (*huáng qí*) and Codonopsis Radix (*dǎng shēn*).

• For severe insomnia, add Albiziae Cortex (*hé huān pí*).

• For bloody, painful urinary dribbling from deficiency or consumption, combine with Internally Tonifying Tangkuei Decoction to Construct the Middle (*dāng guī jiàn zhōng tāng*).

Associated Formula

桂枝甘草龍骨牡蠣湯 (桂枝甘草龙骨牡蛎汤))

Cinnamon Twig, Licorice, Dragon Bone, and Oyster Shell Decoction

guì zhī gān cǎo lóng gǔ mǔ lì tāng

SOURCE *Discussion of Cold Damage* (c. 220)

Cinnamomi Ramulus (*guì zhī*) 3g
Glycyrrhizae Radix praeparata (*zhì gān cǎo*) 6g
Fossilia Ossis Mastodi (*lóng gǔ*) 6g
Ostreae Concha (*mǔ lì*) 6g

Decoction. At present, the dosage of the mineral substances is generally increased to about 15-30g. Unblocks the yang, benefits the yin, calms the spirit, and eliminates irritability. Originally used for irritability caused by the improper use of warm-needle acupuncture that scorches the Heart yin and injures the Heart yang. This would occur either because the sweating induced by this technique injured the Heart yang or because the technique itself frightened the patient and

thereby disturbed the spirit. At present, this formula is used for any disorder of the Heart yin and yang in which the spirit drifts upward, irrespective of etiology. Such disorders are most commonly caused by severe sweating or the improper use of hot herbs. The primary symptoms include restlessness, irritability, spontaneous sweating, and palpitations. Compared to Cinnamon Twig Decoction plus Dragon Bone and Oyster Shell (*guì zhī jiā lóng gǔ mǔ lì tāng*), which treats more generalized disharmony between the yin and yang, this formula focuses only on the Heart.

壽胎丸 (寿胎丸)
Fetus Longevity Pill

shòu tāi wán

This formula is used for threatened miscarriage or a history of miscarriage. It was designed specifically to promote the health of the fetus, hence the name.

Source *Essays on Medicine Esteeming the Chinese and Respecting the Western* (1918-1934)

Cuscutae Semen (*tù sī zǐ*) 120g
Taxilli Herba (*sāng jì shēng*) 60g
Dipsaci Radix (*xù duàn*) 60g
Asini Corii Colla (*ē jiāo*) 60g

Method of Preparation Grind the first three ingredients into a fine powder, and dissolve the fourth in water. Combine and form into pills. The normal dose is 6g taken twice a day with warm water.

Actions Stabilizes the Kidneys and calms the fetus

Indications

Soreness and distention of the lower back, a sensation of collapse in the lower abdomen, and vaginal bleeding during pregnancy. Other signs and symptoms include dizziness, tinnitus, weak legs, frequent urination to the point of incontinence, a pale tongue with a white, slippery coating, and a submerged, frail pulse at the rear position.

The mechanism of this disorder revolves around Kidney deficiency. When the Kidneys are deficient, the Penetrating and Conception vessels become unstable, which deprives the fetus of proper nourishment. This leads to restless fetus disorder, which in severe cases can manifest as vaginal bleeding, a sensation of collapse in the lower abdomen, and even miscarriage. The Kidneys govern the bones and produce the marrow, and the brain is the 'sea' of marrow. When the Kidneys are weak, the patient may therefore experience dizziness, tinnitus, and weakness in the legs. The Kidneys (associated with water) also govern the fluids. Kidney deficiency is manifested in a lack of control over the fluids, specifically frequent urination to the point of incontinence. The pale tongue with a white, slippery coating and the submerged, frail pulse at the rear position are also characteristic of weakness of the Kidneys.

Analysis of Formula

This formula focuses on tonifying the Kidneys' ability to control opening and closing and thus safeguard pregnancy. The chief ingredient is Cuscutae Semen (*tù sī zǐ*). Owing to its capacity to tonify and stabilize the Kidneys, Zhang Xi-Chun, the formula's author, considered it to be the foremost herb for the prevention of miscarriage in the entire materia medica. Zhang chose the other three herbs as assistants that are intended to support the action of the chief herb from a number of different angles. Taxilli Herba (*sāng jì shēng*) nourishes the blood, strengthens the bones, and strengthens the fetal qi. Dipsaci Radix (*xù duàn*) tonifies the Kidneys and Liver and strengthens the bones, and is credited by Zhang with the ability to hold things together. Asini Corii Colla (*ē jiāo*) enriches the yin and nourishes the blood, stops bleeding, and calms the fetus. The formula thus treats both the root and the branch of this disorder.

Cautions and Contraindications

This formula focuses on tonifying deficiency. It is unsuitable where threatened miscarriage is due to heat or stagnation.

Commentary

This formula is designed to prevent a threatened miscarriage. However, it is also quite commonly used to prevent problems during pregnancy in women with deficient Kidneys who have suffered miscarriages in the past. Whereas classical texts generally focus treatment of threatened miscarriage on the mother, the early 20th-century physician Zhang Xi-Chun specifically designed this formula to promote the health of the fetus. In his own clinical experience, he had observed that the health and vitality of the mother was not a good predictor of whether or not a miscarriage would occur. He thus changed the approach and composed a formula that treated the fetus rather than the mother. For this purpose, he selected herbs credited with the ability to calm the fetus in classical texts such as *Divine Husbandman's Classic of the Materia Medica*, but reinterpreted their actions.

Biomedical Indications

With the appropriate presentation, this formula may be used to treat a variety of biomedically-defined disorders including threatened miscarriage, infertility, and hypertension.

Modifications

- For qi deficiency, add Ginseng Radix (*rén shēn*). (source text)
- For collapse of the gathering qi, add Astragali Radix (*huáng qí*). (source text)
- For reduced appetite, add dry-fried Atractylodis macrocephalae Rhizoma (*chǎo bái zhú*). (source text)
- For a generalized sensation of cold, add Psoraleae Fructus (*bǔ gǔ zhī*). (source text)
- For feverishness, add Rehmanniae Radix (*shēng dì huáng*). (source text)
- To strengthen the effect of the formula, add Eucommiae Cortex (*dù zhòng*). This is a very common modification.
- For vaginal bleeding, add charred Artemisiae argyi Folium (*jiāo ài yè*).
- For incontinence of urine, add Alpiniae oxyphyllae Fructus (*yì zhì rén*) and Sepiae Endoconcha (*hǎi piāo xiāo*).

Section 5

....

FORMULAS THAT SECURE IRREGULAR UTERINE BLEEDING AND STOP VAGINAL DISCHARGE

The formulas in this section are indicated for chronic, unremitting uterine bleeding and vaginal discharge due to the inability of the qi in the lower burner to contain essence. This differentiates them from formulas that focus on the actual causes of uterine bleeding or vaginal discharge, such as heat in the qi or blood, qi stagnation or blood stasis, qi and blood deficiency, or yin and yang deficiency. Although the volume of blood or discharge is generally insubstantial, it does not let up and is usually pale in color. Accompanying signs and symptoms include palpitations, shortness of breath, weakness and soreness of the lower back, a pallid complexion, pale tongue, and a deficient, thin, and frail pulse. To treat these patterns, substances that secure irregular uterine bleeding and stop vaginal discharge are usually combined with herbs that focus on the underlying causes, including those that:

- Strengthen the Spleen and augment the qi, such as Astragali Radix (*huáng qí*) and Atractylodis macrocephalae Rhizoma (*bái zhú*)
- Strengthen the Spleen and dry dampness, such as Atractylodis Rhizoma (*cāng zhú*) and Citri reticulatae Pericarpium (*chén pí*)
- Clear heat, drain fire, and leach out dampness, such as Scutellariae Radix (*huáng qín*), Phellodendri Cortex (*huáng bǎi*), and Plantaginis Semen (*chē qián zǐ*)
- Dispel blood stasis, such as Sepiae Endoconcha (*hǎi piāo xiāo*) and Rubiae Radix (*qiàn cǎo gēn*)
- Ascend and disperse, such as Bupleuri Radix (*chái hú*)
- Stop bleeding, such as charred Trachycarpi Petiolus (*zōng lǘ tàn*) and Galla chinensis (*wǔ bèi zǐ*).

固衝湯 （固冲汤）
Stabilize Gushing Decoction

gù chōng tāng

This formula treats the gushing of blood from the uterus that is due to the instability of the Penetrating (literally 'gushing') vessel, hence the name.

Source *Essays on Medicine Esteeming the Chinese and Respecting the Western* (1918-1934)

dry-fried Atractylodis macrocephalae Rhizoma *(chǎo bái zhú)* 30g
Astragali Radix *(huáng qí)* 18g
Corni Fructus *(shān zhū yú)* 24g
Paeoniae Radix alba *(bái sháo)* 12g
calcined Fossilia Ossis Mastodi *(duàn lóng gǔ)* 24g
calcined Ostreae Concha *(duàn mǔ lì)* 24g
Sepiae Endoconcha *(hǎi piāo xiāo)* 12g
charred Trachycarpi Petiolus *(zōng lǘ tàn)* 6g
Galla chinensis *(wǔ bèi zǐ)* 1.5g
Rubiae Radix *(qiàn cǎo gēn)* 9g

Method of Preparation Decoction. The two calcined substances are cooked first for approximately one hour. Galla chinensis *(wǔ bèi zǐ)* is ground into a powder, divided into two portions, and taken with the strained decoction.

Actions Augments the qi, strengthens the Spleen, stabilizes the Penetrating vessel, and stops bleeding

Indications

Uterine bleeding or profuse menstrual bleeding in which the blood is thin and pale that either gushes out or continuously trickles out. Accompanying signs and symptoms include palpitations, shortness of breath, a pale tongue, and a deficient and big or thin and frail pulse.

Uterine bleeding or profuse menstrual bleeding can arise from many causes including heat, blood stasis, Liver and Kidney deficiency, or Spleen deficiency. The early 20th-century author of this formula, Zhang Xi-Chun, emphasized uterine bleeding "caused by instability of qi transformation in the Kidney organ, [leading] to leakage of the Penetrating and Conception vessels." In another passage, Zhang defined the physiology and interconnections between these systems in gynecology even more widely:

> A person's sea of blood is called the Penetrating [vessel]. It is located on both sides of the blood chamber [i.e., the Womb], and both [of these systems] are connected with each other. Above, it is subordinated to the Stomach yang brightness vessel. Below, it connects to the Kidney lesser yin vessel. The Conception vessel takes charge of it, the Governing vessel contains it, and the Girdle vessel restrains it.

Because deficiency or instability of the Penetrating vessel or 'sea of blood' involves many different physiological systems, it is usually a chronic disorder implicating the Kidney, Spleen, Stomach and blood deficiency. In such cases, the blood will be thin and pale, and will either suddenly gush out or continuously trickle out. In both cases, the bleeding is incessant and uncontrolled. Loss of blood leads to qi and blood deficiency, which is reflected in the palpitations, shortness of breath, pale tongue, and deficient, big or thin, and frail pulse.

Analysis of Formula

The stability of the Penetrating vessel or 'sea of blood' ensures the regularity of the menstrual cycle. The Penetrating vessel itself, however, is dependent, in turn, on a multitude of other physiological systems for its own health. In acute conditions, the general rule is to focus on the manifestations. This formula achieves this by stabilizing, binding up, and stopping the bleeding. It also simultaneously treats the root cause by tonifying the Kidneys and strengthening the Spleen and Stomach.

The chief ingredient is sweet, sour, and warming Corni Fructus *(shān zhū yú)*. It tonifies the Kidneys and benefits the Liver but also has a binding action on the Penetrating and Conception vessels. According to Zhang Xi-Chun, "It strongly restrains and holds in the primal qi, stimulates vigor (精神 *jīng shén*), and secures leakage." It is supported by four deputies. The synergistic combination of calcined Fossilia Ossis Mastodi *(duàn lóng gǔ)* and calcined Ostreae Concha *(duàn mǔ lì)* is frequently used to secure leakage. While it focuses on stabilizing the Penetrating vessel, this combination also works with the chief herb in attending to what Zhang Xi-Chun regarded as the main cause of this pattern: deficiency of original qi in the lower burner. Both ingredients are calcined because Zhang believed that this process further strengthened their astringent, binding properties. The other two deputies, dry-fried Atractylodis macrocephalae Rhizoma *(chǎo bái zhú)* and Astragali Radix *(huáng qí)*, augment the qi and strengthen the Spleen. This combination is particularly effective in helping the Spleen govern the blood and stabilize the Penetrating vessel, especially with the rather large dosage used here.

The instability of the Penetrating vessel and the injury to the yin and blood from chronic blood loss are treated by the assistant, Paeoniae Radix alba *(bái sháo)*. Together with the chief ingredient, Corni Fructus *(shān zhū yú)*, this herb nourishes the yin and blood of the Liver and Kidneys and exerts an astringent, binding effect on the blood. The other assistants include Sepiae Endoconcha *(hǎi piāo xiāo)*, charred Trachycarpi Petiolus *(zōng lǘ tàn)*, and Galla chinensis *(wǔ bèi zǐ)*, all of which restrain leakage and stop bleeding. Because of the importance of quickly stopping the bleeding, the dosage of these ingredients is accordingly rather large. However, there is an attendant risk that blood stasis will form. The final assistant, Rubiae Radix *(qiàn cǎo gēn)*, both stops bleeding and invigorates the blood, and is therefore able to prevent the formation of blood stasis.

Cautions and Contraindications

This formula is inappropriate for cases in which the bleeding is so severe that it leads to an abandoned disorder characterized by profuse sweating, cold limbs, and a pulse that is faint to the point of being imperceptible. In such cases, either modify the formula or prescribe Unaccompanied Ginseng Decoction (*dú shēn tāng*) until the condition has stabilized.

Commentary

This is one of five formulas from the gynecology section of *Essays on Medicine Esteeming the Chinese and Respecting the Western* that focuses on the Penetrating vessel. Its author, the influential modern physician Zhang Xi-Chun, followed Qing-dynasty interpretations of the *Inner Classic* in placing the greatest importance on regulating the functions of this system in the treatment of various gynecological disorders. In a brief passage attached to another formula, Zhang outlines the basic principles that should orient such treatment: "Infertility in women is frequently due to the Penetrating vessel. If it is constrained, one regulates it; if it is deficient, one tonifies it; if it has been assaulted by wind, one dispels that; if it has been conquered by dampness, one leaches it out."

The present formula employs a strategy of 'binding tonification' (澀補 *sè bǔ*) to treat a fairly critical condition that goes beyond ordinary patterns of irregular uterine bleeding. In late imperial and early modern China, irregular uterine bleeding was commonly interpreted as being due to 'gushing down' of Liver qi into the lower burner. This, in turn, was caused by constraint due to anger or other factors blocking the physiological ascent of the Liver qi and leading to a concurrent reversal of its flow. In such cases, a treatment strategy aimed at raising the Liver qi and opening areas of constraint—pursued with variants of Tonify the Middle to Augment the Qi Decoction (*bǔ zhōng yì qì tāng*)—would be appropriate. The present pattern is more serious inasmuch as heavy bleeding has also led to abandonment of qi. This means that one must now focus on 'holding in and tonifying the lower [burner] primal [qi]' (收補下元 *shōu bǔ xià yuán*) to stop the bleeding. In his essay, "[My] Interpretation of Primal Qi" (元氣詮 *yuán qì quán*), Zhang elaborated:

> To help [in situations] where the primal qi is about to be lost, it is insufficient to rely [solely] on herbs to tonify the qi. Instead, I give first place to herbs that bind and tonify, such as Corni Fructus (*shān zhū yú*), Fossilia Ossis Mastodi (*lóng gǔ*), and Ostreae Concha (*mǔ lì*), and use herbs that tonify the qi to assist them. ... In cases of loss below, I use Ginseng Radix (*rén shēn*) and Astragali Radix (*huáng qí*) as appropriate assistants. In cases of incessant lower burner diarrhea, it is appropriate to also add Atractylodis macrocephalae Rhizoma (*bái zhú*) in order to stop the diarrhea. This is [my] strategy for providing temporary relief in an emergency.

This passage clearly shows that commentators who claim that Atractylodis macrocephalae Rhizoma (*bái zhú*) and Astragali Radix (*huáng qí*) should be considered the chief ingredients, based on the adage "To treat the blood, first treat the Spleen," are incorrect.

The use of this formula has been expanded to include black, tarry stools in patients with Spleen deficiency. While the author believed that it should work within a couple of days, many modern practitioners consider 5-7 days the normal length of treatment. Because the formula focuses on securing excessive bleeding, it is neither warming nor cooling. Where a patient presents with clear signs of heat or cold, the formula should be adjusted accordingly.

Comparisons

➤ Vs. Restore the Spleen Decoction (*guī pí tāng*)

Both formulas are used in treating excessive menstruation from deficient Spleen qi failing to govern the blood. The difference is that Stabilize the Gushing Decoction (*gù chòng tang*) is used when the condition requires an astringent, binding effect, as in critical conditions characterized by severe, acute blood loss that exhausts the lower burner primal qi, as well as in more chronic disorders where the Kidneys and Liver have become severely depleted. Once the bleeding has stopped, however, a formula that targets the root cause should be used. Restore the Spleen Decoction (*guī pí tāng*) is used for chronic but less severe bleeding with signs of Heart blood deficiency.

➤ Vs. Stabilize the Menses Pill (*gù jīng wán*); see PAGE 446

➤ Vs. Pregnancy Panacea (*shēn líng dān*); see PAGE 447

Biomedical Indications

With the appropriate presentation, this formula may be used to treat a variety of biomedically-defined disorders including dysfunctional uterine bleeding, excessive bleeding postpartum, and bleeding peptic ulcer.

Modifications

• For relatively hot conditions, add Rehmanniae Radix (*shēng dì huáng*). (source text)
• For relatively cold conditions, add Aconiti Radix lateralis praeparata (*zhì fù zǐ*). (source text)
• Where the condition arises following a fit of anger, add Bupleuri Radix (*chái hú*). (source text)
• If the problem has not improved significantly after two days, substitute Asini Corii Colla (*ē jiāo*) for charred Trachycarpi Petiolus (*zōng lǘ tàn*). (source text)
• For severe blood loss with cold extremities, a faint pulse, and other signs of imminent abandonment, increase the dosage of Astragali Radix (*huáng qí*) and add Ginseng Radix (*rén shēn*) and Aconiti Radix lateralis praeparata (*zhì fù zǐ*).

固經丸 （固经丸）
Stabilize the Menses Pill
gù jīng wán

Source *Essential Teachings of [Zhu] Dan-Xi* (1481)

prepared Testudinis Plastrum (*zhì guī bǎn*) 30g
dry-fried Paeoniae Radix alba (*chǎo bái sháo*) 30g
dry-fried Scutellariae Radix (*chǎo huáng qín*) 30g
Ailanthi Cortex (*chūn pí*) 22.5g
dry-fried Phellodendri Cortex (*chǎo huáng bǎi*) 9g
Cyperi Rhizoma (*xiāng fù*) 7.5g

Method of Preparation Grind the ingredients into a powder and form into pills with wine. Take 9g twice a day with warm water. May also be prepared as a decoction with a proportionate reduction in the dosage of the ingredients.

Actions Enriches the yin, clears heat, stops bleeding, and stabilizes the menses

Indications

Continuous menstruation or uterine bleeding that alternates between trickling and gushing of blood. The blood is very red and may contain dark-purple clots. Accompanying signs and symptoms include a sensation of heat and irritability in the chest, abdominal pain, dark urine, a red tongue, and a rapid, wiry pulse.

This pattern is due to heat that enters the Penetrating and Conception vessels, causing the blood to become hot and move recklessly. This can be due to Liver qi constraint and is usually accompanied by yin deficiency. Such patterns are characterized by continuous menstruation or uterine bleeding that alternates between trickling and gushing of blood. When the bleeding is due to the reckless movement of hot blood, its color is very red. Heat from constraint tends to congeal the blood, so there may also be dark-purple clots. Liver heat disturbs the flow in the Penetrating and Conception vessels, which produces a sensation of heat and irritability in the chest, and abdominal pain. The dark urine, red tongue, and rapid, wiry pulse are characteristic of heat in the Liver. Yin deficiency usually precedes this disorder and is aggravated by the loss of blood.

Analysis of Formula

Treatment of bleeding due to heat that causes the blood to move recklessly requires that one attend to the root cause of the heat. In the present case, it is not due to heat in the blood, but rather to excess yang qi arising from or leading to a deficiency of yin essence. For this reason, the formula combines substances that tonify yin with those that drain heat in order to restore equilibrium between the yin and yang. The chief ingredients are salty, sweet, and cooling Testudinis Plastrum (*guī bǎn*), which tonifies the yin essence and directs the fire downward, and sour, bitter, and cooling Paeoniae Radix alba

(*bái sháo*), which preserves the yin and nourishes the blood. The deputies are the bitter, cooling herbs Scutellariae Radix (*huáng qín*), which drains heat from the upper burner and blood to stop the bleeding, and Phellodendri Cortex (*huáng bǎi*), which drains damp-heat from the lower burner. Together with the chief ingredients, they control the fire (yang) by directing it downward, as well as by fortifying the water (yin) itself.

One of the assistants, Cyperi Rhizoma (*xiāng fù*), is an acrid substance that regulates the qi and relieves Liver constraint. Using only a small amount ensures that its warming nature does not add to the fire. The other assistant, Ailanthi Cortex (*chūn pí*), is a bitter, astringent substance that binds up the blood and prevents an abandoned disorder from developing, which is otherwise likely with long-term blood loss. It is considered to be of less importance than the other ingredients because, if the heat is cleared and the yin is enriched, the blood will resume its normal movement in the channels and the bleeding will stop of its own accord. The use of an astringent, binding substance only serves to hasten this effect. The wine used in the preparation of the pills acts as an envoy, which leads the other substances into the blood and prevents the astringent nature of the sour ingredients from causing blood stasis.

Cautions and Contraindictions

This formula is astringent in nature. It is contraindicated in patterns characterized by heat due to blood stasis.

Commentary

This type of uterine bleeding was first mentioned in *Basic Questions* (Chapter 7) where it is attributed to "deficient yin and belligerent yang." Many commentators consider dark purple clots to be a key marker for this pattern. The deficient yin aspect of the presentation is not obvious because it underlies the heat. However, as the composition of the formula reflects, addressing the yin deficiency is an essential part of the treatment. (For a more detailed discussion of Zhu Dan-Xi's approach to the treatment of such pathologies, see the discussion of Great Tonify the Yin Pill (*dà bǔ yīn wán*) and Hidden Tiger Pill (*hǔ qián wán*) in Chapter 8.)

The use of the warming, acrid herb Cyperi Rhizoma (*xiāng fù*) in a formula intended to drain excess heat has attracted much attention. Commentators point to three different functions to explain this usage. First, it resolves constraint. This, as noted in *Record of Challenges [to the Classics]*, was a chief concern of the formula's author: "Zhu Dan-Xi's [approach] to the treatment of [any] disorder did not go beyond the three [categories of] qi, blood, and phlegm. All three often occur together with constraint." A second, related purpose for the inclusion of Cyperi Rhizoma (*xiāng fù*) is to prevent such constraint from transforming into fire and thereby aggravating the existing yang excess. As explained by Wang Fu in *Collectanea of Investigations from the Realm of Medicine*: "[As long as] Liver qi is not constrained, there will be no fire. [The presence of] fire [conversely implies that] Liver qi is constrained. Therefore, Cyperi Rhizoma (*xiāng fù*) is used to break it up." Finally, a small amount of an acrid, warming substance such as Cyperi Rhizoma (*xiāng fù*)—but also the alcohol used to make the pills—prevents blood stasis, which would aggravate the bleeding.

Later generations of physicians expanded the use of this formula to the treatment of vaginal discharge, dysenteric disorders, seminal emissions, and heat in the five centers.

Comparison

➤ Vs. Stabilize Gushing Decoction (*gù chōng tāng*)

Both formulas treat excessive uterine bleeding. However, Stabilize the Menses Pill (*gù jīng wán*) is indicated for bleeding due to yang excess against a background of yin deficiency. Typically, the blood is dark red and contains clots. There will also be other signs of heat such as irritability, restlessness, or heat in the five centers. Stabilize Gushing Decoction (*gù chōng tāng*), on the other hand, is indicated for sudden and profuse uterine bleeding accompanied by signs of qi and blood deficiency, such as pallor and palpitations. Although with appropriate modification this formula can also treat heat-type patterns, its focus is on securing blood loss by binding and tonifying the source qi in the lower burner.

Biomedical Indications

With the appropriate presentation, this formula may be used to treat a variety of biomedically-defined disorders including dysfunctional uterine bleeding and chronic pelvic inflammatory disease.

Alternate names

Ailanthus Root Bark Pill to Stabilize the Menses (*chūn bái gù jīng wán*) in *Concise Medical Guidelines*; Stabilize the Menses Decoction (*gù jīng tāng*) in *Ye Xi-Chun's Case Histories*

Modifications

• For more severe yin deficiency characterized by menstruation that lingers on with scanty, red blood, malar flush, hot palms and soles, dry throat and mouth, a red tongue with little coating, and a thin, fast pulse, remove Scutellariae Radix (*huáng qín*) and Cyperi Rhizoma (*xiāng fù*) and add Lycii Cortex (*dì gǔ pí*) and Rehmanniae Radix praeparata (*shú dì huáng*).

• For severe bleeding, add Sanguisorbae Radix (*dì yú*) and Agrimoniae Herba (*xiān hè cǎo*), or add Sepiae Endoconcha (*hǎi piāo xiāo*), Rubiae Radix (*qiàn cǎo gēn*), Fossilia Ossis Mastodi (*lóng gǔ*), and Ostreae Concha (*mǔ lì*).

震靈丹 (震灵丹)

Pregnancy Panacea

shēn líng dān

This formula stems from the Tang dynasty *Daoist Canon* (道藏 *Daò zàng*). Its original name was Purple Gold Special Pill (紫金丹 *zǐ jīn dān*). Replete with Daoist connotations, the name hints at its ability to prolong life. From there it entered mainstream Chinese medical practice where its name was changed to match its new clinical usage. The character 震 (read as *shēn*) is interchangeable with 娠, which means pregnancy. This suggests that even though the formula was indicated for deficiency in both men and women, it was thought to be particularly useful in gynecology.

Source   *Formulary of the Pharmacy Service for Benefiting the People in the Taiping Era* (1107)

Limonitum (*yǔ yú liáng*) .120g
Fluoritum (*zǐ shí yīng*) .120g
Halloysitum rubrum (*chì shí zhī*) 120g
Haematitum (*dài zhě shí*) 120g
Olibanum (*rǔ xiāng*) 60g
Myrrha (*mò yào*) 60g
Trogopterori Faeces (*wǔ líng zhī*) 60g
Cinnabaris (*zhū shā*) 30g

Method of Preparation   Grind all but the last ingredient into a powder, mix with water and 120g of ground glutinous rice, and form into pills. Coat the pills with Cinnabaris (*zhū shā*). Take one large pill (approximately 9-12g) each day on an empty stomach with warm water or wine. The mineral ingredients are often calcined before being ground to strengthen their astringent properties. Due to the unacceptable toxicity of Cinnabaris (*zhū shā*), this ingredient is no longer used. As early as *Discussion of Illnesses, Patterns, and Formulas Related to the Unification of the Three Etiologies*, this formula was listed without this substance, suggesting that it does not require substitution.

Actions   Stabilizes uterine bleeding and transforms blood stasis

Indications

Continuous uterine bleeding of purplish-red or dark-purple blood with clots, pain and tenderness in the lower abdomen that diminishes with the passage of the clots, a dark-purple tongue that may have purple spots, and a submerged, thin, and wiry pulse.

This is uterine bleeding due to cold from deficiency of the Conception and Penetrating vessels, which causes the blood to stray from the channels. The blood collects in the lower burner where stasis develops. This leads to continuous vaginal bleeding with purplish blood and clots together with lower abdominal pain and tenderness. When the clots pass, the qi in the lower abdomen is temporarily unblocked and the pain diminishes. The dark-purple tongue (which may also have purple spots) and the wiry pulse reflect the stasis of blood. The submerged, thin qualities of the pulse reflect cold from deficiency in the Conception and Penetrating vessels.

Analysis of Formula

To stop the bleeding, one must warm the Womb and stabilize the Conception and Penetrating vessels. And because there is also blood stasis, one must transform the stasis or the condition will worsen. Warming Halloysitum rubrum (chì shí zhī) and neutral Limonitum (yǔ yú liáng) are both astringent substances that excel at stopping bleeding and discharge. Accordingly, they can be regarded as the chief ingredients in this formula. Haematitum (dài zhě shí) enters the Liver, directs rebelliousness downward, and stops bleeding. Fluoritum (zǐ shí yīng) warms the Womb, settles the Heart, and calms the spirit. Serving as deputies, these substances support the chief ingredients by warming the Womb and stabilizing the lower parts of the body. Olibanum (rǔ xiāng), Myrrha (mò yào), and Trogopterori Faeces (wǔ líng zhī) are acrid and warming substances, and are therefore useful for invigorating the blood and transforming stasis. They also regulate the qi and alleviate pain. Glutinous rice augments the qi of the Lungs and Spleen and warms the middle burner. Here it mildly addresses the deficiency that underlies this condition. Originally, Cinnabaris (zhū shā) was used to help calm the spirit, which is often disturbed by the bleeding and pain. All of these substances serve as assistants.

Cautions and Contraindications

This formula should not be used in cases of cold from deficiency in the absence of blood stasis. It is contraindicated during pregnancy or in cases with damp-heat.

Commentary

The term 靈丹 líng dān in the name of this formula translates as 'panacea,' hinting at both the efficacy attributed to the formula as well as its Daoist origins. Indeed, the source text notes that "It treats qi and blood deficiency in women, irregular uterine bleeding [associated with] deficiency harm, discharges [associated with] chronic cold, and infertility. Those who take it will be cured without fail."

The Daoist origins of this formula are also evident in its reliance on mainly mineral substances. From a medical perspective, their sinking nature allows them to move directly to the lower burner. This downward movement is balanced by the acrid, warming nature of the other ingredients. This formula treads a narrow path between stabilizing the lower part of the body and simultaneously transforming blood stasis. This is accomplished by combining warm mineral substances that are astringent in nature with acrid, stasis-transforming resins and animal products. This blending of diverse medicinals makes the formula's composition extremely harmonious in spite of the potent, one-sided action of some of its individual constituents. This combination of effects was noticed by the Qing-dynasty physician Ye Tian-Shi, who described its use in *Case Records as a Guide to Clinical Practice* as "un-blocking and therefore thrusting out [pathogens] from the lower [burner]; binding, and therefore securing the lower [burner]." Such a combination of actions fit well with Ye Tian-Shi's understanding of how conditions of deficiency in the extraordinary vessels should be approached, and its modern usage owes much to his ideas.

The source text also recommends this formula for vaginal discharge due to cold from deficiency with blood stasis and for severe depletion of the true source qi in men due to overindulgence in sex and work, which causes excess above and deficiency below. Symptoms of the latter disorder include periumbilical pain, generalized aches and pains, lightheadedness, vertigo, and disorientation. Because many of the minerals in this formula also stop diarrhea, its use has been expanded to include chronic diarrhea with a similar presentation. Other modern indications consistent with both the source text and Ye Tian-Shi's reinterpretation include retained placenta and hematuria from deficiency.

Comparison

➤ Vs. Stabilize Gushing Decoction (gù chōng tāng)

Both formulas treat irregular uterine bleeding due to conditions of deficiency associated with the extraordinary vessels in the lower burner. However, Stabilize Gushing Decoction (gù chōng tāng) focuses specifically on binding the Penetrating vessel. It is indicated for sudden and severe bleeding associated with Kidney deficiency. Pregnancy Panacea (shēn líng dān), on the other hand, treats both blood stasis and cold in the lower burner associated with deficiency of the extraordinary vessels. Its use is indicated for more chronic conditions that need to be treated over a longer period of time.

Biomedical Indications

With the appropriate presentation, this formula may be used to treat a variety of biomedically-defined disorders including dysfunctional uterine bleeding and pelvic inflammatory disease.

Alternate name

Purple-Gold Special Pill (zǐ jīn dān) in *Formulary of the Pharmacy Service for Benefiting the People in the Taiping Era*

完帶湯 （完带汤）

End Discharge Decoction

wán dài tāng

Source *Fu Qing-Zhu's Women's Disorders* (1826, but written in 17th century)

earth-fried Atractylodis macrocephalae Rhizoma
(tǔ chǎo bái zhú) 30g

dry-fried Dioscoreae Rhizoma (chǎo shān yào) 30g

Ginseng Radix (rén shēn) 6g

prepared Atractylodis Rhizoma (zhì cāng zhú) 9g

Citri reticulatae Pericarpium (chén pí) 1.5g

wine-fried Plantaginis Semen (jiǔ chǎo chē qián zǐ) 9g

wine-fried Paeoniae Radix alba (jiǔ chǎo bái sháo) 15g

Bupleuri Radix (chái hú) 1.8g

charred Schizonepetae Spica (jīng jiè suì tàn) 1.5g

Glycyrrhizae Radix (gān cǎo) .3g

Method of Preparation　Decoction. At present, Codonopsis Radix (dǎng shēn) is usually substituted for Ginseng Radix (rén shēn) at 2-3 times its dosage.

Actions　Tonifies the middle burner, strengthens the Spleen, transforms dampness, and stops vaginal discharge

Indications

Profuse vaginal discharge that is white or pale yellow in color, thin in consistency, not particularly foul-smelling, and usually continuous. Accompanying signs and symptoms include fatigue, lethargy, a shiny, pale complexion, loose stools, a pale tongue with a white coating, and a soggy and frail or moderate pulse.

In the opinion of the formula's author, vaginal discharge (白帶 bái dài) is particularly associated with the functions of the Liver, Spleen, and Girdle vessel (帶脈 dài mài). The Girdle vessel wraps around the lower trunk like a belt, securing all the channels that traverse the area. It has a particularly close relationship with the Spleen and Liver. When there is dysfunction of the Girdle vessel, it is unable to secure the channels and there is a discharge from the lowest part of the trunk in women, the vagina. The Spleen governs transformation and transportation. When the Spleen qi is deficient, these processes are inhibited and the fluids accumulate internally in the form of dampness. The dampness gradually becomes turbid, which obstructs and thereby further weakens the Spleen. The turbid dampness seeps downward and is discharged through the vagina.

The Liver governs the free-flowing or spreading functions of the body. When the flow of Liver qi is impaired, it fails to distribute ministerial fire to the middle burner, which further weakens the Spleen, thereby increasing the dampness. Vaginal discharge due to Spleen deficiency and dampness is profuse, white or pale yellow in color, and thin in consistency. Because there is no heat, the discharge will not be foul-smelling. When the Spleen qi is deficient, it cannot provide the body with proper nourishment and there is fatigue and lethargy. Too little qi and blood rise to the face, which gives it a shiny, pale appearance. Loose stools are a classic sign of Spleen qi deficiency compounded by dampness, which impedes the Spleen's ability to raise the qi and fluids upward. The tongue and pulse signs also reflect Spleen deficiency with dampness.

Analysis of Formula

This formula is based on the idea that this type of vaginal discharge will cease when the Spleen is strong and the dampness diminishes. For this, it uses large dosages of herbs that tonify the qi and dry dampness to focus on the main manifestation. It combines these with herbs that dredge and soften the Liver to ensure that yang qi ascends freely, thereby supporting those functions of the qi dynamic that are most crucial to the process of qi transformation in the middle burner. The chief herbs are Atractylodis macrocephalae Rhizoma (bái zhú) and dry-fried Dioscoreae Rhizoma (chǎo shān yào). Working synergistically, they strengthen the Spleen, augment the qi, drain dampness, and bind up the essence. Both herbs are thought to enter the extraordinary vessels, allowing them to support the Girdle vessel in its task of securing the channels. The deputies are Ginseng Radix (rén shēn), which strongly tonifies the source qi and strengthens the Spleen, Atractylodis Rhizoma (cāng zhú), which is very effective in drying dampness, wine-fried Plantaginis Semen (jiǔ chǎo chē qián zǐ), which leaches out dampness through the urine, and Paeoniae Radix alba (bái sháo), which softens the Liver and regulates the Spleen, allowing the Liver qi to spread in such a manner that it strengthens rather than constrains Spleen function. The chief and deputy herbs tonify without interfering with the resolution of dampness; they also treat the pathogenic influence without injuring the normal qi.

The assistant herbs focus on the qi dynamic. Citri reticulatae Pericarpium (chén pí) moves and regulates the Spleen qi to ensure that the tonifying will not cause stagnation. Bupleuri Radix (chái hú) opens areas of constraint and, in concert with the herbs that augment the qi, facilitates the ascent of the clear yang. This assists Spleen physiology but also balances the downward-moving nature of those herbs that leach out dampness. Charred Schizonepetae Spica (jīng jiè suì tàn) has a special use in Fu's formulas, as discussed in the COMMENTARY below. Basically, he uses it to smooth the interpenetration of qi and blood, and thereby the harmonious interaction of Liver and Spleen. The envoy, Glycyrrhizae Radix (gān cǎo), assists the chief herbs in tonifying the middle burner and harmonizes the actions of the other ingredients.

The famous modern physician Yue Mei-Zhong provided an interesting explanation for the large difference in dosage between the chief and assistant herbs. The chief herbs are tonics that have a still and quiet nature. The assistants are herbs that induce movement and whose actions are focused on certain channels (primarily the Spleen and Liver, but also the Penetrating and Girdle vessels). They push and move the actions of the quiet herbs in such a way that their tonifying properties are increased, and their side effects are moderated. Because they serve this auxiliary role in the formula, their dosage is accordingly smaller.

Cautions and Contraindications

This formula should not be used if the discharge is dark yellow, contains blood, and is thick, sticky, and foul-smelling, and the patient has a yellow tongue coating and a wiry pulse. This pattern is one of Liver constraint that has transformed into heat or damp-heat. The use of this formula in treating that disorder will only make it worse.

Commentary

In the source text, the author of this formula, Fu Qing-Zhu, attributes the disorder to Liver constraint and qi deficiency that injures the Spleen and causes dampness (earth) to descend.

White vaginal discharge [reflects] an overabundance of dampness while fire is debilitated. When the Liver is constrained and the qi is frail, Spleen earth suffers damage, and the damp qi of earth sinks downward. [The pathodynamic involved here] is Spleen essence that is not conserved because it cannot be transformed into nutritive [qi] and blood that [would then] become the menses. Instead, it changes into a slippery white substance that directly leaks from the vagina unable to be contained by natural means. The treatment strategy consists of strongly tonifying the qi of the Spleen and Stomach, and relying for assistants on substances that dredge the Liver. By preventing wind-wood closing off [the movement of qi] in the earth of the middle [burner], earth qi can ascend naturally to the heavens above. When the Spleen qi is strengthened and the damp qi reduced, disorders [characterized by] white vaginal discharge cannot exist.

Fu Qing-Zhu's approach to the treatment of discharge represented a development of older strategies initially appearing in the Jin-Yuan era. Under the influence of Li Dong-Yuan's doctrines regarding Spleen and Stomach physiology, vaginal discharge (viewed as a sinking down of Spleen essence in the manner analyzed by Fu) was then widely treated with variations of Tonify the Middle to Augment the Qi Decoction (*bǔ zhōng yì qì tāng*). In the Ming dynasty, this approach was further developed by Miao Xi-Yong, who suggested that a number of more specific additions be made to this formula for the treatment of discharge. In *Extensive Notes on Medicine*, Miao explained:

White vaginal discharge generally represents Spleen deficiency. When the Liver is constrained, Spleen earth suffers damage. [The pathodynamic involved here] is Spleen essence that is not conserved because it cannot be transformed into nutritive [qi] and blood. Instead, it flows down as a slippery white substance. This is due to wind-wood constraining the earth of the middle [burner]. The strategy [for treating this] should be to lift Liver qi, tonify the Spleen, and assist the primal [qi]. Tonify the Middle to Augment the Qi Decoction (*bǔ zhōng yì qì tāng*), with the addition of such [herbs] as Ziziphi spinosae Semen (*suān zǎo rén*), Poria (*fú líng*), Dioscoreae Rhizoma (*shān yào*), Phellodendri Cortex (*huáng bǎi*), Atractylodis Rhizoma (*cāng zhú*), and Ophiopogonis Radix (*mài mén dōng*), is a suitable [formula].

The influence of Miao Xi-Yong on Fu Qing-Zhu's thinking is obvious. However, Fu did not simply plagiarize Miao's ideas—copying entire passages from other texts is an acceptable practice in Chinese writing—but developed them in a new and different direction. This can be seen most particularly in Fu's use of charred Schizonepetae Spica (*jīng jiè suì tàn*), which is an ingredient in many of the gynecological formulas for which he became famous. Although there is some debate among physicians as to its precise function, Fu's own commentaries indicate that he used it "to unblock the vessels and collaterals," and "to lead the blood in the vessels," in other words, to use the Liver's function of dredging and regulating to harmonize the flow of qi and blood. Reflecting the importance attributed to Liver function in gynecology, Fu Qing-Zhu's End Discharge Decoction (*wán dài tāng*) thus focuses in equal measures on Spleen, Stomach, and Liver functions, while staying true to Li Dong-Yuan's and Miao Xi-Yong's emphasis on enabling the clear yang to ascend. As Fu noted in his discussion:

This formula represents a strategy of treating the Spleen, Stomach, and Liver channels simultaneously. It contains tonification within dispersion, and places elimination in [a generally] ascending [formula]. Opening and raising the qi of Liver wood [ensures] that Liver blood does not become dry. How could it then overcome Spleen earth? By tonifying and augmenting the base of Spleen earth, Spleen qi will not become damp. What difficulty could there then be in separating and eliminating pathogenic water? With regard to tonifying the Spleen and simultaneously tonifying the Stomach, this arises from the interior-exterior [relationship between these organs]. If the Spleen does not have [the support] of a strong Stomach, a frail Spleen cannot be made to flourish [again]. This is how directly tonifying the Stomach will secondarily also tonify the Spleen.

This is a very commonly-used formula for vaginal discharge due to Spleen deficiency, a condition that is quite prevalent. In one sense, this is not strictly a formula that stabilizes and binds because it does not contain significant amounts of astringent, binding substances. It is included in this chapter because it does treat the leakage of fluids by improving the normal functions of the body, rather than attacking a pathogenic influence. The use of this formula has accordingly been expanded to include all kinds of problems associated with Spleen deficiency and turbid dampness such as diarrhea, edema during menstruation or pregnancy, headache, and dizziness.

Comparisons

➢ Vs. CHANGE YELLOW [DISCHARGE] DECOCTION (*yì huáng tāng*); see PAGE 451

➢ Vs. EIGHT-INGREDIENT FORMULA FOR VAGINAL DISCHARGE (*bā wèi dài xià fāng*); see PAGE 698

Biomedical Indications

With the appropriate presentation, this formula may be used to treat a wide variety of biomedically-defined disorders including preeclampsia, otitis media, tinnitus, impotence, and subdural hematoma. It is also used for many kinds of inflammatory disorders such as rhinitis, chronic gastritis, hepatitis, colitis, chronic bacillary dysentery, chronic pyelonephritis, and nephritis with proteinuria.

Modifications

- To strengthen the effect of the formula, add calcined Fossilia Ossis Mastodi *(duàn lóng gǔ)* and calcined Ostreae Concha *(duàn mǔ lì)*.

- For chronic problems with very thin discharge, add Cervi Cornu degelatinatum *(lù jiǎo shuāng)* and Morindae officinalis Radix *(bā jǐ tiān)*.

- For soreness of the lower back, add Taxilli Herba *(sāng jì shēng)*, Eucommiae Cortex *(dù zhòng)*, and Cibotii Rhizoma *(gǒu jǐ)*.

- For lower abdominal and hypochondriac pain, add Corydalis Rhizoma *(yán hú suǒ)* and Cyperi Rhizoma *(xiāng fù)*.

- For pain and a feeling of cold in the lower abdomen, add Linderae Radix *(wū yào)*, Foeniculi Fructus *(xiǎo huí xiāng)*, and Zingiberis Rhizoma praeparatum *(páo jiāng)*.

Associated Formula

清帶湯 （清带汤）

Clear Discharge Decoction

qīng dài tāng

SOURCE *Essays on Medicine Esteeming the Chinese and Respecting the Western* (1918-1934)

Dioscoreae Rhizoma *(shān yào)* 30g
Fossilia Ossis Mastodi *(lóng gǔ)* 18g
Ostreae Concha *(mǔ lì)* 18g
Sepiae Endoconcha *(hǎi piāo xiāo)* 12g
Rubiae Radix *(qiàn cǎo gēn)* 9g

Strengthens the Spleen, binds up, and stops vaginal discharge. For Spleen deficiency with a profuse, thin, clear or red, and continuous vaginal discharge accompanied by soreness and weakness of the lower back, very pale complexion, a pale tongue with a white coating, and a submerged, thin pulse. This formula is very binding but also moves and regulates the blood. It was composed by the modern physician Zhang Xi-Chun to treat discharge he considered to be due to the inability of the Penetrating and Conception vessels to contain the essences. Hence, he focused treatment on securing excessive leakage from these vessels but, in accordance with their nature as vessels that imply movement, added herbs that invigorate the circulation of blood without causing further leakage. The author suggested that the formula be further modified to match the presentation. For bloody

discharge, he added Paeoniae Radix alba *(bái sháo)* and Sophorae flavescentis Radix *(kǔ shēn)*, and for white discharge, Atractylodis macrocephalae Rhizoma *(bái zhú)* and Cervi Cornu degelatinatum *(lù jiǎo shuāng)*.

易黃湯 （易黄汤）

Change Yellow [Discharge] Decoction

yì huáng tāng

This formula changes a yellow vaginal discharge into no discharge, hence the name.

Source *Fu Qing-Zhu's Women's Disorders* (1826, but written in 17th century)

dry-fried Dioscoreae Rhizoma *(chǎo shān yào)* 30g
dry-fried Euryales Semen *(chǎo qiàn shí)* 30g
Phellodendri Cortex *(huáng bǎi)* .6g
Plantaginis Semen *(chē qián zǐ)* .3g
Ginkgo Semen *(bái guǒ)* . . . .[crush] 10 kernels

Method of Preparation Decoction

Actions Strengthens the Spleen, dries dampness, clears heat, and stops vaginal discharge

Indications

Long-term, unremitting vaginal discharge that is yellowish-white in color, viscous, and fishy-smelling. Accompanying signs and symptoms include a pale-yellow complexion, dizziness, a sensation of heaviness in the head, reduced appetite, occasional loose stools, delayed menstruation with pale blood, a pale tongue with a thin, white coating, and a soft, slippery pulse that may be submerged.

According to the formula's author, this is damp-heat of the Conception vessel (see the COMMENTARY below). To align this diagnosis with the current emphasis on organ patterns, modern textbooks have redefined this as Spleen or Kidney qi deficiency with dampness in which the dampness becomes constrained, transforms into damp-heat, and pours downward. This manifests as a pale-yellow complexion, dizziness, a sensation of heaviness in the head, reduced appetite, and occasional loose stools. When the blood is deficient (whether due to Spleen, Kidney, or Penetrating vessel deficiency), the complexion becomes pale yellow, and the periods are late and with pale blood. The tongue and pulse signs reflect the combination of deficiency (pale tongue and soft and submerged pulse) and dampness (slippery pulse). Because the heat is mild and due to constraint, it is manifested only in the color and odor of the discharge.

Analysis of Formula

This is an elegantly designed formula that balances substances that tonify and bind up with those that clear and drain damp-heat. The chief herbs are dry-fried Dioscoreae Rhizoma *(chǎo shān yào)*, which strengthens the Spleen and stabilizes the Penetrating vessel and the essence, and dry-fried Euryales Semen *(chǎo qiàn shí)*, which tonifies the Kidneys and Spleen, as well as binding up the discharge. According to *Seeking Accuracy in the Materia Medica*: "The yin [tonifying properties] of Dioscoreae Rhizoma *(shān yào)* are primary [in the use of that herb] and exceed those of Euryales Semen *(qiàn shí)*. The astringent [properties] of Euryales Semen *(qiàn shí)* [however] are stronger than those of Dioscoreae Rhizoma *(shān yào)*." According to Fu Qing-Zhu, "they excel at tonifying deficiency of the Conception vessel, but are also able to promote water metabolism." The deputy is Ginkgo Semen *(bái guǒ)*, which helps to stabilize the lower burner and restrain the discharge. The assistants are bitter and cooling Phellodendri Cortex *(huáng bǎi)*, which enters the Kidneys and drains damp-heat excess from the lower burner, and sweet and cooling Plantaginis Semen *(chē qián zǐ)*, which leaches dampness primarily through the urine. As the damp-heat is dissipated, the discharge will stop. Working together, the various ingredients bind up the discharge without causing stagnation, and eliminate damp-heat without overly draining the patient.

Cautions and Contraindications

If the presentation does not closely match that described above, this formula may be inappropriate. Nor should it be used in cases without damp-heat, or in those with severe damp-heat.

Commentary

This formula treats yellow discharge (黃帶 *huáng dài*), described in the source text as resembling the color of dark tea. Reflecting the importance attached by Qing-dynasty gynecology to extraordinary vessel function, the formula's author, Fu Qing-Zhu, defined this disorder as a pathology of the Conception vessel:

> Yellow discharge is damp-heat of the Conception vessel. [In terms of its] basic [physiological function,] the Conception vessel is unable to contain water. So how can it be that damp qi enters into it and transforms into yellow discharge? [Those who cannot answer this question by themselves] do not understand that the Girdle vessel's overflow connects with the Conception vessel. The Conception vessel goes straight up to the lips and teeth. Within the lips and teeth is the original unceasing source [of fluid] that [thereby] communicates with the Conception vessel below in the transformation of essence. As long as the Conception vessel is not entangled by hot qi, the fluids in the mouth are entirely transformed into essence, which [then] enters the Kidneys. However, if pathogenic heat is lodged within the lower burner, the body fluids are no longer transformed into essence but, conversely, become dampness. Dampness is the qi of earth. [Let us therefore revise this pathology]. What truly invades the water is [pathogenic] heat, or fire qi that has been generated by wood. The color of water is generally black

and that of fire is red. In the present context, where dampness and fire combine, [the resulting substance] seeks to turn red but is unable to do so, yet can also not turn back to become black. The outcome of this torment is that it produces a yellow fluid. [This fluid] is thus not the product of the transformation of water and fire, but of dampness. Thus, when previous generations [of physicians] identified yellow discharge as Spleen damp-heat and [then] only treated the Spleen, they [obviously] could not cure it completely. The reason is that they did not understand that the true water and true fire combine to produce cinnabar pathogenic qi, [also known as] primal pathogenic qi [terms indicating that pathogenic damp-heat], which harasses the area between the Conception vessel and the uterus, and transforms the [normally] dark [fluids] into a [yellow] colored [discharge]. How could one cure it by just treating the Spleen? The appropriate strategy is to tonify the deficiency of the Conception vessel and to clear the flaring of Kidney fire. Most likely [this will work].

In accordance with this interpretation, Fu Qing-Zhu uses the ingredients in this formula in a somewhat different manner than can be deduced from contemporary textbooks. He argues that both Euryales Semen *(qiàn shí)* and Dioscoreae Rhizoma *(shān yào)* tonify deficiency of the Conception vessel as well as promote water metabolism. He views Ginkgo Semen *(bái guǒ)* as guiding the formula into the Conception vessel, and Phellodendri Cortex *(huáng bǎi)* as draining excess fire from both the Kidneys and the Conception vessel.

In clinical practice, Fu's analysis is important for two reasons. First, it allows this formula to be used in women who do not have signs of Spleen deficiency, as would be required if one sees it as acting primarily on the Spleen. Second, the focus on the Conception vessel implies that inappropriate use can lead to menstrual irregularities such as delayed menstruation, reduced bleeding, or even amenorrhea.

Comparisons

➢ Vs. End Discharge Decoction *(wán dài tāng)*

Both formulas were composed by the famous Qing-dynasty gynecology expert Fu Qing-Zhu to treat patterns characterized by excessive discharge due to dampness. However, End Discharge Decoction *(wán dài tāng)* treats a white, odorless discharge caused by deficiency of the Girdle vessel accompanied by signs that indicate middle burner deficiency. By contrast, Change Yellow [Discharge] Decoction *(yì huáng tāng)* treats a yellow or dark brown discharge that is also odorless, but sticky, and is accompanied by signs of deficiency and damp-heat in the lower burner.

➢ Vs. Damp-Heat Excess Patterns without Deficiency

These patterns will be characterized by yellow discharge that may have a relatively light color or be thick like cottage cheese. In any case, these discharges tend to have an offensive odor and are usually accompanied by itching with a burning sensation. Such problems require formulas like Gentian Decoction to Drain the Liver (*lóng dǎn xiè gān tāng*), discussed in Chapter 4, or Two-Marvel Powder (*èr miào sǎn*), discussed in Chapter 16.

Biomedical Indications

With the appropriate presentation, this formula may be used to treat a variety of biomedically-defined disorders including cervicitis, cervical erosion, vaginitis, trichomoniasis, and chronic pelvic inflammatory disease.

Modifications

- For darker (almost tea-like in color) and more profuse discharge, add Sophorae flavescentis Radix (*kǔ shēn*), Coptidis Rhizoma (*huáng lián*), and Sepiae Endoconcha (*hǎi piāo xiāo*).
- For severe Spleen qi deficiency, add Astragali Radix (*huáng qí*), Ginseng Radix (*rén shēn*), and Cimicifugae Rhizoma (*shēng má*).

Alternate name

Reduce Yellow [Discharge] Decoction (*tuì huáng tāng*) in *Records of Pattern Discrimination*

Comparative Tables of Principal Formulas

■ FORMULAS THAT STABILIZE THE EXTERIOR AND STOP SWEATING

Formula Name	Diagnosis	Indications	Remarks
Oyster Shell Powder (*mǔ lì sǎn*)	Unstable protective qi and constrained heat at the level of the nutritive qi	Spontaneous sweating that worsens at night, palpitations, easily startled, shortness of breath, irritability, general debility, lethargy, a pale-red tongue, and a thin, frail pulse	Stops sweating without any tonifying actions.

■ FORMULAS THAT SECURE THE LUNGS AND STOP COUGHING

Formula Name	Diagnosis	Indications	Remarks
Nine-Immortal Powder (*jiǔ xiān sǎn*)	Lung qi and yin deficiency	Chronic, unremitting cough with wheezing, a shiny-white complexion, shortness of breath, spontaneous sweating, and a deficient, rapid pulse	Treats both the branch and root equally.

■ FORMULAS THAT BIND UP THE INTESTINES AND SECURE ABANDONED CONDITIONS

Common symptoms: long-term, persistent diarrhea, abdominal pain, pale tongue, slow pulse

Formula Name	Diagnosis	Indications	Remarks
True Man's Decoction to Nourish the Organs (*zhēn rén yǎng zàng tāng*)	Spleen and Kidney yang deficiency	Unremitting diarrhea (which may contain pus and blood), mild, persistent abdominal pain that responds favorably to local pressure or warmth, lethargy, reduced appetite, soreness of the lower back, a pale tongue with a white coating, and a slow, thin pulse	Treats both the branch and the root.
Peach Blossom Decoction (*táo huā tāng*)	Injury to the collaterals of the Intestines with Spleen and Kidney yang deficiency	Chronic dysenteric disorders with dark blood and pus in the stool, abdominal pain that responds favorably to local pressure or warmth, a pale tongue, and a pulse that is slow and frail or faint and thin	Focuses on the manifestation.
Four-Miracle Pill (*sì shén wán*)	Insufficient fire at the gate of vitality with Spleen and Kidney yang deficiency	Daybreak diarrhea (possibly with abdominal pain), poor appetite, inability to digest food, lower back soreness, cold limbs, fatigue, a pale tongue with a thin, white coating, and a submerged, slow, and forceless pulse	Also for other types of leakage due to insufficient fire at the gate of vitality.

...cont.

Formula Name	Diagnosis	Indications	Remarks
Halt the Carts Pill (*zhù chē wán*)	Long-term Intestinal damp-heat with damage to both yin and yang	Discharge of blood and pus (which may be mixed up) from the bowels that comes and goes, tenesmus, continuous abdominal pain, irritability of the chest, a red tongue with little coating, and a thin, rapid pulse	For both chronic and intermittent dysenteric disorders.
Benefit the Yellow Powder (*yì huáng sǎn*)	Spleen and Stomach deficiency with qi stagnation	Pediatric abdominal pain and distention, vomiting, unremitting diarrhea, and no desire for food	Also for childhood nutritional impairment with fatigue, yellow complexion, grossly bloated abdomen, and wasting of the body.

■ FORMULAS THAT SECURE THE ESSENCE AND STOP ENURESIS

Common symptoms: frequent urination to the point of incontinence and/or spermatorrhea, pale tongue, frail pulse

Formula Name	Diagnosis	Indications	Remarks
Metal Lock Pill to Stabilize the Essence (*jīn suǒ gù jīng wán*)	Kidney deficiency leading to instability of the gate of essence	Chronic spermatorrhea, impotence, fatigue and weakness, sore and weak limbs, lower back pain, tinnitus, a pale tongue with a white coating, and a thin, frail pulse	Also used for diarrhea while moving, profuse uterine bleeding, and urinary incontinence.
Mantis Egg-Case Powder (*sāng piāo xiāo sǎn*)	Kidney and Heart qi deficiency	Frequent urination, gray and cloudy urine, disorientation, forgetfulness, a pale tongue with a white coating, and a thin, slow, and frail pulse	Incontinence characterized by being aware of the urge to urinate, but unable to suppress it.
Restrict the Fountain Pill (*suō quán wán*)	Cold from deficiency of the Kidneys	Frequent, clear, and prolonged urination or enuresis, a pale tongue with a white coating, and a submerged, frail pulse	Usually combined with other formulas.
Cinnamon Twig Decoction plus Dragon Bone and Oyster Shell (*guì zhī jiā lóng gǔ mǔ lì tāng*)	Deficient yin and yang, with floating of deficient yang above and draining of yin essence below	Spermatorrhea (in men) or dreaming of sexual intercourse (in women), lower abdominal contraction and pain, occasionally watery diarrhea, dizziness, palpitations, insomnia and dream-disturbed sleep, loss of hair, and a hollow, slightly tight pulse	Also for a wide variety of disorders associated with nervous excitability including palpitations, sleep disturbances, and oversensitivity to external stimuli.
Fetus Longevity Pill (*shòu tāi wán*)	Kidney deficiency leading to instability of the Penetrating and Conception vessels	Lower back soreness, a sensation of collapse in the lower abdomen, vaginal bleeding during pregnancy, dizziness, tinnitus, weak legs, frequent urination, a pale tongue with a white, slippery coating, and a submerged, frail pulse at the rear position	Also commonly used to prevent problems during pregnancy in women with deficient Kidneys.

■ FORMULAS THAT SECURE IRREGULAR UTERINE BLEEDING AND STOP VAGINAL DISCHARGE

Common symptom: loss of fluids through the vagina

Formula Name	Diagnosis	Indications	Remarks
Stabilize Gushing Decoction (gù chōng tāng)	Instability of the Penetrating vessel	Uterine bleeding or profuse menstrual bleeding of thin, pale blood that gushes or continuously trickles out, palpitations, shortness of breath, a pale tongue, and a deficient, big or thin, frail pulse	Also used to treat black, tarry stools in patients with Spleen deficiency.
Stabilize the Menses Pill (gù jīng wán)	Heat in the Penetrating and Conception vessels causing blood to move recklessly	Continuous bleeding (alternating between trickling and gushing), very red blood that may contain dark-purple clots, a sensation of heat and irritability in the chest, abdominal pain, dark urine, a red tongue, and a rapid, wiry pulse	Also for vaginal discharge, dysenteric disorders, seminal emissions, and heat in the five centers.
Pregnancy Panacea (shēn líng dān)	Cold from deficiency of the Conception and Penetrating vessels with blood stasis	Continuous uterine bleeding of purplish-red or dark-purple blood with clots, pain and tenderness of the lower abdomen that diminishes with the passage of clots, a dark-purple tongue that may have purple spots, and a submerged, thin, and wiry pulse	Often used for more chronic conditions requiring treatment over a longer period of time.
End Discharge Decoction (wán dài tāng)	Spleen deficiency with dampness and Liver qi constraint	Profuse, thin, white or pale-yellow vaginal discharge, fatigue, a shiny, pale complexion, loose stools, a pale tongue with a white coating, and a soggy and frail or moderate pulse	This is deficiency of the Girdle vessel. Also for diarrhea, edema during menstruation or pregnancy, headache, and dizziness.
Change Yellow [Discharge] Decoction (yì huáng tāng)	Spleen or Kidney qi deficiency with damp-heat from constraint	Long-term, unremitting yellowish-white, viscous, and fishy-smelling vaginal discharge, pale-yellow complexion, heaviness in the head, reduced appetite, loose stools, delayed menses with pale blood, a pale tongue with a thin, white coating, and a soft, slippery pulse that may be submerged	This is damp-heat of the Conception vessel.

守神劇

Chapter 10 Contents

Formulas that Calm the Spirit

....

Formulas that Calm the Spirit

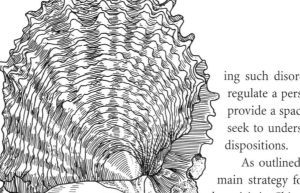

'Spirit' in Chinese medicine denotes the nonphysical aspects of a person's being. Unlike in the West, these are not seen as being separate and qualitatively different from the body. Rather, as Zhou Xue-Hai writes in *Random Notes while Reading about Medicine*: "The five spirits are the dispositions of blood and qi. Elation, anger, pondering, sadness, and fear have their foundation in the [personal] mandate of heaven. A person who does not possess these dispositions will be dull-witted, their personality dead." Disturbances of the spirit, then, are regarded as manifestations of disorders that prevent a person from living their life in a manner appropriate to who they are.

Chinese medicine offers many different ways to treat such disorders. These include changes in diet and lifestyle, emotional counter-therapy (where one excessive emotion is treated by generating other emotions, following the doctrine of the five phases), and counseling, as well as herbal medicine. Indeed, as the 17th-century physician Ye Tian-Shi noted in *Case Records as a Guide to Clinical Practice*: "Prescribing medicines draws on the function of herbs. I am afraid that these may not [be enough to] make the patient happy." Formulas that calm the spirit thus should not be confused with psychoactive drugs in the biomedical sense of the term. Nor are they substitutes for treatment that seeks to enable a person to devise autonomous strategies for overcoming difficulties in living. Nevertheless, the formulas discussed in this chapter can play an important supportive function in treat-

ing such disorders. For in seeking to regulate a person's qi and blood, they provide a space from which they may seek to understand and develop their dispositions.

As outlined by Zhou Xue-Hai, the main strategy for treating disorders of the spirit in Chinese medicine is to calm them:

The multiple transmutations of spirit disorders cannot be fathomed, and they are also the most difficult to treat [among all the various types of illness]. To do this, it is essential to know about their roots and branches. Generally speaking, for the spirit to be in charge [of its functions,] it needs to be regulated; and in order for it to be regulated, it needs to be calm.

This strategy was first described in *Basic Questions* (Chapter 74): "Calm [disorders] with palpitations and anxiety."

Like all other disorders in Chinese medicine, those of the spirit can be sorted into two major types, deficiency and excess. Here, these refer both to the branch (manifestations) and to the root. Manifestations of deficiency include palpitations with anxiety, forgetfulness, disorientation, and insomnia. Generally, such patterns are due to deficiency or constraint of qi and blood, preventing the expression of the spirit and thereby causing it to become agitated. The method of treating this type of disorder is to tonify and harmonize the qi and blood. Manifestations of excess include a feeling of being overstressed, manic behavior, bad temper, and agitation. Such patterns are due to excess heat, uncontrolled yang, blood stasis, phlegm, and severe qi stagnation. The strategy for treating this type of disturbance is to sedate and calm the spirit.

In practice, the manner in which disturbances of the spirit present clinically tends to be complex and often involves aspects of both deficiency and excess. A combination of treatment strategies is therefore utilized in most cases. Furthermore, because disturbances of the spirit occur as a result of imbalances of qi and blood, they often occur in contexts where formulas not discussed in this chapter are more appropriate. For example, yang brightness heat can cause manic behavior that should be treated by purging (Chapter 4); phlegm can veil the orifices, which should be opened (Chapter 11); rebellious qi can present with severe irritability and insomnia (Chapter12); blood stasis can lead to insanity and forgetfulness (Chapter 13); and deficiency of various types can result in palpitations, disorientation, or insomnia (Chapter 8).

Historically, the formulas in this chapter come from many different periods in the history of Chinese medicine, reflecting the different preoccupations of their authors regarding the spirit and its treatment. Han-dynasty formulas from *Discussion of Cold Damage* and *Essentials from the Golden Cabinet* generally emphasize regulating the nutritive and protective qi, be it by draining fire, harmonizing the middle burner, or enriching blood. From the Tang dynasty onward, and especially during the Jin-Yuan period, fire became a main concern of Chinese physicians, and this is reflected in their attempts to calm the spirit. A greater focus on organ systems (rather than qi and blood) led to formulas being designed to specifically treat the Heart as the organ most closely associated with both fire and the spirit. Phlegm disorders also attracted closer attention, while discussions of the ministerial fire and its interaction with the Heart or sovereign fire brought into play the relationship between the Heart and Kidneys. These trends continued throughout the Ming and into the Qing epoch. Intertwined with the emergence of warm pathogen disorders as a major concern for physicians during this time, yin deficiency was accorded great attention, and so was the Liver, which many physicians now viewed as the most important organ in treating all kinds of internal medicine disorders. From the Republican period onward, and well into post-Maoist China, concepts borrowed from Western medicine, such as neurasthenia or nervous exhaustion, became tremendously important in China and Chinese medicine. As always, these changes not only stimulated the composition of new formulas, they also influenced the interpretation and usage of existing ones. For example, the organ systems again became regarded as paramount; consequently, almost all the formulas in this chapter are currently defined as treating predominantly the Heart and the Liver.

Many of the formulas in this chapter contain metals or other heavy substances that are toxic or which readily injure the digestive system. Proper precautions must therefore be taken. Substitutes should be used for toxic substances like Cinnabaris *(zhū shā)*. For reasons of historical accuracy, we have included such substances in the listing of formula constituents and in the discussions of formula compositions. Suggestions for how these might be substituted are provided wherever appropriate. However, for the time being, such suggestions remain provisional and are open to revision by the Chinese medicine community. Heavy substances should be broken up; when used in decoctions, they are generally cooked for 30-60 minutes before adding the other ingredients.

Section 1

....

FORMULAS THAT NOURISH THE HEART (BLOOD AND YIN) AND CALM THE SPIRIT

Disturbances of the spirit due to deficiency of the qi, blood, and yin usually manifest as palpitations, irritability, and insomnia. The Heart and Liver are the organ systems most often involved in such pathologies, although the Spleen, Stomach, and Kidneys also often require attention The proper strategy is to tonify and regulate the qi, enrich the yin, and nourish the blood. Typical herbs used for this purpose are Ziziphi spinosae Semen *(suān zǎo rén)*, Platycladi Semen *(bǎi zǐ rén)*, and Polygalae Radix *(yuǎn zhì)*. These are usually combined with three other types of ingredients, depending on the precise nature of the pattern to be treated:

- Those that enrich the yin and nourish the blood more generally, such as Ophiopogonis Radix *(mài mén dōng)*, Rehmanniae Radix *(shēng dì huáng)*, Rehmanniae Radix praeparata *(shú dì huáng)*, Asini Corii Colla *(ē jiāo)*, and Lycii Fructus *(gǒu qǐ zǐ)*, where such deficiency is the root of a spirit disorder

- Those that augment the qi, such as Ginseng Radix *(rén shēn)* and Glycyrrhizae Radix *(gān cǎo)*, in order to enable the Heart to direct the qi and blood downward and thereby control the spirit

- Those that clear fire and drain heat, such as Fritillariae Bulbus *(bèi mǔ)*, Coptidis Rhizoma *(huáng lián)*, and Anemarrhenae Rhizoma *(zhī mǔ)*, when deficiency of blood and yin is accompanied by yang excess.

Note that while the formulas in this group can be taken over a longer period of time than those that settle and sedate, they are not intended to replace tranquilizers, and must also be adjusted regularly should the pattern change as the result of treatment.

天王補心丹 (天王补心丹)

Emperor of Heaven's Special Pill to Tonify the Heart

tiān wáng bǔ xīn dān

According to the Ming-dynasty physician Zhang Jie-Bin, this formula can be traced to the Daoist canon. It is said that once, when the Buddhist monk Zhi Gong was exhausted from the chanting of scriptures, he was given this formula in a dream by the Heavenly King Deng. The Qing-dynasty writer Wang Ang claims differently, that the formula was revealed by the Heavenly King to the eminent Buddhist monk Dao Xuan (596~667). Dao Xuan is famous for a visionary experience toward the end of his life in which he received instructions from the gods. Although both accounts are mythological, they refer to this formula's magical effect in treating exhaustion from too much thinking.

Source   *Fine Formulas for Women with Annotations and Commentary* (Ming dynasty, 16th century)

Rehmanniae Radix *(shēng dì huáng)* 120g
Ginseng Radix *(rén shēn)* 15g
Asparagi Radix *(tiān mén dōng)* 30g
Ophiopogonis Radix *(mài mén dōng)* 30g
Scrophulariae Radix *(xuán shēn)* 15g
Salviae miltiorrhizae Radix *(dān shēn)* 15g
Poria *(fú líng)* 15g
Polygalae Radix *(yuǎn zhì)* 15g
wine-washed Angelicae sinensis Radix *(jiǔ xǐ dāng guī)* 30g
Schisandrae Fructus *(wǔ wèi zǐ)* .30g
Platycladi Semen *(bǎi zǐ rén)* 30g
dry-fried Ziziphi spinosae Semen *(chǎo suān zǎo rén)* 30g
Platycodi Radix *(jié gěng)* 15g
Cinnabaris *(zhū shā)* 15g

Method of Preparation   Grind the ingredients into a powder and form into pills with honey. Coat the pills with Cinnabaris *(zhū shā)*. The source text advises to take 6-9g on an empty stomach with either boiled water or a decoction of Longan Arillus *(lóng yǎn ròu)*. At present, the usual dosage is 9g taken 2-3 times a day on an empty stomach with warm water. Codonopsis Radix *(dǎng shēn)* is usually substituted for Ginseng Radix *(rén shēn)* at 2-3 times its dosage. Also prepared as a decoction with an appropriate reduction in dosage. *Note:* Due to the unacceptable toxicity of Cinnabaris *(zhū shā)*, it should no longer be used. Some commercial formulations substitute Acori tatarinowii Rhizoma *(shí chāng pǔ)* or Coptidis Rhizoma *(huáng lián)*, or other heavy, settling medicinals such as Fossilia Ossis Mastodi *(lóng gǔ)* or Fossilia Dentis Mastodi *(lóng chǐ)*.

Actions   Enriches the yin, nourishes the blood, clears heat, and calms the spirit

Indications

Irritability, palpitations with anxiety, fatigue, insomnia with very restless sleep, inability to think or concentrate for even short periods of time, nocturnal emissions, forgetfulness, dry stools, a red tongue with little coating, and a thin, rapid pulse.

There may also be sores of the mouth and tongue, low-grade fever, and night sweats.

This is yin and blood deficiency leading to a restless state of mind. From an organ systems perspective, this pattern can also be viewed as Heart and Kidneys failing to properly communicate. The Heart governs the blood and stores the spirit, and its fire normally descends to meet with the Kidneys. The Kidneys store the essence and will, and Kidney water normally rises to meet with the Heart. When the Heart and Kidneys communicate harmoniously, fire and water balance each other, and the essence and Heart are sufficient. Under such circumstances, the spirit and will are calm and settled.

Basic Questions, Chapter 43, notes that "When the yin qi is quiet, the spirit is stored. When it is restless, it withers away." Excessive thinking or deliberation stirs the ministerial fire. In addition, chronic yang excess depletes the blood and yin, and deficient blood deprives the Heart of nourishment, which causes palpitations with anxiety and forgetfulness. As the yin becomes deficient, it is no longer able to balance and control the yang. This turns into fire, ascends to the Heart, and causes irritability, insomnia with very restless sleep, and an inability to think or concentrate for even short periods of time. Night sweats and nocturnal emissions occur when the spirit rushes upward and the essence is lost downward. Disorders of the Heart are manifested in the tongue; Heart fire may therefore manifest as sores in the mouth and tongue. Dry stools, a red tongue with little coating, and a thin, rapid pulse are common signs of yin and blood deficiency. The irritability, restlessness, and insomnia prevent the patient from getting enough sleep, which over time leads to fatigue.

Analysis of Formula

This formula addresses a pattern of mixed excess and deficiency based on a principle expounded in *Divine Pivot* (Chapter 71): "Tonify what is deficient and drain what is excessive, thereby regulating excess and deficiency." It primarily focuses on enriching the yin and nourishing the blood, while secondarily calming the spirit and clearing heat. The chief herb, Rehmanniae Radix *(shēng dì huáng)*, nourishes the yin and clears heat. It enriches the Kidney yin (water), which is then able to control the disturbance of the spirit due to fire. It is also effective in nourishing the blood. There are three deputies: Asparagi Radix *(tiān mén dōng)*, Ophiopogonis Radix *(mài mén dōng)*, and Scrophulariae Radix *(xuán shēn)*, all of which enrich the yin and clear heat from deficiency. In various classical texts, all of these herbs are noted for their efficacy in calming the spirit.

There are four groups of assistants. Salviae miltiorrhizae Radix *(dān shēn)* and Angelicae sinensis Radix *(dāng guī)* tonify the blood to nourish the Heart without causing stasis; Platycladi Semen *(bǎi zǐ rén)* and Polygalae Radix *(yuǎn zhì)* calm the spirit; Ginseng Radix *(rén shēn)* and Poria *(fú líng)* assist the Heart qi; and Ziziphi spinosae Semen (suān zǎo rén) and Schisandrae Fructus (wǔ wèi zǐ) prevent the leakage of Heart qi and yin fluids. Working together, these eight assistants support those functions of the Heart that have been damaged by worry, thinking, and mental exertion. The envoy is Platycodi Radix (jié gěng), which conducts the actions of the other herbs upward toward the upper burner, the abode of the spirit. Cinnabaris (zhū shā) anchors and calms the wayward spirit.

Cautions and Contraindications

Because the ingredients in this formula are cold and rich, it should be used with caution in those with a weak and deficient Spleen and Stomach.

Commentary

This formula was first listed by the influential Ming-dynasty imperial physician Xue Ji, in his revision of a Song-dynasty work on gynecology. Xue Ji may have assimilated the formula from Daoist sources or based it on formulas from Sun Si-Miao. Its original actions read:

> Makes the heart tranquil, guards the spirit, augments the blood, secures the essence, fortifies one's energy, strengthens the resolve, and causes people not to forget. It clears the three burners, transforms phlegm and saliva, dispels irritability heat, eliminates fright palpitations, treats dry throat, and fosters and nourishes the Heart spirit.

With their emphasis on clearing the three burners and promoting fluid metabolism (a function that includes the transformation of phlegm), these indications reflect that the generation of body fluids is key to the successful treatment of this disorder. In fact, the chief and deputy herbs constitute what would later become Increase the Fluids Decoction (zēng yè tāng), discussed in Chapter 15. Thus, the prominent Qing-dynasty writer Wang Ang points out that many herbs in this formula not only tonify the Heart, but also support the Lung's ability to move the blood and govern the fluids:

> Rehmanniae Radix (shēng dì huáng) and Scrophulariae Radix (xuán shēn) are herbs of the north. They tonify water in order to control fire. This is the intention for selecting them to benefit [this pattern]. Salviae miltiorrhizae Radix (dān shēn) and Angelicae sinensis Radix (dāng guī) generate Heart blood. Blood is generated by means of qi. Ginseng Radix (rén shēn) and Poria (fú líng) augment the Heart qi. Ginseng Radix (rén shēn) combined with Ophiopogonis Radix (mài mén dōng) and Schisandrae Fructus (wǔ wèi zǐ) comprise Generate the Pulse Powder (shēng mài sǎn). While the Heart governs the blood, the Lungs are the canopy of the Heart that faces the one hundred vessels. Tonifying the Lungs generates the pulse, whereby the heavenly qi is directed downward.

Expanded Usage

Later generations of physicians expanded the use of this formula from just women to all patients suffering from this pattern. Wang Ang described the pathogenesis of the symptoms associated with this disorder: "Both the essence and will of humans are stored in the Kidneys. When the essence is insufficient, the will and qi become weak and are unable to communicate above with the Heart. This leads to erratic emotions and forgetfulness." Wang also recommended that the pill be taken regularly by those who read or study a lot. Contemporary physicians—based on the passage in Basic Questions (Chapter 74) that "All painful, itchy sores concern the Heart"—use this formula in treating chronic or recurrent urticaria, chronic conjunctivitis, and mouth ulcers. Whatever the external manifestation, the following key symptoms (reflecting the damage to the yin fluids that defines the underlying pathodynamic) should be present when prescribing this formula: dry stools, a dry mouth, a red tongue with little coating, and a fine pulse.

Differences among Commentators

Commentators also raise two issues of wider interest. The first concerns the role and function of Platycodi Radix (jié gěng), which some physicians specifically link to the Heart. Dissecting the Secrets of Sustaining Life, for instance, states that this formula "uses Platycodi Radix (jié gěng) as the envoy that carries all herbs into the Heart and [thereby] prevents them from descending too quickly." Jottings from Repeated Celebration Hall notes that this herb "dissipates constraint of the Heart qi," while Comprehensive Outline of the Materia Medica indicates its use for "ulcers of the mouth and tongue, and red, swollen, and painful eyes." This use of Platycodi Radix (jié gěng) is of interest in relation to other formulas introduced in this book, such as Drive Out Stasis from the Mansion of Blood Decoction (xuè fǔ zhú yū tāng), discussed in Chapter 13.

Another topic is the mode of action whereby the formula calms the spirit. Most classical and contemporary texts refer to its action on the Heart's spirit, and some also mention that it firms the Kidneys' resolve. The Qing-dynasty writer Wang Zi-Jie took a wider view. In Selected Annotations to Ancient Formulas from the Garden of Crimson Snow, he argued that the formula acts on all aspects of the spirit stored in the five yin organs:

> Tonifying the Heart implies tonifying the Heart's function. [The Heart's function] is that it stores the [Heart] spirit. But what this spirit utilizes are the ethereal and corporeal souls, the intention, knowledge, essence, and resolve. By tonifying this function, the Heart is able to take responsibility for things. Chapter 8 of Divine Pivot states 'what comes and goes with the spirit is the ethereal soul.' Angelicae sinensis Radix (dāng guī), Platycladi Semen (bǎi zǐ rén), and Salviae miltiorrhizae Radix (dān shēn) are moving herbs that can delight the ethereal soul. 'That which the heart recalls is the intention.' Ginseng Radix (rén shēn) and Poria (fú líng) are herbs that regulate the middle [burner] and preserve the intention. 'Dealing with things by way of deliberation is called knowl-

edge.' By using Ziziphi spinosae Semen *(suān zǎo rén)*, one quiets excessive movement and [thereby] benefits knowledge. 'What comes and goes with the essence is called the corporeal soul.' Using calming herbs like Asparagi Radix *(tiān mén dōng)*, Ophiopogonis Radix *(mài mén dōng)*, and Schisandrae Fructus *(wǔ wèi zǐ)* thus calms the corporeal soul. 'What is created at conception is referred to as the essence.' Using herbs that fill the lower [burner] such as Rehmanniae Radix *(shēng dì huáng)* and Polygalae Radix *(yuǎn zhì)* settles the essence [preventing its leakage]. 'What the intention preserves is called resolve.' Using Polygalae Radix *(yuǎn zhì)* and Platycodi Radix *(jié gěng)* generates movement from stillness and [thereby] unblocks the resolve. In this manner, the yang of the spirit moves and generates intention by way of the actions of the ethereal soul. When intention connects with what is outside [of a person,] knowledge is produced. The yin of the spirit becomes quiet and produces essence by way of the actions of the corporeal soul. When essence settles in the middle burner, it generates resolve. What the spirit can accomplish is unlimited. Hence, [the name of this formula] refers to tonifying the Heart.

Comparisons

➤ Vs. Restore the Spleen Decoction *(guī pí tāng)*

Both formulas are designed for treating conditions marked by insomnia, palpitations, and forgetfulness. However, Restore the Spleen Decoction *(guī pí tāng)* is indicated for concurrent qi and blood deficiency marked by reduced appetite, loose stools, a pale tongue, and a thin, frail pulse. Emperor of Heaven's Special Pill to Tonify the Heart *(tiān wáng bǔ xīn dān)*, on the other hand, is for blood and yin deficiency with irritability, a red tongue with little coating, and a thin, rapid pulse. Both types of patient will tend to think and worry a lot. However, those with Spleen/Heart deficiency tend to have thoughts that turn around in one's mind but do not necessarily lead to action, while those with yin deficiency tend to be more agitated, resulting in much activity that is not, however, completed. Note that the symptom of loose stools by itself is not enough to differentiate these two patterns, as some patients with blood and yin deficiency will also present with loose stools. In addition, Restore the Spleen Decoction *(guī pí tāng)* can be used to treat patterns of bleeding associated with the Spleen failing to contain the blood.

➤ Vs. Prepared Licorice Decoction *(zhì gān cǎo tāng)*; see page 358.

Biomedical Indications

With the appropriate presentation, this formula may be used to treat a variety of biomedically-defined disorders including perimenopausal syndrome, chronic urticaria, apthous ulcers, cardiac disease, and nervous exhaustion. It is especially useful for patients who have taken tranquilizers or sleeping pills for so long that they have ceased to have any effect.

Modifications

- For severe palpitations and restless sleep due to blood deficiency, add Longan Arillus *(lóng yǎn ròu)* and Polygoni multiflori Caulis *(yè jiāo téng)*.

- For more severe insomnia due to floating yang, add Fossilia Dentis Mastodi *(lóng chǐ)* and Magnetitum *(cí shí)*.

- For severe dry mouth and throat, add Dendrobii Herba *(shí hú)*.

- For mouth and tongue sores, add Nelumbinis Plumula *(lián zǐ xīn)*.

- For seminal emissions or premature ejaculation, add Rosae laevigatae Fructus *(jīn yīng zǐ)*, Euryales Semen *(qiàn shí)*, and Ostreae Concha *(mǔ lì)*

- For bedwetting, enuresis, and premature ejaculation, add Mantidis Oötheca *(sāng piāo xiāo)*.

- For mouth ulcers, add Coptidis Rhizoma *(huáng lián)* and Moutan Cortex *(mǔ dān pí)*.

- For toothache, add Clear the Stomach Decoction *(qīng wèi tāng)*.

- For dizziness and vertigo, add Chuanxiong Rhizoma *(chuān xiōng)* and Angelicae dahuricae Radix *(bái zhǐ)*.

Associated Formulas

養心湯 （养心汤）

Nourish the Heart Decoction from *Comprehensive Collection*

yǎng xīn tāng

Source *Systematic Great Compendium of Medicine Past and Present* (1556)

Angelicae sinensis Radix *(dāng guī)* 9g
Rehmanniae Radix *(shēng dì huáng)* 9g
Rehmanniae Radix praeparata *(shú dì huáng)* 9g
Poriae Sclerotium pararadicis *(fú shén)* 9g
Ginseng Radix *(rén shēn)* 12g
Ophiopogonis Radix *(mài mén dōng)* 12g
Ziziphi spinosae Semen *(suān zǎo rén)* 12g
Platycladi Semen *(bǎi zǐ rén)* 6g
Glycyrrhizae Radix praeparata *(zhì gān cǎo)* 3g
Schisandrae Fructus *(wǔ wèi zǐ)* 6g

Decoct with the addition of Junci Medulla *(dēng xīn cǎo)* and Nelumbinis Semen *(lián zǐ)*. At present, Codonopsis Radix *(dǎng shēn)* is usually substituted for Ginseng Radix *(rén shēn)* at 2-3 times its dosage. Nourishes the Heart and calms the spirit. For patients with a weak constitution or debility in the wake of illness, palpitations with anxiety, insomnia, and forgetfulness. In contrast to the principal formula, this is more for deficient blood disorders without deficiency of yin fluids. This will be reflected in a wan and withered complexion, a tongue that is only slightly red and not as dry, and a pulse that is deficient and frail rather than fine. Compared to the principal formula, this one focuses more on the blood and essence and somewhat less on enriching the body fluids.

養心湯 (养心汤)

Nourish the Heart Decoction from *Indispensable Tools*

yǎng xīn tāng

SOURCE   *Indispensable Tools for Pattern Treatment* (1602)

Astragali Radix (*huáng qí*) 4.5g
Poriae Sclerotium pararadicis (*fú shén*) 4.5g
Poria (*fú líng*) 4.5g
Pinelliae massa fermentata (*bàn xià qū*) 4.5g
Angelicae sinensis Radix (*dāng guī*) 4.5g
Chuanxiong Rhizoma (*chuān xiōng*) 4.5g
ginger juice Polygalae Radix (*jiāng zhī yuǎn zhì*) 3g
dry-fried Ziziphi spinosae Semen (*suān zǎo rén*) 3g
Cinnamomi Cortex (*ròu guì*) 3g
Platycladi Semen (*bǎi zǐ rén*) 3g
Schisandrae Fructus (*wǔ wèi zǐ*) 3g
Ginseng Radix (*rén shēn*) 3g
Glycyrrhizae Radix praeparata (*zhì gān cǎo*) 1.5g

Decoct with the addition of 5 slices of Zingiberis Rhizoma recens (*shēng jiāng*) and 2 pieces of Jujubae Fructus (*dà zǎo*), beginning with approximately a half-liter (about 2.1 cups) of water and cooking until half that amount of liquid remains. Preferably taken before meals. Augments the qi, tonifies and harmonizes the blood, nourishes the Heart and calms the spirit, and transforms phlegm. For the treatment of Heart blood deficiency with disquiet, apprehensiveness, being easily frightened, anxiety, palpitations, insomnia, and dream-disturbed sleep. In contrast to the principal formula, this also acts to transform phlegm, and the majority (but by no means unanimous) opinion is that this formula is more for deficient blood disorders without yin deficiency.

This formula also appeared in *Fine Formulas for Women with Annotations and Commentary* and was subsequently recorded in other well-known texts including *Women's Diseases According to Fu Qing-Zhu* and *Essential Teachings of [Zhu] Dan-Xi*.

柏子養心湯 (柏子养心汤)

Arborvitae Seed Pill to Nourish the Heart

bǎi zǐ yǎng xīn wán

SOURCE   *Compilation of Materials of Benevolence for the Body* (1549)

Platycladi Semen (*bǎi zǐ rén*) 120g
Lycii Fructus (*gǒu qǐ zǐ*) 90g
Ophiopogonis Radix (*mài mén dōng*) 30g
Angelicae sinensis Radix (*dāng guī*) 30g
Acori tatarinowii Rhizoma (*shí chāng pǔ*) 30g
Poriae Sclerotium pararadicis (*fú shén*) 30g
Scrophulariae Radix (*xuán shēn*) 60g
Rehmanniae Radix praeparata (*shú dì huáng*) 60g
Glycyrrhizae Radix (*gān cǎo*) .15g

Grind the ingredients into a powder and form into small pills with honey. Nourishes the Heart, calms the spirit, and tonifies the Kidney yin. For disorientation, severe, continuous palpitations, dream-disturbed sleep, forgetfulness, and night sweats due to disharmony between the Heart and Kidneys. In contrast to the principal formula, this focuses more on moistening and nourishing the blood and less on clearing heat from deficiency. Platycladi Semen (*bǎi zǐ rén*), the

chief herb in this formula, is particularly indicated for the treatment of palpitations. As noted in *Transforming the Significance of Medicinal Substances*:

> Its fragrant qi vents the Heart, its moist body enriches the blood. Combined with Poriae Sclerotium pararadicis (*fú shén*), Ziziphi spinosae Semen (*suān zǎo rén*), Rehmanniae Radix (*shēng dì huáng*), and Ophiopogonis Radix (*mài mén dōng*), it is a substance that clears even though it is turbid. It focuses on the treatment of deficiency timidity of the Heart spirit, fright palpitations and panicky throbbing, a wan and withered complexion, dandruff, and itchy skin. All of these [effects are due] to its ability to nourish the blood.

酸棗仁湯 (酸枣仁汤)

Sour Jujube Decoction

suān zǎo rén tāng

Source   *Essentials from the Golden Cabinet* (c. 220)

Ziziphi spinosae Semen (*suān zǎo rén*) 12-18g
Poria (*fú líng*) 6g
Anemarrhenae Rhizoma (*zhī mǔ*) 6g
Chuanxiong Rhizoma (*chuān xiōng*) 6g
Glycyrrhizae Radix (*gān cǎo*) .3g

Method of Preparation   Decoction. The source text advises to decoct Ziziphi spinosae Semen (*suān zǎo rén*) first. This is no longer commonly done, although some physicians, like the contemporary classical formula expert Huang Huang, think that the original mode of preparation can significantly increase the efficacy of the formula. In any case, the seeds should be crushed before decoction in order to facilitate extraction of the active ingredients.

Actions   Nourishes the blood, calms the spirit, clears heat, and eliminates irritability

Indications

Irritability, inability to sleep, palpitations, night sweats, dizziness and vertigo, dry throat and mouth, a dry tongue, and a wiry or thin, rapid pulse.

The patterns treated by this formula belong to disease categories known in the literature as deficiency overwork (虛勞 *xū láo*) and deficiency irritability (虛煩 *xū fán*). If the former refers to possible etiologies, the latter emphasizes symptomatology and pathodynamic. The specific conjunction of both denotes the conditions for which this formula is most appropriate. Deficiency irritability refers to a subjective sensation of irritability although the surface of the body does not feel hot. Other symptoms include lightheadedness, pain in the head and eyes, a dry mouth and throat without thirst, and insomnia with a clear mind when the patient lies in bed. All of these symptoms indicate the presence of heat and thus of excess. However, unlike cases of irritability defined as excess, the heat has not taken on any form by way of causing fluids or substances such as phlegm or stools to congeal. Such a disorder often occurs in the wake of overwork, exhaustion, old age, or illness, hence the name 'deficiency overwork.' In the present pattern, it is the result of Liver deficiency reflected in blood deficiency, constraint, and internal fire.

The Liver stores the blood and carries the ministerial fire. When the Liver is deficient, it leads to blood deficiency and stasis. This can manifest as a failure in its function to store the spirit and regulate the coming and going of the ethereal soul. This causes inability to sleep along with palpitations. Inability to sleep is more serious than simple insomnia and is characterized by both failure to fall asleep and early waking. This lack of nourishment is accompanied by fire from constraint, which moves upward into the chest and disturbs the Heart, thereby exacerbating the symptoms. Pathogenic fire in combination with blood deficiency causes night sweats, a dry mouth and throat, and a dry tongue. However, because the body does not feel hot, deficiency irritability cannot be explained by pathogenic heat alone. Rather, it is the subjective experience of constraint reflecting the disorganized qi distribution within the Triple Burner resulting from Liver deficiency. Moreover, the deficient Liver cannot restrain the yang, which rises and manifests as dizziness and vertigo. The wiry or thin, rapid pulse is typical of Liver blood deficiency with constraint and internal fire.

Analysis of Formula

The type of deficiency irritability treated by this formula is a complex pattern combining Liver deficiency with blood stasis, qi constraint, and pathogenic fire. Accordingly, this formula utilizes a strategy of tonifying the Liver, particularly the Liver blood, invigorating the blood, clearing the heat, and promoting water metabolism. The chief ingredient, sweet, sour, and bland Ziziphi spinosae Semen *(suān zǎo rén)*, nourishes the Liver while calming the spirit. According to *Miscellaneous Records of Famous Physicians,* this herb "focuses on Heart irritability with inability to sleep ... deficiency sweating, and irritability with thirst. It tonifies the middle [burner] and augments the Liver qi." In *Renewed Materia Medica,* the early 19th-century writer Ye Gui noted that it "calms the Liver to regulate the qi, moistens the Liver to nourish the yin, warms the middle to facilitate water metabolism, restrains the qi to stop sweating, strengthens the resolve to settle angry outbursts, enhances the hearing and brightens the eyes." This complex set of actions matches up well with the pathodynamic of this condition.

The deputy is acrid, warming, and aromatic Chuanxiong Rhizoma *(chuān xiōng)*, which regulates the Liver blood by encouraging it to flow freely, calming the spirit by providing them with their natural abode. This may seem odd at first because normally we think of the spirit's abode as being disturbed by too much activity. The analogy often used is that of a fish (the spirit) becoming restless when the temperature of the water (its abode) rises. However, the fish will also become restless if the water becomes too turbid or too stagnant, requiring the use of an opening or unblocking rather than a cooling or calming strategy. This ingredient also has a complex of actions within the Liver system, as summarized in *Comprehensive Outline of the Materia Medica*: "This is an herb [for treating] the qi within the blood. When the Liver suffers from hypertonicity (急 jí), use acrid [herbs] to tonify it. Hence, it is appropriate for cases of blood deficiency. Acrid [herbs] are used for dispersion. Hence, it is [also] appropriate for cases of constraint." The combination of one astringent and one dispersing herb is very effective in nourishing and regulating the Liver while calming the spirit.

The assistant herbs are sweet and bland Poria *(fú líng)*, which calms the spirit and tonifies the Spleen and Stomach, along with bitter, sweet, and cooling Anemarrhenae Rhizoma *(zhī mǔ)*, which drains heat to preserve the yin and thus, by protecting the Stomach from dryness, indirectly enriches the fluids. Like most of the other herbs in this formula, the envoy, Glycyrrhizae Radix *(gān cǎo)*, also fulfills several different functions at once. First, complementing the action of Poria *(fú líng)*, it tonifies the middle burner and augments the qi to ensure the harmonious dispersion of qi and blood. Second, as a sweet substance, it relaxes hypertonicity of the Liver. When used together with an herb like Ziziphi spinosae Semen *(suān zǎo rén)*, it follows the principle of combining "sour and sweet [flavors] to transform [the effect of a formula] toward [the generation or protection of] yin." Third, it regulates the actions of the other herbs and harmonizes the middle burner.

Cautions and Contraindications
Use with caution in cases with loose stools.

Commentary

Important Considerations when Treating Insomnia

Sleep is not a passive state of complete stillness, but, like any other physiological activity, is a process. *Divine Pivot* (Chapter 71) elaborates:

> During the day, the protective qi moves through the yang [aspects]. At night, it moves through the yin. If the protective qi only moves through the yang [because it is] unable to enter into the yin, the yin will be deficient and the eyes will not be able to close.

Yin deficiency, in this context, does not denote a lack of yin substance but rather an insufficient penetration of nutritive yin by the protective yang. This can result from many different types of disharmony. One of these is yin or blood deficiency characterized by an inability of the yin to anchor the yang. But there are many others. These include phlegm obstructing the Triple Burner (one of the hinges between the yin and yang, the nutritive and protective qi); disruption of the downward-directing function of the Stomach qi, which prevents the yang from entering into the yin; blood stasis in the collaterals, which prevents the protective yang from entering into the nutritive yin; exuberant heat causing the yang to become hyperactive and the yin to become insufficient; or even yang deficiency with cold in the nutritive aspect repelling the protective yang and causing it to float to the surface. In treating insomnia, it is therefore of the utmost importance to ensure not only that the yin fluids and blood are sufficient, but that their penetration by the protective yang is not obstructed. For this reason, herbs such as Chuanxiong Rhizoma (*chuān xiōng*), Aconiti Radix lateralis praeparata (*zhì fù zǐ*), Cinnamomi Cortex (*ròu guì*), or Pinelliae Rhizoma praeparatum (*zhì bàn xià*), all of which facilitate the movement of nutritive qi, are thus frequently added to prescriptions that nourish the blood, enrich the fluids, or drain heat.

The present formula is no exception. Although the chief ingredient focuses on nourishing the blood and calming the spirit, it does contain, in Chuanxiong Rhizoma (*chuān xiōng*) and Poria (*fú líng*), two herbs that invigorate the blood, move the qi, and promote fluid metabolism. In *Expounding on the [Essentials from] the Golden Cabinet*, the contemporary physician Jin Shou-Shan explained their contribution to the effectiveness of this formula:

> The true marvel of this formula lies [in its use] of the two herbs Poria (*fú líng*) and Chuanxiong Rhizoma (*chuān xiōng*). When overabundant yang caused by yin deficiency stews the fluids into phlegm, such phlegm will obstruct the middle [burner causing] Gallbladder qi to be agitated. This is one of the causes whereby irritability and insomnia are produced. Poria (*fú líng*) dispels phlegm without being dry. Chuanxiong Rhizoma (*chuān xiōng*) soothes the qi of the Liver and Gallbladder. When dry phlegm is completely transformed, the Gallbladder qi can also be soothed. The yin fluids will be filled [again,] and the irritability heat will then be resolved.

Other commentators, like the Qing-dynasty writer Xu Bin, author of *Discussion and Annotation of the Essentials from the Golden Cabinet*, identified constraint as a key factor in the pathogenesis of the pattern treated by Sour Jujube Decoction (*suān zǎo rén tāng*):

> Insomnia [here] is due to fire along with the [flow of] qi, which also becomes unsmooth, and this, going over its bounds, encroaches on the Heart. Overabundance of Heart fire thus truly arises from Liver qi constraint, which prevents the ethereal soul from being calm. [It is because of such constraint] that wood can generate fire.

Because constraint can manifest in underactivity as well as in overactivity, this formula should be viewed as regulatory in nature rather than tranquilizing or sedative. It has thus been used by Kampo physicians in Japan to treat cases of hypersomnia. Another application is its use in treating insomnia associated with mild pain, or even for the treatment of pain itself, such as trigeminal neuralgia, angina pectoris, migraine,

and other types of headache. The formula's indication for these conditions again arises from its conjunction of acrid opening (which opens the stagnation that causes pain), cooling (particularly useful where pain is due to or accompanied by inflammation), and calming of the spirit.

Effects on the Liver

Rather than just treating blood deficiency, Sour Jujube Decoction (*suān zǎo rén tāng*) thus adjusts many different aspects of Liver function. It tonifies and invigorates the Liver blood, smoothes the qi while also constraining excessive dispersion, promotes water metabolism to remove obstructions from the Triple Burner, and clears heat from constraint. Unlike formulas such as Rambling Powder (*xiāo yáo sǎn*), which focus on the qi even as they also tonify the Liver blood, Sour Jujube Decoction (*suān zǎo rén tāng*) focuses on the blood and fluids and thereby also succeeds in harmonizing the qi. The pattern it treats often arises in the wake of an illness or exhaustion from overwork. Although there is some depletion of blood and essence, this is not yet severe, and the disorder is functional rather than organic, involving both excess and deficiency. Typically, therefore, patients will find it difficult to sleep even though they are tired or even exhausted. Insomnia, furthermore, will be accompanied by signs of restlessness, irritability, nervousness and impatience, as well as night sweats, palpitations, and thirst.

Because of its ability to harmonize and regulate Liver function, Sour Jujube Decoction (*suān zǎo rén tāng*) has been used as a model around which formulas to tonify the Liver have been built. For example, the contemporary physician Chen Chao-Zu recommends four types of modification, all of which focus on the movement of qi and blood:

- For patterns with more severe dryness, reduce the dosage of Chuanxiong Rhizoma (*chuān xiōng*) and add Rehmanniae Radix (*shēng dì huáng*), Ophiopogonis Radix (*mài mén dōng*), and Scrophulariae Radix (*xuán shēn*).
- For blood stasis, add Angelicae sinensis Radix (*dāng guī*), Paeoniae Radix rubra (*chì sháo*), and Persicae Semen (*táo rén*);
- For dampness causing qi stagnation, add Pinelliae Rhizoma praeparatum (*zhì bàn xià*), Polygalae Radix (*yuǎn zhì*), and Acori tatarinowii Rhizoma (*shí chāng pǔ*).
- For more pronounced heat, add Gardeniae Fructus (*zhī zǐ*), Sojae Semen praeparatum (*dàn dòu chǐ*), and Gypsum fibrosum (*shí gāo*).

Questions Regarding Dosage, Preparation, and Modifications

As with many classical formulas, some physicians increase the dosage of individual ingredients far beyond the amount indicated in contemporary textbooks. The literature contains many cases where a dosage of up to 80g of the main herb Ziziphi spinosae Semen *(suān zǎo rén)* has been used, and an occasional case with a dosage as high as 200g. While some physicians argue that the herb should be used fresh because it is then thought to be cooling, others prefer to use the prepared (dry-fried) variety, which is warming and binding. In practice, one can select the mode of preparation that best meets the requirements of a given case. It is also important to note that because of its regulatory and unblocking functions, this formula can be modified in many different ways by adding either warming, opening, cooling, or binding herbs. The Tang-dynasty physician Sun Si-Miao, for instance, added Zingiberis Rhizoma *(gān jiāng)* and Ophiopogonis Radix *(mài mén dōng)* to treat insomnia and irritability following purgation or vomiting. For other examples, see MODIFICA- TIONS below. It is also possible to combine this formula with others that open constraint or regulate the qi, such as Pinellia and Magnolia Bark Decoction *(bàn xià hòu pò tāng)*, Minor Bupleurum Decoction *(xiǎo chái hú tāng)*, or Warm Gallbladder Decoction *(wēn dǎn tāng)*.

Comparisons

➤ Vs. RESTORE THE SPLEEN DECOCTION *(guī pí tāng)*

Both formulas can be used for treating conditions marked by insomnia, palpitations, and irritability. However, Restore the Spleen Decoction *(guī pí tāng)* focuses on tonifying the Heart and Spleen by strengthening the functions of the middle burner in order to generate blood. When blood is sufficient, the Heart is nourished and the spirit is calmed. For this reason, it is most appropriate for treating patterns where insomnia is accompanied by symptoms of middle burner qi and blood deficiency such as fatigue, particularly after eating, loose stools, bloating, forgetfulness, and palpitations. While Sour Jujube Decoction *(suān zǎo rén tāng)* also has blood-tonifying properties, these are rather mild. Its strength lies in harmonizing the Liver qi and blood when that organ has become debilitated through illness or overwork. It is thus particularly suitable for insomnia accompanied by fatigue, irritability, and impatience, as well as excessive sweating.

➤ Vs. SETTLE THE EMOTIONS PILL *(dìng zhì wán)*; SEE PAGE 467.

➤ Vs. COPTIS AND ASS-HIDE GELATIN DECOCTION *(huáng lián ē jiāo tāng)*; SEE PAGE 470.

➤ Vs. LICORICE, WHEAT, AND JUJUBE DECOCTION *(gān mài dà zǎo tāng)*; SEE PAGE 473.

Biomedical Indications

With the appropriate presentation, this formula may be used to treat a wide variety of biomedically-defined disorders. These can be divided into the following groups:

- Disorders marked primarily by an increase in sympathetic tone or other neurological imbalances such as insomnia, hypersomnia, sleep walking, nervous exhaustion, paroxysmal tachycardia, hypertension, perimenopausal syndrome, general anxiety disorder, depression, schizophrenia, and hepatolenticular degeneration
- Disorders marked by pain, including trigeminal neuralgia, migraine, and angina pectoris

This formula has also been used for chronic hepatitis.

Modifications

- For deficient Heart and Gallbladder qi manifesting as dream-disturbed sleep, waking up at night terrified, palpitations, a pale tongue body, and a wiry, thin pulse, add Codonopsis Radix *(dǎng shēn)* and Fossilia Ossis Mastodi *(lóng gǔ)*.
- For night sweats, add Ostreae Concha *(mǔ lì)* and Schisandrae Fructus *(wǔ wèi zǐ)*.
- For more pronounced irritability and heat, add Gardeniae Fructus *(zhī zǐ)* and Forsythiae Fructus *(lián qiáo)*.
- For severe fire from deficiency, remove Chuanxiong Rhizoma *(chuān xiōng)* and add Ecliptae Herba *(mò hàn lián)*, Ligustri lucidi Fructus *(nǚ zhēn zǐ)*, and Paeoniae Radix alba *(bái sháo)*.
- For night sweats due to constraint, add Mori Folium *(sāng yè)*, Moutan Cortex *(mǔ dān pí)*, Talcum *(huá shí)*, and Ostreae Concha *(mǔ lì)*.
- For dizziness due to more pronounced phlegm-dampness, add Pinelliae Rhizoma *(bàn xià)* and Bambusae Caulis in taeniam *(zhú rú)*.
- For qi deficiency, add Ginseng Radix *(rén shēn)*, Ophiopogonis Radix *(mài mén dōng)*, and Schisandrae Fructus *(wǔ wèi zǐ)*.
- For insomnia associated with pain, add Paeoniae Radix *(sháo yào)* and Angelicae sinensis Radix *(dāng guī)*.

定志丸
Settle the Emotions Pill
dìng zhì wán

The name of this formula is literally 'settle the resolve.' Here the word *zhì* refers to all the emotions that are ultimately governed by the Heart.

Source   *Important Formulas Worth a Thousand Gold Pieces* (650)

Ginseng Radix *(rén shēn)* 90g
Poria *(fú líng)* 90g
Acori tatarinowii Rhizoma *(shí chāng pǔ)* 60g
Polygalae Radix *(yuǎn zhì)* 60g

Method of Preparation   The source text advises to grind the ingredients into a powder and form into small pills with honey, taking 6g three times a day. At present, it is usually prepared as a decoction with approximately 10 percent of the dosage specified above. Codonopsis Radix *(dǎng shēn)* is usually substituted for Ginseng Radix *(rén shēn)* at 2-3 times its dosage.

Actions   Tonifies the Heart qi, strengthens the resolve, and calms the spirit

Indications

Feeling apprehensive, easily frightened, worried, disheartened, or incessant laughter and glee, together with fright palpitations and forgetfulness. Dizziness and a pale tongue with a white tongue coating may be other manifestations of this pattern.

This is Heart qi deficiency and constraint caused by phlegm turbidity. The Heart qi has the task of focusing the spirit. Deficiency of Heart qi is characterized by apprehensiveness, indicating a subjective awareness of one's inability to carry out a task. Such patients find it difficult to cope with change, and their spirits easily become disoriented. This results in a state of anxiety or being easily frightened, as well as palpitations. If the Heart spirit fails to focus on the tasks at hand, it cannot convert experience into memory, leading to forgetfulness. This may manifest as forgetting names or events, mixing up words, speaking words in the wrong order, or simply finding it difficult to commit anything to memory. Other signs of qi deficiency include being disheartened or worried, or lacking in drive. In severe cases, the spirit loses its moorings such that it is no longer rooted in the will. This is due to the Heart being unable to carry out its task of directing fire downward. Under these circumstances, joy, which is the emotion associated with the Heart, is no longer controlled, leading to incessant laughter and giddiness. Dizziness and a white tongue coating reflect phlegm turbidity, while a pale tongue reflects qi deficiency.

Analysis of Formula

Qi deficiency invariably is accompanied by some qi stagnation. This formula therefore combines the strategy of tonifying with that of moving the qi. The Heart governs the blood vessels. The qi moving in the blood vessels is the nutritive qi. Dampness and phlegm arise upon stagnation of nutritive qi. Thus, the formula focuses on the nutritive qi and combines the elimination of dampness and transformation of phlegm with the regulation of qi.

Deficient qi is the root of this disorder. Accordingly, the chief herb is sweet, slightly bitter, and slightly warming Ginseng Radix *(rén shēn)*. This herb powerfully tonifies the primal qi of all five yin organs, while also benefiting the Heart qi and calming the spirit. The *Divine Husbandman's Classic of the Materia Medica* notes that "it governs tonification of

the five yin organs, quiets the consciousness, settles the ethereal and corporeal souls, arrests palpitations with anxiety, expels pathogenic qi, brightens the eyes, opens the Heart, and strengthens the resolve." These actions are complemented by those of the deputy, bland and neutral Poria *(fú líng)*, which quiets the Heart and calms the spirit. It is specifically indicated for palpitations, insomnia, or forgetfulness due to Heart insufficiency or internal obstruction of turbid phlegm. Together, these two herbs focus on the Heart to tonify its qi, promoting the elimination of dampness and, via the fluid-enriching action of Ginseng Radix *(rén shēn)*, ensure that the physiological fluids are not damaged.

The assistants are acrid, slightly warming, and drying Polygalae Radix *(yuǎn zhì)* and acrid, bitter, aromatic, and slightly warming Acori tatarinowii Rhizoma *(shí chāng pǔ)*. The former disseminates, drains, unblocks, and thrusts outward (to assist in the free movement of the Heart qi), opens constraint, and guides the Kidney qi upward to reach the Heart, thereby reestablishing harmonious communication between the Heart and Kidneys. The latter opens the orifices, dislodges phlegm, removes filth, and quiets the spirit. These two herbs are often used in combination, relying on their acrid quality to disperse constraint and their bitter quality to drain and direct downward, thereby transforming phlegm and opening the orifices.

Cautions and Contraindications

This formula is acrid and warming and thus should not be used without modification to treat patterns involving deficiency of blood or yin.

Commentary

This is the most famous of a family of formulas for treating phlegm obstructing the qi transformation of the Heart and is built around the synergistic pairing of Polygalae Radix *(yuǎn zhì)* and Acori tatarinowii Rhizoma *(shí chāng pǔ)*, first attributed to the Tang-dynasty physician Sun Si-Miao. Its origins go back further to a formula named Small Pills to Settle the Emotions (定志小丸 *dìng zhì xiǎo wán*), composed of the same ingredients but with slightly different dosages, attributed to the Daoist scholar Chen Ming in *Arcane Essentials from the Imperial Library*. Like the present formula, its indications extended from mild patterns of unsettled Heart qi to attacks of mania and dizziness. Quoted almost verbatim, or with some further elucidation, these indications have been repeated down through the ages. Here is a representative example from the late-Ming-dynasty writer Fu Ren-Xu in *Scrutiny of the Precious Jade Case*:

> [This formula treats] insufficiency of the five yin organs [manifesting as] absentmindedness, fright palpitations, sadness and sorrow, [being prone to] errors and forgetfulness, frightful or dream-disturbed sleep, being filled with dread such that one is unable to be calm, [as well as] emotional outbursts at any time.

The pathodynamic underlying this presentation is helpfully explained in *Comprehensive Medicine According to Master Zhang:*

> Palpitations are what is referred to as panicky throbbing, which is anxious pulsations below the Heart with a swooshing beat and intense panic and throbbing. These are not caused by being startled, but constitute a spontaneous stirring of the Heart that cannot be calmed and so are called palpitations. When there is Heart deficiency with water stoppage, then [the water will] seep into the chest. Heart fire abhors water that is upwardly encroaching, so that it cannot calm down by itself [anymore].

Modern Issues

In contemporary Chinese medical practice, this formula and its variations are often prescribed for anxiety and insomnia due to Gallbladder and Heart deficiency. However, by emphasizing deficiency, this interpretation does not fully take into account the phlegm turbidity that is such an important aspect of the underlying pathodynamic. This has led to use of the formula in the treatment of epileptic disorders. In clinical practice, the relative dosage of the qi-tonifying herbs Ginseng Radix *(rén shēn)* and Poria *(fú líng)*, along with that of Polygalae Radix *(yuǎn zhì)* and Acori tatarinowii Rhizoma *(shí chāng pǔ),* which open the Heart orifices and disperse stagnation, can be adjusted depending on whether qi deficiency or damp-phlegm excess are, respectively, root or branch.

Another common indication of this formula is nearsightedness, as explained by Zhang Bin-Cheng in *Convenient Reader of Established Formulas:*

> [This formula] treats [conditions] where the eyes can perceive [things that] are close but not those that are far away. [The Song-dynasty physician] Wang Hai-Cang [i.e., Wang Hao-Gu] said: The ability of the eyes to see [what is] close depends on their having water. Their ability to see [what is] distant depends on their having fire. If one cannot see [what is] distant, this is due to lack of fire. The appropriate strategy is to tonify the Heart. The Heart is the minister governing the entire body. It is the abode of the primal qi. Even though the eyes are the orifices of the Liver, the Heart, too, attaches itself to the eyes. How is this? When the eyes perceive the characteristic quality [of something] and judge it to be good or bad, this [type of] complete knowing comes from the Heart. Therefore, when the Heart lacks the power to perceive distant [things], how can one cure this by way of a strategy [aimed at] enriching water and softening the Liver?

Comparison

➢ Vs. SOUR JUJUBE DECOCTION *(suān zǎo rén tāng)*

Both formulas treat insomnia and anxiety associated with patterns of deficiency. However, Sour Jujube Decoction *(suān zǎo rén tāng)* focuses on Liver blood deficiency with qi con-

straint, while Settle the Emotions Pill *(dìng zhì wán)* focuses on Heart qi deficiency with stagnation due to phlegm turbidity. For this reason, Sour Jujube Decoction *(suān zǎo rén tāng)* is appropriate for patterns characterized by irritability and restlessness accompanied by heat, sweating, and signs of dryness. Settle the Emotions Pill *(dìng zhì wán),* on the other hand, is indicated for patterns characterized by anxiety, confusion, forgetfulness, and an inability to concentrate.

Biomedical Indications

With the appropriate presentation, this formula may be used to treat a variety of biomedically-defined disorders including general anxiety disorder and obsessive-compulsive disorders, myopia, and seizures.

Modifications

- For severe palpitations, add Fossilia Ossis Mastodi *(lóng gǔ)* and Succinum *(hǔ pò).*
- For upward rebellion of phlegm, add Pinelliae Rhizoma praeparatum *(zhì bàn xià)* and Bambusae Succus *(zhú lì).*
- For Heart blood deficiency, add Angelicae sinensis Radix *(dāng guī)*, Ziziphi spinosae Semen *(suān zǎo rén),* and Longan Arillus *(lóng yǎn ròu).*

Variations

定志丸

Settle the Emotions Pill from the Yang family
dìng zhì wán

SOURCE   *Yang Family Formulas* (1178)

Add Fossilia Dentis Mastodi *(lóng chǐ)*, Ziziphi spinosae Semen *(suān zǎo rén)*, Ferri Frusta *(shēng tiě luò)*, Ophiopogonis Radix *(mài mén dōng)*, and Cinnabaris *(zhū shā)*, Olibanum *(rǔ xiāng)*, Moschus *(shè xiāng)*, and Succinum *(hǔ pò)* and decoct with juice extracted from Rehmanniae Radix *(shēng dì huáng)* for more severe fright palpitations, disorientation, restlessness and insomnia. The source text recommends it for "all (types of) Heart diseases." When used today, modifications should be made to reflect the cost and toxicity of some of these ingredients, particularly Cinnabaris *(zhū shā)*, which must be replaced.

定志丸

Settle the Emotions Pill from *Wondrous Lantern*
dìng zhì wán

SOURCE   *Wondrous Lantern for Peering into the Origin and Development of Miscellaneous Diseases* (1773)

Add Poriae Sclerotium pararadicis *(fú shén)*, Atractylodis macrocephalae Rhizoma *(bái zhú)*, Ophiopogonis Radix *(mài mén dōng)*, and Cinnabaris *(zhū shā)* for more severe restlessness and insomnia. Cinnabaris *(zhū shā)* is no longer used, due to its unacceptable toxicity.

Associated Formulas

琥珀多寐丸
Succinum Pill for Promoting Sleep
hǔ pò duō mèi wán

SOURCE *Systematic Great Compendium of Medicine Past and Present* (1556)

Succinum (*hǔ pò*)
Saigae tataricae Cornu (*líng yáng jiǎo*)
Ginseng Radix (*rén shēn*)
Poriae Sclerotium pararadicis (*fú shén*)
Polygalae Radix (*yuǎn zhì*)
Glycyrrhizae Radix (*gān cǎo*)

The source text advises to grind equal amounts of the six herbs into a fine powder and make into pills with honey and pig's blood. The pills are then coated with gold foil and taken with a decoction prepared from Junci Medulla (*dēng xīn cǎo*). At present, the pig's blood and gold foil are omitted, and usually Naemorhedi Cornu (*shān yáng jiǎo*) is substituted for Saigae tataricae Cornu (*líng yáng jiǎo*). Calms the Heart, quiets the spirit, clears heat, and extinguishes fire. For Liver yang harassing the Heart characterized by forgetfulness, disorientation, insomnia, fright palpitations, or panicky throbbing. In contrast to the principal formula, this one treats patterns where hyperactive Liver yang harasses the Heart, leading to a breakdown in its qi transformation. Succinum (*hǔ pò*) specifically enters the blood level to transform stasis and settle the ethereal and corporeal souls, while Naemorhedi Cornu (*shān yáng jiǎo*) or Saigae tataricae Cornu (*líng yáng jiǎo*) clears Liver fire and extinguishes wind from hyperactive yang, allowing this formula to treat both the root and branches of the pattern.

龍齒清魂散 （龙齿清魂散）
Dragon Tooth Powder to Clear the Ethereal Soul
lóng chǐ qīng hún sǎn

SOURCE *Comprehensive Medicine According to Master Zhang* (1695)

Fossilia Dentis Mastodi (*lóng chǐ*) 15g
Poriae Sclerotium pararadicis (*fú shén*) 10g
Polygalae Radix (*yuǎn zhì*) 15g
Ginseng Radix (*rén shēn*) 15g
Angelicae sinensis Radix (*dāng guī*) 15g
Ophiopogonis Radix (*mài mén dōng*) 10g
Cinnamomi Cortex (*ròu guì*) 10g
Glycyrrhizae Radix praeparata (*zhì gān cǎo*) 10g
Corydalis Rhizoma (*yán hú suǒ*) 30g
Asari Radix et Rhizoma (*xì xīn*) 5g

Grind the herbs into a fine powder and take 10-15g twice daily with a decoction made from Zingiberis Rhizoma recens (*shēng jiāng*) and Jujubae Fructus (*dà zǎo*). Tonifies the Heart, calms the spirit, invigorates the blood, and moves stasis. For Heart qi deficiency accompanied by blood stasis manifesting with palpitations, restlessness, laughing and crying uncontrollably, a lusterless complexion, a dark tongue body, and a deficient, rough pulse. This pattern is said to occur in women following birth, when the qi and blood are naturally weakened. In contrast to Succinum Pill for Promoting Sleep (*hǔ pò duō mèi wán*), this formula is indicated for patterns of blood stasis

due to cold in the lower burner, while the latter formula treats hyperactive Liver yang (which is invariably associated with heat) invading the Heart and causing its blood to become static.

孔子枕中丹
Special Pill from Confucius' Pillow
Kǒng zi zhěn zhōng dān

SOURCE *Important Formulas Worth a Thousand Gold Pieces* (650)

Testudinis Plastrum (*guī bǎn*)
Acori tatarinowii Rhizoma (*shí chāng pǔ*)
Polygalae Radix (*yuǎn zhì*)
Fossilia Ossis Mastodi (*lóng gǔ*)

Grind equal amounts of the ingredients into a powder and take 3g twice daily after meals with hot water or yellow rice or millet wine. If the herbs are made into pills by mixing the powder with honey, the dosage is increased to 6g twice daily. Opens the Heart, augments the intelligence, and calms the spirit. For lack of interaction between the Heart and Kidneys and phlegm-fire harassing the interior, characterized by forgetfulness and insomnia. In contrast to the principal formula, which focuses on unblocking stagnation of the Heart qi caused by phlegm turbidity, this formula clears heat from deficiency and directs fire downward, thereby regulating the qi and transforming the phlegm. Testudinis Plastrum (*guī bǎn*) tonifies yin essence without being cloying, while Fossilia Ossis Mastodi (*lóng gǔ*) directs fire downward without being drying. This formula is therefore particularly suitable for treating patterns characterized by yin deficiency and phlegm, where both sweet, tonifying herbs such as Rehmanniae Radix praeparata (*shú dì huáng*) and bitter, cooling herbs such as Coptidis Rhizoma (*huáng lián*) would be contraindicated. The source text notes that, taken long-term, this formula can improve the clarity of one's understanding, while *Medical Formulas Collected and Analyzed* adds that it improves one's memory. If the Heart fire is cleared and the phlegm transformed, one's attention will become more focused and one's sense of discrimination will be sharpened. This may also be linked to the function of the Small Intestine (the yang organ associated with the Heart) in separating the clear from the turbid.

The original name of this formula was Pillow Formula of the Great Sage Confucius (孔子大聖枕中方 *Kǒng zi dà shèng zhěn zhōng fāng*). This was shortened to its present name by Wang Ang, author of *Medical Formulas Collected and Analyzed*, although the older version is still in use. The late Qing-dynasty physician Fei Bo-Xiong recommended that the following herbs be added if the formula is to be used long-term: Angelica sinensis radix (*dāng guī*), Paeoniae Radix (*sháo yào*), Salviae miltiorrhizae Radix (*dān shēn*), and Platycladi Semen (*bǎi zǐ rén*).

妙香散
Marvelously Fragrant Powder
miào xiāng sǎn

SOURCE *Formulary of the Pharmacy Service for Benefiting the People in the Taiping Era* (1148)

Ginseng Radix (*rén shēn*) 15g
Dioscoreae Rhizoma (*shān yào*) 30g

Astragali Radix (*huáng qí*) 30g
Poria (*fú líng*) 30g
Poriae Sclerotium pararadicis (*fú shén*) 30g
Polygalae Radix (*yuǎn zhì*) 30g
Cinnabaris (*zhū shā*) 9g
Aucklandiae Radix (*mù xiāng*) 75g
Moschus (*shè xiāng*) 3g
Platycodi Radix (*jié gěng*) 15g
Glycyrrhizae Radix praeparata (*zhì gān cǎo*) 15g

Grind the ingredients into a powder and take in 6g doses with warm wine. Nourishes the Heart and calms the spirit. For Heart qi deficiency characterized by anxiety, apprehensiveness, worry, and distress with palpitations, insomnia, forgetfulness, nocturnal emissions, spontaneous sweating, a pale tongue body, and a deficient pulse. At present, Codonopsis Radix (*dǎng shēn*) is usually substituted for Ginseng Radix (*rén shēn*) at 2-3 times its dosage. In contrast to the principal formula, this is indicated for a condition with more restlessness and generalized qi deficiency.

黃連阿膠湯 （黄连阿胶汤）
Coptis and Ass-Hide Gelatin Decoction

huáng lián ē jiāo tāng

Source   *Discussion of Cold Damage* (c. 220)

Coptidis Rhizoma (*huáng lián*) 12g
Scutellariae Radix (*huáng qín*) 6g
Asini Corii Colla (*ē jiāo*) . . . . . (dissolve in strained decoction) 9g
Paeoniae Radix (*sháo yào*) 6g
Egg yolk (*jī zi huáng*) . . . . . . (stir into strained decoction) 2 yolks

Method of Preparation   Decoction. At present, Paeoniae Radix alba (*bái sháo*) is the form of Paeoniae Radix (*sháo yào*) used, and the dosage of Coptidis Rhizoma (*huáng lián*) is usually reduced by one-third to one-half. The strained decoction should be allowed to cool down before stirring in the egg yolks.

Actions   Enriches the yin, causes fire to descend, eliminates irritability, and calms the spirit

Indications

Irritability with a sensation of heat in the chest, insomnia, palpitations with anxiety, a red tongue with a dry, yellow coating, and a thin, rapid pulse. There may also be sores on the tongue or in the mouth.

This is a so-called heat transformation (熱化 *rè huà*) pattern in the lesser yin warp of a cold damage disorder. The lesser yin corresponds to the Kidneys, which govern the fluids and store the essence, and the Heart, which governs the blood vessels. When pathogenic heat enters the lesser yin, it consumes the yin fluids, blood, and essence. This results in a pattern characterized by excess heat at the qi level (the heat pathogen usually enters via the Stomach or Intestines) combined with deficiency of yin and blood. The presence of qi-aspect pathogenic heat is reflected in the red tongue with a dry, yellow coating, while the thin, rapid pulse indicates

that the yin has already been damaged. Lesser-yin water (the Kidneys) is no longer able to properly control lesser-yin fire (the Heart). This leads to a sensation of heat in the chest and symptoms of a disturbed spirit: palpitations with anxiety, irritability, and insomnia characterized by an inability of the patient to calmly lie down. Sores in the mouth and on the tongue are also a sign of pathogenic heat in the Heart.

Analysis of Formula

To treat a pattern characterized by heat excess and blood deficiency whose symptoms predominantly manifest in the Heart lesser yin, this formula utilizes a strategy of directing fire downward by means of bitter, cooling herbs while simultaneously nourishing the yin and blood with sweet, salty, and sour substances. The chief ingredients are the bitter, cooling Coptidis Rhizoma (*huáng lián*), which directly clears fire from the Heart and thereby calms the spirit, and the sweet and neutral Asini Corii Colla (*ē jiāo*), which indirectly controls the Heart fire by enriching the yin and nourishing the blood. Together, they facilitate interaction between water and fire to effectively treat the root and branch of this pattern. The deputies are bitter and cooling Scutellariae Radix (*huáng qín*), which drains heat from the upper burner and the Intestines to assist Coptidis Rhizoma (*huáng lián*) in directing fire downward, and sour and cooling Paeoniae Radix alba (*bái sháo*), which assists Asini Corii Colla (*ē jiāo*) in enriching and retaining the yin to harmonize the functions of the qi and also both of the heat-draining herbs in controlling the yang. The assistant and envoy is sweet and balanced egg yolk (*jī zi huáng*), which enters the Heart and Kidneys, tonifies the yin and blood, and resolves heat toxicity. It assists the heat-draining herbs in eliminating the pathogen while protecting against their drying properties, but also acts in concert with the blood-tonifying substances to enrich the yin.

Commentary

Like Gardenia and Prepared Soybean Decoction (*zhī zǐ chǐ tāng*), discussed in Chapter 4, and Sour Jujube Decoction (*suān zǎo rén tāng*), discussed above, this formula treats a form of deficiency irritability (虛煩 *xū fán*). This is a disorder characterized by symptoms like vexation, restlessness, insomnia, and subjective sensations of fullness in the chest indicating the presence of pathogenic heat. Such heat represents a local excess, but unlike patterns where the heat has led to clumping of body fluids or other substances, it has 'no form.' 'Deficiency' in this context thus does not refer primarily to deficiency of qi or essence, but functions as a designator that refers to a class of disorders in which the pathodynamic does not manifest with palpable excess or fullness.

In the conditions treated by this formula, the heat will tend to be of external origin (including alcohol, sugar, or other foodstuffs that generate heat). Hence, even though the patient will show signs of blood and yin deficiency, these are secondary. To treat patterns characterized by yin and blood deficiency and empty fire, one should select a formula like Ass-Hide Gelatin and Egg Yolk Decoction *(ē jiāo jī zi huáng tāng)* or Major Arrest Wind Pearls *(dà dìng fēng zhū)*, discussed in Chapter 14. These formulas retain the yin- and blood-tonifying ingredients of Coptis and Ass-Hide Gelatin Decoction *(huáng lián ē jiāo tāng)* but combine them with salty and cooling substances that clear heat without damaging the yin.

The particular combination of excess heat and deficiency of essence treated by this formula is reflected in a strategy often said to embody the principle of draining the south (i.e., fire) while tonifying the north (i.e., water) first outlined in the *Classic of Difficulties*. Its distinguishing characteristics are a capacity for draining damp-heat pathogens from the body while simultaneously enriching the yin and tonifying the blood. In the type of cold damage disorders for which this formula was first composed, such pathogens enter the body primarily via the mouth and lodge in the Stomach and Intestines.

Later Usages

The scope of this formula has been expanded by later writers to include qi-aspect heat penetrating to the blood aspect, bleeding disorders, and dysenteric disorders due to heat toxin. A passage in the 19th-century Japanese work *Expansion of the Categorized Collected Formulas* notes:

> It treats all kinds of patterns involving loss of blood, chest palpitations, body fever, abdominal pain and mild dysentery, a dry tongue, burnt lips, irritability and restlessness with inability to lie down, bodily exhaustion, a complexion drained of blood or, alternatively, a red, flushed complexion.

In clinical practice, the following pointers provided by the contemporary physician Huang Huang in *One-Hundred Classic Formulas*, based on a review of both Chinese and Japanese sources, will prove useful in determining when this formula is appropriate:

- The tongue will be red, indicating the presence of heat.
- The pulse will be thin and rapid, indicating the presence of both heat and yin deficiency.
- The skin will tend to be dry and may show signs of flaking or chafing, but there will also be redness, particularly in the face.
- There will often be bleeding or a tendency to bleed, indicating heat stirring the blood to move recklessly.

Comparison

➤ Vs. Sour Jujube Decoction *(suān zǎo rén tāng)*

Both formulas treat irritability and insomnia. Comparing the indications of these formulas in their source texts, the dif-

ferences between them become clear. Coptis and Ass-Hide Gelatin Decoction *(huáng lián ē jiāo tāng)* is for irritability when the patient is unable to lie down, that is, when he is so irritable that he cannot even tolerate lying in bed. This is due to the yang failing to enter the yin, and the treatment strategy focuses on draining fire from the Heart and enriching the yin and blood. Sour Jujube Decoction *(suān zǎo rén tāng)* is for irritability with insomnia in which the patient is able to lie in bed, but cannot sleep. This occurs when deficient Liver blood is unable to nourish the Heart, and the treatment strategy focuses on tonifying and harmonizing the Liver.

➤ Vs. Polyporus Decoction *(zhū líng tāng)*; see PAGE 731

Biomedical Indications

With the appropriate presentation, this formula may be used to treat a variety of biomedically-defined disorders including nervous exhaustion, the recuperative stage of an infectious disease, autonomic dystonia, erectile dysfunction, apthous ulcers, and hypertension.

Alternate name

Coptis and Egg Yolk Decoction *(huáng lián jī zi tāng)* in *Thorough Understanding of Cold Damage*

Modifications

- For severe yin deficiency with injured fluids and a dry throat, add Scrophulariae Radix *(xuán shēn)*, Ophiopogonis Radix *(mài mén dōng)*, and Dendrobii Herba *(shí hú)*.
- For heat in the five centers, add Gardeniae Fructus *(zhī zǐ)* and Lophatheri Herba *(dàn zhú yè)*.
- For feverishness with dark urine, add Junci Medulla *(dēng xīn cǎo)*, Tetrapanacis Medulla *(tōng cǎo)*, and Imperatae Rhizoma *(bái máo gēn)*.
- For purpura or bleeding of the gums, add Ligustri lucidi Fructus *(nǚ zhēn zǐ)*, Ecliptae Herba *(mò hàn lián)*, Moutan Cortex *(mǔ dān pí)*, and Rehmanniae Radix *(shēng dì huáng)*.
- For dysenteric disorders with abdominal pain and pus and blood in the stool, remove the egg yolk *(jī zi huáng)*.

Associated Formula

交泰丸

Grand Communication Pill

jiāo tài wán

Source   *Comprehensive Medicine According to Master Han* (1522)

Coptidis Rhizoma *(huáng lián)* 15g
Cinnamomi Cortex *(ròu guì)* 1.5g

Grind the ingredients into a powder and form into pills with honey. Also prepared as a decoction with the dosage reduced by one-half to two-thirds. Reestablishes harmonious communication between the

Heart and Kidneys. For irritability, restlessness, severe, continuous palpitations, coolness of the lower limbs, and great difficulty in falling asleep due to disharmony between the Heart and Kidneys. This formula is used for internally-generated disorders in which the Kidney yang is unable to provide a base for the Heart yang. By contrast, the principal formula is best used in treating the lingering effects of an externally-contracted febrile disease where there is Kidney yin deficiency.

甘麥大棗湯 （甘麦大枣汤）
Licorice, Wheat, and Jujube Decoction
gān mài dà zǎo tāng

Source　*Essentials from the Golden Cabinet* (c. 220)

Glycyrrhizae Radix *(gān cǎo)* 9g
Tritici Fructus *(xiǎo mài)* 9-15g
Jujubae Fructus *(dà zǎo)* . . . . 10 pieces

Method of Preparation　Decoction. Many physicians believe that it should be taken long-term to achieve the best effect.

Actions　Nourishes the Heart, calms the spirit, harmonizes the middle burner, and relaxes hypertonicity

Indications

Disorientation, frequent attacks of melancholy and crying spells, inability to control oneself, restless sleep (sometimes with night sweats), and frequent bouts of yawning. In severe cases, the behavior and speech become abnormal.

This is called restless organ disorder (臟躁 *zàng zào*), an emotional condition that is generally due to excessive worry, anxiety, or pensiveness. This injures the Heart spirit and unsettles the ethereal and corporeal souls. The pathodynamic underlying this disorder is outlined in Chapter 11 of *Essentials from the Golden Cabinet*:

> [Patients manifesting with] pathogenic weeping that causes the ethereal and corporeal souls to be unsettled are deficient in qi and blood. [Disorders characterized by] qi and blood deficiency pertain to the Heart. Patients with Heart qi deficiency are [full] of fears. When they close their eyes wanting to sleep, they dream of going far away, [indicating] that their essence and spirit are dispersing, and their ethereal and corporeal souls are moving chaotically.

Patients who have suffered recent or recurring blood loss, which can further injure the blood and qi, such as women who have recently given birth, also can suffer from this condition. It is therefore listed in the source text under 'miscellaneous disorders of women.'

Not only is the cause of this disorder primarily emotional, its manifestations are also of an emotional nature. As explained above, this is due to the ethereal and corporeal souls losing their mooring and the spirit being lost. The souls are literally 'lost,' implying that they become detached from the conventions of normal behavior and are no longer controlled by the rules and etiquette that govern ordinary human interaction. In the early stages of such a disorder, the patient is mentally disoriented, anxious, impulsive, and suffers from fitful sleep. During attacks, they often feel extremely upset or depressed to the point of uncontrollable crying, manic behavior, or severe disorientation. More severe cases will present with frequent attacks of unusual behavior, especially those relating to a loss of self-control (crying, yawning, etc.). One explanation for the yawning is that it reflects the frustrated attempt of the yang (which has been almost extruded from the body due to deficiency of the yin) to reintegrate with the body. Note that while the source text mentions attacks of yawning as one of the indications for this formula, many modern practitioners believe that attacks of moaning or deep sighing occur more frequently in this type of patient. The insomnia and night sweats (sweat, like blood, being associated with the Heart) reflect that this condition is primarily one of Heart deficiency.

Analysis of Formula

According to Chapter 8 of *Divine Pivot*, the ethereal and corporeal souls come and go with the spirit and essence. In order to guide the drifting souls back toward a more normal attachment to the body, this formula focuses on tonifying the nutritive qi with sweet substances while simultaneously inhibiting the unrestrained dispersal of the souls. The chief herb, sweet and salty Tritici Fructus *(xiǎo mài)*, is light in weight, reaching outward to the exterior, yet also enters the Heart channel where it conserves the fluids of the Heart. According to the *Inner Classic*, wheat is the cereal associated with the Heart; Sun Si-Miao thought that it nourished the Heart qi. This ability, more commonly used to treat spontaneous sweating and night sweats, is utilized here to control the dispersal of the ethereal and corporeal souls. The deputies are sweet Glycyrrhizae Radix *(gān cǎo)*, which nourishes the Heart, tonifies the qi, and harmonizes the middle burner, and Jujubae Fructus *(dà zǎo)*, which augments the qi and moistens internal dryness. Although both of these herbs are generally understood to be tonifying, they also clear heat. *Records of Thoughtful Differentiation of Materia Medica*, for instance, observes of Glycyrrhizae Radix *(gān cǎo)* that it "is yellow in the middle, with a reddish bark," and thus

> certainly an herb of the Spleen and Heart channels. … Its effects are completely due to its sweetness, by which it tonifies, by which it moderates. Whenever the sage [Zhang] Zhong-Jing prescribed it in formulas, he used it in its prepared form to tonify or moderate urgency, but in its unprepared form to drain fire—yet even this 'draining' involved the idea of moderation.

Because the herb is used here in its unprepared form, this implies that its focus is on draining excess rather than tonifying deficiency. Likewise, *Divine Husbandman's Classic of the Materia Medica* states of Jujubae Fructus *(dà zǎo)* that "it governs pathogenic qi in the Heart and abdomen, quiets the middle, nourishes the Spleen, and assists the twelve channels."

By combining three simple and readily available herbs, this formula thus achieves a remarkable effect: it guides the floating souls back within the bounds of normal behavior, allowing the patient to feel at ease with herself once again. If the efficacy of such 'kitchen medicine' may be difficult to accept because only powerful remedies are considered capable of treating unusual disorders, physicians throughout the ages have been aware that it is precisely this simplicity that generates the effect. The spirit is yang in nature, but, unlike qi, does not attach to any substance. It is difficult to influence with herbs alone and requires the most subtle of treatment strategies. And what could be more subtle then pacifying the wayward soul by means of herbs that nourish the nutritive yin, governed by the Heart and therefore rooting the spirit?

Commentary

While in the source text this formula is discussed under the heading of 'miscellaneous women's disorders,' it is equally applicable to men as well as children.

Which Organ is Restless?

There has been some discussion by later commentators about the meaning of 'organ' in the term restless organ disorder. Some, like the 18th-century writer You Yi in *Personal Standards for the Essentials from the Golden Cabinet*, believed that it refers to the Womb, and specifically to the deficiency of blood in that organ. However, this type of problem is also seen, if less frequently, in men. Others, such as You's contemporary, Wu Qian, editor of *Golden Mirror of the Medical Tradition*, believed that it refers to the Heart. Wu argued that when the Heart is tranquil, the spirit is properly stored; but when that organ loses its tranquility, the spirit becomes disorderly. This explanation fits more closely with the purpose of the formula, which focuses on the Heart. In *Elaborating on the Subtleties of the Golden Cabinet*, the modern physician Cao Ying-Fu argued that the Lungs were the main root of this disorder because the Lungs are associated with melancholia and crying, which are prominent symptoms. In fact, all of the yin organs can be involved, depending on the specific case. Besides the Heart, the Spleen can be injured by overwork or obsessive deliberation; fire from Liver constraint is often implicated in hyperactive yang; and qi deficiency also affects the Kidneys and Lungs. This is the view taken by the Qing-dynasty author Xu Bin, who writes in *Discussion and Annotation of the Essentials from the Golden Cabinet* that "[the term] organ refers to all of the five yin organs."

Controversy over Pathodynamic

Commentators similarly disagree with respect to the path-odynamic responsible for producing the symptoms of this disorder. Some, including the Yuan-dynasty writer Zhao Li-ang-Ren in *Elucidating the Meaning of Discussion of Formulas from the Golden Cabinet*, argued that the symptoms are caused by Liver deficiency and subsequent constraint that also affects the Lung and results in a state where the person is sad and cries. Although this explanation accords with some of the actions attributed to Tritici Fructus (*xiǎo mài*), it is difficult to reconcile overall with the formula's emphasis on controlling floating yang by nourishing the nutritive yin. The opening and unblocking actions of a formula like Rambling Powder (*xiāo yáo sǎn*) would appear to be much more consistent with the logic of Zhao's argument.

Other physicians, including You Yi and Pu Fu-Zhou, thus believed that a pathology of the Womb was not the effect but rather the cause of this disorder. You's argument in *Personal Standards for the Essentials from the Golden Cabinet* is representative of this view:

> Restless organ disorder is exactly what Chen [Zi-Ming] was referring to by blood deficiency of the Womb that is affected by wind and transforms into fire. In blood deficiency [causing] restless organ [disorder,] internal fire harasses [the Heart,] causing the spirit to be uneasy. [This manifests] as sorrow damage with a desire to cry.

Neither of these positions clearly explains why constraint of the ministerial fire should lead to the symptoms of restless organ disorder and how this pathology differs from that of a Sour Jujube Decoction (*suān zǎo rén tāng*) pattern. Wu Qian and the editors of *Golden Mirror of the Medical Tradition* resolve this by simply defining the disorder as a disturbance of the seven emotions that prevents the Heart from being tranquil. A similar but slightly more elaborate analysis is offered by Chen Nian-Zu in *Simple Annotation of the Essentials from the Golden Cabinet*:

> The yin organs pertain to yin. Agitation is due to yin deficiency that is exploited by fire. There is no need to restrict this to any particular yin organ because, irrespective of which one is agitated, the symptoms will be the same. However, the [specific symptoms] of sorrow damage [accompanied] by a desire to cry … are due to a Heart disorder. Observing [that a patient who] frequently yawns indicates a Kidney disorder. [From this, one can conclude] that when the five emotions generate fire, its movement can be linked to the Heart; and that when the yin organs are damaged, this will invariably exhaust the Kidneys.

This argument, despite explaining some aspects of the condition, would logically lead to the selection of formulas such as Emperor of Heaven's Special Pill to Tonify the Heart (*tiān wáng bǔ xīn dān*) or Coptis and Ass-Hide Gelatin Decoction (*huáng lián ē jiāo tāng*), rather than to the present formula. Another perspective, which can be traced back at least to Ye Tian-Shi, views this as being due to problems affecting the Liver and Stomach. As Ye wrote in *Selections of Formulas and Cases from the Hall of Longevity*:

I shall discuss the strategy of sedating the Liver and calming the Stomach by using Licorice, Wheat, and Jujube Decoction (*gān mài dà zǎo tāng*) [as an example. This formula] employs Tritici Fructus (*xiǎo mài*) to sedate rebelliousness, and Jujubae Fructus (*dà zǎo*) and Glycyrrhizae Radix (*gān cǎo*) to augment what is deficient. [In doing so,] it follows the *Inner Classic [Divine Pivot,* Chapter 63]*, which says that when the Liver suffers from hypertonicity, one should immediately take sweet [medicinals] in order to relax it.

Based on this interpretation, Ye Tian-Shi modified Licorice, Wheat, and Jujube Decoction (*gān mài dà zǎo tāng*) to treat a wide variety of clinical problems. Among other examples:

- For palpitations and disordered affect, add Poria (*fú líng*), Platycladi Semen (*bǎi zǐ rén*), Paeoniae Radix alba (*bái sháo*), and Nelumbinis Semen (*lián zǐ*)

- For irritability, insomnia, or fright palpitations involving damage to the Heart yin fluids, add Ophiopogonis Radix (*mài mén dōng*), Paeoniae Radix alba (*bái sháo*), and Fossilia Ossis Mastodi (*lóng gǔ*)

- For thirst indicating damage to the Stomach yang fluids, add Ophiopogonis Radix (*mài mén dōng*) and Paeoniae Radix alba (*bái sháo*)

- For Liver deficiency wind with tics and spasms, add Asini Corii Colla (*ē jiāo*), Paeoniae Radix alba (*bái sháo*), Rehmanniae Radix (*shēng dì huáng*), Fossilia Ossis Mastodi (*lóng gǔ*), and Ostreae Concha (*mǔ lì*)

A careful reading of Ye Tian-Shi's analysis of this formula in the light of his clinical usage suggests that he viewed it as being able to control rebellious yang. A disoriented ethereal soul detaching from the body, internal wind, and hyperactive yang are all types of rebelliousness generically linked to Liver, Stomach, and Penetrating vessel pathologies. From this perspective, this formula gently tonifies the nutritive yin in order to control the aberrant yang.

Applications in Clincal Practice

Not only Ye Tian-Shi, but other physicians, too, have widely expanded the range of applications of this formula. The contemporary physician and author of *Treatment Strategies and Formulas in Chinese Medicine*, Chen Chao-Zu, conceives of this formula as relaxing the blood vessels, as these are muscular and as such are governed by the Liver. They are therefore amenable to treatment by sweet relaxation and admirable formulas, such as this one. Chen writes: "By means of this formula, we can make out the subtlety of the ancient formulas. They are as different from contemporary formulas that focus on the treatment of symptoms as heaven is from earth."

It follows that use of this formula is not limited to the treatment of women. It is very useful, for instance, in pediatrics. Possible applications reported in the literature include incessant sobbing and weeping, hyperactivity, bed-wetting—combined with Mantidis Oötheca (*sāng piāo xiāo*), Cuscutae Semen (*tù sī zǐ*), and Alpiniae oxyphyllae Fructus (*yì zhì rén*)—lack of appetite, and night sweats.

Ingredient Issues

While the source text specifies the use of Tritici Fructus (*xiǎo mài*), some contemporary texts list Tritici Fructus levis (*fú xiǎo mài*) instead. The difference between these two herbs is that, when placed in water, the former sinks to the bottom while the latter floats (浮 *fú*). Being essentially the same substance, both herbs are sweet and cooling and enter into the Heart. However, Tritici Fructus (*xiǎo mài*) is believed to focus more on nourishing, while Tritici Fructus levis (*fú xiǎo mài*) is light in weight and thus travels the exterior where it clears heat from constraint and restrains sweating.

With regard to the preparation of this formula, it is important to note that the pre-Song literature advises that Tritici Fructus (*xiǎo mài*) changes its nature in the process of cooking. The famous alchemist Tao Hong-Jing, for instance, notes that when used as a pill, it treats hot disorders, but when it is cooked in a broth, it becomes warming. The *Tang Materia Medica* likewise observes:

> When Tritici Fructus (*xiǎo mài*) is used in a decoction, [care must be taken] that its skin/shell is not broken. It is said that when the shell is broken, it becomes warming. This is why noodles [made from wheat] are unable to eliminate heat and stop irritability.

Furthermore, many contemporary physicians use considerably higher dosages than those listed above. These can reach 25-45g for Glycyrrhizae Radix (*gān cǎo*), 60-100g for Tritici Fructus (*xiǎo mài*), and 30g for Jujubae Fructus (*dà zǎo*).

Comparisons

➤ Vs. Sour Jujube Decoction (*suān zǎo rén tāng*)

Both formulas are used in treating irritability and insomnia occurring in deficient patients and both have an astringent effect that is also used to treat excessive sweating. However, Sour Jujube Decoction (*suān zǎo rén tāng*) focuses on tonifying and regulating the Liver, specifically Liver blood. To this end, it combines sour and sweet tonification with acrid, moving, and cold draining herbs. This formula is altogether more mild. It focuses on tonifying the nutritive yin associated with the Spleen and the Heart by means of sweet herbs that are also cooling. Because sweet herbs fill up or soften the yin, they are able to control the yang, extending their action from the Spleen and the Heart to the Liver.

➤ Vs. Lily Bulb and Rehmannia Decoction (*bǎi hé dì huáng tāng*); *see* page 221

Biomedical Indications

With the appropriate presentation, this formula may be used to treat a variety of biomedically-defined disorders. These can be divided into the following groups:

- Neuropsychiatric disorders including general anxiety disorder, hysteria, schizophrenia, epilepsy, night terrors in children, attention deficit hyperactivity disorder, sleep walking, and nervous exhaustion

- Spasmodic disorder including spasmodic coughs, Parkinson's disease, gastric spasms, spasms of the extremities, and migraines

- Disorders of the electrical system of the heart such as sinus tachycardia and ectopic heartbeats.

This formula has also been used for treating premenstrual tension and perimenopausal syndrome.

Alternate names

Jujube Decoction (*dà zǎo tāng*) and Wheat, Licorice, and Jujube Decoction (*mài gān dà zǎo tāng*) in *Formulas of Universal Benefit from My Practice*; Wheat Decoction (*xiǎo mài tāng*) in *Discussion of Illnesses, Patterns, and Formulas Related to the Unification of the Three Etiologies*; Licorice Decoction (*gān cǎo tāng*) in *Fine Formulas for Women*

Modifications

- For irritability with a sensation of heat in the chest and other signs of more severe Heart yin deficiency, add Lilii Bulbus (*bǎi hé*) and Platycladi Semen (*bǎi zǐ rén*).

- For insomnia with a thin, wiry pulse from Liver blood deficiency, add Ziziphi spinosae Semen (*suān zǎo rén*).

- For constipation, add Sesami Semen nigrum (*hēi zhī má*) and Polygoni multiflori Radix (*hé shǒu wū*).

- For enuresis, add Mantidis Oötheca (*sāng piāo xiāo*), Alpiniae oxyphyllae Fructus (*yì zhì rén*), and Cuscutae Semen (*tù sī zǐ*).

- For palpitations, shortness of breath, loss of appetite, a swollen, tooth-marked tongue, and a thin, frail pulse, combine with Restore the Spleen Decoction (*guī pí tāng*).

- For sinus arrhythmias and a choppy pulse, add Codonopsis Radix (*dǎng shēn*) and Fluoritum (*zǐ shí yīng*).

- For mild cases of schizophrenia, add Cinnamomi Ramulus (*guì zhī*), Fossilia Ossis Mastodi (*lóng gǔ*), and Ostreae Concha (*mǔ lì*).

Associated Formula

半夏秫米湯 (半夏秫米汤)

Pinellia and Millet Decoction

bàn xià shú mǐ tāng

Source *Divine Pivot* (probably later Han dynasty)

Pinelliae Rhizoma praeparatum (*zhì bàn xià*)
Setariae Fructus (*shú mǐ*)

This decoction is one of the few formulas mentioned in the *Inner Classic*, as it is noted in Chapter 71 of *Divine Pivot*. It dispels phlegm and clears away filth and establishes communication between the yin and yang. It is used to treat insomnia due to phlegm and dampness obstructing the middle burner, which obstructs the qi dynamic and results in the yang being unable to enter the yin. The sweet, cool nature of Setariae Fructus (*shú mǐ*) balances the acrid, warm nature of Pinelliae Rhizoma praeparatum (*zhì bàn xià*) and harmonizes the middle burner, with an emphasis on directing downward. This allows the yang to enter the yin at night and therefore resolves insomnia. Note that some commentators follow Li Shi-Zhen who identified 秫米 *shú mǐ* as sorghum (Sorghum Fructus). In present-day China, both types of grain are commonly used. While it can be used by itself, it is commonly combined with other medicinals or with Grand Communication Pill (*jiāo tài wán*) for a more complete effect on both the Triple Burner and the Heart-Kidney axis.

Note that Setariae Fructus (*shú mǐ*) is sweet and slightly cold and enters the Lung, Stomach, and Large Intestine channels. It harmonizes the Stomach and calms the spirit, dispels wind and eliminates dampness, while also resolving toxicity and helping sores close. The normal dosage is 9-15g, either in a decoction or as a porridge.

Section 2

FORMULAS THAT SEDATE AND CALM THE SPIRIT

The formulas in this section are used for patients who have suffered sudden, terrifying experiences that disturb their spirits, in whom the Heart yang is ascendant with upward-blazing of Heart fire or the Liver yang becomes hyperactive. This results in such disturbances of the spirit as severe anxiety or phobia, restlessness, and uncontrolled emotions (usually manifested in bouts of laughter or crying). Because these are relatively excessive conditions, a strategy that sedates is appropriate.

The chief ingredients in these formulas are usually heavy minerals that are said to 'weigh down' or anchor the ascendant Heart yang such as Magnetitum (*cí shí*), Margaritiferae Concha usta (*zhēn zhū mǔ*), or Ferri Frusta (*shēng tiě luò*). Depending on the precise pattern, four other types of ingredients are commonly added:

- When fire is an important root cause, add herbs that drain heat and clear fire such as Coptidis Rhizoma (*huáng lián*), Scutellariae Radix (*huáng qín*), or Forsythiae Fructus (*lián qiáo*).

- For the deficiency that almost invariably accompanies hyperactive yang, add herbs that enrich the yin and nourish the blood such as Rehmanniae Radix (*shēng dì huáng*),

Rehmanniae Radix praeparata *(shú dì huáng)*, or Angelicae sinensis Radix *(dāng guī)*.

- To restore normal consciousness, add herbs that regulate the qi, transform phlegm, and open the orifices such as Citri reticulatae Pericarpium *(chén pí)*, Fritillariae Bulbus *(bèi mǔ)*, Polygalae Radix *(yuǎn zhì)*, or Acori tatarinowii Rhizoma *(shí chāng pú)*.
- To facilitate digestion of the heavy minerals used as chief ingredients, add herbs that guide out food stagnation.

It is important to remember that some of the minerals originally used in these formulas may contain unacceptably high levels of heavy metals. From a traditional perspective, these should not be taken for long periods of time, not only because of their toxicity, but because they also readily injure the Stomach qi. At present, especially in the West, these ingredients are illegal and appropriate substitutions must be made.

朱砂安神丸
Cinnabar Pill to Calm the Spirit

zhū shā ān shén wán

Source *Clarifying Doubts about Injury from Internal and External Causes* (1247)

aqueous trituration of Cinnabaris *(shuǐ fēi zhū shā)* 15g
Coptidis Rhizoma *(huáng lián)* 18g
Angelicae sinensis Radix *(dāng guī)* 7.5g
Rehmanniae Radix *(shēng dì huáng)* 7.5g
Glycyrrhizae Radix praeparata *(zhì gān cǎo)* 16.5g

Method of Preparation Grind the four herbs together and form into pills that are covered with Cinnabaris *(zhū shā)*. Take in 6-9g doses, either once before bedtime or twice daily. May also be prepared as a decoction with a proportionate reduction in dosage. If prepared as a decoction, the Cinnabaris *(zhū shā)* was originally taken with the strained decoction. Due to the unacceptable toxicity of Cinnabaris *(zhū shā)*, it is no longer used (see COMMENTARY below for a discussion of possible substitutes).

Actions Sedates the Heart, calms the spirit, drains fire, and nourishes the yin

Indications

Insomnia, continuous palpitations, a sensation of irritability and heat in the chest, a desire to vomit without result, dream-disturbed sleep, a tongue that is red at the tip, and a thin, rapid pulse. In some cases, the patient also develops a rancorous disposition.

This is vigorous Heart fire injuring the blood and yin. The scorching from Heart fire depletes the blood and yin, which in turn deprives the Heart of nourishment. The combination of heat and deficiency disturbs the serenity of the spirit, which manifests as insomnia and continuous palpitations. Another way of looking at this is that the uprising of Heart fire prevents the Heart from rooting in the Kidneys,

which is necessary to house the spirit. The spirit therefore has no place to reside during the yin time of the day (the nighttime), and insomnia results. The internal movement of fire in the Heart not only aggravates the palpitations, but also gives rise to a sensation of heat and irritability in the chest, a desire to vomit without result, and a tongue with a red tip. This process of heat disturbing the spirit and disrupting the flow of qi in the chest may also lead to the development of a rancorous disposition. The combination of heat and deficiency is clearly reflected in the thin, rapid pulse.

Analysis of Formula

This formula calms the spirit primarily by clearing heat from the Heart, but also tonifies the deficiency of yin and blood that is the secondary aspect of this pattern. The chief ingredient, sweet and slightly cooling Cinnabaris *(zhū shā)*, enters the Heart channel and can sedate excessive yang activity by way of its heavy nature. It calms the spirit and also clears fire from the Heart. The deputy ingredient, bitter and cooling Coptidis Rhizoma *(huáng lián)*, strongly drains excess heat from the Heart and works synergistically with the chief ingredient to reinforce both of its actions. Together, they address both the branch and root of this disorder. The assistant ingredients are acrid, sweet, and warming Angelicae sinensis Radix *(dāng guī)*, which enters the Heart, Liver, and Spleen channels, and sweet, bitter, and strongly cooling Rehmanniae Radix *(shēng dì huáng)*, which enters the Heart, Liver, and Kidneys. Together, they nourish the blood and replenish the yin to tonify those aspects of the body that have been injured by the Heart fire and prevent further injury. The latter ingredient also helps clear fire from the nutritive and blood aspects. The envoy, Glycyrrhizae Radix praeparata *(zhì gān cǎo)*, harmonizes the actions of the other ingredients while protecting the Stomach from the harsh effects of the chief and deputy ingredients.

Cautions and Contraindications

Note that Cinnabaris *(zhū shā)* is no longer used and that appropriate substitutions must be made. Even though this formula contains yin-enriching herbs, it is not indicated for patients where yin deficiency is the primary problem. It is cooling in nature and thus, to avoid damaging the middle burner yang, should not be taken for long periods of time.

Commentary

The author of this formula, Li Dong-Yuan, is one of the masters of the Jin-Yuan period. Variations of this formula appear in different books attributed to him. In the source text, *Clarifying Doubts about Injury from Internal and External Causes*, this formula is simply known as Calm the Spirit Pill *(ān shén wán)*. The hierarchy of ingredients was slightly different than that presented above. There, Coptidis Rhizoma *(huáng lián)* is designated as the chief ingredient because of its actions in relieving irritability and eliminating the damp-heat that was thought to precipitate the condition. The deputy ingredients, Glycyrrhizae Radix (*gān cǎo*) and Rehmanniae Radix (*shēng dì huáng*), are said to drain fire and tonify the qi as a means of enriching the yin and generating blood. In the latter function, they are assisted by Angelicae sinensis Radix (*dāng guī*). The ability of Cinnabaris (*zhū shā*) to clear fire and calm the spirit is related to its function of anchoring or 'weighing down' the floating fire. Some later commentators follow this reading and designate Coptidis Rhizoma (*huáng lián*), or Coptidis Rhizoma (*huáng lián*) and Cinnabaris (*zhū shā*), as the chief ingredients. Following this interpretation, it is possible to substitute other medicinals for Cinnabaris (*zhū shā*), which can no longer be used today because of its toxicity. Appropriate candidates would include Magnetitum (*cí shí*), Margaritiferae Concha usta (*zhēn zhū mǔ*), Margarita (*zhēn zhū*), Fossilia Ossis Mastodi (*lóng gǔ*), Fossilia Dentis Mastodi (*lóng chǐ*), Ostreae Concha (*mǔ lì*), or Fluoritum (*zǐ shí yīng*).

According to the source text, the symptoms treated by this formula are due to "fire lurking in the blood above the diaphragm that rises and flourishes, [making it] impossible to be calm." The formula "holds down the floating movement of yin fire in order to nourish the source qi of the upper burner." This is another example where the term 'yin fire' denotes all kinds of internal fire to Li Dong-Yuan, not just that from qi deficiency (see also the discussion of Tonify the Middle to Augment the Qi Decoction (*bǔ zhōng yì qì tāng*) in Chapter 8). However, all such pathological fire consumes the qi and must therefore be eliminated. In the present case, this is achieved by directing it downward and guiding its excess out of the body via the bowels and urine. Where yin fire arises from qi constraint, the opposite strategy is employed: constraint is opened up and the physiological fire is directed from below to above. In each case, the focus is therefore not only on treating a symptom pattern, but ultimately on re-establishing the normal ascending and downward-directing functions of the qi dynamic.

In clinical practice, this formula is thought to be particularly effective in treating the palpitations and anxiety that occur during dreams. The thin pulse indicates that this is not just a condition of excess, but is caused, in fact, by 'yin fire.' Such fire does not enter the body from the outside but is caused by internal factors. In the 16th-century *Investigations of Medical Formulas*, Wu Kun singles out worry, sadness, and excessive thinking as being particularly important. These prevent the qi from being directed downward and thereby damage the middle burner's function of producing blood. This implies that once the symptoms have been successfully treated, these underlying issues must be addressed to effect a more long-term solution to the problem.

Comparisons

➤ Vs. Magnetite and Cinnabar Pill (*cí zhū wán*); *see* page 478

➤ Vs. Iron Filings Drink (*shēng tiě luò yǐn*); *see* page 479

➤ Vs. Mother-of-Pearl Pill (*zhēn zhū mǔ wán*); see page 481

Biomedical Indications

With the appropriate presentation, this formula may be used to treat a variety of biomedically-defined disorders including neurasthenia, depression, anxiety neurosis, panic attacks, and mitral valve prolapse.

Alternate names

Pill for Calming the Spirit (*ān shén wán*) in *Secrets from the Orchid Chamber*; Cinnabar Pill (*zhū shā wán*) in *Prescriptions for Universal Benefit*; Coptis Pill for Calming the Spirit (*huáng lián ān shén wán*) in *Synopsis for Protecting Infants*; Pill for Calming Sleep (*ān qǐn wán*) in *Guide to Pregnancy and Childbirth*

Modifications

• For severe insomnia, add Nelumbinis Plumula (*lián zǐ xīn*), Polygalae Radix (*yuǎn zhì*), and Poriae Sclerotium pararadicis (*fú shén*).

• For controlling the up-flaring of Heart yang, add Magnetitum (*cí shí*), Fossilia Dentis Mastodi (*lóng chǐ*), or Ostreae Concha (*mǔ lì*).

• For severe irritability with a sensation of heat in the chest, add Gardeniae Fructus (*zhī zǐ*) and Sojae Semen praeparatum (*dàn dòu chǐ*).

• For a sensation of heat and pressure in the chest with nausea, and perhaps some difficulty in swallowing, add Trichosanthis Fructus (*guā lóu*) and Bambusae Caulis in taeniam (*zhú rú*).

• For a redder tongue tip and dark, scanty urine, add Lophatheri Herba (*dàn zhú yè*) and Junci Medulla (*dēng xīn cǎo*).

磁硃丸
Magnetite and Cinnabar Pill
cí zhū wán

Source   *Important Formulas Worth a Thousand Gold Pieces* (650)

Magnetitum (*cí shí*)	60g
Cinnabaris (*zhū shā*)	30g
Massa medicata fermentata (*shén qū*)	120g

Method of Preparation   Grind the ingredients into a powder and form into small pills with honey. Take 6g twice a day.

Actions   Heavily sedates and calms the spirit, weighs down the yang, and improves the vision and hearing

Indications

Palpitations, insomnia, tinnitus, and diminished acuity of hearing and vision. Also used for seizures.

This is ascendant Heart yang with lack of communication between the Heart and the Kidneys. Under normal conditions, the Heart in the upper burner governs the downward-directing of (sovereign) fire and its transformation into essence. The Kidneys in the lower burner store the essence and govern their transformation into (ministerial) fire. In this way, fire and water mutually generate and control each other. This ensures the controlled diffusion of yang qi to the sensory organs, with the Heart above regulating the release of essence and qi from the Kidneys below, while the Kidneys root the spirit residing in the Heart. This is explained by Wang You-Yuan in *Discussion of Famous Physicians' Formulas Past and Present*: "The Kidneys alone store the essence. Therefore, the water of the spirit [神水 *shén shuǐ*; this term can also refer to saliva] develops in the Kidneys. The Heart is the illuminating fire [离照 *lí zhào*; 离 *lí* is sometime used to refer to the fire at the gate of vitality, hence this term brings into play the relationship between sovereign and ministerial fire]. Therefore, the brightness of the spirit develops in the Heart." Thus, when communication is lost between the Heart and Kidneys, Heart yang ascends excessively, depriving the spirit of its calm place of abode. This leads to palpitations and insomnia. It also prevents the essence in the Kidneys from ascending harmoniously to nourish the ears and eyes, diminishing the acuity of hearing and vision. In very severe cases, the uncontrolled upsurge of qi that this lack of communication implies may manifest as internal wind and seizures, as the Kidneys and Liver are said to have the same source.

Analysis of Formula

This formula aims to restore the normal physiological communication between Heart and Kidneys, primarily by pacifying the hyperactive yang. The idea is to root the floating qi once more in the Kidneys, restoring the physiological balance between above and below, water and fire. The chief ingredient, salty, cold, and heavy Magnetitum (*cí shí*), enters the Kidneys, anchors and calms the spirit, weighs down the yang while nourishing the yin, and improves the acuity of hearing and vision. *Comprehensive Outline of the Materia Medica* notes that it "treats all disorders of the Kidneys, while unblocking the ears and brightening the eyes." *Seeking Accuracy in the Materia Medica* says that it "enters the Kidneys to sedate the yin, preventing the dragon [i.e., ministerial] fire from rising upward out of the yin." The deputy, Cinnabaris (*zhū shā*), sedates and calms the spirit, and clears heat from the Heart. Cinnabaris (*zhū shā*) is red and corresponds to the fire phase, like the Heart; Magnetitum (*cí shí*) is black and corresponds to the water phase, like the Kidneys. Together, they anchor the spirit and pacify the floating Heart yang so that it can interact

with the Kidneys. In this manner, the fire in the Heart is controlled and the essence in the Kidneys is able to rise, which gradually resolves the condition.

One assistant, Massa medicata fermentata (*shén qū*), strengthens the Spleen and Stomach and aids digestion. Not only does it prevent injury to the Stomach qi from the heavy metals, it also helps disseminate their actions throughout the body. Focusing on the middle burner, the fulcrum of the qi dynamic, it also plays an active role in stabilizing the normal ascending and descending of the essence and fire. The other assistant, honey, serves as the filler for the pills and also tonifies the middle burner.

Cautions and Contraindications

This formula should not be used without significant modification for problems with visual or auditory acuity associated with fire from Liver and Kidney deficiency. In patients with a weak digestive system, the dosage should be reduced and carefully monitored. At present, the heavy metal toxicity of Cinnabaris (*zhū shā*) renders its use obsolete and requires substitution.

Commentary

In the source text, the emphasis of this formula is on treating problems with visual and auditory acuity. It was only during the Qing dynasty that physicians like Ke Qin and Chen Nian-Zu emphasized its role in treating seizures, mania, and epilepsy, from which its modern usage in treating insomnia and palpitations arose. Even today, however, the original indications are still the distinguishing symptoms for this formula, and it continues to be one of the most important formulas for treating visual problems due to internal injury, particularly when the pattern is lack of communication between the Heart and Kidneys. In *Selected Annotations to Ancient Formulas from the Garden of Crimson Snow*, Wang Zi-Jie outlines the pathodynamic at the root of this disorder and explains why the formula is so well-suited to its treatment:

> Sun Si-Miao, Ni Wei-De, and Li Dong-Yuan all say that dilated pupils are due to Heart fire encroaching on the Lungs and ascending into the brain to scorch the marrow. As the nature of fire is to disperse, the pupils dilate. Ni states that acrid, heating [medicines] are contraindicated. Li states that cold and cooling [medicines] are contraindicated. Sun Si-Miao states that [this formula] benefits the power of the eyes. No [other] common formula is as good as this one.

The use of this formula in the treatment of tinnitus, deafness, and aural hallucinations is also due to its ability to control 'upward rushing of deficient yang' (虛陽之上奔 *xū yáng zhī shàng bēn*). The yang referred to in this quotation from Wang You-Yuan is the ministerial fire, while deficiency refers to the Kidneys' inability to organize its harmonious ascent. Like all other commentators, Wang here points to a breakdown of the qi dynamic as the root cause. Thus, even though the texts speak of fire and water, pronounced signs of heat or cold need not be present to diagnose this pattern.

The original name of this formula was Massa Medicata Fermentata Pill (*shén qū wán*), which is also the ingredient with the highest dosage. Some physicians, such as Ni Wei-De, therefore point to this herb as the true fulcrum of the formula. Wang Zi-Jie links its use to alchemical techniques expounded in the Song dynasty Daoist classic, *Awakening to the Real*. Ke Qin, too, expounds its virtues in *Golden Mirror of the Medical Tradition*:

> Massa medicata fermentata (*shén qū*) pushes out the old and creates space for the new. Connecting with the Heart spirit above and reaching the resolve [stored in the] Kidneys below, it generates know-how. Furthermore, food is assimilated to the yin, but its strength is emitted [through] the yang. Guarding one's diet is thus all [one needs to take care of]. This is the strategy by which the *Inner Classic* treats mania. When [harbored] food is eliminated, one clearly knows what to do, and the essence spirit is regulated. This is the intended use of Massa medicata fermentata (*shén qū*).

Comparison

➤ Vs. Cinnabar Pill to Calm the Spirit (*zhū shā ān shén wán*)

Both of these formulas treat disordered spirit associated with Heart excess patterns manifesting with symptoms such as agitation, irritability, restlessness, palpitations, insomnia, and dream-disturbed sleep. However, Cinnabar Pill to Calm the Spirit (*zhū shā ān shén wán*) focuses on cooling the flaring Heart fire that is damaging the blood and yin fluids. Besides the symptoms outlined above, this type of fire is experienced as disorientation, a sensation of fullness in the chest or of heat flushes, and even occasional vomiting or retching. Magnetite and Cinnabar Pill (*cí zhū wán*), on the other hand, focuses on directing the floating yang downward to anchor it in the Kidneys. It is thus primarily used to reconnect the Heart and Kidneys, with symptoms such as mania, tinnitus, deafness, or epilepsy. It is also an important formula for eye disorders presenting with blurred vision.

Biomedical Indications

With the appropriate presentation, this formula may be used to treat a wide variety of biomedically-defined disorders. These can be divided into the following groups:

- Disorders of the eyes including cataracts, optic nerve atrophy, and disorders of the vitreous humor or lens
- Psychoneurological problems including some types of neural deafness, aural vertigo, epilepsy, tinnitus, and visual hallucinations associated with schizophrenia.

This formula has also been used in the treatment of hypertension.

Alternate names

Vision Improving Pill with Magnetite (*míng mù cí shí wán*) in *Classified Compilation of Medical Prescriptions*; Magnetite Pill (*cí shí wán*) in *Comprehensive Recording of Sagely Beneficence*; Highly Valuable Medicated Leaven Pill (*qiān jīn shén qū wán*) in *Discussion of Illnesses, Patterns, and Formulas Related to the Unification of the Three Etiologies*; Magnetite and Cinnabar Pill (*cí shén wán*) in *Introduction to Medicine*

Modifications

- For seizures with abundant phlegm, add Pinelliae Rhizoma praeparatum (*zhì bàn xià*), Arisaema cum Bile (*dǎn nán xīng*), and Haematitum (*dài zhě shí*).

- For concurrent Liver and Kidney yin deficiency, combine with Six-Ingredient Pill with Rehmannia (*liù wèi dì huáng wán*).

- For phlegm-heat in the chest, take with Warm Gallbladder Decoction (*wēn dǎn tāng*).

- For seizures with abundant mucus, add Pinelliae Rhizoma praeparatum (*zhì bàn xià*), Arisaema cum Bile (*dǎn nán xīng*), and Haematitum (*dài zhě shí*).

- For irritability, fever, and severe insomnia, add Gardeniae Fructus (*zhī zǐ*) and Nelumbinis Plumula (*lián zǐ xīn*).

- For severe palpitations, add Fossilia Dentis Mastodi (*lóng chǐ*) and Mauritiae/Cypraeae Concha (*zǐ bèi chǐ*).

生鐵落飲 (生铁落饮)

Iron Filings Drink

shēng tiě luò yǐn

Source   *Awakening of the Mind in Medical Studies* (1732)

Ferri Frusta (*shēng tiě luò*)	15-60g
Arisaema cum Bile (*dǎn nán xīng*)	3g
Fritillariae Bulbus (*bèi mǔ*)	9g
Scrophulariae Radix (*xuán shēn*)	4.5g
Asparagi Radix (*tiān mén dōng*)	9g
Ophiopogonis Radix (*mài mén dōng*)	9g
Forsythiae Fructus (*lián qiào*)	3g
Uncariae Ramulus cum Uncis (*gōu téng*)	4.5g
Salviae miltiorrhizae Radix (*dān shēn*)	4.5g
Poria (*fú líng*)	3g
Poriae Sclerotium pararadicis (*fú shén*)	3g
Citri reticulatae Pericarpium (*chén pí*)	3g
Acori tatarinowii Rhizoma (*shí chāng pǔ*)	3g
Polygalae Radix (*yuǎn zhì*)	3g
Cinnabaris (*zhū shā*)	0.9g [add at end]

Method of Preparation   Decoction. The source text does not specify the dosage for Ferri Frusta (*shēng tiě luò*). It is first decocted in 5 cups of water that is reduced to 3 cups over a period of three hours, then the other ingredients are added. At present, the cooking period for Ferri Frusta (*shēng tiě luò*) is generally reduced to 45 minutes. Note that due to the unacceptable toxicity of Cinnabaris *(zhū shā)*, it is considered obsolete; other heavy, settling medicinals such as Fossilia Ossis Mastodi *(lóng gǔ)* or Fossilia Dentis Mastodi *(lóng chǐ)* may be substituted.

Actions Sedates the Heart, eliminates phlegm, clears fire, and calms the spirit

Indications

Restless agitation, bad temper, severe and throbbing headache, insomnia, extreme emotional instability, manic behavior, shouting, yelling at people for no apparent reason, reddish eyes, a scarlet tongue with a yellow, greasy coating, and a wiry, rapid pulse.

This is manic behavior due to phlegm-fire agitating the Heart. Emotional constraint in people with a robust constitution manifests in stagnation of yang qi that transforms into heat, accompanied by an accumulation of stagnant fluids that transform into phlegm. Phlegm and heat clump and under certain circumstances 'explode' upward as phlegm-fire. Because of its excess nature, such a pattern is also known as 'yang brightness phlegm-fire.' The explosion upward leads to a severe, throbbing headache. It disturbs the spirit and manifests as restless agitation, bad temper, and insomnia. Phlegm-fire veils the sensorium (i.e., the orifices of the Heart and spirit), leading to extreme emotional instability, manic behavior, shouting, and yelling at people for no apparent reason. The reddish eyes, scarlet tongue with a yellow, greasy coating, and the wiry, rapid pulse reflect the combination of ascendant yang, fire, and phlegm.

Analysis of Formula

To effectively treat acute manic behavior from phlegm fire harassing the upper burner, one should use a strategy of sedating the Heart and calming the spirit, flushing away phlegm, and clearing fire. The chief ingredients in this formula are Ferri Frusta *(shēng tiě luò)*, which enters the Liver channel to treat anger and mania, and Cinnabaris *(zhū shā)*, which enters the Heart. Both strongly anchor and weigh down the spirit.

The deputies are of three types. The first group clears heat and flushes out phlegm. It consists of bitter and cooling Arisaema cum Bile *(dǎn nán xīng)*, an important herb for dispelling wind-phlegm and treating seizures, and bitter, sweet, and cooling Fritillariae Bulbus *(bèi mǔ)*, which enters the upper burner to clear Heart fire and disperse Lung constraint. The second group eliminates phlegm, opens the sensory orifices, and calms the spirit. It includes acrid and slightly warming Acori tatarinowii Rhizoma *(shí chāng pǔ)*, which is said to direct qi downward and thus works well together with acrid, bitter, and slightly warming Polygalae Radix *(yuǎn zhì)*, which is said to raise the qi. Bland and sweet Poriae Sclerotium pararadicis *(fú shén)*, which drains

dampness and thereby deprives phlegm of its source, also belongs to this group. The third type of deputies clears Heart fire and relieves irritability. It includes bitter and slightly cooling Forsythiae Fructus *(lián qiáo)*, which is light and opens constraint in the upper burner; bitter and slightly cooling Salviae miltiorrhizae Radix *(dān shēn)*, which clears heat from the blood aspect and prevents blood stasis; sweet and slightly cooling Uncariae Ramulus cum Uncis *(gōu téng)*, which dispels wind-heat and settles fright; and bitter, sweet, salty, and cooling Scrophulariae Radix *(xuán shēn)*, which enters the Kidneys, clears floating heat, and, according to *Miscellaneous Records of Famous Physicians,* is said "to govern [the treatment] of mania [characterized by] extreme confusion and the inability to recognize people." Working together, the deputies support the function of the chief ingredients by ordering the pathologies of the fluid metabolism that manifest as phlegm: opening stagnation through acrid and bitter dispersal to promote the unhindered diffusion of fluids; clearing fire from the protective, nutritive, and blood aspects to prevent the clumping of fluids and heat that produces phlegm; and dispelling wind in order to regularize the movement of qi.

The assistants further consolidate these effects. One group, comprised of Poria *(fú líng)* and Citri reticulatae Pericarpium *(chén pí)*, treats phlegm at its source by improving the function of the Spleen and qi. The other group, comprised of Ophiopogonis Radix *(mài mén dōng)* and Asparagi Radix *(tiān mén dōng)*, nourishes the yin to replenish the physiological fluids.

Commentary

This is a rather effective formula in treating the manic behavior associated with phlegm-fire. Cheng Guo-Peng, author of the source text, notes that most people who take it for twenty-odd days will be cured. He also states that if there is also constipation, the patient should first be given Flushing Away Roiling Phlegm Pill *(gǔn tán wán)*.

Historically, this is one of the few formulas that can be traced back to the *Inner Classic. Basic Questions,* Chapter 26, recommends the use of a decoction made from Ferri Frusta *(shēng tiě luò)* to treat 'yang inversion' (陽厥 *yáng jué*), a condition characterized by mania and anger due to sudden, strong upward-flushing of qi.

Comparison

➤ Vs. Cinnabar Pill to Calm the Spirit *(zhū shā ān shén wán)*

Both of these formulas treat disordered spirit associated with patterns of Heart fire excess. However, Cinnabar Pill to Calm the Spirit *(zhū shā ān shén wán)* treats Heart fire patterns with secondary yin or blood deficiency. This is a type of yin fire arising from internal causes, specifically disordered emotions, and the formula focuses on guiding yang fire excess downward by means of bitter, cooling, and heavy settling substances. Iron Filings Drink (*shēng tiě luò yǐn*), on the other hand, is primarily indicated for patterns where phlegm-fire agitating the Heart leads to manic behavior. For this purpose, the formula combines herbs that transform and dispel phlegm with substances that sedate the Heart and cool the fire. No bitter, cooling substances are used as these might further inhibit the qi dynamic.

Biomedical Indications

With the appropriate presentation, this formula may be used to treat a variety of biomedically-defined disorders including some psychiatric diseases and epilepsy.

Modifications

- For thirst with a desire to drink, and parched mouth and lips, add Gypsum fibrosum (*shí gāo*), Anemarrhenae Rhizoma (*zhī mǔ*), and Dendrobii Herba (*shí hú*).
- For pronounced irritability and insomnia due to phlegm-heat, add Coptidis Rhizoma (*huáng lián*), Rehmanniae Radix (*shēng dì huáng*), Bambusae Caulis in taeniam (*zhú rú*), and Aurantii Fructus immaturus (*zhǐ shí*).
- For red eyes and a thick, yellow tongue coating, add Saigae tataricae Cornu (*líng yáng jiǎo*).
- For abdominal distention accompanied by a sense of fullness, constipation, and a dry tongue coating, combine with Regulate the Stomach and Order the Qi Decoction (*tiáo wèi chéng qì tāng*).

珍珠母丸
Mother-of-Pearl Pill
zhēn zhū mǔ wán

Source   *Formulas of Universal Benefit from My Practice* (1132)

Margaritiferae Concha usta (*zhēn zhū mǔ*) 21-30g
Fossilia Dentis Mastodi (*lóng chǐ*) 15g
dry-fried Angelicae sinensis Radix (*chǎo dāng guī*) 45g
Rehmanniae Radix praeparata (*shú dì huáng*) 45g
Ginseng Radix (*rén shēn*) 30g
dry-fried Ziziphi spinosae Semen (*chǎo suān zǎo rén*) 30g
Platycladi Semen (*bǎi zǐ rén*) 30g
[Bubali Cornu (*shuǐ niú jiǎo*) . . . . 30-60g]
Poriae Sclerotium pararadicis (*fú shén*) 15g
Aquilariae Lignum resinatum (*chén xiāng*) 15g

Method of Preparation   Grind the ingredients into a powder and form into very small pills with honey. The pills were originally coated with Cinnabaris (*zhū shā*), but this is no longer done due to the toxicity of this substance. Take at

noon and before going to bed. The original text calls for 15g of Rhinocerotis Cornu (*xī jiǎo*), which is no longer used, primarily due to the endangered status of the rhinoceros. Also, Codonopsis Radix (*dǎng shēn*) is usually substituted for Ginseng Radix (*rén shēn*) at 2-3 times its dosage. Originally, 0.9-1.5g of Margarita (*zhēn zhū*) was used instead of Margaritiferae Concha usta (*zhēn zhū mǔ*). The latter is now substituted because it is much less expensive.

Actions   Enriches the yin, nourishes the blood, sedates the Heart, calms the spirit, calms the Liver, and anchors the yang

Indications

Irritability, restless sleep, occasional palpitations with anxiety, dizziness, and a thin, wiry pulse.

This is concurrent blood and yin deficiency with ascendant Liver yang. When the yin and blood are insufficient, the yang loses its control and becomes hyperactive. Rushing upward, it harrasses the upper burner, causing dizziness. Internally, the uncontrolled movement of yang qi is experienced as irritability. Entering the Heart, it leads to palpitations, restless sleep, and anxiety. The thin, wiry pulse reflects deficiency of yin and blood complicated by the excess condition of hyperactive Liver yang.

Analysis of Formula

While blood and yin deficiency are the true root of this pattern, this formula primarily seeks to control the hyperactive yang. To this end, it combines heavy, settling ingredients aimed at calming the spirit and anchoring the yang with herbs that nourish the blood and enrich the yin. The chief ingredients are salty and cooling Margaritiferae Concha usta (*zhēn zhū mǔ*) and astringent and slightly cooling Fossilia Dentis Mastodi (*lóng chǐ*). By means of their heavy nature, these substances calm the Liver, sedate the spirit, and anchor the errant yang. They are supported by three deputies: sweet, sour, and balanced Ziziphi spinosae Semen (*suān zǎo rén*), sweet and acrid Platycladi Semen (*bǎi zǐ rén*), and sweet and bland Poriae Sclerotium pararadicis (*fú shén*). Because of their ability to nourish the Heart and regulate its physiology, these herbs are commonly used together in formulas that calm the spririts. They do so primarily by harmonizing the physiology and nature of the nutritive qi and blood on which the Heart depends for its nourishment.

This function is further supported by the three assistants: sweet, acrid, and warming Angelicae sinensis Radix (*dāng guī*), sweet, rich, and slightly warming Rehmanniae Radix praeparata (*shú dì huáng*), and sweet, slightly bitter, and slightly warming Ginseng Radix (*rén shēn*). Together, these herbs tonify the qi, nourish the blood, and enrich the yin. They thereby assist the chief ingredients in anchoring the yang, while providing the spirit with an abode. Bitter, salty, and cooling Bubali Cornu (*shuǐ niú jiǎo*) and acrid, bitter, and warming Aquilariae Lignum resinatum *(chén xiāng)* comprise a second group of assistants that regulate the qi dynamic. Bubali Cornu *(shuǐ niú jiǎo)* clears heat from the nutritive qi and settles fright, while Aquilariae Lignum resinatum *(chén xiāng)* directs the qi from the upper into the lower burner, facilitating the transformation of hyperactive yang into physiological qi. The small amount of Cinnabaris *(zhū shā)*, which is used to coat the pills, serves as an envoy that focuses the action of the entire formula on the spirit.

Note that, due to its endangered status, Rhinocerotis Cornu *(xī jiǎo)* is not used at present; Bubali Cornu *(shuǐ niú jiǎo)* is substituted, with a much larger dosage. Also, the endangered status of Aquilariae Lignum resinatum *(chén xiāng)* can make it difficult to obtain, as a certificate of cultivation is needed for importation.

Overall, therefore, this formula is very balanced. According to Ran Xue-Feng in *Annotated Fine Formulas from Generations of Famous Physicians*, "it uses moistening in order to tonify, and tonification in order to unblock. Nurturing the generating dynamic for the good offices of the normal qi, this is the mildest formula among those that sedate and calm the spirit."

Cautions and Contraindications

This formula contains a number of cloying ingredients and is therefore contraindicated in the treatment of insomnia, fright palpitations, and similar conditions in those with patterns of phlegm-dampness or phlegm-heat.

Commentary

This formula was composed by the Song-dynasty physician Xu Shou-Wei. It is listed in the source text as treating windstroke with the following pattern:

> When a wind pathogen is received in the interior due to [preexisting] deficiency of the Liver channel, the ethereal soul disperses [and cannot be] conserved. The presentation is one of fright palpitations.

In Chinese medicine, fright palpitations are defined as those caused by sudden shock and fright, such as witnessing or hearing something horrible or frightening, especially when it is completely unexpected. Ordinary palpitations may also be accompanied by anxiety, but there the causation is reversed, that is, palpitations reflect a state of nervousness in which one becomes more easily frightened, rather than fright causing the palpitations.

Most commentators have followed Xu Shou-Wei's interpretation and define Liver deficiency producing internal

wind as the pathodynamic underlying this pattern. Based on their own clinical experience, later physicians added other symptoms to this pattern. *One-Hundred Questions on Women's Disorders*, for instance, prescribes its for the treatment of "red-colored urine [with urination] that is neither rough nor painful," suggesting the presence of internal heat. This is likely, as the Liver carries the ministerial fire, which by its nature is hot. In contemporary texts such as *Annotated Fine Formulas from Generations of Famous Physicians* by Ran Xue-Feng, this is further linked to nervous system disorders. In *Six Texts Summarizing the Medicine of Xu Ling-Tai*, the Qing-dynasty scholar-physician Xu Da-Chun attributes this pathodynamic to:

> Liver deficiency with blazing heat [in which] the overwhelming heat engenders wind. [The wind] prevents the Heart qi from directing downward [and the Liver] from storing the ethereal soul. Restless sleeping and dreaming ensue, generating [a pattern characterized by] fright palpitations and insomnia.

Comparison

➤ Vs. Cinnabar Pill to Calm the Spirit *(zhū shā ān shén wán)*

Both of these formulas treat disordered spirit associated with fire excess and blood deficiency leading to such symptoms as agitation, irritability, restlessness, palpitations, insomnia, and dream-disturbed sleep. However, Cinnabar Pill to Calm the Spirit *(zhū shā ān shén wán)* focuses on the Heart, whereas Mother-of-Pearl Pill *(zhēn zhū mǔ wán)* focuses on the Liver. This is reflected in symptoms such as dizziness and a thin, wiry pulse. The pulse in patterns for which Cinnabar Pill to Calm the Spirit *(zhū shā ān shén wán)* is indicated will, instead, tend to be thin and rapid.

Biomedical Indications

With the appropriate presentation, this formula may be used to treat a variety of biomedically-defined disorders including epilepsy and cataracts.

....

Alternate names

Mother-of-Pearl Pill *(zhēn zhū mǔ wán)* in *Synopsis for Protecting Infants*; Mother-of-Pearl Special Pill *(zhēn zhū dān)* in *Additions to the Essential Teachings of [Zhu] Dan-Xi*

....

Modification

• For a more severe presentation, add Magnetitum *(cí shí)*, Ostreae Concha *(mǔ lì)*, or Fossilia Ossis Mastodi *(lóng gǔ)*.

Comparative Tables of Principal Formulas

■ FORMULAS THAT NOURISH THE HEART (BLOOD AND YIN) AND CALM THE SPIRIT

Common symptoms: irritability, sleep disturbances, palpitations with anxiety, thin and rapid pulse

Formula Name	Diagnosis	Indications	Remarks
Emperor of Heaven's Special Pill to Tonify the Heart (*tiān wáng bǔ xīn dān*)	Yin and blood deficiency with the Heart and Kidneys failing to communicate	Irritability, palpitations, anxiety, insomnia with very restless sleep, inability to concentrate, nocturnal emissions, dry stools, a red tongue with little coating, and a thin, rapid pulse	Focuses on treating irritability. Also for apthous ulcers, recurrent urticaria, and chronic conjunctivitis.
Sour Jujube Decoction (*suān zǎo rén tāng*)	Liver blood deficiency with constraint and internal fire	Irritability, inability to sleep, palpitations, night sweats, dizziness and vertigo, dry throat and mouth, dry tongue, and a wiry or thin, rapid pulse	This is deficiency irritability, often arising in the wake of an illness or exhaustion from overwork. Also for pain such as trigeminal neuralgia and migraine.
Settle the Emotions Pill (*dìng zhì wán*)	Heart qi deficiency and constraint caused by phlegm turbidity	Apprehensiveness, easily frightened, worried, incessant laughter and glee, fright palpitations, forgetfulness, dizziness, and a pale tongue with a white coating	Also for near-sightedness.
Coptis and Ass-Hide Gelatin Decoction (*huáng lián ē jiāo tāng*)	Heat excess and blood deficiency in the Heart lesser yin warp	Irritability with a sensation of heat in the chest, insomnia, palpitations, anxiety, possible mouth or tongue sores, a red tongue with a dry, yellow coating, and a thin, rapid pulse	This is a heat transformation pattern at the lesser yin warp. Also for bleeding disorders, or dysenteric disorders due to heat toxin.
Licorice, Wheat, and Jujube Decoction (*gān mài dà zǎo tāng*)	Qi and yin deficiency of the Heart and Spleen	Disorientation, frequent attacks of melancholy and crying spells, inability to control oneself, restless sleep (sometimes with night sweats), frequent yawning, and in severe cases, abnormal behavior and speech	This is called restless organ disorder.

■ FORMULAS THAT SEDATE AND CALM THE SPIRIT

Common symptoms: upward-wafting spirit with severe irritability, palpitations, insomnia with dream-disturbed sleep, red tongue, and usually a wiry and rapid pulse

Formula Name	Diagnosis	Indications	Remarks
Cinnabar Pill to Calm the Spirit (*zhū shā ān shén wán*)	Vigorous Heart fire injuring the blood and yin	Insomnia, continuous palpitations, a sensation of irritability and heat in the chest, a desire to vomit without result, dream-disturbed sleep, a tongue that is red at the tip, and a thin, rapid pulse	Especially useful for palpitations and anxiety that occur during dreams. Focuses on guiding yang fire excess downward.
Magnetite and Cinnabar Pill (*cí zhū wán*)	Ascendant Heart yang with lack of communication between the Heart and Kidneys	Palpitations, insomnia, tinnitus, and diminished acuity of hearing and vision	Also for epilepsy and cataracts. Focuses on directing floating yang downward to anchor it in the Kidneys.
Iron Filings Drink (*shēng tiě luò yǐn*)	Phlegm-fire agitating the Heart	Restless agitation, severe and throbbing headache, insomnia, extreme emotional instability, yelling at people for no reason, red eyes, a scarlet tongue with a yellow, greasy coating, and a wiry, rapid pulse	Focuses on transforming and dispelling phlegm.
Mother-of-Pearl Pill (*zhēn zhū mǔ wán*)	Concurrent blood and yin deficiency with ascendant Liver yang	Irritability, restless sleep, occasional palpitations with anxiety, dizziness, and a thin, wiry pulse	This is the mildest of the sedating formulas. Focuses on the Liver.

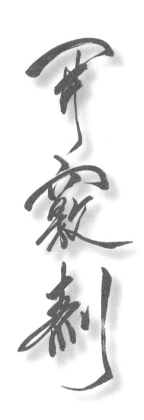

Chapter 11 Contents

Formulas that Open the Sensory Orifices

Formulas that Open the Sensory Orifices 11

THE FORMULAS IN this chapter aromatically open the sensory orifices associated with the spirit or Heart, which in Chinese medicine are said to be closed when there is a loss of consciousness or coma. A passage in Chapter 8 of *Basic Questions* observes, "The heart holds the office of emperor and is the issuer of spirit clarity (神明 *shén míng*)." In Chinese medicine, 'spirit clarity' corresponds to consciousness, so loss of consciousness can occur whenever a pathogen penetrates into the Pericardium, which envelops and protects the Heart, resulting in a veiling of the sensory orifices, which are referred to as the orifices of the Heart (心竅 *xīn qiào*).

Loss of consciousness may be due either to excess or deficiency. When the problem is one of excess, it is known as a 'closed disorder' (閉證 *bì zhèng*) in which pathogens obstruct and veil the sensory orifices. It is the treatment of these disorders that is the subject of this chapter. When the problem is one of deficiency, it is called an abandoned disorder (脫證 *tuō zhèng*), which manifests as loss of consciousness with excessive sweating, cold extremities, bowel and urinary incontinence, flaccidity, open mouth and eyes, and a frail or faint pulse. The formulas for treating abandoned disorders are discussed in Chapters 6 and 9.

Closed disorders are of two types, hot and cold. The hot-type closed disorder is due to pathogenic heat or heat toxin sinking into the Pericardium, and is treated by clearing the heat to open the sensory orifices. The cold-type closed disorder is due to pathogenic cold and constrained qi generating turbid phlegm, which veils the orifices of the Heart. It is treated by warming the cold and unblocking the qi to open the sensory orifices.

Before using these formulas to open the sensory orifices, one should first determine whether the disorder is deficient or excessive in nature. If the pathogenic influences predominate and are excessive in nature, with such manifestations as clenched jaw, clenched fists, rigid limbs, and a forceful pulse in addition to loss of consciousness or mental confusion, one may proceed to use these formulas. For yang brightness-organ disorders with delirious speech and partial or complete loss of consciousness, the strategy of draining the accumulation of heat (see Chapter 2) should be used instead of opening the orifices. For yang brightness-organ disorders that also involve pathogenic heat sinking into the Pericardium, one may elect between first opening the orifices or draining the accumulation of heat, or proceeding with both methods simultaneously.

Even when the clinical presentation is appropriate for these formulas, they should only be used short-term for treating the acute symptoms. If used long-term, their dispersing properties can readily injure the normal qi.

Historically, while the treatment strategy for this type of disorder can be traced back to Chapter 74 of *Basic Questions*, which says that, under appropriate conditions, disorders can be opened up or discharged (開之發之 *kāi zhī fā zhī*), it is not until the Tang dynasty that formulas were specifically designed for this type of problem. While formulas in Sun Si-Miao's *Supplement to the Thousand Ducat Formulas* and Wang Tao's *Arcane Essentials from the Imperial Library* have been superseded by those of later physicians, they are the earliest extant examples of this type of prescription.

This category of formulas is generally prepared in the form of pills, powders, or injectable concentrates, for two reasons. First, they must be immediately available in emergencies when there is no time to prepare a decoction. Second, they cannot tolerate the heat of decoction because their constituents are quite volatile, and the heat will diminish their potency.

The treatment of unconscious patients requires special means of administration. Traditionally, the pills were placed in the mouth to dissolve or powders were insufflated through the nose. In modern times, other methods have been devised, namely, administering through a nasogastric tube directly into the stomach or preparing the medicine in such a way that it can be given intravenously.

Section 1

FORMULAS THAT CLEAR HEAT AND OPEN THE SENSORY ORIFICES

The formulas in this section are used for hot-type closed disorders in which the pathogenic heat or heat toxin sinks into the Pericardium causing high fever, irritability and restlessness, a red face, a yellow tongue coating, heavy breathing, delirious speech, spasms, convulsions, and loss of consciousness. These formulas are appropriate for treating wind-stroke, the accumulation of phlegm, and other disorders presenting with these manifestations.

The core ingredients of these formulas are those that aromatically clear heat and open the sensory orifices such as Bovis Calculus *(niú huáng)*, Moschus *(shè xiāng)*, and Borneolum *(bīng piàn)*.

Given the importance of heat in these disorders, along with the acidity or the aromatic ingredients (which can be drying), it is important to include medicinals that clear heat. These can be bitter and cold to resolve toxicity such as Coptidis Rhizoma *(huáng lián)* and Scutellariae Radix *(huáng qín)*; acrid and cold to treat blazing fire without drying the fluids such as Gypsum fibrosum *(shí gāo)* and Glauberitum *(hán shuǐ shí)*; or cooling purgatives to treat any excess in the yang organs such as Rhei Radix et Rhizoma *(dà huáng)* and Natrii Sulfas *(máng xiāo)*.

Because these patients are often very irritable and their spirits are somewhat unmoored, it is important to use medicinals that sedate and calm such as Succinum *(hǔ pò)*, Magnetitum *(cí shí)*, and Margaritiferae Concha usta *(zhēn zhū mǔ)*.

Because these conditions often have an aspect of internally-generated wind, medicinals are often added to extinguish wind and stop tremors. These include Saigae tataricae Cornu *(líng yáng jiǎo)*, Gastrodiae Rhizoma *(tiān má)*, and Uncariae Ramulus cum Uncis *(gōu téng)*.

When the sensory orifices are veiled by phlegm, one should add medicinals that clear heat and transform phlegm such as Arisaema cum Bile *(dǎn nán xīng)* and Fritillariae cirrhosae Bulbus *(chuān bèi mǔ)*.

萬氏牛黃清心丸 (万氏牛黄清心丸)
Wan's Cattle Gallstone Pill to Clear the Heart
Wàn shì niú huáng qīng xīn wán

This formula clears the Heart and opens the sensory orifices with Bovis Calculus *(niú huáng)* as its chief ingredient. It is drawn from a book by Wan Quan and bears this name to differentiate it from other formulas with a similar name.

Source *Essential Teachings about Pox and Rashes Passed down in Medical Lineages* (1568)

Bovis Calculus *(niú huáng)*	0.75g
Cinnabaris *(zhū shā)*	4.5g
Coptidis Rhizoma *(huáng lián)*	15g
Scutellariae Radix *(huáng qín)*	9g
Gardeniae Fructus *(zhī zǐ)*	9g
Curcumae Radix *(yù jīn)*	6g

Method of Preparation The source text advises to grind the ingredients into a powder and form into millet-sized pills with flour and snow that has fallen during the twelfth month of the Chinese calendar. Seven or eight pills are taken with a decoction of Junci Medulla *(dēng xīn cǎo)*. At present, the ingredients are ground into a powder and formed into 1.5g pills with honey. Two pills are taken 2-3 times daily, with a reduction in dosage for children. Note that due to the unacceptable toxicity of Cinnabaris *(zhū shā)*, it should no longer be used.

Actions Clears heat, resolves toxicity, opens up the orifices, and calms the spirit

Indications

Fever, irritability and restlessness, generalized sense of unease, delirious speech, impaired consciousness, and in some cases childhood convulsions or the closed type of wind-stroke. The tongue will be scarlet red and the pulse thin and rapid or wiry and rapid.

This is pathogenic heat sinking into the interior and entering the Pericardium. While heat entering the Lungs is viewed as a normal transmission (順傳 *shùn chuán*), this is regarded as an abnormal transmission (逆傳 *nì chuán*), at least since the time of Ye Tian-Shi. The distinction between normal and abnormal here refers to the more serious nature of the latter compared to the former. It also refers to the difference between Lung patterns, which relate to qi, and Pericardium patterns, which relate to blood. Pathogenic heat in this pattern penetrates from the qi into the nutritive and blood aspect to harass the spirit and block the orifices of the Heart. This manifests as fever along with irritability, restlessness, and a generalized sense of unease that can progress to delirious speech and impaired consciousness. From an organ perspective, it involves both the Heart and Liver, as noted in the source text: "When the Heart transmits heat to the Liver, wind and fire contend with each other." In terms of warm pathogen disorder theory, where the focus is on the Pericardium rather than the Heart, the connection between these organs is established both via the blood and the terminal yin. The intense heat affecting two organs that focus on the blood manifests as a scarlet red tongue. Depending on the intensity of the heat vis-à-vis the wind, the pulse will be either thin and rapid or wiry and rapid.

Analysis of Formula

This formula treats impaired consciousness from heat affecting the Heart and Pericardium. It does this by focusing on clearing and resolving toxic heat in the Pericardium with aromatic medicinals that open the sensory orifices, assisted by others that sedate jitteriness and calm the spirit.

The chief ingredient is the aromatic, bitter, and cooling Bovis Calculus *(niú huáng),* which excels at clearing intense heat from the Heart and Liver while also venting pathogens from the Pericardium. At the same time, this medicinal excels at dislodging phlegm, opening the orifices, extinguishing wind, and stopping tremors. Three of the deputies—Coptidis Rhizoma *(huáng lián),* Scutellariae Radix *(huáng qín),* and Gardeniae Fructus *(zhī zǐ)*—are bitter, cold herbs that are good at clearing heat, draining fire, and resolving toxicity. They are used here to aid the chief ingredient in clearing heat from the Heart and resolving toxicity. *New Compilation of Materia Medica* states that Coptidis Rhizoma *(huáng lián)* "enters the Heart and Pericardium where it is the ultimate at draining fire. It is also able to enter the Liver. While it can guide into both of these channels, it is especially entrusted [to guide other herbs] to enter the Heart." Because this formula emphasizes clearing heat and opening the orifices, Coptidis Rhizoma *(huáng lián)* has by far the largest dosage among these heat-clearing, fire-draining herbs. The last deputy is bitter and cooling Curcumae Radix *(yù jīn),* which also enters the Heart and Liver channels. It is good at cooling the blood, clearing the Heart, promoting proper movement of qi, and opening up areas of constraint. It helps Bovis Calculus *(niú huáng)* to clear the Heart and open the orifices. Together, these medicinals clear heat, resolve toxicity, open the sensory orifices, and calm the spirit.

Cautions and Contraindications

Do not use in abandoned disorders or for any problem that is not due to clogging and overabundance. Due to the intense bitter and cold nature of this formula, it should not be taken long-term.

Commentary

In this formula, the clearing of heat and draining of fire is the foundation; opening the orifices and calming the spirit is of secondary importance. It can be viewed as a modification of Coptis Decoction to Resolve Toxicity *(huáng lián jiě dú tāng)* from *Arcane Essentials from the Imperial Library.* The ingredient in that formula that drained heat from the lower burner, Phellodendri Cortex *(huáng bǎi),* has been replaced with medicinals that enter the Heart channel to clear heat, open the sensory orifices, and calm the spirit. In turn, this formula is the basis upon which the Qing physician Wu Ju-Tong developed Calm the Palace Pill with Cattle Gallstone *(ān gōng niú huáng wán),* which is the following entry.

Appropriate Presentation for this Formula

In the source text, this formula is prescribed for "Heart heat with impaired consciousness." This indication was expanded, especially by the warm pathogen disease current. For example, in the early 20th-century work *Convenient Reader of Established Formulas,* it is noted that this formula should be used:

> [f]or a warm pathogen sinking internally such that the heat enters the Pericardium, phlegm and mucus clogs and obstructs, with such conditions as impaired consciousness, delirious speech, sudden collapse, locked jaw, as well as acute fright wind in children.

Identification

There is a very complex formula by the same name in *Formulary of the Pharmacy Service for Benefiting the People in the Taiping Era.* It is based on Dioscorea Pill (薯蕷丸 *shǔ yù wán)* from *Essentials from the Golden Cabinet,* and contains 29 ingredients. That formula, which focuses more on clearing the Heart, transforming phlegm, and dispelling wind, is also used in the present day and is known as Cattle Gallstone Pill to Clear the Heart from the *Formulary (niú huáng qīng xīn wán -[jú fāng]).* To avoid confusion, the formula discussed in this entry is commonly referred to as Wan's Cattle Gallstone Pill to Clear the Heart *(Wàn shì niú huáng qīng xīn wán).*

Discussing the various formulas called Cattle Gallstone Pill to Clear the Heart *(niú huáng qīng xīn wán),* Wang Zi-Jie in *Selected Annotations to Ancient Formulas from the Garden of Crimson Snow* notes:

> For treating impaired consciousness from a warm pathogen sinking internally into the enveloping collaterals [i.e., Pericar-

dium], only the one by Wan is marvelous. When a warm-heat pathogen enters into the collaterals of the Pericardium, the pathogen has gone into the interior. The aroma of plants is only able to thrust out [the pathogen] from the exterior; it is unable to vent [it] from the interior. It is necessary to use a substance with a concealed aroma, such as Bovis Calculus (*niú huáng*), that can penetrate through the Pericardium and connect with the consciousness (神明 *shén míng*). Still, it is always appropriate to match these [medicinals] with substances that can assist them.

Comparison

> ➤ Vs. Calm the Palace Pill with Cattle Gallstone (*ān gōng niú huáng wán*)

Both of these formulas treat heat entering the Pericardium with resulting fever and changes in consciousness. Wan's Cattle Gallstone Pill to Clear the Heart (*Wàn shì niú huáng qīng xīn wán*) is slightly weaker than Calm the Palace Pill with Cattle Gallstone (*ān gōng niú huáng wán*), which is used in emergencies; the former is used for milder disorders. Furthermore, while Wan's Cattle Gallstone Pill to Clear the Heart (*Wàn shì niú huáng qīng xīn wán*) focuses on clearing heat and resolving toxicity with such symptoms as fever, irritability, and restlessness, Calm the Palace Pill with Cattle Gallstone (*ān gōng niú huáng wán*) is better at calming the spirit and opening the sensory orifices with such symptoms as high fever, delirium, and semiconsciousness.

Biomedical Indications

With the appropriate presentation, this formula may be used to treat a variety of biomedically-defined disorders including viral encephalitis, meningitis, pertussis, measles-induced pneumonia, and aphthous ulcers.

Alternate names

Wan's Cattle Gallstone Pill to Clear the Heart (*Wàn shì niú huáng qīng xīn wán*) in *Collected Treatises of [Zhang] Jing-Yue*; Wan's Cattle Gallstone Pill (*Wàn shì niú huáng wán*) in *Simple and Appropriate Medical Formulas*; Cattle Gallstone Pill (*niú huáng wán*) in *Precious Mirror of Patterns and Treatments*

Modifications

• For pox and sores when the lesions are a normal color and are not painful, but the person is irritable and ill at ease and has an aversion to heat, take the pills with a decoction of Junci Medulla (*dēng xīn cǎo*). (source text)

• For maculopapular rashes with fever, twitching, and normal urination, take the pills with Guide Out the Red Powder (*dǎo chì sǎn*). (source text)

• For fever and delirium as if one sees ghosts, take the pills with Guide Out the Red Powder (*dǎo chì sǎn*). (source text)

安宮黃牛丸（安宫牛黄丸）
Calm the Palace Pill with Cattle Gallstone
ān gōng niú huáng wán

The palace is a compound in which the emperor resides. It is used here as a metaphor for the Pericardium, which surrounds and shields the sovereign organ (the Heart) in the same manner as a palace surrounds and protects the emperor. This formula clears heat from the Pericardium, which calms the Heart's spirit.

Source *Systematic Differentiation of Warm Pathogen Diseases* (1798)

Bovis Calculus (*niú huáng*) 30g
[Bubali Cornu (*shuǐ niú jiǎo*) . . . . .60g]
Moschus (*shè xiāng*) 7.5g
Coptidis Rhizoma (*huáng lián*) .30g
Scutellariae Radix (*huáng qín*) .30g
Gardeniae Fructus (*zhī zǐ*) 30g
Realgar (*xióng huáng*) 30g
Borneolum (*bīng piàn*) 7.5g
Curcumae Radix (*yù jīn*) 30g
Cinnabaris (*zhū shā*) 30g
Margarita (*zhēn zhū*) 15g

Method of Preparation Grind the ingredients into a powder and form into pills with honey. The pills should be 3g in weight and are traditionally coated with gold leaf, although this is not the modern practice. Take one 3g pill 2-3 times daily (depending on the severity of the condition and the strength of the patient) with warm water. The source text advises that children take one-half pill at a time, which has been refined at present to one-quarter pill for children under 3 and one-half pill for those 4-6 years of age. If the patient is comatose, the formula may be administered via a nasogastric tube.

Note that the original text specifies 30g of Rhinocerotis Cornu (*xī jiǎo*), which is no longer used, primarily due to the endangered status of the rhinoceros. At present, due to their heavy metal content, neither Cinnabaris (*zhū shā*) nor Realgar (*xióng huáng*) should be used.

Actions Clears heat, resolves toxicity, dislodges phlegm, opens the sensory orifices, and calms the spirit

Indications

High fever, irritability and restlessness, delirious speech, impaired consciousness, the sound of phlegm in the throat, a dry mouth, a parched tongue that is red or scarlet, and a rapid pulse. Also for coma due to wind-stroke or childhood convulsions with a similar presentation, and for stiffness of the tongue and frigid extremities.

This is a serious abnormal progression of a warm-febrile disease. The pathogenic heat sinks into the Pericardium and disturbs the spirit causing high fever, irritability and restlessness, delirious speech, impaired consciousness or coma. As noted in Chapter 71 of *Divine Pivot*, "All the pathogenic influences that [appear to be] in the Heart are in the collateral of the Heart's wrap [i.e., the Pericardium]." The blazing heat in the interior scorches and condenses the fluids, which leads not only to a red or scarlet tongue and a rapid pulse, but also to phlegm that can be heard in the throat, veils the sensory orifices, and impairs the consciousness. As stated by Zhang Bing-Cheng in *Convenient Reader of Established Formulas,* "Presentations of warm pathogens sinking internally must include sticky, greasy, filthy turbidity lingering in the midst of the diaphragm." This turbid phlegm aggravates the impaired consciousness due to heat. This is one type of serious phlegm-heat and can lead to a loss of consciousness.

This pattern may also be viewed as a hot-type closed disorder due to phlegm-heat obstructing the orifices of the Heart. This often occurs in cases of childhood convulsions or coma due to wind-stroke. Because the Heart 'opens' through the tongue, the tongue may become stiff, making speech difficult. The internal obstruction from pathogenic heat sinking deep into the body may confine the yang qi in the interior. When the yang qi is unable to reach the extremities, they become very cold. This combination of impaired consciousness, stiff tongue, and very cold extremities (distal to the elbow) is called 'limb collapse' (肢厥 *zhī jué*).

Analysis of Formula

This formula is designed to clear heat and resolve toxicity in the Pericardium. Its focus is on aromatically opening the orifices, while secondarily dislodging phlegm and calming the spirit. This will result in clearing of the heat toxin, opening of the sensory orifices, transforming of the turbid phlegm, and calming of the spirit.

One of the chief ingredients, bitter, cool, and aromatic Bovis Calculus *(niú huáng)*, is very effective in clearing heat from both the Heart and Liver channels. Its aromatic properties vent heat to the exterior by way of the collaterals of the Pericardium. In addition, this ingredient resolves toxicity and dislodges phlegm to open the sensory orifices, extinguish wind, and stop the spasms, tremors, or convulsions. It thereby addresses all the major aspects of this condition. The second chief ingredient, Moschus *(shè xiāng)*, aromatically opens up the orifices and revives the spirit as it penetrates all twelve channels of the body. As noted in *Comprehensive Outline of the Materia Medica,* it "runs and scurries everywhere as it is able to unblock all the orifices that have difficulties and open up clogs and snags in the channels and collaterals." Its strong aromatic nature is essential in treating a disorder in which the sensory orifices are veiled by phlegm. The two chief ingredients are a strong combination for clearing the Heart and opening up the orifices.

The deputies focus on clearing heat. Salty, cold Bubali Cornu *(shuǐ niú jiǎo)* enters the nutritive and blood levels and plays an important role in clearing fire and heat from the Heart, Liver, and Stomach channels. It clears heat from the

Heart, calms the spirit, cools the blood, and resolves toxicity. Its cool, aromatic properties quickly vent pathogenic heat from the Pericardium. Coptidis Rhizoma *(huáng lián)*, which focuses on Heart fire, Scutellariae Radix *(huáng qín)*, which focuses on clearing heat from the Gallbladder and Lungs, and Gardeniae Fructus *(zhī zi)*, which clears and disperses heat from constraint in the Heart and Triple Burner, all work together to conduct the heat downward, assisting Bovis Calculus *(niú huáng)* in clearing and draining heat toxin from the Pericardium.

The other set of deputies help Moschus *(shè xiāng)* in aromatically clearing away turbidity. Acrid and bitter Borneolum *(bīng piàn)* is highly aromatic, scurries everywhere, and is good at unblocking the orifices. Acrid and bitter Curcumae Radix *(yù jīn)* opens up and directs downward; its aromatic nature allows it to disseminate and thrust out as a means of moving the qi and releasing areas of constraint. These deputies unblock the orifices and disperse the heat from constraint, thereby helping the chief ingredients vent heat through the collaterals of the Pericardium.

There are three assistants. Margarita *(zhēn zhū)* clears heat from both the Heart and Liver channels and is effective at sedating and moving phlegm downward. The other two assistants are generally considered obsolete. Realgar *(xióng huáng)* dislodges phlegm and resolves toxicity, thus helping to open the sensory orifices by draining the turbid phlegm. Cinnabaris *(zhū shā)* clears heat from the Heart. Honey serves as an envoy by harmonizing the Stomach and regulating the middle burner. The gold leaf coating on the pills also serves as an envoy by calming the spirit.

The general effect of this formula is concisely described in the source text as "leading the pathogenic fire to be dispersed by way of the dispersing [action] of all the aromatic [substances]."

Cautions and Contraindications

Contraindicated during pregnancy. This formula should only be used for hot-type closed disorders. Because it is extremely cold and aromatic, its use should be discontinued once the desired effect occurs and should not be taken long-term.

Commentary

Both phlegm and heat are very strong in these patterns. In such cases, unless the turbid phlegm is eliminated, it will be difficult to clear the heat. It is therefore common to combine ingredients for clearing heat with others that dislodge and drain turbid phlegm.

The author of this formula, Wu Ju-Tong, succinctly summarized its actions: "The aromatic [ingredients] of this formula transform turbidity and benefit all the orifices; the salty and cold [ingredients] protect the Kidney water and calm the body of the Heart; the bitter and cold [ingredients] unblock the fire in the yang organs and drain the Heart." Note that, as with many of his other formulas, Wu's composition of this formula was heavily influenced by the clinical experiences and work of Ye Tian-Shi.

Wu also noted that this formula could be used for heat causing other problems, including 'flying corpse' (飛屍 *fēi shī)*, which refers to people becoming seriously ill so quickly that it appears that some pathogen has flown at them, spasms that lead to a loss of consciousness in adults and children, any of the five types of epilepsy, as well as noxious attack (惡中 *è zhòng)*. This last condition was earlier defined in *Indispensable Tools for Pattern Treatment*:

> Sudden, frigidly cold hands and feet, goose pimples, cyanotic face and head, and disturbed mental state from suddenly being accosted by an abnormal qi. There may be jumbled speech and crazy talk, locked jaw, or even dizziness with falling down such that the person does not recognize other people.

It is this note from Wu that provided the basis for later practitioners to expand the use of this formula to include certain types of insanity, with the appropriate signs and symptoms.

Contemporary Usage

This is the model formula for clearing heat and opening the orifices in acute cases. The main clinical markers are impaired consciousness, delirious speech, high fever, irritability and restlessness, a red or scarlet tongue, and a rapid pulse. It is widely used in China today, to the point where it has been developed into a liquid that can be given intravenously. The commercial formulations use artificial forms of the very expensive medicinals such as Moschus (*shè xiāng*), and most do not include gold leaf or the obsolete medicinals Cinnabaris (*zhū shā*) and Realgar (*xióng huáng*). Instead, they may add substitutes such as Haliotidis Concha (*shí jué míng*). It is often given to patients whose conditions are deteriorating, but who have not yet become comatose or delirious.

Comparisons

➤ Vs. Wan's Cattle Gallstone Pill to Clear the Heart (*Wàn shì niú huáng qīng xīn wán*), see page 488.

➤ Vs. Purple Snow Special Pill (*zǐ xuě dān*), see page 492.

➤ Vs. Greatest Treasure Special Pill (*zhì bǎo dān*), see page 495.

Biomedical Indications

With the appropriate presentation, this formula may be used to treat a wide variety of biomedically-defined disorders. These can be divided into the following groups:

- Acute infections of the central nervous system such as viral encephalitis (including type B) and viral meningitis

- Other central nervous system disorders such as cerebrovascular accidents, schizophrenia, epilepsy, or hepatic encephalopathy

- Acute infections such as upper respiratory tract diseases, tonsillitis, sinusitis, otitis media, pneumonia, asthma, acute icteric hepatitis, acute pancreatitis, toxic dysentery, acute nephritis, and epidemic hemorrhagic fevers.

This formula has also been used in the treatment of hepatic cancer, uremia, leukemia, septicemia, and Kawasaki disease.

Alternate names

Cattle Gallstone Pill (*niú huáng wán*) in *Systematic Differentiation of Warm Pathogen Diseases*; Newly-Revised Cattle Gallstone Pill to Clear the Heart (*xīn dìng niú huáng qīng xīn wán*) in *Revised and Expanded Popular Guide to the Discussion of Cold Damage*; Pill for Calming the Palace (*ān gōng wán*) in *National Collection of TCM Patent Formulas*

Modifications

- For patients with a deficient pulse, take with a decoction of Ginseng Radix (*rén shēn*). (source text)

- For patients with an excessive pulse, take with a decoction of Lonicerae Flos (*jīn yín huā*) and Menthae haplocalycis Herba (*bò hé*). (source text)

- For patients with high fevers, take with Purple Snow Special Pill (*zǐ xuě dān*).

Variation

牛黄承氣湯 （牛黄承气汤）

Cattle Gallstone Decoction to Order the Qi

niú huáng chéng qì tāng

Source *Systematic Differentiation of Warm Pathogen Diseases* (1798)

Dissolve two pills of the principal formula and add 9g of powdered Rhei Radix et Rhizoma (*dà huáng*). For heat entering the Pericardium with delirious speech and loss of consciousness, constipation, and thirst due to a concurrent yang brightness organ-stage disorder. Take one-half of this mixture first, then follow with the other half if there is no effect.

紫雪丹

Purple Snow Special Pill

zǐ xuě dān

After processing, this formula is purple and frost-like in appearance and possesses a very cold, 'frosty' nature, hence the name.

Source *Arcane Essentials from the Imperial Library* (752)

Gypsum fibrosum (*shí gāo*)	1500g
Glauberitum (*hán shuǐ shí*)	1500g
Talcum (*huá shí*)	1500g
Bubali Cornu (*shuǐ niú jiǎo*)	500g
Saigae tataricae Cornu (*líng yáng jiǎo*)	150g

Moschus (shè xiāng) 37.5g
Scrophulariae Radix (xuán shēn) 500g
Magnetitum (cí shí) 1500g
Cimicifugae Rhizoma (shēng má) 250-300g
Glycyrrhizae Radix praeparata (zhì gān cǎo) 240g
Aucklandiae Radix (mù xiāng) 150g
Aquilariae Lignum resinatum (chén xiāng) 150g
Caryophylli Flos (dīng xiāng) .30g
Cinnabaris (zhū shā) 90g
Natrii Sulfas (máng xiāo) 5000g
Nitrum (xiāo shí) 96g
Gold (huáng jīn) 3000g

Method of Preparation Traditionally, the mineral ingredients were crushed into small pieces and boiled in water three times. The herbal ingredients were then boiled three times with the minerals to produce a syrup. Powdered Natrii Sulfas (máng xiāo) and Nitrum (xiāo shí) were mixed into this syrup, which was then dried and powdered. The horns were filed and powdered; Cinnabaris (zhū shā) was processed in water to remove impurities and then powdered; Moschus (shè xiāng) was powdered. All of these powders were then sifted together to produce the final formula.

The process is very similar today. Note that the original text provides for 150g of Rhinocerotis Cornu (xī jiǎo), which is no longer used, primarily due to the endangered status of the rhinoceros. Cinnabaris (zhū shā) is also removed due to its heavy metal content, and gold is omitted, mostly because of its expense. While the original source calls for 青木香 qīng mù xiāng, it is generally agreed that the herb referred to is Aucklandiae Radix (mù xiāng) or Dolomiaeae Radix (chuān mù xiāng), and not the present-day Aristolochiae Radix (qīng mù xiāng). This last herb is, in any case, no longer used because it contains aristolochic acid.

Take in 1.5-3g doses 1-2 times daily with cool, boiled water, preferably after meals. For children, the dosage is reduced substantially based on the age and size of the child.

Actions Clears heat, opens the sensory orifices, controls spasms and convulsions, and extinguishes wind

Indications

High fever, irritability and restlessness, delirious speech, impaired consciousness, muscle twitches, spasms, convulsions, thirst, parched lips, dark urine, constipation, a scarlet red tongue with a dry, yellow coat, and a forceful, wiry, and rapid pulse. Also used for febrile convulsions in children.

This is blazing heat sinking into the Pericardium and generating internal movement of Liver wind. It usually occurs in the advanced stage of a warm-febrile disease. The heat sinks into the interior of the body where it disturbs the Heart's spirit and impairs consciousness. In relatively mild cases, the changes in consciousness can be limited to irritability, restlessness, a sense of unease, an ongoing desire to sleep, and delirious speech. If more severe, there can be a loss of consciousness and an inability to be aroused. The blazing heat injures the fluids and leads to high fever, thirst, parched lips, dark urine, and constipation.

The blazing heat can stir Liver wind which, in turn, can further fan the flames of the heat. As noted in *Basic Questions* (Chapter 71), "Wind moves when it is vigorous." This leads to twitches, spasms, and, particularly in children, convulsions. These symptoms, combined with the disturbance of consciousness, are known as 'tetanic collapse' (痙厥 jìng jué).

Analysis of Formula

Cool, aromatic Bubali Cornu (shuǐ niú jiǎo) both ascends and disperses. It enters the nutritive and blood levels, and is an important substance for clearing fire and heat from the Heart and Liver channels. It clears heat from the nutritive level, cools the blood, and resolves toxicity. Because of its active nature, it can be cold without retarding movement, making it useful for venting heat through the collaterals of the Pericardium. Saigae tataricae Cornu (líng yáng jiǎo) is particularly useful for draining Liver fire and is an important substance for cooling the Liver and extinguishing wind. Together, these two animal horns treat the heat in the Heart and Liver channels and effectively resolve the spasms, convulsions, and impaired consciousness. The intensely aromatic properties of Moschus (shè xiāng) enable it to open the orifices of the Heart and restore consciousness. As these three ingredients together clear heat, open the sensory orifices, and extinguish wind, they are viewed as the chief ingredients.

Gypsum fibrosum (shí gāo) is an important substance for clearing fire and heat from the qi level, causing the heat to recede and encouraging the generation of fluids. It thereby eliminates irritability and alleviates thirst. Glauberitum (hán shuǐ shí) likewise clears heat and drains fire to eliminate irritability and alleviate thirst. The slippery quality of Talcum (huá shí) enables it to conduct heat downward so that it can be eliminated through the urine. Together, these three minerals are regarded as deputies in the formula for their ability to clear and drain heat from the qi level.

Sweet, bitter, and slightly cold Scrophulariae Radix (xuán shēn) conducts fire downward, enriches the yin, and cools the blood. It is combined with sweet, acrid, and slightly cold Cimicifugae Rhizoma (shēng má) to strengthen its ability to clear heat and resolve toxicity while also venting the pathogen. These herbs are also regarded as deputies because of their effect on the heat.

Aucklandiae Radix (mù xiāng), Aquilariae Lignum resinatum (chén xiāng), and Caryophylli Flos (dīng xiāng) promote the movement of qi and assist Moschus (shè xiāng) in opening the orifices. Magnetitum (cí shí) sedates the Heart and calms the spirit, which strengthens the formula's action in eliminating irritability. Natrii Sulfas (máng xiāo) and Nitrum (xiāo shí) also drain heat and dissipate clumps, especially when combined with Scrophulariae Radix (xuán shēn). This strong, heat-clearing action is called 'removing the firewood from under the cauldron.' These are all regarded as assistants.

Today, the envoy is Glycyrrhizae Radix praeparata *(zhì gān cǎo)*, which helps resolve toxicity, harmonize the Stomach, and protect it from injury by the heavy mineral ingredients. Traditionally, gold *(huáng jīn)*, which weighs upon and sedates the spirit, was also regarded as an envoy.

Taken together, as noted in Zhang Shan-Lei's *Annotated and Corrected Master Yan's Discussion of Formulas for Children,* "Whenever qi and fire are extremely overabundant and there are a variety of symptoms from ascending without descending, this [formula] is especially appropriate."

Cautions and Contraindications

Contraindicated during pregnancy and used with caution in the weak and debilitated. The use of this formula should be discontinued as soon as the symptoms of impaired consciousness improve. Overuse of the formula can easily injure the source qi and exhaust the yin, which, in severe cases may lead to marked sweating, nausea and vomiting, cold extremities, a frozen affect, dyspnea, palpitations, dizziness, and vertigo. While taking this formula, spicy, rich, or greasy foods should be avoided.

Commentary

This is a very commonly used formula for treating high fevers with changes in consciousness and signs of internal wind, from mild twitching to full-blown convulsions. Because the condition is due to intense interior heat, there will be constipation, a scarlet red tongue with a dry, yellow coating, and a rapid, forceful pulse. It uses ingredients for clearing heat that are sweet and cold, instead of bitter and cold. This is done to avoid injury to the fluids from the bitter ingredients, which are drying in nature, and is recommended in treating patterns of vigorous heat and injury to the fluids with such manifestations as spasms and convulsions.

Origin and Variations of the Formula

The earliest known version of this formula is from the early Tang-dynasty work *Formulas of Su Gong* (蘇恭方 *Sū Gōng fāng),* recorded in *Arcane Essentials from the Imperial Library.* There are similar formulas found in other works. In fact, according to the recent *Formulas* edited by Li Fei, there exist more than 50 variations of this particular formula. Some modifications are designed to emphasize certain specific aspects or actions. An example is the increase in dosage of Moschus *(shè xiāng)* in the version of the formula found in *Formulary of the Pharmacy Service for Benefiting the People in the Taiping Era,* which increases its effect in opening the orifices. At other times, the goal appears to be a simplification of the formula, as in the version found in *Golden Mirror of the Medical Tradition,* which omits Magnetitum *(cí shí)*, Talcum *(huá shí)*, Caryophylli Flos *(dīng xiāng)*, Nitrum *(xiāo shí)*, and Moschus *(shè xiāng),* while adding Borneolum *(bīng*

piàn). As noted above, for over 30 years, the official formulation in China has omitted the use of gold, and substitutes an extract from Bubali Cornu *(shuǐ niú jiǎo)* for Rhinocerotis Cornu *(xī jiǎo)*.

Controversy over Chief Ingredients

Similarly, commentators have expressed a variety of opinions regarding the chief ingredients in the formula, reflecting different views about the nature of its principal indications. The source text says that the formula is designed to treat "toxin from leg qi that has spread everywhere, both internally and externally" and "toxins from minerals, herbs, and heating medicinals." Before the early Qing dynasty, the formula was therefore always viewed as one that cleared heat and drained fire; thus, the minerals Gypsum fibrosum *(shí gāo)*, Glauberitum *(hán shuǐ shí)*, Talcum *(huá shí)*, and Nitrum *(xiāo shí)* were regarded as the chief ingredients. An example of this approach is reflected in Xu Da-Chun's *Patterns and Treatment of Miscellaneous Disorders*:

> When toxin invades the channels and yang organs, heat obstructs the consciousness (神明 *shén míng*) so there is out of control mania and disorderly restlessness as well as pain in the Heart and abdomen. This formula expels and directs toxic miasmas downward, protects the Heart and calms the spirit, and excels at treating all patterns of obstruction and clumping from excessive fire.

Physicians of the warm pathogen current held a different opinion. In *Case Records as a Guide to Clinical Practice,* Ye Tian-Shi prescribes the formula for impaired consciousness with tremors or convulsions from "a warm pathogen being obstructed internally with clogging up of heat that extends throughout the three burners." This emphasizes the orifice-opening actions of the formula; thus, in texts such as *Convenient Reader of Established Formulas,* the chief ingredients are Moschus *(shè xiāng)*, Cinnabaris *(zhū shā)*, Nitrum *(xiāo shí)*, and Natrii Sulfas *(máng xiāo)*. At present, this formula is primarily used for heat sinking into the Pericardium with stirring of internal wind due to a variety of acute infectious diseases; the chief ingredients are accordingly those listed above: Bubali Cornu *(shuǐ niú jiǎo)*, Moschus *(shè xiāng)*, and Saigae tataricae Cornu *(líng yáng jiǎo)*.

Comparisons

➢ Vs. Calm the Palace Pill with Cattle Gallstone *(ān gōng niú huáng wán)*, see page 490.

➢ Vs. Greatest Treasure Special Pill *(zhì bǎo dān)*, *see* page 495

Biomedical Indications

With the appropriate presentation, this formula may be used to treat a variety of biomedically-defined disorders includ-

ing acute encephalitis, acute meningitis, severe pneumonia, measles, scarlet fever, diphtheria, acute tonsillitis, febrile convulsions, folliculitis, furuncles, and epilepsy.

Alternate names

Purple Snow Powder (zǐ xuě sǎn) in *Nationwide Collection of TCM Patent Formulas*

Modifications

- For dysenteric disorders with high fever, muscle twitches, and impaired consciousness, take with Pulsatilla Decoction (*bái tóu wēng tāng*).

- For septicemia with furuncles, take with Five-Ingredient Drink to Eliminate Toxin (*wǔ wèi xiāo dú yǐn*).

- For acute encephalitis or meningitis with high fever, irritability and restlessness, and neck stiffness, take with White Tiger Decoction (*bái hǔ tāng*).

- For acute encephalitis or meningitis with repeated attacks of nausea and vomiting, take with Minor Decoction [for Pathogens] Stuck in the Chest (*xiǎo xiàn xiōng tāng*).

- For acute encephalitis or meningitis with delirious speech, follow this formula with Clear Epidemics and Overcome Toxicity Drink (*qīng wēn bài dú yǐn*).

- For acute encephalitis or meningitis with pronounced muscle twitches and spasms of the extremities, follow this formula with Antelope Horn and Uncaria Decoction (*líng jiǎo gōu téng tāng*).

- For measles with high fever, thirst, and a dark-purple rash, take with Rhinoceros Horn and Rehmannia Decoction (*xī jiǎo dì huáng tāng*).

- For insanity, take with Clear the Palace Decoction (*qīng gōng tāng*).

- For tetanic collapse, take with Three-Shell Decoction to Restore the Pulse (*sān jiǎ fù mài tāng*).

至寶丹（至宝丹）
Greatest Treasure Special Pill
zhì bǎo dān

Like treasures, the ingredients of this formula are both very effective and very expensive, hence the name.

Source *Fine Formulas by Su and Shen* (1075)

[Bubali Cornu (*shuǐ niú jiǎo*) . . . . . 300g]
Bovis Calculus (*niú huáng*) 0.3g
Eretmochelydis Carapax (*dài mào*) 30g
Borneolum (*bīng piàn*) 0.3g
Moschus (*shè xiāng*) 0.3g
Benzoinum (*ān xī xiāng*) 45g
Cinnabaris (*zhū shā*) 30g
Succinum (*hǔ pò*) 30g
Realgar (*xióng huáng*) 30g

Method of Preparation Separately grind each ingredient into a powder and then sift together. Cinnabaris (*zhū shā*) and Realgar (*xióng huáng*) were water-refined to remove impurities. Originally, 50 pieces of silver leaf and 25 pieces of gold leaf were ground into a powder and added to the other ingredients. An additional 25 pieces of gold leaf were used to coat the pills. At present, these two ingredients are no longer used. Also, originally, one 3g pill was taken with a decoction of Ginseng Radix (*rén shēn*). At present, the dose is one 3g pill taken 1-3 times daily with warm water. May also be administered by grinding into a powder and dissolving in warm water. The dosage is half or less for children. If the patient is unconscious, the formula may be administered by nasogastric tube.

Note that the original text specified 30g of Rhinocerotis Cornu (*xī jiǎo*), which is no longer used, primarily due to the endangered status of the rhinoceros. In addition, at present, neither Cinnabaris (*zhū shā*) nor Realgar (*xióng huáng*) should be used due to their heavy metal content.

Actions Clears heat, opens the sensory orifices, transforms turbidity, and resolves toxicity

Indications

Fever, irritability and restlessness, delirious speech, impaired consciousness to the point of coma, copious sputum with labored and raspy breathing, spasms, convulsions, a red or deep-red tongue with a foul, greasy, yellow coating, and a slippery, rapid pulse.

This is a closed disorder from phlegm-heat. It is usually associated with summerheat-stroke, wind-stroke, or the advanced stage of a warm-febrile disease when heat sinks into the Pericardium and turbid phlegm veils the orifices of the Heart. When heat sinks into the Pericardium, it causes disorientation by disturbing the spirit and gives rise to fever, irritability and restlessness, delirious speech, or partial loss of consciousness. The vigorous, blazing heat scorches the fluids and causes them to condense into phlegm. Heat and phlegm accentuate each other and completely veil the orifices of the Heart, further disturbing the spirit and impairing the consciousness. As the phlegm increases, the impairment of consciousness becomes even more severe with such manifestations as loss of consciousness or coma.

Phlegm also obstructs the pathways of qi, giving rise to copious sputum and rough breathing accompanied by raspy sounds due to sputum in the throat. Extreme heat may generate internal wind, which manifests as spasms or convulsions. The tongue is the 'sprout' of the Heart; when heat enters the Heart and the nutritive level, the tongue becomes red or deep red. The foul, greasy, yellow tongue coating and slippery, rapid pulse are indicative of phlegm-heat.

Similar presentations also occur in children with phlegm-heat causing fright collapse (驚厥 *jīng jué*).

Analysis of Formula

This formula focuses on clearing heat and resolving toxicity affecting the Pericardium and aromatically opening the sensory orifices, while also dislodging phlegm and draining turbidity. One of the chief ingredients, Bubali Cornu (*shuǐ niú jiǎo*), clears heat from the nutritive level and cools the blood. Its cool, aromatic properties make it useful for treating heat that affects the collaterals of the Pericardium. The other chief ingredient, Moschus (*shè xiāng*), is highly aromatic and scurries everywhere, penetrating all the channels; it is good for unblocking all the orifices of the body. These two medicinals work well together to clear heat and open the sensory orifices.

Benzoinum (*ān xī xiāng*) is highly aromatic and penetrates the sensory orifices, clears away filth, and transforms turbidity. Together with Borneolum (*bīng piàn*), which is likewise highly aromatic, opens the sensory orifices, and clears away filth, they comprise a pair of deputies that assist Moschus (*shè xiāng*). The other deputies, Bovis Calculus (*niú huáng*) and Eretmochelydis Carapax (*dài mào*), assist Bubali Cornu (*shuǐ niú jiǎo*) by entering the Heart and Liver channels to sedate the Heart, calm the spirit, clear heat, resolve toxicity, extinguish wind, and settle spasms and convulsions. The concealed aroma of Bovis Calculus (*niú huáng*) is particularly helpful in dislodging phlegm and opening the sensory orifices.

Realgar (*xióng huáng*) eliminates phlegm and resolves toxicity. It acts as an assistant to Bovis Calculus (*niú huáng*) in breaking up phlegm and opening the orifices. The other assistants, Succinum (*hǔ pò*), along with Cinnabaris (*zhū shā*) and gold and silver leaf in the original formulation, sedate the Heart and calm the spirit, resolving the irritability and impairment of speech and consciousness.

Cautions and Contraindications

Contraindicated during pregnancy. This formula contains many drying, aromatic ingredients that have a tendency to consume the yin and fluids. It should therefore not be used in treating cases with significant yin deficiency.

Commentary

Usage

In the source text, this formula is prescribed for a wide variety of complaints including cold damage, postpartum dizziness and disorientation, sudden turmoil disease, and sudden attacks by a variety of toxins, including noxious-stroke (中惡 *zhòng è*), which is sudden collapse with abdominal pain following exposure to extremely noxious and foul odors, such as those emanating from rotten food or dead bodies.

At present, this formula is generally prescribed for closed disorders due to phlegm-heat with fever, irritability and restlessness, impaired consciousness and delirium, abundant phlegm and rough breathing, with a scarlet tongue that has a yellow, greasy, coating and a slippery, rapid, and forceful pulse. Usually there are accompanying twitches, spasms, or even convulsions.

While this is an extremely useful formula for acute disorder, it is important to remember that it should only be used when clearly indicated. As noted in *Selected Annotations to Ancient Formulas from the Garden of Crimson Snow,* the formula:

> Treats Heart organ impaired consciousness and is a formula that penetrates to the interior from the exterior. ... Therefore, when heat enters the collaterals of the Pericardium, the tongue is scarlet, and consciousness is impaired, this special pill is used by putting it into a cold and cooling decoction. It is able to dispel the yin and raise the yang such that consciousness will immediately unfold. No other medicine can reach this [problem]. If, at the beginning of the disease, there is a headache and afterward consciousness becomes impaired with aphasia, this is Liver deficiency with the ethereal soul rising to the vertex. At this time, Ostreae Concha (*mǔ lì*) should be used to rescue [the patient] from rebellion and direct things downward. This is not [the type of impaired consciousness] that Greatest Treasure Special Pill (*zhì bǎo dān*) can awaken.

Controversy over Chief Ingredients

In the opinion of many modern commentators, the primary actions of this formula are transforming phlegm and opening the orifices, rather than clearing heat. The three chief ingredients are therefore considered to be Moschus (*shè xiāng*), Borneolum (*bīng piàn*), and Benzoinum (*ān xī xiāng*), all of which are aromatic substances that open the sensory orifices. In turn, Bubali Cornu (*shuǐ niú jiǎo*), Bovis Calculus (*niú huáng*), and Eretmochelydis Carapax (*dài mào*) are the deputy ingredients for clearing heat and resolving toxicity. Since the ability of the formula to open the sensory orifices is stronger than its ability to clear heat, it may be combined with other cool or cold decoctions to reliably open up closed disorders with intense heat and to revive the spirit.

Origin and Variations of the Formula

The earliest know version of this formula was composed by the Song-dynasty physician Zheng Gan, as recorded in *Fine Formulas by Su and Shen.* There have been variant formulas since that time, some altering the dosages and others the ingredients. For example, the version in the 16th-century *Compendium of the Rules of Conduct for Physicians* adds Ginseng Radix (*rén shēn*), Bambusae Concretio silicea (*tiān zhú huáng*), and Arisaema cum Bile (*dǎn nán xīng*) to treat all types of closure of the sensory orifices. As noted above, for over 30 years the official formulation in China has omitted gold and silver foil, and substituted Bubali Cornu (*shuǐ niú jiǎo*) for Rhinocerotis Cornu (*xī jiǎo*).

Comparisons

➤ Vs. Calm the Palace Pill with Cattle Gallstone (*ān gōng niú huáng wán*) and Purple Snow Special Pill (*zǐ xuě dān*)

Together with the principal formula, these are the three most commonly used formulas for clearing heat and opening the sensory orifices. They are referred to as the 'three treasures of warm pathogen diseases' (溫病三寶 *wēn bìng sān bǎo*). They have been differentiated from each other at least since the *Systematic Differentiation of Warm Pathogen Diseases*.

Formulas Ranked in Order of Coldness	Strengths	Most Appropriate Presentation
1. Calm the Palace Pill with Cattle Gallstone (*ān gōng niú huáng wán*)	Clears heat and resolves toxicity	Very intense pathogenic heat with high fever and impaired consciousness
2. Purple Snow Special Pill (*zǐ xuě dān*)	Extinguishes wind and stops spasms	High fevers with spasms and convulsions
3. Greatest Treasure Special Pill (*zhì bǎo dān*)	Aromatically opens the sensory orifices	Impaired consciousness with a fever, abundant phlegm, labored breathing

Biomedical Indications

With the appropriate presentation, this formula may be used in treating such biomedically-defined disorders as acute encephalitis, acute meningitis, cerebrovascular accident, pediatric and adult seizure disorders, hepatic coma, toxic dysentery, and heat-stroke.

Modifications

- For serious cases with deficiency of normal qi, take with a decoction of Ginseng Radix (*rén shēn*). (source text)
- For intense phlegm-heat, take with Infantis Urina (*tóng biàn*) and Zingiberis Rhizomatis Succus (*jiāng zhī*). (source text)
- To increase the effects of the formula, take with a decoction made of Acori tatarinowii Rhizoma (*shí chāng pǔ*) and Lonicerae Flos (*jīn yín huā*).

回春丹
Special Pill to Restore Life
huí chūn dān

The name of the formula is literally 'return to spring special pill.' In nature, all living things wither during the winter and return to life during the spring. This formula is used for treating acute childhood convulsions. Its action is compared to "raising up the dead and bringing them back to life," just as the return of spring restores life to the dead.

Source *Medicinal Teachings from the Respectfully Decorated Hall* (late 18th century)

Bovis Calculus (*niú huáng*) 12g
Bambusae Concretio silicea (*tiān zhú huáng*) 37.5g
Fritillariae cirrhosae Bulbus (*chuān bèi mǔ*) 37.5g
Arisaema cum Bile (*dǎn nán xīng*) 60g
Moschus (*shè xiāng*) 12g
Uncariae Ramulus cum Uncis (*gōu téng*) 24g
Scorpio (*quán xiē*) 37.5g
Gastrodiae Rhizoma (*tiān má*) 37.5g
Bombyx batryticatus (*bái jiāng cán*) 37.5g
Cinnabaris (*zhū shā*) 0.3-1.8g
Rhei Radix et Rhizoma (*dà huáng*) 60g
Citri reticulatae Pericarpium (*chén pí*) 37.5g
Pinelliae Rhizoma praeparatum (*zhì bàn xià*) 37.5g
Amomi Fructus rotundus (*bái dòu kòu*) 37.5g
Santali albi Lignum (*tán xiāng*) 37.5g
Aucklandiae Radix (*mù xiāng*) 37.5g
Aurantii Fructus (*zhǐ ké*) 37.5g
Aquilariae Lignum resinatum (*chén xiāng*) 37.5g
Glycyrrhizae Radix (*gān cǎo*) 26.25g

Method of Preparation Grind the ingredients into a powder and form into very small pills, each weighing about 0.09g. The dose is one pill taken 2-3 times daily for children under one year of age, and two pills taken 2-3 times daily for those one to two years of age. Larger doses are used in adults. Take with warm water. Some of the prepared formulations are in powdered form. If the patient is unconscious, the formula may be administered by nasogastric tube. Note that due to its heavy metal content, Cinnabaris (*zhū shā*) should no longer be used.

Actions Opens the sensory orifices, arrests spasms and convulsions, clears heat, and transforms phlegm

Indications

Fever, impaired consciousness, childhood convulsions, irritability and restlessness. The child may also have wheezing, nausea, night crying, vomiting milk, diarrhea, abdominal pain, excessive secretion of mucus and saliva, and sounds of mucus in the throat.

This is childhood convulsions (小兒急驚 *xiǎo ér jí jīng*), which are due to phlegm-heat entering the Pericardium and veiling the orifices of the Heart. The yin, yang, qi, and blood in children are immature, their organs are not fully developed, their skin is thin, and their pores and interstices lack the normal amount of tension. For these reasons, children are quite susceptible to invasion by externally-contracted pathogenic influences. Because children are growing, they tend to be relatively yang, so that an invasion of cold quickly transforms into heat. Hot pathogenic influences likewise transform into fire more quickly, which then enters the terminal yin warp, both stirring Liver wind and being transmitted to the Pericardium. As a result, when children are affected by the invasion of external cold or heat, it is likely to cause high fever. The extreme heat transforms the fluids into phlegm. This commonly leads to phlegm-heat, which moves upward to veil the orifices and manifests as impaired consciousness or even loss of consciousness.

This disorder can be summed up in four words: heat, phlegm, wind, and convulsions. The pathogenic heat disturbs the Heart, which causes irritability. Phlegm clogs the Lungs and inhibits the dissemination of Lung qi, which leads to wheezing. Phlegm also obstructs the qi pathways, which produces the sound of mucus in the throat. In infants and young children, the Spleen commonly tends toward insufficiency. When food is not well-digested, the transportive and transformative functions of the Spleen and Stomach may be injured. This upsets the ascending and descending functions (the qi mechanisms) of the middle burner, leading to nausea, crying at night, vomiting milk, and diarrhea. Spleen deficiency also generates dampness, which causes the fluids to stagnate and further contributes to the problem of phlegm. As the transportive and transformative functions of the Spleen weaken, food accumulates. The accumulation of food produces stagnation and abdominal pain. The disruption of fluid metabolism and the qi mechanisms causes excessive secretion of mucus and saliva and the sound of mucus in the throat, which may be one of the first signs of the impending spasms and convulsions. Also, in infants and children, the Liver commonly tends toward surplus, such that pathogenic heat readily stirs internal wind, which manifests as spasms and convulsions that are characteristic of childhood convulsions. Note that this formula can also be used to treat adults with the proper presentation.

Analysis of Formula

To treat a complicated pattern where exuberance of phlegm-heat blocks the sensory orifices, which then engenders Liver wind to produce childhood convulsions, this formula employs an equally complex strategy. It opens the sensory orifices, arrests spasms and convulsions, clears heat, and transforms phlegm.

One of the chief ingredients is bitter, cool, and aromatic Bovis Calculus (niú huáng), which enters the Heart and Liver channels. It clears heat, resolves toxicity, clears away phlegm, opens the sensory orifices, extinguishes wind, and controls spasms and convulsions. It thereby addresses all of the major aspects of this disorder. It is combined with the other chief ingredient, Moschus (shè xiāng), which is highly aromatic and opens the sensory orifices; in Discussion of Medicinal Properties, it is specifically indicated for childhood convulsions and seizures.

One of the deputies, Uncariae Ramulus cum Uncis (gōu téng), enters both the Liver and Pericardium channels, and is an important substance for extinguishing Liver wind, clearing heat, and resolving spasms and convulsions. In concert with three other deputies, Scorpio (quán xiē), Gastrodiae Rhizoma (tiān má), and Bombyx batryticatus (bái jiāng cán), it has a strong effect in extinguishing wind and controlling spasms and convulsions. Together, they comprise one set of deputy ingredients. The other set strengthens the formula's ability to transform phlegm. It is comprised of Fritillariae cirrhosae Bulbus (chuān bèi mǔ) and Arisaema cum Bile (dǎn nán xīng), which together clear heat and transform phlegm; Pinelliae Rhizoma praeparatum (zhì bàn xià), which redirects rebellious qi downward, and stops the vomiting; and Bambusae Concretio silicea (tiān zhú huáng), which, in addition to clearing heat and transforming phlegm, also cools the Heart and controls spasms and convulsions.

Rhei Radix et Rhizoma (dà huáng), which clears heat and drains fire, is the last of the deputies. In addition, its purgative action removes accumulation and stagnation, which enables it to eliminate the accumulation of phlegm-heat from the Stomach and Intestines. The strategy here is to use a purgative to indirectly clear heat from the upper part of the body by reducing the accumulation of heat in the lower part of the body. This is known as 'removing the firewood from under the cauldron.'

Among the assistant ingredients, Citri reticulatae Pericarpium (chén pí) and Pinelliae Rhizoma praeparatum (zhì bàn xià) harmonize the Stomach, transform phlegm, direct rebellious qi downward, and stop vomiting. Amomi Fructus rotundus (bái dòu kòu) promotes the movement of qi, reduces focal distention, transforms turbid dampness, and stops vomiting. Santali albi Lignum (tán xiāng) and Aucklandiae Radix (mù xiāng) are useful for moving the qi of the Stomach and Intestines, regulating and smoothing the functions of the Stomach and Intestines in order to restore the normal ascending and descending functions of the Spleen and Stomach. Aurantii Fructus (zhǐ ké) eases stagnation in the middle burner and reduces distention, while Aquilariae Lignum resinatum (chén xiāng) directs qi downward so that phlegm will descend. If the flow of qi is smooth, then the phlegm can be reduced, which will discourage the further generation of phlegm-heat. Once the phlegm-heat is eliminated, the orifices will open and the patient will recover. Glycyrrhizae Radix (gān cǎo) serves as the envoy by clearing heat and regulating and harmonizing the actions of the other ingredients.

Cautions and Contraindications

Contraindicated during pregnancy. This formula is used for acute childhood convulsions associated with a pattern of excess and is inappropriate for chronic childhood convulsions due to waning of the Spleen and Kidney yang. If this diagnosis cannot be clearly made in a specific case, it is best not to use the formula.

Commentary

This is an important formula for childhood convulsions. The key indications are fever, irritability, restlessness, impaired consciousness, sudden collapse, vomiting, and diarrhea. Not only does it have the capability of calming down a very serious, urgent condition in children, but it shows how a wide variety of ingredients can be well-crafted into one formula.

In this case, there are four groups of ingredients that are integrated into a whole; those that:

1. Clear the Heart and open the sensory orifices
2. Clear heat and transform phlegm
3. Extinguish wind and stop spasms, and
4. Regulate the qi and harmonize the Stomach.

All four groups are necessary because, by definition, acute childhood convulsions must be due to an externally-contracted pathogen that invades a child who has preexisting phlegm from food stagnation that has transformed into heat, which then stirs up Liver wind.

Because this formula eliminates wind, transforms phlegm, regulates qi, and harmonizes the Stomach, its use has been expanded to include indigestion, vomiting, diarrhea, and coughing in children whenever the presentation involves stagnation and heat.

Note that not all of the available prepared medicines by this name have the same formulation. In particular, they often reduce the dosage or number of acrid, warm substances as a means of avoiding making the fire and subsequent wind worse.

Biomedical Indications

With the appropriate presentation, this formula may be used in treating such biomedically-defined disorders as acute encephalitis, acute meningitis, measles, scarlet fever, diphtheria, septicemia, pediatric seizure disorder, seizure disorder, and severe, acute gastroenteritis.

Alternate name

Pediatric Special Pill to Restore Life *(ér kē huí chūn dān)* in *Medicinal Doctrine from the Hall of Respect and Learning*

Modifications

• To strengthen the effects of clearing heat and pacifying the Liver, take with a decoction of Uncariae Ramulus cum Uncis *(gōu téng)* and Menthae haplocalycis Herba *(bò hé)*. (source text)

• To simultaneously clear and resolve half-exterior, half-interior pathogenic heat, take with a decoction made of Bupleuri Radix *(chái hú)* and Scutellariae Radix *(huáng qín)*. (source text)

• For bloody dysenteric diarrhea, take with a decoction of Crataegi Fructus *(shān zhā)* and Sanguisorbae Radix *(dì yú)*. (source text)

• For dysenteric diarrhea with pus, take with a decoction of Citri reticulatae Pericarpium *(chén pí)* and Crataegi Fructus *(shān zhā)*. (source text)

• For watery diarrhea, take with a decoction of Poria *(fú líng)* and Plantaginis Semen *(chē qián zǐ)*. (source text)

Associated Formula

抱龍丸 （抱龙丸）

Embrace the Dragon Pill

bào lóng wán

SOURCE *Craft of Medicines and Patterns for Children* (1119)

Bambusae Concretio silicea *(tiān zhú huáng)* 30g
Realgar *(xióng huáng)* . . . . [aqueous triturated] 3g
Cinnabaris *(zhū shā)* 15g
Moschus *(shè xiāng)* 15g
Arisaema cum Bile *(dǎn nán xīng)* 120g

The above ingredients are ground into a fine powder and made into small pills with licorice juice that are then taken with warm water. The dosage ranges from one-quarter of a pill in infants who are 3 months or less up to 3-5 pills for adults.

Clears heat, transforms phlegm, opens the sensory orifices, and calms the spirit. This was originally for acute convulsions in children and is still primarily used in that context. This is the historical antecedent to the principal formula. Embrace the Dragon Pill *(bào lóng wán)* is relatively simple and focuses on clearing heat, transforming phlegm, opening the sensory orifices, and calming the spirit. The principal formula, by contrast, has more ingredients for this last action, while adding those that extinguish wind, stop spasms, regulate the qi, harmonize the Stomach, and drain heat. As such, the principal formula is indicated for more severe conditions, particularly those with concurrent gastrointestinal problems.

Section 2

FORMULAS THAT WARM AND OPEN THE SENSORY ORIFICES

The formulas in this section are used for cold-type closed disorders associated with wind-stroke, cold-stroke, or loss of consciousness due to the accumulation of phlegm. These conditions manifest in such signs and symptoms as sudden collapse, clenched jaw, loss of consciousness, ashen face, cold body, a white tongue coating, and a slow pulse.

The core ingredients in these formulas are intensely acrid, aromatic, and warm substances that open the sensory orifices such as Styrax (sū hé xiāng), Moschus (shè xiāng), and Benzoinum (ān xī xiāng).

Given the importance of internal cold in these disorders, it is often important to add aromatic substances that disperse internal cold such as Caryophylli Flos (dīng xiāng) and Piperis longi Fructus (bì bá).

For these disorders, the qi dynamic is often disrupted, requiring the use of substances that regulate the qi such as Aucklandiae Radix (mù xiāng), Cyperi Rhizoma (xiāng fù), and Aquilariae Lignum resinatum (chén xiāng).

In part to avoid further damage to the qi from the harsh medicinals, and in part to assist in the transformation of turbid phlegm, herbs that strengthen the qi and dry dampness are often used, such as Atractylodis macrocephalae Rhizoma (bái zhú).

蘇合香丸 (苏合香丸)
Liquid Styrax Pill

sū hé xiāng wán

Source   *Arcane Essentials from the Imperial Library* (752)

Styrax (sū hé xiāng)	15g
Moschus (shè xiāng)	30g
Borneolum (bīng piàn)	15g
Benzoinum (ān xī xiāng)	30g
Aucklandiae Radix (mù xiāng)	30g
Santali albi Lignum (tán xiāng)	30g
Aquilariae Lignum resinatum (chén xiāng)	30g
Olibanum (rǔ xiāng)	15g
Caryophylli Flos (dīng xiāng)	30g
Cyperi Rhizoma (xiāng fù)	30g
Piperis longi Fructus (bì bá)	30g
[Bubali Cornu (shuǐ niú jiǎo)	200g]
Cinnabaris (zhū shā)	30g
Atractylodis macrocephalae Rhizoma (bái zhú)	30g
Chebulae Fructus (hē zǐ)	30g

Method of Preparation   Grind the ingredients into a powder and form into pills with honey. Take one 3g pill 1-2 times daily with warm water. The dosage for children is reduced according to the age and size of the child. If the patient is unconscious, the formula may be administered by nasogastric tube. Note that the original text calls for 30g of Rhinocerotis Cornu (xī jiǎo), which is no longer used, primarily due to the endangered status of the rhinoceros. Also, because of its heavy metal content, Cinnabaris (zhū shā) should no longer be used.

Actions   Warms and aromatically opens the sensory orifices, promotes the movement of qi, and transforms turbidity

Indications

This formula is for three conditions with a similar pathodynamic:

1. Sudden collapse, loss of consciousness, and clenched jaw

2. Fullness, pain, and a sensation of cold in the chest and abdomen, which may signal the impending sudden loss of consciousness or coma

3. Abdominal pain and focal distention in the chest, an urge to vomit and defecate without doing either, which, in severe cases, can lead to sudden loss of consciousness or coma.

All of the above are accompanied by a pale complexion, purple lips, excessive mucus and saliva, cold extremities, a pale tongue with a slippery, greasy coating, and a submerged, slippery pulse.

This formula is used for treating a variety of acute closed disorders due to excessive cold. The first group of indications represents wind-stroke from damp-cold and turbid phlegm or some sort of miasmic pestilence (瘴癘 *zhàng lì*) veiling the sensory orifices and disturbing the spirit with sudden collapse, loss of consciousness, clenching of the jaw, and, in severe cases, coma.

The second group of indications represents acute disorders involving constrained qi leading to sudden collapse or a crippling attack of damp-cold obstruction. The former is known as qi-stroke (中氣 *zhòng qì*) and the latter as cold-stroke (中寒 *zhòng hán*). Both manifest with fullness, pain, and a sensation of cold in the chest and abdomen, sudden loss of consciousness, and coma.

The third group of indications represents the fierce qi of epidemic sudden turmoil disorder, which obstructs and stagnates the qi mechanisms. This leads to abdominal pain and focal distention in the chest, and an urge to vomit and defecate without being able to do either. When severe, the qi mechanisms become rebellious and disordered, which disturbs the spirit and leads to sudden loss of consciousness and coma.

The yin (cold) nature of these disorders is manifested in the pale complexion, purple lips, excessive mucus and saliva, cold extremities, pale tongue with a slippery, greasy coating, and a submerged, slippery pulse. The pathogenic influences interrupt the proper functioning of the organs, 'closing' them up. Alternatively, sudden anger may induce the qi to rebel upward, as anger causes the qi to ascend. Because qi is the commander of the blood, when qi ascends, so too will the blood. Qi and blood may both become rebellious and disturb the spirit. This leads to sudden loss of consciousness and coma, as phlegm follows the upward movement of qi and veils the sensory orifices.

Analysis of Formula

In the disorders for which this formula is indicated the presence of damp-cold leads to constrained qi and turbid phlegm. This requires a strategy that combines substances which aromatically open the sensory orifices (the chief ingredients) with those that dispel cold, regulate the qi, and penetrate through and transform turbidity (the deputies and assistants). The chief ingredients include Styrax (*sū hé xiāng*), which, in *Encountering the Sources of the Classic of Materia Medica* is said to:

> vent the various orifices and organs and clear away all abnormal qi. Whenever there is qi collapse (氣厥 *qì jué*) from phlegm accumulation, one must first use this to open and guide out. Regulating the qi is the foundation for treating phlegm.

Another chief ingredient is Benzoinum (*ān xī xiāng*), which is also especially useful for penetrating through the turbidity surrounding the sensory orifices, opening closed disorders, and restoring consciousness. The remaining chief ingredients are Moschus (*shè xiāng*) and Borneolum (*bīng piàn*), which break up turbidity, open the sensory orifices, and unblock the channels and collaterals throughout the body. All of these ingredients are powerful medicinals for treating wind and phlegm affecting the head.

The deputies, Aucklandiae Radix (*mù xiāng*), Santali albi Lignum (*tán xiāng*), Aquilariae Lignum resinatum (*chén xiāng*), Olibanum (*rǔ xiāng*), Caryophylli Flos (*dīng xiāng*), and Cyperi Rhizoma (*xiāng fù*), are acrid, dispersing, warm, and moving in nature. Together, they promote the movement of qi, direct rebellious qi downward, open up areas of constraint, dispel cold, and transform turbidity. Santali albi Lignum (*tán xiāng*) specifically treats both chest and abdominal pain as well as sudden turmoil disorder. Because directing the qi downward will cause the phlegm to descend, restoring the orderly flow of qi will help resolve the symptoms of phlegm disturbing the spirit. The strong, aromatic properties of the chief and deputy ingredients release and eliminate the constraint and stagnation affecting the qi and blood. Olibanum (*rǔ xiāng*) promotes the movement of qi and invigorates the blood, which facilitates the unimpeded circulation of qi and blood, and thereby helps alleviate pain. The final deputy, Piperis longi Fructus (*bì bá*), reinforces the actions of warming the middle burner, dispelling cold, arresting pain, and opening up areas of constraint.

The remaining ingredients in the original formula are regarded as assistants. Bubali Cornu (*shuǐ niú jiǎo*) resolves toxicity. Although cold in nature, its clear, aromatic properties enable it to penetrate the turbidity without causing stagnation. Atractylodis macrocephalae Rhizoma (*bái zhú*) tonifies the qi, strengthens the Spleen, dries dampness, and transforms turbidity. Together with Chebulae Fructus (*hē zǐ*), which restrains the leakage of qi, it prevents the acrid, aromatic properties of the other ingredients from consuming or dispersing the normal qi. Originally, Cinnabaris (*zhū shā*) was used to sedate the Heart and calm the spirit.

As this discussion shows, this formula has two distinguishing features: (1) a very strong effect in moving the qi, opening the sensory orifices, and clearing away turbid filth by the synergistic use of several acrid, warm, and aromatic dispersing substances; and (2) the ability to ameliorate the dangers of overly dispersing through the use of tonifying, restraining, cold, and heavy substances.

Cautions and Contraindications

Contraindicated during pregnancy or for hot closed disorders. Because the formula is very acrid and aromatic and thus has a very dispersing effect, the dosage should be carefully monitored.

Commentary

This is the representative warm formula for opening the sensory orifices and is typically used whenever pathogenic cold, turbid filth, or intense qi constraint blocks the orifices, leading to sudden loss of consciousness and trismus, accompanied by a white tongue coating and a slow pulse. The distinctive characteristic of this formula is its use of many aromatic substances that open the sensory orifices, transform turbidity, and promote the movement of qi. It is most commonly used in treating wind-stroke, cold-stroke, qi-stroke, and collapse from disorders involving phlegm. It may also be used for the so-called 'dry' sudden turmoil disorder in which the patient has a strong urge to vomit and defecate, but is unable to do either. It is especially useful when this condition progresses to loss of consciousness.

The wide applicability of this formula was described by the Ming-dynasty writer Wang Ken-Tang in *Indispensable Tools for Pattern Treatment*:

> While commonly wind-stroke, qi-stroke, food [stagnation]-stroke, cold-stroke, heat-stroke, damp-stroke, and noxious-stroke are differentiated, whenever one observes sudden collapse, loss of consciousness; or clogging and obstruction by phlegm and spittle with a [gurgling] sound in the throat; deviation of the mouth and eyes, paralysis of the hands and feet; or hemiplegia, or [all the] six pulse positions being submerged and hidden, or floating and flourishing under the fingers; Liquid Styrax Pill (*sū hé xiāng wán*) mixed with sesame oil, Zingiberis Rhizomatis Succus (*jiāng zhī*), or Bambusae Succus (*zhú lì*) can be used.

Expanded Usage

When used in treating partial or total loss of consciousness due to diseases such as encephalitis, the formula is taken when the fever has receded but the patient is still stuporous. Recently, its scope has been expanded to include painful obstruction of the chest due to qi stagnation, congealing due to cold, and turbid phlegm obstructing the collaterals. For painful obstruction of the chest, it is only used to treat the manifestation. At present, simplified versions of this formula are often used for coronary heart disease.

History

The earliest known citation for this formula is found in *Arcane Essentials from the Imperial Library*, where it is attributed to the now-lost *Buddhist Formulas of Wide Benefit to Open the Primal* (玄宗開元廣濟方 *Xuān Zōng kāi yuán guǎng jì fāng*). There it had the name Atractylodes Pill (吃力伽丸 *chī lì gā wán*). It was given the name Liquid Styrax Pill (*sū hé xiāng wán*) in the Song-dynasty text *Fine Formulas by Su and Shen*, which has continued to be used ever since. There have been other formulas by the same name with similar, but not identical, formulations.

The fact that the original name of this formula was an alternate name for Atractylodis macrocephalae Rhizoma (*bái zhú*) underscores the fact that when attacking an intense pathogen, in this case cold, turbid filth affecting the sensory orifices, it is important that one not neglect the normal qi. Another example of a similar concept is the harshly purging formula from *Discussion of Cold Damage*, Ten-Jujube Decoction (*shí zǎo tāng*).

Comparison

➢ Vs. Open the Gate Powder (*tōng guān sǎn*), see page 501.

Biomedical Indications

With the appropriate presentation, this formula may be used to treat a variety of biomedically-defined disorders including cerebrovascular accident, encephalitis, hysteria, epilepsy, hepatic coma, postconcussion syndrome, angina pectoris, and allergic rhinitis.

Alternate names

Styrax Pill (*ān xī xiāng*) in *Treasury Classic*; Atractylodes macrocephalae Pill (*bái zhú wán*) in *Fine Formulas by Su and Shen*; Atractylodes Pill (*qǐ lì gā wán*) in *Prescriptions of Universal Benefit*; Liquid Styrax Pill (*sū hé wán*) in *Red Water and Dark Pearls*

Modifications

- For those who are weak or debilitated, take with a decoction of Ginseng Radix (*rén shēn*).
- For those with very pronounced signs of phlegm, take with Zingiberis Rhizomatis Succus (*jiāng zhī*), and Bambusae Succus (*zhú lì*).
- For changes in the sensory orifices due to epilepsy, take with a decoction of Acori tatarinowii Rhizoma (*shí chāng pǔ*) and Curcumae Radix (*yù jīn*).

- For angina pectoris due to qi stagnation, blood stasis, or the congealing of cold, either reduce the dosage or remove Bubali Cornu (*shuǐ niú jiǎo*), Moschus (*shè xiāng*), and Cinnabaris (*zhū shā*), add a very small amount (0.03 gram) of Bufonis Venenum (*chán sū*), and increase the dosage of Piperis longi Fructus (*bì bá*).

通關散（通关散）
Open the Gate Powder

tōng guān sǎn

The name of this formula is derived from its ability to induce sneezing, and its rather strong actions in opening the gate of the jaw and the sensory orifices.

Source   *Important Formulas Worth a Thousand Gold Pieces* (650)

Gleditsiae Fructus abnormalis (*zhū yá zào*)
Asari Radix et Rhizoma (*xì xīn*)

Method of Preparation   Grind equal portions of the ingredients into a powder and administer by blowing a small amount of the powder into the nose. Only a very small amount of powder should be used to avoid inhalation of the powder into the lungs.

Actions   Unblocks the gate (jaw) and opens the sensory orifices

Indications

Sudden collapse, loss of consciousness, clenched jaw, extreme difficulty in breathing, a pale, ashen complexion, and obstruction by abundant phlegm and spittle.

This is phlegm collapse (痰厥 *tán jué*) caused by abundant phlegm blocking the qi and causing collapse. It usually occurs after an irregular and overindulgent diet or overwork that damages the Spleen, leading to the collection of dampness and the production of phlegm. This particular type is an excessive, closed disorder that occurs when a sudden attack of turbid qi, usually from exposure to extremely foul smells or a violent emotional outburst, causes the qi mechanisms to become rebellious and disordered. This in turn disturbs the spirit and results in sudden constraint and a 'closing' of the functional activities of qi known as 'noxious-stroke' (中惡 *zhòng è*). Turbid phlegm follows the rebellious qi upward, obstructing the sensory orifices and causing loss of consciousness, clenched jaw, and extreme difficulty in breathing. The surfeit of phlegm in the sensory orifices may also manifest as foaming at the mouth.

Analysis of Formula

The strategy here is to induce sneezing as an emergency measure to open the jaw and the sensory orifices by using herbs specifically targeted to this task. In this formula, the warm, acrid, and scurrying Gleditsiae Fructus abnormalis (*zhū yá zào*), which scours out phlegm, opens the sensory orifices, and revives the spirit (i.e., restores consciousness), is used for its strong irritating quality. As noted in *Essentials of the Materia Medica,* this herb "unblocks the gates of the orifices above and below and is able to [cause] vomiting up of phlegm and spittle. Once it stimulates the nose, there will immediately be a sneeze." Warm, acrid, and dispersing Asari Radix et Rhizoma *(xì xīn)* unblocks the channels and is particularly effective in unblocking the nose. Both ingredients unblock the jaw ('gate') and open the sensory orifices. It is important to remember that the desired effect of the formula here is to induce sneezing; as such, any other functions that the ingredients might serve, such as transforming phlegm, are not relevant, particularly given the small dosages.

Cautions and Contraindications

Contraindicated during pregnancy and for loss of consciousness due to abandoned-type disorders. It is also contraindicated for loss of consciousness due to hypertensive crisis, cerebral hemorrhage, or traumatic cranial injuries, as it stimulates blood circulation in the head. Remember that this formula is intended only for temporary, emergency use in treating acute collapse. Once consciousness has been restored, or indeed once sneezing has been induced, use of this formula should be discontinued.

Commentary

This formula can be understood as going through the orifice of the Lungs (the nose) to stimulate that organ that governs the qi of the entire body. Because the sneezing allows the Lung qi to be disseminated and unblocked, it relieves any obstructions to the qi dynamic, unblocks all of the orifices, and restores consciousness.

This is an acute, life-threatening disorder, and the treatment must focus exclusively on treating the manifestation as quickly as possible. The strategy is therefore to restore consciousness. Once this is accomplished, further treatment based on the patient's condition and differentiation of patterns may be undertaken.

Comatose collapsing disorders are of two types, closed and abandoned. Both types are associated with a variety of etiological factors including disharmonies of the qi, blood, phlegm, and food stagnation. The use of this formula is appropriate when impaired consciousness or coma is part of a pattern of rebellious qi and obstruction due to turbid phlegm. Its warm and aromatic ingredients make it particularly suitable for treating a closed disorder with cold excess.

This method of treatment is known as stimulating the nose to induce sneezing and is based on the relationship between the nose, the Lungs, and the qi. The Lungs govern the qi, and the nose is the orifice of the Lungs. When the Lung qi is obstructed, obstruction of all the sensory orifices may follow, which in this pattern manifests as clenched jaw and loss of consciousness. When sneezing is induced, it unblocks and disseminates the Lung qi, thereby restoring the functional activities of qi, reviving the spirit, and restoring consciousness.

History

This formula can be traced back to *Important Formulas Worth a Thousand Gold Pieces,* where it was prescribed for people who had hung themselves. It does not have a name in that text. It was assigned its present usage in the Song-dynasty text *Effective Medical Formulas Arranged by Category by Master Zhu,* where it is mentioned that Pinelliae Rhizoma *(bàn xià)* may also be used. Its present name first appears in the Ming-dynasty text *Additions to the Teachings of [Zhu] Dan-Xi.*

There have been many modifications of this formula over time. For example, the formula in *Golden Mirror of the Medical Tradition* adds Pinelliae Rhizoma *(bàn xià)*, Arisaematis Rhizoma *(tiān nán xīng)*, and Menthae haplocalycis Herba *(bò hé)*. Note that Centipedae Herba *(é bù shí cǎo)* is added to the formula in the official Chinese *Pharmacopeia.*

Comparison

➢ Vs. Liquid Styrax Pill *(sū hé xiāng wán)*

Both of these formulas can be used to treat such problems as qi collapse, phlegm collapse, and noxious-stroke. Liquid Styrax Pill *(sū hé xiāng wán)* is a complex formula that can be orally ingested a few times a day, and once absorbed, can aromatically transform turbidity, warm and open up the sensory orifices, and promote movement of qi to stop pain. Open the Gate Powder *(tōng guān sǎn),* however, is insufflated and, while its ability to open the orifices is immediate, should only be used once.

Biomedical Indications

With the appropriate presentation, this formula may be used to treat a variety of biomedically-defined disorders including hysteria, psychosis, anaphylactic shock, chronic rhinitis, and sinusitis.

Alternate name

Open the Gate Powder *(kāi guān sǎn)* in *Collection of Empirical Formulas*

Modifications

• To increase the efficacy of opening the sensory orifices, add Moschus *(shè xiāng)* and Menthae haplocalycis Herba *(bò hé)*.

• For excessive sputum and saliva, add Alumen *(míng fán)*.

• To more quickly revive from loss of consciousness, combine with acupuncture at points GV-26 *(shuǐ gōu)* and LI-4 *(hé gǔ)*.

Comparative Tables of Principal Formulas

■ FORMULAS THAT CLEAR HEAT AND OPEN THE SENSORY ORIFICES

Common symptoms: phlegm-heat veiling the sensory orifices with high fever, irritability and restlessness, delirious speech, disturbances of consciousness, red or deep-red tongue, and a rapid pulse

Formula Name	Diagnosis	Indications	Remarks
Wan's Cattle Gallstone Pill to Clear the Heart (*Wàn shì niú huáng qīng xīn wán*)	Pathogenic heat sinking into the interior and entering the Pericardium	Fever, irritability, restlessness, delirious speech, impaired consciousness, a scarlet-red tongue, and a thin and rapid or wiry and rapid pulse	Also for childhood convulsions or closed-type wind-stroke. Focuses on clearing and resolving toxic heat in the Pericardium.
Calm the Palace Pill with Cattle Gallstone (*ān gōng niú huáng wán*)	Warm-febrile disease sinking into the Pericardium with turbid phlegm veiling the orifices	High fever, irritability, restlessness, delirious speech, impaired consciousness, the sound of phlegm in the throat, dry mouth, a parched tongue that is red or scarlet, and a rapid pulse	Also for coma due to wind-stroke or childhood convulsions. Focuses on clearing heat and opening the orifices in acute cases.
Purple Snow Special Pill (*zǐ xuě dān*)	Blazing heat sinking into the Pericardium and generating internal movement of Liver wind	High fever, irritability, restlessness, delirious speech, impaired consciousness, muscle twitches, spasms, convulsions, thirst, dark urine, constipation, a scarlet-red tongue with a dry, yellow coating, and a forceful, wiry, and rapid pulse	Also used for febrile convulsions in children. Focuses on clearing heat and extinguishing wind.
Greatest Treasure Special Pill (*zhì bǎo dān*)	Heat sinking into the Pericardium, and turbid phlegm veiling the orifices of the Heart	Fever, irritability, restlessness, delirious speech, impaired consciousness to the point of coma, copious sputum, labored and raspy breathing, spasms, convulsions, a red or deep-red tongue with a foul, greasy, yellow coating, and a slippery, rapid pulse	This is a closed-type disorder from phlegm-heat. Focuses on opening the orifices and transforming phlegm.
Special Pill to Restore Life (*huí chūn dān*)	Childhood convulsions due to phlegm-heat entering the Pericardium and veiling the orifices of the Heart	Fever, impaired consciousness, childhood convulsions, irritability and restlessness; the child may also have wheezing, night crying, abdominal pain, excessive secretion of mucus and saliva, and sounds of mucus in the throat	Also for indigestion, vomiting, diarrhea, and coughing in children whenever the presentation involves stagnation and heat.

■ FORMULAS THAT WARM AND OPEN THE SENSORY ORIFICES

Common symptoms: sudden collapse, loss of consciousness, clenched jaw, pale complexion, excessive phlegm or mucus

Formula Name	Diagnosis	Indications	Remarks
Liquid Styrax Pill (*sū hé xiāng wán*)	Cold-dampness and turbid phlegm veiling the sensory orifices	Sudden collapse, loss of consciousness, clenched jaw, fullness, pain, and a sensation of cold in the chest and abdomen, pale complexion, purple lips, excessive mucus, cold extremities, a pale tongue with a slippery, greasy coating, and a submerged, slippery pulse	For a variety of acute closed disorders due to excessive cold.
Open the Gate Powder (*tōng guān sǎn*)	Phlegm collapse caused by abundant phlegm blocking the qi and causing collapse	Sudden collapse, loss of consciousness, clenched jaw, extreme difficulty in breathing, a pale, ashen complexion, and obstruction by abundant phlegm and spittle	Only for temporary, emergency use in treating acute collapse.

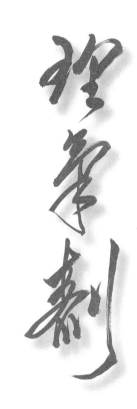

Chapter 12 Contents

Formulas that Regulate the Qi

Formulas that Regulate the Qi

12

WHEN PATHOLOGICAL CHANGE occurs in any area, organ, or channel, it is usually the flow of qi that is affected first. Thus the adage, "In its initial stage, disease resides in the qi." This statement refers to stagnation of qi: the local accumulation of nonfunctional qi that manifests as constraint, clumping, or rebellion. There are many causes for such stagnation, including emotional disturbances, irregular eating habits, trauma, and externally-contracted pathogenic influences. Long-term qi deficiency may also lead to qi stagnation. Conversely, qi stagnation over time will invariably lead to disorders of other bodily functions and systems. Blood stasis, phlegm obstruction, food stagnation, and deficiency disorders are typical sequelae of qi stagnation. This was noted in Chapter 39 of *Basic Questions*: "Myriad disorders are generated through qi."

Qi stagnation causes the ascending and descending (or upward- and downward-directing) functions of the qi dynamic (氣機 *qì jī*) to break down. The primary clinical manifestations of such pathology are pain and distention. This is reflected in another adage: "Lack of free passage results in pain." Facilitating the ascending and descending functions of the qi dynamic in order to unblock (通 *tōng*) the proper flow of qi is therefore the primary objective of the formulas in this chapter. They are said to regulate the qi (理氣 *lǐ qì*) by opening up areas of constraint and smooth the normal movement of the qi dynamic. This includes facilitating the ascent of the clear, directing the turbid downward, and reversing rebellion.

A specific category of formulas that regulate the qi was first introduced by the Qing-dynasty physician Wang Ang in *Medical Formulas Collected and Analyzed*. At present, however, most of the formulas included in this category are considerably older. The largest group comes from Zhang Zhong-Jing's late-Han-dynasty work *Discussion of Cold Damage and Miscellaneous Diseases*. This seminal text focused on regulating the movement and diffusion of qi and essence throughout the body. Only much later, especially during the Jin and Yuan periods, did physicians begin to center their treatment strategies more specifically on the ascent and descent of qi. It is from this period that most of the other formulas in this chapter are taken.

Historically, commentators distinguish between two major types of formulas for regulating the qi. The first promotes the smooth movement of qi, unblocks stagnation, and is used for treating pain and distention. The second type directs rebellious or abnormal flow of qi downward and is used for treating such problems as vomiting, belching, hiccup, and some forms of coughing or wheezing. These are the strategies discussed in this chapter. There are other formulas that also open up constraint or clumping due to qi stagnation and treat pain, such as those that release the exterior (Chapter 1), harmonize the qi (Chapter 3), and warm the interior (Chapter 6). However, while these formulas treat patterns that include pain as a recurrent symptom, their main objective is to regulate the body's yang qi: by venting pathogens that constrain the diffusion of yang toward the exterior, causing fluids or heat to accumulate, or by boosting the body's own internal fire to overcome an excess of yin.

By contrast, the formulas in this chapter focus on the dynamic and moving functions of the broader category of qi. Traditionally, these functions have been associated with the Lungs as the ruler of qi. Thus, Chapter 74 of *Basic Questions*, which discusses the nineteen basic pathodynamic processes that underlie all human disease, states: "All qi rushing and constraint can be attributed to the Lungs." The qi referred to in this passage accumulates in the chest, and its dispersal throughout the body is regulated and controlled through the rhythms bestowed upon it by the Lungs. This is different from the hot yang qi or ministerial fire that permeates the body from its source in the lower burner, whose bold nature is directed and governed by the Liver. It is with respect to pathologies of this particular qi that the same chapter of *Basic Questions* states: "All rebellion and [up-] flushing can be attributed to fire," and "All cold with contracture and tautness can be attributed to the Kidneys."

Beginning in the Ming dynasty, Chinese physicians began to associate all types of qi stagnation and constraint with the Liver. This was accompanied by a tendency to focus on internal (i.e., emotional) rather than external (i.e., environmental) factors as the cause of stagnation. The assimilation into Chinese medicine of the connection between emotional disorders and nervous function posited by late 19th- and early 20th-century Western medicine further reinforced these tendencies, as Chinese physicians interpreted the functions of the nervous system in Western medicine as matching those of the Liver in Chinese medicine. This has led to a tendency in modern times to conflate emotional problems with patterns of Liver qi stagnation and of defining the Liver as the most important organ involved in the regulation of qi. This can be seen as a narrowing of the more complex treatment strategies available in the Chinese medical literature. This issue comes up repeatedly in the COMMENTARY sections of individual formulas in this chapter.

In regulating the qi, it is important to distinguish deficiency from excess. Stagnation is regarded as a form of excess. It is the temporary accumulation of qi in a part of the body where it is not being properly disseminated. When this occurs, the appropriate strategy is to promote the movement of qi. If, instead, the qi is tonified, the stagnation will increase and the patient's condition will worsen. Conversely, promoting the movement of qi when it is deficient will only serve to aggravate the deficiency. When the qi is both stagnant and deficient (a relatively common occurrence), both aspects must be addressed.

Because qi stagnation readily leads to secondary pathologies such as blood stasis, phlegm obstruction, dampness, or food stagnation, it may be necessary to include herbs that address such problems in formulas that regulate the qi. This requires careful pattern differentiation, paying meticulous attention to primary and secondary pathodynamics and their interrelationships.

The main ingredients of the formulas in this chapter are invariably acrid and bitter as well as warming or drying. When improperly used, they can readily injure the fluids and scatter the qi. They should therefore be prescribed only with the utmost caution in patients with both qi stagnation and depleted fluids; they must also be discontinued once the condition improves.

Section 1

FORMULAS THAT PROMOTE THE MOVEMENT OF QI

The formulas in this section are used for treating areas of blocked or stagnant qi, the primary symptom of which is usually pain and distention. The particular manifestations depend upon the location of the blockage or stagnation.

- In the chest, qi stagnation causes chest and back pain, coughing, and shortness of breath. This is treated with herbs such as Citri reticulatae Pericarpium (*chén pí*), Magnoliae officinalis Cortex (*hòu pò*), Pinelliae Rhizoma praeparatum (*zhì bàn xià*), or Allii fistulosi Bulbus (*cōng bái*).

- In the Spleen and Stomach, it causes epigastric and abdominal pain and distention, belching, acid reflux, and irregular bowel movements. This is treated with qi-moving herbs such as Citri reticulatae Pericarpium (*chén pí*), Magnoliae officinalis Cortex (*hòu pò*), Aucklandiae Radix (*mù xiāng*), or Amomi Fructus (*shā rén*).

- Constraint of the ascent of Liver qi manifests as pain and distention in the chest and hypochondria. This is treated with herbs such as Cyperi Rhizoma (*xiāng fù*), Citri reticulatae viride Pericarpium (*qīng pí*), Toosendan Fructus (*chuān liàn zǐ*), or Curcumae Radix (*yù jīn*).

- In the lower burner, qi stagnation can cause painful urinary dysfunction, bulging disorders, irregular menstruation, or dysmenorrhea. Important herbs that promote the movement of qi in this area include Cyperi Rhizoma (*xiāng fù*), Toosendan Fructus (*chuān liàn zǐ*), Foeniculi Fructus (*xiǎo huí xiāng*), Linderae Radix (*wū yào*), and Aquilariae Lignum resinatum (*chén xiāng*).

Clinically, herbs that promote the movement of qi are usually combined with one of more herbs from the following five categories:

1. Herbs that invigorate the blood such as Chuanxiong Rhizoma *(chuān xiōng)*, Angelicae sinensis Radix *(dāng guī)*, Corydalis Rhizoma *(yán hú suǒ)*, Curcumae Rhizoma *(é zhú)*, or Sparganii Rhizoma *(sān léng)*. These are necessary because of the close interaction between qi and blood in instigating and regulating their mutual flow.

2. Herbs that warm the interior such as Cinnamomi Cortex *(ròu guì)*, Zingiberis Rhizoma *(gān jiāng)*, Alpiniae officinarum Rhizoma *(gāo liáng jiāng)*, or Alpiniae katsumadai Semen *(cǎo dòu kòu)*. These are useful where internal cold obstructs the qi dynamic, or where qi stagnation leads to dampness and phlegm, which in turn obstruct the rising of clear yang.

3. Herbs that clear heat from constraint such as Gardeniae Fructus *(zhī zǐ)*, Moutan Cortex *(mǔ dān pí)*, or Prunellae Spica *(xià kū cǎo)*. These are indicated where qi stagnation constrains the diffusion of yang qi or ministerial fire, leading to local symptoms of heat or inflammation.

4. Herbs that transform phlegm such as Pinelliae Rhizoma praeparatum *(zhì bàn xià)*, Arisaematis Rhizoma praeparatum *(zhì tiān nán xīng)*, Trichosanthis Fructus *(guā lóu)*, and Fritillariae Bulbus *(bèi mǔ)*. These are useful where qi stagnation blocks the descent of turbid yin, leading to the accumulation of congealing fluids that become phlegm.

5. Herbs that enrich the yin and nourish the blood such as Lycii Fructus *(gǒu qǐ zǐ)* and Paeoniae Radix alba *(bái sháo)*. These are helpful where qi stagnation has damaged the yin blood, or where the drying action of the main qi-regulating herbs risks damaging the yin blood.

Based on a precise analysis of the disease dynamic in each case, many other types of herbs may be added to formulas that move the qi. Where obstruction of the middle or lower burner qi leads to the generation of dampness, herbs that strengthen the Spleen and expel dampness, such as Atractylodis Rhizoma *(cāng zhú)*, Poria *(fú líng)*, or Alismatis Rhizoma *(zé xiè)*, may be used. Where chronic qi stagnation is complicated by blood stasis and phlegm obstruction, leading to clumping and the formation of lumps, substances that soften masses, such as Eckloniae Thallus *(kūn bù)*, Sargassum *(hǎi zǎo)*, or Laminariae Thallus *(hǎi dài)*, may be used. If qi deficiency is a prominent aspect of the pattern, one may choose to include qi-tonifying herbs such as Ginseng Radix *(rén shēn)* or Atractylodis macrocephalae Rhizoma *(bái zhú)*.

越鞠丸
Escape Restraint Pill
yuè jū wán

There are two explanations for the name of this formula. The first interprets the character 越 *yuè* to mean escape from or the surmounting of difficulties, and the character 鞠 *jū* to mean something that is crooked or bent, a common term for qi that has become constrained and does not flow as it should. This formula resolves many types of stagnation or clumping caused by long-term constraint. It thereby allows the qi to escape the bonds that bend it out of shape, hence the name. A second explanation is based on Li Shi-Zhen's claim that these characters refer to the ancient names for Chuanxiong Rhizoma *(chuān xiōng)* and Gardeniae Fructus *(zhī zǐ)*, respectively.

Source *Essential Teachings of [Zhu] Dan-Xi* (1481)

Atractylodis Rhizoma *(cāng zhú)*
Chuanxiong Rhizoma *(chuān xiōng)*
Cyperi Rhizoma *(xiāng fù)*
Gardeniae Fructus *(zhī zǐ)*
Massa medicata fermentata *(shén qū)*

Method of Preparation Grind equal amounts of the ingredients into a fine powder and form into pills with water. Take 6-9g with warm water. May also be prepared as a decoction with 6-12g of each ingredient.

Actions Promotes the movement of qi and releases constraint

Indications

Focal distention and a stifling sensation in the chest and abdomen, fixed pain in the hypochondria, belching, vomiting, acid reflux, mild coughing with copious sputum, reduced appetite, and indigestion.

According to Zhu Dan-Xi, the formula's author, this treats various types of constraint due to stagnant qi. In Chinese medicine, the term constraint (鬱 *yù*) has the meaning of something being pent-up and unable to move or change. It refers in particular to pathologies of the qi dynamic, as explained by Zhu Dan-Xi's disciple, Dai Yuan-Li: "Constraint is something clumped and fused (結聚 *jié jù*) and unable to escape [from this predicament]. It should ascend but cannot ascend. It should descend but cannot descend. It should transform but cannot transform." Irregular eating habits, exposure to excessive cold or heat, and inordinate joy, anger, or anxiety can disrupt the normal flow of qi and thereby give rise to this condition.

Zhu Dan-Xi differentiated six types of constraint based on the aspect of physiology that was most affected—qi, fire, blood, phlegm, dampness, and food—but viewed all of these as arising primarily from qi stagnation. When qi stagnates in the middle burner, which is the fulcrum of the qi dynamic and thus central to the pattern, this leads to focal distention and a stifling sensation in the chest and abdomen. Disrupting the transformative processes of middle burner physiology gives rise to dampness, phlegm, and food stagnation. Manifestations include bloating, indigestion, mild coughing with copious sputum, reduced appetite, nausea, and vomiting. Qi stagnation transforming into fire manifests as a bitter taste in the mouth and acid reflux. When qi stagnation leads to blood stasis, it manifests as a stabbing, fixed pain in the chest and hypochondria.

Analysis of Formula

Because the principal dysfunction is one of stagnant or constrained qi, this formula focuses on promoting the movement of qi, particularly on unblocking the ascending and descending functions of the qi dynamic in the middle burner. According to the source text, there are two chief herbs in this formula. The first is aromatic and acrid Atractylodis Rhizoma *(cāng zhú),* which promotes the ascending functions of the middle burner, dries dampness, and transforms phlegm. It is used to release the constraint of qi, dampness, and phlegm and addresses the symptoms of focal distention in the chest and copious sputum. The other chief ingredient is acrid and warming Chuanxiong Rhizoma *(chuān xiōng),* a blood-invigorating herb that releases constrained blood and thus resolves the fixed pain. It also reinforces the qi-moving action of the other chief herb. Both of these herbs direct the qi upward, underscoring the primary importance attributed to this function by Li Dong-Yuan, whose thinking strongly influenced Zhu Dan-Xi. In *Essential Teachings of [Zhu] Dan-Xi,* Zhu explains:

> When qi and blood rush harmoniously, the myriad disorders do not arise. But should one of them become constrained, all kinds of disorders are generated. Thus, of all the disorders of the human body, a majority arise from constraint. Atractylodis Rhizoma *(cāng zhú)* and Chuanxiong Rhizoma *(chuān xiōng)* comprehensively resolve all [such] constraint. One adds other herbs [to this combination] according to the presenting symptoms. All constraint involves the middle burner. I use Atractylodis Rhizoma *(cāng zhú)* and Chuanxiong Rhizoma *(chuān xiōng)* to open and lift its [own] qi so it can direct the qi [dynamic] upward.

The two chief herbs are supported by a single deputy, Cyperi Rhizoma *(xiāng fù).* Extremely effective at resolving problems due to constrained qi, this herb is said to enter the blood aspect of the qi. This means that while, as an acrid and warming herb, Cyperi Rhizoma *(xiāng fù)* naturally directs the qi upward, it also directs it downward, being, in fact, a key herb in the treatment of gynecological disorders. It thereby complements the two chief herbs in unblocking the qi dynamic. This synergism is highlighted by Zhu Dan-Xi in his explanation of the principles that guide the formula's composition:

> This formula and its herbs [thereby effectively] combine upward- and downward-directing. If one wishes to direct upward, one must first direct downward. If one wishes to direct downward, one must first direct upward. Atractylodis Rhizoma *(cāng zhú)* is strongly acrid and martial [in its action]. Securing the Stomach and strengthening the Spleen, it is able to enter into all channels, dredging and draining dampness in the yang brightness, unblocking the vessels [while also] securing them. Cyperi Rhizoma *(xiāng fù)* is an herb that accelerates the qi within the yin and that drives the qi downward most rapidly. One herb ascending, the other descending, they are able to disperse constraint and [thereby] balance [the qi dynamic]. As a terminal yin herb, Chuanxiong Rhizoma *(chuān xiōng)* truly

reaches into the three burners, moving upward into the head and eyes and downward into the sea of blood. It has the ability to unblock the qi and blood of the yin and yang.

The remaining herbs serve as assistants. Gardeniae Fructus *(zhī zǐ)* clears heat from all three burners and resolves the fire from constraint, and with it, the acid reflux. Massa medicata fermentata *(shén qū)* relieves constraint caused by food stagnation and harmonizes the Stomach. It is helpful in treating the nausea and vomiting, reduced appetite, and stifling sensation in the epigastrium.

Cautions and Contraindications

Although this formula can be modified in many ways, it is contraindicated in cases of stagnation due to deficiency. To treat such conditions, one should begin with a base formula such as Six-Gentlemen Decoction with Aucklandia and Amomum *(xiāng shā liù jūn zǐ tāng).*

Commentary

This is a very effective formula for treating qi stagnation (particularly of the middle burner) and its sequelae, including heat, blood stasis, phlegm, and food stagnation.

Location of the Disorder

Many modern textbooks define this disorder as being primarily Liver qi stagnation, based on the theory that the Liver is the most important organ in regulating the qi. Accordingly, Cyperi Rhizoma *(xiāng fù)* is designated as the chief herb, and the gastrointestinal symptoms that characterize the pattern are due to Liver wood overcoming Spleen earth. However, many classical and modern commentators believe that this interpretation is unnecessarily restrictive. As the well-known 20th-century physician Qin Bo-Wei explains in *[Qin] Qian-Zhai's Lecture Notes on Medicine:*

> This formula belongs to those general formulas that master the moving of qi and the resolving of constraint. It is not principally a formula for Liver qi [stagnation]. ... When researching and using formulas, one must set out getting to know them via the doctrines and experience of previous generations. Zhu Dan-Xi clearly pointed out that, in respect to this formula [one must look to the statement in *Basic Questions:*] "All qi rushing and constraint can be attributed to the Lungs." He also reckoned that constraint disorders are generally located in the middle burner where the Spleen and Stomach have lost their ascending and descending [functions]. If one mistakenly believes that resolving constraint is [a matter of] soothing the Liver, then one has lost its original intention.

Brief History of Constraint in Chinese Medicine

Qin Bo-Wei's view of this issue is supported by an analysis of treatment strategies for constraint in Chinese medicine. Like many medical concepts, the term constraint (鬱 *yù*) appeared in very early nonmedical texts such as *Rites of Zhou,* where its meaning is that of "a tone that does not carry." The notion of something being hindered in its dynamic was applied to the body in the 3rd-century B.C. text *Annals of Master Lu,* which states that "[when] the essence does not flow, the qi [becomes] pent-up." Chapter 71 of *Basic Questions* integrated this concept into its five-phase doctrine of qi transformation when it listed five types of constraint and their corresponding treatment strategies. These strategies—defined by way of simple mnemonics like "For wood constraint, thrust it out" or "For fire from constraint, discharge it"—were quickly integrated into herbal medicine, where they became guiding principles in the treatment of externally-contracted cold damage disorders. Formulas from *Discussion of Cold Damage,* such as Ephedra Decoction *(má huáng tāng),* Minor Bupleurum Decoction *(xiǎo chái hú tāng),* or Major Bluegreen Dragon Decoction *(dà qīng lóng tāng),* all treat constraint of yang qi due to external invasion of cold.

A second phase in the understanding of constraint disorders began in the Song dynasty, as physicians focused increasingly on internal causes of disease. Chen Yan was the first to specifically link constraint to emotional problems. Likewise, when the Yuan-dynasty writer Wang Lü noted in *Discourse on Tracing Back to the Medical Classics* that "[c]onstraint has the meaning of [something] stagnating and of [something] being blocked," he was no longer thinking primarily of the body's yang qi, but rather of the ascending and descending functions of the qi dynamic. Because Jin-Yuan era physicians paid increasing attention to this dynamic, regarding it as the fulcrum of all physiological and pathological processes, its constraint naturally became a topic of great concern. Thus, by the time *Essential Teachings of [Zhu] Dan-Xi* was published in 1481, its author was able to state that, "of all disorders of the human body, a majority arise from constraint."

Zhu's Six Types of Constraint

Zhu Dan-Xi's doctrine of the six types of constraint (六鬱 *liù yù*) was explained by his disciple Dai Yuan-Li:

> Qi constraint [is characterized by] chest and flank pain, and a submerged, rough pulse. Dampness constraint [is characterized] by pain that moves throughout the entire body, or by joint pain that gets worse when the weather is cold or dank, and a submerged and thin pulse. Phlegm constraint [is characterized] by a cough that occurs with activity, and a submerged, slippery pulse in the distal position. Heat constraint [is characterized] by an indistinct stifling sensation in the chest, red urine, and a submerged and rapid pulse. Blood constraint [is characterized] by a lack of power in the four limbs, no inability to eat, but red stools, and a submerged pulse. Food constraint [is characterized] by acid reflux, a twisted abdomen with an inability to eat, a balanced pulse at ST-9 *(rén yíng),* and an exuberant pulse at the wrist.

In this six-fold classification, qi constraint can be viewed as reflecting stagnation of the gathering qi, governed by the

Lungs. Fire arises from constraint of the yang qi whose ascent is directed by the Liver. Dampness and phlegm are pathologies caused by stagnation of the nutritive qi produced in and associated with the middle burner. Food stagnation, too, reflects a breakdown of middle burner function, while blood constraint, as defined by Zhu Dan-Xi, is not so much the impairment of its movement leading to pain, but rather a failure in its generation and in its function of nourishing the muscles and sinews. Viewed from this perspective, this formula effectively addresses various types of qi stagnation and relieves secondary pathologies.

Later Understandings of Constraint

Zhu Dan-Xi's understanding of constraint moved in a new direction from the Ming dynasty onward. Taking up Chen Yan's proposed linkage of constraint and the emotions, physicians now defined constraint itself as a condition where a person was unable to express his feelings, leading to stagnation and the manifestation of physical symptoms. The difference between the old and new understandings of constraint was expressed by Zhang Jie-Bin in *Collected Treatises of [Zhang] Jing-Yue*:

> Regarding constraint of the five qi [elaborated in the *Inner Classic*], this can occur in all types of disorders. In such a case, constraint is caused by a disorder [i.e., something causing stagnation of qi]. However, with respect to emotional constraint, these all arise from within the Heart-mind. In such a case, [a person] becomes ill because of constraint.

Around the same time, the Ming-dynasty writer Zhao Xian-Ke suggested that Rambling Powder *(xiāo yáo sǎn),* a formula for treating Liver qi stagnation (discussed in Chapter 3), could be substituted for all other formulas and treatment strategies used for constraint by previous generations of physicians. Although a close reading of Zhao's argument in *Thread through Medicine* shows that he was actually concerned with the release of external pathogens, his argument was quickly assimilated into the more powerful discourse on emotional constraint. In *Case Records as a Guide to Clinical Practice,* the influential Qing-dynasty physician Ye Tian-Shi attempted to reconcile the different views:

> Whatever causes constraint leads to qi stagnation. Qi stagnating for a long time invariably transforms into heat. This heat from constraint consumes the body fluids, which then no longer flow [properly]. The mechanism of ascending and descending deviates from its norm. In the initial stages, damage occurs in the qi aspect. In chronic conditions, it extends to the blood aspect. If protracted, this results in exhaustion from constraint, [which is] a severe illness. ... [Vulgar physicians] do not know that constraint is due to hidden emotions that bend one's intentions rather than [allowing them to be] expressed directly. As a result, the upward- and downward-directing of qi, its opening and closing, and [therefore the entire] qi dynamic no longer function freely.

While Ye Tian-Shi himself emphasized that using Escape Restraint Pill (yuè jū wán) requires a careful and precise pattern differentiation that does not accept the simple equation between constraint and Liver disharmonies, the association between constraint and emotional disorders became ever more entrenched. Even today, constraint is almost invariably interpreted as having at least some emotional aspect, and the term is rarely used in connection with the resolution of external pathogens.

Controversy over the Chief Ingredient

Because this formula treats constraint whether or not due to emotional causes, it focuses on the middle burner (Spleen and Stomach) but also involves failure of the clear to ascend (Liver) and of the turbid to descend (Lungs), and this, in turn, can manifest in a myriad of patterns all of which have qi stagnation as their root, it is wise to be flexible about the use of this formula in the clinic. This is underscored by the late-Qing-dynasty physician Fei Bo-Xiong in *Discussion of Medical Formulas*:

> All constraint disorders must first of all be qi disorders. For when the qi flows freely, how could there be constraint? The commentaries on this formula say that it rules treatment of the six types of constraint. But how could these six types of constraint all be present at once? One needs to understand that when the ancients set down a formula, they did so only to outline a general strategy. In the case of qi constraint, Cyperi Rhizoma (xiāng fù) is the chief ingredient. In the case of dampness constraint, Atractylodis Rhizoma (cāng zhú) is the chief ingredient. In the case of blood constraint, Chuanxiong Rhizoma (chuān xiōng) is the chief ingredient. In the case of food constraint, Massa medicata fermentata (shén qū) is the chief ingredient. In the case of fire constraint, Gardeniae Fructus (zhī zǐ) is the chief ingredient. Furthermore, one adjusts the dosages and makes substitutions in accordance with the location of the disorder. Any formula [that one composes should always] take up the intentions of the ancients without getting stuck in [precisely how they wrote down] the formula. One should study any formula book with this perspective in mind.

In contemporary clinical practice, this formula is used for treating all types of disorders whose origins can be traced to constraint of the qi dynamic; this gives it a very wide scope of application. In addition to emotional constraint (often identified today with depression) associated with the physical symptoms outlined above, these include insomnia, plum-pit qi (梅核氣 méi hé qì), and restless organ (臟躁 zàng zào) disorder. The formula is also used to treat angina and pain associated with inflammatory disorders of the digestive tract and for gynecological conditions such as irregular or painful menstruation, and infertility in overweight women with accumulation of dampness and phlegm.

Comparisons

➤ Vs. Rambling Powder (xiāo yáo sǎn); see PAGE 123

➤ Vs. Pinellia and Magnolia Bark Decoction (bàn xià hòu pò tāng); see PAGE 518

➤ Vs. Galangal and Cyperus Pill (liáng fù wán); see PAGE 522

Biomedical Indications

With the appropriate presentation, this formula may be used to treat a wide variety of biomedically-defined disorders. These can be divided into the following groups:

- Digestive disorders including peptic ulcer, irritable bowel syndrome, chronic gastritis, biliary tract infections, gallstones, and chronic hepatitis

- Neuropsychiatric disorders such as intercostal neuralgia, migraine, globus hystericus, epilepsy, cerebral thrombosis, and some types of neuroses, including depression.

It has also been used in the treatment of dysmenorrhea, hypocalcemia, coronary artery disease, and pelvic inflammatory disease.

....

Alternate names

Ligusticum and Atractylodes Pill (xióng zhú wán) in *Teachings of (Zhu) Dan-Xi*; Chuanxiong and Atractylodes Pill (xiōng cāng wán) in *Essential Teachings of [Zhu] Dan-Xi*; Escape Crookedness Pill (yuè qū wán) in *Medicine Path of Song-Ya*

....

Modifications

- If stagnant qi predominates, add Curcumae Radix (yù jīn), Aucklandiae Radix (mù xiāng), and Linderae Radix (wū yào).

- If Liver fire predominates, remove Atractylodis Rhizoma (cāng zhú) and add Paeoniae Radix alba (bái sháo) and Moutan Cortex (mǔ dān pí).

- If blood stasis predominates, add Persicae Semen (táo rén) and Carthami Flos (hóng huā).

- If phlegm predominates, add Pinelliae Rhizoma praeparatum (zhì bàn xià) and Arisaematis Rhizoma praeparatum (zhì tiān nán xīng).

- If dampness predominates, add Magnoliae officinalis Cortex (hòu pò) and Poria (fú líng).

- If food stagnation predominates, add Crataegi Fructus (shān zhā) and Hordei Fructus germinatus (mài yá).

- For concurrent cold in the middle burner, remove Gardeniae Fructus (zhī zǐ) and add Evodiae Fructus (wú zhū yú) and Zingiberis Rhizoma (gān jiāng).

- For severe bloating and distention, add Citri reticulatae viride Pericarpium (qīng pí), Citri reticulatae Pericarpium (chén pí), Aurantii Fructus immaturus (zhǐ shí), and Arecae Semen (bīng láng).

Associated Formulas

排氣飲 （排气饮）

Discharge Gas Drink

pái qì yǐn

Source *Practical Established Formulas* (1761)

Citri reticulatae Pericarpium (*chén pí*) 4.5g
Cyperi Rhizoma (*xiāng fù*) 6g
Linderae Radix (*wū yào*) 6g
Magnoliae officinalis Cortex (*hòu pò*) 3g
Aucklandiae Radix (*mù xiāng*) 3g
Aurantii Fructus (*zhǐ ké*) 4.5g
Pogostemonis/Agastaches Herba (*huò xiāng*) 4.5g
Alismatis Rhizoma (*zé xiè*) 3g

Regulates the qi, dries dampness, and resolves food stagnation. For epigastric and abdominal bloating and distention resulting from disruption in the flow of qi from obstruction due to dampness, rebellious qi, and food stagnation. In contrast to the principal formula, this focuses more on the bloating and gas by promoting the movement of qi and resolving food stagnation in the middle burner.

達鬱湯 （达郁汤）

Thrust Out Constraint Decoction

dá yù tāng

Source *Wondrous Lantern for Peering into the Origin and Development of Miscellaneous Diseases* (1773)

Bupleuri Radix (*chái hú*)
Cimicifugae Rhizoma (*shēng má*)
Cyperi Rhizoma (*xiāng fù*)
Chuanxiong Rhizoma (*chuān xiōng*)
Tribuli Fructus (*cì jí lí*)
Mori Cortex (*sāng bái pí*)
Perillae Caulis (*zǐ sū gěng*)

Decoction. The source text does not specify dosages. For emotional constraint manifesting with nausea and vomiting and a submerged pulse. This is an example of modifying Escape Restraint Pill (*yuè jū wán*) to treat emotional disorders according to the adage, "For wood constraint, thrust it out," from the *Inner Classic*. Like the principal formula, emphasis is placed on regulating the ascending and descending functions. The root cause, however, is defined here as failure of Liver wood to ascend due to emotional causes. This requires an out-thrusting strategy, represented here by the inclusion of Bupleuri Radix (*chái hú*) and Cimicifugae Rhizoma (*shēng má*), both of which open the qi dynamic to allow pathogenic qi to be thrust out toward the exterior. The formula is indicated where Liver wood becomes constrained by excessive sadness, melancholy, or pensiveness.

通氣散 （通气散）

Unblock the Qi Powder

tōng qì sǎn

Source *Correction of Errors among Physicians* (1830)

Bupleuri Radix (*chái hú*) 30g
Cyperi Rhizoma (*xiāng fù*) 30g

Chuanxiong Rhizoma (*chuān xiōng*) 15g

Grind the ingredients into a powder and take in 9g doses followed by warm water twice a day. Spreads and regulates the Liver qi and opens up the sensory orifices. For acute, severely diminished hearing where the patient "cannot even hear thunder" due to emotional upset or an externally-contracted condition.

女神散

Goddess Powder

nǚ shén sǎn

Source *Formulary and Mnemonics from 'No Mistake' Pharmacy* (1956)

Angelicae sinensis Radix (*dāng guī*) 3-4g
Chuanxiong Rhizoma (*chuān xiōng*) 3g
Atractylodis macrocephalae Rhizoma (*bái zhú*) 3g
Cyperi Rhizoma (*xiāng fù*) 3-4g
Cinnamomi Ramulus (*guì zhī*) 2-3g
Scutellariae Radix (*huáng qín*) 2-4g
Ginseng Radix (*rén shēn*) 1.5-2g
Arecae Semen (*bīng láng*) 2-4g
Coptidis Rhizoma (*huáng lián*) 1-2g
Aucklandiae Radix (*mù xiāng*) 1-2g
Caryophylli Flos (*dīng xiāng*) 0.5-1g
Glycyrrhizae Radix (*gān cǎo*) 1-1.5g
Rhei Radix et Rhizoma (*dà huáng*) 0.5-1g

Decoction. This is a Japanese formula transmitted within the family of the 19th-century Kampo physician Asada Sōhaku who made it available to a wider public. According to some sources, it was originally created to treat stress in soldiers fighting at the front, although in contemporary practice, it is used primarily as a woman's remedy to treat what is known in Kampo as disorders of the 'blood pathways' (血の道 *chi no michi*). The term describes presentations characterized by the presence of psychosomatic symptoms that trouble the patient but cannot be attributed to organic illness. Although such presentations are claimed to be more frequent in women, the original usage of this formula indicates that they are, in fact, not gender specific. Common symptoms include depression, anxiety, and nervous tension accompanied by hot flushes, dizziness, heavy-headedness, palpitations, abdominal distention, nausea, fatigue, and insomnia. The tongue may have a white coating with a red tip, and the pulse is excessive and floating. In women, one may also observe menstrual irregularity, or an association of symptoms with the menstrual cycle. In modern Chinese medical terms, the formula treats qi stagnation with heat constraint and clumping that occurs in the context of qi and blood deficiency.

In contrast to the principal formula, Goddess Powder (*nǚ shén sǎn*) focuses more strongly on draining heat by unblocking the Stomach and Intestines. In the clinic, the presence of strong internal heat from constraint is experienced as hot flushes, but also as a burning-hot sensation along the spine and back. Constipation, irritability, and insomnia, too, are common presenting symptoms. As a result, the formula is frequently used in the treatment of menopausal syndrome, premenstrual tension, pre- and postpartum neuroses or depression, and similar psychosomatic disorders. In Japan, the formula is often given for several months. During pregnancy, and if constipation is not a major part of the presentation, Rhei Radix et Rhizoma (dà huáng) should be omitted.

Note: This formula is also known as Calm the Nutritive Decoction (安營湯 ān yíng tāng).

柴胡疏肝散

Bupleurum Powder to Dredge the Liver

chái hú shū gān sǎn

Source   *Indispensable Tools for Pattern Treatment* (1602)

vinegar-fried Citri reticulatae Pericarpium (cù chǎo chén pí) . . . 6g
Bupleuri Radix (chái hú) 6g
Chuanxiong Rhizoma (chuān xiōng) 4.5g
dry-fried Aurantii Fructus (chǎo zhǐ ké) 4.5g
Paeoniae Radix (sháo yào) 4.5g
Glycyrrhizae Radix praeparata (zhì gān cǎo) 1.5g
Cyperi Rhizoma (xiāng fù) 4.5g

Method of Preparation   Administer before meals in one dose with 2 cups of water boiled down to eight-tenths of a cup.

Actions   Spreads the Liver qi, harmonizes the blood, and alleviates pain

Indications

Flank pain, a stifling sensation in the chest causing one to heave deep sighs, suppressed emotions and feelings of frustration that easily give rise to anger, belching, abdominal distention and fullness, alternating fever and chills, and a wiry pulse.

This is constraint and clumping of the Liver qi. The Liver likes to thrust outward and resists being curbed or constrained. Its channel spreads through the flanks and chest above and the lower abdomen and groin below. When the dredging and discharging functions of the Liver are constrained, which can easily happen in situations where one cannot 'speak one's mind,' or where one is forced to do things against one's will, the Liver qi stagnates and clumps. This manifests as hypochondriac and flank pain, a stifling sensation in the chest, causing one to heave deep sighs and a tendency to vent one's frustration through anger. When the Liver qi stagnates and does not ascend as it should, it starts to flow horizontally (instead of vertically upward) to invade the Stomach and Spleen. This causes distention and fullness of the abdomen. When Liver qi constraint blocks the circulation of yang qi, the person often begins to feel cold. As the constraint is suddenly released, the pent-up heat floods the Triple Burner, leading to sensations of fever or heat. A wiry pulse reflects the stagnation of Liver qi.

Analysis of Formula

This formula is a modification of Frigid Extremities Powder (sì nì sǎn) to which Cyperi Rhizoma (xiāng fù), Citri reticulatae Pericarpium (chén pí), and Chuanxiong Rhizoma (chuān

xiōng) have been added. The chief herb is acrid, bitter, and slightly cooling Bupleuri Radix (chái hú). It enters the Liver and Gallbladder channels to facilitate the Liver's out-thrusting functions by dredging constraint and clumping. It is supported by two deputies: bitter, acrid, and balanced Cyperi Rhizoma (xiāng fù), which enters the Liver channel to regulate its qi, and the acrid Chuanxiong Rhizoma (chuān xiōng), whose powerful qi enters the qi and blood aspects of the Liver to open constraint and stop pain. Together, these two deputies support the chief herbs in resolving constraint and stagnation in the Liver channel, move its qi, and stop pain. There are two groups of assistants. Citri reticulatae Pericarpium (chén pí) and Aurantii Fructus (zhǐ ké) regulate the qi of the Stomach and Intestines. Directing qi downward, they facilitate the discharge of the buildup of qi excess from the chest and middle burner that manifests in sensations of fullness and distention. They also balance any excessive ascending that might result form a sudden release of Liver qi. The other group of assistants is comprised of the sweet herbs Paeoniae Radix (sháo yào) and Glycyrrhizae Radix (gān cǎo). Together, they nourish the blood to soften the Liver, relaxing hyperactivity to stop the pain. Their sweetness and moisture also balance the drying action of the chief and deputy herbs. Glycyrrhizae Radix (gān cǎo) serves the additional role of envoy to harmonize the various actions of the seven ingredients in this formula.

Cautions and Contraindications

This formula is aromatic, acrid, and drying. It readily injures the qi and yin, and is therefore contraindicated for long-term use or in patients with Liver qi stagnation-type pain due to qi or yin deficiency.

Commentary

Through the direct and straightforward manner in which it focuses on Liver qi stagnation, this formula has become the key script for treating this disorder. Its range of application has been expanded to cover all patterns due to Liver qi stagnation. This includes various types of abdominal pain, premenstrual syndrome or dysmenorrhea, and back pain. A key marker for its use is the nature of the pain, which tends to come and go, depending on the patient's emotional state and level of energy. This indicates that the pain is not due to external causes. The pain is generally relieved by activity and therefore may be worse at night than during the day. This distinguishes it from conditions of deficiency. Finally, the wiry pulse, location, and muscle-hypertonicity mark the condition as one of Liver excess.

The source text does not indicate which type of Paeoniae Radix (sháo yào) should be used. Most commentators think that Paeoniae Radix alba (bái sháo) is more appropriate, given its ability to soften the Liver and work in conjunction with

Glycyrrhizae Radix *(gān cǎo)* to achieve this effect. However, a minority, represented by the text *Casual Notes on Medicine*, argue that Paeoniae Radix rubra *(chì sháo)* should be used because of its ability to clear heat from constraint at the blood level.

This formula was composed by the Ming-dynasty physician Ye Wen-Ling, who used it to treat 'flank pain.' It was popularized by Zhang Jie-Bin, who included it in his enormously influential work, *Collected Treatises of [Zhang] Jing-Yue.* Because of the popularity of this book, many later commentators erroneously attributed authorship of the formula to Zhang.

Comparisons

➢ Vs. FRIGID EXTREMITIES POWDER *(sì nì sǎn)*

Both formulas are able to treat Liver qi stagnation. However, Frigid Extremities Powder *(sì nì sǎn)* focuses on constraint of the yang qi in the abdomen failing to reach and warm the extremities. In modern TCM texts, this is often described as being due to a Liver/Spleen disharmony. Bupleurum Powder to Dredge the Liver *(chái hú shū gān sǎn)*, on the other hand, focuses solely on the Liver channel, moving its qi, resolving constraint, and opening up clumps. It is thus better for patterns characterized by qi stagnation-type pain in areas traversed by the Liver channel.

➢ Vs. AUGMENTED LINDERA DECOCTION *(jiā wèi wū yào tāng)*; see PAGE 536

Biomedical Indications

With the appropriate presentation, this formula may be used to treat a variety of biomedically-defined disorders including hepatitis, chronic cholecystitis, chronic gastritis, peptic ulcers, and intercostal neuralgia.

Alternate names

Bupleurum Powder to Soothe the Liver *(chái hú shū gān sǎn)* in *Newly Compiled Book of Empirical Formulas*; Bupleurum Decoction to Dredge the Liver *(chái hú shū gān tāng)* in *Essentials for Those Who Do Not Know Medicine*

Modifications

• For more severe flank pain, add Angelicae sinensis Radix *(dāng guī)*, Curcumae Radix *(yù jīn)*, and Linderae Radix *(wū yào)*.

• For thirst, a red tongue, and other signs indicating the presence of excess heat, add Toosendan Fructus *(chuān liàn zǐ)*, Scutellariae Radix *(huáng qín)*, and Gardeniae Fructus *(zhī zǐ)*.

• For vomiting or diarrhea due to Liver qi attacking the Stomach horizontally, add Pinelliae Rhizoma praeparatum *(zhì bàn xià)* and Poria *(fú líng)*.

疏肝湯（疏肝汤）
Dredge the Liver Decoction
shū gān tāng

Source *Restoration of Health from the Myriad Diseases* (1587)

Coptidis Rhizoma *(huáng lián)*
(fried in Evodiae Fructus *[wú zhū yú]* extract) 6g
Bupleuri Radix *(chái hú)* 4.5g
Angelicae sinensis Radix *(dāng guī)* 4.5g
Citri reticulatae viride Pericarpium *(qīng pí)* 3g
Persicae Semen *(táo rén)* .3g
Aurantii Fructus *(zhǐ ké)* .3g
Chuanxiong Rhizoma *(chuān xiōng)* 2.1g
Paeoniae Radix alba *(bái sháo)* 2.1g
Carthami Flos *(hóng huā)* 1.5g

Method of Preparation Decoction. Imbibe at a time distant from meals. These small dosages are typical of the source text. Modern practitioners generally increase the dosages slightly, except for Coptidis Rhizoma *(huáng lián)*.

Actions Dredges the Liver, regulates the qi, dispels stasis, relieves pain, invigorates the blood, and clears the heat

Indications

The source text cites this formula for treatment of "pain beneath the left [side of the] ribcage, Liver accumulation pertaining to the blood [aspect], damage to qi from anger, or [rib] pain resulting from knocks and bruises." The source text also indicates that a wiry pulse is characteristic of this pattern.

These symptoms are indicative of pain in the Liver channel from stagnation of qi and blood. As stated in the source text, the stagnation could be brought on by internal damage from the emotions or could be the result of trauma.

Analysis of Formula

As this formula addresses pain in areas related to the Liver, it aims to promote the proper movement of qi and blood and to dredge the Liver. Heat-clearing is added to clear the heat generated by constraint. Bupleuri Radix *(chái hú)*, Aurantii Fructus *(zhǐ ké)*, and Citri reticulatae viride Pericarpium *(qīng pí)* work together to regulate the Liver qi, dredge the Liver, and resolve constraint. Carthami Flos *(hóng huā)*, Angelicae sinensis Radix *(dāng guī)*, Persicae Semen *(táo rén)*, and Chuanxiong Rhizoma *(chuān xiōng)* move the blood and dispel stasis, thereby working with the qi-regulating agents to relieve the pain. The early Qing-dynasty text *Complete Treatise for Benefiting Society* summarizes the use of this combination of qi-regulating and blood-moving herbs by noting that, "for pain [in the] left ribs, Bupleuri Radix *(chái hú)* is chief and Citri reticulatae viride Pericarpium *(qīng pí)* and Chuanxiong Rhizoma *(chuān xiōng)* are deputies." From this perspective, the other blood-invigorating herbs are assistants.

Another assistant is Paeoniae Radix alba (bái sháo), which works with Bupleuri Radix (chái hú) and Angelicae sinensis Radix (dāng guī) to soothe and nourish the Liver; it also moderates pain. The final assistant is Coptidis Rhizoma (huáng lián), which clears heat that arises from constrained Liver qi.

The use of Chuanxiong Rhizoma (chuān xiōng) and Paeoniae Radix alba (bái sháo), both of which are pain-relieving herbs, underscores the formula's emphasis on treating pain.

Cautions and Contraindications

This formula is inappropriate if the patient presents without Liver constraint or pain from blood stasis. And because the formula contains blood-moving agents, caution should be exercised if internal bleeding is suspected.

Commentary

In *Restoration of Health from the Myriad Diseases*, this formula is found in the section on rib pain. While pain beneath the left ribs is the symptom mentioned in the source text, later texts are less specific and cite the presence of constraint as the main indication. For example, the Qing-dynasty work *Personal Standards for Internal Medicine* states that the formula treats "Liver constraint rib pain with occasional deep sighs and difficulty in rotating [the body]." Since heaving deep sighs and difficulty with rotation are well-known indications of Liver qi constraint, the message of this passage is clearly that Liver constraint is the primary marker for use of this formula.

Other formulas mentioned in the source text for treatment of rib pain in various locations and causes include Tangkuei, Gentian, and Aloe Pill (dāng guī lóng huì wán) for treatment of pain in both flanks owing to damp-heat in the Liver channel, and Trichosanthes Fruit and Unripe Bitter Orange Decoction (guā lóu zhǐ shí tāng) for pain from phlegm clumped beneath the ribs. For bitter taste with distention of the ribs, it suggests Minor Bupleurum Decoction (xiǎo chái hú tāng) with the addition of Coptidis Rhizoma (huáng lián) and Gardeniae Fructus (zhī zǐ).

Biomedical Indications

With the appropriate presentation, this formula may be used to treat a variety of biomedically-defined disorders including intercostal neuralgia, traumatic injury to the ribs, or pancreatitis.

Alternate name

Powder to Dredge the Liver (shū gān sǎn) in *Achieving Longevity by Guarding the Source*

Modifications

• If pain is severe, add Corydalis Rhizoma (yán hú suǒ).

• For constipation, add Rhei Radix et Rhizoma (dà huáng). This is especially important for acute traumatic pain.

枳實薤白桂枝湯（枳实薤白桂枝汤）

Unripe Bitter Orange, Chinese Garlic, and Cinnamon Twig Decoction

zhǐ shí xiè bái guì zhī tāng

Source   *Essentials from the Golden Cabinet* (c. 220)

Trichosanthis Fructus (guā lóu) 12g
Allii macrostemi Bulbus (xiè bái) .9g
Aurantii Fructus immaturus (zhǐ shí) 12g
Magnoliae officinalis Cortex (hòu pò) 12g
Cinnamomi Ramulus (guì zhī) 3g

Method of Preparation   The source text advises to first decoct Aurantii Fructus immaturus (zhǐ shí) and Magnoliae officinalis Cortex (hòu pò) with 5 cups of water until 2 cups remain. The dregs are then removed and the remaining three ingredients added to the decoction. This is then brought to a boil for a short period of time. The final decoction is divided into three portions and taken warm. At present, it is usually prepared by boiling all five ingredients together.

Actions   Unblocks the yang, dissipates clumps, expels phlegm, and directs the qi downward

Indications

Fullness and pain in the chest or a stabbing pain that radiates from the chest to the back, wheezing, coughing, shortness of breath, focal distention in the chest that feels like a flow of qi proceeding from the flanks to the area around the heart, a white, greasy tongue coating, and a submerged, wiry, or tight pulse.

This is painful obstruction of the chest with severe clumping of qi that results in focal distention and pain. It is a form of yang deficiency. The chest is located above and associated with yang. When the yang of the chest is not properly animated, yin from below usurps its place. Physiologically, this is due to the yang of the chest being unable to disperse the fluids throughout the body, and especially to direct them downward to the lower burner. Instead, they congeal and form phlegm. The phlegm accumulates and obstructs the normal flow of qi. This causes a deep aching in the chest or pain that radiates from the chest to the back. The circulation in the Lungs is also disrupted, giving rise to coughing, wheezing, and shortness of breath. Yin rebelling upward to usurp the place of yang is subjectively experienced as a flushing sensation that proceeds from the flanks (the area associated with the Liver and Gallbladder, which are responsible for circulating the qi and fluids from below to above) to the area around the heart. The thick, greasy tongue coating is another indication of turbid phlegm in the chest. The pulse reflects obstruction in the chest and the lack of animation of the yang. This is a pattern in which the clinical presentation is one of excess, but the underlying cause is deficiency.

Analysis of Formula

Because this formula treats the manifestation rather than the root of painful obstruction of the chest, all of its ingredients focus on unblocking the clear yang by eliminating turbid yin. For this purpose, it combines herbs that focus on the chest with those that direct downward and break up clumping. The chief herbs are sweet and cold Trichosanthis Fructus (*guā lóu*), which expels phlegm and unbinds the chest, and Allii macrostemi Bulbus (*xiè bái*), which warms and thus unblocks the yang to promote the movement of qi and alleviate pain. This combination of herbs, one of which disperses clumps of phlegm and the other unblocks the qi mechanism, is very effective in treating this type of painful obstruction of the chest. The deputies are Aurantii Fructus immaturus (*zhǐ shí*), which directs the qi downward, breaks up clumping, gets rid of focal distention, and eliminates fullness; and Magnoliae officinalis Cortex (*hòu pò*), which also directs the qi downward and eliminates fullness, but also dries dampness and transforms phlegm. Acting synergistically, this combination supports the chief in unblocking the yang and transforming the phlegm. The assistant is Cinnamomi Ramulus (*guì zhī*), which unblocks the yang, disperses cold, directs rebellious qi downward, and calms flushing.

Cautions and Contraindications

This formula is warm, drying, and dispersing. It should not be used for cases of chest pain due to Lung consumption or phlegm-heat in the chest, nor should it be used long-term.

Commentary

This is one of a number of formulas for the treatment of painful obstruction of the chest introduced by Zhang Zhong-Jing. Its basic pathodynamic is defined in *Essentials of the Golden Cabinet* as "feeble yang and wiry yin (陽微陰弦 *yáng wēi yīn xián*)." Ostensibly reflecting the pulse that accompanies all of the patterns of this disorder, the passage has been interpreted by most commentators to mean that turbid yin occupies the place vacated by feeble yang qi in the chest. The former constitutes the branch, the latter the root. Because this is a potentially life-threatening disorder, all of Zhang Zhong-Jing's formulas for painful obstruction of the chest focus on the treatment of the branch. This is achieved by a strategy aimed at dissipating obstruction to unblock the yang, supported by the secondary goal of dispelling phlegm and dispersing clumping. For this purpose, all of Zhang Zhong-Jing's formulas combine Trichosanthis Fructus (*guā lóu*) with Allii macrostemi Bulbus (*xiè bái*) and then add a variety of assistant herbs, depending on the manifestations. The reasoning behind this choice of herbs is most clearly explained by Zhou Yan in *Records of Thoughtful Differentiation of Materia Medica*:

> The strength of Trichosanthis Fructus (*guā lóu*) lies in its ability to guide out phlegm and move the turbid downward. Therefore, one cannot treat clumping or focal distention of the chest without [it]. However, it guides out by facilitating movement and is unable to expel [pathogens] to get rid of them. Its nature is gentle. Lacking the benefit of hardness, its downward-directing is bereft of power. ... Trichosanthes Fruit, Chinese Garlic, and Wine Decoction (*guā lóu xiè bái bái jiǔ tāng*) [and its derivative formulas] thus employ bitter, acrid, fast-moving substances that promote [the qi dynamic] such as Allii macrostemi Bulbus (*xiè bái*), white Chinese wine (*bái jiǔ*), Cinnamomi Ramulus (*guì zhī*), and Magnoliae officinalis Cortex (*hòu pò*). Without diminishing the strong points [of the chief ingredient], they thereby complement its deficiencies.

As outlined by Zhou Yan, Trichosanthes Fruit, Chinese Garlic, and Wine Decoction (*guā lóu xiè bái bái jiǔ tāng*), which is listed below, serves as a base formula to be modified according to the actual pattern. Unripe Bitter Orange, Chinese Garlic, and Cinnamon Twig Decoction (*zhǐ shí guā lóu guì zhī tāng*) and Trichosanthes Fruit, Chinese Garlic, and Pinellia Decoction (*guā lóu xiè bái bàn xià tāng*), which is also listed below, are two possible variations. This formula is a reminder, too, that not all cases of painful obstruction of the chest are due to blood stasis.

Biomedical Indications

With the appropriate presentation, this formula may be used to treat a wide variety of biomedically-defined disorders including esophageal spasms, angina pectoris, chronic obstructive pulmonary disease, intercostal neuralgia, costochondritis, and hyperventilation disorders.

Alternate names

Unripe Bitter Orange and Chinese Garlic Decoction (*zhǐ shí xiè bái tāng*) in *Introduction to Medicine*; Trichosanthes Fruit, Chinese Garlic, and Cinnamon Twig Decoction (*guā lóu xiè bái guì zhī tāng*) in *Personal Standards for the Essentials from the Golden Cabinet*

Modifications

- For severe cold with pain radiating from the chest to the back that intensifies upon exposure to cold, add Aconiti Radix lateralis praeparata (*zhì fù zǐ*) and Zingiberis Rhizoma (*gān jiāng*).
- For intercostal neuralgia, add Frigid Extremities Powder (*sì nì sǎn*).
- For angina pectoris, add Salviae miltiorrhizae Radix (*dān shēn*), Paeoniae Radix rubra (*chì sháo*), Chuanxiong Rhizoma (*chuān xiōng*), and Carthami Flos (*hóng huā*).

Associated Formulas

栝蔞薤白白酒湯 （栝蒌薤白白酒汤）

Trichosanthes Fruit, Chinese Garlic, and Wine Decoction
guā lóu xiè bái bái jiǔ tāng

SOURCE *Essentials from the Golden Cabinet* (c. 220)

Trichosanthis Fructus (*guā lóu*) 12g
Allii macrostemi Bulbus (*xiè bái*) 9-12g
White wine (*bái jiǔ*) 30-60ml

Decoction. Often prepared with equal amounts of wine and water. In patients where ingestion of wine is contraindicated, the amount of wine may be reduced or omitted altogether. Unblocks the yang, promotes the movement of qi, and expels phlegm. This is the formula for a simple painful obstruction of the chest disorder that is characterized by pain in the chest that often radiates to the upper back, wheezing, cough with copious sputum, shortness of breath, a thick, greasy tongue coating, and a pulse that is either submerged and wiry or tight.

栝蔞薤白半夏湯 （栝蒌薤白半夏汤）

Trichosanthes Fruit, Chinese Garlic, and Pinellia Decoction

guā lóu xiè bái bàn xià tāng

Source   *Essentials from the Golden Cabinet* (c. 220)

Trichosanthis Fructus (*guā lóu*) 12g
Allii macrostemi Bulbus (*xiè bái*) 9g
Pinelliae Rhizoma praeparatum (*zhì bàn xià*) 9-12g
White wine (*bái jiǔ*) 30-60ml

Add in cases of painful obstruction of the chest where the pain is so severe that the patient is unable to lie down comfortably. Most commentators agree that this indicates that the accumulation of phlegm is more severe; consequently, the other symptoms that characterize the Trichosanthes Fruit, Chinese Garlic, and Wine Decoction pattern (pain radiating to the back, wheezing, and cough) will also be more severe. A slightly different view was offered by the 17th-century physician Xu Bin in *Discussion and Annotation of the Essentials from the Golden Cabinet*. Xu argued that this pattern is a joint disorder combining both painful obstruction of the chest (defined by cold-type pain with little phlegm) and propping thin mucus (defined by phlegm but no pain).

半夏厚樸湯 （半夏厚朴汤）
Pinellia and Magnolia Bark Decoction
bàn xià hòu pò tāng

Source   *Essentials from the Golden Cabinet* (c. 220)

Pinelliae Rhizoma praeparatum (*zhì bàn xià*) 9-12g
Magnoliae officinalis Cortex (*hòu pò*) 9g
Poria (*fú líng*) 12g
Zingiberis Rhizoma recens (*shēng jiāng*) 15g
Perillae Folium (*zǐ sū yè*) 6g

Method of Preparation   Decoction. At present, only 9g of Zingiberis Rhizoma recens (*shēng jiāng*) is generally used.

Actions   Promotes the movement of qi, dissipates clumps, directs rebellious qi downward, and transforms phlegm

Indications

A feeling of something caught in the throat that can neither be swallowed nor ejected, a stifling sensation in the chest and hypochondria, a moist or greasy, white tongue coating, and a wiry, slow or wiry, slippery pulse. There may also be coughing and vomiting.

This condition is known as plum-pit qi (梅核氣 *méi hé qì*) and is the result of emotional upset due to circumstances that the patient figuratively cannot swallow. The qi thereupon becomes constrained and the Lungs and Stomach lose their ability to move the qi downward. This, in turn, leads to problems with the transportation and transformation of fluids, which leads to the formation of phlegm. The phlegm clashes with the qi and ultimately lodges in the throat. The obstruction of the qi mechanism by phlegm is also manifested in the stifling sensation in the chest and hypochondria. In severe cases, there will also be coughing or vomiting. The moist or greasy tongue coating, and the slow and wiry or slippery and wiry pulse, are signs of constrained qi and phlegm-dampness.

Analysis of Formula

This formula treats a pattern where the stagnation of qi and formation of phlegm are mutually reinforcing: If the qi is not moved, the phlegm obstruction cannot be resolved; if the phlegm is not transformed, the qi cannot be moved. The appropriate strategy for dealing with such a pattern is to simultaneously open the qi dynamic (primary) and transform the phlegm (secondary).

As indicated in its name, the two bitter, acrid, warming, and downward-directing herbs, Pinelliae Rhizoma praeparatum (*zhì bàn xià*) and Magnoliae officinalis Cortex (*hòu pò*), serve as joint chiefs in this formula. The former transforms phlegm, dissipates clumps, directs rebellious qi downward, and harmonizes the Stomach. It thereby addresses all the major aspects of this condition. The latter eliminates the stifling sensation and assists the other chief herb in dissipating the clumps and directing the rebellious qi downward. The capacity of Pinelliae Rhizoma praeparatum (*zhì bàn xià*) to disperse clumping and direct rebellious qi downward assists Magnoliae officinalis Cortex (*hòu pò*) in regulating the qi. Conversely, the ability of Magnoliae officinalis Cortex (*hòu pò*) to regulate the qi and dry dampness supports Pinelliae Rhizoma praeparatum (*zhì bàn xià*) in transforming the phlegm.

The first deputy, sweet, bland Poria (*fú líng*), leaches out dampness and assists Pinelliae Rhizoma praeparatum (*zhì bàn xià*) in transforming phlegm. The second deputy, acrid, light, warm, and dispersing Perillae Folium (*zǐ sū yè*), reinforces the ability of Magnoliae officinalis Cortex (*hòu pò*) to regulate the qi and break up stagnation. Entering the Lungs, which govern the throat, the place where the main symptom is located, this herb also serves as the envoy. It also helps focus the action of the formula on the Lung channel and relieves coughing, should it occur. The assistant, Zingiberis Rhizoma recens (*shēng jiāng*), helps the chief herbs harmonize the Stomach and thereby stops the vomiting.

Cautions and Contraindications

This formula is comprised of warm, acrid, or fragrant substances, which are drying and dispersing in nature and can readily injure the yin and fluids. Thus, the formula is appropriate only in cases of constrained qi and phlegm. It is contraindicated in patients presenting with a flushed face, a bitter taste in the mouth, and a red tongue with scanty coating.

Commentary

This is an important formula that can be used to treat a wide range of disorders presenting with both somatic and psychoemotional symptoms.

Plum-Pit Qi

In the source text, this formula is recommended for women who feel as if a piece of roasted meat were stuck in their throats. The Tang-dynasty work *Important Formulas Worth a Thousand Gold Pieces* further described this sensation as "something that can neither be expectorated nor swallowed." This implies that the pattern treated by this formula is not phlegm constraining the dispersion of qi (in which case expectorating or swallowing the phlegm would bring relief), but rather constrained qi preventing the fluids from moving downward, whereupon they clump with the stagnant qi and transform into phlegm. This condition, which, according to *Golden Mirror of the Medical Tradition* may also be experienced in men, has come to be known as plum-pit qi. This frequently equates to what in biomedicine is known as globus hystericus.

In *One-Hundred Classic Formulas*, the contemporary scholar Huang Huang argues that a close reading of the source text allows us to extend the meaning of the term plum-pit qi beyond such narrow correspondences. He notes that the reference to *roasted* meat is deliberate rather than accidental. This means that the sensation experienced in the throat may also be of a burning nature or accompanied by dryness, itching, or numbness. However, there will be no signs of heat such as local redness or swelling, which allows us to differentiate this pattern from similar presentations involving heat, fire, or toxin.

A pattern of qi constraint with concurrent phlegm is not the only cause of plum-pit qi, but it is by far the most common one. Other causes include fire from constraint, hyperactive yang associated with yin deficiency, as well as qi and blood deficiency. Other useful formulas include Frigid Extremities Powder *(sì nì sǎn)*, Bupleurum, Cinnamon Twig, and Ginger Decoction *(chái hú guì jiāng tāng)*, Bupleurum Plus Dragon Bone and Oyster Shell Decoction *(chái hú jiā lóng gǔ mǔ lì tāng)*, Cinnamon Twig Decoction plus Dragon Bone and Oyster Shell *(guì zhī jiā lóng gǔ mǔ lì tāng)*, and Poria, Cinnamon Twig, Atractylodes, and Licorice Decoction *(líng guì zhú gān tāng)*. A thorough differentiation is essential before the present formula can be prescribed.

Commentaries Regarding Etiology and Pathodynamic

During the Song dynasty, commentators elaborated in greater detail on the causes of this pattern, attributing it mainly to emotional disorders. *Discussion of Illnesses, Patterns, and Formulas Related to the Unification of the Three Etiologies* noted that "when [the experience and expression of] elation and anger is not regulated, or when sadness and pensiveness combine as they frequently do to generate sadness and [unwarranted] fear, or when one is at times shaken by anxiety, the qi of the organs is [no longer] balanced," causing illness that, besides plum-pit qi, manifests with symptoms that include "chills and fever, distention and fullness of the chest and abdomen, and a rushing [of qi] into the two flanks."

Simple Book of Formulas was even more precise in its analysis: "The qi [generated by] elation, anger, grief, pensiveness, sadness, fear, and fright clumps to produce phlegm and oral mucus that feels like broken cotton wadding or a plum pit lodged in the throat that can neither be expectorated nor swallowed. This is [a manifestation of a dysfunction of] the seven qi." It also listed a number of systemic symptoms generated by the same pathodynamic, including "focal distention and fullness of the central abdomen, [an awareness of] qi not moving smoothly, an abundance of phlegm and oral mucus clogging [the chest and causing] rebellious qi and acute wheezing, or vomiting due to rebellion and nausea caused by phlegm and thin mucus accumulating in the middle burner, and also morning sickness during pregnancy." Both texts slightly modified the original formula, creating new prescriptions listed below.

Expanded Usage

Based on a clear understanding of the formula's mode of action and of the pathodynamic it seeks to correct, it is used in contemporary practice to treat problems of the respiratory system such as coughing, dyspnea, fullness of the chest, and even the later stages of acute infectious disorders; and gastrointestinal disorders such as nausea and vomiting, travel or motion sickness, and abdominal fullness.

Japanese physicians have extended the formula's range of indications even further to include obstruction of the qi dynamic with accumulation of phlegm fluids in all three burners, as well as more severe emotional disorders. *Collection of Orally Transmitted Explanations of Medical Formulas*, for instance, added manifestations such as "pain due to loss of regulation of all the various qi, pain in the hands and feet, or unbearable wrenching pain in the abdomen and chest, or reduced and rough urination, as in painful urinary dysfunction." Other contemporary Japanese usages include the treatment of paroxysmal psychosomatic symptoms such as anxiety, depressed moods, insomnia and palpitations that are accompanied by abdominal discomfort and bloating, nausea, a tendency to develop edema, expectoration of thin sputum, or irregular menstruation. All of these manifestations have in common an obstruction of the qi dynamic centered on the downward-directing function of the Lungs and Stomach, causing the fluids to stagnate and transform into phlegm mucus, which in turn inhibits the ascent of the clear yang. This is a typical example of how emotional disorders are related to a pathodynamic that does not primarily involve the Liver.

Composition

In terms of its composition, this formula is a modification of two smaller formulas also listed in *Essentials from the Golden Cabinet:*

- Minor Pinellia Decoction *(xiǎo bàn xià tāng)* consists of Pinelliae Rhizoma praeparatum *(zhì bàn xià)* and Zingiberis Rhizoma recens *(shēng jiāng)* and treats propping thin mucus in the epigastrium with vomiting but no thirst.

- Minor Pinellia plus Poria Decoction *(xiǎo bàn xià jiā fú líng tāng)* consists of Pinelliae Rhizoma praeparatum *(zhì bàn xià)*, Zingiberis Rhizoma recens *(shēng jiāng)*, and Poria *(fú líng)*. It also treats propping thin mucus with vomiting and focal distention in the epigastrium, but also dizziness and palpitations.

The present formula adds two more qi-regulating herbs—Magnoliae officinalis Cortex *(hòu pò)* and Perillae Folium *(zǐ sū yè)*—to the latter formula, shifting its focus from the transformation of thin mucus to the downward-directing of qi. While the use of Magnoliae officinalis Cortex *(hòu pò)* does not require much further explanation, that of Perillae Folium *(zǐ sū yè)* is more interesting. Most commentators think that its acrid, dispersing action facilitates the resolution of constraint that is the root of the pattern treated by this formula. However, in *Discussion and Annotation of the Essentials from the Golden Cabinet,* Xu Bin provides a somewhat different explanation:

> Perillae Folium *(zǐ sū yè)* has an acrid flavor and an aromatic qi. Its color is purple, and its nature is warming. It is able to enter the yin to harmonize the blood, and to guide the qi into the blood. Therefore, in cases of blood loss, if one combines it with Phaseoli Semen *(chì xiǎo dòu)* and takes it as pills it can prevent the blood from moving recklessly.
> In the summer, when summerheat has injured the Heart yin, this formula can direct summerheat constraint downward. Used for plum-pit qi, it therefore harmonizes the qi and blood, preventing [the qi] from floating upward again.

Given the emphasis *Essentials from the Golden Cabinet* placed throughout on the harmonization of qi and blood as a key strategy, as well as the sympathetic magic that pervades all of Chinese medicine, Xu Bin's analysis opens another window on understanding the otherwise somewhat enigmatic use of Perillae Folium *(zǐ sū yè)* in this formula.

Comparison

➤ Vs. ESCAPE RESTRAINT PILL *(yuè jū wán)*

Both formulas treat patterns of qi constraint due to unbalanced emotions. In both cases, this leads to stagnation of the qi dynamic such that its ascending and descending functions are no longer working smoothly. Invariably, this manifests with localized sensations of fullness that tend to come and go, that improve with movement or distraction, and that are aggravated by rest or further emotional distress. In general, Escape Restraint Pill *(yuè jū wán)* focuses on the middle burner to regulate both ascent and descent while also drying dampness. Pinellia and Magnolia Bark Decoction *(bàn xià hòu pò tāng)*, by contrast, focuses on the upper burner to facilitate the downward-direction of qi and the transformation of phlegm. Furthermore, Escape Restraint Pill *(yuè jū wán)* contains the bitter, cooling herb Gardeniae Fructus *(zhī zǐ)*, which clears fire from constraint, suggesting that this formula is indicated for patients with strong yang qi or ministerial fire. Pinellia and Magnolia Bark Decoction *(bàn xià hòu pò tāng)*, on the other hand, contains warming and dispersing Zingiberis Rhizoma recens *(shēng jiāng)*, which warms the Stomach to move fluids, suggesting that this formula is indicated for patients with constitutional yin (i.e., water) excess.

Biomedical Indications

With the appropriate presentation, this formula may be used to treat a wide variety of biomedically-defined disorders. These can be divided into the following groups:

- Disorders marked by a sensation of something stuck in the throat including glomus hystericus, neuroses, neurogenic vomiting, irritable bowel syndrome, hysteria, psychosis, epilepsy, depression, perimenopausal syndrome, and Parkinson's disease
- Disorders of the throat and surrounding structures including laryngitis, tonsillitis, edema of the vocal cords, goiter, hyperthyroidism, and cervical spine syndrome
- Digestive disorders including esophageal strictures, esophageal spasms, gastritis, and indigestion
- Respiratory disorders including bronchitis and emphysema.

The formula has also been used in the treatment of morning sickness, Ménière's disease, and vertebrobasilar insufficiency.

Modifications

- For severe cases of stagnant qi with the above presentation, add Bupleuri Radix *(chái hú)*, Curcumae Radix *(yù jīn)*, Cyperi Rhizoma *(xiāng fù)*, and Citri reticulatae viride Pericarpium *(qīng pí)*.

- For vomiting, add Amomi Fructus *(shā rén)*, Caryophylli Flos *(dīng xiāng)*, and Amomi Fructus rotundus *(bái dòu kòu)*.

- For a severe stifling sensation in the chest, add Curcumae Radix *(yù jīn)* and Aurantii Fructus *(zhǐ ké)*.

- For chest pain, add Trichosanthis Fructus *(guā lóu)* and Allii macrostemi Bulbus *(xiè bái)*.

- For abdominal distention, add Amomi Fructus *(shā rén)* and Aucklandiae Radix *(mù xiāng)*.

- For hypochondriac pain, add Toosendan Fructus *(chuān liàn zǐ)* and Corydalis Rhizoma *(yán hú suǒ)*.

- For pain and swelling in the throat, add Scrophulariae Radix *(xuán shēn)* and Platycodi Radix *(jié gěng)*.

Associated Formulas

大七氣湯 (大七气汤)

Major Seven-Emotions Decoction

dà qī qì tāng

SOURCE *Discussion of Illnesses, Patterns, and Formulas Related to the Unification of the Three Etiologies* (1174)

Pinelliae Rhizoma praeparatum *(zhì bàn xià)* 150g
Poria *(fú líng)* 120g
Perillae Folium *(zǐ sū yè)* 60g
ginger-fried Magnoliae officinalis Cortex
(*jiāng chǎo hòu pò*) 90g

The source text advises to grind the herbs into a coarse powder and decoct 12g with 1 cup of water and 7 slices of Zingiberis Rhizoma recens *(shēng jiāng)*. Moves the qi, directs rebellion downward, transforms phlegm, and disperses clumping. The source text is specific in indicating this formula for a pattern due to problems caused by the seven emotions, and expanded its use to obstruction of the qi dynamic in the middle and upper burners by qi constraint and phlegm obstruction.

———————

四七湯 (四七汤)

Four-Ingredient Decoction for the Seven Emotions

sì qī tāng

SOURCE *Simple Book of Formulas* (1191)

Pinelliae Rhizoma praeparatum *(zhì bàn xià)* 150g
Poria *(fú líng)* 120g
Perillae Folium *(zǐ sū yè)* 60g
Magnoliae officinalis Cortex *(hòu pò)* 90g

The source text advises to grind the herbs into a coarse powder and decoct 12g with 1 cup of water, 7 slices of Zingiberis Rhizoma recens *(shēng jiāng)*, and 1 piece of Jujubae Fructus *(dà zǎo)*. Moves the qi, directs rebellion downward, transforms phlegm, and disperses clumping. The source text is specific in indicating this formula for a pattern due to problems caused by any of the seven emotions. Unlike the principal formula, it also harmonizes the Stomach. It is thus milder and more suitable for long-term use. Note that the literature

includes several other formulas by the same name but with different ingredients, and somewhat different indications.

———————

小七氣湯 (小七气汤)

Minor Seven-Emotions Decoction

xiǎo qī qì tāng

SOURCE *Formulary of the Pharmacy Service for Benefiting the People in the Taiping Era* (1107)

Ginseng Radix *(rén shēn)* 3g
Cinnamomi Cortex *(ròu guì)* 3g
Pinelliae Rhizoma praeparatum *(zhì bàn xià)* 3g
Glycyrrhizae Radix praeparata *(zhì gān cǎo)* 1.5g

The source text advises to decoct the herbs together with 3 slices of Zingiberis Rhizoma recens *(shēng jiāng)*. Tonifies the qi, warms the middle burner, resolves constraint, and transforms phlegm. For clumping or constraint caused by imbalance of the seven emotions characterized by colicky pain in the chest and abdomen or drum distention. In *Revision of the Subtle Discussions on Caring for Life,* the Ming-dynasty physician Li Zhong-Zi recommended this formula for treating chronic constraint due to long-term emotional problems. In *Discussion of Medical Formulas,* the Qing-dynasty physician Fei Bo-Xiong likewise noted that it was eminently suitable for constraint patterns characterized by cold from deficiency.

In *Medical Formulas Collected and Analyzed,* the Qing-dynasty scholar Wang Ang changed the name of the formula to Four-Ingredient Decoction for the Seven Emotions *(sì qī tāng)*. Due to the popularity of Wang Ang's work, this is the name now generally used for this formula, which has caused it to be confused with the above formula by the same name. Moreover, there are other formulas by the same name with different ingredients.

厚樸溫中湯 (厚朴温中汤)

Magnolia Bark Decoction for Warming the Middle

hòu pò wēn zhōng tāng

SOURCE *Clarifying Doubts about Damage from Internal and External Causes* (1247)

ginger Magnoliae officinalis Cortex *(jiāng hòu pò)* . . . 30g (9-15g)
Alpiniae katsumadai Semen *(cǎo dòu kòu)* 15g (6-9g)
Citri reticulatae Pericarpium *(chén pí)* 30g (9-15g)
Aucklandiae Radix *(mù xiāng)* 15g (6-9g)
Zingiberis Rhizoma *(gān jiāng)* 2.1g (1.5-6g)
Poria *(fú líng)* 15g (9-12g)
Glycyrrhizae Radix praeparata *(zhì gān cǎo)* 15g (3-9g)

Method of Preparation The source text advises to grind the ingredients into a powder and take 15g as a draft with 3 pieces of Zingiberis Rhizoma recens *(shēng jiāng)* before meals. May also be prepared as a decoction with the dosage specified in parentheses and the addition of 3 pieces of Zingiberis Rhizoma recens *(shēng jiāng)*.

Actions Promotes the movement of qi, eliminates fullness, dries dampness, and warms the middle burner

Indications

Epigastric and abdominal distention and fullness, loss of appetite, fatigue in the extremities, loose diarrhea, and a white, slippery tongue coating. There may also be abdominal pain and vomiting of clear liquid.

This is damp-cold injuring the Spleen and Stomach either due to inappropriate clothing or the consumption of damp-cold food or drink. Li Dong-Yuan, the formula's author, wrote in the source text that "Food and drink that one is not used to, or heat and cold that do not suit one, damage the Spleen and Stomach." Cold tends to congeal, and dampness is cloying in nature. When the two combine and attack the Spleen and Stomach, they obstruct the qi dynamic of the middle burner. This interferes with the ascending and descending functions of these organs, which is manifested as epigastric and abdominal distention and fullness, loss of appetite, fatigue in the extremities, and loose diarrhea. The etiology of this condition is discussed in Chapter 5 of *Basic Questions*: "The cold qi gives rise to turbidity. ... When the turbid qi is above, there will be distention in the upper abdomen." The tongue coating reflects the presence of damp-cold in the interior. If the cold is particularly severe, there may also be abdominal pain and vomiting of clear liquid.

Analysis of Formula

This formula dispels patterns where damp-cold has obstructed the qi dynamic of the middle burner, with distention and pain being the two key symptoms. Thus, it focuses primarily on moving the qi and eliminating fullness, and only secondarily warms the middle burner and dries dampness. For this reason, bitter, acrid, and warming Magnoliae officinalis Cortex *(hòu pò)* and Citri reticulatae Pericarpium *(chén pí)* are the chief herbs. Magnoliae officinalis Cortex *(hòu pò)* warms the middle burner, dries dampness, promotes the descent of qi, and expands the chest. It is one of the most important herbs in the materia medica for the treatment of abdominal fullness. Citri reticulatae Pericarpium *(chén pí)* is one of the most frequently used herbs to move the qi, particularly in the upper and middle burners. It also dries dampness and harmonizes the middle burner. The deputy, Alpiniae katsumadai Semen *(cǎo dòu kòu)*, warms the middle burner, disperses cold, and dries dampness. It strongly reinforces the actions of the chief herbs.

The assistant herbs can be divided into three groups. The first consists of Aucklandiae Radix *(mù xiāng)*, which helps the chief herbs promote the movement of qi, expand the chest, and stop the pain. The second group consists of Zingiberis Rhizoma *(gān jiāng)* and Zingiberis Rhizoma recens *(shēng jiāng)*, which warm the Spleen, harmonize the Stomach, and disperse cold. The third group consists of Poria *(fú líng)* and Glycyrrhizae Radix *(gān cǎo)*. These herbs address the damp aspect of this disorder by strengthening the Spleen, leaching

out dampness, and harmonizing the functions of the middle burner. In concert with Zingiberis Rhizoma recens *(shēng jiāng)*, Glycyrrhizae Radix *(gān cǎo)* also harmonizes and focuses the actions of the other herbs on the middle burner.

Cautions and Contraindications

Because this formula contains bitter, acrid, and warming medicinals, it is contraindicated in patients who present with abdominal distention or pain together with qi deficiency or insufficiency of Stomach yin.

Commentary

Although the name of this formula suggests that it may be a variation of Regulate the Middle Pill *(lǐ zhōng wán)*, discussed in Chapter 6, its true antecedent is Magnolia Bark, Fresh Ginger, Pinellia, Licorice, and Ginseng Decoction (厚樸半夏生薑甘草人參湯 *hòu pò bàn xià shēng jiāng gān cǎo rén shēn tāng)*. That formula was first cited in paragraph 66 of *Discussion of Cold Damage*, where it is indicated for "abdominal fullness and distention following sweating [treatment]." Sweating damages the qi and fluids by dispersing them to the exterior. For this reason, the formula uses Ginseng Radix *(rén shēn)*, an herb that tonifies the qi and enriches the fluids, albeit with a dosage of only 3g, which is significantly less than the 15g prescribed for the two main herbs in that formula, Magnoliae officinalis Cortex *(hòu pò)* and Zingiberis Rhizoma recens *(shēng jiāng)*.

By contrast, in the pattern for which Magnolia Bark Decoction for Warming the Middle *(hòu pò wēn zhōng tang)* is indicated, damp-cold entering the body from the exterior obstructs the qi. This implies that the stagnation is stronger and comes about from the congealing of body fluids, rather than from deficiency. For this reason, the formula omits Ginseng Radix *(rén shēn)* but adds more herbs that move the qi, warm, and dry. As reflected in the dosages—30g for both of the chief herbs, as opposed to approximately 2g for Zingiberis Rhizoma *(gān jiāng)*—the focus is clearly on regulating the qi. Warming the middle burner is merely an adjunctive strategy. Accordingly, the formula can also be used for cold attacking the Stomach with epigastric pain, vomiting, and distention in the chest and hypochondria, as noted by Qin Bo-Wei in *Medical Lecture Notes of [Qin] Qian-Zhai*:

> Cold [type] Stomach pain refers to Stomach pain caused by raw food and drink or cold that directly affects the Stomach [from outside. It is characterized] by sudden pain in the stomach cavity, responds favorably to palpation, and a desire for warm drinks or soup. The pain is unremitting and is generally accompanied by vomiting of clear fluids, aversion to cold, and coldness of the hands and feet. The pulse appears submerged and slow, and the tongue has a greasy, white coating. [As] this type of Stomach pain is due to contraction of cold, it is a pattern of excess. To treat it, one employs the strategy of warming the middle and dispersing cold, using Magnolia Bark Decoction

for Warming the Middle (*hòu pò wēn zhōng tāng*). If one is also not careful about eating and drinking, this can lead to stagnation of food and cold combining [with each other, leading to a pattern characterized] by even more severe pain, one can [then] add herbs like Crataegi Fructus (*shān zhā*) and Massa medicata fermentata (*shén qū*) to assist the digestive [process].

Like many formulas that regulate the qi, Magnolia Bark Decoction for Warming the Middle (*hòu pò wēn zhōng tāng*) focuses on the middle burner as the fulcrum of the qi dynamic. In *Treatment Strategies and Formulas in Chinese Medicine*, the contemporary physician Chen Zao-Chu suggests that its efficacy can be increased by adding herbs that enter the Lungs, such as Perillae Folium (*zǐ sū yè*) and Armeniacae Semen (*xìng rén*), as well as those that enter the Liver, such as Cyperi Rhizoma (*xiāng fù*) and Citri reticulatae viride Pericarpium (*qīng pí*). The former improves the functions of the Lungs in directing qi downward from the upper burner. The latter assists the Liver in directing the clear yang upward from its source at the gate of vitality in the lower burner. Mobilizing the entire qi dynamic in this manner allows the formula to be used for fullness and distention of the Triple Burner.

Comparisons

➢ Vs. GALANGAL AND CYPERUS PILL (*liáng fù wán*)

Both formulas warm the middle, regulate the qi, and reduce pain. However, Magnolia Bark Decoction for Warming the Middle (*hòu pò wēn zhōng tang*) is best for patterns where cold and dampness cause qi stagnation in the Spleen and Stomach. By contrast, Galangal and Cyperus Pill (*liáng fù wán*) focuses instead on patterns that involve stagnation and disharmony of Liver and Stomach qi.

➢ Vs. REGULATE THE MIDDLE PILL (*lǐ zhōng wán*); see PAGE 259

Modifications

• For severe epigastric pain, add Salviae miltiorrhizae Radix (*dān shēn*).

• For food stagnation, add Crataegi Fructus (*shān zhā),* Hordei Fructus germinatus (*mài yá),* and Massa medicata fermentata (*shén qū*).

• For hypochondriac pain and acid reflux, combine with Left Metal Pill (*zuǒ jīn wán*).

良附丸

Galangal and Cyperus Pill

liáng fù wán

Source *Small Collection of Fine Formulas* (1842)

Alpiniae officinarum Rhizoma (*gāo liáng jiāng*)
Cyperi Rhizoma (*xiāng fù*)

Method of Preparation Wash equal amounts of the first herb in wine and the second in vinegar. Bake and then grind the herbs into a fine powder and form into pills with ginger juice. Take in 6g doses 2-3 times a day with water. May also be prepared as a decoction, most commonly using 9g of each ingredient.

Actions Warms the middle burner, dispels cold, promotes the movement of qi, and alleviates pain

Indications

Epigastric pain that responds favorably to warmth, a stifling sensation in the chest, hypochondriac pain, painful menstruation, and a white tongue coating.

The epigastrium pertains to the Stomach and the hypochondria to the Liver. Where both areas are painful, the problem is both in the Liver and the Stomach, the etiology of which can be manifold. Here it is due to stagnation of Liver qi with cold congealing in the Stomach. Both of these problems obstruct the flow of qi and thereby cause pain in their respective areas. When there is cold in the Stomach, the tongue coating will be white and the pain will respond favorably to warmth. The stagnant qi produces a stifling sensation in the chest. The stagnation of Liver qi can also cause painful menstruation.

Analysis of Formula

This condition requires both warming the Stomach and promoting the movement of qi. Acrid, warming Alpiniae officinarum Rhizoma (*gāo liáng jiāng*) enters the Stomach, warms the middle, disperses cold, and stops pain. Washing it in wine augments its capacity to disperse and unblock stagnation. Acrid and slightly bitter Cyperi Rhizoma (*xiāng fù*) enters the qi aspect of the Liver and the Triple Burner channel to regulate their qi, thereby unblocking the movement of qi in all of the twelve primary and eight extra channels. It also excels at relieving constraint. Washing it in vinegar limits its powerful acrid dispersion action from damaging the qi dynamic. Each herb complements the other, and together they address both aspects of this disorder. Ginger juice warms and harmonizes the Stomach.

Cautions and Contraindications

Contraindicated in patients with heat in the Liver and Stomach, or where there is bleeding. The formula is also contraindicated during pregnancy as it enters the Liver, Stomach, and eight extraordinary vessels where its strong qi-moving properties may induce miscarriage.

Commentary

This formula is indicated for epigastric and hypochondriac pain that responds favorably to warmth and is accompanied by a white tongue coating. According to the modern physician Qin Bo-Wei in *[Qin] Qian-Zhai's Lecture Notes on Medicine*, "it is effective in treating qi [stagnation] pain of the Liver and Stomach that tends toward cold."

The source text states that this disorder is caused either by external invasion of cold into the Stomach or by uncontrolled anger causing the Liver qi to rebel and stagnate. In the first case, a dosage of 6g of Alpiniae officinarum Rhizoma (*gāo liáng jiāng*) and 3g of Cyperi Rhizoma (*xiāng fù*) is recommended. In the second case, the dosages are reversed, with 3g of Alpiniae officinarum Rhizoma (*gāo liáng jiāng*) and 9g of Cyperi Rhizoma (*xiāng fù*). Where cold and anger contribute equally, an equal dosage of 4.5g of both ingredients should be used.

Later generations of physicians have expanded the indications of this formula to include painful menstruation, as well as more severe epigastric pain, by variously adding herbs that regulate the qi, invigorate the blood, or warm the middle.

Comparisons

➤ Vs. Escape Restraint Pill (*yuè jū wán*)

Escape Restraint Pill (*yuè jū wán*) focuses on promoting the movement of qi and relieving constraint, while Galangal and Cyperus Pill (*liáng fù wán*) focuses more on warming the middle burner and dispelling cold.

➤ Vs. Other Commonly-Used Formulas for Epigastric and/or Hypochondriac Pain

- Galangal and Cyperus Pill (*liáng fù wán*)—for pain due to qi stagnation with congealed cold
- Minor Construct the Middle Decoction (*xiǎo jiàn zhōng tāng*)—for pain due to cold from deficiency
- Bupleurum Powder to Dredge the Liver (*chái hú shū gān sǎn*)—for pain due to pure qi stagnation
- Pinellia Decoction to Drain the Epigastrium (*bàn xià xiè xīn tāng*)—for pain due to a cold-heat complex

➤ Vs. Magnolia Bark Decoction for Warming the Middle (*hòu pò wēn zhōng tāng*); see page 521

Biomedical Indications

With the appropriate presentation, this formula may be used to treat a variety of biomedically-defined disorders including chronic gastritis, peptic ulcer, and primary dysmenorrhea.

Alternate name

Galangal and Cyperus Pill for Relieving Pain (*zhǐ tòng liáng fù wán*) in *Collected Formulas from the Crane Feeding Pavilion*

Modifications

- If the cold aspects are more severe, increase the dosage of Alpiniae officinarum Rhizoma (*gāo liáng jiāng*) and add Zingiberis Rhizoma (*gān jiāng*).

- If the stagnant qi aspects are more severe, increase the dosage of Cyperi Rhizoma (*xiāng fù*) and add Citri reticulatae viride Pericarpium (*qīng pí*), Aquilariae Lignum resinatum (*chén xiāng*), and Aucklandiae Radix (*mù xiāng*).

- For painful menstruation, add Angelicae sinensis Radix (*dāng guī*).

- For peptic ulcer due to cold from deficiency, combine with Astragalus Decoction to Construct the Middle (*huáng qí jiàn zhōng tāng*).

金铃子散 （金铃子散）

Melia Toosendan Powder

jīn líng zǐ sǎn

Source   *Formulary of the Pharmacy Service for Benefiting the People in the Taiping Era* (1107)

Toosendan Fructus (*chuān liàn zǐ*) 30g
Corydalis Rhizoma (*yán hú suǒ*) 30g

Method of Preparation   Grind the ingredients into a fine powder and take in 9g doses with wine or water. May also be prepared as a decoction with a proportionate reduction in the dosage of the ingredients.

Actions   Spreads Liver qi, drains heat, invigorates the blood, and alleviates pain

Indications

Intermittent epigastric and hypochondriac pain, hernial pain, or menstrual pain that is aggravated by the ingestion of hot food or beverage, and is accompanied by irritability, a bitter taste in the mouth, a red tongue with a yellow coating, and a wiry or rapid pulse.

This is Liver constraint transforming into heat. The Liver is responsible for regulating the dispersion of ministerial fire from the gate of vitality throughout the body. It is "yin in essence but manifests through its yang functions"—implying not only that its ability to regulate the yang qi is a function of its capacity to store yin blood, but also that it likes spreading and abhors constraint. Its channel passes through the hypochondria, the abdomen, and around the genitals. Thus, when Liver function is disrupted, the qi and blood will not flow smoothly and there will be pain—hypochondriac, epigastric, abdominal, genital, and/or menstrual. The Liver prefers orderliness and regularity; Liver dysfunction is thus accompanied by intermittent pain that follows the swell of emotion. Liver constraint readily transforms into heat as the ministerial fire stagnates. This is manifested as irritability and heat-aggravated pain, a wiry or rapid pulse, a bitter taste in the mouth, and a red tongue with a yellow coating.

Analysis of Formula

Constraint of Liver qi transforming into fire should be treated by a strategy of dredging and regulating the Liver qi, supported by invigorating the blood. This strategy is consistent with the nature and function of the Liver, as well as with the relationship between the qi and blood. Because qi is the commander of blood, its constraint invariably impedes the flow of blood. Bitter and cooling Toosendan Fructus (*chuān liàn zǐ*), the chief herb, enters the Liver, Stomach, and Small Intestine channels. It clears heat from the chest, hypochondrium, and groin by draining it through the urine. When the heat has been drained, and the fire constraint resolved, the Liver qi can once again carry out its regulating function. Bitter, acrid, and warming Corydalis Rhizoma (*yán hú suǒ*) invigorates the blood by moving the qi. Li Shi-Zhen praised its actions in *Comprehensive Outline of the Materia Medica*, noting that "it is able to move qi stagnation of the blood and blood stagnation within the qi. Therefore, it specifically focuses on pain throughout the entire body, both above and below. Hitting the mark by using [this herb] is so sublime that it cannot be expressed in words." Acting as both assistant and envoy, it thus reinforces the actions of the chief herb.

Cautions and Contraindications

Use with caution during pregnancy. This formula is inappropriate for pain from Liver qi constraint in the context of cold conditions.

Commentary

The formula's original indications were "heat inversion Heart pain (熱厥心痛 *rè jué xīn tòng*) that is intermittent [in character] and has become chronic." As such, it can be viewed as an alternative to the treatment strategies for heart pain provided in *Essential Formulas from the Golden Cabinet*, which focus on cold. Various commentators have interpreted 'Heart' here in both the narrow sense (i. e., referring to the heart organ), and in the wider sense (i.e., as a body region that encompasses the chest, but also the Stomach). 'Inversion' refers to a sudden upward-rushing of qi. In the present case, this is hot or yang qi rushing upward from the Liver channel into a body region where it does not belong and where it thus constitutes an excess. The intermittent character of the pain indicates that it is a manifestation of qi stagnation, while the fact that it has become chronic implies that this stagnation has also affected the blood. This explains the specific combination of herbs in this formula. Toosendan Fructus (*chuān liàn zǐ*) was used by Jin-dynasty physicians such as Zhang Yuan-Su as a specific herb for "heat inversion Heart pain," while Corydalis Rhizoma (*yán hú suǒ*) is listed in the earlier *Grandfather Lei's Discussion of Herb Preparation* as treating "unbearable Heart pain." In *Six Texts Summarizing the Medicine of Xu Ling-Tai*, the Qing-dynasty commentator Xu Da-Chun provides the following explanation:

When heat lurks in the terminal yin, wood and fire qi are constrained and the yang [of these channels no longer] extends, so there is heat inversion Heart pain that comes and goes irregularly. Toosendan Fructus (*chuān liàn zǐ*) specifically enters the terminal yin and transforms lurking heat in order to eliminate dampness. Corydalis Rhizoma (*yán hú suǒ*) specifically acts on the blood aspect, invigorating the blood vessels by regulating the blood.

Xu Da-Chun's analysis emphasizes the ability of Toosendan Fructus (*chuān liàn zǐ*) to guide out excess fire via the urine. This is a very different approach to resolving qi constraint than the use of acrid, warming herbs that move the qi. For this reason, the formula became extremely popular among Qing-dynasty physicians like Ye Tian-Shi, who were searching for a strategy to treat Liver qi constraint for a southern Chinese clientele whom they considered to be prone to deficiency of yin and excess of yang. Averse to the use of bitter, drying herbs that would further damage the yin as well as to the use of exterior-resolving herbs like Bupleuri Radix (*chái hú*) that might further facilitate the rising of yang and generation of wind, Melia Toosendan Powder (*jīn líng zǐ sǎn*) offered an excellent alternative. Zhang Lu, another Qing-dynasty physician, argued that this formula was at least as effective as Sudden Smile Powder (*shī xiào sǎn*)—another frequently used formula for the treatment of Stomach and Heart pain—without the inconvenience of its foulness and bad smell.

Given the enormous influence of these physicians, Melia Toosendan Powder (*jīn líng zǐ sǎn*) thus became the formula of choice for treating Liver qi constraint due to excess ministerial fire, especially where this was combined with a tendency to yin deficiency. Its range of application was also extended to other types of pain associated with the Liver channel, such as bulging qi, menstrual pain, and urinary obstruction in children, as well as to disorders of the yin and yang Linking vessels, by Shen Jin-Ao in *Wondrous Lantern for Peering into the Origin and Development of Miscellaneous Diseases*. Some modern writers, like Chen Chao-Zu in *Treatment Strategies and Formulas in Chinese Medicine*, even go as far as recommending it for all types of pain, irrespective of location or causation. This attitude is summarized in *Selected Annotations to Ancient Formulas from the Garden of Crimson Snow*: "Although this is a small formula, its synergism is divine. It has the power to effect cures without a hitch. Do not disregard it as being bland."

In contemporary usage, the pain-relieving properties of this formula are employed whenever Liver constraint turns into fire. This includes conditions such as gall stones or kidney stones, characterized by severe pain, obstruction, and inflammation.

This formula is often attributed to *Collection of Writings on the Mechanisms of Illness, Suitability of Qi, and the Safeguarding of Life as Discussed in the Basic Questions*. Although this is the oldest extant texts listing this formula, *Pocket Prescriptions* states that the formula was previously published in *Formulary of the Pharmacy Service for Benefiting the People in the Taiping Era*. Even if the current version of the latter text no longer lists the formula, one must assume that it was deleted in the course of transmission. Hence, it still should be regarded as the source text.

Comparisons

➤ Vs. Left Metal Pill *(zuǒ jīn wán)*

Left Metal Pill *(zuǒ jīn wán)* is used for Liver fire that attacks the Stomach. This disrupts the descending function of the Stomach, which manifests as vomiting or belching of sour fluids. The Stomach is thus the location of this pathology and the target of the formula. Melia Toosendan Powder *(jīn líng zǐ sǎn)*, on the other hand, is indicated for fire constraint that affects the qi dynamic and secondarily leads to blood stasis. It targets the qi and the blood rather than a specific organ.

➤ Vs. Augmented Rambling Powder *(jiā wèi xiāo yáo sǎn)*

Both of these formulas can be used to treat Liver qi constraint transforming into fire. However, Augmented Rambling Powder *(jiā wèi xiāo yáo sǎn)* is better suited for patients where such constraint is due to qi and blood deficiency. By contrast, Melia Toosendan Powder *(jīn líng zǐ sǎn)* is primarily indicated for excess fire causing constraint, particularly where this occurs against a background of constitutional yin deficiency. Linking Decoction *(yī guàn jiān)*, discussed in Chapter 8, is thus a natural extension of this formula.

Biomedical Indications

With the appropriate presentation, this formula may be used to treat a variety of biomedically-defined disorders including peptic ulcer, chronic gastritis, hepatitis, and cholecystitis.

Alternate name

Melia Toosendan Powder *(jīn líng sǎn)* in *Wondrous Lantern for Peering into the Origin and Development of Miscellaneous Diseases*

Modifications

- For epigastric pain due to heat, add Scutellariae Radix *(huáng qín)* and Paeoniae Radix alba *(bái sháo)*.

- For painful menstruation, add Cyperi Rhizoma *(xiāng fù)*, Salviae miltiorrhizae Radix *(dān shēn)*, Carthami Flos *(hóng huā)*, and Leonuri Herba *(yì mǔ cǎo)*.

- For bulging disorders of the lower abdomen, add Citri reticulatae Semen *(jú hé)*. If there are also significant signs of cold, add Evodiae Fructus *(wú zhū yú)* and Foeniculi Fructus *(xiǎo huí xiāng)*.

- For gall stones or kidney stones, add Lysimachiae Herba *(jīn qián cǎo)*, Gigeriae galli Endothelium corneum *(jī nèi jīn)*, Curcumae Radix *(yù jīn)*, and Lygodii Spora *(hǎi jīn shā)*.

- For pain in the chest, epigastrium, flanks, or abdomen, combine with Frigid Extremities Powder *(sì nì sǎn)*.

- For pain in terminal yin patterns, combine with Mume Pill *(wū méi wán)*.

Associated Formulas

奔豚丸

Running Piglet Pill

bēn tún wán

SOURCE *Awakening of the Mind in Medical Studies* (1732)

Toosendan Fructus *(chuān liàn zǐ)* 30g
Poria *(fú líng)* 45g
Citri reticulatae Semen *(jú hé)* 45g
Litchi Semen *(lì zhī hé)* 24g
Foeniculi Fructus *(xiǎo huí xiāng)* 21g
Aucklandiae Radix *(mù xiāng)* 21g

Cook the ingredients with sugar and form into pills. Take 6g with salted water. Dispels cold, directs rebellious qi downward, warms the yang, and regulates the qi. For Kidney accumulation (腎積 *shèn jī*) due to cold in the lower burner. The cold obstructs the flow of qi in the lower burner, which impairs the qi transformation and leads to an accumulation of fire from the gate of vitality, which periodically discharges upward through flushing. All of this manifests as periumbilical palpitations followed by an upsurge of qi from the abdomen to the sternum as the patient becomes unnerved. Accompanying symptoms include cold limbs and body, a white, greasy tongue coating, and a wiry, tight pulse. Based on a passage in Chapter 56 of the *Classic of Difficulties*, this is also known as 'running piglet disorder,' hence the name of the formula.

延胡索湯 (延胡索汤)

Cordyalis Decoction

yán hú suǒ tāng

SOURCE *Formulas to Aid the Living* (1253)

dry-fried Corydalis Rhizoma *(chǎo yán hú suǒ)* 15g
wine-fried Angelicae sinensis Radix *(jiǔ chǎo dāng guī)* 15g
dry-fried Typhae Pollen *(chǎo pú huáng)* 15g
Paeoniae Radix rubra *(chì sháo)* 15g
Cinnamomi Cortex *(ròu guì)* 15g
Curcumae longae Rhizoma *(jiāng huáng)* 90g
Olibanum *(rǔ xiāng)* 90g
Myrrha *(mò yào)* 90g
Aucklandiae Radix *(mù xiāng)* 90g
Glycyrrhizae Radix praeparata *(zhì gān cǎo)* 7.5g

Grind the herbs into a coarse powder and prepare as a draft by decocting 12g with 200ml of water and 7 slices of Zingiberis Rhizoma recens *(shēng jiāng)* until 140ml remain. Discard the dregs and take warm before meals. Invigorates the blood, moves the qi, alleviates pain. For qi stagnation and blood stasis in women due to damage by any one of the seven emotions, manifesting as chest and abdominal pain radiating downward into the lower back and flanks, or upward into the upper back and arms. Also for attacks of piercing pain felt along the spine and severe spasms. All of these pains will be stabbing in nature. The menses will be late or irregular. Can also be used for any type of pain due to simultaneous qi and blood stagnation. In contrast to the principal formula, which treats qi constraint affecting the circulation of blood due to fire excess, this formula focuses to an equal extent on qi stagnation and blood stasis. It is therefore widely used in gynecology to treat all kinds of pain. Contraindicated during pregnancy.

四磨湯 （四磨汤）
Four Milled-Herb Decoction

sì mò tāng

The herbs in this formula were originally milled before decocting, hence the name.

Source   *Formulas to Aid the Living* (1253)

Ginseng Radix *(rén shēn)* 3-6g
Arecae Semen *(bīng láng)* 9g
Aquilariae Lignum resinatum *(chén xiāng)* 3-6g
Linderae Radix *(wū yào)* 6-9g

Method of Preparation   The source text does not give dosages and advises to finely grind the herbs together, make into a quick draft in a small bowl that is brought to a boil 3-5 times, and taken warm. At present, it is prepared as a decoction, generally with the dosages above.

Actions   Promotes the movement of qi, directs rebellious qi downward, expands the chest, and dissipates clumping

Indications

An irritable, stifling sensation in the chest and diaphragm together with labored breathing, wheezing, epigastric focal distention and fullness, and a loss of appetite. The tongue coating is often white and the pulse is wiry.

This is qi excess in the upper burner due to stagnation of the qi dynamic, which thereupon loses its ability to ascend and descend, leading to rebellion and clumping of qi, especially in the upper and middle burners. Causation is attributed to emotional disorders, in particular to excessive pensiveness, anger, worry, and/or grief. The Lungs have lost their ability to direct the qi downward, causing labored breathing and wheezing. This impacts the ability of the Liver qi to ascend, causing it to stagnate, which manifests as an irritable, stifling sensation in the chest and diaphragm. Rebellious qi also impairs the Stomach's harmony and descending function, leading to epigastric focal distention and a loss of appetite. The white tongue coating is indicative of cold, suggesting that this condition does not occur in patients with yang qi excess. The wiry pulse reflects qi stagnation.

Analysis of Formula

This formula treats severe qi stagnation that has led to rebellion and clumping. Besides moving the qi to unblock the stagnation, it also directs the qi downward, expands the chest, and dissipates clumping. The chief herb is acrid, warming, and penetrating Linderae Radix *(wū yào)*. Although it has a particular affinity for the lower burner, it is said to enter all twelve channels where it promotes both the ascent and descent of qi. Acrid, mobilizing, and dispersing Aquilariae Lignum resinatum *(chén xiāng)* acts as deputy. It smoothes the flow of qi, directing it downward from the Lungs to the Kidneys. Working synergistically with the chief herb, this combination effectively disperses the stagnation that is the root of this pattern, while also putting down the rebellion that is its branch. Acrid, warming, and draining Arecae Semen *(bīng láng)* serves as the first assistant. It strongly promotes the downward movement of qi, breaks up stagnation and clumping, and thereby eliminates the irritable, stifling, and full sensations. Strong, acrid dispersion and breaking up of stagnation can readily injure the qi and damage the fluids. For this reason, sweet and tonifying Ginseng Radix *(rén shēn)*, which augments the source qi but also enriches the fluids, is added as the second assistant. No specific envoy is needed because the qi-regulating herbs all act on the qi dynamic—the main target of this formula—with the downward-directing of the rebellion clearly being more important than the upward-directing of qi from below.

Cautions and Contraindications

This formula is designed for treating an acute condition, and should therefore not be taken long-term. It is also inappropriate for patients who have significant deficiency of normal qi, reflected in part by fatigue and a frail pulse.

Commentary

This is another formula for the treatment of qi stagnation caused by emotional excess. Although some texts include it in the category of formulas that direct rebellious qi downward, its primary function is that of regulating a disordered qi dynamic.

Primary Organs Involved

Modern textbooks invariably link the etiology and pathodynamic of the pattern for which this formula is indicated to Liver qi stagnation. The modern physician Qin Bo-Wei, a major force in the systematization of Chinese medicine in contemporary China, likewise noted in *[Qin] Qian-Zhai's Lecture Notes on Medicine* that it "governs the treatment of Liver qi rebelling horizontally, invading the Lungs above and the Spleen and Stomach to the sides." Most premodern writers focus instead on the qi circulation between the Lungs and Kidneys. The Qing-dynasty writer Wang You-Yuan is typical:

Breathing out is yang, breathing in is yin. If the Lung yang is flourishing, it clears and clarifies by moving [qi] downward, returning it to the Kidney yin. When the qi is thus received and contained it is not pathologically dispersed nor does it rebel. If the normal qi is debilitated, pathogenic qi invariably becomes overabundant. If one is firm [in forcing the patient] to get rid of [their addictions] to sensual pleasure and a debauched lifestyle while breaking up stagnation, the pathogenic qi is unable to lurk. The formula uses Ginseng Radix (rén shēn) to tonify the normal qi and Aquilariae Lignum resinatum (chén xiāng) for it to be grasped in the Kidneys. [Once this has been accomplished] one can then use Arecae Semen (bīng láng) and Linderae Radix (wū yào) to guide out [the rebellious pathogenic qi] in accordance [with the manifestations]. This is what is meant by needing to guard against deficiency in cases of excess, and first tonifying if one wishes to drain.

The four herbs [in this formula] all have a thick flavor. Grinding them [into a fine powder allows] these flavors to be fully released. Boiling [the powder allows] the extending [action] of their qi [also] to be released. [Their] flavor and qi thus both available, the [formula's] effects are achieved in perfect coordination. Taking [the powder] together with Special Pill to Nourish the Normal Qi (養正丹 yǎng zhèng dān) is an even more excellent [way of administering it].

The original formula tonifies the Lung qi to nourish the normal [qi] and warms the Kidney qi [so that when the qi] is pressed down, it can be contained and returned to its root. Acute wheezing is thus quickly [brought under control].

Wang's explanation appears to be quite apt, especially as none of the herbs used in the formula have a specific affinity to the Liver, whereas Aquilariae Lignum resinatum (chén xiāng)— considered by some commentators, including Qin Bo-Wei, to be the chief ingredient—is a specific herb for guiding qi into the Kidneys and the gate of vitality. This explanation is also consistent with the intentions of the source text, which relates its use to Special Pill to Nourish the Normal Qi (yǎng zhèng dān). Two formulas by this name are listed in the pre-Song formularies and would have been available to the author of Formulas to Aid the Living. Both contain warming minerals such as Sulfur (liú huáng) and have the function of assisting the yang in order to disperse cold. This has led the modern scholar Fan Qiao-Ling, in her recent book Formulas, to conclude that Yan Yong-He composed this formula to treat rebellion caused by severe qi stagnation arising from cold from deficiency.

Role of Ginseng Radix (rén shēn)

The analysis presented in Discussion of Blood Patterns by the early modern physician Tang Zong-Hai reaches the same conclusion, but by another route:

[This formula] uses Ginseng Radix (rén shēn) to enrich the Lungs by way of tonifying the qi of the mother [i.e., earth]. It uses Aquilariae Lignum resinatum (chén xiāng), which enters the Kidneys, in order to grasp the qi at its root. Only then does it employ Arecae Semen (bīng láng) and Linderae Radix (wū yào) to treat the branch. Draining excess and tonifying

deficiency truly is a sublime method for regulating the grasping of rebellious qi. The Lungs are yang. But their capacity for accepting the qi and moving it downward depends entirely on the yin fluids. Therefore, [the formula] employs Ginseng Radix (rén shēn) in order to generate fluids. The Kidneys are yin. But their capacity for transforming qi and moving it upward depends entirely on the true yang. Therefore, [the formula] employs Aquilariae Lignum resinatum (chén xiāng) in order to secure the yang. As it sinks deeply into the water, it is able to truly grasp the yang within the water.

The analyses of the commentators cited here suggest that the primary function of Ginseng Radix (rén shēn) in this formula is not to balance the harsh drying effects of the qi-moving ingredients, but to tonify a deficiency of qi that lurks in the background of the pattern. In Convenient Reader of Established Formulas, the Qing-dynasty physician Zhang Bing-Chen suggests replacing Ginseng Radix (rén shēn) with Aurantii Fructus (zhǐ ké) if such a deficiency does not exist. A number of other physicians made similar substitutions, creating new formulas that have also become widely used. Some of these are listed under ASSOCIATED FORMULAS below.

In Comprehensive Medicine According to Master Zhang, the Qing-dynasty writer Zhang Lu notes that, following administration of this formula, bubbles should appear in the stool. This indicates that the qi excess is being eliminated, whereupon the chest symptoms should ease.

Biomedical Indications

With the appropriate presentation, this formula may be used to treat a variety of biomedically-defined disorders including bronchial asthma, emphysema, gastritis, and postsurgical adhesions.

Alternate name

Four Milled-Herbs Drink (sì mó yǐn) in Formulas Categorized by the Strategems of Pattern Treatment

Variation

六磨湯 (六磨汤)
Six Milled-Herb Decoction
liù mò tāng

SOURCE Indispensable Tools for Pattern Treatment (1602)

Remove Ginseng Radix (rén shēn) and add Aucklandiae Radix (mù xiāng), Aurantii Fructus (zhǐ ké), and Rhei Radix et Rhizoma (dà huáng) for constipation, belching, and abdominal distention and pain.

Associated Formula

五磨飲子 (五磨饮子)
Five Milled-Herb Decoction
wǔ mò yǐn zi

SOURCE Concise Medicine (1587)

Aucklandiae Radix (*mù xiāng*) 6g
Aquilariae Lignum resinatum (*chén xiāng*) 6g
Arecae Semen (*bīng láng*) 9g
Aurantii Fructus immaturus (*zhǐ shí*) 9g
Linderae Radix (*wū yào*) 9g

Originally milled with white wine, this formula is now commonly prepared as a decoction. Promotes the movement of qi and directs upward-rebelling qi downward. For epigastric and abdominal distention and pain, or wandering pain. The source text also prescribes it for a disorder called 'qi inversion' (氣厥 *qì jué*), where a sudden, extremely intense bout of anger causes sudden death. The Ming-dynasty physician Wu Kun has analyzed this pathodynamic in *Investigations of Medical Formulas:* "When one gets angry, the qi ascends. When the qi ascends, the upper burner qi becomes excessive and [no longer] moves [downward]. The lower burner qi [instead] rebels and [no longer permits] inhalation. Hence, [the person] suddenly dies." In contrast to the principal formula, this is stronger in promoting the movement of qi, and has no action in augmenting the qi. It is used for a rather severe condition in persons of robust health.

天台烏藥散（天台乌药散）
Top-Quality Lindera Powder

tiān tái wū yào sǎn

The literal translation of this formula's name is 'Lindera Powder from Tiantai.' Tiantai is a mountain in Zhejiang province and here refers to the area where the highest quality of this herb can be found.

Source *Comprehensive Recording of Sagely Beneficence from the Zhenghe Era* (1117)

Linderae Radix (*wū yào*) 15g
Aucklandiae Radix (*mù xiāng*) 15g
dry-fried Foeniculi Fructus (*chǎo xiǎo huí xiāng*) 15g
Citri reticulatae viride Pericarpium (*qīng pí*) 15g
dry-fried Alpiniae officinarum Rhizoma (*chǎo liáng jiāng*) . . .15g
Arecae Semen (*bīng láng*) . . . . 2 pieces (12-15g)
Toosendan Fructus (*chuān liàn zǐ*) . . . . 10 pieces (12-15g)
Crotonis Fructus (*bā dòu*) . . . . 70 pieces (15g)

Method of Preparation Dry-fry Toosendan Fructus (*chuān liàn zǐ*) and Crotonis Fructus (*bā dòu*) together until they turn black. Discard the latter ingredient and grind the former together with the remaining ingredients into a powder. Take 3g as a warm draft before meals, often followed by a small amount of wine. For more severe symptoms, dry-fried Zingiberis Rhizoma recens (*chǎo shēng jiāng*) can be added when preparing the draft, and the wine can be heated.

Actions Promotes the movement of qi, spreads the Liver qi, scatters cold, and alleviates pain

Indications

Lower abdominal pain radiating to the testicles, swollen or distended testicles, a pale tongue with a white coating, and either a submerged and slow or a wiry pulse.

This is a qi-type bulging disorder. Most bulging disorder patterns are characterized by symptoms in the area traversed by the Liver channel, which passes around and connects with the external genitalia. This particular presentation is due to qi stagnation in the Liver channel, usually associated with the invasion of cold. The stagnation obstructs the flow to the testicles and results in pain. If cold is a major aspect of the pattern, the patient will present with a localized sensation of cold and hardness. The tongue and pulse signs reflect the internal ascent of cold.

This formula also treats pain from cold qi congealing and clumping in the lower abdomen, as well as menstrual pain and mobile abdominal masses with the same etiology.

Analysis of Formula

This formula treats qi stagnation associated with cold in the lower abdomen, particularly in the area traversed by the Liver channel. Accordingly, it is designed around a strategy of regulating and moving the qi in order to disperse cold, break up clumping, and alleviate pain. This follows a principle outlined in *Appendices to the Golden Cabinet:*

> When the qi gathers [in one place,] it clogs things up. When the qi disperses, things open up. This means that to ease the pain, just disperse the gathered-up qi. Therefore, in treating bulging disorders, one must first treat the qi.

The chief herb is warm, acrid Linderae Radix (*wū yào*), which promotes the movement of qi, disperses the constrained Liver qi, scatters the cold, and thereby alleviates pain. It is very effective in treating pain due to cold, and is therefore considered superior to Cyperi Rhizoma (*xiāng fù*) in treating Liver qi constraint associated with cold. The deputies include Foeniculi Fructus (*xiǎo huí xiāng*), which warms the lower burner and scatters cold; Alpiniae officinarum Rhizoma (*gāo liáng jiāng*), which also scatters cold and alleviates pain; Citri reticulatae viride Pericarpium (*qīng pí*), which regulates the qi and disperses constrained Liver qi; and Aucklandiae Radix (*mù xiāng*), which promotes the movement of qi and alleviates pain. The deputies strengthen the actions of the chief herb. Arecae Semen (*bīng láng*), one of the assistants, conducts the qi downward, removing stagnation and breaking up solid obstructions in the lower burner. The bitter, cold properties of Toosendan Fructus (*chuān liàn zǐ*) are substantially reduced by cooking it with Crotonis Fructus (*bā dòu*), however its ability to soothe the Liver is actually strengthened by this process. What remains of its cold properties have the effect of slightly moderating the warm properties of the other herbs.

Cautions and Contraindications

Contraindicated in patients with damp-heat. Tonifying herbs, such as Ginseng Radix (*rén shēn*) or Astragali Radix (*huáng qí*), should not be added to this formula, as they will counteract the treatment strategy and can lead to lingering stagnation of pathogenic qi in the Liver channel.

Commentary

This is one of the representative formulas for the treatment of bulging disorder and qi stagnation due to cold. It is usually associated with the Liver channel, although classical texts also make frequent references to Small Intestine bulging disorder when discussing this formula.

Background of Bulging Disorders

The term 'bulging disorder' is very old. In the classical period it had a fairly general meaning. For example, in the Han-dynasty text *Elucidations of the Signs and Explications of the Graphs*, it is said that "Bulging refers to abdominal pain." Discussions of bulging in the *Inner Classic* clearly associate its etiology and pathodynamic with cold. For example, a passage in Chapter 48 of *Basic Questions* explains: "Bulging is due to cold and qi clumping and accumulating" while Chapter 55 notes that, "For disorders located in the lower abdomen with abdominal pain and an inability to urinate or defecate, the name of the disorder is called bulging." The early-7th-century encyclopedia *Discussion of the Origins of the Symptoms of Disease* provides a similar but more systematic explanation:

> [This disorder] is caused by yin qi accumulating in the interior. This cold qi tussles and clumps, but does not disperse. With the yin and yang organs [concurrently] being deficient and frail, the wind pathogens and cool qi battle with the normal qi, causing abdominal pain with interior tension. Hence, it is referred to as cold bulging abdominal pain.

Accordingly, the formulas prescribed for the treatment of bulging disorder in early texts such as *Essentials from the Golden Cabinet* focused primarily on cold when treating abdominal pain and bulging. The pathology had been defined as a disorder of the Conception vessel in Chapter 60 of *Basic Questions*, but was also associated with other channels traversing the lower abdomen: the Small Intestine, Bladder, Kidney, and Liver. While these associations persist, from the Jin-Yuan period onward, bulging disorder came to be more closely associated with pain or swelling of the testicles, and thus with the Liver channel. For example, in *Correct Transmission of Medicine*, the Ming-dynasty physician Yu Tuan notes: "Bulging refers to acute pain extending from the testicles into the lower abdomen. In some cases, the pain is in the testicles, in others next to the acupuncture point GB-27 (*wǔ shū*). In both cases, it [involves] the terminal yin Liver channel." By and large, this association has remained dominant to this day. The term bulging disorder no longer occurs in many contemporary internal medicine textbooks, and its presentation has been subsumed under the pattern of cold invading the Liver channel.

Because the nature of cold is to contract and congeal, and qi that has stagnated cannot disseminate, depending on the part of the body involved, different patterns can develop. As previously noted, Chapter 60 of *Basic Questions* referred to seven types of bulging disorders. Over the centuries, physicians devised several other nosological systems to distinguish among these patterns, none of which has succeeded in displacing the others. In clinical practice, the most important differentiation is that between heat and cold, and between the type of physiological substance (qi, blood, or fluids) primarily affected by the constraint. A differentiation based on the organs and channels involved (primarily the Liver, Small Intestine, Bladder, and Kidneys) is less commonly used, as the same herbs tend to be used in any case. In the present formula, for instance, Toosendan Fructus (*chuān liàn zǐ*) enters both the Liver and Small Intestine channels, while Linderae Radix (*wū yào*), Foeniculi Fructus (*xiǎo huí xiāng*), Aucklandiae Radix (*mù xiāng*), and even Citri reticulatae viride Pericarpium (*qīng pí*) can be used for all kinds of lower abdominal pain due to qi stagnation.

Qi-type bulging (氣疝 *qì shàn*) is characterized by intermittent pain or by pain and swelling that is not fixed, sometimes affecting the right side and testicle, other times the left. Blood-type bulging (血疝 *xuè shàn*), on the other hand, will present with more strictly localized pain or swelling that endures for many years. The swelling tends to be hard and immovable, and will not be accompanied by distention or edema. If the fluids are primarily affected, leading to water-type bulging (水疝 *shuǐ shàn*), swelling and edema will be prominent, but the pain will be less pronounced. The skin tends to be edematous, too, without being hot to the touch. This presentation is often associated with Spleen deficiency and dampness, or with the inability of deficient fire at the gate of vitality to transform the fluids. Cold-type bulging (寒疝 *hán shàn*) is associated with cold sensations and pain that respond favorably to the local application of heat and by a tendency to curl up. Conversely, hot-type bulging (熱疝 *rè shàn*) presents with the subjective sensation of heat, an aversion to touch, and a desire to extend the leg on the affected side.

History of Formula

The creation of this formula is widely attributed to the Jin-dynasty master Li Dong-Yuan, who first listed a formula with the name Top-Quality Lindera Powder (*tiān tái wū yào sǎn*) in his book *Illumination of Medicine*. However, a formula named Lindera Powder (*wū yào sǎn*), which contains the same ingredients in identical dosages, was already included in the Northern Song formulary *Comprehensive Recording of Sagely Beneficence from the Zhenghe Era*, where it was indicated for bulging qi with pain extending from the testicles into the lower abdomen. Li Dong-Yuan expanded these indications to include menstrual pain and mobile abdominal masses in women. In *Systematic Differentiation of Warm Pathogen Diseases*, the Qing-dynasty physician Wu Ju-Tong further expanded its indications to include severe pulling pain in the flanks and back.

Use of Crotonis Fructus (bā dòu)

There has been considerable controversy over whether Crotonis Fructus *(bā dòu)* should be used in this formula. Some modern authorities, including the editors of the 1979 edition of the Chinese national textbook on formulas, believe that it should not be used because it is too toxic. However, most commentators agree with the late-19th-century physician Wu Ju-Tong, who observed: "The brilliant aspect [of this formula] is its use of the qi and flavor of Crotonis Fructus *(bā dòu)*, but not its substance. This allows it to lead the qi medicines to scatter the formless cold, which is drained through the rectum by the actions of Arecae Semen *(bīng láng)*." The method of preparation whereby an herb known to be toxic or associated with significant side effects is dry-fried with a complementary herb on which it thereby bestows its desired actions, but not its potentially harmful excess, is commonly used in Chinese medicine.

Comparisons

➣ Vs. Tᴀɴɢᴇʀɪɴᴇ Sᴇᴇᴅ Pɪʟʟ *(jú hé wán)*; see ᴘᴀɢᴇ 530

➣ Vs. Wᴀʀᴍ ᴛʜᴇ Lɪᴠᴇʀ Dᴇᴄᴏᴄᴛɪᴏɴ *(nuǎn nuǎn gān jiān)*; see ᴘᴀɢᴇ 532

Biomedical Indications

With the appropriate presentation, this formula may be used to treat a variety of biomedically-defined disorders including orchitis, epididymitis, primary dysmenorrhea, irritable bowel syndrome, peptic ulcer, and gastritis.

Modifications

• To enhance the overall effect of this formula, add Citri reticulatae Semen *(jú hé)* and Litchi Semen *(lì zhī hé)*.

• For severe cold, add Evodiae Fructus *(wú zhū yú)* and Cinnamomi Cortex *(ròu guì)*.

• For blood stasis, add Carthami Flos *(hóng huā)* and Persicae Semen *(táo rén)*.

• For menstrual pain, add Angelicae sinensis Radix *(dāng guī)*, Chuanxiong Rhizoma *(chuān xiōng)*, and Cyperi Rhizoma *(xiāng fù)*.

• For mobile abdominal masses, add Aurantii Fructus immaturus *(zhǐ shí)*, Magnoliae officinalis Cortex *(hòu pò)*, Curcumae Rhizoma *(é zhú)*, or Sparganii Rhizoma *(sān léng)*.

Associated Formula

導氣湯（导气汤）
Conduct the Qi Decoction
dǎo qì tāng

Sᴏᴜʀᴄᴇ *Medical Formulas Collected and Analyzed* (1682)

Toosendan Fructus *(chuān liàn zǐ)*. 12g
Aucklandiae Radix *(mù xiāng)*. 9g
Foeniculi Fructus *(xiǎo huí xiāng)*. 6g
Evodiae Fructus *(wú zhū yú)*. 3g

Promotes the movement of qi, spreads Liver qi, scatters cold, and alleviates pain. For cold-type bulging disorders. In contrast to the principal formula, this is simpler in composition and has a milder effect.

橘核丸
Tangerine Seed Pill
jú hé wán

Sᴏᴜʀᴄᴇ *Formulas to Aid the Living* (1253)

Citri reticulatae Semen *(jú hé)* .30g
dry-fried Toosendan Fructus *(chǎo chuān liàn zǐ)* 30g
Aucklandiae Radix *(mù xiāng)* .15g
dry-fried Persicae Semen *(chǎo táo rén)* 30g
dry-fried Corydalis Rhizoma *(chǎo yán hú suǒ)* 15g
Cinnamomi Cortex *(ròu guì)* 15g
Akebiae Caulis *(mù tōng)* 15g
ginger-fried Magnoliae officinalis Cortex *(jiāng chǎo hòu pò)* .15g
dry-fried Aurantii Fructus immaturus *(chǎo zhǐ shí)* 15g
Sargassum *(hǎi zǎo)* 30g
Eckloniae Thallus *(kūn bù)* 30g
Laminariae Thallus *(hǎi dài)* 30g

Method of Preparation Grind the ingredients into a fine powder and form into pills with wine. The normal dosage is 6-9g taken 1-2 times daily on an empty stomach with salt, wine, or broth. May also be prepared as a decoction with a proportionate reduction in the dosage of the ingredients.

Actions Promotes the movement of qi, alleviates pain, softens hardness, and dissipates clumps

Indications

Unilateral testicular swelling with colicky pain reaching to the umbilicus, or a rock-like hardness and swelling of the scrotum, or oozing of a yellow fluid from the scrotum. In severe cases, abscess and ulceration may also occur.

This is a protuberant bulging disorder (癲疝 *tuí shàn*) due to damp-cold invading the Liver channel. The Liver channel connects with the external genitalia where it can be blocked by damp-cold. Initially, this causes the testicles to swell. If the condition persists for any period of time, there will be a gradual congealing of dampness and a transformation into phlegm, as well as qi stagnation and stasis of blood. This manifests as a rock-like hardness of the testicles and a colicky pain that reaches to the umbilicus. Long-term blockage from damp-cold will eventually transform into heat and produce redness, swelling, wetness, and itching of the scrotum, or the oozing of a yellow fluid. In severe cases, there will also be abscess and ulceration.

Analysis of Formula

This formula treats damp-cold that has transformed into phlegm and generated stagnation of qi and stasis of blood. Such conditions tend to be present in the body for a long time before being brought to the attention of a physician. The formula thus adopts a complex strategy to address all the various aspects of this pattern. It promotes the movement of qi, invigorates the blood, softens hardness, and dissipates clumping in order to treat the branch. In addition, it employs the secondary strategies of dispersing cold and eliminating dampness, which treat the root.

The chief herb in this formula is bitter and acrid Citri reticulatae Semen (jú hé). It promotes the movement of qi and dissipates clumps and is especially effective in treating the pain associated with bulging disorders. There are four deputies. Toosendan Fructus (chuān liàn zǐ) and Aucklandiae Radix (mù xiāng) are effective qi-moving herbs that reinforce the actions of the chief herb. Because blood stasis is an important aspect of this condition, Persicae Semen (táo rén) and Corydalis Rhizoma (yán hú suǒ) are added to invigorate the blood and dissipate clumps. The latter herb is also very effective in promoting the movement of qi and thereby alleviating the pain. In concert with the chief herb, the deputies disperse the constraint and stagnation of qi and blood in the Liver channel.

The remaining herbs serve as assistants and envoys. Cinnamomi Cortex (ròu guì) warms the Kidneys and the Liver. Here it disperses cold from the lower burner and assists the blood-invigorating ingredients. Akebiae Caulis (mù tōng) unblocks the blood vessels (particularly in the lower burner) and eliminates dampness, thereby reducing the pain and swelling and providing the damp-phlegm in the scrotum with a route of exit. Magnoliae officinalis Cortex (hòu pò) directs the qi downward and dries the dampness, which assists the other herbs in dissipating the hard clumps. Aurantii Fructus immaturus (zhǐ shí) enhances the ability of the chief and deputy herbs to promote the movement of qi and break up clumps and accumulation. Sargassum (hǎi zǎo), Eckloniae Thallus (kūn bù), and Laminariae Thallus (hǎi dài) soften hardness and dissipate clumps.

Cautions and Contraindications

This formula should not be used for soft scrotal or other swellings. If the swellings have ulcerated, appropriate topical applications must also be used.

Commentary

Yan Yong-He, the author of this formula, recommended it for the treatment of any pattern associated with protuberant bulging disorder. He defined such patterns as due to Kidney deficiency, which permits the invasion of wind-cold into the organ. This deficiency may be due to external pathogens, emotional disorders, bad hygiene, overwork, or other causes. Secondarily, this leads to stagnation in the channels that traverse the external genitals, the Liver, and also the Stomach, which is traditionally charged with nourishing the 'ancestral sinew' (宗筋 zōng jīn), that is, the penis. Modern textbooks interpret this to mean that both the Kidneys (the testicles are regarded as the 'external Kidneys') and the Liver are involved in the pathogenesis of this disorder.

In clinical practice, this interpretation is less important than is a clear understanding of the action of the formula and of the specific type of bulging disorder that it treats. This was underscored by Fei Bo-Xiong in Discussion of Medical Formulas:

> This is a special prescription for the treatment of protuberant bulging disorder. It combines the strategies of regulating the qi, breaking up blood [stasis], softening hardness, and moving water. From this one can deduce that using it to treat those suffering from painful [bulging disorder] would be a mistake.

To increase the efficacy of the formula in stubborn cases, the source text recommends adding Sal Ammoniac (náo shā). For patients with ulceration of the scrotum, the medicine should also be applied externally.

Comparison

➤ Vs. Top-Quality Lindera Powder (tiān tái wū yào sǎn)

While both formulas treat bulging disorders, the patterns for which they are indicated differ. Top-Quality Lindera Powder (tiān tái wū yào sǎn) treats qi-type bulging disorder characterized by pain in the lower abdomen radiating to the testicles. This pattern is caused by cold obstructing the flow of qi in the Liver channel or the Small Intestine and Bladder. By contrast, Tangerine Seed Pill (jú hé wán) treats a mixed water- and blood-type bulging disorder characterized by unilateral testicular swelling or a rock-like hardness and swelling of the scrotum. Pain can, but need not, be present and in any case will not be the most prominent symptom. This pattern is caused by dampness transforming into phlegm and creating blood stasis and qi stagnation. Both formulas can also be used in gynecology with a similar presentation related to the ovaries rather than the testes.

Biomedical Indications

With the appropriate presentation, this formula may be used to treat a variety of biomedically-defined disorders including hydrocele, orchitis, testicular tuberculosis, and epididymitis.

Alternate name

Tangerine Seed Pill for Bulging Qi *(jú hé shàn qì wán)* in *Nationwide Collection of TCM Patent Formulas*

Modifications

- To promote the diuretic action of the formula and thereby eliminate dampness more effectively, add Alismatis Rhizoma *(zé xiè),* Poria *(fú líng),* or Polyporus *(zhū líng).*

- For severe blood stasis and pain, add Sparganii Rhizoma *(sān léng)* and Curcumae Rhizoma *(é zhú).*

- For severe cold with intense pain, increase the dosage of Cinnamomi Cortex *(ròu guì)* and Aucklandiae Radix *(mù xiāng).* Alternatively, add Foeniculi Fructus *(xiǎo huí xiāng)* and Evodiae Fructus *(wú zhū yú).*

- If damp-cold transforms into heat with redness and swelling of the scrotum or a yellow, oozing exudate and scanty, dark urine, remove Cinnamomi Cortex *(ròu guì)* and add Plantaginis Semen *(chē qián zǐ),* Alismatis Rhizoma *(zé xiè),* and Smilacis glabrae Rhizoma *(tǔ fú líng).* If the heat is severe, add Scutellariae Radix *(huáng qín),* Phellodendri Cortex *(huáng bǎi),* and Gentianae Radix *(lóng dǎn cǎo).*

暖肝煎
Warm the Liver Decoction

nuǎn gān jiān

This formula is used for treating bulging disorders due to cold in the Liver channel, hence the name.

Source *Collected Treatises of [Zhang] Jing-Yue* (1624)

Angelicae sinensis Radix *(dāng guī)* 6g
Lycii Fructus *(gǒu qǐ zǐ)* 9g
Foeniculi Fructus *(xiǎo huí xiāng)* 6g
Cinnamomi Cortex *(ròu guì)* 3g
Linderae Radix *(wū yào)* 6g
Aquilariae Lignum resinatum *(chén xiāng)* 3g
Poria *(fú líng)* 6g
Zingiberis Rhizoma recens *(shēng jiāng)* . . . . 3-5 slices

Method of Preparation Aquilariae Lignum resinatum *(chén xiāng)* is ground into a powder, and the other herbs are decocted. The decoction is taken warm with the powder being dissolved into the decoction. Because of its greater availability, Aucklandiae Radix *(mù xiāng)* is often substituted for Aquilariae Lignum resinatum *(chén xiāng)* with the same dosage, but added toward the end of the decocting process.

Actions Warms the Liver and Kidneys, promotes the movement of qi, and alleviates pain

Indications

Lower abdominal pain that is sharp, localized, and is aggravated by the local application of cold, accompanied by a pale tongue (especially on the sides and root), and a submerged, tight pulse. Also used for swelling, distention, and pain of the scrotum.

This is a cold-type bulging disorder occurring against a background of Liver deficiency. If the Liver blood is deficient and its yang is unable to move the qi and blood, cold from deficiency causes the qi to stagnate. The pain is therefore sharp and localized in the lower abdomen and is aggravated by the local application of cold. The same mechanism can also lead to swelling, distention, and pain of the scrotum as the fluids are not moved by the qi and congeal in the presence of cold. The deficiency of Liver blood is reflected in the pale color of the tongue, especially in those parts that reflect the Liver and its mother organ, the Kidneys. The submerged aspect of the pulse reflects the interior nature of the disorder, while the tight aspect reflects the presence of cold in the Liver, and the resulting stagnation.

Analysis of Formula

This formula treats a mixed pattern of deficiency and excess, where the stagnation of Liver qi is caused by and coexists with the deficiency of Liver yang and blood. Not only do the Liver and Kidneys share the same source, but from a five phase perspective, a deficient child (wood/Liver) is treated by tonifying the mother (water/Kidneys). For these reasons, nourishing the Liver blood and yang is supported by warming the Kidneys and gate of vitality. These tonifying strategies are complemented by dispersing cold and facilitating the movement of Liver qi by means of acrid, warming substances.

Foeniculi Fructus *(xiǎo huí xiāng)* and Cinnamomi Cortex *(ròu guì)* are the two chief herbs in the formula. The former warms the Liver and disperses cold from the lower abdomen and thereby directly treats the manifestations. The latter is acrid, sweet, and very warming, entering the Liver, Kidneys, and gate of vitality to generate the production of yang at its source.

There are two different groups of deputies, each composed of a pair of synergistic herbs. The first is the combination of Angelicae sinensis Radix *(dāng guī)* and Lycii Fructus *(gǒu qǐ zǐ),* two blood-nourishing herbs that tonify the Liver and augment the Kidneys, once more attending to mother and child organs at the same time. The second group consists of the acrid, warming, and qi-moving herbs Linderae Radix *(wū yào)* and Aquilariae Lignum resinatum *(chén xiāng).* Together, they enhance the actions of the chief herbs by promoting the movement of qi and alleviating pain, especially in the lower abdomen. The assistant is Poria *(fú líng),* which leaches out dampness and strengthens the Spleen to eliminate the yin excess that invariably accompanies yang deficiency. Zingiberis Rhizoma recens *(shēng jiāng),* the envoy, scatters cold and harmonizes the Stomach. In concert with Poria *(fú líng),* it is particularly effective in treating the nausea and loss of appetite that often accompany this condition (usually secondary to the intense pain).

In this manner, the root of the disorder is treated by warming and tonifying the Liver and Kidneys, and the branch by promoting the movement of qi and dispersing the cold.

Cautions and Contraindications

Contraindicated in patients with heat, redness, swelling, and pain of the scrotum due to damp-heat pouring down into the lower burner.

Commentary

The analysis of this formula and its indications given above are derived from contemporary Chinese medical textbooks that tend to attribute this type of bulging disorder to cold obstructing the Liver channel. However, the author of the source text, Zhang Jie-Bin, presents a different approach. Zhang states that this formula was composed to treat "sudden or severe pain from bulging disorder … [in a pattern] that is not characterized by the presence of excess pathogenic [qi] yet is of a cold nature." Like other physicians, he observed many different types of bulging disorder, but he was clear that:

> Cold-type bulging disorder can cause the most severe pain. It is most often caused by contracting cold pathogenic qi or by habitually [eating] raw foods. It generally occurs in those [patients] who like warmth and are averse to cold, [whose] pulse is wiry and thin, [whose] hands, feet, and tip of the nose are generally cold [to the touch], and [who] do not have any heat signs in their stool or urine.

For Zhang Jie-Bin, deficiency thus constituted an important background factor in the etiology and presentation of the patterns that define this formula's scope of action:

> [This pattern occurs] because of excessive sexual desires, or because of harm from overwork, or from pent-up anger, or following the consumption of damp foods and alcoholic drinks. Having no idea about what to be wary of, when they contract a cold pathogen, the yin [from the outside] seeks out the yin [in the inside] and flows into and clumps in the Conception and Penetrating vessels, the seas of qi and blood. Flowing downward into the yin parts, it then generates all types of bulging disorders.

In his understanding of the pathodynamic of bulging disorders, Zhang Jie-Bin follows the original definition of bulging qi advanced in Chapter 60 of *Basic Questions*: "When the Conception vessel causes illness, in men there is clumping internally and there are the seven [types of] bulging disorders. In women, there are discharges as well as conglomerations and gatherings (瘕聚 *jiǎ jù*)." This was reiterated in Chapter 20 of *Classic of Difficulties*: "When the Conception vessel gives rise to illness, one suffers from internal clumps (結 *nèi jié*). In men, this gives rise to the seven [types of] bulging disorders; in women, to concretions and accumulations." The Qing-dynasty writer Chen Jin-Ao elaborates on this pathodynamic in *Wondrous Lantern for Peering into the Origin and Development of Miscellaneous Diseases*: "If the Conception vessel gives rise to illness, this is not illness that comes from the yin, but in reality [it refers to problems] that arise because there is no yang in the yin." If yin here is understood to refer to the blood, and yang to the qi, in particular the yang qi or ministerial fire generated in the gate of vitality, then disorders of the Conception vessel refer to illness caused by failure of the yang qi to mobilize and move the yin blood. Naturally, this occurs more readily when these resources are depleted by inappropriate habits and lifestyles, and when a person's essence-blood has become depleted.

This perspective, the particular choice of herbs in this formula, makes eminent sense. Many of the herbs in this formula, for instance, are regularly used by gynecologists and other physicians who wish to address disorders of the extraordinary vessels. Foeniculi Fructus (*xiǎo huí xiāng*) is said to enter the Conception vessel, tonify the gate of vitality, and warm the cinnabar field (丹田 *dān tián*). Cinnamomi Cortex (*ròu guì*), likewise, tonifies the ministerial fire at the gate of vitality, and warms the Conception vessel. Aquilariae Lignum resinatum (*chén xiāng*) enters the gate of vitality. Angelicae sinensis Radix (*dāng guī*) and Lycii Fructus (*gǒu qǐ zǐ*) are important herbs for tonifying the blood and essence of the Conception and Penetrating vessels. Even Poria (*fú líng*) is used by some physicians to direct herbs into the Stomach channel, and so, at least indirectly, into the Penetrating vessel.

Because the Liver stores the blood, is associated with the sea of blood, and is closely connected physiologically to the functions of the Conception vessel, naming the formula Warm the Liver Decoction (*nuǎn gān jiān*) is not inconsistent with this interpretation. In fact, as shown in the discussion of Resolve the Liver Decoction (*jiě gān jiān*) below, Zhang Jie-Bin often named his formulas after the branch of the treatment, rather than the root. This understanding extends the formula's applications to the treatment of dysmenorrhea due to cold and deficiency of the Conception and Penetrating vessels, and makes it a base formula for the treatment of Liver yang deficiency patterns in contemporary practice.

Comparison

➤ Vs. Top-Quality Lindera Powder *(tiān tái wū yào sǎn)*

Both formulas treat bulging disorders characterized by acute abdominal pain that may radiate into the testes. This is caused by qi stagnation and clumping of qi and fluids following the invasion of cold pathogenic qi. However, Top-Quality Lindera Powder (*tiān tái wū yào sǎn*) treats patterns of excess in patients with strong constitutions. Warm the Liver Decoction (*nuǎn gān jiān*), on the other hand, treats mixed patterns of excess and deficiency, where a cold pathogen causes qi stagnation in a patient whose essence, blood, and yang are deficient. For this reason, Top-Quality Lindera Powder (*tiān tái wū yào sǎn*) focuses entirely on dispersing stagnation by means of acrid, warming herbs, whereas Warm the Liver Decoction *(nuǎn gān jiān)* also tonifies the fire at the gate of vitality and nourishes the sea of blood.

Biomedical Indications

With the appropriate presentation, this formula may be used to treat a variety of biomedically-defined disorders including varicocele, hydrocele, and inguinal hernia.

Modifications

- For more severe cold, add Evodiae Fructus *(wú zhū yú)*, Zingiberis Rhizoma *(gān jiāng)*, and Aconiti Radix lateralis praeparata *(zhì fù zǐ)*. (source text)
- For abdominal pain, add Cyperi Rhizoma *(xiāng fù)*.
- For pain of the scrotum, add Litchi Semen *(lì zhī hé)* and Citri reticulatae Semen *(jú hé)*.
- For severe pain of the lower abdomen, add Corydalis Rhizoma *(yán hú suǒ)* and Toosendan Fructus *(chuān liàn zǐ)*.
- For the treatment of Liver yang deficiency patterns, combine with Frigid Extremities Powder *(sì nì sǎn)*.

Associated Formula

解肝煎

Resolve the Liver Decoction

jiě gān jiān

SOURCE *Collected Treatises of [Zhang] Jing-Yue (1624)*

Citri reticulatae Pericarpium *(chén pí)* 4.5g
Pinelliae Rhizoma praeparatum *(zhì bàn xià)* 4.5g
Magnoliae officinalis Cortex *(hòu pò)* 4.5g
Poria *(fú líng)* 4.5g
Perillae Folium *(zǐ sū yè)* 3g
Paeoniae Radix alba *(bái sháo)* 3g
Amomi Fructus *(shā rén)* 2.1g

Decoct with 3-5 slices of Zingiberis Rhizoma recens *(shēng jiāng)* and take warm. Smoothes the movement of qi, harmonizes the middle burner, transforms dampness, and calms the fetus. For Liver constraint and qi stagnation characterized by fullness, distention, and pain in the chest and flanks, diarrhea, or restless fetus. Although this formula resolves Liver qi constraint, its focus is on regulating the qi dynamic of the middle burner. In terms of five-phase doctrine, it thus treats a pattern where earth excess constrains the transformations of wood qi via the control cycle. This is explained in a commentary by the modern physician Qin Bo-Wei in *[Qin] Qian-Zhai's Lecture Notes on Medicine*:

> Although this formula is called Resolve the Liver [Decoction], apart from Paeoniae Radix alba *(bái sháo)*, [which] nourishes the Liver, and Perillae Folium *(zǐ sū yè)*, which aromatically dredges its qi, it only contains substances that transform dampness, move the qi, and regulate the Spleen and Stomach. Because [in this pattern] Spleen and Stomach dampness obstruct the qi [causing it] to stagnate, which impacts the spreading of Liver qi, in order to treat the root, one must focus on the middle burner. Therefore, the formula does not employ Bupleuri Radix

(chái hú) to dredge the Liver but Perillae Folium *(zǐ sū yè)*, relying on its ability to smoothe Liver constraint while also being able to harmonize the Spleen and Stomach. If the Spleen and Stomach are [sufficiently] strong to transport [qi and blood,] then the Liver qi expands naturally. Therefore, resolving the Liver implies resolving what constrains the Liver and not treating the Liver directly.

啟膈散 （启膈散）

Open Up the Diaphragm Powder

qǐ gé sǎn

Source *Awakening of the Mind in Medical Studies (1732)*

Glehniae/Adenophorae Radix *(shā shēn)* 9g
Salviae miltiorrhizae Radix *(dān shēn)* 9g
Poria *(fú líng)* 3g
Fritillariae cirrhosae Bulbus *(chuān bèi mǔ)* 4.5g
Curcumae Radix *(yù jīn)* 1.5g
Amomi Pericarpium *(shā rén ké)* 1.2g
Nelumbinis Calyx *(hé yè dì)* 3g
Oryzae Testa *(chǔ tóu kāng)* 1.5g

Method of Preparation Decoction. The source text does not specify which type of Glehniae/Adenophorae Radix *(shā shēn)* should be used. Practitioners, therefore, must use their own discretion in prescribing Glehniae Radix *(běi shā shēn)* or Adenophorae Radix *(nán shā shēn)*. Both herbs moisten dryness, but the former is better suited for enriching the yin, while the latter is better for transforming phlegm. The use of Oryzae Testa (杵頭糠 *chǔ tóu kāng)* is first mentioned in *Comprehensive Outline of the Materia Medica*, where it is described as sweet, acrid, and warming, and as entering the Stomach and Large Intestine to open the Stomach and direct the qi downward. Nelumbinis Calyx (荷葉蒂 *hé yè dì)* is described as being bitter and astringent, with a balanced nature. It enters the Spleen, Stomach, and Liver to strengthen the Spleen, expel dampness, direct the Spleen qi upward, and stimulate its yang functions.

If these herbs are unavailable, practitioners should make appropriate substitutions. One suggestion is to substitute Nelumbinis Folium *(hé yè)* for Nelumbinis Calyx *(hé yè dì)*. For Oryzae Testa *(chǔ tóu kāng)*, possible substitutions include Inulae Flos *(xuán fù huā)* together with Setariae (Oryzae) Fructus germinatus *(gǔ yá)*, or Evodiae Fructus *(wú zhū yú)* together with Citri sarcodactylis Fructus *(fó shǒu)*.

Actions Regulates the qi, opens constraint, moistens dryness, and transforms phlegm

Indications

Swallowing that is accompanied by a choking sensation, or the feeling of esophageal constriction or blockage, focal distention of the chest and diaphragm, or distention that is accompanied by indistinct pain and relieved by belching, dry retching, or spitting up of phlegm or oral mucus. These primary symptoms may be accompanied by difficult bowel movements, a dry mouth and throat, gradual emaciation, a red tongue with a white coating, and a thin, wiry pulse.

This is dysphagia-occlusion (噎膈 *yē gé*). Chronic qi constraint leads to clumping of qi such that the body fluids are no longer dispersed throughout the body but collect and transform into phlegm. This robs the qi dynamic of its lubrication but also obstructs the vessels and collaterals. This is experienced as dryness of the mouth and throat, occlusion of the esophagus, and indistinct pain. Stagnation of the qi dynamic manifests as focal distention in the chest and diaphragm. As the Stomach's downward-directing function becomes impeded, vomiting, spitting up of phlegm and oral mucus, and dry retching result. Desiccation of the yang fluids eventually affects the blood, causing the stools to become dry and difficult, the mucous membranes to dry up, and the body to take on an emaciated appearance. The red tongue indicates damage to the body fluids, the white coating the presence of phlegm. The thin pulse, likewise, reflects deficiency of yin fluids, while its wiry quality points to phlegm and qi stagnation.

Analysis of Formula

This formula treats stagnation of the qi dynamic causing the body fluids to congeal as phlegm, which deprives the organism of physiological fluids and leads to dryness. While qi stagnation is generally treated by means of acrid, warming herbs, such a strategy is clearly contraindicated in this case. Instead, the formula adopts a strategy of moistening dryness to resolve constraint, while simultaneously transforming the phlegm and opening up the clumping. This is reflected in the synergism between the two chief herbs, Glehniae/Adenophorae Radix (*shā shēn*) and Fritillariae cirrhosae Bulbus (*chuān bèi mǔ*). The former clears Stomach heat and enriches without being cloying. The latter resolves constraint and transforms phlegm without being drying. Together, these two herbs effectively open the qi dynamic of the upper burner when it has become clogged by phlegm.

Curcumae Radix (*yù jīn*), which facilitates the movement of qi to open up constraint while also dispelling blood stasis to disperse clumping, and Amomi Fructus (*shā rén*), which moves the qi to promote the qi dynamic of the middle burner and harmonizes the Stomach to stop vomiting and retching, serve as deputies. The remaining herbs are all assistants. Poria (*fú líng*) leaches out dampness and transforms phlegm and gently supports the middle burner in its production of blood without being drying. Salviae miltiorrhizae Radix (*dān shēn*) invigorates the blood, eliminates stasis, and thereby assists the dispersion of clumping that has penetrated to the blood aspect. Nelumbinis Calyx (*hé yè dì*) directs the yang upward and strengthens the Spleen's transportive and transformative functions to dispel dampness and harmonize the Stomach. Oryzae Testa (*chǔ tóu kāng*) opens the Stomach, directs the qi downward, and is a specific herb for the treatment of occlusion. Together, the assistants effectively facilitate the downward-directing of turbid phlegm and support the ascent of the clear yang to unblock the qi dynamic and eliminate

pathogenic excess without causing further dryness. Although the formula does not contain any specific envoys, this function is covered by the complementary synergism developed between the two herbs Nelumbinis Calyx (*hé yè dì*) and Oryzae Testa (*chǔ tóu kāng*), which focus on the ascending and descending functions of the qi dynamic , with the diaphragm as its fulcrum.

Cautions and Contraindications

Although this formula moistens dryness, its focus is on regulating the qi dynamic and transforming phlegm. It is contraindicated in cases of occlusion due to blood stasis characterized by an inability to swallow food or vomiting up of blood; in yin deficiency patterns with desiccated fluids characterized by a tongue without coating; and in qi and yang deficiency patterns accompanied by weight loss and fading spirits.

Commentary

The Chinese medical disease category dysphagia-occlusion describes a range of conditions characterized by sensations of obstruction and occlusion of the esophagus that are accompanied by vomiting or retching. The Qing-dynasty physician Cheng Guo-Peng composed this formula in response to what he perceived as being shortcomings in traditional strategies for treating dysphagia-occlusion. Cheng wrote:

> Ancient formulas for treating dysphagia-occlusion generally rely on medicinals that stop vomiting. They disregard [the fact] that vomiting is a symptom of dampness, for which drying is the suitable [treatment strategy]. Dysphagia-occlusion is a symptom of dryness that is best [treated] by moistening. … The symptoms of dysphagia-occlusion do not go beyond the four words 'dry withering [of the] gastric cavity' (胃脘干槁 *wèi wǎn gān gǎo*). If withering [occurs] in the upper [part of the] gastric cavity, fluids [still] pass but food enters only with difficulty. If withering [occurs] in the lower [part of the] gastric cavity, food enters but is vomited [up again] after some time. If the Stomach is withered and one administers drying herbs, will this not aggravate the dryness rather than effect a cure? This is why Major and Minor Pinellia Deoctions (*dà xiǎo bàn xià tāng*) are contraindicated in [the treatment of] dysphagia-occlusion. Instead, one should use Open Diaphragmatic Occlusion Powder (*qǐ gē sǎn*) to open the gate and assist it [by following up] with Four-Gentlemen Decoction (*sì jūn zǐ tāng*) to regulate the Spleen and Stomach.

One of the other formulas suggested by Cheng Guo-Peng in the treatment of dysphagia-occlusion was Rambling Powder (*xiāo yáo sǎn*). This underscores the importance he accorded to the regulation of the qi dynamic and the middle burner in the treatment of this disorder.

Biomedical Indications

With the appropriate presentation, this formula may be used to treat a variety of biomedically-defined disorders including esophagitis, esophageal diverticulum, and the early stages of esophageal cancer.

Modifications

- For pronounced rebellion of Stomach qi with belching and dry retching, add Inulae Flos (*xuán fù huā*), Haematitum (*dài zhě shí*), and a few drops of Zingiberis Rhizomatis Succus (*jiāng zhī*).

- For spitting up of phlegm and oral mucus, add Pinelliae Rhizoma praeparatum (*zhì bàn xià*) and Citri reticulatae Pericarpium (*chén pí*).

- For qi constraint transforming into fire, remove Amomi Pericarpium (*shā rén ké*) and add Coptidis Rhizoma (*huáng lián*), Gardeniae Fructus (*zhī zǐ*), and Sophorae tonkinensis Radix (*shān dòu gēn*).

- For constipation, add Rhei Radix et Rhizoma (*dà huáng*) and Raphani Semen (*lái fú zǐ*). This should only be done for a brief period to avoid further damage to the qi dynamic.

加味烏藥湯（加味乌药汤）
Augmented Lindera Decoction

jiā wèi wū yào tāng

Source　*Fine Formulas of Wonderful Efficacy* (1470)

Linderae Radix (*wū yào*)	30g
Amomi Fructus (*shā rén*)	30g
Aucklandiae Radix (*mù xiāng*)	30g
Corydalis Rhizoma (*yán hú suǒ*)	30g
dry fried Cyperi Rhizoma (*chǎo xiāng fù*)	60g
Glycyrrhizae Radix (*gān cǎo*)	45g

Method of Preparation　Grind equal amounts of the ingredients into a coarse powder and prepare a draft using 20g of the powder and 3 pieces of Zingiberis Rhizoma recens (*shēng jiāng*).

Actions　Promotes the movement of qi, invigorates the blood, regulates the menses, and alleviates pain

Indications

For dysmenorrhea with scanty, dark menstrual blood with clots. Pain occurs before the onset of menstruation or during the early part of menstruation. Lower abdominal pain will be accompanied by distention, which is more pronounced than the pain. There may also be premenstrual symptoms such as swollen and painful breasts. The tongue is normal with a white coating, and the pulse is wiry and tight.

This is dysmenorrhea due to qi stagnation, which causes blood stasis. Menstruation depends not only on the accumulation of blood in the Womb, but also on the downward movement of qi that guides the blood downward and out of the body. Qi stagnation in the lower abdomen is experienced as pain and distention. The fact that distention is more severe than pain indicates that qi stagnation rather than blood stasis is the root cause of this pattern. This is also the reason why the symptoms occur premenstrually or during the early part

of menstruation. However, because the flow of blood is also impeded, menstruation may be scanty, with dark menstrual blood. The uterus and sea of blood in the lower abdomen connect with the Liver and Stomach channels through the Conception and Penetrating vessels. Failure of the qi to move the blood in the uterus below may thus lead to qi excess above manifesting in distended, swollen, and painful breasts, as these are traversed by the Liver and Stomach channels. The tongue is normal, indicating that the disorder is in the qi rather than the blood. The white coating suggests cold as a possible cause of the stagnation. The wiry and tight qualities of the pulse reflect the same pathodynamic.

Analysis of Formula

This formula employs acrid and warming herbs that facilitate the movement of qi in order to promote the smooth flow of menstrual blood. Acrid, warming Linderae Radix (*wū yào*), which gives the formula its name, is the chief herb. It smoothes the flow of qi, disperses cold, and alleviates pain. It directs rebellious qi downward to help relieve the excess symptoms in the chest, disperses cold to address the cause of the stagnation, and alleviates pain to treat the symptoms. Acrid, aromatic, and neutral Cyperi Rhizoma (*xiāng fù*) serves as the deputy, complementing the functions of the chief herb in multiple ways. It specifically treats disorders due to qi clumping, but also enters the blood aspect to move blood that has become static due to qi stagnation. If Linderae Radix (*wū yào*) is better at directing the qi downward, Cyperi Rhizoma (*xiāng fù*) is better at raising and lifting the qi. If the former is better at eliminating cold, the latter is better at resolving constraint due to emotional factors. Their combination thus addresses the blockage of qi within both the qi and blood levels, releases constraint from both the Liver and Gallbladder, directs rebellious qi in the chest and abdomen downward, and warms the flow of qi, which has been slowed by pathogenic cold.

With the exception of Glycyrrhizae Radix (*gān cǎo*), all of the other herbs serve as assistants. Amomi Fructus (*shā rén*) and Aucklandiae Radix (*mù xiāng*) focus on the qi dynamic of the middle burner, the Spleen and the Stomach, because of its focal role in the ascent and descent of qi. Bitter and acrid Aucklandiae Radix (*mù xiāng*) promotes the movement of qi and stops pain. Acrid, warming, and aromatic Amomi Fructus (*shā rén*) also promotes the movement of qi and transforms dampness. Together with Aucklandiae Radix (*mù xiāng*), it reduces distention and alleviates pain while also strengthening the Spleen. Because qi moves not just the blood but also the fluids, qi stagnation is widely accompanied by dampness and water accumulation. This conjunction of symptoms, often found in premenstrual syndrome, is effectively addressed by this combination of herbs. Zingiberis Rhizoma recens (*shēng jiāng*) warms the Stomach to disperse cold, supporting the warming, dispersing action of the chief herbs and the regulation of the middle burner by the other assistants. The fourth assistant, Corydalis Rhizoma (*yán hú suǒ*), moves the qi to invigorate the blood, regulating the menses and alleviating pain. Sweet, cooling, and relaxing Glycyrrhizae Radix (*gān cǎo*) serves as envoy to moderate the acrid, warming actions of the other herbs and harmonize the diverse functions of the various ingredients.

Cautions and Contraindications

Contraindicated for dysmenorrhea due to Liver and Kidney deficiency, where the pain is generally worse after or during the later stages of menstruation.

Commentary

The original name of this formula was Augmented Lindera Decoction (加味烏沉湯 *jiā wèi wū chén tāng*). This was a modification of Lindera Decoction (烏藥湯 *wū yào tāng*), a formula from Li Dong-Yuan's *Secrets from the Orchid Chamber*, which consisted of Linderae Radix (*wū yào*), Cyperi Rhizoma (*xiāng fù*), Aucklandiae Radix (*mù xiāng*), Angelicae sinensis Radix (*dāng guī*), and Glycyrrhizae Radix (*gān cǎo*). Substituting Toosendan Fructus (*chuān liàn zǐ*) and Amomi Fructus (*shā rén*) for Angelicae sinensis Radix (*dāng guī*) replaced the earlier formula's blood-nourishing action with a much stronger emphasis on the regulation of qi as a means of moving the blood. The new formula was later included under its present name in the important gynecological work, *Comprehensive Outline on Benefiting Yin*, where it became a key formula in the treatment of painful periods and premenstrual symptoms.

Once more, it is notable that, while modern textbooks attribute this pattern primarily to Liver qi stagnation, the dynamic developed by the herbs in this formula is actually more complex. Moving qi excess from the upper to the lower body, where it can enter the Womb and the Penetrating and Conception vessels, may be considered at least as important here as the regulation of Liver qi and blood.

Comparisons

➤ Vs. Rambling Powder (*xiāo yáo sǎn*) and Bupleurum Powder to Dredge the Liver (*chái hú shū gān sǎn*)

All three of these formulas can be used to treat dysmenorrhea and premenstrual symptoms such as breast distention. Bupleurum Powder to Dredge the Liver (*chái hú shū gān sǎn*) and Augmented Lindera Decoction (*jiā wèi wū yào tāng*) both treat patterns of excess. However, the former focuses more specifically on the Liver channel, on the flanks, and on the ascent of qi, while the latter focuses on the qi dynamic in the lower burner, the Womb and Conception vessels, and on the descent of qi. Rambling Powder (*xiāo yáo sǎn*) treats a pattern of mixed deficiency and excess, where qi stagnation occurs as a consequence of blood and qi deficiency.

Biomedical Indications

With the appropriate presentation, this formula may be used to treat a variety of biomedically-defined disorders including dysmenorrhea, amenorrhea, and chronic pelvic inflammatory disease.

Modifications

- For pronounced cold or to use this formula in the treatment of bulging disorder, add Foeniculi Fructus (*xiǎo huí xiāng*) and Evodiae Fructus (*wú zhū yú*).

- For more severe blood stasis with dark, scanty menstruation and clotting, add Typhae Pollen (*pú huáng*) and Trogopterori Faeces (*wǔ líng zhī*).

Section 2

....

FORMULAS THAT DIRECT REBELLIOUS QI DOWNWARD

The formulas in this section are used for treating rebellious Lung or Stomach qi. The normal flow of qi in these organs is downward. When it rebels upward, the flow is reversed. In the case of rebellious Lung qi, this manifests in such symptoms as coughing and wheezing, and is treated with herbs such as Perillae Fructus (*zǐ sū zǐ*), Mori Cortex (*sāng bái pí*), Armeniacae Semen (*xìng rén*), Magnoliae officinalis Cortex (*hòu pò*), Peucedani Radix (*qián hú*), or Farfarae Flos (*kuǎn dōng huā*). In the case of rebellious Stomach qi, it manifests in such symptoms as vomiting or belching, and is treated with herbs such as Pinelliae Rhizoma praeparatum (*zhì bàn xià*), Inulae Flos (*xuán fù huā*), Haematitum (*dài zhě shí*), Bambusae Caulis in taeniam (*zhú rú*), Caryophylli Flos (*dīng xiāng*), or Kaki Calyx (*shì dì*).

In practice, herbs that focus on directing rebellious qi downward are most often combined with herbs that strengthen other aspects of the qi dynamic or that focus on particular symptoms. These include:

- Herbs that tonify and augment, like Ginseng Radix (*rén shēn*), Angelicae sinensis Radix (*dāng guī*), Glycyrrhizae Radix praeparata (*zhì gān cǎo*), or Jujubae Fructus (*dà zǎo*). This is necessary, first, because rebellious qi often develops against a background of deficiency, and second, because herbs that direct the qi downward may themselves damage the qi dynamic because of their one-sided nature.

- Herbs that warm the Kidneys and facilitate its role in grasping the qi or that regulate the function of the Penetrating and Conception vessels, such as Angelicae sinensis Radix (*dāng guī*), Cinnamomi Cortex (*ròu guì*), Aquilariae Lignum resinatum (chén xiāng), or Schisandrae Fructus (wǔ wèi zǐ). Focusing on the physiological functions that anchor qi in the lower burner, these herbs greatly assist in the control of rebellion.

- Herbs that stop coughing, such as Schisandrae Fructus (wǔ wèi zǐ) or Ginkgo Semen (bái guǒ). These herbs focus on a symptom, but in doing so, also help to regulate the qi.

In diagnosing patterns characterized by rebellion, the practitioner should ascertain whether the disorder is one of excess or deficiency, heat or cold, or a combination of factors. The formulas discussed here are generally indicated for relatively acute conditions and should not be prescribed long-term.

Regulating the qi and directing the qi downward are mutually dependent and mutually reinforcing actions. Thus, many formulas listed in the first section of this chapter contained herbs that direct the qi downward, such as Aquilariae Lignum resinatum (chén xiāng) or Magnoliae officinalis Cortex (hòu pò), or qi-moving herbs that also direct the qi downward, such as Linderae Radix (wū yào) or Amomi Fructus (shā rén). The formulas in this section, on the other hand, invariably contain qi-regulating herbs, such as Citri reticulatae Pericarpium (chén pí) or Pinelliae Rhizoma praeparatum (zhì bàn xià). Likewise, formulas that regulate the qi, such as Four Milled-Herb Decoction (sì mò tāng) or Pinellia and Magnolia Bark Decoction (bàn xià hòu pò tāng), also direct the qi downward, while formulas like Tangerine Peel and Bamboo Shavings Decoction from Formulas that Aid the Living (jú pí zhú rú tāng) and Minor Pinellia Deoction (xiǎo bàn xià tāng) also regulate the qi dynamic of the middle burner, and Perilla Fruit Decoction for Directing Qi Downward (sū zǐ jiàng qì tāng) also smoothes the interaction between the qi and blood.

蘇子降氣湯 (苏子降气汤)

Perilla Fruit Decoction for Directing Qi Downward

sū zǐ jiàng qì tāng

Source *Important Formulas Worth a Thousand Gold Pieces* (650)

Perillae Fructus (zǐ sū zǐ) 75g (9-12g)
Pinelliae Rhizoma praeparatum (zhì bàn xià) 75g (6-9g)
Citri reticulatae Pericarpium (chén pí) 45g (6-9g)
Angelicae sinensis Radix (dāng guī) 45g (6-9g)
Glycyrrhizae Radix (gān cǎo) 60g (3-4.5g)
Magnoliae officinalis Cortex (hòu pò) 30g (3-6g)
Peucedani Radix (qián hú) 30g (6-9g)
Cinnamomi Cortex (ròu guì) 45g (1.5-3g)

Method of Preparation The source text advises to grind the ingredients into a fine powder and take 6g as a draft with the addition of 2 slices of Zingiberis Rhizoma recens (shēng jiāng) and 3 pieces of Jujubae Fructus (dà zǎo). Many contemporary formularies list the ingredients and dosages set forth in *Formulary of the Pharmacy Service for Benefiting the People in the Taiping Era* rather than those in the source text. That version omits Citri reticulatae Pericarpium (chén pí), but adds 5 leaves of Perillae Folium (zǐ sū yè) to the preparation of the draft. At present, the formula is usually prepared as a decoction with the dosages indicated in parentheses and with the addition of the ingredients mentioned at the top of this paragraph.

Actions Directs rebellious qi downward, arrests wheezing, stops coughing, and warms and transforms phlegm-cold

Indications

Coughing and wheezing with watery, copious sputum, a stifling sensation in the chest and diaphragm, shortness of breath marked by relatively labored inhalation and smooth exhalation, and a white tongue coating that is either slippery or greasy. There may also be pain and weakness of the lower back and legs, edema of the extremities, and fatigue.

This condition is referred to as 'abundance above and deficiency below' (上盛下虛 shàng shèng xià xū). 'Abundance above' refers to excessive pathogenic qi obstructing the clarifying, downward-directing functions of the Lungs. This interferes with the normal circulation of qi and fluids. The Lung qi becomes constrained and rebels upward while the fluids transform into phlegm, which manifests as coughing and wheezing with copious, watery sputum together with a stifling sensation in the chest. 'Deficiency below' refers primarily to deficiency of normal qi below, disabling the Kidneys' function of grasping the qi, which manifests as wheezing and shortness of breath characterized by rather labored inhalation. It may also include yang deficiency with pain and weakness of the lower back and legs, and a disturbance of water metabolism (water failing to transform into qi), which manifests as edema. This condition often occurs in patients with constitutionally deficient yang (the root) with internal phlegm who contract external wind-cold, which transforms into phlegm-cold (the branch) and obstructs the circulation of the Lung qi.

Analysis of Formula

This formula takes into account the pathodynamic both above and below. Where the condition is acute, however, one must necessarily focus on the branches; thus, the primary strategy here is to direct the rebellious qi downward, stop the coughing and wheezing, and expel the phlegm. Warming the fire at the gate of vitality and supporting the lower burner functions of grasping the qi is of secondary importance.

Acrid, warming, and moistening Perillae Fructus (zǐ sū zǐ) directs rebellious qi downward, expels phlegm, stops the coughing, and arrests the wheezing. As a seed, it has a sinking nature, and because it contains oils, it moistens the bowels. Facilitating the functions of the Large Intestine as well as the Lungs, it is a primary herb for controlling rebellious Lung qi and is therefore the chief herb in this formula. Acrid, warming, and drying Pinelliae Rhizoma praeparatum (*zhì bàn xià*) combines with acrid, warming, bitter, and downward-directing Magnoliae officinalis Cortex (*hòu pò*) to support the chief herb in directing the qi downward and transforming the phlegm. They are regarded as deputies. Acrid, warming, bitter, and drying Citri reticulatae Pericarpium (*chén pí*) assists Pinelliae Rhizoma (*bàn xià*) in transforming the phlegm and regulating the qi. Acrid and bitter Peucedani Radix (*qián hú*) assists Magnoliae officinalis Cortex (*hòu pò*) in directing the qi downward and is a special herb for expelling phlegm. Although it has a cool nature, when it is combined with the warm herbs in this formula, only its phlegm-transforming and qi-directing properties are evident. In concert with the chief and deputies herb, these assistants effectively treat the exuberant pathogenic qi above.

To treat the deficiency below, two other assistants are used. Cinnamomi Cortex (*ròu guì*) warms the fire at the gate of vitality and directs the floating yang back to its source, thereby facilitating the Kidneys' ability to grasp the qi. Its yang-warming action also helps to dispel cold. The functions of the other assistant, Angelicae sinensis Radix (*dāng guī*), are complex and still much debated (see COMMENTARY below). First, one of its ancient functions—treating the cough from rebellious qi—mentioned in *Divine Husbandman's Classic of the Materia Medica* but rarely utilized at present, is drawn upon in this formula. Second, this condition represents an acute aggravation of a chronic disorder. Chronic disorders often lead to deficiency or 'devitalization' of the blood. This herb is therefore used to harmonize the qi and blood. This has the effect of conducting errant aspects of the body back to their respective sources, and here has a positive influence on the qi-grasping function of the Kidneys. Finally, this herb is used to prevent injury to the yin and qi from the acrid, dry properties of many of the other ingredients.

The remaining herbs serve as envoys. Zingiberis Rhizoma recens (*shēng jiāng*) and Perillae Folium (*zǐ sū yè*) (if this is included) disperse cold and improve circulation in the Lungs. Glycyrrhizae Radix (*gān cǎo*) and Jujubae Fructus (*dà zǎo*) harmonize the middle burner, which helps resolve the phlegm. They also harmonize the actions of the other ingredients, which is especially important in a formula with so many different types of herbs.

Cautions and Contraindications

Inappropriate for treating Lung and Kidney deficiency in the absence of an externally-contracted pathogenic influence and in cases of wheezing and a productive cough due to heat in the Lungs.

Commentary

Origins

This is a good example of how the indications and usage of a formula can change over time and of the issues that this raises. Furthermore, even though the formula was recommended by the Tang-dynasty physician Sun Si-Miao as early as the year 650, the principles underlying its composition are still debated by commentators today, suggesting that empirical usage as much as theoretical understanding inform its use in practice.

Under the name Perilla Decoction (*zī sū zǐ tāng*), the formula was first listed in the chapter on 'wind poison leg qi' (風毒腳氣 *fēng dú jiǎo qì*) in Sun Si-Miao's *Important Formulas Worth a Thousand Gold Pieces*, where it is prescribed for the treatment of "frail legs with rising of qi" (弱腳上氣 *ruò jiǎo shàng qì*), an acute presentation of a wider disease category known as 'leg qi' (腳氣 *jiǎo qì*). This condition was first discussed in *Emergency Formulas to Keep Up One's Sleeve*, where it is defined as an accumulation of dampness that generates heat and spreads throughout the legs. This can arise from the penetration of external dampness and pathogenic wind into the body as well as from dietary irregularities, specifically the eating of rich food and drink. The disorder presents with symptoms that include numbness, aching and weakness of the feet and legs, or alternatively, acute cramping, edema, muscle wasting, or fever. In acute cases, the dampness and pathogenic wind can enter into the abdomen to attack the Heart. In such cases, one observes insensitivity in the lower abdomen, vomiting, inability to eat, palpitations, dyspnea, a stifling sensation in the chest, disorientation, and disordered speech. Treatment focuses on dispelling dampness, supported by strategies that eliminate wind, clear heat, and regulate the movement of qi and blood.

Four centuries later, the formula appeared (with minor modifications) under the new name Perilla Fruit Decoction for Directing Qi Downward (*sū zǐ jiàng qì tāng*) in the government-sponsored *Formulary of the Pharmacy Service for Benefiting the People in the Taiping Era*. By then, it also had a significantly expanded set of indications:

> [This formula] treats upward attack of deficient yang in men and women. The qi [neither] ascends nor descends [manifesting as] abundance above and deficiency below. The diaphragm is clogged with excessive phlegm, the throat is obstructed, there is coughing, deficiency irritability leading [to a desire for] drink, dizziness, and lightheadedness, lower back pain with weak legs, fatigue with a desire to curl up, … diarrhea in response to cold or hot weather, the bowels are closed by wind, obstructed urine or bowels, floating edema of the extremities, and lack of appetite.

The same text notes that, if taken regularly, "it can clear the spirit and smooth the qi, harmonize the five yin organs, move stagnant qi, promote drinking and eating, and eliminate damp qi."

Changes in Usage

In part, the enormous influence of the *Formulary of the Pharmacy Service for Benefiting the People in the Taiping Era* is responsible for this formula's enduring popularity, and its definition of the corresponding pattern as 'abundance above and deficiency below' became widely accepted. However, while the description of this pattern in the *Formulary of the Pharmacy Service for Benefiting the People in the Taiping Era* still alludes to a more widespread disorder of the qi dynamic, by the Qing era it had been narrowed down to just coughing and wheezing. This is described by the Suzhou physician Zhang Lu, an astute observer of the changing medical practices of his time, in *Extension of the Important Formulas Worth a Thousand Gold Pieces:*

> The pathology of leg qi [is defined as] turbid qi that attacks upward. … Overall, [this formula] focuses on directing and draining rebellious qi. Hence, the *Formulary of the Pharmacy Service for Benefiting the People in the Taiping Era* renamed it Perilla Fruit Decoction for Directing Qi Downward (*sū zǐ jiàng qì tāng*). Later generations [of physicians] used it to treat deficient yang attacking upward with clogging due to abundance of phlegm and oral mucus, [obstruction of] Lung qi with wheezing and fullness. Taking it causes the qi to be directed downward and thereby calms [these symptoms]. From this, one can see that in using a formula one must select [the pattern] for which it is suited. One must not narrowly focus on what type of disorder it mainly treats.

Physicians also adapted the formula to its new indications. In *Indispensable Tools for Pattern Treatment*, the Ming-dynasty physician Wang Ken-Tang, for instance, suggested replacing Cinnamomi Cortex (*ròu guì*) with Aquilariae Lignum resinatum (*chén xiāng*) in order to strengthen the formula's focus on the downward-directing of qi. Wang's modification became so popular that some later formularies, such as Wang Ang's influential *Medical Formulas Collected and Analyzed*, accepted it as the standard formula. Arisaematis Rhizoma praeparatum (*zhì tiān nán xīng*) was added in *Concise Medical Guidelines* to further dry the dampness. Other changes were also suggested, such as adding herbs to simultaneously clear the wind pathogen from the exterior.

Some physicians, however, were more cautious regarding these changes in indication. In *Discussion of Medical Formulas*, the late-Qing physician Fei Bo-Xiong warned:

> This formula has become popular for treating clogging from dampness and phlegm with discomfort in the middle [burner] gastric [cavity]. I am rather suspicious that it is too drying, especially where commentators focus on its treatment of deficient yang attacking upward with symptoms such as wheezing, coughing, and spitting of blood. This is like adding firewood to the fire. In my opinion, this will court immediate disaster.

Use of Angelicae sinensis Radix (*dāng guī*)

Focusing this formula on the treatment of wheezing and coughing, especially where it is linked to Kidney deficiency, has made it difficult to explain the inclusion of Angelicae sinensis Radix (*dāng guī*). Even if *Divine Husbandman's Classic of the Materia Medica* recommended this herb for coughing due to rebellious qi, it is not an herb that enters the Kidneys. Rather, as explained by Zhang Xi-Chun in *Essays on Medicine Esteeming the Chinese and Respecting the Western*, it achieves its purposes by regulating the qi dynamic:

> [This] is the primary herb for generating blood and invigorating blood, but it also disseminates and unblocks the qi aspect, inducing the qi and blood to return [to their proper place], hence the name [of the herb, which is literally] 'state of return.' Its power can raise because it is strong and steady in action, and warm; it can direct downward because its flavor is rich and acrid; internally, it moistens the organs because of its concentrated fluids and sweetness.

From this perspective, viewing the formula as warming and regulating the qi dynamic, rather than tonifying the Kidneys, provides a better understanding of its mode of action. This has allowed contemporary physicians to considerably extend its range of indications beyond the treatment of wheezing, dyspnea, and asthma. Based on the clinical experience of the contemporary physician Yue Mei-Zhong, the following indications stand out:

- Plum-pit qi due to deficiency below and excess above (where Angelicae sinensis Radix (*dāng guī*) is thought to have a purpose similar to that attributed to Perillae Folium (*zǐ sū yè*) in Pinellia and Magnolia Bark Decoction (*bàn xià hòu pò tāng*), discussed perviously). In this case, Yue suggests reducing the dosage of Cinnamomi Cortex (*ròu guì*) and adding Cinnamomi Ramulus (*guì zhī*) in order to control upflushing and unblock the yang.

- Painful obstruction of the chest. For patterns caused by the inability of yang to expand due to constraint by turbid dampness, Yue suggests adding herbs such as Cinnamomi Ramulus (*guì zhī*), Acori tatarinowii Rhizoma (*shí chāng pǔ*), and Allii macrostemi Bulbus (*xiè bái*). For patterns where phlegm constraint is prominent, Yue suggests adding herbs like Trichosanthis Fructus (*guā lóu*), Fritillariae Bulbus (*bèi mǔ*), and Eriobotryae Folium (*pí pá yè*), and removing Cinnamomi Cortex (*ròu guì*); and for Heart and Lung qi stagnation and blood stasis, adding Aucklandiae Radix (*mù xiāng*), Curcumae Radix (*yù jīn*), Corydalis Rhizoma (*yán hú suǒ*), and Aurantii Fructus immaturus (*zhǐ shí*).

- For esophageal obstruction by phlegm-dampness, Yue suggests adding Inulae Flos (*xuán fù huā*) and Haematitum (*dài zhě shí*) to pacify the phlegm qi; Amomi Fructus rotundus (*bái dòu kòu*) and Eriobotryae Folium (*pí pá yè*) to open the chest and abdomen; and Persicae Semen (*táo rén*) and Armeniacae Semen (*xìng rén*) to enrich dryness of the blood.

Comparison

➤ Vs. Minor Bluegreen Dragon Decoction (*xiǎo qīng lóng tāng*)

While both formulas are used for coughing and wheezing associated with cold and congested fluids, Perilla Fruit Decoction for Directing Qi Downward (*sū zǐ jiàng qì tang*) is indicated specifically for a condition of excess above and deficiency below, while Minor Bluegreen Dragon Decoction (*xiǎo qīng lóng tāng*) is indicated for externally-contracted wind-cold in patients with chronic Spleen deficiency and congested fluids.

Biomedical Indications

With the appropriate presentation, this formula may be used to treat a variety of biomedically-defined disorders including chronic bronchitis, emphysema, bronchial asthma, cardiac asthma, and morning sickness.

....

Alternate names

Decoction for Directing Qi Downward (*jiàng qì tāng*) in *Prescriptions for Universal Benefit*; Perilla Fruit Drink for Directing Qi Downward (*sū zǐ jiàng qì yǐn*) in *Restoration of Life from the Groves of Medicine*; Perilla Fruit Decoction (*sū zǐ tāng*) in *Collected Treatises of [Zhang] Jing-Yue*

....

Modifications

• For concurrent exterior cold, add Ephedrae Herba (*má huáng*) and Armeniacae Semen (*xìng rén*).

• For less severe cold, substitute Menthae haplocalycis Herba (*bò hé*) for Perillae Folium (*zǐ sū yè*).

• For more sputum and coughing, add Citri reticulatae Pericarpium (*chén pí*).

• For qi deficiency, add Codonopsis Radix (*dǎng shēn*) and Schisandrae Fructus (*wǔ wèi zǐ*).

• For urinary difficulty, add Plantaginis Semen (*chē qián zǐ*).

• For greater difficulty in inhalation without lower back pain, remove Cinnamomi Cortex (*ròu guì*) and add Aquilariae Lignum resinatum (*chén xiāng*).

定喘湯（定喘汤）
Arrest Wheezing Decoction

dìng chuǎn tāng

Source   *Multitude of Marvelous Formulas for Sustaining Life* (1550)

dry-fried Ginkgo Semen (*chǎo bái guǒ*) . . . . 21 pieces (9g)
Ephedrae Herba (*má huáng*) .9g
Perillae Fructus (*zǐ sū zǐ*) 6g
Glycyrrhizae Radix (*gān cǎo*) 3g
Farfarae Flos (*kuǎn dōng huā*) 9g
Armeniacae Semen (*xìng rén*) 4.5g
prepared Mori Cortex (*zhì sāng bái pí*) 9g
dry-fried Scutellariae Radix (*chǎo huáng qín*) 4.5g
Pinelliae Rhizoma praeparatum (*zhì bàn xià*) 9g

Method of Preparation   Decoction. The source text advises not to use ginger in preparing the decoction, and that there is no specific regime for taking the decoction.

Actions   Disseminates and redirects the Lung qi, arrests wheezing, clears heat, and transforms phlegm

Indications

Coughing and wheezing with copious, thick, and yellow sputum, labored breathing, a greasy, yellow tongue coating, and a slippery, rapid pulse. There may also be simultaneous fever and chills.

This is wheezing caused by wind-cold constraining the exterior and phlegm-heat smoldering in the interior. This usually occurs in patients with a constitutional tendency toward excessive phlegm who also contract wind-cold. When this occurs, the Lung qi is obstructed, its directional flow is disrupted, and the constrained qi transforms into heat. This gives rise to wheezing with thick, yellow sputum that is difficult to expectorate. The greasy, yellow coating on the tongue and the slippery, rapid pulse are also signs of heat and phlegm. Depending on how long this process takes, the patient may still show symptoms of an exterior condition, notably simultaneous fever and chills.

Analysis of Formula

Although this formula is designed to treat a mixed pattern of interior and exterior excess, the main pathodynamic is the obstruction of the Lung qi's descending function by phlegm-heat. For this reason, the main strategy is one of disseminating and directing the Lung qi downward, assisted by the draining of heat and the transformation of phlegm. Acrid and warming Ephedrae Herba (*má huáng*) unblocks and redirects the Lung qi, arrests wheezing, and releases the exterior. Sweet, bitter, and astringent Ginkgo Semen (*bái guǒ*) transforms phlegm, contains the leakage of Lung qi, arrests wheezing, and prevents Ephedrae Herba (*má huáng*) from causing excessive dispersion and depletion. The complementary actions of these chief herbs in dispersing and binding greatly enhances the ability of the formula to arrest wheezing.

Mori Cortex (*sāng bái pí*) drains the Lungs and stops wheezing. Scutellariae Radix (*huáng qín*) clears heat and transforms phlegm. Together, they act as deputies to eliminate phlegm-heat from the Lungs, arrest the wheezing, and stop the coughing. Armeniacae Semen (*xìng rén*) reinforces the actions of Ephedrae Herba (*má huáng*) in expanding the Lungs and arresting the wheezing. The other assistants, Perillae Fructus *(zǐ sū zǐ)*, Pinelliae Rhizoma praeparatum *(zhì bàn xià)*, and Farfarae Flos *(kuǎn dōng huā)*, support the chief and deputy herbs in directing the rebellious qi downward, arresting the wheezing, and expelling phlegm. The envoy, Glycyrrhizae Radix *(gān cǎo)*, harmonizes the actions of the other ingredients in the formula.

Cautions and Contraindications

Inappropriate in cases of externally-contracted wind-cold that present with an absence of sweating and internal phlegm-heat. Also inappropriate in cases of chronic asthma with qi deficiency and a frail pulse.

Commentary

The indication for this formula in the source text simply says 'asthma' (哮喘 *xiào chuǎn*) without specifying either a pattern or a pathodynamic. This was added about 30 years later by the Ming-dynasty physician Wu Kun, who included a discussion of Arrest Wheezing Decoction *(dìng chuǎn tāng)* in *Investigations of Medical Formulas*:

> This formula masters Lung deficiency with contracted cold leading to rebellious qi, diaphragmatic heat, and wheezing. Wheezing (哮 *xiào*) refers to the thick sounds. For disorders due to exterior-contracted excess, it is appropriate to use herbs [that focus on the] exterior. Dyspnea (喘 *chuǎn*) refers to breathing that is hurried. It is a sign of Lung deficiency, and it is appropriate to use herbs [that focus on the] interior. If cold fetters the exterior, the yang qi is unable to thrust outward, causing rebellious qi. The qi joins with the diaphragm, producing yang within yang, and thus leading to heat. In this formula, Ephedrae Herba *(má huáng)*, Armeniacae Semen *(xìng rén)*, and Glycyrrhizae Radix *(gān cǎo)* are acrid and sweet discharging and dispersing substances. They are able to dredge the exterior and [thereby] arrest the wheezing. Ginkgo Semen *(bái guǒ)*, Farfarae Flos *(kuǎn dōng huā)*, and Mori Cortex *(sāng bái pí)* are substances that clear metal [in order to] protect the Lungs. They are able to calm the interior and arrest the dyspnea. Perillae Fructus *(zǐ sū zǐ)* is able to direct the qi downward. Pinelliae Rhizoma praeparatum *(zhì bàn xià)* is able to disperse the rebellion, and Scutellariae Radix *(huáng qín)* is able to eliminate the heat.

Most commentators since have accepted Wu Kun's interpretation, and modern textbooks generally define the pattern for which this formula is indicated as 'wheezing due to wind-cold fettering the exterior with phlegm-heat collecting in the interior.' The problem with this view, however, is the use of a strongly astringent substance like Ginkgo Semen *(bái guǒ)* as deputy. Astringents would normally be contraindicated in patterns of exterior excess as they inhibit dispersion of the yang qi, thus further aggravating its constraint. Some commentators, such as Wang Xu-Gao in *Six Texts on Medicine by Wang Xu-Gao,* have tried to solve this contradiction by suggesting a reduction in its dosage. Others suggest that the

presence of pathogenic qi in the exterior is not a necessary condition for prescribing this formula. In *Discussion of Medical Formulas*, the late-Qing-dynasty physician Fei Bo-Xiong provided a convincing argument for this position:

> To treat phlegm it is necessary to first regulate the qi. If one does not dredge and discharge, [the phlegm] will become sticky and obstinate and not afford free passage. This is the intention of using Ephedrae Herba *(má huáng)* in this formula.

This accords well with the use of Ephedrae Herba *(má huáng)* in other formulas such as Ephedra, Apricot Kernel, Gypsum, and Licorice Decoction *(má xìng shí gān tāng)*. In this way, the formula can be understood to treat wheezing and panting characterized by the presence of phlegm, a yellow tongue coating, and a rapid pulse, irrespective of the presence of exterior symptoms.

Comparisons

➤ Vs. Other Formulas for Lung Heat with Rebellious Qi

- Ephedra, Apricot Kernel, Gypsum, and Licorice Decoction *(má xìng shí gān tāng)* (see page 184) treats patterns characterized by clear phlegm.

- Maidservant from Yue's Decoction plus Pinellia *(Yuè bì jiā bàn xià tāng)* (see page 185) treats patterns characterized by severe facial edema and rebellion such that the eyes appear as if they were popping out of their sockets.

- Arrest Wheezing Decoction *(dìng chuǎn tāng)* treats patterns characterized by thick, sticky phlegm.

➤ Vs. Drain the White Powder *(xiè bái sǎn)*

Both formulas treat patterns characterized by symptoms such as phlegm, coughing, or wheezing. Drain the White Powder *(xiè bái sǎn)* is used for treating a mixed pattern of heat from both excess and deficiency, but focuses on draining heat. One of its key symptoms is skin that feels burning hot to the touch, indicating the presence of heat in the Lungs. Arrest Wheezing Decoction *(dìng chuǎn tāng)*, on the other hand, treats phlegm-heat in the Lungs and focuses on regulating the qi and eliminating phlegm. The key symptoms therefore are wheezing accompanied by thick, sticky phlegm.

➤ Vs. Minor Bluegreen Dragon Decoction *(xiǎo qīng lóng tāng)*

Both formulas treat patterns characterized by wheezing complicated by the presence of cold in the exterior. Minor Bluegreen Dragon Decoction *(xiǎo qīng lóng tāng)*, however, focuses on patterns with cold and thin fluids in the interior, manifesting with a white tongue coating or a wet tongue and a floating, tight pulse. Arrest Wheezing Decoction (*dìng chuǎn tāng*), on the other hand, treats patterns with phlegm-heat in the interior, manifesting with a yellow tongue coating and a rapid pulse.

Biomedical Indications

With the appropriate presentation, this formula may be used to treat a variety of biomedically-defined disorders including chronic bronchitis, bronchial asthma, and bronchiolitis.

Alternate names

Arrest Wheezing Decoction Worth a Thousand Gold Pieces (*qiān jīn dìng chuǎn tāng*) in *Achieving Longevity by Guarding the Source*; Gingko Decoction for Arresting Wheezing (*bái guǒ dìng chuǎn tāng*) in *Li's Mirror of Medicine*; Decoction Worth a Thousand Pieces of Gold (*qiān jīn tāng*) in *Wondrous Lantern for Peering into the Origin and Development of Miscellaneous Diseases*

Modifications

- For thick, yellow sputum that is difficult to expectorate, add Arisaema cum Bile (*dǎn nán xīng*), Trichosanthis Pericarpium (*guā lóu pí*), and Peucedani Radix (*qián hú*).

- For a severe, stifling sensation in the chest, add Aurantii Fructus immaturus (*zhǐ shí*) and Magnoliae officinalis Cortex (*hòu pò*).

- For more heat in the Lungs, add Gypsum fibrosum (*shí gāo*) and Houttuyniae Herba (*yú xīng cǎo*).

- For sputum that is deep-seated and difficult to expectorate together with a reduced appetite, add Raphani Semen (*lái fú zǐ*) and Sinapis Semen (*bái jiè zǐ*).

Associated Formula

神秘湯 (神秘汤)

Mysterious Decoction

shén mì tāng

SOURCE *Arcane Essentials from the Imperial Library* (752)

Ephedrae Herba (*má huáng*) 6g
Armeniacae Semen (*xìng rén*) 6g
Magnoliae officinalis Cortex (*hòu pò*) 6g
Citri reticulatae Pericarpium (*chén pí*) 3g
Glycyrrhizae Radix praeparata (*zhì gān cǎo*) 3g
Bupleuri Radix (*chái hú*) 3g
Perillae Folium (*zǐ sū yè*) 3g

Disperses wind-cold, directs qi downward, and releases constraint. For wheezing and an unproductive cough with an uncomfortable sensation in the chest and hypochondria, difficult breathing (especially when lying down), and a rough sound in the throat. In Japan, this formula is used for wheezing in people who have a constitutional presentation like that for which Minor Bupleurum Decoction (*xiǎo chái hú tāng*) is indicated.

旋覆代赭湯 (旋覆代赭汤)

Inula and Hematite Decoction

xuán fù dài zhě tāng

Source   *Discussion of Cold Damage* (c. 220)

Inulae Flos (*xuán fù huā*) 9g
Haematitum (*dài zhě shí*) 3g (9-15g)
Pinelliae Rhizoma praeparatum (*zhì bàn xià*) 9g
Zingiberis Rhizoma recens (*shēng jiāng*) 15g (6-9g)
Ginseng Radix (*rén shēn*) 6g
Glycyrrhizae Radix praeparata (*zhì gān cǎo*) 9g (3-6g)
Jujubae Fructus (*dà zǎo*) . . . . .12 pieces (4 pieces)

Method of Preparation   Decoct the ingredients in approximately 10 cups of water until 6 cups remain. Strain, discard the dregs, and boil the liquid again until 3 cups remain. Divide into three doses and take one dose warm three times per day. The average dosages recommended in contemporary Chinese textbooks are noted in parentheses. Codonopsis Radix (*dǎng shēn*) is also commonly substituted for Ginseng Radix (*rén shēn*) at 2-3 times its dosage.

Actions   Directs rebellious qi downward, transforms phlegm, augments the qi, and harmonizes the Stomach

Indications

Unremitting belching, hiccup, regurgitation, nausea or vomiting, hard epigastric focal distention, a white, slippery tongue coating, and a wiry, deficient pulse.

This is phlegm turbidity obstructing the interior together with weak, deficient Stomach qi. The Stomach is charged with the reception and digestion of food, and the tendency of its qi is to move downward. The Spleen and Stomach are also responsible for the transformation and transportation of dampness, raising the pure, and eliminating the turbid downward. When this process is impaired by the deficiency of qi in the middle burner, dampness can accumulate and ultimately give rise to phlegm, which obstructs the middle burner and manifests as hard, focal distention in the epigastrium. When fluids accumulate and transform into phlegm and thin mucus, it constrains the Stomach qi and causes it to rebel upward with such symptoms as unremitting belching, hiccup, and vomiting. The white, slippery tongue coating and the wiry, deficient pulse reflect the deficiency of qi in the middle burner and the presence of phlegm turbidity.

Analysis of Formula

This formula focuses on the branch of a mixed pattern of excess and deficiency, that is, rebellious Stomach qi, while also attending to its root, deficiency of middle burner qi with accumulation of phlegm fluids. For this purpose, it employs a strategy of directing the rebellion downward, transforming phlegm, and augmenting the middle burner qi. The chief ingredient is bitter, acrid, salty, and slightly warming Inulae Flos (*xuán fù huā*), a substance that enters the Lungs, Stomach, and Large Intestine. Even though it is a flower, its bitter nature is able to drive rebellious qi downward, while its acrid saltiness allows it to dissolve phlegm. Bitter, sweet, and slightly cooling Haematitum *(dài zhě shí),* which enters the Heart, Liver, and Stomach, serves as the deputy. It has a sinking nature and strongly suppresses rebellious qi. Its original dosage is a third that of the chief ingredient, indicating that its role is subordinated to that of the chief herb. Strengthening the downward-directing rather than the phlegm-transforming action of Inulae Flos *(xuán fù huā)* is a reflection of the fact that the primary focus of this formula is on subduing rebellion in order to control the symptoms of belching, hiccup, and vomiting.

While the chief and deputy herbs treat the branches, the assistant ingredients attend to the root. Pinelliae Rhizoma praeparatum *(zhì bàn xià)* and Zingiberis Rhizoma recens *(shēng jiāng)* warm and harmonize the Stomach and direct the qi downward, thereby dispelling the phlegm and dispersing the focal distention. Ginseng Radix *(rén shēn),* Glycyrrhizae Radix praeparata *(zhì gān cǎo),* and Jujubae Fructus *(dà zǎo)* work together to tonify the deficient qi and strengthen the Spleen and Stomach. By supporting the middle qi, they assist in its recovery and help protect it against further harm from the dispersing properties of the other ingredients in the formula.

Commentary

The source text prescribes this formula for the belching and hard epigastric focal distention that may follow the use of sweating, vomiting, or purging methods. While this identifies the pattern, it does not clearly elaborate the underlying pathodynamic, which was left to later commentators. The first to do so was the Jin-dynasty scholar Cheng Wu-Ji. In *Annotation and Explanation of the Discussion of Cold Damage,* Cheng wrote that it treated "frail stomach qi that is not yet harmonized [after having been exhausted by the use of a dispersing or draining formula leading to] deficient qi and rebellion." It was only during the Ming dynasty that commentators also included phlegm obstruction in their explanation. An example is Fang You-Zhi in *Systematic Differentiation of the Discussion of Cold Damage:*

> [The term] released [in the source text] refers to [the fact] that the major pathogen has already been dispersed. Hard epigastric focal distention and unremitting belching [imply] that the normal qi has not yet [fully] recovered. The Stomach qi is still frail, and lurking thin mucus makes it rebel. … Therefore, the seven [ingredients] have the intended function of nourishing the normal qi while dispersing the remaining pathogen.

Owing to Fang You-Zhi's reputation as a commentator on *Discussion of Cold Damage,* this interpretation gained widespread acceptance and has remained authoritative to the present day. Later generations of physicians have expanded

the use of the formula to include the condition described above, irrespective of its etiology. It is also used in treating regurgitation and vomiting of saliva due to cold in the Stomach. However, as the early modern physician Tang Zong-Hai noted in *Discussion of Blood Patterns,* a correct diagnosis of the underlying pathodynamic is essential to ensure its effectiveness:

> Anyone knows that this formula treats belching and hiccup. They do not know, however, that there are many kinds of hiccup. If the Stomach [qi] is cut off, how could there be no hiccup? For fire hiccup, [one of the] Order the Qi Decoctions *(chéng qì tāng)* is appropriate. For cold hiccup, Regulate the Middle Pill *(lǐ zhōng wán)* plus Caryophylli Flos *(dīng xiāng)* and Kaki Calyx *(shì dì)* is appropriate. For static blood and stagnation hiccup, Major Bupleurum Decoction *(dà chái hú tāng)* plus Persicae Semen *(táo rén)* and Moutan Cortex *(mǔ dān pí)* is appropriate. This formula is for treating hiccup due to phlegm fluids. This is different from all the other types of hiccup. One cannot use this formula just because one sees hiccup.

Because the primary function of Inulae Flos *(xuán fù huā)* and Haematitum *(dài zhě shí)* is to drive the rebellious qi downward, with appropriate modifications, the formula can also be used for coughing and wheezing, plum-pit qi, vomiting during pregnancy, dizziness due to rebellious Stomach qi with phlegm turbidity, and constipation due to turbid yin not being directed downward.

Controversies

Even today, many issues regarding the use of this formula remain contentious. One example is whether Inulae Flos *(xuán fù huā)* should be considered the sole chief herb in the formula or whether this designation should be shared with Haematitum *(dài zhě shí).* An even more important issue is how to approach the low dosage of Haematitum *(dài zhě shí)* prescribed in the source text. One common explanation is that this is due to the deficiency of Stomach qi, the thought being that a high dose of a mineral substance might hurt its recovery. Another common explanation is that its nature as a mineral allows it to exert its downward-directing influence at a lower dose than the flower Inulae Flos *(xuán fù huā).* Some commentators also note the rather large dosage of Zingiberis Rhizoma recens *(shēng jiāng)* and argue that this represents a strategy whereby Zhang Zhong-Jing sought to amplify the downward-directing action of Haematitum *(dài zhě shí)* without increasing the amount of the substance itself.

Whatever the explanation, the low dosage is at variance with most contemporary practice, partly due to the influence of the modern physician Zhang Xi-Chun who used Haematitum *(dài zhě shí)* as a principal herb for all patterns in which rebellious Stomach qi needed to be directed downward. Zhang Xi-Chun did not think that its bitter, cooling properties damaged the Stomach, but believed instead that they nourished both the qi and blood. In present-day China, the ratio of the dosage of Inulae Flos (xuán fù huā) and Haematitum (dài zhě shí), which is 3:1 in the source text, is commonly 2:3 or even 1:3.

Many modern practitioners of the classic formulas current insist that the original dosage of all the ingredients must be adhered to. Liu Du-Zhou, for example, has written that, without a relatively large dose of Zingiberis Rhizoma recens (shēng jiāng), the phlegm turbidity cannot be dispersed. Furthermore, too large a dosage of Haematitum (dài zhě shí) will direct the qi all the way into the lower burner and have no effect on focal distention in the middle burner. Practitioners must use their own discretion in selecting a dosage that is appropriate to their patient's condition.

Comparisons

➤ Vs. Fresh Ginger Decoction to Drain the Epigastrium (shēng jiāng xiè xīn tāng)

Both formulas are used in treating firm epigastric focal distention and rebellious Stomach qi. Fresh Ginger Decoction to Drain the Epigastrium (shēng jiāng xiè xīn tāng) is indicated for a complex of fluid accumulation and heat characterized by dry heaves that have a foul odor, the sound of fluid in the hypochondria, very loud borborygmus, and diarrhea. Inula and Hematite Decoction (xuán fù dài zhě tang), on the other hand, is indicated for phlegm turbidity obstructing the qi mechanism with no signs of heat.

➤ Vs. Clove and Persimmon Calyx Decoction (dīng xiāng shì dì tāng); see PAGE 548

➤ Vs. Major Pinellia Decoction (dà bàn xià tāng); see PAGE 550

Biomedical Indications

With the appropriate presentation, this formula may be used to treat a wide variety of biomedically-defined disorders. These can be divided into the following groups:

- Diseases with belching or hiccup as the primary symptom including functional stomach disorders, chronic gastritis, gastroptosis, gastrectasis, peptic ulcer, chronic hepatitis, postsurgical hiccup, or morning sickness
- Diseases marked by dysphagia including incomplete pyloric obstruction, spasm of the gastroesophageal junction, esophageal cancer, gastric cancer, morning sickness, sequelae of meningitis, or Ménière's disease.

This formula has also been used for hypertension, Ménière's disease, bronchial asthma, bronchiectasis, and globus hystericus.

Alternate names

Inula and Haematite Stone Decoction (xuán fù dài zhě shí tāng) in Prescriptions for Universal Benefit; Haematite and Inula Decoction

(dài zhě xuán fù tāng) in Medical Formulas Collected and Analyzed; Inula Flower and Haematite Stone Decoction (xuán fù huā dài zhě shí tang) in Categorized Collected Formulas

Modifications

- For patients without Stomach qi deficiency, remove Ginseng Radix (rén shēn), Jujubae Fructus (dà zǎo), and Glycyrrhizae Radix praeparata (zhì gān cǎo).
- For copious sputum, a greasy tongue coating, and other signs of predominant dampness, add Citri reticulatae Pericarpium (chén pí), Magnoliae officinalis Cortex (hòu pò), and Poria (fú líng).
- For cold from deficiency in the Stomach, substitute Zingiberis Rhizoma (gān jiāng) for Zingiberis Rhizoma recens (shēng jiāng) or add Evodiae Fructus (wú zhū yú) and Caryophylli Flos (dīng xiāng).
- For food stagnation, add Aurantii Fructus immaturus (zhǐ shí) or Aurantii Fructus (zhǐ ké).
- For heat in the Stomach, add Scutellariae Radix (huáng qín), Coptidis Rhizoma (huáng lián), and Bambusae Caulis in taeniam (zhú rú).
- For heat from deficiency presenting with a red tongue with little coating, add Bambusae Caulis in taeniam (zhú rú), Ophiopogonis Radix (mài mén dōng), Eriobotryae Folium (pí pá yè), and Kaki Calyx (shì dì).
- For persistent vomiting, add Citri reticulatae Pericarpium (chén pí) and Poria (fú líng).
- For coughing and wheezing, add Mori Cortex (sāng bái pí) and Fritillariae cirrhosae Bulbus (chuān bèi mǔ).
- For Ménière's disease, add Zingiberis Rhizoma (gān jiāng), Evodiae Fructus (wú zhū yú), and Aurantii Fructus (zhǐ ké).

橘皮竹茹湯 (橘皮竹茹汤)

Tangerine Peel and Bamboo Shavings Decoction

jú pí zhú rú tāng

Source   Essentials from the Golden Cabinet (c. 220)

Citri reticulatae Pericarpium (chén pí) 9-12g
Bambusae Caulis in taeniam (zhú rú) 9-12g
Ginseng Radix (rén shēn) 3g
Zingiberis Rhizoma recens (shēng jiāng) 18g (6-9g)
Glycyrrhizae Radix (gān cǎo) 15g (3-6g)
Jujubae Fructus (dà zǎo) . . . . .30 pieces (5 pieces)

Method of Preparation   Decoction. At present, the dosage of some of the ingredients is commonly reduced, as indicated in the parentheses.

Actions   Directs rebellious qi downward, stops hiccup, augments the qi, and clears heat

Indications

Hiccup, nausea, dry heaves, or retching. While in some texts a tender, red tongue and a deficient, rapid pulse are given as diagnostic indicators, they do not have to be present for this formula to be used. Also for vomiting resulting from debility following a prolonged illness.

Hiccup may be a manifestation of either cold or heat, excess or deficiency, but is always due to up-flushing of qi. The condition for which this formula is indicated arises when there is qi stagnation and constraint due to long-term Stomach deficiency or when vomiting, diarrhea, or other causes have injured the Stomach qi. Under these circumstances, the Stomach is unable to perform its functions of absorption and digestion. The mechanisms controlling the direction of qi flow are disrupted. Qi accumulates in the area of the diaphragm, while the fluids are no longer harmoniously dispersed. This causes an imbalance between yin and yang, with the qi being expelled upward or manifesting in spasms of the diaphragm. Hiccup, dry heaves, or retching ensues. The tender, red tongue and the deficient, rapid pulse reflect a combination of heat from constraint and deficiency in the Stomach.

Analysis of Formula

Stomach deficiency requires tonification, heat requires clearing, and rebellious qi requires redirection. Hiccup or dry heaves, the main symptoms here, are problems that require prompt attention. For this reason, directing the rebellious qi downward is the primary focus of the formula. The chief herbs are therefore acrid, bitter, and warming Citri reticulatae Pericarpium *(chén pí),* which harmonizes the Stomach and stops hiccup, and sweet, cooling Bambusae Caulis in taeniam *(zhú rú),* which clears heat, calms the Stomach, and stops the hiccup. Due to the acute nature of the symptoms, a rather large dosage of both herbs is used.

One of the deputy herbs is Ginseng Radix *(rén shēn).* Its qi-tonifying action complements the action of Citri reticulatae Pericarpium *(chén pí),* providing tonification in the midst of regulation. The other deputy is Zingiberis Rhizoma recens *(shēng jiāng),* a warm herb that is very effective in harmonizing the functions of the Stomach and stopping vomiting. When combined with the cool Bambusae Caulis in taeniam *(zhú rú),* it reinforces the downward flow of Stomach qi and prevents the cool herbs from injuring the Spleen. The assistants are Glycyrrhizae Radix *(gān cǎo)* and Jujubae Fructus *(dà zǎo).* They assist Ginseng Radix *(rén shēn)* in augmenting the qi. Glycyrrhizae Radix *(gān cǎo)* also serves as the envoy that harmonizes the various actions of the other herbs in the formula.

This formula integrates herbs with very different properties into a harmonious whole. The qi-regulating Citri reticulatae Pericarpium *(chén pí)* is combined with the qi-tonifying Ginseng Radix *(rén shēn)* to tonify in the midst of regulating, so that movement is encouraged without injuring the qi. The cool Bambusae Caulis in taeniam *(zhú rú)* is combined with the warm Zingiberis Rhizoma recens *(shēng jiāng)* so that warming occurs in the midst of cooling, thereby strengthening the formula's regulatory effect on the Stomach and enhancing its ability to direct the rebellious qi downward. These combinations serve to make this a very effective formula.

Cautions and Contraindications

This formula is contraindicated in cases of heat from excess or cold from deficiency.

Commentary

Usage

The indication for this formula in the source text simply reads "eructation and rebellion (噦逆 *yuě nì*)." It was left to later commentators to specify the actual pathodynamic and pattern with the goal of enabling a more precise differential diagnosis and, therefore, its effective deployment in clinical practice. As always, this has allowed for a number of different interpretations centered around two core problems.

The first concerns the actual condition for which the formula is indicated. Some commentators, such as Cheng Wu-Ji and Wang Ken-Tang, took the term 噦逆 *yuě nì*, which by the Song does not seem to have been in much use anymore, to mean 呃逆 *è nì*, or hiccup. Others, such as Li Dong-Yuan, defined it as meaning 干嘔 *gān ǒu*, or retching. Modern textbooks have embraced both interpretations, and physicians use this formula for both conditions.

Pathodynamic

A second and more important topic of debate concerns the nature of the underlying pathodynamic, which modern textbooks define to be heat in the Stomach against a background of deficient Stomach qi. This interpretation dates back at least to the Ming. In *Collected Treatises of [Zhang] Jing-Yue,* for instance, Zhang Jie-Bin noted that, "following vomiting and diarrhea, the Stomach is deficient and the diaphragm hot, causing hiccup." Wu Kun, another Ming-dynasty physician, was even more specific in *Investigations of Medical Formulas:*

> Following a severe illness, the qi of the middle burner is generally deficient. If some remaining pathogen avails itself of this deficiency to enter into the interior, the pathogenic and normal qi will contend with each other, which invariably leads to an upward-surging of qi. This leads [to the manifestation] of hiccup. [If] the pulse becomes deficient and large, deficient implies that the normal qi is frail, while large [indicates] the presence of pathogenic heat.

These interpretations appear to be based partly on clinical experience, and partly on an understanding of the use of herbs in this formula. Not all commentators concur, however. They note that, besides Bambusae Caulis in taeniam *(zhú rú)*, there are no cooling herbs in the formula. Given the high dosage of Citri reticulatae Pericarpium *(chén pí)* and Zingiberis Rhizoma recens *(shēng jiāng)*, two warming and drying ingredients, the overall effect is balanced. Furthermore, the focus of the heat-clearing action of Bambusae Caulis in taeniam *(zhú rú)* is to cancel out the acrid, warming effects of these two ingredients in order to prevent damaging the feeble Stomach qi (an organ that is considered to be averse to dryness), and not to treat pathogenic heat. This is the argument made by the Qing-dynasty physician Wei Nian-Ting in *Original Meaning of Formulas Discussed in Essentials from the Golden Cabinet,* as well as the contemporary expert Chen Chao-Zu in his *Treatment Strategies and Formulas in Chinese Medicine.* Chen, moreover, points out that the original dosages of Glycyrrhizae Radix *(gān cǎo)* and Jujubae Fructus *(dà zǎo)* are also quite large. In his opinion, this reflects the treatment principle, "When the Liver suffers from hypertonicity, quickly take sweet medicinals to relax it." He then elaborates:

> There are two reasons for relating the analysis [of this formula] to the Liver system. (1) Hiccup is not rebellion of Stomach qi, but a spasm of the diaphragm. The Liver governs the muscle-sinews of the entire body. Therefore, the structure [of the diaphragm] is discussed in relation to the Liver and Gallbladder system. Hence, [defining this disorder] in relation to the Liver system represents a more precise definition of the location of the disorder. (2) Clinical observation [tells us] that hiccup may be due to cold, heat, deficiency, excess, qi stagnation, blood stasis, the congealing of phlegm, and obstruction by dampness. Besides emphasizing the elimination of causes responsible for the hiccup [in the first place], the formulas used [to treat these patterns] all contain Paeoniae Radix *(sháo yào)*, Glycyrrhizae Radix *(gān cǎo)*, and Jujubae Fructus *(dà zǎo)* to soften the Liver and relax hypertonicity. For instance, Frigid Extremities Powder *(sì nì sǎn)*, Major Bupleurum Decoction *(dà chái hú tāng)*, and True Warrior Decoction *(zhēn wǔ tāng)* can all treat hiccup, and all contain Paeoniae Radix *(sháo yào)*. Hence, from the perspective of treatment, [this disorder] also should be related to the Liver.

It is perhaps possible to reconcile these different views by following the analysis of Cao Ying-Fu, one of the most prominent experts in the use of Zhang Zhong-Jing's formulas during the early part of the 20th century. In *Elaborating on the Subtleties of the Golden Cabinet,* Cao writes:

> This formula is named [after the ingredients] Citri reticulatae Pericarpium *(chén pí)* and Bambusae Caulis in taeniam *(zhú rú)*. Citri reticulatae Pericarpium *(chén pí)* is used to dredge the qi that has stopped above the diaphragm, impeding [the qi dynamic]. Bambusae Caulis in taeniam *(zhú rú)* is used to dredge [the resulting] constraint of Gallbladder fire. In this way, they are able to stop hiccup. Hiccup, after all, arises from qi above the diaphragm that is not being dispersed and Gallbladder fire—having been constrained by this undispersed qi—flushing upward. The reason, finally, why this qi has not been dispersed to the outside is that the qi of the middle burner is deficient. Therefore, one knows that in this formula Citri reticulatae

Pericarpium *(chén pí)* and Bambusae Caulis in taeniam *(zhú rú)* treat the branches, while Jujubae Fructus *(dà zǎo)*, Zingiberis Rhizoma recens *(shēng jiāng)*, Glycyrrhizae Radix *(gān cǎo)*, and Ginseng Radix *(rén shēn)* treat the root. Alternatively, even if Citri reticulatae Pericarpium *(chén pí)* and Bambusae Caulis in taeniam *(zhú rú)* on their own are sufficient to treat hiccup, how could one guarantee that it might not return?

Cao Ying-Fu's notion of qi stagnation above the diaphragm leading to constraint of yang in the Gallbladder, which requires dispersion and cooling to control the symptoms, and sweet nourishment to treat the root, encompasses all the other viewpoints outlined above. Without modification, this formula should not be used to treat hiccup or retching associated with excess heat and constrained fluids, where Pinellia Decoction to Drain the Epigastrium *(bàn xià xiè xīn tāng)* provides a better alternative, or excess cold with constrained fluids, where Evodia Decoction *(wú zhū yú tāng)* would be the better choice.

Comparison

➤ Vs. Clove and Persimmon Calyx Decoction *(dīng xiāng shì dì tāng)*; *see* PAGE 548

Biomedical Indications

With the appropriate presentation, this formula may be used to treat a variety of biomedically-defined disorders including morning sickness, incomplete pyloric obstruction, gastritis, or recalcitrant postsurgical hiccup.

Alternate names

Inula and Haematite Stone Decoction *(xuán fù dài zhě shí tāng)* in *Prescriptions for Universal Benefit*; Haematite and Inula Decoction *(dài zhě xuán fù tāng)* in *Medical Formulas Collected and Analyzed*; Inula Flower and Haematite Stone Decoction *(xuán fù huā dài zhě shí tang)* in *Categorized Collected Formulas*

Modifications

* For yin deficiency with thirst, a red tongue with a scanty, dry coating, and a thin, rapid pulse, add Ophiopogonis Radix *(mài mén dōng)*, Dendrobii Herba *(shí hú)*, and Phragmitis Rhizoma *(lú gēn)*.
* For patterns of excess heat with a yellow tongue coating, add Coptidis Rhizoma *(huáng lián)*.
* For patients without qi deficiency, remove Ginseng Radix *(rén shēn)*.
* For concurrent phlegm, add Pinelliae Rhizoma praeparatum *(zhì bàn xià)* and Poria *(fú líng)*.

Associated Formulas

橘皮湯（橘皮汤）

Tangerine Peel Decoction

jú pí tāng

SOURCE   *Essentials from the Golden Cabinet* (c. 220)

Citri reticulatae Pericarpium *(chén pí)* 12g
Zingiberis Rhizoma recens *(shēng jiāng)* 18g

Warms the Stomach, unblocks the yang, and stops vomiting. For conditions of rebellious qi due to cold in the Stomach with vomiting and cold hands and feet. At present, the dosage of Zingiberis Rhizoma recens *(shēng jiāng)* is generally reduced by one-half.

橘皮竹茹湯（橘皮竹茹汤）

Tangerine Peel and Bamboo Shavings Decoction from *Formulas to Aid the Living*

jú pí zhú rú tāng

SOURCE   *Formulas to Aid the Living* (1253)

Poria rubra *(chì fú líng)* 30g
Citri reticulatae Pericarpium *(chén pí)* 30g
Eriobotryae Folium *(pí pá yè)* 30g
Ophiopogonis Radix *(mài mén dōng)* 30g
Bambusae Caulis in taeniam *(zhú rú)* 30g
Pinelliae Rhizoma praeparatum *(zhì bàn xià)* 30g
Ginseng Radix *(rén shēn)* 15g
Glycyrrhizae Radix praeparata *(zhì gān cǎo)* 15g

Grind the ingredients into a coarse powder, add 5 pieces of Zingiberis Rhizoma recens *(shēng jiāng)*, and decoct. Directs rebellious qi downward, stops vomiting, harmonizes the Stomach, and clears heat. For heat in the Stomach with severe thirst, vomiting, and loss of appetite. In contrast to the principal formula, which is for heat in the Stomach with Stomach qi deficiency, this formula is indicated for deficiency of both the qi and yin.

新制橘皮竹茹湯（新制橘皮竹茹汤）

Newly-Formulated Tangerine Peel and Bamboo Shavings Decoction

xīn zhì jú pí zhú rú tāng

SOURCE   Systematic Differentiation of Warm Pathogen Diseases (1798)

Citri reticulatae Pericarpium *(chén pí)* 9g
Bambusae Caulis in taeniam *(zhú rú)* 9g
Kaki Calyx *(shì dì)* . . . . 7 pieces (9g)

Decoct the ingredients and add 3 teaspoons of ginger juice to the strained decoction. Directs rebellious qi downward, clears heat, and stops hiccup. For hiccup due to heat in the Stomach without Stomach qi deficiency.

丁香柿蒂湯（丁香柿蒂汤）

Clove and Persimmon Calyx Decoction

dīng xiāng shì dì tāng

Source   *Symptom, Cause, Pulse, and Treatment* (1706)

Caryophylli Flos *(dīng xiāng)* 3-6g
Kaki Calyx *(shì dì)* 6-9g

Ginseng Radix *(rén shēn)* 3-6g
Zingiberis Rhizoma recens *(shēng jiāng)* 6-9g

Method of Preparation   Decoction. At present, Codonopsis Radix *(dǎng shēn)* is usually substituted for Ginseng Radix *(rén shēn)* at 2-3 times its dosage. The dosages are not specified in the source text.

Actions   Augments the qi, warms the middle burner, directs rebellious qi downward, and stops hiccup

Indications

Hiccup, belching, or vomiting with a stifling sensation in the epigastrium, focal distention of the chest, a pale tongue with a white coating, and a submerged, slow pulse

This is hiccup, belching, or vomiting due to cold from deficiency in the Stomach. Chronic disease or improper treatment may injure the yang qi of the Spleen and Stomach, which leads to cold from deficiency in the middle burner. This disrupts the ascending and descending functions of the middle burner. As a result, the Stomach qi, which normally descends, instead rebels upward and manifests as hiccup, belching, or vomiting. The stifling sensation and focal distention are due to cold that obstructs the middle burner and upsets the qi mechanism. The white tongue coating and the submerged, slow pulse are indicative of cold from deficiency.

Analysis of Formula

Warming the middle burner and directing the rebellious qi downward are the primary functions of this formula. The warm, aromatic Caryophylli Flos *(dīng xiāng)* warms the Stomach, dispels cold, and directs the flow of qi downward, stopping the hiccup and belching. It thereby addresses both of the major goals of the formula and is accordingly one of the chief herbs. The other is bitter, astringent Kaki Calyx *(shì dì)*, which is a major herb for stopping hiccup and belching. The combination of these two herbs is very effective in directing the rebellious qi due to Stomach cold downward.

The deputy herb is Zingiberis Rhizoma recens *(shēng jiāng)*. It is so effective in warming the Stomach and directing rebellious qi downward that it is sometimes referred to as a 'sage-like' medicine for vomiting. Here it supports and enhances the actions of the chief herbs. The assistant is Ginseng Radix *(rén shēn)*, which strongly augments the qi and is effective in tonifying the deficient aspects of this disorder. It also prevents the dispersing properties of the other herbs from further injuring the normal qi.

Commentary

This formula, first published in 1641, is actually a combination of two much older formulas: Kaki Cash Powder (蒂錢 散 *dì qián sǎn*)—consisting of Caryophylli Flos *(dīng xiāng)*, Kaki Calyx *(shì dì)*, and Ginseng Radix *(rén shēn)*—from

Concise Formulas to Aid the Multitudes; and Smooth the Qi Decoction (順氣湯 *shùn qì tāng*)—consisting of Caryophylli Flos (*dīng xiāng*), Kaki Calyx (*shì dì*), and Zingiberis Rhizoma recens (*shēng jiāng*)—from *Formulas to Protect Life and the Most Treasured Family Possession*. The latter text claims that, "For treating hiccup, [this formula] is divinely effective."

This implies that its function is rooted in the ability of the two chief herbs to order the qi dynamic. Whereas most commentators focus on the Stomach as the location of this disorder, in *Collectania of Investigations from the Realm of Medicine*, the Qing-dynasty writer Wang Fu takes a broader view:

> Caryophylli Flos (*dīng xiāng*) warms the Kidneys and the gate of vitality below and treats up-flushing of the Penetrating vessel's cold qi. In the middle, it warms the Spleen and Stomach, eliminating accumulated foulness from deep[-seated] cold and harbored [food] clogging [the qi dynamic]. Above, it drains Lung pathogens, eliminating upper burner wind, cold, dampness, and heat. Kaki Calyx (*shì dì*) is bitter, astringent, and cooling. Its astringency allows it to tonify Lung qi [by way of] restraining [its excessive dispersion] so that it is able to accept the Stomach qi's upward transport without being spent on dispersion. Its bitterness allows it to direct the Lung qi downward and drain it in order to calm the upper burner's heat from deficiency without this leading to rebellious up-flushing. Caryophylli Flos (*dīng xiāng*) naturally [works] from below to above, focusing on dispelling cold. Kaki Calyx (*shì dì*) naturally [works] from above to below, in order to drain heat. [Together,] they balance hot and cold so that above and below do not mutually resist each other.

Wang Fu's interpretation of the synergism between the formula's two chief herbs refers to an understanding in Chinese medicine that hiccup is not, like vomiting, a simple rebellion of Stomach qi, but is rather the manifestation of a more complex disease process. This is elaborated upon by Chen Yuan-Xi in *Gathering of Songs for Golden Cabinet Formulas*: "All hiccup patterns involve a disorder of cold and heat, where the contention between the two qi causes [the symptom to] occur." Having explained how this applies to Tangerine Peel and Bamboo Shavings Decoction (*jú pí zhú rú tāng*), discussed above, where Stomach deficiency (i.e., cold) causes constraint of Gallbladder qi (i.e., heat), Chen then identifies that formula as a model for Clove and Persimmon Calyx Decoction (*dīng xiāng shì dì tāng*). Following Wang Fu's analysis, cold in the present pattern can be understood as referring to deficiency of the fire at the gate of vitality, which impedes the Stomach's digestive functions and allows cold and food to accumulate. Heat, on the other hand, refers to yang above caused by up-flushing of the Penetrating vessel.

Later physicians have extended the use of this formula in three different ways. They added herbs like Citri reticulatae Pericarpium (*chén pí*) and Pinelliae Rhizoma praeparatum (*zhì bàn xià*) to further enhance the formula's ability to direct rebellion downward and transform phlegm; they added qi-regulating herbs like Citri reticulatae Pericarpium (*chén pí*) and Citri reticulatae viride Pericarpium (*qīng pí*) to augment the formula's ability to overcome qi stagnation in the middle burner; and they added warming herbs like Zingiberis Rhizoma (*gān jiāng*), Alpiniae officinarum Rhizoma (*gāo liáng jiāng*), and Foeniculi Fructus (*xiǎo huí xiāng*) to further focus the formula's ability to disperse cold on both the middle and lower burners.

Comparisons

➤ Vs. Evodia Decoction (*wú zhū yú tāng*)

Clove and Persimmon Calyx Decoction (*dīng xiāng shī dì tang*) treats hiccup due to cold from deficiency in the Stomach and utilizes the twin strategies of warming the Stomach and tonifying. By contrast, Evodia Decoction (*wú zhū yú tāng*) is used for cold from deficiency in the Liver and Stomach with vomiting upon ingestion of food, indeterminate gnawing hunger, acid reflux, dry heaves or spitting of clear fluids, and sometimes headache at the vertex. The strategy here is to warm the Liver and Stomach while directing the rebellious qi downward.

➤ Vs. Inula and Haematite Decoction (*xuán fù dài zhě tāng*) and Tangerine Peel and Bamboo Shavings Decoction (*jú pí zhú rú tāng*)

All three formulas treat hiccup, belching, or retching due to weak Stomach qi failing to transform the fluids and move the qi. They all contain Ginseng Radix (*rén shēn*) to tonify the Stomach qi and augment the fluids and Zingiberis Rhizoma recens (*shēng jiāng*) to warm and harmonize the yang and stop nausea.

Inula and Haematite Decoction (*xuán fù dài zhě tāng*) focuses on directing the Stomach qi downward, and on transforming the phlegm fluids. A key marker in diagnosis is hard focal distention in the epigastrium. Tangerine Peel and Bamboo Shavings Decoction (*jú pí zhú rú tāng*) focuses on resolving constraint and relaxing tightness in the diaphragm. A key diagnostic marker for the use of this formula is that both heat and cold symptoms can be present, but neither is very pronounced. Clove and Persimmon Calyx Decoction (*dīng xiāng shì dì tāng*) focuses on patterns characterized by cold in the Stomach that ultimately stems from deficient fire at the gate of vitality and involves the Penetrating vessel.

Biomedical Indications

With the appropriate presentation, this formula may be used to treat a variety of biomedically-defined disorders including postoperative spasms of the diaphragm, morning sickness, and neurological hiccup.

Modifications

- To strengthen the effect of the formula, add Citri reticulatae Pericarpium *(chén pí)* and Bambusae Caulis in taeniam *(zhú rú)*.

- For more severe cold together with phlegm due to qi constraint, add Alpiniae officinarum Rhizoma *(gāo liáng jiāng)*, Aquilariae Lignum resinatum *(chén xiāng)*, and Pinelliae Rhizoma praeparatum *(zhì bàn xià)*.

Variation

柿蒂湯 (柿蒂汤)

Persimmon Calyx Decoction

shì dì tāng

SOURCE *Formulas to Aid the Living* (1253)

Remove Ginseng Radix *(rén shēn)* for patients with fullness in the chest and persistent belching.

大半夏湯 (大半夏汤)

Major Pinellia Decoction

dà bàn xià tāng

Source *Essentials from the Golden Cabinet* (c. 220)

Pinelliae Rhizoma praeparatum *(zhì bàn xià)* 15-30g
Ginseng Radix *(rén shēn)* 9g
Honey 9-15g

Method of Preparation The source text advises to first take 12 cups of water, add the honey, and stir 240 times, then decoct until 2.5 cups of liquid remain. While this is still done at present, more commonly it is decocted in the normal manner and divided into two doses.

Actions Harmonizes the Stomach, augments the qi, and nourishes what has become dry

Indications

Vomiting long after eating, after which the patient feels better, a sense of firm fullness in the epigastrium, fatigue, weakness, lusterless complexion, emaciation, and either dried stool that can be like sheep droppings or scanty, loose stools. The tongue is usually pale with either little coating or a thin, white coating, and the pulse is thin and weak or deficient and lax.

This is Stomach reflux (胃反 *wèi fǎn)*, a condition noted in *Essentials from the Golden Cabinet* as being marked by vomiting in the evening the food eaten in the morning, or vomiting in the morning the food eaten in the evening. The underlying problem is viewed as cold from deficiency of the middle burner, usually brought on by irregular eating habits, a proclivity for cold foods, as well as physical or mental overwork. When there is deficiency of Spleen and Stomach qi along with a listless middle burner yang, the body does not have the ability to digest food and drink, which ends

up sitting in the Stomach instead of being transformed and moved downward. This can lead to a sense of a firm fullness in the epigastrium if the problem progresses to the point where dampness builds up in the middle burner and becomes phlegm or thin mucus.

Over a period of time this food will disrupt the normal downward-directing functions of the Stomach qi, which will rebel upward and lead to vomiting. Because the vomiting ejects stagnant food, the patient feels better afterwards. Repeated instances of this over a long period of time causes both a lack of nutrition as well as exhaustion of the fluids, leading to a state where both the qi and yin are deficient. This will manifest as emaciation and severe constipation where any stool passed resembles sheep droppings. The qi and yin deficiency will also manifest as a pale red tongue with little coating and a thin, weak pulse. If the problem affects the Spleen and Stomach more intensely, there will be fatigue, weakness, a lusterless complexion, and loose, scanty stools. In this case, the tongue will be pale with a white (perhaps slippery) coating and the pulse will be deficient and lax.

Analysis of Formula

Treating a condition that arises in the course of chronic or long-term illness, this formula employs a strategy of addressing both the root and branch by harmonizing the Stomach and directing rebellious qi downward while also augmenting the qi and moistening the dryness. The chief herb is Pinelliae Rhizoma praeparatum *(zhì bàn xià)*, used in a large dosage to harmonize the Stomach, stop vomiting, dry dampness, transform phlegm, and open up areas of constraint and disperse clumps. This deals with both the main symptom of this condition, the vomiting, as well as one important aspect of its pathogenesis, phlegm and thin mucus in the middle burner. The deputy is Ginseng Radix *(rén shēn)*, which augments the qi and strengthens the Spleen and Stomach. This herb treats the underlying root issue while Pinelliae Rhizoma praeparatum *(zhì bàn xià)* focuses on the branch. In addition, this combination allows Pinelliae Rhizoma praeparatum *(zhì bàn xià)* to acridly disperse without consuming the qi. The assistant is honey, which tonifies the middle, generates fluids, and benefits the Stomach. The sweet, soothing actions of honey also ameliorate the acrid, drying aspects of Pinelliae Rhizoma praeparatum *(zhì bàn xià)*, which otherwise might further damage the fluids.

This combination of medicinals is appropriate for either of the manifestations above. If there is Spleen and Stomach deficiency and weakness with exhausted fluids and dry Intestines, as well as rebellious Stomach qi, they harmonize the Stomach, redirect rebellious qi downward, augment the qi and strengthen the Spleen, and moisten and enrich the fluids. If there is Spleen and Stomach deficiency and weakness with obstruction of the middle burner by phlegm and thin mucus, such that the qi dynamic is constrained and clumped, they dry the dampness, transform the phlegm, augment the qi and and tonify, while opening up areas of constraint and dispersing clumps.

Commentary

The description of Stomach reflux can be found in the same chapter of *Essentials from the Golden Cabinet* from which this formula is drawn. The discussion goes into some detail about the pathodynamic through an analysis of the dorsal pedis pulse, which is floating and choppy:

> Because it is floating, there is deficiency and because it is choppy, there is damage to the Spleen. Because the Spleen is damaged it does not grind down the food, thus food eaten in the evening is vomited up in the morning and food eaten in the morning is vomited up in the evening. The harbored food is not transformed and this is called Stomach reflux.

The combination of a cold Stomach, which is unable to properly break down foodstuffs, and a damaged, dry Spleen, which is unable to transport the essence of food and drink, leads to the main manifestation of this condition: food that is undigested and then later vomited back up.

This formula has been used by many generations of physicians to treat phlegm and thin mucus disorders, especially when they involve vomiting, however long after eating. One example is found in the 12th-century work, *Discussion of Illnesses, Patterns, and Formulas Related to the Unification of the Three Etiologies*, which prescribes this formula for:

> Lack of movement of the Heart qi, which becomes constrained and produces oral and thin mucus that aggregates and clumps and does not disperse. [This manifests as] focal distention and firmness in the epigastrium, gurgling sounds in the Intestines, and vomiting right after eating.

There has been some discussion over the years about the problem that this formula addresses. Instead of viewing it as a deficient and weak Spleen and Stomach with injury to the fluids and rebellious qi, some commentators, such as the early Ming writer Zhao Yi-De, have understood it as treating a deficient and weak Spleen and Stomach with rebellious qi due to stoppage of thin mucus. Others, including Xu Da-Chun, consider the problem to be a combination of a stoppage of thin mucus with injured fluids. These approaches, however, do not seem to take all the ingredients of the formula into account. The inclusion of honey is hard to understand if there is simply Spleen and Stomach deficiency. And while Ginseng Radix *(rén shēn)* is mentioned in the works of Zhang Zhong-Jing for the treatment of damaged fluids, it is more commonly used in simple formulas to tonify the middle burner.

To some extent, later generations of physicians made these arguments moot by adjusting the formula to fit how they understood the pathodynamic. For example, the formula was often modified by adding Atractylodis macrocephalae Rhizoma *(bái zhú)* and Zingiberis Rhizoma recens *(shēng jiāng)*. These additions were explained by Zhang Lu in *Extension of the Important Formulas Worth a Thousand Gold Pieces:*

> The addition of Atractylodis macrocephalae Rhizoma *(bái zhú)* and Zingiberis Rhizoma recens *(shēng jiāng)* not only assists Ginseng Radix *(rén shēn)* and Pinelliae Rhizoma praeparatum *(zhì bàn xià)* in dispelling phlegm, but also helps disperse any stagnation from the honey.

When this formula is used to treat problems due to phlegm, besides the addition of these two herbs, the honey is omitted to prevent it from causing fullness in the middle burner, and other herbs that strengthen the transportive and transformative functions of the middle burner, such as Poria *(fú líng)* and Cinnamomi Ramulus *(guì zhī)*, are added.

Comparisons

➤ Vs. Inula and Haematite Decoction *(xuán fù dài zhě tāng)*

Both formulas augment the qi and tonify while harmonizing the Stomach and redirecting rebellious qi downward. In addition, both contain Ginseng Radix *(rén shēn)* and Pinelliae Rhizoma praeparatum *(zhì bàn xià)*. Inula and Haematite Decoction *(xuán fù dài zhě tāng)* has Inulae Flos *(xuán fù huā)* as the chief herb and thus has the extra ability to transform phlegm and direct downward; it is used for rather severe cases of Stomach reflux or those with more significant phlegm obstruction.

➤ Vs. Minor Pinellia Decoction *(xiǎo bàn xià tāng)*

Minor Pinellia Decoction *(xiǎo bàn xià tāng)* consists of Pinelliae Rhizoma praeparatum *(zhì bàn xià)* and Zingiberis Rhizoma recens *(shēng jiāng)* and treats propping thin mucus in the epigastrium with vomiting but no thirst. It thus focuses on dispersing excess fluids, whereas Major Pinellia Decoction *(dà bàn xià tāng)* moistens. In contrast to Major Pinellia Decoction *(dà bàn xià tāng)* patterns where there is a regular interval between eating and vomiting, no such regular relationship is found in Minor Pinellia Decoction *(xiǎo bàn xià tāng)* patterns.

➤ Vs. Rhubarb and Licorice Decoction *(dà huáng gān cǎo tāng)*

Both formulas treat patterns characterized by vomiting and dry stools. However, in Rhubarb and Licorice Decoction *(dà huáng gān cǎo tāng)* patterns, the vomiting occurs immediately upon eating and is caused by excess heat. In Major Pinellia Decoction *(dà bàn xià tāng)* patterns, the vomiting occurs a considerable time after eating and is associated with deficiency of qi and dryness.

Biomedical Indications

With the appropriate presentation, this formula may be used to treat a variety of biomedically-defined disorders. These can be divided into the following groups:

- Disorders marked by recurrent vomiting including pyloric spasms, partial obstruction of the pylorus, peptic ulcers, gastritis, morning sickness, chemotherapy-induced vomiting, and gastric cancer
- Other miscellaneous disorders including habitual constipation, chronic pharyngitis, chronic tonsillitis, chronic bronchitis, and asthma.

Modifications

- For more intense vomiting, add Inulae Flos (*xuán fù huā*) and Haematitum (*dài zhě shí*).
- For more severe cold from deficiency of the Spleen and Stomach marked by cold extremities, add Evodiae Fructus (*wú zhū yú*) and Caryophylli Flos (*dīng xiāng*).
- For chronic diseases with exhausted blood and stools resembling sheep droppings, add Angelicae sinensis Radix (*dāng guī*), Cannabis Semen (*huǒ má rén*), and Pruni Semen (*yù lǐ rén*).
- For damage to the yin from fire due to constraint manifesting as blood in the stools along with a dry mouth and a bitter taste, add Scutellariae Radix (*huáng qín*), Ophiopogonis Radix (*mài mén dōng*), and Bletillae Rhizoma (*bái jí*).
- For belching and vomiting related to emotional upset, add Linderae Radix (*wū yào*) and Citri reticulatae viride Pericarpium (*qīng pí*).

Associated Formulas

小半夏湯 （小半夏汤）

Minor Pinellia Decoction

xiǎo bàn xià tāng

SOURCE *Essentials from the Golden Cabinet* (c. 220)

Pinelliae Rhizoma praeparatum (*zhì bàn xià*) 9g
Zingiberis Rhizoma recens (*shēng jiāng*) 9g

Decoction. Alleviates and removes thin mucus, harmonizes the Stomach, directs rebelliousness downward, and stops vomiting. For phlegm and thin mucus tarrying in the interior causing such symptoms as nausea, vomiting, hiccup, sudden turmoil disorder, focal distention in the epigastrium, and insomnia. This formula combines the acrid, drying, and downward-directing Pinelliae Rhizoma praeparatum (*zhì bàn xià*) as the chief herb with the acrid, warming, and dispersing Zingiberis Rhizoma recens (*shēng jiāng*) as deputy. Pinelliae Rhizoma praeparatum (*zhì bàn xià*) eliminates water and dampness, both by drying and by dispersing; and through its ability to direct the qi downward, it harmonizes the Stomach and stops nausea, hiccup, and a sensation of fullness in the epigastrium. Zingiberis Rhizoma recens (*shēng jiāng*), which Sun Si-Miao referred to as a

'sage-like medicinal' in the treatment of vomiting owing to its ability to disperse the accumulation of thin mucus in the epigastrium that causes the qi to rebel upward, complements and supports the action of the chief herb.

When combined and used as a decoction, the two ingredients comprise an important formula for the treatment of nausea and vomiting in morning sickness, travel sickness, and vomiting in the course of acute illness. It can also be used in patients for whom taking an herbal decoction elicits vomiting to settle the Stomach before treating with decoctions appropriate to the presenting pattern.

Minor Pinellia Deoction (*xiǎo bàn xià tāng*) focuses specifically on the treatment of thin mucus and is thus unsuitable if the above symptoms arise from different causes. In *Formulary and Mnemonics from 'No Mistake' Pharmacy*, the Japanese physician Asada Sōhaku notes that a cold area on the back in the area of the 7th and 8th thoracic vertebrae is often indicative of this pattern. Other important clinical markers include vomiting that is aggravated by the intake of fluids, absence of thirst, and a wet, white, slippery tongue coating. In the clinical experience of the contemporary Chinese physician Huang Huang, many patients for whom this formula is indicated suffer from allergies. In his opinion, one should therefore begin treatment with a relatively low dosage of Pinelliae Rhizoma praeparatum (*zhì bàn xià*), which is slightly toxic, and then increase it as appropriate. When used to treat insomnia, however, a large dosage of Pinelliae Rhizoma praeparatum (*zhì bàn xià*) is necessary. As the Qing-dynasty physician Wu Ju-Tong explained, "30g directs rebelliousness downward, 60g calms the sleep."

Compared to the principal formula, which focuses on vomiting associated with obstruction and deficiency, this formula only treats excess. One important distinguishing feature is that in the pattern for which Minor Pinellia Decoction (*xiǎo bàn xià tāng*) is indicated, vomiting occurs quite quickly after the intake of food or drink. In Major Pinellia Decoction (*dà bàn xià tāng*) patterns, on the other hand, vomiting occurs a considerable time after eating.

小半夏加茯苓湯 （小半夏加茯苓汤）

Minor Pinellia plus Poria Decoction

xiǎo bàn xià jiā fú líng tāng

SOURCE *Essentials from the Golden Cabinet* (c. 220)

Pinelliae Rhizoma praeparatum (*zhì bàn xià*) 15g
Zingiberis Rhizoma recens (*shēng jiāng*) 24g
Poria (*fú líng*) 9g

Decoction. Harmonizes the Stomach, stops vomiting, and guides water to move downward into the lower burner. For water tarrying in the Stomach manifesting as sudden vomiting of thin mucus or clear fluids, absence of thirst, a white, slippery tongue coating, and a wiry pulse. There may also be palpitations and focal distention in the epigastrium.

This is a variation of Minor Pinellia Decoction (*xiǎo bàn xià tāng*), and like that formula is indicated for vomiting due to thin fluids accumulating in the Stomach. However, as the source text notes, this formula is indicated for "people with thin mucus" (飲家 *yǐn jiā*); in other words, the presence of fluids here is habitual or constitutional. For this reason, vomiting is sudden, that is, it can occur almost immediately after the intake of food or drink, and there are other signs of systemic fluid accumulation in the diaphragmatic area such as palpitations (due to water/yin accosting fire/yang) and focal distention. Another crucial sign of differentiation is that "people with thin mucus" frequently feel thirsty, even though drinking of fluids may then cause vomiting. As Xu Bin explained in *Discussion and Annotation of the Essentials from the Golden Cabinet*, the habitual presence of pathological thin mucus damages the physiological fluids. This is why such patients feel thirsty. The remedy is to guide out excess fluids via the Bladder, hence the use of Poria (*fú líng*) in this formula. If, instead, one were to use either bitter, cooling herbs or acrid, tonifying, and warming herbs, these would both aggravate the thirst.

With appropriate modifications, this formula is used to treat conditions such as morning sickness, pericarditis, hypertension, Stomach pain, and excess sweating.

乾薑人參半夏丸 (干姜人参半夏丸)
Ginger, Ginseng, and Pinellia Pill
gān jiāng rén shēn bàn xià wán

SOURCE *Essentials from the Golden Cabinet* (c. 220)

Zingiberis Rhizoma (*gān jiāng*) 3g
Ginseng Radix (*rén shēn*) 3g
Pinelliae Rhizoma praeparatum (*zhì bàn xià*) 6g

Grind the ingredients into a powder and form into pills with ginger juice and water. The normal dosage is 3-6 grams. May also be decocted with the addition of Zingiberis Rhizoma recens (*shēng jiāng*). Warms and tonifies the middle burner, directs rebellious qi downward, and stops vomiting. For vomiting due to pregnancy or cold from deficiency in the Spleen and Stomach. While both this and the principal formula contain Pinelliae Rhizoma praeparatum (*zhì bàn xià*) and Ginseng Radix (*rén shēn*), this formula focuses more on warming the middle and dispelling cold in patients with phlegm and thin mucus; it is especially appropriate for morning sickness. By contrast, the principal formula is able to generate fluids and moistens; it is particularly apt for those with Stomach reflux where the fluids have been damaged.

. . . .

Comparative Tables of Principal Formulas

■ FORMULAS THAT PROMOTE THE MOVEMENT OF QI

Common symptoms: pain and distention

Formula Name	Diagnosis	Indications	Remarks
Escape Restraint Pill (*yuè jū wán*)	Constraint due to stagnant qi	Focal distention, a stifling sensation in the chest and abdomen, fixed pain in the hypochondria, belching, acid reflux, mild coughing with copious sputum, reduced appetite	Focuses on unblocking the ascending and descending functions of the qi dynamic in the middle burner.
Bupleurum Powder to Dredge the Liver (*chái hú shū gān sǎn*)	Constraint and clumping of the Liver qi	Flank pain, a stifling sensation in the chest, sighing, easily angered, belching, abdominal distention and fullness, alternating fever and chills, and a wiry pulse	Also treats various types of abdominal pain, dysmenorrhea, and back pain.
Dredge the Liver Decoction (*shū gān tāng*)	Stagnation of qi and blood	Pain beneath the left ribcage, damage to qi from anger, or rib pain resulting from knocks and bruises; a wiry pulse	For stagnation due to internal damage from the emotions or as the result of trauma.
Unripe Bitter Orange, Chinese Garlic, and Cinnamon Twig Decoction (*zhǐ shí xiè bái guì zhī tāng*)	Painful obstruction of the chest with severe clumping of qi	Fullness and pain in the chest or a stabbing pain that radiates from the chest to the back, wheezing, coughing, shortness of breath, a white, greasy tongue coating, and a submerged, wiry, or tight pulse	Focuses on unblocking the clear yang by eliminating turbid yin.
Pinellia and Magnolia Bark Decoction (*bàn xià hòu pò tāng*)	Constrained qi and phlegm-dampness	A feeling of something caught in the throat, a stifling sensation in the chest and hypochondria, a moist or greasy, white tongue coating, and a wiry, slow or wiry, slippery pulse	This condition is known as plum-pit qi (*méi hé qì*). In severe cases, there will also be coughing or vomiting.
Magnolia Bark Decoction for Warming the Middle (*hòu pò wēn zhōng tāng*)	Damp-cold injuring the Spleen and Stomach	Epigastric and abdominal distention and fullness, loss of appetite, fatigue in the extremities, diarrhea, and a white, slippery tongue coating	If the cold is particularly severe, there may also be abdominal pain and vomiting of clear liquid.
Galangal and Cyperus Pill (*liáng fù wán*)	Stagnation of Liver qi with cold congealing in the Stomach	Epigastric pain, a stifling sensation in the chest, hypochondriac pain, painful menstruation, and a white tongue coating	Pain responds favorably to warmth.

cont.

Formula Name	Diagnosis	Indications	Remarks
Melia Toosendan Powder (*jīn líng zǐ sǎn*)	Liver constraint transforming into heat	Intermittent epigastric and hypochondriac pain, hernial pain, or menstrual pain, irritability, bitter taste, a red tongue with a yellow coating, and a wiry or rapid pulse	Pain is aggravated by the ingestion of hot food or beverages.
Four Milled-Herb Decoction (*sì mò tāng*)	Qi excess in the upper burner due to stagnation of the qi dynamic	Irritability, a stifling sensation in the chest, labored breathing, wheezing, epigastric focal distention and fullness, loss of appetite, a white tongue coating, and a wiry pulse	Focuses on regulating a disordered qi dynamic.
Top-Quality Lindera Powder (*tiān tái wū yào sǎn*)	Cold invading the Liver channel and causing qi stagnation	Lower abdominal pain radiating to the testicles, swollen or distended testicles, a pale tongue with a white coating, and a submerged and slow or wiry pulse	May be localized sensations of cold and hardness. Also for menstrual pain and mobile abdominal masses.
Tangerine Seed Pill (*jú hé wán*)	Damp-cold invading the Liver channel	Unilateral testicular swelling with colicky pain reaching to the umbilicus, or a rock-like hardness and swelling of the scrotum, or oozing of a yellow fluid from the scrotum	In severe cases, abscess and ulceration may also occur.
Warm the Liver Decoction (*nuǎn gān jiān*)	Stagnation of Liver qi with deficiency of Liver yang and blood	Lower abdominal pain that is sharp, localized, and is aggravated by the local application of cold, a pale tongue (especially on the sides and root), and a submerged, tight pulse	This is a cold-type bulging disorder. Also used for swelling, distention, and pain of the scrotum.
Open Up the Diaphragm Powder (*qǐ gé sǎn*)	Stagnation of the qi dynamic with both phlegm and dryness	Sensation of choking or constriction while swallowing, focal distention of the chest, difficult bowel movements, dry mouth and throat, a red tongue with a white coating, and a thin, wiry pulse	Distention may be relieved by belching, dry retching, or spitting up of phlegm.
Augmented Lindera Decoction (*jiā wèi wū yào tāng*)	Dysmenorrhea due to qi stagnation, which causes blood stasis	Dysmenorrhea with scanty, dark menstrual blood and clots, lower abdominal distention accompanied by pain, premenstrual breast distention, a normal tongue with a white coating, and a wiry, tight pulse	Pain occurs before the onset of menstruation or during the early part of menstruation.

■ FORMULAS THAT DIRECT REBELLIOUS QI DOWNWARD

Common symptoms (first two formulas): coughing and wheezing

Formula Name	Diagnosis	Indications	Remarks
Perilla Fruit Decoction for Directing Qi Downward (*sū zǐ jiàng qì tāng*)	Congested fluids with Kidney deficiency	Coughing and wheezing with watery, copious sputum, a stifling sensation in the chest and diaphragm, labored inhalation, and a slippery or greasy, white tongue coating	One type of abundance above and deficiency below.
Arrest Wheezing Decoction (*dìng chuǎn tāng*)	Wind-cold constraining the exterior and phlegm-heat in the interior	Coughing and wheezing with copious, thick, and yellow sputum, labored breathing, a greasy, yellow tongue coating, and a slippery, rapid pulse	There may also be simultaneous fever and chills.

Common symptoms (next four formulas): hiccup, nausea, or vomiting

Formula Name	Diagnosis	Indications	Remarks
Inula and Haematite Decoction (*xuán fù dài zhě tāng*)	Phlegm turbidity obstructing the interior with deficient Stomach qi	Unremitting belching, hiccup, regurgitation, nausea or vomiting, hard epigastric focal distention, a white, slippery tongue coating, and a wiry, deficient pulse	Focuses on directing rebellious qi downward and transforming phlegm fluids.

cont. ↘

Formula Name	Diagnosis	Indications	Remarks
Tangerine Peel and Bamboo Shavings Decoction (jú pí zhú rú tāng)	Stomach deficiency with heat from constraint	Hiccup, nausea, dry heaves, or retching, possibly a tender, red tongue and a deficient, rapid pulse	Also for vomiting due to debility after a prolonged illness. Focuses on directing rebellious qi downward by resolving constraint.
Clove and Persimmon Calyx Decoction (dīng xiāng shì dì tāng)	Cold from deficiency in the Stomach	Hiccup, belching, or vomiting, a stifling sensation in the epigastrium, focal distention of the chest, a pale tongue with a white coating, and a submerged, slow pulse	Focuses on directing rebellious qi downward and warming the middle burner.
Major Pinellia Deoction (dà bàn xià tāng)	Cold from deficiency of the middle burner	Vomiting (which brings relief) a long time after eating, fullness in the epigastrium, fatigue, emaciation, dried or scanty, loose stools, a pale tongue with little coating or a thin, white coating, and a thin, weak or deficient, lax pulse	For Spleen and Stomach deficiency with either exhausted fluids or phlegm and thin mucus.

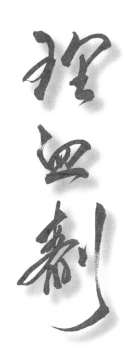

Chapter 13 Contents

Formulas that Regulate the Blood

Formulas that Regulate the Blood

13

THE FORMULAS IN this chapter focus on treating the blood (血 xuè). 'Blood' in Chinese medicine is a physiological essence whose nature is similar but not identical to that of blood in biomedicine. Most importantly, blood in Chinese medicine, like everything else in the organism, is not primarily defined in terms of its structural composition, but in terms of its function. That is why blood, like qi, can be regulated. Such regulation encompasses improving its dynamic, but also its quality, as one determines the other. Blood that has become too thick moves in a sluggish manner, while sluggish movement invariably leads to a thickening of the substance.

The formulas in this chapter have the ability to treat the blood directly. In this, they differ from other formulas—such as those that clear heat, warm the interior, or moisten dryness—that also have an effect on the blood, but achieve this effect indirectly, that is, via the regulation of yang qi or the enrichment of body fluids. This chapter divides formulas that regulate the blood into two large groups: those that invigorate the blood and dispel blood stasis, and those that stop bleeding. Externally-applied formulas that focus on blood stasis are discussed in Chapter 21.

Section 1

FORMULAS THAT INVIGORATE THE BLOOD AND DISPEL BLOOD STASIS

Formulas that invigorate the blood and dispel blood stasis are used in treating patterns of blood stagnation and blood stasis, which represent progressive stages in the impairment and blockage of the flow of blood. When the movement of blood in the channels and collaterals is merely impaired or sluggish, but not yet at a standstill, the condition may be termed 'blood stagnation' (血滞 xuè zhì). However, if, for various reasons, the flow of blood becomes more completely blocked or static, the condition is termed 'blood stasis' (血瘀 xuè yū). This process is described as one of congealing, which in traditional Chinese medicine has been metaphorically compared to the process of silt deposition in the channel-bottom of a sluggish river. Many contemporary textbooks no longer distinguish between these two terms, however, and simply apply the term blood stasis to all problems of blood circulation.

Ideas regarding the nature and treatment of blood stasis in Chinese medicine have a long history, but some of the most commonly prescribed formulas are of relatively recent origin. The *Inner Classic*, for instance, does not talk about 'blood stasis' but discusses problems of blood circulation by means of a vocabulary that refers to the qualitative degeneration of blood as an entity of physiological function, as much as it does to its movement. Pathological states characterized by noxious blood (惡血 *è xuè*), lingering blood (留血 *liú xuè*), or blood excess (血實 *xuè shí*) occur when the relationship between qi and blood is not harmonized; they can be regulated by means of treatment strategies that encompass dredging (決 *jué*), reducing (削 *xuē*), dispersing (散 *sǎn*), and attacking (攻 *gōng*). Although the *Inner Classic* does not directly link these strategies to formulas, one of the few prescriptions listed in the text—Four [Parts] Sepia and One [Part] Rubia Pill (四烏賊骨一蘆茹丸 *sì wū zéi gǔ yī lú rú wán*)—can be regarded as one of the earliest blood-regulating formulas in the history of Chinese medicine. For more on this, see the COMMENTARY under the entry for Stabilize Gushing Decoction (*gù chōng tāng*), discussed in Chapter 9.

The term 'static blood' (瘀血 *yū xuè*) itself appears for the first time in Chapter 16 of *Essentials from the Golden Cabinet*. Its author, the late-Han-dynasty physician Zhang Zhong-Jing, composed a number of formulas for its treatment and outlined key diagnostic markers that have proven their value until the present day. These include dryness of the mouth with no desire to drink, a subjective sensation of fullness in the lower abdomen, and dryness and discoloration of the skin. Later physicians added new formulas and discussed the pathophysiology of blood stasis in more detail, but it was not until the Qing dynasty that two more radical innovations redefined the field. The first was the distinction between stagnation in the channels and collaterals, which was elaborated by Ye Tian-Shi in the early 18th century. Ye attributed stagnation in the channels primarily to qi, and that of stagnation in the collaterals as centered primarily on blood. He argued that stasis of blood in the collaterals requires the use of substances that are acrid but not drying, and suggested that animal medicinals are eminently suitable for this purpose.

A more radical path of innovation was charted by the 19th-century physician Wang Qing-Ren. Based on anatomical observations, Wang proposed to overhaul the entire anatomy of the *Inner Classic* and defined the treatment of blood stasis as the cornerstone of a medicine based on these new definitions. Wang's revolutionary spirit and his focus on blood, a substance that was more easily aligned to biomedical understandings of the body than qi, has contributed to the enormous popularity of his works in contemporary China. Readers will find a more detailed analysis of Wang's innovation in the COMMENTARY to his flagship formula, Drive Out Stasis from the Mansion of Blood Decoction (*xuè fǔ zhú yū tāng*).

Later writers who made significant contributions to the contemporary treatment of blood pathologies include the modern physicians Tang Zong-Hai, who wrote a text dedicated to the treatment of bleeding patterns, and Zhang Xi-Chun, whose contribution to the understanding of blood stasis and its treatment was already influenced by Western anatomy and physiology. In contemporary China, this influence has become ever stronger.

In Chinese medicine, the term 'blood stasis' implies more than blood that has congealed and no longer flows as it should. It denotes all blood that has become noxious (惡 *è*), that is, blood that impedes physiological functions. Key signs and symptoms of such stasis include palpable, immobile masses, abscesses and ulcers, loss of hair or brittle hair, purple lips, dark discoloration of the sclera, purple spots on the tongue or a darkish tongue, and a choppy, submerged, tight, or wiry pulse. In practice, however, the use of blood-invigorating formulas covers a far wider spectrum of clinical signs and symptoms. Wang Qing-Ren, for example, lists fifty different symptoms that can be treated with just one of his formulas. This is because blood, like qi, is the essential foundation of all physiological processes, and its disorders will thus be reflected in almost every body system.

Patterns of blood stasis are qualified and differentiated in terms of the various yin and yang organs involved; the etiological factors of cold, heat, deficiency, and excess; different qualities of disharmony expressed in terms of acute, chronic, mild, and severe; and unusual symptoms such as swelling, pain, and urgency.

Prominent among the etiological factors that contribute to the occurrence of blood stagnation or stasis are the following:

- Qi disharmony, including both deficient and stagnant qi, may lead to blood stagnation since 'qi is the commander of the blood' and 'qi leads the blood.' When the qi is unable to properly move the blood, it may stagnate in the channels. Such is the case in poststroke hemiplegia, which occurs as a result of qi deficiency and blood stagnation leading to obstruction of the channels by blood stasis. Herbs that tonify the qi, such as Ginseng Radix (*rén shēn*), Codonopsis Radix (*dǎng shēn*), Astragali Radix (*huáng qí*), and Polygonati Rhizoma (*huáng jīng*), can be used in formulas for these conditions. Chronic qi stagnation may produce patterns of blood stagnation with various degrees of severity as the loss of proper qi circulation begins to influence the harmonious movement of blood. For this reason, these formulas often contain herbs that regulate the qi such as Aurantii Fructus (*zhǐ ké*), Linderae Radix (*wū yào*), Dalbergiae odoriferae Lignum (*jiàng xiāng*), or Cyperi Rhizoma (*xiāng fù*).

- Blood deficiency is also intrinsically related to blood stasis. Blood that is deficient readily becomes static and, in turn, static blood interferes with the production of new blood. Without the production of new blood, it is very difficult to dispel blood stasis. This can lead to a vicious cycle. For this reason, it is very common to include herbs that tonify the blood in these formulas, such as Angelicae sinensis Radix (*dāng guī*), Rehmanniae Radix praeparata (*shú dì huáng*), Paeoniae Radix alba (*bái sháo*), Polygoni multiflori Radix (*hé shǒu wū*), and Asini Corii Colla (*ē jiāo*).

- Cold inhibits the free movement of blood and will gradually produce blood stasis with such manifestations as delayed menstruation with clots, fixed abdominal masses, and amenorrhea, any of which may be accompanied by abdominal distention and pain. The warming herbs used in these circumstances include Evodiae Fructus (*wú zhū yú*), Cinnamomi Ramulus (*guì zhī*), Cinnamomi Cortex (*ròu guì*), Zingiberis Rhizoma (*gān jiāng*), and Foeniculi Fructus (*xiǎo huí xiāng*).

- Heat influences the blood when it occurs in organs that have an intimate relationship with the blood or when it enters the nutritive or blood levels of the body. This may produce blood stagnation by 'steaming' or drying the blood, which causes it to thicken, and by the tendency of thickened blood to become stagnant and congeal. Heat may also induce the reckless movement of blood such that it leaves the vessels and produces rash, nosebleed, vomiting or spitting up blood, coughing up blood, and blood in the urine or stool. When bleeding occurs internally, the blood may become congealed in the tissues outside of the vessels. The cooling herbs that are commonly used in these circumstances include Moutan Cortex (*mǔ dān pí*), Paeoniae Radix rubra (*chì sháo*), Rehmanniae Radix (*shēng dì huáng*), and Scrophulariae Radix (*xuán shēn*).

Other etiologies of blood stasis include traumatic injury, the birthing process, and surgery. Because of the variety of etiological factors and clinical manifestations, the practitioner must be flexible in adapting the formula to fit the particular circumstances of the case.

It is important to remember that, because the properties of this class of formulas are quite strong for attacking firm and congealed conditions in order to break up and drain them, they should be prescribed with caution in the weak or elderly, or in patients with patterns of deficiency. And because some of the formulas strongly invigorate the blood and dispel blood stasis, they are contraindicated during pregnancy and in most cases involving excessive menstrual bleeding. Nor should they be used in patients with bleeding diathesis or any active hemorrhagic disorder.

桃核承氣湯（桃核承气汤）

Peach Pit Decoction to Order the Qi

táo hé chéng qì tāng

This is one in a family of formulas that order the qi as a means of expelling accumulation and clumping. It is named after one of its chief ingredients, Persicae Semen (*táo rén*) or peach pit.

Source   *Discussion of Cold Damage* (c. 220)

Persicae Semen (*táo rén*) . . . . 50 pieces (12-15g)
Rhei Radix et Rhizoma (*dà huáng*) 12g
Cinnamomi Ramulus (*guì zhī*) 6g
Natrii Sulfas (*máng xiāo*) . . . . [add to strained decoction] 6g
Glycyrrhizae Radix praeparata (*zhì gān cǎo*) 6g

Method of Preparation   Decoction. The source text advises to bring the strained decoction to a boil once more after Natrii Sulfas (*máng xiāo*) has been added. This is generally not done today. The source text also specifies that it should be drunk warm in three doses per day before meals. If the formula is effective, the stools should become slightly loose. Wine-treated Rhei Radix et Rhizoma (*jiǔ zhì dà huáng*) is often used to accentuate the blood-invigorating action of the formula.

Actions   Drains heat and breaks up blood stasis

Indications

Acute lower abdominal pain, smooth urination, night fevers, delirious speech, irritability, restlessness and thirst, and a submerged, full, or choppy pulse. In more severe cases, there may be manic behavior. Women will usually experience dysmenorrhea or amenorrhea.

This is blood buildup (蓄血 *xù xuè*) in the lower burner caused by the accumulation of blood stasis and heat. The source text attributes this condition to the transmission of an externally-contracted pathogenic influence into the lower burner. The static blood and heat obstruct the lower burner and cause acute lower abdominal pain. The buildup of blood disturbs the lower burner but does not disrupt the transformation of the Bladder qi, so urination is normal. Because the heat is in the blood level, there is feverishness at night. The Heart governs the blood and is the organ from which the clarity of spirit emanates. Here the retained heat rises and disturbs the spirit, producing abnormal and chaotic manifestations of the spirit such as delirious speech, irritability, restlessness, and thirst, or, in more severe cases, manic behavior. Moreover, the accumulation and stasis of blood in the lower abdomen inhibits blood circulation and causes amenorrhea or dysmenorrhea in women.

Analysis of Formula

This is a modification of Regulate the Stomach and Order the Qi Decoction (*tiáo wèi chéng qì tāng*) to which Persicae Semen (*táo rén*) and Cinnamomi Ramulus (*guì zhī*) have been added. This changes it from a formula that purges clumping of heat and stools to one that breaks up and expels blood stasis. The chief ingredients are Persicae Semen (*táo rén*), which breaks up and eliminates blood stasis, and Rhei Radix et Rhizoma (*dà huáng*), which attacks and purges accumulations and cleanses pathogenic heat. By attacking the blood stasis and guiding it out of the body, the pathogenic heat is left without anything to which it can attach, and is thereby more easily cleansed or washed away. The ability of the deputy ingredient, Cinnamomi Ramulus (*guì zhī*), to warm the sinews, unblock the vessels, and dispel retained blood from the lower burner effectively unblocks the circulation of blood in the vessels and assists Persicae Semen (*táo rén*) in breaking up and eliminating blood stasis. One of the assistants, Natrii Sulfas (*máng xiāo*), softens areas of hardness and dispels accumulation. This helps Rhei Radix et Rhizoma (*dà huáng*) in moving the stool, draining heat, and eliminating blood stasis. Serving as both an assistant and envoy, Glycyrrhizae Radix praeparata (*zhì gān cǎo*) protects the Stomach and calms the middle burner by moderating the harsh properties of the other ingredients in the formula.

This formula thus effectively combines the draining of heat with the breaking up of blood stasis. Taking the formula should cause mild diarrhea or loose stools. These signs indicate that the pathogenic heat and stasis are being eliminated.

Cautions and Contraindications

Contraindicated during pregnancy. If there are still exterior symptoms, the exterior should first be released before using this formula.

Commentary

Original Usage

In *Discussion of Cold Damage* this formula is indicated for a greater yang-warp disorder with blood stasis in the lower burner. This condition later became known as 'blood buildup' (蓄血 *xù xuè*). In this situation, the source text tells us, there are three possibilities:

1. If the blood descends (either of its own accord or following treatment), the heat will follow the blood, and there will be recovery.

2. If the exterior has not been released, one should not proceed to purge, but must first release the exterior.

3. If the exterior has been released but there is still acute clumping (and pain) in the lower abdomen, then one may purge.

It is the third scenario for which this formula is indicated. The pathodynamic here is that contraction of external cold in a person with strong yang qi causes that qi to become constrained in the interior. This is known as 'heat transformation.' If the heat penetrates into the blood aspect, it will cause

blood stagnation. Because exterior cold is the original cause, this must be expelled first in order to restore the qi dynamic. Depending on the presentation, this can be achieved with a formula such as Ephedra Decoction (*má huáng tāng*) or Cinnamon Twig Decoction (*guì zhī tāng*). Once the exterior has been resolved, the qi in the interior will also begin to move, thereby eliminating the clumping. Only when this does not happen must the clumping itself be purged.

Controversies

There has been much debate regarding both the pathodynamic that leads to this pattern and also the precise location of blood buildup in the lower burner. These issues, in turn, are tied to a third question, namely, the function of the warming herb Cinnamomi Ramulus (*guì zhī*) in a formula designed to eliminate heat. One view, represented by the 11th-century commentator Cheng Wu-Ji in *Annotation and Explanation of the Discussion of Cold Damage*, is that "pathogenic heat in the greater yang channel has not been resolved and [therefore] follows the [greater yang] channel into its [associated] bowel, causing heat to clump in the Bladder." In *Writings on the Esteemed Discussion*, the Ming-dynasty physician Yu Chang likewise argued that "acute clumping in the lower abdomen indicates that the blood of the Bladder builds up and does not move." Although this interpretation explains how the retention of an external pathogen leads to blood stasis in the lower burner, it conflicts with several other key symptoms, most specifically, the fact that urination is not impeded and the absence of blood in the urine. Likewise, while these authors can explain the use of Cinnamomi Ramulus (*guì zhī*) as an herb that guides the formula into the Bladder, they do not take into account that the formula is specifically designed to eliminate pathogens via the bowels.

Another idea, adopted by a number of physicians over time, was to take a broader approach to the meaning of the term 'Bladder' in this context. For example, in his *Investigations of Medical Formulas*, the Ming-dynasty writer Wu Kun argued that the blood buildup occurs not in the Bladder, but in the lower burner. He did not locate it precisely, leaving space for later interpreters to offer a number of different views. In *Collected Writings on Renewal of the Discussion of Cold Damage*, Ke Qin maintained that it was the Intestines, while in *Discourse on Tracing Back to the Source of [the Discussion] of Cold Damage*, Qian Huang located it even more precisely in the ileum (回腸 *huí cháng*).

Other commentators have looked at different structures. In *Simple Annotation of the Discussion of Cold Damage*, the Qing-dynasty physician Chen Nian-Zu suggested the Womb, while in *Records of Experiences with Classic Formulas*, the modern physician Cao Ying-Fu reasoned that both the Intestines and the Womb were possible locations. In *Treatment Strategies and Formulas in Chinese Medicine*, the contemporary physician Chen Chao-Zu defined it functionally as the blood aspect of the Liver channel.

In this manner, each writer offered his own reasons why the source text's reference to "heat clumping the Bladder" could be extended to other organs. Some claimed that the text had been corrupted, while others argued that the term 'Bladder' referred not to an organ, but to a body region—specifically the lower abdomen—in part relying on the *Inner Classic,* where the term Bladder is often matched with the Triple Burner, as in Chapter 8 of *Divine Pivot.*

Usage

If these diverse readings cannot ultimately be reconciled, nor in fact proven, the use of the formula in the clinic supports the wider interpretation of the second group of writers. Over the centuries, the formula has been used to treat any pattern linked to the accumulation of heat and blood stasis in the lower burner. These include traumatic injury with intractable pain or difficulty in passing urine or stool; pain and distention of the head, red eyes, and toothache that results from blood stagnation due to the presence of vigorous fire; nosebleed, vomiting, or coughing up blood due to reckless movement of hot blood; gynecological disorders such as hot flushes, amenorrhea, irregular menstruation, dysmenorrhea, prolonged lochia, and even infertility; fixed, lower abdominal pain; and severe wheezing and distention of the chest. The wide scope of this formula in the modern clinic is reflected in the BIOMEDICAL INDICATIONS below.

Besides symptoms that point to heat excess and blood stasis more generally, the following key markers will be helpful in diagnosing this formula's pattern:

- The abdominal symptoms are acute and there is fixed pain that increases with pressure, usually in the lower abdomen. Some Japanese Kampo physicians locate such hypersensitivity predominantly in the left lower quadrant; others argue that the distinguishing feature is that resistance is experienced on very superficial palpation and that, compared to other patterns of blood stasis, areas of tenderness do not have distinct boundaries.

- The head will usually be hot, or there will be other symptoms of up-flushing such as headache, neck and shoulder stiffness, dizziness, or tinnitus.

- The lower body or extremities may be cold, even though the patient feels subjectively hot.

- If the spirit is disturbed, the manifestations will be irritability, restlessness, anxiety or insomnia, and, in severe cases, delirious speech or manic behavior.

- If there is bleeding, the blood will be very dark purple with clots. The tongue will have dark purple spots, and the pulse will be submerged and choppy.

Issues Related to the Use of Cinnamomi Ramulus (*guì zhī*)

Commentators have also fiercely debated the function of Cinnamomi Ramulus (*guì zhī*) in this formula. Some say that it disperses blood, others that it serves as an envoy that guides the formula into the Bladder, or that it moves the qi in order to move the blood, or that it resolves the exterior. At least one important commentator, Wang Ken-Tang in *Indispensable Tools for Pattern Treatment,* states that Cinnamomi Cortex (*ròu guì*) should be used instead of Cinnamomi Ramulus (*guì zhī*).

One useful approach is to look at this question from the source text itself, that is, to see how Cinnamomi Ramulus (*guì zhī*) is used elsewhere in the writings of Zhang Zhong-Jing. As discussed in the entry on Cinnamon Twig Decoction (*guì zhī tāng*) in Chapter 1, this herb focuses on the nutritive qi, facilitating its movement and dispersion by means of its acrid, warming nature. The nature of yang qi is to ascend (from the lower to the upper burner) and that of yin blood to descend (from the Heart to the Liver). Warming the qi to move the blood, Cinnamomi Ramulus (*guì zhī*) is said both to ascend and to direct downward. In the present formula, herbs such as Rhei Radix et Rhizoma (*dà huáng*) and Persicae Semen (*táo rén*) guide Cinnamomi Ramulus (*guì zhī*) into the blood aspect of the lower burner where it assists in ordering the qi and breaking up clumping by dispersing cold. As noted by the late 19th-century physician Tang Zong-Hai in *Discussion of Blood Patterns:*

> Cinnamomi Ramulus (*guì zhī*) reports to the Liver channel's wood fire qi as to a superior. [If one uses it when] Liver qi is hyperactive, one will observe [symptoms of yang qi] blazing [upward]. Clumped Liver qi [on the other hand] is moved when encountering [this herb]. Therefore, it can sometimes be indicated and sometimes be contraindicated in [the treatment] of blood [aspect] patterns. This formula avails itself of its acrid, dispersing [nature, but by means of] Natrii Sulfas (*máng xiāo*), Rhei Radix et Rhizoma (*dà huáng*), and Persicae Semen (*táo rén*) directly moves downward into the lower burner to break up clumping and facilitate the movement of blood. The only two paths of exit for static blood are the urine and the bowels. [Hence, while] Natrii Sulfas (*máng xiāo*) and Rhei Radix et Rhizoma (*dà huáng*) guide it out via the bowels, Cinnamomi Ramulus (*guì zhī*) simultaneously [facilitates] qi [transformation] and thereby urination. These were [Zhang Zhong-Jing's] intentions in the first place.

Comparisons

➤ Vs. APPROPRIATE DECOCTION (*dǐ dàng tāng*); *see* PAGE 564

➤ Vs. CINNAMON TWIG AND PORIA PILL (*guì zhī fú líng wán*); *see* PAGE 585

➤ Vs. RHUBARB AND GROUND BEETLE PILL (*dà huáng zhè chóng wán*); *see* PAGE 596

Alternate name

Peach Kernel Decoction to Order the Qi *(táo rén chéng qì tāng)* in *Classified Compilation of Medical Prescriptions*

....

Biomedical Indications

With the appropriate presentation, this formula may be used to treat a wide variety of biomedically-defined disorders. These can be divided into the following groups:

- Disorders of the lower abdomen including intestinal obstruction, acute pelvic inflammatory disease, leiomyoma, difficult childbirth, retained placenta, prolonged lochia, posttubal ligation syndrome, ectopic pregnancy, perimenopausal syndrome, cystitis, benign prostatic hypertrophy, prostatitis, gonorrhea urethritis, hemorrhagic fever with renal syndrome, and ulcerative colitis

- Neurological disorders including traumatic headache, cerebral contusion, sequelae of brain trauma, headache from subarachnoid hemorrhage, recalcitrant migraine, and trigeminal neuralgia

- Psychiatric disorders including schizophrenia, hysterical psychosis, reactive psychosis, and epilepsy

- Congestive and inflammatory conditions affecting the face and head including acute conjunctivitis, hordeolum, blepharitis, pterygium, facial acne, brandy nose, and gingivitis with bleeding

- Vascular disorders including cerebrovascular disease, atherosclerosis, hypertension, myocardial infarction, and varicose veins

- Skin disorders including urticaria, seborrheic dermatitis, erysipelas, scarlet fever, allergic purpura, and exudative eczema.

This formula has also been used for treating pancreatitis, hemoptysis from tuberculosis, asthma, periodic epistaxis during menstrual periods, hepatic coma, chronic renal insufficiency, purulent mastitis, bone spurs, Keshan syndrome, and pinworms.

Modifications

- For irregular menstruation or dysmenorrhea, add Angelicae sinensis Radix *(dāng guī)* and Carthami Flos *(hóng huā)*.

- For concurrent qi stagnation, add Cyperi Rhizoma *(xiāng fù)*, Linderae Radix *(wū yào)*, Citri reticulatae viride Pericarpium *(qīng pí,)* and Aucklandiae Radix *(mù xiāng)*.

- For more severe obstruction from blood stasis due to posthemorrhagic retention of blood, traumatic injury, impairment of circulation, difficult defecation, or bowel obstruction with continuous, stabbing abdominal pain, thirst, fever, and a choppy pulse, add Paeoniae Radix rubra *(chì sháo)* and Notoginseng Radix *(sān qī)*.

- For nosebleed or spitting up blood of a purple or dark color accompanied by a stifling sensation in the chest, add Rehmanniae Radix *(shēng dì huáng)* and Imperatae Rhizoma *(bái máo gēn)*.

- For prolonged lochia, hard fullness in the lower abdomen, or severe wheezing and distention of the chest, combine with Sudden Smile Powder *(shī xiào sǎn)*.

Associated Formula

下瘀血湯 （下瘀血汤）

Purge Static Blood Decoction

xià yū xuè tāng

Source   *Essentials from the Golden Cabinet* (c. 220)

Tabanus *(méng chóng)* . . . . 20 bodies, feet removed (9-12g)
Persicae Semen *(táo rén)* . . . . 20 pieces (6-9g)
Rhei Radix et Rhizoma *(dà huáng)* 6g

The source text states that the ingredients are ground and made into four pills with honey, with each pill decocted in 1 cup of wine until 0.8 cup is left. At present, the ingredients are ground (using the dosages in parentheses) and made into 9-15g pills with honey. One pill is taken daily with a small amount of wine. Alternatively, it can be taken as a decoction. The honey ameliorates the harshness of the ingredients and spreads out their actions over time. Decocting in wine helps guide the effects of the formula into the blood aspect.

This formula drives out stasis and drains the heat. It was originally used for abdominal pain during pregnancy due to what was considered to be dried blood below the umbilicus. At present, it is used much more often for similar problems postpartum. It is also an important formula for amenorrhea due to blood stasis as well as chronic lower abdominal inflammatory disorders in both men and women such as pelvic inflammatory disease, prostatitis, and lower back disc disease.

In contrast to the principal formula, it is used for piercing pain in the lower abdomen that gets worse with pressure and may be accompanied by palpable masses. And unlike the principal formula, its presentation does not include any signs of disrupted spirit or mania-like symptoms.

抵當湯 （抵当汤）

Appropriate Decoction

dǐ dàng tāng

Commentators offer four different explanations for the name of this formula. Ke Qin interprets it to mean "directly reaching (抵達 *dǐ dá*) the appropriate (當 *dàng*) location of attacking [the blood stasis]." Fang You-Zhi reads 抵當 *dǐ dàng* as 恰當 *qià dàng*, which means 'appropriate,' implying that this formula is the most suitable strategy for treating this pattern. Yamada Seichin, in *Collection on the Discussion of Cold Damage*, states that 抵當 *dǐ dàng* is another name for Hirudo *(shuǐ zhì)*, the chief substance in the formula. One of the earliest commentators on the *Discussion of Cold Damage*, Cheng Wu-Ji, interprets 抵當 *dǐ dàng* literally as meaning to ward off or resist blood stasis. However, given that the herbs in this formula attack rather than protect against stasis, this interpretation seems the least accurate. The name used here attempts a synthesis of the three other explanations, given that the word 'appropriate' in English means suitable, apposite, and pertinent (as an adjective), but can also be read as capturing, conquering, and taking over (as a verb).

Source   *Discussion of Cold Damage* (c. 220)

Hirudo *(shuǐ zhì)* 30g (9-12g)
Tabanus *(méng chóng)* 30g (9-12g)
Persicae Semen *(táo rén)* . . . . 20 pieces (6-9g)
wine-washed Rhei Radix et Rhizoma *(jiǔ xǐ dà huáng)* 9g

Method of Preparation   Decoct with 5 cups of water until 3 cups remain. Divide into three portions and take warm. If the first dose fails to induce a bowel movement, take another dose.

Actions   Breaks up and dispels blood stasis

Indications

Firmness and distention of the lower abdomen, smooth urination, manic behavior, forgetfulness, black stools that are easy to expel, and a submerged and slow-irregular pulse. In women, there may also be delayed menstruation or amenorrhea. Also treats jaundice.

This is blood buildup in the lower burner caused by clumping of heat and blood. The heat causes the blood to become thick, slowing its flow and causing stasis. This becomes apparent in the firmness and distention of the lower abdomen. Because the stasis is at the level of the blood and not the qi, urination is not impeded and the stools are easy to expel. Black stools, delayed menstruation, or amenorrhea, however, indicates that the movement and generation of blood is abnormal. The Heart is the organ that governs the generation of blood and harbors the spirit. When the static heat flushes upward to harass the Heart spirit, this leads to manic behavior. Blood stasis impeding the production of new blood, on the other hand, is reflected in forgetfulness. The submerged pulse identifies this as an interior problem, while its slowness and irregularity reflect blood stasis. Jaundice is a sign of damp-heat. This can occur when yang brightness excess heat (rather than greater yang cold that has transformed into heat) is the root cause of the problem.

Analysis of Formula

The symptoms that characterize the pattern treated by this formula indicate that the stasis is severe, and that the momentum of the disorder is progressing. In this situation, mild purgation is no longer appropriate, and attacking with strong-acting, stasis-breaking substances is the appropriate strategy. For this purpose, the formula employs two animal medicinals as chief ingredients. Salty, bitter, neutral, and slightly toxic Hirudo *(shuǐ zhì)* enters the Liver channel and, in the words of the *Divine Husbandman's Classic of the Materia Medica*, "expels noxious blood and static blood." In *Essays on Medicine Esteeming the Chinese and Respecting the Western*, Zhang

Xi-Chun observes that this substance has the special characteristic of entering only the blood aspect, allowing it to expel static blood without damaging the qi. Slightly bitter and slightly cooling Tabanus *(méng chóng)* also enters the Liver channel and is even stronger than Hirudo *(shuǐ zhì)* in breaking up blood stasis. Amplifying each other's characteristics, these two substances have a synergy that makes this one of the strongest blood stasis-expelling formulas. The addition of Rhei Radix et Rhizoma *(dà huáng)* and Persicae Semen *(táo rén)* further reinforces this effect. Rhei Radix et Rhizoma *(dà huáng)* also opens the bowels, following the momentum of the pathology (i.e., the downward movement of heat and its clumping in the lower burner) to create a route for the heat to leave the body, as noted in *Basic Questions* (Chapter 5): "Draining downward is guiding out and exhausting [what is stagnating internally]."

Cautions and Contraindications

This formula is indicated only for excess-type blood stasis patterns in the lower burner. It should not be prescribed in case of deficiency or during pregnancy.

Commentary

This formula treats late-stage blood buildup in the lower burner, where heat has substantially dried up the blood and caused palpable hardness.

Use of Animal Substances

Because this is a deep-seated condition located entirely at the blood level, the formula uses animal substances to break up stasis. Many physicians agree with Ke Qin, quoted in the *Golden Mirror of the Medical Traditions*: "When static blood is indicated by signs such as these, only harsh prescriptions are capable of reaching the lair [of the pathogen] and are appropriate for carrying out the weighty task [of flushing it out]." In *Selected Annotations to Ancient Formulas from the Garden of Crimson Snow*, the Qing-dynasty commentator Want Zi-Jie explains why this is so:

> Blood buildup belongs to [disorders characterized] by dead yin. The true qi moves [normally] but can [no longer] enter into it. Therefore, herbs alone are unable to treat this pathogen. One must use those nimble creatures that have a liking for blood in order to guide [the static blood] out. [Medicinals made from] flying [creatures] move through the yang collaterals. [Those made from creatures] that live under water move through the yin collaterals. [In this formula, Tabanus *(méng chóng)* and Hirudo *(shuǐ zhì)*] thus guide Persicae Semen *(táo rén)* toward attacking the blood, and Rhei Radix et Rhizoma *(dà huáng)* to purge heat to break the merciless clumping of blood. It is truly an appropriate formula for carrying out a difficult [task]. There is no need to fear the venomous nature of these medicinals.

Wang Zi-Jie's theory regarding the ability of animal substances to enter the collaterals has been especially influential.

It was further developed by the Qing-dynasty physician Ye Tian-Shi, who used animal substances to treat stasis of the collaterals; and it features prominently in the work of contemporary physicians such as Zhang Ci-Gong and Zhu Liang-Chun, who argue that many chronic conditions can only be helped by means of formulas containing such substances. Influenced by these theories, the formula is used in contemporary China to treat disorders that are now associated with blood stasis such as the sequelae of stroke, abnormal blood lipids, or epilepsy. When this formula is prescribed for long-term use or less acute manifestations, it is usually given as a pill.

Comparisons

➤ Vs. Peach Pit Decoction to Order the Qi (*táo hé chéng qì tāng*)

Both of these formulas treat blood buildup in the lower burner due to clumping of blood and heat by breaking up the stasis and draining heat primarily through the bowels. Symptoms shared by both patterns include lower abdominal fullness and distention, manic behavior, and a submerged, rough pulse. However, while Peach Pit Decoction to Order the Qi (*táo hé chéng qì tāng*) is used for treating the early stages of blood buildup, Appropriate Decoction (*dǐ dàng tāng*) is used for the later stages of this disorder. Thus, while the abdomen in the former pattern is tense, painful when pressed, and accompanied by a subjective sensation of clumping or fullness, in the latter there will be palpable hardness with defined borders. Other differences include signs of yang qi constraint (i.e., remnants of qi aspect symptoms) in the former, such as flushing accompanied by cold extremities or constipation, while in the latter, dark stools that can be passed easily indicate that the disorder is now located solely at the blood level. For this reason, Peach Pit Decoction to Order the Qi (*táo hé chéng qì tāng*) focuses more strongly on also ordering the qi, while Appropriate Decoction (*dǐ dàng tāng*) is much stronger in terms of breaking up blood stasis.

➤ Vs. Rhubarb and Ground Beetle Pill (*dà huáng zhè chóng wán*); *see* page 596

Biomedical Indications

With the appropriate presentation, this formula may be used to treat a wide variety of biomedically-defined disorders. These can be divided into the following groups:

• Gynecological and obstetrical disorders including acute pelvic inflammatory disease, leiomyoma, endometriosis, dysmenorrhea, amenorrhea, retained placenta, and postpartum thrombophlebitis

• Genitourinary disorders including benign prostatic hypertrophy, acute prostatitis, testicular tuberculosis, and acute urinary retention

• Circulatory disorders including angina pectoris, cerebrovascular disease, and cor pulmonale

• Neuropsychiatric disorders including schizophrenia, mania, and epilepsy.

This formula has also been used in the treatment of icteric hepatitis, chronic colitis, habitual constipation, and schistosomiasis.

血府逐瘀湯 (血府逐瘀汤)
Drive Out Stasis from the Mansion of Blood Decoction
xuè fǔ zhú yū tāng

A passage in Chapter 17 of *Basic Questions* observes that, "The vessels are the mansions of the blood." The 18th-century physician Wang Qing-Ren borrowed the name to denote the area above the diaphragm that formed an enclosed space or 'mansion' that he believed was filled with blood. This formula treats the symptoms that Wang Qing-Ren attributed to blood stasis in this area.

Source   *Correction of Errors among Physicians* (1830)

Persicae Semen (*táo rén*) 12g
Carthami Flos (*hóng huā*) 9g
Angelicae sinensis Radix (*dāng guī*) 9g
Chuanxiong Rhizoma (*chuān xiōng*) 4.5g
Paeoniae Radix rubra (*chì sháo*) 6g
Achyranthis bidentatae Radix (*niú xī*) 9g
Bupleuri Radix (*chái hú*) 3g
Platycodi Radix (*jié gěng*) 4.5g
Aurantii Fructus (*zhǐ ké*) 6g
Rehmanniae Radix (*shēng dì huáng*) 9g
Glycyrrhizae Radix (*gān cǎo*) 6g

Method of Preparation   Decoction. While the original text simply calls for 牛膝 *niú xī*, most often Cyathulae Radix (*chuān niú xī*) is used instead of Achyranthis bidentatae Radix (*niú xī*).

Actions   Invigorates the blood, dispels blood stasis, spreads the qi of the Liver, and unblocks the channels

Indications

Pain in the chest and hypochondria, chronic, stubborn headache with a fixed, piercing quality, chronic, incessant hiccup, a choking sensation when drinking, dry heaves, depression or low spirits accompanied by a sensation of warmth in the chest, palpitations, insomnia, restless sleep, irritability, extreme mood swings, evening tidal fever, a dark red tongue, dark spots on the sides of the tongue, dark or purplish lips, complexion, or sclera, and a choppy or wiry, tight pulse

This is blood stasis in the 'mansion of blood' (血府 *xuè fǔ*) with impairment of blood flow in the area above the diaphragm. The stasis of blood obstructs the movement of qi in the chest, which manifests as pain in the chest and hypochondria. The obstruction also prevents the clear yang from ascending to the head, causing a chronic, stubborn headache. Blockage of the flow of blood in the channels from localized blood stasis produces a characteristic fixed and piercing type of headache pain. If blood stasis obstructs the Stomach, the Stomach qi may rebel upward and manifest as incessant hiccup, a choking sensation when drinking, or dry heaves.

Long-term blood stasis tends to transform into heat, and constrained qi tends to transform into fire. Blood stasis may also obstruct the blood vessels and prevent nourishment from reaching the Heart. This combination of stasis, heat, and mal-nourishment of the Heart may cause depression or low spirits accompanied by a sensation of warmth in the chest, palpitations, insomnia, restless sleep, irritability, extreme mood swings, and evening tidal fever. The dark red tongue, dark spots on the sides of the tongue, dark or purplish appearance of the lips, complexion, or sclera, and the choppy or wiry, tight pulse are all typical signs of chronic blood stasis and constrained Liver qi.

Analysis of Formula

This formula is a variation on the combination of Four-Substance Decoction with Safflower and Peach Pit (*táo hóng sì wù tāng*) and Frigid Extremities Powder (*sì nì sǎn*). The chief herbs are those which invigorate the blood and dispel blood stasis, particularly in the upper part of the body: Persicae Semen (*táo rén*), Carthami Flos (*hóng huā*), and Chuanxiong Rhizoma (*chuān xiōng*). Two of the deputies, Paeoniae Radix rubra (*chì sháo*) and Angelicae sinensis Radix (*dāng guī*), also invigorate the blood, although their focus is lower in the body. The latter also nourishes the blood and moistens. This, along with the functions of another deputy, Rehmanniae Radix (*shēng dì huáng*), which cools the blood and clears heat, enables the formula to dispel blood stasis without injuring the yin and blood. The final deputy, Cyathulae Radix (*chuān niú xī*), improves the circulation by eliminating blood stasis and inducing the downward movement of blood.

The assistant herbs include Bupleuri Radix (*chái hú*), which smoothes the flow of Liver qi, relieves constraint, and raises the clear yang. In concert with the other assistants, Platycodi Radix (*jié gěng*) and Aurantii Fructus (*zhǐ ké*), it expands the chest and promotes the movement of qi. By relieving qi stagnation in the chest, these herbs promote the movement of qi and thereby facilitate the movement of blood. The envoy, Glycyrrhizae Radix (*gān cǎo*), regulates and harmonizes the actions of the other herbs.

The value of this formula is that it not only invigorates the blood and transforms stasis in the blood level, but also relieves constraint in the qi level. It invigorates the blood without consuming it, and dispels blood stasis while encouraging the production of new blood. It facilitates the upward and downward flow of qi and harmonizes the circulation of blood, following the adage, "If the qi circulates, then the blood will circulate."

The dosage of particular herbs in this formula may be adjusted based on the relative importance of blood stasis versus qi stagnation in the particular patient.

Cautions and Contraindications

Because the actions of this formula in invigorating the blood and dispelling blood stasis are very strong, it is contraindicated during pregnancy and in most cases that involve excessive menstrual bleeding as well as in the weak or debilitated. It is also contraindicated in cases with bleeding diathesis or any active hemorrhagic disorder.

Commentary

Wang Qing-Ren

The early 19th-century physician Wang Qing-Ren was, without doubt, one of the most innovative physicians in the history of Chinese medicine. Inquisitive and reflecting the pervasive critical attitude that Qing-dynasty scholars had developed regarding the sources of their tradition, Wang Qing-Ren is widely credited with having reintroduced a focus on anatomy into medical debates, well before the large-scale influx of Western medicine into China. Given the legal and moral context of his time, however, his investigations were limited to observing the bodies of children who had died in epidemics and were buried in shallow graves and then dug up by dogs, of criminals that had been executed, and of dissected animals. This allowed him to criticize the portrayal of the body as depicted in the Han-dynasty medical classics. However, his own alternative model was soon after shown to be equally flawed by Western anatomical texts. Among his anatomical findings was a pool of blood that was located at the bottom of the chest and above the diaphragm. He posited that this is the spot where the essential fluids were transformed into blood, and thus called it the 'mansion of blood' (血府 *xuè fǔ*).

Wang's Approach to Medicine

Wang could not find any anatomical evidence for the connections through which classical texts linked various organ systems. On the other hand, he felt that the various qi- and blood-carrying and producing structures that he noted were clearly interconnected with the organs. Based on this observation, he posited that deficiency and stagnation of qi and blood were the underlying causes of all disease:

> Making decisions regarding the treatment of disease is rooted in understanding the qi and blood. Whether one discusses externally-contracted [disorders] or [those due to] internal damage, it is essential to establish which of these [two] substances is damaged in [each] patient at the onset of a disorder. [At the onset,] what is damaged are not the organs, nor the sinews and bones, nor the skin and flesh, but in each case the qi and blood.

In line with his emphasis on anatomy, Wang argued that pulse diagnosis was unreliable and that only those symptoms that could be directly observed and linked to the distribution of qi and blood counted as evidence. For blood stasis, for instance, he listed fifty different symptoms derived from his own clinical experience. Interestingly, he did not include inspection of the tongue, one of the most commonly used methods for diagnosing blood stasis today. He furthermore arranged these symptoms into three primary groups according to the system in which the blood stasis was mainly located: the exterior (encompassing the head, skin, and blood vessels), the mansion of blood (the chest above the diaphragm), and the abdomen (below the diaphragm). For the mansion of blood, he provided this analysis:

> When the blood in the mansion of blood [becomes] static [and therefore] is no longer vigorous, this is most difficult to diagnose. Fever in the latter half of the day that becomes more severe during the first half of the night, abates during the latter half of the night, and [completely] disappears during the first half of the day indicates blood stasis in the mansion of blood. With a milder blood stasis, these four stages are not [clearly] separated. The [patient becomes] feverish only during the two periods before and after sunset. If it is even milder, the fever occurs only during one of these periods. In all cases [of blood stasis,] I am saying that internal fever is accompanied by a hot body.

Relationship between the Qi and Blood

Chinese medicine has long understood that any problem affecting the flow of qi will end up affecting the blood and vice versa, as reflected in the adage, "Blood is the mother of qi, and qi the commander of blood" (血為氣之母;氣為血之帥 *xuè wéi qì zhī mǔ; qì wéi xuè zhī shuài*). In the early 17th century, Wang Ken-Tang wrote in *Indispensable Tools for Pattern Treatment* that "if you want to adjust the blood, first adjust the qi." About a hundred years later, Wu Cheng wrote in *Collection of Versatility* that, "for blood stagnation caused by qi, first move the qi; for qi stagnation caused by blood stasis, invigorating the blood is most important."

Almost all of Wang Qing-Ren's formulas focus on regulating the distribution of qi and blood in the body, paying close attention to the interconnection between the two systems. Blood stasis, for instance, will invariably lead to stagnation of qi. Because qi is hot by nature, this is experienced as fever and body heat. Qi stagnation, likewise, can cause blood stasis. But in this case, the blood congeals because it does not receive the warmth of the qi. These insights are clearly reflected in Wang Qing-Ren's formulas for treating blood stasis. All of them move the qi as well as invigorate the blood. But in each case, the nature of the pathology is responded to by carefully adjusting both the nature and the dosage of the various herbs that act on the qi and blood. Drive Out Stasis from the Mansion of Blood Decoction (*xuè fǔ zhú yū tāng*), for instance, treats blood stasis that leads to qi stagnation. It thus uses a large dosage of blood-invigorating, nourishing, and cooling herbs and a relatively small dosage of herbs that facilitate the qi dynamic and are cooling or neutral in temperature. Drive Out Stasis from the Lower Abdomen Decoction (*shào fù zhú yū tāng*), one of the associated formulas described below and designed to treat blood stasis caused by cold, facilitates the movement of qi with acrid and warming herbs.

Modern Usage

Modern physicians value the clinical experience embodied in Wang Qing-Ren's formulas, but reject the anatomical conjectures on which they are based. This has led to the curious situation where, in order to explain the effectiveness of this formula, some contemporary commentators have gone back to Chapter 17 of *Basic Questions* where the (blood) vessels are defined as mansions of the blood. This allows them to argue that this formula unblocks the blood vessels. However, in doing so, they disregard the fact that Wang Qing-Ren categorically stated that "The blood vessels are not the mansion of blood."

At present, this formula is most commonly used to treat chest pain due to blood stasis, which is accompanied by a dark red tongue and a choppy or wiry, tight pulse. It is also used for problems of blood stasis in children, usually when fever, pain, and difficulty in sleeping develop after trauma. It is indicated for literally dozens of disorders that can be attributed to blood stasis in the vessels. In addition to the characteristic pain and tongue and pulse signs described above, other guidelines for its use include that the condition be chronic and accompanied by heat in the palms and soles due to long-term stasis transforming into heat. Furthermore, the skin is usually dry or even scaly.

Comparisons

➤ Vs. Revive Health by Invigorating the Blood Decoction (*fù yuán huó xuè tāng*); *see* page 573

➤ Vs. Inula Decoction (*xuán fù huā tāng*); *see* page 577

Biomedical Indications

With the appropriate presentation, this formula may be used to treat a wide variety of biomedically-defined disorders. These can be divided into the following groups:

- Cardiac and vascular disorders including coronary artery disease, rheumatic valvular heart disease, hypertension, and cor pulmonale
- Structural disorders of the chest including intercostal neuralgia, costochondritis, and thoracic strains
- Neurological and psychiatric disorders including postconcussion syndrome, migraine, trigeminal neuralgia, depression, and psychosis.

This formula has also been used in the treatment of perimenopausal syndrome, primary dysmenorrhea, chronic hepatitis, peptic ulcers, and urticaria.

Modifications

- For headache, add Viticis Fructus *(màn jīng zǐ)* and Tribuli Fructus *(cì jí lí)*.
- For pain in the hypochondria from an enlarged liver, add Salviae miltiorrhizae Radix *(dān shēn)*, Curcumae Radix *(yù jīn)*, Tabanus *(méng chóng)*, and Aspongopus *(jiǔ xiāng chóng)*.
- For immobile subcostal and abdominal masses, add Curcumae Radix *(yù jīn)* and Salviae miltiorrhizae Radix *(dān shēn)*.
- For amenorrhea or dysmenorrhea, remove Platycodi Radix *(jié gěng)* and add Cyperi Rhizoma *(xiāng fù)*, Leonuri Herba *(yì mǔ cǎo)*, and Lycopi Herba *(zé lán)*.
- For rheumatic valvular heart disease, remove Cyathulae Radix *(chuān niú xī)* and Platycodi Radix *(jié gěng)* and add herbs that support the normal qi as required. For example, for insomnia or restless sleep, add Ziziphi spinosae Semen *(suān zǎo rén)*; for qi deficiency, add Codonopsis Radix *(dǎng shēn)*; for yang deficiency, also remove Bupleuri Radix *(chái hú)* and add Aconiti Radix lateralis praeparata *(zhì fù zǐ)* and Cinnamomi Ramulus *(guì zhī)*.
- For angina pectoris due to coronary artery disease, increase the dosage of Carthami Flos *(hóng huā)* and Chuanxiong Rhizoma *(chuān xiōng)* and add Salviae miltiorrhizae Radix *(dān shēn)*.

Associated Formulas

通竅活血湯 （通窍活血汤）

Unblock the Orifices and Invigorate the Blood Decoction

tōng qiào huó xuè tāng

Source   *Correction of Errors among Physicians* (1830)

Paeoniae Radix rubra *(chì sháo)* 3g
Chuanxiong Rhizoma *(chuān xiōng)* 3g
Persicae Semen *(táo rén)* 9g
Carthami Flos *(hóng huā)* 9g
Allii fistulosi Bulbus *(cōng bái)* 3g
Jujubae Fructus *(dà zǎo)* . . . . 7 pieces
Zingiberis Rhizoma recens *(shēng jiāng)* 9g
Moschus *(shè xiāng)* . . . . [add with a small amount of white wine to the strained decoction] 0.15g

Invigorates the blood, dispels blood stasis, and opens up the orifices. For accumulation of blood stasis in the head, face, and upper part of the body with such symptoms as headache and vertigo, chronic tinnitus, hair loss, dark purple complexion, darkness around the eyes, and 'brandy' nose. Also for childhood nutritional impairment with progressive emaciation, abdominal distention, purplish discoloration of the sinews, tidal fever, and other chronic disorders that arise from the accumulation of blood stasis internally, including the exhaustion of blood in women and deficiency from overwork in men.

Although this formula is commonly interpreted to focus on the head and face, its author, Wang Qing-Ren, stated that it is able "to unblock the blood pipes" (通血管 *tōng xuè guǎn*). He also noted that the bluish blood vessels that become visible on the skin are a distinguishing sign for blood stasis in the blood pipes. Contemporary commentators such as the Shaanxi College of TCM therefore interpret the term 'unblocking the orifices' (通竅 *tōng qiào*) to mean not just the sensory organs of the head, but more generally the small apertures through which the blood enters and exits as it circulates through the body.

Comparison

➤ Vs. Inula Decoction *(xuán fù huā tāng)*; *see* page 577

膈下逐瘀湯 （膈下逐瘀汤）

Drive Out Stasis Below the Diaphragm Decoction

gé xià zhú yū tāng

Source   *Correction of Errors among Physicians* (1830)

dry-fried Trogopterori Faeces *(chǎo wǔ líng zhī)* 9g
Angelicae sinensis Radix *(dāng guī)* 9g
Chuanxiong Rhizoma *(chuān xiōng)* 6g
Persicae Semen *(táo rén)* 9g
Moutan Cortex *(mǔ dān pí)* 6g
Paeoniae Radix rubra *(chì sháo)* 6g
Linderae Radix *(wū yào)* 6-12g
Corydalis Rhizoma *(yán hú suǒ)* 3g
Glycyrrhizae Radix *(gān cǎo)* 9g
Cyperi Rhizoma *(xiāng fù)* 4.5g
Carthami Flos *(hóng huā)* 9g
Aurantii Fructus *(zhǐ ké)* 4.5g

Invigorates the blood, dispels blood stasis, promotes the movement of qi, and alleviates pain. For blood stasis in the area below the diaphragm with palpable abdominal masses accompanied by fixed pain, or abdominal masses that are visible when lying down. Also for chronic diarrhea and daybreak diarrhea. Through his anatomical studies, Wang Qing-Ren discovered that all the organs, with the exception of the heart and lungs, are located below the diaphragm. This formula therefore treats blood stasis within these organs. The most important diagnostic marker are palpable abdominal masses, although it is important to remember that other pathologies (such as qi stagnation, phlegm, or dampness) can also cause these masses. This formula is also commonly used to treat amenorrhea and painful periods.

少腹逐瘀湯 （少腹逐瘀汤）

Drive Out Stasis from the Lower Abdomen Decoction

shào fù zhú yū tāng

Source   *Correction of Errors among Physicians* (1830)

dry-fried Foeniculi Fructus *(chǎo xiǎo huí xiāng)* 1.5g
dry-fried Zingiberis Rhizoma *(chǎo gān jiāng)* 0.6g
Corydalis Rhizoma *(yán hú suǒ)* 3g
Angelicae sinensis Radix *(dāng guī)* 9g
Chuanxiong Rhizoma *(chuān xiōng)* 3g

Myrrha (mò yào) 3g
Cinnamomi Cortex (ròu guì) 3g
Paeoniae Radix rubra (chì sháo) 6g
Typhae Pollen (pú huáng) 9g
dry-fried Trogopterori Faeces (chǎo wǔ líng zhī) 6g

Invigorates the blood, dispels blood stasis, warms the menses, and alleviates pain. For blood stasis accumulating in the lower abdomen caused by cold characterized by palpable masses that may or may not be painful, or lower abdominal pain without palpable masses, or lower abdominal distention, or lower back pain and lower abdominal distention during menstruation, or frequent menstruation (3-5 times per month) with dark or purple menstrual blood (usually with clots), or abnormal uterine bleeding accompanied by lower abdominal soreness and pain.

This formula is basically a combination of Four-Substance Decoction with Safflower and Peach Pit (táo hóng sì wù tāng) and Sudden Smile Powder (shī xiào sǎn). It is particularly indicated for cold from deficiency leading to blood stasis. Thus, in addition to signs of blood stasis, there will also be symptoms of cold. These include an aversion to cold, low or depressed mood, cold extremities, white discharges, and a pale tongue. Recently, this formula has been successfully used in the treatment of cirrhosis of the liver with edema with the addition of Rehmanniae Radix (shēng dì huáng), Cyperi Rhizoma (xiāng fù), Linderae Radix (wū yào), Persicae Semen (táo rén), Carthami Flos (hóng huā), and Luffae Fructus Retinervus (sī guā luò).

身痛逐瘀湯 (身痛逐瘀汤)

Drive Out Stasis from a Painful Body Decoction

shēn tōng zhú yū tāng

SOURCE *Correction of Errors among Physicians* (1830)

Gentianae macrophyllae Radix (qín jiāo) 3g
Chuanxiong Rhizoma (chuān xiōng) 6g
Persicae Semen (táo rén) 9g
Carthami Flos (hóng huā) 9g
Glycyrrhizae Radix (gān cǎo) 6g
Notopterygii Rhizoma seu Radix (qiāng huó) 3g
Myrrha (mò yào) 6g
Angelicae sinensis Radix (dāng guī) 9g
dry-fried Trogopterori Faeces (chǎo wǔ líng zhī) 6g
Cyperi Rhizoma (xiāng fù) 3g
Cyathulae Radix (chuān niú xī) 9g
Pheretima (dì lóng) 6g

Invigorates the blood, promotes the movement of qi, dispels blood stasis, unblocks the collaterals, unblocks painful obstruction, and alleviates pain. For painful obstruction due to the obstruction of qi and blood in the channels and collaterals with such symptoms as shoulder pain, arm pain, lower back pain, leg pain, or other chronic aches and pains of the body. While the principal formula promotes the movement of qi and especially unblocks the flow in the chest and hypochondria, this formula works on the entire body, which makes it particularly useful in treating painful obstruction of the extremities and joints. The source text notes that this formula is often effective when conventional formulas for treating painful obstruction have failed.

癲狂夢醒湯 (癫狂梦醒汤)

Decoction to Wake from the Nightmare of Insanity

diān kuáng mèng xǐng tāng

SOURCE *Correction of Errors among Physicians* (1830)

Persicae Semen (táo rén) 24g
Bupleuri Radix (chái hú) 9g
Cyperi Rhizoma (xiāng fù) 6g
Akebiae Caulis (mù tōng) 6g
Paeoniae Radix rubra (chì sháo) 9g
Pinelliae Rhizoma praeparatum (zhì bàn xià) 6g
Arecae Pericarpium (dà fù pí) 9g
Citri reticulatae viride Pericarpium (qīng pí) 6g
Citri reticulatae Pericarpium (chén pí) 9g
Mori Cortex (sāng bái pí) 9g
Perillae Fructus (zǐ sū zǐ) 12g
Glycyrrhizae Radix (gān cǎo) 6g

Decoction. Invigorates the blood, transforms stasis, regulates the qi, and transforms phlegm. For qi stagnation and blood stasis complicated by phlegm obstruction manifesting as mania that persists for an extended period of time, agitation, restlessness, incoherent speech, and constant anger. If severe, the condition will manifest like a yang brightness excess pattern with a fondness for climbing up to high places, singing, and taking off one's clothes, and a great variety of other odd and bizarre behaviors. There will also be obvious symptoms of blood stasis such as a dark complexion, pain and fullness of the chest and flanks, headache, palpitations, a purple tongue, or stasis spots on the tongue body, and a wiry and fine, or a rough and fine pulse. In contrast to the principal formula, where stasis of blood constrains the ministerial fire causing symptoms of heat, here the qi stagnation causes accumulation of fluids, which transform into phlegm and obstruct the blood.

補陽還五湯 (补阳还五汤)

Tonify the Yang to Restore Five [-Tenths] Decoction

bǔ yáng huán wǔ tāng

'Five' refers to five-tenths of the body's primal or yang qi, which the author of the formula, Wang Qing-Ren, believed was lost when one suffered hemiplegia.

Source *Correction of Errors among Physicians* (1830)

Astragali Radix (huáng qí) 120g
Angelicae sinensis Radix (dāng guī) 6g
Chuanxiong Rhizoma (chuān xiōng) 3g
Paeoniae Radix rubra (chì sháo) 4.5g
Persicae Semen (táo rén) 3g
Carthami Flos (hóng huā) 3g
Pheretima (dì lóng) 3g

Method of Preparation Decoction. This formula calls for the use of the branch-roots of Angelicae sinensis radicis Cauda (dāng guī wěi), which have a stronger blood-invigorating action than other parts of the plant.

Actions Tonifies the qi, invigorates the blood, and unblocks the channels

Indications

Sequelae of wind-stroke including hemiplegia, paralysis, and atrophy of the lower limbs, facial paralysis, slurred speech, drooling, dry stools, urinary frequency or incontinence, a white tongue coating, and a moderate pulse. The source text also prescribes the formula for atrophy disorders with the same underlying mechanism.

This is qi deficiency leading to blood stasis obstructing the channels. This impairs the movement of qi and the provision of nourishment by the blood. The sinews, blood vessels, muscles, and flesh are thereby deprived of nourishment, which manifests as hemiplegia, paralysis, and atrophy of the lower limbs, and facial paralysis. The deficiency of qi and stasis of blood likewise deprive the tongue of its nourishment and strength, which manifests as slurred speech and drooling. Deficiency of yang qi inhibits the descent of the Stomach qi and obstructs the qi of the yang organs. This results in the passage of dry stools because of the extended transit time through the yang organs and thus the increased absorption of fluids from the stool. And because it is the transforming function of qi that stabilizes and retains the fluids, the deficiency of qi also accounts for the urinary frequency or incontinence. The white tongue coating and moderate pulse are indicative of qi deficiency. Atrophy disorder characterized by weakness or flaccidity of the muscles can be due to the same pathodynamic.

Analysis of Formula

When qi deficiency is the cause of blood stasis, deficiency is the root and excess is the branch of the disorder. In such cases, simply tonifying the qi will not fully eliminate the stasis of blood. Accordingly, this formula strongly tonifies the qi, while relying on a smaller dosage of ingredients that invigorate the blood to dispel the stasis in the vessels and collaterals. This approach eliminates blood stasis without injuring the normal qi. The chief ingredient is Astragali Radix *(huáng qí)*, which strongly tonifies the primal qi. The dosage of this herb is five times as much as that of all the other herbs added together. This indicates that tonifying the qi is the clear priority in treating this pattern.

All of the other herbs focus on the blood. Angelicae sinensis radicis Cauda *(dāng guī wěi)*, Chuanxiong Rhizoma *(chuān xiōng)*, and Paeoniae Radix rubra *(chì sháo)* invigorate the blood and harmonize the nutritive qi. Because they tonify as well as move, they serve as deputies in the formula. The assistants, Persicae Semen *(táo rén)*, Carthami Flos *(hóng huā)*, and Pheretima *(dì lóng)*, invigorate the blood, dispel blood stasis, and unblock the channels. Pheretima *(dì lóng)* is especially useful for unblocking and invigorating the channels and collaterals. In concert with Astragali Radix *(huáng qí)*, it moves the qi throughout the body.

Cautions and Contraindications

Because this formula breaks up and eliminates blood stasis, it is contraindicated immediately after a stroke when the cause is cerebral hemorrhage. Until the etiology is established and cerebral hemorrhage has been ruled out, one should refrain from using this formula.

The contemporary physician Zhang Xi-Chun argues that the formula should only be used if the pulse is empty and forceless. It is therefore contraindicated in wind-stroke patients who have a big and forceful, or firm, wiry, and forceful pulse, or in cases of yin deficiency and hot blood, or during pregnancy.

Before using this formula one must be sure that the patient has regained clear consciousness, the body temperature is normal, there is no hemorrhage, and the pulse is moderate. Herbal therapy may be required long-term, as its effects are generally slow and incremental.

Commentary

This formula is another example of Wang Qing-Ren's approach to the treatment of disease based on his revision of classical anatomy and physiology, discussed above in the COMMENTARY to Drive Out Stasis from the Mansion of Blood Decoction *(xuè fǔ zhú yū tāng)*. As explained there, Wang focused on the interaction of qi and blood as the key to treating any disorder. Tonify the Yang to Restore Five-Tenths Decoction *(bǔ yáng huán wǔ tāng)* applies this approach to the treatment of hemiplegia, paralysis, atrophy disorders, and similar symptoms.

Wang Qing-Ren's Conception of Hemiplegia

Previous generations of physicians had attributed hemiplegia to wind-stroke. This was thought to be caused either by wind entering into the vessels, collaterals, and ultimately organs from without—the so-called 'true wind-stroke' (真中風 *zhēn zhòng fēng*)—or by internal wind due to heat, yin deficiency, Liver yang excess, or similar pathologies, often accompanied by phlegm—the so-called 'wind-type stroke' (類中風 *lèi zhòng fēng*). Wang rejected these ideas as incompatible with his anatomical studies and declared that the treatment strategies derived from them were not very effective in clinical practice. In his opinion, hemiplegia and paralysis were due to qi deficiency, which deprived the muscles of the nourishment from blood: "When the primal qi is deficient, it no longer reaches into the blood vessels. Without qi, the blood vessels stop [moving blood, which leads to] stasis." In Wang's writings, the primal qi and yang are different terms used to describe the same substance: "Primal qi is fire, fire is primal qi. This fire is the source of life in the human body."

Wang's anatomical findings convinced him that this qi was produced in the 'mansion of qi' (most likely the greater omentum) from which it was distributed throughout the body via the 'protective qi main pipe' (衛總管 *wèi zǒng guǎn*). Running parallel to the 'nutritive qi main pipe' (榮總管 *róng zǒng guǎn*), qi moved the blood while blood was the substance on which qi acted by means of its warmth and dynamic. That these structures branched symmetrically into smaller vessels that supplied both sides of the body convinced Wang that hemiplegia was due to qi deficiency:

> The primal qi is stored in the qi pipes, which distribute it throughout the body with the left and right sides [each] receiving half. [The capacity] of a person to walk, sit, move, or turn depends entirely on this primal qi. If the primal qi is sufficient, [these actions] have power. If it is insufficient, they lack power. If it is cut off, one dies. [If we imagine that a person possesses] ten parts of primal qi and two parts are exhausted so that eight remain, then each side [of the body] gets four parts. [This is still sufficient] for no disease to occur. If five parts are exhausted and five parts remain, then each side of the body only gets two-and-a-half parts. At this stage, even though hemiplegia may not necessarily occur, there will be symptoms of qi exhaustion. However, because it does not hurt or itch, a person may be unaware of it. As soon as the primal qi becomes exhausted, the vessels and collaterals naturally empty. Given these empty spaces, it is unavoidable that the qi will move to merge on one side. If the two-and-a-half parts [of qi] on the right side move toward the left, the right side will have no qi. Conversely, if the two-and-a-half parts [of qi] on the left side move toward the right, the left side will have no qi. If there is no qi, one cannot move. Being unable to move is called hemiplegia.

Wang Qing-Ren gave a similar explanation for paralysis (where the lower part of the body is deprived of qi) and the other symptoms for which this formula is indicated.

Connections to the Tradition

The appropriate therapeutic strategy here is to tonify the qi and invigorate the blood. The very large dosage of Astragali Radix (*huáng qí*) used for this purpose demonstrates that Wang, despite positioning himself as a radical innovator, in this case used an approach that is deeply rooted in tradition. As Zhang Xi-Chun noted in his comment on this formula in *Essays on Medicine Esteeming the Chinese and Respecting the Western*, "This formula uses 120g of Astragali Radix (*huáng qí*) to harshly tonify the qi aspect. This is [based] on Li Dong-Yuan's doctrine regarding the importance of qi."

The use of Astragali Radix (*huáng qí*) for hemiplegia and similar disorders goes back at least to the 17th-century text, *Indispensable Tools for Pattern Treatment*. In this work, Wang Ken-Tang observed:

> Although there are many causes for sudden falling and hemiplegia patterns, there is none that is not due to the failure of the true qi to circulate [as it should]. Therefore, Astragali Radix (*huáng qí*) is the chief herb that must be employed [in treating such patterns]. Saposhnikoviae Radix (*fáng fēng*) must be used as deputy. Astragali Radix (*huáng qí*) supports the true qi, while Saposhnikoviae Radix (*fáng fēng*) transports the support of true qi by Astragali Radix (*huáng qí*) around the entire body. It also has the power to treat wind.

Wang Qing-Ren borrowed this strategy without acknowledging its source. In his instructions regarding the use of Tonify the Yang to Restore Five[-Tenths] Decoction (*bǔ yáng huán wǔ tāng*), Wang recommends that in the early stages of hemiplegia, it may be useful to add Saposhnikoviae Radix (*fáng fēng*) for up to five days. He also recommends to gradually increase the dosage of Astragali Radix (*huáng qí*) over a number of days. Most often, therefore, contemporary physicians begin with a dosage of 30-60g or even lower, and increase this until they achieve the desired effect. Wang also admonishes that once the symptoms have disappeared, one must continue taking the formula once or twice a week in order to ensure that the symptoms do not recur.

If the use of Astragali Radix (*huáng qí*) is borrowed from Wang Ken-Tang, the relative dosage of qi and blood herbs in Wang Qing-Ren's formulas reflects the influence of Li Shi-Zhen. In *Comprehensive Outline of the Materia Medica*, Li had claimed that herbs like Carthami Flos (*hóng huā*) and Persicae Semen (*táo rén*) "invigorate the blood [when used] in small doses, but break up blood [stasis when used] in large doses." Thus, formulas such as Drive Out Stasis from the Mansion of Blood Decoction (*xuè fǔ zhú yū tāng*) contain large amounts of blood-regulating herbs, while Tonify the Yang to Restore Five [-Tenths] Decoction (*bǔ yáng huán wǔ tāng*) makes do with much smaller amounts. Wang Qing-Ren applied the same principle to his use of qi tonics, which accords with popular sayings such as "Astragali Radix (*huáng qí*) invigorates [the blood] in small doses and tonifies [the qi] in large doses," and "Astragali Radix (*huáng qí*) directs [the qi] upward in small doses, and directs [the blood] downward in large doses."

Modern Usage

In clinical practice, using a large dose of warming, qi-tonifying substances poses a theoretical risk of raising the blood pressure, although this formula is generally not thought to have this effect. Still, some contemporary physicians argue that Gypsum fibrosum (*shí gāo*) and Haematitum (*dài zhě shí*) should be added to this formula to counteract its effect in raising blood pressure. Moreover, modern physicians have expanded its use to a range of conditions not indicated in the source text, including edema due to qi deficiency and blood stasis. For edema, the contemporary writer Chen Chao-Zu recommends combining this formula with True Warrior Decoction (*zhēn wǔ tāng*), discussed in Chapter 16. Other modern uses of the formula are noted in the BIOMEDICAL INDICATIONS below.

Biomedical Indications

With the appropriate presentation, this formula may be used to treat a wide variety of biomedically-defined disorders. These can be divided into the following groups:

- Disorders with weakness or loss of function including poststroke hemiplegia and other sequelae, cerebrovascular disease, sequelae of poliomyelitis, and Bell's palsy

- Neuropsychiatric disorders including a variety of neuralgias, epilepsy, and neuroses

- Vascular diseases including coronary artery disease, hypertension, cor pulmonale, thromboangiitis obliterans, thrombophlebitis, and varicose veins.

It has also been used for chronic nephritis, diabetes, benign prostatic hypertrophy, and sciatica.

Modifications

- For a predominance of cold, add Aconiti Radix lateralis praeparata (*zhì fù zǐ*).

- For a predominance of Spleen and Stomach deficiency, add Codonopsis Radix (*dǎng shēn*) and Atractylodis macrocephalae Rhizoma (*bái zhú*).

- For profuse sputum, add Pinelliae Rhizoma praeparatum (*zhì bàn xià*) and Bambusae Concretio silicea (*tiān zhú huáng*).

- For marked slurred speech, add Acori tatarinowii Rhizoma (*shí chāng pú*) and Polygalae Radix (*yuǎn zhì*).

- For pronounced facial paralysis, add Typhonii Rhizoma praeparatum (*zhì bái fù zǐ*), Bombyx batryticatus (*bái jiāng cán*), and Scorpio (*quán xiē*).

- For mild, chronic hemiplegia, add Hirudo (*shuǐ zhì*) and Tabanus (*méng chóng*).

- To focus the treatment on paralysis of the lower extremities, add Eucommiae Cortex (*dù zhòng*) and Achyranthis bidentatae Radix (*niú xī*).

- For epigastric focal distention and labored breathing, add Linderae Radix (*wū yào*) and Citri reticulatae viride Pericarpium (*qīng pí*).

- For reduced appetite and a stifling sensation in the chest, add Aurantii Fructus (*zhǐ ké*) and Citri reticulatae Pericarpium (*chén pí*).

- For a wiry, deficient, and rapid pulse with irritability and insomnia, add Gardeniae Fructus (*zhī zǐ*) and dry-fried Ziziphi spinosae Semen (*chǎo suān zǎo rén*).

Associated Formula

舒經活血湯 （舒经活血汤）

Relax the Channels and Invigorate the Blood Decoction

shū jīng huó xuè tāng

SOURCE *Restoration of Health from the Myriad Diseases* (1587)

Paeoniae Radix alba (*bái sháo*) 4.5g
Angelicae sinensis Radix (*dāng guī*) 3.6g
Chuanxiong Rhizoma (*chuān xiōng*) 1.8g
Rehmanniae Radix (*shēng dì huáng*) 3g

Persicae Semen (*táo rén*) 3g
Atractylodis Rhizoma (*cāng zhú*) 3g
Poria (*fú líng*) 2.1g
Achyranthis bidentatae Radix (*niú xī*) 3g
Clematidis Radix (*wēi líng xiān*) 3g
Stephaniae tetrandrae Radix (*hàn fáng jǐ*) 1.8g
Notopterygii Rhizoma seu Radix (*qiāng huó*) 1.8g
Saposhnikoviae Radix (*fáng fēng*) 1.8g
Gentianae Radix (*lóng dǎn cǎo*) 1.8g
Angelicae dahuricae Radix (*bái zhǐ*) .1.8g
Citri reticulatae Pericarpium (*chén pí*) 3g
Glycyrrhizae Radix (*gān cǎo*) 1.2g

Take as a decoction with the addition of 3 pieces of Zingiberis Rhizoma recens (*shēng jiāng*). Unblocks and relaxes the channels and invigorates the blood. For blood stasis and wind-dampness in the channels and collaterals characterized by muscle aches, joint pain, radiating pain in the leg, numbness in the lower extremities, and pain in the trunk and extremities. In contrast to the principal formula, which is indicated for deficiency, this formula is indicated for disorders that are predominantly excessive in nature.

Comparison

> Vs. BONESETTER'S PURPLE-GOLD SPECIAL PILL (*zhèng gǔ zǐ jīn dān*); see PAGE 575

復元活血湯 （复元活血汤）

Revive Health by Invigorating the Blood Decoction

fù yuán huó xuè tāng

This formula invigorates the blood and dispels blood stasis as a means of generating new blood and thereby reviving the health of the patient. This is expressed in *Convenient Reader of Established Formulas*: "[This formula] gets rid of what one should be rid of, and generates what should be generated. Thus, the pain is naturally soothed and health is naturally revived."

Source   *Illumination of Medicine* (Jin dynasty)

Angelicae sinensis Radix (*dāng guī*) 9g
Persicae Semen (*táo rén*) . . . . 50 pieces (9-15g)
Carthami Flos (*hóng huā*) 6g
prepared Manitis Squama (*páo shān jiǎ*) 6g
wine-prepared Rhei Radix et Rhizoma (*jiǔ zhì dà huáng*) 30g
Trichosanthis Radix (*tiān huā fěn*) 9g
Bupleuri Radix (*chái hú*) 15g
Glycyrrhizae Radix (*gān cǎo*) 6g

Method of Preparation   The source text advises to coarsely grind the herbs and take 30g as a draft in a mixture of three parts water and one part wine. Strain the decoction before consuming, and take warm before meals. At present, it is usually prepared as a decoction. Loose stools following administration of the formula is regarded as a positive sign. Once loose stools and a diminution of the pain have occurred, one should not take any more of the formula.

Actions   Invigorates the blood, dispels blood stasis, spreads the Liver qi, and unblocks the channels

Indications

Excruciating pain associated with traumatic injury, especially in the chest, hypochondria, or flanks.

This is traumatic physical injury that results in blood leaving the vessels. The overflow of blood from the vessels remains localized and forms an internal obstruction, which causes pain. This formula is primarily used in treating such pain in the chest, hypochondria, or flanks, which are traversed by the Liver and Gallbladder channels. In addition, because the Liver stores the blood, it should be treated irrespective of which channel is injured and causes blood stasis. The impairment of circulation in the hypochondria and flanks due to the stasis of blood in turn causes the qi to stagnate. This combination of severe blood stasis and qi stagnation results in excruciating pain.

Analysis of Formula

Among the chief ingredients are Angelicae sinensis Radix *(dāng guī)*, Persicae Semen *(táo rén)*, Carthami Flos *(hóng huā)*, and Manitis Squama *(chuān shān jiǎ)*. All are very effective for invigorating the blood, dispelling blood stasis, reducing swelling, alleviating pain, and unblocking the channels. Manitis Squama *(chuān shān jiǎ)* is particularly effective in breaking up stasis of blood and unblocking the channels. The last of the chief ingredients, Rhei Radix et Rhizoma *(dà huáng)*, is treated with wine to enhance its three-fold action in treating this condition: (1) to cleanse the coagulation of static and decayed blood downward, pushing out the stale blood to make way for the new; (2) to strengthen the actions of the chief ingredients in invigorating the blood and dispelling blood stasis; and (3) to relax the middle burner and direct the qi downward in order to assist in unblocking the ascending and descending movements in the thorax that remove the constrained qi and stasis of blood. Treating this herb with wine and decocting it together with the other ingredients reduces its purgative action.

The deputy, Trichosanthis Radix *(tiān huā fěn)*, is described in various classical materia medica as able to treat traumatic physical injury because of its ability to promote the growth of new tissue and reduce swelling. In its dual capacity as an assistant ingredient, it enters the blood level and helps reduce the stasis of blood and disperse the accumulations that cause swelling. It also clears heat and moistens dryness, both of which may result from the chronic constraint of qi and blood. Another assistant, Bupleuri Radix *(chái hú)*, spreads the Liver qi, promotes the movement of qi, and guides the other herbs into the Liver channel in order to treat pain and distention in the chest, hypochondria, or flanks. With Rhei Radix et Rhizoma *(dà huáng)*, this combination provides one ascending and one descending herb in order to restore the functional activities of qi. The envoy, Glycyrrhizae Radix *(gān cǎo)*, relaxes spasms and alleviates pain, and regulates and harmonizes the functions of the other ingredients.

Cautions and Contraindications

Contraindicated during pregnancy. If administering this formula leads to diarrhea without a complete cure, one should switch to a different formula.

Commentary

This formula was composed by Li Dong-Yuan to treat severe pain in the flanks caused by injury from falling from a height. Since then, it has become established as one of the most important formulas for the treatment of traumatic injury. Its use is indicated under the following conditions: the problem must be due to trauma; the pain must be in the chest, hypochondria, or flanks; and the pathology must be one of blood stasis, that is, the pain should be fixed and should increase with pressure. The pulse is usually choppy, wiry, and/or submerged.

Controversies

There are various interpretations of the functions and interactions of the ingredients in this formula. For example, some commentators feel that only Rhei Radix et Rhizoma *(dà huáng)* and Persicae Semen *(táo rén)*, which together invigorate the blood and eliminate stasis, should be designated as the chief ingredients. In this view, the relatively large dosage of Rhei Radix et Rhizoma *(dà huáng)* signals its primary role in moving the blood, while Angelicae sinensis Radix *(dāng guī)*, Carthami Flos *(hóng huā)*, and Manitis Squama *(chuān shān jiǎ)* merely assist the two chief ingredients in performing these functions. Others believe that Bupleuri Radix *(chái hú)* and Angelicae sinensis Radix *(dāng guī)*, or Rhei Radix et Rhizoma *(dà huáng)* and Bupleuri Radix *(chái hú)*, should be regarded as the chief ingredients. Yet another opinion holds that the sole purpose of Bupleuri Radix *(chái hú)* is to guide the other herbs into the Liver channel, rather than to spread the Liver qi itself. The analysis above follows that of Fei Bo-Xiong in *Discussion of Medical Formulas*:

> The primary strategy for treating traumatic injury is to break up [blood] stasis. The second [most important] strategy is to move the qi, followed by generating new [blood and tissue]. This formula is especially fine because it adds one or two herbs that move the qi.

Usage

Contemporary physicians have expanded the use of this formula to treat severe pain not directly caused by trauma, but in the area traversed by the Liver and Gallbladder channels, such as headache or postherpetic neuralgia. In combination with Seven-Thousandths of a Tael Powder *(qī lí sǎn)*, it is also used to facilitate the healing of fractures.

Comparisons

➤ Vs. Drive Out Stasis from the Mansion of Blood Decoction (*xuè fǔ zhú yū tāng*)

Both of these formulas treat chest and flank pain due to blood stasis, primarily by invigorating the blood and transforming stasis, and secondarily by moving and regulating the qi. For this reason, the basic structure of their composition is similar, combining herbs that transform and dispel blood stasis with those that unblock the ascending and downward-directing functions of the qi dynamic. Their differences are as follows: Revive Health by Invigorating the Blood Decoction (*fù yuán huó xuè tāng*) strongly dispels stasis and relieves pain in the treatment of traumatic injury or other pathologies that cause blood to accumulate, with a primary focus on the flanks and diaphragmatic area. Drive Out Stasis from the Mansion of Blood Decoction (*xuè fǔ zhú yū tāng*), on the other hand, invigorates the blood and transforms stasis to resolve static blood, with a primary focus on the chest and vessels.

➤ Vs. Seven-Thousandths of a Tael Powder (*qī lí sǎn*); see PAGE 574

Biomedical Indications

With the appropriate presentation, this formula may be used to treat a variety of biomedically-defined disorders including traumatic injury, soft tissue injury, intercostal neuralgia, costochondritis, and acute lower back sprain.

Alternate name

Decoction to Invigorate Blood due to Damage of the Source (*shāng yuán huó xuè tāng*) in *Fine Formulas of Wonderful Efficacy*; Regenerative Powder for Invigorating Blood and Alleviating Pain, (*zài shēng huó xuè zhǐ tòng sǎn*) in *Marvelous Formulas for Traumatic Injuries*; Revive Health Decoction (*fù yuán tāng*) in *Achieving Longevity by Guarding the Source*; Decoction to Revive Health by Unblocking the Qi (*fù yuán tōng qì tāng*) in *Precious Mirror of Patterns and Treatments*; Notopterygium Decoction for Reviving Health (*fù yuán qiāng huó tāng*) in *Medical Formulas Collected and Analyzed*; Tangkuei Decoction for Reviving Health (*dāng guī fù yuán tāng*) in *Six Texts Summarizing the Medicine of Xu Ling-Tai*

Modifications

• For especially intense pain, add Notoginseng Radix (*sān qī*), Olibanum (*rǔ xiāng*), Myrrha (*mò yào*), and Corydalis Rhizoma (*yán hú suǒ*).

• For severe qi stagnation, add Curcumae Radix (*yù jīn*), Citri reticulatae viride Pericarpium (*qīng pí*), and Aurantii Fructus (*zhǐ ké*).

• For constipation, add Natrii Sulfas (*máng xiāo*).

Associated Formula

柴胡細辛湯 (柴胡细辛汤)

Bupleurum and Asarum Decoction

chái hú xì xīn tāng

SOURCE *Lecture Notes on Traditional Chinese Traumatology* (1963)

Bupleuri Radix (*chái hú*) 6g
Asari Radix et Rhizoma (*xì xīn*) 3g
Menthae haplocalycis Herba (*bò hé*) 4.5g
Angelicae sinensis radicis Cauda (*dāng guī wěi*) 9g
Eupolyphaga/Stelophaga (*tǔ biē chóng*) 9g
Salviae miltiorrhizae Radix (*dān shēn*) 9g
Pinelliae Rhizoma praeparatum (*zhì bàn xià*) 4.5g
Chuanxiong Rhizoma (*chuān xiōng*) 9g
Lycopi Herba (*zé lán*) 9g
Coptidis Rhizoma (*huáng lián*) 3g

Decoction. The source text does not list amounts for individual herbs, which are taken from secondary contemporary texts. Dispels stasis, promotes the production of new blood and tissue, regulates and harmonizes ascending and directing downward. This is a modern formula designed specifically for the treatment of concussion, cerebral contusion headache, and similar traumas accompanied by headache, dizziness, and nausea. This is reflected in the formula's composition, which includes light herbs such as Menthae haplocalycis Herba (*bò hé*) and Asari Radix et Rhizoma (*xì xīn*) that dispel wind pathogens and thus help the formula to focus on the head; the diuretic Lycopi Herba (*zé lán*) for the reduction of edematous swellings in the brain and meninges; and the combination of Pinelliae Rhizoma praeparatum (*zhì bàn xià*) and Coptidis Rhizoma (*huáng lián*)—that is, the core of Pinellia Decoction to Drain the Epigastrium (*bàn xià xiè xīn tāng*)—which directs the Stomach qi downward, drains heat, and opens constraint, all of which cause nausea and vomiting.

七厘散

Seven-Thousandths of a Tael Powder

qī lí sǎn

This is a dispersing formula that was originally designed for external application, but which may also be taken internally. Each dose was measured as 'seven-thousandths of a tael,' hence the name.

Source *Collection for the Common Pursuit of Longevity* (1762)

Daemonoropis Resina (*xuè jié*) 30g
Carthami Flos (*hóng huā*) 4.5g
Olibanum (*rǔ xiāng*) 4.5g
Myrrha (*mò yào*) 4.5g
Moschus (*shè xiāng*) 0.36g
Borneolum (*bīng piàn*) 0.36g
Catechu (*ér chá*) 7.5g
floating Cinnabaris (*shuǐ fēi zhū shā*) 3.6g

Method of Preparation Grind the ingredients into a fine powder and store in an airtight container. For internal use, each dose is 0.22-1.5g taken with yellow wine or warm water. For external use, mix with wine and apply to the affected area. Apply externally for bleeding. *Note:* Due to the unacceptable toxicity of Cinnabaris (*zhū shā*), this ingredient should no longer be used.

Actions Invigorates the blood, dispels blood stasis, promotes the movement of qi, reduces swelling, and alleviates pain and bleeding

Indications

Bruising, swelling, and pain accompanying traumatic injuries such as broken bones and torn sinews, and bleeding due to lacerations.

Traumatic injury causes stasis of blood and stagnant qi, which obstructs free movement and produces swelling and pain. If there is injury to the blood vessels, there may also be bleeding.

Analysis of Formula

The chief ingredient, Daemonoropis Resina (*xuè jié*), dispels blood stasis and alleviates pain. Its astringent quality also enables it to stop bleeding. Carthami Flos (*hóng huā*) serves as a deputy by invigorating the blood and dispelling stasis. The remaining ingredients are regarded as assistants. Olibanum (*rǔ xiāng*) and Myrrha (*mò yào*) dispel blood stasis, promote the movement of qi, reduce swelling, and alleviate pain. This combination is particularly effective in promoting the movement of qi and invigorating the blood. The acrid, aromatic properties of Moschus (*shè xiāng*) and Borneolum (*bīng piàn*) eliminate blockage from the channels, assisting those ingredients that invigorate the blood and dispel blood stasis. Catechu (*ér chá*) is a cool, astringent substance that clears heat and assists Daemonoropis Resina (*xuè jié*) in stopping the bleeding and generating new tissue. Because traumatic injury can be startling or frightening, it may cause disorder of the qi and confusion or panic. This is embodied in the adage, "Fright leads to disorder of the qi." For this reason, Cinnabaris (*zhū shā*) is added to relieve the fright and calm the spirit.

Cautions and Contraindications

Because this formula contains ingredients that both move and expel, it may consume the qi and induce abortion. It is therefore contraindicated during pregnancy.

Commentary

The qi and blood are mutually dependent in that qi is the basis for the movement of blood throughout the body. Even with mild traumatic injuries, the movement of qi and blood will be impaired, the channels may be damaged, and the blood may spill out of the blood vessels. This causes the stasis of qi and blood and the resulting swelling and pain. To promote the circulation of blood, it is therefore necessary to move the qi.

This is a very commonly used formula for trauma because of its multifaceted action, which makes it suitable for both external and internal use. Not only does it eliminate blood stasis, promote the movement of qi, reduce swelling, and alleviate pain, it also has the ability to clear heat, help generate new tissue, and stop bleeding. It may be used externally for the pain of blood stasis due to traumatic injury,

to promote the healing of fractures, and with relatively good effect for the bleeding that may occur as a result of traumatic injury. It may also be used for various internal medical disorders that manifest with pain due to blood stasis (such as chest pain), for vomiting of blood, for burns, and for nonspecific toxic swellings.

Comparison

➤ Vs. Revive Health by Invigorating the Blood Decoction (*fù yuán huó xuè tāng*)

Both formulas treat traumatic injury leading to stasis of blood and stagnation of qi. Revive Health by Invigorating the Blood Decoction (*fù yuán huó xuè tāng*) focuses on invigorating the blood, dispelling stasis, dredging the Liver, and unblocking the collaterals. It is indicated for severe pain in areas traversed by the Liver and Gallbladder channels, particularly in the flanks and chest. By contrast, Seven-Thousandths of a Tael Powder (*qī lí sǎn*) stops bleeding and generates the production of new tissue, in addition to invigorating the blood and dispersing stasis. For this reason, it is specific for trauma accompanied by swelling or bleeding. In further contrast to the other formula, it can be used both internally and externally.

Biomedical Indications

With the appropriate presentation, this formula may be used to treat a variety of biomedically-defined disorders including traumatic injury due to falls, fractures, contusions, strains, lacerations, or burns.

Modification

• For injuries that involve fractures, add Notoginseng Radix (*sān qī*), Eupolyphaga/Stelophaga (*tǔ biē chóng*), and Pyritum (*zì rán tóng*).

Associated Formulas

跌打丸

Trauma Pill
diē dǎ wán

Source   *Nationwide Collection of TCM Patent Formulas* (1962)

Angelicae sinensis Radix (*dāng guī*) 30g
Chuanxiong Rhizoma (*chuān xiōng*) 30g
Olibanum (*rǔ xiāng*) 60g
Myrrha (*mò yào*) 30g
Daemonoropis Resina (*xuè jié*). 30g
Eupolyphaga/Stelophaga (*tǔ biē chóng*) 30g
Ephedrae Herba (*má huáng*). 60g
Pyritum (*zì rán tóng*) 30g

Grind the ingredients into a powder and form into pills with honey. Take one or two 3g pills twice daily with wine or warm water. This formula invigorates the blood, transforms blood stasis, harmonizes the nutritive qi, reduces swelling, and alleviates pain. It is for traumatic injuries such as sprain with bruising, swelling, and distended aches and pain at a fixed location.

The presence of blood stasis following a traumatic injury or sprain obstructs the movement of qi and blood in the area of the trauma. This causes local bruising, swelling, and distended aches and pains. The principal formula stops bleeding and generates the production of new tissue in addition to invigorating the blood and dispersing stasis; it is therefore specifically indicated for trauma accompanied by swelling or bleeding. By contrast, Trauma Pill *(diē dǎ wán)* focuses on reducing swelling and alleviating pain by including warmer, acrid herbs that move the protective qi to the surface of the body.

正骨紫金丹
Bone-Setter's Purple-Gold Special Pill

zhèng gǔ zǐ jīn dān

Source *Golden Mirror of the Medical Tradition* (1742)

Caryophylli Flos *(dīng xiāng)* 37.5g
Aucklandiae Radix *(mù xiāng)* .37.5g
Daemonoropis Resina *(xuè jié)* .37.5g
Catechu *(ér chá)* 37.5g
prepared Rhei Radix et Rhizoma *(zhì dà huáng)* 37.5g
Moutan Cortex *(mǔ dān pí)* 18g
Carthami Flos *(hóng huā)* 37.5g
Angelicae sinensis radicis Caput *(dāng guī tóu)* 75g
Nelumbinis Semen *(lián zǐ)* 75g
Poria *(fú líng)* 75g
Paeoniae Radix alba *(bái sháo)* 75g
Glycyrrhizae Radix *(gān cǎo)* 12g

Grind the herbs into a powder and form into honey pills. Take 9g per dose with either yellow wine or Infantis Urina *(tóng biàn)*. This formula invigorates the blood, dispels stasis, moves the qi, and alleviates pain. It is mostly used to treat second- and third-stage trauma. After the swelling and inflammation of the first stage of trauma have decreased, stasis is a main theme, both due to the trauma itself and to the inactivity that is typical during recovery. The second stage is characterized by a yellow-purple color and pain and stiffness in the affected area. After time, the site of the trauma is susceptible to invasion by wind, dampness, and cold, which may combine with the deficiency and stasis in the area. This is third-stage trauma; it presents as painful obstruction.

This formula's dispersing actions make room for the regenerated tissue, known as 'expelling the old to engender the new.' The formula does not have a strong ability to dispel wind-dampness or to expel cold. If signs of wind-dampness such as aching and stiffness appear, or if the condition is aggravated by cold and relieved by warmth, treatment will be enhanced with the addition of agents to dispel wind-dampness and expel cold, as noted below.

Cautions and Contraindications

This formula is unsuitable for pregnant women.

Comparison

➢ Vs. Relax the Channels and Invigorate the Blood Decoction *(shū jīng huó xuè tāng)*

Of these two formulas, Bonesetter's Purple-Gold Special Pill

(zhèng gǔ zǐ jīn dān) is better able to support the normal qi to encourage healing, particularly in second-stage trauma where stagnation from wind, dampness, and cold are less of a factor. For third-stage trauma where painful obstruction is prominent, Relax the Channels and Invigorate the Blood Decoction *(shū jīng huó xuè tāng)* is often a better choice because it contains more agents to dispel wind-dampness.

Modifications

- To enhance the ability to heal traumatized bones and sinews, add Pyritum *(zì rán tóng)*, Dipsaci Radix *(xù duàn)*, and Eucommiae Cortex *(dù zhòng)*.
- For more significant pain, add Olibanum *(rǔ xiāng)* and Myrrha *(mò yào)*.
- For persistent heat and swelling, add Forsythiae Fructus *(lián qiáo)*, Taraxaci Herba *(pú gōng yīng)*, and Paeoniae Radix rubra *(chì sháo)*.
- For aching and stiffness, or conditions that are aggravated by exposure to wind or dampness, add agents to dispel wind-dampness such as Clematidis Radix *(wēi líng xiān)* and Acanthopanacis Cortex *(wǔ jiā pí)*.
- For cold in the channels, add Cinnamomi Cortex *(ròu guì)*, Aconiti Radix lateralis praeparata *(zhì fù zǐ)*, or Cinnamomi Ramulus *(guì zhī)*.

旋覆花湯 (旋覆花汤)
Inula Decoction

xuán fù huā tāng

Source *Essentials from the Golden Cabinet* (c. 220)

Inulae Flos *(xuán fù huā)* 9g
Allii fistulosi Bulbus *(cōng bái)* . . . . .14 stalks
New crimson *(xīn jiàng)* . . . . small amount

Method of Preparation Decoction. For a brief discussion of the meaning of 新絳 *xīn jiàng*, literally 'new crimson,' see the COMMENTARY below. At present, the most common understanding is that it refers to Rubiae Radix *(qiàn cǎo gēn)* with a dosage of 6-9g.

Actions Unblocks the yang, expands the chest, dredges stasis, and transforms clumps

Indications

A sensation of fullness, distention, or even pain in the chest that is improved with massage. When nonsymptomatic, the patient prefers to drink warm beverages. The pulse is wiry and large. The formula is also used to treat uterine bleeding during the second half of pregnancy.

This is Liver fixation (肝著 *gān zhuó*), a pattern first discussed in Chapter 11 of *Essentials from the Golden Cabinet*. The root of this disorder is obstruction of the qi dynamic in the chest. This prevents qi from entering into the blood, causing it to become constrained in the collaterals. Obstruction of qi in the chest is experienced as a sensation of fullness, distention, or even pain. The source text notes that this feeling makes the patient want to have their chest stepped on (i.e., that it improves with pressure or massage). This feeling is not constant, and when nonsymptomatic, the patient will show a preference for warm beverages. This indicates that even though the obstruction manifests at the blood level, its root is at the qi level, and more specifically that it is due to yang constraint. The pulse is wiry, indicating stagnation, and large, indicating that this is a channel-level problem, not an organ-level problem.

Uterine bleeding in the second half of pregnancy due to blood stasis (rather than deficiency) occurs when a woman's qi is unable to move the increasing amount of yin fluids and blood that are accumulating in her body. Such patterns can also be treated with this formula.

Analysis of Formula

This formula treats relatively superficial blood stasis lodged in the collaterals by invigorating the blood, moving the qi, and warming the yang. The chief herb is warming and slightly salty Inulae Flos (xuán fù huā). Although it is a flower and therefore light in nature, it is able to direct the qi downward. Here it is used to unblock the collaterals, facilitating the downward flow of qi and blood that have accumulated in the chest. Acrid and warming Allii fistulosi Bulbus (cōng bái) serves as a deputy. Its fragrance transforms turbidity and opens painful obstruction, and it is a specific herb for unblocking the yang qi and dispersing clumping in the collaterals. Rubiae Radix (qiàn cǎo gēn) enters the Liver channel to invigorate the blood and transform stasis. It serves as both assistant and envoy, focusing the action of the qi-moving herbs on the blood level, thereby enabling the formula to achieve its objectives of unblocking the collaterals and opening the qi dynamic. When the formula is used to treat uterine bleeding, the ability of the herb to invigorate the blood while also stopping bleeding is also drawn upon.

Commentary

This formula treats a very distinctive pattern where the movement of blood from the chest to the lower burner has become blocked. The underlying pathodynamic is described in a useful, if anachronistic, manner by Tang Zong-Hai in *Discussion of Blood Patterns*:

> The Liver governs the blood. Liver fixation is [a pattern] where the blood becomes sticky because it is not dispersed. The blood is generated in the Heart and comes together in the Liver. From the membranous separation in the anterior chest, it descends into the Womb. Presently, it has become fixed in this membrane in the anterior chest. Therefore, the person [suffering from this pattern] feels like having his chest stepped on in order to unblock it.

Tang Zong-Hai was strongly influenced by Wang Qing-Ren. He thus uses Wang's concept of the mansion of blood from the early 19th century—discussed above in the COMMENTARY to Drive Out Stasis from the Mansion of Blood Decoction (xuè fǔ zhú yū tāng)—to explain a formula from the late Han period, whose author, Zhang Zhong-Jing, most certainly did *not* conceive of a membrane in the chest that stored the blood. Nevertheless, his analysis does capture the essence of the pathodynamic and helps to differentiate this pattern from the one for which Wang Qing-Ren's formula is indicated (see COMPARISONS below).

Clinically, this formula is useful for treating any pattern characterized by blood stasis affecting the Liver and related organs (including the Womb or sea of blood) due to stagnation of qi in the chest. This stagnation may be due to internal causes (including sadness or overexertion) or arise from externally-contracted pathogens, such as cold or dampness, that transform into phlegm and obstruct the yang qi in the chest. Other physicians use the formula to treat patterns where the Liver assails the Lungs, that is, where coughing is viewed as arising from Liver constraint. The famous Qing-dynasty physician Ye Tian-Shi used this formula as a model for treating blood stasis in the collaterals, drawing inspiration from its combination of acrid, warming herbs that do not dry the blood. In Ye's view, stasis in the collaterals leads to very chronic conditions that do not respond well to formulas that forcefully break up or dispel stasis, as over time the desiccated blood becomes increasingly dry. Such conditions therefore require an approach that softens as well as moves and dispels, and that, above all, does not induce further dryness. This formula provides just such a strategy, to which other herbs can be added depending on the nature and location of the stasis.

New Crimson (新絳 xīn jiàng)

There has been some controversy about the nature of new crimson (新絳 xīn jiàng). This appears to have been cloth-dyed with a red liquid derived from various herbs. The 5th-century writer Tao Hong-Jing claims that it is Rubiae Radix (qiàn cǎo gēn) and most modern commentators have followed his interpretation. Others think the dye was produced from Rubiae Radix (qiàn cǎo gēn), Sappan Lignum (sū mù), and Croci Stigma (fān hóng huā) and therefore believe that any of these herbs can be used here, as well as Carthami Flos (hóng huā). Ye Tian-Shi often added herbs such as Angelicae sinensis Radix (dāng guī), Salviae miltiorrhizae Radix (dān shēn), or Persicae Semen (táo rén) to prescriptions based on this formula. All of these substitutions can be considered in clinical practice.

Comparisons

➤ Vs. Drive Out Stasis from the Mansion of Blood Decoction (xuè fǔ zhú yū tāng)

Both formulas treat blood stasis in the area of the chest. However, Drive Out Stasis from the Mansion of Blood Decoction (*xuè fǔ zhú yū tāng*) treats a pattern where blood stasis causes qi stagnation. This is reflected in symptoms of heat (e.g., fever, restlessness, agitation, a hot body) caused by constraint of the yang qi. Inula Decoction (*xuán fù huā tāng*), on the other hand, treats a pattern where a relative deficiency of yang qi leads to blood stasis. This is reflected in a desire for warm beverages and an absence of heat signs. Furthermore, because blood stasis is the root and qi stagnation the branch, the blood stasis symptoms will be relatively more severe and pronounced in Drive Out Stasis from the Mansion of Blood Decoction (*xuè fǔ zhú yū tāng*) patterns, but have an on-again, off-again quality in patterns for which Inula Decoction (*xuán fù huā tāng*) is indicated.

➤ Vs. Unblock the Orifices and Invigorate the Blood Decoction (*tōng qiào huó xuè tāng*)

Both formula treat blood stasis in the collaterals and use Allii fistulosi Bulbus (*cōng bái*) to unblock the yang. However, Unblock the Orifices and Invigorate the Blood Decoction (*tōng qiào huó xuè tāng*) treats patterns where blood stasis is primary and relatively more severe. For this reason, it uses a larger number of medicinals that break up blood stasis. Furthermore, whereas Inula Decoction (*xuán fù huā tāng*) focuses on directing the blood downward and on symptoms in the chest and uterus, Unblock the Orifices and Invigorate the Blood Decoction (*tōng qiào huó xuè tāng*) is especially indicated for treating symptoms in the upper body and head.

Biomedical Indications

With the appropriate presentation, this formula may be used to treat a variety of biomedically-defined disorders including chronic or persistent hepatitis, cirrhosis, coronary artery disease, cor pulmonare, and threatened abortion.

Modifications

- For coughing of blood, add Agrimoniae Herba (*xiān hè cǎo*), Asini Corii Colla (*ē jiāo*), Notoginseng Radix (*sān qī*), and Bletillae Rhizoma (*bái jí*).
- For nausea and vomiting, add Bambusae Caulis in taeniam (*zhú rú*) and Phragmitis Rhizoma (*lú gēn*).
- For pain and distention, add Curcumae Radix (*yù jīn*), Citri reticulatae Vascular (*jú luò*), Linderae Radix (*wū yào*), Aspongopus (*jiǔ xiāng chóng*), and Arecae Semen (*bīng láng*).
- For cold obstructing the qi of the chest and preventing the yang from rising, add Pinelliae Rhizoma praeparatum (*zhì bàn xià*) and Allii macrostemi Bulbus (*xiè bái*).
- For long-term constraint transforming into heat, add Trichosanthis Pericarpium (*guā lóu pí*) and Houttuyniae Herba (*yú xīng cǎo*).

溫經湯 （温经汤）

Flow-Warming Decoction

wēn jīng tāng

This formula treats disorders related to menstruation using warming herbs as the chief ingredients. In this interpretation, the character 經 *jīng* refers to the expression 月經 *yuè jīng* (lit. 'monthly flow'), hence the name. Another interpretation is that the character 經 *jīng* does not refer to the menses, but to the extraordinary vessels, particularly the Conception and Penetrating vessels. The formula adjusts the function of these vessels, again using a warming strategy. For a more in-depth analysis of this question, see the COMMENTARY below.

Source   *Essentials from the Golden Cabinet* (c. 220)

Evodiae Fructus (*wú zhū yú*) 9g
Cinnamomi Ramulus (*guì zhī*) 6g
Angelicae sinensis Radix (*dāng guī*) .6g
Chuanxiong Rhizoma (*chuān xiōng*) .6g
Paeoniae Radix (*sháo yào*) 6g
Asini Corii Colla (*ē jiāo*)
  [dissolve in the strained decoction] 6g
Ophiopogonis Radix (*mài mén dōng*) 9g
Moutan Cortex (*mǔ dān pí*) 6g
Ginseng Radix (*rén shēn*) 6g
Glycyrrhizae Radix (*gān cǎo*) 6g
Zingiberis Rhizoma recens (*shēng jiāng*) 6g
Pinelliae Rhizoma praeparatum (*zhì bàn xià*) 6g

Method of Preparation   Decoction. At present, Paeoniae Radix alba (*bái sháo*) is the form of Paeoniae Radix (*sháo yào*) that is generally used, and Codonopsis Radix (*dǎng shēn*) is usually substituted for Ginseng Radix (*rén shēn*) at 2-3 times its dosage.

Actions   Warms the vessels, dispels cold, nourishes the blood, and dispels blood stasis

Indications

Mild, persistent uterine bleeding, irregular menstruation (either early or late), extended or continuous menstrual flow, bleeding between periods, pain, distention, and cold in the lower abdomen, infertility, dry lips and mouth, low-grade fever at dusk, and warm palms and soles. The tongue body may be purplish, and the pulse fine and rough. This formula is also used to treat infertility in women.

This is deficiency and cold of the Conception and Penetrating vessels together with obstruction due to the stasis of blood. The Penetrating vessel is the sea of blood, and the Conception vessel is responsible for the well-being of the fetus. Both of these channels begin in the lower abdomen and have a very strong relationship to the menses. When the vessels are deficient and cold, the blood becomes static and the qi stagnates. This manifests as mild, persistent uterine bleeding, irregular menstruation (either early or late), extended or continuous menstrual flow, bleeding between periods, lower abdominal pain, distention, cold, and infertility. When the stasis of blood obstructs the channels, the blood cannot remain in its normal pathways, and the Penetrating and Conception vessels become destabilized, causing early menstruation. Cold, stagnant blood can impede the menstrual flow and cause delayed menstruation. When the essence and blood are destabilized due to the inability of deficient qi to govern the blood, the flow will be extended or continuous. And when the Penetrating and Conception vessels are not properly regulated, blood may spill out of the Womb between periods. The purple tongue, as well as the fine and rough pulse, are both indicative of blood stasis. Cold in the Conception and Penetrating vessels leading to stasis of blood is also a common cause of infertility in women.

Perhaps more difficult to understand are those symptoms which are characteristic of heat. These may be due either to deficiency of blood or obstruction. *Classic of Difficulties* (Chapter 22) notes that the blood governs moistening. In this condition, the presence of blood stasis impedes the production of new blood. This results in a lack of moisture in the body, which manifests as dry lips and mouth. The low-grade fever at dusk and warm palms and soles may be attributed to deficiency and stasis of blood. One part of the blood is composed of fluids that are responsible for moistening and cooling. Deficient blood deprives the body of moisture, and the stasis of blood obstructs the dissemination of fluids throughout the body. At the same time, blood stasis also constrains the body's yang qi, giving rise to heat that is particularly noticeable at dusk and during the first part of the night (see the COMMENTARY in the entry for Drive Out Stasis from the Mansion of Blood Decoction *(xuè fǔ zhú yū tāng)* for a detailed explanation).

Analysis of Formula

The principal etiological factors in this pattern are deficiency and cold. However, since the pattern involves elements of both deficiency and excess as well as heat and cold, it is inadvisable to use the method of dispelling blood stasis alone; instead, it should be combined with warming and nourishing. In Chapter 62 of *Basic Questions* there is a discussion of methods for regulating menstruation: "Qi and blood like warmth and have an aversion to cold because cold inhibits circulation and warmth reduces and eliminates [stagnation]." This is the rationale underlying the addition of the strategy of warming the menses and dispelling cold to the strategy of nourishing the blood and dispelling blood stasis. The expectation is that once the blood is warmed it will circulate and that the improved circulation will in turn serve to reduce the obstruction due to stasis. For this reason, the formula combines warming, tonifying, heat-clearing, and blood-invigorating strategies into an organic whole that attends to the various functions and pathologies of the Conception and Penetrating vessels.

The chief herbs are acrid, bitter, and heating Evodiae Fructus *(wú zhū yú)*, which enters the Liver and Kidney channels to disperse cold and stop pain, and acrid, sweet, and warming Cinnamomi Ramulus *(guì zhī)*, which enters the nutritive qi to improve circulation in the blood vessels and disperse cold. Together, these two herbs are extremely effective in treating conditions of blood stasis due to cold. Angelicae sinensis Radix *(dāng guī)* and Chuanxiong Rhizoma *(chuān xiōng)*, and to some extent Paeoniae Radix alba *(bái sháo)*, serve as deputies that invigorate the blood, dispel blood stasis, nourish the blood, and regulate the menses. Angelicae sinensis Radix *(dāng guī)* and Paeoniae Radix alba *(bái sháo)* also function with Asini Corii Colla *(ē jiāo)* and Ophiopogonis Radix *(mài mén dōng)* to nourish the blood, tonify the yin, and regulate the Liver. Of this group, Asini Corii Colla *(ē jiāo)* and Ophiopogonis Radix *(mài mén dōng)* focus on nourishing the yin, moistening dryness, and clearing heat from deficiency. Complementing Evodiae Fructus *(wú zhū yú)* and Cinnamomi Ramulus *(guì zhī)*, they also prevent the warming and drying properties of the chief herbs from damaging the body fluids and blood.

Moutan Cortex *(mǔ dān pí)* both assists the chief herbs in dispelling blood stasis and facilitating the menses, and clears heat from deficiency from the blood level. Ginseng Radix *(rén shēn)*, Glycyrrhizae Radix *(gān cǎo)*, Zingiberis Rhizoma recens *(shēng jiāng)*, and Pinelliae Rhizoma praeparatum *(zhì bàn xià)* tonify the qi and harmonize the Spleen and Stomach to strengthen the source of production and transformation so that yang can produce yin and the blood may be sufficient. Glycyrrhizae Radix *(gān cǎo)* also harmonizes the actions of the various herbs in the formula.

Together, the herbs in this formula warm and unblock the blood vessels by dispelling cold, tonifying and nourishing the blood and qi to stabilize the root of the disorder, moderately dispel blood stasis so that new blood may be produced, and thereby relieve problems of menstrual irregularity and infertility.

Cautions and Contraindications

Contraindicated in cases with abdominal masses due to blood stasis from excess.

Commentary

This formula was originally indicated for the treatment of cold from deficiency of the Penetrating and Conception vessels with internal obstruction due to blood stasis producing mild, persistent uterine bleeding. The etiology was considered to be blood stasis in the aftermath of a miscarriage. The formula has since been used primarily in the treatment of irregular menstruation and infertility.

The distinguishing characteristics of this pattern are symptoms of cold in the lower burner and lower extremities accompanied by warm palms, dry mouth and lips, and low-grade fever at dusk, or up-flushing of heat. Such a presentation is similar to that of yin deficiency, but there are some clear differences. For example, here only the mouth and lips are parched, not the mouth and throat, and there is no desire to drink; in addition, the low-grade fever does not begin in the afternoon, but only at dusk. There are also signs that are totally incompatible with yin deficiency, such as cold in the lower abdomen. This presentation rarely includes abdominal masses; however, should they occur secondary to cold from deficiency, the use of this formula is still appropriate.

Composition

In terms of its composition, this formula can be viewed as a combination of three other formulas by Zhang Zhong-Jing. The first and most fundamental of these is Ass-Hide Gelatin and Mugwort Decoction *(jiāo ài tāng)*, discussed below, which itself served as the model for Four-Substance Decoction *(sì wù tāng)*, discussed in Chapter 8. Because both of these formulas tonify the blood, it can be implied that blood deficiency is the root cause of the present pattern. The other two formulas are Evodia Decoction *(wú zhū yú tāng)*, discussed in Chapter 6, and Ophiopogonis Decoction *(mài mén dōng tāng)*, discussed in Chapter 15. The fact that these two formulas both focus on the leg arm brightness Stomach, that is, the middle burner yang, has led to much discussion among commentators.

Three somewhat different views can be distinguished. The first argues that harmonizing the Stomach and facilitating the transporting functions of the Spleen ensures that the tonifying herbs in the formula do not cause stagnation. A second group of commentators argues that directing the Stomach qi downward by means of Pinelliae Rhizoma praeparatum *(zhì bàn xià)* opens the Penetrating and Conception vessels and thereby regulates the menses. The contemporary physician Wang Mian-Zhi, an expert in formula composition from Beijing, is representative of this view. In *Lecture Notes on Formulas,* Wang explains:

> There exist different explanations regarding Pinelliae Rhizoma praeparatum *(zhì bàn xià)* [in this formula]. Generally speaking, Pinelliae Rhizoma praeparatum *(zhì bàn xià)* harmonizes the Stomach. [However,] in the present case, [its function] must be understood in relation to the vessels. The yang brightness channel and the Penetrating vessel come together at ST-30 (氣衝 *qì chōng*, lit. 'qi thoroughfare'). Therefore, one can say that directing [qi in] the yang brightness downward implies directing the Penetrating and Conception vessels. One aspect [of its function therefore] is to stimulate the Stomach qi, facilitating the qi-tonifying and blood-nourishing herbs to treat deficiency more effectively. At the same time, using Pinelliae Rhizoma praeparatum *(zhì bàn xià)* to unblock the yang brightness and Evodiae Fructus *(wú zhū yú)* to unblock the terminal yin also unblocks the Penetrating and Conception vessels. In this way, one can dispel stasis.

A third view focuses on the ability of these formulas and their ingredients to facilitate fluid metabolism by drying dampness and regulating the qi. This view is linked to another problem of interpretation relating to a passage in the source text, which says that it is indicated for "downward facilitation" (下利 *xià lì*). Because this term is commonly used to mean diarrhea, most commentators think that this is a transcription error, and that the true text must have been "downward bleeding" (下血 *xià xuè*). The contemporary physician Cheng Men-Xue has a somewhat different view, explained in his *Formulas in Verse from the Scholar's Studio in Two Volumes:*

> *Golden Mirror of the Medical Tradition* changed 'downward facilitation' into 'downward bleeding,' and most commentators have followed this. This interpretations also accords with what Zhu Dan-Xi says. Initially, I believed this. However, continuing to think about it, I [became convinced] that 'downward facilitation' actually means 'vaginal discharge' (帶下 *dài xià*). Blood stasis in the lower burner that is not dispelled inhibits the distribution of body fluids and the generation of new blood. Thus, one can use [this formula] for strong vaginal discharge, irregular uterine bleeding that does not stop, or late periods. [According to *Classic of Difficulties*,] disorders of the Conception vessel in women are characterized by vaginal discharge and fixed abdominal masses. When the blood in the Penetrating vessel is blocked and does not move, the essence and yin fluids of the yang brightness diminish and are no longer able to moisten the yin. The Conception vessel governs the gestational membranes [Womb] and fetus, while the Penetrating vessel is the sea of blood. Stasis of blood in the lower abdomen pertains to the Conception and Penetrating vessels. [The fact that] it is listed for vaginal discharges that are really due to blood disorders is the most sublime aspect of this formula by [Zhang] Zhong-Jing. … Arguing that this formula tonifies both the qi and blood, most commentators do not grasp the true intention [of Zhang Zhong-Jing's principles of formula composition]. They do not understand that [Ginseng Radix *(rén shēn)*, Ophiopogonis Radix *(mài mén dōng)*, Pinelliae Rhizoma praeparatum *(zhì bàn xià)*, and Glycyrrhizae Radix *(gān cǎo)*] correspond to Ophiopogonis Decoction *(mài mén dōng tāng)*, which is the principal formula for unblocking and tonifying the yang brightness. The menses exit from the Penetrating vessel, but belong to the yang brightness [in terms of their production]. Therefore, Ophiopogonis Decoction *(mài mén dōng tāng)* is employed here as an assistant in order to treat the root. This intention is even more profound.

Cheng Men-Xue's analysis helps explain the contemporary usage of the formula, which extends to a range of disorders not mentioned in the source text. These include problems associated with dryness, thickening and cracking of the skin or mucous membranes due to the failure of blood to moisten as well as its use in men (see BIOMEDICAL INDICATIONS below). In clinical practice, the following three markers help to differentiate patterns for which this formula is indicated:

- The presence of signs and symptoms indicating blood deficiency and internal cold such as a pale complexion, aversion to cold or cold extremities, loose stools, increased urination, a pale, puffy tongue body, and a thin, forceless pulse

- The presence of heat or dryness signs such as dry and cracked lips or mucous membranes, a dry mouth, hot hands and feet, and feverish sensations, together with the above

- Abdominal fullness or muscle tension, but a generally soft and forceless abdomen.

Furthermore, the formula can be utilized very flexibly in order to match its composition to the complexity of the presenting signs and symptoms. For instance, if blood deficiency is pronounced, the dosage of Angelicae sinensis Radix (*dāng guī*), Paeoniae Radix (*sháo yào*), and Asini Corii Colla (*ē jiāo*) can be increased, and Rehmanniae Radix praeparata (*shú dì huáng*) may be added. If blood stasis is pronounced, the dosage of Chuanxiong Rhizoma (*chuān xiōng*) and Moutan Cortex (*mǔ dān pí*) can be increased, and Persicae Semen (*táo rén*) and Cyperi Rhizoma (*xiāng fù*) added. If cold is pronounced, the dosage of Cinnamomi Ramulus (*guì zhī*), Evodiae Fructus (*wú zhū yú*), and Zingiberis Rhizoma recens (*shēng jiāng*) can be increased. Furthermore, in *Guide to Clinical Usage of Classical Formulas*, the contemporary classical formula expert Liu Du-Zhou suggests increasing the dosage of Ophiopogonis Radix (*mài mén dōng*) in order to enrich the fluids of the Stomach and Intestines, unblock the Lungs and Heart, and reduce potential side effects such as dizziness, irritability, and dry throat arising from the harsh, drying nature of Evodiae Fructus (*wú zhū yú*) in patients with blood deficiency. Finally, if the formula is used to treat dysfunctional uterine bleeding, such bleeding may initially *increase* as the old and static blood is being expelled. This should not be interpreted as a worsening of the condition. If the diagnosis is correct, the bleeding will gradually cease.

Comparisons

➢ Vs. Generating and Transforming Decoction (*shēng huà tāng*); see page 582

➢ Vs. Ass-Hide Gelatin and Mugwort Decoction (*jiāo ài tāng*); see page 612

Biomedical Indications

With the appropriate presentation, this formula may be used to treat a wide variety of biomedically-defined disorders. These can be divided into the following groups:

- Gynecological disorders including dysfunctional uterine bleeding, uterine hypoplasia, endometrial hyperplasia, endometriosis, leiomyoma, dysmenorrhea, amenorrhea, polycystic ovaries, infertility (including blocked uterine tubes), habitual miscarriage, threatened abortion, perimenopausal syndrome, senile vaginitis

- Male urogenital disorders including erectile dysfunction, oligospermia, and benign prostatic hypertrophy.

This formula has also been used in the treatment of hernias, schistosomiasis, eczema, chilblains, psoriasis (particularly of the hands), coronary artery disease, sciatica, rheumatoid arthritis, chronic gastritis, and chronic cholecystitis.

Alternate names

Flow-Regulating Decoction (*tiáo jīng tāng*) in *Straight Direction from [Yang] Ren-Zhai*; Major Flow-Regulating Decoction (*dà wēn jīng tāng*) in *Additions to the Essential Teachings of [Zhu] Dan-Xi*; Minor Flow-Warming Decoction (*xiǎo wēn jīng tāng*) in *Discussions of Blood Patterns*

Modifications

- For more severe lower abdominal cold and pain, remove Ophiopogonis Radix (*mài mén dōng*) and Moutan Cortex (*mǔ dān pí*), add Foeniculi Fructus (*xiǎo huí xiāng*) and Artemisiae argyi Folium (*ài yè*), and substitute Cinnamomi Cortex (*ròu guì*) for Cinnamomi Ramulus (*guì zhī*).

- For more severe qi stagnation, add Cyperi Rhizoma (*xiāng fù*) and Linderae Radix (*wū yào*).

- For mild, persistent uterine bleeding of pale-colored blood, remove Moutan Cortex (*mǔ dān pí*) to reduce the cooling action and add Zingiberis Rhizoma praeparatum (*páo jiāng*), Artemisiae argyi Folium (*ài yè*), and Rehmanniae Radix praeparata (*shú dì huáng*).

- For qi deficiency, add Astragali Radix (*huáng qí*).

- For persistent bleeding after miscarriage, remove Glycyrrhizae Radix (*gān cǎo*) and add Salviae miltiorrhizae Radix (*dān shēn*), Leonuri Herba (*yì mǔ cǎo*), and Achyranthis bidentatae Radix (*niú xī*).

- For chronic endometritis, add Olibanum (*rǔ xiāng*) and Notoginseng Radix (*sān qī*).

Associated Formulas

溫經湯 （温经汤）

Flow-Warming Decoction from *Fine Formulas for Women*
wēn jīng tāng

Source   *Fine Formulas for Women* (1237)

Angelicae sinensis Radix (*dāng guī*)..........................6g
Chuanxiong Rhizoma (*chuān xiōng*)...........................6g
Cinnamomi Cortex (*ròu guì*)...................................6g
vinegar-fried Curcumae Rhizoma (*cù chǎo é zhú*)..............6g
Moutan Cortex (*mǔ dān pí*)...................................6g
Ginseng Radix (*rén shēn*)...................................10g
Achyranthis bidentatae Radix (*niú xī*).....................10g
Glycyrrhizae Radix (*gān cǎo*)..............................10g

Decoction. Warms the channels, tonifies deficiency, transforms stasis, and alleviates pain. For cold with deficiency in the sea of blood characterized by irregular periods, periods that do not flow smoothly, lower abdominal pain, and a submerged, tight pulse. Compared to the principal formula, this variation focuses more strongly on breaking up stasis and less on heat from constraint or deficiency. It is thus more appropriate for cold-type blood stasis characterized by more severe pain.

艾附暖宮丸

Mugwort and Cyperus Pill to Warm the Palace

ài fù nuǎn gōng wán

SOURCE   *Straight Directions from [Yang] Ren-Zhai* (1264)

Artemisiae argyi Folium (*ài yè*) 90g
vinegar-fried Cyperi Rhizoma (*cù chǎo xiāng fù*) 180g
Evodiae Fructus (*wú zhū yú*) 60g
Chuanxiong Rhizoma (*chuān xiōng*) 60g
Wine-fried Paeoniae Radix alba (*jiǔ chǎo bái sháo*) 60g
Astragali Radix (*huáng qí*) 60g
Zanthoxyli Pericarpium (*huā jiāo*) 60g
Dipsaci Radix (*xù duàn*) 45g
wine-fried Rehmanniae Radix (*jiǔ chǎo shēng dì huáng*) 30g
Cinnamomi Cortex (*ròu guì*) 15g

The above ingredients are ground into a fine powder and made into small pills with rice vinegar (to strengthen its blood-invigorating action). The normal dosage is 6g of pills taken before meals with a dilute solution of vinegar. Patients are prohibited from getting angry or ingesting raw or cold substances.

This formula warms the vessels and comforts the Womb while also nourishing and invigorating the blood. It is for cold of the Womb in women with thin vaginal discharge, a sallow and wan complexion, achy limbs, fatigue and lack of strength, reduced appetite, occasional abdominal pain, and infertility. Also for second- or third-trimester pregnancy with a cold, painful sensation in the lower abdomen, abdominal distention, and a pale tongue with a white coating. Compared to the principal formula, this focuses more on warming the vessels and dispelling cold.

生化湯（生化汤）

Generating and Transforming Decoction

shēng huà tāng

The name of this decoction reflects the principle that blood stasis must be transformed before new blood can be generated. This is especially important after birth, as explained by Tang Zong-Hai in *Discussion of Blood Patterns*: "Being able to transform blood stasis is that through which one generates [the new. Therefore, this formula] is often used postpartum." A somewhat different explanation is offered by Lu Mao-Xiu in *Medical Texts from Bettering the World Studio*: "The Heavens are referred to as great. Giving birth (生 *shēng*) is also referred to as a great transformation (大化 *dà huà*). Giving Birth Decoction [the English translation that matches this reading] takes its name from this."

Source   *Fu Qing-Zhu's Women's Disorders* (17th century, published in 1826)

Angelicae sinensis Radix (*dāng guī*) 24g
Chuanxiong Rhizoma (*chuān xiōng*) 9g
Persicae Semen (*táo rén*) . . . . 14 pieces (6-9g)

Zingiberis Rhizoma praeparatum (*páo jiāng*) 1.5g
Glycyrrhizae Radix praeparata (*zhì gān cǎo*) 1.5g

Method of Preparation   The source text advises to prepare as a decoction with a mixture of equal parts of yellow wine and the urine of boys under 12 years of age. At present, it is usually decocted with water, with the optional addition of wine.

Actions   Invigorates the blood, transforms and dispels blood stasis, warms the menses, and alleviates pain

Indications

Retention of the lochia accompanied by cold and pain in the lower abdomen, a pale purple tongue or a pale tongue with purple spots, and a thin, submerged, and choppy pulse.

This pattern is due to cold that takes advantage of the deficiency of normal qi and blood during the postpartum period to enter the abdomen. It is this cold that produces the stasis of blood, such that static blood is retained within the Womb. This manifests as retention of the lochia characterized by discharge of turbid and decaying blood through the vagina. At first, there are small, purple-red clots, and then only the seeping of a dark red fluid.

Cold is a yin pathogenic influence whose nature it is to restrain and contract; blood stasis due to cold from deficiency produces pain and cold in the lower abdomen. The pale, purple tongue or pale tongue with purple spots, and the thin, submerged, and choppy pulse are classic signs of blood stasis due to cold from deficiency.

Analysis of Formula

In the period immediately after childbirth it is almost inevitable that the nutritive qi and blood will be deficient, a condition that requires tonification and nourishment. Here, however, this condition is complicated by abdominal pain due to the stasis of blood. In such cases, a strategy that only tonifies without invigorating the blood cannot hope to eliminate the retained blood, while a strategy that simply disperses the stasis without tonifying will not be conducive to the generation of new blood. That is why this formula combines a strategy of generating new blood while simultaneously transforming blood stasis. This is based on the adage, "If the stasis of blood is not transformed, new blood cannot be generated." If this method is followed, the generation of new blood will not cause further blood stasis, nor will the transformation of stasis injure the nutritive qi. It is therefore an effective approach to this particular pattern of disharmony.

This dual treatment strategy is embodied in the chief herb: acrid, sweet, and warming Angelicae sinensis Radix (*dāng guī*). Used in a large dosage (i.e., 24g), it tonifies and invigorates the blood, transforms blood stasis, and generates new blood. When the blood is abundant, the blood vessels will be full and the circulation of blood will be smooth and unimpeded. This will lead to the dispersal of blood stasis.

Chuanxiong Rhizoma *(chuān xiōng)* invigorates the blood and promotes the movement of qi, while Persicae Semen *(táo rén)* invigorates the blood and dispels stasis. These two herbs serve as the deputies in the formula.

One of the assistants, Zingiberis Rhizoma praeparatum *(páo jiāng),* enters the blood and dispels cold, warms the menses, and alleviates pain. The warm, blood-entering properties of Zingiberis Rhizoma praeparatum *(páo jiāng)* assist Chuanxiong Rhizoma *(chuān xiōng)* and Persicae Semen *(táo rén)* in warming and unblocking blood stasis. This herb also assists Glycyrrhizae Radix praeparata *(zhì gān cǎo)* in warming the middle burner and alleviating pain. The other assistant, yellow wine, helps the other ingredients warm and dispel cold. In its dual role as an envoy, Glycyrrhizae Radix praeparata *(zhì gān cǎo)* also regulates and harmonizes the actions of the other ingredients. The urine of boys under 12 years of age is said to nourish the yin, direct fire downward, and dispel blood stasis. It is therefore useful in treating patterns of blood stasis.

Cautions and Contraindications

Contraindicated in cases with blood stasis due to heat in the blood or postpartum hemorrhage because the warm, blood-invigorating nature of these herbs tends to aggravate such conditions. It is also contraindicated during pregnancy or in cases with bleeding diathesis or any active hemorrhagic disorder. With respect to postpartum use, if there is already normal discharge of lochia and only slight abdominal pain, this formula may be too harsh in its action of breaking up blood stasis and should therefore be modified.

Commentary

This has long been one of the most widely used formulas for postpartum recovery in Chinese medicine. Its composition can be interpreted as a reaction against treatment strategies that had emerged in the Jin-Yuan era. At that time, some physicians, like Zhu Dan-Xi, emphasized tonifying the qi and blood before anything else could be undertaken; others, like Zhang Cong-Zheng, focused exclusively on attacking methods. By combining generation of blood with transformation of stasis, this formula effectively attempted a synthesis.

At present, its composition is widely attributed to the famous Qing-dynasty gynecologist Fu Qing-Zhu, although he was most definitely an important popularizer rather than the original author. Earlier references can be found in Zhang Jie-Bin's *Collected Treatises of [Zhang] Jing-Yue,* however, it is likely that the formula can be traced back to the Song dynasty. Zhang's advice: "Regardless of whether a woman is pregnant or has just given birth, in all cases it is good to take this medicine." He also suggested it could be used to hasten delivery, and for miscellaneous disorders involving qi and blood deficiency and stagnation, internal damage from food, fever, and excessive sweating.

Over time, this became the base formula for almost all postpartum conditions. This included not only cases of retained placenta, but also postpartum convulsions, malarial fevers, and shortness of breath. Indeed, during the 19th century, use of this formula after birth became almost axiomatic, and even those unable to afford a physician prescribed it for themselves or their family members. Wang Shi-Xiong became so alarmed by such overprescribing that he called it "a formula of death." He went on:

> In treating the illnesses of a large number of people, it will certainly be a miraculous method for those whose bodies are cold. But as soon as it is taken by those with blood heat or those who concurrently suffer from warm or hot qi, then in [severe] cases, it will rapidly bring about a warmth disorder, and in [mild] cases, postpartum disorders [that were not there before] will gradually form. And although people will know that these are commonly seen illnesses, they will not know that they arose in large part because of Generating and Transforming Decoction *(shēng huà tāng)* … For several hundred years, women have been harmed by this formula.

Even contemporary Chinese medical textbooks warn against automatically prescribing this formula, suggesting that its appeal has not waned. This means that the formula should not be used unless all three of the key markers are present in the presenting pattern: obstruction due to blood stasis, deficient blood, and cold.

On the other hand, as long as these symptoms are present, it can also be used as a foundational formula for a variety of gynecological problems.

Comparisons

➤ Vs. Flow-Warming Decoction *(wēn jīng tāng)*

Both are important gynecological formulas that can be used in treating postpartum patterns characterized by cold and blood stasis. However, Flow-Warming Decoction *(wēn jīng tāng)* focuses on warming and opening the qi dynamic, and less on breaking up blood stasis. At the same time, it is able to clear heat from constraint. Generating and Transforming Decoction *(shēng huà tāng),* on the other hand, emphasizes unblocking the stasis by means of warming the blood, while also generating new blood. It is thus indicated for more severe signs of blood stasis without heat.

➤ Vs. Sudden Smile Powder *(shī xiào sǎn); see* page 592

Biomedical Indications

With the appropriate presentation, this formula may be used to treat a variety of biomedically-defined disorders including pain from uterine involution, prolonged lochia, retained placenta, bleeding postmiscarriage, ectopic pregnancy, leiomyoma, endometriosis, and infertility.

Modifications

• For postpartum application in which there is already discharge of lochia and only slight abdominal pain, remove Persicae Semen *(táo rén)*.

- For more severe retention of blood and consequently more intense abdominal pain, add Typhae Pollen *(pú huáng)*, Trogopterori Faeces *(wǔ líng zhī)*, and Corydalis Rhizoma *(yán hú suǒ)*.

- For more severe cold characterized by severe cold and pain in the lower abdomen, add Cinnamomi Cortex *(ròu guì)*.

- For feverishness associated with blood stasis, add Moutan Cortex *(mǔ dān pí)* and Paeoniae Radix rubra *(chì sháo)*.

- For marked postpartum qi deficiency with profuse sweating due to loss of blood, add Ginseng Radix *(rén shēn)* and Astragali Radix *(huáng qí)*.

- For failure of the uterus to resume to its normal size postpartum, add Leonuri Herba *(yì mǔ cǎo)*.

Associated Formula

芎歸調血飲 (芎归调血饮)

Chuanxiong and Tangkuei Drink to Regulate the Blood

xiōng guī tiáo xuè yǐn

SOURCE *Restoration of Health from the Myriad Diseases* (1587)

Angelicae sinensis Radix *(dāng guī)* 6-9g
Chuanxiong Rhizoma *(chuān xiōng)* 4.5-9g
Atractylodis macrocephalae Rhizoma *(bái zhú)* 6-9g
Poria *(fú líng)* 6-9g
Rehmanniae Radix praeparata *(shú dì huáng)* 6-9g
Citri reticulatae Pericarpium *(chén pí)* 6-9g
Cyperi Rhizoma *(xiāng fù)* 6-9g
charred Zingiberis Rhizoma *(gān jiāng)* 3-6g
Leonuri Herba *(yì mǔ cǎo)* 6-9g
Moutan Cortex *(mǔ dān pí)* 6-9g
Glycyrrhizae Radix *(gān cǎo)* 3-6g

The source text provides no dosages and instructs to coarsely grind the above ingredients and cook with 1 slice of Zingiberis Rhizoma recens *(shēng jiāng)* and 1 piece of Jujubae Fructus *(dà zǎo)*. The dosages specified above are the editors' suggestions based on similar formulas in the source text.

Tonifies the qi and blood, moves the blood, regulates the qi, and transforms stasis to generate the new. This formula treats a wide variety of postpartum disorders characterized by deficiency of qi and blood and weakened Spleen and Stomach. These include prolonged lochia, excessive postpartum bleeding, puerperal fever, spontaneous sweating, dry mouth, Heart irritability, abdominal pain, flank distention and fullness, dizziness, blurry vision, and tinnitus. In modern-day Japan and Taiwan, the formula is also used in the treatment of menstrual irregularities marked by both deficiency and blood stasis as well as the sequelae of trauma or surgery.

This formula and the principal formula have very similar indications. Chuanxiong and Tangkuei Drink to Regulate the Blood *(xiōng guī tiáo xuè yǐn)* tonifies and regulates both the blood and qi, whereas Generating and Transforming Decoction *(shēng huà tāng)* focuses more on the blood, both by tonifying it and promoting its movement. Chuanxiong and Tangkuei Drink to Regulate the Blood *(xiōng guī tiáo xuè yǐn)* is more appropriate for postpartum patients with blood deficiency and stasis accompanied by middle burner deficiency and qi stagnation.

Modifications

There are approximately thirty sets of modifications listed in the source text. A small selection is provided here:

- For postpartum diarrhea from Spleen deficiency, add Ginseng Radix *(rén shēn)*, Atractylodis Rhizoma *(cāng zhú)*, Magnoliae officinalis Cortex *(hòu pò)*, Amomi Fructus *(shā rén)*, Polyporus *(zhū líng)*, Akebiae Caulis *(mù tōng)*, Arecae Pericarpium *(dà fù pí)*, and dry-fried Paeoniae Radix alba *(chǎo bái sháo)*; and remove Rehmanniae Radix praeparata *(shú dì huáng)*, Chuanxiong Rhizoma *(chuān xiōng)*, Linderae Radix *(wū yào)*, Leonuri Herba *(yì mǔ cǎo)*, and Moutan Cortex *(mǔ dān pí)*.

- For the postpartum woman who returns to her daily work too quickly and suffers from fever and aversion to cold, add Ginseng Radix *(rén shēn)* and Astragali Radix *(huáng qí)*.

- For incessant postpartum bleeding from blood deficiency and blood heat, add Ginseng Radix *(rén shēn)*, Astragali Radix *(huáng qí)*, Rehmanniae Radix *(shēng dì huáng)*, dry-fried Gardeniae Fructus *(chǎo zhī zǐ)*, Schizonepetae Herba *(jīng jiè)*, Asini Corii Colla *(ē jiāo)*, and Mume Fructus *(wū méi)*; and remove Leonuri Herba *(yì mǔ cǎo)*, Moutan Cortex *(mǔ dān pí)*, and Linderae Radix *(wū yào)*. If the bleeding is severe, use charred Sanguisorbae Radix *(dì yú tàn)* .

- For postpartum headache, body aches and fever, and aversion to cold, add Ginseng Radix *(rén shēn)* and Astragali Radix *(huáng qí)* and remove Chuanxiong Rhizoma *(chuān xiōng)*, Moutan Cortex *(mǔ dān pí)*, and Leonuri Herba *(yì mǔ cǎo)*.

桂枝茯苓丸

Cinnamon Twig and Poria Pill

guì zhī fú líng wán

Source *Essentials from the Golden Cabinet* (c. 220)

Cinnamomi Ramulus *(guì zhī)* . . . . (9-12g)
Poria *(fú líng)* . . . . (9-12g)
Paeoniae Radix *(sháo yào)* . . . . (9-15g)
Moutan Cortex *(mǔ dān pí)* . . . . (9-12g)
Persicae Semen *(táo rén)* . . . . (9-12g)

Method of Preparation The source text advises to grind equal amounts of the ingredients into a powder, form into pills the size of rabbit droppings with the addition of honey, and take three times daily before meals. At present, the formula is either prepared as a decoction with the dosage specified in parentheses, or the ingredients are ground into a powder and formed into pills with honey, and taken in 3-6g doses each day with warm water.

Actions Invigorates the blood, transforms blood stasis, and reduces fixed abdominal masses.

Indications

Mild, persistent uterine bleeding of purple or dark blood during pregnancy accompanied by abdominal pain that increases with pressure.

This pattern (described in the source text) represents a form of restless fetus disorder due to blood stasis. The stasis of blood in the Womb disturbs the fetus by obstructing the flow of blood and thereby depriving the fetus of nourishment. When the flow of blood is obstructed in its normal pathways it may spill out, causing mild, persistent uterine bleeding of purple or dark blood.

Later generations of physicians have expanded the indications of this formula to include such problems as immobile masses in the lower abdomen with pain and tenderness, abdominal spasms and tension, amenorrhea with abdominal distention and pain, dysmenorrhea, and retention of the lochia. All of these problems are accompanied by a dark tongue with purple stasis spots and a submerged and choppy pulse. These symptoms are caused by a combination of qi stagnation, blood stasis, dampness, and phlegm obstruction. Under normal circumstances, the qi, blood, and body fluids of a person dynamically interact to facilitate their unhindered movement through the body. If, for various reasons, the movement of one of these substances is impeded, it will affect all the others, and, in due course, immobile abdominal masses are generated. Because blood stasis and phlegm-dampness are pathogens with form, these masses are palpable, while pain and tenderness will be fixed in location. When such stagnation affects the Penetrating and Conception vessels, the period becomes irregular or ceases altogether. Retention of the lochia is also due to the same factors. The pulse and tongue signs reflect the underlying pathodynamic.

Analysis of Formula

This formula was designed by Zhang Zhong-Jing for treating blood stasis during pregnancy. This is a rather delicate situation that requires the utmost care and refinement of strategy. Blood stasis and fixed abdominal masses must be reduced and dispersed if one is to stop the abnormal bleeding that occurs and that threatens the normal development of the fetus. However, a too-forceful attempt to reduce and disperse the stasis may also harm the fetus or risk abortion. The strategy underlying this formula therefore utilizes a relatively mild treatment to reduce the fixed abdominal masses without threatening the well-being of the fetus. This is achieved partly by combining herbs that disperse stasis indirectly by facilitating qi transformation rather than directly attacking it, and partly by using a low dose of pills rather than a decoction.

The chief herbs are Cinnamomi Ramulus (guì zhī) and Poria (fú líng). The acrid, warm properties of Cinnamomi Ramulus (guì zhī) unblock the blood vessels and reduce the stasis of blood by promoting circulation. The ability of Poria (fú líng) to leach downward can help promote the downward circulation of blood in cases of blood stasis. It also nourishes the qi of the Heart and Spleen, quiets the Heart, and calms the spirit, all of which help to calm the fetus. Because phlegm-

dampness may contribute to the formation of masses or the blockage and stasis of blood, Poria (fú líng) is used to transform phlegm and promote urination. This is especially useful if there is edema or phlegm-dampness complicating the blood stasis. Both herbs enter the greater yang and are frequently used together to promote its qi transformation, causing the clear yang and fluids to ascend throughout the body (including the blood) while draining turbidity out through the urine.

Paeoniae Radix (sháo yào) is the deputy herb, the particular type of which is dictated by the nature of the condition. Paeoniae Radix rubra (chì sháo) promotes the circulation of blood to alleviate stasis, while Paeoniae Radix alba (bái sháo) relaxes spasms and alleviates abdominal pain; if necessary, both forms of the herb may be used. Furthermore, the Divine Husbandman's Classic of the Materia Medica notes that this herb also "promotes urination." Nourishing the yin while draining dampness, it thus facilitates the action of the chief herbs in regulating the blood. Fixed abdominal masses are a symptom of constraint, which may transform into heat. The assistants transform blood stasis and clear heat due to constraint. Moutan Cortex (mǔ dān pí) and Persicae Semen (táo rén) cool and invigorate the blood, break up and dispel blood stasis, reduce fixed abdominal masses, and disperse accumulation. The use of honey in making the pills moderates the harshness of those herbs that dispel blood stasis; it may therefore be regarded as an envoy.

Cautions and Contraindications

Use with extreme caution during pregnancy or postpartum and only when there is a confirmed diagnosis of blood stasis producing this pattern.

Commentary

The original indication of this formula was the treatment of a very specific pattern during pregnancy. With the advent of modern biomedical management of complications during pregnancy, it is no longer frequently used for this purpose. Moreover, its scope has been expanded from the treatment of women to both sexes, giving it a wide range of potential applications. These can be summarized under the following headings:

- Disorders of menstruation such as short or long cycles, amenorrhea, dysmenorrhea, uterine bleeding, infertility, premenstrual syndrome, etc.
- Fixed abdominal masses as a category that includes not only problems such as uterine fibroids and ovarian cysts, but also pelvic inflammatory disorders and endometriosis
- Lack of regulation between the nutritive and protective qi, manifesting as hot flushes accompanied by cold feet, headaches, neck and shoulder stiffness, dizziness, eczema, etc.

• Circulatory disorders in the widest sense such as chilblains, hematomas, and the prevention of cerebrovascular accidents, but also painful obstruction patterns manifesting as sciatica, lower back pain, and joint pains.

The common thread among these various patterns is the formula's ability to regulate the circulation of qi, blood, and body fluids that has become blocked by the penetration of cold into the lower burner. This has three consequences. First, it inhibits the qi transformation of the Bladder, causing dampness and eventually phlegm to accumulate. Second, it congeals the blood, thereby slowing its movement. Third, it inhibits the diffusion of physiological yang qi from the gate of vitality leading to symptoms of heat constraint and up-flushing of yang. Both phlegm-dampness and heat constraint contribute to the blood stasis: the former by increasing the water portion of the blood, the latter by drying up the yin portion of the blood. This pathology occurs more easily, of course, in patients with preexisting phlegm-dampness (i.e., an excess of water over fire, yin over yang). It will not, however, occur in patients with weak fire at the gate of vitality (i.e., Kidney yang deficiency), as such patients will not produce symptoms of yang excess. Because this pathology is complex, its resolution may require that the formula be taken over a long period, perhaps for many months.

In practice, the following pointers are helpful in diagnosing a Cinnamon Twig and Poria Pill (*guì zhī fú líng wán*) pattern:

• Resistance and tenderness in the lower abdomen on palpation (some Japanese physicians think that this will be more pronounced on the left); alternatively, patients themselves may have a subjective feeling of fullness in the abdomen; if a mass is palpated, this will tend to be soft and movable and painful to the touch.

• The simultaneous presence of cold and heat signs, such as cold below and heat above, or inflammation aggravated by cold, but none of the signs of dryness associated with Flow-Warming Decoction (*wēn jīng tāng*) and Tangkuei and Peony Powder (*dāng guī sháo yào sǎn*) patterns, both of which include signs of blood deficiency.

• Systemic signs of blood stasis, such as a darkish complexion, dark rings under the eyes, increased pigmentation, and stasis spots on the tongue.

• Other typical signs of impediments to fluid and blood circulation, such as dizziness, vertigo, spots in front of one's eyes, and shoulder stiffness or pain.

Due to its balanced composition and mild-acting nature, this formula is suitable for long-term use, especially if taken in the form of pills. The honey used in the original preparation is believed to aid the sustained release of ingredients over a period of time.

Comparison

> ➢ Vs. Peach Pit Decoction to Order the Qi
(*táo hé chéng qì tāng*)

Both of these formulas treat excess patterns with blood stasis in the lower abdomen with an etiology that involves both cold and heat, typically with cold pathogenic qi leading to blood stasis in the lower burner. This prevents the yang qi from connecting with the blood, so that it moves upward instead to cause symptoms like flushing or restlessness. The difference is that Peach Pit Decoction to Order the Qi (*táo hé chéng qì tāng*) treats patterns that are relatively more yang or hot in nature that tend toward dryness, with symptoms that, as a result, are both more changeable and more severe such as flushed face, nosebleeds, mania, or more indistinct and moveable boundaries of tenderness on palpation of the abdomen. The pulse will be submerged, full, or choppy, the tongue coating may be yellow, and the patient may be thirsty. Cinnamon Twig and Poria Pill (*guì zhī fú líng wán*) patterns, on the other hand, also involve the accumulation of water and are thus more yin in nature. This is reflected in a more stable symptomatology and fixed areas of tenderness on palpation. The pulse will be deep, slow, and tight, any tongue coating will usually be white, and the patient will generally not be thirsty, even if there are other heat signs.

Biomedical Indications

With the appropriate presentation, this formula may be used to treat a wide-variety of biomedically-defined disorders. These can be divided into the following groups:

• Obstetrical and gynecological disorders marked by masses or bleeding including primary dysmenorrhea, dysfunctional uterine bleeding or leiomyoma, cervical erosion, endometritis, polycystic ovaries, chronic salpingitis, chronic pelvic inflammatory disease, endometriosis, habitual miscarriage, ectopic pregnancy, retained placenta, prolonged lochia, and postpartum urinary retention

• Various types of nodular disorders including fibrocystic breasts, benign prostatic hypertrophy, intestinal polyps, postvasectomy pain with localized nodules, thyroid hypertrophy, granulomas, cystic acne, vocal cord nodules, nodular vasculitis, and hemorrhoids

• Vascular disorders including thrombophlebitis of the lower extremities, hypertension, coronary heart disease, chronic congestive heart failure, and pelvic congestion syndrome

• Neuropsychiatric disorders including schizophrenia, epilepsy, neuroses, and recalcitrant insomnia

• Ophthalmic disorders including iritis, central serous retinopathy, choroidal hemorrhage, and conjunctivitis.

This formula has also been used for treating chronic gastritis, hepatoma, appendicitis, orchitis, nephrotic syndrome, anemia, and ulcerations of the lower extremities.

Alternate Names

Fight for Life Pill (*duó mìng wán*) in *Fine Formulas for Women*; Moutan Pill (*mǔ dān wán*) and Fight for Life Pill (*duó mìng wán*), both in *Prescriptions for Universal Benefit*; Life-Preserving Special Pill Handed Down by an Immortal (*xiān chuán bǎo mìng wán*) and Pill to Pacify Prayers (*ān ráng wán*), both in *Essential Teachings on Pregnancy and Childbirth*

Modifications

• For more severe blood stasis, add Rhei Radix et Rhizoma (*dà huáng*).

• For chronic accumulation and clumps that have generated fixed abdominal masses, add Ostreae Concha (*mǔ lì*), Trionycis Carapax (*biē jiǎ*), Salviae miltiorrhizae Radix (*dān shēn*), Olibanum (*rǔ xiāng*), Myrrha (*mò yào*), and Gigeriae galli Endothelium corneum (*jī nèi jīn*).

• For heavy menstrual bleeding or irregular uterine bleeding, add Trogopterori Faeces (*wǔ líng zhī*), Typhae Pollen (*pú huáng*), and Crinis carbonisatus (*xuè yú tàn*).

• For severe pain, add Corydalis Rhizoma (*yán hú suǒ*), Olibanum (*rǔ xiāng*), and Myrrha (*mò yào*).

• For pronounced discharge due to dampness, add Coicis Semen (*yì yǐ rén*), Angelicae dahuricae Radix (*bái zhǐ*), and Plantaginis Semen (*chē qián zǐ*).

• For amenorrhea due to blood stasis, add Chuanxiong Rhizoma (*chuān xiōng*), Carthami Flos (*hóng huā*), Cyperi Rhizoma (*xiāng fù*), and Leonuri Herba (*yì mǔ cǎo*).

• For blood stasis in the Womb characterized by dysmenorrhea, small amounts of blood, clotting, and pain that is reduced as clots are discharged, add Angelicae sinensis Radix (*dāng guī*), Chuanxiong Rhizoma (*chuān xiōng*), Linderae Radix (*wū yào*), Cyperi Rhizoma (*xiāng fù*), and Achyranthis bidentatae Radix (*niú xī*).

• For prolonged lochia, add Angelicae sinensis Radix (*dāng guī*), Leonuri Herba (*yì mǔ cǎo*), and Zingiberis Rhizoma praeparatum (*páo jiāng*).

• For patients with pronounced blood deficiency, combine with Tangkuei and Peony Powder (*dāng guī sháo yào sǎn*).

Associated Formulas

折衝飲 （折冲饮）

Drink to Turn Back the Penetrating [Vessel]
zhé chòng yǐn

SOURCE *Formulas from the Discussion on Women's Precious Delivery* (1851)

Moutan Cortex (*mǔ dān pí*) 3g (6g)
Cinnamomi Ramulus (*guì zhī*) 3g (5g)
Angelicae sinensis Radix (*dāng guī*) 5g (6-9g)
Persicae Semen (*táo rén*) 5g (6-9g)
Corydalis Rhizoma (*yán hú suǒ*) 3g (6-9g)
Achyranthis bidentatae Radix (*niú xī*) 3g (6-9g)
Carthami Flos (*hóng huā*) 2g (3-6g)
Chuanxiong Rhizoma (*chuān xiōng*) 3g (6g)
Paeoniae Radix rubra (*chì sháo*) 3g (6-9g)

Decoction. Because this was originally intended for treatment of discharge of clotted blood during the second to third trimester of pregnancy, the dosages are small so as not to cause miscarriage. The dosages in parentheses are those most commonly used at present for the modern indications.

This formula transforms accumulations and dispels stasis, nourishes and invigorates the blood, adjusts the menses, and relieves pain. It is indicated for blood stasis in the lower abdomen with such symptoms as irregular menstruation, painful menstruation (with pain in the abdomen or lower back), blood stasis abdominal accumulations, amenorrhea or postpartum or postmiscarriage bleeding or pain. Compared to the principal formula, this is a powerful blood-moving and stasis-dispersing formula that is unsuitable for long-term use unless modified to protect from dispersal of qi and exhaustion of blood. At present, it is also contraindicated during pregnancy. It takes a straightforward approach to the dispersal of blood stasis accumulations in the lower abdomen and is also used for blood stasis in the lower burner that gives rise to pelvic inflammatory disease, inflammation of the fallopian tubes, uterine leiomyoma, miscellaneous abdominal masses, endometritis, or dysfunctional uterine bleeding.

Because the treatment of entrenched disorders such as uterine leiomyoma requires an extended time, care must be taken to avoid an excess of dispersal and drainage of the patients' qi and blood. The first option is to alternate use of the formula with a tonic such as Eight-Treasure Decoction (*bā zhēn tāng*). The second approach is to modify the formula by adding agents to tonify the qi and blood such as Codonopsis Radix (*dǎng shēn*), Astragali Radix (*huáng qí*), Ligustri lucidi Fructus (*nǚ zhēn zǐ*), and Rehmanniae Radix praeparata (*shú dì huáng*).

Modifications

• For menstrual disorders exhibiting severe blood stasis with cramping pain, clotted menstrual blood, and pain of fixed location that dislikes pressure, add Sparganii Rhizoma (*sān léng*) and Curcumae Rhizoma (*é zhú*).

• For menstrual irregularity, add Artemisiae anomalae Herba (*liú jì nú*).

• For painful menstruation, add Typhae Pollen (*pú huáng*) and Cyperi Rhizoma (*xiāng fù*).

• For postpartum blood stasis disorders, combine with Generating and Transforming Decoction (*shēng huà tāng*).

• For pelvic inflammatory disease, add Sargentodoxae Caulis (*hóng téng*) and Phellodendri Cortex (*huáng bǎi*).

牛膝散

Achyranthes Powder

niú xī sǎn

SOURCE   *Formulas from Benevolent Sages Compiled during the Taiping Era* (992)

Achyranthis bidentatae Radix (*niú xī*) 30g (9g)
Cinnamomi Ramulus (*guì zhī*) 30g (9g)
Paeoniae Radix rubra (*chì sháo*) 15g (6-9g)
Angelicae sinensis Radix (*dāng guī*) 15g (4-6g)
Aucklandiae Radix (*mù xiāng*) 15g (6-9g)
Moutan Cortex (*mǔ dān pí*) .15g (6-9g)
Corydalis Rhizoma (*yán hú suǒ*) 15g (6-9g)
Chuanxiong Rhizoma (*chuān xiōng*) 15g (6-9g)
Persicae Semen (*táo rén*) 15g (6-9g)

The source text advises to grind the above ingredients into a powder and take 3g per dose mixed in warmed rice wine before meals. The amounts in parentheses are the editors' suggestions for decoction.

This formula invigorates the blood, disperses stasis, adjusts the menses, and relieves pain. In the source text, this formula is used for inhibited menses with periumbilical or lower abdominal pain. This formula, which antedates Drink to Turn Back the Penetrating [Vessel] (*zhé chōng yǐn*) by hundreds of years, uses the qi-regulating herb Aucklandiae Radix (*mù xiāng*) in place of the blood-moving herb Carthami Flos (*hóng huā*). The two formulas can treat the same disorders, with Achyranthes Powder (*niú xī sǎn*) being slightly more effective for moving qi in the abdomen, while Drink to Turn Back the Penetrating [Vessel] (*zhé chōng yǐn*) more adept at dispelling abdominal blood stasis.

當歸芍藥散 （当归芍药散）

Tangkuei and Peony Powder

dāng guī sháo yào sǎn

Source   *Essentials from the Golden Cabinet* (c. 220)

Angelicae sinensis Radix (*dāng guī*) 9g
Paeoniae Radix (*sháo yào*) 48g
Poria (*fú líng*) 12g
Atractylodis macrocephalae Rhizoma (*bái zhú*) 12g
Alismatis Rhizoma (*zé xiè*) 24g
Chuanxiong Rhizoma (*chuān xiōng*) 24g

Method of Preparation   The source text advises to grind the ingredients into a powder and take 3-6g with a little wine and warm water three times a day. At present, it is usually prepared as a decoction with a reduction in the dosage of Paeoniae Radix (*sháo yào*), Alismatis Rhizoma (*zé xiè*), and Chuanxiong Rhizoma (*chuān xiōng*) by one-half to two-thirds. Paeoniae Radix alba (*bái sháo*) is the form of Paeoniae Radix (*sháo yào*) most commonly used.

Actions   Nourishes the Liver blood, spreads the Liver qi, strengthens the Spleen, and resolves dampness

Indications

Continuous, cramping pain of the abdomen that is not severe, urinary difficulty, and slight edema (primarily of the lower limbs). Such pain can occur during pregnancy or with a variety of gynecological disorders.

This is abdominal pain due to disharmony between the Liver and Spleen characterized by both blood stasis and qi stagnation due to dampness. The Liver stores the blood and dredges the qi. The stronger the Liver blood, the better it is able to control the Liver qi. The stronger the Liver qi, the better it is able to regulate the qi dynamic, a process that includes upward diffusion of clear yang as well as downward draining of turbid fluids. When the Liver blood and qi are insufficient, dampness accumulates, the qi stagnates, and the blood becomes static. This is reflected in continuous cramping pain (a wind-like pain that reflects its root in a Liver disorder), which is, however, not as severe as pain from qi stagnation, cold, or blood stasis (reflecting its deficient nature). The Liver is closely connected to the sea of blood in the lower abdomen; it governs women's physiology. Thus, such symptoms occur more readily (but not exclusively) in women, both in relation to the menstrual cycle and during pregnancy. When the Liver overcontrols the Spleen, the metabolism of water is disrupted, which gives rise to internally-generated dampness. Dampness contributes to the abdominal pain by causing stagnation. It also causes urinary difficulty and edema, primarily in the lower limbs where it tends to collect.

Analysis of Formula

This formula treats pain due to a mixed pattern of deficiency and excess where Liver and Spleen deficiency are complicated by blood stasis and stagnating dampness. This requires a primary strategy of nourishing the blood and softening the Liver in order to relax hypertonicity, supported by augmenting the Spleen qi in order to facilitate transportation and transformation, and invigorating the blood and dispelling dampness in order to unblock the yang. The chief herb in this formula, with the highest relative dosage, is sour, bitter, and slightly cooling Paeoniae Radix alba (*bái sháo*). Entering the Liver and Spleen, it nourishes blood, softens the Liver, and moderates spasmodic abdominal pain; but it is also able to unblock the blood vessels and promote water metabolism. It thus addresses all of the diverse aspects of the pathodynamic that underlies this pattern. The deputies are acrid and warming Chuanxiong Rhizoma (*chuān xiōng*), which enters into the sea of blood to dispel stasis and invigorate the blood, and sweet, bland, and cooling Alismatis Rhizoma (*zé xiè*), which enters into the Kidneys and Bladder to promote water metabolism and leach out dampness. Together, they support the chief herb in opening constraint by dredging the vessels and collaterals. Acrid, sweet, and warming Angelicae sinensis Radix (*dāng guī*), which nourishes and invigorates the blood, supports Paeoniae Radix alba (*bái sháo*) in harmonizing the Liver and Chuanxiong Rhizoma (*chuān xiōng*) in invigorating the blood. Two other assistants, Poria (*fú líng*) and Atractylodis macrocephalae Rhizoma *(bái zhú)*, tonify the qi and leach out dampness. The combination of Paeoniae Radix alba *(bái sháo)* and Atractylodis macrocephalae Rhizoma *(bái zhú)* is often used in treating concurrent problems of the Liver and Spleen. This is because tonifying the Spleen as the source of postnatal qi also tonifies the Liver qi, while softening the Liver prevents its qi from overacting on the Spleen. The warm, acrid property of rice wine facilitates flow and disperses. A small amount of wine encourages the free flow of Liver qi and promotes urination, thereby reinforcing both of the formula's functions. It is regarded as the envoy ingredient.

Cautions and Contraindications

At present, it is recommended that this formula be used with caution during pregnancy, specifically because too high a dosage of Chuanxiong Rhizoma *(chuān xiōng)* can affect the fetus, particularly in mothers who have deficient and weak Kidney qi.

Commentary

Appropriate Type of Pain

Abdominal pain has many causes. The classical usage of this formula is for the treatment of sustained pain (疞痛 *xiū tòng)*. This pain is milder but more continuous than that for which Ass-Hide Gelatin and Mugwort Decoction *(jiāo ài tāng)* is indicated, and there is no bleeding. Its pathodynamic is described by the Ming-dynasty physician Xu Bin in *Discussion and Annotation of the Essentials from the Golden Cabinet*:

> Sustained pain denotes continuous pain. It is not like the gripping pain of cold-type bulging disorder, nor the stabbing pain of qi or blood [stagnation]. Insufficiency of the normal qi allows yin to encroach on yang so that water qi prevails over earth. Spleen [qi] is constrained and unable to extend but seeks to [overcome] the constraint by extending itself. This dysregulation of the Spleen qi manifests as continuous pain.

However, the Chinese characters 疞痛 can also be read as *jiáo tòng*, which means hypertonic or 'tense pain.' Some commentators, like the contemporary physician Yue Mei-Zhong, utilize this definition in their understanding of the formula's clinical presentation:

> The pattern [treated by] this formula [presents with] hypertonicity and pain of the central abdomen that may extend upward to the epigastrium or the chest. There may be urinary difficulty. Pain may prevent bending forward or backward. On abdominal diagnosis, the abdomen along the sides of the umbilicus (i.e., the rectus abdominus muscle) will be tender and hypertonic. Alternatively, pressing on the left will shift [fluid] to the right and vice versa. [This feels] as if there were something in the abdomen, but there are no lumps. This [pattern] belongs to blood and water stopping and stagnating.

Yet another translation of the characters 疞痛 is 'slight pain.'

There is no agreement among commentators regarding the correct interpretation of the term in the present context. Rather than seeking for the right solution, it may thus be more useful clinically to follow the analysis of the contemporary physician Huang Huang in *One-Hundred Classic Formulas*, who states that this formula treats all kinds of pain extending from cramping to aching, provided that it fits into the overall manifestation of the pattern for which this formula is indicated.

Expanded Usage

Although the location of the pain in the central abdomen around the umbilicus defines this as being primarily a Spleen pathology, its nature (hypertonicity of the abdominal wall) also refers to Liver wood. In Chinese medicine, the physiological functions of the Liver with regard to qi are referred to as 'dredging and draining.' This implies a keeping open of the channels that relies, on the one hand, on the dispersion of qi and blood from the lower to the upper burner, and, on the other, a draining of excess yin water from the body. This formula achieves both of these functions by combining herbs that tonify the qi, invigorate the blood, and drain fluids. This is outlined, once more, by Yue Mei-Zhong, who states that the ingredients of this formula:

> Used together, dredge the blood that has stagnated and become static, but also disperse constrained built-up water. If after taking it the urine becomes [dark] like blood, or the stools become watery, this means that the medicine has fastened onto the disorder, which is excellent. To treat hardness, it needs to be taken long-term.

Understanding the functions of the formula in this way has widely extended its scope of application. The Song-dynasty text *Discussion of Illnesses, Patterns, and Formulas Related to the Unification of the Three Etiologies* observes: "Taken regularly, it facilitates unimpeded [movement through the] blood vessels to prevent abscesses and sores, eliminates phlegm, nourishes the Stomach, brightens the eyes, and benefits the yang fluids." For many gynecologists, this formula has thus become the preferred choice for treating gynecological problems due to deficiency that involve blood stasis and water buildup, including the treatment of infertility, malposition of the fetus, edema, pain or bleeding during pregnancy, dysmenorrhea, and irregular menstruation. Because it focuses on the blood aspects of Liver dysfunction and the damp aspects of Spleen dysfunction, many practitioners prefer to use it instead of Frigid Extremities Powder *(sì nì sǎn)* or Rambling Powder *(xiāo yáo sǎn)* in cases of Liver/Spleen disorders when the pain is not accompanied by distention.

Viewing pain that involves both blood stasis and water buildup as the key problem treated by this formula has resulted in the expansion of its scope of action to other problems in women, and then to the treatment of similar problems in men. Pain invariably will be the main symptom, although this can occur anywhere in the body and not just the abdomen. Water buildup may manifest in any number of ways, including excessive discharges or dryness resulting from dampness obstructing (as in allergic rhinitis); dizziness, nausea, heavy-headedness and reduced urination indicating accumulation of thin mucus (as in Ménière's disease); sensations of fullness and obstruction in the chest and epigastrium from thin mucus (as in coronary heart disease); swellings in the abdomen or increased sweating from the lower body (as in ovarian cysts or hydrocele); and constipation or urinary difficulty indicating obstruction of the qi dynamic by dampness in the lower abdomen.

This combination of pain and fluid accumulation is thus a key marker for the formula's use in clinical practice. These symptoms may be accompanied by cold (either a subjective aversion to cold or coldness of the extremities), fatigue (indicating deficiency), and some kind of visible edema (often around the eyes).

Issues Relating to Paeoniae Radix (sháo yào)

The action of the formula can further be modified by adjusting the relative dosage of its ingredients. This includes making a judgment with regard to the type of Paeoniae Radix (sháo yào) to be used, as the source text did not yet distinguish between Paeoniae Radix alba (bái sháo) and Paeoniae Radix rubra (chì sháo). Depending on what type of Paeoniae Radix (sháo yào) one uses, or in which combination one combines the two types, one can accentuate one or more of the following effects:

- Relaxing hypertonicity and alleviating the pain
- Nourishing the blood and softening the Liver
- Invigorating the blood and unblocking the vessels
- Promoting fluid metabolism.

Paeoniae Radix alba (bái sháo) is considered superior at achieving the first and second of these goals, as its sour and sweet tastes focus on preserving the yin as a means of controlling the yang. The cold, unblocking, and draining nature of Paeoniae Radix rubra (chì sháo) is more appropriate where the latter goals are considered to be of primary importance. Furthermore, because of its blood-invigorating properties, Paeoniae Radix rubra (chì sháo) should only be used with care if this formula is prescribed during pregnancy.

Comparisons

➤ Vs. Rambling Powder (xiāo yáo sǎn) and Frigid Extremities Powder (sì nì sǎn)

All of these formulas treat patterns characterized by blood deficiency, qi stagnation, and dampness. Historically, Tangkuei and Peony Powder (dāng guī sháo yào sǎn) is the older

formula, and many later commentators thus view Rambling Powder (xiāo yáo sǎn) as either a modification of it, or a combination of it and Frigid Extremities Powder (sì nì sǎn). All three formulas can be used in the treatment of abdominal pain, particularly in the context of gynecological disorders and of combined Liver and Spleen, and qi and blood patterns. Among the three, Frigid Extremities Powder (sì nì sǎn) focuses mainly on qi stagnation. It thus treats relatively severe abdominal pain and colic accompanied by symptoms such as bloating and cold extremities. Tangkuei and Peony Powder (dāng guī sháo yào sǎn) focuses on blood deficiency and dampness. It thus treats milder but often more persistent pain accompanied by edema or other signs of excess water. Rambling Powder (xiāo yáo sǎn) treats qi stagnation, blood and qi deficiency, and dampness patterns. Although it does treat pain, its focus is on resolving constraint and tonifying.

Biomedical Indications

With the appropriate presentation, this formula may be used to treat a wide variety of biomedically-defined disorders. These can be divided into the following groups:

- Obstetrical and gynecological disorders including dysfunctional uterine bleeding, perimenstrual migraines, endometritis, polycystic ovaries, threatened miscarriage, habitual miscarriage, pre-eclampsia, postpartum depression, perimenopausal syndrome, uterine leiomyoma, breast hyperplasia, and infertility
- Disorders marked by pain including chronic gastritis, peptic ulcers, cholecystitis, urinary tract stones, intestinal obstruction, gout, coronary artery disease, vascular headaches, trigeminal neuralgia, sciatica, and rheumatoid arthritis
- Skin disorders marked by a lack of luster including acne, chilblains, eczema, urticaria, varicose veins, and psoriasis
- Swellings from congestive heart disease, renal disease, ascites from cirrhosis, postconcussion syndrome, Ménière's disease, thrombotic stroke, and allergic rhinitis.

This formula has also been used for the treatment of tension, hypotension, cystitis, benign prostatic hypertrophy, appendicitis, hemorrhoids, conjunctivitis, beriberi, and senile dementia.

Alternate Names

Tangkuei and Peony Decoction (dāng guī sháo yào tāng) in *Formulas to Aid the Living*; Tangkuei and Poria Powder (dāng guī fú líng sǎn) in *Prescriptions for Universal Benefit*

Modifications

- For relatively cold presentations, add Cinnamomi Ramulus (guì zhī) and Evodiae Fructus (wú zhū yú).
- For relatively hot presentations, add Moutan Cortex (mǔ dān pí) and Gardeniae Fructus (zhī zǐ).

- For habitual miscarriage, remove Alismatis Rhizoma (zé xiè) and add Cimicifugae Rhizoma (shēng má), Asini Corii Colla (ē jiāo), Astragali Radix (huáng qí), and Artemisiae argyi Folium (ài yè).

- For threatened miscarriage, add Amomi Fructus (shā rén), Eucommiae Cortex (dù zhòng), Dipsaci Radix (xù duàn), Artemisiae argyi Folium (ài yè), and Scutellariae Radix (huáng qín).

- For abdominal pain during pregnancy, reduce the dosage of Chuanxiong Rhizoma (chuān xiōng) and add Perillae Caulis (zǐ sū gěng), Boehmeriae Radix (zhū má gēn), Eucommiae Cortex (dù zhòng), and Taxilli Herba (sāng jì shēng).

- For edema during menstruation due to Kidney qi deficiency, add Curculiginis Rhizoma (xiān máo) and Epimedii Herba (yín yáng huò).

- For dysmenorrhea, add Cyperi Rhizoma (xiāng fù), Corydalis Rhizoma (yán hú suǒ), and Toosendan Fructus (chuān liàn zǐ).

- For rather severe dampness with edema and amenorrhea, combine with Five-Ingredient Powder with Poria (wǔ líng sǎn).

- For hepatomegaly, add Aucklandiae Radix (mù xiāng), Curcumae Radix (yù jīn), and Aurantii Fructus immaturus (zhǐ shí).

- For epigastric pain, add Trogopterori Faeces (wǔ líng zhī) and Aucklandiae Radix (mù xiāng).

- For abdominal pain accompanied by acid reflux, add Sepiae Endoconcha (hǎi piāo xiāo) and Arcae Concha (wǎ léng zǐ).

- For pain in the flanks, add Curcumae Radix (yù jīn) and Toosendan Fructus (chuān liàn zǐ).

- For numbness and painful obstruction of the lower extremities, add Zingiberis Rhizoma (gān jiāng), Stephaniae tetrandrae Radix (hàn fáng jǐ), and Astragali Radix (huáng qí).

- For red and painful eyes, add Plantaginis Semen (chē qián zǐ).

Associated Formulas

當歸散 （当归散）

Tangkuei Powder

dāng guī sǎn

SOURCE *Essentials from the Golden Cabinet* (c. 220)

Angelicae sinensis Radix (dāng guī) 48g
Scutellariae Radix (huáng qín) 48g
Paeoniae Radix alba (bái sháo) 48g
Chuanxiong Rhizoma (chuān xiōng) 48g
Atractylodis macrocephalae Rhizoma (bái zhú) 24g

The source text advises to grind the ingredients into a powder and take in 3-6g doses with a little rice wine. At present, it is usually prepared as a decoction with approximately one-fifth of the specified dosage. Tonifies the blood, strengthens the Spleen, clears heat, and calms a restless fetus. For thin women with long-standing blood and yin deficiency who develop problems during pregnancy such as restless fetus disorder. The source text recommends that the formula be taken regularly during pregnancy as a preventative measure.

連珠飲 （连珠饮）

String of Pearls Drink

lián zhū yǐn

SOURCE *Formulary and Mnemonics from 'No Mistake' Pharmacy* (1956)

Poria (fú líng) 5g
Cinnamomi Ramulus (guì zhī) 4g
Angelicae sinensis Radix (dāng guī) 3g
Chuanxiong Rhizoma (chuān xiōng) 3g
Paeoniae Radix alba (bái sháo) 3g
Rehmanniae Radix praeparata (shú dì huáng) 3g
Atractylodis macrocephalae Rhizoma (bái zhú) 3g
Glycyrrhizae Radix (gān cǎo) 2g

Tonifies and regulates the blood, promotes water metabolism, and leaches out dampness. For palpitations and dizziness, especially on standing up. This is a combination of Four-Substance Decoction (sì wù tāng) and Poria, Cinnamon Twig, Atractylodis, and Licorice Decoction (líng guì zhú gān tāng) that was first used by the famous 19th-century Japanese physician Honma Souken to treat blood deficiency complicated by the presence of water toxin in the body. Besides the main symptoms of palpitations and dizziness, there will be edema (usually mild and commonly constitutional), tinnitus, dyspnea, hot flushes, sweating, or headache. Also for irregular uterine bleeding and postpartum disorders, hemorrhoids, and jaundice.

宣鬱通經湯 （宣郁通经汤）

Diffuse Constraint and Unblock the Channels Decoction

xuān yù tōng jīng tāng

SOURCE *Fu Qing-Zhu's Women's Disorders* (17th century, published in 1826)

Paeoniae Radix alba (bái sháo) 15g
Angelica sinensis radix (dāng guī) 15g
Moutan Cortex (mǔ dān pí) 15g
Gardeniae Fructus (zhī zǐ) 9g
Sinapis Semen (bái jiè zǐ) 6g
Bupleuri Radix (chái hú) 3g
Cyperi Rhizoma (xiāng fù) 3g
Curcumae Radix (yù jīn) 3g
Scutellariae Radix (huáng qín) 3g
Glycyrrhizae Radix (gān cǎo) 3g

Decoction. Softens the Liver, releases constraint, dredges the channels, and drains fire. For Liver qi constraint transforming into fire causing dysmenorrhea that is characterized by pain before the onset of the periods, and periods with dark red clots. The symptoms are usually chronic, without a distinctive cause marking the onset of the disorder. This pattern can be due to constraint from emotional causes or to cold transforming into heat. It occurs more often in young women. Although there is some blood deficiency, pain preceding the onset of periods indicates that the pathodynamic is primarily one of qi-level constraint. Unlike the presentation for which Augmented Rambling Powder (jiā wèi xiāo yáo sǎn), discussed in Chapter 3, is indicated, here there are no symptoms of qi deficiency.

失笑散
Sudden Smile Powder

shī xiào sǎn

Before taking this formula, the patient for whom it is indicated has pain so severe that it is difficult to tolerate. After taking the formula, the pain disappears so fast that it brings a sudden smile to the face.

Source   *Materia Medica Arranged According to Pattern* (1108)

Trogopterori Faeces (wǔ líng zhī) 6g
Typhae Pollen (pú huáng) 6g

Method of Preparation   Grind the above into a fine powder and take mixed with warm, white wine or vinegar. Also prepared as a decoction.

Actions   Invigorates the blood, dispels blood stasis, disperses accumulation, and alleviates pain

Indications

Irregular menstruation, dysmenorrhea, retention of the lochia, postpartum abdominal pain, acute, colicky pain in the lower abdomen, severe pain in the middle abdomen, or epigastric pain.

This is retention of blood stasis that obstructs the vessels that serve the lower abdomen. As a result, the menstrual blood is unable to flow in accordance with its normal periodicity and there is irregular menstruation and dysmenorrhea. Soon after giving birth, the surplus of blood should leave the channels; however, if the blood becomes static and is retained in the form of lochia, it will obstruct the lower abdomen and cause acute spasms in the collaterals. This results in the rather severe abdominal pain symptoms described above.

Analysis of Formula

Sweet and warm substances that break up blood stasis and promote the movement of blood are required for treating this condition. Sweet and warming Trogopterori Faeces (wǔ líng zhī) enters the Liver blood aspect to remove obstruction from the blood vessels, disperse the retained blood, and alleviate pain. Sweet and neutral Typhae Pollen (pú huáng) also enters the Liver blood aspect. It is used because it not only strongly promotes the circulation of blood, but also stops bleeding. White wine warms the menses and promotes the circulation of blood, while vinegar transforms blood stasis and promotes the circulation of blood. The use of either substance enhances the blood-invigorating and pain-alleviating actions of the formula.

Typhae Pollen (pú huáng) is used in its raw form to promote blood circulation and eliminate blood stasis, and in its honey-fried form to stop bleeding owing to its astringent qualities. In treating hemorrhage due to retention of blood stasis, one may use a mixture of equal parts of the raw and honey-fried forms.

Cautions and Contraindications

Contraindicated during pregnancy because of the ability of Typhae Pollen (pú huáng) to cause uterine contractions, as well as the general action of the formula in dispelling blood stasis. Additionally, Trogopterori Faeces (wǔ líng zhī) can readily injure the Stomach qi and should therefore be used with caution in cases with Stomach deficiency.

Commentary

Development of Usage

The source text prescribes this formula for "Small Intestine qi" (小腸氣 *xiǎo cháng qì*), that is, severe lower abdominal pain, and also recommends it as being effective for treating women. From there, it was assimilated into the Song-dynasty work, *Formulary of the Pharmacy Service for Benefiting the People in the Taiping Era*, with its indications expanded to include postpartum epigastric and abdominal pain that is so severe that the patient wants to die. This text also notes that other medicines are ineffective in treating this condition but that it can be cured immediately when this formula is taken. By the Ming, its usage had been further expanded to include pain from blood stasis in other parts of the trunk, in men as well as women. In *Comprehensive Outline of the Materia Medica*, the famous physician Li Shi-Zhen wrote that this combination:

> is able to treat all the various types of Heart and abdominal pain, lower abdominal pain, Small Intestine bulging qi, in men and women, old people, and children. Any kind of pain [where other formulas prove ineffective] can be mobilized and alleviated with it. It is especially effective in women, pregnant women, and postnatal women [suffering from] heart pain, lower abdominal pain, or qi and blood [stagnation] pain.

Recently, it has been widely used as a foundation for formulas that treat angina pectoris and integrated into formulas for abnormal blood lipids.

Pathodynamic

The principal disorder is caused by the formation of blood stasis due to obstruction of the blood vessels. The stasis of blood in turn generates further obstruction and stagnation, and the problem may therefore worsen if not treated properly. Although the formula may be generally utilized in treating this pattern with such diverse clinical complaints as epigastric pain and dysmenorrhea, its efficacy in treating such patterns is linked in *Six Texts Summarizing the Medicine of Xu Ling-Tai* to the physiology of the Conception and Penetrating vessels:

> With blood stasis in the Heart and Spleen, the Stomach qi does not properly transform so there is a lessening of the ability of the Conception and Penetrating vessels to store up and discharge. Therefore, there is profuse uterine bleeding below and Heart pain above.

In *Collectanea of Investigations from the Realm of Medicine*, Wang Fu explains the pathodynamic from a slightly different perspective:

> Blood stasis remaining from pregnancy and other types of blood stasis are not the same. Lodging in the Conception and Penetrating vessels, it rebels, moving into the Pericardium collaterals [and] unable to overflow into other channels. … Typhae Pollen (*pú huáng*) and Trogopterori Faeces (*wǔ líng zhī*) harmonize the Penetrating and Conception vessels below, while above they move in the arm terminal yin and lesser yin. Their nature is balanced. They dispel stasis and thereby are able to tonify. The formula refers to a sudden smile because [one cannot but be delighted realizing that] by using such mild herbs, one can get rid of a dangerous disorder.

Another interesting feature of this formula is that it combines an herb that invigorates the blood with one that stops bleeding. While these actions may be viewed as essentially antagonistic, clinical practice confirms that the combination of these two sharply contrasting actions may produce a useful synthesis, particularly in cases where there is both bleeding and stasis of blood.

Comparison

➤ Vs. Generating and Transforming Decoction (*shēng huà tāng*)

Both of these formulas invigorate the blood and dispel blood stasis and are used in treating internal obstruction due to blood stasis leading to prolonged lochia with lower abdominal pain. However, Generating and Transforming Decoction (*shēng huà tāng*) has a tonifying action that complements its attacking aspects and is used for postpartum cold that congeals the blood. By contrast, Sudden Smile Powder (*shī xiào sǎn*) has no tonifying action and is used only to dispel blood stasis and alleviate pain. For this reason, it is used in treating more severe postpartum abdominal pain. It is also used for abdominal pain and Heart pain, for which Generating and Transforming Decoction (*shēng huà tāng*) is not indicated.

Biomedical Indications

With the appropriate presentation, this formula may be used to treat a variety of biomedically-defined disorders including chronic gastritis, peptic ulcer, endometriosis, prolonged lochia, dysfunctional uterine bleeding, and coronary artery disease.

Alternate names

Broken Bowstring Powder (*duàn gōng xián sǎn*) in *Fine Formulas by Su and Shen*; Sudden Smile Syrup (*shī xiào gāo*) in *Treasury Classic*; Empirical Sudden Smile Powder (*jīng yàn shī xiào sǎn*) in *Appendices to the Golden Cabinet*

Modifications

- For concurrent cold, add Zingiberis Rhizoma praeparatum (*páo jiāng*), Artemisiae argyi Folium (*ài yè*), Foeniculi Fructus (*xiǎo huí xiāng*), and Linderae Radix (*wū yào*).
- For severe qi stagnation, add Cyperi Rhizoma (*xiāng fù*) or take with Melia Toosendan Powder (*jīn líng zǐ sǎn*).
- For irregular menstruation due to a pattern of blood stasis and blood deficiency, combine with Four-Substance Decoction (*sì wù tāng*).
- For angina pectoris from blood stasis, add 15g each of Chuanxiong Rhizoma (*chuān xiōng*), Paeoniae Radix rubra (*chì sháo*), and Carthami Flos (*hóng huā*), and 30g of Salviae miltiorrhizae Radix (*dān shēn*).

Associated Formula

手拈散

Pinch Powder

shǒu niān sǎn

Source   *Essential Teachings of [Zhu] Dan-Xi* (1481)

Corydalis Rhizoma (*yán hú suǒ*)
Trogopterori Faeces (*wǔ líng zhī*)
Tsaoko Fructus (*cǎo guǒ*)
Myrrha (*mò yào*)

Grind equal amounts of the ingredients into a powder and take in 6g doses with water. Invigorates the blood, dispels blood stasis, promotes the movement of qi, and alleviates pain. For epigastric and abdominal pain due to qi stagnation and blood stasis. This formula's ability to alleviate pain is stronger than that of the principal formula, and it is used in treating cold disorders.

活絡效靈丹 (活络效灵丹)
Fantastically Effective Pill to Invigorate the Collaterals
huó luò xiào líng dān

Source   *Essays on Medicine Esteeming the Chinese and Respecting the Western* (1918-1934)

Angelicae sinensis Radix (*dāng guī*) 15g
Salviae miltiorrhizae Radix (*dān shēn*) 15g
Olibanum (*rǔ xiāng*) 15g
Myrrha (*mò yào*) 15g

Method of Preparation   Decoction. Alternatively, the ingredients may be ground into a powder and divided into four equal portions that are taken with warm wine.

Actions   Invigorates the blood, dispels blood stasis, unblocks the collaterals, and alleviates pain

Indications

Pain in various locations such as the heart, stomach, abdomen, back, leg, or arm, bruising and swelling due to traumatic injury, rheumatic pain, fixed abdominal masses, internal or external ulceration, a dark tongue or one with stasis spots, and a wiry or rough pulse

The painful conditions that characterize the pattern treated by this formula are due to qi stagnation and blood stasis obstructing the collaterals. The collaterals are the passageways for the circulation of blood. They are smaller than the channels and, according to a doctrine elaborated by the Qing-dynasty physician Ye Tian-Shi, long-term disorders often reside there. Because they traverse the entire body and are found in every organ, stasis of blood in the collaterals can cause symptoms in the exterior as well as the interior of the body. Under normal circumstances, the qi impels the movement of blood within the collaterals so that they remain free of obstruction. However, if the blood becomes static and the qi stagnates due to traumatic injury, or pathogens penetrate into the blood aspect, or there is internal damage, the blood vessels can no longer accommodate the circulation of blood and pain will ensue, in accordance with the adage, "If there is blockage, pain will follow." Such pain is usually stabbing in nature and fixed in location. More severe obstruction from blood stasis will manifest as fixed abdominal masses. Internal or external ulcerations may occur if toxin accumulates due to blood stasis. A dark tongue or one with stasis spots, and a wiry or rough pulse are common signs of blood stasis.

Analysis of Formula

To transform the stasis and facilitate the flow of blood in the collateral vessels, this formula utilizes substances that invigorate the blood and unblock the collaterals. This is consistent with the strategies of using the attacking method to treat retention and the reducing method to treat hard masses. Sweet, acrid, and warming Angelicae sinensis Radix *(dāng guī)*, the chief ingredient, invigorates and nourishes the blood and alleviates pain. Bitter, draining, and slightly cooling Salviae miltiorrhizae Radix *(dān shēn)* strengthens the blood-invigorating action of Angelicae sinensis Radix *(dāng guī)*, eliminates blood stasis, cools the blood, and reduces ulcerations. Olibanum *(rǔ xiāng)* and Myrrha *(mò yào)* invigorate the blood, dispel blood stasis, promote the movement of qi, and alleviate pain. Both are aromatic substances frequently used in the treatment of traumatic injury. According to Zhang Xi-Chun, the formula's author, the former moves and regulates the qi, while the latter transforms stasis to regulate the blood. Zhang Bin-Cheng, another late-Qing author, writes about their interaction in *Convenient Reader of Established Formulas*: "Together, they disseminate the pores [by means of their] fragrant, aromatic [nature], unblock and spread the nutritive and protective [qi], and are thus miraculous medicinals to treat fixed pain." The warm wine serves as envoy, facilitating the dispersing effects of the other ingredients and focusing their actions on the blood vessels. With the removal of stasis, the flow of blood in the collaterals is facilitated, and the pain is thus relieved.

Cautions and Contraindications

Contraindicated during pregnancy.

Commentary

This formula was originally designed for treating either fixed abdominal masses that result from the stasis of blood or pain that results from obstruction to the flow of blood through the collaterals. The actions of this formula in eliminating blood stasis and alleviating pain are quite strong, and it is therefore also effective in treating the bruising, swelling, and pain associated with traumatic injury. All of the herbs in this formula are frequently used in external medicine. Angelicae sinensis Radix *(dāng guī)*, for instance, reduces swelling and alleviates pain, pushes out pus, and generates the growth of new tissue by means of its warming and tonifying actions. Olibanum *(rǔ xiāng)* and Myrrha *(mò yào)* open the collaterals, reduce swelling, alleviate pain, and promote healing. Salviae miltiorrhizae Radix *(dān shēn)*, meanwhile, adds a cooling action that reduces the inflammation associated with such problems.

The indications for this formula are accordingly extremely wide, and the best results are achieved by means of its flexible application in the clinic. Specific problems are addressed by the modifications formed by adding and subtracting ingredients. These modifications direct the actions of invigorating the blood, dispelling blood stasis, and alleviating pain to particular parts of the body.

Biomedical Indications

With the appropriate presentation, this formula may be used to treat a variety of biomedically-defined disorders including angina pectoris, cerebral thrombosis, postconcussion syndrome, sciatica, restless leg syndrome, pelvic inflammatory disease, ectopic pregnancy, and arthritis as well as traumatic injury.

Modifications

- For pain in the lower extremities, add Angelicae pubescentis Radix *(dú huó)* and Achyranthis bidentatae Radix *(niú xī)*.
- For pain in the upper extremities, add Notopterygii Rhizoma seu Radix *(qiāng huó)*, Curcumae longae Rhizoma *(jiāng huáng)*, and Forsythiae Fructus *(lián qiáo)*.

- For abdominal pain in women, add Persicae Semen (*táo rén*) and Trogopterori Faeces (*wǔ líng zhī*).
- For red, swollen, hot, and painful ulcerations, add Lonicerae Flos (*jīn yín huā*), Forsythiae Fructus (*lián qiáo*), and Anemarrhenae Rhizoma (*zhī mǔ*).
- For deep-rooted yin-type ulcerations, add Cinnamomi Cortex (*ròu guì*) and Cervi Cornus Colla (*lù jiǎo jiāo*).
- For nonhealing ulcerations, add Astragali Radix (*huáng qí*), Anemarrhenae Rhizoma (*zhī mǔ*), and Glycyrrhizae Radix (*gān cǎo*).
- For abscesses of the internal organs, add Notoginseng Radix (*sān qī*) and Arctii Fructus (*niú bàng zǐ*).
- For fixed abdominal masses, add Paeoniae Radix rubra (*chì sháo*), Persicae Semen (*táo rén*), Curcumae Rhizoma (*é zhú*), and Sparganii Rhizoma (*sān léng*).

丹參飲 （丹参饮）
Salvia Drink
dān shēn yǐn

Source *Compendium of Songs on Modern Formulas* (1801)

Salviae miltiorrhizae Radix (*dān shēn*)..................30g
Santali albi Lignum (*tán xiāng*) 3g
Amomi Fructus (*shā rén*) 3g

Method of Preparation Decoction

Actions Invigorates the blood, dispels blood stasis, promotes the movement of qi, and alleviates pain

Indications

Abdominal or epigastric pain that may radiate upward accompanied by signs and symptoms of blood stasis and qi stagnation.

This is blood stasis and qi stagnation that has accumulated in the middle burner where it causes abdominal or epigastric pain that may radiate upward.

Analysis of Formula

The primary action of this formula is to invigorate the blood, and its secondary action is to regulate the qi. Despite its simple composition of moderate herbs, it is quite effective in treating Stomach pain due to stagnant qi and blood stasis. Salviae miltiorrhizae Radix (*dān shēn*) is bitter and slightly cold and can be used in a large dosage without injuring the qi and blood. It serves as the chief herb to invigorate the blood, transform blood stasis, and alleviate pain. Because qi stagnation often accompanies blood stasis, the deputy, Santali albi Lignum (*tán xiāng*), warms the middle burner and regulates the qi, while the assistant, Amomi Fructus (*shā rén*), promotes the movement of qi, relaxes the middle burner, disperses the stifling sensation of constraint in the chest, and al-

leviates pain. Together, these three ingredients unblock the qi and blood to restore its smooth and unimpeded flow, thereby resolving the pain.

The relative dosage of blood-invigorating to qi-regulating herbs in this formula is five to one. Although it is both cooling and warming, the former action is clearly more important. This reflects that the formula focuses on blood stasis patterns, even as it regulates the qi in order to treat them.

Cautions and Contraindications

Contraindicated during pregnancy and in cases with bleeding diathesis or any active hemorrhagic disorder.

Commentary

The source text notes that the use of warm herbs is inappropriate for treating this particular type of epigastric pain. This comment not only suggests that the formula itself is slightly cold, but also that the type of epigastric pain that radiates upward is usually associated with a pattern of blood stasis involving some heat. The source text also observes that this formula is particularly effective in treating chest and epigastric pain in women. Although today the formula is used primarily in treating epigastric pain, it may also be used in treating the dysmenorrhea and flank pain associated with this pattern of disharmony.

Biomedical Indications

With the appropriate presentation, this formula may be used to treat a variety of biomedically-defined disorders including angina pectoris, hepatitis, pancreatitis, cholecystitis, chronic gastritis, peptic ulcer, and primary or secondary dysmenorrhea.

Modifications

- For angina pectoris and dyspnea associated with coronary artery disease, combine with Trichosanthis Fruit, Chinese Chive, and Pinellia Decoction (*guā lóu xiè bái bái jiǔ tāng*).
- For stomach pain and distention, or for pain radiating to the flanks associated with nausea and vomiting and a purplish tongue body, combine with Frigid Extremities Powder (*sì nì sǎn*) or Melia Toosendan Powder (*jīn líng zǐ sǎn*) and add Haematitum (*dài zhě shí*) and Inulae Flos (*xuán fù huā*).
- For painful obstruction of the chest with stabbing pain radiating to the back that is accompanied by shortness of breath, add Paeoniae Radix rubra (*chì sháo*), Chuanxiong Rhizoma (*chuān xiōng*), Carthami Flos (*hóng huā*), Crataegi Fructus (*shān zhā*), and Aurantii Fructus (*zhǐ ké*).
- For pain in the flanks due to blood stasis in the collaterals, add Curcumae Radix (*yù jīn*) and Olibanum (*rǔ xiāng*).

大黃蟅蟲丸（大黃蟅虫丸）

Rhubarb and Ground Beetle Pill

dà huáng zhè chóng wán

Source　*Essentials from the Golden Cabinet* (c. 220)

steamed Rhei Radix et Rhizoma *(shú dà huáng)* 300g
Eupolyphaga/Stelophaga *(tǔ biē chóng)* 30g
Persicae Semen *(táo rén)* 60g
Toxicodendri Resina *(gān qī)* 30g
Holotrichia *(qí cáo)* * 60g
Hirudo *(shuǐ zhì)* 60g
Tabanus *(méng chóng)* 60g
Scutellariae Radix *(huáng qín)* 60g
Armeniacae Semen *(xìng rén)* 60g
Rehmanniae Radix *(shēng dì huáng)* 300g
Paeoniae Radix *(sháo yào)* 120g
Glycyrrhizae Radix *(gān cǎo)* 90g

Method of Preparation　Grind the ingredients into a powder and form into pills with the addition of honey. The source text prescribes five pills the size of a small bean three times a day. At present, Paeoniae Radix alba *(bái sháo)* is most commonly used for Paeoniae Radix *(sháo yào)* and the dose is one 3g pill taken 1-3 times daily with wine or warm water. May also be prepared as a decoction with a proportionate reduction in the dosage of the ingredients.

Actions　Breaks up and dispels blood stasis and generates new blood

Indications

Emaciation, abdominal fullness, loss of appetite, rough, dry and scaly skin, a dull and dark appearance of the eyes, amenorrhea, and tidal fever.

These symptoms are characteristic of a group of disorders known as the 'five consumptions' (五癆 *wǔ láo*), first described in Chapter 23 of *Basic Questions:* "Long-term gazing damages the blood; long-term lying down damages the qi; long-term sitting damages the flesh; long-term standing damages the bones; long-term walking damages the sinews. These are the damages that [lead to] the five consumptions." The precise pattern treated by this formula is defined in the source text as "damage to the circulation of nutritive and protective qi in the channels with accumulation of dry blood (干血 *gān xuè*) in the interior." The pathogenesis of dry blood is two-fold: (1) stasis of blood causes constraint, which transforms into heat, and (2) injury to the yin and blood inhibits the moistening of the muscles and skin. This manifests as rough and dry, scaly skin and other symptoms of malnourishment throughout the body.

* Holotrichia (蠐螬 *qí cáo*) is the immature form of *Holotrichia diomphalia* (Bates), known as the northeast giant black chafer. It is a salty, slighty warm, toxic, blood-invigorating substance that breaks up stasis and disperses clumps while stopping pain, and also resolves toxicity. The normal dosage in pills and powders is 2-5g per day. It should not be given to pregnant women or debilitated patients.

Rough, dry, and scaly skin and the dull and dark appearance of the eyes are typical signs of internal accumulation of static blood. Injury to the yin and blood prevents nourishment from reaching upward to the eyes, which consequently appear dull and dark. Amenorrhea and tidal fever may result from either the injury to the yin and blood, or the obstruction from accumulation of blood.

Analysis of Formula

Although the term 'consumption' suggests severe deficiency, this formula focuses on a pattern characterized primarily by excess (i.e., dry blood) that secondarily gives rise to signs of deficiency. Thus, the strategy it utilizes is one of dispelling stasis to facilitate the generation of new blood.

One of the chief ingredients, Rhei Radix et Rhizoma *(dà huáng)*, eliminates blood stasis by attacking and purging, while simultaneously cooling the blood and clearing heat. It has the ability to break up abdominal masses and accumulations, pushing out the stale blood to allow generation of new blood. The other chief ingredient, Eupolyphaga/Stelophaga *(tǔ biē chóng)*, attacks and purges the accumulation of blood, eliminates blood stasis, and breaks up blood that has aggregated into fixed abdominal masses. The deputies are Persicae Semen *(táo rén)*, Toxicodendri Resina *(gān qī)*, Holotrichia *(qí cáo)*, Hirudo *(shuǐ zhì)*, and Tabanus *(méng chóng)*. They assist the chief ingredients by invigorating the blood, unblocking the channels, and breaking up and eliminating blood stasis, thereby reducing the fixed abdominal masses.

There are four assistants. Scutellariae Radix *(huáng qín)* is matched with Rhei Radix et Rhizoma *(dà huáng)* to clear heat from the Liver due to blood stasis. Armeniacae Semen *(xìng rén)* is matched with Persicae Semen *(táo rén)* to moisten dryness. In association with the blood-invigorating and purgative herbs, their actions of breaking up blood stasis and directing qi downward encourage the elimination of blood stasis. In addition, the combination of Scutellariae Radix *(huáng qín)* and Armeniacae Semen *(xìng rén)* is helpful in relieving the heat from constraint that may accompany this disorder. Rehmanniae Radix *(shēng dì huáng)* and Paeoniae Radix alba *(bái sháo)* nourish the blood and yin. The envoy, Glycyrrhizae Radix *(gān cǎo)*, harmonizes the middle burner, tonifies deficiency, and regulates and harmonizes the actions of the other herbs. It also helps prevent injury to the normal qi from the harsh properties of those herbs that are used in breaking up blood stasis. Moreover, Rehmanniae Radix *(shēng dì huáng)*, Paeoniae Radix alba *(bái sháo)*, and Glycyrrhizae Radix *(gān cǎo)* comprise a group of herbs that tonify deficiency and generate blood, thereby providing a tonifying dimension to this formula to counterbalance its attacking aspect. Taking the pills with wine in effect adds another envoy ingredient that enhances the actions of the other herbs.

Cautions and Contraindications

Contraindicated during pregnancy.

Commentary

This formula is primarily used in treating concurrent blood stasis and consumption. While blood stasis may occur as a result of long-term deficiency, it is also the case that severe blood stasis may inhibit the generation of new blood and thereby prevent the renewal of primal qi. The strategy underlying this formula addresses the latter situation by focusing on the elimination of blood stasis as a means of promoting the generation of new blood, and thus primal qi. This has been emphasized by almost all commentators on the source text. Tang Zong-Hai's analysis in *Discussion of Blood Patterns* is representative of this consensus: "Where dry blood is not being dispelled, the physiology whereby new blood is generated [has broken down]. Therefore, even though one almost exclusively sees deficiency, [treatment] must generally focus on dispelling dry blood." However, because a patient suffering from consumption is extremely deficient, it is inadvisable to use an attacking method, which may be too violent in its action. For this reason, the formula is prescribed in pill form to moderate its dispelling action.

Additionally, this strategy has served as a model that was expanded by later generations of physicians to other types of patterns. Ye Tian-Shi's predilection for using animal substances to treat blood stasis in the collaterals and extraordinary vessels (both of which he defined as chronic problems) can be directly traced to this formula. Zhang Xi-Chun's method for treatment of consumption, represented by formulas such as All-Inclusive Decoction for Fostering the True (*shí quán yù zhēn tāng*) (*see* ASSOCIATED FORMULA below), openly acknowledges Zhang Zhong-Jing's influence.

Although commentators describe the composition of the formula as being so balanced that not one herb can be changed without diminishing its efficacy, Toxicodendri Resina (*gān qī*) is known to produce allergic reactions in sensitive individuals. Additionally, it is not allowed to be used for medicinal purposes in many countries, including the United States. One possible substitute is Daemonoropis Resina (*xuè jié*).

Comparisons

➤ Vs. PEACH PIT DECOCTION TO ORDER THE QI (*táo hé chéng qì tāng*) AND APPROPRIATE DECOCTION (*dǐ dàng tāng*)

All three formulas invigorate the blood and eliminate stasis by draining it via the bowels, and all use Rhei Radix et Rhizoma (*dà huáng*) for this purpose. However, while Rhubarb and Ground Beetle Pill (*dà huáng zhè chóng wán*) treats a pattern of 'dry blood,' the other two formulas treat 'blood buildup' patterns. Blood buildup in the lower burner is due to excess heat entering the blood aspect where it clumps with the blood. This is a condition of excess characterized by lower abdominal pain, night fevers, delirious speech, irritability, restlessness and thirst, and a submerged, full, or choppy pulse. In more severe cases there may be manic behavior. The initial stages of such a pattern are purged with Peach Pit Decoction to Order the Qi (*táo hé chéng qì tāng*). More chronic patterns, characterized by more severe psychological symptoms as well as the passing of dark stools, are treated with Appropriate Decoction (*dǐ dàng tāng*). In these latter patterns, the blood has already become dry. For this reason, animal substances are used to dissolve this 'noxious' blood, but the emphasis is still on draining heat and clumping. Rhubarb and Ground Beetle Pill (*dà huáng zhè chóng wán*) reverses this priority because consumption due to dry blood is a mixed pattern of excess and deficiency where blood stasis gives rise to heat from constraint, dryness, and deficiency. This pattern is characterized by emaciation, abdominal fullness, loss of appetite, rough, dry, and scaly skin, a dull and dark quality in the eyes, amenorrhea, and tidal fever, indicating that the stasis is in the vessels and collaterals. To treat this problem one must use a larger number of animal substances, even though the way to eliminate the noxious blood from the body is still via the bowels.

Biomedical Indications

With the appropriate presentation, this formula may be used to treat a wide variety of biomedically-defined disorders including chronic hepatitis, alcoholic liver disease, fibrosis of the liver, cirrhosis of the liver, hepatic neoplasms, organomegaly, tubercular peritonitis, uterine leiomyoma, chronic myelogenous leukemia, esophageal varices, postsurgical adhesions, diabetes, psoriasis, and thrombocytopenic purpura.

Alternate name

Rhubarb and Ground Beetle Pill to be Used in Women's Diseases (*fù kē dà huáng zhè chóng wán*) in *Collected Formulas from the Crane Feeding Pavilion*

Modifications

• For cirrhosis of the liver, add Bupleuri Radix (*chái hú*).

• For Spleen deficiency, use together or alternate with Six-Gentlemen Decoction with Aucklandia and Amomum (*xiāng shā liù jūn zǐ tāng*).

• For severe qi and blood deficiency, use together or alternate with Eight-Treasure Decoction (*bā zhēn tāng*), All-Inclusive Great Tonifying Decoction (*shí quán dà bǔ tāng*), or Restore the Spleen Decoction (*guī pí tāng*).

• For the treatment of uterine fibroids that occur against a background of lower burner cold, combine with Drive Out Stasis from the Lower Abdomen Decoction (*shào fù zhú yū tāng*) or Flow-Warming Decoction (*wēn jīng tāng*).

- For lumps and swellings in the flanks and chest with distention and pain, combine with Rambling Powder *(xiāo yáo sǎn)*.

Associated Formula

十全育真湯 (十全育真汤)

All-Inclusive Decoction for Fostering the True

shí quán yù zhēn tāng

SOURCE *Essays on Medicine Esteeming the Chinese and Respecting the Western* (1918-1934)

Ginseng Radix *(rén shēn)* 12g
Rehmanniae Radix *(shēng dì huáng)* 12g
Dioscoreae Rhizoma *(shān yào)* 12g
Anemarrhenae Rhizoma *(zhī mǔ)* 12g
Scrophulariae Radix *(xuán shēn)* 12g
Fossilia Ossis Mastodi *(lóng gǔ)* 12g
Ostreae Concha *(mǔ lì)* 12g
Salviae miltiorrhizae Radix *(dān shēn)* 6g
Curcumae Rhizoma *(é zhú)* 4.5g
Sparganii Rhizoma *(sān léng)* 4.5g

Decoction. For deficiency consumption characterized by a wiry, rapid, fine, and minute pulse, rough, dry and scaly skin, emaciation, and inability to sustain one's physical strength by eating. There can also be sweating on exertion, coughing, panting, inappropriate chills and fevers, many confused dreams, and seminal emissions. This formula, designed by the modern physician Zhang Xi-Chun, focuses on deficiency consumption associated with yin deficiency. Usually corresponding to the biomedical disease category tuberculosis, this is the type of disorder with which the term 'deficiency consumption' came to be associated in the late imperial period. Drawing on Zhang Zhong-Jing's approach to deficiency and consumption, Zhang Xi-Chun not only emphasized tonifying the yin and qi, but also breaking up the blood stasis by means of herbs such as Curcumae Rhizoma *(é zhú)*, Sparganii Rhizoma *(sān léng)*, and Salviae miltiorrhizae Radix *(dān shēn)*. He argued that not only blood stasis caused by overwork and exhaustion, but also that due to traumatic injury, sudden exertion of too much force, bleeding, or improper medical treatment itself could lead to deficiency. All of these conditions can be treated with this formula.

Section 2

FORMULAS THAT STOP BLEEDING

The formulas in this section are used when blood leaves the vessels and causes such manifestations as vomiting of blood, nosebleed, coughing of blood, blood in the stool, blood in the urine, excessive menstruation, or uterine bleeding. Patterns with bleeding may be further differentiated in accordance with the various yin and yang organs involved; the etiological factors of cold, heat, deficiency, and excess; the location of the bleeding; and whether the disorder is acute or chronic.

Because bleeding is a common symptom, it is not surprising that discussion of this problem goes back to the *Inner Classic*, which provides some basic differentiation. For example, a passage in Chapter 66 of *Divine Pivot* states: "When the yang collaterals are damaged, the blood overflows externally; when the blood overflows externally, there are nosebleeds. When the yin collaterals are damaged, the blood overflows internally; when the blood overflows internally, there is bleeding from behind." In *Essentials from the Golden Cabinet*, at the end of the Han era, two basic types of bleeding disorders were described: the first due to cold from deficiency and the second to overabundant heat.

By the time of Zhu Dan-Xi, the importance of a relatively complex approach to these problems was clearly articulated. In *Essential Teachings of [Zhu] Dan-Xi*, Zhu specifically observed that, "When using medicinals for the blood, one cannot alone use [those that] promote its movement or alone use [those that] stop it." This multifaceted approach became the norm, as typified by a passage in *Introduction to Medicine* by the Ming-dynasty writer Li Ting:

> To cool the blood, one must first clear the qi; once one knows from which channel the blood has come, use that channel's qi-clearing herbs. When the qi is cleared, the blood will automatically return to the channel. If there is static blood that has congealed and stagnated, one should first get rid of the stasis and then regulate the qi.

The most common causes of bleeding as the primary symptom are the reckless movement of hot blood, where the blood is forced out of the vessels, and qi and yang deficiency, where the body is unable to retain the blood within the vessels.

Not all formulas that treat bleeding are found in this chapter. When treating the root cause is more important than dealing with the manifestation of bleeding, formulas from the appropriate chapters should be used. For example, formulas for treating the reckless movement of hot blood when bleeding is not the primary symptom are discussed in Chapter 4 on clearing heat; formulas for bleeding due to blood or qi deficiency when tonifying is the primary strategy are discussed in Chapter 8 with the other tonics; when bleeding is regarded as a stage in the development of an abandoned disorder, the formulas in Chapter 9 for stabilizing and binding abnormal leakage are used; and finally, when bleeding is due to blood stasis, the appropriate formulas are found in the first section of this chapter, on invigorating the blood.

The core ingredients of these formulas are those that treat the manifestation by directly stopping the bleeding such as Cirsii Herba *(xiǎo jì)*, Platycladi Cacumen *(cè bǎi yè)*, charred Trachycarpi Petiolus *(zōng lǘ tàn)*, Chebulae Fructus *(hē zǐ)*, and Terra flava usta *(zào xīn tǔ)*. Depending on the specific cause of the bleeding, there will be other primary ingredients:

- When blazing heat forces the blood to move recklessly with bleeding of bright red blood and symptoms such as a dry throat, red face and eyes, dry stools, dark and scanty urine, a yellow tongue coating, and a rapid pulse, choose herbs that drain heat and cool the blood such as Rehmanniae Radix (shēng dì huáng), Moutan Cortex (mǔ dān pí), and Gardeniae Fructus (zhī zǐ).

- When qi and yang deficiency are unable to govern the blood, leading to chronic bleeding of pale blood accompanied by such signs and symptoms as cold extremities, a wan complexion, a pale tongue with a white coating, and a submerged and forceless pulse, choose appropriate warming and tonifying herbs such as Zingiberis Rhizoma (gān jiāng), Ginseng Radix (rén shēn), and Astragali Radix (huáng qí).

In addition to these core ingredients, depending on the circumstance, there are a number of other types of herbs that commonly assist in making these formulas effective:

- Because bleeding by its very nature expends and injures the blood and yin, herbs that tonify the blood and enrich the yin are sometimes used, such as Angelicae sinensis Radix (dāng guī), Rehmanniae Radix praeparata (shú dì huáng), and Asini Corii Colla (ē jiāo).

- One of the dangers of stopping bleeding is the development of static blood. To prevent this, it is common for a small amount of herbs that invigorate the blood to be included, among them Moutan Cortex (mǔ dān pí) or Chuanxiong Rhizoma (chuān xiōng).

- Because qi is the commander of the blood, when there is bleeding in a given direction, it is common to include herbs that promote the movement of qi in the opposite direction. For example, if there is bleeding from above (such as nosebleed, vomiting of blood, or coughing up of blood), herbs that direct the qi downward, such as Achyranthis bidentatae Radix (niú xī), Haematitum (dài zhě shí), or Ostreae Concha (mǔ lì), are used. When there is bleeding from below (such as bleeding from the rectum or uterine bleeding), herbs that cause the qi to ascend, such as Schizonepetae Herba (jīng jiè), Cimicifugae Rhizoma (shēng má), and Astragali Radix (huáng qí), are used.

Note that when used to stop bleeding, many herbs are either dry-fried or charred to increase their astringent properties.

The proper strategy for treating chronic bleeding is to focus on both the source or root of the disorder as well as its manifestations. For sudden, massive hemorrhage, the emphasis should clearly be on treating the manifestations, in concert with biomedical management. When severe blood loss causes the collapse of qi, one should first strongly tonify the source qi in order to rescue the collapsed qi, which is a dangerous condition.

十灰散
Ten Partially-Charred Substances Powder
shí huī sǎn

Source   *Miraculous Book of Ten Remedies for Consumption* (1348)

Cirsii japonici Herba sive Radix (dà jì) . . . . (9g)
Cirsii Herba (xiǎo jì) . . . . (15g)
Nelumbinis Folium (hé yè) . . . . (9g)
Platycladi Cacumen (cè bǎi yè) . . . . (9g)
Imperatae Rhizoma (bái máo gēn) . . . . (30g)
Rubiae Radix (qiàn cǎo gēn) . . . . (12g)
Gardeniae Fructus (zhī zǐ) . . . . (12g)
Rhei Radix et Rhizoma (dà huáng) . . . . (9g)
Moutan Cortex (mǔ dān pí) . . . . (9g)
Trachycarpi Petiolus (zōng lǘ pí) . . . . (6g)

Method of Preparation   Partially char equal amounts of the herbs (usually in a vacuum to preserve their properties), then grind into a fine powder. The normal dosage is 9-15g of the powder mixed with prepared Chinese ink that is ground with lotus root juice or Japanese radish (daikon) juice instead of water. This should be taken after meals. May also be prepared as a decoction in water with the dosage specified in parentheses.

Actions   Cools the blood, stops bleeding, clears heat, and drains fire

Indications

Nosebleed or vomiting, spitting, or coughing up of bright red blood. These symptoms usually occur as acute bleeding disorders with sudden onset. The tongue is red and the pulse is rapid.

This is fire blazing in the middle and upper burners that injures the blood vessels, a form of reckless movement of hot blood that spills out of the channels. From an organ perspective, the key here is the Liver, which both stores and regulates the blood. When there is blazing Liver fire, the fire flares upward. This causes the qi to also rebel upward, and the blood then follows. Reckless movement of hot blood damages the collaterals and the blood overflows above, leading to blood emerging from the nose or mouth. This understanding goes back to Chapter 66 of *Divine Pivot*, where it states: "When the yang collaterals are damaged, the blood overflows externally; when the blood overflows externally, there are nosebleeds."

When blazing Liver fire flares and scorches and damages the Lung collaterals, there will be nosebleed or coughing of blood. When the Liver fire attacks the Stomach, it breaks the blood vessels of the Stomach, leading to vomiting or spitting up of blood. The red tongue and rapid pulse also reflect the underlying blazing fire.

Analysis of Formula

This is a pattern of vigorous heat and fire, which forces the reckless movement of hot blood. Treatment requires directly draining the heat in concert with stopping the bleeding. The two chief herbs, sweet, cooling Cirsii japonici Herba sive Radix *(dà jì)* and Cirsii Herba *(xiǎo jì)*, are both good at cooling the blood and stopping bleeding, while also dispelling stasis. As noted in *Essays on Medicine Esteeming the Chinese and Respecting the Western*, they "are able to clear heat from the blood to stop the reckless movement of blood." Furthermore, according to *Rectification of the Meaning of Materia Medica*, their focus is to "move downward to guide out the stasis." This makes them particularly apt for bleeding from above.

The four deputies, Nelumbinis Folium *(hé yè)*, Platycladi Cacumen *(cè bǎi yè)*, Imperatae Rhizoma *(bái máo gēn)*, and Rubiae Radix *(qiàn cǎo gēn)*, act together to cool the blood and stop bleeding. The other deputy, Trachycarpi Petiolus *(zōng lǘ pí)*, is added for its astringent properties, which are very effective at stopping bleeding. Together with the chief herbs, the deputies clear the heat that is the source of this problem while also stopping the bleeding.

The bleeding will not stop unless the heat is cleared and the fire is drained, which is done directly by two of the assistants: Gardeniae Fructus *(zhī zǐ)* drains heat via the urine and Rhei Radix et Rhizoma *(dà huáng)* via the stool. In this manner, the thrust of the upward rebellion is reversed, enabling the qi and fire to descend, the Liver to properly store the blood, and the blood to stay within its normal channels. And because there is a possibility that the use of cooling, astringent herbs can lead to blood stasis, the final assistant in the formula, Moutan Cortex *(mǔ dān pí)*, is matched with Rhei Radix et Rhizoma *(dà huáng)* to cool the blood and eliminate blood stasis. This enables the formula to clear the heat and stop the bleeding without causing stasis of blood.

This formula is traditionally prepared in a rather unique manner. Not only are the ingredients partially charred, they are also mixed with special sweet and cooling liquids to enhance their actions. Preparing the powdered formula with lotus root juice enhances its ability to stop bleeding and disperse blood stasis, while radish juice enhances the downward movement of qi, thus reinforcing the actions of those herbs that conduct the heat downward. Chinese ink helps to cool the blood, stop the bleeding, and transform the blood stasis.

Cautions and Contraindications

This formula treats the manifestation of this problem and should thus be discontinued as soon as the bleeding stops. It should be prepared in advance and the patient must lie quietly during treatment. In severe cases, it may be necessary to combine biomedical and Chinese treatments.

Commentary

The aim of this formula is to quickly stop the bleeding. Once this has been achieved, it is important to determine the cause and treat accordingly. In view of its pathophysiology, this will most likely involve clearing fire from the Liver or yang brightness warp as well as enriching the yin that has been damaged by the heat.

The preparation of this formula involves charring the outer layer of the herbs. This makes them more astringent and thereby strengthens their ability to stop bleeding, but does not otherwise affect their natural properties. Many of the herbs not only possess strong blood-cooling and heat-clearing properties, they also have the specific ability to alleviate acute bleeding in the upper part of the body. One of the distinctive aspects of this formula is its ability to treat upper-body hemorrhage by conducting the heat downward. The basic pathophysiology of this was described in the 17th-century text *Extensive Notes on Medicine* by Miao Xi-Yong:

> When there is a surplus of qi, there is fire. When the qi descends, the fire immediately descends. When the fire descends, the blood does not ascend. As the blood follows the movement of the qi, there is then no problem with [blood] overflowing from the upper orifices.

History

The source text is a Yuan-dynasty book that focuses on the treatment of Lung consumption (肺癆 *fèi láo*), which presents similarly to the biomedically-defined disease of pulmonary tuberculosis. The formula's author, Ge Qian-Sun, noted that "Generally, when blood gets hot, it moves, when it gets cold, it congeals, and when it sees black, it stops." While not explicitly stated in this text, the reference to black is understood as referring to five-phase theory where the color of water (black) overcomes blood, which is the color of fire (red). This is the source of the concept in Chinese medicine that charred medicinals are useful for stopping bleeding, a concept that has been frequently used since that time.

Ink

Above we have translated the term 京墨 *jīng mò*, which literally means 'capital ink,' as 'prepared Chinese ink.' The modern formula scholar, Li Fei, has researched this and established that the term refers to a specific type of ink that was used in the imperial palace and was made from the lampblack produced from the soot of pine branches, along with either a gelatin or some type or gluten, often with the addition of aromatic substances. Modern inks are usually made from a different process and cannot be used as a substitute for the traditional pine lampblack-based materials.

Comparison

➤ Vs. FOUR-FRESH PILL *(sì shēng wán)*; see PAGE 601

Biomedical Indications

With the appropriate presentation, this formula may be used to treat a variety of biomedically-defined disorders including

pulmonary tuberculosis, bronchiectasis, acute hemorrhagic esophagitis or gastritis, bleeding peptic ulcer, hemorrhagic febrile diseases, and dysfunctional uterine bleeding.

Modification

- For cases with more intense fire and heat in the blood, prepare as a decoction because in this form, its ability to clear heat, cool the blood, and conduct heat downward is even stronger. When prepared as a decoction, Rhei Radix et Rhizoma *(dà huáng)* and Gardeniae Fructus *(zhī zǐ)* are designated as the chief herbs, and often Achyranthis bidentatae Radix *(niú xī)* and Haematitum *(dài zhě shí)* are added to lead the hot blood downward.

四生丸
Four-Fresh Pill
sì shēng wán

Source   *Yang Family Formulas* (1178)

fresh Platycladi Cacumen *(shēng cè bǎi yè)* . . . . (12g)
Rehmanniae Radix recens *(xiān dì huáng)* . . . . (15-24g)
fresh Nelumbinis Folium *(shēng hé yè)* . . . . (9-12g)
fresh Artemisiae argyi Folium *(shēng ài yè)* . . . . (6-9g)

Method of Preparation   The source text advises to grind equal amounts of the ingredients into a paste and form into pills. May also be prepared as a decoction, or the juice of the crushed, raw herbs may be taken cool or warm with the dosage specified in parentheses.

Actions   Cools the blood and stops bleeding

Indications

Coughing, spitting, or vomiting of blood or nosebleed, particularly of bright-red blood. Accompanying signs and symptoms include a dry mouth and throat, a red or deep red tongue, and a wiry, rapid or forceful, wiry, and rapid pulse.

These are all upper-burner manifestations of heat in the blood. As noted in *Collected Treatises of [Zhang] Jing-Yue*, "When bleeding is observed from the mouth and nose, it is usually because the yang is overabundant and the yin deficient. The two [resulting] fires compel the blood to move recklessly from the orifices." When heat enters the blood level, it may cause the blood to move recklessly and spill out of the blood vessels, which manifests as coughing, spitting, or vomiting of bright-red blood, or nosebleeds. The pulse becomes wiry, rapid, and forceful. Heat may also injure the fluids, producing dryness in the mouth and throat, and a red or deep-red tongue body.

Analysis of Formula

Focusing on bleeding from the orifices of the upper body, this formula employs a strategy of cooling the blood and stopping bleeding. Platycladi Cacumen *(cè bǎi yè)*, the chief herb, cools the blood and stops bleeding. It is combined with the deputy, Rehmanniae Radix *(shēng dì huáng)*, which clears heat and cools the blood, and thereby enhances the chief herb's ability to stop bleeding. The deputy also treats injury to the yin by nourishing the yin and thereby generating fluids. One assistant is Nelumbinis Folium *(hé yè)*, which clears heat, cools the blood, and stops bleeding while also dispersing stasis. The other assistant is Artemisiae argyi Folium *(ài yè)*, which, although acrid and warm, is not drying and serves to enhance the overall effect of the formula in stopping bleeding, while also helping to prevent the cooling nature of the other ingredients from leading to any form of stasis.

This formula is notable for enriching in the midst of clearing so that no further damage is done to the blood. Similarly, there is dispersing in the midst of clearing, so that cooling of the blood does not lead to any form of constraint. Finally, there is warming in the midst of clearing, so that the Stomach is not adversely affected. Of all the formulas that clear heat to stop bleeding, this is the most balanced and least harsh.

Three of the herbs, Platycladi Cacumen *(cè bǎi yè)*, Rehmanniae Radix *(shēng dì huáng)*, and Nelumbinis Folium *(hé yè)*, are cool or cold in nature, but are matched with a warm herb, Artemisiae argyi Folium *(ài yè)*, which warms the channels and scatters cold. This is an example of using an ingredient with properties that are opposite those of the principal ingredients to moderate their effect when they might otherwise be too strong.

Cautions and Contraindiations

Even with its well-balanced composition, this formula should only be used acutely and should be discontinued once the bleeding has stopped. Prolonged use increases the chances of developing blood stasis.

Commentary

One of the distinctive features of this formula is the optional use of fresh (unprocessed) herbs to strengthen its action in cooling the blood. This is particularly helpful when treating those types of bleeding caused by the reckless movement of hot blood.

History

This formula first appeared in the 12th-century work *Yang Family Formulas*, in which it was called Four-Flavors Pill (四味丸 *sì wèi wán);* none of the ingredients was fresh. In the next century, the formula was listed in *Fine Formulas for Women* under its present name, where fresh leaves were specified. However, because at the present time it is rare for fresh herbs to be used, some modern writers (including Li Fei and the other editors of the standard textbook on formulas) have suggested that Four-Flavors Pill *(sì wèi wán)* should again become the standard name.

Variations in Preparation

Some practitioners prefer to prepare the formula as a decoction using stir-baked rather than fresh ingredients, with the exception of Rehmanniae Radix (*shēng dì huáng*), which is used in its raw form. In that case, a larger dosage of dry-friend Artemisiae argyi Folium (*chǎo ài yè*) may be utilized. Artemisiae argyi Folium (*ài yè*) contains a volatile oil that stimulates the gastrointestinal tract. A small amount of this herb in the decoction can increase the appetite, while a large amount may cause symptoms of acute gastroenteritis. Dry-frying has the effect of vaporizing this oil, which permits the use of a larger dosage while avoiding its unfavorable side effects. Research has also demonstrated that dry-friend Artemisiae argyi Folium (*chǎo ài yè*) has a stronger action in stopping bleeding than does its raw form.

Comparisons

➤ Vs. Ten Partially-Charred Substances Powder (*shí huī sǎn*)

Both formulas treat similar conditions of bleeding affecting the upper part of the body. Four-Fresh Pill (*sì shēng wán*) is for conditions that are less severe and with less bleeding than those treated by Ten Partially-Charred Substances Powder (*shí huī sǎn*), which is stronger at stopping bleeding. By contrast, Four-Fresh Pill (*sì shēng wán*) has a stronger effect on cooling the blood.

➤ Vs. Small Thistle Drink (*xiǎo jì yǐn zi*); see page 604

Biomedical Indications

With the appropriate presentation, this formula may be used to treat a variety of biomedically-defined disorders including pulmonary tuberculosis, bronchiectasis, peptic ulcer, acute gastritis, hypertension, dysfunctional uterine bleeding, gingivitis, and periodontitis.

Modifications

• To strengthen the effect of the formula, add Nelumbinis Nodus rhizomatis (*ǒu jié*), Imperatae Rhizoma (*bái máo gēn*), Cirsii japonici Herba sive Radix (*dà jì*), Cirsii Herba (*xiǎo jì*), and Agrimoniae Herba (*xiān hè cǎo*).

• For severe coughing or spitting of blood, add Coptidis Rhizoma (*huáng lián*), Rhei Radix et Rhizoma (*dà huáng*), Rubiae Radix (*qiàn cǎo gēn*), and powdered Notoginseng Radix (*sān qī*).

• For dysfunctional uterine bleeding, combine with Ass-Hide Gelatin and Mugwort Decoction (*jiāo ài tāng*).

• For bleeding peptic ulcer, combine with Yellow Earth Decoction (*huáng tǔ tāng*).

Associated Formulas

寧血湯 （宁血汤）
Quiet the Blood Decoction
níng xuè tāng

Source   *Traditional Chinese Ophthalmology* (c. 1970)

Agrimoniae Herba (*xiān hè cǎo*)	15g
Ecliptae Herba (*mò hàn lián*)	15g
Rehmanniae Radix (*shēng dì huáng*)	15g
charred Gardeniae Fructus (*zhī zǐ tàn*)	6g
Paeoniae Radix alba (*bái sháo*)	15g
Bletillae Rhizoma (*bái jí*)	9g
Ampelopsis Radix (*bái liàn*)	6g
Platycladi Cacumen (*cè bǎi yè*)	15g
Asini Corii Colla (*ē jiāo*)	15g
Imperatae Rhizoma (*bái máo gēn*)	15g

Cools the blood and stops bleeding. For hemorrhage in the anterior chamber of the eye due to trauma, or chorioretinitis with repeated hemorrhage, accompanied by red lips and cheeks, bitter taste, dry throat, dizziness, tinnitus, lumbar soreness, spontaneous emissions, a sensation of heat in the palms and soles, a deep-red tongue with a scanty coating, and a wiry, thin, and rapid pulse.

順經湯 （顺经汤）
Smooth the Menses Decoction
shùn jīng tāng

Source   *Women's Diseases According to Fu Qing-Zhu* (17th century, published in 1826)

Angelicae sinensis Radix (*dāng guī*)	15g
Rehmanniae Radix praeparata (*shú dì huáng*)	15g
Paeoniae Radix alba (*bái sháo*)	6g
Moutan Cortex (*mǔ dān pí*)	15g
Poria (*fú líng*)	9g
Glehniae/Adenophorae Radix (*shā shēn*)	9g
Schizonepetae Herba (*jīng jiè*)	9g

Nourishes the yin, moistens the Lungs, clears heat, and cools the blood. For Lung and Kidney yin deficiency leading to blazing fire from deficiency characterized by vomiting or spitting of blood or nosebleeds accompanied by abdominal pain that occurs just before or during menstruation. This is one type of inverted menses (倒經 *dào jīng*).

咳血方
Coughing of Blood Formula
ké xuè fāng

Source   *Essential Teachings of [Zhu] Dan-Xi* (1481)

Indigo naturalis (*qīng dài*)	(6-9g)
Gardeniae Fructus (*zhī zǐ*)	(9g)
Trichosanthis Semen (*guā lóu rén*)	(9g)
Costaziae Os (*fú hǎi shí*)	(9g)
Chebulae Fructus (*hē zǐ*)	(6-9g)

> **Method of Preparation**   The source text advises to grind the ingredients into a powder and form into pills with honey and ginger juice. The pills are dissolved in the mouth, which focuses their actions on the Lungs. Dosage is not specified in the source text. May also be prepared as a decoction with the dosage indicated in parentheses.

> **Actions**   Clears fire, transforms phlegm, preserves the Lungs, and stops coughing and bleeding

Indications

Coughing of blood-streaked sputum, thick sputum that is difficult to expectorate, bitter taste, irritability and easily-provoked anger, constipation, red cheeks, a red tongue with a yellow coating, and a wiry, rapid pulse.

Expectoration of thick sputum streaked with blood is a symptom that is common to many patterns of disharmony. The pattern here is one of Liver fire attacking and scorching the Lungs. The Liver and Lungs are physiologically related in several ways. The Liver channel courses through the chest and lower rib cage, with a branch ascending into the Lungs. The Liver promotes the ascending and spreading of qi, while the Lungs govern the descending and dissemination of qi. The coordination of these functions between the Liver and Lungs ensures the orderly, uninhibited flow of qi throughout the thorax. However, if the motivating action of the Liver qi becomes excessive and transforms into fire, the qi and fire may rebel upward into the Lungs. This scorches the Lung fluids, which congeal and form phlegm. When subjected to more fire, thick sputum is formed that is difficult to expectorate. Phlegm obstructs the proper circulation of Lung qi, which produces coughing, while fire scorches and injures the collaterals of the Lungs, which leads to coughing with blood-streaked sputum. The bitter taste in the mouth, irritability, easily-provoked anger, constipation, red cheeks, red tongue with a yellow coating, and wiry, rapid pulse are all indicative of Liver fire. In the parlance of the five phases, the Lungs (metal) are rebelling against the violation by the Liver (wood). The ancients therefore described this pattern as 'Liver fire punishing the Lungs' or a 'disorder of violation' of metal by wood.

Analysis of Formula

This formula treats a condition where Liver fire scorches the Lungs. In this case, the root of the problem is in the Liver, as once the Liver fire has been cleared, the blood will not move recklessly and the Lungs will be calm. For this reason, the two chief ingredients are focused primarily on clearing Liver fire. Both salty, cold Indigo naturalis *(qīng dài)* and bitter, cold Gardeniae Fructus *(zhī zǐ)* clear the Liver, drain fire, and cool the blood. Indigo naturalis *(qīng dài)* also disperses the fire from constraint and thereby prevents Liver fire from scorching the Heart and Lungs. To stop bleeding of this type, it is advisable to direct the qi downward, since the blood will

follow the qi. In addition to its other functions, Gardeniae Fructus *(zhī zǐ)* conducts the qi downward, thereby clearing heat from the Heart and relieving the irritability. *Medical Formulas Collected and Analyzed* describes the synergistic actions of these two herbs:

> Indigo naturalis *(qīng dài)* drains the Liver, regulates the blood, and scatters fire from constraint in the five yin organs. Gardeniae Fructus *(zhī zǐ)* cools the Heart and clears the Lungs while leading the pathogenic heat to travel downward. These two [herbs] are used to treat fire.

Coughing will persist as long as there is phlegm, and as long as there is coughing, the blood cannot be calm. Sweet, cold Trichosanthis Semen *(guā lóu rén)* and salty, neutral Costaziae Os *(fú hǎi shí)* serve as deputies that cool and transform the hot phlegm and reduce the fire. The former focuses more on moistening the Lungs and stopping coughing while the latter has the effect of softening what is hard. Bitter, sour, astringent, and neutral Chebulae Fructus *(hē zǐ)* serves both as an assistant and an envoy to cool the Lungs while containing any leakage of Lung qi and stopping the coughing.

Cautions and Contraindications

This formula should not be given to patients with Spleen deficiency or Lung and Kidney yin deficiency.

Commentary

If the coughing is not alleviated, one generally cannot expect the bleeding to stop. Similarly, the formula emphasizes the elimination of phlegm, since coughing as a rule will not be alleviated until this is accomplished. The choice of Chebulae Fructus *(hē zǐ)* is important in this regard as it acts both to relieve coughing as well as to transform phlegm.

Allowing the pills to slowly dissolve in the mouth enables the medicine to be assimilated locally and prolongs its effect in treating the coughing up of blood. Furthermore, when the acute bleeding has ceased, the source text recommends the use of tonifying formulas such as Eight-Treasure Decoction *(bā zhēn tāng)* to stabilize the condition and prevent its recurrence.

Indirect or Direct Treatment of Bleeding

The location of the primary symptom or manifestation is in the Lungs, but the root of this disorder lies in the Liver. To treat the root of this disorder, the underlying strategy of the formula is thus to drain Liver fire. This assumes that the Lungs will thereupon return to a calm, tranquil state. Many commentators have praised this formula for omitting herbs that directly stop bleeding, as the simultaneous treatment of the root and indirect resolution of the branch is considered to be more elegant; this is one reason why it is regarded as a model formula. This view was expressed in *Medical Formulas Collected and Analyzed*: "[It] does not use herbs that treat bleeding; once the fire recedes, the bleeding will stop by itself."

This, however, is overstating the case because the formula does contain herbs that stop bleeding. For example, in *Comprehensive Outline of the Materia Medica*, among the indications of Indigo naturalis *(qīng dài)* are vomiting and spitting up of blood. Gardeniae Fructus *(zhī zǐ)* is said to "treat vomiting of blood, nosebleeds, bloody dysenteric disorders, bloody diarrhea, painful bloody urinary dribbling, and static blood from trauma." Similarly, in the 8th-century text *Materia Medica of Ri Hua-Zi*, Chebulae Fructus *(hē zǐ)* is said to stop bloody diarrhea from Intestinal wind as well as vaginal discharge with profuse uterine bleeding.

Change in Ingredients

The source text calls for Notarchi Filamentum (海粉 *hǎi fěn*). This is a salty, cold medicinal that enters the Kidney channel and is used to clear heat, nourish the yin, soften hardness, and reduce phlegm. However, since at least the time of Wang Ang's *Medical Formulas Collected and Analyzed*, Costaziae Os *(fú hǎi shí)* has been used instead because it is much easier to obtain and has a very similar set of functions.

Biomedical Indications

With the appropriate presentation, this formula may be used to treat a variety of biomedically-defined disorders including pulmonary tuberculosis and bronchiectasis.

Alternate name

Lung Bleeding Pill *(fèi xuè wǎn)* in *Essential Teachings of [Zhu] Dan-Xi*

Modifications

- For severe coughing, add Armeniacae Semen *(xìng rén)*. (source text)
- For nosebleeds, substitute Artemisiae annuae Herba *(qīng hāo)* and Moutan Cortex *(mǔ dān pí)* for Chebulae Fructus *(hē zǐ)* and Costaziae Os *(fú hǎi shí)*.
- For coughing with profuse sputum, add Fritillariae thunbergii Bulbus *(zhè bèi mǔ)*, Bambusae Concretio silicea *(tiān zhú huáng)*, and Eriobotryae Folium *(pí pá yè)*.
- For vigorous fire that injures the yin, add Glehniae/Adenophorae Radix *(shā shēn)* and Ophiopogonis Radix *(mài mén dōng)*.
- For nosebleeds, remove Chebulae Fructus *(hē zǐ)* and Costaziae Os *(fú hǎi shí)* and add Artemisiae annuae Herba *(qīng hāo)*, Scutellariae Radix *(huáng qín)*, and Moutan Cortex *(mǔ dān pí)*.
- For profuse sputum and a greasy tongue coating, take with Sweet Wormwood and Scutellaria Decoction to Clear the Gallbladder *(hāo qín qīng dǎn tāng)*.

小薊飲子（小蓟饮子）
Small Thistle Drink
xiǎo jì yǐn zi

Source *Formulas to Aid the Living* (1253)

Cirsii Herba *(xiǎo jì)* 9-15g
Nelumbinis Nodus rhizomatis *(ǒu jié)* 9-15g
dry-fried Typhae Pollen *(chǎo pú huáng)* 9-15g
Rehmanniae Radix *(shēng dì huáng)* 9-18g
Talcum *(huá shí)* 9-15g
Akebiae Caulis *(mù tōng)* 9-15g
Lophatheri Herba *(dàn zhú yè)* 9-15g
Gardeniae Fructus *(zhī zǐ)* 9-15g
Angelicae sinensis Radix *(dāng guī)* 9-15g
Glycyrrhizae Radix praeparata *(zhì gān cǎo)* 9-15g

Method of Preparation The source text advises to coarsely grind the ingredients and take as a draft in 15g doses. At present, it is usually prepared as a decoction with approximately one-quarter of the specified dosage of Rehmanniae Radix *(shēng dì huáng)*, and one- to two-thirds the dosage of the other herbs. It is also common to substitute either unprepared Glycyrrhizae Radix *(gān cǎo)* or Glycyrrhizae Radix tenuis *(gān cǎo shāo)* for Glycyrrhizae Radix praeparata *(zhì gān cǎo)*.

Actions Cools the blood, stops bleeding, promotes urination, and unblocks painful urinary dribbling

Indications

Painful bloody urinary dribbling (with blood in the urine and urinary frequency, urgency, burning, and pain) or simple blood in the urine, accompanied by thirst, irritability, a red tongue with a thin, yellow coating, and a rapid, forceful pulse.

This is static heat accumulating in the lower burner where it injures the blood collaterals and causes the blood to seep downward into the Bladder, from which it is excreted in the urine. If blood in the urine is accompanied by pain, it is called 'painful bloody urinary dribbling.' Urinary frequency, urgency, burning, and pain are due to the obstruction of the lower burner and Bladder functions by the accumulation of heat. Thirst, irritability, a red tongue with a thin, yellow coating, and a rapid, forceful pulse are also indicative of the accumulation of heat in the lower burner. Blood in the urine from this process may also occur without pain.

Analysis of Formula

To adequately treat this condition, a formula must focus on cooling the blood and stopping bleeding as well as promoting urination and treating painful urinary dribbling. Sweet, cooling Cirsii Herba *(xiǎo jì)* is the chief ingredient as it is both quite capable of cooling the blood to stop bleeding—particularly in the urine—and also promoting urination by clearing damp-heat from the Bladder. The three deputies are Typhae Pollen *(pú huáng)*, Nelumbinis Nodus rhizomatis *(ǒu jié)*, and Rehmanniae Radix *(shēng dì huáng)*. These herbs cool the blood and stop bleeding, and also transform stasis and nourish the yin. In this way, they not only strengthen the chief ingredient's ability to stop urinary bleeding, but make it unlikely that the process of stopping bleeding will lead to blood stasis or that promotion of urination will injure the yin.

With heat clumping in the Bladder, the momentum of the disease is downward. The first group of assistants follows this momentum to help get rid of the pathogen via the urine. The cold, slippery properties of Talcum *(huá shí)* enable it to clear heat, promote urination, and unblock painful urinary dribbling. Its slipperiness soothes the urinary passageways and allows heat to pass out through the Bladder. Akebiae Caulis *(mù tōng)*, Lophatheri Herba *(dàn zhú yè)*, and Gardeniae Fructus *(zhī zǐ)* clear and drain fire and heat from the Heart, Lungs, and Triple Burner, eliminating the heat by conducting it downward. Together, they conduct the pathogenic heat out of the body via the urine and unblock painful urinary dribbling.

Urinary bleeding itself can injure the blood, and the use of herbs that stop bleeding can lead to stasis. The final assistant in this formula is Angelicae sinensis Radix *(dāng guī)*, which nourishes and harmonizes the blood, leading it back into the channels and preventing the formation of blood stasis. Its warm nature also moderates the cool and cold properties of the other herbs.

Glycyrrhizae Radix praeparata *(zhì gān cǎo)* serves as the envoy. It relieves spasmodic pain and harmonizes the middle burner, and reconciles the disparate actions of the other herbs in the formula. Where there is more heat, manifested by urethral pain, this herb can be replaced with Glycyrrhizae Radix tenuis *(gān cǎo shāo)*, which drains fire and treats damp-heat pouring downward into the Bladder.

Cautions and Contraindications

Contraindicated during pregnancy. Because the ingredients are primarily cold and unblocking, this formula is inappropriate for use in chronic conditions or for urinary dribbling due to deficiency of the normal qi.

Commentary

The primary strategy underlying Small Thistle Drink *(xiǎo jì yǐn zi)* is to cool the blood and stop the bleeding, and secondarily to drain the fire and unblock painful urinary dribbling. There are also substrategies: some of the ingredients used for the primary strategy of cooling the blood and stopping the bleeding also transform blood stasis, while nourishing the yin is an aspect of some of the ingredients used in the secondary strategy of draining the fire and unblocking painful urinary dribbling. It is therefore a well-rounded formula for treating blood in the urine due to excess heat.

Controversies

As early as *Essentials from the Golden Cabinet,* painful urinary dribbling was defined as heat in the lower burner. Many writers view the pathogenesis of this problem as did Zhang Bing-Cheng in *Convenient Reader of Established Formulas:*

> As to the disorder of painful bloody urinary dribbling, all cases arise from an accumulation of heat in the Heart and Small Intestine. The Heart is the yin organ that generates blood, and the Small Intestine is the yang organ that transmits and conducts. When the Heart transfers heat to the Small Intestine and the Small Intestine transfers the heat to the Bladder, can it be that [the heat] does not force the blood to seep downward and make for a case of painful urinary dribbling?

This formula can be seen as a variation of Guide Out the Red Powder *(dǎo chì sǎn)*, which is the standard formula for guiding out excess Heart fire via the Small Intestine. This led Zhang to describe Gardeniae Fructus *(zhī zǐ)*, Lophatheri Herba *(dàn zhú yè)*, and Akebiae Caulis *(mù tōng)* as the chief herbs, because their ability to clear Heart fire "cleared the source" of the problem. Taking a slightly different view, the sixth edition of the textbook on formulas in the People's Republic of China regarded Rehmanniae Radix *(shēng dì huáng)* as the chief ingredient: "The dosage of Rehmanniae Radix *(shēng dì huáng)* is large, it cools the blood and stops bleeding, and nourishes the yin and clears heat."

Li Fei and the other editors of the advanced text *Formulas* disagree with these arguments. They point out that not only is Cirsii Herba *(xiǎo jì)* found in the name of the formula, but its main focus is stopping the bleeding. As such, the cool, moistening nature of this herb that enters the blood aspect and clears heat clumped in the blood aspect of the lower burner, while also promoting urination, makes it an ideal chief ingredient in a formula to treat urinary bleeding due to heat.

Comparisons

➤ Vs. Four-Fresh Pill *(sì shēng wán)*

Both formulas focus on cooling the blood and stopping bleeding. However, Four-Fresh Pill *(sì shēng wán)* enriches in the midst of clearing heat and is primarily used for reckless movement of hot blood leading to bleeding from the upper part of the body. Small Thistles Drink *(xiǎo jì yǐn zi)* additionally transforms stasis, drains fire, and unblocks painful urinary dribbling and thus is used for bleeding in the lower part of the body via the urethra.

➤ Vs. Powder for Five Types of Painful Urinary Dribbling *(wǔ lín sǎn)*

Both formulas are used to treat painful bloody urination. Small Thistle Drink *(xiǎo jì yǐn zi)* is used for conditions where there is more blood in the urine and the heat is relatively intense.

➤ Vs. Eight-Herb Powder for Rectification (*bā zhèng sǎn*); *see* PAGE 715

Biomedical Indications

With the appropriate presentation, this formula may be used to treat a variety of biomedically-defined disorders including acute urinary tract infection, renal calculi, renal tuberculosis, polycystic kidneys, renal cysts, sickle cell disease, hydronephrosis, and benign prostatic hypertrophy.

Alternate names

Small Thistle Decoction (*xiǎo jì tāng*) in *Correct Transmission of Medicine*; Small Thistle Drink (*xiǎo jì yǐn*) in *Displays of Enlightened Physicians*

Modifications

• For more intense heat and stasis with marked rough urination and burning pain, add Pyrrosiae Folium (*shí wěi*), Persicae Semen (*táo rén*), Taraxaci Herba (*pú gōng yīng*), and Phellodendri Cortex (*huáng bǎi*).

• For injury to the qi and yin, remove Akebiae Caulis (*mù tōng*) and Talcum (*huá shí*) and add Codonopsis Radix (*dǎng shēn*), Astragali Radix (*huáng qí*), and Asini Corii Colla (*ē jiāo*).

• For severe pain, add Succinum (*hǔ pò*) and Lygodii Herba (*jīn shā téng*).

• For acute nephritis, add Spirodelae Herba (*fú píng*), Imperatae Rhizoma (*bái máo gēn*), Lonicerae Flos (*jīn yín huā*), and Forsythiae Fructus (*lián qiáo*).

槐花散

Sophora Japonica Flower Powder

huái huā sǎn

Source *Formulas of Universal Benefit from My Practice* (1132)

dry-fried Sophorae Flos (*chǎo huái huā*) . . . . (12g)
Platycladi Cacumen (*chǎo bǎi yè*) . . . . (12g)
Schizonepetae Spica (*jīng jiè suì*) . . . . (6g)
bran-fried Aurantii Fructus (*fū chǎo zhǐ ké*) . . . . (6-9g)

Method of Preparation The source text advises to grind equal amounts of the ingredients into a powder and take in 6g doses mixed with boiled water or thin rice gruel, preferably before meals on an empty stomach. At present, it is usually prepared as a decoction with the dosage specified in parentheses.

Actions Cools the Intestines, stops bleeding, disperses wind, and promotes the movement of qi

Indications

Bright-red bleeding from the rectum during defecation that typically precedes (but may also follow) the passage of stool, blood in the stools, hemorrhoids with either bright-red or dark-red bleeding, a red tongue body, and a wiry, rapid or soggy, rapid pulse.

This condition involves either the lodging of wind-heat or the accumulation of damp-heat in the Intestines and Stomach where it forms toxin. Both processes obstruct the blood level of these organs and lead to blood in the stool, or passing of stool accompanied by bleeding. Blood in the stool is traditionally divided into two categories: Intestinal wind (腸風 *cháng fēng*) due to wind-heat trapped in the Intestines, and toxin in the yin organs (臟毒 *zàng dú*) from turbid damp-heat in the Intestines.

Intestinal wind occurs when the two yang pathogens, wind and heat, are trapped in the Intestines, injuring the blood collaterals and pushing blood into the Intestines. This usually results in bright-red bleeding that precedes defecation or is present in the stools.

With toxin in the yin organs, damp-heat collects and clumps in the Intestines and also damages the blood collaterals. The turbid dampness aspect has a tendency to obstruct the qi dynamic, leading to stagnation and stasis of qi and blood. This commonly manifests as dark blood, either mixed in with the stools or after defecation. In both case, the tongue will be red and the pulse rapid. With wind-heat, the pulse will have a tendency to be wiry, while it will be soggy or slippery when damp-heat is involved.

Analysis of Formula

In order to treat rectal bleeding from either wind-heat or damp-heat, this formula employs a strategy of clearing the Intestines and cooling blood as well as stopping bleeding. The chief herb, bitter and cold Sophorae Flos (*huái huā*), clears damp-heat from the Intestines, drains heat and clears the Intestines, cools the blood, and also stops bleeding. It is an important herb for Intestinal bleeding due to heat. The bitter, astringent, and slightly cold nature of the deputy, Platycladi Cacumen (*cè bǎi yè*), assists the chief herb in cooling the blood and stopping the bleeding. It is also able to dry dampness without injuring the yin, making it an excellent choice for clearing the heat associated with this condition. The other deputy, Schizonepetae Spica (*jīng jiè suì*), disperses wind and enters the blood level to stop the bleeding.

The assistant herb is Aurantii Fructus (*zhǐ ké*), which promotes the movement of qi and thereby relaxes the Intestines. The moderate action of this herb is focused on the Intestines, the locus of this disorder. It enters the blood level and regulates the qi within the blood. Its downward-directing functions are matched with the ascending action of Schizonepetae Spica (*jīng jiè suì*). It adds some ascending qualities that ameliorate the downward-directing aspects of the other ingredients, helping restore proper functioning to the qi dynamic and aiding in the reduction and separation of the pathogens. Because the qi is the 'commander' of the blood, the unimpeded movement of qi facilitates the smooth flow of the blood. Thus, "By regulating the qi, the blood will be regulated," and one can thereby avoid the stasis of blood that may occur when only herbs that stop bleeding are used.

Cautions and Contraindications

Because this formula consists of cold herbs, it should not be used long-term and should be used with caution in patients with cold from deficiency of the middle burner.

Commentary

One of the unique aspects of this formula is its combination of apparently antagonistic, yet complementary therapeutic strategies. The strategy of restraint in stopping the bleeding and stabilizing the blood is combined with the strategies of clearing damp-heat, dispersing wind, and promoting the movement of qi. Promoting the movement of qi is a counterpoint to the basic strategy of stopping the bleeding, while clearing damp-heat is a counterpoint to stabilizing the blood. These complementary actions are required to achieve the objective of stopping the bleeding, while at the same time avoiding the retention of damp-heat that can obstruct the flow in the Intestines. This formula clears the Intestines, cools the blood, and disperses wind in order to resolve the source of the disorder. When the wind, heat, dampness, and toxin are resolved, the symptom of blood in the stools will usually be relieved.

It is important to remember that this formula only addresses the manifestations of this disorder. After it has been used, one must still address the root problem.

Comparison

➤ Vs. YELLOW EARTH DECOCTION (*huáng tǔ tāng*); *see* PAGE 610

Biomedical Indications

With the appropriate presentation, this formula may be used to treat a variety of biomedically-defined disorders including amebic dysentery, ulcerative colitis, hemorrhoids, anal fissure, and rectal prolapse.

Alternate name

Sophora Japonica Flower Decoction (*huái huā tāng*) in *Indispensable Tools for Pattern Treatment*

Modifications

* To enhance the formula's ability to stop bleeding, substitute charred Schizonepetae Herba (*jīng jiè tàn*) for Schizonepetae Spica (*jīng jiè suì*).
* For severe heat in the Large Intestine, add Coptidis Rhizoma (*huáng lián*) and Phellodendri Cortex (*huáng bǎi*).

* For vigorous Liver heat pouring downward to the Intestines, add Sophorae flavescentis Radix (*kǔ shēn*), Scutellariae Radix (*huáng qín*), Gardeniae Fructus (*zhī zǐ*), and Indigo naturalis (*qīng dài*).
* For chronic or profuse rectal bleeding, add Sanguisorbae Radix (*dì yú*) and Sepiae Endoconcha (*hǎi piāo xiāo*).
* For chronic bleeding causing blood and qi deficiency, add such herbs as Angelicae sinensis Radix (*dāng guī*), Ginseng Radix (*rén shēn*), Astragali Radix (*huáng qí*), Puerariae Radix (*gé gēn*), and Cimicifugae Rhizoma (*shēng má*).
* For bleeding hemorrhoids, add Sanguisorbae Radix (*dì yú*) and Scutellariae Radix (*huáng qín*).
* For ulcerative colitis, substitute Paeoniae Radix alba (*bái sháo*) for Aurantii Fructus (*zhǐ ké*) and add Sanguisorbae Radix (*dì yú*), Bletillae Rhizoma (*bái jí*), Sepiae Endoconcha (*hǎi piāo xiāo*), and Scutellariae Radix (*huáng qín*).
* For amebic dysentery, combine with Pulsatilla Decoction (*bái tóu wēng tāng*).

Associated Formulas

槐角丸

Sophora Japonicae Fruit Pill

huái jiǎo wán

SOURCE *Formulary of the Pharmacy Service for Benefiting the People in the Taiping Era* (1107)

dry-fried Sophorae Fructus (*chǎo huái jiǎo*) 500g
Saposhnikoviae Radix (*fáng fēng*) 250g
Sanguisorbae Radix (*dì yú*) 250g
wine-washed Angelicae sinensis Radix (*jiǔ xǐ dāng guī*) 250g
Scutellariae Radix (*huáng qín*) 250g
bran-fried Aurantii Fructus (*fū chǎo zhǐ ké*) 250g

Grind the herbs into a powder and form into pills with wine. Take in 9g doses with warm water. May also be prepared as a decoction with a proportionate reduction in dosage. Clears heat from the Intestines, stops bleeding, disperses wind, and regulates the qi. For bleeding hemorrhoids or rectal prolapse associated with Intestinal wind with hot toxin or damp-heat. In contrast to the principal formula, this has a stronger effect in clearing heat and stopping bleeding. At present, it is used primarily for treating bleeding hemorrhoids. Note that historically, the principal formula is a modification of this formula.

地榆散

Sanguisorba Powder

dì yú sǎn

SOURCE *Traditional Chinese Internal Medicine* (c.1970)

Sanguisorbae Radix (*dì yú*)
Rubiae Radix (*qiàn cǎo gēn*)
Scutellariae Radix (*huáng qín*)
Coptidis Rhizoma (*huáng lián*)
Gardeniae Fructus (*zhī zǐ*)
Poria (*fú líng*)

Grind equal amounts of the ingredients into a powder and take in 6-9g doses. Cools the blood, stops bleeding, clears heat, and dispels dampness. For accumulation and 'steaming' of damp-heat accompanied by bloody stools with fresh, red blood, bowel movements preceded by bleeding, difficult defecation, a bitter taste, a yellow, greasy tongue coating, and a soggy, rapid pulse.

乙字湯（乙字汤）

Decoction 'B'

yǐ zì tāng (otsuji tō)

<small>SOURCE</small> *Trivial Comments on Medical Matters* (1820)

Angelicae sinensis Radix *(dāng guī)* 6g
Bupleuri Radix *(chái hú)* 5g
Scutellariae Radix *(huáng qín)* 3g
Glycyrrhizae Radix *(gān cǎo)* 3g
Cimicifugae Rhizoma *(shēng má)* 1g
Rhei Radix et Rhizoma *(dà huáng)* 1g

Clears heat and drains stagnation, cools the blood and resolves toxicity. For Intestinal wind, bleeding hemorrhoids or fistulas, prolapsed rectum, uterine bleeding, bleeding during childbirth, or blood-stasis abdominal pain. It may also address itching or pain in or around the vagina owing to heat stasis.

This formula was devised by the Japanese physician Hara Nanyō, who was active in the late 18th and early 19th centuries. It addresses two main categories of disorders due to stasis and heat in the lower body: hemorrhoids or other lesions of the lower portion of the intestinal tract, and uterine bleeding. Similar to the principal formula, it only treats the branch; thus, successful use requires follow-up treatment of the root.

Compared to the principal formula, which has a stronger effect at clearing heat and stopping bleeding, Decoction 'B' *(yǐ zì tāng)* is stronger at treating stasis and also can direct the yang upward.

Modifications

- If heat is prominent, add Phellodendri Cortex *(huáng bǎi)*, Houttuyniae Herba *(yú xīng cǎo)*, and Rehmanniae Radix *(shēng dì huáng)*.

- If stasis is extreme with hard swellings and pain, add Persicae Semen *(táo rén)* and Moutan Cortex *(mǔ dān pí)*.

- For damp-heat, add Phellodendri Cortex *(huáng bǎi)* and a large dosage (30g) of Coicis Semen *(yì yǐ rén)*.

- To increase the formula's ability to stop bleeding, add Sanguisorbae Radix *(dì yú)*.

- For vaginal itching, add Lonicerae Flos *(jīn yín huā)* and Forsythiae Fructus *(lián qiáo)*.

- For painful hemorrhoids, add Aurantii Fructus *(zhǐ ké)*, Linderae Radix *(wū yào)*, and Cyperi Rhizoma *(xiāng fù)*.

- For weak patients or those with loose stools or diarrhea, remove Rhei Radix et Rhizoma *(dà huáng)*.

- For heat-stasis vaginal itching or pain, add Paeoniae Radix rubra *(chì sháo)*, Tetrapanacis Medulla *(tōng cǎo)*, and Phellodendri Cortex *(huáng bǎi)*.

柏葉湯（柏叶汤）

Arborvitae Twig Decoction

bǎi yè tāng

<small>Source</small> *Essentials from the Golden Cabinet* (c. 220)

Platycladi Cacumen *(cè bǎi yè)* 9g
Zingiberis Rhizoma *(gān jiāng)* 9g
Artemisiae argyi Folium *(ài yè)* . . . . 3 handfuls (9-12g)

Method of Preparation   Decoction. The source text recommends adding strained horse feces to the decoction. At present, either nothing is added or Infantis Urina *(tóng biàn)*, the urine of boys under 12 years of age, is used.

Actions   Warms the yang and stops bleeding

Indications

Unremitting vomiting or spitting up of blood or nosebleeds accompanied by a wan complexion, a pale tongue with a thin coating, and a deficient, rapid, and forceless pulse.

This is cold from deficiency affecting the middle qi, resulting in the failure of the Spleen qi to govern the blood, often attributed to overwork. Because the main symptom is a constant, but variable, vomiting or spitting up of blood, it is thought that there is an aspect of ascendant Liver yang that induces the upward-movement of uncontrolled blood. The variability in the amount of the bleeding may be related to a fluctuation in both the degree of Spleen deficiency (related to overwork) and the intensity of the rebellious qi. Although this pattern involves an aspect of ascendant yang, examination should reveal a clear predominance of Spleen qi deficiency, which is failing to hold in the blood. This will be accompanied by characteristic signs of cold from deficiency of the middle burner including a wan complexion, pale tongue with a thin coating, and a deficient, slow, and forceless pulse.

Analysis of Formula

To treat a complex pattern where middle burner cold and ascendant Liver yang combine to cause vomiting or spitting up of blood, this formula employs a strategy of warming the yang, cooling the blood and causing it to descend, and stopping the bleeding. Bitter, astringent, and slightly cold Platycladi Cacumen *(cè bǎi yè)*, the chief herb, has a cooling and descending nature that conducts the blood downward and thereby reverses its reckless, upward movement. It enters the Liver and Lungs, the two channels most involved in the bleeding. Zingiberis Rhizoma *(gān jiāng)*, the deputy, warms the channels, reinforces the yang, and stops the bleeding. Li Shi-Zhen considered this herb to be particularly useful for encouraging the blood herbs to enter the blood, and the qi herbs to enter the qi. He recommended it whenever there was bleeding with yang deficiency. Artemisiae argyi Folium *(ài yè)*, the assistant herb, warms and protects the yang of the middle burner, enabling the Spleen qi to govern the blood.

Cautions and Contraindications

Do not use this formula in cases due to yin deficiency.

Commentary

The source text limits the application of this formula to un-remitting vomiting of blood. Its use has since been expanded to include any type of bleeding in the upper part of the body associated with yang deficiency. The structure of the formula combines both cooling and warming strategies by clearing and redirecting downward the effects of Liver fire, and warming the Spleen yang. Despite this duality, it remains clearly in the category of formulas that emphasize warming the yang in order to govern the blood.

In *Personal Standards for the Essentials from the Golden Cabinet*, the Qing commentator You Yi wrote about the specific problems addressed by this formula:

> When blood encounters heat, it disseminates and moves about, [and] so usually to stop bleeding, cooling herbs are used. Still, there are also cases where blood can move improperly due to qi deficiency accompanied by cold such that the yin and yang do not conserve each other and the nutritive qi is made deficient and is scattered. This is what Zingiberis Rhizoma *(gān jiāng)* and Artemisiae argyi Folium *(ài yè)* are used for. If the blood overflows above, then warming medicines cannot control its floating, ascendant momentum, and it requires the control of Platycladi Cacumen *(cè bǎi yè)* to redirect it downward.

Ingredients

In its original form, this formula called for the addition of horse feces to the decoction, which are strained through a cloth and allowed to clarify by settling. This produces a slightly warm fluid that conducts the blood downward and is one method of "using turbid substances to conduct turbidity out" (以濁導濁 *yǐ zhuó dǎo zhuó*). However, because the quality of this substance varies depending upon its source and the level of nourishment provided to the horse, if this type of substance is deemed necessary, it is usually replaced by Infantis Urina *(tóng biàn)*.

At present, to strengthen the formula's ability to stop bleeding, Zingiberis Rhizoma praeparatum *(páo jiāng)* is commonly substituted for Zingiberis Rhizoma *(gān jiāng)*, and the other two ingredients are usually used in their charred forms.

Comparison

➤ Vs. YELLOW EARTH DECOCTION *(huáng tǔ tāng)*; see PAGE 610

Biomedical Indications

With the appropriate presentation, this formula may be used to treat a variety of biomedically-defined disorders including acute hemorrhagic esophagitis, hemorrhagic gastritis, bleed-ing from peptic ulcer, bronchiectasis, hemoptysis from tuber-culosis, and hypertension-related epistaxis.

Modifications

- For profuse vomiting of blood, add Ophicalcitum *(huā ruì shí)*, charred Nelumbinis Nodus rhizomatis *(ǒu jié tàn)*, and charred Trachycarpi Petiolus *(zōng lǘ tàn)*.
- For profuse spitting up of blood, add Asini Corii Colla *(ē jiāo)* and Bletillae Rhizoma *(bái jí)*.
- For more pronounced qi deficiency, add Ginseng Radix *(rén shēn)* and Notoginseng Radix *(sān qī)*.
- For Spleen and Kidney yang deficiency, add Ginseng Radix *(rén shēn)*, Curculiginis Rhizoma *(xiān máo)*, and Epimedii Herba *(yín yáng huò)*.
- For concurrent blood deficiency, combine with Four-Substance Decoction *(sì wù tāng)*.

黃土湯（黃土汤）
Yellow Earth Decoction
huáng tǔ tāng

This formula is named after its chief ingredient, Terra flava usta *(zào xīn tǔ)*, which resembles yellow earth.

Source   *Essentials from the Golden Cabinet* (c. 220)

Terra flava usta *(zào xīn tǔ)* 18g
Rehmanniae Radix *(shēng dì huáng)* 9g
Asini Corii Colla *(ē jiāo)* 9g
Atractylodis macrocephalae Rhizoma *(bái zhú)* 9g
Aconiti Radix lateralis praeparata *(zhì fù zǐ)* 9g
Glycyrrhizae Radix *(gān cǎo)* 9g
baked Aconiti Radix lateralis *(bāo fù zǐ)* 9g
Scutellariae Radix *(huáng qín)* 9g

Method of Preparation   The source text recommends decocting in 8 cups of water until 3 cups remain, and then taking warm in two doses. At present, it is taken as a decoction with Terra flava usta *(zào xīn tǔ)* being decocted for 30-40 minutes before add-ing the other ingredients, and Asini Corii Colla *(ē jiāo)* being melted into the warm, strained decoction. Terra flava usta *(zào xīn tǔ)* is commonly prescribed in a larger dosage (30-60g), or it is replaced with Halloysitum rubrum *(chì shí zhī)* at 3-4 times its dosage.

Actions   Warms the yang, strengthens the Spleen, nourishes the blood, and stops bleeding

Indications

Blood in the stool, vomiting or spitting up blood, nosebleeds, or abnormal uterine bleeding of dark or pale blood accompa-nied by cold extremities, a wan complexion, general fatigue, a lack of taste and no particular thirst, a pale tongue with a white coating, and a submerged, thin, and forceless pulse.

This is Spleen yang deficiency, also known as middle burner cold from deficiency, which is characterized by the failure of the Spleen qi to govern the blood. The uncontrolled blood overflows its vessels and either moves upward, causing incessant vomiting or spitting up of blood or nosebleeds, or downward, causing blood in the stools and abnormal uterine bleeding. The dark or pale blood, cold extremities, wan complexion, general fatigue, pale tongue with a white coating, and submerged, thin, and forceless pulse are indicative of cold and deficiency of the Spleen.

Analysis of Formula

This formula simultaneously treats the manifestation (bleeding) and the root (cold from deficiency) by warming the yang, strengthening the Spleen, nourishing the blood, and stopping the bleeding. The chief ingredient, acrid, warm, and astringent Terra flava usta *(zào xīn tǔ)*, warms the middle, gathers and binds, and stops the bleeding. When there is bleeding from deficient Spleen qi and yang, in order to get good results, one must include medicinals that warm the yang and strengthen the Spleen, thereby restoring the ability of the Spleen and Stomach qi to govern the blood. The deputies, Atractylodis macrocephalae Rhizoma *(bái zhú)* and Aconiti Radix lateralis praeparata *(zhì fù zǐ)*, perform this function.

However, the use of such warming and acrid herbs poses a problem when there is bleeding, as they accentuate the depletion of the blood and yin that occurs just from the loss of blood itself. In addition, their warming nature can incite the reckless movement of blood that can lead to further bleeding. This is why Rehmanniae Radix *(shēng dì huáng)* and Asini Corii Colla *(ē jiāo)*, which nourish the yin and blood and stop bleeding, are chosen as assistants. Long-term blood loss can lead to Liver yin and blood deficiency, which risks the development of internal heat. The addition of the third assistant, cold and bitter Scutellariae Radix *(huáng qín)*, clears Liver heat and also cools the blood to prevent this from occurring, especially in concert with Rehmanniae Radix *(shēng dì huáng)*. In addition, the three cooling assistants ameliorate the warm, drying nature of Atractylodis macrocephalae Rhizoma *(bái zhú)* and Aconiti Radix lateralis praeparata *(zhì fù zǐ)*. Those herbs, in turn, moderate the cloying, greasy, yin- and blood-tonifying herbs in the formula.

The envoy, Glycyrrhizae Radix *(gān cǎo)*, harmonizes the middle burner and the actions of the other herbs in the formula.

Cautions and Contraindications

Contraindicated in cases of bleeding from excess heat. Also, this formula should not be used where external pathogens are present.

Commentary

In *Essentials from the Golden Cabinet,* this formula is indicated for 'distant bleeding,' defined as bleeding from the rectum that follows the passage of stool. Its use has been expanded over time to include vomiting of blood or nosebleed, among other types of bleeding. For example, *Comprehensive Medicine According to Master Zhang* cites a passage in Chapter 66 of *Divine Pivot:* "When the yin collaterals are damaged, the blood overflows internally; when the blood overflows internally, there is bleeding from behind." Zhang then specifically states that this formula can be used for bleeding prior to defecation as well as postpartum dysenteric disorders. The early 20th-century physician Zhang Xi-Chun noted that the formula is indicated for "all bleeding disorders from a deficient Spleen and Stomach yang that is unable to govern the blood." The cardinal symptoms of this pattern are profuse bleeding of dark-colored blood, the absence of pain accompanying the bleeding, and general fatigue. This formula simultaneously treats the root of the disorder, cold from deficiency, as well as the branch, which includes the various bleeding symptoms. It is used in treating a pattern of chronic, severe bloody stools that is typically accompanied by chronic diarrhea due to Spleen yang deficiency.

Because the Spleen and Stomach are the source of qi and blood, when the Spleen is deficient, the Liver may be deprived of the nourishment of blood, which may cause the generation of heat during treatment with warm and acrid herbs. This is the rationale, when treating patterns of cold from deficiency, for combining herbs that nourish the yin and blood with cooling herbs. This approach had a large impact on later writers, inspiring similar formulas in such books as *Important Formulas Worth a Thousand Gold Pieces, Yun Qi-Zi's Collection for Safeguarding Life,* and *Prescriptions of Universal Benefit.*

Ingredients

Terra flava usta *(zào xīn tǔ)* was traditionally derived from the center of an earthen double-wok wood-burning cooking stove after long use. Not only is standardization of this substance quite difficult, but it is very hard to procure at the present time. The preferred substitute, at least since the time of Chen Nian-Zu in the early 19th century, is Halloysitum rubrum *(chì shí zhī)*, which has been shown to be effective in these circumstances, particularly when, from a biomedical perspective, the problem is due to bleeding from the upper digestive tract. When this substance is used in this context, it is best to grind it into a fine powder, *not* put it into a separate cheesecloth bag but just add it in with the other ingredients, and *not* filter the strained decoction.

There has been some discussion about the rationale for including Scutellariae Radix *(huáng qín)* in this formula. One view is that it is used here to clear heat and drain fire, as noted by Tang Zong-Hai in *Discussion of Blood Patterns:* "When the blood is damaged, the yin becomes deficient and the fire stirs, so Scutellariae Radix *(huáng qín)* is used to clear the fire." Another view is that it is primarily a corrective assistant, controlling the warmth and dryness of Aconiti Radix lateralis praeparata *(zhì fù zǐ)* and Atractylodis macrocephalae Rhizoma *(bái zhú)*. This view was stated by You Yi in *Personal Standards for the Essentials from the Golden Cabinet:* "Considering that acrid, warm substances can, in turn, lead to harm with bleeding disorders, one uses the bitterness and cold of Scutellariae Radix *(huáng qín)* to prevent them from overdoing it." Yet another perspective, discussed by Huang Huang in *One-Hundred Classical Formulas*, is that Scutellariae Radix *(huáng qín)* excels at stopping bleeding and is used here for that purpose alone. The ANALYSIS OF FORMULA section above includes both interpretations, as they are not mutually exclusive.

Comparisons

> Vs. RESTORE THE SPLEEN DECOCTION *(guī pí tāng)*

Both formulas strengthen the Spleen and nourish the blood, and both are used to treat bleeding due to the Spleen's failure to govern the blood. However, Restore the Spleen Decoction *(guī pí tāng)* focuses more on the Spleen qi, with herbs such as Ginseng Radix *(rén shēn)* and Astragali Radix *(huáng qí)*, and also emphasizes treatment of the root. By contrast, Yellow Earth Decoction *(huáng tǔ tāng)* focuses more on the Spleen yang, with Aconiti Radix lateralis praeparata *(zhì fù zǐ)*, along with a treatment principle that address both the root and the branch.

> Vs. SOPHORA JAPONICA FLOWER POWDER *(huái huā sǎn)*

Both formulas treat blood in the stool. However, Sophora Japonica Flower Powder *(huái huā sǎn)* focuses on treating problems due to wind-heat or damp-heat, while Yellow Earth Decoction *(huáng tǔ tāng)* focuses on bleeding from a listless Spleen yang that fails to govern the blood. Traditionally, the bleeding from heat and stasis was thought to occur closer to the anus, in part because of its urgency and the fact that it preceded defecation, and was therefore called 'near bleeding' (近血 *jìn xuè*), while bleeding that was due to deficiency was thought to occur farther up the digestive tract, since it followed defecation, and was therefore called 'distant bleeding' (遠血 *yuǎn xuè*).

> Vs. ARBORVITAE TWIG DECOCTION *(bǎi yè tāng)*

Both formulas treat bleeding due to yang deficiency of the middle burner. However, while Arborvitae Twig Decoction *(bǎi yè tāng)* treats problems that also have an element of upward-rebelling Stomach qi (hence vomiting or spitting up of blood), Yellow Earth Decoction *(huáng tǔ tāng)* treats those with downward-sinking Spleen qi along with more significant blood deficiency. Also, at present, Arborvitae Twig Decoction *(bǎi yè tāng)* is usually taken as a component of a larger formula to treat an appropriate condition, while Yellow Earth

Decoction *(huáng tǔ tang)*, with its intertwining functions of warming, clearing, tonifying, and plugging, is thought to be more comprehensive and is commonly used as a treatment for bleeding from yang deficiency.

Biomedical Indications

With the appropriate presentation, this formula may be used to treat a variety of biomedically-defined disorders including chronic hemorrhagic gastritis and peptic ulcer.

Alternate names

Hidden Dragon Liver Decoction *(fú lóng gān tāng)* in *Discussion of Illnesses, Patterns, and Formulas Related to the Unification of the Three Etiologies*; Hidden Dragon Liver Powder *(fú lóng gān sǎn)* in *Pulse, Causes, Symptoms, and Treatment*; Yellow Earth Powder *(huáng tǔ sǎn)* in *Master He's Discussion on Aiding the Living*

Modifications

* To enhance the ability of the formula to stop bleeding, substitute charred Scutellariae Radix *(huáng qín tàn)* for Scutellariae Radix *(huáng qín)*.
* For more severe hemorrhaging, add Notoginseng Radix *(sān qī)*, Bletillae Rhizoma *(bái jí)*, and Artemisiae argyi Folium *(ài yè)*.
* For severe qi deficiency, add Codonopsis Radix *(dǎng shēn)*.
* For loose stools, substitute charred Scutellariae Radix *(huáng qín tàn)* or dry-fried Astragali Radix *(chǎo huáng qí)* for Scutellariae Radix *(huáng qín)*. One may also moderate the effect of the bitter, cold ingredients by adding Zingiberis Rhizoma praeparatum *(páo jiāng)*.

膠艾湯 (胶艾汤)
Ass-Hide Gelatin and Mugwort Decoction
jiāo ài tāng

Source *Essentials from the Golden Cabinet* (c. 220)

Asini Corii Colla *(ē jiāo)* . . . . . [dissolve in strained decoction] 6g
Artemisiae argyi Folium *(ài yè)* 9g
Rehmanniae Radix *(shēng dì huáng)* 12g
Angelicae sinensis Radix *(dāng guī)* 9g
Chuanxiong Rhizoma *(chuān xiōng)* 6g
Paeoniae Radix *(sháo yào)* .12g
Glycyrrhizae Radix *(gān cǎo)* 6g

Method of Preparation The source text advises to decoct in 5 parts water and 3 parts rice wine and take in three doses over the course of a day. At present, it is usually prepared as a decoction with water. Paeoniae Radix alba *(bái sháo)* is the form of Paeoniae Radix *(sháo yào)* that is generally used.

Actions Nourishes the blood, stops bleeding, regulates menstruation, and calms the fetus

Indications

Abdominal pain with uterine bleeding, excessive menstruation, menstruation with constant spotting, postpartum bleeding, or bleeding during pregnancy. The blood is pale and thin without clots, and is accompanied by weakness and soreness of the lower back, a dull complexion, a pale tongue with a thin, white coating, and a thin, frail pulse.

This pattern is one of injury and deficiency of the Penetrating and Conception vessels with a tendency toward cold. Both vessels arise from the Womb; the former is the 'sea' of blood, and the latter controls the Womb and fetus. When these vessels are injured, deficient, and cold, the blood leaves the vessels and bleeding occurs, accompanied by abdominal pain and weakness and soreness of the lower back. When the Penetrating vessel fails to supply sufficient blood to the Womb during pregnancy, the Womb weakens and bleeding occurs together with restlessness of the fetus and abdominal pain, particularly when there is also cold. The deficient nature of the bleeding is reflected in its pale, thin quality and the absence of clots. Blood deficiency that tends toward cold is reflected in the dull complexion, the pale tongue with a thin, white coating, and the thin, frail pulse.

Analysis of Formula

This is an important formula for treating abnormal uterine bleeding as well as a restless fetus. The main focus of the formula is on stopping the bleeding, but it also needs to nourish the blood, regulate the menses, and calm the fetus. The chief ingredients are therefore sweet, neutral Asini Corii Colla (*ē jiāo*), which tonifies the blood and stops bleeding, and bitter, acrid, warming Artemisiae argyi Folium (*ài yè*), which warms the Womb, calms the restless fetus, and stops uterine bleeding. This is a commonly-used combination for both abnormal uterine bleeding and bleeding during pregnancy.

However, bleeding is just the manifestation of this disorder, the root of which is injury to the deficient Penetrating and Conception vessels. Thus, one must also tonify the blood and stabilize these vessels. The deputy ingredients, Rehmanniae Radix (*shēng dì huáng*), Angelicae sinensis Radix (*dāng guī*), Chuanxiong Rhizoma (*chuān xiōng*), and Paeoniae Radix alba (*bái sháo*), tonify the blood and regulate the menses, while also invigorating the blood. The latter function is very important because in bleeding disorders, especially chronic ones, it is just as important to prevent the development of blood stasis as it is to tonify the blood. This is particularly true here, as there is a danger of inadvertently causing blood stasis when using herbs that stop bleeding. For a detailed discussion of the functions and interactions of these four herbs, see Four-Substance Decoction (*sì wù tāng*) in Chapter 8.

Glycyrrhizae Radix (*gān cǎo*), the assistant ingredient, harmonizes the actions of the other ingredients, and potentiates the ability of Asini Corii Colla (*ē jiāo*) to stop the bleed-

ing. Also, in concert with Paeoniae Radix alba (*bái sháo*), it is useful for treating abdominal pain. The function of rice wine, the envoy, is to reinforce the moving actions of the other warming ingredients, namely, Artemisiae argyi Folium (*ài yè*), Angelicae sinensis Radix (*dāng guī*), and Chuanxiong Rhizoma (*chuān xiōng*), and thereby prevent the development of blood stasis.

Cautions and Contraindications

Do not use this formula when there is abnormal uterine bleeding due to heat.

Commentary

This is a very useful formula for treating abnormal uterine bleeding, excessive menstruation, or bleeding during pregnancy when the diagnosis is blood deficiency that tends toward cold. The cardinal symptoms are pale, thin blood accompanied by weakness, low backache, a complexion that lacks normal luster, a pale tongue, and a fine pulse. Furthermore, because this formula not only tonifies but also invigorates the blood, some degree of stasis, such as tenderness on palpation of the lower abdomen even though the abdomen itself is weak and soft, or sensations of heat or restlessness in the extremities resulting from stasis, are frequently present.

Historical Impact

This formula has also had a profound effect on how bleeding has been treated in Chinese medicine, particularly uterine bleeding. Over the centuries, there have been many modifications of this formula, themselves often called Ass-Hide Gelatin and Mugwort Decoction (*jiāo ài tāng*). In general, these variations have taken one of four forms, which have become the main modifications to this formula:

1. Addition of more warming herbs such as Zingiberis Rhizoma (*gān jiāng*)

2. Addition of more herbs that specifically stop bleeding such as Halloysitum rubrum (*chì shí zhī*) or Sanguisorbae Radix (*dì yú*)

3. Addition of qi tonics such as Astragali Radix (*huáng qí*) to help the Spleen qi contain the blood

4. Addition of heat-clearing herbs such as Scutellariae Radix (*huáng qín*) to prevent the development of heat in the blood.

While Ass-Hide Gelatin and Mugwort Decoction appears to be a variation of Four-Substance Decoction (*sì wù tāng*), it should be remembered that it predates the latter by approximately six-hundred years and is, in fact, the base formula from which Four-Substance Decoction (*sì wù tāng*) was developed.

Importance of Wine

As noted above, the wine in this formula is generally thought to be used for its ability to disseminate, promote movement, and disperse cold. In *Commentary on the Classic of Materia Medica*, Zou Shu says of wine:

> It cannot be said that it does not move the blood and dispel stasis. ... In the two texts *Discussion of Cold Damage* and *Essentials from the Golden Cabinet*, there are three instances when water and wine are used together: Prepared Licorice Decoction *(zhì gān cǎo tāng)* uses seven cups of wine and eight of water; Tangkuei Decoction for Frigid Extremities plus Evodia and Fresh Ginger *(dāng guī sì nì jiā wú zhū yú shēng jiāng tāng)* uses six cups each of wine and water; Ass-Hide Gelatin and Mugwort Decoction *(jiāo ài tāng)* uses three cups of wine and five of water.
>
> Here it can be seen that in yin-tonifying formulas, this [combination] unblocks the retarding and stagnating nature of the herbs; while in cold-dispersing formulas, this [combination] breaks up the congealed knots due to lurking cold. In addition, there are differences of severity in the use [of this combination].

Comparison

➢ Vs. Flow-Warming Decoction *(wēn jīng tāng)*

Both formulas treat irregular menstruation and abnormal uterine bleeding from injury and deficiency of the Penetrating and Conception vessels. Ass-Hide Gelatin and Mugwort Decoction *(jiāo ài tāng)* is primarily a tonic that stops up by nourishing and that contains some blood-invigorating actions within its general effect of tonification. It is used for conditions of blood deficiency that tend toward cold, and is especially useful for calming a restless fetus. By contrast, Flow-Warming Decoction *(wēn jīng tāng)* is a formula that primarily uses herbs that warm and invigorate the blood, and that contains some tonics and heat-clearing herbs within its general effect of warming. It is used for conditions of blood stasis that tend toward cold and is especially useful in treating irregular menstruation.

Biomedical Indications

With the appropriate presentation, this formula may be used to treat a variety of biomedically-defined disorders including dysfunctional uterine bleeding, threatened miscarriage, habitual miscarriage, postpartum uterine bleeding, prolonged lochia, bleeding peptic ulcer, bleeding hemorrhoids, and idiopathic thrombocytopenic purpura.

Alternate names

Tangkuei Decoction *(dāng guī sǎn)* in *Prescriptions of Universal Benefit*; Ass-Hide Gelatin and Mugwort with Four-Substance Decoction *(jiāo ài sì wù tāng)* in *Introduction to Medicine*; Ass-Hide Gelatin and Mugwort Decoction *(ē jiao qí ài tāng)* in *Displays of Enlightened Physicians*; Mugwort and Rehmannia Decoction *(ài yè dì huáng tāng)* in *Collection on Birth and Pregnancy*

Modifications

- For restless fetus disorder, add Zingiberis Rhizoma *(gān jiāng)*.
- For concurrent qi deficiency, add Codonopsis Radix *(dǎng shēn)* and Astragali Radix *(huáng qí)*.
- For bleeding during pregnancy with lower back pain, remove Chuanxiong Rhizoma *(chuān xiōng)* and add Atractylodis macrocephalae Rhizoma *(bái zhú)*, Eucommiae Cortex *(dù zhòng)*, and Taxilli Herba *(sāng jì shēng)*.
- For concurrent Spleen deficiency failing to govern the blood, take with Restore the Spleen Decoction *(guī pí tāng)*.

Associated Formula

丁香膠艾湯 （丁香胶艾汤）

Clove, Ass-Hide Gelatin, and Mugwort Decoction

dīng xiāng jiāo ài tāng

Source   *Secrets from the Orchid Chamber* (1336)

Rehmanniae Radix praeparata *(shú dì huáng)* 0.9g
Paeoniae Radix alba *(bái sháo)* 0.9g
Chuanxiong Rhizoma *(chuān xiōng)* 1.2g
Caryophylli Flos *(dīng xiāng)* 1.2g
Artemisiae argyi Folium *(ài yè)* 3g
Angelicae sinensis Radix *(dāng guī)* 3.6g
Asini Corii Colla *(ē jiāo)* . . . . [dissolve in strained decoction] 1.8g

Nourishes the blood, warms the Womb, and stops bleeding. For persistent uterine bleeding with an ice-cold sensation in the lower abdomen due to blood deficiency and cold. There may also be profuse, thin vaginal discharge, occasional bleeding of bright-red blood, or a slightly flooding pulse at the right proximal position.

Comparative Tables of Principal Formulas

■ FORMULAS THAT INVIGORATE THE BLOOD AND DISPEL BLOOD STASIS

Common symptoms: pain is fixed and usually severe

Formula Name	Diagnosis	Indications	Remarks
Peach Pit Decoction to Order the Qi *(táo hé chéng qì tāng)*	Blood buildup in the lower burner caused by the accumulation of blood stasis and heat	Acute lower abdominal pain, smooth urination, night fevers, delirious speech, irritability, restlessness, and thirst, dysmenorrhea or amenorrhea in women, and a submerged, full, or choppy pulse	In severe cases, there may be manic behavior. Focuses on draining heat and breaking up blood stasis.
Appropriate Decoction *(dǐ dàng tāng)*	Blood buildup in the lower burner caused by clumping of heat and blood	Firmness and distention of the lower abdomen, smooth urination, manic behavior, forgetfulness, black stools that are easy to expel, delayed menstruation or amenorrhea in women, and a submerged and slow-irregular pulse	Also treats jaundice. For late-stage blood buildup in the lower burner where heat has dried the blood, causing palpable hardness.
Drive Out Stasis from the Mansion of Blood Decoction *(xuè fǔ zhú yū tāng)*	Blood stasis in the 'mansion of blood' with impairment of blood flow in the area above the diaphragm	Pain in the chest and hypochondria, chronic, fixed headache, incessant hiccup, dry heaves, depression accompanied by a sensation of warmth in the chest, palpitations, insomnia, irritability, evening tidal fever, dark-red tongue with dark spots on the sides, dark or purplish lips, complexion, or sclera, and a choppy or wiry, tight pulse	Focuses on invigorating the blood and relieving qi constraint.
Tonify the Yang to Restore Five [-Tenths] Decoction *(bǔ yáng huán wǔ tāng)*	Qi deficiency leading to blood stasis obstructing the channels	Sequelae of wind-stroke including hemiplegia, paralysis, and atrophy of the lower limbs, facial paralysis, slurred speech, drooling, dry stools, urinary frequency or incontinence, a white tongue coating, and a moderate pulse	Also for atrophy disorders.
Revive Health by Invigorating the Blood Decoction *(fù yuán huó xuè tāng)*	Traumatic physical injury that results in blood leaving the vessels	Excruciating pain associated with traumatic injury, especially in the chest, hypochondria, or flanks	Also used to treat severe pain not caused by trauma but in the area traversed by the Liver and Gallbladder channels such as headache or postherpetic neuralgia.
Seven-Thousandths of a Tael Powder *(qī lí sǎn)*	Traumatic injury causing stasis of blood and stagnant qi	Bruising, swelling, and pain accompanying traumatic injuries such as broken bones and torn sinews, and bleeding due to lacerations	Also used externally for pain, bleeding, and to promote the healing of fractures.
Inula Decoction *(xuán fù huā tāng)*	Liver fixation caused by obstruction of the qi dynamic in the chest	A sensation of fullness, distention, or even pain in the chest that improves with massage, a preference for warm beverages during asymptomatic periods, and a wiry and large pulse	Also used to treat uterine bleeding during the second half of pregnancy.
Flow-Warming Decoction *(wēn jīng tāng)*	Deficiency and cold of the Conception and Penetrating vessels together with obstruction due to the stasis of blood	Mild, persistent uterine bleeding, irregular menstruation, bleeding between periods, pain, distention, and cold in the lower abdomen, dry lips and mouth, low-grade fever at dusk, a tongue body that may be purplish, and a fine and rough pulse	Also used to treat infertility in women.
Generating and Transforming Decoction *(shēng huà tāng)*	Blood stasis in the Womb resulting from cold with deficient blood	Retention of the lochia accompanied by cold and pain in the lower abdomen, a pale purple tongue or a pale tongue with purple spots, and a thin, submerged, and choppy pulse	Used for a variety of gynecological problems. Focuses on unblocking stasis by warming the blood, while also generating new blood.

Formula Name	Diagnosis	Indications	Remarks
Cinnamon Twig and Poria Pill (guì zhī fú líng wán)	Restless fetus disorder due to blood stasis in the Womb	Mild, persistent uterine bleeding of purple or dark blood during pregnancy accompanied by abdominal pain that increases with pressure	Also for immobile masses in the lower abdomen with pain and tenderness or similar problems, accompanied by a dark tongue with purple stasis spots and a submerged and choppy pulse.
Tangkuei and Peony Powder (dāng guī sháo yào săn)	Liver and Spleen disharmony characterized by both blood stasis and qi stagnation due to dampness	Continuous cramping pain of the abdomen that is not severe, urinary difficulty, and slight edema (primarily of the lower limbs)	For various gynecological problems due to deficiency that involve blood stasis and water buildup including infertility, edema, pain or bleeding during pregnancy, and dysmenorrhea.
Sudden Smile Powder (shī xiào săn)	Retention of blood stasis that obstructs the vessels that serve the lower abdomen	Irregular menstruation, dysmenorrhea, retention of the lochia, postpartum abdominal pain, acute, colicky pain in the lower abdomen, severe pain in the middle abdomen, or epigastric pain	Focuses on dispelling blood stasis and alleviating pain. Also modified to treat angina pectoris.
Fantastically Effective Pill to Invigorate the Collaterals (huó luò xiào líng dān)	Pain due to qi stagnation and blood stasis obstructing the collaterals	Pain in various locations such as the heart, stomach, abdomen, back, leg, or arm, bruising and swelling due to traumatic injury, rheumatic pain, fixed abdominal masses, internal or external ulceration, a dark tongue or one with stasis spots, and a wiry or rough pulse	More for long-term problems. Modified to direct the actions of the formula to particular parts of the body.
Salvia Drink (dān shēn yĭn)	Blood stasis and qi stagnation that has accumulated in the middle burner	Abdominal or epigastric pain that may radiate upward accompanied by signs and symptoms of blood stasis and qi stagnation	Particularly useful for epigastric, flank, or menstrual pain in women. Also modified to treat angina pectoris.
Rhubarb and Ground Beetle Pill (dà huáng zhè chóng wán)	Damage to the circulation of nutritive and protective qi in the channels with accumulation of dry blood in the interior	Emaciation, abdominal fullness, loss of appetite, rough, dry, and scaly skin, a dull and dark appearance of the eyes, amenorrhea, and tidal fever	Primarily used in treating concurrent conditions of blood stasis and consumption.

■ FORMULAS THAT STOP BLEEDING

Common symptoms: bleeding, either acute or chronic

Formula Name	Diagnosis	Indications	Remarks
Ten Partially-Charred Substances Powder (shí huī săn)	Fire blazing in the middle and upper burners that injures the blood vessels	Nosebleeds, vomiting, spitting, or coughing up of bright red blood, red tongue, and a rapid pulse; symptoms usually occur as acute bleeding disorders with sudden onset	This is a form of reckless movement of hot blood that spills out of the channels. Focuses on draining heat and quickly stopping bleeding.
Four-Fresh Pill (sì shēng wán)	Upper-burner manifestations of heat in the blood	Coughing, spitting, or vomiting of blood or nosebleeds (particularly of bright-red blood), dry mouth and throat, red or deep-red tongue, and a wiry, rapid or forceful, wiry, and rapid pulse	The most balanced and least harsh of all the formulas that clear heat to stop bleeding.

cont. ↘

Formula Name	Diagnosis	Indications	Remarks
Coughing of Blood Formula (ké xuè fāng)	Liver fire attacking and scorching the Lungs	Coughing of blood-streaked sputum, thick sputum that is difficult to expectorate, bitter taste, irritability and easily-provoked anger, constipation, red cheeks, a red tongue with a yellow coating, and a wiry, rapid pulse	Focuses on treating both the root (Liver fire) as well as the branch (coughing with blood-streaked sputum) of this disorder.
Small Thistle Drink (xiǎo jì yǐn zi)	Static heat accumulating in the lower burner where it injures the blood collaterals	Painful bloody urinary dribbling (with blood in the urine and urinary frequency, urgency, burning, and pain) or simple blood in the urine, accompanied by thirst, irritability, a red tongue with a thin, yellow coating, and a rapid, forceful pulse	A well-rounded formula for treating blood in the urine due to excessive heat.
Sophora Japonica Flower Powder (huái huā sǎn)	Either the lodging of wind-heat or the accumulation of damp-heat in the Intestines and Stomach where it forms toxin	Bright-red bleeding from the rectum during defecation that typically precedes (but may also follow) the passage of stool, blood in the stools, hemorrhoids with either bright-red or dark-red blood, a red tongue body, and a wiry, rapid or soggy, rapid pulse	Focuses on clearing the Intestines and cooling blood as well as stopping bleeding.
Arborvitae Twig Decoction (bǎi yè tāng)	Cold from deficiency affecting the middle qi	Unremitting vomiting or spitting up of blood or nosebleeds accompanied by a wan complexion, a pale tongue with a thin coating, and a deficient, rapid, and forceless pulse	This is failure of the Spleen qi to govern the blood along with ascendant yang. Also for any type of bleeding in the upper part of the body associated with yang deficiency.
Yellow Earth Decoction (huáng tǔ tāng)	Spleen yang deficiency, also known as middle burner cold from deficiency	Blood in the stool, vomiting or spitting up blood, nosebleeds, or abnormal uterine bleeding of dark or pale blood accompanied by cold extremities, wan complexion, fatigue, lack of taste, no thirst, pale tongue with a white coating, and a submerged, thin, and forceless pulse	This is failure of the Spleen qi to govern the blood along with blood deficiency.
Ass-Hide Gelatin and Mugwort Decoction (jiāo ài tāng)	Injury and deficiency of the Penetrating and Conception vessels with a tendency toward cold	Abdominal pain with uterine bleeding, excessive menstruation, menstruation with constant spotting, postpartum bleeding, or bleeding during pregnancy, pale and thin blood without clots accompanied by weakness and soreness of the lower back, dull complexion, pale tongue with a thin, white coating, and a thin, frail pulse	Especially useful for restless fetus disorder.

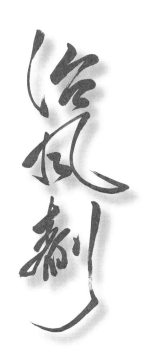

Chapter 14 Contents

Formulas that Expel Wind

Formulas that Expel Wind

FORMULAS THAT EXPEL wind are used to treat patterns dominated by wind-type symptoms. Such disorders were first described in classical texts like *Basic Questions*. Chapter 42 of that work is devoted entirely to this subject. Observations like "Wind likes to move and frequently changes [its manifestation]" attests to the wide variety of problems and bewildering array of symptoms associated with wind. The adage that "Wind is the leader of all diseases" reflects the status attributed to its disease-causing powers. Even today, most textbooks on internal medicine begin with a chapter on externally-contracted disorders (which includes wind), followed by a discussion of wind-stroke and its treatment. A similar distinction between external and internal wind is used to organize the formulas in this chapter into those that dredge and disperse external wind and those that pacify and extinguish internal wind.

External wind refers to the wind that enters the body from outside, as described in *Divine Pivot*, Chapter 46: "When the flesh is not firm and the interstices and pores are sparse, one is prone to wind disorders." This type of wind can attack any level of the body including the skin, the muscle layer, the channels, the sinews, the bones, and the organs. It is usually accompanied by another pathogenic influence such as cold, heat, dryness, or dampness. The formulas for external wind in this chapter treat disorders in which wind is the primary pathogenic influence and whose manifestations are characteristic of wind: rapid in onset, changeable, or affecting move-

ment. Because wind is a yang pathogen, it often causes problems that affect the upper part of the body, particularly the head. Symptoms that are characteristic of external wind include itching, numbness of the skin and flesh, headaches, deep source nasal congestion, muscular spasms, difficulty in moving the joints, and asymmetrical appearance or strength.

Internally-generated wind arises when the internal organs, primarily the Liver and Kidneys, lose the ability to exercise control over the yang qi, which by its nature is wild and readily transforms into pathogenic wind. This was first discussed in Chapter 74 of *Basic Questions*: "The various wind [manifestations such as] loss of consciousness and dizziness are all attributed to the Liver." Internal stirring of wind may arise from Kidney or Liver yin deficiency, ascendant Liver yang, blood deficiency, or heat excess. Its most common presentations include dizziness, vertigo, tremors, loss of muscle tone, and, in severe cases, convulsions, difficulty in speaking, and sudden loss of consciousness with facial asymmetry or hemiplegia.

External and internal wind can mutually produce or combine with each other, making the boundary between the categories somewhat fuzzy. For instance, external wind may penetrate into the organs or provoke the stirring of internal wind. Internal wind, on the other hand, may disrupt the protective yang, which then leads to the contraction of external wind. The terminology, moreover, is not always precise. Facial asymmetry and hemiplegia, for instance, are regarded as indications of wind-stroke (中風 *zhòng fēng*). Initially, physicians generally believed that this was caused by external wind penetrating into the channels in patients with deficient blood and qi. From the Song dynasty onward, the same symptoms were increasingly understood to arise from internal causes involving fire, phlegm, yin deficiency, and ascendant yang. To avoid confusion, the latter condition is often referred to as wind-type stroke (類中風 *lèi zhòng fēng*), although some writers have tried to reconcile the two views into a single doctrine. Wind-stroke may also refer, however, to exterior conditions characterized by fever, headache, sweating, and a floating, moderate pulse. For the sake of clarity, in this text, 中 風 *zhòng fēng* in these situations is translated as wind attack; see, for example, the discussion of Cinnamon Twig Decoction (*guì zhī tāng*) in Chapter 1. Today, the term wind-stroke usually refers to conditions with loss of muscle control or paralysis, and is divided into channel-stroke (a relatively mild condition with no loss of consciousness) and organ-stroke (with loss of consciousness). Some of the formulas that treat acute, severe wind-stroke are discussed in Chapter 11 in connection with opening the sensory orifices.

External wind is generally treated by dispersion with the goal of dispelling it externally. Internal wind, on the other hand, is treated with herbs that calm, extinguish, and sedate, as well as those that tonify the yin and regulate the Liver. Accurate diagnosis is essential to avoid complications resulting from the use of inappropriate formulas. Some conditions may involve both external and internal wind, in which case the treatment must deal with both aspects. However, because herbs that scatter and disperse wind are usually warm and dry in nature and can readily injure the fluids or generate fire, they must be used with great care in cases of yin deficiency or ascendant yang. If necessary, they must be combined with sweet, cooling herbs that enrich the fluids. In addition, since it is unusual for wind to invade the body alone—more commonly, it is accompanied by other pathogenic influences such as cold or dryness—proper treatment requires that each pathogenic influence be addressed. Because wind is sometimes a secondary rather than a primary factor in a pattern, therefore, not all of the formulas that treat wind are found in this chapter.

Section 1

FORMULAS THAT DREDGE AND DISPERSE EXTERNAL WIND

External wind invades the body when the normal qi is deficient, the interstices and pores are open, or the protective qi is weak. Manifestations will vary according to the strength of the pathogenic influence, the combination of pathogenic influences involved, and the individual constitution of the patient. Some of the formulas in this section are used for treating external wind that enters the flesh, channels, sinews, joints, and bones, and is characterized by rashes, dizziness, numbness, difficulty in movement, and joint pain. Other formulas treat disorders in which external wind induces internal stirring of wind. In such cases, the pathogenic wind first attacks the head and face and then progresses into the channels where it gives rise to muscular tetany with clenched jaw, spasms of the lips, stiffness, opisthotonus, facial paralysis, and other disturbances involving muscle spasms. Formulas for treating internal stirring of Liver wind due to heat entering the terminal yin channel, or the sequelae of wind-stroke from wind attacking the channels and collaterals, are also discussed in this chapter. Exterior conditions develop when externally-contracted wind settles in the exterior and muscle layer.

Formulas that dredge and disperse external wind are composed primarily of acrid ingredients that expel the pathogen to the exterior. This is an example of treating like with like. Representative herbs used for this purpose include Schizonepetae Herba (*jīng jiè*), Saposhnikoviae Radix (*fáng fēng*), Ephedrae Herba (*má huáng*), Chuanxiong Rhizoma (*chuān xiōng*), Angelicae dahuricae Radix (*bái zhǐ*), Menthae haplocalycis Herba (*bò hé*), and Aconiti Radix praeparata (*zhì chuān wū*). Depending on the presentation and the underlying pathodynamic, they are typically combined with four other types of ingredients in the formulas discussed below. These are:

1. Substances that drain heat and clear fire such as Scutellariae Radix (*huáng qín*), Gypsum fibrosum (*shí gāo*), Anemarrhenae Rhizoma (*zhī mǔ*), or Rehmanniae Radix (*shēng dì huáng*). These herbs are added both to moderate the effect of the acrid wind-dispersing herbs on the body's own yang qi, preventing them from stirring up internal wind, and to treat symptoms that arise because wind itself readily transforms into heat.

2. Substances that eliminate wind-phlegm from the channels such as Arisaematis Rhizoma praeparatum (*zhì tiān nán xīng*), Sinapis Semen (*bái jiè zǐ*), and Bombyx batryticatus (*bái jiāng cán*). These herbs are added when external wind penetrating into the channels and collaterals impairs their fluid metabolism to produce phlegm, or where preexisting phlegm combines with external wind.

3. Substances that invigorate the blood and eliminate stasis such as Myrrha (*mò yào*), Olibanum (*rǔ xiāng*), or Pheretima (*dì lóng*). Like phlegm, blood stasis can be a product of wind entering the vessels and collaterals, or, by impeding

the normal circulation of qi and blood, blood stasis can facilitate the penetration of wind from the exterior.

4. Herbs that nourish the blood such as Angelicae sinensis Radix (*dāng guī*), Rehmanniae Radix praeparata (*shú dì huáng*), Paeoniae Radix alba (*bái sháo*), or Cannabis Semen (*huǒ má rén*). Wind, a yang pathogenic factor, readily generates dryness and damages the blood. On the other hand, deficient blood in the vessels and collaterals creates a space into which wind can enter. In both cases, tonifying the blood is an essential aspect of treatment.

小續命湯 (小续命汤)
Minor Extend Life Decoction

xiǎo xù mìng tāng

The indication of this formula in the source text is "wind stroke [where the patient] is on the point of death." Being able to save a person at such a point of crisis warrants the name 'extend life.' An entire family of formulas with similar composition was in use during the Sui and Tang dynasties. To distinguish this formula from a very similar one with a somewhat stronger action, it was called 'minor.' (See the COMMENTARY for a more extensive discussion.)

Source *Formulas with Short Articles* (Eastern Jin, 4th century)

Ephedrae Herba (*má huáng*). 30g (3-6g)
Chuanxiong Rhizoma (*chuān xiōng*) 30g (3-6g)
Stephaniae tetrandrae Radix (*hàn fáng jǐ*) 30g (6-12g)
Armeniacae Semen (*xìng rén*). 30g (9-12g)
Saposhnikoviae Radix (*fáng fēng*). 45g (9-12g)
Zingiberis Rhizoma recens (*shēng jiāng*) . . . . .150g (9-12 pieces)
Ginseng Radix (*rén shēn*) 30g (3-6g)
Aconiti Radix lateralis praeparata (*zhì fù zǐ*) . . . . .1 piece (9-15g)
Cinnamomi Cortex (*ròu guì*) 30g (3-6g)
Paeoniae Radix (*sháo yào*). 30g (6-12g)
Scutellariae Radix (*huáng qín*) 30g (4.5-9g)
Glycyrrhizae Radix (*gān cǎo*) 30g (3-6g)

Method of Preparation The source text advises to grind all but the last ingredient into a coarse powder. Cook Ephedrae Herba (*má huáng*) first by bringing the water to a boil three times, each time removing the foam. Add the other herbs, strain, and divide into three doses. At present, it is usually prepared as a decoction with the dosage indicated in parentheses. Boil Aconiti Radix lateralis praeparata (*zhì fù zǐ*) 30-60 minutes before adding the other ingredients. Codonopsis Radix (*dǎng shēn*) is usually substituted for Ginseng Radix (*rén shēn*) with 2-3 times its dosage. Paeoniae Radix alba (*bái sháo*) is the form of Paeoniae Radix (*sháo yào*) that is used. In modern formulations, Cinnamomi Ramulus (*guì zhī*) is sometimes substituted for Cinnamomi Cortex (*ròu guì*). This is done to strengthen the exterior-releasing action of the formula, and, in combination with Paeoniae Radix alba (*bái sháo*), to regulate the nutritive and protective qi. Sometimes the formula is prepared as a tincture.

Actions Warms the channels, unblocks the yang qi, dispels wind, and supports the normal qi

Indications

Hemiplegia, asymmetry of the face, slow and slurred speech. Usually accompanied by fever and chills, a pale tongue with a thin, white coating, and a deficient, floating pulse. In severe cases, there is loss of consciousness. The formula is also used for the treatment of pain from wind-damp painful obstruction.

This is wind-stroke due to invasion of wind from the exterior into the channels. When the protective qi is weak and the interstices and pores are left open, external wind readily invades the body. When the channels are weak, the normal qi will also be weak and cannot prevent the pathogenic influences from invading the channels. This produces a form of wind-stroke known as 'channel-stroke.' Wind causes movement; cold causes contraction. When wind-cold enters the channels, it causes an irregular flow of qi and blood that manifests as spasms, hemiplegia, or facial asymmetry. If the pathogenic influences invade the collaterals, the tongue will become stiff, which impairs speech. If wind penetrates to the deeper levels of the body and affects the organs, there will be organ-stroke with loss of consciousness. Fever and chills, a pale tongue with a thin, white coating, and a floating pulse are signs of wind in the exterior.

This same pathodynamic can cause pain from wind-damp painful obstruction, for which this formula is also indicated.

Analysis of Formula

The type of wind-stroke treated by this formula is a pattern thought to be due to excess wind in the exterior that arises against a background of qi deficiency. For this reason, the formula combines acrid, warming herbs that disperse exterior wind with those that augment the qi and warm the yang. The chief herbs, warm and acrid Ephedrae Herba (*má huáng*), Chuanxiong Rhizoma (*chuān xiōng*), Stephaniae tetrandrae Radix (*hàn fáng jǐ*), Armeniacae Semen (*xìng rén*), Saposhnikoviae Radix (*fáng fēng*), and Zingiberis Rhizoma recens (*shēng jiāng*), facilitate the flow of qi in the channels and conduct the pathogenic influences out of the body. Codonopsis Radix (*dǎng shēn*), one of the deputies, augments the qi, while the other deputies, Aconiti Radix lateralis praeparata (*zhì fù zǐ*) and Cinnamomi Cortex (*ròu guì*), reinforce the yang. The deputies work with the blood-regulating assistants, Paeoniae Radix alba (*bái sháo*) and Chuanxiong Rhizoma (*chuān xiōng*), to support the normal qi in dispelling the pathogenic influences. When wind is trapped in the exterior and the qi does not flow smoothly in the interior, there will be constraint, which readily transforms into heat. Bitter, cold Scutellariae Radix (*huáng qín*), another assistant, is especially effective in treating this type of heat. The envoy, Glycyrrhizae Radix (*gān cǎo*), harmonizes the actions of the other herbs.

Cautions and Contraindications

This formula is contraindicated for both wind-stroke due to internal stirring of Liver wind and hot painful obstruction.

Commentary

This is a modification of Combined Cinnamon Twig and Ephedra Decoction (*guì zhī má huáng gè bàn tāng*) with Ginseng and Aconite Accessory Root Decoction (*shēn fù tāng*).

History

Prior to the Song dynasty, wind-stroke (a form of cerebrovascular accident in the biomedical sense) was viewed as being a consequence of the invasion of external wind. Its pathogenesis was thus essentially the same as that of superficial wind-cold invasion, also known as 'wind attack' (中風 *zhòng fēng*). This explains why the same treatment strategy, and therefore the same herbs and formulas, were employed in treating both of these conditions. Conceptually, this is warranted since both conditions are characterized by sudden onset, rapid development of symptoms that often appear unpredictable, and symptoms such as muscle aches, cramping, or paralysis that involve the sinews and muscles and thus, by extension, the Liver as the organ system resonating internally with wind-wood. These symptoms are related to Liver wood not only because the Liver governs the sinews, but also via the ethereal soul, which moves away from the body in dreams that characterize feverish disorders, or detaches itself from the body altogether at the time of death.

In fact, the various Extend Life Decoctions (*xù mìng tāng*) are derived from Return the Ethereal Soul Decoction (還魂湯 *huán hún tāng*). This is the original name of the formula, discussed in Chapter 1, that is now known as Three-Unbinding Decoction (*sān ǎo tāng*). It consists of Ephedrae Herba (*má huáng*), Armeniacae Semen (*xìng rén*), and Glycyrrhizae Radix (*gān cǎo*) and is prescribed in Chapter 23 of *Essentials from the Golden Cabinet* for the treatment of "[someone on the point of] sudden death" (卒死 *cù sǐ*). This can be taken to refer to 'sudden stroke' (卒中 *cù zhòng*), which, in turn, is a synonym for wind-stroke in ancient medical texts. According to Zhang Lu in *Extension of the Important Formulas Worth a Thousand Gold Pieces*, the difference between wind attacking the exterior and wind-stroke is that the latter occurs against a background of severe internal deficiency. In such cases, the protective qi is too weak to secure the ethereal soul. This explains the addition of Ginseng and Aconite Accessory Root Decoction (*shēn fù tāng*) to what is otherwise an exterior-releasing formula.

From the Song dynasty onward, physicians began to conceive of wind-stroke as primarily an internally-generated condition. Liu Wan-Su, for instance, attributed it to "sudden and severe Heart fire," while Zhu Dan-Xi defined it as "arising from dampness and phlegm generating heat." The Ming-dynasty physician Wang Fu suggested that "true wind-stroke" (真中風 *zhēn zhòng fēng*), referring to externally-contracted wind, be differentiated from "wind-type stroke" (類中風 *lèi zhòng fēng*), referring to wind generated by internal fire. Other physicians, such as Zhang Jie-Bin, went so far as to propose that what had previously been described as wind-stroke was, in fact, "not wind" (非風 *fēi fēng*). Other physicians, such as Fei Bo-Xiong, attempted to reconcile these different views, differentiating between "strike into the collaterals" (中絡 *zhòng luò*) and "strike into the channels" (中經 *zhòng jīng*), both due to external wind, and "strike into the yang organs" (中腑 *zhòng fǔ*) and "strike into the yin organs" (中藏 *zhòng zāng*), both due to internal wind. Minor Extend Life Decoction (*xiǎo xù mìng tang*) is primarily used for treating the former. Translated into the language of biomedicine, this is taken to mean acute-stage, nonhemorrhagic cerebrovascular accidents, that is, those caused by thrombosis, embolism, and, in particular, vascular spasm. In *Annotated Fine Formulas from Generations of Famous Physicians*, the contemporary physician Ran Xiao-Feng attributes the efficacy of the formula in these cases to its blood-invigorating and antispasmodic properties.

Zhang Hui-Wu, a senior physician from Henan, uses the formula to treat hemiplegia that is not accompanied by high blood pressure, suggesting a clinically useful method of differentiating patterns for which this formula is indicated from those discussed in the second section of this chapter. This formula is also used for wind-cold-damp painful obstruction, particularly in the upper body.

Modification for the Six Warps

In *Medical Formulas Collected and Analyzed*, the Qing-dynasty writer Wang Ang recommended "Old Yi's [Zhang Yuan-Su's] strategy for modification according to a six channel [differentiation]," a helpful tool for modifying the formula in clinical practice. This works as follows:

- In greater yang channel wind-stroke where lack of sweating and aversion to cold are the main symptoms, one should double the dosage of Ephedrae Herba (*má huáng*), Armeniacae Semen (*xìng rén*), and Saposhnikoviae Radix (*fáng fēng*) in the original formula in order to strengthen its ability to promote sweating, and to open and disseminate in order to expel wind. This is called Ephedra Extend Life Decoction (*má huáng xù mìng tāng*). In greater yang channel wind-stroke where sweating and aversion to wind are the main symptoms, one should double the dosages of Cinnamomi Ramulus (*guì zhī*), Paeoniae Radix alba (*bái sháo*), and Armeniacae Semen (*xìng rén*) in the original formula in order to strengthen its ability to resolve the muscles, harmonize the nutritive and protective qi, and disseminate the Lungs. This is called Cinnamon Twig Extend Life Decoction (*guì zhí xù mìng tāng*).

- In yang brightness channel wind-stroke where lack of sweating, fever, and no aversion to cold are the main symptoms, one should remove Aconiti Radix lateralis praeparata *(zhì fù zǐ)* from the original formula and add Gypsum fibrosum *(shí gāo)* and Anemarrhenae Rhizoma *(zhī mǔ)* in order to strengthen its ability to clear and drain the yang brightness. This is called White Tiger Extend Life Decoction *(baí hǔ xù mìng tāng)*. In yang brightness channel wind-stroke where body fever with sweating and no aversion to wind are the main symptoms, one should add Puerariae Radix *(gé gēn)* to the original formula and double the dosage of Scutellariae Radix *(huáng qín)* in order to strengthen its ability to clear the yang brightness while simultaneously resolving the muscles. This is called Kudzu Extend Life Decoction *(gé gēn xù mìng tāng)*.

- In greater yin channel wind-stroke where lack of sweating and a cold body are the main symptoms, one should double the dosage of Aconiti Radix lateralis praeparata *(zhì fù zǐ)* in the original formula and add Zingiberis Rhizoma *(gān jiāng)* and Glycyrrhizae Radix *(gān cǎo)* in order to strengthen its ability to warm and tonify the Spleen yang and disperse yin cold. This is called Aconite Extend Life Decoction *(fù zǐ xù mìng tāng)*.

- In lesser yin channel wind-stroke where the absence of both sweating and fever are the main symptoms, one should double the dosage of Cinnamomi Ramulus *(guì zhī)*, Aconiti Radix lateralis praeparata *(zhì fù zǐ)*, and Glycyrrhizae Radix *(gān cǎo)* in the original formula in order to strengthen its ability to warm and tonify Kidney yang and disperse yin cold. This is called Cinnamon and Aconite Extend Life Decoction *(guì fù xù mìng tāng)*.

- Where the symptoms of six channel wind-stroke are mixed up and not clear but related to the lesser yang and terminal yin channels , characterized by such clinical manifestations as spasmodic contractions of the extremities or numbness, one should add Notopterygii Rhizoma seu Radix *(qiāng huó)* and Forsythiae Fructus *(lián qiáo)* in order to also take these symptoms into account. This is called Notopterygium and Lonicera Extend Life Decoction *(qiāng lián xù mìng tāng)*.

Biomedical Indications

With the appropriate presentation, this formula may be used to treat a variety of biomedically-defined disorders including central and peripheral facial paralysis, cerebrovascular accident and its sequelae, urticaria, and rheumatoid arthritis.

Modifications

- For disorientation, add Poriae Sclerotium pararadicis *(fú shén)* and Polygalae Radix *(yuǎn zhì)*. (source text)

- For irritable pain in the bones and fever, remove Aconiti Radix lateralis praeparata *(zhì fù zǐ)* and increase the dosage of Paeoniae Radix alba *(bái sháo)*. (source text)

- For facial asymmetry, add Scolopendra *(wú gōng)*.

- For excessive sweating and an aversion to wind, substitute Astragali Radix *(huáng qí)* for Ephedrae Herba *(má huáng)*.

- For pain in the joints that worsens at night, add Angelicae sinensis Radix *(dāng guī)*, Persicae Semen *(táo rén)*, and Astragali Radix *(huáng qí)*.

Associated Formulas

大續命湯（大续命汤）

Major Extend Life Decoction

dà xù mìng tāng

SOURCE *Arcane Essentials from the Imperial Library* (752)

Ephedrae Herba *(má huáng)*	9g
Cinnamomi Ramulus *(guì zhī)*	9g
Ginseng Radix *(rén shēn)*	9g
Angelicae sinensis Radix *(dāng guī)*	9g
Chuanxiong Rhizoma *(chuān xiōng)*	4.5g
Armeniacae Semen *(xìng rén)*	9g
Zingiberis Rhizoma *(gān jiāng)*	9g
Glycyrrhizae Radix *(gān cǎo)*	9g
Gypsum fibrosum *(shí gāo)*	9g

Supports the normal qi, clears heat, and disperses wind. For external wind invading the channels with qi and blood deficiency, or internal stirring of Liver wind with the production of heat characterized by flaccid hemiplegia and aphasia. The patient is unable to recognize friends or identify the source of pain. There are also dry stools, low-grade fever, malar flush, a yellow, greasy or yellow, thin tongue coating, and a wiry, forceful or slippery, rapid pulse. There may also be stiffness with an inability to rotate the trunk.

烏藥順氣散（乌药顺气散）

Lindera Powder to Smooth the Flow of Qi

wū yào shùn qì sǎn

SOURCE *Formulary of the Pharmacy Service for Benefiting the People in the Taiping Era* (1107)

Ephedrae Herba *(má huáng)*	60g
Citri reticulatae Pericarpium *(chén pí)*	60g
Linderae Radix *(wū yào)*	60g
Bombyx batryticatus *(bái jiāng cán)*	30g
Chuanxiong Rhizoma *(chuān xiōng)*	30g
Aurantii Fructus *(zhǐ ké)*	30g
Glycyrrhizae Radix *(gān cǎo)*	30g
Angelicae dahuricae Radix *(bái zhǐ)*	30g
Platycodi Radix *(jié gěng)*	30g
Zingiberis Rhizoma praeparatum *(páo jiāng)*	15g

Grind the ingredients into a powder and take as a draft in 9g doses with Zingiberis Rhizoma recens *(shēng jiāng)* and Jujubae Fructus *(dà zǎo)*. Disperses wind and opens up the channels (especially in the extremities). For wind attacking the extremities characterized by joint pain, numbness, headache, and dizziness. In severe cases, there may be hemiplegia or difficulty in walking, aphasia, and spasms. May also be used for cold attacking the chest and axillae (common in the elderly) characterized by stabbing pain in the flanks, epigastric and abdominal distention, vomiting, diarrhea, and borborygmus.

烏頭湯 （乌头汤）

Aconite Decoction

wū tóu tāng

SOURCE   *Essentials from the Golden Cabinet* (c. 220)

Aconiti Radix praeparata *(zhì chuān wū)* 9-12g
Ephedrae Herba *(má huáng)* 9g
Paeoniae Radix alba *(bái sháo)* 9g
Astragali Radix *(huáng qí)* 9g
Glycyrrhizae Radix praeparata *(zhì gān cǎo)* 9g

The source text advises to grind the ingredients into a coarse powder and prepare as a decoction. At present, it is simply prepared as a decoction without grinding the ingredients. Cook Aconiti Radix praeparata *(zhì chuān wū)* with honey for 40-60 minutes to reduce its toxicity before adding the other ingredients. Warms the channels, disperses wind, and alleviates pain. For long-term invasion of the channels by wind-cold-dampness leading to severe obstruction of the sinews, vessels, and joints characterized by intense pain and severely restricted motion in the joints, particularly those of the hands and feet. Also for leg qi due to damp-cold.

三生飲 （三生饮）

Drink from Three Unprepared Ingredients

sān shēng yǐn

The name of this formula refers to the three main ingredients in this formula. They are not, as is usual, prepared to reduce their toxicity, but are used in their unprepared form to increase their efficacy in the treatment of a life-threatening condition.

Source   *Simple Book of Formulas* (1191)

Arisaematis Rhizoma *(tiān nán xīng)* 30g
Aconiti Radix *(chuān wū)* 15g
Aconiti Radix lateralis *(fù zǐ)* 15g
Aucklandiae Radix *(mù xiāng)* 7.5g

Method of Preparation   Grind the herbs into a coarse powder and prepare 15g as a draft by boiling in 2 cups of water together with 10 slices of Zingiberis Rhizoma recens *(shēng jiāng)* until about half of the liquid has evaporated. At present, it is usually prepared as a decoction with an appropriate reduction in dosage. (See CAUTIONS AND CONTRAINDICATIONS below.)

Actions   Dispels wind, transforms phlegm, disperses cold, and assists the yang

Indications

Loss of consciousness, overabundant and congested phlegm, halting and sluggish speech, and inversion frigidity of the ex-

tremities. Also for deviation of the mouth and eyes or hemiplegia with a white tongue coating, and a submerged, hidden pulse.

This is sudden wind-stroke in a person with constitutional yang deficiency and phlegm-dampness. Such people are often obese, with a history of over-consumption of rich, greasy food. Obstruction of the interstices and pores by phlegm-dampness combined with a deficiency of yang qi in the exterior predisposes a person to the invasion of wind from the exterior. Wind entering the body from the outside combines with phlegm-dampness in the interior to obstruct the sensory orifices. This causes one to fall down suddenly and become unconscious. Phlegm congestion and sluggish speech are other manifestations of this pathodynamic. Overabundance of wind-phlegm in the interior obstructs the channels and collaterals, leading to deviation of the mouth and eyes and hemiplegia. The white tongue coating reflects the overabundance of phlegm-dampness, while the submerged, hidden pulse expresses the almost complete obstruction of the qi dynamic.

Analysis of Formula

The appropriate strategy for treating wind-phlegm blocking the channels and orifices (i.e., an interior cold excess pattern) is to expel the wind, transform the phlegm, disperse the cold, and assist the yang. For this purpose, the formula relies on the three unprepared herbs for which it is named: Arisaematis Rhizoma *(tiān nán xīng)*, Aconiti Radix lateralis *(fù zǐ)*, and Aconiti Radix *(chuān wū)*. Acrid and warming Arisaematis Rhizoma *(tiān nán xīng)* is the most important herb in the Chinese materia medica for dispelling wind-phlegm from the channels and collaterals. The late 17th-century work *New Compilation of Materia Medica* specifically notes that "other dispersing herbs do not have the harsh power of Arisaematis Rhizoma *(tiān nán xīng)*. When the jaw is clenched in wind-stroke, it must be used because it breaks open the 'gate' and goes directly in." Acrid and strongly warming Aconiti Radix *(chuān wū)* dispels cold-dampness and disperses wind. It is an essential ingredient in all formulas for severe wind-cold-damp painful obstruction and wind-stroke due to the same pathogens. Aconiti Radix lateralis *(fù zǐ)* is the accessory root tuber of the same plant as Aconiti Radix *(wū tóu)* and is thus very similar in function. However, by tonifying the fire at the gate of vitality, it also disperses internal cold and revives the yang. Usually, these three ingredients are prepared to reduce their toxicity. However, in this formula, they are used in their unprepared form to maximize their effect in a potentially life-threatening situation. Some degree of protection against potential side effects is, nevertheless, supplied by Zingiberis Rhizoma recens *(shēng jiāng)*, one of two assistants in the formula, as this herb is normally used when processing the chief ingredients into their prepared form. The other assistant, acrid and fragrant Aucklandiae Radix *(mù xiāng)*, regulates the qi and thereby ensures that the turbid phlegm is more easily dispelled.

Cautions and Contraindications

This formula is potentially highly toxic and must therefore be used with extreme caution. To reduce its potential side effects, the three main herbs should be decocted together with Zingiberis Rhizoma recens *(shēng jiāng)* for at least an hour or more. In general, the decoction is safe to use when it no longer irritates the mucous membranes in the mouth. Once the intended effect has been achieved, use of the formula should be immediately discontinued. It is absolutely contraindicated in patterns characterized by yin or blood deficiency, heat or fire, or ascendant Liver yang.

Commentary

The consensus among commentators is that this formula is based on Aconite Decoction *(wū tóu tāng)*. As discussed above, that formula, originally listed in *Essentials from the Golden Cabinet*, is used for long-term invasion of the channels by wind-cold-dampness. In order to deal with an acute and potentially life-threatening condition, the potency of that formula is increased here by adding warming herbs that assist the yang and dispel phlegm, while removing its qi-tonifying ingredients. There are several unresolved issues with respect to these modifications. In *Selected Annotations to Ancient Formulas from the Garden of Crimson Snow*, the Qing-dynasty physician Wang Zi-Jie argued that the formula's name refers to three types of unprepared Aconite. The famous Ming-dynasty imperial physician Xue Ji, on the other hand, argued in *Summary of Internal Medicine* that Ginseng Radix *(rén shēn)* must also be included in the formula in order to tonify the primal qi. This view was supported by Ke Qin in *Golden Mirror of the Medical Tradition*, who raised an even more important point in the process:

> Wind is a yang pathogen. Wind without cold [therefore] cannot seriously harm a person. Only if wind also carries cold does the harm begin to be severe. If the cold is mild and located in the exterior, it is appropriate for promoting sweating in order to drive out the pathogens. If the cold is severe and enters into the interior, it is impossible to fully help [a patient] unless one warms the middle and tonifies the deficiency. This [formula] therefore picks three very acrid and very heating substances and [uses] them [in their] unprepared [form]. It assists their [action] by adding Aucklandiae Radix *(mù xiāng)*, thereby mobilizing the qi in the strongest and most acute manner. In truth, [therefore] this is not a strategy for treating wind but for treating cold.

In *Annotated Fine Formulas from Generations of Famous Physicians*, the contemporary physician Ran Xue-Feng took up this argument and sought to integrate it with a biomedical perspective:

> [Symptoms such as] deviation of the mouth and eyes, hemiplegia, and unconsciousness, which for generations have been commonly known as wind-stoke, are in reality not wind at all. They are pathological changes of the cerebral sensory and motor nerves. Eighty to ninety percent of these disorders are associated with heat due to qi and fire ascending and floating, and they come on very suddenly. One sees very few [cases] associated with cold.

Some textbooks thus group this formula under the categories of warming the interior or transforming wind-phlegm. In clinical practice, its use may also be considered for cases of severe dizziness due to wind-cold-phlegm.

Biomedical Indications

With the appropriate presentation, this formula may be used to treat a variety of biomedically-defined disorders including stroke, epilepsy, and facial paralysis.

Modification

- For patterns with a pulse that is not only submerged and hidden, but also frail, add Ginseng Radix *(rén shēn)* to augment the primal qi.

川芎茶調散 (川芎茶调散)

Chuanxiong Powder to Be Taken with Green Tea

chuān xiōng chá tiáo sǎn

Source *Formulary of the Pharmacy Service for Benefiting the People in the Taiping Era* (1107)

Menthae haplocalycis Herba *(bò hé)*. 240g
Chuanxiong Rhizoma *(chuān xiōng)* 120g
Angelicae dahuricae Radix *(bái zhǐ)* 60g
Notopterygii Rhizoma seu Radix *(qiāng huó)* 60g
Asari Radix et Rhizoma *(xì xīn)* 30g
Schizonepetae Herba *(jīng jiè)* 120g
Saposhnikoviae Radix *(fáng fēng)*. 45g
Glycyrrhizae Radix praeparata *(zhì gān cǎo)* 60g

Method of Preparation Grind the ingredients into a fine powder and take 6g twice daily after meals with green tea. May also be prepared as a decoction by reducing the dosage of the ingredients by about 90 percent. Do not cook for more than 10 minutes.

Actions Disperses wind and alleviates pain

Indications

Headache in any part of the head, which may be accompanied by fever and chills, dizziness, nasal congestion, a thin, white tongue coating, and a floating pulse.

This is headache due to externally-contracted wind. The head is the meeting place of the yang channels. When wind invades the body, it follows the course of the channels upward to the head and eyes, obstructing the clear yang qi, and causing headache and dizziness. This pattern is referred to in Chapter 29 of *Basic Questions*: "Injury from wind is suffered first in the upper body." When wind attacks the exterior, the mutual regulation of the nutritive and protective qi is impaired, which leads to chills. When wind invades the exterior, it battles with the normal qi, which produces fever. The normal qi forces the pathogenic influence outward, which is manifested as a floating pulse. The Lungs are the most superficial of the organs and are therefore most easily affected by wind. Because the nose is governed by the Lungs, this leads to nasal congestion.

Analysis of Formula

In order to dispel exterior wind from the head and stop pain, one should select so-called 'wind herbs' (風藥 *fēng yào*). The reason is explained by Wang Ang in *Medical Formulas Collected and Analyzed*: "For headaches one must employ wind herbs because only wind is able to reach upward to the vertex of the head." The so-called wind herbs are acrid, warm, and ascending in nature and thereby embody the nature of wind within themselves. The present formula relies on three such herbs as chiefs: Chuanxiong Rhizoma (*chuān xiōng*) alleviates headaches along the lesser yang and terminal yin channels (temporal and vertex), Notopterygii Rhizoma seu Radix (*qiāng huó*) along the greater yang channel (occipital), and Angelicae dahuricae Radix (*bái zhǐ*) along the yang brightness channel. In combination, these three herbs treat headache in any part of the head. If the pain is localized, the dosage of the corresponding herb can be increased accordingly.

Four deputies aid the chief herbs by dispersing wind from the head and releasing the exterior. Schizonepetae Herba (*jīng jiè*) and Saposhnikoviae Radix (*fáng fēng*) comprise a frequently used synergistic combination that disperses wind from both the exterior and the channels. Menthae haplocalycis Herba (*bò hé*), which some commentators regard as the chief herb of the formula (see COMMENTARY below), disperses wind from the exterior, benefits the head and eyes, and clears heat from constraint. The final deputy, Asari Radix et Rhizoma (*xì xīn*), scatters cold, alleviates pain, and is especially effective in treating headaches along the lesser yin channel, such as orbital headaches.

The assistant herb here is the green tea that is used to swallow the powder, an essential constituent of this formula. Bitter and cool, it causes the clear yang to ascend and directs the turbid yin downward, helps to clear the head and eyes, and moderates the undesirable side effects caused by the warm, drying properties of some of the other ingredients. Glycyrrhizae Radix (*gān cǎo*), the envoy, cools, detoxifies, and harmonizes the actions of the other herbs in the formula.

Cautions and Contraindications

This formula contains a relatively large number of warm, acrid substances and is therefore inappropriate for treating headache from ascendant Liver yang due to Liver and Kidney deficiency, and for headache due to qi and blood deficiency. It should be administered in small doses and cooked no more than 1-3 minutes when taken as a powder.

Commentary

History

Viewed from the perspective of the herbs it contains, this formula is distinctly acrid and warm, characteristics it shares with most other prescriptions listed in *Formulary of the Pharmacy Service for Benefiting the People in the Taiping Era*. In terms of its genealogy, however, Chuanxiong Powder to be Taken with Green Tea (*chuān xiōng chá tiáo sǎn*) belongs to a distinct lineage of heat-clearing formulas. For example, *Essential Subtleties on the Silver Sea*, which probably contains some Tang-dynasty material, even though it was likely compiled in the 16th century, contains a formula by the same name that was indicated for hot tears and damp, macerated orbits. This formula does not use Asari Radix et Rhizoma (*xì xīn*) and Angelicae dahuricae Radix (*bái zhǐ*), but, instead, includes Haliotidis Concha (*shí jué míng*), Gypsum fibrosum (*shí gāo*), Equiseti hiemalis Herba (*mù zéi*), and Chrysanthemi Flos (*jú huā*). Later on, physicians like Zhu Dan-Xi in the 13th century and Cheng Guo-Peng in the 17th century again modified the formula by adding cold and cooling herbs; the formula was then used in the treatment of headache and nasal discharge.

Debates about the Chief Herb and Indications

This genealogy brings into focus some of the reasons for the historical debates that attach to this formula's indications and composition. The analysis above follows the consensus of contemporary Chinese textbooks, which generally view the formula as treating wind-cold headaches. Many classical writers, however, believed that because of its large dosage, Menthae haplocalycis Herba (*bò hé*) should be regarded as the chief herb in this formula and that the formula was accordingly best suited for the treatment of wind-heat headaches. The late 17th-century physician Zhang Lu-Xuan, for instance, noted in *Comprehensive Medicine According to Master Zhang* that Chuanxiong Powder to Be Taken with Green Tea (*chuān xiōng chá tiáo sǎn*) should be used for headache due to wind that has gradually transformed into fire. His contemporary, Wang Ang, wrote in *Medical Formulas Collected and Analyzed* that it was intended for wind-heat in the upper part of the body.

One possible resolution of these differences is to follow the source text, which notes that this is a well-balanced formula that can be used for treating any externally-contracted wind disorder where headache is the principal symptom. A second possibility is to examine the various commentaries for underlying agreement. Most commentators, for instance, concur that this formula treats not only acute, but also chronic headaches that are caused by the lingering of wind in the body. This type of headache, which occurs at irregular intervals and is often resistant to treatment, is called 'wind in the head' (頭風 *tóu fēng*).

Tracking down Wind

Classical treatment strategies aimed at eliminating wind that has been retained in the body for a long time require the use of herbs that have the special ability to 'track down wind' (*soū fēng* 搜風). Because wind, by its very nature, is elusive and difficult to grasp, it can penetrate and hide everywhere, in the most superficial areas of the skin as well as in the interior of the body in organs like the Intestines and Bladder. Over time, this wind also invades the Liver and exhausts its essence, further aggravating the chronicity of the problem. To dispel this type of wind, an herb must be able to penetrate into all of these places and clear heat constraint from both excess and deficiency. Menthae haplocalycis Herba (*bò hé*) is one such herb.

According to Wang Fu in *Collectanea of Investigations from the Realm of Medicine*:

> Menthae haplocalycis Herba (*bò hé*) … is light and hollow and therefore floats upward. Above it clears wind-heat in the head and eyes. On the sides, it tracks down damp-heat in the skin. In the middle, it expels deficiency wind from the Liver and Gallbladder. Below, it eliminates blood heat from the Bowels and gestation membranes.

In *Convenient Reader of Materia Medica*, Zhang Bing-Cheng likewise emphasizes that in this formula, Menthae haplocalycis Herba (*bò hé*) is used to "pursue wind and disperse heat." He also reminds his readers that two other herbs in the formula—Chuanxiong Rhizoma (*chuān xiōng*) and Schizonepetae Herba (*jīng jiè*)—enter the Liver and remove constraint from within the blood, while Glycyrrhizae Radix (*gān cǎo*) "is a harmonizing herb that relaxes the middle," a standard treatment strategy for treating Liver constraint from deficiency. This connection to the Liver is further thrown into relief by the Qing-dynasty scholar-physician Xu Da-Chun, who was working from an edition of the source text that includes Cyperi Rhizoma (*xiāng fù*) in the formula instead of Asari Radix et Rhizoma (*xì xīn*). In *Six Texts Summarizing the Medicine of Xu Ling-Tai* , Xu pointed out that "Cyperi Rhizoma (*xiāng fù*) regulates the qi and blood in the interior, while on the exterior it can spread out through the skin and hair and pierce through pathogens [lurking] in the interstices."

Taken together, these commentaries define quite precisely the specific pathology for which this formula is indicated, namely, headache and dizziness due to external wind-cold that have remained in the body for some time and upset the balance of qi and blood organized by the Liver. It should be differentiated, on one hand, from headache and dizziness due to acute and superficial invasion of external wind-cold or wind-heat into the channels and collaterals, and, on the other, from internal wind due to depletion of yin or blood.

Biomedical Indications

With the appropriate presentation, this formula may be used to treat a variety of biomedically-defined disorders including upper respiratory tract infection, migraine headache, tension headache, neurogenic headache, and acute and chronic rhinitis or sinusitis. Some reports also mention its usefulness in treating postconcussion headache.

Alternate names

Tea Mediated Powder (*chá tiáo sǎn*) in *Effective Formulas from Generations of Physicians*; Tea Mediated Decoction (*chá tiáo tāng*) in *Classified Compilation of Medical Prescriptions as Coming from the Empirical Efficacious Formulas*; Chuanxiong Drink to Be Taken with Green Tea (*chuān xiōng chá tiáo yǐn*) in *Collection of Versatility*

Modifications

- For wind-cold headache, remove Menthae haplocalycis Herba (*bò hé*) and add Zingiberis Rhizoma recens (*shēng jiāng*) and Perillae Folium (*zǐ sū yè*).
- For wind-heat headache, remove Notopterygii Rhizoma seu Radix (*qiāng huó*) and Asari Radix et Rhizoma (*xì xīn*) and add Chrysanthemi Flos (*jú huā*) and Viticis Fructus (*màn jīng zǐ*).
- For chronic headache, add Carthami Flos (*hóng huā*), Persicae Semen (*táo rén*), Bombyx batryticatus (*bái jiāng cán*), and Scorpio (*quán xiē*).
- To alter the focus of the formula in addressing headache along specific channels, add the following: Ligustici Rhizoma (*gǎo běn*) for greater yang (occipital) headache; Bupleuri Radix (*chái hú*) for lesser yang (temporal) headache; Puerariae Radix (*gé gēn*) for yang brightness (frontal) headache; and Evodiae Fructus (*wú zhū yú*) and Pheretima (*dì lóng*) for terminal yin (vertex) headache.

Variations

菊花茶調散 （菊花茶调散）

Chrysanthemum Powder to Be Taken with Green Tea
jú huā chá tiáo sǎn

Source *Medical Formulas Collected and Analyzed* (1682)

Add 120g of Chrysanthemi Flos (*jú huā*) and 45g of Bombyx batryticatus (*bái jiāng cán*) for headache and dizziness primarily due to wind-heat.

川芎茶調散 （川芎茶调散）

Chuanxiong Powder to Be Taken with Green Tea from
Awakening of the Mind

chuān xiōng chá tiáo sǎn

Source   *Awakening of the Mind in Medical Studies* (1732)

Chuanxiong Rhizoma (*chuān xiōng*) . . . . . . [mixed with alcohol] 30g
Schizonepetae Herba (*jīng jiè*) 30g
Angelicae dahuricae Radix (*bái zhǐ*) 30g
Platycodi Radix (*jié gěng*) . . . . [fried] 30g
Glycyrrhizae Radix (*gān cǎo*) 30g
Scutellariae Radix (*huáng qín*) . . . . [fried with alcohol] 30g
Fritillariae cirrhosae Bulbus (*chuān bèi mǔ*) 30g
Gardeniae Fructus (*zhī zǐ*) 60g

Grind into a fine powder. Take 6g after meals three times daily together with aged, good-quality green tea. Treats chronic nasal discharge that is transparent in color. The root cause here is cold that was not dispersed and has transformed into heat. In contrast to the principal formula, this variation focuses on obstruction of the Lung channel due to chronic wind-cold that has transformed into heat.

蒼耳子散 （苍耳子散）

Xanthium Powder

cāng ér zǐ sǎn

Source   *Formulas to Aid the Living* (1253)

Xanthii Fructus (*cāng ěr zǐ*) 7.5g (6-9g)
Magnoliae Flos (*xīn yí huā*) 15g (3-6g)
Angelicae dahuricae Radix (*bái zhǐ* 30g (6-9g)
Menthae haplocalycis Herba (*bò hé*) . . [add near end] 1.5g (3-6g)

Method of Preparation   The source text advises to grind the herbs into a fine powder and take in 6g doses with a tea made from Allii fistulosi Bulbus (*cōng bái*) and green tea. Today it is often prepared as a decoction with the dosage indicated in parentheses.

Actions   Disperses wind, alleviates pain, and unblocks the nose

Indications

Copious, purulent, and even foul-smelling nasal discharge, nasal obstruction, dizziness, frontal headache, a normal or thin, white or greasy, white tongue coating.

This condition is known as 'deep-source nasal congestion' (鼻淵 *bì yuān*) or 'seepage from the brain' (腦漏 *nǎo lòu*). It usually appears after an unresolved case of the common cold where an external wind pathogen remains in the body and obstructs the protective qi. Because protective qi is governed by the Lungs, such obstruction readily manifests in its external orifice, the nose. Obstruction of the yang brightness channel, which traverses the nose, causes frontal headache and dizziness. Heat engendered from constraint and fluids that are not directed downward by the Lungs combine to produce profuse, foul-smelling nasal discharge. A normal or

white tongue coating indicates, however, that the heat constraint is not pronounced.

Analysis of Formula

In order to unblock deep-source nasal congestion, this formula employs a strategy of dispelling wind and unblocking the orifices. The chief herbs, Xanthii Fructus (*cāng ěr zǐ*) and Magnoliae Flos (*xīn yí huā*), are acrid and warm, unblock the nasal passages, and are frequently used in treating profuse nasal discharge. The deputy, acrid, warming, and aromatic Angelicae dahuricae Radix (*bái zhǐ*), releases the exterior and opens up the orifices, disperses wind-dampness, and promotes the discharge of pus. The assistant, acrid and cooling Menthae haplocalycis Herba (*bò hé*), releases wind-heat from the exterior and clears the eyes and head. Its light nature guides the other ingredients to the head, a function supported by Allii fistulosi Bulbus (*cōng bái*), which is regarded as one of the envoys. The other envoy is green tea, which clears the head and directs the qi downward to balance the ascending and acrid nature of most of the other ingredients.

Commentary

Since its first publication in the Song dynasty, commentators have prescribed this formula for nasal discharge caused by wind-heat. Wang Ang even listed it as a formula that drains fire. Given that its three key herbs are acrid, warm, and drying, and that Menthae haplocalycis Herba (*bò hé*), which is acrid and cool, was originally used only in a very small dosage, this interpretation appears highly problematic; indeed, it is increasingly rejected by contemporary writers. The famous contemporary physician Ran Xue-Feng, for instance, writes in *Annotated Fine Formulas from Generations of Famous Physicians*: "This formula clears [heat] and is light and therefore relies on acrid opening." Somewhat earlier, the Qing-dynasty commentator Zhang Bing-Cheng had emphasized that the formula's heat-clearing properties were due to its ascending and dispersing nature. This argument, outlined in *Convenient Reader of Established Formulas*, brought into play a treatment principle first explained in the *Inner Classic*: "For fire from constraint, discharge it." The idea is that, where heat is caused by constraint, especially if it is due to cold, dispersal of such constraint by means of acrid herbs will also clear the fire. This is clearly the treatment strategy followed in this formula.

In fact, the source text states that the symptoms characterizing this pattern are caused by wind-cold. However, it also says that the wind-cold has combined with an excess of qi already present in the nose. This, in turn, is attributed to Liver blood deficiency with Lung qi excess. Although the formula does not treat these underlying causes, the explanation helps us define more precisely the type of patient for whom this formula is indicated. External cold causing constraint will tend to occur in those who are both prone to the invasion of external pathogens and have a tendency toward relatively excess qi. Those with blood deficiency fulfill both of these conditions. In clinical practice, this pattern must therefore be differentiated from those caused by the invasion of external wind-heat or by Liver and Gallbladder fire.

The nature of the nasal discharge will help make this differentiation. Patterns due to cold transforming into heat are characterized by turbid nasal discharge; external wind-heat patterns are characterized by clear nasal discharge; and patterns due to Liver and Gallbladder fire typically involve one side of the nose more than the other and are characterized by yellow discharge.

A novel use of the formula has been suggested by Ran Xue-Feng in *Annotated Fine Formulas from Generations of Famous Physicians*:

This formula clears [fire by means of] light [herbs] and simultaneously unblocks [by means of] acrid [herbs]. Any formula can be connected [to different patterns] and any medicinal can be used for another purpose. Qi and blood travel upward together. They either interpenetrate each other, or they lose each other. What Western medicine calls cerebral congestion, cerebral anemia, thrombosis, or blood clots all resemble [in terms of their pathodynamic, the pattern] for which this formula is intended, and therefore can be treated by it in modifiedied form. It guides the clear yang qi to the location of the disorder through the power of its herbs.

Biomedical Indications

With the appropriate presentation, this formula may be used to treat a variety of biomedically-defined disorders including acute or chronic sinusitis and acute, chronic, or allergic rhinitis.

Alternate names

Angelicae and Magnolia Flower Powder (*zhǐ yí sǎn*) in *Introduction to Medicine*; Angelica and Magnolia Flower Powder (*zhǐ xīn sǎn*) in *Selected Annotations to Ancient Formulas from the Garden of Crimson Snow*; Magnolia Flower Decoction (*xīn yí sǎn*) in *Collection Picked by Immortals*; Xanthium Herb Powder (*cāng ér cǎo sǎn*) in *Manual of the Art of Benevolence*; Xanthium Powder (*cāng ér zǐ sǎn*) in *Small Collection of Fine Formulas*

Modifications

- For severe nasal obstruction, add Centipedae minimae Herba (*é bù shí cǎo*) and Asari Radix et Rhizoma (*xì xīn*).

- For concurrent fever and heat in the Lungs, add Scutellariae Radix (*huáng qín*) and Houttuyniae Herba (*yú xīng cǎo*).

- For bloody nasal discharge or nosebleed, add Rubiae Radix (*qiàn cǎo gēn*) and Rehmanniae Radix (*shēng dì huáng*).

- For more severe dizziness and headache, add Chrysanthemi Flos (*jú huā*) and Fructus Tribuli Terrestris (*bái jí lí*).

Associated Formula

辛夷散

Magnolia Flower Powder

xīn yí sǎn

Source *Formulas to Aid the Living* (1253)

Magnoliae Flos (*xīn yí huā*)
Chuanxiong Rhizoma (*chuān xiōng*)
Akebiae Caulis (*mù tōng*)
Asari Radix et Rhizoma (*xì xīn*)
Saposhnikoviae Radix (*fáng fēng*)
Notopterygii Rhizoma seu Radix (*qiāng huó*)
Ligustici Rhizoma (*gǎo běn*)
Cimicifugae Rhizoma (*shēng má*)
Angelicae dahuricae Radix (*bái zhǐ*)
Glycyrrhizae Radix praeparata (*zhì gān cǎo*)

Grind equal amounts of the ingredients into a fine powder and take 6g with tea after meals. Disperses wind-cold and unblocks the nasal passages. For nasal congestion and pain, persistent, copious nasal discharge, loss of smell, and headache due to wind-cold.

大秦艽湯 (大秦艽汤)

Major Large Gentian Decoction

dà qín jiāo tāng

Source *Collection of Writings on the Mechanism of Disease, Suitability of Qi, and the Safeguarding of Life as Discussed in Basic Questions* (1186)

Gentianae macrophyllae Radix (*qín jiāo*) 90g
Glycyrrhizae Radix (*gān cǎo*) 60g
Chuanxiong Rhizoma (*chuān xiōng*) 60g
Angelicae sinensis Radix (*dāng guī*) 60g
Paeoniae Radix alba (*bái sháo*) 60g
Asari Radix et Rhizoma (*xì xīn*) 15g
Notopterygii Rhizoma seu Radix (*qiāng huó*) 30g
Saposhnikoviae Radix (*fáng fēng*) 30g
Scutellariae Radix (*huáng qín*) 30g
Gypsum fibrosum (*shí gāo*) 60g
Angelicae dahuricae Radix (*bái zhǐ*) 30g
Atractylodis macrocephalae Rhizoma (*bái zhú*) 30g
Rehmanniae Radix (*shēng dì huáng*) 30g
Rehmanniae Radix praeparata (*shú dì huáng*) 30g
Poria (*fú líng*) 30g
Angelicae pubescentis Radix (*dú huó*) 60g

Method of Preparation The source text advises to grind the ingredients into a powder and take warm in 30g doses as a decoction. Today it is usually prepared as a regular decoction with an appropriate reduction in dosage.

Actions Expels wind, clears heat, nourishes and invigorates the blood

Indications

Deviation of the mouth and eyes, difficulty speaking due to stiffness of the tongue, an inability to move one's arms and legs or numbness and lack of sensation in the hands and feet. Often accompanied by chills and fever, muscle spasms, aching joints, a white or yellow tongue coating, and a pulse that is either floating and tight or wiry and thin.

This is early- or middle-stage wind-stroke in the channels. This arises when wind invades a person with deficiency of the channels. When the pathogen enters the channels and collaterals of the face, it obstructs the flow of qi and blood. The muscle-sinews thereby lose nourishment, their functions fail, and they relax. On the other hand, those places where the blood and qi can still penetrate become excessive, which leads to hypertonicity. Areas of excessive relaxation are pulled toward those of hypertonicity, causing deviation of the mouth and eyes. If the wind pathogen invades the channels of the tongue, another muscle and therefore prone to such invasion, it stiffens, causing difficulty in speaking. Invasion of wind into the superficial collaterals is experienced as numbness and a lack of sensation in the hands and feet, while obstruction of the major channels leads to an inability to move one's arms and legs. Because wind is extremely mobile, this type of pathology is not limited to a specific channel but spreads throughout an entire area. Clinically, symptoms of obstruction in the channels and collaterals are therefore often accompanied by systemic signs indicating that a pathogen is disrupting the normal function of one or more of the yang warps. When it affects the greater yang, there will be fever and chills, muscle spasms, aching joints, and a pulse that is floating and tight; for the lesser yang, alternating fever and chills, a white tongue coating, and a wiry and thin pulse; for the yang brightness, fever with no chills, and a yellow tongue coating.

Analysis of Formula

The appropriate strategy for treating wind in the channels and collaterals obstructing the movement of qi and blood is to focus on dispelling wind and unblocking the channels, while also augmenting the qi, and nourishing and invigorating the blood. The chief herb is therefore bitter and acrid Gentianae macrophyllae Radix (qín jiāo). It dispels wind from the channels, unblocks the flow of nutrients to the sinews and muscles, and thereby eliminates the obstruction. Unlike other wind-expelling herbs, which are usually drying, its bitterness does not dry excessively, and its nature is relatively harmonious. The deputies are Notopterygii Rhizoma seu Radix (qiāng huó), Angelicae pubescentis Radix (dú huó), Saposhnikoviae Radix (fáng fēng), Asari Radix et Rhizoma (xì xīn), and Angelicae dahuricae Radix (bái zhǐ). All of these herbs are acrid and warming and therefore able to disperse and unblock, assisting Gentianae macrophyllae Radix (qín jiāo) in its task of dispelling the wind and opening the channels. Moreover, each of the deputies has an affinity for a specific channel, or focuses on a specific supplementary task. Angelicae dahuricae

Radix (bái zhǐ) enters the yang brightness; Saposhnikoviae Radix (fáng fēng) tracks down wind in any of the channels; Notopterygii Rhizoma seu Radix (qiāng huó) and Angelicae pubescentis Radix (dú huó) focus on the greater yang, while also combining to reach both the upper and lower halves of the body; and Asari Radix et Rhizoma (xì xīn) is particularly suitable for dispelling wind from the small collaterals.

The assistants can be divided into three groups. The first, consisting of Rehmanniae Radix praeparata (shú dì huáng), Angelicae sinensis Radix (dāng guī), Paeoniae Radix alba (bái sháo), and Chuanxiong Rhizoma (chuān xiōng), comprises the blood-tonifying formula Four-Substance Decoction (sì wù tāng). Its inclusion in this formula has three interrelated purposes. First, nourishing the blood is a necessary strategy for nourishing the muscle sinews and thereby promoting their normal function; second, wind, a yang pathogen, readily dries out the blood, depriving the muscles and skin of moisture and nourishment; and third, the chief and deputies in this formula are also very drying, which could easily cause further damage to the blood unless they were counterbalanced by other, blood-tonifying herbs. The second group of assistants consists of Atractylodis macrocephalae Rhizoma (bái zhú), Poria (fú líng), and Glycyrrhizae Radix (gān cǎo), which comprises three-fourths of the formula Four-Gentlemen Decoction (sì jūn zǐ tāng). Tonifying the qi facilitates both the production and movement of blood. Filling the vessels and collaterals, this effectively supports the elimination of wind to the outside, while guarding against damage to the normal qi from excessive dispersal. The third group of assistants consists of Scutellariae Radix (huáng qín), Gypsum fibrosum (shí gāo), and Rehmanniae Radix (shēng dì huáng), which clear and drain heat from both the qi and blood aspects. This is necessary because constraint of the yang qi due to wind readily transforms into fire, a tendency aggravated by the acrid, warming nature of the wind herbs in the formula. Glycyrrhizae Radix (gān cǎo), finally, serves as the envoy to balance and moderate the diverse actions of the many different herbs in this complex formula.

Cautions and Contraindications

This formula is very acrid and warming. It is unsuitable for treating conditions due to internal wind.

Commentary

The original indications of this formula are set out in the source text:

> As for wind-stroke, there are no physical manifestations associated with the six warps externally and there is no obstruction of stool and urine internally. [Instead], the arms and legs cannot move and the tongue is stiff so that one cannot speak. This is due to the blood being frail and unable to nourish the sinews.

The composition of the formula thus reflects efforts by physicians of the Jin-Yuan era to move away from the six-warp framework of *Discussion of Cold Damage* that governed the treatment of external pathogens at the time. Conceptually, it seeks to come to terms with a pattern dominated by wind symptoms, but missing those indicators that could clearly link this manifestation to one or more of the six warps, or, in fact, to an interior organ pattern. The solution was to combine herbs that disperse wind with those that tonify the blood and qi. This strategy was severely criticized several centuries later by the influential Ming-dynasty physician Zhang Jie-Bin in *Collected Treatises of [Zhang] Jing-Yue*:

> Although [Major] Large Gentian Decoction (*dà qín jiāo tāng*) contains blood nourishing herbs, half of it is comprised of cooling and dispersing medicinals. Now how does it work to use dispersing [medicinals] in the absence of an external pathogen in the six warps? How does it work to use cooling [medicinals] in the absence of a major pathogen obstructing and plugging [internally]? With so much dispersion and cooling, how can the result be able to nourish the blood and qi in order to strengthen the sinews and bones?

Zhang's critique reflects the rejection by Ming- and Qing-dynasty physicians of approaches to the treatment of wind-stroke that perceived wind to be contracted from the outside. More often, therefore, the formula is used today not for the treatment of cerebrovascular accidents, but for facial paralysis, numbness of the hands and feet due to wind obstruction, as well as wind-damp-cold painful obstruction.

Biomedical Indications

With the appropriate presentation, this formula may be used to treat a variety of biomedically-defined disorders including Bell's palsy, thrombotic strokes, and rheumatoid arthritis.

Alternate name

Large Gentian Decoction (*qín jiāo tāng*) in *Revised and Annotated Fine Formulas for Women*

Modifications

* For dampness in the environment, add Zingiberis Rhizoma recens (*shēng jiāng*). (source text)
* For epigastric focal distention, add Aurantii Fructus immaturus (*zhǐ shí*). (source text)
* If there are no signs of heat, remove Gypsum fibrosum (*shí gāo*), Scutellariae Radix (*huáng qín*), and Rehmanniae Radix (*shēng dì huáng*).
* If there are no clear exterior signs, remove Asari Radix et Rhizoma (*xì xīn*), Angelicae dahuricae Radix (*bái zhǐ*), and Saposhnikoviae Radix (*fáng fēng*).
* For facial paralysis, add Scolopendra (*wú gōng*) and Scorpio (*quán xiē*).

小活絡丹（小活络丹）

Minor Invigorate the Collaterals Special Pill

xiǎo huó luò dān

Source *Formulary of the Pharmacy Service for Benefiting the People in the Taiping Era* (1107)

Aconiti kusnezoffii Radix praeparata (*zhì cǎo wū*) 180g
Aconiti Radix praeparata (*zhì chuān wū*) 180g
Arisaematis Rhizoma praeparatum (*zhì tiān nán xīng*) 180g
Myrrha (*mò yào*) 66g
Olibanum (*rǔ xiāng*) 66g
Pheretima (*dì lóng*) 180g

Method of Preparation Grind the ingredients into a powder and form into pills with honey. Take twice a day in 3g doses on an empty stomach with wine or a decoction made of Schizonepetae Herba (*jīng jiè*).

Actions Dispels wind, eliminates dampness, transforms phlegm, invigorates the blood, unblocks the collaterals, and alleviates pain

Indications

Chronic pain, weakness, and numbness (especially in the lower extremities) due to wind-stroke. Also for fixed or migrating pain in the bones and joints with reduced range of motion due to wind-cold-damp painful obstruction. In both conditions, the symptoms are aggravated by cold. The tongue coating is white and moist.

After the onset of wind-stroke, wind, dampness, phlegm, and lifeless blood obstruct the channels and collaterals. This leads to persistent numbness and weakness in the extremities. In severe cases, the obstruction causes severe pain. Although its pathogenesis is quite different, wind-cold-damp painful obstruction presents with similar symptoms. The white, moist tongue coating reflects the presence of interior cold.

Analysis of Formula

To treat obstruction of the channels and collaterals by wind-cold-damp pathogens, blood stasis, and phlegm this formula employs strategies first outlined in Chapter 74 of *Basic Questions*: "Attack what lingers" and "Move what has strayed." The chief ingredients, Aconiti kusnezoffii Radix praeparata (*zhì cǎo wū*) and Aconiti Radix praeparata (*zhì chuān wū*), are among the strongest herbs in the materia medica for warming the channels and dispersing wind, cold, and dampness. Acrid, hot, and toxic, Aconiti kusnezoffii Radix praeparata (*zhì cǎo wū*) searches out wind, overcomes dampness, disperses cold, stops pain, and unbinds areas constrained by phlegm. Aconiti Radix praeparata (*zhì chuān wū*) quickly and powerfully warms and unblocks the channels and drives out wind, dampness, and cold. Together, these two potent herbs are particularly effective in treating this type of disorder. The deputy, Arisaematis Rhizoma praeparatum (*zhì tiān nán xīng*), too, is a strongly warming and intensely acrid substance. While its actions are similar to those of Pinelliae Rhizoma praeparatum *(zhì bàn xià)*, it also enters the Liver channel, and this special quality enables it to move within the channels and collaterals. Thus, it is particularly good at eliminating wind-phlegm. Two of the assistants, Myrrha *(mò yào)* and Olibanum *(rǔ xiāng)*, invigorate the blood and increase the flow in the channels. In *Essays on Medicine Esteeming the Chinese and Respecting the Western*, Zhang Xi-Chun observes that:

> [Used together, the two herbs] form an important combination that disseminates and unblocks the organs, and dredges channels and collaterals. … The power of this combination to unblock the flow of blood also treats wind-cold-damp painful obstruction, which causes numbness throughout the body and unresponsive extremities.

The other assistant, salty and cooling Pheretima *(dì lóng)*, clears heat, unblocks, and promotes movement in the channels and collaterals. Although this is a cooling substance, the many warming herbs in this formula allow its piercing nature to be exploited here to treat cold painful obstruction. Wine serves as the envoy by strengthening the blood-invigorating action of the formula. This is preferred when cold is the main pathogen. Alternatively, if wind symptoms are predominant, a decoction of Schizonepetae Herba *(jīng jiè)* is used to take the pills, which focuses the formula on dispersing wind.

Cautions and Contraindications

Because this formula is quite harsh, warming, and drying, it should only be prescribed for individuals with a relatively strong constitution. It is contraindicated in those with yin deficiency or during pregnancy.

Commentary

Like Drink from Three Unprepared Ingredients *(sān shéng yǐn)*, discussed above, this formula is based on Aconite Decoction *(wū tóu tāng)* from *Essentials from the Golden Cabinet*. This, however, is an even more intensely dispersing formula, whose mode of preparation was accordingly changed from a decoction to a pill. In the source text, its indications read:

> [Treats] all types of wind pathogens and turbid toxic qi [occurring in] men with qi deficiency of the original organ or women with long-standing cold in the Spleen and blood. These linger and stagnate in the vessels and collaterals, spread to the hands and feet, and cause contraction of the sinew vessels. They may also emerge as red swellings, make walking difficult, the waist and legs feel heavy, or pain on raising the legs. Gushing upward, [they cause] drum distention of the abdomen and flanks, focal distention or a stifling sensation in the chest and diaphragm, and reduced appetite. Or they gush into the Heart, [causing] stifling and confusion. It also [treats] any kind of wandering, wind-type pain, or pain all over the body.

The Ming-dynasty physician Wu Kun extended this already broad range of indications to the sequelae of wind-stroke, and the Qing-dynasty writer Zhang Lu to cold-damp painful obstruction. The underlying pathodynamic in each case is a combination of stubborn phlegm and lifeless blood obstructing the channels and collaterals. Although this is often caused by an invasion of wind, it is a very different problem than wind-damp-cold painful obstruction. This difference is explained by Zhang Bin-Cheng in *Convenient Reader of Established Formulas*:

> This formula treats wind-stroke with long-term numbness of the hands or feet that does not improve, [as well as] phlegm-dampness and lifeless blood in the channels and collaterals characterized by one or two painful spots in the arms or legs. When wind lingers in the channels and is not eliminated, the body fluids, qi, and blood in the collaterals become mixed up with each other [rather than staying] separate. As the protective qi no longer flows along its normal path, the blood in the collaterals congeals and no longer moves, while the body fluids clump and turn into phlegm. Numbness, the inability to use [the limbs], and pain in the arms and legs are all due to this dampness, phlegm, and lifeless blood in the collaterals. However, a strategy for treating the collaterals is more difficult [to execute] than treating the yin or yang organs. Because no decoction is able to flush them out, one must use violent substances prepared as pills in order to search for and drive out these pathogens.

The original name of this formula was simply Invigorate the Collaterals Special Pill *(huó luò dān)*. Because the Qing-dynasty scholar-physician Xu Da-Chun promoted a formula composed of 50 ingredients known as Major Invigorate the Collaterals Special Pill *(dà huó luò dān)*, which is commonly used today (although containing too many toxic medicinals to be used in the West), the term 'Minor' was appended by contemporary textbook writers to avoid any possible confusion.

Biomedical Indications

With the appropriate presentation, this formula may be used to treat a variety of biomedically-defined disorders including hemiplegia after cerebrovascular accident, rheumatoid arthritis, osteoarthritis, bone spurs, and peripheral nervous disorders.

Modifications

- For damp-predominant disorders, add Atractylodis Rhizoma *(cāng zhú)*, Stephaniae tetrandrae Radix *(hàn fáng jǐ)*, and Coicis Semen *(yì yǐ rén)*.
- For wind-predominant disorders, add Gentianae macrophyllae Radix *(qín jiāo)* and Saposhnikoviae Radix *(fáng fēng)*.
- For severe cold, increase the dosage of Aconiti Radix praeparata *(zhì chuān wū)* and Aconiti kusnezoffii Radix praeparata *(zhì cǎo wū)*.
- For disabling pain, increase the dosage of Olibanum *(rǔ xiāng)* and Myrrha *(mò yào)*.
- For Liver and Kidney deficiency, combine with Pubescent Angelica and Taxillus Decoction *(dú huó jì shēng tāng)*.

牽正散 （牽正散）

Lead to Symmetry Powder

qiān zhèng sǎn

This formula restores symmetry to the face.

Source *Yang Family Formulas* (1178)

Typhonii Rhizoma praeparatum *(zhì bái fù zǐ)*
Bombyx batryticatus *(bái jiāng cán)*
Scorpio *(quán xiē)*

Method of Preparation The source text advises to grind equal amounts of the ingredients into a fine powder and take in 3g doses with hot wine. Today, it is usually taken with warm water. It may also be prepared as a decoction with 6g of each ingredient.

Actions Dispels wind, transforms phlegm, and stops spasms

Indications

Sudden facial paralysis with deviation of the eyes and mouth and facial muscle twitch.

This is sequelae of channel-stroke with symptoms confined to the head and face, a condition that occurs when deficient normal qi and unstable protective qi allow pathogenic wind to invade the channels and collaterals. This causes movement of turbid phlegm that, in concert with the pathogenic wind, results in wind-phlegm obstructing the channels and collaterals of the head and face. Wind-phlegm obstructing the channels and collaterals of the head and face interferes with the supply of nourishment to the muscles, which causes a loss of muscle function manifested as muscle flaccidity and a flat, expressionless demeanor. Those areas that are unaffected (i.e., where the qi and blood circulate freely) will have relatively healthy muscle tone. The imbalance in muscle tone causes the face to draw to one side, with deviation around the eyes and mouth (facial paralysis). This was first described in Chapter 5 of *Essentials from the Golden Cabinet*: "Where there is pathogenic qi contrarily, there is laxity, and where there is normal qi, it is hypertonic. The [areas of] normal qi pull on those of the pathogenic, causing deviation and paralysis." Wind may also cause facial muscle twitch.

Analysis of Formula

To treat facial paralysis due to wind-phlegm obstructing the channels and collaterals, one must dispel the wind, transform the phlegm, and unblock the collaterals. The chief ingredient, acrid, warm Typhonii Rhizoma praeparatum *(zhì bái fù zǐ)*, dispels wind and transforms phlegm. It thereby stops the spasms, and is particularly effective in eliminating wind from the head and face. The deputy, Bombyx batryticatus *(bái jiāng cán)*, extinguishes internal wind, dispels external wind, and transforms phlegm. It also eliminates wind-phlegm and unblocks the collaterals. The assistant, Scorpio *(quán xiē)*, extinguishes wind and stops spasms, and is especially effec-tive in unblocking the collaterals, arresting wind, and thereby alleviating the facial paralysis. When combined with Bombyx batryticatus *(bái jiāng cán)*, the actions of both ingredients are markedly strengthened. The envoy, hot wine, focuses the actions of the other ingredients on the head and face.

Cautions and Contraindications

This formula contains toxic substances and should therefore not be taken in large doses, long-term, or during pregnancy. Because the formula is composed primarily of acrid and warm ingredients, it is most appropriate for treating wind-phlegm disorders due primarily to damp-cold. It is contraindicated for paralysis due to internal Liver wind or qi deficiency and blood stasis.

Commentary

One of the methods for categorizing wind-stroke is the distinction between channel-stroke (wind attacking the channels and collaterals) and organ-stroke (direct attack on the organs). The major difference is that organ-stroke is marked by at least a transient loss of consciousness or loss of function of the internal organs, such as incontinence. This formula is most commonly used in treating the former, that is, facial paralysis following a cerebrovascular accident, but may also be used for facial paralysis due to external or internal wind. The distinctive feature in each case, as the Ming-dynasty physician Wu Kun noted in *Investigations of Medical Formulas*, is that "deviation of the mouth and eyes is not accompanied by any other symptoms."

With regard to the underlying pathodynamic, most commentators identify the leg yang brightness channel, which encircles the mouth and lips, and the leg greater yang channel, a branch of which reaches the inner canthus of the eye, as being primarily involved. The yang brightness channel is associated with the interior and the production of turbid phlegm from both dampness and heat. The greater yang channel is associated with the exterior and therefore is easily attacked by wind from the outside. Under the right conditions, these pathogenic factors combine to produce the pattern treated by this formula. For the same reason, the formula can be used to treat channel-stroke irrespective of whether the primary cause is internal or whether the wind was contracted externally. In the early stages, when external symptoms may still be prominent, one may add Saposhnikoviae Radix *(fáng fēng)*, Angelicae dahuricae Radix *(bái zhǐ)*, and Notopterygii Rhizoma seu Radix *(qiāng huó)* to focus the formula more on dispelling wind to the exterior. On the other hand, in very chronic and stubborn cases, one may instead add such herbs as Gastrodiae Rhizoma *(tiān má)*, Pheretima *(dì lóng)*, Scolopendra *(wú gōng)*, Carthami Flos *(hóng huā)*, and Persicae Semen *(táo rén)* to focus on dispelling phlegm and driving out lifeless blood from the channels.

Biomedical Indications

With the appropriate presentation, this formula may be used to treat a variety of biomedically-defined disorders including facial spasms, migraines, sequelae of cerebrovascular accident, Bell's palsy, trigeminal neuralgia, and peripheral neuritis.

Alternate names

Wind Dispelling Powder (qū fēng sǎn) in Secret Formulas from the Court of Lu; Three Miracle Powder (sān shén sǎn) in Collection Picked by Immortals

Modifications

• For facial paralysis due to rheumatic disorder, facial neuritis, or simply to strengthen the effect of the formula, add Scolopendra (wú gōng) and Gastrodiae Rhizoma (tiān má).

• For Bell's palsy, add powdered Aconiti Radix praeparata (zhì chuān wū), Aconiti kusnezoffii Radix praeparata (zhì cǎo wū), Pinelliae Rhizoma praeparatum (zhì bàn xià), Clematidis Radix (wēi líng xiān), Bletillae Rhizoma (bái jí), Citri reticulatae Pericarpium (chén pí), and ginger juice. Apply topically to the affected area.

止痙散 （止痉散）

Stop Spasms Powder

zhǐ jìng sǎn

Source   *Chinese Medical Treatment for Epidemic Encephalitis B* (1955)

Scorpio (quán xiē)
Scolopendra (wú gōng)

Method of Preparation   Grind equal amounts of the ingredients into a powder. Take in 0.9-1.5g doses 2-4 times a day with warm water.

Actions   Extinguishes wind, relieves spasms, and alleviates pain

Indications

Muscle twitches of the extremities, rigidity and spasms of the entire body to the point of opisthotonus (a tetanic spasm in which the spine and extremities are so extended that the body rests on the head and heels), trismus, or convulsions. In severe cases, there is loss of consciousness. The formula is also used for the treatment of stubborn headaches, migraine, and joint pain.

This is heat entering the terminal yin channel. Vigorous heat generates wind, which leads to internal stirring of Liver wind characterized by the indications above. When accompanied by a loss of consciousness, it is called 'tetanic collapse' (痙厥 jìng jué).

Analysis of Formula

To treat the acute manifestations of wind generated by heat, this formula focuses on treating the manifestations by means of extinguishing wind and relieving spasms. Salty, acrid, neutral, and toxic, Scorpio (quán xiē) has a piercing, opening nature that enters the Liver channel to strongly extinguish internal wind, halt spasms, unblock the collaterals, search out externally-contracted wind lodged internally, and stop pain. Scolopendra (wú gōng) is acrid, warm, toxic, and enters the Liver channel. By nature, it excels at traveling and piercing, with a strong ability to track down wind and stop spasms and convulsions. Mutually enhancing, the two substances powerfully relieve spasms. Scorpio (quán xiē) excels at extinguishing wind, while Scolopendra (wú gōng) is more effective at searching out wind. They can be used for wind due to high fever leading to seizures and convulsions, as well as for stopping pain due to spasms.

Cautions and Contraindications

Because the ingredients in this formula are toxic, it should not be taken in large doses, long-term, or during pregnancy.

Commentary

This formula was devised by physicians in Hebei during an epidemic of encephalitis B in the early 1950s. In Chinese medicine, this disorder is most often treated as a wind-warmth or summerheat-warmth disorder. In these disorders, a warm pathogen enters the body from outside, usually via the Lungs. If from there it enters directly into the terminal yin, this is considered a very serious development. The terminal yin channels are associated with wind, which is very easily stirred up by heat. Wind, in turn, increases fire by mobilizing the body's own yang qi. At this level, essentially a blood aspect disorder, one must first deal with the manifestations, that is, extinguish the wind, before attempting to eliminate the pathogen. This is why only two herbs are used, which focus entirely on extinguishing the wind and relieving the spasms. In a less acute stage of the disorder, or once the fever has abated and the body has cooled, these herbs may be combined with Glycyrrhizae Radix (gān cǎo) and Paeoniae Radix alba (bái sháo), which soften the Liver to reduce hypertonicity.

At present, this formula is often modified by adding other ingredients or formulas to treat intractable headache (including severe migraines), joint pain, and especially painful obstruction due to wind-cold. One specific use described in *Traditional Chinese Medical Therapeutics for Women's Diseases* is for puerperal eclampsia with sudden convulsions, loss of consciousness, ophistotonus, and lockjaw in women after having given birth; this is associated with such symptoms as facial flushing, fever, and a floating, wiry, and forceful pulse. This is interpreted as wind entering from the exterior, to which a woman in the immediate postnatal period is especially prone due to blood loss when giving birth. To treat this pattern, Angelicae pubescentis Radix (*dú huó*) and Schizonepetae Herba (*jīng jiè*) are added to the basic formula.

Biomedical Indications

With the appropriate presentation, this formula may be used to treat a variety of biomedically-defined disorders including encephalitis B, meningitis, tetanus, pediatric epilepsy, cluster headache, and migraine.

Modifications

- For acute febrile diseases with heat generating internal stirring of wind, add Mori Folium (*sāng yè*), Chrysanthemi Flos (*jú huā*), Gentianae Radix (*lóng dǎn cǎo*), Uncariae Ramulus cum Uncis (*gōu téng*), and Gastrodiae Rhizoma (*tiān má*), or combine with Antelope Horn and Uncaria Decoction (*líng jiǎo gōu téng tāng*).

- For paralysis as a sequelae of encephalitis, combine with Major Arrest Wind Pearls (*dà dìng fēng zhū*).

- For chronic childhood convulsions due to prolonged diarrhea and chronic Spleen deficiency, take with Aconite Accessory Root Pill to Regulate the Middle (*fù zǐ lǐ zhōng wán*).

- For muscle twitches and spasms due to tetanus, combine with True Jade Powder (*yù zhēn sǎn*).

玉真散
True Jade Powder

yù zhēn sǎn

In medieval China, 'true jade' refers to the immortals, the celestial beings who reside in heaven with the Jade Emperor. The efficacy attributed to this formula, which brings those on the edge of death back to life, is so outstanding that it could have been composed by the immortals, hence the name.

Source   *Orthodox Lineage of External Medicine* (1617)

Typhonii Rhizoma praeparatum (*zhì bái fù zǐ*)
Arisaematis Rhizoma praeparatum (*zhì tiān nán xīng*)
Notopterygii Rhizoma seu Radix (*qiāng huó*)
Angelicae dahuricae Radix (*bái zhǐ*)
Saposhnikoviae Radix (*fáng fēng*)
Gastrodiae Rhizoma (*tiān má*)

Method of Preparation   The source text advises to grind equal amounts of the ingredients into a powder and take in 6g doses with hot wine. Today the ingredients are ground into a powder, sifted and mixed evenly, and taken in 3g doses with hot wine. May also be prepared as a decoction, or the powder may be applied externally to the affected area.

Actions   Dispels wind, transforms phlegm, relieves muscular tetany, and alleviates pain

Indications

Stiffness and spasms of the jaw, closed mouth, lip spasms, deviation of the eyes, rigidity of the entire body to the point of opisthotonus, and a wiry, tight pulse.

This is a type of muscular tetany (痙 *jìng*), a disorder marked by a stiff and tense neck and jaw, spasms of the extremities, and possibly opisthotonus. Here the muscular tetany is due to wind and toxin invading the body through a wound or ulceration, a disorder known as 'wind due to incised wounds' (破傷風 *pò shāng fēng*).

Chen Shi-Gong, author of *True Lineage of External Medicine*, explained the pathogenesis of this disorder: "When the skin is broken, pathogenic wind and toxin may make a surprise attack and enter the channels and collaterals, gradually penetrating to the interior." For this reason, wind that results from incised wounds is classified as a condition due to external wind. Wind moves and changes rapidly. Once it reaches the mouth, it advances through the channels and causes stiffness and spasms of the jaw, closed mouth, lip spasms, deviation of the eyes, and rigidity of the entire body to the point of opisthotonus. The wiry, tight pulse reflects the obstruction from wind.

Analysis of Formula

The appropriate strategy for treating wind that has entered the body from outside is to expel it, while also treating the spasms that are the main manifestations of the pattern. For this purpose, the formula uses herbs that disperse wind and unblock the channels and collaterals with those that extinguish internal wind. One of the chief ingredients, acrid, sweet, and warm Typhonii Rhizoma praeparatum (*zhì bái fù zǐ*), dries dampness, transforms phlegm, dispels wind, and stops spasms, especially those of muscular tetany. It also enters the Liver and Stomach channels, and is thus very effective in dispelling wind from the head and face. The other chief ingredient, acrid, warm Arisaematis Rhizoma praeparatum (*zhì tiān nán xīng*), eliminates wind-phlegm from the channels and collaterals, arrests muscle twitches, and stops spasms.

The deputies, Notopterygii Rhizoma seu Radix (*qiāng huó*), Angelicae dahuricae Radix (*bái zhǐ*), and Saposhnikoviae Radix (*fáng fēng*), disperse wind and dispel the pathogenic influences. In concert with the chief ingredients, they dispel wind from the channels and collaterals and vent the pathogenic influences through the exterior. The assistant, sweet and slightly warm Gastrodiae Rhizoma (*tiān má*), enters the Liver channel to extinguish Liver wind and relieve spasms. This is important, as externally-contracted wind can easily stir up internal wind. The envoy, hot wine, unblocks the channels and collaterals.

Cautions and Contraindications

This formula usually contains the untreated forms of Typhonii Rhizoma praeparatum (zhì bái fù zǐ) and Arisaematis Rhizoma praeparatum (zhì tiān nán xīng), both of which are very toxic. Dosage should therefore be carefully monitored, and the formula should not be taken long-term or during pregnancy. The acrid, drying ingredients in this formula readily injure the fluids and exhaust the qi, and should not be used for advanced-stage muscular tetany (a pattern of fluid injury and qi collapse). Severe hemorrhaging due to trauma may lead to blood deficiency, which prevents the blood from nourishing the sinews, and then to spasms. In such cases, the formula should be modified to focus on nourishing the blood and relaxing the sinews, rather than on dispelling wind.

Commentary

Wind entering the channels will manifest along the course of the affected channel. Wind in the yang brightness channel—which traverses the mouth and lips, enters the gums, and winds around the corners of the mouth and the lips—causes stiffness and spasms in the jaw and lips. Wind in the leg terminal yin channel—which connects with the tissues surrounding the eyes—causes deviation of the eyes. Wind in the leg greater yang channel, which meets the Governing vessel at GV-14 (dà zhuī) and divides to run along both sides of the spine, as well as the Governing vessel, which traverses the midline of the back, causes full-body rigidity, or opisthotonus.

This formula is based on one by the same name from *Formulas of Universal Benefit from My Practice*, which consists of Arisaematis Rhizoma praeparatum (zhì tiān nán xīng) and Saposhnikoviae Radix (fáng fēng). This formula strengthens the actions of the latter by adding ingredients that disperse wind to the exterior, while simultaneously extinguishing internal wind.

Biomedical Indications

With the appropriate presentation, this formula may be used to treat a variety of biomedically-defined disorders such as neurotoxic clostridial disease, including tetanus and botulism, as well as posttraumatic pain.

Alternate names

True Jade Special Pill (yù zhēn dān) in *Supplemented Collections on Patterns and Treatments*; Jade Normalizing Powder (yù zhèng sǎn) in *The Collection of Excellent, Efficacious Formulas*; Jade Constancy Powder (yù zhēn sǎn) in *New Edition of Mei's Collected Empiric Formulas*; Typhonium Powder (bái fù sǎn) in *Unusually Effective Empirical Formulas*

Modifications

- To strengthen the wind-dispelling action of the formula and to stop spasms, prepare as a decoction and add Cicadae Periostracum (chán tuì) and Schizonepetae Herba (jīng jiè).

- For the symptoms associated with tetanus, add Scorpio (quán xiē), Scolopendra (wú gōng), and Bombyx batryticatus (bái jiāng cán).

Associated Formula

五虎追風散 （五虎追风散）

Five-Tiger Powder to Pursue Wind

wǔ hǔ zhuī fēng sǎn

SOURCE *Collection of Experiential and Secret Chinese Medical Formulas from Shanxi Province* (1956)

Cicadae Periostracum (chán tuì) 30g
Arisaematis Rhizoma praeparatum (zhì tiān nán xīng) 6g
Gastrodiae Rhizoma (tiān má) 6g
dry-fried Bombyx batryticatus (chǎo jiāng cán) 6g
Scorpio (quán xiē) 3g

In the source text, a mixture of 1.5g of ground Cinnabaris (zhū shā) and 60ml of yellow wine are added to the strained decoction. Cinnabaris (zhū shā) is no longer used due to its heavy metal content. Expect good results if administration of the formula induces sweating on the palms, soles, and sternum; if sweating does not occur, continue administering for up to three days. Eliminates wind-phlegm, relieves spasms and twitches, and alleviates pain. For stiffness and spasms of the jaw, muscle twitches, and rigidity of the entire body to the point of opisthotonus. In contrast to the principal formula, which focuses on dispelling wind, this formula focuses on relieving spasms.

Because this formula contains toxic Cinnabaris (zhū shā), it is contraindicated during pregnancy and should not be taken in large doses or long-term. Nor should it be decocted, as heating this substance increases the risk of mercury poisoning. This formula was devised by Shi Chuan-En, a contemporary physician from Shanxi province.

消風散 （消风散）

Eliminate Wind Powder from *Orthodox Lineage*

xiāo fēng sǎn

Source *Orthodox Lineage of External Medicine* (1617)

Schizonepetae Herba (jīng jiè) 3g
Saposhnikoviae Radix (fáng fēng) .3g
Arctii Fructus (niú bàng zǐ) 3g
Cicadae Periostracum (chán tuì) 3g
Atractylodis Rhizoma (cāng zhú) 3g
Sophorae flavescentis Radix (kǔ shēn) 3g
Akebiae Caulis (mù tōng) 1.5g
Gypsum fibrosum (shí gāo) 3g
Anemarrhenae Rhizoma (zhī mǔ) .3g
Rehmanniae Radix (shēng dì huáng) 3g
Angelicae sinensis Radix (dāng guī) 3g
Sesami Semen nigrum (hēi zhī má) 3g
Glycyrrhizae Radix (gān cǎo) 1.5g

Method of Preparation   Decoction. May be taken orally on an empty stomach or applied topically. Allow decoction to cool before applying topically. At present, 2-3 times the above dosages are generally used.

Consumption of foods that are thought to stimulate the stirring of wind (發物 *fā wù*), such as alcohol, coffee, spicy foods, and seafood, as well as smoking, may interfere with the actions of the herbs and should be avoided while taking this formula.

Actions   Disperses wind, eliminates dampness, clears heat, and cools the blood

Indications

Weepy, itchy, red skin lesions over a large part of the body, a yellow or white tongue coating, and a forceful, floating, and rapid pulse.

This is wind rash (風疹 *fēng zhěn*) or damp rash (濕疹 *shī zhěn*). It is caused by wind-heat or wind-dampness that invades the body and contends with preexisting damp-heat. It then becomes trapped between the flesh, skin, interstices, and pores, and settles in the blood vessels. Unable to drain internally or vent externally, it transforms into wind toxin. The presence of wind, the primary pathogenic influence, is reflected in the itchiness and the floating pulse. Bleeding that occurs after excoriation is called 'seepage of blood pearls' and is an indication of heat in the blood. This type of seepage is caused by damp-heat trapped between the flesh and the interstices and pores. The combination of heat in the blood and damp-heat gives rise to toxin. The tongue coating varies according to the level of penetration of the heat: when the heat is superficial, the tongue coating will remain white; a slightly deeper level of penetration produces a yellow coating. The forceful, rapid pulse indicates internal heat and toxin. Disorders of this nature, where the pathogenic influence is trapped between layers of the body, are often difficult to treat.

Analysis of Formula

A complex condition such as wind or damp rash requires a complex treatment strategy. To dispel the pathogenic qi to the exterior, the formula disperses wind, eliminates dampness, and clears heat. Because the disease process is located in the blood vessels, it includes herbs that nourish and invigorate the blood and that moisten dryness; this is in accordance with the adage, "To treat wind, first treat the blood; when the blood moves, the wind will naturally be extinguished." Itching, a sign of wind, is relieved by dispersing the wind. The chief herbs, Schizonepetae Herba *(jīng jiè)*, Saposhnikoviae Radix *(fáng fēng)*, Arctii Fructus *(niú bàng zǐ)*, and Cicadae Periostracum *(chán tuì)*, unblock the interstices and pores and disperse external wind. The first group of deputies treats the seepage of fluids. Atractylodis Rhizoma *(cāng zhú)* dries dampness; Sophorae flavescentis Radix *(kǔ shēn)* clears damp-heat; and Akebiae Caulis *(mù tōng)* drains damp-heat through the urine. Sophorae flavescentis Radix *(kǔ shēn)* also kills parasites and resolves toxicity, and is an effective remedy

for itchiness from damp-heat. The second group of deputies, Gypsum fibrosum *(shí gāo)* and Anemarrhenae Rhizoma *(zhī mǔ)*, clears qi-aspect fire, which helps drain the heat from the interior and prevents the condition from advancing to a deeper level.

The assistant ingredients address the blood aspects of this disorder. Rehmanniae Radix *(shēng dì huáng)* cools the blood; Angelicae sinensis Radix *(dāng guī)* nourishes and invigorates the blood; and Sesami Semen nigrum *(hēi zhī má)* nourishes the blood and moistens. All of these herbs assist the blood as a means of extinguishing the wind. The envoy, Glycyrrhizae Radix *(gān cǎo)*, clears heat, resolves toxicity, and harmonizes the actions of the other herbs.

Cautions and Contraindications

Because this formula is primarily dispersing in nature, it should not be used in cases with marked qi or blood deficiency.

Commentary

This is one of three formulas by the same name (the other two are noted in ASSOCIATED FORMULAS below). Its source has been attributed to the *Golden Mirror of the Medical Tradition*. It is one of the most important base formulas for skin disorders in contemporary Chinese medicine. Its original indications read:

> [This formula] is effective for pernicious wind-dampness invading the blood, causing sores and burrows (瘡疥 *chuāng jiè*) that itch mercilessly, as well as wind-heat dormant papules (癮疹 *yǐn zhěn*) in adults and children that are spread all over the body in patchy, small macules, which come and go.

These indications make it clear that wind-dampness and wind-heat at the blood level are the basic pathodynamics for which this formula should be used, but that parasites, too, can be a cause. Note that 疥瘡 *jiè chuāng* in contemporary Chinese refers to scabies, and Sophorae flavescentis Radix *(kǔ shēn)* is an important herb for killing parasites in the skin. Better results can often be achieved if treatment also involves the topical application of the herbs.

Blood Aspect of the Formula

Herbs that treat the blood are essential to this formula, for several reasons. First, the location of the disorder itself is within the blood vessels and at the blood level. Second, the adage, "To treat wind, first treat the blood; when the blood moves, the wind will naturally be extinguished," implies that blood stasis—rather than blood deficiency—is an important secondary cause. This is due to wind and heat damaging the blood yin, while dampness obstructs its movement. The use of herbs that expel wind and dry dampness may further aggravate these problems. For this reason, the blood-aspect herbs in this formula focus on moving and dispelling pathogens from the blood rather than on tonification. According to *Seeking Accuracy in the Materia Medica*, the actions of Rehmanniae Radix *(shēng dì huáng)* "are directed at cooling heat and draining fire, cooling the blood, and dissolving stagnation." Angelicae sinensis Radix *(dāng guī)* invigorates the movement of blood, and in ancient times, Sesami Semen nigrum *(hēi zhī má)* was thought to make phlegm slippery and thus more easily expelled, thereby cooling the blood and resolving toxicity. All three of these herbs also promote bowel movements, suggesting that elimination of pathogens from the blood via the stool is an important aspect of treating skin disorders.

Biomedical Indications

With the appropriate presentation, this formula may be used to treat a variety of biomedically-defined disorders including urticaria, eczema, psoriasis, drug rash, contact dermatitis, Schönlein-Henoch purpura, tinea infection, and diaper rash.

Alternate name

Cool Blood and Eliminate Wind Powder *(liáng xuè xiāo fēng sǎn)* in *Great Compendium of External Medicine*

Modifications

- For severe wind-heat and toxin, add Lonicerae Flos *(jīn yín huā)*, Forsythiae Fructus *(lián qiáo)*, Taraxaci Herba *(pú gōng yīng)*, and Chrysanthemi indici Flos *(yě jú huā)*.

- For severe heat in the blood, add Moutan Cortex *(mǔ dān pí)*, Paeoniae Radix rubra *(chì sháo)*, and Arnebiae/Lithospermi Radix *(zǐ cǎo)*.

- For severe dampness, add Coicis Semen *(yì yǐ rén)*, Dictamni Cortex *(bái xiān pí)*, and Kochiae Fructus *(dì fū zǐ)*.

- For severe wind, add Agkistrodon/Bungarus *(bái huā shé)*, Scorpio *(quán xiē)*, and Spirodelae Herba *(fú píng)*.

Associated Formulas

消風散 （消风散）

Eliminate Wind Powder from *Formulary of the Pharmacy Service*

xiāo fēng sǎn

SOURCE *Formulary of the Pharmacy Service for Benefiting the People in the Taiping Era* (1107)

Schizonepetae Spica *(jīng jiè suì)*	60g
Menthae haplocalycis Herba *(bò hé)*	60g
Notopterygii Rhizoma seu Radix *(qiāng huó)*	60g
Saposhnikoviae Radix *(fáng fēng)*	60g
Chuanxiong Rhizoma *(chuān xiōng)*	60g
Cicadae Periostracum *(chán tuì)*	60g
Bombyx batryticatus *(bái jiāng cán)*	60g
Poria *(fú líng)*	60g
Citri reticulatae Pericarpium *(chén pí)*	15g
Magnoliae officinalis Cortex *(hòu pò)*	15g
Ginseng Radix *(rén shēn)*	60g

Grind the ingredients into a powder and take in 6g doses with green tea. For stubborn conditions, take three times a day. Disperses wind-dampness and regulates the qi. Codonopsis Radix *(dǎng shēn)* is usually substituted for Ginseng Radix *(rén shēn)* at 2-3 times its dosage. For wind-dampness in the channels characterized by headache, dizziness, vertigo, nasal congestion, numbness of the skin, itchiness, and rashes. In contrast to the principal formula, this focuses on treating wind-dampness and regulating the qi.

消風散 （消风散）

Eliminate Wind Powder from *Effective Formulas*

xiāo fēng sǎn

SOURCE *Effective Formulas from Generations of Physicians* (1345)

Gypsum fibrosum *(shí gāo)*	30g
Chrysanthemi Flos *(jú huā)*	30g
Chuanxiong Rhizoma *(chuān xiōng)*	30g
Saposhnikoviae Radix *(fáng fēng)*	30g
Notopterygii Rhizoma seu Radix *(qiāng huó)*	30g
Schizonepetae Spica *(jīng jiè suì)*	30g
Angelicae sinensis Radix *(dāng guī)*	30g
Angelicae dahuricae Radix *(bái zhǐ)*	30g
Glycyrrhizae Radix *(gān cǎo)*	15g
Saigae tataricae Cornu *(líng yáng jiǎo)*	30g
Sojae Semen germinatum *(dà dòu juǎn)*	30g

Grind the ingredients into a powder and take after meals in 12g doses with 1.5g of good-quality green tea. Disperses wind, clears heat, and dissipates clumps. For vertigo during pregnancy, diminished vision, and swelling under the jaws and in the neck.

四物消風飲 （四物消风饮）

Eliminate Wind Drink with the Four Substances

sì wù xiāo fēng yǐn

SOURCE *Golden Mirror of the Medical Tradition* (1742)

Rehmanniae Radix *(shēng dì huáng)*	9g
Angelicae sinensis Radix *(dāng guī)*	6g
Schizonepetae Herba *(jīng jiè)*	4.5g
Saposhnikoviae Radix *(fáng fēng)*	4.5g
Paeoniae Radix rubra *(chì sháo)*	3g
Chuanxiong Rhizoma *(chuān xiōng)*	3g
Dictamni Cortex *(bái xiān pí)*	3g
Cicadae Periostracum *(chán tuì)*	3g
Menthae haplocalycis Herba *(bò hé)*	3g
Angelicae pubescentis Radix *(dú huó)*	2.1g
Bupleuri Radix *(chái hú)*	2.1g
Jujubae Fructus *(dà zǎo)*	2 pieces

Nourishes the blood and expels wind. For rashes (such as urticaria and psoriasis) from wind-dampness. In contrast to the principal formula, this variation focuses more on moistening and invigorating the blood, as well as on expelling wind-dampness.

當歸飲子 (当归饮子)

Tangkuei Drink

dāng guī yǐn zi

SOURCE *Formulas to Aid the Living* (1253)

Angelicae sinensis Radix (*dāng guī*)	30g
Paeoniae Radix alba (*bái sháo*)	30g
Chuanxiong Rhizoma (*chuān xiōng*)	30g
dry-fried Tribuli Fructus (*chǎo cì jí lí*)	30g
Saposhnikoviae Radix (*fáng fēng*)	30g
Rehmanniae Radix (*shēng dì huáng*)	30g
Polygoni multiflori Radix (*hé shǒu wū*)	15g
Schizonepetae Herba (*jīng jiè*)	30g
Astragali Radix (*huáng qí*)	15g
Glycyrrhizae Radix praeparata (*zhì gān cǎo*)	15g

Grind the herbs into a coarse powder and prepare 12g as a draft by boiling with 5 slices of Zingiberis Rhizoma recens (*shēng jiāng*). At present, it is often taken as a decoction using one-third to one-half the listed dosages. Nourishes the blood, moistens dryness, dispels wind, and alleviates itching. For external wind that has lodged in the body for a long time and has damaged the blood, or for those with a blood-deficient constitution who contract a wind pathogen leading to itchiness that worsens at night and may or may not be accompanied by rash and flaking skin. The tongue will tend to be pale with a thin coating, and the pulse thin and wiry. This is an important formula in contemporary China for chronic itching skin disorders due to deficiency of blood. In contrast to the principal formula, it focuses more strongly on nourishing blood deficiency and wind that arises in the context of deficiency. Eliminate Wind Powder from the *Orthodox Lineage* (*xiāo fēng sǎn*), on the other hand, focuses on dispelling wind-damp-heat toxins from the blood vessels.

Note that this formula uses Rehmanniae Radix (*shēng dì huáng*) and not Rehmanniae Radix praeparata (*shú dì huáng*), thus emphasizing the importance of cooling the blood while simultaneously tonifying it. The use of Rehmanniae Radix (*shēng dì huáng*) also helps to cool heat in the Heart. The *Inner Classic* states that "painful or itching sores all pertain to the heart"; in practice, herbs such as Albiziae Cortex (*hé huān pí*), Polygoni multiflori Caulis (*yè jiāo téng*), and Ziziphi spinosae Semen (*suān zǎo rén*) that nourish the Heart and quiet the spirit are often added to formulas that treat itching.

風引湯 (风引汤)

Wind-Drawing Decoction

fēng yǐn tāng

'Wind-drawing' is an ancient name for a disorder that resembles epilepsy and similar seizures in modern biomedicine. This formula is indicated for the treatment of such disorders, hence the name.

Source *Essentials from the Golden Cabinet* (c. 220)

Rhei Radix et Rhizoma (*dà huáng*)	120g
Zingiberis Rhizoma (*gān jiāng*)	120g
Fossilia Ossis Mastodi (*lóng gǔ*)	120g
Cinnamomi Ramulus (*guì zhī*)	90g
Glycyrrhizae Radix (*gān cǎo*)	60g
Ostreae Concha (*mǔ lì*)	60g

Glauberitum (*hán shuǐ shí*)	180g
Talcum (*huá shí*)	180g
Halloysitum rubrum (*chì shí zhī*)	180g
Kaolinitum (*bái shí zhī*)*	180g
Fluoritum (*zǐ shí yīng*)	180g
Gypsum fibrosum (*shí gāo*)	180g

Method of Preparation Grind the herbs into a coarse powder and fill a soft leather pouch with three pinches of the powder. This is then decocted with 3 cups of water, bringing it to a boil three times. One cup per dose is taken warm. Today it is prepared as a decoction with an appropriate reduction in dosage.

Actions Extinguishes and pacifies wind with heavy medicinals, clears heat, and calms the spirit

Indications

Sudden collapse where the person falls to the ground, convulsions with upturned eyeballs, deviation of the mouth and eyes, gurgling sounds in the throat, irritability and restlessness, or mental confusion, a red tongue, and a forceful, wiry, and/or rapid pulse. Also for hemiplegia and hemilateral withering.

This pattern is seen in seizures, wind-stroke, or child fright wind caused by exuberant heat and stirring of internal Liver wind. Heat can be contracted from the exterior or arise from internal causes. Entering the Liver, it leads to the sudden stirring of Liver yang, which transforms into wind. Unable to balance the sudden up-rushing of qi, the patient collapses, and falls to the ground. Their eyeballs are turned up, and the extremities thrash about due to uncontrollable muscle contractions, indicating that the Liver system is the location of this pathology. The sudden stirring of internal wind disturbs the fluid metabolism and generates phlegm that is carried to the upper burner and head. This manifests as gurgling sounds in the throat and foaming at the mouth. Phlegm also clouds the Heart orifices leading to confusion, irritability, mental confusion, and loss of consciousness. The red tongue and forceful, wiry pulse that may also be rapid reflect the exuberance of heat and wind.

Analysis of Formula

To treat stirring of internal wind due to exuberance of heat, this formula employs a strategy of clearing heat and extinguishing and pacifying wind with heavy herbs. Because wind and heat unsettle the spirit, this is helped by calming the spirit. Gypsum fibrosum (*shí gāo*), Glauberitum (*hán shuǐ shí*), and Talcum (*huá shí*) are three cooling mineral substances that clear fire and drain heat to eliminate the underlying cause of this pattern. They are assisted by bitter and cooling Rhei Radix et Rhizoma (*dà huáng*), which directs the qi downward and drains heat through the bowels. Together, these four in-

---

* Kaolinitum (白石脂 *bái shí zhī*) is sweet and neutral and enters the Large Intestine channel. It stops bleeding, stabilizes abandoned disorders, absorbs dampness and sores. The normal dosage in decoctions is 9-12g, but it is often used in pills and topically.

gredients counteract the upward-moving momentum of fire and thereby effectively treat the root. Several other mineral and animal substances, all of them heavy in nature, are used to pacify the wind: Fossilia Ossis Mastodi (*lóng gǔ*), Ostreae Concha (*mǔ lì*), Halloysitum rubrum (*chì shí zhī*), Kaolinitum (*bái shí zhī*), and Fluoritum (*zǐ shí yīng*). Among these, Fossilia Ossis Mastodi (*lóng gǔ*), Ostreae Concha (*mǔ lì*), and Fluoritum (*zǐ shí yīng*) also calm the spirit, while the astringent nature of Halloysitum rubrum (*chì shí zhī*) and Kaolinitum (*bái shí zhī*) counterbalances the draining nature of Rhei Radix et Rhizoma (*dà huáng*) and the heaviness of the mineral and animal substances. Cinnamomi Ramulus (*guì zhī*) dispels heat from the muscle layer and, together with Glycyrrhizae Radix (*gān cǎo*), protects the yang of the Heart, assisting in the ascent of the clear yang, while also directing turbid yin downward. Acrid, warming, and sweet Zingiberis Rhizoma (*gān jiāng*) protects the middle burner from the excessive coldness of the cooling ingredients. Glycyrrhizae Radix (*gān cǎo*) cools and resolves toxicity, but also harmonizes the many actions of this complex formula.

Cautions and Contraindications

This is a draining formula and must not be prescribed for cases of Liver yang associated with blood or yin deficiency.

Commentary

History

This formula is listed in Chapter 5 of *Essentials from the Golden Cabinet*, which tersely notes that "it dispels heat [and treats] paralysis and epilepsy." Many commentators have questioned the authenticity of this passage. They argue that the formula's composition (combining cooling and warming substances) and the wording of the indications are more characteristic of Song-dynasty formulas and that there is a contradiction between the formula's name (which refers to wind) and indications (paralysis) and the lack of wind-dispersing ingredients normally used to treat such symptoms. For example, in *Essays on Medicine Esteeming the Chinese and Respecting the Western,* Zhang Xi-Chun observed: "The words after this formula are exceedingly concise and appear not to be from the pen of [Zhang] Zhong-Jing. [Other] formularies suspect that it was added by later generations and that is why the ingredients are impure."

However, based on work done by the contemporary physician Ding Guang-Di and others, this is currently accepted as a Han-dynasty formula. In a historical record there is a statement that in the year 308 a physician named Zhang Si-Wei successfully used the formula to treat an epidemic wind disorder leading to seizures in both adults and children. Furthermore, Huang-Fu Shi-An (215-282) noted that it was a Zhang Zhong-Jing formula, although under the alternate name of Fluoritum Decoction (*zǐ shí yīng tāng*).

Pathodynamic

Most contemporary textbooks follow the Ming-dynasty physician Zhao Yi-De, writing in *Two Commentaries on the Classic of the Golden Cabinet and Jade Coffer,* who defined the pattern as one of exuberant fire transforming into wind:

> Wind, if it is external [contracted] takes charge of the terminal yin, and, if internal [generated,] pertains to Liver wood. Above it manifests in the channels of the arm, below in the channels of the leg, and in the middle as lesser yang ministerial fire. Accordingly, wind that develops spontaneously internally is, in fact, produced [from] the same [source] as fire and heat. Once wind is generated, it invariably harms the middle [burner] earth. Earth governs the four extremities. When the earth is diseased and the four extremities lose their function, the yin fluids accumulate and become phlegm. Paralysis is due to the wind pathogen carrying phlegm into the four extremities. Epilepsy is caused by wind-heat leading to hypertonicity of the sinews and vessels, while internally it resonates [and disrupts] the Heart ruler.

This interpretation accepts the indications of the source text literally. While it provides an explanation of the disease dynamic that might cause paralysis, it does not explain the absence of herbs that would disperse wind from the channels and collaterals. The modern physician Lu Yuan-Lei has therefore argued that the term 癱 *tān*, paralysis, in the source text was a corruption of the term 癲 *diān*, meaning convulsions. If that is the case, then the formula is not designed to treat wind in the channels and collaterals after all, but rather excess heat causing the upward-rushing of Liver yang. In *Essays on Medicine Esteeming the Chinese and Respecting the Western,* another modern physician, Zhang Xi-Chun, provides an analysis of the formula's action based on this perspective:

> *Essentials from the Golden Cabinet* states that Wind Drawing Decoction (*fēng yǐn tāng*) eliminates heat [to treat] paralysis and epilepsy. Since paralysis is a name that implies [the presence of] heat, the cause of the disorder was understood to be heat. Basically, however, this pattern is [due to] the brain being filled up with blood. The formula uses six mineral ingredients, most of which are cold or cooling. Although it contains the acrid, warming Zingiberis Rhizoma (*gān jiāng*) and Cinnamomi Ramulus (*guì zhī*), they are combined with Rhei Radix et Rhizoma (*dà huáng*), Gypsum fibrosum (*shí gāo*), Glauberitum (*hán shuǐ shí*), and Talcum (*huá shí*) [all of which are strongly cooling]. This mixture of ingredients has again and again [been explained] by means of a doctrine [that emphasizes] cooling. (If one examines this issue meticulously, then Cinnamomi Ramulus (*guì zhī*) and Zingiberis Rhizoma (*gān jiāng*) would not at all be appropriate). Moreover, the nature of all minerals is to sink. By its nature, Rhei Radix et Rhizoma (*dà huáng*), too, excels at directing downward. Basically [therefore these ingredients] are able to guide the blood that has rebelled upward and move it downward again. Furthermore, combining Fossilia Ossis Mastodi (*lóng gǔ*) and Ostreae Concha (*mǔ lì*) with Fluoritum (*zǐ shí yīng*) is excellent for restraining the gushing of qi,

and if this is combined with Cinnamomi Ramulus *(guì zhī)*, it is excellent for pacifying the Liver qi. If the gushing Liver qi does not move upward, the blood that fills [the brain] above will naturally be directed downward gradually. Hence, although the formula's name refers to wind drawing, it does not actually use herbs that dispel wind. This makes it clear that [the formula] is not indicated for heat [causing] paralysis and seizures but for wind-stroke. Because later generations of physicians did not understand the intention of the formula's [composition], they mostly explained it in the wrong way

The contemporary physician Ran Xue-Feng takes up Zhang Xi-Chun's argument and extends it to the treatment of stroke. His interpretation also discusses more fully the role of the warming herbs Cinnamomi Ramulus *(guì zhī)* and Zingiberis Rhizoma *(gān jiāng)* in the formula, which is of great importance in the clinic:

What the ancients referred to as wind disorders are what [we] moderns call brain disorders. … The sedating, downward-directing [action] of the formula's six mineral [ingredients], with Fossilia Ossis Mastodi *(lóng gǔ)* and Ostreae Concha *(mǔ lì)* anchoring [aberrant yang], and Rhei Radix et Rhizoma *(dà huáng)* driving [pathogenic qi] downward and draining it, is entirely consistent with this. However, on the basis of this interpretation of the pattern, I did not understand why the formula also used Cinnamomi Ramulus *(guì zhī)* and Zingiberis Rhizoma *(gān jiāng)*, because, from what I knew, there was nothing in the pattern that would call for them. After a long time, I suddenly gained insight. … In this formula, Cinnamomi Ramulus *(guì zhī)* strengthens the Heart, increasing the oxygenation of the blood. Zingiberis Rhizoma *(gān jiāng)* restores the pulse, and in addition, seeks to support the fountainhead of the pulse.

In this disorder, the pathogens are blazing and the qi is overly abundant. It is an excess [type of disorder reflected] in an excessive pulse. Sedating, anchoring, driving downward, and draining is the correct [strategy]. Why then also use Cinnamomi Ramulus *(guì zhī)* and Zingiberis Rhizoma *(gān jiāng)*? If this [process] is not restrained for a long period, the Heart function will decline, with the result that the pulse and breathing no longer match. The danger [of this condition] is that suddenly the pulse is cut off, and one has to worry that one sedates, anchors, drives down, and drains not only the pathogenic, but also the normal qi. In this context, the addition of Cinnamomi Ramulus *(guì zhī)* and Zingiberis Rhizoma *(gān jiāng)* [allows], on the one hand, to sedate the pathogenic qi so that it does not rebel upward again, while, on the other, to also stimulate the middle burner qi in order to promote transportation. In this manner, the formula calms the nervous system and returns the pulse while also controlling rebelliousness. How can one provide help in this type of pattern unless one conforms [in one's prescribing] to the most profound levels of scholarship? Hence, if later [commentators] argued to reduce the dosage of Cinnamomi Ramulus *(guì zhī)* and Zingiberis Rhizoma *(gān jiāng)*, or even leave them out altogether, they did not understand why this cannot be done. Without Cinnamomi Ramulus *(guì zhī)* and Zingiberis Rhizoma *(gān jiāng)*, one can only treat superficial cases of wind-stroke. With both herbs, one can also treat serious cases. Those learned [in Chinese medicine] should deeply ponder the reasons for why this is so.

Biomedical Indications

With the appropriate presentation, this formula may be used to treat a variety of biomedically-defined disorders including epilepsy, stroke, childhood febrile convulsions, schizophrenia, and hysterical psychosis.

Alternate names

Boiled Powder with Fluoritum *(zǐ shí zhǔ sǎn)* in *Important Formulas Worth a Thousand Gold Pieces*; Fluoritum Decoction *(zǐ shí tāng)* in *Arcane Essentials from the Imperial Library*; Decoction for Induced Wind *(yǐn fēng tāng)* in *Formulas from the Imperial Pharmacy*; Fluoritum Powder *(zǐ shí sǎn)* in *Prescriptions of Universal Benefit*; Seizures Decoction *(diān xián tāng)* in *Prescriptions of Universal Benefit*

Modifications

- For seizures, add Bambusae Succus *(zhú lì)*, Arisaema cum Bile *(dǎn nán xīng)*, and Acori tatarinowii Rhizoma *(shí chāng pú)*.
- For wind-stroke, add Magnetitum *(cí shí)*, Haematitum *(dài zhě shí)*, and Achyranthis bidentatae Radix *(niú xī)*.
- For child fright wind, add Saigae tataricae Cornu *(líng yáng jiǎo)*, Uncariae Ramulus cum Uncis *(gōu téng)*, and Scorpio *(quán xiē)*.

Section 2

FORMULAS THAT PACIFY AND EXTINGUISH INTERNAL WIND

The formulas in this section are used for treating conditions with internal stirring of Liver wind. Such disorders are most commonly due to Liver and Kidney yin deficiency, or ascendant Liver yang. They are typically characterized by headache, dizziness, blurred vision, and tinnitus, and, in more severe case, by irritability, vomiting, palpitations with anxiety, and muscle twitches.

Further progression of these patterns may lead to wind-stroke with tremors, muscular tetany, sudden loss of consciousness, facial paralysis, hemiplegia, and aphasia. Wind due to extreme heat is characterized by convulsions, opisthotonus, or febrile convulsions in children. Wind generated by blood deficiency is characterized by dizziness, blurred vision, tinnitus, numbness in the extremities, and, in severe cases, by loss of consciousness or convulsions.

To treat these patterns, the formulas in this section rely on herbs that calm the Liver and extinguish wind such as Saigae tataricae Cornu *(líng yáng jiǎo)*, Uncariae Ramulus cum Uncis *(gōu téng)*, Gastrodiae Rhizoma *(tiān má)*, Haematitum (*dài zhě shí*), Fossilia Ossis Mastodi (*lóng gǔ*), and Ostreae Concha (*mǔ lì*). Depending on the pathodynamic, these are combined with ingredients from one or more of the following groups:

- Substances that clear fire and drain heat such as Gardeniae Fructus (*zhī zǐ*), Gypsum fibrosum (*shí gāo*), Scutellariae Radix (*huáng qín*), Glauberitum (*hán shuǐ shí*), or Talcum (*huá shí*). This is important where blazing fire stirs up internal wind.

- Substances that enrich yin and nourish blood such as Rehmanniae Radix (*shēng dì huáng*), Paeoniae Radix alba (*bái sháo*), Scrophulariae Radix (*xuán shēn*), Testudinis Plastrum (*guī bǎn*), or Asini Corii Colla (*ē jiāo*). This is necessary in cases where external or internal fire has depleted the essence, leading to yin deficiency with yang excess, or where internal wind is associated with blood deficiency.

- Substances that calm the spirit such as Poriae Sclerotium pararadicis (*fú shén*), Polygoni multiflori Caulis (*yè jiāo téng*), Fossilia Ossis Mastodi (*lóng gǔ*), or Ostreae Concha (*mǔ lì*). Whether viewed in terms of the close relationship between the ethereal soul and the spirit, or from a five-phase perspective where wood excess invariably damages fire, disorders of the spirit such as irritability, agitation, or even loss of consciousness are common consequences of wind disorders and must be addressed. For this purpose, but also in order to control the upward-rushing of Liver yang, substances that extinguish wind are frequently either themselves heavy in nature, for example, Haliotidis Concha (*shí jué míng*), Haematitum (*dài zhě shí*), or Ostreae Concha (*mǔ lì*); or they are combined with substances that can anchor the aberrant yang, such as Testudinis Plastrum (*guī bǎn*) and Trionycis Carapax (*biē jiǎ*).

羚角鉤藤湯 (羚角钩藤汤)
Antelope Horn and Uncaria Decoction

líng jiǎo gōu téng tāng

Source   *Revised Popular Guide to the Discussion of Cold Damage* (Qing dynasty)

Saigae tataricae Cornu (*líng yáng jiǎo*) 4.5g
Uncariae Ramulus cum Uncis (*gōu téng*) 9g
Mori Folium (*sāng yè*) 6g
Chrysanthemi Flos (*jú huā*) 9g
Paeoniae Radix alba (*bái sháo*) 9g
Rehmanniae Radix (*shēng dì huáng*) 15g
Fritillariae cirrhosae Bulbus (*chuān bèi mǔ*) 12g
Bambusae Caulis in taeniam (*zhú rú*) 15g
Poriae Sclerotium pararadicis (*fú shén*) 9g
Glycyrrhizae Radix (*gān cǎo*) 2.4g

Method of Preparation   The source text advises to prepare as a decoction, cooking Saigae tataricae Cornu (*líng yáng jiǎo*) with Bambusae Caulis in taeniam (*zhú rú*) before the other

ingredients, and adding Uncariae Ramulus cum Uncis (*gōu téng*) near the end. At present, the decoction is prepared by cooking Saigae tataricae Cornu (*líng yáng jiǎo*) for an hour before adding the other ingredients, or adding it as a powder to the strained decoction. Although not as effective, for ethical reasons either Naemorhedi Cornu (*shān yáng jiǎo*) or Margaritiferae Concha usta (*zhēn zhū mǔ*) should be substituted for Saigae tataricae Cornu (*líng yáng jiǎo*), with a ten-fold increase in dosage.

Actions   Cools the Liver, extinguishes wind, increases the fluids, and relaxes the sinews

Indications

Persistent high fever, irritability, restlessness, dizziness, vertigo, twitching and spasms of the extremities, a deep-red, dry, or burnt tongue with prickles, and a wiry, rapid pulse. In severe cases, there may also be impaired or actual loss of consciousness.

This is heat excess in the Liver channel stirring up internal wind. When pathogenic heat enters the terminal yin stage, it generates vigorous heat in the Liver channel that causes internal stirring of wind. Heat excess in the interior causes persistent high fever. Heat harassing the spirit causes irritability and restlessness. When heat causes internal stirring of wind, the wind and fire are joined in battle, which manifests as dizziness and vertigo.

Vigorous heat scorching the fluids generates phlegm and aggravates the symptoms of dizziness and vertigo. The Liver governs the sinews; extreme heat in the Liver channel that injures the fluids and consumes the blood will deprive the sinews of nourishment, causing twitching and spasms in the extremities, which may progress to rigidity of the neck and jaw. This is called muscular 'tetany' (痙 *jìng*). In severe cases, the presence of phlegm may lead to a condition called 'tetanic collapse' (痙厥 *jìng jué*) characterized by impaired or actual loss of consciousness. Severe heat injuring the fluids produces a burnt tongue with prickles, while heat in the Liver channel produces a wiry, rapid pulse.

Analysis of Formula

This formula treats overabundance of heat in the Liver channel stirring wind, a pattern with a momentum that can quickly deteriorate and that requires urgent attention. For this reason, the formula focuses on treating the manifestations by calming the Liver and extinguishing wind, while secondarily enriching the yin and clearing the heat.

Salty, cold Saigae tataricae Cornu (*líng yáng jiǎo*), one of the chief ingredients, enters the Liver and Heart channels where it pacifies the Liver, extinguishes wind, and clears heat. The other chief ingredient, bitter and slightly cold Uncariae Ramulus cum Uncis (*gōu téng*), enters the arm (Pericardium) and leg (Liver) terminal yin channels. The arm terminal yin channel governs the ministerial fire; the leg terminal yin channel governs wind. Spasms, convulsions, dizziness, and vertigo are all disorders caused by the interaction of wind (associated with wood) and fire. Uncariae Ramulus cum Uncis (*gōu téng*) restores the proper relationship between the Pericardium (fire) and Liver (wood). By this means, the wind is extinguished and the fire is cleared. The deputies are bitter, sweet, and cooling Mori Folium (*sāng yè*) and sweet, bitter, and cooling Chrysanthemi Flos (*jú huā*). They dispel wind and clear heat from the Liver and Lungs. Light in nature, their intention is to vent the pathogen via the protective aspect, an important strategy in the treatment of damp-warm disorders. In doing so, they strengthen the wind-extinguishing action of the formula.

Wind and fire readily provoke one another, which exhausts the yin and scorches the fluids. Two of the assistant ingredients, Paeoniae Radix alba (*bái sháo*) and Rehmanniae Radix (*shēng dì huáng*), nourish the yin and increase the fluids and thereby soften the Liver and relax the sinews. Fritillariae cirrhosae Bulbus (*chuān bèi mǔ*) and Bambusae Caulis in taeniam (*zhú rú*), two other assistants, clear heat and transform phlegm. Poriae Sclerotium pararadicis (*fú shén*), another assistant, addresses the irritability and restlessness caused by heat harassing the spirit. The envoy, Glycyrrhizae Radix (*gān cǎo*), regulates and harmonizes the actions of the other ingredients. The combination of sour Paeoniae Radix alba (*bái sháo*) and sweet Glycyrrhizae Radix (*gān cǎo*) strengthens the yin, relaxes the sinews, and moderates the painful spasms.

Cautions and Contraindications

Contraindicated in cases with wind due to internal deficiency.

Commentary

This is the representative formula for treating overabundance of heat in the blood aspect causing the stirring of internal wind. The key symptoms of this pattern are high fever and spasms. Traditionally, this was thought to be due to the contraction of external pathogenic heat penetrating into the blood aspect. Although formulas for treating such patterns have been around since the Tang era, it was only from the late Ming onward that physicians formulated clear treatment principles in accordance with the emergent paradigm of warm pathogen disorders. In *Discussion of Warm-Heat Pathogen [Disorders]*, the famous and influential physician Ye Tian-Shi outlined the strategies that are reflected in the composition of this formula:

> [When a warm pathogen] enters into the nutritive [aspect] it is still possible to vent the heat and turn it [back] toward the qi aspect with substances like Rhinocerotis Cornu (*xī jiǎo*), Scrophulariae Radix (*xuán shēn*), and Saigae tataricae Cornu (*líng yáng jiǎo*). When it enters the blood, one must fear it consuming the blood and moving the blood. It therefore is essential to directly cool and disperse the blood with substances

like Rehmanniae Radix (*shēng dì huáng*), Moutan Cortex (*mǔ dān pí*), Asini Corii Colla (*ē jiāo*), and Paeoniae Radix rubra (*chì sháo*).

In light of these principles, it is clear that the formula seeks to vent heat via the qi aspect while simultaneously reducing it in the interior through a combined strategy of cooling, moistening, and unblocking at the blood level. (This strategy is discussed in detail in Chapter 4 in the section on Formulas that Clear Nutritive-Level Heat and Cool the Blood.) Venting heat requires that the qi dynamic is open and affords a passageway out of the body for the pathogenic heat that is being pushed out from the blood. If the qi dynamic is obstructed, manifested primarily as constipation, then it is essential to first open this up by means of downward-draining, combining substances such as Bubali Cornu (*shuǐ niú jiǎo*) and Coptidis Rhizoma (*huáng lián*) with one of the Order the Qi Decoctions (*chéng qì tāng*). In *Treatment Strategies and Formulas in Chinese Medicine,* the contemporary physician Chen Chao-Zu also recommends adding herbs such as Forsythiae Fructus (*lián qiáo*), Lonicerae Flos (*jīn yín huā*), Isatidis Folium (*dà qīng yè*), and Isatidis/Baphicacanthis Radix (*bǎn lán gēn*) to augment the formula's capacity for clearing toxic heat from both the qi and blood aspects. To more effectively stop spasms, he also suggests increasing the dosage of Paeoniae Radix alba (*bái sháo*) and Glycyrrhizae Radix (*gān cǎo*).

While the type of infectious diseases for which the formula was originally composed (including epidemic encephalitis and meningitis) is nowadays treated primarily with biomedicine, this formula still retains its clinical utility. As noted by Qin Bo-Wei in *Medical Lecture Notes of [Qin] Qian-Zhai:*

> Among Liver disorders, Liver heat [causing] wind and yang to rebel upward is due to the same pathodynamic [as overabundance of heat in the blood aspect stirring wind]. Therefore, it is commonly used for the treatment of severe cases of Liver yang, where it can be combined with substances that anchor and sedate [aberrant yang], such as Haliotidis Concha (*shí jué míng*).

Comparisons

➢ Vs. Sedate the Liver and Extinguish Wind Decoction (*zhèn gān xī fēng tāng*); *see* page 646, and Gastrodia and Uncaria Drink (*tiān má gōu téng yǐn*); *see* page 649

➢ Vs. Major Arrest Wind Pearls (*dà dìng fēng zhū*); *see* page 653

➢ Vs. Ass-Hide Gelatin and Egg Yolk Decoction (*ē jiāo jī zi huáng tāng*); *see* page 654

Biomedical Indications

With the appropriate presentation, this formula may be used to treat a very wide variety of biomedically-defined disorders. These can be divided into the following groups:

- Acute infectious diseases that affect the central nervous system such as encephalitis and meningitis as well as dysentery and pneumonia

- Cardiovascular diseases that affect the central nervous system such as cerebrovascular disease, cerebrovascular accidents, and eclampsia.

This formula has also been used for facial spasms and hysterical psychosis.

Modifications

- For severe heat, add Isatidis Folium (*dà qīng yè*), Isatidis/ Baphicacanthis Radix (*bǎn lán gēn*), Prunellae Spica (*xià kū cǎo*), and Haliotidis Concha (*shí jué míng*).

- For persistent, high fever with severe wasting and injury to the fluids, add Scrophulariae Radix (*xuán shēn*), Asparagi Radix (*tiān mén dōng*), Ophiopogonis Radix (*mài mén dōng*), Dendrobii Herba (*shí hú*), and Asini Corii Colla (*ē jiāo*).

- For impaired consciousness with gurgling sounds in the throat, add Bambusae Concretio silicea (*tiān zhú huáng*), Bambusae Caulis in taeniam (*zhú rú*), and the juice of Zingiberis Rhizomatis Succus (*jiāng zhī*).

- For severe tics or spasms, add Scorpio (*quán xiē*), Scolopendra (*wú gōng*), and Bombyx batryticatus (*bái jiāng cán*).

- For heat primarily in the qi level, add Gypsum fibrosum (*shí gāo*).

- For heat primarily in the nutritive and blood levels, add Bubali Cornu (*shuǐ niú jiǎo*) and Moutan Cortex (*mǔ dān pí*).

- For heat trapped in the interior with impaired or loss of consciousness, take with Purple Snow Special Pill (*zǐ xuě dān*) or Calm the Palace Pill with Cattle Gallstone (*ān gōng niú huáng wán*).

- For hypertension, add Achyranthis bidentatae Radix (*niú xī*) and Tribuli Fructus (*cì jí lí*).

Associated Formula

鉤藤飲 （钩藤饮）

Uncaria Decoction

gōu téng yǐn

Source   *Golden Mirror of the Medical Tradition* (1742)

Uncariae Ramulus cum Uncis (*gōu téng*) 9g
Saigae tataricae Cornu (*líng yáng jiǎo*) 0.3g
Scorpio (*quán xiē*) 0.9g
Ginseng Radix (*rén shēn*) 3g
Gastrodiae Rhizoma (*tiān má*) 6g
Glycyrrhizae Radix praeparata (*zhì gān cǎo*) 1.5g

Grind Saigae tataricae Cornu (*líng yáng jiǎo*), or today one of its substitutes, into a powder and take with the strained decoction.

Clears heat and extinguishes wind. For 'heavenly hook disorder' (天 钓 *tiān diào*), a form of childhood convulsions first mentioned in *Family Secrets for Nursing Infants*. The disorder is characterized by the eyes suddenly turning upward (as if 'hooked' by heaven), high fever, clenched jaw, hyperextension of the head and neck, and drooling (in cases with qi deficiency). There may also be palpitations. It is attributed to externally-contracted wind-heat leading to pathogenic phlegm-heat clogging the upper burner and obstructing the diffusion of Heart qi. The source text recommends reducing the dosage of Ginseng Radix (*rén shēn*) in patterns characterized by severe internal heat and abundant phlegm. In contrast to the principal formula, this treats wind due to severe heat with qi deficiency.

鎮肝熄風湯 （镇肝熄风汤）

Sedate the Liver and Extinguish Wind Decoction

zhèn gān xī fēng tāng

Source   *Essays on Medicine Esteeming the Chinese and Respecting the Western* (1918-1934)

Achyranthis bidentatae Radix (*niú xī*) 30g
Haematitum (*dài zhě shí*) 30g
Fossilia Ossis Mastodi (*lóng gǔ*) 15g
Ostreae Concha (*mǔ lì*) 15g
Testudinis Plastrum (*guī bǎn*) 15g
Scrophulariae Radix (*xuán shēn*) 15g
Asparagi Radix (*tiān mén dōng*) 15g
Paeoniae Radix alba (*bái sháo*) 15g
Artemisiae scopariae Herba (*yīn chén*) 6g
Toosendan Fructus (*chuān liàn zǐ*) 6g
Hordei Fructus germinatus (*mài yá*) 6g
Glycyrrhizae Radix (*gān cǎo*) 4.5g

Method of Preparation   Decoction.

Actions   Sedates the Liver, extinguishes wind, nourishes the yin, and anchors the yang

Indications

Dizziness, vertigo, a feeling of distention in the eyes, tinnitus, feverish sensation in the head, headache, irritability, flushed face (as if intoxicated), and a wiry, long, and forceful pulse. There may also be frequent belching, progressive motor dysfunction of the body or development of facial asymmetry that occurs over a period of a few hours to a few days, severe dizziness and vertigo, sudden loss of consciousness, mental confusion with moments of clarity, and an inability to fully recover after loss of consciousness.

This is wind-type stroke caused by excessive gushing upward of qi that, in turn, leads to congestion of blood in the brain. Though primarily due to ascendant Liver yang, the underlying pathodynamic implies a more complex conjunction of factors, as explained by the formula's author, Zhang Xi-Chun:

This [disorder] is caused by Liver wood losing its balance with wind arising from the Liver. This is aggravated by the Lungs failing to direct qi downward, the Kidneys failing to contain [qi], and the qi of the Penetrating [vessel] and the Stomach also rebelling upward. As a consequence, there is too much upward movement in the qi dynamic of all the organs. This, in turn, leads to too much blood pouring upward into the brain.

This pathology is a common precursor to wind-stroke. Wind and Liver yang ascending to attack the head causes dizziness, vertigo, a distended sensation in the eyes, tinnitus, a feverish sensation in the head, headache, irritability, and flushed face. Liver and Stomach disharmony may develop and cause the Stomach qi to rebel, manifested as frequent belching. Ascendant Liver yang may cause the blood to follow the rebellious qi upward. Depending on the individual's constitution and other factors, this can lead to severe dizziness and vertigo, sudden loss of consciousness, and mental confusion, or a more gradual, progressive motor dysfunction that can lead to hemiplegia and other symptoms of wind-stroke. The wiry, long, and forceful pulse reflects the vigorously ascending qi and yang.

Analysis of Formula

This elegantly designed formula is an excellent example of simultaneously treating both the manifestation and the root of a disorder. The chief and deputy ingredients directly sedate the Liver and anchor the yang to extinguish the wind; the assistant ingredients nourish the yin and the fluids, which softens and moistens the Liver so that the wind indirectly dies out of its own accord.

The relatively large dosage of Achyranthis bidentatae Radix *(niú xī)*, the chief ingredient, conducts the circulation of blood downward, separating the blood from the ascendant yang. Sweet, bitter and sour, it not only moves, but also tonifies, nourishing the Liver and Kidneys to treat both the root and manifestations of this pattern. The deputy, bitter and sweet Haematitum *(dài zhě shí)*, has a heavy nature that enables it to direct the qi downward and control its rebelliousness. It calms the Liver, anchors the yang, directs the Stomach qi downward, and pacifies the rebellious qi in the Penetrating vessel. The other deputies are the heavy Fossilia Ossis Mastodi *(lóng gǔ)* and Ostreae Concha *(mǔ lì)*. In Zhang Xi-Chun's opinion, they "are able to restrain fire and extinguish wind" and are thus especially suitable for treating the sudden stirring of Liver fire and Liver wind. Together, the chief and deputy ingredients make a powerful combination for sedating the Liver, extinguishing the wind, anchoring the yang, and directing the rebellious qi downward.

Among the assistants, Testudinis Plastrum *(guī bǎn)*, Scrophulariae Radix *(xuán shēn)*, Asparagi Radix *(tiān mén dōng)*, and Paeoniae Radix alba *(bái sháo)* clear heat, nourish the yin, and enrich the fluids. This treats the ascendant Liver yang at the root, which indirectly extinguishes the wind.

As explained in the source text, via two of these assistants, the formula also mobilizes the controlling relationship between metal and wood: "Scrophulariae Radix *(xuán shēn)* and Ophiopogonis Radix *(mài mén dōng)* are used to clear the Lung qi. If the clearing and clarifying qi within the Lungs moves downward, it naturally sedates and controls Liver wood." The other assistants, Artemisiae scopariae Herba *(yīn chén)*, Toosendan Fructus *(chuān liàn zǐ)*, and Hordei Fructus germinatus *(mài yá)*, smooth the movement of Liver qi and drain Liver yang excess. This reinforces the actions of pacifying, controlling, and sedating the Liver yang. Among these, according to Zhang, the bitter, acrid, and cooling Artemisiae scopariae Herba *(yīn chén)* "is most able to handle the smoothing of Liver wood's nature, while also excelling at draining Liver heat … making it an essential herb for clearing and cooling the brain." To Hordei Fructus germinatus *(mài yá)* Zhang attributed the function of "excelling in smoothing Liver wood's nature so that it does not become constrained," while Toosendan Fructus *(chuān liàn zǐ)* "excels at guiding the Liver qi to spread downward, as well as turning back its contrary force." As explained in the COMMENTARY below, the inclusion of these three assistants is based on Zhang's clinical experience and therefore considered by him to be essential to the formula's efficacy. The envoy, Glycyrrhizae Radix *(gān cǎo)*, regulates and harmonizes the actions of the other ingredients. In concert with Hordei Fructus germinatus *(mài yá)*, it harmonizes the Stomach and adjusts the middle burner, thereby preventing the metals and minerals in the formula from adversely affecting the Stomach.

Cautions and Contraindications

Because this formula contains many enriching, cloying, heavy, and sedating substances that can injure the Spleen yang, it should be used with caution and appropriate modification in cases with Spleen qi deficiency.

Commentary

Context

Zhang Xi-Chun, the author of this formula, is a leading representative of the current of convergence and assimilation (匯通學派 *huì tōng xué paì*) in Chinese medicine. Emerging in the late 19th century, this current was composed of physicians who sought to develop Chinese medicine by assimilating elements from the Western medical tradition. Their goal was not, as was that of physicians in the latter half of the 20th century, to create an entirely new medicine by fusing East and West. Rather, it was an effort to assimilate new knowledge into well-established modes of practice by means of equally well-established methods of scholarship. For this reason, the term 匯通 *huì tōng* (sometimes also written 會通) may be translated more precisely as an assembling (匯合 *huì hé*) of diverse tools in the flexible pursuit (變通 *biàn tōng)* of clinical efficacy. No one was better at this task than Zhang Xi-Chun, and Sedate the Liver and Extinguish Wind Decoction *(zhèn gān xī fēng tāng)* is a typical example of this process in action.

"[This formula]," Zhang begins his discussion, "treats internal wind-stroke patterns (also called wind-type stroke, and referred to by Westerners as cerebral hemorrhage [literally 'cerebral congestion syndrome' 腦充血證 *nǎo chōng xuè zhèng*]), with a pulse that is wiry, long, and forceful (which is referred to in Western medicine as high blood pressure)." He then defines the pathodynamic that causes this pattern as an excessive upward-gushing of the ministerial fire carried and managed by the Liver. "This, in turn, leads to excessive blood pouring upward into the brain. As a consequence, the blood vessels [in the brain] become clogged, straining the nerves. If this is severe, the nerves lose their governing function, resulting in loss of consciousness. Western medicine calls this cerebral hemorrhage. This [knowledge] is derived from dissections and experiments."

Besides the influence of Western medical knowledge on the composition of this formula, it is also rooted in the doctrines of the Jin-dynasty master physician Liu Wan-Su regarding the movement of internal fire. Even further back, Zhang drew inspiration from Wind Drawing Decoction *(fēng yǐn tāng)*, discussed above, which treats wind due to heat by means of mineral substances that subdue rebellious yang, and Rhei Radix et Rhizoma *(dà huáng)*, which drains fire downward. That formula served as a model for Zhang Xi-Chun's Construct Roof Tiles Decoction *(jiàn líng tāng)*, discussed below, from which the present formula was, in turn, developed.

Impact of Context on Composition

It is because of this novel understanding that Achyranthis bidentatae Radix *(niú xī)* was chosen by Zhang Xi-Chun to "guide the blood downward" and as the "key herb for treating the manifestation." The other ingredients treat the root, which—unlike the manifestation—is understood and analyzed entirely in Chinese medical terms. This reflects the core ideological statement that informed the current of convergence and assimilation in all aspects of culture during this period, namely, that "Chinese [traditional culture] serves as the [core] substance while Western [modern knowledge] is used for its [external] applications" (中體西用 *zhōng tǐ xī yòng*).

If Zhang Xi-Chun's thinking—and by implication the composition of this formula—cannot be understood outside of this context, clinical experience constituted an equally important input into the final product. Zhang recounts that his initial attempts at composing a formula for the pattern outlined above did not include the three assistants Artemisiae scopariae Herba *(yīn chén)*, Hordei Fructus germinatus *(mài*

yá), and Toosendan Fructus *(chuān liàn zǐ)*. Although this formula often worked, it would sometimes result in the aggravation of symptoms with patients experiencing "an upward attack of qi and blood" following ingestion of the decoction. Zhang attributed this to the characteristics of the Liver. Like the official in charge of military affairs whose duty it is to maintain order, the Liver becomes fierce if constrained. A strategy that simply sedates and anchors the Liver yang, nourishes the yin, and moistens the fluids thus may overly constrain the Liver, causing its qi to rebel upward even more. For this reason, he added the three qi-regulating ingredients. They prevent the development of Liver constraint and thereby assist in directing the yang downward. Fresh varieties of the ingredients are used if possible because they are more effective in smoothing Liver qi. While there has been some debate that the type of Artemisia used by Zhang Xi-Chun himself may have been Artemisiae annuae Herba *(qīng hāo)* rather than Artemisiae scopariae Herba *(yīn chén)*, the consensus now is that the latter should be used.

Usage

In contemporary practice, this formula is used to treat patients at risk from stroke rather than the sequelae of a stroke. It is also widely employed to treat hypertension. According to Zhang Xi-Chun, there are four key markers that suggest a pattern of impending cerebral hemorrhage:

1. A long and forceful pulse, which will often extend beyond the distal position toward the thenar eminence, or a pulse that is overabundant in the distal position and deficient in the proximal position, or a very rapid pulse

2. Frequent sensations of dizziness, confusion, forgetfulness, headache, deafness, or distention of the eyes

3. An occasional upward-rushing sensation in the epigastrium, or of food being stuck and unable to move downward, or of qi gushing upward from the lower burner, manifesting as hiccup

4. Frequent sensations of irritability and restlessness in the Heart, or of heat in the Heart, or of the ethereal soul drifting away during sleep.

This formula is unsuitable for hypertension due to qi or yang deficiency, wind-cold fettering the exterior, or yin excess. If Liver heat is severe, better results are obtained by combining the formula with Gentian Decoction to Drain the Liver *(lóng dǎn xiè gān tāng)*.

Comparisons

➢ Vs. Antelope Horn and Uncaria Decoction *(líng jiǎo gōu téng tāng)*, see PAGE 643

➢ Vs. Gastrodia and Uncaria Drink *(tiān má gōu téng yǐn)*, see PAGE 649

Biomedical Indications

With the appropriate presentation, this formula may be used to treat a wide variety of biomedically-defined disorders including essential hypertension, renal hypertension, hypertensive encephalopathy, focal disorders of the central nervous system such as aphasia and apraxia, epilepsy, Parkinson's disease, hysterical collapse, vascular headache, trigeminal neuralgia, postconcussion syndrome, recalcitrant hiccup, cerebral arteriosclerosis, coronary artery disease, acute nephritis, perimenopausal syndrome, and puerperal fever.

Modifications

- For a sensation of heat in the chest, add 30g of Gypsum fibrosum *(shí gāo)*. (source text)

- For profuse sputum, add Arisaema cum Bile *(dǎn nán xīng)*. (source text)

- For a proximal pulse that is deficient when pressed hard, add 24g of Rehmanniae Radix praeparata *(shú dì huáng)* and 15g of Corni Fructus *(shān zhū yú)*. (source text)

- For stools that are not well-formed, remove Haematitum *(dài zhě shí)* and Testudinis Plastrum *(guī bǎn)* and add Halloysitum rubrum *(chì shí zhī)*. (source text)

- For headache and dizziness, add Prunellae Spica *(xià kū cǎo)* and Chrysanthemi Flos *(jú huā)*.

- For postpartum fever with vertigo, twitching and spasms of the extremities, a red tongue, and a wiry, rapid pulse, add Chaenomelis Fructus *(mù guā)* and Uncariae Ramulus cum Uncis *(gōu téng)*.

- For hypertension, add Prunellae Spica *(xià kū cǎo)*, Uncariae Ramulus cum Uncis *(gōu téng)*, and Chrysanthemi Flos *(jú huā)*.

- For cerebral vascular disease, add Haliotidis Concha *(shí jué míng)*, Atractylodis Rhizoma *(cāng zhú)*, Citri reticulatae Pericarpium *(chén pí)*, Persicae Semen *(táo rén)*, and Pogostemonis/Agastaches Herba *(huò xiāng)*.

- For coronary artery disease, add Paeoniae Radix rubra *(chì sháo)* and Salviae miltiorrhizae Radix *(dān shēn)*.

Associated Formula

建瓴湯 （建瓴汤）

Construct Roof Tiles Decoction

jiàn líng tāng

SOURCE   *Essays on Medicine Esteeming the Chinese and Respecting the Western* (1918-1934)

Dioscoreae Rhizoma *(shān yào)* 30g
Achyranthis bidentatae Radix *(niú xī)* 30g
Haematitum *(dài zhě shí)* 24g
Fossilia Ossis Mastodi *(lóng gǔ)* 18g
Ostreae Concha *(mǔ lì)* 18g
Rehmanniae Radix *(shēng dì huáng)* 18g

Paeoniae Radix alba *(bái sháo)* 12g
Platycladi Semen *(bǎi zǐ rén)* 12g

The source text advises to decoct with rusty water. This is not usually done today. Sedates and extinguishes Liver wind, enriches the yin, and calms the spirit. For ascendant Liver yang characterized by vertigo, tinnitus and a distended sensation in the ears, palpitations, forgetfulness, irritability, restlessness, insomnia with dream-disturbed sleep, and a wiry, firm, and long pulse. Although this formula is not as powerful in sedating and extinguishing Liver wind as the principal formula, it is more effective in calming the Heart and quieting the spirit. Its author believed the formula functioned like roof tiles by allowing the fluids (primarily the blood) congesting the brain to flow downward like water during rain. Its composition was modeled on Wind Drawing Decoction *(fēng yǐn tāng)*, discussed above, as outlined in the source text: "My humble composition of Construct Roof Tiles Decoction *(jiàn líng tāng)* emphasizes the use of Haematitum *(dài zhě shí)*, Ostreae Concha *(mǔ lì)*, and Fossilia Ossis Mastodi *(lóng gǔ)*, sometimes adding Gypsum fibrosum *(shí gāo)*. Truly, I am plagiarizing here the intention of Wind Drawing Decoction *(fēng yǐn tāng)*."

天麻鉤藤飲 （天麻钩藤饮）

Gastrodia and Uncaria Drink

tiān má gōu téng yǐn

Source   *Deriving New Treatments for Patterns of Miscellaneous Disorders in Chinese Internal Medicine* (1958)

Gastrodiae Rhizoma *(tiān má)* 9g
Uncariae Ramulus cum Uncis *(gōu téng)* 12-15g
Haliotidis Concha *(shí jué míng)* 18-24g
Gardeniae Fructus *(zhī zǐ)* 9g
Scutellariae Radix *(huáng qín)* 9g
Leonuri Herba *(yì mǔ cǎo)* 9-12g
Cyathulae Radix *(chuān niú xī)* 12g
Eucommiae Cortex *(dù zhòng)* 9-12g
Taxilli Herba *(sāng jì shēng)* 9-24g
Polygoni multiflori Caulis *(yè jiāo téng)* 9-30g
Poriae Sclerotium pararadicis *(fú shén)* 9-15g

Method of Preparation   Prepare as a decoction, cooking Haliotidis Concha *(shí jué míng)* first and adding Uncariae Ramulus cum Uncis *(gōu téng)* near the end. The source text does not specify dosage.

Actions   Calms the Liver, extinguishes wind, clears heat, invigorates the blood, and tonifies the Liver and Kidneys

Indications

Headache, dizziness, vertigo, tinnitus, blurred vision, a sensation of heat rushing to the head, insomnia with dream-disturbed sleep, a red tongue, and a wiry, rapid pulse. In severe cases, there may also be numbness, twitching and spasms in the extremities, or hemiplegia.

This is hyperactive Liver yang leading to internal stirring of Liver wind. The Liver pertains to wood and therefore resonates with wind in nature. Its physiological function is to carry the ministerial fire, the body's yang qi. The nature of yang is to ascend, and to move freely. Hence, the Liver is firm and vigorous. This is counterbalanced by its other function, the storage of blood, which provides the Liver with softness and flexibility. Thus, it is said that its essence is yin while its function is yang. Pent-up emotions, qi constraint, constitutional yang excess, heating foods, and excessive habits all can cause the Liver yang to become hyperactive, and indeed often combine to this end. When yang ascends uncontrolled, it eventually loses its connection with yin blood. This is called 'internal wind.' Wind and hyperactive yang disturb the upper body, causing headache, dizziness, vertigo, tinnitus, blurred vision, and a sensation of heat rushing to the head. Ascendant Liver yang affecting the spirit causes insomnia and dream-disturbed sleep. A red tongue and a wiry, rapid pulse are also indicative of ministerial fire excess. At a more advanced stage, wind and hyperactive yang may cause numbness and spasms in the extremities, or hemiplegia.

Analysis of Formula

To control hyperactive yang causing the stirring of internal wind, this formula focuses on calming the Liver and directing the rebellious qi downward. Its composition is also influenced by pharmacological knowledge regarding the action of individual herbs, as well as biomedical treatment strategies for the treatment of high blood pressure. The chief ingredients, sweet and balanced Gastrodiae Rhizoma (tiān má) and sweet and cooling Uncariae Ramulus cum Uncis (gōu téng), are frequently used herbs in the treatment of internal wind. Their calming and cooling action is complemented by that of the deputy, the heavy, salty Haliotidis Concha (shí jué míng). Like many other seashells, it is able to anchor the errant yang and calm the Liver. It is specific for headaches and dizziness due to hyperactive Liver yang because, through its action on the yang qi, it guides blood downward from the head.

The remaining ingredients are regarded as assistants. The first group, bitter and cooling Gardeniae Fructus (zhī zǐ) and Scutellariae Radix (huáng qín), clear heat and drain fire, and prevent the yang from rising in the Liver channel. A second group of assistants acts on the blood. Leonuri Herba (yì mǔ cǎo) invigorates the blood to prevent it from rising to the head with the ascending Liver yang, while Cyathulae Radix (chuān niú xī) has a descending nature that conducts the blood downward. Both herbs are also diuretic in nature, guiding pathogenic qi and fluid out via the urine. Eucommiae Cortex (dù zhòng) and Taxilli Herba (sāng jì shēng) tonify and nourish the Liver and Kidneys in order to strengthen the root. Polygoni multiflori Caulis (yè jiāo téng) and Poriae Sclerotium pararadicis (fú shén) calm the spirit and steady the will, and are symptomatically effective for the restlessness and insomnia that often characterizes patterns of Liver yang excess.

Cautions and Contraindications

This formula should not be used for problems caused by yin deficiency.

Commentary

This formula was composed by the contemporary physician Hu Guang-Ci and first published in 1958 for the treatment of "hypertensive headaches, dizziness, and insomnia." Like Sedate the Liver and Extinguish Wind Decoction (zhèn gān xī fēng tāng), discussed above, it is the product of the assimilation of Western biomedical knowledge into the Chinese medical tradition. By the 1950s and 1960s, vigorous efforts at modernization no longer questioned the utility of biomedical disease categories and frequently accepted them as superordinate to Chinese medical patterns. On the level of treatment, too, pharmacological knowledge and treatment strategies became increasingly important. Guided by recently developed paradigms of pattern differentiation and treatment determination, physicians of Chinese medicine sought to integrate this new knowledge with traditional ideas about body function, illness, and therapy. Gastrodia and Uncaria Drink (tiān má gōu téng yǐn) is one of the most famous products of this process.

Its target is not a Chinese pattern but a biomedical disease, hypertensive headaches. These have been translated into a diagnosis based on traditional concepts of organ disharmony. In this manner, Hu defined these headaches to be "Liver inversion headaches" (肝厥頭痛 gān jué tóu tòng). "Their origin," the source texts further explains, "lies in the inverse rebellion of Liver fire." The appropriate treatment strategy, accordingly, was to subdue the rebelliousness and clear the fire. The formula that Hu composed for this purpose was made up of herbs that implemented these strategies, but that also had been shown to reduce blood pressure. In Hu's words:

> [In view of] contemporary theories regarding [the nature of] hypertensive headaches, this formula employs Scutellariae Radix (huáng qín), Eucommiae Cortex (dù zhòng), Leonuri Herba (yì mǔ cǎo), and Taxilli Herba (sāng jì shēng) because they have been shown experimentally to reduce high blood pressure. This means they have the ability to calm the mind, direct rebelliousness downward, and relax pain.

Furthermore, the biomedical strategy of lowering high blood pressure by means of diuretics was translated into the use of herbs that promote water metabolism; and an attempt was made to relax the smooth muscle in the arterioles and promote the blood flow therein with herbs that invigorate the blood. For arteriosclerosis, the source text also recommended the addition of Rosae rugosae Flos (méi guī huā) and Sargassum (hǎi zǎo) because they contain rutin.

In China, this formula is widely recommended for the treatment of hypertension, although it will only be effective if the presentation matches the pattern. It has had a tremendous influence on attempts to formulate new formulas that closely match biomedical disease categories, but remains one of the few such formulas to date that is widely listed in formula textbooks.

Biomedical Indications

With the appropriate presentation, this formula may be used to treat a variety of biomedically-defined disorders including cerebrovascular disease, transitory ischemic attacks, essential hypertension, renal hypertension, hypertensive encephalopathy, and focal disorders of the higher nervous functions such as aphasia and apraxia, epilepsy, and neurosis.

Comparisons

> ➤ Vs. Antelope Horn and Uncaria Decoction
> *(líng jiǎo gōu téng tāng)* and Sedate the Liver and
> Extinguish Wind Decoction *(zhèn gān xī fēng tāng)*

All of these formulas treat patterns with Liver yang excess and internal wind. Antelope Horn and Uncaria Decoction *(líng jiǎo gōu téng tāng)* focuses on clearing heat and extinguishing wind. It is specific for overabundant heat at the blood level causing Liver wind characterized by high fever and spasms. Sedate the Liver and Extinguish Wind Decoction *(zhèn gān xī fēng tāng)* focuses on directing rebellious qi and blood downward, extinguishing wind, and anchoring errant yang. It is specific for Liver yang excess that is accompanied by deficiency of Liver and Kidney yin characterized by symptoms such as dizziness, syncope, and gushing up of qi and fire. Gastrodia and Uncaria Drink *(tiān má gōu téng yǐn)* focuses on calming the Liver and extinguishing wind. Compared to the other two formulas, its action is relatively mild but it also invigorates the blood, calms the spirit, and promotes water metabolism. It is specific for hypertensive headaches that are accompanied by dizziness and insomnia.

Modifications

- For more severe symptoms, add Saigae tataricae Cornu *(líng yáng jiǎo)*.
- For severe dizziness, add Haematitum *(dài zhě shí)*, Ostreae Concha *(mǔ lì)*, Fossilia Ossis Mastodi *(lóng gǔ)*, or Magnetitum *(cí shí)*.
- For Liver fire, add Gentianae Radix *(lóng dǎn cǎo)*, Prunellae Spica *(xià kū cǎo)*, and Moutan Cortex *(mǔ dān pí)*.
- For constipation, add Rhei Radix et Rhizoma *(dà huáng)*, Natrii Sulfas *(máng xiāo)*, or Tangkuei, Gentian, and Aloe Pill *(dāng guī lóng huì wán)*.
- For Liver and Kidney yin deficiency, add Ligustri lucidi Fructus *(nǚ zhēn zǐ)*, Lycii Fructus *(gǒu qǐ zǐ)*, Paeoniae Radix alba *(bái sháo)*, Rehmanniae Radix *(shēng dì huáng)*, or Polygoni multiflori Radix *(hé shǒu wū)*.

三甲復脈湯 （三甲复脉汤）

Three-Shell Decoction to Restore the Pulse

sān jiǎ fù mài tāng

This is a Qing-dynasty variation of Prepared Licorice Decoction *(zhì gān cǎo tāng)*, also known as Restore the Pulse Decoction *(fù mài tāng)*, from *Discussion of Cold Damage*. It has been modified by adding three ingredients that are shells, hence the name.

Source   *Systematic Differentiation of Warm Pathogen Diseases* (1798)

Glycyrrhizae Radix praeparata *(zhì gān cǎo)* 18g
Rehmanniae Radix *(shēng dì huáng)* 18g
Paeoniae Radix alba *(bái sháo)* 18g
Ophiopogonis Radix *(mài mén dōng)* 15g
Cannabis Semen *(huǒ má rén)* 9g
Asini Corii Colla *(ē jiāo)* 9g
Ostreae Concha *(mǔ lì)* 15g
Trionycis Carapax *(biē jiǎ)* 24g
Testudinis Plastrum *(guī bǎn)* 30g

Method of Preparation   Decoction

Actions   Nourishes the yin, restores the pulse, clears heat, anchors the yang, and extinguishes wind

Indications

Severe palpitations, Heart pain, and a thin, rapid, irregular pulse. These may be accompanied by other symptoms including fever, a flushed face, hot palms and soles, a dry throat, dizziness, tinnitus, spasms, quivering fingers, impaired consciousness, stiffness of the tongue or a deep-red and dry tongue, blackish teeth, and cracked lips.

This is a late-stage warm pathogen disorder where the yin has been injured. This occurs when a warm pathogen has become deeply lodged in the lower burner (i.e., the lesser yin and terminal yin) where it severely injures the true yin. As the yin becomes depleted, it is no longer able to anchor the yang. Hot Liver yang rebels upward and attacks the Heart, which already is deprived of fluids, causing severe palpitations, a thin, rapid, irregular pulse, and in severe cases, Heart pain. Ascendant yang also manifests as a flushed face, dizziness, and tinnitus. Pathogenic heat in a context of fluid deficiency causes feverish palms and soles (i.e., the palms and soles are hotter to the touch than the back of the hands and top of the foot), a dry throat, deep-red and dry tongue, blackish teeth, and cracked lips. The combination of wind and fluid deficiency (where the sinews are undernourished) causes spasms, loss of consciousness, and quivering fingers.

Analysis of Formula

This formula focuses on stopping severe palpitations and Heart pain by anchoring the errant yang, tonifying the true yin, and nourishing the Heart qi and blood. Glycyrrhizae Radix praeparata (zhì gān cǎo) is the chief herb because it tonifies the Heart qi and restores the pulse. Used in a large dosage, it nourishes the Heart and, according to *Materia Medica of Ri Hua-Zi,* "quiets the ethereal soul and settles the corporeal soul." Rehmanniae Radix (shēng dì huáng), also used in a rather large dosage, serves as deputy. Sweet and cooling, enriching and moistening, it restores the Heart yin and tonifies the blood. Together with Glycyrrhizae Radix praeparata (zhì gān cǎo), it fills the vessels with qi and fluids, providing the basis for returning the pulse to its normal state. Paeoniae Radix alba (bái sháo), the second deputy, tonifies the yin while restraining the yang, relaxing the sinews and moderating the Liver. Together with the chief herb, it is an effective combination for treating spasms due to yin deficiency.

Ophiopogonis Radix (mài mén dōng), Cannabis Semen (huǒ má rén), and Asini Corii Colla (ē jiāo) serve as assistants to nourish the yin and blood, and thereby cause the heat due to yin and blood deficiency to recede. Asini Corii Colla (ē jiāo) effectively enriches the yin, tonifies the blood, and moistens dryness. Ophiopogonis Radix (mài mén dōng) moistens dryness in the Stomach and Lungs (upper burner), while Cannabis Semen (huǒ má rén) nourishes the yin and moistens the Intestines (lower burner). Together, these three herbs assist Rehmanniae Radix (shēng dì huáng) in enriching the yin, moistening the dryness, and cooling the heat from deficiency. Ostreae Concha (mǔ lì), Trionycis Carapax (biē jiǎ), and Testudinis Plastrum (guī bǎn), the three shells, make up a second group of assistants. They nourish the yin and anchor the yang. Ostreae Concha (mǔ lì) is especially effective in calming the Liver and sedating the Liver yang; Trionycis Carapax (biē jiǎ) more strongly tonifies the yin, and is cooling at a deeper level, entering the Kidneys to enrich the yin so as to anchor the yang. Testudinis Plastrum (guī bǎn) is particularly strong at nourishing the yin to anchor ascendant Liver yang.

Cautions and Contraindications

This formula should not be used during pregnancy unless Testudinis Plastrum (guī bǎn) and Trionycis Carapax (biē jiǎ) are removed, since these substances are contraindicated during pregnancy. It should also be used with caution in patients with symptoms such as diarrhea due to Spleen yang or Stomach qi deficiency.

Commentary

This is a development of Prepared Licorice Decoction (zhì gān cǎo tāng) from *Discussion of Cold Damage,* discussed in Chapter 8, which is also known as Restore the Pulse Decoction (fù mài tāng). It is used to treat Heart deficiency presenting with a consistently irregular or slow-irregular pulse due to damage of the Heart qi and blood. The Qing-dynasty physician Wu Ju-Tong modified that formula in various ways to

treat patterns due to warm pathogens entering into the lower burner, damaging the true yin. This leads to ascendant yang, the symptoms of which become more severe if there is also pathogenic heat. For this reason, the formula is composed of substances that nourish the yin and essence as a means of anchoring the ascendant yang and cause the heat to recede. This follows Ye Tian-Shi's dictum that when pathogenic heat has entered the blood aspect, the prevention and treatment of wind and blood stasis rather than venting of the pathogen becomes the primary goal of treatment. This is because these secondary pathological processes are so severe that they have potentially fatal consequences and must therefore be addressed first.

Wu Ju-Tong's first modification is Modified Restore the Pulse Decoction (jiā jiǎn fù mài tāng), also discussed in Chapter 8. This formula focuses on nourishing the yin of the Kidneys and Liver without treating wind and ascendant yang directly. To treat patterns where ascendant yang and wind become increasingly severe, Wu Ju-Tong used three variants of Modified Restore the Pulse Decoction (jiā jiǎn fù mài tāng), which he named One-, Two-, and Three-Shell Decoction to Restore the Pulse (yī, èr, sān jiǎ fù mài tāng). The present formula treats the most severe of these conditions, characterized by severe palpitations and even Heart pain. Wu analyzed the pathodynamic that leads to palpitations as ascendant Liver yang entering the Heart. Heart pain constitutes an even more serious condition, which involves the eight extraordinary channels:

> An even more severe [pattern] is characterized by [Heart] pain (because the yin Linking vessel governs Heart pain). In this pattern, heat has damaged the yin over the course of some time. The eight [extraordinary] vessels attach themselves to the Liver and Kidneys. When the Liver and Kidneys become deficient, they affect the yin Linking vessel, leading to Heart pain. This is unlike the Heart pain caused by cold qi residing in the Heart, where one can employ [a strategy] of warming to unblock [the vessels]. Therefore, [this formula] employs Testudinis Plastrum (guī bǎn), which anchors the Kidney qi, tonifies the Conception vessel, and unblocks the yin Linking vessel to stop the Heart pain. It combines these with the two other shells [Ostreae Concha (mǔ lì) and Trionycis Carapax (biē jiǎ)], which track down the pathogenic [heat and wind]. Together, they achieve the [desired] effect.

This pattern can also occur in internal medicine disorders, where ascendant yang is caused by yin deficiency rather than an externally-contracted heat pathogen. On the other hand, when an externally-contracted heat pathogen penetrates the interior causing such symptoms as spasms and loss of consciousness while remaining vigorous, this formula is inappropriate. Such patterns are due to heat excess stirring up internal wind, and therefore should be treated with a formula that focuses on heat excess, for example, Clear the Nutritive-Level Decoction (qīng yíng tāng) with the addition of Saigae tataricae Cornu (*líng yáng jiǎo*), Uncariae Ramulus cum Uncis (*gōu téng*), and Purple Snow Special Pill (*zǐ xuě dān*).

Comparison

➢ Vs. Major Arrest Wind Pearls (*dà dìng fēng zhū*)

Both formulas enrich the yin and extinguish wind in the treatment of internal wind and yin deficiency patterns. The difference is that Major Arrest Wind Pearls (*dà dìng fēng zhū*) focuses on sour, sweet, and salty medicinals that are able to bind up qi and yin in addition to extinguishing wind and enriching the yin. This is useful in life-threatening patterns where the severity of yin deficiency complicated by internal wind suggests that the condition is quickly transforming into a desertion pattern. Three-Shell Decoction to Restore the Pulse (*sān jiǎ fù mài tāng*), on the other hand, employs salty, cooling, sweet, and moistening medicinals to control floating yang, particularly where yin deficiency is accompanied by Heart pain, and a thin and rapid, irregular pulse indicating that stirring of internal wind is focused on the Heart and the vessels.

Biomedical Indications

With the appropriate presentation, this formula may be used to treat a variety of biomedically-defined disorders including encephalitis, meningitis, hypocalcemia, carpopedal spasms, and spasms of the facial muscles.

Variations

一甲復脈湯 （一甲复脉汤）

One-Shell Decoction to Restore the Pulse

yī jiǎ fù mài tāng

Source *Systematic Differentiation of Warm Pathogen Diseases* (1798)

Remove Cannabis Semen (*huǒ má rén*), Trionycis Carapax (*biē jiǎ*), and Testudinis Plastrum (*guī bǎn*) from the principal formula. For sudden diarrhea occurring in the context of a warm pathogen disorder when the patient has been constipated for several days. This indicates damage to the true yin in the lower burner that is unable to contain yang when the stools begin to move. Ostreae Concha (*mǔ lì*) is used because of its ability to bind up the bowels while simultaneously clearing excess pathogenic heat lingering in the interior.

———————

二甲復脈湯 （二甲复脉汤）

Two-Shell Decoction to Restore the Pulse

èr jiǎ fù mài tāng

Source *Systematic Differentiation of Warm Pathogen Diseases* (1798)

Remove Testudinis Plastrum (*guī bǎn*) from the principal formula. For slight stirring of Liver wind with mild trembling of the fingers occurring in the context of a warm pathogen disorder due to damage to the true yin in the lower burner.

大定風珠 （大定风珠）

Major Arrest Wind Pearls

dà dìng fēng zhū

Wu Ju-Tong, the author of this formula, wrote that its name was based on the notion that "the yolk of the chicken egg resembles a pearl in shape, possesses the essence of wood, and is able to extinguish wind." It also relates to the turtle shells, another important ingredient in this formula. Wu Ju-Tong says:

> Turtles also [have shells that are shaped] like pearls. They possess the virtue of the true warrior and [correspond to the trigram] 震 *zhèn* wood. *Zhèn,* [is the image of] thunder. In the human person, it [corresponds to] the Gallbladder. Thunder never occurs without wind. When thundering becomes quiet, the wind also dies down. Hyperactive yang directly ascends to the crown of the head, just as the dragon ascends in the sky. That which controls the dragon is the turtle.

The dragon here represents the ministerial fire or yang qi of the body, carried by the Liver. When this qi detaches from the yin and ascends uncontrollably, it becomes wind. Trionycis Carapax (*biē jiǎ*), and by implication the other shells in this formula, are important medicinals for controlling wind from yin deficiency. The term 'Major' distinguishes this formula from another formula, Minor Arrest Wind Pearls (*xiǎo dìng fēng zhū*), also listed in the source text.

Source *Systematic Differentiation of Warm Pathogen Diseases* (1798)

Egg yolk (*jī zi huáng*) . . . . 2 yolks
Asini Corii Colla (*ē jiāo*) 9g
Paeoniae Radix alba (*bái sháo*) 18g
Glycyrrhizae Radix praeparata (*zhì gān cǎo*) 12g
Schisandrae Fructus (*wǔ wèi zǐ*) 6g
Rehmanniae Radix (*shēng dì huáng*) 18g
Ophiopogonis Radix (*mài mén dōng*) 18g
Cannabis Semen (*huǒ má rén*) 6g
Testudinis Plastrum (*guī bǎn*) 12g
Trionycis Carapax (*biē jiǎ*) 12g
Ostreae Concha (*mǔ lì*) 12g

Method of Preparation Blend the egg yolk into the strained decoction and take warm.

Actions Nourishes the yin and extinguishes wind

Indications

Weariness, muscle spasms with alternating flexion and extension of the extremities, a deficient or frail pulse, and a deep-red tongue with a scanty or peeled coating. Often the patient will appear as if about to go into shock.

This is internal stirring of wind due to yin deficiency, which may be caused by the long-standing retention of pathogenic heat from a warm pathogen disease or by improper treatment involving excessive sweating or purging. Either one of these processes can severely injure the yin. Presently, most of the pathogenic qi has left the body, and the true yin (Kidney water) is nearly exhausted. The injury to the qi and yin from pathogenic heat causes weariness and a deficient or frail pulse. When the Liver, which is the organ associated with wind, becomes malnourished due to injury to the yin and fluids or essence deficiency, Liver wind may arise. Twitches or spasms with alternating flexion and extension of the muscles of the extremities (typical of tonic-clonic spasms or convulsion) are likewise symptoms of wind. The deep-red tongue with a scanty or peeled coating reflects severe injury to the yin and fluids. The severity of this injury is also reflected in the shock-like demeanor of the patient.

Analysis of Formula

Wu Ju-Tong, the author of this formula, described this pattern as characterized by "eighty to ninety percent of the pathogen having been expelled, but with only ten to twenty percent of the true yin left." In this situation, the primary focus of this formula must be to enrich and nourish the yin and fluids. One of the chief ingredients, egg yolk (*jī zǐ huáng*), nourishes the yin and dispels wind. Wu Ju-Tong attributed to it the function of tonifying the middle burner, connecting the Heart and Kidneys, and extinguishing internal wind, being impartial to either yin or yang and thereby able to connect both within a harmonious physiological relationship. It is often combined with the other chief ingredient, Asini Corii Colla (*ē jiāo*), which strongly tonifies the blood and nourishes the yin. *Materia Medica of Ri Hua-Zi* notes that it can "treat any type of wind," an ability emphasized in several other classical texts as well. Together, the two chief ingredients amplify each other's action to powerfully nourish the yin fluids and extinguish wind.

The deputies, Paeoniae Radix alba (*bái sháo*), Glycyrrhizae Radix praeparata (*zhì gān cǎo*), and Schisandrae Fructus (*wǔ wèi zǐ*), are a mix of sweet and sour substances that work in concert to nourish the yin and soften the Liver. The remaining ingredients serve as assistants. Rehmanniae Radix (*shēng dì huáng*) nourishes the yin and increases the fluids. Ophiopogonis Radix (*mài mén dōng*) nourishes the yin and moistens the Lungs. Greasy and cloying Cannabis Semen (*huǒ má rén*) nourishes the yin and moistens dryness. Testudinis Plastrum (*guī bǎn*), Trionycis Carapax (*biē jiǎ*), and Ostreae Concha (*mǔ lì*) enrich the yin to anchor the yang. Ostreae Concha (*mǔ lì*) is especially effective in calming the Liver and sedating the Liver yang. Trionycis Carapax (*biē jiǎ*) more strongly tonifies the yin, and is cooling at a deeper level, entering the Kidneys to enrich the yin so as to anchor the yang. Testudinis Plastrum (*guī bǎn*) is particularly strong at nourishing the yin to anchor the ascendant Liver yang.

Cautions and Contraindications

Because the formula contains many cloying and astringent ingredients that might otherwise trap the pathogen, it is contraindicated in cases of yin and fluid deficiency with vigorous pathogenic qi.

Commentary

This is a modification of Three-Shell Decoction to Restore the Pulse (*sān jiǎ fù mài tāng*), discussed above. By adding two more ingredients—egg yolk (*jī zǐ huáng*) and Schisandrae Fructus (*wǔ wèi zǐ*—it strengthens that formula's ability to enrich the yin and extinguish wind. It is targeted at conditions of severe deficiency complicated by wind excess. In *Case Records as a Guide to Clinical Practice*, Ye Tian-Shi describes the etiology of this disorder: "The Liver is the organ of wind. Decline and consumption of the essence [leads to] the inability of water to restrain wood. With less nourishment, wood is not luxuriant; therefore, Liver yang tends to ascend and internal [stirring] of wind often arises."

This formula controls the symptoms of excess (wind) by nourishing what is deficient (the yin and fluids). This is the only way to deal with a situation where the body's essence has become so severely depleted that any dispersing method is absolutely contraindicated. Hence, although it belongs to a class of formulas that treat internal wind, its ingredients do not address this pathology directly. Rather, it focuses on the root to control the manifestations and should properly be regarded as a formula that rescues abandonment. Viewed from this perspective, the wind here is not a manifestation of excess yang that cannot be contained by the deficient yin, but is rather a sign that yin and yang are beginning to separate. This pathodynamic is addressed by both of the ingredients to which the formula's name refers. In the words of its author, Wu Ju-Tong:

> Egg yolk (*jī zǐ huáng*) is a substance that, following the leg lesser yin, calms all three yin [channels] in the lower burner, while in the upper burner, it helps all of the three arm yin [channels]. Facilitating the interchange between above and below, it calms the yin in its position while establishing a foundation for yang. Its [use] has the intention of treating yin and yang equally, as if in a family. Why would they then abandon each other?

As for the two turtle shells in the formula, they amplify this action from below, as explained in *Detailed Materia Medica*:

> Trionycis Carapax (*biē jiǎ*) is green in color so it enters the Liver, and the illnesses it governs are all those of the blood level of the Liver channel. Testudinis Plastrum (*guī bǎn*) is black in color so it enters the Kidneys, and the illnesses it governs are all those of the blood level of the Kidney channel; it also unblocks the Heart. Both are shelled animals in the yin category, and primarily treat yin channels, each according to its type.

While late-stage fevers with marked trembling of the fingers or limbs, or tonic-clonic convulsions of the feet and hands, are the main indications of this formula, it can also be used in the treatment of internal wind with severe deficiency, or palpitations due to the failure of the Liver to nourish the Heart. Such patterns may be seen in hyperthyroidism or restless leg syndrome. In these cases, the formula should be modified further, as indicated below.

Comparisons

> Vs. Antelope Horn and Uncaria Decoction
> (*líng jiǎo gōu téng tāng*)

Both formulas treat patterns of warm pathogen disorders where heat has penetrated to the blood aspect causing stirring of internal wind. However, Antelope Horn and Uncaria Decoction (*líng jiǎo gōu téng tāng*) treats excess patterns with heat in the blood generating wind, characterized by high fever, irritability, restlessness, dizziness, vertigo, twitching and spasms of the extremities, a deep-red, dry, or burnt tongue with prickles, and a wiry, rapid pulse. By contrast, Major Arrest Wind Pearls (*dà dìng fēng zhū*) treats late-stage deficiency patterns with harm to the true yin, and yang separating from yin, characterized by weariness, muscle spasms with alternating flexion and extension of the extremities, a deficient or frail pulse, and a deep-red tongue with a scanty or peeled coating.

> Vs. Ass-Hide Gelatin and Egg Yolk Decoction
> (*ē jiāo jī zi huáng tāng*); *see* page 655.

> Vs. Three-Shell Decoction to Restore the Pulse
> (*sān jiǎ fù mài tāng*); *see* page 651.

Biomedical Indications

With the appropriate presentation, this formula may be used to treat a variety of biomedically-defined disorders including the sequelae of encephalitis and meningitis, Parkinson's disease, essential tremor, tongue atrophy after radiation treatment, hyperthyroidism, urticaria, coronary artery disease, and restless leg syndrome.

Modifications

- For wheezing and labored breathing with qi deficiency, add Ginseng Radix (*rén shēn*). (source text)
- For spontaneous sweating with qi deficiency, add Fossilia Ossis Mastodi (*lóng gǔ*), Ginseng Radix (*rén shēn*), and Tritici Fructus levis (*fú xiǎo mài*). (source text)
- For palpitations with qi deficiency, add Poriae Sclerotium pararadicis (*fú shén*), Ginseng Radix (*rén shēn*), and Tritici Fructus levis (*fú xiǎo mài*). (source text)
- For muscle spasms in the extremities with phlegm, add Bambusae Concretio silicea (*tiān zhú huáng*) and Fritillariae cirrhosae Bulbus (*chuān bèi mǔ*).
- For concurrent, lingering low-grade fever, add (with discretion) Cynanchi atrati Radix (*bái wēi*) and Lycii Cortex (*dì gǔ pí*).

Associated Formula

小定風珠 (小定风珠)

Minor Arrest Wind Pearls

xiǎo dìng fēng zhū

Source *Systematic Differentiation of Warm Pathogen Diseases* (1798)

Egg yolk (*jī zi huáng*) 1
Asini Corii Colla (*ē jiāo*) 6g
Testudinis Plastrum (*guī bǎn*) 18g
Infantis Urina (*tóng biàn*) .150ml
Mytilus seu Perma (*dàn cài*)* .9g

The source text advises to first decoct Testudinis Plastrum (*guī bǎn*) with Mylilussiccus (*dàn cài*) in 5 cups of water until 2 cups remain before dissolving Asini Corii Colla (*ē jiāo*) in the strained decoction. When this has cooled down, egg yolk (*jī zi huáng*) and Infantis Urina (*tóng biàn*) are added. Enriches the yin, extinguishes the wind, and stops the vomiting. For warm pathogens that have been in the body for a long time and entered the lower burner, causing inversion characterized by vomiting and a thin but still forceful pulse. Wu Ju-Tong, the author of this formula, defines this as a disorder of the Penetrating vessel combining aspects of both excess and deficiency, which are reflected in the pulse. According to the source text, the formula uses the combination of Asini Corii Colla (*ē jiāo*) and egg yolk (*jī zi huáng*) to nourish the yin and extinguish the wind; Testudinis Plastrum (*guī bǎn*) "to tonify the Conception vessel and settle the Penetrating vessel"; Mytilus seu Perma (*dàn cài*) to tonify the Liver and Kidneys, and because of its "ability to tonify the true yang within the yin … as well as anchor the upward movement of the true yang"; and Infantis Urina (*tóng biàn*) "as a turbid fluid that guides [the formula] into the turbid pathways [of the Penetrating vessel]." Compared to the principal formula, it is less tonifying and is indicated for patterns where the yin and essence have not yet been completely exhausted.

阿膠雞子黃湯 (阿胶鸡子黄汤)

Ass-Hide Gelatin and Egg Yolk Decoction

ē jiāo jī zi huáng tāng

Source *Popular Guide to the Discussion of Cold Damage* (Qing dynasty)

Asini Corii Colla (*ē jiāo*) 6g
Egg yolk (*jī zi huáng*) . . . . .2 yolks
Rehmanniae Radix (*shēng dì huáng*) 12g
Paeoniae Radix alba (*bái sháo*) 9g
Glycyrrhizae Radix praeparata (*zhì gān cǎo*) 1.8g
Uncariae Ramulus cum Uncis (*gōu téng*) 6g
Haliotidis Concha (*shí jué míng*) 15g
Ostreae Concha (*mǔ lì*) 12g
Poriae Sclerotium pararadicis (*fú shén*) 12g
Trachelospermi Caulis (*luò shí téng*) 9g

Method of Preparation Blend the egg yolk into the strained decoction and take warm.

Actions Enriches the yin, nourishes the blood, softens the Liver, and extinguishes wind

---

* Mytilus seu Perma (淡菜 *dàn cài*) is salty and warm and enters the Liver and Kidney channels. It tonifies the Liver and Kidneys, augments the essence and blood, and reduces goiters. The normal dosage in decoctions is 9-30g.

Indications

Rigid extremities, muscle spasms and twitches in the extremities, dry mouth, parched lips, a deep-red tongue with a scanty coating, and a thin, rapid pulse. There may also be dizziness and vertigo.

This is blood deficiency and insufficiency of yin fluids that leads to stirring of internal wind. It is a pattern that occurs in the late stages of warm pathogen disorders and is referred to as 'deficiency wind' (虚風 xū fēng). Because the yin and blood have been damaged by the warm pathogen, they are unable to nourish the sinews, leading to yang excess characterized by twitches, spasms, and rigidity in the muscles of the extremities. Muscle twitches, which appear and disappear quickly and involve rapid movements, are associated with wind. The mechanism leading to dizziness and vertigo may be explained in terms of the five phases: when water, which has been damaged by heat, is unable to generate wood, the result is Liver yin and blood deficiency, which leads to internal stirring of wind. The dry mouth and parched lips are indicative of heat injuring the yin and fluids. The deep-red tongue with a scanty coating and the thin, rapid pulse are signs of heat injuring the yin.

Analysis of Formula

The focus of this formula is primarily to nourish the yin and blood, and secondarily to sedate the yang and unblock the channels. The chief ingredients, Asini Corii Colla (ē jiāo) and egg yolk (jī zi huáng), nourish the yin and blood, extinguish wind, and sedate the yang. He Lian-Chen says of this combination: "These two ingredients [belong to medicinals made from the] blood and flesh of sentient beings. They are heavy substances with a thick flavor. They are very capable of providing yin, extinguishing wind, augmenting the yin fluids, and moistening the sinews." The deputies, Rehmanniae Radix (shēng dì huáng), fresh Paeoniae Radix alba (bái sháo), and Glycyrrhizae Radix praeparata (zhì gān cǎo), a combination of sweet and sour substances, soften the Liver to extinguish the wind. The combination of Paeoniae Radix alba (bái sháo) and Glycyrrhizae Radix praeparata (zhì gān cǎo) is very effective in treating painful spasms.

The assistants, Uncariae Ramulus cum Uncis (gōu téng), Haliotidis Concha (shí jué míng), and Ostreae Concha (mǔ lì), sedate the ascendant yang and extinguish wind. These actions are indirectly strengthened by Poriae Sclerotium pararadicis (fú shén), which calms the Liver and the spirit. The envoy, Trachelospermi Caulis (luò shí téng), focuses the actions of the other ingredients on the collaterals and sinews. *Divine Husbandman's Materia Medica* prescribes this formula for wind-heat with lifeless muscles; *Miscellaneous Records of Famous Physicians* states that it nourishes the Kidneys, governs lumbar and sacral pain, fortifies the sinews, and facilitates movement in the joints. Especially when combined with Paeoniae Radix alba (bái sháo) and Glycyrrhizae Radix praeparata (zhì gān cǎo), it is very effective in relaxing the sinews and unblocking the collaterals.

Working synergistically, the ingredients of this formula tonify deficiency (injury to the yin fluids and blood) while also effectively dealing with the excess (internal stirring of wind). In practice, it is essential to distinguish the primary from the secondary aspects of the disorder. The relative dosage of the ingredients should reflect this distinction.

Commentary

The source text does not specify an indication for this formula but merely notes that it represents "a strategy for enriching the yin and extinguishing wind." In *Revised Popular Guide to the Discussion of Cold Damage*, He Lian-Chen defines its pathodynamic more precisely:

> [This is] not true [i.e., external] wind but blood deficiency generating wind. Its real cause is the failure of blood to nourish the sinews [so that] the vessels constrict and the sinews contract, making flexion and extension impossible. Thus, the hands and feet contract. This is similar to stirring of wind [in internal medicine]. Therefore, it is called surreptitious wind due to internal deficiency (內虛暗風 nèi xū àn fēng) and is generally known as Liver wind. This pattern often occurs when a warm pathogen heat disorder remains in the collaterals. In [those cases,] it is due to heat damaging the blood and yin fluids.

This explanation clarifies that use of the formula is not restricted to warm pathogen heat disorders, but that it is equally useful for treating internal medicine patterns characterized by yin and blood deficiency and hyperactive Liver yang with such symptoms as dizziness and tinnitus. Key markers in both cases will be a dry mouth and dry lips, a crimson tongue with little coating, and a thin, rapid pulse.

Historically, the treatment strategies on which this formula is based were first elucidated by the Qing-dynasty physician Ye Tian-Shi in *Case Records as a Guide to Clinical Practice*. To treat patterns characterized by internal wind seizing the collaterals and deficiency wind, Ye recommended strategies like "relaxing the Liver, moistening the blood, and extinguishing wind," and "nourishing the blood to extinguish wind." He also argued that "wind herbs [as well as] cold and cooling [formulas] are strongly contraindicated," as are "hard and drying herbs." Some writers, like the contemporary formula expert Chen Chao-Zu in *Treatment Strategies and Formulas in Chinese Medicine*, argue that the use of Trachelospermi Caulis (luò shí téng) in this formula violates these principles and its use should accordingly be reconsidered.

Comparisons

➢ Vs. Antelope Horn and Uncaria Decoction
   (líng jiǎo gōu téng tāng)

Both formulas were composed by Yu Gen-Chu to treat stirring of Liver wind in the context of warm pathogen disorders and both contain Paeoniae Radix alba (bái sháo), Uncariae Ramulus cum Uncis (gōu téng), Poriae Sclerotium pararadicis (fú shén), Rehmanniae Radix (shēng dì huáng), and Glycyrrhizae Radix (gān cǎo) to relax the Liver, enrich the fluids, clear fire, and extinguish wind. Antelope Horn and Uncaria Decoction (líng jiǎo gōu téng tāng) combines these ingredients with Saigae tataricae Cornu (líng yáng jiǎo), Mori Folium (sāng yè), Chrysanthemi Flos (jú huā), Fritillariae cirrhosae Bulbus (chuān bèi mǔ), and Bambusae Caulis in taeniam (zhú rú), while also specifying that Rehmanniae Radix (shēng dì huáng) and Glycyrrhizae Radix (gān cǎo) should be used fresh. As a result, it is stronger at clearing fire while also transforming phlegm, and is indicated for spasms and convulsions as well as loss of consciousness that occurs during episodes of high fever.

By contrast, Ass-Hide Gelatin and Egg Yoke Decoction (ē jiāo jī zi huáng tang) adds egg yolk (jī zi huáng), Asini Corii Colla (ē jiāo), Ostreae Concha (mǔ lì), Haliotidis Concha (shí jué míng), and Trachelospermi Caulis (luò shí téng), as well as Glycyrrhizae Radix praeparata (zhì gān cǎo). It thus focuses more strongly on nourishing the blood and providing essence, on anchoring the errant yang, and on opening the collaterals and sinew vessels. It is indicated for late-stage warm pathogen and yin deficiency disorders characterized by

muscle spasms, dizziness, a thin and rapid pulse, and other signs of empty wind.

➤ Vs. Major Arrest Wind Pearls (dà dìng fēng zhū)

Both formulas treat internal wind caused by essence and blood deficiency and contain Egg yolk (jī zi huáng), Asini Corii Colla (ē jiāo), Paeoniae Radix alba (bái sháo), Rehmanniae Radix (shēng dì huáng), and Glycyrrhizae Radix (gān cǎo) to provide yin, anchor the errant yang, and extinguish wind. However, Major Arrest Wind Pearls (dà dìng fēng zhū) is indicated for conditions of severe deficiency with yin and yang beginning to separate. For this reason, it does not treat wind directly, but relies entirely on enriching the yin and containing the yang with substances like Testudinis Plastrum (guī bǎn), Trionycis Carapax (biē jiǎ), Ophiopogonis Radix (mài mén dōng), Cannabis Semen (huǒ má rén), and Schisandrae Fructus (wǔ wèi zǐ). Ass-Hide Gelatin and Egg Yolk Decoction (ē jiāo jī zi huáng tāng), on the other hand, directly eliminates wind from the vessel sinews and collaterals with herbs like Uncariae Ramulus cum Uncis (gōu téng) and Trachelospermi Caulis (luò shí téng), even if its main focus is also on nourishing the blood.

Biomedical Indications

With the appropriate presentation, this formula may be used to treat a variety of biomedically-defined disorders including the sequelae of encephalitis and meningitis.

Comparative Tables of Principal Formulas

■ FORMULAS THAT DREDGE AND DISPERSE EXTERNAL WIND

Common symptoms: all arise from an external invasion of wind

Formula Name	Diagnosis	Indications	Remarks
Minor Extend Life Decoction (xiǎo xù mìng tāng)	Wind-stroke due to invasion of wind from the exterior into the channels	Hemiplegia, asymmetry of the face, and slurred speech usually accompanied by fever and chills, pale tongue with a thin, white coating, and a deficient, floating pulse	May be loss of consciousness; also used for pain from wind-damp painful obstruction.
Drink from Three Unprepared Ingredients (sān shēng yǐn)	Sudden wind-stroke in a person with constitutional yang deficiency and phlegm-dampness	Loss of consciousness, overabundant and congested phlegm, halting, sluggish speech, and inversion frigidity of the extremities; also for deviation of the mouth and eyes or hemiplegia, a white tongue coating, and a submerged, hidden pulse	Also for severe dizziness due to wind-cold-phlegm.
Chuanxiong Powder to Be Taken with Green Tea (chuān xiōng chá tiáo sǎn)	Headache due to externally-contracted wind	Headache in any part of the head, which may be accompanied by fever and chills, dizziness, nasal congestion, a thin, white tongue coating, and a floating pulse	Can be modified to treat either wind-heat or wind-cold headache.
Xanthium Powder (cāng ěr zǐ sǎn)	External wind pathogen remaining in the body and obstructing the protective qi	Copious, purulent, foul-smelling nasal discharge, nasal obstruction, dizziness, frontal headache, a normal or thin and white or greasy and white tongue coating	This is known as deep-source nasal congestion.

........cont.↘

Formula Name	Diagnosis	Indications	Remarks
Major Large Gentian Decoction (*dà qín jiāo tāng*)	Early or middle stage wind-stroke in the channels	Deviation of the mouth and eyes, difficulty speaking, inability to move one's arms and legs or numbness in the hands and feet, often with chills and fever, muscle spasms, aching joints, a white or yellow tongue coating, and a floating and tight or wiry and thin pulse	Also used for wind-damp-cold painful obstruction.
Minor Invigorate the Collaterals Special Pill (*xiǎo huó luò dān*)	Obstruction of the channels and collaterals by wind-cold-damp pathogens, blood stasis, and phlegm following wind-stroke	Chronic pain, weakness, and numbness (especially in the lower extremities) due to wind-stroke, aggravation of symptoms by cold, and a moist, white tongue coating	Also for fixed or migrating pain in the bones and joints with reduced range of motion due to wind-cold-damp painful obstruction.
Lead to Symmetry Powder (*qiān zhèng sǎn*)	Channel-stroke from wind-phlegm with symptoms confined to the head and face	Sudden facial paralysis with deviation of the eyes and mouth and facial muscle twitch	Most appropriate for treating wind-phlegm disorders due primarily to damp-cold.
Stop Spasms Powder (*zhǐ jìng sǎn*)	Heat entering the terminal yin channel	Muscle twitches of the extremities, rigidity and spasms of the entire body to the point of opisthotonus, trismus, or convulsions, and in severe cases loss of consciousness	Also used for the treatment of stubborn headaches, migraine, and joint pain.
True Jade Powder (*yù zhēn sǎn*)	Invasion of wind and toxin through a wound or sore	Stiffness and spasms of the jaw, closed mouth, lip spasms, deviation of the eyes, rigidity of the entire body to the point of opisthotonus, and a wiry, tight pulse	This is a type of muscular tetany.
Eliminate Wind Powder from *Orthodox Lineage* (*xiāo fēng sǎn*)	Wind-heat or wind-dampness invading the body and contending with preexisting damp-heat	Weepy, itchy, red skin lesions over a large part of the body, a yellow or white tongue coating, and a forceful, floating, and rapid pulse	This is wind rash or damp rash; also applied topically.
Wind-Drawing Decoction (*fēng yǐn tāng*)	Exuberant heat and stirring of internal Liver wind	Sudden collapse, convulsions, upturned eyeballs, deviation of the mouth and eyes, gurgling sounds in the throat, irritability and restlessness, or mental confusion, a red tongue, and a forceful, wiry and/or rapid pulse	For seizures, wind-stroke, or child fright wind; also for hemiplegia and hemilateral withering.

■ FORMULAS THAT PACIFY AND EXTINGUISH INTERNAL WIND

Common symptoms: dizziness, spasms, and twitches or motor dysfunction of the extremities, impaired consciousness (in severe cases), red tongue

Formula Name	Diagnosis	Indications	Remarks
Antelope Horn and Uncaria Decoction (*líng jiǎo gōu téng tāng*)	Heat excess in the Liver channel stirring up internal wind	Persistent high fever, irritability, restlessness, dizziness, vertigo, twitching and spasms of the extremities, a deep-red, dry, or burnt tongue with prickles, and a wiry, rapid pulse	In severe cases there may also be impaired or actual loss of consciousness.
Sedate the Liver and Extinguish Wind Decoction (*zhèn gān xī fēng tāng*)	Wind-type stroke caused by excessive upward-gushing of qi that, in turn, leads to congestion of blood in the brain	Severe dizziness and vertigo, a feeling of distention in the eyes, tinnitus, headache, flushed face, disorientation, sudden loss of consciousness, motor dysfunction of limbs and trunk or facial paralysis, and a wiry, long, and forceful pulse	More for those at risk from stroke than the sequelae of stroke; also commonly used to treat hypertension.

cont. ↘

Formula Name	Diagnosis	Indications	Remarks
Gastrodia and Uncaria Drink (*tiān má gōu téng yǐn*)	Hyperactive Liver yang leading to internal stirring of Liver wind	Headache, dizziness, vertigo, tinnitus, blurred vision, a sensation of heat rushing to the head, insomnia with dream-disturbed sleep, a red tongue, and a wiry, rapid pulse	Severe cases may have numbness, twitching and spasms in the extremities, or hemiplegia. Especially useful for hypertension.
Three-Shell Decoction to Restore the Pulse (*sān jiǎ fù mài tāng*)	Late-stage warm pathogen disorder where the yin has been injured	Severe palpitations, Heart pain, and a thin, rapid, irregular pulse; may also have fever, flushed face, hot palms and soles, dizziness, tinnitus, spasms, quivering fingers, impaired consciousness, or a deep-red and dry tongue	Focuses on anchoring errant yang and tonifying the true yin.
Major Arrest Wind Pearls (*dà dìng fēng zhū*)	Internal stirring of wind due to yin deficiency	Weariness, muscle spasms, alternating flexion and extension of the extremities, a deficient or frail pulse, and a deep-red tongue with a scanty or peeled coating	Also for patterns of internal wind with severe deficiency or palpitations from the Liver failing to nourish the Heart, as seen in restless leg syndrome or hyperthyroidism.
Ass-Hide Gelatin and Egg Yolk Decoction (*ē jiāo jī zi huáng tāng*)	Blood deficiency and insufficiency of yin fluids that leads to stirring of internal wind	Rigid extremities, muscle spasms and twitches in the extremities, possible dizziness and vertigo, dry mouth, parched lips, a deep-red tongue with a scanty coating, and a thin, rapid pulse	This is deficiency wind occurring in the late stages of a warm pathogen disorder.

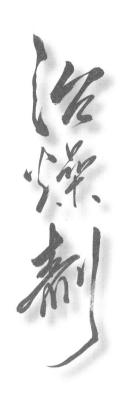

Chapter 15 Contents

Formulas that Treat Dryness

Formulas that Treat Dryness

DRYNESS IS ONE of the six pernicious qi. It specifically damages the body fluids, which impairs their functions of moistening and providing lubrication to the movements of the qi dynamic. Although dryness disorders and their treatment were discussed in the *Inner Classic* and *Essentials of the Golden Cabinet*, it was not until the early Qing dynasty and the publication of Yu Chang's *Precepts for Physicians* that they became more than a passing concern to Chinese physicians. According to Yu:

> Among the nineteen pathodynamics [discussed] in the *Inner Classic*, only dry qi is missing. I specifically want to correct this [omission]. The general principle is that in spring one is damaged by wind, in summer by heat, in late summer by dampness, in autumn by dryness, in winter by cold. … The various [types of] roughness, withering, and desiccation, as well as progressive chapping and erosions, all pertain to dryness.

The publication of Wu Ju-Tong's *Systematic Differentiation of Warm Pathogen Diseases* some two centuries later finally supplied Chinese medicine with the first systematic framework for discussing dryness disorders. Wu Ju-Tong differentiated between internal and external dryness—the former due to internal organ disharmonies, the latter to invasion of pathogenic dryness from the outside—and organized the ensuing patterns according to their location within the three burners.

As a key theoretician of warm pathogen disorders, Wu Ju-Tong was concerned above all with the contraction of dry-ness from the external environment, which he further differentiated into hot and cold types. Until the present day, this opposition has remained the basic scheme according to which these disorders are understood, diagnosed, and treated. Yu Gen-Chu, another Qing-dynasty physician, explained the difference between warm and cool dryness in *Revised Popular Guide to the Discussion of Cold Damage*:

> In the depth of autumn, [the air] begins to cool and the west wind is fierce. The externally-contracted condition that people usually get at this time is wind-dryness, a type of cool-dryness. This condition is milder than the wind-cold of winter. If [in autumn] there are many sunny days and no rain, then the autumnal yang 'basks in the sun.' Warm-dryness is commonly contracted at this time, which is a type of hot-dryness. It is more severe than the wind-warmth disease of spring.

The seasonality of dryness in northern China does not, of course, necessarily correspond to its occurrence in other parts of the world. Moreover, the widespread use of central heating and air conditioning in modern times has become a common cause of dryness, irrespective of the season or locale. Externally-contracted dryness readily injures the Lungs and depletes the fluids. In its early stages, in addition to such typical exterior symptoms as fever and chills, there may also be a dry mouth, sore throat, and either a nonproductive cough or one with scanty sputum.

Opposite of external dryness is internal dryness, which arises from the loss of an organ's essence and depletion of the fluids. It is most commonly associated with improper sweating or purging of a serious illness, severe vomiting, excessive urination, overindulgence in sex, or overconsumption of spicy foods. The clinical presentation of internal dryness is rather complex and will vary depending on the depth of the condition and which organs are affected. The Lungs, Spleen, Kidneys, and Large Intestine are most commonly involved. Internal dryness may also be understood from the perspective of the three burners: dryness in the upper burner leads to a hacking cough and thirst; dryness in the middle burner produces vomiting and belching, with an inability to keep food down; dryness in the lower burner causes dry stools or wasting and thirsting disorders.

Because of the complex relationships among the various organs and body regions, and between the exterior and interior, differentiation of external and internal dryness is not always a simple matter. External dryness may affect the interior, the organs may affect each other, and different parts of the body may interact on many levels. Such differentiation is especially difficult with the Lungs since external dryness almost immediately injures this organ.

It is important to differentiate dryness disorders, where dryness is the root, from other types of disorders that cause damage to the fluid metabolism and deprive the body of moisture, but where dryness is just a manifestation. These are, on the one hand, cold and qi stagnation, and on the other, heat and yin deficiency. Cold and qi stagnation interfere with the body's ability to disperse and disseminate fluids. Because the fluids are not actually damaged, however, dryness in some part of the body will invariably be accompanied by an accumulation or excess of fluids in another. With cold dryness, this is also the case, but symptoms of dryness will be significantly more pronounced. Yin deficiency and heat imply damage to the body fluids and therefore lead to dryness. However, dryness (associated with the Lungs and the yang brightness) primarily indicates a failure of fluids to accomplish their functions of moistening and harmonizing movement. Dry pathologies are thus disorders of the qi dynamic that manifest as coughing, constipation, or rebellious qi. Yin deficiency, on the other hand, indicates an impairment of the yin functions of holding and anchoring the yang, and are thus invariably accompanied by yang excess. Heat disorders, finally, damage the fluids and yin, but yang excess predominates over damage to the yin and fluids in terms of both its pathodynamic and manifestations.

Given the differentiation between internal and external dryness, formulas to treat dryness are generally grouped into two broad categories: those that gently disperse and moisten external dryness, and those that enrich yin and moisten internal dryness. All of these formulas contain enriching, cloying substances that may obstruct the qi dynamic. They also encourage the development of dampness and should there-fore not be used in those with a damp constitution. It is also important that they be used with caution (and appropriate modification) in cases with diarrhea due to Spleen deficiency or where there is marked qi stagnation.

Section 1

FORMULAS THAT GENTLY DISPERSE AND MOISTEN DRYNESS

The formulas in this section are used in treating externally-contracted cool-dryness and warm-dryness. Cool-dryness, which results from the contraction of a wind-cold dry pathogen, impairs the Lungs' functions of diffusing the qi and clarifying by directing downward. This manifests as chills, headache, and a dry mouth and throat. Because patterns of cold-dryness share many characteristics with the more severe wind-cold patterns of winter, they were traditionally referred to as 'lesser cold' (次寒 *cì hán*). Warm-dryness, on the other hand, results from the contraction of dryness in conditions that are warm and where the air lacks moisture. It primarily injures the Lung yang fluids, causing fever, headache, thirst, and irritability. Such patterns share many characteristics with wind-heat patterns but are generally less severe in nature.

The focus of all formulas that gently disperse and moisten dryness is to release the exterior. For this purpose, formulas that treat cool-dryness use light, acrid, warming herbs like Perillae Folium (*zǐ sū yè*), Sojae Semen praeparatum (*dàn dòu chǐ*), and Zingiberis Rhizoma recens (*shēng jiāng*). Formulas that treat warm-dryness use light, acrid, cooling herbs like Mori Folium (*sāng yè*) and Menthae haplocalycis Herba (*bò hé*). Formulas generally combine these chief herbs with three other types of herbs as deputies and assistants. The first group includes herbs that stop coughing and transform phlegm, like Armeniacae Semen (*xìng rén*), Peucedani Radix (*qián hú*), Platycodi Radix (*jié gěng*), and Fritillariae Bulbus (*bèi mǔ*). These symptoms, and the herbs used to treat them, reflect the attack on the Lungs that is typical of exterior dryness disorders. The second group includes herbs that nourish the yin and moisten dryness, like Glehniae/Adenophorae Radix (*shā shēn*), Asini Corii Colla (*ē jiāo*), and Cannabis Semen (*huǒ má rén*). This is necessary because dryness damages the fluids and blood, which must be replenished. The third group is comprised of herbs that clear heat, like Gypsum fibrosum (*shí gāo*), Gardeniae Fructus (*zhī zǐ*), and Forsythiae Fructus (*lián qiáo*). Dryness diminishes the yin but also produces stagnation. It therefore readily transforms into heat. In these situations, it is important to use herbs that clear heat but that are also acrid or that open the qi dynamic.

杏蘇散 (杏苏散)

Apricot Kernel and Perilla Leaf Powder

xìng sū sǎn

Source *Systematic Differentiation of Warm Pathogen Diseases* (1798)

Perillae Folium (*zǐ sū yè*) 6-9g
Peucedani Radix (*qián hú*) 6-9g
Armeniacae Semen (*xìng rén*) 6-9g
Platycodi Radix (*jié gěng*) 6g
Aurantii Fructus (*zhǐ ké*) 6g
Citri reticulatae Pericarpium (*chén pí*) 6g
Poria (*fú líng*) 6-9g
Pinelliae Rhizoma praeparatum (*zhì bàn xià*) 6-9g
Zingiberis Rhizoma recens (*shēng jiāng*) . . . . 2-3 pieces
Jujubae Fructus (*dà zǎo*) . . . . 2-3 pieces
Glycyrrhizae Radix (*gān cǎo*) 3g

Method of Preparation The source text advises to grind the herbs into a powder and take as a draft. At present, it is usually prepared as a decoction.

Actions Gently disperses cool-dryness, disseminates the Lung qi, and transforms thin mucus

Indications

Slight headache, chills without sweating, cough with watery sputum, stuffy nose, dry throat, a dry, white tongue coating, and a wiry pulse

This is externally-contracted cool-dryness interfering with the disseminating, clearing, and downward-directing functions of the Lungs. Headache and chills without sweating indicates cool-dryness attacking the exterior, where it constrains the movement of protective yang. When cool-dryness attacks the Lungs, it disrupts their ability to facilitate the circulation of fluids. This results in the internal accumulation of fluids and produces a type of thin mucus characterized by cough with watery sputum. Since the nose is the sensory orifice of the Lungs and the throat is part of the Lung system, dryness in the Lungs can lead to a stuffy nose and a dry throat. The dry, white tongue coating indicates cool-dryness. The wiry pulse indicates cool-dryness and thin mucus.

Analysis of Formula

The composition of this formula is based on the principle stated in Chapter 74 of *Basic Questions*: "A dry pathogenic qi is treated internally with bitter and warm [herbs], while sweet and acrid [herbs are used] adjunctively." Because the pathogen is located in the upper burner and the exterior, the formula relies primarily on light, acrid, dispersing herbs. They are assisted by those that regulate the disturbed qi dynamic. The chief herbs, therefore, are bitter Armeniacae Semen (*xìng rén*), which disseminates the Lung qi and stops the coughing, and acrid Perillae Folium (*zǐ sū yè*), which releases the exterior cold by promoting moderate sweating. There are

three deputies. The first, Peucedani Radix (*qián hú*), assists the chief herbs by directing the qi downward and releasing the exterior; the second, Platycodi Radix (*jié gěng*), causes the Lung qi to descend and stops the coughing; and the third, Aurantii Fructus (*zhǐ ké*), moves the qi, expands the chest, and stops the coughing by regulating the qi.

To address the problem of thin mucus, the qi dynamic must be regulated and the phlegm transformed. The assistant herbs, Citri reticulatae Pericarpium (*chén pí*), Poria (*fú líng*), and Pinelliae Rhizoma praeparatum (*zhì bàn xià*), regulate the qi of the middle burner, which is the fulcrum of the qi dynamic, and thereby transform the phlegm. The envoys, Zingiberis Rhizoma recens (*shēng jiāng*), Jujubae Fructus (*dà zǎo*), and Glycyrrhizae Radix (*gān cǎo*), harmonize the actions of the other herbs and regulate the nutritive and protective qi. They thereby contribute both to the release of the exterior and the regulation of the middle qi.

Commentary

This formula is a variation of Perilla Leaf and Apricot Kernel Drink (*xìng sū yǐn*), an earlier formula from *Golden Mirror of the Medical Tradition*. That formula was used to treat wind-cold residing in the Lungs, where it caused wheezing. It is composed of Perillae Folium (*zǐ sū yè*), Aurantii Fructus (*zhǐ ké*), Platycodi Radix (*jié gěng*), Puerariae Radix (*gé gēn*), Peucedani Radix (*qián hú*), Citri reticulatae Pericarpium (*chén pí*), Glycyrrhizae Radix (*gān cǎo*), Pinelliae Rhizoma praeparatum (*zhì bàn xià*), Armeniacae Semen (*xìng rén*), and Poria (*fú líng*). Perilla Leaf and Apricot Kernel Drink (*xìng sū yǐn*), in turn, is a variation of Ginseng and Perilla Leaf Drink (*shēn sū yǐn*), discussed in Chapter 1, a Song-dynasty formula used for treating wind-cold disorders with qi deficiency. By the early 18th century, the older formulas appear to have fallen out of favor, for Wu Ju-Tong remarked: "Perilla Leaf and Apricot Kernel Powder (*xìng sū sǎn*) dominates the contemporary treatment of wind-damage cough during [all of the] four seasons." This suggests that Wu Ju-Tong, whose *Systematic Differentiation of Warm Pathogen Diseases* is generally regarded as the source text for this formula, was not himself its author, but merely expanded its scope of application. Wu Ju-Tong also explained how and why cold-dryness produces stagnation:

> Dry qi rises following the autumnal equinox and [comes to an end] before the slight snow [i.e., the 20th solar term and beginning of winter]. It is commanded by the cool qi of yang brightness dryness metal. The *Classic* states, 'The nature of yang brightness is clear discharging from the middle [burner, causing] pain in the right flank and sloppy diarrhea [if it is obstructed]. Internally, it manifests as throat obstruction. Externally, it causes prominent bulging (癩疝 *tuí shàn*). When the great coolness clarifies and kills, the flowers change their appearance, the hairy pests die out, there is discomfort in the chest, the throat is blocked, and one coughs.' According to this

classical text, dryness will cause cool qi to be contracted by the people. As Liver wood receives this pathogen, it transforms into dryness. ... Dry disorders therefore come under [the wider rubric] of cold. They are referred to as lesser cold because these disorders and the contraction of cold are of the same kind.

Wu Ju-Tong thus defines cool-dryness to be a secondary consequence of mild cold. Cold slows down the qi dynamic. This leads to qi stagnation, on the one hand, and the failure of qi transformation with production of pathological fluids on the other. Both prevent physiological fluids from performing their moistening function. This explains why acrid, warming herbs used to unblock the qi dynamic and resolve the exterior can also treat dryness.

Comparisons

➤ Vs. Ginseng and Perilla Leaf Drink *(shēn sū yǐn)*

The principal formula can be seen as a modification of Ginseng and Perilla Leaf Drink *(shēn sū yǐn)*, where Ginseng Radix *(rén shēn)* and Aucklandiae Radix *(mù xiāng)* have been removed and Armeniacae Semen *(xìng rén)* added. Both formulas thus share core characteristics, yet address different pathologies. Ginseng and Perilla Leaf Drink *(shēn sū yǐn)* is warming without being drying, and augments the normal qi without retaining the pathogenic qi. It treats externally-contracted cold in patients with a deficient constitution and damp-phlegm in the interior arising from the failure of qi transformation in the middle burner. Perilla Leaf and Apricot Kernel Powder *(xìng sū sǎn)*, on the other hand, is indicated for pure excess conditions characterized by the simultaneous presence of dryness and thin mucus. Thus, it does not include Ginseng Radix *(rén shēn)* and replaces Aucklandiae Radix *(mù xiāng)*, which is warming, drying, and acts on the middle burner, with Armeniacae Semen *(xìng rén)*, which is bitter, sweet, moistening, and acts on the upper burner. Rather than facilitating the transformation of qi in the Spleen, it thus supports the Lungs, whose control of fluid regulation has been impaired.

➤ Vs. Mulberry Leaf and Apricot Kernel Decoction *(sāng xìng tāng)*; see page 666

➤ Vs. Stop Coughing Powder *(zhǐ sòu sǎn)*; see page 816

Biomedical Indications

With the appropriate presentation, this formula may be used to treat a variety of biomedically-defined disorders including upper respiratory tract infections, acute and chronic bronchitis, and emphysema.

Modifications

- For absence of sweating and a very wiry or tight pulse, add Notopterygii Rhizoma seu Radix *(qiāng huó)*. (source text)

- For diarrhea and a sensation of fullness in the abdomen, add Atractylodis Rhizoma *(cāng zhú)* and Magnoliae officinalis Cortex *(hòu pò)*. (source text)

- For headache involving the supraorbital ridge, add Angelicae dahuricae Radix *(bái zhǐ)*. (source text)

- For pronounced fever, add Scutellariae Radix *(huáng qín)*. Do not use in case of diarrhea with abdominal fullness. (source text)

Associated Formulas

杏前蔥豉湯 （杏前葱豉汤）

Apricot Kernel, Peucedanum, Spring Onion, and Prepared Soybean Decoction

xìng qián cōng chǐ tāng

Source   *Revised and Expanded Discussion of Warm-Heat Pathogen Diseases* (1907)

Armeniacae Semen *(xìng rén)*	9g
Peucedani Radix *(qián hú)*	4.5g
Perillae Caulis *(zǐ sū gěng)*	4.5g
Citri reticulatae Pericarpium *(chén pí)*	2.4g
Sojae Semen praeparatum *(dàn dòu chǐ)*	6g
Aurantii Fructus *(zhǐ ké)*	3g
Platycodi Radix *(jié gěng)*	2.1g
Allii fistulosi Bulbus *(cōng bái)*	3 stalks

Decoction. Disperses the wind, warms the cold, and resolves the exterior. For the initial stages of a cool-dryness disorder characterized by headaches, mild fever, nasal congestion, aversion to wind, chills, absence of sweating, dry skin, a dry and hacking cough, fullness of the chest, stabbing pain in both flanks, a dry and thin white tongue coating, and a pulse that is floating and rough on the right, and floating and wiry or tight on the left. This formula unblocks the protective yang in the exterior that has been fettered by the sudden invasion of coolness. It is a formula that He Lian-Chen, the author of the source text, copied from the case records of the famous Qing-dynasty physician Ye Tian-Shi. Ye used the formula for "patterns that occur when the first cold arrives in the middle of autumn. [These are] characterized by mild fever and coughing, [and] resemble [in their manifestation] the wind-warmth [disorders] that occur in the spring."

蔞薤六仁湯 （蒌薤六仁汤）

Six-Seed Decoction with Trichosanthis and Chinese Garlic

lóu xiè liù rén tāng

Source   *Bases of Medicine* (1861)

Trichosanthis Pericarpium *(guā lóu pí)*	9g
Armeniacae Semen *(xìng rén)*	9g
Amomi Fructus *(shā rén)*	0.9g
Pruni Semen *(yù lǐ rén)*	9g
Allii macrostemi Bulbus *(xiè bái)*	4.5g
Persicae Semen *(táo rén)*	5 pieces
Pini Semen *(sōng zǐ rén)*	40 pieces
Platycladi Semen *(bǎi zǐ rén)*	4.5g

Decoction. Unblocks stagnation and directs the qi downward with the help of acrid and slippery herbs. For the sequelae of exterior wind-cold, where the wind-cold has been eliminated but dryness remains, or Lung painful obstruction, with dryness of the bowels. Such patterns are characterized by abdominal urgency, despondency, painful obstruction of the chest, pain in the diaphragmatic area, and incomplete bowel movements. In severe cases, there may be dry clumping accompanied by abdominal pain. The tongue coating is white and yellow and sore to the touch. The pulse is submerged, excessive, and small on the right, while being wiry, small, and rough on the left. These disorders tend to occur in the autumn in the wake of contraction of wind-cold, when the wind has been eliminated but dryness remains to obstruct the qi dynamic in the upper burner. The formula uses Trichosanthis Pericarpium (*guā lóu pí*) and Allii macrostemi Bulbus (*xiè bái*) as chief herbs that moisten by means of their acrid nature and direct the qi downward by means of their slipperiness.

潤燥滲濕湯 （润燥渗湿汤）

Moisten Dryness and Leach Out Dampness Decoction

rùn zào shèn shī tāng

SOURCE　*Bases of Medicine* (1861)

Citri reticulatae Pericarpium (*chén pí*) 3g
Sinapis Semen (*bái jiè zǐ*) 1.5g
Acori tatarinowii Rhizoma (*shí chāng pǔ*) 3g
Coicis Semen (*yì yǐ rén*) 9g
Arctii Fructus (*niú bàng zǐ*) 4.5g
Angelicae dahuricae Radix (*bái zhǐ*) 3g
Forsythiae Fructus (*lián qiáo*) 2.4g
Talcum (*huá shí*) 16g

Decoction. Aromatically transforms and causes dampness to flow away and moistens dryness. For cool-wind-dryness contracted in the late summer or early autumn, which fetters the exterior and constrains damp-heat in the interior and leads to veiling of the sensory orifices characterized by disorientation and clouding of the consciousness. Other symptoms include coughing of phlegm that is difficult to expectorate, heat in the interior, irritability, incomplete bowel movements, dark urine that is reduced in volume, and a mixed white and yellow tongue coating that seems moist, but turns out to be dry when scraped. The pulse is said to be checked (過 *è*) and indistinct (不顯 *bù xiǎn*) on the right proximal position, and submerged, wiry, and rapid on the left.

　　This formula was composed by the late-Qing-dynasty physician Shi Shou-Tang to deal with the difficult problem of simultaneous dryness in the exterior (Lungs) and dampness in the interior (Spleen). In this situation, simply moistening the Lungs would exacerbate the internal dampness, while transforming the dampness would further injure the body fluids. To avoid this dilemma, Shi combined acrid, moistening seeds like Arctii Fructus (*niú bàng zǐ*) and Sinapis Semen (*bái jiè zǐ*), whose natural slipperiness prevents them from injuring the fluids, even as they open areas of constraint, with sweet, fragrant, and aromatic herbs like Coicis Semen (*yì yǐ rén*), Acori tatarinowii Rhizoma (*shí chāng pǔ*), and Talcum (*huá shí*) that expel dampness by moving downward to support the natural movement of Lung qi without injuring its yin aspect.

桑杏湯 （桑杏汤）

Mulberry Leaf and Apricot Kernel Decoction

sāng xìng tāng

Source　*Systematic Differentiation of Warm Pathogen Diseases* (1798)

Mori Folium (*sāng yè*) 3g
Gardeniae Fructus (*zhī zǐ*) 3g
Sojae Semen praeparatum (*dàn dòu chǐ*) 3g
Armeniacae Semen (*xìng rén*) 4.5g
Fritillariae thunbergii Bulbus (*zhè bèi mǔ*) 3g
Glehniae/Adenophorae Radix (*shā shēn*) 6g
Pyri Exocarpium (*lí pí*) 3g

Method of Preparation　Decoction. The listed dosage is based on the source text. At present, the dosage is increased 2-3 times.

Actions　Clears and disperses warm-dryness

Indications

Moderate fever, headache, thirst, a dry, hacking cough or one with scanty, thick, and sticky sputum, a red tongue with a thin, dry, and white coating, and a floating, rapid pulse (especially on the right).

　　This is externally contracted warm-dryness injuring the Lung qi at a relatively superficial (exterior) level. This type of disorder occurs most often in the early autumn when the warm qi of summer has still not been dispersed, but the autumnal dryness is already prevalent. It is easily contracted because one does not yet wear appropriate clothing or because of a weakened constitution. The same conditions prevail in air-conditioned or centrally-heated environments. Because the Lungs are responsible for respiration and govern the skin, they are the organ most affected by the external environment. When the weather is dry, dryness will affect the Lungs first. At a relatively exterior level, this leads to moderate fever and headache. Disruption in the flow of Lung qi and the scorching effect of warm-dryness causes a dry, hacking cough. Dryness also depletes the Lung fluids, which manifests as thirst, a red tongue, and a dry tongue coating. The floating, rapid pulse indicates a relatively superficial disorder. It is especially floating on the right (qi) side. Both the pulse and symptomatology resemble that of wind-heat, from which this condition must be distinguished.

Analysis of Formula

The treatment of warm-dryness attacking the Lungs requires the use of cool, acrid herbs to release the exterior, and cool, moistening herbs to facilitate the Lung qi's function of clearing and clarifying. One of the chief herbs, light, acrid, cooling, and aromatic Mori Folium (*sāng yè*), excels at clearing and dredging the Lung collaterals as well as resolving wind-heat in the exterior. Because it is also sweet and moistening in nature, it achieves these effects without damaging the Lung yin. Its deputies, Gardeniae Fructus (*zhī zǐ*) and Sojae Semen praeparatum (*dàn dòu chǐ*), release constrained heat. This combination simultaneously prevents the pathogenic influence from penetrating further into the body while helping release it from the exterior.

The other chief herb, bitter, acrid, and moistening Armeniacae Semen (*xìng rén*), causes the Lung qi to direct downward, transforms phlegm, and stops coughs. Compared to Mori Folium (*sāng yè*), which disperses the protective yang in the exterior and controls the Lungs via the Liver, this herb directly focuses on the interior and the Lungs. Together, they have a synergism that regulates and moistens the Lung qi while also dredging the exterior. Armeniacae Semen (*xìng rén*) is assisted by its deputy, Fritillariae thunbergii Bulbus (*zhè bèi mǔ*), which cools and transforms the stagnation that might otherwise cause phlegm to form. As noted in *Rectification of the Meaning of Materia Medica*, Fritillariae thunbergii Bulbus (*zhè bèi mǔ*) "has a bitter taste and a cooling nature, but also contains acrid, dispersing qi." This allows it to clear heat without causing stagnation. The assistants, Glehniae/Adenophorae Radix (*shā shēn*) and Pyri Exocarpium (*lí pí*), nourish the yin and clear heat. Together, they have a cooling and moistening effect.

Cautions and Contraindications

Contraindicated in cases with injury to the yin. Because this formula is composed of light, disseminating herbs, the dosage should not be too large.

Commentary

The important indications for this formula include a dry, hacking cough, a thin, dry, white tongue coating, and a floating, rapid pulse. It may also be used for conditions at this level that affect the collaterals of the Lungs with coughing of blood and for the treatment of respiratory problems caused by working in dry environments.

In composing this formula, Wu Ju-Tong was influenced by Yu Chang's principles of treating dryness by means of sweet, moistening, and slight cooling, which is discussed in more detail in the entry for Clear Dryness and Rescue the Lungs Decoction (*qīng zào jiù fèi tāng*), as well as by Ye Tian-Shi's treatment of autumn dryness, as outlined in his *Differentiating Lurking Pathogens and Externally-Contracted Diseases during Three Seasons*:

> In the depth of autumn at the onset of cool [weather, one observes] each year a pattern characterized by fever and coughing that resembles the wind-warmth pattern of spring. They differ, however, [in that] warmth designates a lesser degree of heat, and coolness a lesser degree of cold. Disorders occurring during the spring are still a remnant of [excessive] closure [of the pores] by winter cold [constraining yang qi in the interior]. Contraction of damage during the autumn occurs during the period that follows the discharge of summer. The character of [these disorders] thus differs in the sense [that the former constitutes an] excess [and the latter a] deficiency. Yet warm pathogens are naturally contracted in the upper [burner], while dryness naturally [also] damages the upper [burner]. Their [inherent] principles thus resemble each other because [in both cases it is] the Lung qi that contracts the disorder [first] … Vulgar physicians who know about heat disorders [in the Lungs] use Drain the White Powder (*xiè bái sǎn*) with additions like Scutellariae Radix (*huáng qín*) or Coptidis Rhizoma (*huáng lián*) [to treat it], unaware that they prolong the suffering by increasing the dryness [by such use of bitter herbs], leading to further complications. [Rather], one should use acrid, cooling, and sweet moistening formulas. The dry qi will then naturally be balanced and cured. One must carefully avoid using bitter and drying [formulas] that cut off and scorch the Stomach juices.

Ye Tian-Shi's linkage of wind-warmth and warm-dryness disorders with the seasonal movements of qi within and outside the body provides a dynamic perspective for the understanding of these disorders that goes beyond modern textbook presentations, where pathogens are treated as entities that possess distinctive qualities. Wind-warmth in spring occurs because the warm yang qi in the body that seeks to rise upward and outward is fettered by cold in the exterior, which is contracted during the winter. Warm-dryness represents a movement into the body of pathogenic qi that follows the spontaneous movement of autumn, and that can easily penetrate into the body because the pores are still open. Once inside, it leads to constraint that transforms into heat and damages the fluids, which already tend to be deficient because they have been depleted by summer-heat. Thus, this formula not only releases the exterior, but also opens constraint in the interior and generates the fluids of both Lungs and Stomach.

Comparisons

➢ Vs. Apricot Kernel and Perilla Leaf Powder (*xìng sū sǎn*)

Both are light formulas that treat externally-contracted dryness. Apricot Kernel and Perilla Leaf Powder (*xìng sū sǎn*) treats cool-dryness where the fluids are constrained but have not been damaged. Thus, one employs acrid and warming herbs to disperse the exterior and the spreading of the fluids. By contrast, Mulberry Leaf and Apricot Kernel Decoction (*sāng xìng tāng*) treats warm-dryness, where the fluids have already been damaged. Thus, one employs sweet, moistening herbs in addition to acrid, cooling herbs that disperse the exterior.

➢ Vs. Mulberry Leaf and Chrysanthemum Drink (*sāng jú yǐn*)

Both formulas are based on light, acrid, and sweet, moistening herbs. Mulberry Leaf and Chrysanthemum Drink (*sāng jú yīn)* is used to treat early-stage wind-heat disorders invading the Lung collaterals that present with fever, headaches, and coughing. Compared to a Mulberry Leaf and Apricot Kernel Decoction *(sāng xìng tāng)* pattern, the fever and other heat symptoms will tend to be more pronounced and the development more rapid due to the presence of wind. For this reason, the formula combines sweet, moistening herbs with a larger number of light, acrid, and cooling herbs that clear heat and disperse wind.

➤ Vs. Clear Dryness and Rescue the Lungs Decoction *(qīng zào jiù fèi tāng)*; see page 668.

➤ Vs. Fritillaria and Trichosanthes Fruit Powder *(bèi mǔ guā lóu sǎn)*; see page 803

Biomedical Indications

With the appropriate presentation, this formula may be used to treat a variety of biomedically-defined disorders including upper respiratory tract infections, acute and chronic bronchitis, and pertussis.

Modifications

- For more pronounced exterior symptoms like aversion to cold, fever, and the absence of sweating, add Schizonepetae Herba *(jīng jiè)* and Menthae haplocalycis Herba *(bò hé)*.

- For nosebleed, increase the dosage of Gardeniae Fructus *(zhī zǐ)* and add Moutan Cortex *(mǔ dān pí)* and Artemisiae annuae Herba *(qīng hāo)*; alternatively, use Imperatae Rhizoma *(bái máo gēn)* and Ecliptae Herba *(mò hàn lián)*.

- For marked sore throat, add Arctii Fructus *(niú bàng zǐ)* and Scrophulariae Radix *(xuán shēn)*.

- For thick, yellow sputum, add Trichosanthis Pericarpium *(guā lóu pí)* and Aristolochiae Fructus *(mǎ dōu líng)*.

- For dryness of the skin and thirst, add Phragmitis Rhizoma *(lú gēn)* and Trichosanthis Radix *(tiān huā fěn)*.

清燥救肺湯 （清燥救肺汤）
Clear Dryness and Rescue the Lungs Decoction

qīng zào jiù fèi tāng

Source *Precepts for Physicians* (1658)

Mori Folium *(sāng yè)*. 9g
Gypsum fibrosum *(shí gāo)*. 7.5g
Ophiopogonis Radix *(mài mén dōng)* 3.6g
Asini Corii Colla *(ē jiāo)* . . . [dissolve in strained decoction] 2.4g
dry-fried Sesami Semen nigrum *(chǎo hēi zhī má)*. 3g
Armeniacae Semen *(xìng rén)*. 2.1g
honey-prepared Eriobotryae Folium *(mì zhì pí pá yè)* 3g
Ginseng Radix *(rén shēn)* 2.1g
Glycyrrhizae Radix *(gān cǎo)* 3g

Method of Preparation Decoction. Glehniae/Adenophorae Radix *(shā shēn)* or Pseudostellariae Radix *(tài zǐ shēn)* is usually substituted for Ginseng Radix *(rén shēn)* with 2-3 times its dosage. While the source text specifies Gypsum praeparatum *(duàn shí gāo)*, which is calcined, almost all contemporary physicians use unprepared Gypsum fibrosum *(shí gāo)*, reserving the use of the calcined version for external application.

Actions Clears dryness and moistens the Lungs

Indications

Headache, fever, hacking cough, wheezing, a dry and parched throat, dry nasal passages, a sensation of fullness in the chest, hypochondriac pain, irritability, thirst, a dry tongue without coating, and a deficient, big, and rapid pulse.

This is warm-dryness attacking the Lungs with damage to both the qi and yin. Invasion of external warm-dryness constrains the protective yang and causes fever. There is no aversion to cold, indicating that the pathogen has already penetrated to the qi level of the upper burner, that is, the Lungs. This causes the Lung qi to rebel, which is reflected in headaches, cough, and wheezing. When the Lung qi is unable to spread, a sensation of fullness in the chest and pain in the hypochondria develops. The presence of dryness is reflected in the dry, hacking cough, dry nasal passages, parched throat, irritability and thirst, and dry tongue without coating. The injury to the Lungs from warm-dryness also causes a mild deficiency of qi, which is reflected in the deficient and big pulse, and of yin, which is reflected in the rapid pulse.

Analysis of Formula

When warm dryness has damaged the Lung qi and yin such that it can no longer effectively direct the qi downward to clear and clarify, the most effective strategy will be to combine clearing heat and dryness, while also nourishing the fluids, and simultaneously tonifying the qi, while directing it downward. The chief herb in this formula is Mori Folium *(sāng yè)*, which clears and disperses dryness from the Lungs. This herb is often described as soft and moist, and because they don't fall off the mulberry trees until after a frost, they are said to acquire the metal qi of autumn. This inspired Yu Chang to include them as the chief herb in this formula. Gypsum fibrosum *(shí gāo)*, the deputy, clears heat from the Lung (and Stomach) channels and thereby relieves thirst. The relatively small dosage of Gypsum fibrosum *(shí gāo)* prevents this ingredient from inhibiting the spreading action of Mori Folium *(sāng yè)*. A second deputy, Ophiopogonis Radix *(mài mén dōng)*, is sweet and cooling. It nourishes the yin by generating yang fluids. It assists the chief herb by preventing damage to yin due to warm-dryness and by protecting the Lungs as the tender organ.

All of the remaining herbs, with the exception of Glycyrrhizae Radix *(gān cǎo)*, serve as assistants. Asini Corii Colla *(ē jiāo)* and Sesami Semen nigrum *(hēi zhī má)* moisten the

Lungs and nourish the Lung yin. These herbs work to counterbalance the heat-clearing and Lung qi-disseminating actions of the other ingredients with a moistening action. Armeniacae Semen *(xìng rén)* and honey-prepared Eriobotryae Folium *(mì zhì pí pá yè),* two of the assistants, cause the Lung qi to descend and also moisten the Lungs. The other two assistants, Ginseng Radix *(rén shēn)* and Glycyrrhizae Radix *(gān cǎo),* augment the qi and harmonize the middle, thereby supplementing the 'mother' (Spleen) to benefit the 'child' (Lungs). Glehniae/Adenophorae Radix *(shā shēn)* or Pseudostellariae Radix *(tài zǐ shēn)* are usually substituted for Ginseng Radix *(rén shēn)* because they are less expensive, and also because they directly nourish the Lung yin and possess a mild, qi-tonifying action. Glycyrrhizae Radix *(gān cǎo)* is also regarded as an envoy because it harmonizes the actions of the other herbs in the formula.

Cautions and Contraindications

This formula contains rich, cloying substances and should therefore be used with caution in patients with Spleen and Stomach deficiency. Although the formula contains tonifying herbs, its principal application is in cases where the pathogenic influence has not been eliminated. It should not be used for cases of deficiency in the absence of exterior signs.

Commentary

This formula was devised by the early Qing-dynasty physician Yu Chang in response to what he perceived to be an important omission from the arsenal of treatment strategies available to him: a formula that adequately addressed conditions of dryness due to heat in the Lungs, causing the Lungs to fail in their task of regulating the qi dynamic. Successful treatment of this condition requires a certain degree of sophistication. Acrid, aromatic substances are inappropriate because they can injure the Lung qi. Bitter, cold herbs are also inappropriate because they can injure the Stomach and the fluids. Only a combination of ingredients that simultaneously clears dryness and heat, nourishes the yang fluids, directs the Lung qi downward, and tonifies the qi can achieve this complex task. In fact, as Yu Chang pointed out in his own commentary, the real focus of the formula is not the Lungs but the Stomach, which he considered to be the source of the body's yang fluids:

> Now, when composing this formula I named it Clear Dryness and Rescue the Lungs Decoction *(qīng zào jiù fèi tāng).* [However, to achieve] this goal, it focuses on the Stomach qi because [according to the doctrine of the five phases] Stomach earth is the mother of Lung metal. Therefore, I did not use Asparagi Radix *(tiān mén dōng)* even though it is able to protect the Lungs. For its taste is bitter and its qi is stagnating, which made me fear that it might damage the Stomach and [cause] phlegm obstruction. I also did not use Anemarrhenae Rhizoma *(zhī mǔ)* because of its bitterness, even though I know that is able to enrich Kidney water and clear Lung metal. Even more so did I

avoid [the use] of bitter, cooling herbs that direct fire downward and that directly treat the pathogen. Lung metal naturally tends toward dryness, because the yin qi stored within it never [can] exceed [its physiological amount] by even a fraction. If [therefore] one were to purge its qi with bitter, cold [herbs or formulas] and [thereby] damage the Stomach, how could the person still manage to survive?

Here, Yu Chang applied an indirect method of treating the Lungs based on the doctrine of the five phases, discussed above in Chapter 6 in the entry for Licorice and Ginger Decoction *(gān cǎo gān jiāng tāng).* There it was applied to the treatment of Lung yang deficiency. Yu Chang extended it to that of dryness.

This formula is usually prescribed for disorders caused by exposure to dry environmental conditions (including seasonal and indoor dryness). Sometimes patients with acute-onset hemiplegia will have signs and symptoms of dryness invading the Lungs. This formula may be helpful for such patients.

Comparisons

➤ Vs. Mulberry Leaf and Apricot Kernel Decoction *(sāng xìng tāng)*

Both of these formulas treat externally-contracted warm-dryness, but differ in terms of the depth of pathogen penetration and therefore the severity of the disorder. Mulberry Leaf and Apricot Kernel Decoction *(sāng xìng tāng)* treats penetration of a warm-dryness pathogen into the protective level. Thus, fever and dryness symptoms are relatively mild. Slight chills is the key symptom indicating its use, as they are indicative of protective-level disorders. By contrast, Clear Dryness and Rescue the Lungs Decoction *(qīng zào jiù fèi tāng)* treats penetration of a warm-dryness pathogen into the Lung qi level. This stage is characterized by an absence of chills, but the presence of high fever and more pronounced dyness, as well as flank and chest pain and fullness (indicating stagnation), and a dry tongue without coating (indicating damage to the body fluids).

➤ Vs. Glehnia and Ophiopogonis Decoction *(shā shēn mài mén dōng tāng); see* PAGE 670.

➤ Vs. Lily Bulb Decoction to Preserve the Metal *(bǎi hé gù jīn tāng); see* PAGE 386

➤ Vs. Fritillaria and Trichosanthes Fruit Powder *(bèi mǔ guā lóu sǎn); see* PAGE 803

Biomedical Indications

With the appropriate presentation, this formula may be used to treat a variety of biomedically-defined disorders including upper respiratory tract infection, influenza, acute and chronic bronchitis, asthma, bronchiectasis, pulmonary tuberculosis, pneumonia, and pertussis; also for some symptoms of lung cancer.

Modifications

- For profuse, thick, and sticky sputum, add Fritillariae cirrhosae Bulbus (*chuān bèi mǔ*) and Trichosanthis Semen (*guā lóu rén*). (source text)
- For blood-streaked sputum, add Rehmanniae Radix (*shēng dì huáng*) and Platycladi Cacumen (*cè bǎi yè*).
- For constipation, add Persicae Semen (*táo rén*) and Cannabis Semen (*huǒ má rén*).
- For hot Lung atrophy, add Mori Cortex (*sāng bái pí*), Phragmitis Rhizoma (*lú gēn*), Indigo naturalis (*qīng dài*), and Gecko (*gé jiè*).

沙參麥門冬湯（沙参麦门冬汤）

Glehnia and Ophiopogonis Decoction

shā shēn mài mén dōng tāng

Source *Systematic Differentiation of Warm Pathogen Diseases* (1798)

Glehniae/Adenophorae Radix (*shā shēn*) 9g
Ophiopogonis Radix (*mài mén dōng*) 9g
Polygonati odorati Rhizoma (*yù zhú*) 6g
Mori Folium (*sāng yè*). 4.5g
Trichosanthis Radix (*tiān huā fěn*) 4.5g
Lablab Semen album (*biǎn dòu*) 4.5g
Glycyrrhizae Radix (*gān cǎo*) 3g

Method of Preparation Decoction. The source text advises to decoct the herbs in 5 cups of water until 2 cups remain. The decoction should be taken twice a day.

Actions Clears and nourishes the Lungs and Stomach, generates fluids, and moistens dryness

Indications

Dry throat, thirst, fever, a hacking cough with scanty sputum, a red tongue with little coating, and a rapid, thin pulse.

This is injury to the Lungs, Stomach, and fluids from dryness. This pattern usually occurs in a constitutionally yin-deficient patient who contracts external cool-dryness during the autumn. The Lungs, the organ associated with dryness/metal, is most easily damaged by the invasion of external pathogens. In someone already suffering from damage to the fluids, the two pathologies combine, with each exacerbating the other. This condition, by definition, involves the Stomach because it is the organ responsible for the generation of body fluids. Deficiency of fluids in the Lungs leads to a dry throat, while deficiency of fluids in the Stomach leads to thirst. The red tongue, the lack of tongue coating, and the thin pulse are other symptoms of fluid deficiency. Fever and a rapid pulse are due to internal heat from yin deficiency. The hacking cough with scanty sputum reflects obstruction of the Lung qi by the invasion of external cool-dryness.

Analysis of Formula

This formula combines sweet and cooling herbs that generate fluids to clear and nourish the Lungs and Stomach. There are three chief herbs: Glehniae/Adenophorae Radix (*shā shēn*), Ophiopogonis Radix (*mài mén dōng*), and Mori Folium (*sāng yè*). Glehniae/Adenophorae Radix (*shā shēn*) is cooling, sweet, and slightly bitter. Despite its moistening nature, it is thought to dredge the Lungs. It is thus ideally suited for conditions where the tonification of Lung yin must be combined with the venting of pathogens to the exterior. Because it more strongly tonifies the Stomach yin, Glehniae Radix (*běi shā shēn*) is the most commonly-used form of this herb in the formula. Ophiopogonis Radix (*mài mén dōng*) is a sweet, cooling substance that enters both the Lungs and Stomach. It combines with Glehniae/Adenophorae Radix (*shā shēn*) to nourish the yin by generating fluids. Mori Folium (*sāng yè*) excels at clearing warm-dryness because of its acrid, cooling nature. In combination with Glehniae/Adenophorae Radix (*shā shēn*) and Ophiopogonis Radix (*mài mén dōng*), it vents the pathogenic heat and expels the dryness while enriching and nourishing the fluids of the Lungs and Stomach.

Polygonati odorati Rhizoma (*yù zhú*) and Trichosanthis Radix (*tiān huā fěn*) serve as deputies. Polygonati odorati Rhizoma (*yù zhú*) nourishes the yin and moistens dryness. It enriches without being cloying. Trichosanthis Radix (*tiān huā fěn*) clears heat and generates yang fluids. Used together, they support the chief herbs in generating fluids and clearing internal heat. Damage to the Stomach yin invariably affects the transportive and transforming functions of the middle burner and eventually damages the Spleen. For this reason, the formula includes Lablab Semen album (*bái biǎn dòu*) as an assistant. Building the Spleen and Stomach to assist the transportation and transformation, this herb ensures that the earth is sufficiently strong to support the generation of metal. Glycyrrhizae Radix (*gān cǎo*) clears heat and harmonizes the middle burner, regulating the functions of the other herbs, and thereby serves as the envoy.

Cautions and Contraindications

This is a representative formula for tonifying while also clearing and nourishing the Lungs and Stomach. It is inappropriate for patterns characterized by heat excess damaging the body fluids.

Commentary

This formula was composed by Wu Ju-Tong and was listed in the section on autumn dryness disorders in the first chapter of *Systematic Differentiation of Warm Pathogen Diseases*. This section of the book systematically analyzes the penetration of dry pathogens into the body. Penetration of pathogens into the protective qi aspect are treated with Mulberry Leaf and Apricot Kernel Decoction (sāng xìng tāng) and Mulberry Leaf and Chrysanthemum Drink (sāng jú yǐn). At this stage, the focus is on venting the heat and moistening the dryness. If the condition progresses to damage the Lung and Stomach yin, usually in a patient with preexisting yin deficiency, one must adapt the treatment strategies accordingly. It is now more important to focus on generating yang fluids in order to ensure that sufficient yin is available to support the unhindered movement of the protective yang, enabling it to vent the pathogen.

From an historical perspective, this formula is a variation of Ophiopogonis Decoction (mài mén dōng tāng), discussed in more detail below. In contemporary practice, its usage has been extended to the treatment of internal medicine disorders, where it is used for conditions characterized by damage to the Lung and Stomach yin such as certain types of wasting and thirsting disorder. Its mild nature makes it especially useful in pediatric practice.

Comparison

➤ Vs. CLEAR DRYNESS AND RESCUE THE LUNGS
  DECOCTION (qīng zào jiù fèi tāng)

These formulas treat similar patterns. Clear Dryness and Rescue the Lungs Decoction (qīng zào jiù fèi tāng) is used when there is exuberant heat damaging the yang fluids and qi. By contrast, Glehnia and Ophiopogonis Decoction (shā shēn mài mén dōng tāng) is indicated for generally milder conditions that are characterized by damage to the body fluids without severe heat.

Biomedical Indications

With the appropriate presentation, this formula may be used to treat a variety of biomedically-defined disorders including pneumonia, bronchitis, pulmonary tuberculosis, chronic gastritis, and diabetes.

Modifications

- For chronic fever and cough, add Lycii Cortex (dì gǔ pí). (source text)

- For more pronounced coughing as the chief presenting symptom, add Fritillariae Bulbus (bèi mǔ) and Armeniacae Semen (xìng rén).

- For blood-streaked sputum, add Agrimoniae Herba (xiān hè cǎo), Bletillae Rhizoma (bái jí), and Asini Corii Colla (ē jiāo).

- For constipation with dry stools, add Trichosanthis Fructus (quán guā lóu) and Cannabis Semen (huǒ má rén).

- For more pronounced thirst due to damage of the Stomach yin, add Pyri Succus (lí zhī).

Section 2

....

FORMULAS THAT ENRICH THE YIN AND MOISTEN DRYNESS

The formulas in this section treat internal dryness where the fluids of the organs have been exhausted and harmed. The most common symptoms of this pattern include cough with scanty sputum, nausea and vomiting, a dry mouth, wasting and thirsting disorder, constipation, dry or cracked skin, a tongue with little coating, and a thin pulse. This condition is often caused by internal disharmonies but may also appear as the sequelae of externally-contracted dryness. The chief herbs used for treating this disorder are those that moisten dryness by enriching the yin and generating fluids such as Ophiopogonis Radix (mài mén dōng), Rehmanniae Radix (shēng dì huáng), and Scrophulariae Radix (xuán shēn). Depending on the context, these herbs are combined with others that augment the qi and harmonize the middle, or that clear heat. Herbs that augment the qi and harmonize the middle, like Atractylodis macrocephalae Rhizoma (bái zhú), Poria (fú líng), Astragali Radix (huáng qí), or Pinelliae Rhizoma praeparatum (zhì bàn xià), support the Spleen and Stomach as the sources of the body's postnatal essence, including the fluids. Herbs that clear heat, like Moutan Cortex (mǔ dān pí), Anemarrhenae Rhizoma (zhī mǔ), and Trichosanthis Radix (tiān huā fěn), are used when internal dryness causing yin deficiency leads to heat, or where heat causes dryness.

When using the formulas in this category, it is important to properly differentiate between internal and external dryness. Prescribing a formula that enriches the yin and moistens dryness for a condition in which the pathogenic influence is still active in the exterior may cause the pathogenic influence to linger or may exacerbate the condition. Conversely, the use of herbs that disperse externally-contracted dryness where the condition is actually one of internal dryness with yin deficiency will aggravate the injury to the qi and yin.

麥門冬湯 （麦门冬汤）
Ophiopogonis Decoction
mài mén dōng tāng

Source *Essentials from the Golden Cabinet* (c. 220)

Ophiopogonis Radix (mài mén dōng) 15-64g
Ginseng Radix (rén shēn) 9g
Nonglutinous rice (jīng mǐ) 6-15g
Jujubae Fructus (dà zǎo) . . . . 12 pieces
Glycyrrhizae Radix (gān cǎo) 6g
Pinelliae Rhizoma praeparatum (zhì bàn xià) 6-9g

Method of Preparation Decoction. The source text advises to divide the decoction into four portions. Three portions are taken during the day and the fourth at night. At present, 3-4 pieces of Jujubae Fructus (*dà zǎo*) are used, rather than the 12 listed above.

Actions Benefits the Stomach, generates fluids, and directs rebellious qi downward

Indications

Coughing, wheezing, shortness of breath, coughing up of phlegm that is difficult to expectorate, or spitting of saliva, a dry and uncomfortable sensation in the throat, dry mouth, heat of the palms and soles, a dry, red tongue with little coating, and a deficient, rapid pulse.

The original indication of this formula is Lung atrophy (肺痿 *fèi wěi*) due to heat. Although the symptoms are primarily related to the Lungs, the condition is actually caused by heat from deficiency in the Stomach, which rises rebelliously and scorches the Lung yin. It may also be understood by reference to the theory of the five phases, wherein the 'mother' (Stomach) transmits the problem to the 'child' (Lungs). Today, the formula is used mainly for two patterns: insufficiency of Lung yin and insufficiency of Stomach yin.

The Lungs are the most delicate of the yin organs and serve as a canopy for the trunk. They depend on the earth (Spleen/Stomach) for nourishment and for some of their fluids. If, over an extended period of time, the Lungs do not receive proper nourishment or moisture, they shrivel up or 'atrophy.' The rebellious qi from the Stomach prevents the Lung qi from descending properly, and results in coughing and wheezing. The scorching of the Lung yin causes shortness of breath and depletes the fluids. The depletion of the fluids leaves only saliva or a thick, viscous sputum that becomes lodged in the throat, causes a dry, uncomfortable sensation, and is difficult to expectorate. The dry mouth and the tongue and pulse signs are classic indications of heat from deficiency leading to internal dryness.

Analysis of Formula

Following the classical precepts of moistening dryness and tonifying the 'mother' in case of deficiency, the focus of this formula is on moistening and nourishing the Stomach earth yin in order to also treat manifestations affecting Lung metal. Only secondarily does it direct the rebellious qi downward. The chief herb, Ophiopogonis Radix (*mài mén dōng*), clears heat from deficiency from the Stomach and generates fluids in the Stomach and Lungs. It is therefore very useful in the treatment of Lung atrophy. The deputy, Ginseng Radix (*rén shēn*), augments the qi, generates fluids, and revives the qi and yin. Ophiopogonis Radix (*mài mén dōng*) and Ginseng Radix (*rén shēn*) form a particularly powerful combination for reviving the qi and yin of the Lungs and Stomach.

The balance of the ingredients are regarded as assistants. Nonglutinous rice, Jujubae Fructus (*dà zǎo*), and Glycyrrhizae Radix (*gān cǎo*) work synergistically with the chief and deputy herbs to assist the Stomach qi and generate fluids. While Glycyrrhizae Radix praeparata (*zhì gān cǎo*) has a relatively stronger action in tonifying the Stomach, its unprepared form is used here because it also improves the condition of the throat. The assistant, Pinelliae Rhizoma praeparatum (*zhì bàn xià*), facilitates the flow of Stomach qi and directs the qi downward. The warm, acrid, drying nature of this herb is moderated by the moistening herbs in the formula and by its relatively low dosage. In fact, adding a small amount of this acrid, dispersing herb to the formula will assist in the distribution of nourishment from the middle burner to the upper burner, and redirect the qi, thereby facilitating the replenishment of fluids in the Lungs.

Cautions and Contraindications

Use with caution in cases with high fever and irritability, where the pathogenic influence remains in the exterior, and the qi and yin have yet to be affected. Contraindicated in cases with dampness or Lung atrophy due to cold from deficiency.

Commentary

Historically, the most common use of this formula has been for Lung atrophy, based on its indication for this purpose in *Emergency Formulas to Keep Up One's Sleeve*. Lung atrophy is marked by incessant coughing and spitting of saliva, a dry throat, and thirst. Other uses in the classical and modern literature include Lung dryness coughing, coughing of blood, and yin deficiency leading to stirring of wind with dizziness and stomach pain accompanied by nausea and vomiting of phlegm (*Case Records as a Guide to Clinical Practice*); wheezing and coughing (*Selected Annotations to Ancient Formulas from the Garden of Crimson Snow*); pulmonary tuberculosis with chronic cough and phlegm in the throat that is difficult to expectorate (*Imperial Han Medicine*); and, more generally, Lung and Stomach yin deficiency patterns (*Formulas by Li Fei*). All of these are, to a greater or lesser extent, interpretations by later commentators of the rather terse definition of the formula's core pattern in the source text: "rebellious fire and ascending of qi leading to obstruction of the throat."

Core Clinical Manifestation and Pathodynamic

As outlined by Chen Nian-Zu in *Simple Annotation of the Essentials from the Golden Cabinet*, the fire underlying this pattern is a type of yin fire caused by internal dysfunction rather than the invasion of external pathogens into the body. This implies that it must be treated by tonification (of yin and qi) and regulation of the qi dynamic, rather than eliminated by means of bitter, cooling or acrid, dispersing herbs. The pathological ascent of qi represents both an effect of this yin fire and damage to the downward-directing functions of the Lungs and Stomach. Commentators agree that, in practice, such rebelliousness may manifest with many different symptoms including nausea, vomiting, hiccup, belching, coughing, wheezing, dysphagia, spitting or vomiting of blood, and blood-streaked coughing.

Differentiation from other patterns with the same symptoms thus requires careful analysis. If contemporary textbooks emphasize Lung and Stomach deficiency (i.e., organ system diagnosis patterns), experts in the usage of classical formulas highlight the presence of key signs and symptoms mentioned in the source text. In the present case, this is 'throat obstruction' (咽喉不利 *yān hóu bù lì*). In *One-Hundred Classic Formulas*, the contemporary writer Huang Huang describes such obstruction as characterized by dryness or itching of the throat, or as phlegm that is difficult to expectorate. In his opinion, this does not imply that there is necessarily very little phlegm, but rather that the presence of phlegm will be accompanied by a sensation of dryness, itchiness, or obstruction in the throat.

The presence of throat obstruction against a background of Lung and Stomach yin deficiency helps to differentiate patterns for which this formula is indicated from similar presentations but a different underlying pathodynamic, such as Pinellia and Magnolia Bark Decoction (*bàn xià hòu pò tāng*), which treats throat obstruction resulting from qi stagnation and excess phlegm. Formulas like Lophatherum and Gypsum Decoction (*zhú yè shí gāo tāng*), on the other hand, which also treat coughing against a background of heat and yin and qi deficiency, present with a stronger degree of heat (as reflected, e.g., in the presence of fever or a flooding pulse) and less or no throat obstruction.

Actions and Synergies between Chief and Deputy Ingredients

This formula may be regarded as a modification of Lophatherum and Gypsum Decoction (*zhú yè shí gāo tāng*), discussed in Chapter 4. The ingredients in the title of that formula are omitted here, and the dosage of Ophiopogonis Radix (*mài mén dōng*) is increased. Some contemporary sources recommend a dosage of as much as 45g or even 70g of this herb, noting that a lesser amount will diminish the formula's efficacy. While such an increase in dosage may partially reflect changes in herb quality, reviewing the actions of the chief ingredient is nevertheless central to understanding the usage of the entire formula. An extended discussion from *New Compilation of Materia Medica* is very useful for this purpose:

> Ophiopogonis Radix (*mài mén dōng*) drains lurking heat from the Lungs and clears heat pathogens from the Stomach. It tonifies consumptive damage of the Heart qi, stops vomiting

of blood, augments the essence, strengthens the yin, relieves irritability, stops thirst, beautifies the complexion, is pleasing to the skin, reduces fever from deficiency, resolves Lung dryness, and stops coughing. It truly should be prescribed as a chief herb, but can also be used as deputy or assistant. Unfortunately, the common people do not know about the marvelous uses of Ophiopogonis Radix (*mài mén dōng*) [anymore]. Gradually, they have used less and less [of it] and no longer achieve results. This is too bad. They do not know that one must use Ophiopogonis Radix (*mài mén dōng*) in large amounts in order to open up its power. [In case of] lurking heat in the Lungs scorching dry the yin fluids in the interior, only a large dosage of Ophiopogonis Radix (*mài mén dōng*) can control the fire. [In case of] fire blazing within the Stomach and depleting its yin, only a large dosage of Ophiopogonis Radix (*mài mén dōng*) can extinguish this fire.

The second key ingredient is Pinelliae Rhizoma praeparatum (*zhì bàn xià*), which, according to the Ming-dynasty physician Wang Zi-Jie, is responsible for the dynamic action of the formula. Whereas all the other ingredients can be viewed as constructing earth in order to tonify metal, and thereby as moistening dryness, the acrid and warming nature of Pinelliae Rhizoma praeparatum (*zhì bàn xià*) directs the qi downward through the hand yang brightness Large Intestine. It thereby facilitates the clarifying and downward-directing movement of the Lungs and opens the Triple Burner so that both the qi and fire can be pacified.

Expanded Clinical Usage

The interaction between the key ingredients Ophiopogonis Radix (*mài mén dōng*) and Pinelliae Rhizoma praeparatum (*zhì bàn xià*)—centered on the treatment of rebellious fire with rising qi, as indicated in the source text—allows for a much wider field of application. In *Discussion of Blood Patterns*, the late 19th-century physician Tang Zong-Hai provided a cogent summary of these possibilities:

> The four herbs Ginseng Radix (*rén shēn*), Nonglutinous rice (*jīng mǐ*), Glycyrrhizae Radix (*gān cǎo*), and Jujubae Fructus (*dà zǎo*) greatly construct the middle burner qi and generate body fluids. The Stomach yang fluids are transported upward to the Lungs. When the Lungs clear [through their directing downward,] fire is naturally calmed; when they are regulated, the qi naturally flows smoothly. Fire and qi that are not rebelling or ascending are satisfactorily calmed in this manner. However, fire and qi that have already rebelled and ascended are not put to task [in this way] and linger on. Therefore, [the formula] employs Ophiopogonis Radix (*mài mén dōng*) as chief in order to clear the fire and Pinelliae Rhizoma praeparatum (*zhì bàn xià*) as assistant in order to regulate the qi. When the fire and qi are directed downward, the body fluids are generated. When the body fluids are generated, fire and qi are naturally directed downward. They flow [as they should] and not in a perverse [manner]. Using this formula to treat cough with dry phlegm is the most [appropriate] symptom [for which its use is indicated]. As it moistens and promotes the Stomach and Lungs, it also treats food stagnation in the diaphragm. It can furthermore

treat upward rebellion of qi in the Penetrating [vessel], carrying phlegm and blood [upward] and interfering with Lung [function]. The Penetrating vessel arises in the uterus and connects with the Kidneys and Liver below, but [unfolds] its true majestic [nature] through the yang brightness. In order to regulate the blood of yang brightness, it enters into the uterus below. When the qi of yang brightness flows smoothly, the qi of the Penetrating vessel also flows smoothly. The blood and water of the uterus also then return to their [natural] abode and do not rebel upward. Comparing this formula to Minor Bupleurum Decoction *(xiǎo chái hú tāng)* is even more enlightening [in this respect]. Minor Bupleurum Decoction *(xiǎo chái hú tāng)* guides the qi of the Penetrating vessel upward by way of the Stomach. This is a strategy for preventing fire from becoming constrained in the lower [burner]. This formula directs the qi of the Penetrating vessel downward by way of the Stomach. This is a strategy for not letting fire ascend and interfere with the upper [burner].

The formula is thus used in the treatment of menstrual disorders, as well as for belching, nausea, or vomiting due to Stomach yin deficiency. It has exerted considerable influence on the development of Chinese medical doctrines. The focus on the preservation of body fluids and on the preservation of the Stomach yin, associated with physicians like Ye Tian-Shi and Xue Sheng-Bai, can be traced to the strategies contained in this formula. It is one of many examples of how the development of warm pathogen treatment strategies must be seen as an extension of those for cold damage disorders.

Comparison

➤ Vs. Precious Jade Syrup *(qióng yù gāo)*; see page 391

Biomedical Indications

With the appropriate presentation, this formula may be used to treat a variety of biomedically-defined disorders including laryngitis, pertussis, bronchiectasis, pneumonia, acute and chronic bronchitis, asthma, hypertension, diabetes, peptic ulcer, reactive lymphoid hyperplasia, and the side effects of radiation therapy.

Modifications

- For severe depletion of the fluids, add Glehniae/Adenophorae Radix *(shā shēn)* and Polygonati odorati Rhizoma *(yù zhú)*.

- For tidal fever, add Stellariae Radix *(yín chái hú)* and Lycii Cortex *(dì gǔ pí)*.

- For severe cough, add Fritillariae cirrhosae Bulbus *(chuān bèi mǔ)* and Trichosanthis Semen *(guā lóu rén)*.

- For oral side effects of radiation therapy with dryness that is worse at night, irritability, a dry tongue, and a rapid and thin pulse, add Chrysanthemi Flos *(jú huā)*, Trichosanthis Radix *(tiān huā fěn)*, Glehniae/Adenophorae Radix *(shā shēn)*, Dioscoreae Rhizoma *(shān yào)*, and Moutan Cortex *(mǔ dān pí)*.

Associated Formula

加味麥門冬湯（加味麦门冬汤）
Augmented Ophiopogonis Decoction
jiā wèi mài mén dōng tāng

Source   *Essays on Medicine Esteeming the Chinese and Respecting the Western* (1918-1934)

Ophiopogonis Radix *(mài mén dōng)* 15g
Ginseng Radix *(rén shēn)* 12g
Pinelliae Rhizoma praeparatum *(zhì bàn xià)* 9g
Dioscoreae Rhizoma *(shān yào)* 12g
Paeoniae Radix alba *(bái sháo)* 9g
Salviae miltiorrhizae Radix *(dān shēn)* 9g
Glycyrrhizae Radix *(gān cǎo)* 6g
Persicae Semen *(táo rén)* 6g
Jujubae Fructus *(dà zǎo)* . . . . .3 pieces

Benefits the Stomach, regulates the Penetrating vessel, and directs rebellious qi and blood downward. For inverted menses (nosebleed or vomiting of blood during the menses). Zhang Xi-Chun, the author of this formula, explained its efficacy by referring to the relationship of the Penetrating vessel to the yang brightness Stomach channel with which it connects superiorly. When the Stomach is deficient, its qi cannot move downward properly to anchor the qi of the Penetrating vessel. This leads to an upward rebellion or 'gushing' of the Penetrating vessel's qi. The blood follows the qi upward, and inverted menses results. It is clear that Zhang Xi-Chun borrowed this idea from Tang Zong-Hai, who had earlier discussed this topic at length (see the discussion of extended clinical usage in the COMMENTARY above).

養陰清肺湯（养阴清肺汤）
Nourish the Yin and Clear the Lungs Decoction
yǎng yīn qīng fèi tāng

Source   *Jade Key to Layered Stories* (18th century)

Rehmanniae Radix *(shēng dì huáng)* .6g
Scrophulariae Radix *(xuán shēn)* 4.5g
Ophiopogonis Radix *(mài mén dōng)* 3.6g
dry-fried Paeoniae Radix alba *(chǎo bái sháo)* 2.4g
Moutan Cortex *(mǔ dān pí)* 2.4g
Fritillariae Bulbus *(bèi mǔ)* 2.4g
Menthae haplocalycis Herba *(bò hé)* 1.5g
Glycyrrhizae Radix *(gān cǎo)* 1.5g

Method of Preparation   Decoction. At present, the dosage is increased 2-3 times. Fritillariae cirrhosae Bulbus *(chuān bèi mǔ)* is generally the species of Fritillariae Bulbus *(bèi mǔ)* used.

Actions   Nourishes the yin, clears the Lungs, improves the condition of the throat, and resolves toxicity

Indications

Development of a white, curd-like membrane in the throat that is difficult to scrape off, swollen and sore throat, fever, dry nasal passages, parched lips, raspy breathing resembling wheezing, a red and dry tongue, and a rapid, usually thin pulse. There may also be coughing.

This is 'white throat' (白喉 *bái hóu*) or diphtherial disorder, which usually develops in those with constitutional yin deficiency and internal clumping of heat who contract epidemic toxin (疫毒 *yì dú*). Epidemic toxin further injures the deficient fluids, and hot epidemic toxin fumes upward, causing the distinctive symptom of a white, curd-like membrane in the throat that is difficult to scrape off. This membrane interferes with breathing and causes it to become raspy. The fever, tongue, and pulse signs are characteristic of heat with yin deficiency. The sore and swollen throat, dry nasal passages, and parched lips are due to hot epidemic toxin and heat (from Kidney and Lung yin deficiency) rising upward. This type of deficiency can also disrupt the qi mechanism of the Lungs, which produces coughing.

Analysis of Formula

The chief herb in this formula is sweet, bitter, and cooling Rehmanniae Radix (*shēng dì huáng.*) It enriches the yin fluids to support the normal qi while cooling the blood and resolving toxicity to dispel the pathogenic qi. Scrophulariae Radix (*xuán shēn*), Ophiopogonis Radix (*mài mén dōng*), and Paeoniae Radix alba (*bái sháo*) serve as deputies and assist the chief herbs in nourishing the yin. Scrophulariae Radix (*xuán shēn*) is salty and cooling, enriches the yin, directs fire downward, resolves toxicity, and improves the condition of the throat. This herb is routinely used in the treatment of sores from yin deficiency, particularly of the throat. Ophiopogonis Radix (*mài mén dōng*) acts on the Lungs, which are connected to the throat as a main pathway of qi. Scrophulariae Radix (*xuán shēn*) focuses on the Kidney yin, while Ophiopogonis Radix (*mài mén dōng*) focuses on the Lung yin. Together, they nourish the upper and lower sources of water. Paeoniae Radix alba (*bái sháo*) preserves and protects the yin.

Moutan Cortex (*mǔ dān pí*), Fritillariae cirrhosae Bulbus (*chuān bèi mǔ*), and Menthae haplocalycis Herba (*bò hé*) act as assistants. Moutan Cortex (*mǔ dān pí*) cools the blood, reduces swelling, and thereby supports the functions of the chief herb. Fritillariae cirrhosae Bulbus (*chuān bèi mǔ*) moistens the Lungs, stops coughing, and clears and transforms phlegm-heat. Together with Moutan Cortex (*mǔ dān pí*) and Paeoniae Radix alba (*bái sháo*), it disperses the swelling in the throat and stops the pain. Menthae haplocalycis Herba (*bò hé*) is added to help vent the pathogenic qi to the exterior. Being acrid, it also provides movement to the qi and thereby facilitates the unclogging of the throat. Glycyrrhizae Radix (*gān cǎo*) resolves toxicity, improves the condition of the throat, and harmonizes the actions of the other herbs in the formula.

Cautions and Contraindications

Diphtheria is a very serious, even life-threatening disease, and extreme care must be exercised in its treatment. In China, this condition is treated with a combination of traditional Chinese herbs and biomedicine, especially in cases with breathing difficulties.

Commentary

This formula is an example for how Chinese medicine has historically adjusted to the appearance of new types of disease. The condition known as diphtherial disorder (lit. 'white throat' 白喉 *bái hóu*) did not appear in China prior to the mid-18th century. Initially, following established treatment strategies for feverish disorders, many physicians treated the condition with acrid, dispersing formulas that release the exterior even though, in terms of its nature—a highly contagious epidemic disorder with distinctive throat symptoms that manifest early in the course of the disease—it did not fit known patterns of cold damage disorders. The 18th-century physician Zheng Hong-Gang was the first to propose an entirely new approach, published posthumously by his son Zheng Han-Jia in *Jade Key to Many Towers.*

Regarding the etiology of diphtherial disorder, Zheng Hong-Gang stated: "This disorder arises from the Lungs and Kidneys in those with deficiency, or in those who have contracted a prevalent dry qi, or who eat too many spicy and hot foods." With regard to treatment, he argued that "In general, one must nourish the yin and clear the Lungs, and combine this with acrid, cooling, and dispersing as the governing [strategy]." Thereafter, Zheng Hong-Gang's approach became established as the most effective in the field. Its continued utility was proven during a serious diphtheria epidemic in Tianjin in 1960 that was treated with a formula based in part on Nourish the Yin and Clear the Lungs Decoction (*yǎng yīn qīng fèi tāng*).

This formula is used for a variety of severe throat infections and other problems. It is advisable to combine it with external applications of a powder painted onto the throat or blown into the throat with the help of a tube. A typical formula for this purpose combines heat-draining, phlegm-transforming, and toxicity-resolving herbs. An example is a mixture of Canarii Fructus (*qīng guǒ*) 6g, Phellodendri Cortex (*huáng bǎi*) 3g, Fritillariae cirrhosae Bulbus (*chuān bèi mǔ*) 3g, Borneolum (*bīng piàn*) 1.5g, Catechu (*ér chá*) 3g, Menthae haplocalycis Herba (*bò hé*) 3g, and Galli Membrana Ovi (*fèng huáng yī*)* 1.5g.

---

* Galli Membrana Ovi (鳳凰衣 *fèng huáng yī*) is bland and neutral, enters the Spleen, Stomach, and Lung channels, and nourishes the yin, clears the Lungs, fills in sores, reduces superficial visual obstruction, and mends bones. The normal dosage is 3-9g. Use with caution in those with Spleen and Stomach deficiency.

Biomedical Indications

With the appropriate presentation, this formula may be used to treat a variety of biomedically-defined disorders including diphtheria, tonsillitis, pharyngitis, and the side effects of radiation therapy to tumors of the head and throat.

Modifications

- For severe constitutional yin deficiency, add Rehmanniae Radix praeparata *(shú dì huáng).* (source text)
- For severe dryness, add Asparagi Radix *(tiān mén dōng),* Anemarrhenae Rhizoma *(zhī mǔ),* and Phragmitis Rhizoma *(lú gēn).*
- For severe swelling and pain in the throat, add Belamcandae Rhizoma *(shè gān),* Platycodi Radix *(jié gěng),* Bombyx batryticatus *(bái jiāng cán),* and Lasiosphaera/Calvatia *(mǎ bó).*
- For marked exterior signs, add Mori Folium *(sāng yè)* and Cicadae Periostracum *(chán tuì).*
- For more pronounced fever, add Forsythiae Fructus *(lián qiáo),* Lonicerae Flos *(jīn yín huā),* and Isatidis/Baphicacanthis Radix *(bǎn lán gēn).*

Associated Formula

四陰煎 （四阴煎）

Four-Yin Decoction

sì yīn jiān

Source *Collected Treatises of [Zhang] Jing-Yue (1624)*

Rehmanniae Radix *(shēng dì huáng)* 6-9g
Ophiopogonis Radix *(mài mén dōng)* 6g
Paeoniae Radix alba *(bái sháo)* 6g
Lilii Bulbus *(bǎi hé)* 6g
Glehniae/Adenophorae Radix *(shā shēn)* 6g
Glycyrrhizae Radix *(gān cǎo)* 3g
Poria *(fú líng)* 4.5g

Decoction. The source text specifies to take the decoction separate from meals. Nourishes the yin, clears heat, protects the Lungs, and stops coughing. For yin deficiency consumption with blazing of the ministerial fire leading to parching of the yang fluids characterized by irritability and thirst, coughing, spitting up blood, spontaneous external bleeding, and severe fever. Compared to the principal formula, this focuses more strongly on nourishing the yin to protect the yang, that is, on the yang rather than the yin fluids. Nourish the Yin and Clear the Lungs Decoction *(yǎng yīn qīng fèi tāng),* on the other hand, focuses on resolving toxins that clog the throat and thus includes acrid, dispersing herbs.

玉液湯 （玉液汤）

Jade Fluid Decoction

yù yè tāng

Jade symbolizes that which is precious and refers to this formula's ability to repair the mechanism by which the body replenishes its fluids. In Daoist longevity practices, the term 'jade spring' (玉泉 *yù quán)* refers to the fluids secreted by the two vessels below the tongue. These fluids are viewed as the origin of the generation of yin essence in the body. Jade is yin in nature and symbolizes the essence that is generated by this formula's actions.

Source *Essays on Medicine Esteeming the Chinese and Respecting the Western (1918-1934)*

Dioscoreae Rhizoma *(shān yào)* 30g
Astragali Radix *(huáng qí)* 15g
Anemarrhenae Rhizoma *(zhī mǔ)* .18g
Trichosanthis Radix *(tiān huā fěn)* .9g
Gigeriae galli Endothelium corneum *(jī nèi jīn)* 6g
Puerariae Radix *(gé gēn)* 4.5g
Schisandrae Fructus *(wǔ wèi zǐ)* 9g

Method of Preparation Decoction.

Actions Augments the qi, generates fluids, moistens dryness, and alleviates thirst

Indications

Excessive thirst that is not quenched by a substantial intake of fluids, frequent, copious, or turbid urine, lassitude, shortness of breath, and a deficient, thin, and weak pulse.

This is one type of wasting and thirsting disorder due to deficiency of the primal qi, which fails to ascend and transport fluids upward. As a result, the Lungs become depleted of fluids, leading to thirst. The Lungs also lose their ability to control the water metabolism, causing frequent, copious, or turbid urine. Lung deficiency also manifests as shortness of breath, while the more generalized deficiency of primal qi is reflected in lassitude and the deficient, weak pulse.

Analysis of Formula

One of the chief ingredients, Dioscoreae Rhizoma *(shān yào),* tonifies the Spleen, stabilizes the Kidneys to stop the frequent urination, and moistens the Lungs and generates fluids to reduce the thirst. The other chief ingredient, Astragali Radix *(huáng qí),* reduces thirst by raising the primal qi, and supports the Lungs' function of dispersing the fluids throughout the body. These herbs work synergistically with each other. The deputy ingredients are Anemarrhenae Rhizoma *(zhī mǔ)* and Trichosanthis Radix *(tiān huā fěn),* which treat thirst by enriching the yin, draining fire, and moistening dryness. Together with the chief herbs, they treat both the root and branch of this pattern.

The remaining ingredients serve as assistants. Gigeriae galli Endothelium corneum *(jī nèi jīn)* supports the transforming and transporting functions of the Spleen to encourage the production of fluids from food. Puerariae Radix *(gé gēn)* raises the clear yang and helps to convey the fluids to the upper burner. Schisandrae Fructus *(wǔ wèi zǐ)* acts to preserve the yin, generate fluids, and stabilize the essence of the Kidneys; not only does this help reduce the flow of urine, but more importantly, it prevents further injury to the Lungs and Kidneys.

Cautions and Contraindications

This formula is indicated for a specific pattern of diabetes characterized by failure of primal qi to ascend. It is unsuitable for patterns characterized by yang brightness excess heat with internal clumping, or insufficiency of ministerial fire.

Commentary

Based on similarities in their clinical presentation, many modern physicians equate wasting and thirsting disorder with the biomedical disease category of diabetes. The present formula is one of the earliest documents of this convergence. It was composed by the early 20th-century physician Zhang Xi-Chun, who belonged to the 'convergence and assimilation current' in Chinese medicine. Physicians affiliated with this current actively sought to utilize Western medical knowledge for the advancement of Chinese medicine. Zhang Xi-Chun was its most influential representative in the domain of actual clinical practice.

Historically, wasting and thirsting disorder had been organized into three main categories based on the location of its root in one of the three burners. Upper burner wasting (上消 *shàng xiāo*), characterized by thirst that cannot be quenched, is attributed to the Lungs' inability to control water. This can be due to Heart or Stomach fire scorching the Lungs, or constitutional deficiencies impairing Lung function. It is treated with formulas like White Tiger plus Ginseng Decoction (*bái hǔ jiā rén shēn tāng*). Middle burner wasting (中消 *zhōng xiāo*), characterized by incessant hunger, is attributed to excess heat in the Spleen and Stomach, and is treated with formulas like Regulate the Stomach and Order the Qi Decoction (*tiáo wèi chéng qì tāng*). Lower burner wasting (下消 *xià xiāo*), characterized by increased urination, is attributed to insufficiency of the ministerial fire with inability of the Kidneys to control the urinary orifice, and is treated with formulas like Kidney Qi Pill (*shèn qì wán*).

Zhang Xi-Chun, who knew some rudimentary Western science, integrated this knowledge into his understanding of Chinese physiology. As a consequence, he formulated a completely new doctrine of wasting and thirsting disorder that focused on the nonascent of primal qi (元氣不升 *yuán qì bù shēng*). He first outlined this doctrine in *Essays on Medicine Esteeming the Chinese and Respecting the Western*:

> Under consideration of chemistry, I have come to realize the principle of treating wasting and thirsting disorder [in a new light] ... when the middle qi in the abdomen of humans is robust and flourishing, the clear yang qi ascends ceaselessly. This qi carries hydrogen along with it in its ascent, which

combines with the oxygen inhaled by the Lungs to transform into water. Moving within the pulmonary alveoli, this [water then] transforms into the body fluids. When the body fluids are abundant, there is no thirst. When there is heat within the body of the Lungs, this is like turning up the heat under a kettle that soon dries up the water [within]. This is how thirst comes about. It is appropriate to treat with substances that clear heat and moisten the Lungs. If [such a condition arises] because of prior heat in the Heart that scorches the Lungs, it is more appropriate to use herbs that clear the Heart [and thereby treat the root]. If there is no heat in the body of the Lungs, [the condition must then be caused by the products of] qi transformation in the abdomen failing to ascend. In this case, hydrogen does not reach the Lungs above to combine with the oxygen inhaled by the Lungs to form water. [In this case,] it is appropriate to use ascending and tonifying herbs in order to tonify the qi transformation and guide [what is then produced] to ascend upward. This is the intention of Jade Fluid Decoction (*yù yè tāng*) that I have humbly drafted.

Although Zhang Xi-Chun emphasized knowledge of chemistry as a key to his understanding of wasting and thirsting disorder, unacknowledged inspiration may have come from within the Chinese medical tradition itself. *Straight Direction from [Yang] Ren-Zhai*, a formulary by the Song-dynasty physician Yang Shi-Ying, for instance, contains a formula named Jade Spring Pill (*yù quán wán*) that is very similar in intention to that of Zhang Xi-Chun's. It, too, focuses on tonification of the primal qi, on generation of fluids, and on the ascent of the clear. Jade Spring Pill (*yù quán wán*) was frequently modified by later authors and incorporated into well-known formularies like the 18th-century work *Wondrous Lantern for Peering into the Origin and Development of Miscellaneous Diseases*. It is very unlikely that a physician of Zhang Xi-Chun's stature would not have known about it.

Jade Fluid Decoction (*yù yè tāng*) is today a popular formula in the treatment of wasting and thirsting disorder. Its two chief herbs, Astragali Radix (*huáng qí*) and Dioscoreae Rhizoma (*shān yào*), were promoted by the influential Beijing physician Shi Jin-Mo as one of the key combinations for the treatment of diabetes. The formula is also used, however, for other conditions that present with thirst and qi deficiency as main symptoms, such as certain types of fever, urinary incontinence, and gastritis.

Biomedical Indications

With the appropriate presentation, this formula may be used to treat a variety of biomedically-defined disorders including diabetes, diabetes insipidus, chronic gastritis, and epidemic hemorrhagic fever.

Modifications

- For more severe qi deficiency manifesting as lassitude, a disinclination to talk, and shortness of breath, add Ginseng

Radix *(rén shēn)* or Panacis quinquefolii Radix *(xī yáng shēn)*.

- For more severe heat leading to severe thirst that cannot be quenched by drinking as well as irritability, add Lophatheri Herba *(dàn zhú yè)* and Gypsum fibrosum *(shí gāo)*.
- For Kidney deficiency manifesting as backache and urinary frequency, add Rehmanniae Radix praeparata *(shú dì huáng)* and Corni Fructus *(shān zhū yú)*.
- For yin deficiency with up-flaring of fire from deficiency, add Scrophulariae Radix *(xuán shēn)*.

Associated Formula

五汁飲 （五汁饮）

Five-Juice Drink

wǔ zhī yǐn

SOURCE *Systematic Differentiation of Warm Pathogen Diseases* (1798)

Pyri Succus *(lí zhī)*
Eleocharitis Succus *(bí qi zhī)*
Phragmitis Rhizomatis Succus *(lú gēn zhī)*
Ophiopogonis Succus *(mài mén dōng zhī)*
Nelumbinis Nodus Succus *(ǒu zhī)*

Roughly equal amounts of the fresh juices are usually taken cold, but may be warmed up for patients averse to cold drinks. The dosage depends on the degree of a patient's thirst. Generates fluids and moistens dryness. For damage to the fluids of the Lungs and Stomach by severe external heat in the course of a warm pathogen disorder. This manifests as thirst, spitting of white, frothy, and sticky saliva, and a general feeling of malaise. The formula can also be used to treat internal medicine disorders with a similar presentation. All of the herbs in this formula are sweet and cooling and are thereby able to reduce fever. Pyri Succus *(lí zhī)*, Ophiopogonis Succus *(mài mén dōng zhī),* and Phragmitis Rhizomatis Succus *(lú gēn zhī)* clear Stomach heat but also move the Intestines. Eleocharitis Succus *(bí qì zhī)* clears heat but also reduces and guides out the phlegm produced by the condensation of fluids. Nelumbinis Nodus Succus *(ǒu zhī)* clears heat and cools the blood.

This formula is a good example of the use of cold juices in clinical practice. The general strategy for treating severe heat damaging the yang fluids of the Lungs and Stomach in the course of feverish disorders is to use sweet, cooling, and acrid formulas like White Tiger Decoction *(bái hǔ tāng)*. In the present pattern, however, the symptoms of damage to the fluids are more pronounced than those of heat. For this reason, it is essential to concentrate on replenishing the fluids in order to quell fire as the primary strategy for ensuring the continued functioning of the qi dynamic. This follows an important maxim in the treatment of warm pathogen disorders: "As long as a portion of body fluids remains, there is an equal portion of the chance to survive."

Outside of East Asia, it is very difficult to obtain most of the fresh juices used in this formula. There are a number of substitutes, including isotonic drinks, a soup made from edible fungi such as white wood ears, or the juices of such fruits and vegetables as radishes, oranges, or grapefruit.

增液湯 （增液汤）

Increase the Fluids Decoction

zēng yè tāng

The source text likens the condition for which this formula is indicated to "the boat [that] stops because there is no water." The word 'boat' refers to the bowels, and 'water' to the fluids that are needed to move the bowels. In effect, this formula increases the fluids to float the boat.

Source *Systematic Differentiation of Warm Pathogen Diseases* (1798)

Scrophulariae Radix *(xuán shēn)* 30g
Ophiopogonis Radix *(mài mén dōng)* 24g
Rehmanniae Radix *(shēng dì huáng)* 24g

Method of Preparation Decoction. According to the source text, this formula must be prescribed in a large dose. It should only be prescribed for acute conditions. If one dose does not induce a bowel movement within 12 hours, prescribe Increase the Fluids and Order the Qi Decoction *(zēng yè chéng qì tāng)*.

Actions Generates fluids, moistens dryness, and unblocks the bowels

Indications

Constipation, thirst, a dry, red tongue, and a thin and slightly rapid, or a weak and forceless pulse.

This is constipation due to exhaustion of the fluids, usually from a warm-febrile disease. When a warm-febrile disease persists for a long time, or occurs in a patient with constitutional yin deficiency, heat will begin to clump at the yang brightness level. This depletes the fluids (especially in the Large Intestine) and leads to constipation. As they become depleted, the fluids are unable to rise to the mouth, causing thirst and a dry tongue. The tongue and pulse signs reflect heat from yin deficiency.

Analysis of Formula

When there is constipation due to exhausted fluids, particularly in the aftermath of a yang brightness disease, one must unblock the stool by increasing the fluids and moistening what is dry. The large dosage of the chief herb, bitter, salty, and cooling Scrophulariae Radix *(xuán shēn)*, nourishes the yin and generates fluids, while moistening what is dried and softening what is hard. In the source text, Wu Ju-Tong notes that it:

> [F]ortifies water to control fire, unblocks the excretions, and starts the Kidney water surging upward toward heaven. It can treat dried up yang fluids, so one does not have to depend on the words of the *[Divine Husbandman's] Classic of the Materia Medica* stating that it mainly treats hot and cold accumulations and conglomerations in the abdomen, to know that it can also resolve hot clumping.

One of the deputies, sweet, cold, and juicy Ophiopogonis Radix *(mài mén dōng),* assists in enriching and moistening the yin, especially of the Stomach and Intestines. The other deputy, bitter, sweet, and cold Rehmanniae Radix *(shēng dì huáng),* nourishes the yin, clears heat, and cools the blood. Used together in relatively large dosages, these three herbs greatly tonify the yin and fluids while moistening and lubricating the intestinal tract and also clearing any heat that remains.

Cautions and Contraindications

It is worth noting that this formula is not a purgative, but promotes evacuation of the bowels by clearing heat and replenishing the fluids. It is not strong enough for conditions with severe dryness; in such cases, Increase the Fluids and Order the Qi Decoction *(zēng yè chéng qì tāng)* is a better choice. Moreover, to be effective, a large dose of this formula must also be used.

Commentary

Constipation as a symptom of yang brightness disorders always has two aspects: clumping of heat and drying up of the yin fluids that moisten the Intestines and facilitate the passage of stool. Where clumping of heat is predominant, indicating the presence of a strong pathogen, one should select from one of the Order the Qi Decoctions *(chéng qì tāng).* If the yin fluids have dried up, leading to a pattern characterized by both deficiency (the lack of fluids) and excess (the presence of hard stool in the bowels that cannot be moved), this formula is indicated. Although simple in its composition, it is still able to attack the clumped heat and prevent further injury to the yin. This is because the herbs that comprise this formula do not merely enrich the fluids, but also promote movement and are indicated for clumping. The formula's author, Wu Ju-Tong, explains:

> I have selected only Scrophulariae Radix *(xuán shēn)* [to function as] chief herb. Its taste is bitter and salty. It is slightly cooling. It fortifies water to control fire. It unblocks the urine and bowels. It arouses Kidney water to rise toward the heavens. It can treat dryness of the yin fluids. These [effects] go without saying. [But the] *Classic of the Materia Medica* also says that it focuses on treating hot cold accummulations within the abdomen. From this one can deduce that it also is able to relieve clumping from heat. Ophiopogonis Radix *(mài mén dōng)* focuses on treating clumping of qi in the Heart and abdomen, on damage of the middle [burner] and the Womb [where] the collateral vessels of the Stomach have been cut off, on severe emaciation, and shortness of breath. Thus, it too is a substance that can tonify and moisten as well as unblock. Hence, it functions as deputy. Rehmanniae Radix *(shēng dì huáng)* also focuses on hot cold accummulations, driving out blood painful obstruction. When used with care, one selects its tonifying [properties] without [the herb] being cloying so that its [action also] extends to the collaterals.

The treatment strategy embodied in this formula is modeled after Wu You-Ke's Order the Qi and Nourish the Nutritive Decoction *(chéng qì yǎng róng tāng),* discussed in Chapter 2, which Wu Ju-Tong admired for its combination of tonifying and downward-draining herbs. Over the years, the use of this formula has been expanded to include any constipation due to yin deficiency, regardless of etiology. Based on the functions of its individual ingredients, the formula is also commonly used for nutritive-level heat with signs of dryness in the middle burner. Used together, more often in various synergistic pairs, and sometimes alone, its three ingredients are found in formulas that treat warm-pathogen disorders or fire toxin at almost any level. They can, for instance, be added to Honeysuckle and Forsythia Powder *(yín qiáo sǎn)* for patients with internal heat due to yin deficiency, even at the onset of such disorders. In addition, they are invariably included in formulas that treat late-stage feverish disorders, including those of the cold-damage type, such as Prepared Licorice Decoction *(zhì gān cǎo tāng),* which contains Ophiopogonis Radix *(mài mén dōng)* and Rehmanniae Radix *(shēng dì huáng).* This attests to the core objective of preserving the fluids and maintaining fluid metabolism in the treatment of all such disorders. First outlined in the treatment strategies of Zhang Zhong-Jing, it is from this observation that the composition of the present formula was derived.

Biomedical Indications

With the appropriate presentation, this formula may be used to treat a variety of biomedically-defined disorders including habitual constipation, sequelae of infectious diseases, hemorrhoids, irritable bowel syndrome, aphthous ulcers, gingivitis, chronic pharyngitis, hyperthyroid conditions, diabetes, chronic pancreatitis, and the oral side effects associated with radiation therapy.

Comparison

> ➤ Vs. Increase the Fluids and Order the Qi Decoction *(zēng yè chéng qì tāng)*

These formulas both treat yang brightness patterns with constipation as the chief symptom that arise in the course of a warm pathogen disorder. Because it incorporates Rhei Radix et Rhizoma *(dà huáng)* and Natrii Sulfas *(máng xiāo),* Increase the Fluids and Order the Qi Decoction *(zēng yè chéng qì tāng)* combines purgation with the tonification of fluids. It is indicated when acute signs of heat clumping, such as rebound tenderness of the abdomen, are accompanied by signs that indicate dessicated fluids, such as a thin pulse. By contrast, Increase the Fluids Decoction *(zēng yè tāng)* must be prescribed only when the heat clumping does not constitute a primary symptom. If its use does not show an immediate effect, this is a sign that the clumping heat must be drained. Thus, one should follow through with a dose of Increase the Fluids and Order the Qi Decoction (*zēng yè chéng qì tāng*).

Modifications

- For a peeled tongue with a shiny coating and parched mouth and lips due to severe Stomach yin deficiency, add Glehniae/Adenophorae Radix (*shā shēn*), Polygonati odorati Rhizoma (*yù zhú*), and Dendrobii Herba (*shí hú*).

- For toothache, add Achyranthis bidentatae Radix (*niú xī*), Moutan Cortex (*mǔ dān pí*), Psoraleae Fructus (*bǔ gǔ zhī*), and Vespae Nidus (*lù fēng fáng*).

- For bleeding hemorrhoids, combine with Sophora Japonica Flower Powder (*huái huā sǎn*).

- For signs of more severe clumped heat, combine with Regulate the Stomach and Order the Qi Decoction (*tiáo wèi chéng qì tāng*).

Comparative Tables of Principal Formulas

■ FORMULAS THAT GENTLY DISPERSE AND MOISTEN DRYNESS

Common symptoms: cough, dry throat, dry tongue (thin or no coating)

Formula Name	Diagnosis	Indications	Remarks
Apricot Kernel and Perilla Leaf Powder (*xìng sū sǎn*)	Externally-contracted cool-dryness	Slight headache, chills without sweating, cough with watery sputum, stuffy nose, dry throat, a dry, white tongue coating, and a wiry pulse	Focuses on dispersing cool-dryness and transforming thin mucus.
Mulberry Leaf and Apricot Kernel Decoction (*sāng xìng tāng*)	Externally-contracted warm-dryness	Moderate fever, headache, thirst, dry, hacking cough or one with scanty, thick, and sticky sputum, a red tongue with a thin, dry, and white coating, and a floating, rapid pulse (especially on the right)	Also for coughing of blood. Focuses on dispersing warm-dryness and generating fluids.
Clear Dryness and Rescue the Lungs Decoction (*qīng zào jiù fèi tāng*)	Warm-dryness attacking the Lungs with damage to both the qi and yin	Headache, fever, hacking cough, wheezing, dry throat and nasal passages, a sensation of fullness in the chest, hypochondriac pain, irritability, thirst, a dry tongue without coating, and a deficient, big, and rapid pulse	Also for acute-onset hemiplegia. Focuses on clearing heat and dryness while nourishing the fluids and tonifying the qi.
Glehnia and Ophiopogonis Decoction (*shā shēn mài mén dōng tāng*)	Injury to the Lungs, Stomach, and fluids from dryness	Dry throat, thirst, fever, hacking cough with scanty sputum, a red tongue with little coating, and a rapid, thin pulse	Focuses on generating fluids in order to clear and nourish the Lungs and Stomach.

■ FORMULAS THAT ENRICH THE YIN AND MOISTEN DRYNESS

Common symptoms: dry, red tongue, thin and/or rapid pulse

Formula Name	Diagnosis	Indications	Remarks
Ophiopogonis Decoction (*mài mén dōng tāng*)	Heat from deficiency of the Stomach scorching the Lung yin (upper and middle burners)	Coughing up difficult-to-expectorate phlegm, spitting of saliva, wheezing, shortness of breath, dry and uncomfortable throat, heat in the palms and soles, a dry, red tongue with little coating, and a deficient, rapid pulse	For insufficiency of either Lung or Stomach yin.
Nourish the Yin and Clear the Lungs Decoction (*yǎng yīn qīng fèi tāng*)	Diphtherial disorder (upper burner)	White, curd-like membrane in the throat that is difficult to scrape off, swollen and sore throat, fever, parched lips, raspy breathing, a red and dry tongue, and a rapid, usually thin pulse	May also have coughing.

cont. ↘

Formula Name	Diagnosis	Indications	Remarks
Jade Fluid Decoction (*yù yè tāng*)	Wasting and thirsting disorder due to deficiency of the primal qi (lower burner)	Excessive thirst that is not quenched by substantial intake of fluids, frequent, copious, or turbid urine, lassitude, shortness of breath, and a deficient, thin, and weak pulse	Also for certain types of fever, urinary incontinence, and gastritis.
Increase the Fluids Decoction (*zēng yè tāng*)	Constipation due to exhaustion of the fluids (lower burner)	Constipation, thirst, a dry, red tongue, and a thin and slightly rapid, or a weak, forceless pulse	Focuses on unblocking the bowels by clearing heat and replenishing the fluids.

寿濕劑

Chapter 16 Contents

Formulas that Expel Dampness

Formulas that Expel Dampness

16

FLUID PHYSIOLOGY AND pathology are at the foundation of Chinese medicine, and Chinese physicians have always been greatly concerned with damp disorders. In Chapter 71 of *Basic Questions,* it is noted that "water constraint [is treated] by breaking it up." Chapter 14 lists sweating, diuresis, and elimination via the stools as three possible routes for eliminating water excess. A passage in Chapter 74 elaborates on the nature of herbs used for these purposes:

> Damp pathogens in the interior are treated with bitter, warming [medicinals] assisted by sour and bland [medicinals] because one can use bitterness [flavor] to dry [dampness] and the bland [flavor] to drain it. If dampness is [more pronounced] above, leading to heat, it is treated with bitter, warming [medicinals] assisted by sweet and acrid [medicinals] to promote sweating and thereby arrest [the disorder].

Zhang Zhong-Jing's *Discussion of Cold Damage* and *Essential Formulas from the Golden Cabinet* offered formulas that translated these strategies into clinical practice. Many of these—Five-Ingredient Powder with Poria *(wŭ líng săn),* Polyporus Decoction from *Comprehensive Recording (zhū líng tāng),* Virgate Wormwood Decoction *(yīn chén hāo tāng),* and True Warrior Decoction *(zhēn wŭ tāng)*—not only continue to be widely used today, but also served as platforms for the development of other formulas and strategies.

By the Tang dynasty, the adage "Drying can eliminate dampness" had become one of the ten exemplary treatment principles in Chen Cang-Qi's *Omissions from the [Classic of the] Materia Medica,* and every epoch in the history of Chinese medicine since then has added to the ever-growing therapeutic arsenal in this group.

The importance accorded to the qi dynamic by the various Jin-Yuan masters imparted a new stimulus to the treatment of damp disorders. Most innovative, without doubt, was Zhang Yuan-Su and Li Dong-Yuan's use of wind medicinals (風藥 *fēng yào*) to assist in the uplifting of middle burner qi and thus the transformation and dispelling of dampness. They also devised the strategy of 'separating and reducing' (分消 *fēn xiāo*), which utilizes the different functions of the Triple Burner vis-à-vis the fluid metabolism as a method for treating complex damp pathologies. This strategy was later taken up by Ye Tian-Shi and other exponents of the warm pathogen disorder current in Chinese medicine, who perfected it as one of the key methods in their treatment of damp-warmth disorders.

Dampness is a yin pathogenic influence that has a heavy, sluggish nature. Damp disorders progress slowly and linger in the body. Internally-generated dampness is usually associated with improper eating habits, overindulgence in alcohol, and obsessive deliberation or other emotional behavior that injures the Spleen. Manifestations include generalized and focal abdominal distention, nausea, vomiting, diarrhea, jaundice, painful urinary dribbling, or edema of the lower extremities. Dampness can also be externally contracted from living in a damp climate or environment, or getting wet from rain or sweat. Manifestations of externally-contracted dampness include chills and fever, a feeling of distention in the head and heaviness in the body, stiffness and pain in the joints, or superficial edema. Because it is not uncommon for conditions of dampness to present with both externally-contracted and internally-generated aspects, it must therefore be approached carefully in each case to gain a full understanding of its etiology and the underlying constitution of the patient.

The word 'water' (水 *shuǐ*) is often used in connection with dampness. Sometimes this word refers to the fluids in general and sometimes specifically to edema or to an accumulation that is more distinct and localized than dampness. The latter usage is reflected in the adage, "Dampness is the permeation of water, while water is the accumulation of dampness." In this text, *shuǐ* is translated as 'edema' when it refers specifically to that condition, but otherwise we have left it simply as 'water.'

Problems with those organs that are most intimately connected with the process of water metabolism in the body often result in damp disorders. The three most important organs are the Kidneys, which are said to govern water, the Spleen, which controls water, and the Lungs, which govern the ascending and descending aspects of water metabolism known as the 'water pathways' (水道 *shuǐ dào*). Among the yang organs, the Triple Burner and the Bladder also have important connections with water metabolism, and therefore with dampness. If the qi is obstructed in the Triple Burner, there is no force behind the metabolism of water; if the Bladder does not function smoothly and urination becomes difficult, the qi mechanisms of the Triple Burner can be affected by the backflow. Because dampness is a heavy, sluggish pathogenic influence that readily hinders and obstructs the qi mechanisms, these formulas often include qi-regulating herbs. The value of such herbs in treating dampness is succinctly stated in *Systematic Differentiation of Warm Pathogen Diseases:* "When the qi [mechanisms] are transformed, dampness will likewise be transformed." For example, when the Bladder qi is obstructed by dampness, these herbs can regulate the Bladder qi and thereby provide an avenue for water and dampness to exit the body.

The principal patterns of externally-contracted dampness are damp-heat and wind-dampness, which are generally conditions of excess. Dampness in the exterior was previously discussed in Chapter 1. Manifestations of damp-heat include jaundice, painful urinary dribbling, and atrophy disorder. It is always important to carefully distinguish both the level (burner) at which the process is active and the pathogenic influence that predominates, and treat accordingly. Wind-dampness is marked by pain (usually of the joints) and is sometimes accompanied by edema. Here it is also important to discern whether wind or dampness predominates. Furthermore, because these conditions lodge primarily in the channels, ensuring the free flow of healthy blood is an im-

portant aspect of treatment. When the flow in the channels is open, the wind has no place to lodge, hence the adage, "When treating wind [disorders], first treat the blood."

In general, the formulas in this chapter are comprised of acrid, aromatic, and warm substances that dry dampness, or sweet, bland substances that leach out dampness. They should be used with extreme caution in cases of yin deficiency and depleted fluids. In patients with debility brought on by disease or pregnancy with edema or other signs of dampness, these formulas must be modified with Spleen-strengthening herbs to protect the normal qi.

Section 1

FORMULAS THAT TRANSFORM DAMPNESS AND HARMONIZE THE STOMACH

When dampness lingers in the interior, stagnation and turbidity ensue. This can be a relatively rapid process. Dampness obstructs the ascent of the clear (governed by the Spleen) and the descent of the turbid (governed by the Stomach), slowing or blocking the transportive function of the Spleen and the Stomach's ability to receive food. This leads to symptoms such as epigastric and abdominal distention and fullness, belching, acid reflux, vomiting, diarrhea, reduced appetite, and fatigue. These symptoms require the use of formulas that dry dampness and harmonize the Stomach. Such formulas rely on bitter and warming herbs that dry dampness, and on aromatic herbs that transform dampness. The most important of these are Atractylodis Rhizoma (*cāng zhú*), Magnoliae officinalis Cortex (*hòu pò*), Pogostemonis/Agastaches Herba (*huò xiāng*), and Amomi Fructus rotundus (*bái dòu kòu*).

Depending on the pattern, the formulas combine these chief herbs with three other types of herbs. Where severe obstruction to the qi dynamic by dampness encumbers the Spleen, herbs that move the qi and awaken the Spleen like Citri reticulatae Pericarpium (*chén pí*), Aucklandiae Radix (*mù xiāng*), and Amomi Fructus (*shā rén*) are added. In order to strengthen the Spleen's functions of transportation and transformation in patterns where deficiency has contributed to the accumulation of dampness, herbs that strengthen the Spleen like Ginseng Radix (*rén shēn*), Atractylodis macrocephalae Rhizoma (*bái zhú*), Glycyrrhizae Radix (*gān cǎo*), and Jujubae Fructus (*dà zǎo*) are used. In patterns where obstruction of the qi dynamic in the interior has facilitated the infiltration of pathogens into the exterior, one adds herbs that resolve the exterior and disperse pathogenic qi such as Angelicae dahuricae Radix (*bái zhǐ*), Perillae Folium (*zǐ sū yè*), Moslae Herba (*xiāng rú*), or Bupleuri Radix (*chái hú*).

平胃散

Calm the Stomach Powder

píng wèi săn

The generally accepted explanation of this formula's name comes from *Collected Treatises of [Zhang] Jing-Yue:* "Calming the Stomach here refers to wanting to put in order (平治 *píng zhì*) that which is unbalanced (不平 *bù píng*)." The term 'Stomach' here is not a reference to the stomach organ, but to the entire digestive system, which removes obstruction and stagnation by elimination via the Intestines.

Source   *Concise Formulas to Aid the Multitudes* (1051)

dry-fried Atractylodis Rhizoma (*chăo cāng zhú*) . . 120g (12-15g)
ginger-fried Magnoliae officinalis Cortex
   (*jiāng chăo hòu pò*) 90g (9-12g)
Citri reticulatae Pericarpium (*chén pí*) 60g (9-12g)
Glycyrrhizae Radix praeparata (*zhì gān căo*) 30g (3-6g)

Method of Preparation   Grind the ingredients into a powder, add Zingiberis Rhizoma recens (*shēng jiāng*) and Jujubae Fructus (*dà zăo*), and take as a draft in 6-9g doses on an empty stomach. May also be prepared as a decoction with the dosage specified in parentheses.

Actions   Dries dampness, improves the Spleen's transportive function, promotes the movement of qi, and harmonizes the Stomach

Indications

Distention and fullness in the epigastrium and abdomen, loss of taste and appetite, a heavy sensation in the limbs, loose stools or diarrhea, easily-fatigued, increased desire to sleep, nausea and vomiting, belching, acid reflux, a swollen tongue with a thick, white, and greasy coating, and a moderate or slippery pulse.

This is dampness stagnating in the Spleen and Stomach. The Spleen is responsible for transforming food into nutrients and for transporting those nutrients throughout the body. It prefers dryness and the smooth flow of qi, and is averse to dampness and stagnation. Overconsumption of raw or cold foods leads to dampness, which encumbers the Spleen and produces turbid dampness. This in turn causes the qi of the middle burner to stagnate, giving rise to distention and fullness throughout the abdomen. The symptoms of loss of taste and appetite, a heavy sensation in the limbs, fatigue, an increased desire to sleep, and loose stools or diarrhea indicate that the Spleen yang is unable to function. The encumbrance of the Spleen allows dampness to flow into the Intestines, which exacerbates the diarrhea. The failure of the Spleen's transportive function prevents the Stomach from receiving and passing the fluids downward. This causes the turbid yin to rise, which is characterized by nausea, vomiting, and acid reflux. The swollen tongue reflects deficient qi, and the tongue coating the presence of turbid dampness. The moderate or slippery quality of the pulse reflects dampness encumbering the Spleen and Stomach.

Analysis of Formula

This formula is designed to treat dampness stagnating in the Spleen and Stomach. For this purpose, it combines strategies to dry dampness and move the Spleen qi with those that harmonize the Stomach. The chief herb, acrid, bitter, and warm Atractylodis Rhizoma (*cāng zhú*), is perhaps the best substance in the materia medica for dispelling dampness and strengthening the transportive function of the Spleen. Because of the importance of these functions in treating this condition, its dosage is rather large. Dampness causes the qi to stagnate. In order to transform dampness, it is thus essential to regulate the qi by removing obstructions to the qi dynamic. The deputy, Magnoliae officinalis Cortex (*hòu pò*), serves this function. Bitter and warming, it moves the qi, disperses fullness, and directs the qi downward; but it is also aromatic and fragrant, and thereby transforms dampness. It works synergistically with the chief herb to dry the dampness and strengthen the Spleen. The assistant herb, Citri reticulatae Pericarpium (*chén pí*), also regulates the qi and harmonizes the Stomach. It assists the deputy in directing rebellious qi downward and eliminating distention. The combination of the deputy and assistant herbs revives the Spleen and improves the appetite. Glycyrrhizae Radix praeparata (*zhì gān căo*), an envoy, tonifies the Spleen. It harmonizes the actions of the other herbs and enhances their Spleen-strengthening properties. The other envoys, Zingiberis Rhizoma recens (*shēng jiāng*) and Jujubae Fructus (*dà zăo*), mildly regulate and harmonize the relationship between the Spleen and Stomach.

Cautions and Contraindications

This formula contains warm, drying herbs that readily injure the yin and blood, and should therefore only be used with significant modification for patients with yin or blood deficiency. Caution must also be exercised when using the formula during pregnancy.

Commentary

This is the most representative and popular formula for the treatment of dampness stagnating in the middle burner. The cardinal symptoms are distention and fullness in the epigastrium and abdomen, and a thick, white, and greasy tongue coating. These symptoms imply that the primary pathology is obstruction of the qi dynamic by dampness. The most appropriate strategy for resolving this problem is to guide out obstruction and open the qi dynamic. Once the qi is regulated, any remaining dampness will naturally be transformed, as explained by Fei Bo-Xiong in *Discussion of Medical Formulas:*

Calm the Stomach Powder (*píng wèi sǎn*) is a sagely formula for treating the Spleen and Stomach. It facilitates the resolution of dampness, transforms focal distention, disperses distention, and harmonizes the middle. It also treats unseasonal epidemics [due to] miasmatic qi. It is drying but not violently [so]. Hence, it is the primary formula for reducing and guiding out.

If, as Fei Bo-Xiong suggests, the primary intention of the formula is to guide out excess and fullness in order to open the qi dynamic, the many diverse uses for which the formula has been employed over the centuries are more easily understood. Besides the treatment of various digestive disorders, these include amenorrhea, the facilitation of labor, insomnia, chronic cough, coronary artery disease, male impotence, and damp-type eczema.

There has long been a debate in the literature about whether the dampness for which this formula is intended is primarily due to excess (as described above) or to Spleen deficiency. Most commentators have argued that if the formula were designed to treat dampness due to Spleen deficiency, Atractylodis macrocephalae Rhizoma (*bái zhú*), which is better suited for strengthening the Spleen, would have been used in place of Atractylodis Rhizoma (*cāng zhú*). For a formula in which this substitution is made to focus more on the deficient aspects of the presentation, see MODIFICATIONS below.

Comparison

➤ Vs. Rectify the Qi Powder Worth More than Gold (*bù huàn jīn zhèng qì sǎn*); *see* PAGE 690

➤ Vs. Patchouli/Agastache Powder to Rectify the Qi (*huò xiāng zhèng qì sǎn*); *see* PAGE 693

Biomedical Indications

With the appropriate presentation, this formula may be used to treat a wide variety of biomedically-defined disorders. These can be divided into the following groups:

- Digestive disorders such as peptic ulcer, chronic gastritis, chronic colitis, irritable bowel syndrome, intestinal obstruction, infantile diarrhea, and infectious hepatitis
- Gynecological disorders such as amenorrhea, premenstrual syndrome, and cervicitis.

This formula has also been used for eczema, pertussis, reduced libido in men, erectile dysfunction, and halitosis.

Alternate names

Universally Venerated Calm the Stomach Powder (*tiān xià shòu bài píng wèi sǎn*) in *Lingnan Formulas for Preserving Health*; Venerated Powder to Calm the Stomach (*shòu bài píng wèi sǎn*) in *Diverse Collection of Famous Formulas*; Miraculously Effective Calm the Stomach Powder (*shén xiào píng wèi sǎn*) in *Master Wan's Family Compilation of Songs for Protecting Life*

Modifications

- For severe cold-dampness with generalized cold and pain, add Cinnamomi Cortex (*ròu guì*) and Zingiberis Rhizoma (*gān jiāng*).
- For damp-heat with a bitter taste in the mouth, a dry throat with no thirst, and a yellow, greasy tongue coating, add Scutellariae Radix (*huáng qín*) and Coptidis Rhizoma (*huáng lián*).
- For food stagnation with severe distention and constipation, add Raphani Semen (*lái fú zǐ*), Arecae Pericarpium (*dà fù pí*), and Aurantii Fructus (*zhǐ ké*).
- For severe vomiting, add Pinelliae Rhizoma praeparatum (*zhì bàn xià*).
- For more Spleen deficiency marked by a loss of appetite with less distention and fullness, substitute Atractylodis macrocephalae Rhizoma (*bái zhú*) for Atractylodis Rhizoma (*cāng zhú*) and add Astragali Radix (*huáng qí*) and Dioscoreae Rhizoma (*shān yào*).
- For delayed labor or fetal death with a similar presentation, add Natrii Sulfas (*máng xiāo*) and Aurantii Fructus immaturus (*zhǐ shí*).
- For stones in the common bile duct, add Artemisiae scopariae Herba (*yīn chén*), Gardeniae Fructus (*zhī zǐ*), and Curcumae Radix (*yù jīn*).

Associated Formulas

香砂平胃散

Cyperus and Amomum Calm the Stomach Powder
xiāng shā píng wèi sǎn

SOURCE   *Golden Mirror of the Medical Tradition* (1742)

Cyperi Rhizoma (*xiāng fù*) 3-6g
Amomi Fructus (*shā rén*) 3-6g
Atractylodis Rhizoma (*cāng zhú*) 12-15g
Citri reticulatae Pericarpium (*chén pí*) 6-9g
Aurantii Fructus (*zhǐ ké*) 9-12g
Paeoniae Radix alba (*bái sháo*) 9-12g
Crataegi Fructus (*shān zhā*) 9-12g
Hordei Fructus germinatus (*mài yá*) 9-12g
Glycyrrhizae Radix (*gān cǎo*) 1.5-3g
Zingiberis Rhizoma recens (*shēng jiāng*) 1.5-3g

Decoction. The source text does not specify dosage. Strengthens the Spleen, reduces food stagnation, moves the qi, and alleviates pain. For food stagnation characterized by abdominal distention and pain, an aversion to eating, vomiting of sour fluids, and diarrhea that does not relieve the abdominal pain.

––––––––––––

香砂平胃散

Aucklandia and Amomum Calm the Stomach Powder
xiāng shā píng wèi sǎn

SOURCE   *Achievements Regarding Epidemic Rashes* (1794)

dry-fried Atractylodis Rhizoma (*chǎo cāng zhú*) 4.5g
Magnoliae officinalis Cortex (*hòu pò*) 3g
Citri reticulatae Pericarpium (*chén pí*) 3g
Aucklandiae Radix (*mù xiāng*) 1.5g
Amomi Fructus (*shā rén*) 2.4g
Glycyrrhizae Radix (*gān cǎo*) 1.5g
Zingiberis Rhizoma recens (*shēng jiāng*) . . . . 1 slice

Decoction. Dries dampness, strengthens the Spleen, moves the qi, and eases the middle. Originally for the aftermath of an unseasonal epidemic disorder where the remnants of heat have not been entirely dispersed and the Stomach and Intestines are deficient and weak. The patient has no appetite but is forced to eat and the resulting food stagnation provides a place to store the heat. The heat and food stagnation combine to cause a disorder known as 'relapse due to poor diet' (食復 *shí fù*). This is characterized by epigastric and abdominal distention, reduced intake, nausea, and vomiting. This formula focuses on opening the qi dynamic in order to vent the lingering heat and guide out the stagnation.

除濕胃苓湯 （除湿胃苓汤）

Eliminate Dampness Decoction by Combining Calm the Stomach and Five-Ingredient Powder with Poria

chú shī wèi líng tāng

Source *Golden Mirror of the Medical Tradition* (1742)

Atractylodis Rhizoma (*cāng zhú*) 3g
Magnoliae officinalis Cortex (*hòu pò*) 3g
Citri reticulatae Pericarpium (*chén pí*) 3g
Polyporus (*zhū líng*) 3g
Alismatis Rhizoma (*zé xiè*) 3g
Poria rubra (*chì fú líng*) 3g
dry-fried Atractylodis macrocephalae Rhizoma
   (*chǎo bái zhú*) 3g
Talcum (*huá shí*) 3g
Saposhnikoviae Radix (*fáng fēng*) 3g
Gardeniae Fructus (*zhī zǐ*) 3g
Akebiae Caulis (*mù tōng*) 3g
Cinnamomi Cortex (*ròu guì*) 0.9g
Glycyrrhizae Radix (*gān cǎo*) 0.9g
Junci Medulla (*dēng xīn cǎo*) 3g

Clears heat and dries dampness in the lower burner, regulates the qi, and harmonizes the middle burner. For fire papules that encircle the waist. This condition usually corresponds to herpes zoster that erupts in the mid- to lower-back region.

分消湯 （分消汤）

Separate and Reduce Decoction

fēn xiāo tāng

Source *Restoration of Health from the Myriad Diseases* (1587)

Atractylodis Rhizoma (*cāng zhú*) 3g
Atractylodis macrocephalae Rhizoma (*bái zhú*) 3g
Poria (*fú líng*) 3g
Citri reticulatae Pericarpium (*chén pí*) 3g
Magnoliae officinalis Cortex (*hòu pò*) 3g

Cyperi Rhizoma (*xiāng fù*) 2.4g
Polyporus (*zhū líng*) 2.4g
Alismatis Rhizoma (*zé xiè*) 2.4g
Aurantii Fructus immaturus (*zhǐ shí*) 3g
Arecae Pericarpium (*dà fù pí*) 2.4g
Amomi Fructus (*shā rén*) 2.1g
Aucklandiae Radix (*mù xiāng*) .0.9g
Junci Medulla (*dēng xīn cǎo*) . . . . 1 piece
Zingiberis Rhizoma recens (*shēng jiāng*) . . . . 1 piece

Promotes urination, promotes the movement of qi, and guides out stagnation. For abdominal fullness and drum-like distention, firm focal distention in the epigastrium, pitting edema and ascites, scanty, yellow urine, and constipation.

不換金正氣散 （不换金正气散）

Rectify the Qi Powder Worth More than Gold

bù huàn jīn zhèng qì sǎn

The original name of this formula was simply Powder Worth More than Gold. The current name is explained in Feng's *Secret Records from the Brocade Purse*: "[This formula] transports the normal qi so that pathogenic qi has no means by which to mount an attack. What could be more valuable? Hence, it is called 'worth more than gold.'" *Investigations of Medical Formulas* adds: "The formula's name [refers to] rectifying the qi. This is because it can rectify that which is not [moving] correctly."

Source *Simple Book of Formulas* (1191)

Magnoliae officinalis Cortex (*hòu pò*)
Atractylodis Rhizoma (*cāng zhú*)
Pogostemonis/Agastaches Herba (*huò xiāng*)
Pinelliae Rhizoma praeparatum (*zhì bàn xià*)
Citri reticulatae Pericarpium (*chén pí*)
Glycyrrhizae Radix (*gān cǎo*)

Method of Preparation Grind equal amounts of all the ingredients into a powder and take in 3-6g doses as a draft before meals with Zingiberis Rhizoma recens (*shēng jiāng*).

Actions Dries dampness, transforms turbidity, directs rebellious qi downward, and stops vomiting

Indications

Vomiting, abdominal distention and fullness, fever and chills. Also used for sudden turmoil disorders characterized by diarrhea and vomiting, and a thick, white, and greasy tongue coating.

The first pattern is damp turbidity obstructing the middle with wind-cold fettering the exterior. When damp turbidity collects in the interior, it obstructs the qi dynamic. This leads to qi stagnation, which manifests as abdominal distention and fullness. It also interrupts the physiological ascending and downward-directing functions centered on the middle burner, causing the Stomach qi to rebel. In the present case, this is exacerbated by external cold, as explained in *String of Pearls from the [Discussion] of Cold Damage*: "When the Stomach qi becomes cold, it rebels." This implies that the vomiting here is relatively severe. Wind-cold fettering the protective yang in the exterior manifests as fever and chills.

Sudden turmoil disorder characterized by vomiting and diarrhea is due to obstruction of the qi dynamic in the middle burner. The thick, greasy, white tongue coating shows that, in the present case, this is caused by cold-dampness and foul turbidity. The clear yang cannot ascend, while the turbid yin fails to be directed downward, leading to an intermingling of clear and turbid qi that manifests as simultaneous diarrhea and vomiting.

Analysis of Formula

The purpose of this formula is to dry dampness, transform turbidity, harmonize the Stomach, stop vomiting, and resolve the exterior by dispersing cold. It can be seen as a variation of Calm the Stomach Powder (*píng wèi sǎn*) to which Pogostemonis/Agastaches Herba (*huò xiāng*) and Pinelliae Rhizoma praeparatum (*zhì bàn xià*) have been added.

The chief herb in this formula is Pogostemonis/Agastaches Herba (*huò xiāng*). Fragrant, acrid, and slightly warming, it enters the Spleen, Stomach, and Lung channels. It is one of the most important herbs in the materia medica for aromatically transforming dampness. Its light, acrid, and warming nature enables it to disperse cold-dampness from the exterior. It is thus ideally suited to treat patterns where obstruction of dampness in the interior is exacerbated by pathogenic qi, especially cold-dampness, fettering the exterior. The deputy herbs are Atractylodis Rhizoma (*cāng zhú*) and Magnoliae officinalis Cortex (*hòu pò*). Atractylodis Rhizoma (*cāng zhú*) excels at drying dampness in the Spleen, but it also moves into the exterior to dispel wind and eliminate dampness. Magnoliae officinalis Cortex (*hòu pò*) directs the qi downward, eliminates fullness, and aromatically transforms turbidity. Its synergistic combination with Atractylodis Rhizoma (*cāng zhú*) increases the ability of both herbs to dry dampness and strengthen the Spleen's transportive functions.

Pinelliae Rhizoma praeparatum (*zhì bàn xià*) excels at directing the qi downward to stop the vomiting, but it also can dry dampness, transform phlegm, and reduce focal distention. Citri reticulatae Pericarpium (*chén pí*) regulates the qi, harmonizes the Stomach, and awakens the Spleen with its aromatic fragrance. Together, these herbs act as assistants. Glycyrrhizae Radix (*gān cǎo*) is the envoy, which supports the middle burner qi and harmonizes the various functions of the formula. Zingiberis Rhizoma recens (*shēng jiāng*), added when preparing the draft, disperses cold from the exterior, harmonizes the Stomach, and stops vomiting.

Cautions and Contraindications

This formula is acrid, bitter, warming, and drying. It readily consumes the blood and body fluids. It is therefore contraindicated for patients suffering from yin deficiency and those with a weak Spleen and Stomach. It should be taken with caution during pregnancy.

Commentary

The original indication of this formula was wind-cold in both the exterior and interior as well as unseasonal epidemic disorders due to miasmatic qi. The specific usage of Magnoliae officinalis Cortex (*hòu pò*) for such disorders is discussed in the entry for Patchouli/Agastache Powder to Rectify the Qi (*huò xiāng zhèng qì sǎn*) below. Later physicians widened the formula's indications to include bloody stools due to wind in the bowels (*Straight Direction from [Yang] Ren-Zhai*); invasion of dampness (*Effective Formulas from Generations of Physicians*); pox and sores due to disharmony between the nutritive and protective qi caused by wind-cold in the exterior and food stagnation in the interior (*Prescriptions of Universal Benefit*); sores due to Spleen qi deficiency in the interior and cold in the exterior (*Collected Treatises of [Zhang] Jing-Yue*); and malarial disorders (*Treatment Decisions Categorized according to Pattern*). A particularly intersting indication that implies an effect on the regulation of fertility was suggested by Xu Da-Chun in *Six Texts Summarizing the Medicine of Xu Ling-Tai*:

> When dampness damages the qi dynamic, the clear and turbid are no longer separated. Accordingly, [this manifests as] incessant diarrhea and as deregulation of the heavenly dew. … The [formula is] taken as a powder (散 *sǎn*) in order to [facilitate] dispersal (散 *sàn*). It is taken with rice water in order to harmonize it. It brings about the transformation of dampness and the regulation of qi so that the Spleen and Stomach have the authority to convert and transform [dampness]. Any [case of] diarrhea will then be cured and all heavenly dew regulated.

Comparison

➤ Vs. Calm the Stomach Powder (*píng wèi sǎn*)

Both formulas dry dampness, harmonize the Stomach, and regulate the qi. Calm the Stomach Powder (*píng wèi sǎn*), with Atractylodis Rhizoma (*cāng zhú*) as the chief herb, is better at drying dampness and strengthening the Spleen's transportive functions. By contrast, Rectify the Qi Powder Worth More than Gold (*bù huàn jīn zhèng qì sǎn*), by merely adding Pogostemonis/Agastaches Herba (*huò xiāng*) and Pinelliae Rhizoma praeparatum (*zhì bàn xià*), disperses wind-cold in the exterior as well as dispelling damp turbidity collecting in the interior. It excels at treating vomiting caused by the conjunction of these pathologies.

➤ Vs. Patchouli/Agastache Powder to Rectify the Qi (*huò xiāng zhèng qì sǎn*); see page 693

Biomedical Indications

With the appropriate presentation, this formula may be used to treat a variety of biomedically-defined disorders including stomach flu and acute gastroenteritis.

Alternate names

Drink to Rectify the Qi and Clear the Muscles (*zhèng qì qīng jī yǐn*) and Agastache Powder to Calm the Stomach (*huò xiāng ān wèi sǎn*), both in *Enumeration of Formulas Omitted from the Inner Classic*; Genuine Rectify the Qi Powder Worth More than Gold (*zhēn fāng bù huàn jīn zhèng qì sǎn*) in *Prescriptions for Universal Benefit*; Agastache Powder to Rectify the Qi (*huò xiāng zhèng qì sǎn*) in *Symptom, Cause, Pulse, and Treatment*

Modifications

- For headache, add Angelicae dahuricae Radix (*bái zhǐ*) and Chuanxiong Rhizoma (*chuān xiōng*).
- For incessant cold-type diarrhea, add Aucklandiae Radix (*mù xiāng*), Chebulae Fructus (*hē zǐ*), and Myristicae Semen (*ròu dòu kòu*).
- For severe abdominal pain, add Zingiberis Rhizoma (*gān jiāng*) and Cinnamomi Cortex (*ròu guì*).
- For vomiting, add Caryophylli Flos (*dīng xiāng*) and Amomi Fructus (*shā rén*).

藿香正氣散 (藿香正气散)

Patchouli/Agastache Powder to Rectify the Qi

huò xiāng zhèng qì sǎn

In its broadest sense, 'rectify the qi' (正氣 *zhèng qì*) implies the capacity to rectify abnormal seasonal qi (四時不正之氣 *sì shí bù zhèng zhī qì*). Besides the six pathogenic qi, there are many other types of abnormal seasonal qi, including 'mountain vapors and miasmatic qi' (山嵐瘴氣 *shān lán zhàng qì*). Because this formula is acrid and warming in nature, it rectifies only the qi that has become abnormal due to the invasion of wind-cold-dampness or miasmatic qi.

Source   *Formulary of the Pharmacy Service for Benefiting the People in the Taiping Era* (1107)

Pogostemonis/Agastaches Herba (*huò xiāng*) 90g (12g)
ginger-fried Magnoliae officinalis Cortex
   (*jiāng chǎo hòu pò*) 60g (9g)
Citri reticulatae Pericarpium (*chén pí*) 60g (9g)
Perillae Folium (*zǐ sū yè*) 30g (6g)
Angelicae dahuricae Radix (*bái zhǐ*) 30g (6g)
Pinelliae Rhizoma praeparatum (*zhì bàn xià*) 60g (9g)
Arecae Pericarpium (*dà fù pí*) 30g (9g)
Atractylodis macrocephalae Rhizoma (*bái zhú*) 60g (12g)
Poria (*fú líng*) 30g (9g)
Platycodi Radix (*jié gěng*) 60g (9g)
Glycyrrhizae Radix praeparata (*zhì gān cǎo*) 75g (3g)

Method of Preparation   Grind the ingredients into a powder and take in 3-6g doses as a draft with 3-6g of Zingiberis Rhizoma recens (*shēng jiāng*) and 1 piece of Jujubae Fructus (*dà zǎo*). May also be prepared as a decoction over a relatively high flame for a short period of time (about 10-20 minutes) with the dosage specified in parentheses. Available in a variety of prepared forms. In China, the more fast-acting liquid preparations are preferred.

Actions   Releases the exterior, transforms dampness, regulates the qi, and harmonizes the middle burner

Indications

Fever and chills, headache, a sensation of fullness and stifling oppression in the chest, pain in the epigastrium and abdomen, nausea and vomiting, borborygmus, diarrhea, loss of taste, a white, greasy tongue coating, and a moderate, soggy pulse. Also for sudden turmoil disorders or malarial disorders with the above symptomatology.

This is externally-contracted wind-cold with concurrent internal injury due to dampness and stagnation. Externally-contracted wind-cold fetters the protective yang, producing fever and chills. The greater yang channels, the most yang aspects of which traverse the head, are the first to be affected by wind-cold, which causes headache. The internal stagnation obstructs the qi dynamic in the middle burner, leading to a sensation of fullness and stifling oppression in the chest and abdominal pain. It also disrupts the normal ascending and downward-directing functions of the middle burner. This causes abdominal pain, nausea, vomiting, borborygmus, and diarrhea. In the present case, this pathology is further exacerbated by wind-cold fettering the exterior and constraining the Lung's dispersing functions. This further disrupts the ascending and downward-directing actions of the qi dynamic, leading to an intermingling of external and internal pathogens. Internal stagnation of dampness causes a loss of taste, and produces a white, greasy tongue coating and a moderate, soggy pulse.

Analysis of Formula

This formula is designed to treat patterns characterized by the contraction of external wind-cold in the context of internal damp turbidity. For this purpose, it relies on a strategy of dispersing the exterior, transforming dampness in the interior, and regulating the qi dynamic. The chief herb, acrid and aromatic Pogostemonis/Agastaches Herba (*huò xiāng*), addresses all the major aspects of this condition. It disperses wind-cold, transforms turbid dampness, revives the Spleen, and stops vomiting. There are two distinct groups of deputy herbs. The first, consisting of Magnoliae officinalis Cortex (*hòu pò*) and Citri reticulatae Pericarpium (*chén pí*), reinforces the actions of the chief herb in the middle burner. Magnoliae officinalis Cortex (*hòu pò*) moves the qi and promotes proper water metabolism to expand the chest and reduce the sensation of fullness and stifling oppression in the chest. Citri reticulatae Pericarpium (chén pí) regulates the qi, transforms dampness, and harmonizes the functions of the middle burner. The second group, consisting of Perillae Folium (zǐ sū yè) and Angelicae dahuricae Radix (bái zhǐ), helps the chief herb dispel externally-contracted cold. Perillae Folium (zǐ sū yè) is a strong, exterior-releasing herb that also harmonizes the middle burner. Angelicae dahuricae Radix (bái zhǐ) is very effective in treating headache.

One of the assistants, Pinelliae Rhizoma praeparatum (zhì bàn xià), harmonizes the Stomach and stops the vomiting. Another assistant, Arecae Pericarpium (dà fù pí), functions like Magnoliae officinalis Cortex (hòu pò) but focuses on the lower burner. Both herbs act upon the qi mechanism in the middle and lower burners and reinforce the actions of the chief herb, which focuses on the upper burner. Internal stagnation of dampness in the middle burner weakens the Spleen's transportive and transformative functions. The assistants Atractylodis macrocephalae Rhizoma (bái zhú) and Poria (fú líng) form a powerful combination for strengthening the Spleen and transforming dampness. The last of the assistants, Platycodi Radix (jié gěng), promotes the proper functioning of the Lungs and the diaphragm, which strengthens the actions of the chief herb. The envoys, Glycyrrhizae Radix praeparata (zhì gān cǎo), Zingiberis Rhizoma recens (shēng jiāng), and Jujubae Fructus (dà zǎo), harmonize the actions of the other herbs and regulate the Spleen and Stomach.

The herbal groupings in this formula have been carefully matched and balanced. Pogostemonis/Agastaches Herba (huò xiāng), Perillae Folium (zǐ sū yè), and Angelicae dahuricae Radix (bái zhǐ) release the exterior. Magnoliae officinalis Cortex (hòu pò), Arecae Pericarpium (dà fù pí), and Citri reticulatae Pericarpium (chén pí) promote the movement of qi internally. Perillae Folium (zǐ sū yè), Angelicae dahuricae Radix (bái zhǐ), and Platycodi Radix (jié gěng) provide an ascending action. Poria (fú líng), Pinelliae Rhizoma praeparatum (zhì bàn xià), and Arecae Pericarpium (dà fù pí) cause the turbid, rebellious qi to descend.

Cautions and Contraindications

Because this formula contains warm and drying herbs, it should not be used without significant modification for conditions of wind-heat or fire due to deficiency.

Commentary

The spectrum of indications for this formula listed in the source text is very broad, encompassing not only headache and diarrhea from cold damage, but also sudden turmoil disorders, mountain forest miasmatic malarial disorders, pre- and postpartum abdominal pain, and childhood nutritional impairment.

This formula treats various types of diarrhea caused by the obstruction of the qi dynamic in the middle burner. The most important of these is 'urgent diarrhea' (飧泄 sūn xiè), the nature of which is explained in *Wondrous Lantern for Peering into the Origin and Development of Miscellaneous Diseases*:

> An overabundance of dampness causes urgent diarrhea. [In fact,] it is only due to dampness. Some wonder if wind, cold, heat, and deficiency cannot also lead to this disorder. If the Spleen is strong and without dampness, these four [pathologies] cannot interfere [with its function]. How could there then be diarrhea?

Sudden Turmoil Disorders

Another type of diarrhea is that of sudden turmoil disorders (霍亂 huò luàn). These are acute conditions characterized by the simultaneous onset of vomiting and diarrhea. They were first described in *Discussion of Cold Damage* and are associated with the penetration of wind-cold-dampness into the body. During the 19th century when cholera was first introduced into China from India, Chinese physicians sought to explain the nature of this new infectious disease by describing it as a type of sudden turmoil disorder. Some contemporary texts therefore equate the two conditions. This is not only historically wrong, but more importantly, clinically misleading, for even if 19th-century physicians called cholera a form of sudden turmoil disorder, they treated it by means of new formulas. Patchouli/Agastache Powder to Rectify the Qi (huò xiāng zhèng qì sǎn) is therefore not a remedy for the biomedically-defined disease of cholera. It is suited for treating those types of sudden turmoil disorders that occur during the summertime, when dampness is the predominant aspect. The cardinal symptoms are abdominal pain, vomiting, and diarrhea, together with signs of an exterior condition.

Miasmic Malarial Disorder

This formula is also used for mild cases of mountain mist miasmic malarial disorder (山嵐瘴瘧 shān lán zhàng nuè). This is thought to be contracted from the mists of the mountains and forests, considered to be damp and hot in nature. Manifestations include intermittent fever and chills, disorientation, and madness with delirious speech or loss of voice. Miasmic disorders were viewed as one type of abnormal seasonal qi, regarded as one of the main causes of epidemic disorders in traditional China. The early 19th-century physician Chen Nian-Zu explained the treatment strategy appropriate for such disorders:

> The qi of [any one of] the four seasons that does not arrive at its proper time enters through the mouth and nose; it is different from the pathogenic qi that injures the channels [and enters through the skin]. Therefore, do not use strong sweating [herbs] to release the exterior, but aromatic substances that promote the proper flow of qi.

In late imperial China, the occurrence of miasmic qi was particularly linked with the southeastern provinces of the country, known collectively as Lingnan 嶺南, whose warm and moist climate was considered unsuitable for the northern Chinese then settling there. It is undoubtedly due to this association that Patchouli/Agastache Powder to Rectify the Qi (*huò xiāng zhèng qì sǎn*) is still one of the most important formulas for treating digestive disorders contracted while traveling, that is, when one encounters qi to which one is not accustomed.

Pogostemonis/Agastaches Herba (*huò xiāng*), the chief in this formula, is one of the main herbs in the materia medica for treating miasmic disorders. *Encountering the Sources of the Classic of Materia Medica* notes: "In all cases of unseasonal epidemic disorders or miasmic malarial disorders, one uses [this herb] to awaken the Spleen and strengthen the Stomach. Then the pathogenic qi naturally has no place where it might lodge, and [the condition] is cured." *Explanation of the Classic of Materia Medica* attributes this capacity not only to its well-known aromatic, dampness-transforming nature, but also postulates a more specific toxicity-resolving effect:

> Pogostemonis/Agastaches Herba (*huò xiāng*) has a qi that is slightly warming. Its constitution is that of the wood qi of early spring. … Its flavor is acrid, sweet, and without toxicity. Possessing the two flavors of metal and earth, it enters into the hand greater yin Lung channel and the foot greater yin Spleen channel. Its qi and flavor are both ascending. … If a damp toxin enters the Spleen, sweetness can resolve such toxicity. Noxious qi is the noxious qi of pathogens. The Lungs govern the qi. Acrid [flavor] can disperse pathogens, hence [it also] governs [the dispersion of noxious qi].

Use in Interior Disorders

Although the formula simultaneously disperses the exterior and regulates the interior, its cold-dispersing and exterior-releasing powers are mild compared to its ability to transform dampness. Hence, it can also be used where no pathogens are present in the exterior. As the Ming-dynasty physician Wu Kun notes in *Investigations of Medical Formulas*: "If there is no wind-cold in the exterior, the two substances [Perillae Folium (*zǐ sū yè*) and Angelicae dahuricae Radix (*bái zhǐ*)] are still able to discharge the Spleen qi." Likewise, the inclusion of Atractylodis macrocephalae Rhizoma (*bái zhú*) and Poria (*fú líng*) in the formula does not imply that patients for whom this formula is indicated need present with marked signs of deficiency. Rather, by augmenting the Spleen's qi, they strengthen its ability to transport and transform and thereby eliminate excess dampness.

Comparisons

➢ Vs. Calm the Stomach Powder (*píng wèi sǎn*)

This formula contains all the ingredients of both Calm the Stomach Powder (*píng wèi sǎn*) and Two-Aged [Herb] Decoction (*èr chén tāng*). Its ability to transform dampness is accordingly stronger than its ability to release exterior conditions. By contrast, Patchouli/Agastache Powder to Rectify the Qi (*huò xiāng zhèng qì sǎn*) focuses more on the exterior and on dispersing pathogenic qi. It is therefore indicated when dampness lodges not only in the greater yin Spleen, but also in the greater yin Lung aspect.

➢ Vs. Rectify the Qi Powder Worth More than Gold (*bù huàn jīn zhèng qì sǎn*)

Both formulas are used for treating sudden turmoil disorders and have many ingredients in common, including Pogostemonis/Agastaches Herba (*huò xiāng*), which serves as the chief herb. However, Rectify the Qi Powder Worth More than Gold (*bù huàn jīn zhèng qì sǎn*), which also contains Atractylodis Rhizoma (*cāng zhú*), is stronger at transforming damp turbidity and is especially good for treating vomiting. Patchouli/Agastache Powder to Rectify the Qi (*huò xiāng zhèng qì sǎn*), on the other hand, is better suited for conditions where the presence of wind-cold in the exterior is pronounced. This is because it contains Perillae Folium (*zǐ sū yè*) and Angelicae dahuricae Radix (*bái zhǐ*), which are able to resolve the exterior.

➢ Vs. Mosla Powder (*xiāng rú sǎn*)

Both of these formulas treat externally-contracted wind-cold in the summertime with internal accumulation of dampness. However, the focus of Mosla Powder (*xiāng rú sǎn*) is on releasing the exterior where the primary symptoms are chills and fever, and the internal accumulation is relatively mild. Conversely, Patchouli/Agastache Powder to Rectify the Qi (*huò xiāng zhèng qì sǎn*) is indicated for severe internal accumulation with only mild exterior symptoms.

➢ Vs. Coptis and Magnolia Bark Drink (*lián pò yǐn*); *see* PAGE 706

Biomedical Indications

With the appropriate presentation, this formula may be used to treat a variety of biomedically-defined disorders including acute gastroenteritis, stomach flu, the common cold contracted during the summer, and urticaria.

Alternate names

Rectify the Qi Powder (*zhèng qì sǎn*) in *Complete Compendium of Cold Damage*; Agastache Decoction to Rectify the Qi (*huò xiāng zhèng qì tāng*) in *Golden Mirror of the Medical Tradition*

Modifications

• For severe wind-cold, increase the dosage of Perillae Folium (*zǐ sū yè*).

- For food stagnation, remove Glycyrrhizae Radix *(gān cǎo)* and Jujubae Fructus *(dà zǎo)* and add Massa medicata fermentata *(shén qū)* and Gigeriae galli Endothelium corneum *(jī nèi jīn)*.
- For severe dampness with a very thick, greasy tongue coating, substitute Atractylodis Rhizoma *(cāng zhú)* for Atractylodis macrocephalae Rhizoma *(bái zhú)*.
- For brief, scanty urination, add Akebiae Caulis *(mù tōng)* and Alismatis Rhizoma *(zé xiè)*.
- For pronounced qi stagnation with adominal distention and pain, add Aucklandiae Radix *(mù xiāng)* and Corydalis Rhizoma *(yán hú suǒ)*.

Associated Formulas

Note: Each of the five modifications of this formula from *Systematic Differentiation of Warm Pathogen Diseases* listed below contains Pogostemonis/Agastaches Herba *(huò xiāng)*, Magnoliae officinalis Cortex *(hòu pò)*, Citri reticulatae Pericarpium *(chén pí)*, and Poria *(fú líng)*. These herbs regulate the middle burner, transform turbid dampness, and treat dampness constrained in the Triple Burner, with an emphasis on the middle burner. The first three modifications treat conditions with some signs of heat. The other two treat cold-dampness.

一加減正氣散 （一加减正气散）

First Modification of Rectify the Qi Powder
yī jiā jiǎn zhèng qì sǎn

SOURCE	*Systematic Differentiation of Warm Pathogen Diseases* (1798)

Pogostemonis/Agastaches Herba *(huò xiāng)* 6g
Magnoliae officinalis Cortex *(hòu pò)* 6g
Armeniacae Semen *(xìng rén)* 6g
Poriae Cutis *(fú líng pí)* 6g
Citri reticulatae Pericarpium *(chén pí)* 3g
Massa medicata fermentata *(shén qū)* 4.5g
Hordei Fructus germinatus *(mài yá)* 4.5g
Artemisiae scopariae Herba *(yīn chén)* 6g
Arecae Pericarpium *(dà fù pí)* 3g

Decoction. Spreads and facilitates the flow of qi in the middle burner, transforms dampness, and reduces food stagnation. For food stagnation and dampness constraining and obstructing the middle burner (causing a loss of control over the ascending and descending functions) characterized by epigastric and abdominal distention and fullness, and gummy stools with irregular defecation.

二加減正氣散 （二加减正气散）

Second Modification of Rectify the Qi Powder
èr jiā jiǎn zhèng qì sǎn

SOURCE	*Systematic Differentiation of Warm Pathogen Diseases* (1798)

Pogostemonis/Agastaches Herba *(huò xiāng)* 9g
Citri reticulatae Pericarpium *(chén pí)* 6g
Magnoliae officinalis Cortex *(hòu pò)* 6g
Poriae Cutis *(fú líng pí)* 9g
Stephaniae tetrandrae Radix *(hàn fáng jǐ)* 9g
Sojae Semen germinatum *(dà dòu juǎn)* 6g
Tetrapanacis Medulla *(tōng cǎo)* 4.5g
Coicis Semen *(yì yǐ rén)* 9g

Decoction. Transforms dampness, regulates the qi, and facilitates the flow of qi in the channels. For a stifling sensation in the epigastrium with loose stools, body aches, a white tongue coating, and an indistinct pulse.

三加減正氣散 （三加减正气散）

Third Modification of Rectify the Qi Powder
sān jiā jiǎn zhèng qì sǎn

SOURCE	*Systematic Differentiation of Warm Pathogen Diseases* (1798)

Pogostemonis/Agastaches Herba *(huò xiāng)* 9g
Poriae Cutis *(fú líng pí)* 9g
Magnoliae officinalis Cortex *(hòu pò)* 6g
Citri reticulatae Pericarpium *(chén pí)* 4.5g
Armeniacae Semen *(xìng rén)* 9g
Talcum *(huá shí)* 15g

Decoction. Regulates the qi, transforms dampness, and clears and drains damp-heat. For long-term internal constraint from dampness that has transformed into damp-heat characterized by a stifling sensation in the epigastrium and a yellow tongue coating.

四加減正氣散 （四加减正气散）

Fourth Modification of Rectify the Qi Powder
sì jiā jiǎn zhèng qì sǎn

SOURCE	*Systematic Differentiation of Warm Pathogen Diseases* (1798)

Pogostemonis/Agastaches Herba *(huò xiāng)* 9g
Magnoliae officinalis Cortex *(hòu pò)* 6g
Poria *(fú líng)* 9g
Citri reticulatae Pericarpium *(chén pí)* 4.5g
Tsaoko Fructus *(cǎo guǒ)* 3g
dry-fried Crataegi Fructus *(chǎo shān zhā)* 15g
Massa medicata fermentata *(shén qū)* 6g

Decoction. Warms the middle burner and transforms dampness. For dampness obstructing the qi level of the middle burner causing an overabundance of yin and subsequent generation of cold. This is characterized by a white, slippery tongue coating and a moderate pulse on the right (qi) side.

五加減正氣散 （五加减正气散）

Fifth Modification of Rectify the Qi Powder
wǔ jiā jiǎn zhèng qì sǎn

SOURCE	*Systematic Differentiation of Warm Pathogen Diseases* (1798)

Pogostemonis/Agastaches Herba (huò xiāng) 6g
Citri reticulatae Pericarpium (chén pí) .4.5g
Poria (fú líng) 9g
Magnoliae officinalis Cortex (hòu pò) 6g
Arecae Pericarpium (dà fù pí) 4.5g
Setariae (Oryzae) Fructus germinatus (gǔ yá) 3g
Atractylodis Rhizoma (cāng zhú) 6g

Decoction. Strengthens the Spleen, benefits the Stomach, warms and transforms cold and dampness. For cold-dampness obstructing the middle burner and injuring the Spleen and Stomach characterized by a stifling sensation in the epigastrium and diarrhea.

六和湯 (六和汤)

Harmonize the Six Decoction

liù hé tāng

See the COMMENTARY below for competing interpretations of the formula's name.

Source　*Formulary of the Pharmacy Service for Benefiting the People in the Taiping Era* (1107)

Ginseng Radix (rén shēn) 30g
Amomi Fructus (shā rén) 30g
Pinelliae Rhizoma praeparatum (zhì bàn xià) 30g
Armeniacae Semen (xìng rén) 30g
Atractylodis macrocephalae Rhizoma (bái zhú) 60g
Pogostemonis/Agastaches Folium (huò xiāng yè) 60g
Lablab Semen album (biǎn dòu) 60g
Poria rubra (chì fú líng) 60g
Chaenomelis Fructus (mù guā) 60g
ginger-fried Magnoliae officinalis Cortex (jiāng chǎo hòu pò)120g
Moslae Herba (xiāng rú) 120g
Glycyrrhizae Radix praeparata (zhì gān cǎo) 30g

Method of Preparation　The source text advises to coarsely grind the ingredients and take 12g of the resulting powder in a small cup-and-a-half of water, along with 3 slices of Zingiberis Rhizoma recens (shēng jiāng) and 1 Jujubae Fructus (dà zǎo). Cook until 80 percent of the liquid remains, discard the dregs, and take without regard to meals. At present, it is taken as a decoction with an appropriate reduction in dosages, divided into three doses a day.

Actions　Strengthens the Spleen, transforms dampness, causes the pure to ascend and the turbid to descend, and harmonizes the functions of the six yang organs

Indications

Chills and fever, absence of sweating, headache, feeling muddled, wheezing from phlegm, cough, a stifling sensation in the chest or a sensation of fullness and distention in the diaphragmatic region, vomiting and diarrhea, lack of strength in the extremities, no desire for food or drink, dark urine that is reduced in volume, and a white, slippery tongue coating.

This is externally-contracted cold during the summer months with internal damage due to dampness. Such con-

ditions readily occur during late summer when damp and hot weather leads to the accumulation of damp-heat in the interior. In this context, even a brief spell of cold weather, or ingestion of cold food or drink (often taken in order to 'cool down'), can lead to contraction of cold in the exterior. This traps the dampness in the interior, while the internal dampness prevents the protective yang from ascending to disperse the pathogen. Constraint of yang qi in the exterior by a cold pathogen manifests as chills and fever without sweating as well as headache. Feeling muddled and a stifling sensation in the chest or diaphragmatic region betray the presence of dampness and distinguish this pattern from the simple contraction of wind-cold. Wheezing, cough, and phlegm indicate constraint of qi and the presence of dampness in the hand greater yin Lung organ. Disruption of the qi dynamic in the middle burner with intermingling of pure and turbid qi leads to vomiting and diarrhea or sudden turmoil disorder. The extremities are associated with the Spleen. Their weakness, combined with no desire for food and drink and a white, slippery tongue coating, indicate qi constraint in the greater yang Spleen due to dampness and turbidity. Dark urine that is reduced in volume is a consequence of damp-heat.

Analysis of Formula

This formula is a combination of Mosla Powder (xiāng rú sǎn), discussed in Chapter 5, and Four-Gentlemen Decoction (sì jūn zǐ tāng), discussed in Chapter 8. Like Mosla Powder (xiāng rú sǎn), this formula contains Moslae Herba (xiāng rú), Magnoliae officinalis Cortex (hòu pò), and Lablab Semen album (bái biǎn dòu). Among these herbs, acrid and warming Moslae Herba (xiāng rú) is regarded as the best herb for dispersing cold fettering the exterior during the summer months, when dampness in the interior is prevalent. It both ascends and directs downward. It facilitates the rise of clear yang to disperse cold from the exterior and the descent of turbid yin so that it can be eliminated via the bowels and bladder. Acrid, bitter, and aromatic Magnoliae officinalis Cortex (hòu pò) moves the qi, transforms stagnation, and eases the middle. Sweet and balanced Lablab Semen album (bái biǎn dòu) reduces summerheat, transforms dampness, strengthens the Spleen qi, and harmonizes the middle. Ginseng Radix (rén shēn), Poria rubra (chì fú líng), and Glycyrrhizae Radix praeparata (zhì gān cǎo) are basically Four-Gentlemen Decoction (sì jūn zǐ tāng), a key formula for tonifying the Spleen and Stomach. When the Spleen qi is strong, summerheat-dampness is naturally transformed and eliminated.

The remaining herbs assist in various ways the therapeutic strategies represented by these two foundational formulas. Pinelliae Rhizoma praeparatum (zhì bàn xià) and Amomi Fructus (shā rén) amplify their ability to harmonize the Stomach to stop the nausea and vomiting. Pogostemonis/Agastaches Folium (huò xiāng yè) supports the dispersal of cold from the exterior, while also aromatically transforming dampness in the middle burner and rectifying the qi dynamic. Bitter, acrid, and oily Armeniacae Semen *(xìng rén)* assists Magnoliae officinalis Cortex *(hòu pò)* in directing downward, but also prevents the acrid nature of that herb from damaging the fluids. Chaenomelis Fructus *(mù guā)* harmonizes the Stomach and soothes the sinews. In conjunction with Pogostemonis/Agastaches Herba *(huò xiāng)* and Zingiberis Rhizoma recens *(shēng jiāng)*, it treats sudden turmoil disorder, vomiting, and diarrhea. Zingiberis Rhizoma recens *(shēng jiāng)*, Jujubae Fructus *(dà zǎo)*, and Glycyrrhizae Radix *(gān cǎo)* combine as envoys to harmonize the Spleen and Stomach and smooth the interaction between the various ingredients in the formula.

Cautions and Contraindications

The majority of herbs in this formula are acrid and warming. The formula is thus contraindicated for sudden turmoil disorder due to damp-heat.

Commentary

This is a widely used formula for expelling summerheat, transforming dampness, strengthening the Spleen, and harmonizing the Stomach. It is suited for mixed patterns where excess dominates over deficiency, dampness over heat, and obstruction of the qi dynamic in the interior over cold fettering qi in the exterior.

Meaning of the Name

There are two competing interpretations of the meaning of the word 'six' in the formula's name. One group of commentators thinks that it refers to the formula's ability to harmonize (i.e., correct) the function of the six yang organs. These organs, responsible for transportation of both the clear and turbid qi throughout the body, stand for the qi dynamic that is harmonized by this formula. The Ming-dynasty physician Wu Kun explains this in *Investigations of Medical Formulas*: "The Spleen and Stomach are the general commander of the six yang organs. Hence, in all disorders where the six yang organs are not regulated, one primarily regulates them through the Spleen and Stomach."

The second interpretation is that 'six' stands for the six pernicious qi. Wang Ang, writing in *Medical Formulas Collected and Analyzed*, is representative of this view:

> 'Harmonizing the six' means harmonizing the six qi. When one says that it harmonizes the six yang organs, does this mean that the five yin organs should not be harmonized? With regard to the six qi of wind, cold, summerheat, dampness, dryness, and fire, these are contracted [especially] often during the summer months. Therefore, one uses all of these herbs to correct [the function] of the Spleen and Stomach in order to resist all pathogens, regularizing and harmonizing [any disorder].

It is possible to synthesize these interpretations by viewing the six yang organs as representing the qi dynamic, which centers on the ascending and downward-directing functions of the Spleen and Stomach. When the qi dynamic is open, the yang qi is able to ascend, dispersing pathogens in the exterior through the pores, while pathogens in the interior can be eliminated via the bowels and urine.

Comparisons

➤ Vs. Patchouli/Agastache, Magnolia Bark, Pinellia, and Poria Decoction *(huò pò xià líng tāng)*

Both formulas were listed for the first time in the same source text for the treatment of sudden turmoil disorder due to cold-dampness damaging the Stomach and Intestines. Patchouli/Agastache, Magnolia Bark, Pinellia, and Poria Decoction *(huò pò xià líng tāng)* is better suited for milder conditions of wind-cold in the exterior or invasion by miasmic qi. By contrast, Harmonize the Six Decoction *(liù hé tāng)* focuses on strengthening the Spleen and regulating the ascending and descending functions of the middle burner. It is indicated for conditions characterized by more severe cold in the exterior and summerheat dampness in the interior.

➤ Vs. Mosla Powder *(xiāng rú sǎn)*

Both formulas treat cold fettering the exterior during the summer months with dampness obstructing the qi dynamic in the interior. The key symptoms for both formulas are thus vomiting and diarrhea accompanied by fever and chills. Mosla Powder *(xiāng rú sǎn)* is relatively better at treating conditions where cold-dampness invades the body from the exterior. Harmonize the Six Decoction *(liù hé tāng)*, on the other hand, is better suited for conditions due to damage from food and drink, where the Spleen and Stomach have been damaged.

➤ Vs. Ginseng, Poria, and White Atractylodes Powder *(shēn líng bái zhú sǎn)*

Both formulas treat complex conditions characterized by qi deficiency of the middle burner accompanied by the presence of dampness. Ginseng, Poria, and White Atractylodes Powder *(shēn líng bái zhú sǎn)* is indicated for patterns characterized by more severe qi deficiency without exterior symptoms. Harmonize the Six Decoction *(liù hé tāng)*, on the other hand, is better suited for patterns where the deficiency is not marked, but pathogens in the exterior may be present.

Biomedical Indications

With the appropriate presentation, this formula may be used to treat a variety of biomedically-defined disorders including summertime colds, bronchitis, and gastroenteritis.

Alternate name

Unite the Six Decoction (*liù hé tāng*) in *Prescriptions for Universal Benefit*

···

Modifications

- For more severe cold fettering the exterior with headache, add Notopterygii Rhizoma seu Radix *(qiāng huó)* and Angelicae dahuricae Radix *(bái zhǐ)*.
- For coughing with phlegm that is not easy to expectorate, add Platycodi Radix *(jié gěng)*, Peucedani Radix *(qián hú)*, Aurantii Fructus *(zhǐ ké)*, and Fritillariae cirrhosae Bulbus *(chuān bèi mǔ)*.
- For borborygmus and severe diarrhea, add Atractylodis Rhizoma *(cāng zhú)* and Chebulae Fructus *(hē zǐ)*.

八味帶下方

Eight-Ingredient Formula for Vaginal Discharge

bā wèi dài xià fāng

Source *Selected Formulas of Famous Physicians* (1781)

Angelicae sinensis Radix *(dāng guī)* 5g
Smilacis glabrae Rhizoma *(tǔ fú líng)* 4g
Chuanxiong Rhizoma *(chuān xiōng)* 3g
Poria *(fú líng)* 3g
Akebiae Caulis *(mù tōng)* 3g
Citri reticulatae Pericarpium *(chén pí)* 2g
Lonicerae Flos *(jīn yín huā)* 2g
Rhei Radix et Rhizoma *(dà huáng)* 05.-1g

Method of Preparation Decoct the above ingredients, adding Rhei Radix et Rhizoma *(dà huáng)* at the end. Rhei Radix et Rhizoma *(dà huáng)* may be removed if the patient's stools are loose. In modern practice, the dosages are frequently larger than those listed here.

Actions Clears heat, resolves toxicity, dispels dampness, and arrests vaginal discharge

Indications

Women who feel subjectively cold due to underlying deficiency but also have damp-heat symptoms such as aching in the lower back, abdominal pain, profuse red, yellow or white vaginal discharge, and itching sores.

This is a situation in which either a condition marked by cold and underlying deficiency has debilitated the body's ability to transform dampness, or that strong pathogenic water or a parasitic pathogen has damaged the body's yang qi. In either case, there is pathogenic water or dampness and heat (resulting from stagnation) collecting in the lower burner and giving rise to the above symptoms. Although not mentioned in the source text, the tongue associated with this pattern would usually be pale, with a white or yellow coating, and the pulse would be slippery and without force.

Anaysis of Formula

This formula takes a multifaceted approach to address all the major components of this condition. Smilacis glabrae Rhizoma *(tǔ fú líng)* is the chief ingredient and facilitates the resolution of dampness while helping the body separate the pure from the impure. Because this agent is sweet (and thus tonifies), it is ideal for conditions such as this one where the collection of dampness is compounded by Spleen deficiency. Historically, Smilacis glabrae Rhizoma *(tǔ fú líng)* is frequently used to address sores in the lower body (such as those associated with sexually transmitted diseases) and other disorders due to damp-heat toxin.

Angelicae sinensis Radix *(dāng guī)* and Chuanxiong Rhizoma *(chuān xiōng)* tonify and move the blood and are frequently used in formulas that treat sores. The inclusion of Poria *(fú líng)*, Akebiae Caulis *(mù tōng)*, and Citri reticulatae Pericarpium *(chén pí)* is intended to increase the chief ingredient's ability to transform damp-heat and dispel water toxin. Here, Poria *(fú líng)* serves a dual purpose since it also supplements the Spleen to assist in its transformation of dampness.

Lonicerae Flos *(jīn yín huā)* and Rhei Radix et Rhizoma *(dà huáng)* both clear heat and resolve toxicity. Rhei Radix et Rhizoma *(dà huáng)* adds the function of moving the stool, thereby helping to clear heat from the lower burner.

Cautions and Contraindications

This formula treats damp-heat disorders with symptoms in the lower burner. It is inappropriate for vaginal discharge in the absence of damp-heat.

Commentary

This formula originates in Japan where it is used to treat damp-heat vaginal discharge. It differs from many other formulas that treat this disorder in that it does not contain astringents such as Ailanthi Cortex *(chūn pí)* or Euryales Semen *(qiàn shí)*. While used to treat vaginal discharge associated with such biomedically-defined diseases as vaginitis, endometriosis, trichomoniasis, and gonorrhea, it also addresses attendant symptoms of lower burner damp-heat such as pain in the abdomen and lower back. The formula's ability to clear heat, resolve toxicity, and drain dampness also make it suitable for treating lower body damp-heat toxic sores or genital itching.

Since this formula treats mostly the branch and only slightly addresses the root deficiency, it is best to follow treatment with a formula that attends more evenly to root and branch, such as Tokoro Drink to Separate the Clear *(bì xiè fēn qīng yǐn)* with the addition of Ailanthi Cortex *(chūn pí)*. As a final step, one may wish to solely address the root deficiency with formulas such as Ginseng, Poria, and White Atractylodes Powder *(shēn líng bái zhú sǎn)* or Six-Gentlemen Decoction *(liù jūn zǐ tāng)*.

Comparisons

➤ Vs. End Discharge Decoction *(wán dài tāng)*

Both formulas treat damp-heat vaginal discharge and Spleen deficiency. Eight-Ingredient Formula for Vaginal Discharge *(bā wèi dài xià fāng)* is better at clearing damp-heat but is less adept than End Discharge Decoction *(wán dài tang)* at supplementing the Spleen. In addition, End Discharge Decoction *(wán dài tāng)* can also treat Spleen deficiency compounded by Liver constraint. Eight-Ingredient Formula for Vaginal Discharge *(bā wèi dài xià fāng)*, on the other hand, is more appropriate for conditions where damp-heat toxin is severe. It can also address genital sores.

Biomedical Indications

With the appropriate presentation, this formula may be used to treat a variety of biomedically-defined disorders including endometriosis, vaginitis, trichomoniasis, and gonorrhea.

Modifications

- For damp-heat genital sores or if vaginal discharge is dark and malodorous, add some or all of the components of Coptis Decoction to Resolve Toxicity *(huáng lián jiě dú tāng)*: Scutellariae Radix *(huáng qín)*, Phellodendri Cortex *(huáng bǎi)*, and Gardeniae Fructus *(zhī zǐ)*.

- If Spleen deficiency is obvious through symptoms such as loose stools, a pale complexion, and fatigue, add small amounts of Atractylodis macrocephalae Rhizoma *(bái zhú)*, Codonopsis Radix *(dǎng shēn)*, and Glycyrrhizae Radix praeparata *(zhì gān cǎo)*. This changes the formula to one that treats the root and branch more equally.

Section 2

. . . .

FORMULAS THAT CLEAR HEAT AND EXPEL DAMPNESS

Conditions of damp-heat develop from the invasion of dampness and heat from the exterior, or from dampness that transforms into heat in the interior. Summerheat invariably contains a degree of dampness. If the dampness in pronounced, or should summerheat invade a person suffering from internal dampness, this leads to summerheat-dampness (暑濕 *shǔ shī*) disorders. Such disorders typically manifest with focal distention, a stifling sensation in the chest or epigastrium, irritability, generalized fever, and a yellow, greasy tongue coating. This presentation implies a predominance of heat over dampness. When warm and damp pathogens combine to invade the body, which usually occurs during the summer season, this causes damp-warmth (濕溫 *shī wēn*). This typically manifests with symptoms like headache, aversion to heat, heaviness or aching of the body, focal distention, a stifling sensation in the chest, lack of appetite, and fever that worsens in the afternoon. Where damp-heat collects in the skin and flesh, this can cause jaundice or a variety of skin disorders characterized by damp discharges. When it inhibits the nourishment of the sinews and muscles, damp-heat can also lead to atrophy disorders. Because dampness is heavy in nature, it tends to move downward in the body or to attack the body from below. Damp-heat in the lower burner causes reduced and dark urination, heaviness of the body, lethargy, and a greasy, yellow tongue coating.

Dampness and heat are antagonistic. One is yang and tends to move upward, the other is yin and tends to move downward. Furthermore, when dampness combines with heat, it can 'weigh down' the heat and make it more difficult to clear. For this reason, formulas that treat damp-heat disorders must rely on a dual strategy of clearing heat and expelling dampness. The most important herbs for this purpose are Talcum *(huá shí)*, Gardeniae Fructus *(zhī zǐ)*, Coicis Semen *(yì yǐ rén)*, and Artemisiae scopariae Herba *(yīn chén)*. Depending on the pattern, these herbs may be combined with four other types of herbs.

The first group is comprised of herbs that disseminate and facilitate the Triple Burner such as Armeniacae Semen *(xìng rén)* for the upper burner, Amomi Fructus rotundus *(bái dòu kòu)* for the middle burner, and Coicis Semen *(yì yǐ rén)* for the lower burner. The Triple Burner is the official that 'keeps the sluice clear' (決瀆之官 *jué dú zhī guān*), ensuring the smooth diffusion of fluids throughout the body and, in particular, their drainage from the upper toward the lower burner. This makes it particularly useful for dispelling dampness in contexts where the use of warm and acrid qi-moving herbs would be inappropriate.

The second group of herbs encompasses those that drain heat downward such as Rhei Radix et Rhizoma *(dà huáng)*. Their use is appropriate if dampness acquires form, which can be drained via the bowels. The third group of herbs, exemplified by Magnoliae officinalis Cortex *(hòu pò)*, Amomi Fructus *(shā rén)*, and Aurantii Fructus immaturus *(zhǐ shí)*, regulates the qi. They are used where dampness causes qi stagnation. The fourth group tonifies the qi and nourishes the blood and includes such herbs as Ginseng Radix *(rén shēn)*, Atractylodis macrocephalae Rhizoma *(bái zhú)*, Glycyrrhizae Radix *(gān cǎo)*, and Angelicae sinensis Radix *(dāng guī)*. They are used because heat readily damages the qi and blood, a tendency aggravated by the use of the bitter, drying, and heat-clearing herbs that must sometimes also be used in these patterns.

三仁湯（三仁汤）

Three-Seed Decoction

sān rén tāng

The three 'seeds' in this formula are apricot kernel *(xìng rén)*, cardamom seed *(bái dòu kòu)*, and Job's tears or pearl barley *(yì yǐ rén)*.

Source   *Systematic Differentiation of Warm Pathogen Diseases* (1798)

Armeniacae Semen *(xìng rén)* 15g
Amomi Fructus rotundus *(bái dòu kòu)* 6g
Magnoliae officinalis Cortex *(hòu pò)* 6g
Pinelliae Rhizoma praeparatum *(zhì bàn xià)* 9g
Coicis Semen *(yì yǐ rén)* 18g
Tetrapanacis Medulla *(tōng cǎo)* 6g
Lophatheri Herba *(dàn zhú yè)* 6g
Talcum *(huá shí)* 18g

Method of Preparation   The source text advises to prepare as a decoction by cooking the herbs in 'billows water' (澜水 *lán shuǐ*, also known as 'sweet-worked water' 甘澜水 *gān lán shuǐ*) until about half of the liquid has evaporated. It is called 'billows water' because the ladling is supposed to resemble wind billowing the waves. The decoction is taken in three doses throughout the day. Billows water is prepared by putting water into a large basin and repeatedly ladling it until there are thousands of water droplets on the surface. At present, it is prepared as a decoction in the standard fashion, with the dosage of the ingredients reduced by one-half to two-thirds.

Actions   Disseminates the qi, facilitates the qi mechanisms, and clears damp-heat

Indications

Headache, chills, afternoon fever, a heavy sensation in the body, generalized pain, pale yellow complexion, a stifling sensation in the chest, loss of appetite, an absence of thirst, a white tongue coating, and a wiry, thin, and soggy pulse.

This is an early-stage damp-warmth disease or summer-heat-warmth disease in which dampness predominates and the pathogenic influences are lodged in the protective and qi levels. Although the chills, headache, and heavy and painful body sensations resemble those of an exterior cold (greater yang warp) condition, the pulse suggests otherwise. Also, the chills here are caused by constriction of the yang from dampness and are much milder than the chills associated with exterior cold. Dampness lodged in the flesh and muscles causes a heavy sensation in the body and generalized pain; it also prevents the clear yang from rising, which manifests as headache, a stifling sensation in the chest, and loss of appetite. When dampness, a yin pathogenic influence, combines with heat, it sequesters the heat in the deeper levels of the body. This manifests as fever in the afternoon, the 'yin within the yang' time of day. The predominance of dampness over heat in this pattern is reflected in the pale yellow complexion, white tongue coating, and soggy pulse.

Analysis of Formula

The treatment of damp-warmth disorders—caused by the invasion of two different pathogens into the body—presents great difficulties in clinical practice. "Dampness is a yin pathogen," Wu Ju-Tong, the author of this formula, notes. "It naturally appears in the late summer. It appears gradually. Its nature is thick [like fog], sticky, and greasy. Unlike cold pathogens that can be resolved with a single dose of a sweating formula, or heat pathogens that can be reduced with a single dose of a cooling formula, [dampness disorders] are therefore difficult [to resolve] speedily." The combination of dampness with heat, a yang pathogen, presents even greater difficulties because attempting to eliminate one will reinforce the other. The new insight into these problems, by physicians such as Ye Tian-Shi and Wu Ju-Tong, was to overcome these obstacles through indirect treatment, that is, facilitating the body's qi dynamic rather than attacking the pathogen directly. This was achieved by focusing on the different functions of the three burners: the upper burner's capacities for moving qi and directing fluids downward; the middle burner's ability to transform dampness; and the lower burner's function of elimination and qi transformation.

"I use Three-Seed Decoction *(sān rén tāng)* to lightly open the upper burner Lung qi," wrote Wu Ju-Tong. "The Lungs govern the qi of the entire body. If the qi is transformed, dampness is also transformed." However, because dampness resonates with earth, treatment of the middle burner is just as important. To quote Wu Ju-Tong again:

> While compared to other warm pathogen disorders, the momentum of damp-warmth is measured, it nevertheless can constitute a serious [problem]. It is least often [observed] in the upper burner, as there the momentum of the disorder is not very obvious. Middle burner [damp-warmth] diseases are the most common. … This is because dampness is a yin pathogen and should be sought out in the middle burner.

The lower burner, finally, needs to be kept open for excess dampness and heat to be eliminated, but also for the upward movement of physiological qi transformation to begin. The fulcrum of that movement is, again, the middle burner. Hence, as the contemporary physician Qin Bo-Wei emphatically stated, "although the formula attends to all three burners at the same time, it really emphasizes [treatment] of the middle burner."

For these reasons, the formula contains three chief ingredients, one for promoting the qi dynamic of each burner. The chief herb for the upper burner is Armeniacae Semen *(xìng rén)*. Bitter and warming, it dredges the Lung qi, opens what is clogged, and facilitates the downward-directing of qi and fluids. The chief ingredient for the middle burner, aromatic and warming Amomi Fructus rotundus *(bái dòu kòu)*, transforms turbid dampness and revives the Spleen. It also treats the upper burner by spreading the qi in the chest. The chief ingredient for the lower burner, Coicis Semen *(yì yǐ rén)*, leaches out dampness through the urine. It also treats the middle burner by strengthening the Spleen.

Because dampness and heat join in obstructing the qi dynamic, three deputy ingredients, Tetrapanacis Medulla *(tōng cǎo)*, Lophatheri Herba *(dàn zhú yè)*, and Talcum *(huá shí)*, are added to resolve dampness by promoting urination. All of these herbs also clear heat. Talcum *(huá shí)* is also able to resolve summerheat. Lophatheri Herba *(dàn zhú yè)* is light and vents pathogenic heat through the exterior in addition to resolving dampness. Tetrapanacis Medulla *(tōng cǎo)* assists in opening and directing the Lung qi downward.

Dampness resonates with earth and most easily obstructs the middle burner. Amomi Fructus rotundus *(bái dòu kòu)* is therefore supported by two assistants with drying properties, Magnoliae officinalis Cortex *(hòu pò)* and Pinelliae Rhizoma praeparatum *(zhì bàn xià)*. These ingredients effectively treat epigastric and abdominal distention due to dampness or phlegm. The original formula uses 'worked water' to decoct the herbs, which acts as an envoy. First described in the *Inner Classic*, 'worked water' is said to prevent the cooking water from assisting the dampness in the body. Its mode of preparation is also said to change the nature of water from salty to sweet, thus directing its focus on the middle rather than the lower burner.

Working together, the ingredients of this formula clear damp-heat from the qi level by unblocking the Lung qi (upper burner), transforming and drying dampness (middle burner), draining dampness (lower burner), and clearing heat.

Contraindications

It is important to prescribe this formula only for damp-warmth or damp-heat disorders where dampness is prominent. Practitioners must be careful to distinguish the presence of these disorders from others with which they share certain symptoms. These include cold damage, yin deficiency, and internal clumping in the Intestines.

Commentary

This formula is an example of the innovative treatment of damp-warmth disorders developed during the Qing dynasty. First listed in Wu Ju-Tong's *Systematic Differentiation of Warm Pathogen Diseases*, its composition was inspired by the case records of the influential physician Ye Tian-Shi. Hua Xiu-Yun, one of the editors of *Case Records as a Guide to Clinical Practice,* has analyzed Ye's approach to the treatment of early-stage damp-warmth disorders:

> The human body is like a microcosm. If we inspect master [Ye Tian-Shi's] treatment strategies, we [note that he treated patterns] of dampness obstructing the upper burner by using [herbs] that open the Lung qi, assisted by bland [herbs] that

leach out [dampness] and promote [the qi transformation] of the Bladder. This is the same principle as opening the upper sluice gate and unlocking the branch canals in order to direct water by utilizing its [inherent] momentum to flow downward.

This strategy was conceived in response to a perceived failure of existing methods to adequately diagnose and treat early-stage damp-warmth disorders. This is expressed most clearly by Wu Ju-Tong himself:

> Hereditary physicians do not understand [that the symptoms with which these disorders present are those of] damp-warmth. They note [that the patient suffers from] headache, chills, a heavy body and pain, think that it [indicates] cold damage, and [employ formulas to induce] sweating. [This] sweating injures the Heart yang. Dampness [furthermore] follows the acrid, warming, exterior-releasing herbs, steaming and fuming. to rebel upward. Veiling the Heart orifices internally, [such treatment] causes impaired consciousness. Veiling the clear orifices above, it causes deafness, heavy eyes, and inability to talk. [Such physicians] notice fullness of the middle burner and lack of appetite. Thinking that this is [clumping] congealing, and stagnating [of the qi dynamic], they vehemently purge it. Mistaken purgation, [however,] damages the yin and severely curbs the ascending of the Spleen yang so that the Spleen qi inversely sinks [downward]. The damp pathogen avails itself of this momentum to flood the interior, causing cavernous diarrhea. [Such physicians] note the afternoon fever. Thinking that it [indicates] yin deficiency, they employ soft herbs to moisten. [But] dampness is [already] a sticky, stagnating yin pathogen [to which they now] add even more soft, moistening yin herbs. The two yin combine, their similar qi assisting each other. Like pouring molten metal into cracks, it creates a momentum that can [no longer] be resolved. …
>
> Damp qi spreads throughout [the body]. Its original nature is shapeless. If one uses large doses of herbs with a turbid, enriching taste, treatment turns into disaster. In my district, lurking summerheat-damp-warmth is commonly called 'autumnal obtuseness' (秋呆子 *qiū dāi zi*) and is treated with strategies from Mr. Tao's *Six Texts on Cold Damage.* I do not know from where this learning comes. When obtuse physicians instead call a condition obtuse, is that not slander?

Wu Ju-Tong is cited at length because he discusses the three most common types of *misdiagnosis* for damp-warmth disorders: cold damage at the greater yang warp, clumping in the middle burner, and yin deficiency. These are related to the three treatment methods—sweating, purgation, and tonification of yin—that are most strongly contraindicated in the treatment of damp-warmth disorders. An examination of case histories of famous physicians demonstrates, however, that exceptions to this general rule do exist. When dampness obstructs the exterior or channels, for instance, acrid herbs like Pogostemonis/Agastaches Herba *(huò xiāng)*, Notopterygii Rhizoma seu Radix *(qiāng huó)*, or Atractylodis Rhizoma *(cāng zhú)* may be used. Or again, when damp-heat consumes the body fluids in the Intestines and causes internal clumping, it may be essential to use a purgative formula to open this obstruction. Finally, when damp-heat damages the body fluids, it may be appropriate to combine herbs like Glehniae/Adenophorae Radix *(shā shēn)*, Ophiopogonis Radix *(mài mén dōng)*, Polygonati odorati Rhizoma *(yù zhú)*, or Phragmitis Rhizoma *(lú gēn)* with formulas that facilitate water metabolism. Still, at the stage of the disorder for which Three-Seed Decoction *(sān rén tāng)* is appropriate, all of these strategies are contraindicated.

Although a relatively new formula in the context of Chinese medicine's long history, Three-Seed Decoction *(sān rén tāng)* quickly established itself as a classic in its own right. Its importance beyond actual clinical usage lies in its embodiment of the very essence of treating damp-warmth disorders. Precisely because it focuses on facilitating the qi dynamic and on enabling "the transformation of qi so that dampness is also transformed," Three-Seed Decoction *(sān rén tāng)* is nowadays employed for the treatment of internal damp-heat as well. Thus, contemporary physicians use this formula for an extremely wide range of conditions including insomnia, tinnitus, night sweats, diarrhea, ear infections, skin disorders, and painful obstruction. In clinical practice, Three-Seed Decoction *(sān rén tāng)* thus provides an effective treatment strategy for a wide range of internal and external conditions due to damp-warmth or damp-heat at the qi level, where dampness is more pronounced than heat. The following key symptoms are indicative of such problems and should therefore be present: a stifling and heavy sensation in the chest, afternoon fever, fatigue, a body that feels heavy, discomfort in the epigastrium and abdomen, a white, greasy tongue coating, and a soggy pulse.

Comparison

➤ Vs. Nine-Herb Decoction with Notopterygium *(jiǔ wèi qiāng huó tāng)*; *see* page 26

➤ Vs. Sweet Dew Special Pill to Eliminate Toxin *(gān lù xiāo dú dān)*; *see* page 704

Biomedical Indications

With the appropriate presentation, this formula may be used to treat a very wide variety of biomedically-defined disorders. These can be divided into the following groups:

- Infectious diseases such as typhoid fever, pyelonephritis, hepatitis, and brucellosis

- Digestive disorders such as gastritis, colitis, and bacillary dysentery.

This formula has also been used for treating arthritis, morning sickness, fever of unknown origin, chronic bronchitis, diabetes, and biliary ascariasis.

Modifications

- For severe headache and aversion to cold, add Pogostemonis/Agastaches Herba *(huò xiāng)* and Perillae Folium *(zǐ sū yè)*.

- For patterns characterized by distinctly more dampness than heat, add Atractylodis Rhizoma *(cāng zhú)*, Acori tatarinowii Rhizoma *(shí chāng pǔ)*, and Tsaoko Fructus *(cǎo guǒ)*.

- For a more severe stifling sensation in the chest and focal distention in the epigastrium, add Peucedani Radix *(qián hú)* and Pogostemonis/Agastaches Herba *(huò xiāng)*.

- For severe fever, dark urine, and a red tongue indicating the presence of more severe heat, add Artemisiae scopariae Herba *(yīn chén)*, Gardeniae Fructus *(zhī zǐ)*, and Scutellariae Radix *(huáng qín)*.

- For strong heat and dampness in the qi aspect leading to patterns characterized by high fever, severe sweating, a heavy body, facial flushing, thirst, and heart irritability, remove Pinelliae Rhizoma praeparatum *(zhì bàn xià)* and Magnoliae officinalis Cortex *(hòu pò)* and add Gypsum fibrosum *(shí gāo)*, Anemarrhenae Rhizoma *(zhī mǔ)*, and Atractylodis Rhizoma *(cāng zhú)*.

- For heat damaging the body fluids leading to patterns characterized by thirst, parched lips, a yellow, dry tongue coating, and redness of the tongue body on the sides of the tip, remove Pinelliae Rhizoma praeparatum *(zhì bàn xià)* and Magnoliae officinalis Cortex *(hòu pò)* and add Ophiopogonis Radix *(mài mén dōng)* and Trichosanthis Radix *(tiān huā fěn)*.

- For malarial disorders, add Artemisiae annuae Herba *(qīng hāo)* and Tsaoko Fructus *(cǎo guǒ)*.

Associated Formulas

藿樸夏苓湯（藿朴夏苓汤）

Patchouli/Agastache, Magnolia Bark, Pinellia, and Poria Decoction

huò pò xià líng tāng

Source *Bases of Medicine* (1861)

Pogostemonis/Agastaches Caulis *(huò xiāng gěng)* 4.5-6g
Pinelliae Rhizoma praeparatum *(zhì bàn xià)* 6-9g
Poria *(fú líng)* 9-12g
Armeniacae Semen *(xìng rén)* 9-12g
Coicis Semen *(yì yǐ rén)* 12-18g
Amomi Fructus rotundus *(bái dòu kòu)* 2.4g
Polyporus *(zhū líng)* 4.5-6g
Sojae Semen praeparatum *(dàn dòu chǐ)* 9g
Alismatis Rhizoma *(zé xiè)* 4.5-6g
Magnoliae officinalis Cortex *(hòu pò)* 2.4-3g
Tetrapanacis Medulla *(tōng cǎo)* . . . . [decocted first] 9-15g

Releases the exterior and transforms dampness. Primarily for early-stage damp-warmth disorders with clear exterior signs characterized by fever and chills, lassitude, a stifling sensation in the chest, a pasty sensation in the mouth, a white, thin tongue coating, and a moderate, soggy pulse. Compared to the principal formula, this is stronger at resolving dampness and releasing the exterior but weaker at clearing heat.

Comparison

➢ Vs. Harmonize the Six Decoction (liù hé tāng); see page 696

黃芩滑石湯 (黄芩滑石汤)

Scutellaria and Talcum Decoction

huáng qín huá shí tāng

Source   *Systematic Differentiation of Warm Pathogen Diseases* (1798)

Scutellariae Radix (*huáng qín*) 9g
Talcum (*huá shí*) 9g
Poriae Cutis (*fú líng pí*) 9g
Arecae Pericarpium (*dà fù pí*) 6g
Amomi Fructus rotundus (*bái dòu kòu*) 3g
Tetrapanacis Medulla (*tōng cǎo*) 3g
Polyporus (*zhū líng*) 9g

Clears heat and resolves dampness. For damp-warmth diseases in the middle burner characterized by fevers that apparently resolve with sweating but then recur, body aches, little or no thirst, a pale yellow and overly-moist tongue coating, and a moderate pulse. In this condition, the dampness is caused by untransformed food that stagnates and leads to heat from constraint. Dampness and heat are equally severe, which is often a difficult problem to resolve. Because the heat is caused by dampness, it cannot be treated by the clearing method. Instead, the formula employs acrid, disseminating herbs to open up areas of stagnation, bitter, draining herbs to eliminate excess heat via the bowels and urine, and bland herbs to leach out dampness.

杏仁滑石湯 (杏仁滑石汤)

Apricot Kernel and Talcum Decoction

xìng rén huá shí tāng

Source   *Systematic Differentiation of Warm Pathogen Diseases* (1798)

Armeniacae Semen (*xìng rén*) 9g
Scutellariae Radix (*huáng qín*) 6g
Coptidis Rhizoma (*huáng lián*) 3g
Citri reticulatae Pericarpium (*chén pí*) 4.5g
Pinelliae Rhizoma praeparatum (*zhì bàn xià*) 9g
Magnoliae officinalis Cortex (*hòu pò*) 6g
Curcumae Radix (*yù jīn*) 6g
Talcum (*huá shí*) 9g
Tetrapanacis Medulla (*tōng cǎo*) 3g

Clears heat and summerheat and resolves dampness. For smoldering damp-heat or damp-summerheat in all three burners characterized by tidal fever, sweating, thirst, a stifling sensation in the chest, nausea, severe diarrhea, scanty urine, and a grayish-white tongue coating.

甘露消毒丹

Sweet Dew Special Pill to Eliminate Toxin

gān lù xiāo dú dān

This formula is also known as the Universal Benefit Special Pill to Resolve Toxicity (*pǔ jǐ jiě dú dān*). In Chinese the term 'sweet dew' refers to the sweet and luscious taste of dew, which comes down from heaven. In a larger sense, it is like 'manna from heaven.' The formula treats epidemic disorders by draining dampness, clearing heat, and eliminating toxins. Thus, although it contains many bitter herbs, its action is like that of manna, capable of benefiting all people.

Source   *Secretly Transmitted Effective Medicine* (1831)

Forsythiae Fructus (*lián qiáo*) 120g (12-15g)
Scutellariae Radix (*huáng qín*) 300g (12-15g)
Menthae haplocalycis Herba (*bò hé*) 120g (6-9g)
Belamcandae Rhizoma (*shè gān*) 120g (9-12g)
Fritillariae cirrhosae Bulbus (*chuān bèi mǔ*) 150g (6-9g)
Talcum (*huá shí*) 450g (18-21g)
Akebiae Caulis (*mù tōng*) 150g (9-12g)
Artemisiae scopariae Herba (*yīn chén*) 330g (24-30g)
Pogostemonis/Agastaches Herba (*huò xiāng*) 120g (9-12g)
Acori tatarinowii Rhizoma (*shí chāng pǔ*) 180g (4-6g)
Amomi Fructus rotundus (*bái dòu kòu*) 120g (10-12g)

Method of Preparation   The source text advises to grind the ingredients into a powder and form into pills and take in 9g doses twice a day with water. At present, it is usually prepared as a decoction with the dosage specified in parentheses.

Note: The term 'special pill' (丹 *dān*) was originally a designation for special preparations intended to enhance longevity, most of which contained cinnabar. Over time, the use of this term was extended to formulas like this one that were valued for their life-prolonging effects.

Actions   Resolves dampness, transforms turbidity, clears heat, and resolves toxicity

Indications

Fever, achy limbs, lethargy, swollen throat, a stifling sensation in the chest, abdominal distention, dark, scanty urine, a white, greasy or yellow, dry tongue coating, and a soggy, rapid pulse. There may also be vomiting and diarrhea, jaundice, or unremitting fever.

This is the early stage of a damp-warmth epidemic disorder (時溫時疫 *shī wēn shí yì*). The problem is in the qi level, with heat and dampness being equally strong and some of the heat manifesting as toxic heat, either due to constraint or because it was contracted as such from the outside. These conditions are caused by pathogenic influences entering the body through the mouth and nose. Since the nose is linked to the Lungs and the mouth to the Stomach, the pathogenic influences first attack these organs. The resulting smoldering damp-heat causes fever, achy limbs, and lethargy. Smoldering damp-heat also constrains the clear yang and disrupts the qi mechanism, causing a stifling sensation in the chest, abdominal distention, and possibly vomiting and diarrhea. Heat surging upward, especially when accompanied by dampness, causes the throat to swell. Depending on the level of penetration and whether dampness or heat predominates, the tongue coating may be white or yellow, greasy or dry. The soggy, rapid pulse is indicative of damp-heat. Dark, scanty urine and diarrhea reflect the preponderance of heat. In severe cases, dampness may confine the heat internally and cause jaundice. Severe damp-heat in the qi level can also lead to unremitting fever.

Analysis of Formula

This formula treats damp-warmth disorders where dampness and heat are equally strong as well as unseasonal epidemic disorders. To treat dampness, one must create a route for it to be expelled from the body. To treat heat, one must drain its excess and disperse its constraint. To treat toxicity, one must drain fire and resolve toxicity. This formula addresses all of these problems in such a manner that each of its component strategies enhances the others. It clears heat without focusing on the use of bitter, cold substances that would inhibit the qi dynamic; it transforms dampness without being overly acrid and drying, which would fan the heat; and it resolves toxicity without impeding the qi dynamic.

The formula contains three chief herbs: Talcum *(huá shí)*, Artemisiae scopariae Herba *(yīn chén)*, and Scutellariae Radix *(huáng qín)*. These three herbs are equally effective at draining heat and facilitating the resolution of dampness. They act on the upper, middle, and lower burners, respectively. Both Talcum *(huá shí)* and Artemisiae scopariae Herba *(yīn chén)* are used to treat jaundice, while Scutellariae Radix *(huáng qín)* clears heat and resolves toxicity. By clearing the upper parts of the body, the qi can flow freely, and by opening the flow in the lower parts of the body, the damp-heat has an avenue by which to exit the body. However, when the middle burner is obstructed by the thick, cloying properties of dampness, one must use aromatic substances to eliminate the turbidity and revive the Spleen. For this purpose, the formula contains three deputies: Acori tatarinowii Rhizoma *(shí chāng pú)*, Amomi Fructus rotundus *(bái dòu kòu)*, and Pogostemonis/Agastaches Herba *(huò xiāng)*. Fragrant and aromatic, these herbs transform dampness, and because they are acrid and warming, they open the qi dynamic.

Four assistants—Akebiae Caulis *(mù tōng)*, Belamcandae Rhizoma *(shè gān)*, Fritillariae cirrhosae Bulbus *(chuān bèi mǔ)*, and Forsythiae Fructus *(lián qiáo)*—support the chief and deputy herbs. Akebiae Caulis *(mù tōng)* clears heat and facilitates the resolution of dampness, assisting Talcum *(huá shí)* and Artemisiae scopariae Herba *(yīn chén)* in guiding damp-heat out though the urine. Belamcandae Rhizoma *(shè gān)* clears and improves the condition of the throat. Fritillariae cirrhosae Bulbus *(chuān bèi mǔ)* clears up-flaring fire

from the Lung channel and collaterals and assists Belamcandae Rhizoma *(shè gān)* in clearing the throat. Forsythiae Fructus *(lián qiáo)* clears heat and resolves toxicity, facilitating the functions of Scutellariae Radix *(huáng qín)*. Acrid and cooling Menthae haplocalycis Herba *(bò hé)* serves as the envoy. Its light and floating nature focuses the action of the assistants on the throat, while aiding the chief and deputies in opening the qi dynamic. As Chen Jia-Mo notes in *Coverage of the Materia Medica*:

> [Menthae haplocalycis Herba *(bò hé)*] drives the qi downward to reduce fullness and distention. It promotes sweating to unblock the joints. It clears the common pathways of the six yang [organs]. It expels all wind generated by heat. It reduces steaming bone [fever] resolving consumption fatigue. It excels in guiding [other herbs] into the nutritive and protective [qi].

Cautions and Contraindications

Contraindicated in cases with significant underlying yin deficiency.

Commentary

The original indication of this formula is a damp-warmth epidemic disorder. Unlike seasonal disorders (時病 *shí bìng*), which are caused by pathogenic qi resonating with the five seasons (i.e., wind, heat, fire, dampness, dryness, and cold), such epidemic disorders are specifically defined as being 'unseasonal' (非時 *fēi shí*). That is, they do not occur as the result of an excess in one of the six pathogenic qi, but are caused by transmission of pestilential qi (癘氣 *lì qì*). As described in Wu You-Ke's *Discussion of Warm Epidemics*, "Epidemics are contractions of pestilential qi [present] in the world [that one picks up] according to the luck of the year, the fortitude of chance, or the ups and downs of the seasons. It is in the nature of such [pestilential] qi that it strikes irrespective of age or physical fitness." In modern Chinese texts they are regarded as endemic infectious disorders (鄉土流行疾病 *xiāng tǔ liú xíng jí bìng*). It follows that 'damp-warmth' in this context refers primarily not to the cause, but to the manifestations, which are heat and dampness at the qi level, with heat predominating.

Another name for this formula that is no longer used is Universal Benefit Special Pill to Resolve Toxicity *(pǔ jǐ jiě dú dān)*. This name resonates with the above indication inasmuch as it can be given to anyone afflicted by such a disorder irrespective of age, constitution, or other factors that would influence the manifestations of a normal seasonal disorder. The influential Qing-dynasty proponent of warm pathogen disorder therapeutics, Wang Shi-Xiong, thus referred to this formula as "the master formula for damp-warmth epidemic disorders" and attributed special efficacy to it. The later Qing-dynasty scholar Wu Jin-Shou attributed its composition to Ye Tian-Shi. Wu claimed to have gained access to hitherto unknown case records of the great master, which he published as *Secretly Transmitted Effective Medicine* in 1831. According to this text, Ye Tian-Shi composed the formula for the treatment of epidemic unseasonal disorders where the pathogenic qi was lodged in the qi level. This is indicated by a pale tongue with a white tongue coating or one that has a burned tip. If, on the other hand, the tongue is dry, crimson in color, glossy, or contracted, it indicates that the body fluids have been damaged and that the pathogen has already entered the nutritive level.

Because the kind of pestilential qi that causes the disorders for which this formula is most suitable enters the body via the nose and mouth, it directly enters the qi aspect, usually at the level of the Triple Burner or the half-interior, half-exterior from which it can vent to the exterior or discharge via the Intestines. In clinical practice, it can thus be taken right at the onset of disorders that have the appropriate manifestations. Typical conditions include damp-heat infectious disorders centered on the upper burner with such symptoms as coughing, sore throat, and swollen lymph glands and tonsils, or even parotitis. It may also be used in treating damp-heat stagnating in the Triple Burner characterized by persistent low-grade fever, sweating, reduced appetite, a sensation of heaviness in the body, bowel dysfunction, simultaneous bitter and sweet tastes in the mouth, and a yellow, greasy tongue coating. Although most practitioners use this formula for conditions in which both heat and dampness are present, some believe that it is more effective in treating conditions in which heat is the predominant factor.

In conditions of damp-heat, the presence of either constipation or diarrhea with difficulty in passing stool are additional clues for locating the disorder. Diarrhea with difficulty in passing stool indicates that the pathogenic influences are in the Stomach or Intestines, while constipation indicates that the damp-heat is in the upper burner or the lesser yang channel.

Biomedical Indications

With the appropriate presentation, this formula may be used to treat a variety of biomedically-defined disorders including acute gastroenteritis, enteric fever, typhoid, mild leptospirosis, infectious hepatitis, cholecystitis, pyelonephritis, allergic purpura, viral myocarditis, and parotitis.

Comparisons

➤ Vs. THREE-SEED DECOCTION (*sān rén tāng*)

Both formulas clear heat and facilitate the resolution of dampness via the Triple Burner. For this purpose, they combine herbs that transform, dry, and resolve dampness with those that clear and drain heat. Both formulas treat damp-warmth disorders where the pathogen is located in the qi level charac-

terized by symptoms like fever that worsens in the afternoon, lethargy, a heavy and aching body, nausea, lack of appetite, diarrhea, reduced urination, and a white and greasy tongue coating. However, Three-Seed Decoction (*sān rén tāng*) focuses on conditions where dampness is more prominent than heat, and where the pathogen is often also in the protective aspect. This is reflected in symptoms like fever and chills and the absence of thirst, which do not occur in patterns for which Sweet Dew Special Pill to Eliminate Toxin (*gān lù xiāo dú dān*) is indicated. Sweet Dew Special Pill to Eliminate Toxin (*gān lù xiāo dú dān*) treats conditions with more severe heat that transforms into toxin and unseasonal epidemic disorders. This is reflected in symptoms like a dry mouth, swelling or pain in the throat, or jaundice.

➤ Vs. UNIVERSAL BENEFIT DRINK TO ELIMINATE TOXIN (*pǔ jì xiāo dú yǐn*)

Both formulas treat disorders of the throat due to heat toxin. Universal Benefit Drink to Eliminate Toxin (*pǔ jì xiāo dú yǐn*) focuses on unseasonal epidemic disorders associated with wind-heat. There, dysfunction of the throat is accompanied by strong fever, thirst, and a powdery, white or yellow tongue coating indicating that massive heat toxin has damaged the fluids. Sweet Dew Special Pill to Eliminate Toxin (*gān lù xiāo dú dān*), on the other hand, focuses on epidemic disorders associated with damp-heat. In such patterns, dysfunction of the throat is accompanied by afternoon fever, thirst but not necessarily a strong desire to drink, and a greasy, white or slightly yellow tongue coating. In *Annotated Fine Formulas from Generations of Famous Physicians*, the contemporary physician Ran Xue-Feng summarizes these differences: "[Both formulas] excel at clearing. The former emphasizes unblocking the exterior, the latter clearing the interior. The former represents the turbid within the clearing [method], the latter the clear within the clearing [method]."

➤ Vs. COPTIS AND MAGNOLIA BARK DRINK (*lián pò yǐn*); see PAGE 706

Alternate names

Universal Benefit Special Pill to Resolve Epidemic Toxins (*pǔ jì jiě yì dān*) in *Warp and Woof of Warm-Heat Diseases*; Universal Benefit Drink to Eliminate Toxin (*pǔ jì xiāo dú yǐn*) in *Continuation of Classified Case Histories by Renowned Physicians*; Sweet Dew Pill to Eliminate Toxins (*gān lù xiāo dú wán*) in *Handbook of Chinese Medicinal Pharmaceutics*

Modifications

• For high fever, thirst, jaundice, body aches, impeded urination and bowel movements indicating that heat and dampness are equally strong, add Gardeniae Fructus (*zhī zǐ*), Rhei Radix et Rhizoma (*dà huáng*), and Imperatae Rhizoma (*bái máo gēn*).

• For unremitting low-grade fever, a stifling sensation in the chest, lack of appetite, tired limbs, a bitter taste, a sticky mouth, reduced urination that is dark in color, and a slippery, rapid pulse, add Gentianae macrophyllae Radix (*qín jiāo*), Lysimachiae Herba (*jīn qián cǎo*), Bupleuri Radix (*chái hú*), and Artemisiae annuae Herba (*qīng hāo*).

• For mumps where dampness is not pronounced, add Indigo naturalis (*qīng dài*) or Isatidis/Baphicacanthis Radix (*bǎn lán gēn*).

• For a swollen throat, add Isatidis/Baphicacanthis Radix (*bǎn lán gēn*), Lonicerae Flos (*jīn yín huā*), and Sophorae tonkinensis Radix (*shān dòu gēn*).

• For macular rashes and bleeding, add Artemisiae annuae Herba (*qīng hāo*), Imperatae Rhizoma (*bái máo gēn*), Cirsii Herba (*xiǎo jì*), or Cirsii japonici Herba sive Radix (*dà jì*).

• For enteric fever, add Sanguisorbae Radix (*dì yú*), Sophorae flavescentis Radix (*kǔ shēn*), and Coptidis Rhizoma (*huáng lián*).

• For pyelonephritis, add Dianthi Herba (*qú mài*), Polygoni avicularis Herba (*biān xù*), Pyrrosiae Folium (*shí wěi*), and Imperatae Rhizoma (*bái máo gēn*).

• For infectious hepatitis, increase the dosage of Artemisiae scopariae Herba (*yīn chén*) and add Gardeniae Fructus (*zhī zǐ*), Phellodendri Cortex (*huáng bǎi*), and Rhei Radix et Rhizoma (*dà huáng*).

連樸飲 (连朴饮)
Coptis and Magnolia Bark Drink

lián pò yǐn

Source *Discussion of Sudden Turmoil Disorders* (1862)

ginger Coptidis Rhizoma (*jiāng huáng lián*) 3g
prepared Magnoliae officinalis Cortex (*zhì hòu pò*) 6g
Gardeniae Fructus (*zhī zǐ*) 9g
dry-fried Sojae Semen praeparatum (*chǎo dòu chǐ*) 9g
Acori tatarinowii Rhizoma (*shí chāng pǔ*) 3g
Pinelliae Rhizoma praeparatum (*zhì bàn xià*) 3g
Phragmitis Rhizoma (*lú gēn*) 60g

Method of Preparation Decoction

Actions Clears heat, transforms dampness, regulates the qi, and harmonizes the middle burner

Indications

Simultaneous vomiting and diarrhea, focal distention and a stifling sensation in the chest and epigastrium, irritability, restlessness, dark, scanty urine, a yellow, greasy tongue coating, and a slippery, rapid pulse.

This is sudden turmoil disorder due to an aggregation of damp-heat smoldering in the body. This causes the clear and turbid fluids to become intermingled, with resulting disrup-tion of the ascending and descending functions of the Spleen and Stomach. The condition is characterized by vomiting and diarrhea and a stifling sensation in the chest and epigastrium. Irritability and restlessness, dark, scanty urine, a yellow, greasy tongue coating, and a slippery, rapid pulse are classic indications of damp-heat.

Analysis of Formula

Vomiting and diarrhea are prominent symptoms of sudden turmoil disorder. This formula aims to remove the obstruction of the qi dynamic that causes these symptoms by clearing heat and dispelling dampness. For this purpose, it employs two chief herbs: bitter and cold Coptidis Rhizoma (*huáng lián*) effectively drains heat and dries dampness in the middle burner; and Magnoliae officinalis Cortex (*hòu pò*) is one of the most effective herbs for transforming dampness and promoting the movement of qi, and also focuses on the middle burner. Together, these two herbs transform dampness, which, in this type of condition, facilitates the clearing of heat. The combination of two of the deputy herbs, Gardeniae Fructus (*zhī zǐ*) and Sojae Semen praeparatum (*dàn dòu chǐ*), clears the constrained heat from the chest and epigastrium. Another deputy, aromatic Acori tatarinowii Rhizoma (*shí chāng pǔ*), transforms dampness and revives the Spleen. The final deputy, Pinelliae Rhizoma praeparatum (*zhì bàn xià*), assists Magnoliae officinalis Cortex (*hòu pò*) in drying dampness and is very effective in directing the rebellious Stomach qi downward, thereby stopping the vomiting. Despite its relatively large dosage, Phragmitis Rhizoma (*lú gēn*) is classified as an assistant herb that aids in clearing and transforming damp-heat, generating fluids, harmonizing the Stomach, and stopping the vomiting.

The name of the formula specifies that this is a 'drink' (飲 *yǐn*). This designation implies either that the herbs are to be decocted for a shorter period of time than with a decoction or that the decoction is to be taken cold. In the present case, it is generally accepted that the latter meaning is implied. Cold has a contracting nature. Taking the decoction cold is thought to enhance the formula's capacity for stopping the symptoms of vomiting and diarrhea. Nevertheless, at present, the decoction is usually taken warm.

Cautions and Contraindications

This formula is indicated only for damp-heat type sudden turmoil disorders. It must not be used where the symptoms that characterize these disorders are due to dampness and cold.

Commentary

Sudden Turmoil Disorders

This is one of several formulas for the treatment of sudden turmoil disorders (霍亂 *huò luàn*) composed by the late

19th-century physician Wang Shi-Xiong. In Chinese medicine the term 'sudden turmoil disorder' refers to acute conditions characterized by the simultaneous onset of vomiting and diarrhea. There are two basic types of this disorder. In the first, known as 'wet sudden turmoil disorder' (濕霍亂 *shī huò luàn*), the body attempts to dispel pathological substances from the Stomach or Intestines by means of vomiting or diarrhea. The second type, known as 'dry sudden turmoil disorder' (乾霍亂 *gān huò luàn*) or 'bowel-gripping granular disorder' (絞腸痧 *jiǎo cháng shā*), is characterized by abdominal cramping, irritability, restlessness, a stifling sensation, and confusion. The patient feels as if he should vomit or pass stools but cannot do so. This formula (and the others discussed in this chapter) are indicated for the first type.

Use of the term 霍亂 *huò luàn* to designate disorders characterized by sudden and intense vomiting and diarrhea goes back at least to the Han dynasty. Zhang Zhong-Jing discussed its treatment in detail in *Discussion of Cold Damage*, and there are many later discussions in the literature, including those by proponents of warm pathogen therapeutics. In modern Chinese, the term 霍亂 *huò luàn* is used as a translation for the biomedical disease 'cholera,' leading many modern physicians to assume that there is an equivalence between sudden turmoil disorders and cholera. In fact, as the historian Kim Taylor has demonstrated, cholera only arrived in China from India in the course of the 19th century. This led to a frantic search for effective treatments. While some physicians went back to the *Discussion of Cold Damage* and other classical texts, others, like Wang Shi-Xiong, argued that new strategies, specifically those derived from warm pathogen therapeutics, which were still quite recent and by no means orthodox at the time, were required. Attaching these new strategies to an established disorder like 霍亂 *huò luàn* enabled Wang Shi-Xiong to more easily convince others of the potential utility of his ideas. Readers should thus be clear that while Wang Shi-Xiong's formulas most certainly were designed to treat cholera, pre-19th-century formulas indicated for 霍亂 *huò luàn* were not.

Focus of the Treatment

This formula focuses on clearing and transforming damp-heat and regulating the ascending and descending functions of the middle burner. It does not treat the diarrhea directly because this is unnecessary, since once the damp-heat is resolved and the qi is regulated, the diarrhea will stop. The focus on the qi dynamic is evident in the various groups of synergistic herbs that act on the ascending and descending functions to build the momentum of the formula. In this sense, it closely resembles the action of Pinellia Decoction to Drain the Epigastrium (*bàn xià xiè xīn tāng*), analyzed in Chapter 3. Both formulas remove damp-heat obstructing the qi dynamic by draining it through the bowels. However, whereas

Pinellia Decoction to Drain the Epigastrium (*bàn xià xiè xīn tāng*) employs sweet and moderate herbs to treat conditions of mixed excess and deficiency, the present formula relies on fragrant and aromatic herbs to treat conditions where heat and dampness are equally pronounced.

Like Pinellia Decoction to Drain the Epigastrium (*bàn xià xiè xīn tāng*), however, its action is not limited to acute conditions. It can be used for all kinds of patterns characterized by damp-heat obstructions of the middle burner that manifest with diarrhea, abdominal distention, belching, or vomiting. Such conditions are not limited to digestive disorders, but also include impotence, infertility, and postviral fatigue syndrome.

Phragmitis Rhizoma (lú gēn)

The relatively large dosage of Phragmitis Rhizoma (*lú gēn*) has led some commentators to suggest that this substance should be regarded as the chief herb. In view of the formula's name and its focus on the regulation of the qi dynamic, this view appears to be off the mark. By clearing heat and facilitating the resolution of dampness from the Lungs and Stomach while simultaneously generating fluids, Phragmitis Rhizoma (*lú gēn*) secures the fluid metabolism. In a condition marked by severe loss of body fluids through vomiting and diarrhea, this is a key strategic objective. This justifies its large dosage without implying that it serves as chief herb in the formula.

Comparisons

➤ Vs. Patchouli/Agastache Powder to Rectify the Qi (*huò xiāng zhèng qì sǎn*)

Both formulas treat sudden turmoil disorder due to obstruction of the qi dynamic in the middle burner. However, Coptis and Magnolia Bark Drink (*lián pò yǐn*) focuses on obstruction due to damp-heat, as reflected in symptoms like restlessness, irritability, and a greasy, yellow tongue coating. By contrast, Patchouli/Agastache Powder to Rectify the Qi (*huò xiāng zhèng qì sǎn*) focuses on conditions where wind-cold fetters the protective yang in the exterior in patients with dampness obstructing the interior, as reflected in symptoms like chills and fever, and a white tongue coating.

➤ Vs. Sweet Dew Special Pill to Eliminate Toxin (*gān lù xiāo dú dān*)

Both formulas treat patterns characterized by an equally strong presence of both dampness and heat pathogens. However, whereas Coptis and Magnolia Bark Drink (*lián pò yǐn*) focuses on the middle burner, as reflected in symptoms like diarrhea, vomiting, and abdominal distention, Sweet Dew Special Pill to Eliminate Toxin (*gān lù xiāo dú dān*) focuses on the upper burner, as reflected in symptoms like sore throat and swollen glands.

Biomedical Indications

With the appropriate presentation, this formula may be used to treat a variety of biomedically-defined disorders including acute gastroenteritis, typhoid, paratyphoid, peptic ulcers, infectious hepatitis, and asthma.

....

Alternate name

Master Wang's Coptis and Magnolia Bark Drink (*wáng shì lián pò yǐn*) in *Lectures on Warm Pathogen Diseases*

....

Modifications

- If diarrhea is more pronounced than vomiting, add Plantaginis Semen (*chē qián zǐ*) and Coicis Semen (*yì yǐ rén*).
- For abdominal fullness and distention, add Tsaoko Fructus (*cǎo guǒ*) or Amomi Fructus rotundus (*bái dòu kòu*).
- For blood in the stools, add Sanguisorbae Radix (*dì yú*) and Rubiae Radix (*qiàn cǎo gēn*).

Associated Formula

蠶矢湯 （蚕矢汤）

Silkworm Droppings Decoction

cán shǐ tāng

SOURCE   *Discussion of Sudden Turmoil* (1862)

Bombycis Faeces (*cán shā*) 9g
Coicis Semen (*yì yǐ rén*) 12g
Sojae Semen germinatum (*dà dòu juǎn*) 12g
Chaenomelis Fructus (*mù guā*) 9g
ginger Coptidis Rhizoma (*jiāng huáng lián*) 6g
Pinelliae Rhizoma praeparatum (*zhì bàn xià*) 3g
wine-fried Scutellariae Radix (*jiǔ chǎo huáng qín*) 3g
Tetrapanacis Medulla (*tōng cǎo*) 3g
Gardeniae Fructus (*zhī zǐ*) 6g
dry-fried Evodiae Fructus (*chǎo wú zhū yú*) 2g

Decoction. The source text advises to decoct the herbs in 'earth syrup' (地漿 *dì jiāng*), which is a mixture of fresh spring water and loess soil, or 'yin yang water' (陰陽水 *yīn yáng shuǐ*), which is a mixture of fresh spring water and boiled water. Both of these preparations are said to facilitate the separation of the clear and turbid. At present, most physicians use ordinary water. The decoction is to be taken cold. Clears heat, promotes the resolution of dampness, causes the clear to ascend, and directs the turbid downward. For damp-heat sudden turmoil disorders characterized by vomiting, diarrhea, cramp, thirst, irritability, restlessness, a thick and dry, yellow tongue coating, and a soggy, rapid pulse.

This is another formula for the treatment of damp-heat type sudden turmoil disorder composed by Wang Shi-Xiong. Compared to Coptis and Magnolia Bark Drink (*lián pò yǐn*), which is best suited for patterns characterized by severe vomiting, this formula addresses patterns presenting with cramps of the leg or abdominal muscles. Wang Shi-Xiong considered the formula's chief herb, Bombycis Faeces (*cán shā*), to be "the most important herb for sudden turmoil disorders." It is able to guide out dampness by directing it downward and to facilitate the transformation of dampness into

clear qi. It also dispels wind. The deputy, Chaenomelis Fructus (*mù guā*), facilitates the resolution of dampness and is an essential herb for cramping. Among the assistants, Coptidis Rhizoma (*huáng lián*), Scutellariae Radix (*huáng qín*), Pinelliae Rhizoma praeparatum (*zhì bàn xià*), and Evodiae Fructus (*wú zhū yú*) combine acrid, opening with bitter, downward-directing actions, embodying a strategy familiar from Pinellia Decoction to Drain the Epigastrium (*bàn xià xiè xīn tāng*), discussed in Chapter 3. Sojae Semen germinatum (*dà dòu juǎn*) and Gardeniae Fructus (*zhī zǐ*) lightly clear heat by venting it via the exterior, while sweet and bland Coicis Semen (*yì yǐ rén*) and Tetrapanacis Medulla (*tōng cǎo*) dispel dampness via the urine.

當歸拈痛湯 （当归拈痛汤）

Tangkuei Decoction to Pry Out Pain

dāng guī niān tòng tāng

The original name of this formula was simply Decoction to Pry Out Pain (*niān tòng tāng*), but this was changed to its current name about a century after its composition (with slight modifications) by the famous physician Li Dong-Yuan. *Supplemental Formulas Omitted from the Inner Classic* explains the origin of the name: "Angelicae sinensis Radix (*dāng guī*) is a medicine that harmonizes the qi and blood. When the qi and blood each has a place to return, there is free flow in the channels and collaterals and the pain ceases. It is like a hand prying it out, so it is referred to in this way."

Source   *Expounding on the Origins of Medicine* (Yuan dynasty)

Notopterygii Rhizoma seu Radix (*qiāng huó*) 15g
Saposhnikoviae Radix (*fáng fēng*) 9g
Cimicifugae Rhizoma (*shēng má*) 3g
Puerariae Radix (*gé gēn*) 6g
Atractylodis macrocephalae Rhizoma (*bái zhú*) 3g
Atractylodis Rhizoma (*cāng zhú*) 9g
Angelicae sinensis radicis Corpus (*dāng guī shēn*) 9g
Ginseng Radix (*rén shēn*) 6g
Glycyrrhizae Radix (*gān cǎo*) .15g
wine-fried Sophorae flavescentis Radix (*jiǔ chǎo kǔ shēn*) 6g
dry-fried Scutellariae Radix (*chǎo huáng qín*) 3g
wine-washed Anemarrhenae Rhizoma (*jiǔ xǐ zhī mǔ*) 9g
Artemisiae scopariae Herba (*yīn chén*) 15g
Polyporus (*zhū líng*) 9g
Alismatis Rhizoma (*zé xiè*) 9g

Preparation   Grind the ingredients into a powder. The source text recommends taking 30g and mixing with 2 cups of water, let it sit for a while, then boil it down to 1 cup and drink after straining and letting it sit for an additional while. Rich foods limit its actions. May also be prepared as a decoction with each ingredient used in accordance with common dosage practice.

Actions   Resolves dampness, clears heat, disperses wind, and stops pain

Indications

Generalized body aches and pains accompanied by irritability, heavy sensation in the shoulders and back, discomfort or a constricted sensation in the area of the chest and diaphragm, aching and painful extremities and joints, especially with unbearable swelling and pain of the lower extremities. The tongue coating will be greasy with a tinge of yellow, and the pulse is usually wiry and rapid, although it can be soggy and moderate or slippery and rapid. Additionally or alternatively, there may be multiple sores, carbuncles, furuncles or abscesses, accompanied by redness, persistent swelling, and possibly itching, pain, fever, or thirst.

This is a pattern of interaction between dampness and heat with the addition of externally-contracted pathogenic wind. The presentation can also be due to wind-dampness transforming into heat as an aspect of long-standing painful obstruction. The complex interaction between wind and damp-heat will flow over into the channels, collaterals, and joints, obstructing the free-flow of qi and blood. This manifests as generalized body aches and pains accompanied by irritability. In addition, most of the painful areas will feel hot to the touch. Dampness is a yin pathogen, and when it predominates, it can lead to a sensation of heaviness in the shoulders and back along with a constricted sensation in the chest and diaphragm. When damp-heat flows down to lodge in the legs, it results in a form of leg qi (腳氣 *jiǎo qì*) with leg cramps and intolerable swelling and pain. With either an acute attack of wind, dampness, and heat, or the chronic retention of damp-heat, there may be a tendency to produce toxin. The wind, dampness, and toxin clog and stagnate in the muscles and skin and enter into the blood aspect. With the presence of heat, this leads to putrefaction and further generation of toxin. This will manifest as various types of sores and abscesses accompanied by redness, a sensation of heat, and swelling, and perhaps itching, pain, fever, or thirst. The tongue and pulse are reflections of dampness and heat, changing as the relative balance of these two pathogens changes.

It is also advisable to examine the tongue proper for the presence of dark or purple spots, as this is an important sign that helps to distinguish both the existence and relative significance of blood stasis in these relatively complex patterns.

Analysis of Formula

This formula treats damp-heat in the interior complicated by the contraction of pathogenic wind. It thus promotes the resolution of dampness, drains and vents heat, courses wind, and disperses constraint. Notopterygii Rhizoma seu Radix (*qiāng huó*) is an acrid, warm herb that strongly releases the exterior and is very effective at dispersing externally-contracted pathogenic wind. It also prevails over dampness, facilitates movement in the joints, and stops pain, all of which are useful here. It is especially helpful for shoulder, upper extremity, and upper back pain. As noted in *Materia Medica for Decoctions*: "Notopterygii Rhizoma seu Radix (*qiāng huó*) has a virile qi and treats wind and dampness interacting in the leg greater

yang. When treating headache, pain in the joints of the extremities, or pain throughout the body, it is indispensable." Artemisiae scopariae Herba (*yīn chén*) is bitter and drains downward. It is effective in clearing and resolving damp-heat by leading them out through the urine. Together, these are the two chief ingredients as they work together to eliminate the dampness and unblock the channels and collaterals.

Three sets of deputies accentuate the actions of clearing heat, draining dampness, and dispersing wind. Both Sophorae flavescentis Radix (*kǔ shēn*) and Scutellariae Radix (*huáng qín*) strongly clear heat and dry dampness. Sophorae flavescentis Radix (*kǔ shēn*) has the ability to clear damp-heat from the lower burner and facilitate urination to help eliminate dampness. Another set of deputies, Alismatis Rhizoma (*zé xiè*) and Polyporus (*zhū líng*), promote urination and leach out dampness, while also slightly clearing heat. They work with Artemisiae scopariae Herba (*yīn chén*) to resolve dampness affecting the lower part of the body. The last set of deputies is comprised of Saposhnikoviae Radix (*fáng fēng*), Cimicifugae Rhizoma (*shēng má*), and Puerariae Radix (*gé gēn*). These cooling, exterior-releasing herbs accentuate the wind-dispersing action of Notopterygii Rhizoma seu Radix (*qiāng huó*).

Atractylodis macrocephalae Rhizoma (*bái zhú*) and Atractylodis Rhizoma (*cāng zhú*) strengthen the Spleen and dry dampness, working simultaneously on both the root and the branch. They improve the functioning of the Spleen, which reduces the generation of dampness, while also drying any dampness that is already present. Another group of assistants, Ginseng Radix (*rén shēn*) and Angelicae sinensis Radix (*dāng guī*), tonifies the qi and blood so that all the clearing, draining, and drying do not harm them. Angelicae sinensis Radix (*dāng guī*) is also moistening and thus ameliorates the rather drying nature of most of the other herbs in the formula. In addition, it has the ability to invigorate the blood and stop pain, which is helpful here. As noted in *Fine Formulas for Women*: "To treat wind, first treat the blood; once the blood moves [properly], the wind will automatically be extinguished." The final assistant is Anemarrhenae Rhizoma (*zhī mǔ*), which, although bitter and cold, is not drying. In the context of this formula, it is able to clear heat and nourish the yin and thus, in one way, aids in treating the symptoms while concurrently helping to prevent the main herbs from damaging the yin. Glycyrrhizae Radix (*gān cǎo*) serves primarily as an envoy to adjust and harmonize the actions of the various groups of herbs. At the same time, it aids Ginseng Radix (*rén shēn*) and Atractylodis macrocephalae Rhizoma (*bái zhú*) in augmenting the qi and strengthening the Spleen.

Cautions and Contraindications

Do not use for painful obstruction due to wind-cold-dampness.

Commentary

This formula is distinct in that it simultaneously treats the exterior and interior and attends to both the pathogens and the normal qi. Focusing on wind externally and on dampness and heat internally, it is a complex formula built for a complex presentation. In the source text, it was used for "disease constituted from damp-heat with irritable and painful joints of the extremities, a feeling of heaviness in the shoulders and upper back, discomfort of the chest and diaphragm, and generalized body aches. When it pours downward into the lower legs, the swelling and pain are unbearable." Later, in *Subtle Import of the Jade Key*, it was indicated for sores of the lower extremities as well

At present, it is most commonly used for wind-damp-heat painful obstruction as well as the early stages of damp-heat leg qi marked by heaviness, swelling, and pain in the joints of the extremities along with a greasy tongue coating (usually white with a tinge of yellow, but may be yellow) and a rapid pulse.

Over the years, and particularly the last 15 years, clinical studies of this formula have helped to systematically expand its use to include many disorders that share the patterns of damp-heat and blood stasis. These include skin disorders involving toxin, which produce rashes, sores, and ulceration, as well as urogenital and gynecological disorders. As a practical matter, the elegant design of this complex formula simultaneously addresses factors of dampness, heat, wind, blood stasis, toxin, and obstruction of the channels and collaterals involving both external and internal pathogenic factors. This facilitates effective treatment of many dermatological problems involving a mix of both internal and external etiologies including both localized, superficial purulent infections as well as skin disorders with allergic or systemic immune-response aspects, when viewed from a biomedical perspective.

Name

The original name of this formula was simply Decoction to Pry Out Pain (拈痛湯 *niān tòng tāng*). It was renamed Tangkuei Decoction to Pry Out Pain (*dāng guī niān tòng tāng*) by Li Dong-Yuan and was included, in a slightly modified form, in his *Secrets from the Orchid Chamber*. In that formula, the dosages of four herbs are different, namely, 9g of dry-fried Scutellariae Radix (*chǎo huáng qín*), 6g of Cimicifugae Rhizoma (*shēng má*), 6g of Atractylodis Rhizoma (*cāng zhú*), and 4.5g of Atractylodis macrocephalae Rhizoma (*bái zhú*); in addition, Glycyrrhizae Radix praeparata (*zhì gān cǎo*) is used. Other, slightly modified versions appear in such texts as *Golden Mirror of the Medical Tradition*. It is also known as Tangkuei Decoction to Stop Pain (當歸止痛湯 *dāng guī zhǐ tòng tāng*).

Comparisons

➤ Vs. Cinnamon Twig, Peony, and Anemarrhena Decoction (*guì zhī sháo yào zhī mǔ tāng*)

Both formulas are used for widespread joint pain. However, Cinnamon Twig, Peony, and Anemarrhena Decoction (*guì zhī sháo yào zhī mǔ tāng*) is used for both generalized aches and pains in all the joints, called panarthralgia (歷節病 *lì jié bìng*), and for leg and foot edema with swollen, painful joints of the lower extremities that are warm to the touch. It primarily focuses on recurrent wind-cold-damp painful obstruction in which it is the localized constraint, rather than systemic, internal damp-heat, that generates the heat. A white, greasy tongue coating may help to distinguish cold-dampness from damp-heat; however, in chronic painful obstruction, one often transforms into the other.

➤ Vs. Disband Painful Obstruction Decoction (*xuān bì tāng*); *see* page 763

Alternate names

Decoction to Pry Out Pain (*niān tòng tāng*) in *Secrets from the Orchid Chamber*; Tangkuei Decoction to Alleviate Pain (*dāng guī zhǐ tòng tāng*) in *The Manual of the Art of Benevolence*; Tangkuei Powder to Pry Out Pain (*dāng guī niān tòng sǎn*) in *Zheng Family Formulas for Women's Diseases Worth Ten Thousand in Gold*

Biomedical Indications

With the appropriate presentation, this formula may be used to treat a wide variety of biomedically-defined disorders. These can be divided into the following groups:

- Neuromuscular disorders such as periarthritis of the shoulder, rheumatoid arthritis, and peripheral neuritis
- Skin diseases such as eczema, urticaria, dermatitis, and impetigo
- Urogenital disorders such as primary dysmenorrhea, irregular menstruation, urinary tract infection, hematuria associated with acute nephritis, renal calculi, pyelonephritis, urinary tract infection, leukorrhea, and prolonged lochia
  This formula has also been used for treating beriberi.

Modifications

- For generalized body aches and pains, add Cinnamomi Ramulus (*guì zhī*) and Paeoniae Radix alba (*bái sháo*).
- For red, swollen, and hot painful obstruction, add Lonicerae Flos (*jīn yín huā*), Forsythiae Fructus (*lián qiáo*), and Gypsum fibrosum (*shí gāo*).
- For purulent skin lesions due to the presence of heat and toxin, add Lonicerae Flos (*jīn yín huā*) and Forsythiae Fructus (*lián qiáo*).
- For intense body pain, add Curcumae longae Rhizoma (*jiāng huáng*) and Erythrinae Cortex (*hǎi tóng pí*).

- For pronounced swelling of the legs, add Stephaniae tetrandrae Radix *(hàn fáng jǐ)* and Chaenomelis Fructus *(mù guā)*.

- For eczema with the presence of wind-heat, add Rehmanniae Radix *(shēng dì huáng)*, Gypsum fibrosum *(shí gāo)*, and Moutan Cortex *(mǔ dān pí)*; with the presence of damp-heat, add Coicis Semen *(yì yǐ rén)*, Magnoliae officinalis Cortex *(hòu pò)*, and Phaseoli Semen *(chì xiǎo dòu)*; with the presence of heat in the blood, add Arnebiae/Lithospermi Radix *(zǐ cǎo)*, Sophorae Flos *(huái huā)*, and Lycii Cortex *(dì gǔ pí)*; with the presence of blood deficiency and wind-dryness, add Polygoni multiflori Radix *(hé shǒu wū)*, Salviae miltiorrhizae Radix *(dān shēn)*, and Scrophulariae Radix *(xuán shēn)*.

- For painful menstruation due to damp-heat and blood stasis, combine with Four-Substance Decoction *(sì wù tāng)* and Sudden Smile Powder *(shī xiào sǎn)*.

- For prolonged lochia, add Akebiae Caulis *(mù tōng)*, Rehmanniae Radix *(shēng dì huáng)*, Moutan Cortex *(mǔ dān pí)*, and Phellodendri Cortex *(huáng bǎi)*.

- For painful urinary dysfunction, add Phellodendri Cortex *(huáng bǎi)*, Dianthi Herba *(qú mài)*, and Akebiae Caulis *(mù tōng)*.

茵陳蒿湯 （茵陈蒿汤）
Virgate Wormwood Decoction

yīn chén hāo tāng

Source   *Discussion of Cold Damage* (c. 220)

Artemisiae scopariae Herba *(yīn chén)* 18g
Gardeniae Fructus *(zhī zǐ)* 9-12g
Rhei Radix et Rhizoma *(dà huáng)* 6g

Method of Preparation   Decoction. The source text advises to first decoct the Artemisiae scopariae Herba *(yīn chén)* by itself in about 12 cups of water until half remains. The other two ingredients are then added and the mixture decocted until the liquid is once again reduced by one-half. The decoction is strained and taken in three doses over the course of a day.

According to *Records of Thoughtful Differentiation of Materia Medica,* this mode of preparation enhances the synergistic effects among the herbs in the formula. Decocting aromatic Artemisiae scopariae Herba *(yīn chén)* by itself first allows its aromatic nature, which resonates with the qi of the muscle layer and exterior, to be extracted. Only then are Rhei Radix et Rhizoma *(dà huáng)* and Gardeniae Fructus *(zhī zǐ)* added; they eliminate damp-heat via the urine and bowels. This mode of preparation thus mirrors the intended actions of the formula.

At present, the dosage of the ingredients is commonly doubled. Depending on how much of a purgative action is required, steamed Rhei Radix et Rhizoma *(shú dà huáng)* may be used, Rhei Radix et Rhizoma *(dà huáng)* may be cooked with the rest of the herbs or may be added near the end of the decocting process.

Actions   Clears heat, resolves dampness, and reduces jaundice

Indications

Whole-body jaundice with a color that resembles a 'fresh tangerine,' slight abdominal distention, urinary difficulty, thirst (with the ability to take only sips), little or no sweating, or sweating only from the head and stopping at the neck, a yellow, greasy tongue coating, and a slippery, rapid pulse

This is yang-type or damp-heat jaundice. It is caused by excess heat in the interior that cannot be released via the skin due to the presence of dampness. This is reflected in the absence of sweating despite of other signs of heat, or in sweating just from the head. Heat and dampness clump and accumulate in the interior to form what is called 'stasis heat'(瘀熱 *yū rè)*. When the stasis heat steams to the exterior, it causes the entire body to turn a bright orange. The obstruction of the qi dynamic by stasis heat causes slight abdominal distention and urinary difficulty. Damp-heat collecting internally prevents the fluids from ascending and produces this particular type of thirst. The tongue and pulse signs reflect the presence of both dampness (greasy and slippery) and heat (yellow and rapid).

Analysis of Formula

To treat yang jaundice where stasis heat has formed by the clumping of heat and dampness in the interior that steams to the skin, one must simultaneously treat the root by draining the heat and promoting the resolution of dampness, and treat the manifestation by reducing the jaundice. The chief herb, Artemisiae scopariae Herba *(yīn chén)*, can be used in treating all types of jaundice, but especially jaundice due to damp-heat. The rather large dosage of this herb increases its efficacy. The deputy, Gardeniae Fructus *(zhī zǐ)*, clears heat from the three burners, and more specifically, drains damp-heat through the urine. The assistant, Rhei Radix et Rhizoma *(dà huáng)*, purges heat, eliminates stasis heat, directs downward, and facilitates the expression of pathogenic toxin retained by the clogging of the qi dynamic by damp-heat. These three herbs thus act synergistically to drain damp-heat and encourage the fading of the jaundice.

According to the source text, administration of the formula should produce a rapid clearing of the jaundice. After just one night, there should be an increase in urination, with the urine turning red in color. This may be accompanied by freed-up bowel movements. These signs indicate that damp-heat is being eliminated via the urine and stool.

Cautions and Contraindications

Unless modified, this formula is contraindicated for yin-type jaundice or jaundice in which dampness predominates (see ASSOCIATED FORMULAS). Rhei Radix et Rhizoma *(dà huáng)* should be used with extreme caution during pregnancy.

Commentary

Jaundice

This is a very effective formula for the treatment of jaundice, especially those types in which damp-heat is the predominant factor. This type of jaundice is commonly referred to as 'yang-type jaundice.' If dampness predominates, its color is dark like that of strong tea. If heat predominates, its color is orange and bright like that of a tangerine. This should be distinguished from yin-type jaundice, where cold and dampness constrain the yang qi. This causes mild damp-heat, which manifests with a pale yellow color like that of a lemon. The presence of dampness in all cases reflects the adage that "Without dampness, jaundice does not arise."

Modern textbooks explain the relationship between cause (dampness) and manifestation (jaundice) as mediated by the dredging function of the Liver qi. As Liver qi is obstructed by dampness, bile seeps into the exterior, turning the skin yellow. Clearly, this is an explanation mediated by biomedicine. Premodern texts, instead, emphasize the connection between dampness and the color yellow via their mutual association with earth in five-phase theory. To give just one example, *Links to the Origins of the Records of Materia Medica* observes: "In jaundice, … dampness holds in and steams the heat. Heat, likewise, thickens the dampness. Both are based in the middle earth damp toxin."

While all jaundice is due to damp-heat, the source of both pathogens and their respective strength varies from case to case, requiring different treatment. Hence, the Han-dynasty works *Discussion of Cold Damage* and *Essentials from the Golden Cabinet* already listed at least six different patterns and formulas for the treatment of jaundice. Of these, Virgate Wormwood Decoction (*yīn chén hāo tāng*) is the most famous. In *Essentials from the Golden Cabinet*, it is prescribed for the treatment of 'food jaundice' (谷瘅 *gǔ dān*), where food that is not properly digested causes a gradual buildup of damp-heat. In *Discussion of Cold Damage*, it is used to treat jaundice arising from stasis heat, which in turn is classified as belonging to the larger class of yang brightness disorders. In this pattern, the heat produced by a relatively strong reaction to an external pathogen (classified as yang brightness) clumps with dampness that is already present in the interior (associated with the greater yin). This requires that the heat be drained from the yang brightness via the stool, and from the greater yin via the urine, and explains the inclusion of both Gardeniae Fructus (*zhī zǐ*) and Rhei Radix et Rhizoma (*dà huáng*) in the formula.

Stasis in this Presentation

Some physicians read the term 'stasis' as referring to severe heat obstructing not only the qi dynamic, but also the circulation of blood. They hold that this provides a better expla-

nation for the use of Rhei Radix et Rhizoma (*dà huáng*)—an herb that can move the blood and break up stasis—in a pattern that does not need to be accompanied by blocked stools. The Ming-dynasty physician Wu You-Ke, who used this formula to treat jaundice occurring in the course of unseasonal epidemic disorders, even went so far as to make Rhei Radix et Rhizoma (*dà huáng*) the chief herb. In the relevant passage from *Discussion of Warm Epidemics*, Wu explained:

> Artemisiae scopariae Herba (*yīn chén*) is a special herb for reducing jaundice. If we compare the patterns [in which it is used,] then the jaundice [treated by Virgate Wormwood Decoction (*yīn chén hāo tāng*)] is due to urinary difficulty. Therefore, one employs Gardeniae Fructus (*zhī zǐ*) to eliminate fire from the bends of the Small Intestine. The stasis heat is then eliminated and urine flows normally. One should view jaundice as the manifestation and urinary difficulty as the root. In determining the cause of urinary difficulty, we [find that] its source is not located in the Bladder but connected to heat transferred from the Stomach group. Therefore, one should view the urinary difficulty as the manifestation and the Stomach group as the root. Thus, it is Rhei Radix et Rhizoma (*dà huáng*) which is specific for attacking [the heat at the root of this condition], while Gardeniae Fructus (*zhī zǐ*) is the secondary herb, followed by Artemisiae scopariae Herba (*yīn chén*) in order of importance.

Based on this analysis, Wu You-Ke adjusted the dosages of the formula to Rhei Radix et Rhizoma (*dà huáng*) 15g, Gardeniae Fructus (*zhī zǐ*) 6g, and Artemisiae scopariae Herba (*yīn chén*) 3g. Although few other physicians share Wu You-Ke's view, many attribute to Rhei Radix et Rhizoma (*dà huáng*) more than a subordinate role. Wu Qian, the influential editor of *Golden Mirror of the Medical Tradition*, for instance, considered Gardeniae Fructus (*zhī zǐ*) to be the envoy and Rhei Radix et Rhizoma (*dà huáng*) the assistant. Physicians also hold very different opinions regarding the manner in which Rhei Radix et Rhizoma (*dà huáng*) should be used. Those who see its role as merely opening the bowels argue that it should be discontinued as soon as the bowel movements become smooth, in order to prevent it from injuring the normal qi if. If this leads to rebound constipation, the herb should be replaced with a mild laxative that is suitable for this condition, such as Gentianae macrophyllae Radix (*qín jiāo*) and Benincasae Semen (*dōng guā zǐ*). Another group of physicians views the inclusion of Rhei Radix et Rhizoma (*dà huáng*) in the formula as essential irrespective of whether the stool is dry or soft, and the abdomen distended or not.

Since its inclusion in *Discussion of Cold Damage*, Virgate Wormwood Decoction (*yīn chén hāo tāng*) has been used as the foundation for many formulas that treat jaundice, including those discussed under ASSOCIATED FORMULAS below. However, because jaundice is a symptom and not the root of the disorder, this formula can be used to treat other manifestations of stasis heat in the interior or of clumping of the yang brightness accompanied by greater yin dampness, such as uterine bleeding, fever of unknown origin, abdominal pain, or mouth ulcers.

Comparison

➢ Vs. Other Formulas that Treat Jaundice

A number of different classical formulas included in this book list jaundice as one of the main symptoms. Besides Virgate Wormwood Decoction (*yīn chén hāo tāng*), these include Virgate Wormwood and Five-Ingredient Powder with Poria (*yīn chén wǔ líng sǎn*) and Gardenia and Phellodendron Decoction (*zhī zǐ bǎi pí tāng*). All of these formulas eliminate damp-heat as the primary cause of jaundice. By comparison with Virgate Wormwood and Five-Ingredient Powder with Poria (*yīn chén wǔ líng sǎn*), Virgate Wormwood Decoction (*yīn chén hāo tāng*) is stronger at clearing heat, which it drains through both the bowels and urine. It is indicated in cases with strong interior heat that has its root in the yang brightness warp. Virgate Wormwood and Five-Ingredient Powder with Poria (*yīn chén wǔ líng sǎn*), on the other hand, is better at promoting the resolution of dampness. It is indicated for patterns where dampness, which has its root in the greater yin and yang warps, predominates.

Virgate Wormwood Decoction (*yīn chén hāo tāng*) and Gardenia and Phellodendron Decoction (*zhī zǐ bǎi pí tāng*) both treat damp-heat jaundice with relatively strong heat. The selection of one over the other is based on the location of the root of the heat. Gardenia and Phellodendron Decoction (*zhī zǐ bǎi pí tāng*) focuses on heat arising from constraint in the muscle layer and qi dynamic that has not yet produced heat stasis in the interior. This is indicated by palpitations and reduced urination, but an absence of abdominal distention. Virgate Wormwood Decoction (*yīn chén hāo tāng*) focuses on stasis heat in the exterior, indicated by abdominal distention or bowel obstruction and sweating from the head only.

Biomedical Indications

With the appropriate presentation, this formula may be used to treat a wide variety of biomedically-defined disorders. These can be divided into the following groups:

- Diseases marked by jaundice such as acute viral hepatitis, cirrhosis, hepatic atrophy, biliary ascariasis, and neonatal jaundice
- Skin diseases marked by pruritus such as eczema, psoriasis, allergic dermatitis, and acne
- Gynecological disorders such as pelvic inflammatory disease, dysfunctional uterine bleeding, vaginitis, and dysmenorrhea

This formula has also been used in the treatment of otitis media, conjunctivitis, and appendicitis.

Alternate names

Virgate Wormwood Powder (*yīn chén sǎn*) in *Arcane Essentials from the Imperial Library*; Heat Cleansing Decoction (*dí rè tāng*) in *Comprehensive Recording of Sagely Beneficence*; Major Virgate Wormwood Decoction (*dà yīn chén tāng*) in *Indispensable Tools for Pattern Treatment*; Virgate Wormwood, Gardenia and Rhubarb Decoction (*yīn chén zhī zǐ dà huáng tāng*) in *Comprehensive Outline on Benefiting Yang*; Virgate Wormwood and Rhubarb Decoction (*yīn chén dà huáng tāng*) in *Symptom, Cause, Pulse, and Treatments*

Modifications

- For high fever and other signs of severe heat, add Gentianae Radix (*lóng dǎn cǎo*), Isatidis/Baphicacanthis Radix (*bǎn lán gēn*), and Polygoni cuspidati Rhizoma (*hǔ zhàng*).
- For fever and chills, add Forsythiae Fructus (*lián qiáo*) and Chrysanthemi indici Flos (*yě jú huā*).
- For difficult and irregular bowel movements with loose stools, add Eupatorii Herba (*pèi lán*).
- For hypochondriac pain and other signs of constrained Liver qi, add Bupleuri Radix (*chái hú*), Toosendan Fructus (*chuān liàn zǐ*), Cyperi Rhizoma (*xiāng fù*), and Paeoniae Radix alba (*bái sháo*).
- For nausea, vomiting, and reduced appetite, add Bambusae Caulis in taeniam (*zhú rú*), Pinelliae Rhizoma praeparatum (*zhì bàn xià*), and Massa medicata fermentata (*shén qū*).
- For cholelithiasis, add Lysimachiae Herba (*jīn qián cǎo*).

Associated Formulas

茵陳四逆湯 （茵陈四逆汤）

Virgate Wormwood Decoction for Frigid Extremities
yīn chén sì nì tāng

Source   *Comprehensive Medicine According to Master Zhang* (1695)

Artemisiae scopariae Herba (*yīn chén*) 4.5g
Zingiberis Rhizoma praeparatum (*páo jiāng*) 4.5g
Aconiti Radix lateralis praeparata (*zhì fù zǐ*) 3g
Glycyrrhizae Radix (*gān cǎo*) 3g

At present, the dosage is usually doubled. Warms the interior, reinforces the yang, resolves dampness, and reduces jaundice. For yin-type or cold-dampness jaundice characterized by a dull complexion with a dark yellow sheen, reduced appetite, lethargy, frigid extremities, and a submerged, thin, and weak pulse. Heat, in this pattern, is secondary to constraint from internal cold. For this reason, the formula focuses on warming the interior and reinforcing the yang.

茵陳朮附湯 （茵陈术附汤）

Virgate Wormwood, Atractylodes, and Aconite Accessory Root Decoction
yīn chén zhú fù tāng

Source   *Awakening of the Mind in Medical Studies* (1732)

Artemisiae scopariae Herba (*yīn chén*) .3g
Atractylodis macrocephalae Rhizoma (*bái zhú*) 6g
Zingiberis Rhizoma (*gān jiāng*) 1.5g

Aconiti Radix lateralis praeparata *(zhì fù zǐ)* 1.5g
Cinnamomi Cortex *(ròu guì)* 0.9g
Glycyrrhizae Radix praeparata *(zhì gān cǎo)* 3g

Warms and strengthens the Spleen, transforms dampness, and reduces jaundice. For yin-type jaundice with Spleen yang deficiency in addition to interior cold.

栀子柏皮湯 (栀子柏皮汤)

Gardenia and Phellodendron Decoction

zhī zǐ bǎi pí tāng

SOURCE *Discussion of Cold Damage* (c. 220)

Gardeniae Fructus *(zhī zǐ)* .15 pieces (9-15g)
Phellodendri Cortex *(huáng bǎi)* 6g
Glycyrrhizae Radix praeparata *(zhì gān cǎo)* 3g

Clears heat, resolves dampness, and reduces jaundice. For fever and jaundice as the sequela of a cold-induced disorder. For cases with more heat than dampness, indicated by symptoms like thirst and palpitations. The heat, however, has not yet penetrated to the yang brightness warp; hence, there is no abdominal distention.

八正散

Eight-Herb Powder for Rectification

bā zhèng sǎn

This formula combines eight herbs that expel pathogenic influences and rectify the function of the lower burner, hence the name.

Source *Formulary of the Pharmacy Service for Benefiting the People in the Taiping Era* (1107)

Akebiae Caulis *(mù tōng)* 3-6g
Talcum *(huá shí)* 12-30g
Plantaginis Semen *(chē qián zǐ)* 9-15g
Dianthi Herba *(qú mài)* 6-12g
Polygoni avicularis Herba *(biǎn xù)* .6-12g
Gardeniae Fructus *(zhī zǐ)* 3-9g
wine-washed Rhei Radix et Rhizoma *(jiǔ xǐ dà huáng)* 6-9g
Junci Medulla *(dēng xīn cǎo)* 3-6g
Glycyrrhizae Radix praeparata *(zhì gān cǎo)* 3-9g

Method of Preparation The source text advises to grind equal amounts of the ingredients into a powder and take as a draft in 9g doses with 1.5-3g of Junci Medulla *(dēng xīn cǎo)*. At present, it is usually prepared as a decoction with the dosage specified.

Actions Clears heat, drains fire, promotes urination, and unblocks painful urinary dribbling

Indications

Dark, turbid, scanty, difficult, and painful urination, a dry mouth and throat, a yellow, greasy tongue coating, and a slippery, rapid pulse. In severe cases, there may be urinary retention and lower abdominal distention and pain.

This is damp-heat collecting in the lower burner, specifically the Bladder, causing painful urinary dribbling or urinary retention. As explained in *Medical Formulas Collected and Analyzed*:

> The promotion and regulation of the waterways is governed by the Triple Burner. Accepting and storing the body fluids so that the qi transformation can issue from it is governed by the Bladder. If the waterways do not transport [the fluids] causing a buildup of water internally [that manifests as] wheezing and distention, or a flooding of the exterior [that manifests as] edema of the skin, then this is a disorder of the Triple Burner. If [having been] received and stored [the body fluids] are not transformed causing all kinds of urinary dribbling, roughness, and pain or urinary retention, then this is a disorder of the Bladder.

Commonly, there is a history of overindulgence in spicy, sweet, or rich foods, or overconsumption of alcohol. Damp-heat in the Bladder manifests as turbid, dark urine that is scanty, difficult to pass, and painful. The urine will become dark red if there is injury to the blood vessels. If especially severe, the patient may be unable to urinate and will experience lower abdominal distention and pain. The presence of heat with accumulation of dampness in the lower burner is reflected in the dry mouth and throat. The tongue and pulse signs are typical of damp-heat.

Analysis of Formula

The formula's name values all of the ingredients equally. Nevertheless, by analyzing the formula's original indications, genealogy, and later usage, one can chart its internal organization according to classical principles of formula composition. Historically, Eight-Herb Powder for Rectification *(bā zhèng sǎn)* is derived from Dianthus Powder *(qú mài sǎn)*, a formula for bloody or painful urinary dribbling that was first listed in the Song-dynasty work *Formulas from Benevolent Sages Compiled during the Taiping Era*. The source text defines Eight-Herb Powder for Rectification *(bā zhèng sǎn)* itself as "treating pathogenic heat in the Heart channel in both children and adults, [as well as] all collections of toxin." Examination of its later usage among physicians shows that the most important herbs in the formula (i.e., those that are never substituted) are Dianthi Herba *(qú mài)*, Polygoni avicularis Herba *(biǎn xù)*, Talcum *(huá shí)*, and Glycyrrhizae Radix *(gān cǎo)*, while Gardeniae Fructus *(zhī zǐ)* and Rhei Radix et Rhizoma *(dà huáng)* are those that are most often dropped.

Combining these different pieces of information, it can be deduced that Dianthi Herba *(qú mài)* and the similarly acting Polygoni avicularis Herba *(biǎn xù)* serve as chief herbs. According to *Thoroughly Revised Materia Medica*, "bitter and cold Dianthi Herba *(qú mài)* directs the Heart fire downward, unblocks the Small Intestine, expels damp-heat from the Bladder, and is an essential herb for the treatment of dribbling disorders." It enters the blood aspect to invigorate the blood and is thus particularly useful in the treatment of bloody and painful urinary dribbling. Polygoni avicularis

Herba *(biǎn xù)* enters the qi aspect to promote urination, unblock painful urinary dribbling, and clear damp-heat. The deputies are Talcum *(huá shí),* Plantaginis Semen *(chē qián zǐ),* and Akebiae Caulis *(mù tōng),* whose main function is to assist the chief ingredients in unblocking the painful urinary dribbling. Among them, bitter and cold Akebiae Caulis *(mù tōng)* clears heat, promotes urination, and is very effective in clearing the obstruction caused by damp stagnation. Talcum *(huá shí)* and Plantaginis Semen *(chē qián zǐ),* meanwhile, are both slippery and thus smooth the passage of urine despite any stagnation along its passage.

The assistant ingredients indirectly treat the painful urinary dribbling by draining heat: Gardeniae Fructus *(zhī zǐ)* drains heat from the three burners through the urine, and Rhei Radix et Rhizoma *(dà huáng)* drains heat through the stool. Junci Medulla *(dēng xīn cǎo),* one of the envoys, guides heat downward. The other envoy, Glycyrrhizae Radix *(gān cǎo),* harmonizes the actions of the other ingredients and relieves the abdominal pain. The combination of Glycyrrhizae Radix *(gān cǎo)* and Talcum *(huá shí)* also helps to alleviate irritability. Sometimes the tips of the root, called Glycyrrhizae Radix tenuis *(gān cǎo shāo),* are used to strengthen the diuretic action of this formula.

In terms of its action, the formula thus focuses in equal measure on clearing the heat, promoting urination, and unblocking obstruction. While the location of the symptoms points to the lower burner, their etiology implicates the upper and middle burners as the source of heat and dampness. For this reason, the formula includes herbs that drain fire from the Heart—Dianthi Herba *(qú mài),* Akebiae Caulis *(mù tōng),* and Junci Medulla *(dēng xīn cǎo)*—clear heat from the Lungs—Plantaginis Semen *(chē qián zǐ)*—clear the Triple Burner—Gardeniae Fructus *(zhī zǐ)*—and unblock the Intestines—Rhei Radix et Rhizoma *(dà huáng).*

Cautions and Contraindications

Long-term use of this formula may cause weakness, lightheadedness, palpitations, and a loss of appetite. It should not be used without significant modification in treating conditions of cold from deficiency, or during pregnancy.

Commentary

The Chinese prescription literature contains numerous formulas for the treatment of urinary dribbling disorders. Eight-Treasure Decoction *(bā zhēn tāng)* is one of the most famous, indicated specifically for the treatment of hot, bloody, and painful urinary dribbling. At present, many formulas for urinary tract infection are based on this formula. However, since urinary tract infection (usually a type of painful urinary dribbling) is not always caused by damp-heat or other forms of excess, indiscriminate use will prove to be ineffectual or even harmful.

The body generally attempts to drain excess heat caused by inappropriate diet, alcohol, or drugs via the skin, bowels, urine, or even blood. This type of excess heat, which always comes from the outside, is different from the heat from constraint that is caused by the stagnation of the body's own yang qi. Excess heat readily turns into toxic heat; it readily combines with the body substances like stool, urine, and blood with which it shares routes of transport and elimination to produce clumping; and it must therefore be drained with bitter and cold herbs, rather than cleared with acrid and sweet ones. From an organ perspective, Heart patterns indicate conditions where such excess heat has penetrated into the blood aspect, causing bleeding and agitation of the spirit. Attempts by the body to drain this heat via the urine lead to damp-heat clumping and stagnating within the lower burner. Hence, the source text prescribes this formula not only for painful and bloody urinary dribbling and urinary retention, but also for heat in the Heart channel characterized by a parched throat, severe thirst, irritability, eye redness and pain, scorched lips, nosebleed, and sores in the mouth, tongue, or throat. The formula should be most effective when used in the treatment of patterns that match this presentation.

The inclusion in this formula of Rhei Radix et Rhizoma *(dà huáng),* an herb more commonly associated with bowel obstruction and yang brightness-warp disorders, underscores the original intention of this formula to drain heat from the lower burner and blood aspect. Rhei Radix et Rhizoma *(dà huáng)* contributes four different actions to the overall effect of the formula. First, it drains damp-heat not only via the stool, but also via the urine. *Materia Medica of Ri Hua-Zi,* for instance, notes that it "promotes [both] urination and bowel [movement]." Similarly, *Secret Essentials of Main Indications,* a no longer extant text quoted in *Expounding on the Origins of Medicine,* emphasizes that it "eliminates lower burner dampness." Second, Rhei Radix et Rhizoma *(dà huáng)* drains excess heat and resolves toxins by guiding them downward. This is useful for counteracting the innate tendency of fire to flare upward, as well as draining it from its source. Third, Rhei Radix et Rhizoma *(dà huáng)* cools the blood and stops bleeding. It enters the blood aspect and enlivens blood where it has become static, but also effectively treats bleeding from the upper body orifices by directing fire downward. Fourth, the use of Rhei Radix et Rhizoma *(dà huáng)* embodies the treatment principle of "treating upper [burner] disorders through the lower [burner]." By draining fire downward and eliminating excess through both the urine and stool, Rhei Radix et Rhizoma *(dà huáng)* removes the source of the heat that is responsible for symptoms like parched throat, severe thirst, irritability, eye redness and pain, scorched lips, nosebleed, and sores in the mouth, tongue, or throat.

All of these actions are directed at eliminating excess heat. The 19th-century physician Fei Bo-Xiong thus suggests providing a substitute for Rhei Radix et Rhizoma (*dà huáng*) in cases of mixed excess and deficiency disorders:

> In [those with] a constitution combining yin deficiency with dampness [and] fire, one should remove Rhei Radix et Rhizoma (*dà huáng*) and add substances like Asparagi Radix (*tiān mén dōng*), Salviae miltiorrhizae Radix (*dān shēn*), Moutan Cortex (*mǔ dān pí*), and Succinum (*hǔ pò*). One must furthermore not use Rhei Radix et Rhizoma (*dà huáng*) where it would damage the primal qi of a patient.

Comparisons

➣ Vs. GUIDE OUT THE RED POWDER (*dǎo chì sǎn*)

Both formulas can be used to treat hot painful urinary dribbling, but their modes of action and indications are quite different. Eight-Herb Powder for Rectification (*bā zhèng sǎn*) strongly unblocks painful urinary dribbling, does not nourish the yin in any way, and focuses on the lower burner (urinary retention along with lower abdominal distention and pain). Guide Out the Red Powder (*dǎo chì sǎn*), on the other hand, focuses on the upper burner (irritability and mouth sores), nourishes the yin, but has a much weaker effect on painful urinary dribbling.

➣ Vs. SMALL THISTLE DRINK (*xiǎo jì yǐn zi*)

Both formulas can be used to treat hot and bloody urinary dribbling due to heat clumping in the lower burner. However, Small Thistle Drink (*xiǎo jì yǐn zi*) focuses on cooling blood to stop bleeding. It is indicated where heat clumping in the Bladder damages the collaterals, leading to bloody urinary dribbling or blood in the urine. Eight-Herb Powder for Rectification (*bā zhèng sǎn*) focuses on draining and clearing damp-heat from the lower burner that accumulates in the Bladder and causes hot painful urinary dribbling.

➣ Vs. OPEN THE GATE PILL (*tōng guān wán*); *see* PAGE 719

➣ Vs. POWDER FOR FIVE TYPES OF PAINFUL URINARY DRIBBLING (*wǔ lín sǎn*); *see* PAGE 716

Biomedical Indications

With the appropriate presentation, this formula may be used to treat a variety of biomedically-defined disorders including glomerulonephritis, cystitis, urethritis, urinary tract calculi, prostatitis, and stomatitis.

Alternate names

Eight-Treasure Powder (*bā zhēn sǎn*) in *Effective Formulas from Generations of Physicians*; Eight-Herb Decoction for Rectification (*bā zhèng tāng*) in *Song Family Secret Texts on Women's Disorders*

Modifications

• For bloody painful urinary dribbling, increase the dosage of Polygoni avicularis Herba (*biān xù*) and add Imperatae

Rhizoma (*bái máo gēn*) and Cirsii Herba (*xiǎo jì*).

• For stony painful urinary dribbling, add Lysimachiae Herba (*jīn qián cǎo*), Lygodii Spora (*hǎi jīn shā*), Pyrrosiae Folium (*shí wěi*), and Achyranthis bidentatae Radix (*niú xī*).

• For cloudy painful urinary dribbling, add Dioscoreae hypoglaucae Rhizoma (*bì xiè*) and Acori tatarinowii Rhizoma (*shí chāng pú*).

• For urinary retention, increase the dosage of Akebiae Caulis (*mù tōng*), Talcum (*huá shí*), and Polygoni avicularis Herba (*biān xù*) and add Phellodendri Cortex (*huáng bǎi*) and Cinnamomi Cortex (*ròu guì*).

• For stomatitis, add Lophatheri Herba (*dàn zhú yè*) and Rehmanniae Radix (*shēng dì huáng*).

Variation

加味八正散

Augmented Eight-Herb Powder for Rectification

jiā wèi bā zhèng sǎn

SOURCE *Essential Teachings of [Zhu] Dan-Xi* (1481)

Add Aucklandiae Radix (*mù xiāng*). Not only does this strengthen the transforming function of the Bladder qi, its acrid, warm nature prevents the cold properties of the other ingredients from injuring the yang qi.

Associated Formulas

清肺飲子（清肺饮子）

Clear the Lungs Drink

qīng fèi yín zi

SOURCE *Secrets from the Orchid Chamber* (1336)

Junci Medulla (*dēng xīn cǎo*) 0.3g
Tetrapanacis Medulla (*tōng cǎo*) 0.6g
Alismatis Rhizoma (*zé xiè*) .1.5g
Dianthi Herba (*qú mài*) 1.5g
Succinum (*hǔ pò*) 1.5g
Polygoni avicularis Herba (*biān xù*) 2.1g
Akebiae Caulis (*mù tōng*) 2.1g
Plantaginis Semen (*chē qián zǐ*) 3g
Poria (*fú líng*) 6g
Polyporus (*zhū líng*) 9g

Grind the herbs into a coarse powder and decoct 15g as a draft. Should not be taken with meals. Clears and drains Lung heat, promotes urination, and unblocks painful urinary dribbling. For painful urinary dribbling or urinary blockage accompanied by thirst. This pattern is due to pathogenic heat in the qi aspect of the upper burner inhibiting the Lung's regulation of the water pathways. If the qi transformation of the upper burner is disordered, the fluids in the lower burner will lack the power to be discharged, accumulating as damp-heat that causes painful urinary dribbling or urinary blockage. Because the clear fluids cannot ascend, the patient feels thirsty. Compared to Eight-Treasure Decoction (*bā zhēn tāng*), this formula treats milder conditions with more pronounced dampness and no heat in the blood aspect.

三金湯（三金汤）

Three-Gold Decoction

sān jīn tāng

SOURCE *Differential Diagnosis in Traditional Chinese Medicine* (1984)

Desmodii styracifolii Herba *(guǎng jīn qián cǎo)* 60g
Malvae Fructus *(dōng kuí guǒ)* 12g
Lygodii Herba *(jīn shā téng)* 30g
Pyrrosiae Folium *(shí wěi)* 9g
Dianthi Herba *(qú mài)* 12g
Gigeriae galli Endothelium corneum *(jī nèi jīn)* 9g

Promotes urination and expels stones. For painful urinary dribbling due to damp-heat in the lower burner characterized by urgent, burning, and painful urination, anuria, or oliguria due to stones in the urinary tract. In contrast to the principal formula, this focuses on stony painful urinary dribbling. This formula originated from the Shuguang Hospital of the Shanghai College of Traditional Chinese Medicine and its name can be attributed to the fact that three of the ingredients' names contain the word gold (金 *jīn*). The specific action of these three herbs—Lysimachiae Herba *(jīn qián cǎo)*, Lygodii Herba *(jīn shā téng)*, and Gigeriae galli Endothelium corneum *(jī nèi jīn)*—is to dissolve stones in both the urinary and bile tracts. Hence, they are frequently combined for this purpose.

五淋散

Powder for Five Types of Painful Urinary Dribbling

wǔ lín sǎn

Source   *Formulary of the Pharmacy Service for Benefiting the People in the Taiping Era* (1107)

Poria rubra *(chì fú líng)* 12-18g
Angelicae sinensis Radix *(dāng guī)* 9-15g
Glycyrrhizae Radix *(gān cǎo)* 3-6g
Paeoniae Radix rubra *(chì sháo)* 9-18g
Gardeniae Fructus *(zhī zǐ)* 6-15g

Method of Preparation   The source text recommends grinding equal amounts of the ingredients into a fine powder and take in 6g doses as a draft. Can also be taken as a decoction, generally with the dosages above.

Actions   Clears heat, cools the blood, promotes urination, and unblocks painful urinary dribbling

Indications

Rough, painful urination that is red or the color of red bean juice, or with multiple tiny stones. Urinary symptoms may be accompanied by acute lower abdominal pain.

This is damp-heat bloody painful urinary dribbling, which is usually due to overindulgence in spicy, sweet, or rich foods, or overconsumption of alcohol. It may also be caused by the penetration of damp-heat from the exterior into the lower burner. If damp-heat pours into the Bladder, the heat damages the collaterals, causing the blood to move recklessly. This leads to rough and painful urinary dribbling. Damp-heat collecting in the Bladder and clumping with the urine may also produce stones through a process of steaming. This manifests as painful urinary dribbling with stabbing pain and the voiding of multiple tiny stones. Damp-heat obstructing the qi dynamic in the lower burner leads to acute lower abdominal pain.

Analysis of Formula

To treat blood in the urine due to reckless movement of blood caused by damp-heat entering into the lower burner blood aspect, this formula employs a combined strategy of clearing the heat, cooling the blood, promoting water metabolism, and unblocking painful urinary dribbling. As reflected in its original name, Gardenia Decoction *(shān zhī zǐ tāng)*, the chief herb in this formula is bitter and cooling Gardeniae Fructus *(zhī zǐ)*. It clears heat from the qi aspect via the Triple Burner and cools and moves the blood. It is thus ideally suited for a pattern characterized by damp-heat leading to reckless movement of the blood. The two deputies are Poria rubra *(chì fú líng)* and Paeoniae Radix rubra *(chì sháo)*. Sweet and bland, Poria rubra *(chì fú líng)* drains damp-heat from the Heart, Small Intestine, and Bladder by promoting urination and unblocking the lower body orifices. Unlike the closely related Poria *(fú líng)*, Poria rubra *(chì fú líng)* does not possess any tonifying properties that would be counterproductive in an excess pattern such as this. Bitter and slighlty cooling Paeoniae Radix rubra *(chì sháo)* enters into the blood aspect to dispel constrained heat, enhancing the efficacy of the chief herb at this level. It also moves the blood, and, according to *Divine Husbandman's Classic of the Materia Medica*, stops abdominal pain and promotes urination. Warming, acrid, and oily Angelicae sinensis Radix *(dāng guī)* serves as the assistant, supporting Paeoniae Radix rubra *(chì sháo)* in moving the blood to dispel stasis and stop the abdominal pain while moderating its cooling nature. It also nourishes the blood to compensate for any blood loss. Glycyrrhizae Radix *(gān cǎo)*, which drains fire, resolves toxicity, and harmonizes the actions of the other ingredients, serves as the envoy.

Cautions and Contraindications

This formula is indicated for excess-type painful urinary dribbling. It should not be used without modification to treat chronic conditions or patterns characterized by deficiency and cold.

Commentary

According to its name, this formula is indicated for all five of the different types of painful urinary dribbling (淋 *lín*). While there are different classification schemes, these are usually considered to be hot, cloudy, bloody, consumptive, and stony. In clinical practice, the present formula is most effective for the heat type, especially if it is accompanied by bleeding. It should be modified for treating other types of painful urinary dribbling, as explained by the contemporary physicians Zhu Liang-Chun and Xue Ban-Ding in *Detailed Explanation of Versified Prescriptions*:

> Viewed from the perspective of each individual herb's [actions] and their combination, this formula will be effective for hot painful urinary dribbling where urination is rough and red [in color. This manifests as] stabbing pain or blood in the urine. The name of this formula—Powder for Five Types of Painful Urinary Dribbling (*wǔ lín sǎn*)—implies that it can, by way of modification through additions and subtractions, be used to treat the five different manifestations of painful urinary dribbling.

Some possible modifications, drawn from the text by Zhu and Xue, are listed later in this entry.

Comparisons

➢ Vs. Eight-Herb Powder for Rectification (*bā zhèng sǎn*)

Both formulas treat painful urinary dribbling caused by damp-heat pouring downward into the Bladder. Powder for Five Types of Painful Urinary Dribbling (*wǔ lín sǎn*) clears heat from constraint in both the qi and blood aspects that causes reckless movement of blood. It is thus best suited for treating excess heat patterns accompanied by blood in the urine. By contrast, Eight-Herb Powder for Rectification (*bā zhèng sǎn*) drains excess heat from the upper and lower burners via both the urine and stool. It is thus indicated for patterns characterized by excess heat that has clumped in the lower burner and manifests as Heart fire in the upper burner.

➢ Vs. Small Thistle Drink (*xiǎo jì yǐn zi*); *see* PAGE 605

Biomedical Indications

With the appropriate presentation, this formula may be used to treat a variety of biomedically-defined disorders including urethritis, cystitis, urinary calculi, gonorrhea, and appendicitis.

Alternate names

Gardenia Decoction (*shān zhī zǐ tāng*) in *Prescriptions of Universal Benefit*; Decoction for Five Types of Painful Urinary Dribbling (*wǔ lín tāng*) in *Medicine is Truly Easy Era*

Modifications

- For visible blood in the urine, add Imperatae Rhizoma (*bái máo gēn*), Cirsii japonici Herba sive Radix (*dà jì*), and Cirsii Herba (*xiǎo jì*).
- For painful urination with blood in the urine, add Rehmanniae Radix (*shēng dì huáng*), Moutan Cortex (*mǔ dān pí*), and Achyranthis bidentatae Radix (*niú xī*).

- For urinary calculi, add Lysimachiae Herba (*jīn qián cǎo*), Lygodii Spora (*hǎi jīn shā*), and Gigeriae galli Endothelium corneum (*jī nèi jīn*).
- For qi stagnation with distention of the lower abdomen, add Linderae Radix (*wū yào*) and Cimicifugae Rhizoma (*shēng má*).
- For turbid urine, add Dianthi Herba (*qú mài*) and Pyrrosiae Folium (*shí wéi*).

Associated Formulas

加味五淋散

Augmented Powder for Five Types of Painful Urinary Dribbling

jiā wèi wǔ lín sǎn

SOURCE *Golden Mirror of the Medical Tradition* (1742)

Poria rubra (*chì fú líng*) 18g
Angelicae sinensis Radix (*dāng guī*) 15g
Glycyrrhizae Radix (*gān cǎo*) 15g
Paeoniae Radix rubra (*chì sháo*) 60g
Gardeniae Fructus (*zhī zǐ*) 60g
Rehmanniae Radix (*shēng dì huáng*) 30g
Alismatis Rhizoma (*zé xiè*) 30g
Plantaginis Semen (*chē qián zǐ*) 30g
Talcum (*huá shí*) 30g
Akebiae Caulis (*mù tōng*) 15g

Decoction. The source text does not specify dosage. Clears heat and resolves dampness. For painful urinary dribbling during pregnancy (子淋 *zǐ lín*) characterized by frequent, rough urination with burning pain, dirty yellow complexion, a dry mouth with no desire to drink, stifling sensation in the chest, reduced appetite, a red tongue with a yellow coating, and a slippery, rapid pulse.

石韋散 (石韦散)

Pyrrosiae Powder

shí wéi sǎn

SOURCE *Supplemented Collections on Patterns and Treatments* (1687)

Pyrrosiae Folium (*shí wéi*) 12g
Malvae Fructus (*dōng kuí guǒ*) .9g
Dianthi Herba (*qú mài*) 9g
Talcum (*huá shí*) 15g
Plantaginis Semen (*chē qián zǐ*) 12g

Grind the herbs into a powder and take 9g with warm water. Clears heat, promotes the resolution of dampness, unblocks painful urinary dribbling, and expels stones. For rough urination accompanied by severe, acute pain in the lower abdomen, and small stones or sand in the urine. The pain ceases once the stones have been expelled. This is stony painful urinary dribbling, which is often caused by damp-heat in the lower burner obstructing the qi dynamic. The formula focuses on the use of herbs like Malvae Fructus (*dōng kuí guǒ*), Plantaginis Semen (*chē qián zǐ*), and Talcum (*huá shí*) that are considered to be slippery and thus able to facilitate the expulsion of stones without aggravating the heat, as would be the case with acrid, qi-moving herbs.

通關丸（通关散）

Open the Gate Pill

tōng guān wán

The term 關 *guān* in the formula's name can be read in two different ways. In its literal translation, it means 'pass' or 'gate.' Opening the gate would then imply unblocking urinary obstruction. It may also be read as a reference to Chapter 12 of *Classic of Difficulties*, where the term 關 *guān* is used to refer to blocked urination.

Source   *Secrets from the Orchid Chamber* (1336)

wine-fried Phellodendri Cortex *(jiǔ chǎo huáng bǎi)* 30g
wine-fried Anemarrhenae Rhizoma *(jiǔ chǎo zhī mǔ)* 30g
Cinnamomi Cortex *(ròu guì)* 1.5g

Method of Preparation   Grind the herbs into a powder, make a paste with water, and form into pills. At present, the dosage is 9g taken once or twice daily. The source text advises to take the pills on an empty stomach.

Actions   Clears heat, enriches the yin, opens urinary obstruction, and promotes urination

Indications

Urinary obstruction, pain in the lower abdomen, rough and painful urination, and absence of thirst.

This is urinary obstruction due to heat collecting in the lower burner and obstructing the qi transformation of the Bladder. This may also manifest as rough and painful urination, or as pain in the abdomen. Because heat in the Bladder and Kidneys steams the fluids upward to the Lungs and Stomach, the patient does not feel thirsty. This sign distinguishes this pattern from similar ones caused by excess heat in the upper or middle burners.

Analysis of Formula

To drain excess or pathogenic heat from the lower burner, one should use bitter and cooling herbs that enter the Bladder and Kidneys. Phellodendri Cortex *(huáng bǎi)*, the chief herb in this formula, fulfills these requirements. It drains fire from excess affecting the Kidneys and clears lower burner damp-heat, effectively removing the cause of urinary obstruction. Phellodendri Cortex *(huáng bǎi)* is often combined with Anemarrhenae Rhizoma *(zhī mǔ)*, the deputy herb in this formula, because their synergy amplifies the primary actions of each herb. Anemarrhenae Rhizoma *(zhī mǔ)* is bitter and cooling, but also moistening, thus preventing damage to the yin by the extreme bitterness of Phellodendri Cortex *(huáng bǎi)*. It enters the Lungs and Stomach from which it directs the 'yin fire' (i.e., internal fire flaring upward from the lower burner) downward toward its source. By contrast, Phellodendri Cortex *(huáng bǎi)* focuses only on the Bladder and Kidneys, from which it effectively drains this fire out of the body.

Acrid and warming Cinnamomi Cortex *(ròu guì)* serves as the assistant. It is used in a small dosage to ensure that the cooling nature of the chief and deputy herbs does not extinguish the physiological fire at the gate of vitality. By promoting the qi dynamic in the lower burner, it anchors the yang qi. This is called "guiding the dragon [i.e., the fire at the gate of vitality] back to the sea [i.e., the lower burner]." Together, the three herbs in this formula thus drain pathogenic heat without injuring the physiological fire, and open urinary blockage without damaging either the yin or yang.

Cautions and Contraindications

The bitter, cooling nature of this formula can easily injure the Spleen qi. It is thus contraindicated for patients with Spleen qi deficiency who suffer from diarrhea or thin stools. Because it drains excess fire from the lower burner, it is also contraindicated for Kidney qi and yin deficiency.

Commentary

This formula was composed by the Jin-dynasty physician Li Dong-Yuan to treat "heat in the blood aspect of the lower burner" characterized by "absence of thirst in spite of severe dryness and urinary obstruction." In this context, the term 'blood aspect' (血分 *xuè fēn*) refers to yin, that is, the lower burner, and not, as in Ye Tian-Shi's later system of diagnosis, to the end-stage in the progression of warm pathogen disorders. This heat causes the qi transformation of the lower burner to break down, which then manifests as urinary obstruction. This is similar to the condition treated by Five-Ingredient Powder with Poria *(wǔ líng sǎn)*, discussed below, where obstruction is caused by the penetration of cold. However, whereas cold leads to a buildup of water (蓄水 *xù shuǐ*), heat steams the fluids in the lower burner upward. This causes a person to feel no particular thirst, even as the Kidneys become dry.

The alternate name of this formula, Enrich the Kidneys Pill (滋腎丸 *zī shèn wán*), has fueled debate among commentators regarding the function of Phellodendri Cortex *(huáng bǎi)* and Anemarrhenae Rhizoma *(zhī mǔ)* in relation to the Kidneys. Some famous physicians of the period, notably Zhu Dan-Xi, referred to this combination as tonifying the Kidney yin. As late as the Qing period, we find statements like the following taken from Wang Ang's influential *Medical Formulas Collected and Analyzed*:

> Phellodendri Cortex *(huáng bǎi)* is bitter, cooling, and slightly acrid. It drains the Bladder [and] ministerial fire, tonifies insufficient Kidney water, and enters the blood aspect of the Kidney channel. Anemarrhenae Rhizoma *(zhī mǔ)* is acrid, bitter, cooling, and slippery. Above, it clears Lung metal and directs fire downward. Below, it moistens Kidney dryness and enriches the yin. Thus, the two herbs accentuate each other's actions. They are an excellent prescription for tonifying water.

The tonifying action on Kidney water mentioned by Wang Ang and others is difficult to understand given the bitter and cooling nature of both herbs, which is drying and draining, and therefore damaging to both the Kidney yin and yang. Following centuries of debate, a consensus has slowly emerged that understands tonification in this case to be a consequence of draining. By draining excess pathogenic heat from the Bladder and Kidneys, Phellodendri Cortex (*huáng bǎi*) and Anemarrhenae Rhizoma (*zhī mǔ*) effectively prevent the heat from injuring the yin. The combination must not be used, however, if the fire is due to deficiency of yin itself. In that case, sweet, cooling herbs like Rehmanniae Radix (*shēng dì huáng*) and Scrophulariae Radix (*xuán shēn*) would be appropriate.

Li Dong-Yuan used variations of this formula to treat internal obstruction of the eye and clouded vision. These conditions are caused by pathogenic fire rising upward from the lower burner and are treated by draining the fire at its source. Later generations of physicians extended the application of this formula even further. In *Precious Mirror of Health*, Li Dong-Yuan's disciple Luo Tian-Yi recommended the formula for "treating lower burner yin deficiency [characterized by] soft and forceless lower back and knees, sweating of the genitals, impotence, and hot feet that are unable to walk." In *Indispensable Tools for Pattern Treatment*, the Ming-dynasty writer Wang Ken-Tang prescribed it for "treating sores [due to] yin deficiency of the Kidney channel [that leads to] fever, thirst, bloody stools, and hot feet." In *Correct Transmission of Medicine*, the Ming-dynasty physician Yu Tuan used it "to treat tinnitus and deafness." *Case Records as a Guide to Clinical Practice* show that Ye Tian-Shi utilized it in the treatment of painful lower extremities due to heat from Kidney yin deficiency as well as for headache, palpitations, paraesthesia, and chronic bulging disorders due to up-flaring of fire. In the case records of Xue Sheng-Bai, this formula is indicated for "Spleen and Lung accumulation heat that causes wheezing in children." In all of these cases, heat in the upper, middle, or lower burners is traced back to excess heat in the lower burner and drained from there.

In practice, the chief and deputy herbs are often washed in alcohol when they are intended to drain up-flaring heat from the upper burner or baked with salt when one wishes to focus more directly on symptoms in the lower burner.

Comparisons

➢ Vs. Great Tonify the Yin Pill (*dà bǔ yīn wán*)

Both formulas use the combination of Phellodendri Cortex (*huáng bǎi*) and Anemarrhenae Rhizoma (*zhī mǔ*) to drain excess heat from the lower burner. However, Great Tonify the Yin Pill (*dà bǔ yīn wán*) combines this pair with herbs that strongly enrich the Kidney yin and essence. It is used to treat patterns where excess heat has already damaged the yin

essence or for mixed excess and deficiency patterns characterized by up-flaring of fire from the lower burner that leads to night sweats or other manifestations of pathological heat. Open the Gate Pill (*tōng guān wán*), on the other hand, treats a pattern of pure excess characterized by urinary obstruction and the absence of thirst.

➢ Vs. Eight-Herb Powder for Rectification (*bā zhèng sǎn*)

Both formulas treat excess heat collecting in the lower burner leading to painful urinary difficulty or urinary obstruction. Eight-Herb Powder for Rectification (*bā zhèng sǎn*) is appropriate when the source of the heat is located in the upper and middle burners, specifically the Heart and Small Intestine. Open the Gate Pill (*tōng guān wán*), on the other hand, is indicated when the source of the heat is located in the lower burner itself. The distinguishing symptom between the two is the presence or absence of thirst.

➢ Vs. Two-Marvel Powder (*èr miào sǎn*); *see* PAGE 720

Biomedical Indications

With the appropriate presentation, this formula may be used to treat a variety of biomedically-defined disorders including benign prostatic hypertrophy, urinary retention, acute pyelonephritis, urinary dysfunction post prostatectomy, and urinary tract infections during pregnancy.

....

Alternate names

Enrich the Kidneys Pill (*zī shèn wán*) in *Secrets from the Orchid Chamber*; Water and Fire Pill (*kǎn lí wán*) in *Displays of Enlightened Physicians*; Anemarrhena and Phellodendron Pill to Enrich the Kidneys (*zhī mǔ huáng bǎi zī shèn wán*) and Pill to Greatly Supplement and Enrich the Kidneys (*dà bǔ zī shèn wán*) in *Compendium of the Rules of Conduct for Physicians*; Discharge the Kidneys Pill (*xiè shèn wán*) in *Complete Collection of Charts and Texts Past and Present*; Open the Gate and Enrich the Kidneys Pill (*tōng guān zī shèn wán*) in *Nationwide Collection of TCM Patent Formulas*; Enrich the Kidneys and Open the Gate Pill (*zī shèn tōng guān wán*) in *Case Histories of Ding Gan-Ren*

....

Modifications

- To strengthen urination by improving the qi dynamic of the upper burner, add Platycodi Radix (*jié gěng*).

- For pronounced damp-heat, add Plantaginis Semen (*chē qián zǐ*), Talcum (*huá shí*), Polyporus (*zhū líng*), and Akebiae Caulis (*mù tōng*).

- For qi deficiency, add Astragali Radix (*huáng qí*) and Atractylodis macrocephalae Rhizoma (*bái zhú*).

- For yin deficiency, add Rehmanniae Radix (*shēng dì huáng*) and Ligustri lucidi Fructus (*nǚ zhēn zǐ*).

- For toxic heat, add *guàn zhòng* (Dryopteridis/Cyrtomii/etc. Rhizoma) and Violae Herba (*zǐ huā dì dīng*).

- For blood stasis, add Succinum (*hǔ pò*).

二妙散

Two-Marvel Powder

èr miào săn

This formula is regarded as a 'marvel' of simplicity (composed of just two herbs) and effectiveness, hence the name.

Source *Essential Teachings of [Zhu] Dan-Xi* (1481)

dry-fried Phellodendri Cortex *(chăo huáng băi)* 9-12g
prepared Atractylodis Rhizoma *(zhì cāng zhú)* 6-9g

Method of Preparation The source text advises to fry equal amounts of both herbs, grind into a powder, and take twice a day with ginger juice. At present, if prepared in this manner, the normal dosage is 3-6g. It may also be prepared as a decoction with the dosage specified.

Actions Clears heat and dries dampness

Indications

For a wide variety of complaints accompanied by scanty, yellow urine and a yellow, greasy tongue coating. Among these complaints are pain in the lower back or extremities (especially the sinews or bones); weakness or atrophy of the lower extremities; red, hot, swollen, and painful feet or knees; a thick, yellow, foul-smelling vaginal discharge; and sores on the lower extremities due to dampness.

These are different presentations of damp-heat lodged in the lower burner. Damp-heat in the sinews and bones of the lower burner causes pain in the lower back and extremities with red, hot, swollen, and painful joints. It may also interfere with the nourishment of the sinews and bones, resulting in weakness or atrophy. Damp-heat lodged in the genital region causes a thick, yellow, and foul-smelling leukorrhea. The urine and tongue signs reflect damp-heat in the lower burner.

Analysis of Formula

This formula dries dampness and drains heat from the lower burner. Phellodendri Cortex *(huáng băi)*, a bitter and cooling herb that directly enters into the lower burner, is the chief ingredient. It focuses on eliminating heat from the yin aspects of the body, drains lower burner heat, and dries dampness. It is complemented by bitter and warm Atractylodis Rhizoma *(cāng zhú)* as deputy. While this herb primarily focuses on the Spleen and middle burner, its inclusion in a formula for damp-heat in the lower burner is one of the 'marvels' alluded to in the formula's name. On one level, Atractylodis Rhizoma *(cāng zhú)* deals with the problem of dampness at its root in the middle burner. Its bitterness dries the dampness that impedes the Spleen's function of transformation, while its acrid, warming nature promotes its transportive function. At another level, acrid, warming, and dispersing Atractylodis Rhizoma *(cāng zhú)* also moderates the bitter, cooling, and downward-directing agency of Phellodendri Cortex *(huáng băi)*. The cooling nature of Phellodendri Cortex *(huáng băi)*,

in turn, prevents the warmth of Atractylodis Rhizoma *(cāng zhú)* from further aggravating pathogenic heat, even as each herb supports the other in drying dampness. Chief and deputy thus constitute an ideally matched, elegant, and powerfully synergistic combination that has become the foundation for many prescriptions for drying and clearing damp-heat lodged in the lower burner.

According to the source text, the powder should be taken with ginger juice, which serves as assistant. It moderates the cooling nature of Phellodendri Cortex *(huáng băi)*, preventing it from damaging the Stomach qi and thereby indirectly aggravating the dampness, while also stimulating the qi dynamic in a more general sense. Despite its apparent simplicity, the formula thus unfolds a complex web of interrelated functions that are reflected in its efficacy.

Commentary

This formula is commonly used as the foundation for larger and more complex formulas, and is very useful in the treatment of atrophy disorders due to damp-heat. *Essential Teachings of [Zhu] Dan-Xi* offers a number of suggestions for further improving its effectiveness: "For qi [deficiency,] add qi [-tonifying] herbs. For those with blood deficiency, add [blood-] tonifying herbs. If the pain is severe, add ginger juice and take it steaming hot." Zhu Dan-Xi's case records reflect how he applied these rules in his own practice. For qi deficiency, he added herbs from Generate the Pulse Powder *(shēng mài săn)* or Four-Gentlemen Decoction *(sì jūn zĭ tāng)*, while for blood deficiency, he drew on Four-Substance Decoction *(sì wù tāng)*. Ginger juice (often combined with bamboo juice) is frequently used in formulas directed at dispelling phlegm-dampness from the channels and collaterals, a usage that can also be found in Zhu Dan-Xi's own cases.

In other passages from *Essential Teachings of [Zhu] Dan-Xi*, there are recommendations for adding herbs like Rhei Radix et Rhizoma *(dà huáng)*, Scutellariae Radix *(huáng qín)*, Coptidis Rhizoma *(huáng lián)*, and Talcum *(huá shí)* for cases of phlegm-heat, and blood-moving herbs in those cases characterized by more severe pain. Later generations of physicians built on these suggestions and expanded the formula in various ways. The most important of the resulting new formulas, some of which became famous in their own right, are listed below.

Cautions and Contraindications

This formula should not be used without modification in cases with Lung heat or Liver and Kidney deficiency.

Comparison

➤ Vs. Open the Gate Pill *(tōng guān wán)*

Both formulas drain damp-heat from the lower burner using Phellodendri Cortex *(huáng băi)* as their chief herb. Open the Gate Pill *(tōng guān wán)* combines Phellodendri Cortex *(huáng bǎi)* with Anemarrhenae Rhizoma *(zhī mǔ)*, which drains heat from the Lungs and Stomach, and also moistens the yin. That formula is therefore indicated for patterns where heat is predominant, where lower burner damp-heat leads to up-flaring of yin fire (reflected in symptoms in the upper part of the body), or where damp-heat is beginning to damage the yin (reflected in a lack of thirst in spite of the heat). Two-Marvel Powder *(èr miào sǎn)*, on the other hand, combines Phellodendri Cortex *(huáng bǎi)* with Atractylodis Rhizoma *(cāng zhú)*, which is acrid and warming and focuses on the Spleen. This formula is therefore indicated for patterns where dampness is predominant, where lower burner damp-heat flows downward (reflected in symptoms in the legs), or where damp-heat is obstructing the qi and blood (indicated by pain). Open the Gate Pill *(tōng guān wán)* combines two bitter, cooling herbs with a small dosage of acrid and warming Cinnamomi Cortex *(ròu guì)*, which focuses on the gate of vitality. This underscores the formula's focus on regulating the physiology of the fire at the gate of vitality. Two-Marvel Powder *(èr miào sǎn)* combines Phellodendri Cortex *(huáng bǎi)* and Atractylodis Rhizoma *(cāng zhú)* with the acrid, warming Zingiberis Rhizoma recens *(shēng jiāng)*, which disperses the yang and opens the pores. This reflects the formula's focus on pathogenic dampness that arises from the middle burner, from which it flows downward to obstruct the channels and collaterals in the lower body.

Biomedical Indications

With the appropriate presentation, this formula may be used to treat a variety of biomedically-defined disorders including osteoarthritis, gout, spasm of the gastrocnemius muscle, and vaginitis.

Alternate names

Two-Marvel Atractylodes and Phellodendron Powder *(èr miào cāng bǎi sǎn)* in *Introduction to Medicine*; Atractylodes and Phellodendron Powder *(cāng bǎi sǎn)* in *Select Treatments for Sores*; Two-Marvel Pill *(èr miào wán)* in *Comprehensive Outline of Medicine*; Atractylodes and Phellodendron Two-Marvel Pill *(cāng bǎi èr miào wán)* in *Symptom, Cause, Pulse, and Treatments*

Modifications

- For pain in the lower back and lower extremities as the major complaint, add Achyranthis bidentatae Radix *(niú xī)*, Chaenomelis Fructus *(mù guā)*, and Acanthopanacis Cortex *(wǔ jiā pí)*.
- For atrophy disorder as the major complaint, add Siegesbeckiae Herba *(xī xiān cǎo)* and Acanthopanacis Cortex *(wǔ jiā pí)*.
- For leg qi as the major complaint, add Coicis Semen *(yì yǐ rén)*, Phaseoli Semen *(chì xiǎo dòu)*, and Arecae Semen *(bīng láng)*.

- For leukorrhea as the major complaint, add Poria rubra *(chì fú líng)* and Euryales Semen *(qiàn shí)*.
- For sores on the lower extremities as the major complaint, add Gentianae Radix *(lóng dǎn cǎo)*, Coicis Semen *(yì yǐ rén)*, and Phaseoli Semen *(chì xiǎo dòu)*.

Associated Formulas

三妙丸

Three-Marvel Pill

sān miào wán

SOURCE   *Fang's Orthodox Lineage of Pulse and Symptoms* (1749)

wine-fried Phellodendri Cortex *(jiǔ chǎo huáng bǎi)* 120g
Atractylodis Rhizoma *(cāng zhú)* 180g
Achyranthis bidentatae Radix *(niú xī)* 60g

The source text advises to grind the ingredients into a powder, mix with flour and form into tiny pills, and take 70 pills on an empty stomach with ginger juice or salted water. At present, it is prepared as a decoction with an appropriate reduction in dosage. Clears heat and dries dampness. For damp-heat lodged in the lower burner with numbness or burning pain in the feet. There may also be weakness in the lower back and extremities.

四妙丸

Four-Marvel Pill

sì miào wán

SOURCE   *Convenient Reader of Established Formulas* (1904)

Phellodendri Cortex *(huáng bǎi)* 240g
Coicis Semen *(yì yǐ rén)* 240g
Atractylodis Rhizoma *(cāng zhú)* 240g
Achyranthis bidentatae Radix *(niú xī)* 240g

The source text advises to grind the ingredients into a powder and take in 6-9g doses 2-3 times daily. At present, it is more commonly prepared as a decoction with an appropriate reduction in dosage. Clears heat and resolves dampness. For atrophy disorder characterized by severe numbness and weakness in the lower extremities with painful and swollen feet.

加味二妙丸

Augmented Two-Marvel Pill

jiā wèi èr miào wán

SOURCE   *Medical Mirror of Past and Present* (Ming dynasty)

Atractylodis Rhizoma *(cāng zhú)* 120g
Phellodendri Cortex *(huáng bǎi)* 60g
Cyathulae Radix *(chuān niú xī)* 30g
Angelicae sinensis radicis Cauda *(dāng guī wěi)* 30g
Stephaniae tetrandrae Radix *(hàn fáng jǐ)* 30g
Dioscoreae hypoglaucae Rhizoma *(bì xiè)* 30g
processed Testudinis Plastrum *(zhì guī bǎn)* 30g

Grind the ingredients into a powder and cook in wine, then form into tiny pills. Should be taken on an empty stomach. Clears heat and resolves dampness. For a sensation of heaviness and discomfort in the extremities with atrophy and loss of strength accompanied by slight edema and numbness, a yellow tongue coating, and a soft, rapid pulse. There will often be a sensation of heat that begins at the dorsum of the foot and slowly progresses up the leg to the waist.

愈帶丸

Cure Discharge Pill

yù dài wán

SOURCE   *Shanghai Municipal Medicine Standards* (1974)

Ailanthi Cortex *(chūn pí)* 90g
Paeoniae Radix alba *(bái sháo)* 30g
charred Alpiniae officinarum Rhizoma *(gāo liáng jiāng huī)* 18g
charred Phellodendri Cortex *(huáng bǎi huì)* 12g

Grind the ingredients to a fine powder and form into pills with 10-20 percent (by weight) being ground glutinous rice. Take in 3-9g doses 1-2 times daily with water. Clears and transforms damp-heat and stops vaginal discharge. For profuse, viscous, fishy-smelling, red-and-white vaginal discharge due to damp-heat. Although this is a condition of excess, this formula contains astringent herbs to control the unremitting, profuse discharge.

中滿分消丸

Separate and Reduce Fullness in the Middle Pill

zhōng mǎn fēn xiāo wán

This formula reduces fullness in the middle burner by separating the various imbalances and addressing each one individually, hence the name.

Source   *Secrets from the Orchid Chamber* (1336)

ginger-fried Magnoliae officinalis Cortex *(jiāng chǎo hòu pò)* .30g
dry-fried Aurantii Fructus immaturus *(chǎo zhǐ shí)* 15g
Curcumae longae Rhizoma *(jiāng huáng)* 3g
dry-fried Scutellariae Radix *(chǎo huáng qín)* 36g
dry-fried Coptidis Rhizoma *(chǎo huáng lián)* 15g
Zingiberis Rhizoma *(gān jiāng)* 6g
Pinelliae Rhizoma praeparatum *(zhì bàn xià)* 15g
dry-fried Anemarrhenae Rhizoma *(chǎo zhī mǔ)* 12g
Alismatis Rhizoma *(zé xiè)* 9g
Polyporus *(zhū líng)* 3g
Poria *(fú líng)* 6g
Atractylodis macrocephalae Rhizoma *(bái zhú)* 3g
Ginseng Radix *(rén shēn)* 3g
Glycyrrhizae Radix praeparata *(zhì gān cǎo)* 3g
Citri reticulatae Pericarpium *(chén pí)* 9g
Amomi Fructus *(shā rén)* 6g

Method of Preparation   Grind the ingredients into a fine powder and steam into small pills. Take in 6-9g doses 2-3 times a day with warm water.

Actions   Strengthens the Spleen, regulates the qi, drains heat, and resolves dampness

Indications

Abdominal distention, firmness with a sensation of fullness and bursting pain in the epigastrium and abdomen, irritability, fever, a bitter taste in the mouth, dark yellow urine, constipation or foul-smelling diarrhea, a yellow, greasy tongue coating, and a wiry, rapid pulse.

This is drum-like abdominal distention (鼓脹 *gǔ zhàng*) due to damp-heat. The transportive function of the Spleen may be impeded by injury from externally-contracted pathogenic influences, emotional problems that generate internal disharmonies, improper diet, overindulgence in sex, or Liver constraint. The disruption of this function prevents the smooth flow of qi, blood, and (especially) fluids. Stagnation of the fluids generates dampness, which in turn leads to qi stagnation and eventually blood stasis. Obstruction of the middle burner from stagnation leads to a pathological intermingling of the clear and the turbid, which inhibits the normal physiological processes and generates heat. The clumping of dampness and heat produces an accumulation of turbidity in the middle burner that manifests as abdominal distention and firmness, and a sensation of fullness and bursting pain in the epigastrium and abdomen.

The upward-steaming of damp-heat and the lingering turbid fluids produces irritability, fever, a bitter taste in the mouth, and thirst with no desire to drink (an important indication of this pattern). Damp-heat lodged in the lower burner leads to dark yellow urine, while damp-heat in the Stomach and Intestines causes constipation or foul-smelling diarrhea. The tongue and pulse signs are likewise indicative of damp-heat.

Analysis of Formula

In order to accomplish the complex task of strengthening the Spleen, regulating the qi, draining heat, and resolving dampness, this formula is composed of three major groups of herbs. The large dosage of the qi-regulating herb Magnoliae officinalis Cortex *(hòu pò)*, coupled with Aurantii Fructus immaturus *(zhǐ shí)*, focuses the formula on removing the obstruction to the flow of qi in the middle burner. In this, they are aided by Curcumae longae Rhizoma *(jiāng huáng)*. These three bitter, warming herbs promote the movement of qi and harmonize the Stomach. The second group includes Scutellariae Radix *(huáng qín)*, Coptidis Rhizoma *(huáng lián)*, Zingiberis Rhizoma *(gān jiāng)*, and Pinelliae Rhizoma praeparatum *(zhì bàn xià)*. This group combines acrid, unbinding herbs with bitter, descending ones in order to drain stagnation from the epigastrium and thereby separate the dampness from the heat. Anemarrhenae Rhizoma *(zhī mǔ)*, another member of this group, primarily clears yang brightness-warp heat, but also enriches the yin to prevent it from being further injured by the progress of the disorder or the actions of the other herbs. The third group, Alismatis

Rhizoma *(zé xiè)*, Polyporus *(zhū líng)*, and Poria *(fú líng)*, leaches out dampness through the urine.

The combination of Poria *(fú líng)*, Atractylodis macrocephalae Rhizoma *(bái zhú)*, Ginseng Radix *(rén shēn)*, and Glycyrrhizae Radix praeparata *(zhì gān cǎo)* is known as Four-Gentlemen Decoction *(sì jūn zǐ tāng)*, which is the basic formula for tonifying the Spleen qi (see Chapter 8). The remaining herbs, Citri reticulatae Pericarpium *(chén pí)* and Amomi Fructus *(shā rén)*, are qi-regulators like those in the first group. Here, however, they serve to regulate and revive (along with the qi-tonifying herbs) the Spleen. Thus, they not only assist in resolving the acute problem, but also help the patient back on the road to health.

Cautions and Contraindications

This formula should only be used for distention due to damp-heat. It should not be used without modification for conditions due to cold.

Commentary

This is a complex formula that is actually an amalgamation of five constituent formulas: Four-Gentlemen Decoction *(sì jūn zǐ tāng)* (Chapter 8), Pinellia Decoction to Drain the Epigastrium *(bàn xià xiè xīn tāng)* (Chapter 3), Two-Aged [Herb] Decoction *(èr chén tāng)* (Chapter 17), Four-Ingredient Powder with Poria *(sì líng sǎn)* (below in this chapter), and Calm the Stomach Powder *(píng wèi sǎn)* (above in this chapter). Among these formulas, Pinellia Decoction to Drain the Epigastrium *(bàn xià xiè xīn tāng)* serves as the foundation. It treats blockage of the qi dynamic in the middle burner due to dampness, phlegm, and heat against a background of Stomach and Spleen deficiency. The present formula addresses the same core problems but is used for patterns in which both excess and deficiency are more pronounced.

Treatment Strategy

The pathological mechanisms underlying this condition were first described in *Basic Questions* (Chapter 74). There it is noted that fullness and swelling from dampness are symptoms of the Spleen, while gross abdominal distention is a symptom of heat. In *Secrets from the Orchid Chamber*, Li Dong-Yuan elaborates on his treatment strategy, using terms first noted in Chapter 14 of *Basic Questions*:

> [Regarding] treatment strategies for abdominal fullness, one should open the ghost gates (鬼門 *guǐ mén*) and cleanse the clear receptacle (淨府 *jìng fǔ*). Opening the ghost gates refers to inducing sweating. Cleansing the clear receptacle refers to promoting urination. Those with abdominal fullness must be drained from the inside. This implies a disorder of the Spleen and Stomach, so one must separate out and reduce the dampness above and below, with the lower burner acting as a sluice. Once the qi and blood sift and transform by themselves, there is no need to [directly] drain the dregs and filth.

Li Dong-Yuan's commentary underscores the emphasis that Jin-Yuan era physicians placed on the treatment of the qi dynamic, which, in its focus on the Triple Burner, prefigures the strategies for the treatment of damp-warmth disorders developed by representatives of the warm pathogen disorder current during the Qing era. The Triple Burner circulates the yang qi and fluids. If one stagnates, the other is also affected. In the present case, the root problem is obstruction of the qi dynamic by dampness (most likely due to inappropriate diet), which then transforms into heat. It is not excess fire. The Qing-dynasty physician Fei Bo-Xiong underscored the importance of this fact:

> To explain what is meant by heat distention, one need not go beyond [understanding that when] the Spleen and Stomach neglect their duties, this results in an accumulation of dampness that [then] transforms into heat. It certainly does not [stem from] excess fire. If [the cause of heat distention was excess fire], how then could water qi move horizontally, and how could turbid yin in turn become exuberant?

Accordingly, the treatment must focus on dispelling dampness rather than draining heat. This task is made easier by exploiting the physiological unity of the Triple Burner, that is, not only by removing obstruction from the Spleen and Stomach, but by simultaneously facilitating water metabolism in the upper and lower burners. Thus, Li Dong-Yuan's formula not only drains the middle burner via the bowels, it also disseminates the Lung qi to facilitate regulation of the water metabolism, and it promotes urination as a means of dispelling dampness via the lower burner. In addition, it strengthens the functions of Spleen and Stomach. Not only does deficiency of these organs give rise to dampness, their functions are also weakened by the various reducing strategies in this formula and are thus in need of augmentation.

Dried Zingiberis Rhizoma recens (gān shēng jiāng)

The list of ingredients in the source text includes dried Zingiberis Rhizoma recens *(gān shēng jiāng)*, while the instructions for preparation simply mention Zingiberis Rhizoma recens *(shēng jiāng)*. This has led to much controversy. Some physicians read dried Zingiberis Rhizoma recens *(gān shēng jiāng)* as Zingiberis Rhizoma *(gān jiāng)*. Textual studies indicate, however, that in late imperial China the terms dried Zingiberis Rhizoma recens *(gān shēng jiāng)* and Zingiberis Rhizoma *(gān jiāng)* were not used interchangeably. Nevertheless, many contemporary physicians prefer to include Zingiberis Rhizoma *(gān jiāng)* because they believe it is more appropriate in the context of this formula.

Biomedical Indications

With the appropriate presentation, this formula may be used to treat a variety of biomedically-defined disorders including

ascites from cirrhosis, icteric infectious hepatitis, and urinary tract infections.

Modifications

- For jaundice due to damp-heat in the Spleen and Stomach, remove Ginseng Radix (*rén shēn*) and Zingiberis Rhizoma (*gān jiāng*) and add Artemisiae scopariae Herba (*yīn chén*), Rhei Radix et Rhizoma (*dà huáng*), and Gardeniae Fructus (*zhī zǐ*).

- For painful, rough urination, add Talcum (*huá shí*), Dianthi Herba (*qú mài*), and Polygoni avicularis Herba (*biān xù*).

- For dark purple blood vessels showing on the abdomen, a dark purple tongue, and a choppy pulse, add Sparganii Rhizoma (*sān léng*), Curcumae Rhizoma (*é zhú*), and Salviae miltiorrhizae Radix (*dān shēn*).

Associated Formula

中滿分消湯 （中满分消汤）

Separate and Reduce Fullness in the Middle Decoction

zhōng mǎn fēn xiāo tāng

SOURCE   *Secrets from the Orchid Chamber* (1336)

Aconiti Radix praeparata (*zhì chuān wū*)	6g
Alismatis Rhizoma (*zé xiè*)	6g
Coptidis Rhizoma (*huáng lián*)	6g
Ginseng Radix (*rén shēn*)	6g
Citri reticulatae viride Pericarpium (*qīng pí*)	6g
Angelicae sinensis Radix (*dāng guī*)	6g
Zingiberis Rhizoma recens (*shēng jiāng*)	6g
Zingiberis Rhizoma (*gān jiāng*)	6g
Ephedrae Herba (*má huáng*)	6g
Bupleuri Radix (*chái hú*)	6g
Litseae Fructus (*bì chéng qié*)	6g
Alpiniae oxyphyllae Fructus (*yì zhì rén*)	15g
Pinelliae Rhizoma praeparatum (*zhì bàn xià*)	15g
Poria (*fú líng*)	15g
Aucklandiae Radix (*mù xiāng*)	15g
Cimicifugae Rhizoma (*shēng má*)	15g
Astragali Radix (*huáng qí*)	15g
Evodiae Fructus (*wú zhū yú*)	15g
Magnoliae officinalis Cortex (*hòu pò*)	15g
Phellodendri Cortex (*huáng bǎi*)	15g
Alpiniae katsumadai Semen (*cǎo dòu kòu*)	15g

Grind the ingredients into a coarse powder and take warm as a draft in 3-9g doses before meals. Warms the middle, moves the qi, opens areas of constraint, and reduces fullness. For drum-like abdominal distention due to cold characterized by a lack of urination or bowel movements, irritability, and vomiting immediately after eating. Other symptoms include yin-type agitation (陰躁 *yīn zào*), restless legs, cold extremities, vomiting up the food one has eaten, cold in the abdomen, and focal distention in the epigastrium. The formula may also be used to treat bulging disorders due to cold, and running piglet disorder.

Section 3

FORMULAS THAT PROMOTE URINATION AND LEACH OUT DAMPNESS

The formulas in this section are used when dampness clogs the water pathways, primarily those associated with urination. Since urination is the principal vehicle for expelling dampness from the body, promoting urination is an effective method for leaching out dampness. The most common signs of dampness affecting urination include edema, urinary obstruction, and painful urinary dribbling. Diarrhea may also appear in cases due to dysfunction of water metabolism.

    The chief herbs used to promote urination and leach out dampness are Poria (*fú líng*), Polyporus (*zhū líng*), Alismatis Rhizoma (*zé xiè*), and *fáng jǐ* (Stephaniae/Cocculi/etc. Radix). Depending on the pattern, they may be combined with deputies and assistants drawn from three other groups of herbs. The first consists of herbs that strengthen the Spleen and facilitate the dispelling of dampness such as Astragali Radix (*huáng qí*) and Atractylodis macrocephalae Rhizoma (*bái zhú*). The second group consists of herbs that warm the yang and promote the transformation of qi, in particular Cinnamomi Ramulus (*guì zhī*). Promoting the qi transformation of the Bladder is an effective way of dispelling water buildup by activating the body's own physiological water metabolism. The third group consists of herbs that nourish the yin such as Asini Corii Colla (*ē jiāo*). Their use is necessary when dampness has caused stagnation that transforms into heat, which then damages the yin.

五苓散

Five-Ingredient Powder with Poria

wǔ líng sǎn

Source   *Discussion of Cold Damage* (c. 220)

Alismatis Rhizoma (*zé xiè*)	15g
Poria (*fú líng*)	9g
Polyporus (*zhū líng*)	9g
Atractylodis macrocephalae Rhizoma (*bái zhú*)	9g
Cinnamomi Ramulus (*guì zhī*)	6g

Method of Preparation   The source text advises to grind the ingredients into a powder, mix with white wine, and take a small spoonful three times a day followed by warm water. It may also be taken as a powder without wine in 3-6 grams doses 1-3 times a day. At present, the formula is generally prepared as a decoction with the dosage given above. If prepared as a decoction, it should not be cooked for more than 10 minutes. If the treatment strategy includes inducing slight sweating, it can be taken with hot water (as a powder) or very warm (as a decoction).

Actions Promotes urination, drains dampness, strengthens the Spleen, warms the yang, and promotes the transforming functions of qi

Indications

(1) Headache, fever, irritability, strong thirst but with vomiting immediately after drinking, urinary difficulty, a floating pulse, and a white tongue coating; (2) edema, generalized sensation of heaviness, diarrhea, urinary difficulty, and possibly vomiting and diarrhea due to sudden turmoil disorder; (3) throbbing pulsations just below the umbilicus, vomiting frothy saliva, vertigo, shortness of breath, and coughing.

The first group of symptoms (the original indications for this formula) are manifestations of water buildup (蓄水 *xù shuǐ*), a greater yang-warp disorder in which the pathogenic influences have not been released from the exterior, but have also penetrated to the greater yang organ, the Bladder. The headache, fever, irritability, and floating pulse indicate an exterior condition. The pathogenic influences attack and disrupt the functions of the Bladder, resulting in urinary difficulty. Disruption of Bladder qi transformation also leads to water retention, which interferes with the upward transportation and downward elimination of fluids. Although this causes strong thirst, fluids cannot be transported downward and are vomited up. This is known as 'water rebellion disorder' (水逆證 *shuǐ nì zhèng*).

The second group of symptoms refers to a pattern of Spleen deficiency that can be described in terms of five-phase theory as earth failing to transport water. This causes internal accumulation of water and dampness that overflows into the muscles and skin and produces edema and a sensation of heaviness. Because the water and dampness are not properly transformed by the Spleen and transported to the Bladder, there may also be diarrhea and urinary difficulty. The effects of the Spleen's failure to transform and transport water may be felt throughout the Triple Burner. This is because the Spleen serves as a pivot in the water pathways of the Triple Burner, providing the key link between the upper and lower burners. In addition to these problems with water metabolism, when the yang of the middle burner is deficient, external pathogenic influences more readily penetrate to the interior. This disrupts the normal function of the Stomach and Intestines, and thereby prevents the clear yang from ascending and the turbid yin from descending. This gives rise to the simultaneous vomiting and diarrhea that are characteristic of sudden turmoil disorders.

The third group of symptoms reflects retention of thin mucus in the lower burner. This causes a throbbing pulsation below the umbilicus as the thin mucus prevents the clear yang from ascending. The stagnation produced by thin mucus leads to an upward rebellion (vomiting) of frothy saliva. When the ascent of clear yang is obstructed, turbid yin cannot move downward, which causes vertigo. If the thin mucus encroaches on the Lungs, there may also be coughing.

Analysis of Formula

This formula treats water buildup in the interior where a pathogen remains in the exterior. For this reason, it combines the promotion of water metabolism, to resolve excess dampness, with the promotion of the qi dynamic, to resolve the exterior. The chief ingredient, sweet, bland, and cold Alismatis Rhizoma (*zé xiè*), leaches out dampness and promotes urination. Its dosage is relatively large, and it is the strongest of the three diuretic herbs in this formula. The cold nature of Alismatis Rhizoma (*zé xiè*), furthermore, enables it to eliminate the heat constraint caused by water buildup or thin mucus obstructing the ascent of yang qi. Note that such constraint occurs even if the original pathogen is cold. One of the deputies, Poria (*fú líng*), is particularly effective in leaching out dampness by promoting urination, strengthening the Spleen, and assisting the yang. The other deputy, bitter Polyporus (*zhū líng*), also eliminates dampness and promotes urination. The chief and deputy ingredients act synergistically to drain dampness, unblock and regulate the urinary pathways, and drain heat from the Bladder.

The Spleen has an aversion to dampness, and the retention of fluids inhibits the Spleen qi's ability to transform and transport fluids. Atractylodis macrocephalae Rhizoma (*bái zhú*), one of the assistants, strengthens the Spleen qi, thereby aiding in the transformation and transportation of fluids, and thus the resolution of dampness. Cinnamomi Ramulus (*guì zhī*) serves as both an assistant and envoy ingredient in this formula. When the retention of dampness impedes the circulation of fluids, the Kidneys and Bladder may be unable to transform them. Cinnamomi Ramulus (*guì zhī*) is therefore used to warm the fire at the gate of vitality, which is like adding firewood under the cauldron. Not only does this assist the Bladder in transforming and discharging urine, it also helps the Spleen qi to raise the clear, thus facilitating the movement and 'steaming' of the fluids by the Kidney yang. In this respect, it serves as an envoy to the Kidneys and Bladder. As an assistant, it also helps to dispel pathogenic influences from the exterior and thereby release the exterior aspects of the greater yang-warp disorder.

Within the formula, certain ingredients work in pairs to reinforce particular actions. Poria (*fú líng*) and Polyporus (*zhū líng*) promote urination; Poria (*fú líng*) and Atractylodis macrocephalae Rhizoma (*bái zhú*) strengthen the Spleen and promote urination; and Cinnamomi Ramulus (*guì zhī*) and Poria (*fú líng*) warm and transform the water and fluids, unblock the yang, and promote urination.

Cautions and Contraindications

In patients with Spleen or Kidney qi deficiency, the dosage and duration of use of this formula must be carefully limited. Symptoms of overdose may include dizziness, vertigo, a bland taste, and reduced appetite. In cases with deficiency, this formula is often combined with others that tonify and nourish the Spleen and Stomach to prevent injury to the normal qi. In cases of urinary difficulty with yin deficiency, it should be modified to protect the yin from further injury. It is not indicated for thirst due to heat excess or from yin deficiency.

Commentary

The primary mechanism common to all of the conditions for which this formula is indicated is the severe accumulation of water in the greater yang warp and the inability of the qi to transform fluids, manifested as urinary difficulty or edema. Another way to put this is that the balance between fluids (water, yin) and qi (fire, yang) has been shifted toward the former. This can occur as a result of invasion of pathogenic wind-cold into the exterior where it fetters the yang qi. It may also reflect a more chronic disorder of qi transformation caused by the interaction of a person's constitution, lifestyle, emotional state, and environmental factors. From an organ perspective, such problems are centered on the Bladder because it is the Bladder from which 'qi transformation issues.' Qi transformation here refers to the process by which the fire at the gate of vitality permeates the body fluids, steaming the clear portion upward and outward to moisten the entire body, while expelling the turbid portion from the body through the urine. If yang and yin no longer interact, water accumulates below and fails to order the yang, which turns into rebellious qi. Because water excess is the root of this pattern, the most effective strategy for restoring a physiological balance between yin and yang is to drain excess fluids (water) through the urine. Yet, at the same time, fire must be tonified in order to guide the yang once more toward the transformation of yin and thereby control the rebelliousness.

Expanded Usage

This formula may therefore be used in treating other problems than those described above. Because it enhances the transformation and transportation of fluids, it can be utilized when the Small Intestine fails in its task of separating the clear from the turbid. It is also useful in treating damp painful obstruction, which is characterized by a sensation of heaviness in the extremities and urinary difficulty. Where an accumulation of fluids known as 'pathogenic water' (水邪 *shuǐ xié*) invades the Lungs and causes coughing and wheezing, the use of this formula will promote urination and thereby eliminate the water and relieve the coughing and wheezing. In each case, the pattern will be characterized by the simultaneous occurrence of

thirst despite fluid intake, reduced urinary output, a floating pulse, a thin, white, and wet tongue coating, and signs of heat or rebelliousness. In *Annotated Fine Formulas from Generations of Famous Physicians*, the modern physician Ran Xue-Feng cogently sums up the nature of this pattern and the character of the formula:

> If one examines this formula, [one notes that] by transforming the qi and moving the water, it stimulates the transformative [functions of the qi] dynamic in a divine fashion. Its extraordinary effectiveness is on a par with that of Cinnamon Twig Decoction (*guì zhī tāng*). ... Qi transforms water and water transforms qi in a continuous transformative dynamic. In case of cold damage [disorders] the qi dynamic becomes constrained and stagnates, and if it does not transform into fire, it will transform into [pathological] water. Water and fire contend with each other. When this happens, the sheen of qi does not moisten and there cannot but be irritability and thirst. In case of the miscellaneous disorders from thin mucus or water qi, there is obstruction from pathogenic water. Where the water does not reach, the qi does not reach; where the qi does not reach, water does not reach. If they rebel to the lower [burner], there are pulsations below the umbilicus. If they rebel to the middle [burner], there is spitting up of frothy saliva. If they rebel to the upper [burner], there is vertigo. Therefore, both *Discussion of Cold Damage* and *Essentials of the Golden Cabinet* employ this formula.

The contemporary physician Nie Hui-Min concisely describes the connections at the base of this formula's broad utility:

> Facilitating the functions of the Bladder facilitates the Triple Burner; facilitating the Triple Burner facilitates the Lung qi. One can see that Five-Ingredient Powder with Poria (*wǔ líng sǎn*) is able to facilitate urination and unblock the water pathways and therefore it can be used for anyone with urinary dysfunction due to internal [stoppage of] water qi. Even when there are no signs of an exterior pattern, it can still be used.

To summarize, the following four pointers are key to the successful use of this formula in the clinic:

1. The presence of excess water and fluids manifesting as outright edema or as thin, watery mucus, a swollen tongue body with slippery tongue coating, reduced urination relative to the intake of fluids, dizziness, etc.

2. Up-rushing of qi that is usually only subjectively experienced by the patient and that can also lead to symptoms such as sensations of fullness or obstruction in the chest, throat, or abdomen. In severe cases, there may be actual pain including headache, or coughing and wheezing. This can also be reflected in a superficial and large pulse.

3. A sensation of heaviness or fuzziness in the head indicating that the turbid is not descending and being eliminated from the lower burner.

4. Up-flushing of heat into the face and upper body due to yang qi separating from yin water. The 'flushing' nature of this heat distinguishes this symptom from the floating

yang of yang deficiency disorders, which tends to be continuous in nature and is also accompanied by signs and symptoms of true cold.

Chief Ingredient

There has been much debate among commentators regarding the identity of the chief ingredient. Given the inclusion of the term 苓 *líng* in the formula's name, the Jin-dynasty scholar Cheng Wu-Ji, the first extant commentator on the *Discussion of Cold Damage,* believed this to be Poria (*fú líng*). Cheng explains his reasoning in *Discussion Illuminating the Principles of Cold Damage*: "[The word] 苓 *líng* implies causation (令 *lìng*) in the sense of issuing a command (號令 *hào lìng*). Unblocking and moving the body fluids and curtailing Kidney pathogens depends on issuing a special command, which is the effect of *[fú líng]*."

In *Selected Annotations to Ancient Formulas from the Garden of Crimson Snow,* the Qing-dynasty writer Wang Zi-Jie supplied a different interpretation of the same term to support his claim that Poria (*fú líng*) and Polyporus (*zhū líng*) jointly fulfill the function of chief herb: "*Líng* 苓 refers to deputy herbs [because they are subjects of a ruler]. But because Poria (*fú líng*) and Polyporus (*zhū líng*) mutually accentuate each other, they can function as chiefs among the five [herbs of which this formula is composed]. Hence, it is called Five *Líng* [Powder]."

The analysis above follows those physicians who accord the position of chief ingredient to Alismatis Rhizoma (*zé xiè*), partly because of its larger dosage, and partly because of its special function. The contemporary physician Ran Xue-Feng outlines this argument in *Annotated Fine Formulas from Generations of Famous Physicians*:

> The composer of this formula only used Alismatis Rhizoma (*zé xiè*) in a large dosage. The [functions of] Alismatis Rhizoma (*zé xiè*) do not exhaust themselves in making the water that has form and substance move downward [into the lower burner]. It also is able to make the water qi that does not move [because it is constrained in the lower burner] ascend to enrich [the upper burner]. Therefore, [in Chinese, the herb is] is called 'moistening' (澤 *zé*) and 'draining' (瀉 *xiè*). Although this is clearly so, most people only know that it drains but do not know that it also moistens. Yet this supplies a somewhat more specific understanding of [why one would] use Alismatis Rhizoma (*zé xiè*) in a larger dosage.

Yet another group of commentators, among them the Qing-dynasty writers Shen Jin-Ao and Shen Shi-Fu, suggest that Cinnamomi Ramulus (*guì zhī*) has the most important functions in the formula, that is, warming the yang to transform water in the interior and mobilizing the protective qi in the exterior to dispel pathogenic wind-cold. Chen Chao-Zu, a contemporary expert on formulas, broadly agrees with this view, arguing that function rather than dosage is the criterion according to which the importance of any individual herb in a formula should be evaluated. From this perspective, Cinnamomi Ramulus (*guì zhī*) is the only herb that addresses both the relative deficiency of yang (by warming and dispersing fire) and the relative excess of yin (by promoting the movement and transformation of water) at the heart of all the various patterns treated by this formula. In *Treatment Strategies and Formulas in Chinese Medicine,* Chen Chao-Zu also advises, however, against placing too much emphasis on assigning herbs into categories rather than on understanding their interactions:

> A complex formula is often composed of three types of herbs: those that eliminate the cause of the disorder, those that regulate the function of the yin and yang organs, and those that circulate and unblock or tonify and refill the qi, blood, body fluids, and essence. Among different herbs, each has its [specific] uses and its synergies with others. In going back to the source [of the efficacy of a formula,] it is therefore unnecessary to order them according to their relative values.

Type of Cinnamon

Another issue among commentators has been the question of whether Cinnamomi Cortex (*ròu guì*) should be substituted for Cinnamomi Ramulus (*guì zhī*). The chief proponent of this view was the influential Qing-dynasty scholar Wang Ang. Others, like Lu Yuan-Lei, the famous modernizer of the Republican era, instead insisted on the use of Cinnamomi Ramulus (*guì zhī*) in Zhang Zhong-Jing's original formula. Still others, like the Qing-dynasty physician Zhang Lu, believed that both could be used according to context. The 19th-century physician Fei Bo-Xiong offered an insightful compromise. He argued that if the formula is used to treat the pattern for which it was originally conceived (i.e., one where the qi dynamic in both the exterior and interior is obstructed), then Cinnamomi Ramulus (*guì zhī*) must be used. If, on the other hand, one uses the formula to treat interior disorders like cold-dampness, a use to which it was put by later generations of physicians, then Cinnamomi Cortex (*ròu guì*) is more appropriate.

Buildups

Both water and blood buildup (蓄血 *xù xuè*) can be traced back to concepts from the *Discussion of Cold Damage.* They are caused by pathogenic influences entering the greater yang organ, the Bladder. Water buildup occurs when the pathogenic influence enters the qi level of the Bladder and prevents the qi from carrying out its transforming function. This leads to urinary difficulty with either normal bowel movements or diarrhea. However, when the pathogenic influence enters the blood level of the Bladder, it obstructs the lower burner and causes incontinence of urine, dark stool, and acute lower abdominal pain. At this level, Peach Pit Decoction to Order the Qi (*táo hé chéng qì tāng*) is indicated (see Chapter 13).

Biomedical Indications

With the appropriate presentation, this formula may be used to treat a wide variety of biomedically-defined disorders. These can be divided into the following groups:

- Urogenital disorders such as glomerulonephritis, pyelonephritis, nephrotic syndrome, early-stage renal insufficiency, cystitis, hydrocele, and benign prostatic hypertrophy
- Disorders affecting the head and neck such as migraine, trigeminal neuralgia, headache from increased intracranial pressure, motion sickness, and Ménière's disease
- Digestive system disorders such as infectious hepatitis, gastrectasis, acute gastroenteritis, acute enteritis, and infantile indigestion
- Disorders involving increased fluid accumulation such as ascites, congestive heart failure, pericardial and pleural effusions, hydrocephalus, and polyhydramnios
- EENT disorders such as central serous retinopathy, glaucoma, catarrhal conjunctivitis, otitis media, allergic rhinitis, aphthous ulcers, and diffuse polyps of the vocal cords
- Dermatological disorders such as flat warts, urticaria, alopecia areata, eczema, and herpes zoster.

This formula has also been used for treating renal hypertension, gestational hypertension, premenstrual syndrome, epilepsy, pertussis, erectile dysfunction, and obesity as well as a wide variety of other disorders.

Comparisons

➤ Vs. WHITE TIGER DECOCTION (*bái hǔ tāng*)

Both of these formulas treat patterns characterized by irritability and thirst. In patterns treated by Five-Ingredient Powder with Poria (*wǔ líng sǎn*), although the patient is thirsty, they either do not want to drink or will vomit what has been drunk. In patterns for which White Tiger Decoction (*bái hǔ tāng*) is indicated, on the other hand, the thirst is intense, even unquenchable, and will usually be for cold beverages.

➤ Vs. MINOR BLUEGREEN DRAGON DECOCTION (*xiǎo qīng lóng tāng*); *see* PAGE 23

➤ Vs. DREDGING AND CUTTING DRINK (*shū záo yǐn zi*); *see* PAGE 96

➤ Vs. POLYPORUS DECOCTION (*zhū líng tāng*); *see* PAGE 731

➤ Vs. FIVE-PEEL POWDER (*wǔ pí sǎn*); *see* PAGE 734

➤ Vs. PORIA, CINNAMON TWIG, ATRACTYLODES, AND LICORICE DECOCTION (*líng guì zhú gān tāng*); *see* PAGE 741

Alternate names

Polyporus Powder (*zhū líng sǎn*) in *Formulas from Benevolent Sages Compiled during the Taiping Era*; Five-Ingredient Decoction with Poria (*wǔ líng tāng*) in *Formulas from the Discussion Illuminating the Yellow Emperor's Basic Questions*; Unprocessed Five-Ingredient Powder with Poria (*shēng liào wǔ líng sǎn*) in *Straight Directions from [Yang] Ren-Zhai*; Five-Ingredient Drink with Poria (*wǔ líng yǐn zi*) in *Effective Medical Formulas Arranged by Category by Master Zhu*

Modifications

- For severe edema, add Mori Cortex (*sāng bái pí*), Citri reticulatae Pericarpium (*chén pí*), and Arecae Pericarpium (*dà fù pí*).
- For cold-damp painful obstruction accompanied by thirst and urinary difficulty, add Notopterygii Rhizoma seu Radix (*qiāng huó*).
- For painful wind obstruction contracted during the summer, add Clematidis Radix (*wēi líng xiān*), Saposhnikoviae Radix (*fáng fēng*), *fáng jǐ* (Stephaniae/Cocculi/etc. Radix), Asari Radix et Rhizoma (*xì xīn*), Chaenomelis Fructus (*mù guā*), Coicis Semen (*yì yǐ rén*), and Xanthii Fructus (*cāng ěr zǐ*).
- For concurrent fever, remove Cinnamomi Ramulus (*guì zhī*) and add Scutellariae Radix (*huáng qín*).
- For damp-heat diarrhea, remove Atractylodis macrocephalae Rhizoma (*bái zhú*) and Cinnamomi Ramulus (*guì zhī*) and add Artemisiae scopariae Herba (*yīn chén*) and Lonicerae Flos (*jīn yín huā*).
- For summerheat diarrhea or sudden turmoil disorder, add Talcum (*huá shí*).
- For lurking summerheat with whole body fever and thirst, take with White Tiger Decoction (*bái hǔ tāng*).
- For both exterior signs and edema, take with Maidservant from Yue's Decoction (*yuè bì tāng*).
- For concurrent edema and qi obstruction due to excessive water retention, take with Five-Peel Drink (*wǔ pí yǐn*).

Variations

四苓散

Four-Ingredient Powder with Poria

sì líng sǎn

SOURCE *Displays of Enlightened Physicians* (Ming dynasty)

Remove Cinnamomi Ramulus (*guì zhī*) for uncomplicated cases of dampness due to Spleen deficiency leading to dampness in the Bladder. This is characterized by loose stools and urinary difficulty.

胃苓湯（胃苓汤）

Calm the Stomach and Poria Decoction

wèi líng tāng

SOURCE *Essential Teachings of [Zhu] Dan-Xi* (1481)

Combine with Calm the Stomach Powder (*píng wèi sǎn*) for the treatment of the following four patterns: (1) watery diarrhea with stools that resemble water and are evacuated frequently; (2) edema that is more pronounced in the lower extremities; (3) dampness obstructing the middle burner characterized by focal distention in the epigastrium and abdomen, reduced appetite, and semi-liquid stools; and (4) dampness obstructing the body's exterior characterized by heaviness of the extremities. These patterns are caused by cold-dampness encumbering the Spleen and the accumulation of fluids. They are usually accompanied by a pale tongue, white tongue coating, and relaxed pulse. The formula can be further modified to address more precisely the cause of the dampness.

茵陳五苓散 (茵陈五苓散)

Virgate Wormwood and Five-Ingredient Powder with Poria

yīn chén wǔ líng sǎn

SOURCE *Essentials from the Golden Cabinet* (c. 220)

Combine two parts powdered Artemisiae scopariae Herba (*yīn chén*) with one part of this formula for jaundice due to damp-heat (dampness predominant) with urinary difficulty and a slightly pale skin tone.

Associated Formulas

茯苓甘草湯 (茯苓甘草汤)

Poria and Licorice Decoction

fú líng gān cǎo tāng

SOURCE *Discussion of Cold Damage* (c. 220)

Poria (*fú líng*) 6g
Cinnamomi Ramulus (*guì zhī*) 6g
Glycyrrhizae Radix praeparata (*zhì gān cǎo*) 3g
Zingiberis Rhizoma recens (*shēng jiāng*) 9g

Warms the yang, transforms thin mucus, unblocks the yang, and disperses pathogenic water. For pathogenic water stopping in the epigastrium in a patient with deficiency of the Spleen and Stomach. Manifestations include epigastric palpitations, cold extremities, no particular thirst, a slippery and white tongue coating, and a wiry pulse. While the principal formula treats water buildup in the lower burner accompanied by thirst and urinary difficulty, this formula is for water buildup in the middle burner accompanied by palpitations.

春澤湯 (春泽汤)

Spring Marsh Decoction

chūn zé tāng

SOURCE *Prescriptions of Universal Benefit* (early 15th century)

Alismatis Rhizoma (*zé xiè*) 9g
Polyporus (*zhū líng*) 6g
Poria (*fú líng*) 6g
Atractylodis macrocephalae Rhizoma (*bái zhú*) 6g
Cinnamomi Ramulus (*guì zhī*) 3g
Ginseng Radix (*rén shēn*) 4.5g
Bupleuri Radix (*chái hú*) 3g
Ophiopogonis Radix (*mài mén dōng*) 4.5g

Augments the qi, promotes urination, and releases lingering summerheat. For lingering summerheat characterized by fever, irritability, thirst, and urinary difficulty. At present, Codonopsis Radix (*dǎng shēn*) is substituted for Ginseng Radix (*rén shēn*) with 2-3 times its dosage.

豬苓湯 (猪苓汤)

Polyporus Decoction

zhū líng tāng

The name of this formula is explained by Wang Zie-Jie in *Selected Annotations to Ancient Formulas from the Garden of Crimson Snow*: "All five [ingredients in this formula] are herbs that promote urination. To symbolize this characteristic, it is named after [the herb] that most strongly promotes [urination]. Hence, it is called Polyporus Decoction (*zhū líng tāng*)."

SOURCE *Discussion of Cold Damage* (c. 220)

Polyporus (*zhū líng*) 3g
Poria (*fú líng*) 3g
Alismatis Rhizoma (*zé xiè*) 3g
Talcum (*huá shí*) 3g
Asini Corii Colla (*ē jiāo*) 3g

Method of Preparation Prepare the first four ingredients as a decoction and dissolve one-half of Asini Corii Colla (*ē jiāo*) into the strained liquid. At present, 2-3 times the original dosage is generally used.

Actions Promotes urination, clears heat, and nourishes the yin

Indications

Urinary difficulty accompanied by fever and thirst with a desire to drink. There may also be diarrhea, cough, nausea, irritability, or insomnia.

According to the source text, this is injury from cold entering the yang brightness or lesser yin warp where it transforms into heat. The heat battles with the water (controlled by the Kidneys, the organ corresponding to the leg lesser yin channel), which leads to clumping of water and heat. Heat also injures the yin (fluids) and disturbs the water pathways, resulting in urinary difficulty. It is also common for this pattern to develop in patients with constitutional yin deficiency and invasion of heat in the lower burner.

Heat gives rise to fever. Obstruction of the qi transformation in the lower burner means that the fluids are not spread throughout the body. Complicated by injury to the fluids, the result is thirst with a desire to drink (in contrast to thirst without a desire to drink, which is characteristic of damp-heat). When fluids cannot be eliminated through the urine, they filter out into the Large Intestine, resulting in diarrhea. If the disturbance to the water pathways affects the flow of qi in the Lungs, there will be coughing. If the disturbance affects the middle burner, there will be nausea. Vigorous heat due to yin deficiency agitates the Heart and leads to irritability and insomnia.

Analysis of Formula

In a pattern dominated by clumping of water and heat, the treatment must focus on promoting urination, while also clearing the heat and nourishing the yin. Polyporus (*zhū* líng), the chief ingredient, strongly reinforces the proper functioning of the water pathways and thereby promotes urination. Poria (fú líng), a deputy, promotes urination, benefits the Spleen, and harmonizes the Stomach. The second deputy, Alismatis Rhizoma (zé xiè), promotes water metabolism, unblocks the deep parts of the water pathways that involve the Kidneys, and aids the chief ingredients in promoting urination. These three herbs aid one another, reinforcing their ability to unblock the waterways, eliminate water dampness, and clear heat. As explained in *Records of Thoughtful Differentiation of Materia Medica*:

> Poria (fú líng), Polyporus (zhū líng), and Alismatis Rhizoma (zé xiè) are all bland, percolating substances. Their use lies entirely in promoting urination. … That these three substances promote urination [also] has the ingenious [effect of promoting] transportation and draining [throughout] the entire qi [dynamic]. If the three substances are not used together in patterns [characterized] by clumping of heat and water—such as those [treated by] Five-Ingredient Powder with Poria (wǔ líng sǎn) and Polyporus Decoction (zhū líng tāng)—the water may not necessarily be eliminated. If water is not eliminated, heat will not be gotten rid of. If heat is not gotten rid off, thirst does not cease, and urination remains obstructed. Thus, in one stroke, they achieve all these effects.

The assistant, Talcum (huá shí), clears heat and unblocks painful urinary dribbling. The combination of these four ingredients clears heat and promotes flow in the water pathways, and is therefore very effective in resolving the clumping of water and heat. Asini Corii Colla (ē jiāo) is a moist substance that enriches the yin (without causing retention of the pathogenic influences) and prevents excessive urination and thus further injury to the yin.

Contraindications

This formula is contraindicated in patients with abundant heat and severely damaged yin fluids because its diuretic power will further aggravate the yin deficiency. This was pointed out as early as *Discussion of Cold Damage* (paragraph 224): "When there is copious sweating and thirst in a yang brightness disorder, one cannot give Polyporus Decoction (zhū líng tāng) because, with copious sweating, the Stomach is dry and Polyporus Decoction (zhū líng tāng) promotes urination."

This formula is also contraindicated in cases with pronounced dampness because Asini Corii Colla (ē jiāo) will aggravate this pathogen.

Commentary

What is special about this formula is its ability to promote urination without injuring the yin, and to stabilize the yin without causing the retention of pathogenic influences. In large part, this is due to the use of Asini Corii Colla (ē jiāo), which is better able to maintain this delicate balance than such substances as Rehmanniae Radix praeparata (shú dì huáng). Unlike those other herbs, Asini Corii Colla (ē jiāo)

not only tonifies the yin and nourishes the blood, it also stops bleeding and moistens the Lungs. The latter is due to its gelatinous nature and also the fact that it is prepared from a hide, which corresponds to the Lungs' governance of the skin. According to some physicians, this gives Asini Corii Colla (ē jiāo) a slippery quality like that of Talcum (huá shí) and thus the ability to promote urination without damaging the yin.

Although this formula tonifies the yin, its main focus is on promoting urination, unblocking the waterways, and clearing heat, that is, on treating excess. The lower abdomen may thus be tense or tender to pressure, a sign that is absent in yin deficiency. Another telling sign of this pattern is a red tongue, which indicates stagnation, with a coating that may be white or absent depending on the patient's constitution. The contemporary physician and teacher Cheng Men-Xue describes this tongue:

> [The tongue body will be] red like paper stained with menstrual flow. It is a dark, dull, dry red. This is very different from the shiny, fresh red [tongue that indicates] heat exuberance. One must distinguish these [two types] in the clinic. Whenever one observes such a tongue accompanied by reduced urination, especially if there is also Heart irritability and insomnia, one can unhesitatingly prescribe [this formula knowing that it] will fit [the pattern].

Given this particular combination of excess and deficiency, the use of this formula was extended by the late-Qing-dynasty physician Tang Zong-Hai to the treatment of phlegm in yin deficient patients. Tang explained his reasoning in *Discussion of Blood Patterns*:

> This formula is specific for enriching the yin and promoting urination. It is effective in all cases of Kidney channel yin deficiency with water flooding that becomes phlegm. It employs Asini Corii Colla (ē jiāo) to moisten dryness and Talcum (huá shí) to clear heat. Combining these enriching and downward-directing substances with all the other herbs [in the formula] accounts for its efficacy in eliminating phlegm. The root of phlegm is in the Kidneys. One controls the Lungs to treat its manifestations. One treats the Kidneys to treat its root.

This formula is also used to treat hot or bloody painful urinary dribbling with lower abdominal fullness and pain. Recently, its use has been further extended to the treatment of diarrhea in infants caused by damp-heat and injury to the yin characterized by reduced urination, dry skin, sunken eyes, and fever that worsens at night.

Clinical Pointers

Given the wide spectrum of potential applications, the key clinical markers for this formula can be summarized as follows:

1. Reduced urination is more a matter of reduced frequency, urinary difficulty, or incomplete voiding. The amount of urine itself is less significant of an indicator.

2. Signs of water excess such as edema, fullness, and resistance to pressure in the lower abdomen, diarrhea, and a white (but dry) tongue coating. Because the edema results from clumping of heat and water in the lower burner rather than from excess water flooding the body, it generally does not affect the respiratory system.

3. Signs that heat has damaged the yin, such as a darkish red tongue, insomnia, and irritability.

Comparisons

➤ Vs. Five-Ingredient Powder with Poria (*wǔ líng sǎn*)

Both formulas treat urinary difficulty due to disturbances of the water pathways by promoting urination. Both formulas contain Poria (*fú líng*), Polyporus (*zhū líng*), and Alismatis Rhizoma (*zé xiè*). The difference is that Five-Ingredient Powder with Poria (*wǔ líng sǎn*) treats a condition where the disease is still active in the exterior by focusing on unblocking the flow of yang to encourage the transformation of qi, while Polyporus Decoction (*zhū líng tāng*) treats pathogenic influences that have transformed into heat in the interior by clearing the heat and nourishing the yin. This difference was succinctly described by Wang Ang in *Medical Formulas Collected and Analyzed*: "Five-Ingredient Powder with Poria (*wǔ líng sǎn*) drains vigorous dampness, hence the use of Cinnamomi Ramulus (*guì zhī*) and Atractylodis macrocephalae Rhizoma (*bái zhú*); Polyporus Decoction (*zhū líng tāng*) drains vigorous heat, hence the use of Talcum (*huá shí*)."

➤ Vs. Coptis and Ass-Hide Gelatin Decoction (*huáng lián ē jiāo tāng*)

Both of these formulas treat patterns characterized by irritability and insomnia due to heat damaging the yin and use Asini Corii Colla (*ē jiāo*) to address this deficiency. However, Coptis and Ass-Hide Gelatin Decoction (*huáng lián ē jiā tāng*) focuses on patterns where both the pathogenic heat and the yin deficiency are relatively pronounced with such symptoms as focal distention in the epigastrium, abdominal pain, irritability and thirst, and palpitations. Polyporus Decoction (*zhū líng tāng*), on the other hand, treats patterns where the momentum of the heat and damage to the yin are less severe, but instead clump with the water in the lower burner leading to the main symptom of obstructed urination.

Biomedical Indications

With the appropriate presentation, this formula may be used to treat a wide variety of biomedically-defined disorders. These can be divided into the following groups:

- Urinary disorders such as cystitis, urethritis, gonorrhea, pyelonephritis, glomerulonephritis, renal calculus, and benign prostatic hypertrophy
- Hemorrhages such as dysfunctional uterine bleeding, he-

maturia, thrombocytopenic purpura, and bleeding secondary to cirrhosis.

This formula has also been used for treating cardiogenic edema, chronic gastritis, epilepsy, insomnia, perimenopausal syndrome, uclerative colitis, ascites, eczema, and upper respiratory infections.

Alternate name

Polyporus Powder (*zhū líng sǎn*) in *Formulas from Benevolent Sages Compiled during the Taiping Era*

Modifications

- For severe thirst from yin deficiency, add Glehniae/Adenophorae Radix (*shā shēn*) and Trichosanthis Radix (*tiān huā fěn*).
- For bloody painful urinary dribbling, add Imperatae Rhizoma (*bái máo gēn*), Dianthi Herba (*qú mài*), and Cirsii Herba (*xiǎo jì*).
- For hot painful urinary dribbling, add Gardeniae Fructus (*zhī zǐ*) and Polygoni avicularis Herba (*biān xù*).

Variation

沈氏豬苓湯 (沈氏猪苓汤)

Polyporus Decoction from Master Shen

Shěn shì zhū líng tāng

SOURCE *Shen's Book for Revering Life* (1773)

Remove Asini Corii Colla (*ē jiāo*) and add Cimicifugae Rhizoma (*shēng má*) for severe diarrhea with urinary difficulty.

Associated Formulas

豬苓湯 (猪苓汤)

Polyporus Decoction from *Comprehensive Recording*

zhū líng tāng

SOURCE *Comprehensive Recording of Sagely Beneficence from the Zhenghe Era* (1117)

Polyporus (*zhū líng*)	30g
Mori Cortex (*sāng bái pí*)	30g
Akebiae Caulis (*mù tōng*)	30g

Grind the ingredients into a powder and take in 9g doses as a draft before meals with 2-3g of Junci Medulla (*dēng xīn cǎo*). Drains and leaches out lower burner dampness. For urinary obstruction with pain and rigidity in the area below the umbilicus.

五苓通關湯 (五苓通关汤)

Five-Ingredients with Poria Decoction to Open the Gate

wǔ líng tōng guān tāng

SOURCE *Case Histories of Cheng Men-Xue* (2002)

Cinnamomi Cortex (*ròu guì*) 0.9g
Anemarrhenae Rhizoma (*zhī mǔ*) 6g
Phellodendri Cortex (*huáng bǎi*) 3g
Polyporus (*zhū líng*) 9g
Poria (*fú líng*) 9g
Alismatis Rhizoma (*zé xiè*) 6g
Talcum (*huá shí*) 13g
Polygoni avicularis Herba (*biǎn xù*) 4.5g

Decoction. Clears heat, promotes the resolution of dampness, unblocks the qi dynamic, and facilitates the dissemination of qi. For hot painful urinary dribbling disorder characterized by reduced urination, difficulty in starting urination, and discomfort in the lower abdomen.

當歸貝母苦參丸 （当归贝母苦参丸）

Tangkuei, Fritillaria, and Sophora Decoction

dāng guī bèi mǔ kǔ shēn wán

SOURCE　*Essentials from the Golden Cabinet* (c. 220)

Angelicae sinensis Radix (*dāng guī*) 12g
Fritillariae Bulbus (*bèi mǔ*) 12g
Sophorae flavescentis Radix (*kǔ shēn*) 12g

The source text recommends grinding the ingredients into a powder and forming into pills the size of an aduki bean with honey. Take 3 pills with water, increasing the dosage up to 10 pills if necessary. Can also be prepared as a decoction with the dosage increased by up to 30g for each ingredient and adding an equal amount of honey to the strained liquid. Drains heat, promotes the resolution of dampness, opens constraint, and nourishes the blood. For patterns characterized by damp-heat pouring into the lower burner accompanied by qi constraint and blood deficiency manifesting as painful urinary dysfunction, urinary difficulty, dark yellow or reddish urine, irritability, a stuffy sensation in the chest, and normal digestion. The tongue coating will tend to be yellow, and the pulse thin, slippery, and rapid.

The original indication of this formula is for urinary difficulty during pregnancy in women whose appetite is normal. However, the text also suggests that the formula can be used to treat men by adding 15g of Talcum (*huá shí*). The formula has been used not only for pregnant women, but for those of both sexes with painful urinary dysfunction. Based on an analysis of the formula's constituents, it will be most appropriate in blood deficient patients who tend toward dryness and thus toward constraint. Angelicae sinensis Radix (*dāng guī*) tonifies the blood and moistens the skin and membranes, while Fritillariae Bulbus (*bèi mǔ*) opens constraint and clears heat; they are widely used when heat or dryness has damaged the mucous membranes. Although Fritillariae Bulbus (*bèi mǔ*) is generally used to treat Lung disorders, the *Divine Husbandman's Classic of the Materia Medica* recommends it for "painful urinary dysfunction [from] pestilential and pathogenic qi." The Lungs, moreover, play an important role in promoting water metabolism, making the choice of this herb less odd than may first appear. Nevertheless, some physicians such as the modern scholar Qin Bo-Wei argued that "difficult urination" in the source text must have been a transcription error and that the correct term should have been "difficult stools." Qin supported his argument with evidence from other

physicians who reported that taking this formula as a decoction can cause the stools to become loose. However, there is little concrete historical evidence that would support Qin's claims. Furthermore, as some physicians point out, the action of decocted Fritillariae Bulbus (*bèi mǔ*) will be different than taking it as a powder made into pills.

The heat-clearing and moistening action of Fritillariae Bulbus (*bèi mǔ*) on the Lungs has inspired some physicians to extend the indications of this formula to the treatment of chronic coughing in yin deficient patients with Lung heat. This accords with the ancient usage of Angelicae sinensis Radix (*dāng guī*) as an herb for coughing, discussed in Chapter 12 in the COMMENTARY to Perilla Fruit Decoction for Directing Qi Downward (*sū zǐ jiàng qì tāng*). Tangkuei, Fritillaria, and Sophora Decoction (*dāng guī bèi mǔ kǔ shēn wán*) is also used today for a wide variety of disorders characterized by inflammation of the mucous membranes and skin that is frequently accompanied by yellow, turbid, or sticky discharges.

This formula and the principal formula are indicated for similar presentations. However, Angelicae sinensis Radix (*dāng guī*) is a much warmer herb than Asini Corii Colla (*ē jiāo*), suggesting that the blood deficiency here is more chronic and constitutional; in other words, that it is this deficiency that predisposes the patient to constraint and secondary inflammation. In a Polyporus Decoction (*zhū líng tāng*) pattern, on the other hand, excess water and heat clump together implying that dryness and yin deficiency are accompanied by signs of actual water excess.

五皮散

Five-Peel Powder

wǔ pí sǎn

This formula is a powder made from the peel or rind of various plants. In Chinese, the term for 'peel' (皮 *pí*) can also mean 'skin.' The formula treats skin edema (皮水 *pí shuǐ*), which is due partly to the obstruction of Lung qi, the organ that governs the skin.

Source　*Treasury Classic* (c. 4th century)

Mori Cortex (*sāng bái pí*) 15g
Zingiberis Rhizomatis Cortex (*shēng jiāng pí*) 6g
Poriae Cutis (*fú líng pí*) 15g
Citri reticulatae Pericarpium (*chén pí*) .9g
Arecae Pericarpium (*dà fù pí*) 15g

Method of Preparation　Grind equal amounts of the ingredients into a coarse powder and take 6-9g as a draft. May also be prepared as a decoction with the dosage specified.

Actions　Resolves dampness, reduces edema, regulates the qi, and strengthens the Spleen

Indications

Generalized edema with a sensation of heaviness, distention, and fullness in the epigastrium and abdomen, labored and heavy breathing, urinary difficulty, a white, greasy tongue coating, and a submerged and moderate pulse.

This is skin edema (皮水 *pí shuǐ*). The development of edema may be attributed to various pathological mechanisms: the invasion of wind disrupting the Lungs' ability to disseminate and move the qi downward; Kidney yang deficiency leading to the accumulation of fluids and dampness; Spleen deficiency with vigorous dampness and qi stagnation; or any combination of these. This formula treats a pattern characterized by vigorous dampness and qi stagnation obstructing the greater yin warp (Lungs and Spleen).

One of the primary functions of the Spleen and Lungs, the transportation of fluids, is inhibited when their qi is obstructed. This leads to internally-generated dampness that further disrupts their functions of transporting and directing downward. It prevents the proper elimination of fluids, which instead spread through the tissues and cause generalized edema. Dampness, a yin pathogen, readily obstructs the qi dynamic leading to qi stagnation and the accumulation of fluids. The generalized sensation of heaviness is indicative of dampness. Distention and fullness in the epigastrium and abdomen reflects qi stagnation in the middle burner (Spleen and Stomach). The dampness and surplus of fluids flood the upper source of the fluids (the Lungs), which causes labored and heavy breathing. The stagnation of fluids prevents the water pathways from fully opening, causing urinary difficulty. The pulse and tongue signs reflect the presence of internal dampness.

Analysis of Formula

Effective treatment of this condition requires regulating the functions of the Spleen and Lungs to prevent dampness from spreading through the tissues, and opening the water pathways to provide an exit for the surplus fluids. Mori Cortex (*sāng bái pí*) promotes urination by directing the Lung qi downward and opening up the water pathways, while Zingiberis Rhizomatis Cortex (*shēng jiāng pí*) transforms dampness and disperses edema. The dispersing and descending actions of these herbs restore the water metabolism function to the Lungs and facilitate the smooth flow of fluids into the Bladder. Poriae Cutis (*fú líng pí*) leaches out dampness, promotes urination, and strengthens the transportive function of the Spleen. If the smooth flow of qi is reestablished, the fluids will follow. Citri reticulatae Pericarpium (*chén pí*) and Arecae Pericarpium (*dà fù pí*) perform this function by eliminating qi stagnation.

Cautions and Contraindications

Although this is a relatively mild formula, Spleen-tonifying herbs should be added for cases with severe Spleen deficiency.

Commentary

The focus of this formula is on leaching out dampness and promoting urination. It is interesting to note that the peel, rind, or 'skin' of the herbs is used to treat skin edema. In tra-

ditional Chinese medicine, the peel or rind is considered to be especially effective in moving water just below the skin.

The classification (chief, deputy, assistant, and envoy) of the herbs in this formula varies depending on the commentator. For this reason, the ingredients have been presented in what appears to be the most logical order. In fact, however, these herbs interact very closely, and it serves no clinical purpose to assign a greater importance to one herb over another.

Most contemporary textbooks analyze this formula exclusively from the perspective of the Spleen's function in transporting fluids. This follows the source text, which recommends this formula for the treatment of edema due to "stagnation of Spleen and Stomach in men and women." However, this is an overly narrow interpretation, as the Lungs' downward-directing function appears to be very important in terms of both the pathodynamic and treatment strategy for this pattern. For example, in *Six Texts Summarizing the Medicine of Xu Ling-Tai*, the influential Qing-dynasty scholar-physician Xu Da-Chun noted that this edema is due to "Spleen and Lung qi stagnation." In *Outline of Medical Formulas,* Li Shou-Ren noted that the formula "is able to promote the [functions] of the Lungs and harmonize [those of the] Spleen."

In *Convenient Reader of Established Formulas,* Zhang Bing-Cheng offered a synthesis of these views by observing that Lung and Spleen pathologies arise from their interconnection via the generation cycle of the five phases:

> [This formula] treats edema and swelling disorders, rising qi with wheezing and urgent [breathing], as well as edema below the waist. All of these are due to the Lungs' [functions] of management and regulation being inhibited leading to water overflowing into the skin as well as causing all of the above symptoms. … Now, the Lungs and Spleen are organs [related to each other as] child and mother. No disorder in a child does not also wear out its mother. Therefore, the symptoms of fullness and swelling are related to Spleen excess. If this were not the case, the Spleen would be able to build and move. If earth flourishes, it naturally controls water. Hence, even if the Lungs' [functions] of management and regulation were inhibited, [the patient] definitely would not suffer from fullness and swelling.

In contemporary practice, this formula is also used to treat edema during pregnancy. For stagnation causing damp-heat, which later transforms into toxin and wind (as in eclampsia), the contemporary physician Liu Yun-Peng combines this formula with Two-Marvel Powder (*èr miào sǎn*) and herbs that resolve toxicity and disperse wind such as Forsythiae Fructus (*lián qiáo*), Lonicerae Flos (*jīn yín huā*), Siegesbeckiae Herba (*xī xiān cǎo*), and Schizonepetae Herba (*jīng jiè*).

Another indication of this formula in contemporary practice is the treatment of acute glomerulonephritis or acute flare-ups of inflammation that become chronic. For this purpose, the contemporary physician Shi Zhen-Cheng combines this formula with Ephedra Decoction (*má huáng tāng*) if aversion to wind and cold are pronounced; with Maidservant from Yue's Decoction (*yuè bì tāng*) if there is pronounced thirst or a yellow tongue coating; and with Five-Ingredient Powder with Poria (*wǔ líng sǎn*) if there is mainly edema.

Comparisons

➤ Vs. Stephania and Poria Decoction (*fáng jǐ fú líng tāng*)

Both formulas treat skin edema. Stephania and Poria Decoction (*fáng jǐ fú líng tāng*) warms and opens the yang to improve qi transformation within the greater yang warp. It is used for cases of skin edema where protective yang is deficient and where fire no longer transforms water, as reflected in fibrillations in the skin and superficial muscles. By contrast, Five-Peel Powder (*wǔ pí sǎn*) focuses on the greater yin warp and on resolving dampness and regulating the qi. It is indicated for cases where the dampness and qi stagnation are relatively strong, but the deficiency is mild.

➤ Vs. Five-Ingredient Powder with Poria (*wǔ líng sǎn*)

Both formulas treat edema characterized by reduced urination and are therefore often combined in practice. However, Five-Ingredient Powder with Poria (*wǔ líng sǎn*) focuses on water buildup in the lower burner that is associated with impairment of qi transformation in the Bladder and greater yang warp. Five-Peel Powder (*wǔ pí sǎn*), on the other hand, focuses on qi stagnation in the Lungs and Spleen, the organs associated with the greater yin warp, which leads to edema because the fluids are not properly transported.

Biomedical Indications

With the appropriate presentation, this formula may be used to treat a variety of biomedically-defined disorders including pre-eclampsia, protein-deficiency edema, ascites from cirrhosis, congestive heart failure, urticaria, and menopausal edema. For chronic glomerulonephritis, larger doses (between 30-60g) of the ingredients may be prescribed.

Alternate name

Five-Peel Drink (*wǔ pí yǐn*) in *Discussion of Illnesses, Patterns, and Formulas Related to the Unification of the Three Etiologies*

Modifications

- For externally-contracted wind with edema above the waist, add Saposhnikoviae Radix (*fáng fēng*), Perillae Folium (*zǐ sū yè*), Schizonepetae Herba (*jīng jiè*), and Angelicae dahuricae Radix (*bái zhǐ*).
- For dampness lodged in the lower burner with edema below the waist, add Stephaniae tetrandrae Radix (*hàn fáng jǐ*) and Plantaginis Semen (*chē qián zǐ*).

- For damp-heat lodged in the lower burner with edema below the waist, add Talcum (*huá shí*), Plantaginis Semen (*chē qián zǐ*), and Coicis Semen (*yì yǐ rén*).
- For internal cold-dampness, add Zingiberis Rhizoma (*gān jiāng*) and Aconiti Radix lateralis praeparata (*zhì fù zǐ*).
- For severe abdominal distention, add Raphani Semen (*lái fú zǐ*) and Magnoliae officinalis Cortex (*hòu pò*).
- For marked signs of Spleen deficiency, add Codonopsis Radix (*dǎng shēn*) and Atractylodis macrocephalae Rhizoma (*bái zhú*).
- For constipation due to accumulation in the Stomach and Intestines, add Rhei Radix et Rhizoma (*dà huáng*) and Aurantii Fructus immaturus (*zhǐ shí*).
- For edema due to pregnancy, add Maydis Stigma (*yù mǐ xū*).
- For edema, add Benincasae Exocarpium (*dōng guā pí*), Plantaginis Herba (*chē qián cǎo*), and Astragali Radix (*huáng qí*).

Variation

五皮飲 （五皮饮）

Five-Peel Drink

wǔ pí yǐn

Source　*Formulary of the Pharmacy Service for Benefiting the People in the Taiping Era* (1107)

Substitute Acanthopanacis Cortex (*wǔ jiā pí*) and Lycii Cortex (*dì gǔ pí*) for Citri reticulatae Pericarpium (*chén pí*) and Mori Cortex (*sāng bái pí*) to focus on the lower burner and nourish the Kidneys. Acanthopanacis Cortex (*wǔ jiā pí*) enters the Kidneys to move the water. Lycii Cortex (*dì gǔ pí*) clears heat from deficiency in the Lungs and Kidneys. This formula does not treat upper burner symptoms like wheezing and shortness of breath. Instead, it is indicated for patterns where edema constrains the Kidney qi and generates heat.

Associated Formula

七皮飲 （七皮饮）

Seven-Peel Drink

qī pí yǐn

Source　*Formulas to Aid the Living* (1253)

Arecae Pericarpium (*dà fù pí*) 15g
Citri reticulatae Pericarpium (*chén pí*) 15g
Poriae Cutis (*fú líng pí*) 15g
Zingiberis Rhizomatis Cortex (*shēng jiāng pí*) 15g
Citri reticulatae viride Pericarpium (*qīng pí*) 15g
Lycii Cortex (*dì gǔ pí*) 15g
Glycyrrhizae Radixcis Cortex (*gān cǎo pí*) 15g

Regulates the qi, strengthens the Spleen, resolves dampness, and reduces swelling. For skin edema with more emphasis on the treatment of abdominal distention and fullness.

防己黃耆湯（防己黄芪汤）

Stephania and Astragalus Decoction

fáng jǐ huáng qí tāng

Source *Essentials from the Golden Cabinet* (c. 220)

Astragali Radix *(huáng qí)* 3.8g (15g)
Stephaniae tetrandrae Radix *(hàn fáng jǐ)* 3g (12g)
Atractylodis macrocephalae Rhizoma *(bái zhú)* 2.3g (9g)
Glycyrrhizae Radix praeparata *(zhì gān cǎo)* 1.5g (6g)
Zingiberis Rhizoma recens *(shēng jiāng)* . . . . 4 pieces (3g)
Jujubae Fructus *(dà zǎo)* . . . . 1 piece (2 pieces)

Method of Preparation   Grind the first four ingredients into a powder and take in 1.5g doses as a draft with the last two ingredients. The measurements used to specify dosage in the source text differ from those used in other formulas in both *Discussion of Cold Damage* and *Essentials from the Golden Cabinet*. Many commentators thus believe they were mistakenly inserted by later copyists. At present, the formula is usually prepared as a decoction with the dosage specified in parentheses. While the source text lists the ingredient *fáng jǐ* (Stephaniae/Cocculi/etc. Radix), at present, only Stephaniae tetrandrae Radix *(hàn fáng jǐ)* is used in Chinese preparations.

The source text states that administration of the formula should be followed by a feeling as if bugs were crawling under the skin as well as an icy-cold sensation from the waist downward. This is interpreted to mean that the protective qi is returning and that the dampness is moving downward into the lower burner and Bladder. The patient should then sit down with a quilt covering both the body and legs in order to induce a slight sweat, which signifies that the normal qi dynamic has been restored, after which the condition will be cured.

Actions   Augments the qi, dispels wind, strengthens the Spleen, promotes urination, and reduces edema

Indications

Sweating, a heavy sensation in the body, superficial edema, urinary difficulty, a pale tongue with a white coating, and a floating pulse.

This is wind-dampness or wind edema (風水 *fēng shuǐ)* caused by deficiency in the exterior and an invasion of wind and dampness. Sweating and an aversion to wind are indicative of unstable protective qi. A heavy sensation in the body is due to dampness in the channels. Superficial edema and a floating pulse indicate that the condition is lodged in the superficial aspects of the body. When wind-dampness invades the body, it first lodges in the greater yang warp. This inhibits the qi dynamic, manifesting as urinary difficulty, which contributes to superficial edema. Exterior deficiency or unstable protective qi is generally related to Lung and Spleen qi deficiency: the Lungs, which control the qi, skin, and body hair, also control the exterior; and the Spleen is the source of movement and transformation. If the Lung qi is deficient, it is no longer able to move the fluids downward to the Bladder. Instead, they accumulate in the skin. If the Spleen qi

is deficient, dampness accumulates in the middle, inhibiting movement of the qi and exacerbating the problems noted above. The pale tongue with a white coating also reflects these deficiencies as well as the obstructive dampness.

Analysis of Formula

The terms 'dampness' and 'water' refer to the same substance in different states of aggregation. Dampness is water that has been dispersed, while water is dampness that has gathered in one place. Although the two conditions are not entirely the same—one manifesting as heaviness of the body and the other as edema—they share many symptoms and the same underlying pathology and can therefore be treated with the same formula.

When pathogenic influences are lodged in the exterior, the appropriate strategy is to release the exterior; if there is superficial edema and the exterior is not released, the edema will persist. However, when the protective qi (which circulates in the exterior) is unstable and not contained, it must also be stabilized. This twin strategy is the focus of the formula. Astragali Radix *(huáng qí)*, one of the chief herbs, is the principal substance in the materia medica for stabilizing the protective qi in cases of deficiency. The other chief herb, acrid, bitter Stephaniae tetrandrae Radix *(hàn fáng jǐ)*, releases the exterior, unblocks the channels, promotes urination, expels dampness, and relieves pain. By combining these herbs, their functions of tonifying the qi and promoting urination are reinforced, and the edema is alleviated without injuring the normal qi. The deputy, Atractylodis macrocephalae Rhizoma *(bái zhú)*, strengthens the Spleen and resolves dampness; it assists Astragali Radix *(huáng qí)* in stabilizing the exterior (protective qi), and Stephaniae tetrandrae Radix *(hàn fáng jǐ)* in resolving the dampness. The assistant, Glycyrrhizae Radix praeparata *(zhì gān cǎo)*, helps tonify the Spleen. The combination of Zingiberis Rhizoma recens *(shēng jiāng)* and Jujubae Fructus *(dà zǎo)*, the envoys in this formula, regulates and harmonizes the nutritive and protective qi to assist in the stabilization of the exterior and the strengthening of the qi and blood.

Cautions and Contraindications

This formula is contraindicated for excess-type edema manifesting as nausea, abdominal distention, loose stools, or other Stomach and Intestinal symptoms. It should also not be used in cases of water dampness constraining the protective yang in the exterior, characterized by an absence of sweating, even though the pulse is also superficial and the patient has an aversion to wind.

Administration of the formula should lead only to slight sweating. A strong sweat would not only be ineffective in removing dampness (a yin pathogen), it would also further weaken the yang qi in the exterior. Thus, the source text states that "it is best to readminister the formula after a lengthy [interval]."

Commentary

This formula exemplifies the simultaneous treatment of manifestation (wind-dampness or wind-edema) and root (exterior deficiency). The cardinal signs and symptoms of wind-dampness at this level and in this type of patient are the same as those for wind edema: floating pulse, heavy sensation in the body, sweating, and frequently an aversion to wind. A commonly-used formula, its application has been expanded to include acute invasion of wind-dampness without edema; edema (usually of the lower extremities) in women with constitutional deficiency; damp-predominant painful obstruction with a heavy sensation in the body and limbs accompanied by numbness; menstrual disorders due to obstruction of the qi dynamic by wind-dampness; and ulcers and sores characterized by deficiency, where the qi is too weak to expel pus and toxins.

This latter use indicates that the main focus of the formula is on augmenting the qi rather than on dispersing the yang. In fact, it is the tonification of the gathering qi in the chest achieved by Astragali Radix *(huáng qí)* that effectively stabilizes the dispersion of yang qi intrinsic to its fiery nature. Located in the chest and upper burner, the primary movement of the gathering qi is downward. Acting as a mover of both water and blood, it leads both substances downward into the Bladder and Liver, respectively. It thereby balances the dispersing nature of the protective yang, which steams upward from the gate of vitality in the lower burner, infusing both the blood and body fluids with its heat. Wind invading from the exterior accelerates this dispersing and centrifugal movement, leading to the characteristic symptoms of sweating and aversion to wind. Because wind is a yang excess, it will be accompanied by a deficiency of yin. Very often, this is a deficiency of nutritive qi or blood, hence the adage, "To treat wind, one must treat the blood." Another possibility of strengthening the yin, however, is that of strengthening yin (downward) movement rather than yin substance. This is the method represented by this and other formulas employing the combination of Astragali Radix *(huáng qí)* and Atractylodis macrocephalae Rhizoma *(bái zhú)* to secure the protective yang.

In *Two Commentaries on the Classic of the Golden Cabinet and Jade Coffer*, Zhao Yi-De thus remarks: "If [this formula treats] the two pathogens of wind and dampness, why does it contain no herbs to disperse wind? … It only firms up the protective. When the normal qi is strong, wind is reduced of its own accord. This is treating [something] by not treating it." In *Discussion of Medical Formulas*, the late-Qing-dynasty scholar-physician Fei Bo-Xiong approached the same problem from another angle:

To eliminate wind, first nourish the blood; to treat dampness, first strengthen the Spleen. This is the specified strategy. The symptoms [that characterize the patterns treated by this formula] are from wind and water encroaching upon each other. This cannot be compared with blood deficiency generating wind. Therefore, one only uses herbs that treat wind, expel water, and strengthen the Spleen and does not have to add blood herbs. Once the water qi has been eliminated and the interstices and pores firmed, the wind can no longer remain of its own accord.

There is, however, an intimate connection between water-dampness and blood, inasmuch as excess dampness constrains the movement of blood. This has led to the use of this formula in the treatment of elevated blood lipids in overweight patients with qi deficiency and dampness presentations. Other modern indications include the treatment of body odor accompanied by severe underarm sweating, as well as the treatment of arthritic patients whose pain responds to biomedical anti-inflammatory treatment but who continue to sweat excessively, experience heaviness of the limbs, and suffer from aversion to wind-cold. All of these indications can be traced back to the combination of Lung and Spleen deficiency and excess dampness that underlies this pattern. Key clinical markers that would suggest the use of this formula thus include a tendency to tire easily or feeling tired all the time, heaviness of the extremities, aversion to wind or drafts, absence of thirst, and a pale and sometimes puffy tongue with a thin, white coating.

Comparisons

➤ Vs. OTHER FORMULAS FOR SUPERFICIAL EDEMA

This formula and Ephedra Decoction plus Atractylodes *(má huáng jiā zhú tāng)*, as well as Ephedra, Apricot Kernel, Coicis, and Licorice Decoction *(má huáng xìng rén yì yǐ gān cǎo tāng)*, discussed in Chapter 1, all treat superficial edema. Ephedra Decoction plus Atractylodes *(má huáng jiā zhú tāng)* is indicated for cold-dampness in the exterior, characterized by edema, aversion to cold, and an absence of sweating. Ephedra, Apricot Kernel, Coicis, and Licorice Decoction *(má huáng xìng rén yì yǐ gān cǎo tāng)* is indicated for wind-dampness fettering the exterior without deficiency, manifesting as edema and aversion to wind, but no sweating. This formula treats wind-dampness in the exterior with qi deficiency characterized by superficial edema, aversion to wind, and the presence of sweating. Although the patterns treated are different, administration of the decoction in all three cases should elicit only a slight sweat.

➤ Vs. STEPHANIA AND PORIA DECOCTION *(fáng jǐ fú líng tāng)*; *see* PAGE 738

Biomedical Indications

With the appropriate presentation, this formula may be used to treat a variety of biomedically-defined disorders includ-

ing rheumatic heart disease, ascites, acute glomerulonephritis, chronic nephritis, rheumatoid arthritis, and lumbar disc disease.

Alternate names

Stephania Decoction (*fáng jǐ tāng*) in *Pulse Classic*; Cocculus Decoction (*mù fáng jǐ tāng*) in *Arcane Essentials from the Imperial Library*; Stephania Decoction (*hàn fáng jǐ tāng*) in *Book to Safeguard Life Arranged according to Pattern*; Dampness Expelling Decoction (*zhú shī tāng*) in *Yongle Encyclopedia*; White Atractylodes Decoction (*bái zhú jiān*) in *Collection Picked by Immortals*; Astragalus and Stephania Decoction (*huáng qí fáng jǐ tāng*) in *Wondrous Lantern for Peering into the Origin and Development of Miscellaneous Diseases*

Modifications

• For abdominal pain, add Paeoniae Radix alba (*bái sháo*). (source text)

• For wheezing, add a small amount (1-3g) of Ephedrae Herba (*má huáng*). (source text)

• For a sense of upward-surging, add Cinnamomi Ramulus (*guì zhī*). (source text)

• For vigorous cold below, add Asari Radix et Rhizoma (*xì xīn*). (source text)

• For severe dampness with a sensation of heaviness in the lower back and legs, add Poria (*fú líng*) and Atractylodis Rhizoma (*cāng zhú*).

• For fullness and pain in the chest and abdomen, add Citri reticulatae Pericarpium (*chén pí*), Aurantii Fructus (*zhǐ ké*), and Perillae Folium (*zǐ sū yè*).

防己茯苓湯 (防己茯苓汤)
Stephania and Poria Decoction
fáng jǐ fú líng tāng

Source *Essentials from the Golden Cabinet* (c. 220)

Stephaniae tetrandrae Radix (*hàn fáng jǐ*) 9g
Astragali Radix (*huáng qí*) 6g
Cinnamomi Ramulus (*guì zhī*) 9g
Poria (*fú líng*) 18g
Glycyrrhizae Radix (*gān cǎo*) 6g

Method of Preparation Decoction

Actions Augments the qi, unblocks the yang, promotes urination, and reduces edema

Indications

Edema that is most pronounced in the extremities, a sensation of heaviness in the body and extremities, fibrillations of the skin and muscles in the extremities, a white, slippery tongue coating, and a superficial pulse.

This is skin edema (皮水 *pí shuǐ*), which does not disappear under pressure from the finger. It usually results from

excess-type disorders that have been improperly treated, from overwork, or from constitutional factors that are harmful to the Spleen yang such that the Spleen is unable to control water. This leads to an accumulation of dampness manifesting as edema. Because the Spleen governs the four extremities, the edema will be more pronounced there. The accumulation of dampness makes the body and extremities feel heavy, and the tongue coating appear slippery. The superficial nature of the pulse reflects the location of the disorder in the skin. The battle between the constrained yang qi and dampness in the exterior becomes visible as fibrillations in the skin and superficial muscles.

Analysis of Formula

Edema due to impairment of the Spleen yang's transportive function should be treated by augmenting the qi, unblocking the yang, promoting urination, and reducing the edema. To that end, this formula employs Poria (*fú líng*) and *fáng jǐ* (Stephaniae/Cocculi/etc. Radix) as its chief herbs. Poria (*fú líng*) filters out dampness to reduce swelling while also strengthening the Spleen to support the normal qi. It thus attends to both the root and branch at the same time. *Fáng jǐ* (Stephaniae/Cocculi/etc. Radix) promotes urination and bowel movement to eliminate water-dampness. In combination with Poria (*fú líng*), it focuses the formula's action on reducing the skin edema. Cinnamomi Ramulus (*guì zhī*), the deputy, unblocks the yang, improves the transformation of qi, and moves water via the urine to facilitate the reduction of edema. Astragali Radix (*huáng qí*), the assistant, augments the qi and strengthens the Spleen. Glycyrrhizae Radix (*gān cǎo*), the envoy, regulates and harmonizes the function of all the ingredients.

Besides their individual functions, the herbs in this formula unfold a complex number of synergistic functions. The combination of bland, percolating Poria (*fú líng*) and yang, warming Cinnamomi Ramulus (*guì zhī*) strongly promotes the qi transformation in the greater yang warp. When combined with Astragali Radix (*huáng qí*), the effects of Cinnamomi Ramulus (*guì zhī*) are focused on the exterior and extremities, where it opens up the yang and unblocks obstruction. In combination, Astragali Radix (*huáng qí*), Poria (*fú líng*), and Glycyrrhizae Radix (*gān cǎo*) strengthen the Spleen and augment the qi, improving the Spleen's transportive function while reducing the dampness that constrains its yang.

Cautions and Contraindications

The formula should not be used for skin edema accompanied by heat constraint. It is also unsuitable for the treatment of edema in the interior characterized by generalized edema and a submerged pulse.

Commentary

This formula focuses on conditions characterized by an excess of water-dampness against a background of yang and qi deficiency. The main symptomatology here is one of stagnation, characterized by the heavy sensation in the body and extremities as well as edema that does not disappear under pressure from the finger. Nevertheless, as with all conditions in which yang (fire) fails to transform yin (water), this yang becomes visible as pathological wind or heat. In the present pattern, where the disorder is located in the extremities, it manifests as fibrillations of the skin and superficial muscles. The combination of Poria (*fú líng*) and Cinnamomi Ramulus (*guì zhī*) is used in many classical formulas to treat throbbing pulsations below the heart or in the lower abdomen due to water excess and yang deficiency. In the present formula, they treat the fibrillations.

Comparisons

➤ Vs. Stephania and Astragalus Decoction
   (*fáng jǐ huáng qí tāng*)

While both formulas eliminate water from the exterior of the body, Stephania and Astragalus Decoction (*fáng jǐ huáng qí tāng*) focuses more strongly on strengthening the qi of the greater yin, while Stephania and Poria Decoction (*fáng jǐ fú líng tāng*) warms and opens the yang to improve the qi transformation within the greater yang warp. Stephania and Astragalus Decoction (*fáng jǐ huáng qí tāng*) thus eliminates dampness not only from the limbs, but also from the interior of the body. Stephania and Poria Decoction (*fáng jǐ fú líng tāng*), by contrast, focuses entirely on the exterior. The qi deficiency treated by Stephania and Astragalus Decoction (*fáng jǐ huáng qí tāng*) manifests as sweating and aversion to wind, while the yang deficiency treated by Stephania and Poria Decoction (*fáng jǐ fú líng tāng*) manifests as a cold body without subjective aversion to wind.

➤ Vs. Five-Peel Powder (*wǔ pí sǎn*); *see* PAGE 734

Alternate names

Cocculus Decoction (*mù fáng jǐ tāng*) in *Arcane Essentials from the Imperial Library*; Stephania Decoction (*fáng jǐ tāng*) in *Comprehensive Recording of Sagely Beneficence*; Poria Decoction (*fú líng tāng*) in *Ji-Feng's Formulas of Universal Benefit*; Stephania Plus Poria Decoction (*fáng jǐ jiā fú líng tāng*) in *Red Water and Dark Pearls*

Modifications

• For more severe Spleen deficiency, add Codonopsis Radix (*dǎng shēn*).

• For Kidney yang deficiency, add Aconiti Radix lateralis praeparata (*zhì fù zǐ*) and Epimedii Herba (*yín yáng huò*).

• For severe edema, add Alismatis Rhizoma (*zé xiè*) and Polyporus (*zhū líng*).

Section 4

FORMULAS THAT
WARM AND TRANSFORM
WATER AND DAMPNESS

The formulas in this section are used in treating patterns of dampness caused by cold, or where cold and dampness clump together. The reasons for this may be yang deficiency or invasion of cold-dampness from the outside. When the Kidney yang is deficient and its qi loses the ability to transform water, the water becomes pathogenic by overflowing and causing edema, or stagnant and giving rise to dampness. Symptoms include urinary difficulty, edema, and lower abdominal numbness. Spleen yang deficiency can give rise to similar problems. Cold-dampness, which has many etiologies, tends to settle in the lower parts of the body. It may lodge in the Intestines, manifesting as thin mucus; or it may cause cloudy painful urinary dribbling, leg qi, or various types of edema.

To treat cold-dampness, the formulas in this chapter rely on chief herbs that warm the yang and promote the resolution of dampness such as Cinnamomi Ramulus (*guì zhī*), Aconiti Radix lateralis praeparata (*zhì fù zǐ*), Poria (*fú líng*), and Atractylodis macrocephalae Rhizoma (*bái zhú*). Depending on the pattern, they may be combined with deputies and assistants that strengthen the Spleen and tonify the Kidneys, or that regulate the qi. Herbs that strengthen the Spleen and tonify the Kidneys include Alpiniae oxyphyllae Fructus (*yì zhì rén*), Atractylodis macrocephalae Rhizoma (*bái zhú*), Glycyrrhizae Radix (*gān cǎo*), Jujubae Fructus (*dà zǎo*), and Aconiti Radix lateralis praeparata (*zhì fù zǐ*). Kidney and Spleen yang is essential in supporting the body's water metabolism and, in turn, is easily damaged by cold-dampness. This makes it essential to ensure its vitality. Herbs that regulate the qi, like Magnoliae officinalis Cortex (*hòu pò*), Linderae Radix (*wū yào*), Aucklandiae Radix (*mù xiāng*), Citri reticulatae Pericarpium (*chén pí*), or Arecae Pericarpium (*dà fù pí*), are used to open the qi dynamic in order to facilitate the dispelling of dampness.

苓桂朮甘湯 (苓桂术甘汤)
Poria, Cinnamon Twig, Atractylodes, and Licorice Decoction

líng guì zhú gān tāng

Source   *Discussion of Cold Damage* (c. 220)

Poria (*fú líng*)	12g
Cinnamomi Ramulus (*guì zhī*)	9g
Atractylodis macrocephalae Rhizoma (*bái zhú*)	6g
Glycyrrhizae Radix praeparata (*zhì gān cǎo*)	6g

Method of Preparation Decoction. The source text specifies that administration of the formula should lead to an increase in urination.

Actions Warms and transforms phlegm and thin mucus, strengthens the Spleen, and resolves dampness

Indications

Fullness in the chest and hypochondria, palpitations, shortness of breath, coughing up clear and watery sputum, and dizziness or vertigo. The tongue is pale and swollen with a white and slippery or greasy coating, and the pulse is usually slippery and either wiry or soggy.

This is thin mucus in the epigastrium. When the Spleen yang is weak it is unable to transform the fluids. This results in thin mucus, which gathers in the area around the diaphragm and obstructs the qi dynamic, causing a sensation of fullness in the chest and hypochondria, shortness of breath, and sometimes the coughing up of clear, watery sputum. The thin mucus blocks the rise of the clear yang and the descent of the turbid yin, which results in dizziness or vertigo. A pale, swollen tongue with a white coating and a soggy pulse reflects Spleen deficiency, while a slippery or greasy coating and a slippery or wiry pulse are signs of thin mucus.

Analysis of Formula

In the source text, the author of this formula, Zhang Zhong-Jing, outlined a guiding principle for the treatment of all thin mucus disorders that has been accepted by physicians ever since: "Disorders [characterized by] thin mucus should be treated by harmonization with warming herbs." This treatment principle applies as well to the present formula, which is aimed at correcting patterns where thin mucus accumulates in the epigastrium due to deficiency of middle burner yang qi. For this purpose, it combines herbs that warm the yang, transform the fluids, build the Spleen, and harmonize the middle burner.

The chief herb, Poria (*fú líng*), strengthens the Spleen and leaches out dampness. It thereby transforms the thin mucus by addressing the root of this disorder: the metabolism of fluids. The deputy, Cinnamomi Ramulus (*guì zhī*), warms the yang and improves the transforming power of the qi, which resolves the thin mucus. Improving the functioning of the qi also assists in directing the rebellious qi downward. The combination of these two herbs—one increasing the circulation of the fluids, the other warming the flow of qi—is an exquisite way of dealing with the lingering of thin mucus due to cold.

Atractylodis macrocephalae Rhizoma (*bái zhú*), the assistant herb, strengthens the transforming and transportive functions of the Spleen, and dries dampness. Together with Cinnamomi Ramulus (*guì zhī*), it even more strongly promotes the Spleen yang so that the excess dampness is more easily resolved. The envoy, Glycyrrhizae Radix praeparata (*zhì*

gān cǎo), augments the qi of the middle burner. It has a mild tendency to cause stagnation, but this is effectively counteracted by Poria (*fú líng*). Cinnamomi Ramulus (*guì zhī*), when combined with Glycyrrhizae Radix (*gān cǎo*), transforms its sweetness into yang through its own acrid, moving nature, while the combination of Poria (*fú líng*), Atractylodis macrocephalae Rhizoma (*bái zhú*), and Glycyrrhizae Radix (*gān cǎo*) strengthens the Spleen to dispel dampness. These multiple synergies ensure that, while there are only four ingredients in the formula, they are well-matched and thus effective in resolving the thin mucus, strengthening the Spleen, and preventing dampness from recurring.

Cautions and Contraindications

This formula is acrid and warming, and is therefore contraindicated for thin mucus occurring as the result of damp-heat or in patterns characterized by yin deficiency and hyperactive Liver yang.

Commentary

Discussion of Cold Damage (Chapter 67) prescribes this formula for cases of injury due to cold caused by the improper use of purgatives or emetics, with such symptoms as fullness in the chest and hypochondria together with vertigo. *Essentials from the Golden Cabinet* recommends it for thin mucus in the epigastric region, which is resolved through the urine. This has been the purpose for which it is most frequently used by later generations of physicians. The combination of Poria (*fú líng*) and Cinnamomi Ramulus (*guì zhī*) is very effective in promoting urination (see the discussion of Five-Ingredient Powder with Poria (*wǔ líng sǎn*) earlier in this chapter).

In Chinese medicine, the term thin mucus (飲 *yǐn*) refers both to a constellation of symptoms and a cause of disease, and is used in both a wider and more narrow sense. In its wider sense, thin mucus is a term for a disorder that can manifest through a range of different patterns, all of which are due to the accumulation of pathological fluids in one of the body cavities (the bowels, the flanks, the chest) or in the extremities. This may be due to the invasion of external pathogens or stem from the dysfunction of internal organs. In its more narrow sense, the term thin mucus defines a subcategory of phlegm. One can further differentiate between deficient and excessive types of thin mucus. This formula is indicated for the deficient type associated with yang deficiency of the Spleen and Kidneys. The excess type is characterized by severe cold in the epigastrium and abdomen and is treated with formulas like Major Construct the Middle Decoction (*dà jiàn zhōng tāng*).

Although from an organ-based perspective, deficient-type thin mucus is associated with Spleen and Kidney yang deficiency, the treatment is directed at harmonizing the fluids and qi dynamic rather than focusing on specific organ functions. As noted above, this was underscored by Zhang Zhong-Jing in *Essentials of the Golden Cabinet* when he noted that thin mucus should be treated by harmonization with warming herbs. Harmonization here implies the regulation of yin and yang, water and fire. The intention is to employ warming herbs like Cinnamomi Ramulus (*guì zhī*) to stimulate the body's own fluid metabolism and thereby create a more physiological balance between yin and yang. Resolving thin mucus through the urine is extremely important in this pattern for another reason: seeking to disperse fluids by promoting sweating will, according to the source text, lead to "pulsation of the vessels and shaking of the body." The reason is that, when excess fluids are located in the interior, mobilizing the yang toward the exterior will lead to a dangerous imbalance between yang on the outside and yin on the inside. Thus, it is by harmonizing water and fire that the formula is able to treat a wide range of vasomotor dysfunctions like dizziness, palpitations, hot flushes, and tinnitus, for which it is specifically indicated. In *Discussion of Blood Patterns*, the 19th-century physician Tang Zong-Hai elaborates:

> Cinnamomi Ramulus (*guì zhī*) tonifies the Heart fire so that is descends to connect with the Kidneys. Poria (*fú líng*) promotes Kidney water so that it does not insult the Heart above. In fact, Poria (*fú líng*) is a Spleen herb. Earth can control water so that water does not insult fire. Cinnamomi Ramulus (*guì zhī*) is a Liver herb that transforms water. The Liver is the child of the Kidneys. In case of excess, one drains the child. The Liver also governs dredging and draining and therefore possesses the function of transforming water qi. [With regard to] tonifying the Heart fire, in [cases of] deficiency, one tonifies the mother. Liver is the mother of Heart fire. Furthermore, Cinnamomi Ramulus (*guì zhī*) is red and enters the Heart. To promote sweating, one uses Cinnamomi Ramulus (*guì zhī*), drawing on the warmth of wood qi to disperse and thrust outward. To direct upward-gushing and rebellion downward, one also uses Cinnamomi Ramulus (*guì zhī*) because the Penetrating vessel connects with the Liver below and with the Kidneys internally. Cinnamomi Ramulus (*guì zhī*) warms the Liver qi to draw it out and warms Kidney water in order to drain it. Whenever cold water attacks the lower burner [leading] the yang of the Penetrating [vessel] to float upward, one can often assist it with Poria (*fú líng*) and Pinelliae Rhizoma praeparatum (*zhì bàn xià*) to achieve success.

Based on such considerations, this formula can be prescribed for any condition marked by cold in the lower burner leading to thin mucus throughout the Triple Burner. The following are examples of the wide range of conditions that can be treated in this manner.

- Cardiovascular disorders: Liu Du-Zhou, the famous contemporary expert on classical formulas, uses Poria, Cinnamon Twig, Atractylodes, and Licorice Decoction (*líng guì zhú gān tāng*) to treat a wide variety of cardiovascular disorders including coronary heart disease, pericarditis, and right heart failure. In Liu's experience, the following signs

are important clinical indicators: a pale and tender tongue with a wet, slippery coating; darkish discoloration or black spots in various areas of the face, indicating water stasis; and a deep, wiry pulse.

- Eye disorders: Lu Yuan-Lei, a modern classical formula expert, recommends the use of this formula with the addition of Plantaginis Semen (*chē qián zǐ*) in the treatment of eye disorders characterized by redness, pain, and excessive gumminess, which he saw as arising from water blocking the Stomach. Japanese Kampo physicians, too, use the formula to treat eye disorders including inflammation, cataract, and retinopathies where there are signs of internal water stagnation.

- Digestive disorders: The famous early-Qing-dynasty physician Ye Tian-Shi employed this formula to treat a wide variety of digestive disorders ranging from pain, distention, and fullness in the Stomach to diarrhea and borborygmi. For this purpose, he flexibly combined it with other formulas that warm the interior, regulate the qi, or tonify the yang.

- Headaches and dizziness: Ye Tian-Shi also used this formula to treat headaches due to internal cold and yang deficiency with accumulation of turbid yin above. Modern indications include Menieres' disease, low blood pressure, and tinnitus.

It is obvious from the above that Poria, Cinnamon Twig, Atractylodes, and Licorice Decoction (*líng guì zhú gān tāng*) treats a pattern and not a disease and that clearly defining this pattern is key to its successful use in the clinic. Based on an analysis of the literature, the following clinical markers will facilitate correctly identifying this pattern:

- Dizziness or spots in front of the eyes when getting up
- Hot flushes, palpitations, tachycardia, nervousness (indicating that the yang qi does not penetrate into the excess yin water)
- Cold abdomen or splashing sounds in the Stomach on palpation (indicating cold in the Stomach and accumulation of thin mucus); or large areas of coldness on the back or along the spine (indicating lack of yang qi in the interior)
- Pale tongue with a slippery, white coating (indicating cold and water) seen together with a submerged and wiry pulse (indicating stagnation of fluids in the interior)
- Periodic nature of the symptomatology, characterized by periods of acute ill-health alternating with others when few or no symptoms are present; symptoms will be aggravated by exhaustion, fatigue, nervous tension, or the contraction of external pathogens, that is, periods when the yang qi has been depleted.
- Visible signs of thin mucus such as increased urination, edema, coughing of thin mucus, or excess saliva.

Comparisons

➤ Vs. Five-Ingredient Powder with Poria *(wǔ líng sǎn)*

Both formulas warm the yang and promote urination via the combination of Poria *(fú líng)*, Atractylodis macrocephalae Rhizoma *(bái zhú)*, and Cinnamomi Ramulus *(guì zhī)*. Five-Ingredient Powder with Poria *(wǔ líng sǎn)* also contains Alismatis Rhizoma *(zé xiè)* and Polyporus *(zhū líng)*, and is thus a more powerful diuretic formula. Its action is focused on the lower burner where it treats water buildup and urinary difficulty. Although symptoms in the upper and middle burners may also be observed, these are usually relieved by urination. By contrast, Poria, Cinnamon Twig, Attractylodes, and Licorice Decoction *(líng guì zhú gān tang)* contains Glycyrrhizae Radix praeparata *(zhì gān cǎo)* and thus focuses on tonifying Spleen earth in addition to harmonizing thin mucus away. It is specific for thin mucus in the epigastrium that insults the Heart, leading to a variety of vasomotor symptoms.

➤ Vs. Licorice, Ginger, Poria, and White Atractylodes Decoction *(gān cǎo gān jiāng fú líng bái zhú tāng)*; *see* PAGE 743

➤ Vs. True Warrior Decoction *(zhēn wǔ tāng)*; *see* PAGE 746

Biomedical Indications

With the appropriate presentation, this formula may be used to treat a wide variety of biomedically-defined disorders. These can be divided into the following groups:

- Disorders affecting the head such as Ménière's disease and basilar insufficiency
- Cardiovascular disorders such as coronary heart disease, hypertension, hypotension, cor pulmonare, mitral valve prolapse, myocarditis, and pericardial effusion
- Gastrointestinal disorders such as gastroptosis, peptic ulcers, chronic gastritis, and functional stomach disorders
- Respiratory disorders such as bronchitis, asthma, pertussis, and pleurisy
- Ophthalmologic disorders such as cataracts, viral conjunctivitis, optic nerve atrophy, and central serous retinopathy.

This formula has also been used for treating nephritis, renal calculus, ascites, pediatric inguinal hernia, hydrocele, and pediatric rhinitis.

Alternate names

Poria, Cinnamon Twig, Atractylodes, and Licorice Decoction *(líng guì zhú gān tāng)* in *Essentials from the Golden Cabinet*; Licorice Decoction *(gān cǎo tāng)* in *Important Formulas Worth a Thousand Gold Pieces*; Poria and White Atractylodes Decoction *(fú líng bái zhú tāng)* in *General Discussion of the Disease of Cold Damage*; Poria Decoction *(fú líng tāng)* in *Comprehensive Recording of Sagely Beneficence*; Poria Powder *(fú líng sǎn)* in *Prescriptions of Universal Benefit*; Poria, White Atractylodes, Cinnamon Twig, and Licorice Decoction *(fú líng bái zhú guì zhī gān cǎo tāng)* in *Complete Compendium of Cold Damage*; Poria, Cinnamon Twig, Licorice, and White Atractylodes Decoction *(fú líng guì gān bái zhú tāng)* in *Systematic Great Compendium of Medicine Past and Present*; Poria, Cinnamon Twig, Atractylodes, and Licorice Decoction *(fú líng guì zhú gān cǎo tāng)* in *Introduction to Medicine*; Poria and Cinnamon Decoction *(líng guì tāng)* in *Restoration of Life from the Groves of Medicine*; Cinnamon Twig, Poria, Atractylodes, and Licorice Decoction *(guì líng zhú gān cǎo tāng)* in *Collected Treatises of [Zhang] Jing-Yue*; Cinnamon Twig, Poria, Atractylodes, and Licorice Decoction *(guì líng zhú gān tāng)* in *Medical Formulas Collected and Analyzed*

Modifications

- For vomiting, add Pinelliae Rhizoma praeparatum *(zhì bàn xià)*.
- For severe belching and vomiting, add Kaki Calyx *(shì dì)* and Amomi Fructus *(shā rén)*.
- For fatigue and lethargy, add Codonopsis Radix *(dǎng shēn)*.
- For focal distention and pain in the epigastrium, add Aurantii Fructus *(zhǐ ké)* and Magnoliae officinalis Cortex *(hòu pò)*.
- For Ménière's disease or vertigo from hypotension, take with True Warrior Decoction *(zhēn wǔ tāng)*.

Associated Formula

變製心氣飲 （变制心气饮）

Modified Formulation of Heart Qi Drink

biàn zhì xīn qì yǐn/hensei shinki-in

SOURCE *Collection of Treasured Essentials*

Cinnamomi Ramulus *(guì zhī)*	3g
Poria *(fú líng)*	5g
Pinelliae Rhizoma praeparatum *(zhì bàn xià)*	2.5g
Akebiae Caulis *(mù tōng)*	4g
Mori Cortex *(sāng bái pí)*	3g
Arecae Semen *(bīng láng)*	4g
Perillae Fructus *(zǐ sū zǐ)*	2g
Trionycis Carapax *(biē jiǎ)*	4g
Glycyrrhizae Radix *(gān cǎo)*	2g
Aurantii Fructus immaturus *(zhǐ shí)*	4g
Evodiae Fructus *(wú zhū yú)*	3g

This formula is indicated for qi constraint and water accumulating in the interior, manifesting as palpitations, rebellious qi and fullness in the epigastrium, focal distention in the chest and flanks, heaviness of the body, and edema; or numbness and painful obstruction; or pulling pain in the feet and legs; or acute stiffness of the back and shoulders; or acid reflux; or urinary difficulty. As in many patterns involving water obstructing the qi dynamic, this may appear as a darkish discoloration of certain areas in the face, particularly below the eyes and on the temples. The patient may also have depressive moods, headache, dizziness, and insomnia. In contemporary Japan and China, the formula is commonly used to treat cardiac failure leading to edema, angina pectoris, and chronic bronchitis.

In terms of its composition, the formula can be understood as a combination of Poria, Cinnamon Twig, Atractylodes, and Licorice Decoction (*líng guì zhú gān tāng*) and Unripe Bitter Orange, Chinese Garlic, and Cinnamon Twig Decoction (*zhǐ shí xiè bái guì zhī tāng*). It warms the yang, transforms stagnation, and promotes water metabolism. The inclusion of Trionycis Carapax (*biē jiǎ*) is intended to soften and dissolve hardness and clumping that may occur as a result of water accumulation. From a biomedical point of view, this encompasses enlargement of the liver and spleen that may occur as a result of cardiac failure.

甘草乾薑茯苓白术湯
（甘草干姜茯苓白术汤）
Licorice, Ginger, Poria, and White Atractylodes Decoction
gān cǎo gān jiāng fú líng bái zhú tāng

Source　*Essentials from the Golden Cabinet* (c. 220)

Glycyrrhizae Radix (*gān cǎo*) .6g
Zingiberis Rhizoma (*gān jiāng*) 12g
Poria (*fú líng*) 12g
Atractylodis macrocephalae Rhizoma (*bái zhú*) 6g

Method of Preparation　Decoction. The source text specifies that administration of the formula should cause the patient to experience a warm sensation in the lower back.

Actions　Warms the Spleen and overcomes dampness

Indications

For a heavy sensation in the body, cold and pain in the lower back, pressure in the lower back as if carrying a heavy weight, normal appetite and absence of thirst, and copious urine. The tongue will be pale with a white, moist coating that may be thick and greasy at the root, and the pulse will be submerged, thin, and moderate.

This is fixed Kidney disorder (腎著 *shèn zhuó*), a type of painful obstruction of the waist and lower back due to cold-dampness. The etiology of this disorder commonly involves internal causes such as overwork and habitual sweating that weaken the normal qi, and the invasion of cold-dampness from the outside. The source text speaks of exposure to rain, walking in water, or sitting in damp places. In modern patients, this might be swimming for too long, or in too cold water, or not toweling off properly. The onset can be both acute and chronic. Dampness in the entire body causes a heavy sensation. As a yin pathogen, it tends to flow downward, settling in the lower back where it obstructs the flow of qi and causes a cold sensation, pain, or pressure. Normal appetite and a lack of any particular thirst indicate that the functions of the middle and upper burners are unimpaired. Copious urination reflects attempts by the body to rid itself of dampness, implying that Kidney function is normal, too, and that the pathogen has settled in the skin and muscle layer.

However, because the lower back is the residence of the Kidneys and because the pain is fixed, the condition is referred to as a fixed Kidney disorder. The tongue and pulse reflect the dampness settling in the lower burner.

Analysis of Formula

This formula treats cold-dampness obstructing the movement of qi and fluids in the skin and muscles, primarily in the lower back. Although the lower back is the seat of the Kidneys, the Kidney organ itself functions normally. It is unnecessary, therefore, to treat the Kidneys directly. Rather, by warming the yang and eliminating the dampness, focusing primarily on the Spleen due to its resonance with both dampness and the flesh, it is possible to effectively treat this disorder.

The main herb for this purpose is acrid and warming Zingiberis Rhizoma (*gān jiāng*). It warms the middle but also drives out wind-damp painful obstruction, effectively addressing both the actual pathology and the background disposition. Because dampness in this pattern is relatively severe, bland Poria (*fú líng*) is added as a deputy. It strengthens the Spleen and promotes urination to eliminate dampness via the urine. The combination of Poria (*fú líng*) and Zingiberis Rhizoma (*gān jiāng*) warms the yang and dispels dampness, removing pathogenic qi without injuring the normal qi. Bitter, sweet, and warming Atractylodis macrocephalae Rhizoma (*bái zhú*) functions as the assistant. It tonifies the Spleen qi even as it dries dampness. In combination with Zingiberis Rhizoma (*gān jiāng*), it effectively tonifies the Spleen yang, while together with Poria (*fú líng*), it assists in dispelling dampness. Glycyrrhizae Radix (*gān cǎo*) harmonizes the function of the other herbs while also contributing to strengthening the Spleen.

Cautions and Contraindications

Heaviness of the body and backache due to damp-heat must not be treated with this formula.

Commentary

Although modern textbooks frequently define fixed Kidney disorder as a type of painful obstruction, it differs from other types of painful obstruction patterns in a number of ways. First, it conjoins only two (rather than three) pathogens—dampness and cold—while wind is absent. Second, cold-dampness here is located in the skin and muscles rather than in the channels and collaterals and is therefore treated via the Spleen. Third, as indicated by the symptoms of heaviness throughout the body and coldness below the waist, the pattern involves more than a local accumulation of dampness. This is explained by Xu Bin in *Discussion and Annotation of the Essentials from the Golden Cabinet:*

[The term] fixed Kidneys expresses [a condition of something] adhering and not moving. As the protective qi issues from the lower burner, the Kidneys being fixed by a pathogen [means] that dampness stagnates the protective qi. Hence, the entire body feels heavy.

The formula thus focuses on promoting yang and dispelling dampness via the urine rather than sweating. Sweating and the use of herbs that dispel wind-dampness would not be an appropriate strategy, in part because of the nature of the pathogen, and in part because the protective yang is hemmed in by dampness.

Over time, physicians have extended the application of this formula to the treatment of Girdle vessel disorders. This is based on a passage in Chapter 29 of *Classic of Difficulties:* "Girdle vessel disorders [are characterized] by abdominal fullness, the lumbar area feels weak and as if one were sitting in water." This closely matches the description of the pattern for Licorice, Ginger, Poria, and White Atractylodes Decoction *(gān cǎo gān jiāng fú líng bái zhú tāng)* in *Essentials from the Golden Cabinet*, which speaks of a sensation "as if one were sitting in water" and "the back being heavy, as if one were carrying a belt containing five-thousand coins." Another important indication is edema during pregnancy, for which *Discussion of Illnesses, Patterns, and Formulas Related to the Unification of the Three Etiologies* recommends the addition of Armeniacae Semen *(xìng rén)*.

Clinically, the key diagnostic markers suggesting use of this formula can thus be summarized as follows:

- Heaviness, coldness, or pain of the abdomen or back. The sensation of cold can be subjective, or may be palpated. Heaviness may manifest as a sensation of numbness or insensitivity. There may also be difficulty in bending from the waist.

- Excess water may manifest as increased urination, diarrhea or soft stools, sweating, saliva, phlegm, discharge or increased secretions from the skin. Due to the underlying cold, these will usually not be malodorous.

- Signs of dampness on the tongue such as a white, moist coating that may be thick and greasy at the root accompanied by a pulse that is submerged, thin, and moderate.

Comparisons

➤ Vs. Regulate the Middle Pill *(lǐ zhōng wán)*

Both formulas combine Zingiberis Rhizoma *(gān jiāng)*, Atractylodis macrocephalae Rhizoma *(bái zhú)*, and Glycyrrhizae Radix *(gān cǎo)*. Regulate the Middle Pill *(lǐ zhōng wán)* adds Ginseng Radix *(rén shēn)* to tonify the middle burner. It focuses on patterns characterized by cold and qi deficiency of the Spleen and Stomach. Licorice, Ginger, Poria, and White Atractylodes Decoction *(gān cǎo gān jiāng fú líng*

bái zhú tang) adds Poria *(fú líng)* to focus the formula on dispelling cold-dampness, particularly from the lower back.

➤ Vs. Poria, Cinnamon Twig, Atractylodes, and Licorice Decoction *(líng guì zhú gān tāng)*

Both formulas contain Poria *(fú líng)*, Atractylodis macrocephalae Rhizoma *(bái zhú)*, and Glycyrrhizae Radix *(gān cǎo)*. Poria, Cinnamon Twig, Atractylodes, and Licorice Decoction *(líng guì zhú gān tāng)* adds Cinnamomi Ramulus *(guì zhī)*, focusing the action of the formula on warming the yang and transforming the fluids to treat thin mucus, particularly in the epigastrium and abdomen. Licorice, Ginger, Poria, and White Atractylodes Decoction *(gān cǎo gān jiāng fú líng bái zhú tāng)*, on the other hand, adds Zingiberis Rhizoma *(gān jiāng)* to focus on warming and dispersing the cold-dampness.

Biomedical Indications

With the appropriate presentation, this formula may be used to treat a wide variety of biomedically-defined disorders including acute lumbar strain, lumbar disc disease, sciatica, renal calculi, chronic pelvic inflammatory disease, benign prostatic hypertrophy, enuresis, acute gastroenteritis, eczema, allergic rhinitis, and chronic bronchitis.

....

Alternate names

Licorice, Ginger, Poria and Atractylodes Decoction *(gān jiāng líng zhú tāng)* in *Essentials from the Golden Cabinet*; Licorice Decoction *(gān cǎo tāng)* in *Arcane Essentials from the Imperial Library*; Decoction for Fixed Kidneys *(shèn zhuó tāng)* in *Supplement to Important Formulas Worth a Thousand Gold Pieces*; Dampness Eliminating Decoction *(chú shī tāng)* in *Discussion of Illnesses, Patterns, and Formulas Related to the Unification of the Three Etiologies*; Poria, Ginger, Atractylodes, and Licorice Decoction *(líng jiāng zhú gān tāng)* in *Categorized Collected Formulas*; Poria, Ginger, White Atractylodes, and Licorice Decoction *(fú líng gān jiāng bái zhú gān cǎo tāng)* in *Extraordinarily Correct Formulas*

....

Modifications

- For chronic backache and discharges in women, add Carthami Flos *(hóng huā)*.

- For older patients with chronic backache and urinary frequency, add Aconiti Radix lateralis praeparata *(zhì fù zǐ)* and Cervi Cornu degelatinatum *(lù jiǎo shuāng)*. Also for incontinence in both boys and girls up to the age of fourteen.

- For more severe cold, add Aconiti Radix lateralis praeparata *(zhì fù zǐ)* and Asari Radix et Rhizoma *(xì xīn)*.

- For more severe dampness, add Alismatis Rhizoma *(zé xiè)*, Atractylodis Rhizoma *(cāng zhú)*, and Coicis Semen *(yì yǐ rén)*.

- For pronounced Spleen deficiency, add Ginseng Radix *(rén shēn)*.

真武湯（真武汤）

True Warrior Decoction

zhēn wǔ tāng

This formula, which warms the yang and promotes urination, is named after one of the four directional spirits of Chinese folklore. The relationship is explained in *Golden Mirror of the Medical Tradition:* "The true warrior is the spirit of the north who manages water. The name has been used for this formula with the meaning of drawing [on these powers] to pacify water." *Simple Explications of Han Formulas* likewise notes: "The name true warrior is entirely due to its pacifying water by anchoring a person's dragon." The term 'dragon' refers to the fire at the gate of vitality. This formula controls water excess by stimulating its transformation by the fire at the gate of vitality. Another name for the formula, which some physicians believe to be its original name, is Tortoise Decoction (玄武湯 *xuán wǔ tāng*). The tortoise is the spirit of the northern sky.

The formula thus belongs to the group of formulas named after the directional spirits of the skies, including Bluegreen Dragon Decoction (*qīng lóng tāng*) and White Tiger Decoction (*bái hǔ tāng*), which were first listed in *Discussion of Cold Damage*. All of these formulas are concerned with the regulation and protection of body fluids.

Source   *Discussion of Cold Damage* (c. 220)

baked Aconiti Radix lateralis (*bāo fù zǐ*) 9g
Atractylodis macrocephalae Rhizoma (*bái zhú*) 6g
Poria (*fú líng*) 9g
Zingiberis Rhizoma recens (*shēng jiāng*) 9g
Paeoniae Radix (*sháo yào*) 9g

Method of Preparation   The source text advises to decoct in 8 cups of water boiled down to 3 cups, and then take in three equal doses. At present, it is usually prepared as a decoction in the usual manner with Paeoniae Radix alba (*bái sháo*) being the most commonly-used form of Paeoniae Radix (*sháo yào*).

Actions   Warms the yang and promotes urination

Indications

Abdominal pain that is aggravated by cold, urinary difficulty, and deep aching and heaviness in the extremities. There may also be generalized edema, loose stools, dizziness, heavy sensation in the head, palpitations, coughing, and vomiting. The tongue is pale or dark and swollen with tooth marks, and has a white, slippery coating. The pulse tends to be submerged, thin, and forceless.

Also for externally-contracted disorders with sweating that does not reduce the fever, palpitations in the epigastrium, dizziness, generalized twitching, the patient feeling unstable on their feet as if they were about to fall, a white, slippery tongue coating, and a submerged, thin, and forceless pulse.

The first presentation is Kidney yang deficiency, or Spleen and Kidney yang deficiency, with retention of pathogenic water. The Kidneys are the yin organ associated with water and fire. They control the process of water metabolism and urina-

tion. When the true yang is deficient, the Kidney qi loses its ability to transform water, which thereupon accumulates as pathogenic water in the lower burner where it causes urinary difficulty. Because this obstructs the qi, it causes abdominal pain that is aggravated by cold.

The Kidneys are the root of the body's yang qi and support the generative and transforming processes of the other organs. For this reason, Kidney yang deficiency is often accompanied by Spleen yang deficiency. The Spleen governs the transformation and transportation of water and dampness. The inability of the Spleen yang to transport water leads to various problems associated with the retention of pathogenic water and dampness. They may flood or spill over into the flesh and skin, producing generalized edema with deep aching and heaviness in the extremities. In the Intestines, this may cause loose stools. Water and dampness prevent the clear yang from ascending and the turbid yin from descending. This veils the sensory orifices and produces dizziness and a heavy sensation in the head. Internal accumulation of cold-dampness obstructs the flow of water and qi and causes abdominal pain. When pathogenic water ascends and affects the Heart, it causes epigastric palpitations; when it attacks the Lungs, it disrupts the Lung qi and produces coughing; and when it attacks the middle burner, it disturbs the Spleen and Stomach and causes vomiting and diarrhea. The pale or dark swollen tongue with tooth marks, the white, slippery tongue coating, and the submerged, thin, and forceless pulse are signs of yang deficiency with internal retention of pathogenic water and dampness.

The second presentation is externally-contracted wind-cold at the greater yang warp. When sweating does not alleviate the fever, the continuous loss of fluids causes the body to wither and severely depletes the yang qi. This deprives the sinews and flesh of nourishment, and the channels and extremities of warmth. As a result, a generalized twitching of the muscles may be observed. The patient also feels weak and unstable, as if she were about to fall. This sensation may range from lightheadedness and positional vertigo to severe dizziness even when lying down.

Analysis of Formula

Because insufficiency of Kidney yang is the root of the condition, this formula focuses on warming and strengthening the fire at the gate of vitality. The chief herb is therefore the very heating and acrid Aconiti Radix lateralis praeparata (*zhì fù zǐ*), which tonifies the fire at the gate of vitality, restores the Kidney yang, and thereby enables the Kidneys to resume their function of transforming water. The deputies, Atractylodis macrocephalae Rhizoma (*bái zhú*) and Poria (*fú líng*), strengthen the Spleen and promote urination. Poria (*fú líng*) also drains the dampness and pathogenic water that has been retained in the body through the urine. Zingiberis Rhizoma recens (*shēng jiāng*), an assistant herb, warms and dispels the pathogenic water and thereby strengthens the actions of the deputy herbs. It disseminates the Lung qi, warms the Stomach, and assists the chief herb by dispelling the dampness that has overflowed into the flesh and skin. Zingiberis Rhizoma recens *(shēng jiāng)*, Atractylodis macrocephalae Rhizoma *(bái zhú)*, and Poria *(fú líng)* thus reinforce the earth (Spleen/Stomach) to control the water (Kidneys), thereby indirectly assisting the chief herb in warming and strengthening the Kidney yang. The other assistant, bitter, sour, and cooling Paeoniae Radix *(sháo yào)*, preserves the yin and alleviates pain. It prevents the dry, hot herbs that promote urination from injuring the yin. According to various commentators, it unfolds a number of other important actions that are discussed in the COMMENTARY that follows.

Commentary

Water is a yin pathogenic factor that requires the assistance of yang in order to be properly transformed. In this case, the source of yang in the gate of vitality must be strengthened in order to reduce the diffusion of yin. Although water is governed by the Kidneys, it is also controlled by the Spleen. Thus, in addition to warming the Kidney yang, one must also address its manifestations (the retention of water and dampness) by using herbs that strengthen the Spleen and benefit dampness.

From a six-warps rather than organ-based perspective, this formula focuses on lesser yin patterns characterized by yang deficiency and water flooding. Lesser yin-warp disorders are characterized by fatigue and lethargy as well as a faint, thin pulse that indicates that the yang qi is failing to move and transform the yin. These symptoms should therefore be present in all patterns treated by this formula. They will be accompanied by symptoms reflecting the flooding of water. In Chinese texts, such flooding is also referred to as water qi (水氣 *shuǐ qì*). Like qi, water penetrates everywhere in the body, hence the symptoms can also occur anywhere. This makes the formula useful for a wide spectrum of potential applications.

Usage

One of the most useful guides to the many patterns for which this formula can be used is provided by the contemporary physician Chen Chao-Zu. In *Treatment Strategies and Formulas in Chinese Medicine*, Chen groups these patterns under eight headings:

1. Lesser yin warp yang deficiency with obstruction and stagnation of phlegm fluids and water-dampness in the lower burner, Kidneys, or Bladder. This may manifest as urinary difficulty or obstruction, tidal flushing of the genitals by dampness, water buildup leading to bulging disorder, clear, watery discharges, seminal emissions, impotence, or gradual weight gain.

2. Stagnation and lingering of excess fluids in the exterior, manifesting as aversion to cold, aches and pains in the body and extremities, or edema. If symptoms of yang deficiency predominate and the exterior is not secured, there will be sweating, the person will easily catch colds and infections, be prone to allergies, or wind erysipelas and dormant papules.

3. Joint disorders of the Kidneys and Spleen, where the ascending and descending functions are disordered. This can manifest as abdominal fullness or pain, nausea, vomiting, diarrhea, or constipation.

4. Clogging and stagnation of the Liver channel manifesting as flank pain, dizziness and vertigo, twitching of the muscles and sinews, atrophy or aching of the muscles, or hiccup.

5. Water qi intimidating the Heart, manifesting as chest painful obstruction, palpitations, and disordered mental and emotional functions.

6. Water flooding the upper source, manifesting as wheezing and coughing.

7. Phlegm fluids and water-dampness attacking the clear yang above, clogging and obstructing the sensory orifices. This may manifest as lightheadedness, a distending or heavy sensation in the head, headaches, hair loss, impaired memory, nasal obstruction with clear nasal mucus, incessant sneezing, impaired visual acuity, or swelling and pain of teeth or gums.

8. Impairment of qi transformation leading to dampness stagnating in the vessels and blood vessels. This may manifest as a husky voice, a sensation of something being stuck in the throat, a puffy tongue body, a greasy white tongue coating, and a pulse that has no fixed form or shape.

Controversies about the Ingredients

Some commentators have questioned the use of Paeoniae Radix *(sháo yào)* in this formula, which is generally taken to be Paeoniae Radix alba *(bái sháo)*. They argue that in patients with yang deficiency and the overflow of water, the sour, binding properties of Paeoniae Radix alba *(bái sháo)* might further aggravate the retention of water. Those who support its inclusion in the formula refer to three important properties of the herb. First, several ancient texts, including *Divine Husbandman's Classic of the Materia Medica*, state that Paeoniae Radix *(sháo yào)* is able to promote urination and move water. This property is enhanced when it is combined with Poria *(fú líng)* and Atractylodis macrocephalae Rhizoma *(bái zhú)*. Second, Paeoniae Radix *(sháo yào)* augments the yin, softens the Liver, and moderates abdominal pain. The Liver is responsible for dredging and draining, which includes keeping open the waterways. Abdominal pain is a symptom in the formula's patterns. Third, while Paeoniae Radix *(sháo yào)* prevents injury to the yin by checking the drying action of the herbs that drain dampness, its own binding nature is moderated by the other herbs in this formula. Rather than causing the pathogenic water to accumulate or stagnate, these synergistic interactions elevate Paeoniae Radix *(sháo yào)* to an essential ingredient. Moreover, because this formula is also indicated for cases in which the protective yang qi is depleted by excessive sweating, Paeoniae Radix alba *(bái sháo)* serves to restrain the sweating in the same manner as it does in Cinnamon Twig Decoction *(guì zhī tāng)*.

Other commentators question why Zingiberis Rhizoma recens *(shēng jiāng)*, rather than the more heating Zingiberis Rhizoma *(gān jiāng)*, is used in a formula intended to mobilize the yang. They point to the combination of Aconiti Radix lateralis praeparata *(zhì fù zǐ)* and Zingiberis Rhizoma *(gān jiāng)* in Frigid Extremities Decoction *(sì nì tāng)*, which is the flagship formula for lesser yin patterns. However, whereas the intention of that formula is to mobilize the yang in the channels for which a heating substance is preferable, the focus of this formula is on moving excessive water qi out of the body. For this purposes, the more acrid and moving (but less heating) Zingiberis Rhizoma recens *(shēng jiāng)* is more appropriate. In fact, Zingiberis Rhizoma recens *(shēng jiāng)* is used in many of Zhang Zhong-Jing's formulas whenever this is the objective.

Comparisons

➤ Vs. Poria, Cinnamon Twig, Atractylodes, and Licorice Decoction *(líng guì zhú gān tāng)*

Both formulas warm the yang, promote water metabolism, include Poria *(fú líng)* and Atractylodis macrocephalae Rhizoma *(bái zhú)*, and are used for internal stoppage of water and qi in patients with yang deficiency, which can lead to a wide variety of problems, including dizziness. However, True Warrior Decoction *(zhēn wǔ tāng)* is for a problem focused on the lower burner and Kidneys, marked by more significant urinary difficulty, edema, a tongue that is swollen, pale, or dark with tooth marks and a white, slippery coating, and a pulse that is submerged, thin, and forceless. By contrast, Poria, Cinnamon Twig, Atractylodes, and Licorice Decoction *(líng guì zhú gān tāng)* is for problems that focus more on the middle burner or Spleen, marked by fullness in the chest and hypochondria, shortness of breath, a tongue that is pale and swollen with a white, greasy coating, and a pulse that is slippery and may be wiry.

➤ Vs. Dredging and Cutting Drink *(shū záo yǐn zi)*; *see* page 96

➤ Vs. Aconite Accessory Root Decoction *(fù zǐ tāng)*; *see* page 749

➤ Vs. Bolster the Spleen Drink *(shí pí yǐn)*; *see* page 751

➤ Vs. Kidney Qi Pill *(shèn qì wán)*; *see* page 399

➤ Vs. Frigid Extremities Decoction *(sì nì tāng)*; *see* page 276

Biomedical Indications

With the appropriate presentation, this formula may be used to treat a very wide variety of biomedically-defined disorders. These can be divided into the following groups:

- Disorders marked by edema and other types of swellings such as congestive heart failure, chronic glomerulonephritis, hyperaldosteronism, hypothyroidism, ascites from cirrhosis, Ménière's disease, chronic pelvic inflammatory disease with effusion, and rheumatoid arthritis with joint effusion

- Disorders marked by dizziness such as hypertension, orthostatic hypotension, carbon monoxide poisoning, basilar insufficiency, and postconcussion syndrome

- Disorders marked by pain such as osteoarthritis, sciatica, lumbar disc disease, piriformis syndrome, trigeminal neuralgia, and postconcussion headache

This formula has also been used for chronic bronchitis, cor pulmonare, essential tremors, facial tics, prostatitis, benign prostatic hypertrophy, allergic rhinitis, chronic sinusitis, scrotal eczema, and prolapsed uterus.

Alternate names

Dark Warrior Decoction *(xuán wǔ tāng)* in *Supplement to Important Formulas Worth a Thousand Gold Pieces;* Secure the Yang Decoction *(gù yáng tāng)* in *Simple Book of Formulas*

Modifications

- For more pronounced Spleen yang deficiency with diarrhea, remove Paeoniae Radix alba *(bái sháo)* and add Zingiberis Rhizoma *(gān jiāng)*.

- For coughing, add Schisandrae Fructus *(wǔ wèi zǐ)*, Asari Radix et Rhizoma *(xì xīn)*, and Zingiberis Rhizoma *(gān jiāng)*.

- For urinary frequency, remove Poria *(fú líng)*.

- For palpitations due to source qi deficiency, add Ginseng Radix *(rén shēn)*.

- For palpitations, wheezing, or coughing with copious, watery sputum, add Asari Radix et Rhizoma *(xì xīn)* and Schisandrae Fructus *(wǔ wèi zǐ)*.

- For unremitting spontaneous sweating due to yang deficiency and instability of the exterior, add Ginseng Radix *(rén shēn)*, Astragali Radix *(huáng qí)*, and Schisandrae Fructus *(wǔ wèi zǐ)*.

- For vomiting due to retention of pathogenic water in the Stomach with no signs of lower burner dysfunction, remove Aconiti Radix lateralis praeparata *(zhì fù zǐ)* to avoid irritation of the Stomach and increase the dosage of Zingiberis Rhizoma recens *(shēng jiāng)*.

- For painful obstruction of the chest, add Trichosanthis Semen *(guā lóu rén)*, Allii macrostemi Bulbus *(xiè bái)*, Cinnamomi Ramulus *(guì zhī)*, and Salviae miltiorrhizae Radix *(dān shēn)*.

- For improper purging that has injured the Spleen yang and caused abdominal distention, add Magnoliae officinalis Cortex *(hòu pò)*, Alpiniae katsumadai Semen *(cǎo dòu kòu)*, and Alismatis Rhizoma *(zé xiè)*.

- For leukorrhea due to cold-dampness, add Cinnamomi Ramulus *(guì zhī)* and Codonopsis Radix *(dǎng shēn)*.

- For urinary difficulty, aching and heaviness in the extremities, and edema, take with Powder for Five Types of Painful Urinary Dribbling *(wǔ lín sǎn)* or Stephania and Astragalus Decoction *(fáng jǐ huáng qí tāng)*.

- For edema due to chronic nephrotic syndrome, add Codonopsis Radix *(dǎng shēn)*, Amomi Fructus *(shā rén)*, Eucommiae Cortex *(dù zhòng)*, Cuscutae Semen *(tù sī zǐ)*, and Epimedii Herba *(yín yáng huò)*.

- For edema due to chronic heart failure with yang deficiency, add Plantaginis Semen *(chē qián zǐ)*, Alismatis Rhizoma *(zé xiè)*, and Stephaniae tetrandrae Radix *(hàn fáng jǐ)*.

- For ascites due to liver cirrhosis with Spleen and Kidney yang deficiency, add Codonopsis Radix *(dǎng shēn)*, Astragali Radix *(huáng qí)*, Morindae officinalis Radix *(bā jǐ tiān)*, Trigonelle Semen *(hú lú bā)*, and Cervi Cornu *(lù jiǎo)*.

- For rheumatoid arthritis, add Cinnamomi Ramulus *(guì zhī)* and Codonopsis Radix *(dǎng shēn)*.

- For chronic bronchitis with Spleen and Kidney yang deficiency, substitute Zingiberis Rhizoma *(gān jiāng)* for Zingiberis Rhizoma recens *(shēng jiāng)*.

附子湯（附子汤）

Aconite Accessory Root Decoction

fù zǐ tāng

Source   *Discussion of Cold Damage* (c. 220)

baked Aconiti Radix lateralis *(bāo fù zǐ)* . . . . 2 pieces (12-18g)
Atractylodis macrocephalae Rhizoma *(bái zhú)* 12g
Ginseng Radix *(rén shēn)* 6g
Poria *(fú líng)* 9g
Paeoniae Radix alba *(bái sháo)* 9g

Method of Preparation   Decoction. The source text advises to decoct using 8 cups of water until 3 cups remain; strain, and divide into three doses over the course of a day. Each dose should be taken warm. At present, Paeoniae Radix alba *(bái sháo)* is the most common form of Paeoniae Radix *(sháo yào)* used; Aconiti Radix lateralis praeparata *(zhì fù zǐ)* is decocted for 30-60 minutes prior to the addition of the other herbs, and the

entire formula should be cooked until the strained decoction can be tasted without any numbing sensation of the tongue.

Actions   Warms the channels, assists the yang, dispels cold, and transforms dampness

Indications

Generalized body pain, aching bones and joints, aversion to cold especially at the back, cold extremities, no thirst, a white, slippery tongue coating, and a submerged, faint, and forceless or a choppy, slow pulse.

Also used for abdominal distention and pain during late pregnancy with aversion to cold. There is lower abdominal pain and cold in which the abdomen feels as chilled as if it were being fanned. These symptoms are accompanied by fever and a wiry pulse.

This is yang deficiency with internal cold-dampness harassing the interior and obstructing the channels. According to the source text, this is one possible manifestation of a lesser yin disorder. The lesser yin warp functions as the 'hinge' of the interior. This conveys an image of movement and change. The lesser yin warp embodies the potential for movement and transformation made possible by the diffusion of yang qi, the fire at the gate of vitality, throughout the entire organism. Among the organs, it relates to the Kidneys and Heart, one located below, the other above. If the Heart and Kidneys communicate with each other, the yang qi is active throughout the body. If the yang qi is deficient and its diffusion blocked by cold-dampness, there will be generalized body pain. Because the Kidneys relate to the bones, this obstruction leads to aching bones and joints. The yang qi is diffused through the Governing vessel, which reaches upward from the coccyx to the neck, and is dispersed on the outside through the greater yang. If cold-dampness obstructs this diffusion, there will be aversion to cold, especially at the back, and the extremities will become cold. The absence of thirst allows the physician to distinguish this pattern from greater yang and yang brightness disorders manifesting with similar symptoms, as discussed in the COMMENTARY below. The slippery tongue coating and the pulse reflect the nature of the pathology.

Essentials of the Golden Cabinet prescribes this formula for abdominal pain during pregnancy due to internal cold. This occurs in yang deficient women whose yang qi is progressively exhausted over the course of the pregnancy. As a result, wind-cold invades the Womb from the outside leading to lower abdominal pain and an aversion to wind. The wiry pulse reflects stagnation due to cold. While there is fever, it is likely to be low-grade, reflecting the floating outward of false yang rather than the constraint of yang in the exterior that is seen in greater yang patterns.

Analysis of Formula

The formula uses a large dosage of Aconiti Radix lateralis praeparata *(zhì fù zǐ)* as its chief herb to warm the interior and disperse cold. Its heating nature penetrates into the gate of vitality to invigorate the yang, while its acridity disperses cold from all twelve channels. As noted by Zhang Jie-Bin: "[Aconiti Radix lateralis praeparata (zhì fù zǐ)] is an essential herb for yin-type patterns. In all cases of cold damage that transmit or transform into [disorders of one of] the three yin [warps] as well as in [direct] cold strike into the yin [warps], if the pulse is submerged, it must be used even if there is high fever." Atractylodis macrocephalae Rhizoma (bái zhú) and Poria (fú líng) are used as deputies to strengthen the Spleen, promote urination, and provide a route for the dampness to exit the body. Sweet and warming Ginseng Radix (rén shēn) functions as an assistant. It strongly tonifies the original qi but also generates fluids, providing the organism with a basis for reestablishing normal physiological functioning. Paeoniae Radix (sháo yào), which is frequently combined with Aconiti Radix lateralis praeparata (zhì fù zǐ) in the treatment of lesser yin disorders, is the second assistant. Although it is cooling and restrains the yin, these actions complement, rather than inhibit, those of the chief herb. Nourishing the yin provides a substratum to which the yang generated by Aconiti Radix lateralis praeparata (zhì fù zǐ) can attach itself, keeping it in the interior and preventing it from dissipating to the outside.

Cautions and Contraindications

If not properly prepared, the main ingredient of this formula is toxic. For this reason, only the prepared form should be used and then cooked appropriately.

Commentary

Although this formula focuses on warming the interior, it is effective in unblocking the channels and stopping pain. It does this by combining a large dosage of Aconiti Radix lateralis praeparata (zhì fù zǐ), which mobilizes the protective yang, with herbs that tonify and regulate the nutritive qi. According to Wang Hu in Extensive Annotations to the Differentiation of Patterns in the Discussion of Cold Damage, "[Aconiti Radix lateralis praeparata (zhì fù zǐ)] not only warms the lesser yin channels, but also travels through the protective qi and thereby treats aversion to cold in the back." This is equivalent to saying that Aconiti Radix lateralis praeparata (zhì fù zǐ) mobilizes the fire at the gate of vitality throughout the entire body. In so doing, it expels the pathogenic cold while promoting movement and the transformation of the body's own substances.

All the other herbs in the formula focus on the Spleen and the nutritive qi. The combination of Ginseng Radix (rén shēn), Atractylodis macrocephalae Rhizoma (bái zhú), and Poria (fú líng) prefigures Four-Gentlemen Decoction (sì jūn zǐ tāng), the most important formula for tonifying the Spleen and Stomach qi. Paeoniae Radix (sháo yào) also enters the Spleen to order and regulate the movement of its qi. The Spleen and Stomach are the root of the postnatal constitu-

tion, and, in particular, of the nutritive qi. The nutritive qi is the most substantive of the various types of qi and its pathology is intimately tied to dampness, as explained by Zhou Xue-Hai in Random Notes while Reading about Medicine:

> The nutritive qi is damp qi. When it follows the vessels, they are made slippery and smooth; when it emits to the skin, it is filled and moistened. … Therefore, the protective qi encompasses heat and cold disorders, the nutritive qi dampness and dryness disorders.

By tonifying the Spleen, dispelling dampness and generating fluids, the deputy and assistant herbs order the quality and movement of the nutritive qi—which in the present case has become too wet—and thereby draw the heating action of Aconiti Radix lateralis praeparata (zhì fù zǐ) to this level.

An explanation that focuses on the formula's action in relation to these different types of qi also holds the key to understanding why Paeoniae Radix (sháo yào) is an essential element in this and similar formulas, such as True Warrior Decoction (zhēn wǔ tāng), discussed above, as well as in the various formulas based on Cinnamon Twig Decoction (guì zhī tāng). By tonifying the Spleen and harmonizing the nutritive qi, Paeoniae Radix (sháo yào) augments the substratum to which the protective qi, mobilized by heating herbs like Aconiti Radix lateralis praeparata (zhì fù zǐ) or Cinnamomi Ramulus (guì zhī), can attach itself. The herb's sourness stabilizes this interpenetration, preventing the protective yang from dispersing to the exterior, while its coolness moderates the heat that would otherwise cause dryness.

The same dynamic—mobilizing the protective qi while harmonizing the nutritive qi—allows this formula to be used to treat lower abdominal pain due to the invasion of wind-cold in pregnancy. Normally, a strongly heating herb like Aconiti Radix lateralis praeparata (zhì fù zǐ) is contraindicated in pregnancy, as it may induce a miscarriage. In the present case, however, its use is necessary because of the presence of cold, while its action is moderated by the tonification of blood and Spleen functions. The Qing-dynasty physician Zhang Lu observed: "[This formula] employs Aconite Accessory Root Decoction (fù zǐ tāng) to warm the Womb. Generations of people have considered Aconiti Radix lateralis praeparata (zhì fù zǐ) to be the most abortifacient of all the herbs. Only [Zhang] Zhong-Jing uses it as a sagely herb for calming the fetus. Were it not for [such a] spirit to have understood [such usage], how could this be attempted lightly?"

Usage

Over time, physicians expanded the use of this formula to a variety of other patterns including wind-stroke, severe painful obstruction patterns, cold damage with high fever but severe fatigue, and exhaustion in the wake of cold damage disorders. In terms of diagnosis, the absence of thirst or any other abnormal symptoms in the mouth such as bitterness and sensitivity to cold in the back is of key significance in differentiating Aconite Accessory Root Decoction (*fù zǐ tāng*) patterns from similar ones occurring in the course of greater yang or yang brightness disorders. Chilliness of the back in greater yang disorders is due to constraint of the yang qi in the exterior. It will be accompanied by fever, headache, and a floating rather than a submerged pulse. There may be thirst as a result of body fluids failing to disperse. In yang brightness disorders, chilliness of the back may occur as a result of constraint of the yang qi in the interior by pathogenic heat. It will be accompanied by fever, sweating, irritability, and thirst.

Comparison

➤ Vs. True Warrior Decoction (*zhēn wǔ tāng*)

Both formulas combine Aconiti Radix lateralis praeparata (*zhì fù zǐ*), Atractylodis macrocephalae Rhizoma (*bái zhú*), Poria (*fú líng*), and Paeoniae Radix (*sháo yào*) to treat lesser yin disorders characterized by cold in the interior. True Warrior Decoction (*zhēn wǔ tāng*) adds Zingiberis Rhizoma recens (*shēng jiāng*) to focus on reducing the edema and treating the flooding of water. By contrast, Aconite Accessory Root Decoction (*fù zǐ tang*) adds Ginseng Radix (*rén shēn*) to tonify the nutritive qi and focus on treating body aches.

Biomedical Indications

With the appropriate presentation, this formula may be used to treat a variety of biomedically-defined disorders including migraine, cluster headache, trigeminal neuralgia, Bell's palsy, piriformis syndrome, rheumatoid arthritis, cervical spine disease, periarthritis of the shoulder, ankylosing spondylitis, lumbar disc disease, essential tremor, chronic nephritis, nephrotic syndrome, cirrhosis, chronic bronchitis, cardiac disease, congestive heart failure, uterine prolapse, and erectile dysfunction.

Modifications

- To improve the formula's capacity for dispelling wind-dampness, add Notopterygii Rhizoma seu Radix (*qiāng huó*), Angelicae pubescentis Radix (*dú huó*), Clematidis Radix (*wēi líng xiān*), and Siegesbeckiae Herba (*xī xiān cǎo*).
- For more severe cold-dampness, add Cinnamomi Ramulus (*guì zhī*) and Aconiti Radix praeparata (*zhì chuān wū*).
- For chronic painful obstruction leading to blood stasis, add Myrrha (*mò yào*) and Olibanum (*rǔ xiāng*).

Associated Formula

甘草附子湯 （甘草附子汤）

Licorice and Aconite Accessory Root Decoction
gān cǎo fù zǐ tāng

Source　*Discussion of Cold Damage* (c. 220)

Glycyrrhizae Radix praeparata (*zhì gān cǎo*) 6g
Aconiti Radix lateralis praeparata (*zhì fù zǐ*) . . . . 2 pieces (12-15g)
Atractylodis macrocephalae Rhizoma (*bái zhú*) 6g
Cinnamomi Ramulus (*guì zhī*) 12g

Decoction. The source text recommends taking the decoction in three doses over the course of the day. Production of a mild sweat soon after taking the decoction indicates that the condition is being resolved.

For deep-seated pain in the bones and joints due to wind-dampness with restriction of movement and aggravation on pressure. Accompanying symptoms include sweating, shortness of breath, inhibited urination, aversion to wind with disinclination to take off one's clothes, or slight edema. A distinguishing feature of the pattern, according to the modern physician Araki Shō in *Medicine Bag of Classic Formulas,* is the presence of constipation, which indicates that wind-dampness has obstructed the qi dynamic. There is no heat, so while the stools are not dry, there will only be a bowel movement every 2–3 days. Although the source text attributes the disorder to wind-dampness, the symptomatology and the formula's composition make it clear that cold is an equally important contributing factor. 'Disinclination to take off one's clothes' is thus often interpreted as aversion to wind and cold in the back due to obstruction of the greater yang.

In contemporary clinical practice, this formula is used to treat severe pain associated with disorders such as acute polyarthritis, brachial neuritis, ankylosing spondylitis, prolapsed intervertebral discs, sciatica, and similar painful inflammatory disorders. It has also been used to treat colds, allergic rhinitis, rheumatic heart disease, chronic coronary insufficiency, and intractable spontaneous sweating.

Unlike the pain treated by Peony and Licorice Decoction (*sháo yào gān cǎo tāng*), one does not normally find muscle spasms associated with this pattern. Maidservant from Yue Decoction plus Atractylodes (*Yuè bì jiā zhú tāng*) similarly treats pain due to wind-cold-dampness, but its associated patterns are distinguished by the presence of heat manifesting as thirst, irritability, or a slippery, rapid pulse.

實脾飲 （实脾饮）

Bolster the Spleen Drink
shí pí yǐn

Source　*Formulas to Aid the Living* (1253)

baked Aconiti Radix lateralis (*bāo fù zǐ*) 30g
Zingiberis Rhizoma praeparatum (*páo jiāng*) 30g
Poria (*fú líng*) 30g
Atractylodis macrocephalae Rhizoma (*bái zhú*) 30g
Chaenomelis Fructus (*mù guā*) 30g
ginger-fried Magnoliae officinalis Cortex (*jiāng chǎo hòu pò*) 30g
Aucklandiae Radix (*mù xiāng*) 30g
Arecae Pericarpium (*dà fù pí*) 30g
Tsaoko Fructus (*cǎo guǒ*) 30g
Glycyrrhizae Radix praeparata (*zhì gān cǎo*) 15g

Method of Preparation　The source text advises to grind the ingredients into a powder and take as a draft in 12g doses with 5 slices of Zingiberis Rhizoma recens (*shēng jiāng*) and 1 piece of Jujubae Fructus (*dà zǎo*). At present, it is usually prepared as a decoction with one-fifth the specified dosage of the ingredients, plus the additional herbs mentioned here. The original formula contains Arecae Semen (*bīng láng*), but because of its harsh actions, Arecae Pericarpium (*dà fù pí*) is usually substituted.

Actions   Warms the yang, strengthens the Spleen, moves the qi, and promotes urination

Indications

Generalized edema that is more severe below the waist, cold extremities, chest and abdominal fullness and distention, a heavy sensation in the body, loss of appetite, absence of thirst, scanty urine, semiliquid, unformed stools, a thick, greasy tongue coating, and a submerged, slow or submerged, thin pulse.

This is yin-type edema due to Spleen and Kidney yang deficiency. The incapacity of the yang qi to transform water leads to internal accumulation of water and dampness. It is the nature of water to descend; when it accumulates, it causes edema that is more severe below the waist. This is almost always pitting edema. When the yang qi is deficient, it impedes the ability of the Spleen to warm the extremities. The accumulation of water and dampness obstructs the qi mechanism, producing chest and abdominal fullness and distention and a heavy sensation in the body. Loss of appetite, absence of thirst, scanty urine, semiliquid, unformed stools, the thick, greasy tongue coating, and the submerged, slow or submerged, thin pulse are all manifestations of Spleen and Kidney yang deficiency and obstruction due to the accumulation of dampness.

Analysis of Formula

This is a representative formula for the treatment of yin-type edema due to Spleen and Kidney yang deficiency. One treats a condition such as this by warming the yang and bolstering the Spleen while simultaneously promoting the water metabolism in order to eliminate the pathogenic water. For this reason, Aconiti Radix lateralis praeparata (*zhì fù zǐ*) and Zingiberis Rhizoma (*gān jiāng*) serve as the chief herbs in the formula. Zingiberis Rhizoma (*gān jiāng*) warms and promotes the movement of Spleen yang to invigorate the transportive processes in the middle burner, and the Spleen yang's ability to transform and transport water and dampness. It is very hot in nature but is not toxic. Because its action is confined primarily to the middle burner, it is used in almost every case involving a cold, deficient Stomach pattern. Aconiti Radix lateralis praeparata (*zhì fù zǐ*), on the other hand, is acrid and very hot in nature. It tends to travel throughout the body unblocking and promoting the movement of yang qi in all twelve channels. It also tonifies the fire at the gate of vitality. It is therefore very effective in overcoming stagnation from the accumulation of yin (water). Together, these herbs work synergistically to warm and nourish the Spleen and Kidneys, supporting the yang and curbing the yin.

The deputies, Poria (*fú líng*) and Atractylodis macrocephalae Rhizoma (*bái zhú*), strengthen the Spleen and resolve dampness by promoting urination. Aromatic Chaenomelis Fructus (*mù guā*), an assistant herb, revives the Spleen, transforms dampness, and promotes urination to strengthen the Spleen's transporting and transforming functions. The other assistants, Magnoliae officinalis Cortex (*hòu pò*), Aucklandiae Radix (*mù xiāng*), Arecae Pericarpium (*dà fù pí*), and Tsaoko Fructus (*cǎo guǒ*), direct the qi downward, guide out stagnation, transform dampness, and circulate the fluid. Arecae Pericarpium (*dà fù pí*) also promotes the movement of qi, promotes urination, and reduces edema. Once the circulation of qi is restored, dampness will be transformed. The envoys, Glycyrrhizae Radix praeparata (*zhì gān cǎo*), Zingiberis Rhizoma recens (*shēng jiāng*), and Jujubae Fructus (*dà zǎo*), regulate and harmonize the other herbs, benefit the Spleen, and harmonize the middle burner.

Cautions and Contraindications

This formula is strongly warming and moving. It is contraindicated for the treatment of any kind of yang-type edema.

Commentary

This is a variation of Aconite Accessory Root Pill to Regulate the Middle (*fù zǐ lǐ zhōng wán*) to which herbs that move the qi, dry dampness, and warm the middle have been added. Focusing on firming the Spleen, it has become the representative formula in the treatment of yin-type edema. The differentiation of yin- and yang-type edema is explained by Zhu Dan-Xi in *Essential Teachings of [Zhu] Dan-Xi*:

> Generally, if swelling of the body [is accompanied by] irritability, thirst, red and rough urination, and bowel blockage, it is yang edema. … If it is not [accompanied] by irritability and thirst, the stools are semiliquid, urination is reduced and is neither rough nor red, then it is yin edema.

A passage in Chapter 74 of *Basic Questions* observes: "All dampness, swelling, and distention pertains to the Spleen." In fact, Spleen earth has an important function in the regulation of water in the body. According to five-phase theory, earth controls water. Within the body, the earth exerts this control via its regulation of the qi dynamic, as explained in *Golden Mirror of the Medical Tradition* : "Qi is the mother of water. Earth is the embankment for water. If qi moves, water moves. If earth is strong, water is regulated. Hence, the reference to bolstering the Spleen." By tonifying the Spleen yang and moving the Spleen qi, the formula effectively supports earth's control over water. It is thus indicated specifically for conditions characterized by exuberance of cold in the interior that impedes the Spleen's functions of transportation and transformation. *Golden Mirror of the Medical Tradition* also notes that, in patterns characterized by more pronounced qi deficiency and less stagnation, the moving herbs may be left out.

Comparison

> ➤ Vs. True Warrior Decoction *(zhēn wǔ tāng)*

Although both formulas warm the Spleen and Kidneys and support the yang in circulating the fluids, each has a different focus. True Warrior Decoction *(zhēn wǔ tāng)* focuses on warming the Kidneys. It warms the yang, preserves the yin, promotes urination, and relaxes spasms. It is thus a very important formula for treating fluid retention due to yang deficiency characterized by abdominal pain and shivering. Bolster the Spleen Drink *(shí pí yǐn)*, on the other hand, focuses on warming the Spleen. Its ability to support the yang and dispel cold is slightly stronger than True Warrior Decoction *(zhēn wǔ tāng)*. It promotes the movement of qi and transforms stagnation, and is therefore an important formula for treating yang deficiency edema characterized by chest and abdominal fullness and distention.

Biomedical Indications

With the appropriate presentation, this formula may be used to treat a variety of biomedically-defined disorders including chronic nephritis, rheumatic valvular heart disease, congestive heart failure, and cirrhosis or other chronic hepatic disorders.

. . . .

Alternate name

Bolster the Spleen Drink *(shí pí yǐn)* in *Indispensable Tools for Pattern Treatment*

. . . .

Modifications

- For qi deficiency characterized by shortness of breath, fatigue, and disinclination to talk, add Codonopsis Radix *(dǎng shēn)* and Astragali Radix *(huáng qí)*.
- For scanty urine and severe edema, add Alismatis Rhizoma *(zé xiè)* and Polyporus *(zhū líng)*.
- For abdominal distention, add Citri reticulatae Pericarpium *(chén pí)* and Amomi Fructus *(shā rén)*.
- In case of proteinuria, add Pyrolae Herba *(lù xián cǎo)* and Euryales Semen *(qiàn shí)*.
- For palpitations, increase the dosage of Aconiti Radix lateralis praeparata *(zhì fù zǐ)* and add Fossilia Ossis Mastodi *(lóng gǔ)* and Magnetitum *(cí shí)*.
- For painful distention of the liver area, add Citri reticulatae viride Pericarpium *(qīng pí)*, Sparganii Rhizoma *(sān léng)*, and Curcumae Rhizoma *(é zhú)*.
- For ascites due to liver cirrhosis, add Codonopsis Radix *(dǎng shēn)*, Alismatis Rhizoma *(zé xiè)*, Curcumae Radix *(yù jīn)*, and Citri reticulatae Pericarpium *(chén pí)*.
- For constipation, add Pharbitidis Semen *(qiān niú zǐ)*.

萆薢分清飲（萆薢分清饮）

Tokoro Drink to Separate the Clear

bì xiè fēn qīng yǐn

This formula is so named because it treats cloudy painful urinary dribbling by strengthening the transforming function of the qi, thereby restoring its ability to separate the clear from the turbid.

Source   *Yang Family Formulas* (1178)

Dioscoreae hypoglaucae Rhizoma *(bì xiè)* 9-12g
Alpiniae oxyphyllae Fructus *(yì zhì rén)* 9g
Linderae Radix *(wū yào)* 9g
Acori tatarinowii Rhizoma *(shí chāng pú)* 9g

Method of Preparation   The source text advises to grind equal amounts of the ingredients into a powder and take as a draft in 12g doses with a small amount of salt. At present, it is usually prepared as a decoction with the dosage specified.

Actions   Warms the Kidneys, promotes the resolution of dampness, separates out the clear, and transforms the turbid

Indications

Urinary frequency with cloudy, dense, milky (resembling rice water), or greasy urine.

This is cloudy painful urinary dribbling (膏淋 *gāo lín*) due to cold from deficiency in the lower burner, which causes turbid dampness to pour downward. When the Kidney qi is deficient and weak, it is unable to stabilize or restrain the water, and thus fails to assist the Bladder in retaining the urine. This leads to frequent urination. The turbid, pale, or whitish appearance of the urine is due to Kidney and Bladder yang unable to separate the clear from the turbid in water. However, it also involves deficiency of the middle burner, which is dependent on the Kidney yang for its functioning, as explained by Zhang Jie-Bin in *Collected Treatises of [Zhang] Jing-Yue*: "In painful urinary dribbling disorders that persist for a long time, pain and roughness [on urination] disappear but a cloudy fluid remains. Painful urinary dribbling [characterized by] white, turbid [urine] is a pattern due to the downward collapse of middle burner qi and instability at the gate of vitality."

Analysis of Formula

Warming the Kidneys assists the Bladder in properly storing and releasing the urine, which in turn alleviates dampness and discharges the turbid water. The chief herb, bitter and neutral Dioscoreae hypoglaucae Rhizoma *(bì xiè)*, enters the Bladder, Liver, and Stomach channels. It excels at eliminating dampness by promoting the separation of the turbid from the pure fluids and directing the turbid fluids out through the Bladder. It is thus one of the most important herbs in the treatment of cloudy urinary difficulty or vaginal discharge.

The deputy, acrid and aromatic Alpiniae oxyphyllae Fructus (*yì zhì rén*), warms the Spleen and Stomach to harmonize the middle, and the Kidney yang to secure the lower burner. It thereby reduces the frequency of urination and stabilizes the qi. Together, the chief and deputy herbs moderate each other's actions so as to restrain the loss of primal qi in the lower burner, while promoting the expulsion of turbid dampness through the urine and thus eliminate the turbid damp qi. The flow of water also requires the movement of qi. Linderae Radix (*wū yào*), an assistant, warms the Kidneys and promotes the movement of qi and the transformation of water. The other assistant, warm and acrid Acori tatarinowii Rhizoma (*shí chāng pú*), transforms turbidity and eliminates dampness and cold from deficiency in the Bladder.

Cautions and Contraindications

This formula should not be used in treating cloudy painful urinary dribbling characterized by milky, turbid urine due to an accumulation of damp-heat in the Bladder.

Commentary

Discussion of the formula in the source text is followed by the sentence, "One [variation of this] formula adds Poria (*fú líng*) and Glycyrrhizae Radix (*gān cǎo*)." Addition of these herbs focuses the action of the formula even more strongly on the middle burner to promote the resolution of dampness and the transformation of turbidity. The addition of salt to the draft guides the formula into the Kidneys.

Most classical and contemporary commentators refer to the pattern treated by this formula as cloudy painful urinary dribbling (膏淋 *gāo lín*) disorder. In clinical practice, these patterns may be due to damp-heat as well as cold-dampness. The present formula focuses on cold-dampness. A variation, Tokoro Drink to Separate the Clear from *Awakening of the Mind in Medical Studies* (*bì xiè fēn qīng yǐn*), discussed as an ASSOCIATED FORMULA below, treats damp-heat patterns. Because the appearance of cloudy urine need not be accompanied by pain, the contemporary physician Ding Xue-Ping differentiates further between painful urinary dribbling (淋 *lín*) and turbid urine (濁 *zhuó*):

> Painful urinary dribbling and turbid urine are really two different patterns. Their causes are different and their treatment [requires] strategies that are not alike. The ancient master Ye Tian-Shi has explained this most conclusively. [He stated]: 'Painful urinary dribbling is attributed to the Liver and Gallbladder. Turbidity is attributed to the Heart and Kidneys.' With respect to the two Tokoro Drink to Separate the Clear (*bì xiè fēn qīng yǐn*) formulas, that from *Essential Teachings of [Zhu] Dan-Xi* focuses on treating the Kidneys. [For this purpose,] it uses herbs specific for warming and containing, assisted by [those] that separate [the clear] and promote resolution [of the turbid]. The formula from *Awakening of the Mind in Medical Studies* instead focuses on treating the Heart. Bitter herbs enter

the Heart. The Small Intestine is the fire yang organ. Without bitter [herbs,] it cannot be unblocked. Thus, in using herbs [the formula] aims at bitter draining, [while those that] separate [the clear] and promote resolution [of the turbid here] function also as assistants and envoys.

If Ding Xue-Ping's perspective differs from the textbook consensus, it nonetheless provides a useful framework for devising treatment strategies in the clinic. One can differentiate between problems of function/movement caused by the stagnation of qi/dampness and blood/heat (attributed to the Liver and Gallbladder, which govern the coursing of qi and blood), and problems of substance caused by the failure of transformation (attributed to the Kidneys and Heart, which govern the transformation of qi and blood).

Note: The term 淋 *lín* is translated as 'painful urinary dribbling' because diseases for which this term is used are marked by both urinary dribbling and pain or discomfort. However, it is important to note that in some of the later stages of these problems, frank pain is no longer present.

Biomedical Indications

With the appropriate presentation, this formula may be used to treat a variety of biomedically-defined disorders including chronic prostatitis, nephrotic syndrome, acute exacerbations of chronic pyelonephritis, chronic pelvic inflammatory disease, and trichomoniasis.

....

Alternate names

In the source text this formula is called Tokoro Powder to Separate the Clear (草薢分清散 *bì xiè fēn qīng sǎn*). It was listed under the present name in *Essential Teachings of [Zhu] Dan-Xi*, from whence its popularity derives. Other names include Powder for Separating the Clear (*fēn qīng sǎn*) in *Formulas to Aid the Living*; Drink for Separating the Clear (*fēn qīng yǐn*) in *Experiential Formulas from the Auspicious Bamboo Hall*; Tokoro Drink (*bì xiè yǐn*) in *Medical Mirror of Past and Present*; and Tokoro Powder (*bì xiè sǎn*) in *Achieving Longevity by Guarding the Source*.

....

Modifications

- To strengthen the actions of draining dampness and transforming turbidity, add Poria (*fú líng*) and Glycyrrhizae Radix (*gān cǎo*).

- For qi deficiency of the middle burner, add Codonopsis Radix (*dǎng shēn*), Atractylodis macrocephalae Rhizoma (*bái zhú*), Poria (*fú líng*), and Glycyrrhizae Radix praeparata (*zhì gān cǎo*).

- For leukorrhea due to cold-dampness, add Aconiti Radix lateralis praeparata (*zhì fù zǐ*), Cinnamomi Cortex (*ròu guì*), Cuscutae Semen (*tù sī zǐ*), Atractylodis Rhizoma (*cāng zhú*), and Poria (*fú líng*).

- For chronic prostatitis with chyluria, add Cuscutae Semen (*tù sī zǐ*), Ligustri lucidi Fructus (*nǚ zhēn zǐ*), Lysimachiae Herba (*jīn qián cǎo*), and Plantaginis Semen (*chē qián zǐ*).

Associated Formula

萆薢分清飲 (萆薢分清饮)

Tokoro Drink to Separate the Clear from *Awakening of the Mind in Medical Studies*

bì xiè fēn qīng yǐn

SOURCE *Awakening of the Mind in Medical Studies* (1732)

Dioscoreae hypoglaucae Rhizoma *(bì xiè)* 6g
dry-fried Phellodendri Cortex *(chǎo huáng bǎi)* 1.5g
Acori tatarinowii Rhizoma *(shí chāng pǔ)* .1.5g
Poria *(fú líng)* 3g
Atractylodis macrocephalae Rhizoma *(bái zhú)* 3g
Salviae miltiorrhizae Radix *(dān shēn)* 4.5g
Plantaginis Semen *(chē qián zǐ)* 4.5g
Nelumbinis Plumula *(lián zǐ xīn)* 2.1g

Clears heat, resolves dampness, and separates the clear from the turbid. For damp-heat seeping into the Bladder which causes turbid urination with cloudy urine that continues to drip after completion, and a yellow, greasy tongue coating. The source of this heat is located in the Heart, from which it penetrates into the Bladder via the Small Intestine.

雞鳴散 (鸡鸣散)

Powder to Take at Cock's Crow

jī míng sǎn

This formula should be taken at daybreak or when the 'cock crows.' At this time of day, the yang increases, the yin diminishes, and the Stomach is empty. The increase in yang assists the body in dispelling cold-dampness, while the empty Stomach increases absorption and thus the laxative effect of the formula.

Source *Effective Medical Formulas Arranged by Category by Master Zhu* (1266)

Arecae Semen *(bīng láng)* . . . . 7 pieces (36-45g)
Chaenomelis Fructus *(mù guā)* 30g
Evodiae Fructus *(wú zhū yú)* 6g
Citri reticulatae Pericarpium *(chén pí)* 30g
Perillae Folium *(zǐ sū yè)* 9g
Platycodi Radix *(jié gěng)* 15g
Zingiberis Rhizoma recens *(shēng jiāng)* 15g

Method of Preparation The source text advises to grind the ingredients into a coarse powder and take upon waking as a draft on an empty stomach. The draft should be prepared by twice cooking the ingredients over a low flame. The liquid from both decoctions is combined into a single daily dose. At present, it is usually prepared as a decoction, reducing the dosage of the ingredients by approximately two-thirds.

Actions Promotes the movement of qi, directs turbidity downward, disseminates and transforms cold-dampness

Indications

Heavy and weak feet and calves with difficulty in walking. There may also be numbness, cold, or pain (or all three) in these areas, or spasms and up-rushing that reaches to the chest and, in severe cases, produces a stifling sensation in the chest and an overwhelming sense of nausea (泛惡 *fàn è*).

This is damp leg qi, which is caused by cold-dampness settling in the legs and feet where it clogs the channels and interrupts the smooth flow of qi and blood. Cold and dampness cause heaviness and weakness, which makes it difficult to walk. Disruption in the flow of qi and blood results in numbness, cold, or pain, depending on the relative strength of the dampness and cold. Sometimes the obstruction of the channels will force the qi upward, causing spasms and up-rushing that reaches to the chest. If the disruption in the flow of qi becomes severe, rebellious qi will develop, causing a stifling sensation in the chest and a particular type of nausea, that is, one accompanied by a sense of things overflowing from the abdomen into the throat.

Analysis of Formula

The type of leg qi treated by this formula is caused by cold-dampness clogging the channels. This requires that warming and transforming the dampness be combined with unblocking the qi dynamic. For this reason, bitter and warming Arecae Semen *(bīng láng)* is the chief herb in the formula. It breaks up stagnation, directs rebellious qi downward, and eliminates lurking pathogens; it is used here to regulate the qi and to expel the obstruction from dampness. One of the deputies, Chaenomelis Fructus *(mù guā)*, also has a descending action; it transforms dampness, relaxes the sinews, and invigorates the collaterals. Mutually reinforcing the other, the chief and deputy drive out dampness through the stool, which effectively ameliorates the edema and pain of damp leg qi. The other deputy, Citri reticulatae Pericarpium *(chén pí)*, regulates the qi and strengthens the Spleen, indirectly resolving the dampness.

Perillae Folium *(zǐ sū yè)*, one of the assistants, disperses wind-cold. The other assistant, Platycodi Radix *(jié gěng)*, unblocks and disseminates the Lung qi. When combined with Citri reticulatae Pericarpium *(chén pí)*, these herbs benefit the flow of Lung qi, which is essential to proper water metabolism. The use of these three herbs illustrates the maxim, "When the qi moves, dampness will move [out]." Evodiae Fructus *(wú zhū yú)*, one of the envoys, disperses cold and causes the turbidity to descend. When combined with Chaenomelis Fructus *(mù guā)*, it treats the nausea and stifling sensation in the chest due to the upsurge of leg qi. The other envoy, Zingiberis Rhizoma recens *(shēng jiāng)*, warms and disperses cold and thereby helps treat the leg qi. Together, the herbs in this formula open the upper burner, clear the lower burner, and spread the middle qi to produce a warming and ventilating action that encourages the elimination of turbidity.

Cautions and Contraindications

This formula should not be used without significant modification in cases of leg qi due to dryness or to damp-heat.

Commentary

Leg qi is generally divided into two types: damp and dry. Damp leg qi is indicated by swelling of the legs; dry leg qi by withering of the flesh. For more detail, see the discussion of leg qi in Chapter 12 under the listing for Perilla Fruit Decoction for Directing Qi Downward (*sū zǐ jiàng qì tāng*). Over time, the name of the disorder has changed. According to the 18th-century physician Wang Zi-Jie in *Selected Annotations to Ancient Formulas from the Garden of Crimson Snow*, it was referred to as 'inversion' (厥 *jué*) in the *Inner Classic*, as 'moderate wind' (緩風 *huǎn fēng*) until the Tang era, and as 'leg qi' from the Song onward. It is caused by wind, cold, dampness, and summerheat assaulting the three yin channels of the legs. Different types of leg qi are differentiated according to the precise combination of pathogens. Treatment in each case focuses on disseminating the pathogens and opening the channels and collaterals: "Leg qi is a disorder [due to] clogging. One treats it by disseminating and unblocking, preventing the qi from becoming clogged." (*Indispensable Tools for Pattern Treatment*) The combination of Evodiae Fructus (*wú zhū yú*), Arecae Semen (*bīng láng*), and Chaenomelis Fructus (*mù guā*), which is known as Evodia Decoction (*wú zhū yú tāng*) and was first listed in the Song-dynasty work *Comprehensive Recording of Sage-like Benefit*, is an essential ingredient in many classical formulas for the treatment of leg qi.

The present formula is designed for leg qi due to wind-dampness or cold-dampness and thus focuses on transforming cold-dampness by warming and on unblocking the qi dynamic. It is most effective if taken during the early stages. It is also used for acute invasion of wind-dampness that pours downward, characterized by fever and chills, severe leg and foot pain, and superficial swelling of the sinews and vessels.

The source text specifies that the draft be taken cold, except during the winter months when it may be taken warm. The cold liquid resonates with the cold nature of the disorder and is thus more easily accepted by the body, as explained by Chen Nian-Zu in *Compendium of Songs on Modern Formulas*: "When using yang to transform yin, one must first confuse [the pathogen to accept the formula] as belonging to its own family. [In this way, the formula] is first accepted and then attacks." Taking the draft should cause black-colored diarrhea, indicating that the pathogen is being expelled. The black color here is associated with the Kidneys and the cold-dampness toxin.

Biomedical Indications

With the appropriate presentation, this formula may be used to treat a variety of biomedically-defined disorders including beriberi and filariasis.

Modifications

- For spontaneous sweating, aversion to wind, and a floating, moderate pulse due to wind-dampness, add Cinnamomi Ramulus (*guì zhī*) and Saposhnikoviae Radix (*fáng fēng*).
- For absence of sweating, body aches and pain, and a submerged, slow pulse due to cold-dampness, add Cinnamomi Cortex (*ròu guì*) and Aconiti Radix lateralis praeparata (*zhì fù zǐ*).
- For damp-heat lodged in the lower burner, remove Evodiae Fructus (*wú zhū yú*) and Zingiberis Rhizoma recens (*shēng jiāng*), and add Three-Marvel Pill (*sān miào wán*).
- For cold-dampness leg qi rushing upward to the Heart with palpitations, a cold and stifling sensation in the chest, and an almost imperceptible pulse, remove Citri reticulatae Pericarpium (*chén pí*), Perillae Folium (*zǐ sū yè*), and Platycodi Radix (*jié gěng*), and add Aquilariae Lignum resinatum (*chén xiāng*), Cinnamomi Cortex (*ròu guì*), Aconiti Radix lateralis praeparata (*zhì fù zǐ*), and Pinelliae Rhizoma praeparatum (*zhì bàn xià*).

Section 5

FORMULAS THAT DISPEL WIND-DAMPNESS

The formulas in this section are used in treating externally-contracted wind-dampness, the presence of which is indicated by pain and sometimes numbness. These conditions are generally known as painful obstruction (痹 *bì*). The nature and location of the pain vary depending on the level of penetration of the pathogenic influences, and whether cold or heat is also involved.

These formulas use chief herbs that expel wind-dampness from the vessels, such as Angelicae pubescentis Radix (*dú huó*), Notopterygii Rhizoma seu Radix (*qiāng huó*), Saposhnikoviae Radix (*fáng fēng*), or Gentianae macrophyllae Radix (*qín jiāo*). Depending on the pattern, they are combined with deputies and assistants from three other groups of herbs.

The first group includes herbs that invigorate the blood such as Chuanxiong Rhizoma (*chuān xiōng*), Cinnamomi Cortex (*ròu guì*), Achyranthis bidentatae Radix (*niú xī*), or Angelicae sinensis Radix (*dāng guī*). Their use is explained in an adage from *Convenient Reader of Established Formulas*: "To treat wind, first treat the blood; when the blood moves, the wind will be extinguished."

The second group includes herbs that tonify qi and nourish the blood such as Ginseng Radix (*rén shēn*), Astragali

Radix *(huáng qí)*, Glycyrrhizae Radix *(gān cǎo)*, Angelicae sinensis Radix *(dāng guī)*, Paeoniae Radix *(sháo yào)*, or Rehmanniae Radix praeparata *(shú dì huáng)*. Their purpose is to support the organism as well as mediate the drying and dispersing actions of the chief herbs.

The third group includes herbs that tonify the Liver and augment the Kidneys such as Eucommiae Cortex *(dù zhòng)*, Taxilli Herba *(sāng jì shēng)*, and Achyranthis bidentatae Radix *(niú xī)*. The Kidneys govern the bones, while the Liver governs the sinews. Where painful obstruction penetrates to the bones and sinews, usually in more chronic patterns that involve weakness of the lower back and knees, it is therefore essential to tonify the Liver blood and Kidney qi.

羌活勝濕湯 （羌活胜湿汤）
Notopterygium Decoction to Overcome Dampness
qiāng huó shèng shī tāng

Source   *Clarifying Doubts about Damage from Internal and External Causes* (1247)

Notopterygii Rhizoma seu Radix *(qiāng huó)* 3g
Angelicae pubescentis Radix *(dú huó)* 3g
Ligustici Rhizoma *(gǎo běn)* 1.5g
Saposhnikoviae Radix *(fáng fēng)* 1.5g
Chuanxiong Rhizoma *(chuān xiōng)* 1.5g
Viticis Fructus *(màn jīng zǐ)* 0.9g
Glycyrrhizae Radix praeparata *(zhì gān cǎo)* 1.5g

Method of Preparation   The source text advises to grind the ingredients into a coarse powder and take as a draft, preferably before meals. This should promote mild sweating. At present, it is usually prepared as a decoction with 2-3 times the specified dosage of each ingredient.

Actions   Expels wind and dampness

Indications

A heavy and painful head, generalized sensation of heaviness, back pain or generalized pain, stiffness of the neck, difficulty in rotating or bending the trunk, mild fever, chills, a white tongue coating, and a floating pulse.

This is painful obstruction with wind-dampness being predominant. The invasion is into the muscle layer and channels only. It is commonly found in those who have caught cold after sweating profusely or who live in a damp environment. The chills, fever, and floating pulse indicate an exterior condition. Wind and dampness clog the interstices and pores and move upward to attack the head, where they cause heaviness and pain. The greater yang channel, the most superficial of the channels, controls the exterior level of the body, so when the pathogen mostly resides here, the shoulders and up-

per back will be painful and the muscles along the spine and in the neck will be stiff. The body may also feel heavy, with difficulty rotating the trunk. If the pathogen resides mainly in the lesser yang and terminal yin channels, the patient will frequently be frightened when lying down (臥而多驚 *wò ér duō jīng)*, as dampness constrains the movement of qi in those channels, making them deficient. Since the condition is superficial, it does not affect the tongue and the coating remains a normal white.

Analysis of Formula

This formula treats invasion by wind-cold-dampness (wind-dampness predominant). For this reason, it focuses on expelling wind and dispelling dampness while also promoting the circulation of blood and qi. Notopterygii Rhizoma seu Radix *(qiāng huó)*, one of the chief herbs, expels wind-dampness from the upper reaches of the greater yang channel. The other chief herb, Angelicae pubescentis Radix *(dú huó)*, expels wind-dampness from the lower reaches of this channel. Together, they are very effective in treating systemic wind-dampness. The deputies, Ligustici Rhizoma *(gǎo běn)* and Saposhnikoviae Radix *(fáng fēng)*, expel wind and dampness from the exterior aspects of the greater yang channel, and reinforce the actions of Notopterygii Rhizoma seu Radix *(qiāng huó)*, especially its ability to treat headache. One of the assistants, Chuanxiong Rhizoma *(chuān xiōng)*, treats the headache and invigorates the blood, which helps relieve the generalized heaviness and pain. The other assistant, Viticis Fructus *(màn jīng zǐ)*, also treats the headache. The envoy, Glycyrrhizae Radix *(gān cǎo)*, harmonizes the actions of the other herbs.

Cautions and Contraindications

Use with caution in patients with constitutional yin deficiency, or for any condition with heat.

Commentary

Composed by Li Dong-Yuan, one of the four great masters of the Jin-Yuan dynasties, Notopterygium Decoction to Overcome Dampness *(qiāng huó shèng shī tāng)* embodies two important treatment strategies found in many of his other formulas and is thus representative of his style. The first is the principle that 'wind overcomes dampness.' For this purpose, Li Dong-Yuan chose a class of herbs that he and his followers refer to as 'wind herbs' (風藥 *fēng yào)*. These are herbs that promote the movement of yang qi throughout the body, are drying, and have an ascending nature. Li Dong-Yuan favored the use of these herbs because, by tonifying the ascending functions of the qi dynamic, they support the transforming and transporting functions of the middle burner, to which he attached considerable importance. This also naturally pertains to the treatment of dampness. According to Wu Kun in *Investigations of Medical Formulas,* "Using wind herbs to treat dampness is like wind moving above damp earth. Before the day has come to an end, the dampness will be gone."

The second strategy is that of "analyzing [patterns] according to the channels, following the [manifestation] of a disorder to compose the formula." In the present pattern, wind-dampness is located predominantly in the greater yang channel. Thus, the wind herbs employed focus on that channel. In other formulas, such as Tonify the Middle to Augment the Qi Decoction *(bǔ zhōng yì qì tāng),* discussed in Chapter 8, they may be used for the purpose of lifting up the Spleen and Gallbladder yang.

Most practitioners use relatively small doses of this formula to produce a mild sweat. This is especially important when treating conditions such as wind-dampness, where profuse sweating could easily injure the yang and the fluids. The formula is also frequently used in treating headaches.

Comparison

➤ Vs. Nine-Herb Decoction with Notopterygium *(jiǔ wèi qiāng huó tāng)*

Both formulas treat systemic wind-dampness. Because Notopterygium Decoction to Overcome Dampness *(qiāng huó shèng shī tāng)* focuses less on releasing the exterior, it is indicated for conditions with mild exterior symptoms and relatively severe generalized pain and heaviness. Nine-Herb Decoction with Notopterygium *(jiǔ wèi qiāng huó tāng),* on the other hand, is better for treating wind-cold-dampness fettering the exterior accompanied by heat from constraint in the interior, characterized by aversion to cold with fever, a bitter taste in the mouth, and slight thirst.

Biomedical Indications

With the appropriate presentation, this formula may be used to treat a variety of biomedically-defined disorders including upper respiratory tract infection, rheumatic fever, and tension headache.

Modifications

- For cold-dampness obstructing the channels with heaviness of the body and lower back, add Stephaniae tetrandrae Radix *(hàn fáng jǐ).*
- For hot, painful joints, add Atractylodis Rhizoma *(cāng zhú),* Phellodendri Cortex *(huáng bǎi),* Stephaniae tetrandrae Radix *(hàn fáng jǐ),* and Coicis Semen *(yì yǐ rén).*
- For severe cases, add Aconiti Radix lateralis praeparata *(zhì fù zǐ).*

蠲痹湯 （蠲痹汤）

Remove Painful Obstruction Decoction

juān bì tāng

This formula is intended to have a rapid effect in treating painful obstruction patterns. As Wang Zi-Jie explained in *Selected Annotations to Ancient Formulas from the Garden of Crimson Snow*: "蠲 *Juān* [means] dispelling the disease quickly. 痹 *Bì* is a dampness disorder. It also means painful."

Source *Yang Family Formulas* (1178)

Notopterygii Rhizoma seu Radix *(qiāng huó)* 45g
Curcumae longae Rhizoma *(jiāng huáng)* 45g
wine-washed Angelicae sinensis Radix *(jiǔ xǐ dāng guī)* 45g
honey-prepared Astragali Radix *(mì zhì huáng qí)* 45g
Paeoniae Radix alba *(bái sháo)* 45g
Saposhnikoviae Radix *(fáng fēng)* .45g
Glycyrrhizae Radix praeparata *(zhì gān cǎo)* 15g

Method of Preparation   The source text advises to coarsely grind the ingredients and take as a draft with 5 pieces of Zingiberis Rhizoma recens *(shēng jiāng)* and 3 pieces of Jujubae Fructus *(dà zǎo).* At present, it is taken as a decoction with 3g of Zingiberis Rhizoma recens *(shēng jiāng)* and approximately a 90 percent reduction in the dosage of the other ingredients. Note that some practitioners use Paeoniae Radix alba *(bái sháo)* in this formula, while others use Paeoniae Radix rubra *(chì sháo).*

Actions   Tonifies and harmonizes the protective and nutritive qi, dispels wind, and eliminates dampness

Indications

A generalized sensation of heaviness in the body, stiffness in the neck, shoulder, and upper back, numbness in the extremities, difficulty in moving, a white tongue coating, and a moderate pulse.

This is painful obstruction in a patient with deficiency of qi and blood. According to the early 7th-century work *Discussion of the Origins of the Symptoms of Disease,* "The three [pathogenic] qi of wind, cold, and dampness arrive separately, combine, and give rise to painful obstruction." Although painful obstruction patterns are thus produced by the intermingling of three different pathogens, one or two usually predominate. In the present case, these are wind and dampness. As a yang pathogen, wind tends to invade more easily if one's nutritive qi or blood is already deficient. Dampness, a yin pathogen, invades if qi is deficient. Moreover, wind dries the blood even further, while dampness obstructs the qi dynamic. When the circulation of qi and blood are impeded, pain, stiffness, and numbness result. In painful obstruction, the impediment is located at the level of the channels and collaterals; thus, there are no signs of internal illness. The presence of wind means that most symptoms are located in the upper body, that is, the back and neck. Dampness, on the other hand, causes stiffness, heaviness, and restricted movement.

Analysis of Formula

This formula treats invasion by wind-cold-dampness (wind-dampness being predominant) due to deficiency of the protective and nutritive qi. For this reason, it focuses on expelling the wind and dispelling the dampness while also augmenting the qi and harmonizing the nutritive and protective qi. Because the focus is on eliminating wind and dispelling dampness to treat pain and stiffness, the chief herbs are Notopterygii Rhizoma seu Radix (qiāng huó) and Saposhnikoviae Radix (fáng fēng). Notopterygii Rhizoma seu Radix (qiāng huó) is specific for dispelling wind-dampness from the upper body. Saposhnikoviae Radix (fáng fēng) opens the yang and dispels dampness without being too drying. Angelicae sinensis Radix (dāng guī) and Paeoniae Radix (sháo yào) serve as deputies to nourish the blood and harmonize the nutritive qi, thereby facilitating the dispelling of the pathogenic qi. They also prevent the acrid and drying nature of the chief herbs from damaging the blood. Astragali Radix (huáng qí) is the third deputy, augmenting the qi and firming up the protective qi. In combination with Saposhnikoviae Radix (fáng fēng), it dispels wind-dampness, while in combination with Angelicae sinensis Radix (dāng guī) and Paeoniae Radix (sháo yào), it harmonizes the nutritive and protective qi.

Curcumae longae Rhizoma (jiāng huáng) acts as assistant in invigorating the blood and moving the qi. It is specific for spasms and pain in the shoulders and upper arms. Together with Paeoniae Radix (sháo yào) and Angelicae sinensis Radix (dāng guī), it helps regulate the blood in accordance with the adage that, "To treat wind, one must first treat the blood, [because] when the blood moves, the wind is naturally extinguished." Glycyrrhizae Radix (gān cǎo) augments the qi and, as envoy, harmonizes the functions of the other herbs. Jujubae Fructus (dà zǎo) and Zingiberis Rhizoma recens (shēng jiāng), which are added when preparing the draft, harmonize the nutritive and protective qi, enhancing the formula's ability to dispel wind and dampness.

Cautions and Contraindications

This formula is warming and tonifying. It is not indicated for patterns of wind-damp-heat painful obstruction.

Commentary

This formula was first listed in the Song-dynasty formulary *Yang Family Formulas*. Several later physicians used it as a blueprint to compose similar formulas published under the same name. Its strategy of tonifying the qi and blood at the same time as dispelling wind-dampness was equally influential. Thus, Wang Zi-Jie referred to it as "the ancestor of [formulas] for treating painful obstruction." In *Discussion of Medical Formulas*, the late-Qing-dynasty physician Fei Bo-Xiong penned a similar eulogy:

If the nutritive and protective qi are not exhausted, from where might wind enter? Those who do not regulate the nutritive and protective qi and [rely on the] excessive use of wind herbs either raise phlegm upward or assist [in the generation of] fire. This formula attends to both the nutritive and protective qi while also being able to dispel wind and promote the resolution of dampness. It is a perfect formula for treating patterns of painful obstruction.

This formula focuses on the upper and middle burner, with symptoms concentrated in the upper body and upper extremities. Thus, as Zhang Bin-Cheng noted in his *Convenient Reader of Established Formulas*, "[As long as] one does not take this formula for disorders of the sinews and bones due to Liver and Kidney deficiency, this formula will produce results like putting a key in a lock."

The formula can also be used externally as a wash or steam bath. Because these applications open the pores, patients should cover themselves up afterwards in order to avoid contracting any new wind-cold pathogens.

Comparison

➤ Vs. Pubescent Angelica and Taxillus Decoction (dú huó jì shēng tāng); see PAGE 759

Biomedical Indications

With the appropriate presentation, this formula may be used to treat a variety of biomedically-defined disorders including periarthritis of the shoulder and rheumatoid arthritis.

Modifications

- For more severe cold, add Cinnamomi Ramulus (guì zhī) and Asari Radix et Rhizoma (xì xīn).
- For more severe dampness, add Atractylodis Rhizoma (cāng zhú), Stephaniae tetrandrae Radix (hàn fáng jǐ), and Coicis Semen (yì yǐ rén).
- For paraesthesia and numbness, indicating that the vessels and collaterals are blocked, increase the dosage of Astragali Radix (huáng qí) and add Cinnamomi Ramulus (guì zhī) and Scorpio (quán xiē).

Associated Formula

蠲痹湯 (蠲痹汤)

Remove Painful Obstruction Decoction from *Awakening of the Mind in Medical Studies*

juān bì tāng

SOURCE *Awakening of the Mind in Medical Studies* (1732)

Notopterygii Rhizoma seu Radix (qiāng huó) 3g
Angelicae pubescentis Radix (dú huó) 3g
Gentianae macrophyllae Radix (qín jiāo) 3g
Mori Ramulus (sāng zhī) 9g

Piperis kadsurae Caulis (*hǎi fēng téng*) 9g

Angelicae sinensis Radix (*dāng guī*) 9g

Chuanxiong Rhizoma (*chuān xiōng*) 2.1g

Olibanum (*rǔ xiāng*) 2.4g

Aucklandiae Radix (*mù xiāng*) 2.4g

Cinnamomi Cortex (*ròu guì*) 1.5g

Glycyrrhizae Radix praeparata (*zhì gān cǎo*) 1.5g

Decoction. At present, the dosage is increased 2-3 times, and Cinnamomi Ramulus (*guì zhī*) is substituted for Cinnamomi Cortex (*ròu guì*). Removes wind-dampness and alleviates painful obstruction. This formula is used for joint pain that increases with cold and diminishes with warmth, possibly accompanied by a sensation of heaviness and numbness in the limbs, a thick, white tongue coating, and a slow and possibly slippery pulse. This is joint pain due to local obstruction of qi from the effects of wind, cold, and dampness. The presence of wind is manifested in the changing position of the pain. The presence of cold is reflected in the response to temperature change, the white tongue coating, and the slippery pulse. The numbness is caused by a combination of wind and dampness. This is an important formula for treating relatively early-stage painful obstruction. It may be modified to focus the actions on whichever pathogenic influence is predominant.

獨活寄生湯 (独活寄生汤)
Pubescent Angelica and Taxillus Decoction
dú huó jì shēng tāng

Source   *Important Formulas Worth a Thousand Gold Pieces* (650)

Angelicae pubescentis Radix (*dú huó*) 9g

Asari Radix et Rhizoma (*xì xīn*) 6g

Saposhnikoviae Radix (*fáng fēng*) 6g

Gentianae macrophyllae Radix (*qín jiāo*) 6g

Taxilli Herba (*sāng jì shēng*) 6g

Eucommiae Cortex (*dù zhòng*) 6g

Achyranthis bidentatae Radix (*niú xī*) 6g

Cinnamomi Cortex (*ròu guì*) 6g

Angelicae sinensis Radix (*dāng guī*) 6g

Chuanxiong Rhizoma (*chuān xiōng*) .6g

Rehmanniae Radix (*shēng dì huáng*) .6g

Paeoniae Radix alba (*bái sháo*) 6g

Ginseng Radix (*rén shēn*) 6g

Poria (*fú líng*) 6g

Glycyrrhizae Radix (*gān cǎo*) 6g

Method of Preparation   Decoction. The source text advises to coarsely grind the ingredients. At present, the normal dosage of Taxilli Herba (*sāng jì shēng*) is 15-30g, but Dipsaci Radix (*xù duàn*) is often substituted for this herb. Codonopsis Radix (*dǎng shēn*) is usually substituted for Ginseng Radix (*rén shēn*), with twice the dosage.

Actions   Expels wind-dampness, disperses painful obstruction, and tonifies deficiency

Indications

Heavy and painful sensations at fixed locations in the lower back and lower extremities accompanied by weakness and stiffness or hypertonicity and immobility, an aversion to cold and attraction to warmth, palpitations, shortness of breath, a pale tongue with a white coating, and a thin, weak, slow pulse. There may also be paresthesias or numbness.

This is painful obstruction with Liver and Kidney deficiency. The lower back and lower extremities are the province of the Kidneys. The knees are the province of the sinews and are therefore associated with the Liver. Chronic painful obstruction can lead to deficiency in these organs. Individuals with Liver and Kidney deficiency are especially prone to problems with the joints in the lower extremities. Kidney yang deficiency is often involved, which is manifested in the aversion to cold and attraction to warmth, palpitations, shortness of breath, pale tongue, and thin, weak pulse. This condition is commonly due to cold-predominant painful obstruction, which is indicated by the fixed pain, white tongue coating, and slow pulse.

Analysis of Formula

This formula treats chronic painful obstruction patterns that commonly involve Kidney and Liver deficiency, as well as insufficiency of both the qi and blood. For this reason, the formula employs a complex strategy of dispelling wind-dampness, stopping pain, augmenting the functions of the Liver and Kidneys, and tonifying the qi and blood. The chief herb, Angelicae pubescentis Radix (*dú huó*), expels wind, dampness, and cold from the lower burner, bones, and sinews. Asari Radix et Rhizoma (*xì xīn*), one of the deputies, scatters cold in the channels and scours out wind-dampness from the sinews and bones to stop the pain. Another deputy, Saposhnikoviae Radix (*fáng fēng*), expels the wind and overcomes dampness. The third deputy, Gentianae macrophyllae Radix (*qín jiāo*), relaxes the sinews and expels the wind and dampness.

The remaining ingredients serve as assistants. Taxilli Herba (*sāng jì shēng*), Eucommiae Cortex (*dù zhòng*), and Achyranthis bidentatae Radix (*niú xī*) expel wind-dampness and tonify the Liver and Kidneys. Achyranthis bidentatae Radix (*niú xī*) also serves as an envoy and directs the actions of the other herbs toward the lower extremities. Cinnamomi Cortex (*ròu guì*) warms and unblocks the channels and fortifies the yang. It thereby opens up the lower back and is an important herb for treating lower back pain.

Angelicae sinensis Radix (*dāng guī*), Chuanxiong Rhizoma (*chuān xiōng*), Rehmanniae Radix (*shēng dì huáng*), and Paeoniae Radix alba (*bái sháo*) serve the important function of nourishing and invigorating the blood. These herbs are more fully discussed under the entry for Four-Substance Decoction (*sì wù tāng*) in Chapter 8. When treating conditions with dampness, especially chronic ones, the Spleen must be strengthened. Ginseng Radix (rén shēn) and Poria (fú líng) serve this purpose. The envoy, Glycyrrhizae Radix praeparata (zhì gān cǎo), tonifies the middle qi and harmonizes the actions of the other herbs in the formula.

Cautions and Contraindications

Contraindicated for painful obstruction marked by strong excess conditions or damp-heat.

Commentary

The pathological mechanism of painful obstruction was first described in Chapter 43 of Basic Questions: "Painful obstruction in the bones causes heaviness; in the blood vessels, [it] causes coagulation and loss of flow; in the sinews, [it] causes contractions with an inability to extend the joints; and in the muscles, [it] causes numbness." Chapter 34 of the same text states: "Deficiency of the nutritive qi causes numbness. Deficiency of the protective qi causes loss of function. Deficiency of both the nutritive and protective qi causes numbness and loss of function." Consequently, this formula focuses on augmenting the qi and nourishing the blood. It thereby illustrates the principle that proper treatment of a chronic disease requires both tonification of the normal qi and dispelling of the pathogenic influences.

This formula is commonly used for chronic painful obstruction, especially in the bones and sinews, and is also used in treating atrophy disorder characterized by wasting of the lower extremities. Many physicians substitute Rehmanniae Radix praeparata (shú dì huáng) for Rehmanniae Radix (shēng dì huáng) because of its stronger tonifying effect on the blood. However, the source text advises to leave out Rehmanniae Radix (shēng dì huáng) if the patient has a tendency toward loose stools.

Because of its ability to tonify and disperse at the same time, the formula has been used more recently to treat a variety of internal medicine conditions ranging from abdominal pain and hepatitis to asthma and impotence. Many contemporary physicians furthermore think that adding herbs to invigorate the blood to this formula enhances its clinical efficacy. This view reflects a tendency, which started in the late Qing era, to place considerable importance on treating blood stasis in cases of painful obstruction. Stagnation of qi and blood had been acknowledged as an important cause in the pathogenesis of painful obstruction for a long time, as the 19th-century writer Lin Pei-Qin explained in the encylopedic Treatment Decisions Categorized According to Pattern:

> All [cases of] painful obstruction … intrinsically [develop] from a primary deficiency of protective and nutritive qi. If the pores and interstices are not firm, wind-cold avails itself of [this] deficiency to assault the interior. The normal qi [then] becomes blocked by the pathogens and is unable to disseminate or move. As it lodges and stagnates, the qi and blood congeal and stagnate, which, over time, causes painful obstruction.

While Qing-dynasty physicians, including Ye Tian-Shi, emphasized the role of blood stasis in the treatment of chronic pain, Lin Pei-Qin's contemporary, Wang Qing-Ren, launched a full-scale attack on older treatment methods. In a discussion entitled "Painful Obstruction Patterns are Characterized by Static Blood," included in his seminal Correction of Errors among Physicians, Wang observed: "Generally, [when] one drives out wind-cold or eliminates damp-heat, it becomes even more difficult to invigorate the already congealing blood." This is because the bitter and warming or cooling nature of the herbs used for this purpose dries up the blood and slows down the qi, thus aggravating any preexisting stasis.

Comparison

➤ Vs. Remove Painful Obstruction Decoction (juān bì tāng)

This formula treats lower-body painful obstruction with Liver and Kidney deficiency, while Remove Painful Obstruction Decoction (juān bì tāng) is for upper-body painful obstruction with deficiency of nutritive and protective qi.

Biomedical Indications

With the appropriate presentation, this formula may be used to treat a variety of biomedically-defined disorders including osteoarthritis, rheumatoid arthritis, sciatica, periarthritis of the shoulder, lumbar disc disease, postpolio syndrome, temporomandibular joint dysfunction, and eczema.

Alternate names

Pubescent Angelica Decoction (dú huó tāng) and Decoction Worth Ten Thousand in Gold (wàn jīn tāng), both in Effective Medical Formulas Arranged by Category by Master Zhu

Modifications

- For severe pain, add Agkistrodon/Bungarus (bái huā shé), Pheretima (dì lóng), and Carthami Flos (hóng huā).
- For severe cold, add Aconiti Radix lateralis praeparata (zhì fù zǐ) and Zingiberis Rhizoma (gān jiāng).
- For severe dampness, add Stephaniae tetrandrae Radix (hàn fáng jǐ) and Atractylodis Rhizoma (cāng zhú).
- For signs of only mild deficiency, remove Ginseng Radix (rén shēn), Paeoniae Radix alba (bái sháo), and Rehmanniae Radix (shēng dì huáng).
- For sequelae of poliomyelitis, add Notoginseng Radix (sān qī), Clematidis Radix (wēi líng xiān), and Chaenomelis Fructus (mù guā).

Associated Formulas

三痹湯 （三痹汤）

Three Painful Obstruction Decoction

sān bì tāng

SOURCE *Fine Formulas for Women* (1237)

Dipsaci Radix (*xù duàn*) 30g
Eucommiae Cortex (*dù zhòng*) 30g
Saposhnikoviae Radix (*fáng fēng*) 30g
Cinnamomi Cortex (*ròu guì*) 30g
Asari Radix et Rhizoma (*xì xīn*) 30g
Ginseng Radix (*rén shēn*) 30g
Poria (*fú líng*) 30g
Angelicae sinensis Radix (*dāng guī*) 30g
Paeoniae Radix alba (*bái sháo*) 30g
Glycyrrhizae Radix (*gān cǎo*) 30g
Gentianae macrophyllae Radix (*qín jiāo*) 15g
Rehmanniae Radix (*shēng dì huáng*) 15g
Chuanxiong Rhizoma (*chuān xiōng*) 15g
Angelicae pubescentis Radix (*dú huó*) 15g
Astragali Radix (*huáng qí*) 30g
Cyathulae Radix (*chuān niú xī*) 30g

The source text advises to grind the herbs into a coarse powder and prepare 15g as a draft by boiling it in 2 cups of water to which 3 slices of Zingiberis Rhizoma recens (*shēng jiāng*) and 1 piece of Jujubae Fructus (*dà zǎo*) has been added. The draft should be taken on an empty stomach. At present, it is prepared as a decoction in the usual manner with one-third to one-half the dosage specified above. Tonifies the Liver and Kidneys, augments the qi, nourishes the blood, expels wind, and overcomes dampness. For Liver and Kidney deficiency with qi and blood stagnation characterized by tremors of the hands and feet. The sinews and bones are soft and weak, and there is also pain due to wind-damp painful obstruction. In contrast to the principal formula, this one focuses on nourishing the qi and blood to extinguish the wind.

大防風湯 （大防风汤）

Major Saposhnikovia Decoction

dà fáng fēng tāng

SOURCE *Formulary of the Pharmacy Service for Benefiting the People in the Taiping Era* (1107)

Chuanxiong Rhizoma (*chuān xiōng*) 45g
Aconiti Radix lateralis praeparata (*zhì fù zǐ*) 45g
Rehmanniae Radix praeparata (*shú dì huáng*) 60g
Atractylodis macrocephalae Rhizoma (*bái zhú*) . . 60g
Saposhnikoviae Radix (*fáng fēng*) 60g
Angelicae sinensis Radix (*dāng guī*) 60g
Paeoniae Radix alba (*bái sháo*) 60g
Astragali Radix (*huáng qí*) 60g
Eucommiae Cortex (*dù zhòng*) 60g
Notopterygii Rhizoma seu Radix (*qiāng huó*) 30g
Ginseng Radix (*rén shēn*) 30g
Glycyrrhizae Radix praeparata (*zhì gān cǎo*) 30g
Achyranthis bidentatae Radix (*niú xī*) 30g

Coarsely grind and take 15g as a draft before meals with 7 slices of Zingiberis Rhizoma recens (*shēng jiāng*) and 1 piece of Jujubae Fructus (*dà zǎo*). Also prepared as a decoction by reducing the dosage of the ingredients by approximately 80 percent. Dispels wind, smooths the flow of qi, invigorates the blood vessels, fortifies the sinews and bones, and eliminates cold-dampness. Originally prescribed for dy-

senteric wind (痢風 *lì fēng*) where the legs are so painful and weakened after a dysenteric disorder that it is very difficult to walk. Also used for crane's-knee wind (鶴膝風 *hè xī fēng*) in which one or both knees become swollen, enlarged, and painful accompanied by atrophy above and below the knee. In this condition, the patient cannot move the knee.

疏風活血湯 （疏风活血汤）

Dredge the Wind and Invigorate the Blood Decoction

shū fēng huó xuè tāng

SOURCE *Precious Mirror of Eastern Medicine* (1613)

Angelicae sinensis Radix (*dāng guī*) 3g
Chuanxiong Rhizoma (*chuān xiōng*) 3g
Clematidis Radix (*wēi líng xiān*) 3g
Angelicae dahuricae Radix (*bái zhǐ*) 3g
Stephaniae tetrandrae Radix (*hàn fáng jǐ*) 3g
Phellodendri Cortex (*huáng bǎi*) 3g
Arisaema cum Bile (*dǎn nán xīng*) 3g
Atractylodis Rhizoma (*cāng zhú*) 3g
Notopterygii Rhizoma seu Radix (*qiāng huó*) 3g
Cinnamomi Ramulus (*guì zhī*) 3g
Carthami Flos (*hóng huā*) 0.9g

Decoct with 5 slices of Zingiberis Rhizoma recens (*shēng jiāng*). For sharp pain in all the joints from wind, dampness, phlegm, and blood stasis. The painful areas can be swollen and/or red. There may also be stiffness, hypertonicity, and paraesthesia. Symptoms are often worse at night. This is originally a Korean formula that is also popular in Japan. It is most often used for aches and pains in the lower back and legs. If the blood stasis is pronounced, more herbs to invigorate the blood should be added.

桂枝芍藥知母湯 （桂枝芍药知母汤）

Cinnamon Twig, Peony, and Anemarrhena Decoction

guì zhī sháo yào zhī mǔ tāng

SOURCE *Essentials from the Golden Cabinet* (c. 220)

Cinnamomi Ramulus (*guì zhī*) 12g
Ephedrae Herba (*má huáng*) 6g
baked Aconiti Radix lateralis (*bāo fù zǐ*) 15g
Anemarrhenae Rhizoma (*zhī mǔ*) 12g
Paeoniae Radix (*sháo yào*) 9g
Atractylodis macrocephalae Rhizoma (*bái zhú*) . . 15g
Saposhnikoviae Radix (*fáng fēng*) 12g
Zingiberis Rhizoma recens (*shēng jiāng*) 15g
Glycyrrhizae Radix (*gān cǎo*) 6g

Method of Preparation　Decoction. Paeoniae Radix alba (*bái sháo*) is the form of Paeoniae Radix (*sháo yào*) that is most often used.

Actions　Unblocks the flow of yang qi, promotes movement (in areas with painful obstruction), dispels wind, eliminates dampness, and clears heat

Indications

Swollen and painful joints (especially of the lower extremities) that are warm to the touch and worsen at night, reduced range of motion in the affected joints, chills, absence of sweating, weight loss, headache, dizziness, shortness of breath, a feeling as if one wants to vomit, a white, greasy tongue coating, and a wiry, slippery pulse.

This is recurrent wind-cold-damp painful obstruction in which localized constraint generates heat. This causes swollen, painful joints that are warm to the touch. Heat from constraint tends to worsen at night when the yin is waxing. At this level of disease, the heat from constraint is confined to the affected joints and does not produce systemic heat signs. When dampness has no way to exit from the body, it tends to accumulate in the lower extremities where it causes edema, stiffness, and a reduced range of motion in the joints. Wind, on the other hand, moves upward, causing headaches and dizziness. When it invades the Stomach, it causes the Stomach qi to rebel, producing a feeling as if one wants to vomit. At this stage there is a predisposition toward internal dampness, indicated by a white, greasy tongue coating and a slippery pulse. The chronic nature of the disorder and the obstruction of the qi dynamic that this involves leads to a loss of appetite and weight. The wiry pulse is a sign of pain and constraint.

Analysis of Formula

This formula treats chronic panarthralgia where pathogenic wind-cold-dampness has lingered in the body for a long time, constrained the qi dynamic, and produced heat from constraint that has, in turn, damaged the yin. For this reason, it combines the strategies of dispelling the wind and elimination of dampness with warming the channels and collaterals as well as nourishing the yin and clearing the heat. The chief herb, Cinnamomi Ramulus *(guì zhī),* warms and unblocks the channels. Ephedrae Herba *(má huáng),* a deputy, strengthens this effect and relieves the relatively superficial swelling. Another deputy, Aconiti Radix lateralis praeparata *(zhì fù zǐ),* warms the channels and relieves pain. Two other deputies, Anemarrhenae Rhizoma *(zhī mǔ)* and Paeoniae Radix alba *(bái sháo),* clear heat and prevent injury to the yin by recurrent painful obstruction. The combination of the chief herb and Paeoniae Radix alba *(bái sháo)* is a common one that harmonizes the functions of the protective and nutritive qi. The less common pairing of Anemarrhenae Rhizoma *(zhī mǔ)* with the chief herb effectively resolves heat from constraint in the joints.

Atractylodis macrocephalae Rhizoma *(bái zhú),* one of the assistants, works with the chief herb to unblock the flow of yang qi and leach out dampness. The other assistant, Saposhnikoviae Radix *(fáng fēng),* strengthens the formula's function of expelling wind and dampness. Warm, acrid

Zingiberis Rhizoma recens *(shēng jiāng),* one of the envoys, strengthens the spreading and mobilizing actions of the other herbs. In concert with the other envoy, Glycyrrhizae Radix praeparata *(zhì gān cǎo),* it harmonizes the actions of the other herbs and regulates the functions of the middle burner.

Commentary

The source text recommends this formula for aches and pains in all the joints, emaciation, severe swelling of the feet, dizziness, shortness of breath, and mild nausea. This condition is called panarthralgia (歷節病 *lì jié bìng)* and is thought to occur in patients with constitutional deficiency of nutritive and protective qi who contract wind-cold-dampness. Some commentators analyze the symptoms of dizziness, shortness of breath, and nausea with a desire to vomit as manifestations of leg qi, which is often accompanied by an up-rushing of qi. Others interpret them to be internal wind. Yet others see them as obstructions of the qi dynamic in all three burners. Most modern physicians simply ignore them altogether, choosing to concentrate on the formula's action on the sinews, bones, and joints.

Thus, this formula is most widely used at present for treating painful obstruction and is modified for either hot or cold conditions. In fact, in its chronic stage, it is quite difficult to differentiate hot from cold painful obstruction because one often transforms into the other. Whether the formula was intended primarily for hot or cold disorders has been a subject of debate for more than fifteen-hundred years. Depending on the point of view, Cinnamomi Ramulus *(guì zhī),* Ephedrae Herba *(má huáng),* Atractylodis macrocephalae Rhizoma *(bái zhú),* Anemarrhenae Rhizoma *(zhī mǔ),* and Aconiti Radix lateralis praeparata *(zhì fù zǐ)* has each been identified as the chief herb in the formula.

Clinically, it is unnecessary that all the pieces of the presentation be there for this formula to be appropriate. It should be considered whenever there are joints that are painful and swollen with localized heat in patients with systemic manifestations of cold from deficiency.

The range of application for this formula has been extended to the treatment of dizziness caused by inner ear disorders. Its efficacy in such cases is explained by its ability to dispel dampness and regulate the qi. Besides other obvious signs of dampness and phlegm, a pale tongue body with a thick, white coating and a wiry, slippery pulse should be present. To more effectively transform phlegm and direct the qi downward, herbs such as Citri reticulatae Pericarpium *(chén pí),* Pinelliae Rhizoma praeparatum *(zhì bàn xià),* and Fossilia Dentis Mastodi *(lóng chǐ)* should be added to the formula.

Comparisons

> Vs. White Tiger Decoction *(bái hǔ tāng)*-Derived Formulas

This formula should be distinguished from White Tiger plus Cinnamon Twig Decoction (*bái hǔ jiā guì zhī tāng*), which is indicated for hot painful obstruction with symptoms of systemic heat. It should also be distinguished from White Tiger plus Atractylodes Decoction (*bái hǔ jiā zhú tāng*), which is indicated for damp painful obstruction that has transformed into systemic heat.

➤ Vs. Tangkuei Decoction to Pry Out Pain (*dāng guī niān tòng tāng*); *see* page 709

Biomedical Indications

With the appropriate presentation, this formula may be used to treat a variety of biomedically-defined disorders including rheumatoid arthritis, connective tissue disorders, gouty arthritis, psoriatic arthritis, periarthritis of the shoulder, sciatica, deep vein thrombosis, erythema nodosum, and cor pulmonare.

Alternate name

Cinnamon Twig, Peony, and Anemarrhena Decoction (*guì sháo zhī mǔ tāng*) in *Shen's Annotated Essentials from the Golden Cabinet*

Modifications

- For severe pain and restricted movement that responds favorably to warmth, increase the dosage of Aconiti Radix lateralis praeparata (*zhì fù zǐ*) and Ephedrae Herba (*má huáng*).
- For a heavy sensation throughout the body which is especially severe in the affected joints, increase the dosage of Atractylodis macrocephalae Rhizoma (*bái zhú*).
- For symptoms that worsen at night, substitute Paeoniae Radix rubra (*chì sháo*) for Paeoniae Radix alba (*bái sháo*).
- For pronounced heat in the joints, increase the dosage of Paeoniae Radix (*sháo yào*) and Anemarrhenae Rhizoma (*zhī mǔ*) and add Mori Ramulus (*sāng zhī*) and Lonicerae Caulis (*rěn dōng téng*).
- For qi deficiency, add Astragali Radix (*huáng qí*).
- For blood and yin deficiency, add Rehmanniae Radix (*shēng dì huáng*) and Achyranthis bidentatae Radix (*niú xī*).
- For more severe dampness, add Coicis Semen (*yì yǐ rén*) and Atractylodis Rhizoma (*cāng zhú*).
- For damp-heat, add Gypsum fibrosum (*shí gāo*) and Phellodendri Cortex (*huáng bǎi*).
- For blood stasis, add Olibanum (*rǔ xiāng*) and Myrrha (*mò yào*).

Associated Formula

薏苡仁湯 (薏苡仁汤)
Coicis Decoction from *Enlightened Physicians*

yì yǐ rén tāng

Source *Displays of Enlightened Physicians* (Ming dynasty)

Ephedrae Herba (*má huáng*). 6g
Angelicae sinensis Radix (*dāng guī*). 9g
Atractylodis Rhizoma (*cāng zhú*). 9g
Coicis Semen (*yì yǐ rén*). 24g
Cinnamomi Ramulus (*guì zhī*). 6g
Paeoniae Radix alba (*bái sháo*). 9g
Glycyrrhizae Radix praeparata (*zhì gān cǎo*). 3g

Disperses swelling in the exterior and treats dry blood in the interior. For swelling and pain in the joints (usually of the hands and feet) as well as numbness and difficulty in moving the joints, usually accompanied by fever. Commonly used for pain and swelling of the joints that has not responded to treatment (or was improperly treated) at the acute stage and is beginning to show chronic signs. The dosage and actions are drawn from Japanese sources, the only ones available to the editors. Available as a prepared medicine with the substitution of Atractylodis macrocephalae Rhizoma (*bái zhú*) for Atractylodis Rhizoma (*cāng zhú*).

宣痹湯 (宣痹汤)
Disband Painful Obstruction Decoction
xuān bì tāng

Source *Systematic Differentiation of Warm Pathogen Diseases* (1798)

fáng jǐ (Stephaniae/Cocculi/etc. Radix) 15g
Armeniacae Semen (*xìng rén*). 15g
Talcum (*huá shí*) 15g
Forsythiae Fructus (*lián qiáo*). 9g
Gardeniae Fructus (*zhī zǐ*). 9g
Coicis Semen (*yì yǐ rén*). 15g
Pinelliae Rhizoma praeparatum (*zhì bàn xià*). 9g
Bombycis Faeces (*cán shā*). 9g
Phaseoli Semen (*chì xiǎo dòu*). 9g

Method of Preparation Decoction. At present, usually Stephaniae tetrandrae Radix (*hàn fáng jǐ*) is used. The dosage of Phaseoli Semen (*chì xiǎo dòu*) is often increased 2-3 times.

Actions Clears and resolves damp-heat, unblocks the channels, and disbands painful obstruction

Indications

Heat and pain in the joints, reduced mobility, fever and shaking chills, a lusterless, yellow complexion, scanty, dark urine, and a gray or yellow and greasy tongue coating.

This is painful obstruction due to the containment of damp-heat primarily in the channels, but also obstructing the qi dynamic. The 'steaming' of damp-heat causes fever and prevents the yang qi from circulating, which leads to shaking chills. Damp-heat obstructing the joints causes heat and pain in the joints with reduced mobility. The lusterless, yellow complexion is a sign of constrained dampness, and the scanty, dark urine indicates vigorous heat. A gray or yellow, greasy tongue coating indicates that both dampness and heat are strong.

Analysis of Formula

To treat damp-heat painful obstruction, this formula focuses on clearing and resolving damp-heat, unblocking the channels, and stopping the pain. Stephaniae tetrandrae Radix *(hàn fáng jǐ)* dispels damp-heat in the upper burner by venting the heat externally. At the same time, it disperses superficial swelling and drains damp-heat through the urine. It also has some ability to dry dampness and strengthen the Spleen, which helps resolve the underlying cause of this condition. Its effect on all three burners, together with its ability to treat painful obstruction, distinguishes it as the chief herb in the formula. Armeniacae Semen *(xìng rén)* regulates the Lungs' function in water metabolism. Coicis Semen *(yì yǐ rén)* and Bombycis Faeces *(cán shā)* both strengthen the Spleen, resolve dampness, and treat painful obstruction. These three herbs serve as the deputies in the formula.

The remaining herbs are regarded as assistants. Pinelliae Rhizoma praeparatum *(zhì bàn xià)* dries dampness and transforms turbidity. Forsythiae Fructus *(lián qiáo)* is very effective in clearing relatively superficial heat. Gardeniae Fructus *(zhī zǐ)*, Talcum *(huá shí)*, and Phaseoli Semen *(chì xiǎo dòu)* assist the chief herb in clearing heat and draining dampness through the urine.

Commentary

The classical understanding of painful obstruction advanced in the *Inner Classic* is that it is caused by the combination of wind, cold, and dampness. Until the Qing era, such patterns were treated primarily with warm, acrid substances that dispel wind, warm cold, and dry dampness. If heat was observed, this was thought to arise from constraint of the yang qi. Even though cooling herbs were used to drain the heat, the acrid and moving herbs formed the core of formulas for painful obstruction patterns. Cinnamon Twig, Peony, and Anemarrhena Decoction *(guì zhī sháo yào zhī mǔ tāng)*, discussed earlier in this chapter, is a typical example of this approach. During the Qing, physicians associated with the warm pathogen disorder current in Chinese medicine developed a new understanding of pathology that allowed for the direct invasion of damp-heat into the body. This led to the development of new treatment strategies that focused on clearing and draining damp-heat via the Triple Burner, as discussed under Three-Seed Decoction *(sān rén tāng)*. The present formula uses this approach and extends it to the treatment of painful obstruction. In clinical practice, it is often prescribed together with Two-Marvel Powder *(èr miào sǎn)*, also discussed above.

Comparison

> Vs. Tangkuei Decoction to Pry Out Pain *(dāng guī niān tòng tāng)*

Both formulas are used to treat damp-heat painful obstruction. In addition to resolving dampness and clearing heat, Tangkuei Decoction to Pry Out Pain *(dāng guī niān tòng tāng)* also disperses wind and is used when there are manifestations of externally-contracted wind. Furthermore, it deals with a more complex presentation that includes both blood stasis as well as blood and qi deficiency. By contrast, Disband Painful Obstruction Decoction *(xuān bì tāng)* focuses equally on both the dampness and heat and is indicated when only these pathogens are involved.

Biomedical Indications

With the appropriate presentation, this formula may be used to treat a variety of biomedically-defined disorders including rheumatic fever, rheumatoid arthritis, gouty arthritis, and connective tissue disorders.

Modification

For severe pain, add Mori Ramulus *(sāng zhī)*, Curcumae longae Rhizoma *(jiāng huáng)*, and Erythrinae Cortex *(hǎi tóng pí)*.

上中下通用痛風丸
(上中下通用痛风丸)
Pill to Treat Painful Wind Anywhere
shàng zhōng xià tōng yòng tòng fēng wán

Source   *Medical Formulas Collected and Analyzed* (1682)

wine-fried Phellodendri Cortex *(jiǔ chǎo huáng bǎi)* 75g (9g)
Atractylodis Rhizoma *(cāng zhú)* 75g (9g)
Arisaematis Rhizoma praeparatum *(zhì tiān nán xīng)* . . 75g (9g)
dry-fried Massa medicata fermentata *(chǎo shén qū)* . . 37.5g (9g)
Chuanxiong Rhizoma *(chuān xiōng)* 37.5g (9g)
Persicae Semen *(táo rén)* 37.5g (9g)
Gentianae Radix *(lóng dǎn cǎo)* 37.5g (3g)
fáng jǐ (Stephaniae/Cocculi/etc. Radix) 37.5g (9g)
Angelicae dahuricae Radix *(bái zhǐ)* 37.5g (9g)
Notopterygii Rhizoma seu Radix *(qiāng huó)* 11g (6g)
wine-fried Clematidis Radix *(jiǔ chǎo wēi líng xiān)* . . 11g (6-9g)
Cinnamomi Ramulus *(guì zhī)* 11g (6-9g)
Carthami Flos *(hóng huā)* 7.5g (3-6g)

Method of Preparation   The source text states to grind the above ingredients, mix with paste and form into pills, and take 37.5g each time. At present, the formula is usually prepared as a decoction with the dosages in parentheses.

Actions   Clears heat, dries dampness, invigorates blood, and dispels wind

Indications

Sore and achy joints, specifically marked by pain that moves from joint to joint.

This is painful wind, a disorder characterized by aching and pain in the joints owing to invasion of wind, cold, and dampness. The formula can treat either acute or chronic joint pain. The channels, as they pass through the narrow confines of the joints, are particularly susceptible to congestion and obstruction to the flow of qi and blood. Since the lack of free flow leads to pain, the main symptoms of the patterns this formula treats are aching and pain in the joints. Wind is thought to aid the damp and cold pathogens penetrate the protective aspect of the body, after which they settle in the joints and cause aching (dampness) and pain (cold). The migration of pain from joint to joint is also indicative of the migratory nature of the wind pathogen.

Analysis of Formula

Although this formula treats disorders due to wind, dampness, and cold, it also addresses the stagnation of qi and blood that accompanies painful wind disorders and the secondary heat that can result from the stagnation of wind, cold, and dampness. As a whole, the formula dispels wind and dampness, disperses cold, moves the blood and qi, and clears heat. Phellodendri Cortex (*huáng bǎi*), Atractylodis Rhizoma (*cāng zhú*), *fáng jǐ* (Stephaniae/Cocculi/etc. Radix), and Gentianae Radix (*lóng dǎn cǎo*) clear heat and dry dampness. Persicae Semen (*táo rén*), Chuanxiong Rhizoma (*chuān xiōng*), and Carthami Flos (*hóng huā*) move the blood. Chuanxiong Rhizoma (*chuān xiōng*) specifically treats the qi within the blood aspect. Arisaematis Rhizoma praeparatum (*zhì tiān nán xīng*) eliminates phlegm. Notopterygii Rhizoma seu Radix (*qiāng huó*), Angelicae dahuricae Radix (*bái zhǐ*), Clematidis Radix (*wēi líng xiān*), and Cinnamomi Ramulus (*guì zhī*) dispel wind and disperse cold, and Massa medicata fermentata (*shén qū*) disperses ingrained accumulation.

Naturally, many of the ingredients serve more than one function in this formula. For example, *Divine Husbandman's Classic of the Materia Medica* notes that Cinnamomi Ramulus (*guì zhī*) facilitates the functioning of the joints. Similarly, Zhu Dan-Xi observed that Platycodi Radix (*jié gěng*) opens and uplifts the blood and qi and, like a boat, transports the herbs, not allowing them to sink. As a group, these herbs remove the causes of joint pain such as wind, dampness, cold, heat, and phlegm, and move the blood and qi to disperse the stagnation.

Commentary

Although the version of this formula that is most commonly used in modern times is taken from *Medical Formulas Collected and Analyzed*, it was Zhu Dan-Xi in *Delving into the Mysteries of the Golden Cabinet* who introduced this combi-nation of herbs and set down its foundations. In his discussion of painful wind, which he described as "moving pain in the four limbs and hundred joints," he laid out the cause of the disorder and the principles of treatment. He posited that wind-heat and wind-dampness penetrate the defenses and combine with blood deficiency and phlegm to bring on this disorder. For treatment, he suggested a foundational group of herbs to dispel wind, clear heat, dry dampness, transform phlegm, and nourish the blood. These are Atractylodis Rhizoma (*cāng zhú*), Arisaematis Rhizoma praeparatum (*zhì tiān nán xīng*), Chuanxiong Rhizoma (*chuān xiōng*), Angelicae dahuricae Radix (*bái zhǐ*), Angelicae sinensis Radix (*dāng guī*), and Scutellariae Radix (*huáng qín*). In addition, he proposed the following additions to the formula based on the location of the joint pain:

- Upper body: Notopterygii Rhizoma seu Radix (*qiāng huó*), Cinnamomi Ramulus (*guì zhī*), Platycodi Radix (*jié gěng*), and Clematidis Radix (*wēi líng xiān*)
- Lower body: Cyathulae Radix (*chuān niú xī*), *fáng jǐ* (Stephaniae/Cocculi/etc. Radix), Akebiae Caulis (*mù tōng*), and Phellodendri Cortex (*huáng bǎi*).

Furthermore, Zhu emphasized that for blood deficiency, one must assist Chuanxiong Rhizoma (*chuān xiōng*) and Angelicae sinensis Radix (*dāng guī*) with Persicae Semen (*táo rén*) and Carthami Flos (*hóng huā*).

This formula is designed for the treatment of painful wind anywhere in the body. Zhu's own name for the formula—Formula for Painful Wind at the Top, Middle, or Bottom (上中下 痛風方 *shàng zhōng xià tòng fēng fāng*)—suggests its universal application. To localize the formula, additions were made to the foundational herbs, including joint-homing Notopterygii Rhizoma seu Radix (*qiāng huó*), downward-moving *fáng jǐ* (Stephaniae/Cocculi/etc. Radix) and Gentianae Radix (*lóng dǎn cǎo*), and shoulder-homing Cinnamomi Ramulus (*guì zhī*). In the complete formula, *fáng jǐ* (Stephaniae/Cocculi/etc. Radix) and Gentianae Radix (*lóng dǎn cǎo*) move downward, Notopterygii Rhizoma seu Radix (*qiāng huó*), Platycodi Radix (*jié gěng*), and Angelicae dahuricae Radix (*bái zhǐ*) move upward, Chuanxiong Rhizoma (*chuān xiōng*) and Clematidis Radix (*wēi líng xiān*) move both upward and downward, Cinnamomi Ramulus (*guì zhī*) moves horizontally, Massa medicata fermentata (*shén qū*), Atractylodis Rhizoma (*cāng zhú*), and Arisaematis Rhizoma praeparatum (*zhì tiān nán xīng*) move to the middle, and Persicae Semen (*táo rén*) and Carthami Flos (*hóng huā*) move throughout the body. The whole body is benefited by all of the herbs because, as *Investigations of Medical Formulas* observes, "the ascending herbs are led downward and the descending herbs are guided to the upper [body]."

Of the causes which Zhu Dan-Xi identifies for this disorder, only blood deficiency is not fully addressed. Angelicae sinensis Radix (*dāng guī*) and Spatholobi Caulis (*jī xuè téng*) are thus useful additions in those cases where blood deficiency is evident.

For acute cases, it is often acceptable to use the formula as is or with slight modifications (see MODIFICATIONS below). For chronic cases, however, the underlying deficiency and stagnation inherent in long-term illness must also be addressed. For this purpose, one can add agents that address the patient's underlying disharmony. For example, if the patient presents with yin deficiency expressed as night sweats, thirst, and a dry, red tongue body, adding herbs such as Ecliptae Herba *(mò hàn lián)*, Ligustri lucidi Fructus *(nǚ zhēn zǐ)*, Moutan Cortex *(mǔ dān pí)*, and Rehmanniae Radix *(shēng dì huáng)* may be advisable. If there is underlying yang deficiency, the patient may benefit from the addition of Drynariae Rhizoma *(gǔ suì bǔ)*, Morindae officinalis Radix *(bā jǐ tiān)*, Epimedii Herba *(yín yáng huò)*, or Curculiginis Rhizoma *(xiān máo)*. In addition, if blood stagnation is extreme, as reflected in localized, sharp pain, the blood-moving agents in the formula can be complemented with others such as Euonymi Ramulus *(guǐ jiàn yǔ)*, Centellae Herba *(jī xuě cǎo)*, or Verbenae Herba *(mǎ biān cǎo)*.

Comparisons

➢ Vs. OTHER FORMULAS FOR PAINFUL OBSTRUCTION

Pill to Treat Painful Wind Anywhere *(shàng zhōng xià tōng yòng tòng fēng wán)* is a commonly used formula for the treatment of migrating painful obstruction. It can also be used, however, in the treatment of other painful obstruction patterns, especially if deficiency is not a major contributing factor. If deficiency is prominent, then formulas such as Pubescent Angelica and Taxillus Decoction *(dú huó jì shēng tāng)* and Three Painful Obstruction Decoction *(sān bì tāng)* are favored because they are better able to supplement the Liver and Kidneys, and the blood and qi. Think of these three formulas on a continuum where Three Painful Obstruction Decoction *(sān bì tāng)* favors root treatment (i.e., tonification), Pubescent Angelica and Taxillus Decoction *(dú huó jì shēng tāng)* treats the root and branch equally, and Pill to Treat Painful Wind Anywhere *(shàng zhōng xià tōng yòng tòng fēng wán)* is focused on treating the branch.

Cautions and Contraindications

Contraindicated during pregnancy. Unsuitable for use in the debilitated, without modifications.

Biomedical Indications

With the appropriate presentation, this formula may be used to treat a variety of biomedically-defined disorders including sciatica pain, trigeminal neuralgia, late-stage trauma, and the joint pain associated with disorders such as osteoarthritis, lupus, and gout.

Modifications

- If blood deficiency is present, add Angelicae sinensis Radix *(dāng guī)* for cold patterns and Spatholobi Caulis *(jī xuè téng)* for warm patterns.
- For hot joint pain with red and swollen joints, add Siegesbeckiae Herba *(xī xiān cǎo)* and Lonicerae Caulis *(rěn dōng téng)*. Replace Chuanxiong Rhizoma *(chuān xiōng)* with Paeoniae Radix rubra *(chì sháo)*. For intense heat, add Gypsum fibrosum *(shí gāo)* and Anemarrhenae Rhizoma *(zhī mǔ)*.
- For phlegm, add Pinelliae Rhizoma praeparatum *(zhì bàn xià)* and Atractylodis macrocephalae Rhizoma *(bái zhú)*.
- For cold pain that is aggravated by cold and is relieved by warmth, add Aconiti Radix lateralis praeparata *(zhì fù zǐ)* and Acanthopanacis Cortex *(wǔ jiā pí)*, and remove Phellodendri Cortex *(huáng bǎi)* and Gentianae Radix *(lóng dǎn cǎo)*.
- For more pronounced dampness, add Coicis Semen *(yì yǐ rén)*, Saposhnikoviae Radix *(fáng fēng)*, and Angelicae pubescentis Radix *(dú huó)*.
- For qi deficiency, add Astragali Radix *(huáng qí)* and Ginseng Radix *(rén shēn)*.
- For joint pain that is restricted to the lower body, add Cyathulae Radix *(chuān niú xī)*, Coicis Semen *(yì yǐ rén)*, Dipsaci Radix *(xù duàn)*, and Akebiae Caulis *(mù tōng)* and remove Notopterygii Rhizoma seu Radix *(qiāng huó)* and Platycodi Radix *(jié gěng)*.
- For gout, add Chaenomelis Fructus *(mù guā)*, Cyathulae Radix *(chuān niú xī)*, and Coicis Semen *(yì yǐ rén)*.
- For damp-heat, add Coicis Semen *(yì yǐ rén)*, Polygoni cuspidati Rhizoma *(hǔ zhàng)*, and Cyathulae Radix *(chuān niú xī)*.
- If wind symptoms such as migrating pain are prominent, increase the dosage of Saposhnikoviae Radix *(fáng fēng)* and add Piperis kadsurae Caulis *(hǎi fēng téng)*.

Comparative Tables of Principal Formulas

■ **FORMULAS THAT TRANSFORM DAMPNESS AND HARMONIZE THE STOMACH**

Common symptoms: abdominal distention or pain, nausea and vomiting, diarrhea, greasy tongue coating, slippery pulse

Formula Name	Diagnosis	Indications	Remarks
Calm the Stomach Powder (*píng wèi sǎn*)	Dampness stagnating in the Spleen and Stomach	Distention and fullness in the epigastrium and abdomen, loss of taste and appetite, heaviness in the limbs, loose stools or diarrhea, fatigue, nausea and vomiting, belching, acid regurgitation, a swollen tongue with a thick, white, and greasy coating, and a moderate or slippery pulse	This is the representative formula for the treatment of dampness stagnating in the middle burner.
Rectify the Qi Powder Worth More than Gold (*bù huàn jīn zhèng qì sǎn*)	Dampness turbidity obstructing the middle with wind-cold fettering the exterior	Vomiting, abdominal distention and fullness, fever and chills	Also for sudden turmoil disorder characterized by diarrhea and vomiting, and a thick, white, and greasy tongue coating.
Patchouli/Agastache Powder to Rectify the Qi (*huò xiāng zhèng qì sǎn*)	Externally-contracted wind-cold with concurrent internal injury due to dampness and stagnation	Fever and chills, headache, sensation of fullness and stifling oppression in the chest, pain in the epigastrium and abdomen, nausea and vomiting, borborygmus, diarrhea, loss of taste, a white, greasy tongue coating, and a moderate, soggy pulse	Also for sudden turmoil disorders or miasmatic malarial disorders with similar symptomatology.
Harmonize the Six Decoction (*liù hé tāng*)	Externally-contracted cold during the summer months with internal damage due to dampness	Chills and fever, no sweating, headache, feeling muddled, wheezing from phlegm, cough, a stifling sensation in the chest or a sensation of fullness and distention in the diaphragm, vomiting and diarrhea, no desire for food or drink, dark urine that is reduced in volume, and a white, slippery tongue coating	Widely used formula for expelling summerheat, transforming dampness, strengthening the Spleen, and harmonizing the Stomach.
Eight-Ingredient Formula for Vaginal Discharge (*bā wèi dài xià fāng*)	Pathogenic water or dampness and heat (heat being the result of stagnation) collecting in the lower burner	Women who feel subjectively cold due to underlying deficiency but also have damp-heat symptoms such as aching in the lower back, abdominal pain, profuse red, yellow, or white vaginal discharge, and itching sores	The tongue will usually be pale, with a white or yellow coating; the pulse is usually slippery and without force.

■ **FORMULAS THAT CLEAR HEAT AND EXPEL DAMPNESS**

Common symptoms: generalized heaviness or pain in the body, fever, abdominal distention or pain, no thirst or thirst with a desire to only sip fluids, scanty or difficult urination, greasy (usually yellow) tongue coating, slippery or soggy pulse

Formula Name	Diagnosis	Indications	Remarks
Three-Seed Decoction (*sān rén tāng*)	Early-stage damp-warmth disease or summerheat-warmth disease lodged in the protective and qi levels (dampness predominant)	Headache, chills, afternoon fever, a heavy sensation in the body, generalized pain, pale yellow complexion, a stifling sensation in the chest, loss of appetite, an absence of thirst, a white tongue coating, and a wiry, thin, and soggy pulse	Focuses on facilitating the qi dynamic in order to transform dampness. Also used by contemporary physicians for the treatment of internal damp-heat.
Sweet Dew Special Pill to Eliminate Toxin (*gān lù xiāo dú dān*)	Early-stage damp-warmth epidemic disorder affecting the qi level (heat and dampness are equally strong)	Fever, achy limbs, lethargy, swollen throat, a stifling sensation in the chest, abdominal distention, dark, scanty urine, a white, greasy or yellow, dry tongue coating, and a soggy, rapid pulse	May also be vomiting and diarrhea, jaundice, unremitting fever, or damp-heat stagnating in the Triple burner. Also for conditions with more severe heat that transforms into toxin.

Formula Name	Diagnosis	Indications	Remarks
Coptis and Magnolia Bark Drink (*lián pò yǐn*)	Sudden turmoil disorder due to an aggregation of damp-heat smoldering in the body	Simultaneous vomiting and diarrhea, focal distention and a stifling sensation in the chest and epigastrium, irritability, restlessness, dark, scanty urine, a yellow, greasy tongue coating, and a slippery, rapid pulse	Focuses on clearing and transforming damp-heat and regulating the ascending and descending functions of the middle burner.
Tangkuei Decoction to Pry Out Pain (*dāng guī niān tòng tāng*)	A pattern of interaction between dampness and heat with the addition of externally-contracted pathogenic wind	Generalized body aches and pains, irritability, heaviness in the shoulders and back, discomfort of the chest and diaphragm, aching and painful extremities and joints, especially with unbearable swelling and pain of the lower extremities, a greasy tongue coating with a tinge of yellow, and a pulse that is usually wiry and rapid, although it can be soggy and moderate or slippery and rapid	Also for a similar presentation due to wind-dampness transforming into heat as an aspect of long-standing painful obstruction. May also be multiple sores, carbuncles, furuncles or abscesses, with redness, persistent swelling, and possibly itching, pain, fever, or thirst.
Virgate Wormwood Decoction (*yīn chén hāo tāng*)	Yang-type or damp-heat jaundice	Whole-body jaundice with a color that resembles a fresh tangerine, slight abdominal distention, urinary difficulty, thirst (with the ability to take only sips), little or no sweating, or sweating only from the head, a yellow, greasy tongue coating, and a slippery, rapid pulse	Focuses on simultaneously treating the root by draining heat and promoting the resolution of dampness, and the manifestation by reducing jaundice.
Eight-Herb Powder for Rectification (*bā zhèng sǎn*)	Damp-heat collecting in the lower burner, specifically the Bladder	Dark, turbid, scanty, difficult, and painful urination, a dry mouth and throat, a yellow, greasy tongue coating, and a slippery, rapid pulse	In severe cases, there may be urinary retention and lower abdominal distention and pain. This is painful urinary dribbling or urinary retention.
Powder for Five Types of Painful Urinary Dribbling (*wǔ lín sǎn*)	Damp-heat bloody painful urinary dribbling	Rough, painful urination that is red or the color of red bean juice, or with multiple tiny stones; urinary symptoms may be accompanied by acute lower abdominal pain	Most effective for heat-type painful urinary dribbling, especially if accompanied by bleeding.
Open the Gate Pill (*tōng guān wán*)	Urinary obstruction due to heat collecting in the lower burner and obstructing the qi transformation of the Bladder	Urinary obstruction, pain in the lower abdomen, rough and painful urination, no thirst	Focuses on draining excess pathogenic heat without injuring the physiological fire at the gate of vitality.
Two-Marvel Powder (*èr miào sǎn*)	Damp-heat lodged in the lower burner	For a wide variety of complaints accompanied by scanty, yellow urine and a yellow, greasy tongue coating; complaints include pain in the lower back or extremities (especially the sinews or bones); weakness or atrophy of the lower extremities; red, hot, swollen, and painful feet or knees; a thick, yellow, foul-smelling vaginal discharge; and sores on the lower extremities due to dampness	Commonly used as the foundation for larger and more complex formulas. Very useful in the treatment of atrophy disorders due to damp-heat.
Separate and Reduce Fullness in the Middle Pill (*zhōng mǎn fēn xiāo wán*)	Drum-like abdominal distention due to damp-heat	Abdominal distention, firmness with a sensation of fullness and bursting pain in the epigastrium and abdomen, irritability, fever, bitter taste, dark yellow urine, constipation or foul-smelling diarrhea, a yellow, greasy tongue coating, and a wiry, rapid pulse	For obstruction of the qi dynamic by dampness, which then transforms into heat. Both excess and deficiency are pronounced.

■ FORMULAS THAT PROMOTE URINATION AND LEACH OUT DAMPNESS

Common symptoms: urinary difficulty and fluid metabolism dysfunction

Formula Name	Diagnosis	Indications	Remarks
Five-Ingredient Powder with Poria (wǔ líng sǎn)	(1) Water buildup; (2) Spleen deficiency; (3) retention of thin mucus in the lower burner	(1) Headache, fever, irritability, strong thirst but with vomiting immediately after drinking, urinary difficulty, a floating pulse, and a white tongue coating; (2) edema, generalized sensation of heaviness, diarrhea, urinary difficulty, and possible vomiting and diarrhea due to sudden turmoil disorder; (3) throbbing pulsations just below the umbilicus, vomiting frothy saliva, vertigo, shortness of breath, and coughing	Used for many disorders of water metabolism marked by problems with the ability of the qi to transform dampness.
Polyporus Decoction (zhū líng tāng)	Clumping of water and heat	Urinary difficulty accompanied by fever and thirst with a desire to drink; may also have diarrhea, cough, nausea, irritability, or insomnia	Also used for diarrhea in infants from damp-heat and injury to the yin.
Five-Peel Powder (wǔ pí sǎn)	Skin edema	Generalized edema with a sensation of heaviness, distention, and fullness in the epigastrium and abdomen, labored and heavy breathing, urinary difficulty, a white, greasy tongue coating, and a submerged and moderate pulse	For patterns of vigorous dampness and qi stagnation obstructing the greater yin warp (Lungs and Spleen). Also used to treat edema during pregnancy.
Stephania and Astragalus Decoction (fáng jǐ huáng qí tāng)	Wind-dampness or wind edema	Sweating, a heavy sensation in the body, superficial edema, urinary difficulty, a pale tongue with a white coating, and a floating pulse	Also used for edema in women of a deficient nature, and some forms of damp-predominant painful obstruction.
Stephania and Poria Decoction (fáng jǐ fú líng tāng)	Skin edema	Edema that is most pronounced in the extremities, a sensation of heaviness in the body and extremities, fibrillations of the skin and muscles in the extremities, a white, slippery tongue coating, and a superficial pulse	For conditions characterized by excess water dampness against a background of yang and qi deficiency.

■ FORMULAS THAT WARM AND TRANSFORM WATER AND DAMPNESS

Common symptoms: sensations of heaviness, cold, aches or pain, urinary dysfunction, a white, slippery, or greasy tongue coating, submerged pulse

Formula Name	Diagnosis	Indications	Remarks
Poria, Cinnamon Twig, Atractylodes, and Licorice Decoction (líng guì zhú gān tāng)	Thin mucus in the epigastrium	Fullness in the chest and hypochondria, palpitations, shortness of breath, coughing up clear and watery sputum, dizziness or vertigo, a pale, swollen tongue with a white, slippery or greasy coating, and a pulse that is usually slippery and either wiry or soggy	Focuses on harmonizing the fluids and qi dynamic. For any condition marked by cold in the lower burner leading to thin mucus throughout the Triple Burner.
Licorice, Ginger, Poria, and White Atractrylodes Decoction (gān cǎo gān jiāng fú líng bái zhú tāng)	Fixed Kidney disorder	Heavy sensation in the body, cold and pain in the lower back, pressure in the lower back as if carrying a heavy weight, normal appetite, absence of thirst, copious urine, pale tongue with a white, moist coating that may be thick and greasy at the root, and a submerged, thin, and moderate pulse	This is a type of painful obstruction of the waist and lower back due to cold-dampness. Also used to treat Girdle vessel disorders.

cont. ↘

Formula Name	Diagnosis	Indications	Remarks
True Warrior Decoction (*zhēn wǔ tāng*)	Kidney yang deficiency, or Spleen and Kidney yang deficiency, with retention of pathogenic water	Abdominal pain that is aggravated by cold, urinary difficulty, deep aching and heaviness in the extremities, a pale or dark, swollen tongue with tooth marks and a white, slippery coating, and a submerged, thin, and forceless pulse	May also be generalized edema, loose stools, dizziness, a heavy sensation in the head, palpitations, coughing, and vomiting. Also for externally-contracted disorders with sweating that does not reduce the fever, and palpitations in the epigastrium.
Aconite Accessory Root Decoction (*fù zǐ tāng*)	Yang deficiency with internal cold-dampness harassing the interior and obstructing the channels	Generalized body pain, aching bones and joints, aversion to cold especially at the back, cold extremities, no thirst, a white, slippery tongue coating, and a submerged, faint, and forceless or choppy, slow pulse	This is one possible manifestation of a lesser yin disorder. Also used for abdominal distention and pain during late pregnancy with aversion to cold.
Bolster the Spleen Drink (*shí pí yǐn*)	Yin-type edema due to Spleen and Kidney yang deficiency	Generalized edema that is more severe below the waist, cold extremities, chest and abdominal fullness and distention, heaviness, loss of appetite, absence of thirst, scanty urine, semiliquid, unformed stools, a thick, greasy tongue coating, and a submerged, slow or submerged, thin pulse	For conditions characterized by exuberance of cold in the interior that impedes the Spleen's functions of transportation and transformation.
Tokoro Drink to Separate the Clear (*bì xiè fēn qīng yǐn*)	Cloudy painful urinary dribbling due to cold from deficiency in the lower burner	Frequent urination with cloudy, dense, milky (resembling rice water), or greasy urine	Focuses on warming the Kidneys to resolve dampness and transform turbidity.
Powder to Take at Cock's Crow (*jī míng sǎn*)	Damp leg qi caused by cold-dampness clogging the channels	Heavy and weak feet and calves with difficulty in walking; may also be numbness, cold, or pain in these areas, or spasms and up-rushing that reaches to the chest and, in severe cases, produces a stifling sensation in the chest and an overflowing sense of nausea	Also used for acute invasion of wind-dampness that pours downward with simultaneous fever and chills and excruciating pain in the lower extremities.

■ FORMULAS THAT DISPEL WIND-DAMPNESS

Common symptoms: sense of heaviness, joint pain

Formula Name	Diagnosis	Indications	Remarks
Notopterygium Decoction to Overcome Dampness (*qiāng huó shèng shī tāng*)	Painful obstruction with wind-dampness predominant	Heavy and painful head, a generalized sensation of heaviness, back pain or generalized pain, stiffness of the neck, difficulty in rotating or bending the trunk, mild fever, chills, a white tongue coating, and a floating pulse	For invasion of wind-cold-dampness into the muscle layer and channels.
Remove Painful Obstruction Decoction (*juān bì tāng*)	Painful obstruction in patients with deficiency of qi and blood	Generalized sensation of heaviness in the body, stiffness in the neck, shoulder, and upper back, numbness in the extremities, difficulty in moving, a white tongue coating, and a moderate pulse	For invasion by wind-cold-dampness due to deficiency of the protective and nutritive qi. Also used externally as a wash or steam bath.
Pubescent Angelica and Taxillus Decoction (*dú huó jì shēng tāng*)	Painful obstruction with Liver and Kidney deficiency	Heavy and painful sensations at fixed locations in the lower back and lower extremities accompanied by weakness and stiffness or hypertonicity and immobility, aversion to cold and attraction to warmth, palpitations, shortness of breath, a pale tongue with a white coating, and a thin, weak, slow pulse	There may also be paresthesias or numbness.

cont. ↘

Formula Name	Diagnosis	Indications	Remarks
Cinnamon Twig, Peony, and Anemarrhena Decoction (*guì zhī sháo yào zhī mǔ tāng*)	Recurrent wind-cold-damp painful obstruction in which localized constraint generates heat	Swollen and painful joints (especially of the lower extremities) that are warm to the touch and worsen at night, reduced range of motion in the affected joints, chills, absence of sweating, weight loss, headache, dizziness, shortness of breath, a feeling as if one wants to vomit, a white, greasy tongue coating, and a wiry, slippery pulse	For patients with constitutional deficiency of nutritive and protective qi who contract wind-cold-dampness. Currently modified to treat either hot or cold conditions.
Disband Painful Obstruction Decoction (*xuān bì tāng*)	Painful obstruction with damp-heat in the channels that also obstructs the qi dynamic	Heat and pain in the joints, reduced mobility, fever and shaking chills, a lusterless, yellow complexion, scanty, dark urine, and a gray or yellow and greasy tongue coating	Focuses equally on both dampness and heat.
Pill to Treat Painful Wind Anywhere (*shàng zhōng xià tōng yòng tòng fēng wán*)	Painful wind with stagnation of qi and blood	Sore and achy joints, specifically marked by pain that moves from joint to joint	For acute or chronic joint pain resulting from the invasion of wind, cold, or dampness.

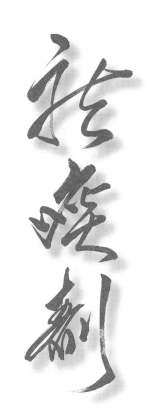

Chapter 17 Contents

Formulas that Dispel Phlegm

Formulas that Dispel Phlegm

PHLEGM IS A DISORDER of the body fluids that have become thick, dense, and turbid, and interfere with the proper flow of qi in the channels, collaterals, Triple Burner, and organ systems. Like static or noxious blood (discussed in Chapter 13), phlegm is thus both the result of pathological processes and a cause of further pathology. It can be caused by externally-contracted pathogens as well as internal damage, and it may affect all parts of the body. Its manifestations are diverse and include coughing and wheezing, nausea, dizziness or vertigo, nodules or lumps, and seizures. As a result, phlegm is implicated in all kinds of disorders, especially those that are difficult to diagnose and difficult to cure.

Like blood, the body fluids are essential to life, and some degree of phlegm will therefore invariably be present in most people. Health thus does not denote the complete absence of phlegm, but rather the ability of the body to transform or, if necessary, eliminate it. Illness only arises if the body fails in this task, as explained by the Qing-dynasty physician Shen Jin-Ao in *Wondrous Lantern for Peering into the Origin and Development of Miscellaneous Diseases*:

> When the *Inner Classic* talks about phlegm and thin mucus, it always [cites] damp earth as its cause. Thus, from birth to death a human being always has phlegm. It is all generated by the Spleen and collects in the Stomach, so that [one can say] that the absence of phlegm in the body cannot enrich and moisten [its physiological processes]. It is only when it materializes [to such an extent] that its movement can [no longer] be fathomed that it becomes harmful.

The same idea is found throughout the classical literature and explains why strategies for the treatment of phlegm do not, on the whole, focus on draining excess but rather on regulating the qi dynamic. These principles were concisely summarized by the Ming-dynasty writer Wang Ken-Tang in *Indispensable Tools for Pattern Treatment*: "Those who are best at treating phlegm treat the qi instead of [directly treating] phlegm. When the qi flows smoothly, all the body's fluids will then flow smoothly." Accordingly, the primary strategy for treating phlegm is to smooth the flow of qi and keep the passageways of qi, blood, and body fluids open. This is known as 'transforming phlegm' (化痰 *huà tán*), which implies an effort to change pathological phlegm back into physiological fluids. The most important formula used for this purpose is Two-Aged [Herb] Decoction *(èr chén tāng)*. Many of the formulas discussed in this chapter are direct modifications or contain key ingredients of this formula, or apply its principles of composition. Those formulas that are not built on Two-Aged [Herb] Decoction *(èr chén tāng)* invariably use other qi-regulating herbs as key ingredients.

Although there may be other contributing factors, the basis of all phlegm is disruption of the transforming and transporting functions of the Spleen. This has been captured in a series of apt analogies by the Ming-dynasty physician Zhang Jie-Bin in *Collected Treatises of [Zhang] Jing-Yue*:

> Phlegm is simply the body fluids, which are themselves nothing but transformations of food and fluids. Since this phlegm is also

a transformed substance, it cannot be classified as untransformed. But transformation, if normal, produces a strong body with flourishing nutritive and protective qi. In this case, [what would in a pathological situation be] phlegm is [still normal] blood and qi. On the other hand, if transformation proceeds abnormally, the organ systems become disordered, the body fluids fail, and qi and blood then produce phlegm. This is exactly like robbers and thieves creating chaos in society: who are they but otherwise good people in a troubled world? The rise of brigands in society must of necessity be the consequence of malady in the governance of the country, just as the appearance of phlegm must result from infirmity of the primal qi. … Strong people can eat and drink whatever they like, in whatever quantities, and everything they eat is duly transformed. We never see it becoming phlegm. … It can be seen that hardly any of the phlegm under heaven is phlegm from excess and also that hardly any phlegm should be attacked. … [To] treat phlegm, we should treat the root. By gradually replenishing the basic root, phlegm will without [direct] treatment eliminate itself.

The second most important strategy for treating phlegm is tonification of the root. Most physicians interpret this as tonifying the transforming and transporting functions of the Spleen and Stomach. For this reason, herbs that strengthen the Spleen are included in almost all of the formulas discussed in this chapter. Some, such as Zhang Jie-Bin cited above, considered the Kidneys to be even more important because of their key role in regulating the fluids. Warming herbs that tonify the ministerial fire at the gate of vitality and thereby augment the Spleen yang are thus also sometimes used to treat phlegm directly, while a more indirect strategy is to tonify the Kidneys with formulas such as Six-Ingredient Pill with Rehmannia *(liù wèi dì huáng wán)* and Kidney Qi Pill *(shèn qì wán),* both discussed in Chapter 8. Other organ systems that are important in the treatment of phlegm are the Triple Burner and the Lungs; this is because of their role in the regulation of water metabolism.

Strategies for treating phlegm must also take into account the nature of its pathogenesis. When Spleen deficiency leads to an accumulation of dampness that transforms into phlegm, the appropriate strategy is to strengthen the Spleen, dry the dampness, and expel the phlegm. When heat from excess scorches the fluids and transforms them into phlegm, one should clear the heat and transform the phlegm. When the Lungs are dry and the yin is deficient and fire from deficiency transforms the depleted fluids into phlegm, one should moisten the Lungs and transform the phlegm. When fire burns up the fluids in the channels and precipitates the formation of rubbery nodules or masses, one should cool the fire and transform the phlegm. When cold injures the upper or middle burners and causes the fluids to congeal, one should warm the cold and transform the phlegm. And when phlegm so severe that it disturbs the qi mechanisms such that tremors or seizures ensue, the proper strategy is to transform the phlegm and extinguish the wind.

Historically, the explanation of these treatment strategies and the classification used to organize the formulas in this chapter mainly occurred after the Song era. The term 'phlegm' (痰 *tán*) does not appear in the *Inner Classic*, and only appears in the compound term 'phlegm and thin mucus' (痰飲 *tán yǐn*) in *Essentials from the Golden Cabinet*. The earliest differentiation between phlegm and thin mucus is attributed to the early 7th-century text *Discussion of the Origins of the Symptoms of Disease*, where it is discussed in the context of pulse diagnosis: "If the pulse is more wiry, it indicates phlegm; floating and thin means thin mucus." The Song-dynasty work *Straight Directions from [Yang] Ren* distinguished between the two categories based on their nature and pathogenesis, defining phlegm as a more dense, thick, and turbid substance produced by excess dryness and warmth, and thin mucus as more clear and thin, produced by excess cold and dampness. Another difference is that thin mucus is perceived to be a more localized phenomenon, while phlegm is often viewed as neither fixed in form nor location. These attributes are summed up by Lin Pei-Qin in *Treatment Decisions Categorized According to Pattern:* "As a rule, clear and thin is thin mucus; thick and turbid is phlegm. Thin mucus accumulates only in the Stomach and Intestines, while phlegm can follow the rise and fall of qi to reach anywhere in the body."

Although these distinctions remain current today, they are less easily made in actual clinical practice. Throughout the classical period, the two terms were thus frequently used interchangeably (sometimes within the same sentence or paragraph), and the realities of the clinic continue to defy today's more stringent efforts at systematization. Dampness, for instance, is a major cause not only of thin mucus but also of phlegm, and thin mucus often manifests with symptoms such as dizziness, insomnia, palpitations, or headache. For all of these reasons, formulas that are used in the treatment of phlegm disorders are found in many other chapters of this book.

Section 1

FORMULAS THAT DRY DAMPNESS AND TRANSFORM PHLEGM

The formulas in this section are used in treating disorders of phlegm-dampness. The most common manifestations are coughing with copious, clear, or white sputum that is easy to expectorate, focal distention, nausea, weakness of the extremities, headache, and palpitations with anxiety. The tongue usually has a white coating that is slippery or greasy, and the pulse is moderate or wiry. The etiology of this disorder is generally attributed to a weakening of the middle burner's transporting and transforming functions that impedes the circulation of fluids, which thereupon accumulate and form phlegm. This was described by Zhang Jie-Bin in *Collected Treatises of [Zhang] Jing-Yue*:

> Phlegm is basically transformed from food and [its production] thus depends on the [relative] vigor and strength of the Spleen and Stomach. In young people during their prime, everything that is eaten is transformed to become qi and blood. Where [under such conditions] is anything left over to become phlegm? However, when the food is not entirely transformed and ten or twenty percent remain, these ten or twenty percent becomes phlegm. If forty percent remain, then these forty percent becomes phlegm.

The Spleen, moreover, prefers dryness and has an aversion to dampness. Excess external dampness or an inappropriate diet contributes to the formation of dampness, and thereby of phlegm. As noted in *Red Water and Dark Pearls*: "Dampness in the Spleen channel becomes phlegm-dampness." Drying the dampness serves to strengthen the transportive function of the Spleen, which in turn will reduce the phlegm.

Thus, the chief herbs used in the formulas discussed in this section are those that dry dampness and transform phlegm such as Pinelliae Rhizoma praeparatum *(zhì bàn xià)*, Arisaematis Rhizoma praeparatum *(zhì tiān nán xīng)*, Sinapis Semen *(bái jiè zǐ)*, and Cynanchi stauntonii Rhizoma *(bái qián)*. These are usually combined with herbs from one or more of the following groups:

- Herbs that regulate the qi such as Citri reticulatae Pericarpium *(chén pí)*, Cyperi Rhizoma *(xiāng fù)*, Aurantii Fructus *(zhǐ ké)*, or Aurantii Fructus immaturus *(zhǐ shí)*. The reasons for this were first explained by the Song-dynasty physician Yan Yong-He in *Formulas to Aid the Living*:

  > A person's qi pathway serves the function of smoothing [the flow of qi]. If this is smooth, the fluids can flow openly, with no chance of a phlegm and thin mucus disorder. But if this regularity is upset, the qi pathway closes off, water and yin occlude in and around the chest and diaphragm, clump, and become phlegm.

- Herbs that strengthen the Spleen and promote water metabolism such as Poria *(fú líng)*, Atractylodis macrocephalae Rhizoma *(bái zhú)*, or Glycyrrhizae Radix *(gān cǎo)*. This is necessary because of the close relationship between Spleen physiology and water metabolism, outlined above.

- Herbs that preserve the fluids, moisten, and tonify the blood such as Mume Fructus *(wū méi)*, Schisandrae Fructus *(wǔ wèi zǐ)*, Ginseng Radix *(rén shēn)*, Angelicae sinensis Radix *(dāng guī)*, or even Rehmanniae Radix praeparata *(shú dì huáng)*. This is necessary because the presence of phlegm obstructs the circulation of physiological fluids and, inasmuch as phlegm represents a failure of fluid

transformation, reduces their amount. Adding such herbs addresses this crucial but often neglected aspect of phlegm disorders and increases the efficacy of these formulas.

二陳湯 (二陈汤)
Two-Aged [Herb] Decoction
èr chén tāng

The name of this formula indicates that the two chief herbs, unlike most other herbs, become more effective when they have been stored for some time because this makes their action less harsh. As noted in *Medical Formulas Collected and Analyzed*: "Aged Citri reticulatae Pericarpium *(chén pí)* and Pinelliae Rhizoma praeparatum *(zhì bàn xià)* are highly valued because there is no worry about their drying and dispersing [natures]. Hence, [the formula] has 'two-aged' in its name."

Source *Formulary of the Pharmacy Service for Benefiting the People in the Taiping Era* (1148)

Pinelliae Rhizoma praeparatum *(zhì bàn xià)* 15g
Citri reticulatae Exocarpium rubrum *(jú hóng)* 15g
Poria *(fú líng)* 9g
Glycyrrhizae Radix praeparata *(zhì gān cǎo)* 4.5g

Method of Preparation The source text advises to coarsely grind the ingredients and take 12g as a draft with 7 pieces of Zingiberis Rhizoma recens *(shēng jiāng)* and 1 piece of Mume Fructus *(wū méi)*. Most modern texts omit these two additions, and substitute Citri reticulatae Pericarpium *(chén pí)* for Citri reticulatae Exocarpium rubrum *(jú hóng)*. When the formula is prepared as a decoction, the dosage of all ingredients is reduced by one-third.

Actions Dries dampness, transforms phlegm, regulates the qi, and harmonizes the middle burner

Indications

Coughing with copious, white sputum that is easily expectorated, focal distention and a stifling sensation in the chest and diaphragm, palpitations, nausea or vomiting, dizziness, a white, moist or greasy tongue coating, and a slippery pulse.

This is a phlegm-dampness pattern, usually caused when the Spleen and Lungs fail to transform and transport the fluids, which thereupon accumulate and form phlegm. The accumulation of phlegm-dampness in turn encumbers the Spleen, which further impedes the transportation of fluids. Phlegm obstructs the qi mechanisms of the middle burner, which manifests as focal distention and a stifling sensation in the chest and diaphragm, and palpitations. Phlegm follows the flow of qi upward to the Lungs, where it interferes with its qi mechanisms and produces coughing. Because the process that generates the phlegm is one caused by excess dampness, the sputum is copious, white, and easily expectorated. Phlegm also interferes with the normal descent of the Stomach qi, which leads to nausea or vomiting. The presence of phlegm in the middle burner obstructs the ascent of the clear yang and causes dizziness. The slippery pulse and the white, moist or greasy tongue coating are indicative of phlegm-dampness.

Analysis of Formula

The preferred strategy for treating phlegm is to strengthen the transportive functions of the Spleen, Stomach, and Lungs by regulating the qi and drying the dampness. One of the chief ingredients, warm, acrid Pinelliae Rhizoma praeparatum (zhì bàn xià), dries dampness, expels phlegm, and causes the rebellious Stomach qi to descend. It thereby provides most of the actions required in treating this disorder. Useful in controlling nausea and vomiting, its main purpose is to open the qi dynamic, as noted by Zhang Shan-Lei:

> The best aspects of Pinelliae Rhizoma (bàn xià) can be summed up in four characters: opening (開 kāi), disseminating (宣 xuān), slippery (滑 huá), and downward-directing (降 jiàng). The reason that it can eliminate turbidity and phlegm is simply its actions in opening, draining, and slipping downward.

The other chief ingredient is Citri reticulatae Exocarpium rubrum (jú hóng), or Citri reticulatae Pericarpium (chén pí), whose fragrance revives the Spleen and facilitates the flow of qi in the middle burner. Its acrid flavor disperses clumped qi, while its bitter warmth disperses cold and dries dampness. By removing the obstruction to the flow of qi, the functions of the Spleen and Stomach are assisted; by dispelling cold dampness, phlegm is eliminated. The restored movement of qi induced by Citri reticulatae Pericarpium (chén pí) promotes the spontaneous resolution of phlegm. The transformation of phlegm by Pinelliae Rhizoma praeparatum (zhì bàn xià) facilitates the smooth flow of qi. Once this occurs, the transportive and transformative functions of the Spleen and Stomach will be restored, and the middle burner will no longer produce phlegm.

The deputy, Poria (fú líng), supports the actions of the chief ingredients by leaching out dampness from the middle burner and strengthening the Spleen. It also resolves the palpitations and dizziness caused by the upward-rising phlegm-dampness. In this manner, it treats the root of the disorder, as explained in Medical Texts from the Bettering the World Studio: "Poria (fú líng) is an herb that focuses on treating phlegm. The root of phlegm is water. Poria (fú líng) is able to move water. Phlegm is a change [in the state of] dampness. Poria (fú líng) is also able to move dampness." The assistant, Glycyrrhizae Radix praeparata (zhì gān cǎo), is used here to tonify the Spleen. Zingiberis Rhizoma recens (shēng jiāng) may be added as an envoy to reinforce the actions of the chief herbs in moving the qi and eliminating the phlegm, harmonizing the Stomach, and controlling the nausea. Mume Fructus (wū méi) counterbalances the dispersing tendencies of the chief ingredients and thereby prevents the dissipation of Lung qi. Its astringent nature also acts to collect the phlegm

together before it can be eliminated, an action referred to by Li Shi-Zhen as "ejecting phlegm" (涌痰 yǒng tán). It also prevents injury to the fluids and, as an expectorant, symptomatically assists in the treatment of coughing.

Cautions and Contraindications

The improper use of this formula can lead to excessive thirst and a dry throat. Without modification, it is contraindicated for cases with cough associated with Lung yin deficiency.

Commentary

This formula serves as the foundation for literally dozens of other formulas that address the problem of phlegm, many of which are discussed elsewhere in this text. The close connection between Spleen deficiency and phlegm is illustrated by the fact that, with the addition of Ginseng Radix (rén shēn) and Atractylodis macrocephalae Rhizoma (bái zhú), this formula is transformed into Six-Gentlemen Decoction (liù jūn zǐ tāng), one of the principal formulas for tonifying the qi. In terms of its functions, however, Two-Aged [Herb] Decoction (èr chén tāng) is a qi-regulating formula and is thus indicated for excess patterns following a famous adage first expressed by Pang An-Chang in Indispensable Tools for Pattern Treatment: "Experts in treating phlegm treat the qi not the phlegm. [Once] the qi is normalized, the fluids of the entire body follow the qi and are also normalized."

History

Historically, this formula can be viewed as a combination of Minor Pinellia plus Poria Deoction (xiǎo bàn xià jiā fú líng tāng) and Pinellia and Magnolia Bark Decoction (bàn xià hòu pò tāng) from Essentials from the Golden Cabinet. Both of these are qi-regulating formulas (discussed in Chapter 12), the former treating phlegm and thin mucus in the epigastrium and diaphragmatic region, and the latter treating qi stagnation leading to phlegm in the throat and chest. Although the present formula was first listed in the Song-dynasty Formulary of the Pharmacy Service for Benefiting the People in the Taiping Era, a similar combination of ingredients used to treat phlegm disorders can be found as early as Sun Si-Miao's Warm Gallbladder Decoction (wēn dǎn tāng) from the Tang dynasty. This suggests that is was used long before. Its modern popularity owes much to the Yuan-dynasty master physician Zhu Dan-Xi, who used this formula as one of the pillars of his medical practice. As Wang Lun-Zeng explained in Miscellaneous Writings of Enlightened Physicians:

> Mr. [Zhu] Dan-Xi's treatment of illness does not go beyond [the three categories of] qi, blood, and phlegm. Thus, he utilized three essential medicinals: to treat the qi, he used Four-Gentlemen Decoction (sì jūn zǐ tāng); to treat the blood, he used Four-Substance Decoction (sì wù tāng); and to treat phlegm, he used Two-Aged [Herb] Decoction (èr chén tāng).

Zhu Dan-Xi created a number of modifications to treat various kinds of phlegm disorders. His influence ensured the widespread use of these formulas. One of his followers, the Qing-dynasty physician Li Yong-Cui, expanded these doctrines into a comprehensive approach that added other herbs to the core formula in line with one or more of the following strategies:

- To treat phlegm disorders on the basis of its manifestation (e.g., wind-phlegm, phlegm-dampness, phlegm-fire, phlegm due to harbored food), one adds herbs that disperse wind, dry dampness, drain fire, etc.

- To treat phlegm disorders on the basis of their location, one can add herbs that guide the formula into specific organs or body regions.

- To treat phlegm disorders on the basis of a patient's constitution, one can add, for example, Cyperi Rhizoma *(xiāng fù)* and Aurantii Fructus *(zhǐ ké)* to treat obese people who have a tendency toward qi stagnation, or Atractylodis Rhizoma *(cāng zhú)* and Coptidis Rhizoma *(huáng lián)* to treat thin people who have a tendency toward phlegm-fire.

- One can also modify the formula in response to the dynamic of specific disease processes. In the treatment of withdrawal-mania, for example, bitter, cooling, and phlegm-dispelling herbs like Coptidis Rhizoma *(huáng lián)*, Scutellariae Radix *(huáng qín)*, Arisaematis Rhizoma praeparatum *(zhì tiān nán xīng)*, and Trichosanthis Fructus *(guā lóu)* are added during the manic phase, while during the withdrawal phase, tonifying and moistening substances like Angelicae sinensis Radix *(dāng guī)*, Rehmanniae Radix *(shēng dì huáng)*, or Ziziphi spinosae Semen *(suān zǎo rén)* may be utilized.

- One can modify the formula as the disorder develops. For example, when a patient has already vomited, one can add Platycodi Radix *(jié gěng)* and Phragmitis Rhizoma *(lú gēn)* to facilitate the upward expulsion of the pathogen. Once the vomiting has ceased, one then adds Amomi Fructus *(shā rén)* and Aucklandiae Radix *(mù xiāng)* in order to harmonize the Stomach.

Place in the Treatment of Phlegm

Other physicians expanded the use of this formula to include such diverse problems as excessive drooling in children, diarrhea, stomach pain, insomnia as well as hypersomnia, menstrual disorders, infertility, and emotional constraint, to name but a few. This diversity is reflected in the MODIFICATIONS and ASSOCIATED FORMULAS below. Some commentators went so far as to recommend this as the basic formula for all phlegm disorders. Fei Bo-Xiong's account in *Discussion of Medical Formulas* is representative of this view:

Phlegm disorders are the harshest and also the most frequent [that we see in practice]. Accumulation of dampness and con-

straint [generating] fire are the main sources whereby phlegm is produced. It can also be due to wind, cold, qi, or food [so that phlegm disorders] emerge in myriad shapes and strange variations that cannot be listed in any systematic fashion. The main strategy for treating phlegm is—where they occur—to dry the dampness, clear the fire, disperse the wind, warm the cold, smooth the qi, and eliminate [the harbored] food. Two-Aged [Herb] Decoction *(èr chén tāng)* is the principal formula. One employs it in order to transform phlegm and regulate the qi, [which it is] capable of doing [by way of] moving the Spleen and harmonizing the Stomach. If the student modifies it according to the presenting symptoms, imposing [treatment according to] the cause of the disorder, then there are no limits to its use.

While Fei's views are widely shared among physicians, others are more circumspect. Writing in *Convenient Reader of Established Formulas*, Zhang Bin-Cheng exemplifies this group by restricting the use of Two-Aged [Herb] Decoction *(èr chén tāng)* to phlegm-dampness:

[In treating] phlegm disorders, the first step is to differentiate them into two groups according to dampness and dryness. Phlegm-dryness is due to fire scorching the Lungs. Here, the scorched fluids turn into phlegm, [producing] cough with little phlegm that is difficult to expel. This should be treated by moistening, directing downward, and clearing metal. Phlegm-dampness is due to dampness encumbering the Spleen yang so that the water fluids accumulate to become phlegm, [producing] cough with copious phlegm that is easy to expel. This should be treated by drying the dampness and promoting earth, which is what this formula does.

Issues Regarding the Use of Pinelliae Rhizoma praeparatum *(zhì bàn xià)*

The concern of physicians like Zhang Bin-Cheng is that Pinelliae Rhizoma praeparatum *(zhì bàn xià)*, the main herb in this formula, is intensely drying and therefore contraindicated in patterns characterized by a lack of body fluids. Traditionally, therefore, Pinelliae Rhizoma praeparatum *(zhì bàn xià)* is said to be contraindicated for patterns characterized by thirst, and many physicians prefer to use herbs like Fritillariae Bulbus *(bèi mǔ)* and Trichosanthis Radix *(tiān huā fěn)* in these cases. In *Investigations of Medical Formulas*, the Ming-dynasty physician Wu Kun presented a more sophisticated differentiation:

There are those who say that Pinelliae Rhizoma praeparatum *(zhì bàn xià)* is not appropriate for phlegm [disorders characterized] by thirst. One therefore should remove the drying of Pinelliae Rhizoma praeparatum *(zhì bàn xià)* [from this formula] and replace it with the moistening of Fritillariae Bulbus *(bèi mǔ)* or Trichosanthis Radix *(tiān huā fěn)*. I say there is a better trick. [If a patient] is thirsty and desires to drink water, then it should be substituted. However, if they are thirsty but do not want to drink, then it is better to use Pinelliae Rhizoma praeparatum *(zhì bàn xià)*. In these cases, phlegm is the root and heat the branch. Thus, when one also observes thirst, this is what is known as extreme dampness transforming into what it [ordinarily] conquers. This is not a true manifestation [of the underlying condition] but only those who understand know this.

Another perspective on this issue is provided by Li Shi-Zhen in *Comprehensive Outline of the Materia Medica*. Regarding the formula's chief ingredient, he observed:

> The reason that Pinelliae Rhizoma *(bàn xià)* governs phlegm and thin mucus with abdominal distention is that it is physically slippery, its flavor is acrid, and its nature is warm: the slipperiness moistens the phlegm, and the acrid warmth disperses and also moistens; thus, it promotes [elimination of] dampness and unblocks stool, facilitates [the proper functioning of the] orifices and drains urination, and thus it is said that 'the acrid mobilizes the qi to transform phlegm'—this is the use of acridity to moisten.

Hence, although it is probably inadvisable to use this formula in cases of yin deficiency characterized by a severe lack of fluids, dryness alone is not a contraindication. This is because phlegm itself generates dryness: partly by obstructing the movement of qi and fluids, and partly by being itself the pathological product of those body fluids that withdraws their moisture from the body. Transforming and eliminating phlegm thus has the ability to moisten, while both Pinelliae Rhizoma praeparatum *(zhì bàn xià)* and Two-Aged [Herb] Decoction *(èr chén tāng)* are often combined with moistening and blood-tonifying herbs such as Angelicae sinensis Radix *(dāng guī)*, Rehmanniae Radix praeparata *(shú dì huáng)*, Lycii Fructus *(gǒu qǐ zǐ)*, or Ziziphi spinosae Semen *(suān zǎo rén)*. See, for example, the associated formula Six-Gentlemen of Metal and Water Decoction *(jīn shuǐ liù jūn jiān)* as well as Ten-Ingredient Warm Gallbladder Decoction *(shí wèi wēn dǎn tāng)*, discussed later in this chapter.

Other Ingredients

That this formula is, at the most fundamental level, for regulating the qi dynamic and fluid metabolism can also be seen in its putatively less important ingredients, the assistant and envoy herbs. Several commentators, such as Chen Nian-Zu in *Compendium of Songs on Modern Formulas* and Tang Zong-Hai in *Discussion of Blood Patterns*, argue that, because all phlegm is a pathological transformation of water, Poria *(fú líng)* should be viewed as the main herb in this formula. Considering just the relative dosage of the ingredients, this is probably incorrect. But it does point to the importance, in the treatment of phlegm disorders, of reordering the fluid metabolism throughout the Triple Burner.

This applies as well to the use of Zingiberis Rhizoma recens *(shēng jiāng)* and Mume Fructus *(wū méi)*. Some writers, such as Wang Ang in *Medical Formulas Collected and Analyzed* and the authors of the 1964 standard textbook *Chinese Medical Formulas*, consider these herbs superfluous. But

others, such as Li Fei and his colleagues in the most recent edition of *Formulas*, instead define them as examplars of the subtleties of classical formula composition in that they focus on the Lungs rather than the Spleen, to add a second prong to the regulation of qi and fluids. The acrid, warming nature of Zingiberis Rhizoma recens *(shēng jiāng)* promotes the qi dynamic and thereby helps to eliminate pathological fluids. According to the early 20th-century writer Zhang Xi-Chun, "This acrid, dispersing power is ideal for opening the phlegm and regulating the qi, alleviating nausea and vomiting." Mume Fructus *(wū méi)* balances this dispersing action by means of its sourness, while compensating for the loss of pathological fluids (through coughing, increased urination, and sweating) by protecting and generating physiological fluids. According to the *Convenient Reader of Materia Medica*, Mume Fructus *(wū méi)* also directly enters the Liver blood, and for this reason is, of course, used in Mume Pill *(wū méi wán)*, Zhang Zhong-Jing's flagship formula for the treatment of terminal yin disorders. Its use here may at first seem odd. But adding a sour, astringent Liver herb that also supports the Stomach yin to an otherwise acrid, moving formula centered on the Lung's regulation of qi and the Spleen's moving and transforming functions represents precisely the kind of balancing and harmonizing that is at the heart of many great formulas.

Comparison

➤ Vs. Guide Out Phlegm Decoction *(dǎo tán tāng)*; *see* PAGE 781

Biomedical Indications

With the appropriate presentation, this formula may be used to treat a wide variety of biomedically-defined disorders including upper respiratory tract infection, chronic bronchitis, emphysema, goiter, chronic gastritis, peptic ulcer, morning sickness, and Ménière's disease.

Modifications

- For damp-heat in the upper burner, add Scutellariae Radix *(huáng qín)*, Gardeniae Fructus *(zhī zǐ)*, Armeniacae Semen *(xìng rén)*, and Platycodi Radix *(jié gěng)*.

- For damp-heat in the middle burner, add Coptidis Rhizoma *(huáng lián)*, Pogostemonis/Agastaches Herba *(huò xiāng)*, Magnoliae officinalis Cortex *(hòu pò)*, and Coicis Semen *(yì yǐ rén)*.

- For damp-heat in the lower burner, add Sophorae flavescentis Radix *(kǔ shēn)*, Phellodendri Cortex *(huáng bǎi)*, and Talcum *(huá shí)*.

- For wind-dampness, add Clematidis Radix *(wēi líng xiān)*, Gentianae macrophyllae Radix *(qín jiāo)*, Xanthii Fructus *(cāng ěr zǐ)*, and Cinnamomi Ramulus *(guì zhī)*.

- For cough with copious sputum due to phlegm-dampness in the interior complicated by the presence of pathogenic qi in the exterior, add Perillae Folium (*zǐ sū yè*) and Armeniacae Semen (*xìng rén*).

- For cough with copious sputum due to externally-contracted cold in the Lungs, add Ephedrae Herba (*má huáng*) or Perillae Folium (*zǐ sū yè*) and Armeniacae Semen (*xìng rén*).

- For vomiting due to cold in the Stomach, add Zingiberis Rhizoma (*gān jiāng*) and Amomi Fructus (*shā rén*).

- For vomiting of clear fluids, add Atractylodis Rhizoma (*cāng zhú*) and Atractylodis macrocephalae Rhizoma (*bái zhú*).

- For chronic phlegm in the channels and flesh leading to rubbery nodules, add Ostreae Concha (*mǔ lì*), Scrophulariae Radix (*xuán shēn*), Eckloniae Thallus (*kūn bù*), and Laminariae Thallus (*hǎi dài*).

- For Spleen and Kidney yang deficiency characterized by coughing of thin, watery sputum, a submerged pulse, and urinary difficulty, add Cinnamomi Cortex (*ròu guì*), and Aconiti Radix lateralis praeparata (*zhì fù zǐ*).

- For insomnia and a desire to sleep during the day that worsens after meals, add Atractylodis macrocephalae Rhizoma (*bái zhú*) and Acori tatarinowii Rhizoma (*shí chāng pú*).

- For severe coughing at night due to a combination of phlegm and blood deficiency, add Angelicae sinensis Radix (*dāng guī*).

- For phlegm-dampness obstructing the womb with irregular menstruation and copious leukorrhea, add Chuanxiong Rhizoma (*chuān xiōng*) and Angelicae sinensis Radix (*dāng guī*).

- For concurrent dryness, substitute Trichosanthis Fructus (*guā lóu*) and Fritillariae cirrhosae Bulbus (*chuān bèi mǔ*) for Pinelliae Rhizoma praeparatum (*zhì bàn xià*).

Associated Formulas

金水六君煎

Six-Gentlemen of Metal and Water Decoction

jīn shuǐ liù jūn jiān

SOURCE *Collected Treatises of [Zhang] Jing-Yue* (1624)

Pinelliae Rhizoma praeparatum (*zhì bàn xià*). 6g
Citri reticulatae Pericarpium (*chén pí*). 4.5g
Poria (*fú líng*). 6g
Glycyrrhizae Radix praeparata (*zhì gān cǎo*). 3g
Angelicae sinensis Radix (*dāng guī*). 6g
Rehmanniae Radix praeparata (*shú dì huáng*). 9-15g

Decoct with 3-7 pieces of Zingiberis Rhizoma recens (*shēng jiāng*). Enriches and nourishes the Lungs and Kidneys, dispels dampness,

and transforms phlegm. For Lung and Kidney yin deficiency with rising phlegm characterized by copious, white sputum that is difficult to expectorate, wheezing, nausea, and a peeled tongue. The sputum may have a salty taste and the throat may be parched. Recently, this formula has been widely used for treating chronic bronchitis in the elderly.

In the pattern for which this formula is indicated, yin deficiency is the root and phlegm is the branch. This can be compared to a sponge that has become too dry to hold any fluid. For this reason, one must enrich the yin with cloying and moistening herbs even though this hinders the expulsion of phlegm. By matching the chief ingredient, moistening Rehmanniae Radix praeparata (*shú dì huáng*), with the deputy, acrid and moving Pinelliae Rhizoma praeparatum (*zhì bàn xià*), at a dosage ratio of two to one, this formula succeeds in tonifying the yin without increasing the dampness, and in transforming the phlegm without further injuring the yin. Removing acrid and dispersing Zingiberis Rhizoma recens (*shēng jiāng*) and astringent Mume Fructus (*wū méi*) from the original formula can also be viewed as a means of achieving this objective.

Some commentators view Zhang Jie-Bin's innovative combination of moistening and drying herbs as most appropriate. For example, in *Convenient Reader of Established Formulas*, Zhang Bin-Cheng noted that "this formula is balanced and achieves its two (objectives) in an appropriate manner." However others, such as Xie Guan in the *Encyclopedia of the Medicine of China*, had fundamental criticisms:

> If this formula employs Rehmanniae Radix praeparata (*shú dì huáng*) as a cooling, moistening [herb] and Angelicae sinensis Radix (*dāng guī*) as an acrid, moistening [herb] together with Two-Aged [Herb] Decoction (*èr chén tāng*) as a prescription for Spleen and Kidney cold from deficiency [causing] water flooding that becomes phlegm, then [its author] does not understand that one cannot treat Lung cold without the combination of Zingiberis Rhizoma (*gān jiāng*) and Asari Radix et Rhizoma (*xì xīn*), and Kidney cold without large [doses] of Zingiberis Rhizoma (*gān jiāng*) and Aconiti Radix lateralis praeparata (*zhì fù zǐ*). If one uses cooling and moistening Rehmanniae Radix praeparata (*shú dì huáng*) and Angelicae sinensis Radix (*dāng guī*) to help [in a pattern characterized by] water and thin mucus, it will [only] result in yin haze spreading throughout the body, with the momentum of water attacking the upper [burner] so that disorders [characterized by] rebellious qi and coughing will get worse day by day.

理中化痰丸

Regulate the Middle and Transform Phlegm Pill

lǐ zhōng huà tán wán

SOURCE *Miscellaneous Writings of Enlightened Physicians* (1549)

Zingiberis Rhizoma (*gān jiāng*)
Ginseng Radix (*rén shēn*)
Atractylodis macrocephalae Rhizoma (*bái zhú*)
Glycyrrhizae Radix praeparata (*zhì gān cǎo*)
Poria (*fú líng*)
Pinelliae Rhizoma praeparatum (*zhì bàn xià*)

The source text does not specify dosage, but simply instructs to grind the ingredients into a powder and form into small pills, 40-50 of which are taken with warm water. At present, equal amounts of the ingredients are used, taken 6-9g at a time. Augments the qi, strengthens the Spleen, and warms and transforms phlegm. For Spleen and Stomach yang deficiency with cold and thin mucus characterized by reduced appetite, loose stools, vomiting of clear fluids, excessive salivation, coughing up watery sputum, a white, slippery tongue coating, and a submerged, slow pulse.

六安煎

Six-Serenity Decoction

liù ān jiān

Source   *Collected Treatises of [Zhang] Jing-Yue* (1624)

Citri reticulatae Pericarpium (*chén pí*) 4.5g
Pinelliae Rhizoma praeparatum (*zhì bàn xià*) 6-9g
Poria (*fú líng*) 6g
Glycyrrhizae Radix (*gān cǎo*) 3g
Armeniacae Semen (*xìng rén*) 3g
Sinapis Semen (*bái jiè zǐ*) 1.5-2.1g

Decoct with 3-7 pieces of Zingiberis Rhizoma recens (*shēng jiāng*). Dries dampness, transforms phlegm, directs rebellious qi downward, and calms wheezing. For the subacute stage of wind-cold disorders presenting with coughing and wheezing with sticky sputum that is difficult to expectorate. The use of a modification of Two-Aged [Herb] Decoction (*èr chén tāng*) in patients with exterior conditions was severely criticized by the Qing-dynasty physician Chen Nian-Zu, who wrote in *Compendium of Songs on Modern Formulas*: "[Some] use this as a formula for resolving the exterior in any of the three yang [warps]. Its ingestion causes the pathogen to linger and generates fever leading to the death [of the patient without the physician] understanding [the reason why]." Accordingly, where phlegm is caused by external wind-cold pathogens obstructing the qi dynamic and water metabolism, they must be expelled first; Two-Aged [Herb] Decoction (*èr chén tāng*) should only be used when no external pathogens remain.

加味二陳湯 (加味二陈汤)

Augmented Two-Aged [Herb] Decoction

jiā wèi èr chén tāng

Source   *Golden Mirror of the Medical Tradition* (1742)

Pinelliae Rhizoma praeparatum (*zhì bàn xià*) 2.4g
Citri reticulatae Pericarpium (*chén pí*) 2.4g
Poria (*fú líng*) 2.4g
Glycyrrhizae Radix (*gān cǎo*) 1.5g
Scutellariae Radix (*huáng qín*) 2.4g
Coptidis Rhizoma (*huáng lián*) 1.5g
Menthae haplocalycis Herba (*bò hé*) 1.5g

Decoct with 3 pieces of Zingiberis Rhizoma recens (*shēng jiāng*). Clears fire, transforms phlegm, harmonizes the Stomach, and directs turbidity downward. For phlegm-fire with incessant, cicada-like tinnitus, hearing loss with occasional deafness, lightheadedness, a sensation of heaviness in the head, a stifling sensation and fullness in the chest and abdomen, coughing with copious sputum, bitter taste, urinary and bowel difficulty, a red tongue with a yellow, greasy coating, and a wiry, slippery pulse.

導痰湯 (导痰汤)

Guide Out Phlegm Decoction

dǎo tán tāng

Source   *Transmitted Trustworthy and Suitable Formulas* (1180)

Pinelliae Rhizoma praeparatum (*zhì bàn xià*) 12g
Citri reticulatae Exocarpium rubrum (*jú hóng*) 3g
Poria (*fú líng*) 3g
Aurantii Fructus immaturus (*zhǐ shí*) 3g
Arisaematis Rhizoma praeparatum (*zhì tiān nán xīng*) 3g

Method of Preparation   Coarsely grind the ingredients and take 12g as a draft with 10 slices of Zingiberis Rhizoma recens (*shēng jiāng*). May also be prepared as a decoction.

Actions   Dries dampness, clears away phlegm, promotes the movement of qi, and opens up areas of constraint

Indications

Fainting or vertigo with headache accompanied by such symptoms as a stifling sensation and focal distention in the chest and diaphragm, reduced appetite, distention and fullness in the hypochondria and flanks, restlessness when sitting or lying down, coughing and wheezing with copious sputum and difficulty breathing, thick and gummy nasal discharge and saliva, a white, greasy tongue coating, and a slippery pulse.

This is collapse due to phlegm (痰厥 *tán jué*), or wind-phlegm, or an accumulation of congested fluids that will not dissipate. The term collapse (厥 *jué*) implies that the yin and yang do not flow smoothly and harmoniously in concert with each other. In the present case, this is due to phlegm obstructing the interior and preventing the proper expansion of the qi dynamic. Vertigo and headache can be caused by the same pathology: phlegm-dampness preventing the clear yang from ascending and the turbid dampness from being directed downward. The obstruction of the qi dynamic is experienced subjectively as a stifling sensation and focal distention in the chest and diaphragm, reduced appetite, distention and fullness in the hypochondria and flanks, restlessness when sitting or lying down, coughing and wheezing with copious sputum and difficulty breathing, thick and gummy nasal discharge and saliva. The white, greasy tongue coating and slippery pulse reflect this pathology.

Analysis of Formula

To open the obstruction of the qi dynamic that is at the heart of the various patterns treated by this formula, Guide Out Phlegm Decoction (*dǎo tán tāng*) focuses on drying dampness and dispelling phlegm, moving the qi and opening constraint. Acrid, warming, and drying Pinelliae Rhizoma praeparatum (*zhì bàn xià*), with a dosage that is four times as much as that of the other herbs, serves as chief because it addresses all of these objectives. It dries dampness, expels phlegm, directs the turbid qi downward, and focuses particularly on the Stomach, chest, and epigastrium, the fulcrum of the qi dynamic and the body region where this kind of obstruction is most visible. Warming and intensely drying Arisaematis Rhizoma praeparatum *(zhì tiān nán xīng)* acts as deputy. More dispersing then Pinelliae Rhizoma praeparatum *(zhì bàn xià)*, this herb also enters the Liver channel, and its special quality enables it to move within the channels and collaterals. Thus, it is particularly good at eliminating wind-phlegm, which here manifests as collapse and headache. Bitter, acrid, and slightly cold Aurantii Fructus immaturus *(zhǐ shí)* breaks up stagnant qi and reduces accumulation. As an assistant, it transforms the phlegm and expels focal distention to treat the fullness in the chest and epigastrium caused by turbid phlegm obstructing and plugging the qi dynamic. Citri reticulatae Pericarpium *(chén pí)* and Poria *(fú líng)* also serve as assistants, entering the Spleen to support its functions of transporting and transformation. Citri reticulatae Pericarpium *(chén pí)* works together with Pinelliae Rhizoma praeparatum *(zhì bàn xià)* and Aurantii Fructus immaturus *(zhǐ shí)* in unblocking the qi dynamic, while Poria *(fú líng)* facilitates the water metabolism to eliminate dampness, the main source of phlegm. Zingiberis Rhizoma recens *(shēng jiāng)* serves as envoy. It reduces the toxicity of Pinelliae Rhizoma praeparatum *(zhì bàn xià)* and Arisaematis Rhizoma praeparatum *(zhì tiān nán xīng)*, based on the concept of 'mutual suppression' (相殺 *xiāng shā*), assists Pinelliae Rhizoma praeparatum *(zhì bàn xià)* in reducing the symptoms of nausea and vomiting, and also helps to stop the coughing and eliminate the phlegm.

Cautions and Contraindications

This formula is intensely drying and moving. It is contraindicated in patterns characterized by yin deficiency or heat.

Commentary

In the source text, this formula was attributed to the Song physician Huang-Fu Dan. It was also included in several other texts of the period, including *Formulas to Aid the Living*, in which Glycyrrhizae Radix *(gān cǎo)* was added. (This expanded formula is mistakenly cited in many contemporary textbooks as the original formula.) The addition of Glycyrrhizae Radix *(gān cǎo)* balances the harshly drying properties of the formula but may lead to some obstruction in the middle burner.

Many of the symptoms treated by this formula, such as headache, dizziness, pain and numbness in the extremities, resemble the manifestations of wind. However, as Wu Yi-Luo points out in *Practical Established Formulas,* they do not denote the presence of wind in the narrow sense, that is, exter-

nal wind that has penetrated into the body from the exterior, nor internal wind due to Liver yang excess or yin deficiency, but rather an obstruction to the qi dynamic. He thus recommends the addition of other qi-regulating herbs such as Aucklandiae Radix *(mù xiāng)* or Cyperi Rhizoma *(xiāng fù)* to further support the function of the formula.

In contemporary practice, this formula is used for asthma and chronic bronchitis provided they are due to phlegm-dampness. In these, as in the conditions listed above, a slippery pulse, greasy tongue coating, and copious phlegm are the key clinical markers.

Comparisons

➤ Vs. Two-Aged [Herb] Decoction *(èr chén tāng)*

Both formulas treat patterns caused by phlegm-dampness obstructing the qi dynamic. But while Two-Aged [Herb] Decoction *(èr chén tāng)* is a base formula that can be modified according to the precise manifestations, Guide Out Phlegm Decoction *(dǎo tán tāng)* is for conditions with more severe phlegm and constriction of qi, which may suddenly discharge as wind causing collapse or manifest with wind-like symptoms such as headache and dizziness.

➤ Vs. Scour Out Phlegm Decoction *(dí tán tāng)*;
   see PAGE 783

Biomedical Indications

With the appropriate presentation, this formula may be used to treat a variety of biomedically-defined disorders including chronic bronchitis, Ménière's disease, and pleurisy.

Modifications

- For pain in the extremities, back, or shoulders, replace Arisaematis Rhizoma praeparatum *(zhì tiān nán xīng)* with Arisaema cum Bile *(dǎn nán xīng)* and add Aucklandiae Radix *(mù xiāng)* and Curcumae longae Rhizoma *(jiāng huáng)*.

- For palpitations, forgetfulness, and insomnia, replace Arisaematis Rhizoma praeparatum *(zhì tiān nán xīng)* with Arisaema cum Bile *(dǎn nán xīng)* and add Acori tatarinowii Rhizoma *(shí chāng pǔ)*.

- For epilepsy with phlegm obstructing the heart orifices, add Chrysanthemi Flos *(jú huā)*, Uncariae Ramulus cum Uncis *(gōu téng)*, Gleditsiae Fructus *(zào jiá)*, Acori tatarinowii Rhizoma *(shí chāng pǔ)*, Bambusae Succus *(zhú lì)*, and Zingiberis Rhizomatis Succus *(jiāng zhī)*.

- For more severe dampness and cold, add Asari Radix et Rhizoma *(xì xīn)* and Zingiberis Rhizoma *(gān jiāng)*.

- For wind-phlegm with headache and dizziness, add Gastrodiae Rhizoma *(tiān má)* and Atractylodis macrocephalae Rhizoma *(bái zhú)*.

滌痰湯 （涤痰汤）

Scour Out Phlegm Decoction

dí tán tāng

Source   *Fine Formulas of Wonderful Efficacy* (1470)

Arisaematis Rhizoma praeparatum *(zhì tiān nán xīng)* 7.5g

Pinelliae Rhizoma praeparatum *(zhì bàn xià)* 7.5g

Poria *(fú líng)* 6g

Aurantii Fructus immaturus *(zhǐ shí)* 6g

Citri reticulatae Exocarpium rubrum *(jú hóng)* 4.5g

Acori tatarinowii Rhizoma *(shí chāng pǔ)* 3g

Ginseng Radix *(rén shēn)* 3g

Bambusae Caulis in taeniam *(zhú rú)* 2.1g

Glycyrrhizae Radix *(gān cǎo)* 2.1g

Method of Preparation   The source text advises to decoct the ingredients with 5 slices of Zingiberis Rhizoma recens *(shēng jiāng)* and to take following meals. At present, the dosage of Zingiberis Rhizoma recens *(shēng jiāng)* is reduced to 3 slices, and Citri reticulatae Pericarpium *(chén pí)* is often substituted for Citri reticulatae Exocarpium rubrum *(jú hóng)*.

Actions   Scours out phlegm, opens the sensory orifices, and tonifies the qi

Indications

Stiffness of the tongue and speech impairment.

These are the cardinal symptoms of this pattern of internal obstruction due to severe phlegm in which the smooth movement of the fluids has been impaired and the fluids have accumulated and formed phlegm that veils the orifices of the Heart. The Heart connects to the tongue. When phlegm veils the Heart orifices, it also obstructs the collaterals of the tongue, leading to stiffness and inability to speak. This generally occurs as a symptom or consequence of wind-stroke when phlegm moves upward under the influence of internal wind. It can also result from excessive accumulation of phlegm that spreads throughout the body.

Analysis of Formula

This formula focuses on scouring phlegm from the collaterals and orifices of the Heart, while also resolving stiffness, relaxing excessive contraction, and supporting the normal qi. Its chief ingredient is acrid, warm, and very drying Arisaematis Rhizoma praeparatum *(zhì tiān nán xīng)*. An important herb for expelling phlegm-dampness and thus removing the root of this disorder, it is also able to disperse wind and thereby treat phlegm turbidity clogging the vessels and collaterals. The deputy is Pinelliae Rhizoma praeparatum *(zhì bàn xià)*, another acrid, warming herb that excels at drying dampness and transforming phlegm, directing the rebellious qi downward, and harmonizing the Stomach.

These two herbs are supported by several groups of assistants. The first is comprised of Citri reticulatae Exocarpium rubrum *(jú hóng)*, which regulates the qi and dries dampness, and Aurantii Fructus immaturus *(zhǐ shí)*, which breaks up stagnation and transforms phlegm. To restore the qi dynamic, this combination embodies the principle of smoothing the flow of qi in order to treat phlegm. The second group of assistants includes Poria *(fú líng)*, which strengthens the Spleen by leaching out dampness, and Ginseng Radix *(rén shēn)*, which supports the normal qi to strengthen the Spleen. The Spleen is widely considered to be the source of phlegm pathologies, so that supporting its normal function prevents the disorder from recurring. The combination of Pinelliae Rhizoma praeparatum *(zhì bàn xià)*, Citri reticulatae Exocarpium rubrum *(jú hóng)*, Poria *(fú líng)*, and Glycyrrhizae Radix *(gān cǎo)* makes up Two-Aged [Herb] Decoction *(èr chén tāng)*, the main formula for treating phlegm-dampness. The third group of assistants consists of Bambusae Caulis in taeniam *(zhú rú)* and Acori tatarinowii Rhizoma *(shí chāng pǔ)*. The former transforms phlegm and is slightly cooling in nature to counteract the warming properties of most of the other ingredients. The latter not only transforms phlegm-dampness, but also aromatically opens up the orifices, directing the formula into the Heart channel to unblock the collaterals of the tongue. Glycyrrhizae Radix *(gān cǎo)* harmonizes the actions of the other ingredients and the functions of the middle burner. Together with Poria *(fú líng)* and Ginseng Radix *(rén shēn)*, it makes up Four-Gentlemen Decoction *(sì jūn zǐ tāng)*, discussed in Chapter 8. Zingiberis Rhizoma recens *(shēng jiāng)* also serves as an assistant, counteracting the toxicity of the chief and deputy ingredients as well as promoting dispersion of qi throughout the Triple Burner.

Overall, this is an especially powerful combination for breaking up stagnant qi, reducing accumulation, directing the qi downward, drying dampness, eliminating phlegm, clearing heat, and dispersing wind-phlegm in the channels.

Cautions and Contraindications

Contraindicated during pregnancy. Use with caution in weak patients.

Commentary

This is a Ming-dynasty formula that combines several older formulas to achieve a new effect: Two-Aged [Herb] Decoction *(èr chén tāng)*, discussed above, the basic formula for drying dampness and transforming phlegm; Four-Gentlemen Decoction *(sì jūn zǐ tāng)*, discussed in Chapter 8, a core formula for tonifying the qi; and Settle the Emotions Pill *(dìng zhì wán)*, discussed in Chapter 10, which treats phlegm obstructing the qi transformation of the Heart. To these has been added a large dosage of Arisaematis Rhizoma praeparatum *(zhì tiān nán xīng)* because of its ability to eliminate wind-phlegm from the channels and collaterals and its specific indication for wind-stroke.

Although there is a tonifying aspect to this formula, the pattern treated is one of acute excess. Accordingly, once the acute symptoms have been resolved, a more moderate and less drying formula should be employed. Any deficiency present is a deficiency of the nutritive qi associated with dampness or dryness disorders as well in the channels and collaterals. Viewed from this perspective, one can interpret the use of Ginseng Radix (*rén shēn*), Glycyrrhizae Radix (*gān cǎo*), and Poria (*fú líng*), all of which enter not only the Spleen but also the Heart, as a means of ensuring an adequate supply of clear nutritive qi to compensate for what has been transformed into pathological phlegm-dampness. Many commentators, nevertheless, consider the use of Arisaematis Rhizoma praeparatum (*zhì tiān nán xīng*) as being too drying and recommend that it be replaced with Arisaema cum Bile (*dǎn nán xīng*), which is bitter, cooling, and moistening in nature.

Several later formulas by the same name go even further and add herbs such as Coptidis Rhizoma (*huáng lián*) or Scutellariae Radix (*huáng qín*). This implies that the patient's constitution is very strong, and that long-term phlegm stagnation has caused the yang qi to become constrained so that it eventually combines with the phlegm and forms phlegm-fire. The inclusion of Bambusae Caulis in taeniam (*zhú rú*) in the original formula can also be interpreted from this perspective,

In contemporary practice, this formula is most commonly used in treating impaired speech following wind-stroke due to phlegm veiling the orifices of the Heart, and thus the tongue. Its efficacy in treating such patterns may be improved by adding other herbs, such as Scorpio (*quán xiē*), that resolve spasms. It can also be used to treat epilepsy with a similar presentation. Based on the actions of its constituent ingredients, its use has been expanded to include wheezing with copious sputum and focal distention and fullness in the chest due to obstruction of the qi in the chest by phlegm, as well as to other problems commonly attributed to phlegm pathologies such as severe dizziness, insomnia, or loss of motor function in disorders such as multiple sclerosis or motor aphasia.

Comparison

➤ Vs. Guide Out Phlegm Decoction (*dǎo tán tāng*)

Both formulas are modifications of Two-Aged [Herb] Decoction (*èr chén tāng*). Guide Out Phlegm Decoction (*dǎo tán tāng*) replaces Mume Fructus (*wū méi*) with Arisaematis Rhizoma praeparatum (*zhì tiān nán xīng*) and Aurantii Fructus immaturus (*zhǐ shí*) to produce a less balanced, but more drying and dispersing formula indicated for severe dizziness or stubborn cough associated with collapse due to phlegm or severe phlegm stagnation. By contrast, Scour Out Phlegm Decoction (*dí tán tāng*) adds Acori tatarinowii Rhizoma (*shí chāng pǔ*), Bambusae Caulis in taeniam (*zhú rú*), and Ginseng

Radix (*rén shēn*) to produce a formula that focuses these dispersing actions on the Heart and that therefore is particularly suitable for opening the Heart orifices and unblocking the collaterals of the tongue.

Biomedical Indications

With the appropriate presentation, this formula may be used to treat a variety of biomedically-defined disorders including cerebrovascular accident, seizure disorder, motor aphasia, bronchial asthma, chronic obstructive pulmonary disease, acute and chronic bronchitis, bronchiectasis, multiple sclerosis, and motor aphasia.

Alternate name

Scour Phlegm Powder (*dí tán sǎn*) in *Standards of the Imperial Archives*

Modifications

- For phlegm that is not hot, remove Bambusae Caulis in taeniam (*zhú rú*) and replace Arisaema cum Bile (*dǎn nán xīng*) with Arisaematis Rhizoma praeparatum (*zhì tiān nán xīng*).
- For severe heat, add Scutellariae Radix (*huáng qín*), Coptidis Rhizoma (*huáng lián*), Zingiberis Rhizomatis Succus (*jiāng zhī*), and Bambusae Succus (*zhú lì*).

茯苓丸

Poria Pill

fú líng wán

Source　*Selected Formulas* (1196)

Poria (*fú líng*)..............6g
Aurantii Fructus (*zhǐ ké*)..............3g
Pinelliae Rhizoma praeparatum (*zhì bàn xià*)..............9g
Natrii Sulfas (*máng xiāo*)..............3g

Method of Preparation　Grind the herbs into a powder, mix with fresh ginger juice to make a paste, and form into small pills. The recommended daily dose is 6g, to be taken with a decoction made from fresh ginger. At present, the pills are also taken with warm water.

Actions　Dries dampness, moves the qi, softens hardness, and transforms phlegm

Indications

Pain in both arms or shoulders with inability to lift the hands. The symptoms are often more pronounced on one side, and then on the other. Also used for numbness in both hands, or for superficial edema in all four extremities. The tongue will tend to have a white, greasy coating, and the pulse will be submerged and thin, or wiry and slippery.

This is phlegm tarrying in the middle burner from which

it overflows into the channels and collaterals. The four extremities resonate with the Spleen. When the transporting and transforming functions of the Spleen are impaired, dampness accumulates in the middle burner and transforms into phlegm. Pain and loss of function is caused by phlegm-dampness overflowing into the channels and collaterals where it obstructs the flow of qi and blood. Spleen qi naturally ascends, thus the symptoms are more pronounced in the arms. The nature of the pathogen becomes apparent in the superficial edema and swelling, greasy tongue coating, and the submerged and thin or wiry and slippery pulse.

Analysis of Formula

To treat phlegm obstructing the vessels and collaterals in the extremities due to phlegm-dampness tarrying in the middle burner and epigastrium, this formula employs a strategy of drying the dampness, moving the qi, softening the hardness, and transforming the phlegm. The chief herb, as in most formulas in this section, is acrid, warming, and drying Pinelliae Rhizoma praeparatum (*zhì bàn xià*), chosen for its ability to transform phlegm and facilitate the downward directing of the qi dynamic. Bland and neutral Poria (*fú líng*) acts as deputy to strengthen the Spleen, leach out dampness, and transform phlegm, attending to both the root and branch of this pattern. Aurantii Fructus (*zhǐ ké*) moves the qi and eases the middle, smoothing the qi dynamic to facilitate the elimination of phlegm. Salty and cooling Natrii Sulfas (*máng xiāo*) softens hardness and moistens dryness, reducing and guiding out lurking phlegm via the bowels. These two ingredients are regarded as assistants. Zingiberis Rhizoma recens (*shēng jiāng*), used both in the preparation of the pills and in the decoction that is taken to swallow them, serves as envoy. It counteracts the toxicity of Pinelliae Rhizoma praeparatum (*zhì bàn xià*), but also supports the chief and deputy herbs in transforming phlegm and dispersing thin mucus.

Cautions and Contraindications

This formula has a strong drying and downward-draining action. It should not be used in patients with weak constitutions. Its use should be discontinued as soon as the symptoms have eased.

Commentary

The traditional literature lists more than fifty different formulas named Poria Pill (*fú líng wán*). Those that treat phlegm-dampness generally contain Pinelliae Rhizoma praeparatum (*zhì bàn xià*), Poria (*fú líng*), and Aurantii Fructus (*zhǐ ké*) or Aurantii Fructus immaturus (*zhǐ shí*). Like most of the formulas in this section, this variation dates from the Song dynasty and can be traced, ultimately, to Minor Pinellia plus Poria Deoction (*xiǎo bàn xià jiā fú líng tāng*) in *Essentials from the Golden Cabinet*, discussed in Chapter 12.

This formula treats palpitations and vomiting, but focuses on thin mucus rather than phlegm. Its core strategy of regulating the qi and promoting the water metabolism, however, is also applicable to the treatment of phlegm-dampness and has thus been assimilated into the present formula. This strategy is combined with draining the lurking phlegm by means of purgation, borrowed from another formula in *Essentials from the Golden Cabinet*, Kansui and Pinellia Decoction (*gān suì bàn xià tāng*). This follows the adages, "Move what lingers" (留者行之 *liú zhě xíng zhī*) and "Disperse what has clumped" (結者散之 *jié zhě sàn zhī*). In the present formula, the harsh and toxic Kansui Radix (*gān suì*) has been replaced by the milder Natrii Sulfas (*máng xiāo*), which is particularly apt at eliminating phlegm-heat from the upper burner and Lungs (i.e., the arms and shoulders). The original formula uses nitre efflorescence (風化硝 *fēng huà xiāo*) rather than Natrii Sulfas (*máng xiāo*). This is the powder that remains when 'clean nitre' has been exposed to the wind, leading to evaporation of its water content. About this ingredient, *Rectification of the Meaning of Materia Medica* observes:

> In winter, placed in a coarse bag and hung from the eaves, its substance gradually turns white; this is nitre efflorescence, which obtains lightness without directing downward, and is an excellent remedy for heavy drinkers in whom old, stubborn phlegm readily forms.

Pathodynamic

The pathodynamic resulting in the present pattern is thus inferred not from the presence of dampness in the middle burner itself, but rather from the nature of signs that accompany the main symptom of pain in the shoulders and arms. Classically, these are the greasy tongue coating, superficial edema or swelling, and the slippery, wiry, and submerged pulse. In practice, a number of other markers can help to make this diagnosis. First, unlike painful obstruction due to wind, dampness, cold, or heat, pain due to lingering phlegm does not change in relation to climatic influences. Second, it tends to be fixed in location, and painful areas are well-circumscribed and often feel cold to the touch, either subjectively to the patient or on palpation or both. There may also be hard or moveable swellings. Third, the onset is likely to be slow and the condition chronic. There may be other signs of phlegm-dampness such as nausea, lack of appetite, dizziness, or palpitations, but these do not have to be present.

This pathology is described and analyzed by Cheng Bin-Cheng in *Convenient Reader of Established Formulas*:

> Phlegm disorders are easy to treat [when the phlegm] is located in the yang organs, but difficult when it is located in the yin organs. It is even more difficult to weed out from the collaterals. All four extremities owe their qi to the Spleen. If the Spleen is diseased so that it cannot transport and transform, phlegm tarries in the middle burner and epigastrium [and once it] has

filled this up overflows into the extremities. This is where it originates. In order to treat it, one must attack it at a time when the normal qi is not yet deficient. When the phlegm from the middle burner and epigastrium has been eliminated so that nothing remains, the Spleen's healthy transporting function will return by itself. [In this manner,] the phlegm in the collaterals can naturally return to the yang organs. Furtively eliminating and silently moving [the formula] thus achieves its effect.

In clinical practice, phlegm obstructing the collaterals often leads to blood stasis and vice versa. In these cases, provided that phlegm is the root, it is useful to add herbs that invigorate the blood and unblock the collaterals such as Pheretima (*dì lóng*), Mori Ramulus (*sāng zhī*), or Cinnamomi Ramulus (*guì zhī*). The formula can also be used for other patterns characterized by excess phlegm in the upper burner and Lungs such as cough, plum-pit qi, or insomnia.

Biomedical Indications

With the appropriate presentation, this formula may be used to treat a variety of biomedically-defined disorders including chronic bronchitis and vascular edema of the upper extremities.

Alternate names

Poria Pill (*fú líng wán*) in *Fine Formulas for Women*; Poria Pill for Reducing Phlegm (*xiāo tán fú líng wán*) in *Discussion of Formulas from Straight Directions from [Yang] Ren-Zhai*; Poria Pill to Guide the Way (*zhǐ mí fú líng wán*) in *Subtle Import of the Jade Key*; Pill Worth a Thousand Pieces of Gold to Guide the Way (*qiān jīn zhǐ mí wán*) in *Introduction to Medicine*; Poria Pill Passed through the Generations (*shì chuán fú líng wán*) in *Indispensable Tools for Pattern Treatment*; Guide the Way Pill with Poria (*fú líng zhǐ mí wán*) in *Collection of Versatility*; Guide the Way Pill (*zhǐ mí wán*) in *Golden Mirror of the Medical Tradition*

Modification

- For the treatment of cough due to phlegm-heat in the upper burner, add Meretricis/Cyclinae Concha (*gé qiào*) and Trichosanthis Fructus (*quán guā lóu*).

Associated Formulas

清濕化痰湯 (清湿化痰汤)

Clear Dampness and Transform Phlegm Decoction

qīng shī huà tán tāng

SOURCE *Achieving Longevity by Guarding the Source* (1615)

Pinelliae Rhizoma praeparatum (*zhì bàn xià*) 4g
Poria (*fú líng*) 4g
Atractylodis Rhizoma (*cāng zhú*) 4g
Arisaematis Rhizoma praeparatum (*zhì tiān nán xīng*) 3g
Scutellariae Radix (*huáng qín*) 3g
Citri reticulatae Pericarpium (*chén pí*) 2.5-3g
Notopterygii Rhizoma seu Radix (*qiāng huó*) 1.5g
Sinapis Semen (*bái jiè zǐ*) 1.5g

Angelicae dahuricae Radix (*bái zhǐ*) 1.5g
Glycyrrhizae Radix (*gān cǎo*) 1-1.5g
Zingiberis Rhizoma recens (*shēng jiāng*) 1-3g
Zingiberis Rhizoma (*gān jiāng*) 1g

Clears phlegm-dampness from the channels. For phlegm-dampness in the channels with joint dysfunction, generalized joint and body aches, tightness in the chest and back, numbness in the limbs, an ice-cold sensation in the mid- to upper back, and a submerged, slippery pulse. The dosage and actions are drawn from Japanese sources, the only ones available to the editors.

二朮湯 (二术汤)

Dual Atractylodes Decoction

èr zhú tāng

SOURCE *Restoration of Health from the Myriad Diseases* (1587)

Atractylodis Rhizoma (*cāng zhú*) 4.5g
Atractylodis macrocephalae Rhizoma (*bái zhú*) 3g
Arisaematis Rhizoma praeparatum (*zhì tiān nán xīng*) 3g
Citri reticulatae Pericarpium (*chén pí*) 3g
Poria (*fú líng*) 3g
Cyperi Rhizoma (*xiāng fù*) 3g
wine-fried Scutellariae Radix (*jiǔ chǎo huáng qín*) 3g
Clematidis Radix (*wēi líng xiān*) 3g
Notopterygii Rhizoma seu Radix (*qiāng huó*) 3g
Glycyrrhizae Radix (*gān cǎo*) 3g
Pinelliae Rhizoma praeparatum (*zhì bàn xià*) 6g

The source text states that the ingredients should be coarsely ground and decocted with an unspecified amount of Zingiberis Rhizoma recens (*shēng jiāng*). At present, 3 slices are generally used.

This formula dries dampness, transforms phlegm, dispels wind, dredges the channels, and relieves pain. The source text states that the formula is for treating pain in the upper arm that is a consequence of phlegm-dampness in the upper burner that moves horizontally to enter the channels and collaterals. At present, this formula is used for periarthritis of the shoulder, frozen shoulder, miscellaneous shoulder pains, and neuralgia of the upper arm. These disorders fit the Chinese medical description of phlegm-dampness obstructing the channels. Usually both the pulse and tongue coating are slippery.

Note that a very similar group of herbs was mentioned in the works of Zhu Dan-Xi, without either prescribed dosages or a formula name. Zhu Dan-Xi intended this formula for treatment of an excess dampness disorder in those who are overweight. In *Essentials of [Zhu] Dan-Xi's Treatment Methods*, differentiation is based on which side the upper arm pain is found:

> If [the affected side is] the left, this belongs to wind-dampness; [treat with] Bupleuri Radix (*chái hú*), Chuanxiong Rhizoma (*chuān xiōng*), Angelicae sinensis Radix (*dāng guī*), Notopterygii Rhizoma seu Radix (*qiāng huó*), Angelicae pubescentis Radix (*dú huó*), Pinelliae Rhizoma praeparatum (*zhì bàn xià*), Atractylodis Rhizoma (*cāng zhú*), [and] Glycyrrhizae Radix (*gān cǎo*). If [the affected side is] the right, this is phlegm-dampness; herbs such as Arisaematis Rhizoma praeparatum (*zhì tiān nán xīng*) and Atractylodis Rhizoma (*cāng zhú*) [are needed].

In *Restoration of Health from the Myriad Diseases,* it is noted that phlegm-dampness in the channels is not the only cause of painful wind in the upper arm or shoulder. There it is suggested that when cold is the cause, Five-Accumulation Powder *(wǔ jī sǎn)* should be used, while if the problem is due to wind, Lindera Powder to Smooth the Flow of Qi *(wū yào shùn qì sǎn)* should be the base formula.

At present, this formula is also used for patients with phlegm-dampness who experience any type of painful obstruction anywhere in the body. Herbs are frequently added to guide the formula to the affected location.

Modifications

- To guide the effects to the lower extremity, add Cyathulae Radix *(chuān niú xī)* and Chaenomelis Fructus *(mù guā).*

- Blood-deficient patients may benefit from the addition of Angelicae sinensis Radix *(dāng guī).*

- If no heat signs are present, add Cinnamomi Ramulus *(guì zhī).*

溫膽湯 （温胆汤）

Warm Gallbladder Decoction

wēn dǎn tāng

The original indication of this formula was a type of deficiency irritability (虛煩 *xū fán)* that develops after a serious illness. This is due to phlegm-heat in the chest and epigastrium constraining the movement of qi in the Triple Burner. The qi disseminated through the Triple Burner is the ministerial fire, whose ascending movement is directed by, and therefore most closely reflected in, the functions of the Gallbladder. The formula succeeds in opening this constraint so that the smooth functioning of the qi dynamic is restored and the warming qi of the Gallbladder is able to expand smoothly once more. Although its formulation has changed over the centuries, the original name has been retained.

Source   *Discussion of Illnesses, Patterns, and Formulas Related to the Unification of the Three Etiologies* (1174)

Bambusae Caulis in taeniam *(zhú rú)*. 6g
Aurantii Fructus immaturus *(zhǐ shí)*. 6g
Pinelliae Rhizoma praeparatum *(zhì bàn xià)*. 6g
Citri reticulatae Pericarpium *(chén pí)*. 9g
Poria *(fú líng)*. 4.5g
Glycyrrhizae Radix praeparata *(zhì gān cǎo)*. 3g

Method of Preparation   Grind the herbs into a powder and prepare as a draft by decocting 12g in 1 cup of water with 5 slices of Zingiberis Rhizoma recens *(shēng jiāng)* and 1 piece of Jujubae Fructus *(dà zǎo).* The liquid is strained and taken before meals. At present, it is usually prepared as a decoction.

Actions   Regulates the qi, transforms phlegm, clears the Gallbladder, and harmonizes the Stomach

Indications

Dizziness, vertigo, nausea or vomiting, insomnia, dream-disturbed sleep with strange or unusual dreams, palpitations, anxiety, indeterminate gnawing hunger, or seizures accompanied by copious sputum, focal distention of the chest, a bitter taste in the mouth, slight thirst, a greasy, yellow tongue coating, and a rapid pulse that is either slippery or wiry.

While the signs and symptoms of this disorder are manifold, the underlying pathodynamic is always the same: disharmony between the Gallbladder and Stomach with phlegm-heat obstructing the qi dynamic. Phlegm in the Stomach leads to focal distention, copious sputum, a greasy tongue coating, and a slippery pulse. Heat in the Gallbladder gives rise to a bitter taste in the mouth, a yellow tongue coating, and either a rapid, slippery or a rapid, wiry pulse. Phlegm-heat in these organs causes constraint that interferes with the rising of the clear yang and manifests as dizziness or vertigo. At the same time, the turbid yin rises in rebellion and manifests as nausea or vomiting. Phlegm-heat disturbs the chest and Heart and causes irritability, insomnia, palpitations, and anxiety. In very severe cases, this can lead to seizures. The obstruction of the qi dynamic in the Stomach by phlegm-heat may also lead to indeterminate gnawing hunger.

Analysis of Formula

To treat disharmony between the Stomach and Gallbladder with phlegm-heat obstructing the qi dynamic, this formula employs a strategy of dispelling the phlegm, regulating the qi, and clearing the heat. The chief ingredient, as in most formulas in this section, is Pinelliae Rhizoma praeparatum *(zhì bàn xià).* Acrid for opening, slippery for directing rebellious qi downward, and bitter for drying dampness, this is the principal substance in the materia medica for transforming phlegm and regulating the Stomach qi. Here, it is joined as a deputy by Bambusae Caulis in taeniam *(zhú rú),* which is sweet and slightly cold. It enters the Stomach to expel heat and stop nausea, and the Gallbladder to calm the spirit, release constraint, and alleviate irritability.

The first group of assistants consists of bitter and cooling Aurantii Fructus immaturus *(zhǐ shí),* which focuses on reversing the flow of rebellious qi and is particularly effective in treating focal distention, and acrid and warming Citri reticulatae Pericarpium *(chén pí),* which dries dampness and expels phlegm while regulating the qi and harmonizing its circulation in the Stomach. Together with the chief and deputy ingredients, these four herbs make an effective combination to treat patterns where phlegm and heat have combined to obstruct the flow of qi in the Stomach, leading to focal distention in the chest and epigastrium, as well as in the Gallbladder, where it causes palpitations, irritability, insomnia, and emotional lability. The other group of assistants, consisting of bland and neutral Poria *(fú líng)* and of sweet and warming Glycyrrhizae Radix praeparata *(zhì gān cǎo),* strengthens the Spleen, leaches out dampness, and harmonizes the functions of the middle burner. These herbs also calm the spirit.

The addition of the envoy, Zingiberis Rhizoma recens *(shēng jiāng)*, to regulate the relationship between the Gallbladder and Stomach and assist the other herbs in stopping the vomiting, is particularly astute. Although it acts to clear heat and transform phlegm, it is not overly cold in nature but is well-balanced for treating the obstruction of the qi dynamic as the core pathology leading to the various patterns treated by this formula.

Commentary

History

The origin of this formula dates back to 6th-century physician Yao Seng-Yuan. Although his original text was later lost, the formula was included in *Arcane Essentials from the Imperial Library* for the following condition: "After a severe illness [when the patient suffers from] irritability and insomnia, it is because of Gallbladder cold (膽寒 *dǎn hán)*." The formula listed is similar to the one described here, but omits Poria *(fú líng)* and contains a much larger dosage (12g) of Zingiberis Rhizoma recens *(shēng jiāng)*. *Important Formulas Worth a Thousand Gold Pieces,* published by Sun Si-Miao during the same period, contains virtually the same formula with identical indications.

'Gallbladder Cold' Deficiency Irritability

The present formula is a modification of the original published in the Song-dynasty text *Discussion of Illnesses, Patterns, and Formulas Related to the Unification of the Three Etiologies* where it is listed as one of several prescriptions for treating deficiency irritability patterns (虛煩證 *xū fán zhèng*). These patterns are due to internal heat from constraint characterized by irritability, a body that does not feel hot to the touch, headache or lightheadedness, a dry mouth or throat with no desire to drink, and insomnia without feeling hot. The term 'deficiency' here does not refer to depletion of the body's normal qi but to the fact that, even though constraint has caused heat to accumulate in the chest and epigastrium, both areas remain soft and pliable to the touch. Any feeling of obstruction is entirely subjective, with no objective evidence of palpable lumps or distention. If the heat constraint is mild, it causes insomnia, characterized by tossing and turning before falling asleep. If it is more severe, there will also be very restless sleep thereafter and the person will have a stifling sensation in the chest. Several such patterns can be differentiated depending on the nature of the underlying pathogen as well as its effects on the qi dynamic. In the present case, accumulation of phlegm-heat hinders the normal physiological diffusion of ministerial fire by way of the lesser yang. This disables the ministerial fire's normal functions of warming and transformation, hence the definition of this pattern as characterized by 'Gallbladder cold.' A description of this pro-

cess is found in *Comprehensive Medicine According to Master Zhang,* written by the Qing-dynasty physician Zhang Lu:

> Failure of the Gallbladder to warm arises when Stomach heat has not been cleared, [causing] tarrying of phlegm and buildup of thin mucus. When this overflows into the tranquil yang organ, the yang qi [distributed by way of the lesser yang] is no longer able to expand smoothly and therefore loses its warming nature.

Zhang Lu's reference to the Gallbladder as the "tranquil yang organ" refers to its function of directing the qi of all the other eleven organs owing to its role in decision-making. To perform this function effectively and efficiently, the Gallbladder must be calm and impartial, not favoring one organ or the other; it is therefore especially prone to even the slightest disturbance in the qi dynamic. This is described by Luo Mei in *Discussion of Famous Physicians' Formulas Past and Present:*

> The Gallbladder is the fair official; the tranquil yang organ. It prefers to be peaceful and quiet and abhors being vexed and worried. It prefers gentleness and abhors constraint. [Resonating with] the virtues of the east and wood, it [embodies] the warm and gentle qi of the lesser yang. In the wake of a serious illness, or in the course of a chronic disorder, or when chills and fevers have just retreated but residual heat in the chest and diaphragm has not yet been entirely cleared, this will invariably damage the mild qi of the lesser yang and cause deficiency irritability.

From that perspective, warming the Gallbladder (as the name of the formula implies) does not refer to tonifying its yang qi, but rather to unblocking the qi dynamic constraint by phlegm and residual heat so that the mild and warming qi of the Gallbladder can again expand. This is explained by Chen Nian-Zu in *Compendium of Songs on Modern Formulas:*

> Two-Aged [Herb] Decoction *(èr chén tāng)* is a prescription for calming the Stomach and dispelling phlegm. By adding Bambusae Caulis in taeniam *(zhú rú)* to clear heat from deficiency above the diaphragm and Aurantii Fructus immaturus *(zhǐ shí)* to dispel phlegm clogging the Triple Burner, the heat is cleared and the phlegm is eliminated and the Gallbladder is thereby naturally calmed and harmonized. This [is what is meant by] warming the Gallbladder. [The term] warming thus really implies cooling (涼 *liáng)*. If there is true cold in someone with a Gallbladder [disorder manifesting with] timidity, this should be treated with [a formula] like Cinnamon Twig Decoction plus Dragon Bone and Oyster Shell *(guì zhī jiā lóng gǔ mǔ lì tāng)* plus Aconiti Radix lateralis praeparata *(zhì fù zǐ)*.

Significance of Formula Name

Modern textbooks attribute the apparent contradiction between the term 'warming' in the formula's name and its indication for phlegm-heat patterns to the more warming nature of the original formula, which contained a large dosage of Zingiberis Rhizoma recens *(shēng jiāng)*. As noted above, a more coherent interpretation is that 'warming' refers to the objective of this formula to reorder a constrained qi dynamic by eliminating the source of constraint. This is reflected in the choice of Bambusae Caulis in taeniam (*zhú rú*) as deputy herb, which focuses on opening constraint rather than draining heat. As Zhang Xi-Chun explained in *Essays on Medicine Esteeming the Chinese and Respecting the Western*:

> As the bark of the bamboo, it is both cooling and directs downward; thus, while cooling the Lungs and facilitating [the removal of] phlegm, it disseminates and unblocks the fluid passageways of the Triple Burner, and below unblocks the Bladder. Therefore, it is an important herb for unblocking and facilitating the flow of urine, similar to bamboo leaves, but superior to the leaves in its power.

Viewed from this perspective, although the formula is cooling in nature, its main purpose is not to drain heat, but to unblock the movement of body fluids within the lesser yang warp whose congealing manifests in the formation of phlegm. This can often be ascertained by way of auscultation, which elicits a splashing sound (indicating the presence of fluids) in the epigastrium or left hypochondriac area. This interpretation helps in understanding the many variations of this formula as well as its wide range of applications in contemporary practice.

With respect to Gallbladder qi constraint, this includes, besides the symptoms already listed above, feelings of apprehension, as well as hypersensitivity to noise, sounds, and smells. With respect to the Triple Burner, the Qing-dynasty physician Ye Tian-Shi recommended it for the treatment of qi-aspect damp-heat characterized by chills and fever, focal distention of the chest, distention of the abdomen, frequent, dark, and scanty urine, and a greasy, yellow tongue coating:

> Pathogens lingering in the Triple Burner [produce patterns] that resemble lesser yang disorders in the cold damage [system of classification]. There, one harmonizes and resolves that which is halfway between the interior and exterior, [while] here, one separates and reduces [pathogens] from the upper or lower burners according to their momentum, flexibly [selecting treatment] strategies according to the [presenting] pattern such as […] that of mobilizing [the qi dynamic] and draining [pathogenic phlegm-heat by means of] Warm Gallbladder Decoction (*wēn dǎn tāng*).

Key Indicators

This formula can be used for a wide variety of conditions provided that the presentation includes symptoms like copious sputum, focal distention of the chest, a bitter taste in the mouth, a yellow, greasy tongue coating, and either a rapid and slippery or rapid and wiry pulse.

Comparisons

> ➤ Vs. Lophatherum and Gypsum Decoction (*zhú yè shí gāo tāng*) and Gardenia and Prepared Soybean Decoction (*zhī zǐ chǐ tāng*)

This formula is particularly useful in treating the irritability, insomnia, depression, and loss of appetite that results from relatively mild constraint of the qi dynamic in the chest and epigastrium. Its pattern is quite different, however, from that of Lophatherum and Gypsum Decoction (*zhú yè shí gāo tāng*), discussed in Chapter 4. Although the latter formula also treats irritability and insomnia from qi constraint, it addresses patterns characterized by qi and yin deficiency as well as phlegm and fire. The cardinal symptoms of that pattern include lassitude, low-grade fever, a dry mouth, thirst, a dark red tongue with little coating, and a deficient, rapid pulse. By contrast, Warm Gallbladder Decoction (*wēn dǎn tāng*) treats deficiency irritability due to constraint from phlegm-heat. This is characterized by the absence of fever, nausea, focal distention, a dry mouth but no thirst, and a greasy tongue coating. Another formula with a similar pattern is Gardenia and Prepared Soybean Decoction (*zhì zǐ chǐ tāng*), also discussed in Chapter 4. That formula treats constraint due to heat, but without deficiency or phlegm. Besides fever, irritability, insomnia with tossing and turning in bed, a stifling sensation in the chest with a soft epigastrium, hunger with no desire to eat, there will be a slightly yellow tongue coating and a slightly rapid pulse, or a strong, floating pulse at the distal position.

Biomedical Indications

With the appropriate presentation, this formula may be used to treat a very wide variety of biomedically-defined disorders. These can be divided into the following groups:

- Cardiovascular diseases such as hypertension, angina, myocarditis, premature atrial contractions, and pericarditis

- Digestive disorders such as chronic gastritis, peptic ulcer, cholecystitis, morning sickness, and chronic hepatitis

- Respiratory disorders such as asthma and chronic bronchitis

- Neuropsychiatric disorders such as depression, severe insomnia, early stage schizophrenia, psychosis, autonomic dystonia, and the sequelae of stroke.

This formula has also been used for treating alopecia, male menopause, tinnitus, and Ménière's disease.

Modifications

- For severe vertigo, add Paeoniae Radix alba (*bái sháo*), Haematitum (*dài zhě shí*), and Scutellariae Radix (*huáng qín*).

- For insomnia, add Succinum (*hǔ pò*), Ziziphi spinosae Semen (*suān zǎo rén*), and Ostreae Concha (*mǔ lì*).

- For a dry mouth and tongue, remove Pinelliae Rhizoma praeparatum (*zhì bàn xià*) and add Ophiopogonis Radix *(mài mén dōng)* and Trichosanthis Radix *(tiān huā fěn)*.

- For tinnitus and hearing loss due to retention of damp-heat in the Gallbladder, add Bupleuri Radix *(chái hú)*, Uncariae Ramulus cum Uncis *(gōu téng)*, Chrysanthemi Flos *(jú huā)*, Acori tatarinowii Rhizoma *(shí chāng pǔ)*, and Tetrapanacis Medulla *(tōng cǎo)*.

- For severe insomnia due to Heart and Gallbladder deficiency (called 'high pillow' or 'no pillow' disorder), add Ginseng Radix *(rén shēn)*, Gypsum fibrosum *(shí gāo)*, Ophiopogonis Radix *(mài mén dōng)*, Longan Arillus *(lóng yǎn ròu)*, and Ziziphi spinosae Semen *(suān zǎo rén)*.

Variation

黃連溫膽湯 （黄连温胆汤）

Warm Gallbladder Decoction with Coptis
huáng lián wēn dǎn tāng

Sᴏᴜʀᴄᴇ *Warp and Woof of Warm-Heat Diseases* (1852)

Add Coptidis Rhizoma *(huáng lián)* for severe phlegm-heat with more restlessness and irritability, and a more intense bitter taste in the mouth.

Comparison

➤ Vs. Mɪɴᴏʀ Dᴇᴄᴏᴄᴛɪᴏɴ [ғᴏʀ Pᴀᴛʜᴏɢᴇɴs] Sᴛᴜᴄᴋ ɪɴ ᴛʜᴇ Cʜᴇsᴛ *(xiǎo xiàn xiōng tāng)*; *see* ᴘᴀɢᴇ 794

Associated Formula

十味溫膽湯 （十味温胆汤）

Ten-Ingredient Warm Gallbladder Decoction
shí wèi wēn dǎn tāng

Sᴏᴜʀᴄᴇ *Indispensable Tools for Pattern Treatment* (1602)

Pinelliae Rhizoma praeparatum *(zhì bàn xià)* 6g
Aurantii Fructus immaturus *(zhǐ shí)* 6g
Citri reticulatae Pericarpium *(chén pí)* 6g
Poria *(fú líng)* 4.5g
Ziziphi spinosae Semen *(suān zǎo rén)* 3g
Polygalae Radix *(yuǎn zhì)* 3g
Schisandrae Fructus *(wǔ wèi zǐ)* 3g
Rehmanniae Radix praeparata *(shú dì huáng)* 3g
Ginseng Radix *(rén shēn)* 3g
Glycyrrhizae Radix praeparata *(zhì gān cǎo)* 1.5g
Zingiberis Rhizoma recens *(shēng jiāng)* . . . . 5 slices
Jujubae Fructus *(dà zǎo)* . . . . 1 piece

Transforms phlegm and calms the Heart. For Heart and Gallbladder deficiency characterized by anxiety and being easily frightened, together with edema of the limbs, loss of taste and appetite, palpitations, irritability, a stifling sensation in the chest, and difficulty in sitting without fidgeting. This formula is for disturbances of the spirit due to Heart and Gallbladder deficiency; it does not contain any heat-clearing ingredients.

香附旋覆花湯 （香附旋覆花汤）

Cyperus and Inula Decoction
xiāng fù xuán fù huā tāng

Sᴏᴜʀᴄᴇ *Systematic Differentiation of Warm Pathogen Diseases* (1798)

Cyperi Rhizoma *(xiāng fù)* 9g
Inulae Flos *(xuán fù huā)* . . . . [wrap in cheesecloth] 9g
Perillae Fructus *(zǐ sū zǐ)* 9g
Citri reticulatae Pericarpium *(chén pí)* 6g
Poria *(fú líng)* 9g
Coicis Semen *(yì yǐ rén)* 15g
Pinelliae Rhizoma praeparatum *(zhì bàn xià)* 15g

Method of Preparation   Decoction

Actions   Strengthens the Spleen, dispels dampness, spreads the Liver qi, and unblocks the channels and collaterals

Indications

Hypochondriac pain with or without coughing, either afternoon fevers without chills or alternating chills and fever, a thickly-coated tongue with swollen edges, and a wiry pulse, especially in the middle position.

This is dampness leading to congested fluids that stagnate in the collaterals of the Liver. When damp-warmth diseases enter this channel, dampness and congested fluids collect in the hypochondria and cause pain. Afternoon fevers without chills, or alternating chills and fever, are signs of a pathogenic influence in the collaterals of the Liver. The accumulation of dampness and congested fluids may also cause the Liver qi to rebel upward and violate the Lungs, which may or may not lead to coughing. This is contrary to the normal relationship between these organs, whereby the Lungs control the Liver. The thickly-coated tongue with swollen edges and the wiry pulse (especially in the middle position) reflect the presence of dampness in the Liver channel.

Analysis of Formula

This formula eliminates phlegm-dampness from the body by unblocking the qi dynamic and promoting water metabolism. The two chief ingredients, Cyperi Rhizoma *(xiāng fù)* and Inulae Flos *(xuán fù huā)*, unblock the Liver collaterals to drive out congested fluids from the hypochondria. Perillae Fructus *(zǐ sū zǐ)* directs the Lung qi downward and expels phlegm. Together with Coicis Semen *(yì yǐ rén)*, which also enters the Lung channel, it strengthens the functions of metal in order to control wood. Citri reticulatae Pericarpium *(chén pí)* and Pinelliae Rhizoma praeparatum *(zhì bàn xià)* dry dampness and revive the Spleen. Together, these ingredients have a very strong effect in directing the qi downward and transforming phlegm; see also the analysis of Two-Aged [Herb] Decoction *(èr chén tāng)* above. Poria *(fú líng)* and Coicis Semen *(yì yǐ rén)* leach out dampness. Strengthening the Spleen's transporting function relieves the congested fluids in the Liver channel. In terms of five-phase thinking, these herbs represent a strategy of firming up earth in order to control water.

Commentary

The classical term for the pathology treated by this formula is 'prodding [or propping] thin mucus' (支飲 *zhī yǐn*). It occurs when dampness enters the body in the course of a lurking summerheat or damp-warmth disorder, accumulates, and gathers in the hypochondria. In its manifestations, this pattern resembles that for which Ten-Jujube Decoction *(shí zǎo tāng)* is indicated, discussed in Chapter 2. However, in that case, water floods the Liver channel due to interior excess, requiring strong purgation. Here, dampness invading from the exterior obstructs the qi dynamic. This is a less severe condition where the appropriate strategy is to unblock the qi dynamic. For this reason, the formula focuses on unblocking the qi dynamic rather than on driving out pathological fluids directly. Nevertheless, as the author of the formula, Wu Ju-Tong, noted in the source text, its use should quickly relieve the symptoms in no more than 3-5 days. Should this not occur, Wu recommended the use of Control Mucus Special Pill *(kòng xián dān)*, also discussed in Chapter 2, to attack the congested fluids directly.

Comparison

➤ Vs. Minor Bupleurum Decoction *(xiǎo chái hú tāng)*

Both formulas are indicated for patterns marked by alternating chills and fever accompanied by pain in the hypochondria and a greasy tongue coating. Furthermore, both patterns may also be characterized by dizziness, a dry mouth with no desire to drink, nausea, and occasional irritability and restlessness. However, when Cyperus and Inula Decoction *(xiāng fù xuán fù huā tāng)* is appropriate, the presence of dampness and thin mucus as the primary pathogen can be elicited from the history and from such symptoms as the swollen edges of the tongue and its thick coating. Moreover, a Minor Bupleurum Decoction *(xiǎo chái hú tāng)* pattern will have pronounced chills, while these will be less pronounced or even absent in the pattern for which Cyperus and Inula Decoction *(xiāng fù xuán fù huā tāng)* is indicated.

Modifications

• For abdominal fullness, add Magnoliae officinalis Cortex *(hòu pò)*.

• For severe pain, add Dalbergiae odoriferae Lignum *(jiàng xiāng)*.

Section 2

FORMULAS THAT CLEAR HEAT AND TRANSFORM PHLEGM

The formulas in this section are used in treating phlegm-heat, a condition that usually arises when dampness or body fluids combine with pathogenic heat, which in turn can be contracted from the exterior or generated by emotional disorders, long-term illness, poor diet, or other internal disharmonies. The Heart is associated with fire, while the Lungs are the tender organ that is most averse to both heat and cold. Thus, these are the two organs most closely affected by phlegm-heat. Common manifestations include coughing of thick, yellow, viscous sputum that is difficult to expectorate, a red and flushed face, a yellow tongue coating, and a rapid pulse. There may also be dizziness, palpitations, impaired consciousness, epilepsy, or spasms. Because heat in this instance is the cause of the phlegm, it too must be addressed to resolve the phlegm. The formulas in this section therefore employ chief herbs that transform phlegm and drain heat. These include Trichosanthis Fructus *(guā lóu)*, Fritillariae Bulbus *(bèi mǔ)*, Bambusae Caulis in taeniam *(zhú rú)*, Arisaema cum Bile *(dǎn nán xīng)*, and Chloriti Lapis/Micae Lapis aureus *(méng shí)*. They are usually combined with deputies and assistants from one of the following groups of ingredients:

• Herbs that strengthen the Spleen and leach out dampness in order to rectify the precondition of this pathology such as Poria *(fú líng)* or Coicis Semen *(yì yǐ rén)*.

• Herbs that drain heat such as Coptidis Rhizoma *(huáng lián)*, Scutellariae Radix *(huáng qín)*, or Rhei Radix et Rhizoma *(dà huáng)*. These herbs address the second cause of phlegm-heat disorder and rectify the qi dynamic by draining pathogenic heat from the body.

• Herbs that regulate the qi such as Citri reticulatae Pericarpium *(chén pí)*, Pinelliae Rhizoma praeparatum *(zhì bàn xià)*, Aquilariae Lignum resinatum *(chén xiāng)*, or Aurantii Fructus immaturus *(zhǐ shí)*. This is important because phlegm disorders invariably arise from the congealing of fluids due to stagnation of qi.

清氣化痰丸 (清气化痰丸)
Clear the Qi and Transform Phlegm Pill
qīng qì huà tán wán

While this formula treats phlegm-heat, its primary objective is to reorder the qi dynamic. As Wu Kun, the author of this formula, explained in the source text: "If qi is not clear, phlegm will result. [This formula] is able to treat phlegm and thereby clears the qi."

Source   *Investigations of Medical Formulas (1584)*

Arisaema cum Bile *(dǎn nán xīng)* 45g
Pinelliae Rhizoma praeparatum *(zhì bàn xià)* 45g
Trichosanthis Semen *(guā lóu rén)* 30g
Scutellariae Radix *(huáng qín)* 30g
Citri reticulatae Pericarpium *(chén pí)* 30g
Armeniacae Semen *(xìng rén)* 30g
Aurantii Fructus immaturus *(zhǐ shí)* 30g
Poria *(fú líng)* 30g

Method of Preparation   Grind the ingredients into a powder and form into pills with ginger juice. Take 6-9g twice a day. May also be prepared as a decoction with a proportionate reduction in dosage.

Actions   Clears heat, transforms phlegm, directs rebellious qi downward, and stops coughing

Indications

Coughing of yellow, viscous sputum that is difficult to expectorate, focal distention and a feeling of fullness in the chest and diaphragm, nausea, a red tongue with a greasy, yellow coating, and a slippery, rapid pulse. In severe cases, there may also be difficulty breathing.

This is internal clumping of phlegm-heat that occurs when fire 'brews' the fluids that have become stagnant due to a relative deficiency in the transporting function of the Spleen. In other words, the Spleen is unable to move the fluids because they are excessive, rather than because the Spleen itself is organically weak. The fire and phlegm interfere with the descending function of the Lung qi, which leads to coughing with sputum that is yellow, viscous, and difficult to expectorate. They also obstruct the qi of the middle burner, which manifests as focal distention and a feeling of fullness in the chest and diaphragm, and perhaps nausea. The tongue and pulse signs reflect the presence of heat and phlegm. If the problem is severe, the obstruction will be so intense that the patient may have difficulty breathing.

Analysis of Formula

This formula combines a strategy of draining heat and transforming phlegm, supporting the clearing of fire with the regulation of qi in order to drain heat from the body and smooth the movement of qi. The logic underlying this approach is succinctly explained by Wang Ang in *Medical Formulas Collected and Analyzed:* "When there is a surfeit of qi, fire results; when there is a surfeit of fluids, phlegm results. Therefore, in treating phlegm, it is necessary first to direct the fire downward, and in treating fire, it is necessary to smooth the flow of qi."

The chief ingredient, Arisaema cum Bile *(dǎn nán xīng),* is a powerful substance used for treating blockage caused by a combination of fire and phlegm. The deputies, Scutel-

lariae Radix *(huáng qín)* and Trichosanthis Semen *(guā lóu rén),* work together to drain Lung fire while transforming and clearing phlegm-heat. They markedly reinforce the actions of the chief ingredient. The other ingredients are regarded as assistants. Aurantii Fructus immaturus *(zhǐ shí)* and Citri reticulatae Pericarpium *(chén pí)* both regulate the qi; combined, they are particularly effective in dispelling the focal distention and dissipating the clumps of phlegm. Poria *(fú líng)* and Pinelliae Rhizoma praeparatum *(zhì bàn xià)* address the source of phlegm (the Spleen), and Armeniacae Semen *(xìng rén)* facilitates the flow of qi in the receptacle of phlegm (the Lungs). Pinelliae Rhizoma praeparatum *(zhì bàn xià)* also strongly assists the chief ingredient in expelling the phlegm that has already formed.

Commentary

This is an important formula for treating phlegm-heat. In can be viewed as a modified combination of Two-Aged [Herb] Decoction *(èr chén tāng)* and Minor Decoction [for Pathogens] Stuck in the Chest *(xiǎo xiàn xiōng tāng).* Its composition can be traced to a similar formula by the Yuan-dynasty master physician Zhu Dan-Xi, who added Scutellariae Radix *(huáng qín)* and Glycyrrhizae Radix *(gān cǎo)* to that combination in order to treat phlegm-heat clogging the upper burner. In *Essential Teachings of [Zhu] Dan-Xi,* Zhu outlined the treatment principle on which this formula is based: "[Most physician] see physical phlegm and treat the phlegm. Expert practitioners do not treat the phlegm, but the qi." This principle was, in turn, a synopsis of an earlier statement by Pang An-Chang, cited in *Indispensable Tools for Pattern Treatment:*

> [Under normal conditions,] phlegm in the body does not reach the upper burner just as water does not flow upward in nature. [Accordingly,] experts at treating phlegm do not treat the phlegm, but the qi. Once the qi is normalized the fluids of the entire body follow the qi and are also normalized.

This suggests that phlegm is a physiological by-product of the digestive process in the middle burner that is normally dispersed via the bowels as part of the ongoing separation of the clear and turbid that characterizes healthy metabolic activity. It becomes visible only when it is carried around the body by pathogens, such as fire. As explained by Zhang Bin-Cheng in *Convenient Reader of Established Formulas:*

> The treatment of phlegm-heat [is discussed by] Wang Ang who said that phlegm-heat disorders are caused by fire. Phlegm [can be regarded as] fire with form, while fire is phlegm without form. Phlegm follows fire as it ascends or directs downward, while fire is guided to move horizontally by phlegm. The [ensuing] mutations produce all kinds of patterns, which are too numerous to be detailed exhaustively. Fire avails itself of the qi [generated by] the five yin organs, phlegm avails itself

of the yin fluids [produced from] the five flavors. If the qi is excessive, it becomes fire; if the yin fluids are excessive, they become phlegm. To treat phlegm, one thus must direct this fire downward, and to treat fire, one must smooth the flow of qi. This formula was composed on the basis of these [principles].

Given these considerations, the use of this formula in clinical practice extends primarily to the treatment of productive cough with yellow sputum. This pattern often occurs during wind-warmth disorders when wind has been dispelled from the exterior but phlegm remains and combines with excess internal heat. This often results from the use of acrid, cooling medicinals (including aspirin and similar antipyretics) that succeed in treating the wind but precipitate the transformation of preexisting dampness into phlegm. The formula can also be used to treat warm-dryness disorders where wind has been dispelled but dryness remains, manifesting as a dry painful throat, cough with yellow sputum, and stabbing pains in the flanks. Other possible patterns include damp-heat obstructing the middle burner leading to nausea, vomiting, and other manifestations of rebellious qi; and phlegm-heat obstructing the Triple Burner, causing insomnia and palpitations.

Biomedical Indications

With the appropriate presentation, this formula may be used to treat a variety of biomedically-defined disorders including pneumonia, acute exacerbations of chronic bronchitis, and bronchiectasis.

Modifications

- For high fever, add Gypsum fibrosum (shí gāo) and Anemarrhenae Rhizoma (zhī mŭ).

- For copious sputum, add Houttuyniae Herba (yú xīng cǎo) and Trichosanthis Radix (tiān huā fěn).

- For gummy sputum, remove Pinelliae Rhizoma praeparatum (zhì bàn xià) and add Benincasae Semen (dōng guā zǐ).

- For more severe heat, add Indigo naturalis (qīng dài) and powdered Meretricis/Cyclinae Concha (gé qiào).

- For nausea and vomiting, replace Trichosanthis Fructus (guā lóu) with Bambusae Caulis in taeniam (zhú rú).

- For palpitations and insomnia, add Succinum (hŭ pò), Ostreae Concha (mŭ lì), and Ziziphi spinosae Semen (suān zǎo rén).

Associated Formulas

清金化痰丸

Clear Metal and Transform Phlegm Pill

qīng jīn huà tán wán

SOURCE *Systematic Instructions on Medicine* (1534)

Scutellariae Radix (huáng qín)	12g
Gardeniae Fructus (zhī zǐ)	12g
Anemarrhenae Rhizoma (zhī mŭ)	15g
Trichosanthis Semen (guā lóu rén)	15g
Fritillariae Bulbus (bèi mŭ)	9g
Ophiopogonis Radix (mài mén dōng)	9g
Citri reticulatae Pericarpium (chén pí)	9g
Poria (fú líng)	9g
Platycodi Radix (jié gěng)	9g
Mori Cortex (sāng bái pí)	9g

Decoction. The source text advises to divide the decoction into three portions, which are taken warm over the course of the day. Clears Lung fire, moistens dryness, and transforms phlegm. For phlegm-heat clogging the Lungs characterized by thick, yellow sputum, a greasy, yellow tongue coating, and a soft and rapid pulse. Although these indications superficially resemble those of the principal formula, the underlying pathodynamic is substantially different. The principal formula treats excess phlegm and heat constraint obstructing the qi dynamic. Thus, it employs a strategy of clearing the qi and transforming the phlegm. This formula, by contrast, treats phlegm-heat clogging the Lung channel and collaterals. Thus, it employs a strategy of clearing the Lungs and transforming the phlegm and therefore contains many more ingredients that directly enter into the Lung channel.

栝樓枳實湯 （栝楼枳实汤）

Trichosanthes Fruit and Unripe Bitter Orange Decoction

guā loú zhǐ shí tāng

SOURCE *Restoration of Health from the Myriad Diseases* (1587)

Trichosanthis Fructus (guā lóu)	3g
Aurantii Fructus immaturus (zhǐ shí)	3g
Platycodi Radix (jié gěng)	3g
Poria (fú líng)	3g
Fritillariae Bulbus (bèi mŭ)	3g
Citri reticulatae Pericarpium (chén pí)	3g
Gardeniae Fructus (zhī zǐ)	3g
Scutellariae Radix (huáng qín)	3g
Angelicae sinensis Radix (dāng guī)	1.8g
Amomi Fructus (shā rén)	1.5g
Bambusae Caulis in taeniam (zhú rú)	0.9g
Aucklandiae Radix (mù xiāng)	1.5g
Glycyrrhizae Radix (gān cǎo)	0.9g

The source text advises to coarsely grind the ingredients and take as a draft with small amounts of Zingiberis Rhizoma recens (shēng jiāng), ginger juice, and Bambusae Succus (zhú lì). Transforms and cools phlegm-heat in the chest. For clumping of phlegm in the chest with sputum that is difficult to expectorate and pain in the chest and diaphragm such that the patient is unable to rotate the trunk. Other symptoms may include a stifling sensation and fullness in the chest, fever and chills, and labored breathing. This formula has a stronger effect on the qi than does the principal formula.

小陷胸湯 （小陷胸汤）

Minor Decoction [for Pathogens] Stuck in the Chest

xiǎo xiàn xiōng tāng

The source text for this formula identifies two types of 陷胸 *xiàn xiōng*, a condition in which something becomes 'stuck in the chest.' Both types are due to a yang pathogenic influence clumping in the chest. The condition for which this formula is indicated is the less severe of the two.

Source   *Discussion of Cold Damage* (c. 220)

Trichosanthis Fructus *(guā lóu)* . . . . . [crush] 1 big fruit (24-30g)
Coptidis Rhizoma *(huáng lián)* 3g
ginger-fried Pinelliae Rhizoma praeparatum *(jiāng bàn xià)*9-12g

Method of Preparation   The source text advises to decoct Trichosanthis Fructus *(guā lóu)* for 20-30 minutes before adding the other herbs. At present, all of the ingredients are usually decocted together.

Actions   Clears heat, transforms phlegm, expands the chest, and dissipates clumps

Indications

Focal distention (with or without nodules) in the chest and epigastrium that are painful when pressed, coughing up yellow and viscous sputum, constipation, a bitter taste, a yellow, greasy tongue coating, and a slippery pulse that is either floating or rapid.

This is clumping in the chest (結胸 *jié xiōng),* which is caused by the sinking of pathogenic heat into the chest and epigastrium (upper and middle burners) where it mixes with phlegm and forms clumps. Phlegm and heat in the epigastrium constrain the qi and disrupt the proper ascending and descending functions of the qi dynamic. This excessive type of constraint leads to focal distention and a stifling sensation accompanied by pain upon pressure. The combination of heat and phlegm forms a gummy mixture that constrains the Lung qi, manifested in the coughing up of yellow, viscous sputum. Constipation and a bitter taste in the mouth are signs of heat in the middle burner. The yellow, greasy tongue coating and slippery pulse that is either floating or rapid are classic signs of phlegm-heat.

Analysis of Formula

To treat clumping of heat and phlegm, this formula employs a complex strategy of draining heat with bitter, cooling herbs, opening the areas of clumping with acrid, dispersing herbs, and directing the qi downward with acrid, bitter, and moistening herbs. The chief herb, sweet and cooling Trichosanthis Fructus *(guā lóu),* cools and transforms phlegm-heat, moistens the Intestines, and directs the turbid phlegm downward. It facilitates the elimination of phlegm-heat via the bowels

without causing stagnation or aggravating the heat. Thus, as *Records of Thoughtful Differentiation of Materia Medica* emphasizes, "The most useful aspect of Trichosanthis Fructus *(guā lóu)* is that it guides phlegm and turbidity downward; thus clumping in the chest and chest painful obstruction cannot be [successfully] treated without it." The deputy, bitter and cooling Coptidis Rhizoma *(huáng lián),* helps the chief herb drain heat and turbidity from the upper and middle burners. Simultaneously, the moistening nature of Trichosanthis Fructus *(quán guā lóu)* prevents the dryness of Coptidis Rhizoma *(huáng lián)* from aggravating the stagnation. The assistant is warm and acrid ginger-fried Pinelliae Rhizoma praeparatum *(jiāng bàn xià),* which is very effective in directing the rebellious qi downward, harmonizing the Stomach, transforming phlegm, eliminating focal distention, and dissipating clumps. Together with the deputy, it treats the obstruction caused by phlegm-heat by utilizing their combination of bitter, downward-directing, and acrid opening natures. Together with the chief herb, it is excellent for treating focal distention of the chest and diaphragm due to clumping of phlegm and heat leading to qi constraint, or for painful obstruction of the chest due to clumping of sticky, thick, and turbid phlegm. Overall, even though there are just three herbs in this formula, they combine on many levels to produce a balanced yet powerful effect.

Cautions and Contraindications

Because this formula can cause loose stools, it is contraindicated in cases with significant Spleen and Stomach deficiency.

Commentary

The source text attributes this disorder to the improper purging of a greater yang (exterior) condition, which causes pathogenic heat to sink into the chest and epigastrium where it mixes with phlegm to form clumps. Although this causes qi stagnation (experienced as focal distention by the patient and as hardness in the epigastric area by the palpating physician), it is not yet severe. Thus, there is pain only on pressure. This is reflected in the pulse, which is superficial, indicating that the stagnation is located in the upper burner, and slippery, indicating the presence of phlegm-turbidity. This is different from the pattern for which Major Decoction [for Pathogens] Stuck in the Chest *(dà xiàn xiōng tāng),* discussed in Chapter 2, is indicated, where the pathogen is lodged more deeply in the body and the clumping of heat and water causes more severe stagnation. There, the entire abdomen is hard and distended, and is so painful that it cannot be touched. The pattern is also different from that for which Drain the Epigastrium Decoction *(xiè xīn tāng),* discussed in Chapter 4, is indicated, where there is focal distention in the epigastrium that is soft to the touch because the stagnation is less severe and there is no clumping. Another important distinction is that the tongue coating is rooted in those conditions for which Minor Decoction [for Pathogens] Stuck in the Chest *(xiǎo xiàn xiōng tāng)* is appropriate. If the coating is rootless, the condition is usually due to deficiency of the middle qi with superimposed damp-heat.

In part because the term chest (胸 *xiōng*) in classical Chinese medicine denotes a body region that encompasses not only the chest itself but also the hypchondriac and epigastric regions, the therapeutic scope of this formula is rather broad. Regardless of the pathogenesis, as long as the patient presents with tender, focal distention of the chest and epigastrium, constipation, and a yellow, greasy tongue coating, the use of this formula is appropriate. Thus, in *Comprehensive Medicine According to Master Zhang*, the Qing-dynasty physician Zhang Lu recommends the formula for the following pattern:

> Whenever [the patient] has a cough with a red face, heat in the chest, abdomen, and flanks, and only the hands and feet are cool with an overflowing pulse, the heat is above the diaphragm. Use Minor Decoction [for Pathogens] Stuck in the Chest *(xiǎo xiàn xiōng tāng)*.

Comparison

➤ Vs. Warm Gallbladder Decoction with Coptis *(huáng lián wēn dǎn tāng)*

Both formulas clear heat and transform phlegm and are used, among other conditions, for chest pain with coughing of yellow, viscous sputum, irritability, dry mouth, a yellow, greasy tongue coating, and a slippery and rapid pulse. Minor Decoction [for Pathogens] Stuck in the Chest *(xiǎo xiàn xiōng tāng)* is better at clearing heat and scouring out phlegm in the upper burner and is used for phlegm-heat in the chest with tenderness in the chest and epigastrium along with constipation. By contrast, Warm Gallbladder Decoction with Coptis *(huáng lián wēn dǎn tāng)* works more on Stomach and Gallbladder phlegm-heat that affects the Heart and is thus marked more by problems such as insomnia or palpitations.

Biomedical Indications

With the appropriate presentation, this formula may be used to treat a wide variety of biomedically-defined disorders. These can be divided into the following groups:

- Digestive disorders such as hepatitis, cholecystitis, pancreatitis, biliary reflux gastritis, peptic ulcer disease, biliary ascariasis, and pyloric obstruction
- Respiratory disorders including upper respiratory tract infections, pleurisy, pneumonia, bronchitis, asthma, bronchiectasis, and spontaneous pneumothorax
- Neuropsychiatric disorders such as cerebrovascular disease, psychosis, and insomnia.

This formula has also been used for coronary artery disease, hypertension, mastitis, nephritis, and intercostal neuralgia.

Alternate name

Decoction [for Pathogens] Stuck in the Chest *(xiàn xiōng tāng)* in *Formulas from Benevolent Sages Compiled during the Taiping Era*

Modifications

- For vomiting, add Bambusae Caulis in taeniam *(zhú rú)* and Zingiberis Rhizoma recens *(shēng jiāng)*.
- For very gummy sputum that cannot be expectorated, add Fritillariae Bulbus *(bèi mǔ)* and Arisaema cum Bile *(dǎn nán xīng)*.
- For severe distention and pain, add Curcumae Radix *(yù jīn)* and Aurantii Fructus immaturus *(zhǐ shí)*.
- For indeterminate gnawing hunger, add Aurantii Fructus immaturus *(zhǐ shí)* and Gardeniae Fructus *(zhī zǐ)*.
- For a high fever and severe cough with or without wheezing, take with Ephedra, Apricot Kernel, Gypsum, and Licorice Decoction *(má xìng shí gān tāng)*.
- For myocardial infarction, add Persicae Semen *(táo rén)*, Carthami Flos *(hóng huā)*, Trogopterori Faeces *(wǔ líng zhī)*, and Typhae Pollen *(pú huáng)*.
- For hepatitis, combine with either Virgate Wormwood Decoction *(yīn chén hāo tāng)* or Major Bupleurum Decoction *(dà chái hú tāng)*.

Associated Formulas

加味小陷胸湯 （加味小陷胸汤）

Augmented Minor Decoction [for Pathogens] Stuck in the Chest

jiā wèi xiǎo xiàn xiōng tāng

Source *Bases of Medicine* (1861)

Trichosanthis Semen *(guā lóu rén)* 15g
ginger-fried Pinelliae Rhizoma praeparatum *(jiāng bàn xià)* 6g
Coptidis Rhizoma *(huáng lián)* 3g
Aurantii Fructus immaturus *(zhǐ shí)* 6g
Magnoliae officinalis Cortex *(hòu pò)* 3g
Poria *(fú líng)* 12g
Citri reticulatae Pericarpium *(chén pí)* 6g

Prepare as a decoction. Clears heat, transforms phlegm, regulates the qi, and promotes fluid metabolism. For clumping in the chest with more pronounced fullness and focal distention.

柴胡陷胸湯 （柴胡陷胸汤）

Bupleurum Decoction [for Pathogens] Stuck in the Chest

chái hú xiàn xiōng tāng

Source *Revised Popular Guide to the Discussion of Cold Damage* (Qing dynasty)

Bupleuri Radix (*chái hú*)..3g

ginger-fried Pinelliae Rhizoma praeparatum (*jiāng bàn xià*).......9g

Coptidis Rhizoma (*huáng lián*).............................2.4g

Platycodi Radix (*jié gěng*).....................................3g

Scutellariae Radix (*huáng qín*).............................4.5g

Trichosanthis Semen (*guā lóu rén*)..........................15g

Aurantii Fructus (*zhǐ ké*)....................................4.5g

Prepare as a decoction and add 4 drops of fresh ginger juice into each strained bowl of the liquid. Clears heat, transforms phlegm, expands the chest and diaphragm, and harmonizes and releases the lesser yang. For lesser yang disorders with fullness and focal distention in the chest and diaphragm that is painful on pressure, a bitter taste in the mouth, a yellow tongue coating, and a wiry, rapid pulse.

響聲破笛丸 （响声破笛丸）

Pill for Restoring Sound to a Broken Flute

xiǎng shēng pò dí wán

SOURCE *Straight Directions from [Yang] Ren-Zhai* (1264)

Forsythiae Fructus (*lián qiáo*)...............................94g

Platycodi Radix (*jié gěng*)...................................94g

Chuanxiong Rhizoma (*chuān xiōng*)........................56g

Amomi Fructus (*shā rén*)....................................56g

Chebulae Fructus (*hē zǐ*)........................[stir-fried] 37g

Multiherb Concoction (*bǎi yào jiān*) *...................75g

Menthae haplocalycis Herba (*bò hé*)........................94g

Rhei Radix et Rhizoma (*dà huáng*)..........................37g

Glycyrrhizae Radix (*gān cǎo*)...............................94g

The source text recommends grinding the ingredients into a powder, mixing with egg white, and forming into pills the size of a bullet (equal to a large marble). The dose is one pill, slowly dissolved in the mouth before bedtime. At present, honey is more commonly used than egg white.

This formula clears heat, cools the throat, dispels phlegm, and disperses accumulations. It treats overuse of the voice leading to an irritated throat and voice loss. The pathodynamic relates to overuse of the voice stressing the local tissues and leading to heat, swelling, and stagnation. Wind may settle in the throat, taking advantage of the temporarily compromised region, and cause further stagnation. At present, this formula is used to treat inflammation of the oral cavity, laryngitis, pharyngitis, esophagitis, and loss of voice from overuse.

Note that there is some controversy relating to the name of this formula. In the source text it was called Sound Sage Broken Flute Pill (響聖破笛丸 *xiǎng shèng pò dí wán*), while the present name is found in *Restoration of Health from the Myriad Diseases*.

---

* Multiherb Concoction (百藥煎 *bǎi yào jiān*) is made up of Galla chinensis (*wǔ bèi zǐ*), tea, and other ingredients. It is sour, astringent, slightly sweet, and neutral. It enters the Heart, Lung, and Stomach channels and moistens the Lungs, transforms phlegm, stops bleeding and diarrhea, and also resolves heat and generates fluids. It is difficult to obtain at present and is usually replaced by Catechu (*ér chá*), which clears heat and transforms phlegm, and is found in prepared versions of this formula made in Taiwan or Japan.

滾痰丸

Flushing Away Roiling Phlegm Pill

gǔn tán wán

The name of this formula is based on the different meanings of the character 滾 *gǔn*. This denotes the rapid flow or bubbling of water, from which is derived the meanings of making water muddy and of removing something by force. Thus, the character refers both to the turbid nature of the pathogen and its removal from the body. Both meanings have been used in the translation here.

Source *Subtle Import of the Jade Key* (1396)

calcined Chloriti Lapis/Micae Lapis aureus (*duàn méng shí*)..30g

wine-washed Rhei Radix et Rhizoma (*jiǔ xǐ dà huáng*).....240g

wine-washed Scutellariae Radix (*jiǔ xǐ huáng qín*).........240g

Aquilariae Lignum resinatum (*chén xiāng*)..................15g

Method of Preparation Grind the ingredients into a powder and form into pills with water. Take in 6-9g doses 1-2 times daily with warm water.

Actions Drains fire and drives out phlegm

Indications

Insanity, palpitations with anxiety; or severe, continuous palpitations that can lead to coma; or coughing and wheezing with thick, viscous sputum; or focal distention and a stifling sensation in the chest and epigastrium; or dizziness, vertigo, and tinnitus. In every case there is constipation, a yellow, thick, and greasy tongue coating, and a slippery, rapid, and forceful pulse. There may also be facial tics, insomnia or extremely strange dreams, sudden, deep pain in the joints that is difficult to describe, nodules in the neck, or a choking sensation.

This is a combination of excess heat and chronic phlegm, or phlegm-fire, which accumulates over a period of time. The occurrence of this pattern may be accompanied by a multitude of symptoms. If the phlegm and heat ascend and veil the sensory orifices, insanity or even coma may result. Insanity (癲狂 *diān kuáng*) is a disorder of the spirit marked by two patterns that may or may not alternate with each other. Withdrawal (癲 *diān*) is a yin disorder characterized by a blunted affect, a dull complexion, incoherent speech, disinterest in food, and in severe cases, a blank stare. Mania (狂 *kuáng*) or manic behavior is a yang disorder marked by restlessness, agitation, continuous shouting or singing, and sometimes violent behavior.

Because phlegm also disturbs the Heart's spirit, it may lead to palpitations with anxiety, severe, continuous palpitations, insomnia, or extremely strange dreams. If it collects in the Lungs, the patient will experience coughing and wheezing with thick, viscous sputum, and when severe, a choking sensation. If the phlegm stays in the chest and epigastrium, it obstructs the qi dynamic and gives rise to a stifling sensation and focal distention in the chest and epigastrium. If the phlegm ascends and disturbs the sensory orifices of the head, there may be dizziness, vertigo, and tinnitus. Phlegm in the channels of the face results in facial tics; phlegm in the channels and joints can lead to sudden, deep pain in the joints that is difficult to describe. Because all of these different symptoms are due to excessive heat and phlegm, they are accompanied by a yellow, thick, and greasy tongue coating, and a slippery, rapid, and forceful pulse.

Analysis of Formula

This is a harsh formula that drives out excess phlegm via the bowels. The chief ingredient is sweet, salty, neutral Chloriti Lapis/Micae Lapis aureus (*méng shí*), which strongly drives phlegm retained in the Stomach and Intestines downward and out of the body. It also directs the qi downward to calm wheezing, arrests palpitations, pacifies the Liver, and suppresses jitteriness and convulsions. *Materia Medica of Combinations* explains that:

> [Because this mineral] is drying and can expel dampness, it is apparently inappropriate for old, stubborn phlegm. But when all other herbs have been employed to moisten and cause the phlegm to slip away downward, there may still remain phlegm lurking at the deepest hidden locations, which has not been reached. Only Chloriti Lapis/Micae Lapis aureusi (*méng shí*) with its harsh ferocity can seek out and sweep clear the root of phlegm from the areas hidden deep in the twists and turns of the bowels.

It is used in its calcined form to ensure that its properties are rapidly dispersed. The deputy is bitter, cold Rhei Radix et Rhizoma (*dà huáng*), which cleanses fire from the upper burner by directing it downward through the Large Intestine in the lower burner. It thereby unblocks the obstruction of the yang organs. Unless the obstruction is removed, there is no clear path for removal of phlegm-fire from the body. This is an important use of Rhei Radix et Rhizoma (*dà huáng*) that follows directly from the analysis of its effects in *Divine Husbandman's Classic of the Materia Medica*, where it is described as an herb that "pushes out the old to create the new, regulates the middle to transform food, and quiets the five yin organs." Expanding on this passage, *Commentary on the Divine Husbandman's Classic of Materia Medica* notes that "It is also good for dampness and heat congealing into phlegm in the middle and lower burners. It expels pathogens to halt their violence, and has a special ability to uproot chaos and restore normality." Working in combination, the chief and deputy herbs thus forcibly drive out the phlegm via the Intestines.

The assistant is bitter and cooling Scutellariae Radix (*huáng qín*), which is also used for clearing fire from the upper burner to prevent it from scorching the fluids and thereby generating more phlegm. The large dosage of Rhei Radix et Rhizoma (*dà huáng*) and Scutellariae Radix (*huáng qín*) is used to thoroughly transform the root of this disorder, and

both herbs are washed in wine in order to direct their action to the upper burner from which they can then exert their downward-directing action via the middle and lower burners. As explained in *Convenient Reader of Established Formulas*, "The bitter, cooling [nature of] Scutellariae Radix (*huáng qín*) is employed [here] to clear the heat from the upper burner, while the bitter, cooling [nature of] Rhei Radix et Rhizoma (*dà huáng*) is used to open a way [for this heat] to be moved downward." Finally, a small amount of bitter, acrid, and warming Aquilariae Lignum resinatum (*chén xiāng*) is used as an assistant to regulate the qi and open constraint, rapidly directing the rebellious qi downward in order to eliminate the phlegm. Its inclusion in this formula follows the principle that, in treating phlegm disorders, it is useful to first regulate the qi, since it is the qi that motivates the movement of fluids in the body. Its warming nature, moreover, slightly buffers the cooling action of the three other ingredients in order to protect the normal qi.

Cautions and Contraindications

Contraindicated during pregnancy and postpartum. Because of the rather strong, harsh properties of this formula, it should not be used in weak individuals or in the absence of excessive heat and chronic, stubborn phlegm.

Commentary

This formula was composed by the Yuan-dynasty physician Wang Gui to treat "phlegm patterns that mutate to produce all kinds of strange symptoms." Its influence is reflected by its inclusion in many of the most influential medical texts of the late imperial period, including those by Zhu Dan-Xi, Wang Ken-Tang, and Zhang Jie-Bin, as well as in *Golden Mirror of the Medical Tradition*. Its strategy of eliminating phlegm by way of purging the Intestines can be traced back to Zhang Zhong-Jing's Kansui and Pinellia Decoction (*gān suì bàn xià tāng*), used for treating lingering thin mucus, and Poria Pill (*fú líng wán*), discussed above, used for treating phlegm tarrying in the middle burner. The efficacy of this strategy is explained by Wang Ken-Tang in *Indispensable Tools for Pattern Treatment*: "A pill made from these [four] ingredients is able to draw together stubborn phlegm from all over the body, gathering it together in one place, and then purging it from there. It [thereby] achieves outstanding results."

Ingredients

As can be ascertained from the analysis of the formula above, much of this efficacy was attributed to the chief ingredient, Chloriti Lapis/Micae Lapis aureus (*méng shí*), as well as the heat-draining nature of the deputy and assistant herbs, which are said to attack the root of phlegm in the body. A somewhat different approach that deserves to be included in its entirety is taken by Ke Qin in *Golden Mirror of the Medical Tradition*:

The Spleen is the source [where] phlegm is generated, and the Lungs are the receptacle that holds the phlegm. This is [an often cited] but rarely examined adage. The Spleen moves the body fluids [assimilated by the] Stomach to irrigate the entire body and also moves water essence upward to the Lungs. How might this congeal and clump to form phlegm? The Kidneys, on the other hand, are the gate of the Stomach. If the gate's door does not work, water collects, overflows, and becomes phlegm. Accordingly, it would be [more] appropriate to say that the Kidneys are the source [where] phlegm is generated. The *Inner Classic* states, 'The assimilated food is turbid, the assimilated qi is clear.' The clear yang is moved to the five yin organs, the turbid yin is returned to the six yang organs. The Lungs are the hand greater yin. It alone assimilates all of the clear qi and does not assimilate anything that has form [and therefore] is turbid. How might [such an organ therefore] be the receptacle that holds phlegm? The Stomach, on the other hand, is the sea of food and drink where the myriad [food]stuffs come together. If it should even slightly fail in its task of transferring the flavors, damp-heat will congeal [into] clumps to become phlegm that attaches itself to the Stomach without being directed downward. Accordingly, it would be more appropriate to speak of the Stomach as the receptacle that holds phlegm. Only Master Wang Gui understood the significance of these [facts]. Thus, when he composed a formula to control old phlegm, he did not involve himself with the Spleen and Lungs but with the duties of the Kidneys and Stomach.

The two yellows [i.e., Scutellariae Radix *(huáng qín)* and Rhei Radix et Rhizoma *(dà huáng)*] and the yellow color within Chloriti Lapis/Micae Lapis aureus *(méng shí)* [mean that these are substances] that enter into the central palace. Scutellariae Radix *(huáng qín)* is able to clear the formless qi within the Stomach. Rhei Radix et Rhizoma *(dà huáng)* is able to wash out matter that has form from within the Stomach. Now even though it is slippery it is also sticky and the nature of phlegm is to easily stick to the curvatures of the Intestines and Stomach. These become its lair. Instead of being purged following the current [of movement within the Intestines,] it ascends around the edges. Therefore, it is referred to as old phlegm. Combining the two yellows with moistening and enriching substances only allows them to directly move and drain [what is stuck in the passages of the Intestines]. Guiding out what is stuck in the curvatures is not the forte [of this combination]. Thus, [the formula's author] selected a mineral to assist them. The dryness of Chloriti Lapis/Micae Lapis aureus *(méng shí)* is able to eliminate the root of dampness, while its ferocious nature is able to wash it from its hiding places in the curvatures so that this foul turbid [filth] is unable to remain [in spite of] its greasy sluggish [nature]. This is where the term flushing away roiling phlegm comes from. Finally, he gave consideration to the door of the gate not being open as this is a set pattern [at the heart of all cases of] old phlegm. Aquilariae Lignum resinatum *(chén xiāng)* has the color of the north and [therefore] is able to guide the qi into the Kidneys. Furthermore, it can unblock stagnation within the Stomach and Intestines. When the Kidney qi flows unhindered, filthy water does not remain [in the body] so that phlegm is not [produced] again. Finally, it makes sure that Chloriti Lapis/Micae Lapis aureus *(méng shí)* does not stick to the Intestines and that the two yellows do not damage the Stomach. By selecting one [herb, the author thus obtained] three benefits, hence the [formula] works like magic.

Usage

In practice, this formula is suitable for a wide variety of disorders characterized by phlegm obstruction in any of the yang organs in those with a strong constitution that causes fire to rise upward. This can vary from childhood convulsions, chest painful obstruction, scrofula, drum-like distention, as well as many others disorders.

Generally, for manic behavior, restlessness, and other abnormal symptoms of the spirit associated with phlegm-fire disorders, it is best to use downward-draining substances that indirectly clear heat from the upper body by reducing the accumulation of heat in the lower body. This is another example of 'removing the firewood from under the cauldron.' When phlegm-fire is drained from the body, the spirit will gradually be restored to a clear state of consciousness. This is the same rationale as that used for formulas like Major Order the Qi Decoction *(dà chéng qì tāng)* in treating manic behavior that occurs in the context of yang brightness organ-warp heat.

Biomedical Indications

With the appropriate presentation, this formula may be used to treat a wide variety of biomedically-defined disorders. These can be divided into the following groups:

- Neuropsychiatric disorders such as anxiety neurosis, manic-depression, schizophrenia, pediatric seizure disorder, epilepsy, viral encephalitis, and stubborn headaches
- Respiratory disorders such as bronchial asthma, acute bronchitis, and chronic obstructive pulmonary disease.

This formula has also been used for treating Ménière's disease, benign paroxysmal positional vertigo, stroke, and hypertension.

Alternate names

Flushing Away Roiling Phlegm Pill with Aquilaria *(chén xiāng gǔn tán wán)* in *Empiric Formulas from the Treasured Scroll Chamber*; Flushing Away Roiling Phlegm Pill with Chlorite *(méng shí gǔn tán wán)* in *Golden Mirror Record of Pox and Rashes*

Associated Formula

竹瀝達痰丸 (竹沥达痰丸)

Bamboo Sap Pill to Thrust Out Phlegm

zhú lì dá tán wán

SOURCE *Multitude of Marvelous Formulas for Sustaining Life* (1550)

Pinelliae Rhizoma praeparatum *(zhì bàn xià)*	60g
Ginseng Radix *(rén shēn)*	30g
Poria *(fú líng)*	60g
Glycyrrhizae Radix praeparata *(zhì gān cǎo)*	30g
Atractylodis macrocephalae Rhizoma *(bái zhú)*	90g
Rhei Radix et Rhizoma *(dà huáng)*	90g
Scutellariae Radix *(huáng qín)*	90g

Aquilariae Lignum resinatum (*chén xiāng*) 15g
Chloriti Lapis/Micae Lapis aureus (*méng shí*) 30g

In the source text, the ingredients are ground into a powder and made into pills with Bambusae Succus (*zhú lì*) and Zingiberis Rhizomatis Succus (*jiāng zhī*). Directs fire downward, drives out phlegm, augments the qi, and supports the normal qi. For stubborn phlegm patterns similar to those described for the principal formula in those with a weaker constitution. This formula is a combination of Flushing Away Roiling Phlegm Pill (*gǔn tán wán*) and Two-Aged [Herb] Decoction (*èr chén tāng*) with Atractylodis macrocephalae Rhizoma (*bái zhú*) replacing Citri reticulatae Pericarpium (*chén pí*).

Section 3

. . . .

FORMULAS THAT TRANSFORM PHLEGM AND DISPERSE CLUMPING

The normal condition of the body fluids, like that of qi, is one of continuous movement, dispersal, and transformation. When this process is disordered, it leads to the accumulation of water, dampness, thin mucus, or phlegm. When phlegm gathers in one location to form nodules, swelling, tumors, and masses this is known as 'clumping and gathering of phlegm toxin' (痰毒結聚 *tán dú jié jù*). The formulas in this section are used to disperse such accumulations by way of transforming phlegm, softening hardness, and restoring the normal circulation and transformation of body fluids. For this reason, they employ, as chief herbs, substances that soften hardness and disperse clumping such as Sargassum (*hǎi zǎo*), Eckloniae Thallus (*kūn bù*), Fritillariae Bulbus (*bèi mǔ*), Prunellae Spica (*xià kū cǎo*), Sinapis Semen (*bái jiè zǐ*), and Cremastrae/Pleiones Pseudobulbus (*shān cí gū*). These are combined with herbs like Pinelliae Rhizoma praeparatum (*zhì bàn xià*), Citri reticulatae Pericarpium (*chén pí*), Trichosanthis Fructus (*guā lóu*), or Arisaematis Rhizoma praeparatum (*zhì tiān nán xīng*), which focus on transforming phlegm and drying dampness. Other herbs are added according to the nature of the pattern and pathodynamic, and may include:

- Acrid, dispersing herbs that regulate the qi such as Cyperi Rhizoma (*xiāng fù*), Linderae Radix (*wū yào*), Citri reticulatae viride Pericarpium (*qīng pí*), or Angelicae pubescentis Radix (*dú huó*), both to treat the qi stagnation that invariably arises when fluid congeals in a particular location and also to address the constraint that often underlies these conditions.

- Herbs that regulate the blood and break up stasis such as Angelicae sinensis Radix (*dāng guī*), Chuanxiong Rhizoma (*chuān xiōng*), Spatholobi Caulis (*jī xuè téng*), Curcumae Rhizoma (*é zhú*), and Sparganii Rhizoma (*sān léng*), es-

pecially where the masses have become hard and rock-like. This is necessary because phlegm invariably causes the blood to stagnate.

Other herbs in these formulas address deeper causes such as qi deficiency, yin deficiency, or fire from constraint that disorder the qi dynamic and cause phlegm to accumulate.

消瘰丸

Reduce Scrofula Pill

xiāo luǒ wán

Source   *Awakening of the Mind in Medical Studies* (1732)

Scrophulariae Radix (*xuán shēn*) 120g
Ostreae Concha (*mǔ lì*) 120g
Fritillariae Bulbus (*bèi mǔ*) 120g

Method of Preparation   Grind the ingredients into a powder and form into pills with honey. Take in 9g doses 2-3 times a day. May also be prepared as a decoction with 9-12g of each ingredient. Note that Fritillariae thunbergii Bulbus (*zhè bèi mǔ*) is generally used because it is more effective in treating nodules than Fritillariae cirrhosae Bulbus (*chuān bèi mǔ*).

Actions   Clears heat, transforms phlegm, softens hardness, and disperses clumping

Indications

Nodules on the neck that are firm and rubbery in consistency accompanied by a dry mouth and throat, red tongue, and a rapid pulse that is slippery or wiry.

In traditional Chinese medicine, nodules on the neck are considered to be a form of scrofula (瘰癧 *luǒ lì*), a disorder marked by nodules on the sides of the neck, or goiter (癭 *yǐng*), in which the nodules are on the midline of the neck. Sometimes a general term, phlegm nodules (痰核 *tán hé*), is used to describe both of these conditions. The source text attributes the nodules treated by this formula to Liver fire being constrained and clumping. Modern textbooks explain the pathogenesis in term of deficiency of Liver and Kidney yin. When water does not nourish wood, the Liver loses its ability to regulate the smooth ascent of ministerial fire, which leads to constraint. Fire from constraint consumes the fluids and produces phlegm. Fire and phlegm coalesce into nodules that are firm and rubbery in consistency. The dry mouth, red tongue, and rapid pulse reflect the presence of heat, while the slippery and/or wiry pulse reflects its coalescence into phlegm.

Analysis of Formula

To successfully treat phlegm nodules due to fire from constraint, one must clear fire and transform phlegm as well as soften hardness and disperse clumping. For this reason, the chief herb in this formula is bitter and slightly cooling Fritillariae Bulbus *(bèi mǔ)*, which clears heat and dissipates the nodules caused by the clumping of phlegm and fire. Salty and slightly cooling Ostreae Concha *(mǔ lì)* acts as deputy. It is very effective in softening and dissipating hard masses or nodules. Bitter, salty, and cooling Scrophulariae Radix *(xuán shēn)* is the second deputy, used to clear fire, moisten yin, and soften hardness. It enriches water to nourish wood, and, in combination with Ostreae Concha *(mǔ lì)*, curbs Liver excess. Together, these three herbs treat both the root and branch of the disorder that gives rise to nodules on the neck.

Cautions and Contraindications

Contraindicated in cases from congealing due to cold as well as for inflamed and ulcerated nodules. Patients should be advised to resolve the emotional problems that may underlie or accompany this condition.

Commentary

The author of this formula, Cheng Guo-Peng, composed it to treat early-stage scrofula, that is, swellings that are rubbery and mobile and that are not inflamed or ulcerating. He considered such scrofula to be a manifestation of a Liver disorder that he described as follows: "Scrofula is a Liver tumor (肝瘤 *gān liú*). The Liver governs the sinews. When the blood in the Liver channel becomes dry, there is fire. The fire causes the sinews to tighten, which generates scrofula." The editors of the Qing-dynasty text *Golden Mirror of the Medical Tradition* allowed for a wider pathogenesis, but also emphasized emotional problems that by then were widely associated with Liver disorders:

> [Various types of] scrofula are named differently according to their form. Although the [factors] that cause this disorder encompass [different] accumulations and clumping of phlegm, dampness, fire, heat, and qi toxin, there is not a single case [that does not involve] as a cause hatred leading to anger, indignation leading to constraint, hidden pent-up [feelings], or plans that have come to nothing.

The emphasis on yin deficiency as a primary cause is a recent innovation. This has led, in many modern textbooks, to the designation of Scrophulariae Radix *(xuán shēn)* as the chief herb in the formula.

The use of this formula has been expanded to include a wide variety of nodular masses associated with phlegm-fire including cervical lymphadenopathy, lymphadenitis, simple goiter, thyroiditis, and hyperthyroidism. Some authors recommend the formula for nodular masses anywhere in the body, provided they are a manifestation of a similar pattern. The early 20th-century physician Zhang Xi-Chun increased the dosage of Ostreae Concha *(mǔ lì)* and added Laminariae Thallus *(hǎi dài)*, Curcumae Rhizoma *(é zhú)*, Sparganii Rhizoma *(sān léng)*, Daemonoropis Resina *(xuè jié)*, Olibanum *(rǔ xiāng)*, Myrrha *(mò yào)*, Astragali Radix *(huáng qí)*, and

Gentianae Radix *(lóng dǎn cǎo)* to create a modified formula that has a stronger softening and fire-draining action, but also invigorates the blood and tonifies the qi. This modified formula is used in contemporary practice to treat cysts and masses along the entire course of the Liver channel, including the ovaries and uterus.

Comparison

➤ Vs. Sargassum Decoction for the Jade Flask *(hǎi zǎo yù hú tāng)*; *see* page 801

Biomedical Indications

With the appropriate presentation, this formula may be used to treat a variety of biomedically-defined disorders including simple goiter, hyperthyroidism, scrofula, and simple lymphadenitis.

Alternate name

Reduce Scrofula Pill *(xiāo lì wán)* in *Great Compendium of Medicine for Sores*

Modifications

- For large and very hard nodules, increase the dosage of Ostreae Concha *(mǔ lì)* and add Eckloniae Thallus *(kūn bù)*, Sargassum *(hǎi zǎo)*, and Prunellae Spica *(xià kū cǎo)*.

- For very hot nodules characterized by sticky contents and a bitter taste in the mouth, increase the dosage of Fritillariae Bulbus *(bèi mǔ)* and add Trichosanthis Fructus *(guā lóu)*.

- For severe dryness of the throat and mouth, increase the dosage of Scrophulariae Radix *(xuán shēn)* and add Anemarrhenae Rhizoma *(zhī mǔ)* and Moutan Cortex *(mǔ dān pí)*.

- For Liver qi stagnation with pain in the chest and hypochondria, add Bupleuri Radix *(chái hú)*, Paeoniae Radix alba *(bái sháo)*, and Citri reticulatae viride Pericarpium *(qīng pí)*.

Associated Formula

夏枯草膏

Prunella Syrup

xià kū cǎo gāo

Source　*Golden Mirror of the Medical Tradition* (1742)

Prunellae Spica *(xià kū cǎo)*	450g
Angelicae sinensis Radix *(dāng guī)*	15g
Paeoniae Radix alba *(bái sháo)*	15g
Scrophulariae Radix *(xuán shēn)*	15g
Linderae Radix *(wū yào)*	15g
Fritillariae thunbergii Bulbus *(zhè bèi mǔ)*	15g
Bombyx batryticatus *(bái jiāng cán)*	15g
Eckloniae Thallus *(kūn bù)*	9g
Platycodi Radix *(jié gěng)*	9g

Citri reticulatae Pericarpium (*chén pí*) 9g
Chuanxiong Rhizoma (*chuān xiōng*) 9g
Glycyrrhizae Radix (*gān cǎo*) 9g
Cyperi Rhizoma (*xiāng fù*) 30g
Carthami Flos (*hóng huā*) 6g
Jujubae Fructus (*dà zǎo*) 240g

Decoct Prunellae Spica (*xià kū cǎo*) until the liquid becomes quite concentrated. Add the other ingredients to the strained liquid and cook over a low flame until the mixture has the consistency of a thick syrup. Promotes the movement of qi, invigorates the blood, transforms phlegm, and dissipates nodules. For hard scrofula from dry blood due to Liver yang excess. This formula has stronger dispersing and heat-clearing actions than the principal formula.

海藻玉壺湯 （海藻玉壶汤）
Sargassum Decoction for the Jade Flask
hǎi zǎo yù hú tāng

The term *yù hú* 玉壺 refers to a wine flask made from jade. A poem by the 5th-century poet Bao Zhao contains the stanza: "Genuine like a thread of red silk, clear like ice in a jade wine flask." The term thus came to symbolize spiritual purity, honesty, and virtue. In the present context, it can be taken to mean that the formula truly delivers the effects it claims for itself by using sargassum as its chief herb.

Source   *Orthodox Lineage of External Medicine* (1617)

Sargassum (*hǎi zǎo*) 3g (9g)
Eckloniae Thallus (*kūn bù*) 3g (9g)
Laminariae Thallus (*hǎi dài*) 1.5g (9g)
Fritillariae thunbergii Bulbus (*zhè bèi mǔ*) 3g (9g)
Pinelliae Rhizoma praeparatum (*zhì bàn xià*) 3g (9g)
Angelicae pubescentis Radix (*dú huó*) 3g (9g)
Chuanxiong Rhizoma (*chuān xiōng*) 3g (6g)
Angelicae sinensis Radix (*dāng guī*) 3g (9g)
Citri reticulatae viride Pericarpium (*qīng pí*) 3g (6g)
Citri reticulatae Pericarpium (*chén pí*) 3g (4.5g)
Forsythiae Fructus (*lián qiáo*) 3g (9g)
Glycyrrhizae Radix (*gān cǎo*) 3g

Method of Preparation   Decoction. At present, the dosage of most of the ingredients is increased to that shown in parentheses.

Actions   Transforms phlegm, softens hard masses, reduces and dissipates goiter

Indications

Masses in the center of the neck that are rock-like in hardness, immobile, cause no change in the color of the skin, and do not ulcerate. The tongue has a thin, greasy coating, and the pulse is wiry and slippery.

Swellings and tumors of the neck are referred to as 'goiter' (瘰瘤 *yǐng liú*) in Chinese medicine. They are thought to be caused by the stagnation of dampness, phlegm, qi, and blood in the area between the skin and flesh on the neck. Swellings that come and go and change in size are attributed to

qi stagnation leading to blood stasis and phlegm-dampness and are known as 'qi goiter.' Swellings that are not painful or ulcerated and do not produce any change in the color of the skin, are known as 'flesh goiter' and are attributed primarily to clogging of phlegm-turbidity. If blood and phlegm stasis are primary, leading to hard masses or nodules, this is called 'rock-like goiter.' In practice, these three types of goiter and the pathological processes that produce them are often difficult to separate from each other; this formula treats all three. The thin, greasy tongue coating reflects the superficial retention of dampness or phlegm. The pulse signs reflect the presence of dampness and phlegm (slippery) together with stagnation and stasis (wiry).

Analysis of Formula

To treat hard swellings and goiter due to qi stagnation and the congealing of phlegm, this formula not only transforms the phlegm and moves the qi, but also softens masses, reduces, and dissipates. The chief ingredients in this formula are Sargassum (*hǎi zǎo*), Eckloniae Thallus (*kūn bù*), and Laminariae Thallus (*hǎi dài*). All three of these salty substances effectively soften and dissolve masses. The deputy, Fritillariae thunbergii Bulbus (*zhè bèi mǔ*), clears heat and dissipates nodules. It acts synergistically with the chief ingredients.

Those ingredients that affect specific aspects of this disorder are regarded as assistants: warm and drying Pinelliae Rhizoma praeparatum (*zhì bàn xià*) and Angelicae pubescentis Radix (*dú huó*) expel phlegm; Chuanxiong Rhizoma (*chuān xiōng*) and Angelicae sinensis Radix (*dāng guī*) invigorate the blood and relieve stasis; and Citri reticulatae viride Pericarpium (*qīng pí*) and Citri reticulatae Pericarpium (*chén pí*) promote the movement of qi and relieve constraint. The accumulation of phlegm, stagnant qi, and static blood often generates heat from constraint. Forsythiae Fructus (*lián qiáo*) is therefore added to clear this type of heat, even though there are as yet no external signs of the heat. The envoy, Glycyrrhizae Radix (*gān cǎo*), harmonizes the actions of the other herbs and resolves toxicity, especially when combined with Forsythiae Fructus (*lián qiáo*).

Cautions and Contraindications

Contraindicated in cases where the swelling has ulcerated. The formula strongly regulates the qi and should not be used without modification for patients with significant deficiency.

Commentary

In traditional Chinese medicine, swellings of the neck (particularly in the center) that go up and down with swallowing are called goiter (瘰 *yǐng*), even if they are not associated with the thyroid gland. This formula is also used for treating superficial tumors in other parts of the body. It is designed for relatively acute disorders that are excessive in nature. If it is possible to ascertain the primary pathodynamic (i.e., qi, phlegm-dampness, or blood stasis) the formula should be modified accordingly (see below). For disorders of deficiency, tonifying ingredients should be added. To be effective, the formula must be taken over several months.

While Sargassum *(hǎi zǎo)* and Glycyrrhizae Radix *(gān cǎo)* are traditionally thought to be mutually incompatible, they are in fact often combined for treating goiter in both classical and modern formulas.

Comparison

➤ Vs. Reduce Scrofula Pill *(xiāo luǒ wán)*; see PAGE 799

Both Sargassum Decoction for the Jade Flask *(hǎi zǎo yù hú tāng)* and Reduce Scrofula Pill *(xiāo luǒ wán)* treat swellings of the neck, including goiter. However, Reduce Scrofula Pill *(xiāo luǒ wán)* treats patterns characterized by ascending fire that carries phlegm upward where it congeals in the area of the neck. For this reason, it focuses on clearing heat as well as softening hardness and transforming phlegm. Sargassum Decoction for the Jade Flask *(hǎi zǎo yù hú tāng)*, by contrast, treats patterns characterized by qi stagnation and phlegm-turbidity congealing to form nodules and swelling. For this reason, it focuses on regulating the qi, dispersing clumping, and transforming phlegm. Thus, Reduce Scrofula Pill *(xiāo luǒ wán)* is better at clearing fire and nourishing the yin, while Sargassum Decoction for the Jade Flask *(hǎi zǎo yù hú tāng)* excels at opening stasis and stagnation.

Biomedical Indications

With the appropriate presentation, this formula may be used to treat a variety of biomedically-defined disorders including simple goiter, hyperthyroidism, benign tumors of the thyroid, fibrocystic breasts, polycystic ovaries, and multiple furuncles.

Modifications

- For pronounced qi stagnation and masses that change in size (i.e., qi goiter), add Bupleuri Radix *(chái hú)* and Cyperi Rhizoma *(xiāng fù)*.
- For pronounced phlegm-dampness with soft stools and masses that are not painful or ulcerated, and do not produce any change in the color of the skin (i.e., flesh goiter), add Atractylodis macrocephalae Rhizoma *(bái zhú)*, Dioscoreae Rhizoma *(shān yào)*, and Lablab Semen album *(bái biǎn dòu)*.
- For very hard and firm masses (i.e., rock-like goiter), add Paeoniae Radix rubra *(chì sháo)*, Vespae Nidus *(lù fēng fáng)*, Curcumae Rhizoma *(é zhú)*, Sparganii Rhizoma *(sān léng)*, and Rhei Radix et Rhizoma *(dà huáng)*.
- For a stifling sensation in the chest, add Cyperi Rhizoma *(xiāng fù)* and Curcumae Radix *(yù jīn)*.

- For a rapid pulse, palpitations, and a tendency to sweat, add Poriae Sclerotium pararadicis *(fú shén)* and Ziziphi spinosae Semen *(suān zǎo rén)*.
- For tremors of the tongue, add Uncariae Ramulus cum Uncis *(gōu téng)* and Paeoniae Radix alba *(bái sháo)*.
- For excessive hunger, add Gypsum fibrosum *(shí gāo)* and Anemarrhenae Rhizoma *(zhī mǔ)*.
- For irregular menstruation, add Cervi Cornus Colla *(lù jiǎo jiāo)*, Cistanches Herba *(ròu cōng róng)*, Leonuri Herba *(yì mǔ cǎo)*, and Cuscutae Semen *(tù sī zǐ)*.

Associated Formulas

化痰消核丸

Transform Phlegm and Reduce Nodules Pill
huà tán xiāo hé wán

SOURCE *Treatment Strategies and Formulas in Chinese Medicine* (1975)

Astragali Radix *(huáng qí)*	40g
Spatholobi Caulis *(jī xuè téng)*	24g
Sinapis Semen *(bái jiè zǐ)*	15g
Poria *(fú líng)*	15g
Pinelliae Rhizoma praeparatum *(zhì bàn xià)*	12g
Citri reticulatae Pericarpium *(chén pí)*	10g
Linderae Radix *(wū yào)*	15g
Cyperi Rhizoma *(xiāng fù)*	10g
Cremastrae/Pleiones Pseudobulbus *(shān cí gū)*	10g
Sargassum *(hǎi zǎo)*	15g
Eckloniae Thallus *(kūn bù)*	15g
Glycyrrhizae Radix *(gān cǎo)*	3g

Grind the herbs into a fine powder and make into large pills weighing 10g each by mixing with honey. Take three pills daily. Can also be prepared as a decoction. Supports the normal qi, strengthens the Spleen, transforms phlegm, and disperses clumping. For impaired Spleen transportation leading to clumping of phlegm and the generation of nodules. These tend to be soft and rubbery without change in the color of the skin or ulceration and are known by a few different names in Chinese medicine, including 'flesh goiter' or 'phlegm nodules.' In contrast to the principal formula, this one, composed by the contemporary physician Ai Ru-Di, combines herbs that tonify the qi and invigorate the blood with those that regulate qi and transform phlegm. It is useful not only for patients with obvious qi deficiency, but also for the long-term use needed to successfully treat these types of disorders.

Section 4

FORMULAS THAT MOISTEN DRYNESS AND TRANSFORM PHLEGM

This type of formula is used in treating phlegm-dryness that manifests as viscous, sticky sputum that is difficult to expectorate, dryness of the mouth and throat, and often a raspy voice. Dryness can penetrate directly from the exterior to damage the body fluids, although more often, fire is the primary cause. In a dry environment, patients tending toward yang excess are most likely to develop dry pathologies. This type of pathology also occurs as fire from constraint, often due to emotional causes, which damages the body fluids. Because the Lungs are responsible for directing the body fluids downward and yet are also the 'tender organ,' they are the first to suffer from such a disorder. Damage to the Lungs' clearing and downward-directing functions by dryness causes the fluids to stagnate, while fire condenses them and thereby reduces their volume. In patients with yang excess, the fluids are already relatively deficient. Together, this process produces phlegm-dryness. In addition to the symptoms outlined above, the pulse will tend to be thin and slippery, and the tongue coating will be thick but dry. This helps to distinguish patterns of dryness from those of yin deficiency that often present with similar symptoms. The difference is that yin deficiency invariably implies yang excess. Thus, there will be signs of fire from deficiency such as heat in the five centers or night sweats, which are absent in patterns of dryness. On the other hand, patterns of dryness are often accompanied by stagnation of fluids, that is, phlegm, which does not occur as readily in yin deficiency patterns where the fluids are completely lacking.

In the treatment of phlegm-dryness, emphasis is thus placed on moistening the Lungs and transforming phlegm using such herbs as Fritillariae Bulbus (bèi mǔ) and Trichosanthis Fructus (guā lóu). Bitter, cooling substances and those that are very moist and cloying, on the other hand, are to be avoided. The former damages the Spleen and Stomach; the latter causes the qi and fluids to stagnate. Both conditions will tend to aggravate the production of phlegm. Thus, yin-tonifying substances such as Asparagi Radix (tiān mén dōng), Ophiopogonis Radix (mài mén dōng), or Rehmanniae Radix praeparata (shú dì huáng) are generally contraindicated to treat phlegm-dryness. Instead, two other groups of herbs are frequently added to the formulas in this section:

• Herbs that regulate the qi and disseminate the Lungs such as Citri reticulatae Pericarpium (chén pí), or Platycodi Radix (jié gěng). Facilitating the Lungs' clearing and downward-directing functions, these ingredients disperse the accumulation of phlegm, unblock the qi dynamic, and reinstate the normal dissemination of body fluids.

• Herbs that clear heat and nourish yin such as Trichosanthis Radix (tiān huā fěn) or Dendrobii Herba (shí hú). Clearing heat without inhibiting the qi dynamic, moistening the yin without generating phlegm, these herbs are used where heat has damaged the fluids.

貝母栝樓散 (贝母栝楼散)

Fritillaria and Trichosanthes Fruit Powder

bèi mǔ guā lóu sǎn

Source　*Awakening of the Mind in Medical Studies* (1732)

Fritillariae Bulbus (bèi mǔ) 4.5g
Trichosanthis Fructus (guā lóu) 3g
Trichosanthis Radix (tiān huā fěn) 2.4g
Poria (fú líng) 2.4g
Citri reticulatae Exocarpium rubrum (jú hóng). 2.4g
Platycodi Radix (jié gěng) 2.4g

Method of Preparation　Decoction. Fritillariae cirrhosae Bulbus (chuān bèi mǔ) is the form of Fritillariae Bulbus (bèi mǔ) that is generally used because it moistens better than Fritillariae thunbergii Bulbus (zhè bèi mǔ). Because of the relative expense of this herb, it is often administered as a powder with an appropriate reduction in dosage (usually 1/5th of the raw herb) to be taken with the strained decoction

Actions　Moistens the Lungs, clears heat, regulates the qi, and transforms phlegm

Indications

Cough with deep-seated sputum that is difficult to expectorate, wheezing, a dry and sore throat, a red and dry tongue with white coating, and a rapid and thin but strong or slippery pulse.

This condition is caused by dryness in the Lungs that injures the fluids and causes phlegm. This type of phlegm is referred to as 'phlegm-dryness' and is manifested as coughing with deep-seated sputum that is difficult to expectorate. The phlegm interrupts the flow of Lung qi, which results in coughing and wheezing. The dry pathogenic influence attacking the Lungs also causes a dry, sore throat. The red and dry tongue with white coating and the rapid and thin but strong or slippery pulse reflect the presence of dryness and phlegm in the Lungs.

Analysis of Formula

According to Cheng Guo-Peng, the author of this formula, "Phlegm-dampness is usually generated in the Spleen, while phlegm-dryness is usually generated in the Lungs." Applying a treatment principle first outlined in *Basic Questions* (Chapter 74), "Moisten that which is dry," the formula focuses on moistening the Lungs to unblock constraint, transform phlegm, and clear heat. It also adds herbs that strengthen the Spleen, because all disorders of phlegm are rooted in the dysfunction of fluid metabolism and are therefore helped by supporting the transporting and transforming functions of the Spleen.

The actions of Fritillariae Bulbus (bèi mǔ), the chief herb, encompass all of the primary aspects of this formula: moistening the Lungs, opening constraint, transforming phlegm, and stopping the coughing. It also clears heat and directs Heart fire downward, thus treating one of the key causes of phlegm-dryness outlined by Zhang Bin-Cheng in *Convenient Reader of Established Formulas*: "Phlegm-dryness is due to fire scorching Lung metal when the scorched fluids become phlegm." It is assisted by the deputy, Trichosanthis Fructus *(guā lóu)*, which clears heat, moistens dryness, regulates the qi, and leads turbid phlegm downward in order to remove the obstruction from the chest and diaphragm. The remaining herbs serve as assistants. Trichosanthis Radix *(tiān huā fěn)* clears heat, generates fluids, and transforms phlegm. It thus tonifies the physiological body fluids without generating more phlegm. The combination of Poria *(fú líng)*, which strengthens the Spleen, and Citri reticulatae Exocarpium rubrum *(jú hóng)*, which regulates the qi, is used here to support the Spleen's functions of transportation and transformation. This is important in treating phlegm-dryness because a healthy Spleen will transport physiological fluids to the Lungs to ensure their moistening, while assisting in the transformation of pathological dampness and phlegm. This is one form of the strategy of 'nurturing earth [Spleen] to generate metal [Lungs].' Platycodi Radix *(jié gěng)* encourages the proper flow of Lung qi and treats problems of the throat. All of these herbs reinforce the actions of the chief herb.

Cautions and Contraindications

Contraindicated for cough due to yin deficiency.

Commentary

Context in Tradition

This formula was composed by the 18th-century physician Cheng Guo-Peng for the treatment of phlegm-dryness. Previously, such disorders had been differentiated according to a scheme based on the five organ systems. Li Zhong-Zi's analysis of phlegm-dryness in *Required Readings from the Medical Tradition* is a typical example of this earlier system:

> [Phlegm associated with] the Lung channel is called phlegm-dryness. [This pattern manifests with] a rough pulse, white complexion, ascending qi [that leads to] wheezing and urgent [breathing], shivering with fever and chills, sadness, worry, and unhappiness, and phlegm that is rough and difficult to expectorate.

Cheng Guo-Peng proposed to replace this system with a new and simplified scheme that differentiated only between phlegm-dampness (easy to bring up and associated with the Spleen) and phlegm-dryness (difficult to bring up and associated with the Lungs). Each of these two disorders was then further differentiated into patterns of excess or deficiency. In terms of treatment, Cheng suggested Two-Aged

[Herb] Decoction *(èr chén tāng)* and Six-Gentlemen Decoction *(liù jūn zǐ tāng)* as key formulas for the treatment of phlegm-dampness, and this formula and Six Flavor Pill with Rehmannia *(liù wèi dì huáng wán)* as the basic formulas for phlegm-dryness. This formula can thus be regarded as a variation of Two-Aged [Herb] Decoction *(èr chén tāng)* with the substitution of herbs that moisten and transform phlegm such as Fritillariae Bulbus *(bèi mǔ)* and Trichosanthis Radix *(tiān huā fěn)*, for the acrid, warming Pinelliae Rhizoma praeparatum *(zhì bàn xià)*.

Ingredients

Although the source text does not specify the type of Fritillariae Bulbus *(bèi mǔ)* to be used, it is generally assumed that Fritillariae cirrhosae Bulbus *(chuān bèi mǔ)* rather than Fritillariae thunbergii Bulbus *(zhè bèi mǔ)* is the better choice. Although both herbs cool and transform phlegm-heat and alleviate cough, Fritillariae cirrhosae Bulbus *(chuān bèi mǔ)* is bitter but also sweet, which moistens the Lungs. It is thus better for the dry cough treated by this formula. Moreover, in *Treatment Strategies and Formulas in Chinese Medicine*, the contemporary physician Chen Chao-Zu suggests adding Armeniacae Semen *(xìng rén)* in order to improve the formula's downward-directing function and to double the original dosages for an even better effect.

Comparisons

➤ Vs. Mulberry Leaf and Apricot Kernel Decoction *(sāng xìng tāng)* and Clear Dryness and Rescue the Lungs Decoction *(qīng zào jiù fèi tāng)*

Fritillaria and Trichosanthes Fruit Powder *(bèi mǔ guā lóu sǎn)*, Mulberry Leaf and Apricot Kernel Decoction *(sāng xìng tāng)*, and Clear Dryness and Rescue the Lungs Decoction *(qīng zào jiù fèi tāng)* all treat dryness patterns with herbs that moisten the Lungs and stop coughing. However, Fritillaria and Trichosanthes Fruit Powder *(bèi mǔ guā lóu sǎn)* focuses on phlegm obstructing the Lungs and thus equally emphasizes the transformation of phlegm and the moistening of dryness. The other two formulas are indicated for warm pathogen dryness disorders, and thus combine the clearing of heat with the moistening of dryness. Mulberry Leaf and Apricot Kernel Decoction *(sāng xìng tāng)* treats patterns of dryness in the exterior that constrain the Lung qi and cause coughing. Accordingly, its main focus is on venting the exterior, and its ability to transform phlegm is not very pronounced. Clear Dryness and Rescue the Lungs Decoction *(qīng zào jiù fèi tāng)* treats patterns of dryness that have penetrated deeper into the Lungs and damaged the fluids. Thus, in addition to clearing heat and moistening dryness, it also enriches the fluids.

➤ Vs. Lily Bulb Decoction to Preserve the Metal *(bǎi hé gù jīn tāng)*; see PAGE 386

Biomedical Indications

With the appropriate presentation, this formula may be used to treat a variety of biomedically-defined disorders including pneumonia and pulmonary tuberculosis.

Modifications

• For severe coughing and wheezing, add Armeniacae Semen *(xìng rén)*, Eriobotryae Folium *(pí pá yè)*, and Farfarae Flos *(kuǎn dōng huā)*.

• For a concurrent exterior condition, add Mori Folium *(sāng yè)*, Armeniacae Semen *(xìng rén)*, Peucedani Radix *(qián hú)*, and Arctii Fructus *(niú bàng zǐ)*.

• For hoarseness and blood-streaked sputum, remove Citri reticulatae Exocarpium rubrum *(jú hóng)* and add Glehniae/Adenophorae Radix *(shā shēn)*, Ophiopogonis Radix *(mài mén dōng)*, Phragmitis Rhizoma *(lú gēn)*, and Agrimoniae Herba *(xiān hè cǎo)*.

• For more severe dryness and sore throat, add Scrophulariae Radix *(xuán shēn)*, Ophiopogonis Radix *(mài mén dōng)*, and Anemarrhenae Rhizoma *(zhī mǔ)*.

Associated Formulas

二母散

Fritillaria and Anemarrhena Powder

èr mǔ sǎn

SOURCE   *Investigations of Medical Formulas* (1584)

Fritillariae Bulbus *(bèi mǔ)*
Anemarrhenae Rhizoma *(zhī mǔ)*

Grind equal amounts of the two herbs into a powder and take 6-9g as a draft. Clears heat, transforms phlegm, moistens the Lungs, and stops coughing. Used for either a cough with copious, yellow, thick sputum, or a hacking cough due to dryness and heat in the Lungs.

清肺湯 (清肺汤)

Clear the Lungs Decoction

qīng fèi tāng

SOURCE   *Restoration of Health from the Myriad Diseases* (1587)

Poria *(fú líng)* 3g
Platycodi Radix *(jié gěng)* 3g
Schisandrae Fructus *(wǔ wèi zǐ)* .... [7 fruits] 2g
Citri reticulatae Pericarpium *(chén pí)* 3g
Angelicae sinensis Radix *(dāng guī)* 3g
Asparagi Radix *(tiān mén dōng)* 2g
Ophiopogonis Radix *(mài mén dōng)* 2g
Gardeniae Fructus *(zhī zǐ)* 2g
Scutellariae Radix *(huáng qín)* 5g
Mori Cortex *(sāng bái pí)* 3g

Fritillariae Bulbus *(bèi mǔ)* 3g
Armeniacae Semen *(xìng rén)* 2g
Glycyrrhizae Radix *(gān cǎo)* 1g

Decoct the ingredients with Zingiberis Rhizoma recens *(shēng jiāng)* and Jujubae Fructus *(dà zǎo)*. The source text does not specify dosage for these two ingredients, but typically 3 slices of Zingiberis Rhizoma recens *(shēng jiāng)* and 2 pieces of Jujubae Fructus *(dà zǎo)* are used. At present, if yin-deficiency dry cough is prominent, Fritillariae cirrhosae Bulbus *(chuān bèi mǔ)* is more commonly used, but if phlegm is present, Fritillariae thunbergii Bulbus *(zhè bèi mǔ)* will be more effective.

This formula clears the Lungs, transforms phlegm, relieves coughing, drains fire, and moistens dryness. It is indicated when fire has damaged the Lung yin resulting in coughing, particularly chronic, incessant coughing, chronic hoarseness, or throat lesions. The fire here can be anything from a chronic Liver fire pattern to a secondary pathogen, as long as it damages the Lung yin. Often, the primary and secondary sources of fire coexist. For example, a pattern of chronic Liver stagnation may lead to Liver fire directly affecting the Lungs and simultaneously affect the Spleen such that it can no longer properly disseminate the fluids. Regardless of the cause, over time, damage to the Lung yin reduces the Lungs' ability to disseminate the qi and move the fluids. Together with the heat, this will cause phlegm. Furthermore, the obstructing nature of constrained Lung qi compounded by the presence of fire in its substantial (phlegm) and insubstantial forms, results in symptoms such as hoarseness and incessant cough. If the fire is extreme, it can also manifest as throat lesions.

Note that this formula is contraindicated for patients with exterior disorders. Because many of the herbs in this formula are sweet, cold, and cloying, it should be used with caution or modified in cases with Spleen deficiency or food stagnation. Failure to do so may result in indigestion or diarrhea.

Modifications

• For cough with afternoon fevers, add Anemarrhenae Rhizoma *(zhī mǔ)*, Phellodendri Cortex *(huáng bǎi)*, Rehmanniae Radix *(shēng dì huáng)*, Paeoniae Radix alba *(bái sháo)*, and Bambusae Succus *(zhú lì)*, and remove Scutellariae Radix *(huáng qín)* and Armeniacae Semen *(xìng rén)*. (source text)

• For phlegm-fire cough with red face, fever, and blood-streaked sputum, add Paeoniae Radix alba *(bái sháo)*, Rehmanniae Radix *(shēng dì huáng)*, Asteris Radix *(zǐ wǎn)*, Asini Corii Colla *(ē jiāo)*, and Bambusae Succus *(zhú lì)*, and remove Schisandrae Fructus *(wǔ wèi zǐ)*, Armeniacae Semen *(xìng rén)*, Fritillariae thunbergii Bulbus *(zhè bèi mǔ)*, and Platycodi Radix *(jié gěng)*. (source text)

• For chronic cough with sore throat and raspy voice, add Menthae haplocalycis Herba *(bò hé)*, Rehmanniae Radix *(shēng dì huáng)*, Asteris Radix *(zǐ wǎn)*, and Bambusae Succus *(zhú lì)*, and remove Fritillariae Bulbus *(bèi mǔ)*, Armeniacae Semen *(xìng rén)*, and Schisandrae Fructus *(wǔ wèi zǐ)*. (source text)

- For severe sore throat or sore throat lesions, add Anemarrhenae Rhizoma *(zhī mǔ)* and Isatidis/Baphicacanthis Radix *(bǎn lán gēn)*, and remove the warm herbs in the formula such as Citri reticulatae Pericarpium *(chén pí)* and Angelicae sinensis Radix *(dāng guī)*.
- For phlegm that is difficult to expectorate, add Trichosanthis Fructus *(guā lóu)*, Aurantii Fructus immaturus *(zhǐ shí)*, and Bambusae Succus *(zhú lì)*, and remove Schisandrae Fructus *(wǔ wèi zǐ)*. (source text)
- For constipation, add Trichosanthis Fructus *(guā lóu)*.

清肺飲 （清肺饮）

Clear the Lungs Drink

qīng fèi yǐn

SOURCE *Medical Formulas Collected and Analyzed* (1682)

Armeniacae Semen *(xìng rén)* 3g
Fritillariae Bulbus *(bèi mǔ)* 3g
Poria *(fú líng)* 3g
Platycodi Radix *(jié gěng)* 1.5g
Glycyrrhizae Radix *(gān cǎo)* 1.5g
Schisandrae Fructus *(wǔ wèi zǐ)* 1.5g
Citri reticulatae Exocarpium rubrum *(jú hóng)* 1.5g

Take as a decoction with Zingiberis Rhizoma recens *(shēng jiāng)* and administer apart from meals. At present, the dosages above are modified based on the nature and origin of the cough. Transforms phlegm, disseminates the Lung qi, and relieves coughing. This formula treats phlegm-dampness in the Lungs that impairs the normal downward movement of Lung qi and causes it to rebel upward as a productive cough in a patient with heat (either internally generated or externally contracted) and a deficient Spleen that fails to transform dampness. It is well-balanced and can be used as a base formula to treat cough from a wide variety of causes. The source text provides an extensive list of modifications, selections from which are given below.

Modifications

From *Medical Formulas Collected and Analyzed:*

- "If, in the springtime, [one suffers] damage by wind [and resultant] phlegm-cough [with] clear nasal discharge, it is suitable to clear [heat] and release [pathogens from the exterior]. Add Menthae haplocalycis Herba *(bò hé)*, Saposhnikoviae Radix *(fáng fēng)*, Bupleuri Radix *(chái hú)*, Perillae Folium *(zǐ sū yè)*, and dry-fried Scutellariae Radix *(chǎo huáng qín)*."
- "[In the] summer, [when there is] a good deal of fire and heat, one should clear [heat and encourage qi to] descend. Add Mori Cortex *(sāng bái pí)*, Ophiopogonis Radix *(mài mén dōng)*, Scutellariae Radix *(huáng qín)*, Anemarrhenae Rhizoma *(zhī mǔ)*, and Gypsum fibrosum *(shí gāo)*."
- "[In the] fall, [when there is a lot of] dampness and heat, one should clear heat and promote [the resolution of]

dampness. Add Atractylodis Rhizoma *(cāng zhú)*, Mori Cortex *(sāng bái pí)*, Saposhnikoviae Radix *(fáng fēng)*, Gardeniae Fructus *(zhī zǐ)*, and Scutellariae Radix *(huáng qín)*."
- "[In the] winter, [when there is a] surplus of wind and cold, one should release [pathogens from the] exterior and move the phlegm. Add Ephedrae Herba *(má huáng)*, Cinnamomi Ramulus *(guì zhī)*, Zingiberis Rhizoma *(gān jiāng)*, Zingiberis Rhizoma recens *(shēng jiāng)*, Pinelliae Rhizoma praeparatum *(zhì bàn xià)*, and Saposhnikoviae Radix *(fáng fēng)*."
- "[For] fire cough, add Indigo naturalis *(qīng dài)*, Trichosanthis Fructus *(guā lóu)*, and Costaziae Os *(fú hǎi shí)*."
- "[For] food-accumulation phlegm, add Cyperi Rhizoma *(xiāng fù)*, Crataegi Fructus *(shān zhā)*, and Aurantii Fructus immaturus *(zhǐ shí)*."
- "[For] phlegm-dampness, remove Fritillariae Bulbus *(bèi mǔ)* and add Pinelliae Rhizoma praeparatum *(zhì bàn xià)* and Arisaematis Rhizoma praeparatum *(zhì tiān nán xīng)*."
- "[For] phlegm-dryness, add Trichosanthis Fructus *(guā lóu)*, Anemarrhenae Rhizoma *(zhī mǔ)*, and Asparagi Radix *(tiān mén dōng)*."
- "Cough before noon pertains to Stomach fire. One should clear [heat from] the Stomach. Add Gypsum fibrosum *(shí gāo)* and Coptidis Rhizoma *(huáng lián)*."
- "Cough after noon pertains to yin deficiency. One should enrich the yin and direct fire downward. Add Chuanxiong Rhizoma *(chuān xiōng)*, Angelicae sinensis Radix *(dāng guī)*, Paeoniae Radix alba *(bái sháo)*, Rehmanniae Radix *(shēng dì huáng)*, Anemarrhenae Rhizoma *(zhī mǔ)*, Dioscoreae Rhizoma *(shān yào)*, Ophiopogonis Radix *(mài mén dōng)*, Asparagi Radix *(tiān mén dōng)*, Bambusae Succus *(zhú lì)*, and Zingiberis Rhizomatis Succus *(jiāng zhī)*."
- "[For] cough at dusk [owing to] fire floating to the Lungs, one should not use cool herbs. Choose Galla chinensis *(wǔ bèi zǐ)*, Schisandrae Fructus *(wǔ wèi zǐ)*, and Chebulae Fructus *(hē zǐ)* to preserve [the Lung yin] and [cause the qi to] descend."
- "Consumptive cough presents with blood; it is usually [owing to the] Lungs receiving a heat pathogen. One should add herbs such as Angelicae sinensis Radix *(dāng guī)*, Paeoniae Radix alba *(bái sháo)*, Asini Corii Colla *(ē jiāo)*, Asparagi Radix *(tiān mén dōng)*, Farfarae Flos *(kuǎn dōng huā)*, and Asteris Radix *(zǐ wǎn)*."
- "Chronic cough [stems from] Lung deficiency. Add Ginseng Radix *(rén shēn)* and Astragali Radix *(huáng qí)*. If [there is] Lung heat, one may replace Ginseng Radix *(rén shēn)* with Glehniae/Adenophorae Radix *(shā shēn)*."

Section 5

FORMULAS THAT WARM AND TRANSFORM PHLEGM-COLD

The formulas in this section are used in treating patterns dominated by the presence of phlegm-cold and thin mucus. Such patterns are characterized by symptoms such as coughing of clear, thin, and white sputum, a stifling sensation or focal distention or clogging in the chest, reduced appetite, reduced digestive functions, a sensation of cold in the body, a white, slippery tongue coating, and a slippery pulse. The basic pathodynamic underlying such disorders is aptly summarized in *Introduction to Medicine*: "Phlegm has its source in the Kidneys, is moved by the Spleen, and resides in the Lungs." Deficiency of ministerial fire associated with Kidney yang inhibits the Spleen's ability to transform and transport the body fluids, which accumulate and become phlegm and thin mucus. Thin mucus tends to manifest in the Lungs because the Spleen transports the nutritive qi upward to the Lungs, while the Lungs are charged with moving the fluids downward from the upper burner to the Bladder via the Triple Burner. The end result of this process is summarized by Ye Tian-Shi in *Case Records as a Guide to Clinical Practice*: "When yin is overabundant and yang is deficient, water qi overflows to become thin mucus." Treatment strategies for such patterns follow the adage in *Essentials from the Golden Cabinet*: "For phlegm and thin mucus disorders, one should employ warming herbs to harmonize [the imbalance]."

The chief herbs in the formulas discussed in this section are warming and enter the Lungs to transform the phlegm. Typical examples are Zingiberis Rhizoma (*gān jiāng*), Asari Radix et Rhizoma (*xì xīn*), and Sinapis Semen (*bái jiè zǐ*). These are generally combined with ingredients from one of the following categories:

- Herbs that warm the yang qi such as Aconiti Radix praeparata (*zhì chuān wū*), Zanthoxyli Pericarpium (*huā jiāo*), Cinnamomi Ramulus (*guì zhī*), or Aconiti Radix lateralis praeparata (*zhì fù zǐ*). These herbs warm the Spleen and Kidney yang in order to promote fluid metabolism and strengthen qi transformation.
- Herbs that stop coughing and wheezing such as Ephedrae Herba (*má huáng*), Armeniacae Semen (*xìng rén*), Asteris Radix (*zǐ wǎn*), and Farfarae Flos (*kuǎn dōng huā*). Promoting the Lungs' functions of dissemination and directing downward, these herbs address one of the chief symptoms of the patterns treated by these formulas, and in doing so also promote fluid metabolism.
- Astringent herbs, such as Schisandrae Fructus (*wǔ wèi zǐ*), that counterbalance the acrid, dispersing nature of the chief

and deputy ingredients. The synergism between acrid, dispersing and sour, binding actions mirrors the Lungs' regulation of opening and closing and is thus regularly employed in formulas that disseminate Lung qi.
- Herbs that expel harbored food, such as Raphani Semen (*lái fú zǐ*), that also promote the Spleen's transformative functions. This is especially useful in those, such as the elderly, with weak digestive systems, or in those who regularly overeat and thus tax the Spleen's transformative functions, leading to accumulation of phlegm and thin mucus.

苓甘五味薑辛湯 (苓甘五味姜辛汤)
Poria, Licorice, Schisandra, Ginger, and Asarum Decoction
líng gān wǔ wèi jiāng xīn tāng

Source *Essentials from the Golden Cabinet* (c. 220)

Poria (*fú líng*) 12g
Glycyrrhizae Radix (*gān cǎo*) 9g
Zingiberis Rhizoma (*gān jiāng*) 9g
Asari Radix et Rhizoma (*xì xīn*) 9g
Schisandrae Fructus (*wǔ wèi zǐ*) 6-12g

Method of Preparation Decoction. At present, the dosages of Asari Radix et Rhizoma (*xì xīn*) and Schisandrae Fructus (*wǔ wèi zǐ*) are frequently reduced by half.

Actions Warms the Lungs and transforms congested fluids

Indications

Coughing with profuse sputum that is thin, watery, and white accompanied by a feeling of discomfort in the chest and diaphragm, a white, slippery tongue coating, and a wiry, slippery pulse.

This is cold, thin mucus due to yang deficiency and ascendant yin. The presence of cold, thin mucus in the upper burner may be due to yang deficiency of the Spleen, which impairs the transporting and transforming functions of the middle burner. This leads to stagnation of fluids that ascend and manifest as thin mucus. It may also be due to external cold penetrating into the Lungs and impeding their ability to disseminate the fluids, which collect and form thin mucus. Cold, thin mucus disrupts the directional mechanisms of the Lung qi, which results in wheezing and coughing with profuse, thin, and watery sputum. The thin mucus and rebellious qi in the Lungs causes a feeling of discomfort in the chest and diaphragm. The tongue coating is white because of the presence of cold, and slippery because of the collection of fluids. The pulse is slippery for the same reason, and wiry because of the stagnant qi.

Analysis of Formula

This formula treats cold, thin mucus by means of the core strategy for treating such patterns set out in *Essentials from the Golden Cabinet*: "For phlegm and thin mucus disorders, one should employ warming herbs to harmonize [the imbalance]." However, it adjusts this strategy to the specific location of the pathogen in the Lungs by attending to that organ's regulation of opening and closing. The chief herb is acrid, warming Zingiberis Rhizoma *(gān jiāng)*, which warms the Lungs, disperses cold, and transforms thin mucus. It also warms the Spleen yang to eliminate dampness. The deputy is acrid and warming Asari Radix et Rhizoma *(xì xīn)*, which focuses on warming and dispersing cold from the Lungs to transform thin mucus. Aromatic and piercing, it successfully opens up the clumped qi, thereby assisting the chief herb in unblocking constraint to facilitate the normal dissemination of Lung qi and the dispelling of pathogenic cold and thin mucus. The assistants are bland and neutral Poria *(fú líng)* and sour and binding Schisandrae Fructus *(wǔ wèi zǐ)*. The former strengthens the Spleen and leaches out dampness and thereby treats the problem at its source; the latter restrains the leakage of Lung qi and prevents its depletion by the dispersing actions of the other herbs. A similar synergism also applies to the combination of Schisandrae Fructus *(wǔ wèi zǐ)* and Zingiberis Rhizoma *(gān jiāng)*. The envoy, Glycyrrhizae Radix *(gān cǎo)*, harmonizes the middle burner and the actions of the other herbs in the formula.

Commentary

In the source text this formula is prescribed for patients suffering from coughing and congestion of the chest who, after taking Minor Bluegreen Dragon Decoction *(xiǎo qīng lóng tāng)*, react with rebellious qi ascending from the lower burner, urinary difficulty, and more severe congestion of fluids in the head, extremities, and upper burner. This is interpreted to mean that they were too deficient to tolerate the strong dispersing action of that formula. To treat this reaction, the source text prescribes Cinnamon Twig, Poria, Schisandra, and Licorice Decoction *(guì líng wǔ wèi gān cǎo tāng)*, discussed below as an associated formula. This should settle the rebellious qi, but without easing the cough and fullness in the chest. It is at this final point in the treatment process that the present formula is indicated. This sequence shows that Poria, Licorice, Schisandra, Ginger, and Asarum Decoction *(líng gān wǔ wèi jiāng xīn tāng)* was designed to treat a pattern characterized by cold from deficiency as the root, with thin mucus as the manifestation. This explains why its composition is both quite similar to, and yet also very distinct from, Minor Bluegreen Dragon Decoction *(xiǎo qīng lóng tāng)*.

Both formulas treat thin mucus in the Lungs. As explained above, warming is the basic strategy for all thin mucus disorders. This is because warming is essential to promote the movement of fluids constrained by cold. However, the dispersing nature of acrid, warming herbs (promoting the Lungs' opening functions) conflicts with the downward directing of qi and fluids (the Lungs' closing functions). For this reason,

Zhang Zhong-Jing frequently combined acrid herbs, whose dispersing properties open the Lungs, with sour astringent herbs, whose restraining qualities preserve the Lung qi. Thus, the dispersing herbs open the Lungs without risk of exhausting its qi, while the astringent ones close the Lungs without risk of mistakenly trapping the pathogenic qi. While Minor Bluegreen Dragon Decoction *(xiǎo qīng lóng tāng)* focuses on the exterior and regulates fluid metabolism by dispersing fluids to the exterior as sweat, this formula focuses on the interior and regulates fluid metabolism by promoting urination.

This formula is most suitable for treating cold obstructing the movement of fluids within the Lungs. It warms the interior to open the obstruction of Lung qi, but also promotes the water metabolism to drain excess fluids via the urine. In such patterns, the patient is usually not thirsty because there is already too much fluids congesting the qi dynamic. However, precisely because of this congestion, the diffusion of physiological fluids is also inhibited, which, under some conditions, can manifest as thirst. This must not be confused with thirst due to yin deficiency, in which case the tongue coating would not be white and slippery. A submerged, weak pulse finally helps to distinguish this as a pattern of deficiency, and to differentiate it from patterns of excess with similar symptoms, for which Ephedrae Herba *(má huáng)*-based formulas are indicated.

Biomedical Indications

With the appropriate presentation, this formula may be used to treat a variety of biomedically-defined disorders including chronic bronchitis, chronic asthma, and chronic obstructive pulmonary disease.

Alternate names

Schisandra and Asarum Decoction *(wǔ wèi xì xīn tāng)* in *Ji-Feng's Formulas of Universal Benefit*; Poria, Licorice, Schisandra, Ginger, and Asarum Decoction *(líng gān wèi jiāng xīn tāng)* in *Prescriptions of Universal Benefit*; Cinnamon, Schisandra, and Licorice minus Cinnamon plus Ginger and Asarum Decoction *(guì zhī wǔ wèi gān cǎo qù guì jiā jiāng xīn tāng)* in *Comprehensive Medicine According to Master Zhang*

Modifications

- For profuse sputum with nausea, add Pinelliae Rhizoma praeparatum *(zhì bàn xià)*.

- For abdominal distention, add Citri reticulatae Pericarpium *(chén pí)* and Aurantii Fructus *(zhǐ ké)*.

- For debilitated patients, add Cordyceps *(dōng chóng xià cǎo)*.

- For severe coughing with facial edema, add Armeniacae Semen *(xìng rén)*.

- For persistent coughing, add Asteris Radix *(zǐ wǎn)* and Farfarae Flos *(kuǎn dōng huā)*.

- For facial flushing due to heat in the yang brightness warp, add Rhei Radix et Rhizoma (*dà huáng*).

Associated Formulas

桂苓五味甘草湯（桂苓五味甘草汤）

Cinnamon Twig, Poria, Schisandra, and Licorice Decoction

guì líng wǔ wèi gān cǎo tāng

SOURCE *Essentials from the Golden Cabinet* (c. 220)

Cinnamomi Ramulus (*guì zhī*) 12g
Poria (*fú líng*) 12g
Schisandrae Fructus (*wǔ wèi zǐ*) 12-15g
Glycyrrhizae Radix (*gān cǎo*) 9g

Preserves the Lungs, transforms congested fluids, and directs the qi downward. For yang deficiency with congested fluids manifested as coughing with profuse, thin, and white sputum, cold hands and feet, palpitations, dizziness, occasional attacks of qi rushing upward from the lower abdomen to the chest, a pale tongue with a white, slippery coating, and a submerged, wiry pulse that is forceless at the proximal position. In contrast to the principal formula, this is intended more for cases with underlying Kidney yang deficiency with coughing in the aftermath of a relatively recent, externally-contracted cold disorder.

苓甘五味加薑辛半夏杏仁湯（苓甘五味加姜辛半夏杏仁汤）

Poria, Licorice, and Schisandra plus Ginger, Asarum, Pinellia, and Apricot Kernel Decoction

líng gān wǔ wèi jiā jiāng xīn bàn xià xìng rén tāng

SOURCE *Essentials from the Golden Cabinet* (c. 220)

Poria (*fú líng*) 6g
Glycyrrhizae Radix (*gān cǎo*) 4.5g
Schisandrae Fructus (*wǔ wèi zǐ*) 4.5g
Zingiberis Rhizoma (*gān jiāng*) 4.5g
Asari Radix et Rhizoma (*xì xīn*) 4.5g
Pinelliae Rhizoma (*bàn xià*) 6g
Armeniacae Semen (*xìng rén*) 6g

Warms the interior, transforms fluids, dissipates qi, and promotes the water metabolism. For obstruction of Lung qi due to cold accompanied by edema in the extremities characterized by shortness of breath, wheezing, coughing of thin, white sputum, aversion to cold, heaviness of the body, edema, increased urination but no thirst, fatigue, a white tongue coating, and a thin, submerged pulse. In contrast to the principal formula, this variation is less astringent due to the lower dosage of Schisandrae Fructus (*wǔ wèi zǐ*), but stronger at directing the Lung qi downward to promote water metabolism. Like the principal formula, it is indicated for patterns of deficiency where the use of Ephedrae Herba (*má huáng*)-based formulas would be inappropriate.

冷哮丸

Cold Asthma Pill

lěng xiào wán

SOURCE *Comprehensive Medicine According to Master Zhang* (1695)

Ephedrae Herba (*má huáng*) 30g
Aconiti Radix (*zhì chuān wū*) 30g
Asari Radix et Rhizoma (*xì xīn*) 30g
Zanthoxyli Pericarpium (*huā jiāo*) 30g
Alumen (*bái fán*) 30g
Gleditsiae Fructus abnormalis (*zhū yá zào*) 30g
Pinelliae Rhizoma (*bàn xià*) 30g
Arisaematis Rhizoma (*tiān nán xīng*) 30g
Armeniacae Semen (*xìng rén*) 30g
Glycyrrhizae Radix (*gān cǎo*) 30g
Asteris Radix (*zǐ wǎn*) 60g
Farfarae Flos (*kuǎn dōng huā*) 60g

Grind the herbs into a fine powder and make into pills with Zingiberis Rhizomatis Succus (*jiāng zhī*) and Massa medicata fermentata (*shén qū*). The normal dose is 3-6g taken with a decoction made from Zingiberis Rhizoma recens (*shēng jiāng*). Vomiting up old phlegm after taking the pills is considered a positive sign. After several days of taking the pills, treatment should be switched to tonifying the Spleen and Lungs.

Disperses cold and flushes out phlegm. For cold contracted via the back manifesting as asthma and coughing, clumping and accumulation of stubborn phlegm, focal distention and fullness of the chest and diaphragm, and inability to breathe when lying down. This formula is very warming and drying and is thus unsuitable for deficient patients.

三子養親湯（三子养亲汤）

Three-Seed Decoction to Nourish One's Parents

sān zǐ yǎng qīn tāng

The three seeds refer to the ingredients of this formula, all of which are small seeds. The seeds are used to treat problems commonly encountered in old age, and thus to 'nourish one's parents.' As explained in *Comprehensive Medicine According to Master Han*: "The three seeds [used in this formula] come from [any] vegetable garden. Their nature is balanced and their fragrance is penetrating. They are excellent condiments for food and drink when taking care of one's parents."

Source *Extensive Essentials of Miscellaneous Diseases* (1856)

Sinapis Semen (*bái jiè zǐ*) 6-9g
Perillae Fructus (*zǐ sū zǐ*) 6-9g
Raphani Semen (*lái fú zǐ*) 6-9g

Method of Preparation Decoction. The seeds are washed, lightly fried, crushed, and then placed in a cheesecloth bag before decocting. The source text specifies a maximum dosage of 9g of the powder, and notes that the relative dosage of the herbs in the formula should be adjusted according to the actual pattern. Care should be used not to decoct the powder for too long. The drink is taken in place of tea.

Actions Directs the qi downward, transforms phlegm, and reduces harbored food

Indications

Coughing and wheezing, copious sputum, focal distention in the chest, loss of appetite, digestive difficulties, a white, greasy tongue coating, and a slippery pulse

This is phlegm clogging the Lungs with qi stagnation. This pattern is caused by harbored food and often occurs in the elderly whose digestive systems are becoming weaker. Harbored food is both a cause and an effect of Spleen deficiency and can lead to qi stagnation and the production of phlegm. Phlegm clogging the Lungs disturbs the Lung qi, which manifests as coughing and wheezing. This disturbance, together with the obstruction caused by phlegm and harbored food, gives rise to focal distention in the chest. The harbored food and deficiency of the Spleen suppresses the appetite and causes digestive difficulties. The white tongue coating reflects the presence of cold, and the greasy tongue coating and slippery pulse are signs of harbored food and phlegm.

Analysis of Formula

Although the symptoms of the pattern treated by this formula are often caused by a weak digestive system, it focuses entirely on the manifestations of wheezing and coughing. For this purpose, it warms and transforms phlegm-cold and moves the qi, following the adage that, in treating phlegm, one must regulate the qi. Sinapis Semen *(bái jiè zǐ)* is intensely acrid and warm, with the distinctive ability to penetrate the yin and restore movement to the yang. It enters and warms the Lungs, regulates the qi, and expels phlegm. Perillae Fructus *(zǐ sū zǐ)* directs the Lung qi downward and thereby stops the coughing and wheezing. Raphani Semen *(lái fú zǐ)* is acrid, sweet, and neutral. It enters the Lung channel to direct the qi downward and transform phlegm, and mobilizes the Spleen channel to promote the flow of Spleen qi and reduce harbored food. Aromatic, warm, acrid, and moistening, Perillae Fructus *(zǐ sū zǐ)* excels at directing rebellious qi downward. This action disperses phlegm and calms wheezing, while moistening and facilitating Intestinal movement. All three herbs are acrid and warming in nature and are thus able to transform phlegm-cold. Because of their close interactions, it serves no purpose to distinguish one from the other as chief, deputy, or assistant.

Commentary

The source text prescribes this formula for elderly patients with much phlegm and qi excess in the upper burner. The underlying pathodynamic was lucidly discussed by Wu Kun in *Investigations of Medical Formulas:*

> This formula governs [patterns characterized by] an overabundance of phlegm and qi excess in the elderly. Phlegm does not move of its own accord, but only if moved by qi. Thus, if qi ascends, phlegm also ascends. If qi descends, phlegm also descends. If qi moves, phlegm also moves. If qi stagnates, phlegm

also stagnates. In this formula, Raphani Semen *(lái fú zǐ)* is able to consume the qi, Perillae Fructus *(zǐ sū zǐ)* is able to direct the qi downward, and Semen Sinapis Albae *(bái jiè zǐ)* is able to promote the qi [dynamic]. If qi is consumed, pathogenic qi cannot be excessive. If qi is directed downward, phlegm cannot rebel upward. If the qi [dynamic] is promoted, [stagnation in] the diaphragm is eased of its own accord. Why would one then still worry about phlegm?

Usage and Adaptation

This condition is often seen in those with long-standing middle burner qi and blood deficiency, a generally more sedentary lifestyle, and often bad dietary habits or overeating. For this reason, the formula is often used for the elderly, but that does not mean that its use should be limited to this group. The formula is useful for treating chronic cough and wheezing in younger patients, too, especially where phlegm is difficult to bring up. Provided it is appropriately combined with heat-clearing or moistening herbs, it can even be used for phlegm that has transformed into heat. It is also suitable for other manifestations of phlegm obstructing the qi dynamic of the upper and middle burners.

Similar formulas can be found in other sources. For example, *Symptom, Cause, Pulse, and Treatment* contains a formula that focuses on treating nausea and bloating due to harbored food, by replacing Perillae Fructus *(zǐ sū zǐ)* with Crataegi Fructus *(shān zhā)*. Similarly, *Achieving Longevity by Guarding the Source* combines this formula with Two-Aged [Herb] Decoction *(èr chén tāng)* to focus even more strongly on transforming phlegm.

While this formula does increase the level of energy by promoting the qi dynamic of the upper and middle burners, it is important to remember that it addresses the branch and not the root of this disorder. The formula is not a tonic and should not be taken long-term. If it is, its mobilizing actions may injure the qi of the middle burner. This was aptly described by the famous Yuan-dynasty physician, Zhu Dan-Xi: "Whenever herbs that promote [flow] are overused in the treatment of phlegm, it may result in Spleen qi deficiency that can readily lead to the generation of phlegm." Contemporary physicians therefore usually add Atractylodis Rhizoma *(cāng zhú)*, Atractylodis macrocephalae Rhizoma *(bái zhú)*, and Glycyrrhizae Radix *(gān cǎo)* for deficiency conditions. Even more appropriate for long-term use in cases of qi deficiency complicated by phlegm is a formula such as Six-Gentlemen Decoction *(liù jūn zǐ tāng)*.

Comparison

➤ Vs. Preserve Harmony Pill *(bǎo hé wán)*; *see* page 828

Biomedical Indications

With the appropriate presentation, this formula may be used to treat a variety of biomedically-defined disorders including

acute and chronic bronchitis, bronchial asthma, emphysema, pediatric asthma, and spasms of the diaphragm.

Alternate name

Three-Seed Decoction (*sān zǐ tāng*) in *Achieving Longevity by Guarding the Source*

Modifications

- For severe cold, increase the dosage of Sinapis Semen (*bái jiè zǐ*).
- For severe coughing and wheezing, increase the dosage of Perillae Fructus (*zǐ sū zǐ*).
- For severe harbored food, increase the dosage of Raphani Semen (*lái fú zǐ*).
- For hard, firm stools, add honey to the strained decoction.
- For copious, watery sputum and nausea and vomiting due to Spleen yang deficiency, add Pinelliae Rhizoma praeparatum (*zhì bàn xià*), Zingiberis Rhizoma (*gān jiāng*), and Amomi Fructus (*shā rén*).
- For severe wheezing with a stifling sensation in the chest and difficulty in expectorating, add Armeniacae Semen (*xìng rén*) and Magnoliae officinalis Cortex (*hòu pò*).
- For concurrent wind-cold, add Peucedani Radix (*qián hú*) and Perillae Folium (*zǐ sū yè*).
- For phlegm-cold, add Cinnamomi Cortex (*ròu guì*) and Aconiti Radix lateralis praeparata (*fù zǐ*).

Associated Formula

痰飲丸 (痰饮丸)

Phlegm and Thin Mucus Pill

tán yǐn wán

Source   *Shaanxi New Medicine* (1972)

Atractylodis Rhizoma (*cāng zhú*) 90g
Atractylodis macrocephalae Rhizoma (*bái zhú*) 90g
Raphani Semen (*lái fú zǐ*) 90g
Cinnamomi Cortex (*ròu guì*) 30g
Zingiberis Rhizoma (*gān jiāng*) 30g
Aconiti Radix lateralis praeparata (*fù zǐ*) 45g
Glycyrrhizae Radix (*gān cǎo*) 45g
Perillae Fructus (*zǐ sū zǐ*) 60g

Grind the herbs into a fine powder and make into pills with water. The normal dosage is 6g taken twice daily. This formula warms the Lungs, disperses cold, regulates the qi, and transforms phlegm. It is indicated for cough due to phlegm-cold with coughing of thin sputum, stertorous breathing, and a white tongue coating. All symptoms are made worse by cold.

This is a modern formula first formulated in the early 1970s for the treatment of chronic bronchitis. It can be viewed as a combination of Aconite Accessory Root Pill to Regulate the Middle (*fù zǐ lǐ zhōng wán*) and Three-Seed Decoction to Nourish One's Parents (*sān zǐ yǎng qīn tāng*), and is used for treating both the root and branch

of phlegm-cold in the Lungs. Clinically, a white tongue coating, copious, thin mucus, and aggravation by cold are key markers for the use of this formula. It may also be used as a decoction, adding other herbs as needed in response to the precise pattern.

Modifications

- For even more pronounced cold signs, add Asari Radix et Rhizoma (*xì xīn*) and Ephedrae Herba (*má huáng*).
- For coughing, add Asteris Radix (*zǐ wǎn*) and Farfarae Flos (*kuǎn dōng huā*).
- For stertorous breathing, add Platycodi Radix (*jié gěng*) and Aurantii Fructus (*zhǐ ké*).

Section 6

FORMULAS THAT TRANSFORM PHLEGM AND EXTINGUISH WIND

The formulas in this section are used for treating disorders due to wind and phlegm. There are two basic types of wind-phlegm disorders: external and internal. The first occurs when externally-contracted wind (usually invading as wind-cold) invades a person who is constitutionally prone to phlegm-dampness. External and internal pathogens combine to constrain the flow of qi in the Lungs. The principal symptoms are chills and fever, indicating constraint of qi in the exterior, and coughing with sputum that may not be easily expectorated, indicating qi constraint from phlegm. The main formula discussed in this section, Stop Coughing Powder (*zhǐ sòu sǎn*), and its variants are used to treat coughing from constraint of Lung qi by wind-cold and phlegm. The principal strategy for treating such disorders is to open the constraint of the Lung qi and transform phlegm. The herbs used are light and moderate in action, as these resonate best with the nature of the Lungs: Asteris Radix (*zǐ wǎn*), Farfarae Flos (*kuǎn dōng huā*), and Cynanchi stauntonii Rhizoma (*bái qián*) are typical examples. These are combined with light and acrid herbs like Schizonepetae Herba (*jīng jiè*) that dispel wind cold from the exterior.

By contrast, internal wind-phlegm disorders occur when a patient with a constitutional tendency toward phlegm suffers internal stirring of Liver wind. The phlegm follows the wind upward and disturbs the head and sensory orifices. Such disorders are quite common and reflect the close physiological relationship between the Spleen and Liver. The Spleen relies on the Liver's ability to dredge and drain in order to facilitate its function of transforming dampness and controlling water. The Liver, on the other hand, relies on the power of the Spleen qi to manage the ascent of qi. If Liver wood overdominates Spleen earth, it disrupts the Spleen's transporting and transforming functions, leading to the formation of phlegm. This was succinctly summarized in *Collection of Medical Writings following the Work of Others*: "When wind is generated, it invariably conjoins with the momentum of wood to overcome earth. [This causes] earth disorders characterized by the accumulation of yin fluids and the generation of phlegm." This leads to such symptoms as dizziness, vertigo, headache, and in more severe cases, to seizures or loss of consciousness. Formulas that treat wind-phlegm thus use herbs that dry dampness and transform phlegm, such as Pinelliae Rhizoma *(bàn xià)*, Arisaematis Rhizoma *(tiān nán xīng)*, or Poria *(fú líng)*, as chief herbs. If there is heat, herbs that clear and transform phlegm-heat, such as Fritillariae Bulbus *(chuān bèi mǔ)* or Arisaema cum Bile *(dǎn nán xīng)*, may be used. These are combined with herbs that extinguish wind and calm the Liver, such as Gastrodiae Rhizoma *(tiān má)*, Scorpio *(quán xiē)*, or Bombyx batryticatus *(jiāng cán)*, as well as with herbs that strengthen the Spleen and leach out dampness, such as Poria *(fú líng)* or Atractylodis macrocephalae Rhizoma *(bái zhú)*. These latter herbs, used generally as deputies or assistants, address the root of wind-phlegm disorders by regulating and harmonizing the relationship between the Liver and Spleen.

半夏白朮天麻湯 (半夏白术天麻汤)

Pinellia, White Atractylodes, and Gastrodia Decoction

bàn xià bái zhú tiān má tāng

Source   *Awakening of the Mind in Medical Studies* (1732)

Pinelliae Rhizoma praeparatum *(zhì bàn xià)* 4.5g
Gastrodiae Rhizoma *(tiān má)* 3g
Atractylodis macrocephalae Rhizoma *(bái zhú)* 9g
Citri reticulatae Exocarpium rubrum *(jú hóng)* 3g
Poria *(fú líng)* 3g
Glycyrrhizae Radix *(gān cǎo)* 1.5g
Zingiberis Rhizoma recens *(shēng jiāng)* . . . . 1 slice
Jujubae Fructus *(dà zǎo)* . . . . 2 pieces

Method of Preparation   Decoction. At present, the dosage of every ingredient except Atractylodis macrocephalae Rhizoma *(bái zhú)* is usually doubled.

Actions   Strengthens the Spleen, dispels dampness, transforms phlegm, and extinguishes wind

Indications

Dizziness or vertigo (possibly severe), headache, a stifling sensation in the chest, nausea or vomiting, copious sputum, a white, greasy tongue coating, and a wiry, slippery pulse.

This is wind-phlegm, also known as an upward disturbance of wind-phlegm. This condition develops more readily in those who overwork, overindulge in rich foods, or otherwise lead an irregular lifestyle. These activities injure the Spleen and Stomach and impair their functions of transforming food, which in turn leads to an accumulation of dampness that often transforms into phlegm. Because the clear yang in such patients is weak, it is relatively easy for the phlegm to obstruct its rise. When Spleen earth is deficient, Liver wood becomes dominant. Its qi ascends as wind, carrying the turbid phlegm along the course of the lesser yang Gallbladder and Triple Burner channels to the head. Veiling the clear yang and disturbing the sensory orifices, it manifests as dizziness, vertigo, or headache. A distinctive feature of these head symptoms is that the head feels heavy and clouded. The stifling sensation in the chest and the nausea or vomiting are manifestations of phlegm obstructing the mechanisms of qi in the chest and epigastrium. (The latter symptom is also a sign of rebelliously ascending qi.) The copious sputum, white, greasy tongue coating, and wiry, slippery pulse all reflect the presence of phlegm, wind, and stagnation.

Analysis of Formula

To treat wind-phlegm this formula employs a strategy of strengthening the Spleen and drying dampness to treat the root, and of transforming phlegm and extinguishing wind to treat the branch. The two chief herbs are acrid and warming Pinelliae Rhizoma praeparatum *(zhì bàn xià)*, which dries dampness, transforms phlegm, and directs rebellious qi downward, to treat the nausea and vomiting, and sweet, neutral, moist, and slightly tonifying Gastrodiae Rhizoma *(tiān má)*, which enters the Liver channel to nourish the yin fluids, calm the Liver, and extinguish wind. Together, these herbs constitute an ideal combination for treating the problem at hand. While Pinelliae Rhizoma praeparatum *(zhì bàn xià)* is able to direct the turbid yin downward and thereby control rebellious qi, its acrid nature could easily stir up even more wind. This is compensated for by the moistening character of Gastrodiae Rhizoma *(tiān má)*, which extinguishes wind but on its own would be insufficiently strong to settle the Spleen and Stomach. Thus, as the 13th-century physician Li Dong-Yuan observed in *Discussion of the Spleen and Stomach*: "Headache due to phlegm rebelling in the leg greater yin [channel and organ] cannot be treated without Pinelliae Rhizoma praeparatum *(zhì bàn xià)*; spots before the eyes and vertigo are due to internal movement of wind from deficiency and cannot be eliminated without Gastrodiae Rhizoma *(tiān má)*."

The deputy, Atractylodis macrocephalae Rhizoma *(bái zhú)*, reinforces the actions of the main ingredients in treating phlegm. Its sweet warmth tonifies the Spleen earth, its bitterness dries dampness, and its aromatic quality supports the transportive and transformative functions of the Spleen. It promotes water metabolism, yet also generates fluids and thereby addresses the fluid disharmony that is at the heart of this disorder. One of the assistants, Poria *(fú líng)*, strengthens the Spleen and leaches out dampness. Together with the deputy, this gives the formula the capability of simultaneously treating the branch and the root. The other assistant is Citri reticulatae Pericarpium *(chén pí)*, which regulates the qi by directing excessive qi downward, transforming and eliminating phlegm. The envoys are Glycyrrhizae Radix *(gān cǎo)*, which harmonizes the actions of the other herbs and mildly regulates the functions of the middle burner, and the combination of Zingiberis Rhizoma recens *(shēng jiāng)* and Jujubae Fructus *(dà zǎo)*, which is added to the decoction to harmonize the Stomach and Spleen.

Cautions and Contraindications

Contraindicated for vertigo from either ascendant Liver yang or blood deficiency.

Commentary

This is another variation of Two-Aged [Herb] Decoction *(èr chén tāng)*. It was composed by the 18th-century Qing-dynasty physician Cheng Guo-Peng, drawing on an earlier formula by the same name in *Discussion of the Spleen and Stomach*. The source text outlines its indications in the context of a more general discussion of the pathophysiology of dizziness:

> Vertigo refers to darkening of the vision with dizziness [or a sensation as if] the head was spinning around. The ancients called this spinning of the head with spots before the eyes. Among [the patterns in which this disorder can be found] is internal movement of Liver fire. [This pattern is referred to] in the *Inner Classic* when it states: All wind [disorders], [sudden] falling down, and dizziness belong to Liver wood. It is governed by Rambling Powder *(xiāo yáo sǎn)*. [Another pattern] is dampness and phlegm clogging [the sensory orifices] and trapping [the qi dynamic. This pattern is referred to in medical] texts when they state that spinning of the head with spots before the eyes cannot be eliminated without [the combination of] Pinelliae Rhizoma *(bàn xià)* and Gastrodiae Rhizoma *(tiān má)*. It is governed by Pinellia, White Atractylodes, and Gastrodia Decoction *(bàn xià bái zhú tiān má tāng)*. [Yet another pattern] is qi deficiency complicated by phlegm. [This pattern is referred to in medical] texts as the clear yang not ascending and the turbid yin not descending, leading to [a sensation of] heaviness above/in the head and weakness/lightness below/in the legs. It is governed by Six-Gentlemen Decoction *(liù jūn zǐ tāng)*. [Furthermore, there is the pattern] of insufficient Kidney water with flaring of empty fire, which is governed by Six-Ingredient Pill with Rehmannia *(liù wèi dì huáng wán)*. [Finally, there is the pattern] of sapped fire at the gate of vitality with true yang floating upward, which is governed by Kidney Qi Pill *(shèn qì wán)*.

The source text contains another formula by the same name. It is composed of the same ingredients with slightly different dosages for some—Atractylodis macrocephalae Rhi-zoma *(bái zhú)* 6g only, and Jujubae Fructus *(dà zǎo)* 1 piece only—plus the addition of 9g of Viticis Fructus *(màn jīng zǐ)*. This formula is weaker in terms of its ability to strengthen the Spleen, but focuses more strongly on clearing obstruction from the head and eyes, and is indicated for phlegm inversion headaches.

Biomedical Indications

With the appropriate presentation, this formula may be used to treat a variety of biomedically-defined disorders including Ménière's disease, hypertension, tubercular meningitis, and benign positional vertigo.

Modifications

- For severe headache, add Viticis Fructus *(màn jīng zǐ)*.
- For severe vertigo, add Bombyx batryticatus *(bái jiāng cán)* and Arisaema cum Bile *(dǎn nán xīng)*.
- For ascendant Liver yang, add Uncariae Ramulus cum Uncis *(gōu téng)* and Haematitum *(dài zhě shí)*.
- For more pronounced phlegm-dampness, add Alismatis Rhizoma *(zé xiè)* and Cinnamomi Ramulus *(guì zhī)*.
- For weakness, add Codonopsis Radix *(dǎng shēn)* and Astragali Radix *(huáng qí)*.
- For tubercular meningitis, add Scorpio *(quán xiē)*, Pheretima *(dì lóng)*, and Bombyx batryticatus *(bái jiāng cán)*. To be successful, the formula must be taken long-term, and for no less than 3 months.

Associated Formulas

半夏白朮天麻湯 (半夏白术天麻汤)

Pinellia, White Atractylodes, and Gastrodia Decoction from *Discussion of the Spleen and Stomach*

bàn xià bái zhú tiān má tāng

SOURCE *Discussion of the Spleen and Stomach* (13th century)

Phellodendri Cortex *(huáng bǎi)* 1g
Zingiberis Rhizoma *(gān jiāng)* 1g
Gastrodiae Rhizoma *(tiān má)* 2.5g
Atractylodis Rhizoma *(cāng zhú)* 2.5g
Poria *(fú líng)* 2.5g
Astragali Radix *(huáng qí)* 2.5g
Alismatis Rhizoma *(zé xiè)* 2.5g
Ginseng Radix *(rén shēn)* 2.5g
Atractylodis macrocephalae Rhizoma *(bái zhú)* 5g
Massa medicata fermentata *(shén qū)* 5g
Pinelliae Rhizoma *(bàn xià)* 7.5g
Hordei Fructus germinatus *(mài yá)* 7.5g
Citri reticulatae Pericarpium *(chén pí)* 7.5g

Grind the herbs into a coarse powder and prepare 25g as a draft by boiling in a cup of water. Take warm before meals. Transforms phlegm, extinguishes wind, augments the qi, and benefits the Stomach. For phlegm inversion headaches or upward disturbance of wind-phlegm characterized by distending and stifling headache, vertigo and spots before the eyes, mild nausea, irritability, a stifling sensation in the chest, reluctance to speak, coldness of the extremities, inability to lie down, a pale tongue with a white, greasy coating, and a wiry pulse.

This formula reflects Li Dong-Yuan's emphasis on tonifying the Spleen and Stomach yang in order to promote the qi dynamic, as well as his concern for yin fire and damp-heat as secondary pathologies arising from qi constraint. Compared to the principal formula, this one thus focuses more strongly on tonifying the qi in order to facilitate ascent of the clear yang as well as draining damp-heat and reducing stagnation as a means of directing turbid phlegm downward. It is particularly indicated for mixed patterns of deficiency and excess characterized by such symptoms as an apparently strong build in a person who is easily fatigued, fluctuating blood pressure (sometimes high, sometimes low), constant headache but being tired, feeling cold but also suffering from hot flushes, etc. This is the version of the formula used by most contemporary practitioners in Japan, where it is believed that it should be used for several months in order to be effective.

鉤藤散 （钩藤散）

Uncaria Powder

gōu téng sǎn

SOURCE　*Formulas of Universal Benefit from My Practice* (1132)

Gypsum fibrosum (*shí gāo*) 5-7g
Uncariae Ramulus cum Uncis (*gōu téng*) 3g
Citri reticulatae Pericarpium (*chén pí*) 3g
Pinelliae Rhizoma (*bàn xià*) 3g
Ophiopogonis Radix (*mài mén dōng*) 3g
Poria (*fú líng*) 3g
Ginseng Radix (*rén shēn*) 2g
Saposhnikoviae Radix (*fáng fēng*) 2g
Chrysanthemi Flos (*jú huā*) 2g
Glycyrrhizae Radix (*gān cǎo*) 1g
Zingiberis Rhizoma recens (*shēng jiāng*) 1g

Decoction. Extinguishes wind, transforms phlegm, strengthens the Spleen, and enriches the fluids. For wind-phlegm against a background of qi and yin deficiency characterized by headaches (often starting in the morning and persisting throughout the day), dizziness, hot flushes, a tongue with red edges and a greasy coating, and a soft but wiry and perhaps rapid pulse. Other symptoms include tinnitus, insomnia, muscle tension in the neck and shoulders, lack of appetite, abdominal bloating, and bloodshot eyes. This formula is used in modern Japanese Kampo to treat raised blood pressure and dizziness, particularly in older patients with arteriosclerosis. The dosages listed here are those used in Japan.

Historically, this formula can be viewed as a combination of Lophatherum and Gypsum Decoction (*zhú yè shí gāo tāng*) and Two-Aged [Herb] Decoction (*èr chén tāng*), plus herbs to extinguish and disperse wind. Compared to the principal formula, it focuses more strongly on clearing heat, extinguishing wind, and enriching the fluids, rather than on transforming phlegm and draining dampness. It is a useful formula for conditions where wind-phlegm combines with yin and qi deficiency.

定癇丸 （定痫丸）

Arrest Seizures Pill

dìng xián wán

Source　*Awakening of the Mind in Medical Studies* (1732)

Gastrodiae Rhizoma (*tiān má*) 30g
Fritillariae cirrhosae Bulbus (*chuān bèi mǔ*) 30g
Pinelliae Rhizoma praeparatum (*zhì bàn xià*) 30g
Poria (*fú líng*) 30g
Poriae Sclerotium pararadicis (*fú shén*) 30g
Arisaema cum Bile (*dǎn nán xīng*) 15g
Acori tatarinowii Rhizoma (*shí chāng pǔ*) 15g
Scorpio (*quán xiē*) 15g
Bombyx batryticatus (*bái jiāng cán*) 15g
Succinum (*hǔ pò*) 15g
Junci Medulla (*dēng xīn cǎo*) 15g
Citri reticulatae Pericarpium (*chén pí*) 21g
Polygalae Radix (*yuǎn zhì*) 21g
Salviae miltiorrhizae Radix (*dān shēn*) 60g
Ophiopogonis Radix (*mài mén dōng*) 60g
Cinnabaris (*zhū shā*) . . . . [refine with water] 9g

Method of Preparation　Grind the ingredients into a powder and form into pills by decocting with 120g of Glycyrrhizae Radix (*gān cǎo*), one small bowl (100ml) of Bambusae Succus (*zhú lì*), and a glass (50ml) of ginger juice. The normal dose is 6g taken with warm water, morning and night. Note that due to the unacceptable toxicity of Cinnabaris (*zhū shā*), it should no longer be used.

Actions　Scours out phlegm, opens the sensory orifices, clears heat, and extinguishes wind

Indications

Sudden loss or clouding of consciousness together with falling down, upward-rolling of the eyes, deviation of the mouth, spitting up of mucus with a loud, raspy sound, and in severe cases, tonic-clonic convulsions, sudden shrieking, or incontinence of stool or urine. The tongue coating is white and greasy, and the pulse is usually wiry and slippery. These attacks may or may not be preceded by prodromal signs such as recurrent vertigo, weakness, and a stifling sensation in the chest.

This condition is known as seizure disorder (癇證 *xián zhèng*) and arises from a combination of wind and phlegm. More common in children, it is attributed to emotional factors, improper eating habits, irregular lifestyle, overwork, trauma, or one's inherited constitution. These factors may cause phlegm to accumulate, which may lead to the prodromal signs. Phlegm clogging the qi dynamic leads to qi constraint that is invariably accompanied by fire. If such constraint reaches a 'critical mass,' it discharges upward in the form of wind that carries the phlegm with it and obstructs the channels and sensory orifices. This results in a sudden disruption of consciousness with accompanying symptoms of wind (vertigo, tonic-clonic seizures) and phlegm (loud, raspy sounds due to mucus in the throat). The tongue coating reflects the presence of phlegm, as does the slippery pulse. The wiry aspect of the pulse is a sign of Liver wind.

Analysis of Formula

This formula treats the acute phase of a seizure disorder when wind-phlegm is obstructing the channels and sensory orifices. To treat this obstruction, it combines a strategy of scouring out phlegm and opening the sensory orifices with clearing heat and extinguishing wind. The chief herb is Bambusae Succus (zhú lì). Sweet and very cooling, with an especially slippery nature, according to *Extension of the Materia Medica,* it is able to "mobilize the orifices to dredge out phlegm and restore open communication between the inside and the outside." Bitter and cooling Arisaema cum Bile (dǎn nán xīng) serves as deputy to clear fire and transform phlegm, settle fright, stop seizures, and amplify the ability of the chief herb to open the orifices by scouring out phlegm.

Most of the other herbs are regarded as assistants. Cooling and bitter Fritillariae cirrhosae Bulbus (chuān bèi mǔ) causes the qi to descend, transforms phlegm-heat, and possesses a moistening action that prevents the dry properties of the other herbs in the formula from injuring the yin. Acrid and warming Pinelliae Rhizoma praeparatum (zhì bàn xià) dries dampness, transforms, and directs rebellious qi downward. According to *Essentials of the Materia Medica,* together with Zingiberis Rhizomatis Succus (jiāng zhī), it "unblocks the clarity of the spirit and expels the foul noxious [qi]" and thereby addresses the root cause of this disorder. Bambusae Succus (zhú lì) also benefits from the mobilizing action of ginger juice, without which it cannot mobilize the channels and collaterals. Ginger juice also protects the Stomach and itself excels at scouring phlegm and unblocking the orifices. Acrid, bitter, and warming Citri reticulatae Pericarpium (chén pí) dries dampness, directs the qi downward, and excels at opening its stagnation. Bland, sweet, and neutral Poria (fú líng) dries dampness by promoting water metabolism and strengthens the Spleen, which is regarded as the source of phlegm. Together, these herbs comprise Two-Aged [Herb] Decoction (èr chén tāng), and as such have the function of supporting the chief and deputy herbs through their ability of transforming phlegm.

A second group of assistants addresses wind. Sweet and neutral Gastrodiae Rhizoma (tiān má) extinguishes Liver wind and also slightly moistens. Salty, acrid, neutral, and toxic Scorpio (quán xiē) enters the Liver channel to strongly extinguish internal wind, halt spasms, and unblock the collaterals. Acrid, salty, and neutral Bombyx batryticatus (bái jiāng

cán) disperses, softens areas of hardness, transforms phlegm, and dries dampness. Moreover, several writers, among them Zhang Shan-Lei, say that it "clears, clarifies, and directs fire downward."

A third group of assistants addresses the Heart, which governs the clarity of the spirit that is affected when the sensory orifices become obstructed by phlegm. Sweet and slightly bitter Ophiopogonis Radix (mài mén dōng), bitter and slightly cooling Salviae miltiorrhizae Radix (dān shēn), and sweet and bland Poriae Sclerotium pararadicis (fú shén) clear heat from the Heart, while sweet and neutral Succinum (hǔ pò) and sweet and cooling Cinnabaris (zhū shā) sedate the Heart. Together, these five ingredients are very effective in calming the spirit. Salviae miltiorrhizae Radix (dān shēn) also has the effect of unbinding the constrained qi in the chest, which is helpful in resolving the accumulation of phlegm. Aromatic, acrid, bitter, and warming Acori tatarinowii Rhizoma (shí chāng pú) transforms phlegm and turbid dampness and harmonizes the Stomach. Together with acrid, bitter, and slightly warming Polygalae Radix (yuǎn zhì), which facilitates the flow of Heart qi and expels phlegm, it transforms turbid phlegm and opens the sensory orifices. Glycyrrhizae Radix (gān cǎo) harmonizes the disparate actions of the other herbs and helps meld them into a balanced formula for scouring out phlegm and extinguishing wind.

Cautions and Contraindications

This formula has no significant heat-clearing or tonifying properties and should therefore not be used without modification for seizures associated with Liver fire with phlegm-heat, Liver and Kidney yin deficiency, or Spleen and Stomach deficiency.

Effective treatment of seizures may require long-term use of formulas such as this one. However, because the formula is draining, its use should be alternated with tonifying formulas like Placenta Pill (hé chē wán), analyzed in the COMMENTARY below. If the normal qi is deficient, the source text also advises to add 9g of Ginseng Radix (rén shēn) to the formula.

Commentary

Seizure disorders can be mild or severe, of acute onset or of long duration. They are usually rather mild in the beginning, but after many recurrences, the normal qi steadily weakens while the accumulation of phlegm grows steadily larger. This leads to more frequent and severe attacks. During the period of frequent attacks, it is important to focus on the manifestations by scouring out the phlegm and extinguishing the wind. That is what this formula seeks to accomplish. Once the frequency of seizures has noticeably declined, the source text recommends to switch to Placenta Pill (hé chē wán), which tonifies the essence as well as transforms phlegm in order to address the cause of the disorder.*

Various other techniques, too, may be utilized to treat the root of the disorder. These include correcting the diet, calming the mind, and the use of herbal formulas to strengthen the Spleen, nourish the Heart, or tonify the Liver and Kidneys. The formula can also be used for insanity (癲狂 *diān kuáng*, also translated as withdrawal-mania) provided this is due to the same pathodynamic.

While the formula is well-balanced between hot and cold substances, some consider it more appropriate for patterns that are slightly more hot in nature. Although the formula employs acrid, warming substances to scour out phlegm and regulate the qi, the balance of ingredients leans toward cooling and heat-clearing substances. This is because the underlying pathodynamic invariably involves constraint of Liver yang or ministerial fire. This dynamic is explained in *Comprehensive Outline of Medicine*:

> Mania and seizures [are due to] phlegm pathologically rebelling upward. When pathological qi rebels upward, the qi in the head becomes chaotic. When the qi in the head has become chaotic, the channel pathways close [because they become] clogged. The sensory orifices [thereupon] become blocked. Hence, the ear no longer hears sounds. The eyes do not recognize people, one becomes muddled, dizzy, loses consciousness, and falls to the ground.

The qi that rebels upward here is the clear yang, whose ascent is managed and controlled by the Liver. By nature, this qi is hot and wild. When constrained, it readily becomes rebellious, ascends uncontrollably, and transforms into wind. This requires clearing of fire and extinguishing of wind. This analysis also concurs with the discussion of seizures in the source text. Cheng Guo-Peng dismissed attempts by previous writers to categorize seizures into organ types according to the nature of the sound emitted by the patient (e.g., a barking sound would indicate a Lung pathology because the dog was classified as corresponding to metal). Instead, Cheng argued that all seizures were caused by the same pathological process and therefore amenable to treatment by the same formula.

Biomedical Indications

With the appropriate presentation, this formula may be used to treat a variety of biomedically-defined disorders including epilepsy and multi-infarct dementia.

Modification

- For weak patients, add Ginseng Radix (*rén shēn*). (source text)

---

* Placenta Pill (紫河車丸 *hé chē wán*): Hominis Placenta (*zǐ hé chē*) 1 entire placenta, Poriae Sclerotium pararadicis (*fú shén*) 30g, Poria (*fú líng*) 30g, Polygalae Radix (*yuǎn zhì*) 30g, Ginseng Radix (*rén shēn*) 15g, and Salviae miltiorrhizae Radix (*dān shēn*) 21g. The ingredients are ground into a fine powder and made into pills with honey. The normal dose is 9g taken every morning with some water.

止嗽散

Stop Coughing Powder

zhǐ sòu sǎn

Source   *Awakening of the Mind in Medical Studies* (1732)

Platycodi Radix (*jié gěng*) 960g
Schizonepetae Herba (*jīng jiè*) 960g
Asteris Radix (*zǐ wǎn*) 960g
Stemonae Radix (*bǎi bù*) 960g
Cynanchi stauntonii Rhizoma (*bái qián*) 960g
Glycyrrhizae Radix (*gān cǎo*) 360g
Citri reticulatae Pericarpium (*chén pí*) 480g

Method of Preparation   Grind the ingredients into a powder and take 9g after meals and before bedtime with warm water. May also be prepared as a decoction with a proportionate reduction in dosage.

Actions   Stops coughing, transforms phlegm, disperses the exterior, and disseminates the Lung qi

Indications

Coughing with or without slight chills and fever, an itchy throat, phlegm that is difficult to expectorate, a thin, white tongue coating, and a moderate, floating pulse.

This formula treats the cough that occurs as the sequela to externally-contracted wind-cold. The pathogen has largely been dispelled from the exterior but the cough persists. The fact that the exterior has not yet been completely resolved is reflected in the itchy throat and the slight chills and fever. The main pathodynamic, however, is now located in the Lungs, whose qi has become constrained by the inward penetration of the wind-cold pathogen. This is reflected in the coughing, which can be interpreted as an effort by the body to unblock the qi constraint. Constraint of Lung qi inhibits the physiological spreading out of the body fluids, which then congeal to become phlegm that is difficult to expectorate. The thin, white tongue coating and the moderate, floating pulse indicate that the pathogenic influence has not penetrated deeply.

Analysis of Formula

To treat coughing due to Lung qi constraint when the exterior has yet to be entirely resolved requires a strategy of transforming the phlegm and disseminating the Lungs assisted by mild dispersion of the exterior. The chief herbs, Asteris Radix (*zǐ wǎn*) and Stemonae Radix (*bǎi bù*), are both bitter substances said to be warming without causing heat as well as moistening without being cold, and are therefore effective in stopping coughs and transforming phlegm in both acute and chronic disorders. The deputies, Cynanchi stauntonii Rhizoma (*bái qián*) and Platycodi Radix (*jié gěng*), focus on opening constraint of Lung qi, the former by directing its qi downward, the latter by facilitating its dissemination. In attending to the cause of the cough, these herbs effectively support the action of the chief ingredients. One of the assistants, Citri reticulatae Pericarpium (chén pí), regulates the qi to transform phlegm, while the other, Schizonepetae Herba (jīng jiè), gives the formula a slight, exterior-releasing action that helps eliminate the lingering pathogenic influence. The envoy, Glycyrrhizae Radix (gān cǎo), harmonizes the actions of the other herbs, and together with Schizonepetae Herba (jīng jiè) and Platycodi Radix (jié gěng), is very effective in treating throat disorders due to externally-contracted wind.

Cautions and Contraindications

This formula has a tendency to dry and should therefore not be used in treating coughs associated with yin deficiency. It was designed for treating wind-cold and should not be used, without modification, in treating coughs due to heat in the Lungs.

Commentary

This is an effective, well-balanced formula for treating the very common problem of lingering cough due to an externally-contracted disorder. With modification, it can be used in treating the sequelae of a wide variety of disorders, as shown below. Its author, the early 18th-century physician Cheng Guo-Peng, explained:

> In composing this formula, I selected common herbs [none of which has any particularly strong actions]. Nevertheless, when administered [for the pattern that they treat] these seven herbs are extremely effective.
>
> One might ask: How can it be that these light and mild herbs can be so comprehensively effective? To this I respond that I came to this formula only after great care and deliberation. Based on its essence, the Lungs pertain to metal and fear fire, so that too much heat causes coughing. Because of their nature, the Lungs are dry and averse to cold, so that too much cold also causes coughing. As the Lungs are the tender organ, they cannot withstand the effects of attacking prescriptions. Furthermore, as they govern the skin and body hair, they most easily contract pathogens. If one does not disperse the exterior, pathogenic qi remains without being released.
>
> The Classic states that slight shivers and slight coughing indicate contraction of cold. Like a petty thief, one need only open the door, push it out, and it will be gone. Physicians who do not understand this mistakenly use clearing, cooling, sour, and astringent prescriptions. Inevitably, they shut the door and trap the thief. The thief who wants to get out now cannot do so through the door, and so must break out to escape. This [is the cause of] cough and a flushed complexion. The Lungs have two openings. The first is the nose, the second the throat. The nose is valued for being open and not closed. The throat [instead] should stay closed rather than open. Now the nasal orifices are blocked so the orifice of the throat will be forced open. Can one ignore this? This formula warms and moistens in a balanced manner, being neither too warming nor too cooling, thus one need not worry about it being too attacking [in nature], yet it

> definitely has the force to open the door and expel the thief. Thereby, the pathogen lodging [in the Lungs] is easily dispersed and the Lung qi calmed. How can using it not be effective?

Strictly speaking, therefore, this formula is not directed primarily at transforming phlegm, but at unblocking qi constraint in the Lungs. This is most directly apparent in its use of Schizonepetae Herba (jīng jiè), which facilitates "opening the door" in order to eliminate the pathogenic wind-cold that is at the root of the problem. If, nevertheless, the formula is widely perceived to be one that transforms wind-phlegm, this is because the symptoms of phlegm clogging the Lungs are those that are most immediately apparent. Clinically, the formula is used by some physicians to treat patterns where no exterior pathogen remains at all, but the symptoms of phlegm-dampness clogging the interior are more pronounced. In that case, Schizonepetae Herba (jīng jiè) is replaced with herbs such as Armeniacae Semen (xìng rén), Inulae Flos (xuán fù huā), or Perillae Fructus (zǐ sū zǐ).

Comparisons

➢ Vs. Apricot Kernel and Perilla Leaf Powder (xìng sū sǎn)

Both formulas treat coughing due to an externally-contracted pathogen and combine herbs that resolve the exterior with those that transform phlegm and regulate the qi. The difference is that Apricot Kernel and Perilla Leaf Powder (xìng sū sǎn) focuses on externally-contracted cold-dryness in the exterior, while Stop Coughing Powder (zhǐ sòu sǎn) focuses on wind-cold constraining the Lung qi. The cold in the first pattern tends to be more severe, and the pathogen is still predominantly in the exterior. For this reason, Apricot Kernel and Perilla Leaf Powder (xìng sū sǎn) combines the more acrid and warming Perillae Folium (zǐ sū yè) with Two-Aged [Herb] Decoction (èr chén tāng), a drying and qi-regulating formula that powerfully transforms phlegm. Stop Coughing Powder (zhǐ sòu sǎn), on the other hand, is composed of lighter and less acrid herbs that are neither excessively warming nor cooling in order to gently promote the movement of qi in the Lungs and dispel wind from the exterior. For this reason, it is more suitable for patterns of wind-cold, where coughing rather than chills and fever is the main symptom.

➢ Vs. Inula Powder (jīn fèi cǎo sǎn); see page 33

Biomedical Indications

With the appropriate presentation, this formula may be used to treat a variety of biomedically-defined disorders including upper respiratory tract infection, acute bronchitis, chronic bronchitis, pertussis, and the early stages of viral and mycoplasmic pneumonia.

Modifications

* For early stages of wind-cold, take with a decoction of Zingiberis Rhizoma recens (shēng jiāng). (source text)

* For headache, stuffy nose, chills, and fever due to wind-cold, add Saposhnikoviae Radix (fáng fēng), Perillae Folium (zǐ sū yè), and Zingiberis Rhizoma recens (shēng jiāng).

* For thirst, irritability, and dark urine due to summerheat attacking the Lungs, add Coptidis Rhizoma (huáng lián), Scutellariae Radix (huáng qín), and Trichosanthis Radix (tiān huā fěn).

* For thick, sticky sputum from dampness transforming into phlegm, add Pinelliae Rhizoma praeparatum (zhì bàn xià), Poria (fú líng), Mori Cortex (sāng bái pí), Zingiberis Rhizoma recens (shēng jiāng), and Jujubae Fructus (dà zǎo).

* For a dry, nonproductive cough, remove Schizonepetae Herba (jīng jiè) and Citri reticulatae Pericarpium (chén pí) and add Trichosanthis Fructus (guā lóu), Fritillariae Bulbus (bèi mǔ), Anemarrhenae Rhizoma (zhī mǔ), and Platycladi Semen (bǎi zǐ rén).

* For sore throat, painful eyes, and more severe fever than chills due to wind-heat, add Chrysanthemi Flos (jú huā), Mori Folium (sāng yè), Menthae haplocalycis Herba (bò hé), Scutellariae Radix (huáng qín), and Arctii Fructus (niú bàng zǐ).

* For copious sputum, reduced appetite, a stifling sensation in the chest, and a white, greasy tongue coating, take with Two-Aged [Herb] Decoction (èr chén tāng).

Associated Formula

降氣化痰湯 （降气化痰汤）

Direct Qi Downward and Transform Phlegm Decoction

jiàng qì huà tán tāng

SOURCE *Systematic Instructions on Medicine* (1534)

Perillae Fructus (zǐ sū zǐ) 4.5g
Peucedani Radix (qián hú) 3g
Pinelliae Rhizoma (bàn xià) 3g
Poria (fú líng) 3g
Citri reticulatae Pericarpium (chén pí) 3g
Mori Cortex (sāng bái pí) 3g
Armeniacae Semen (xìng rén) 3g
Platycodi Radix (jié gěng) 3g
Glycyrrhizae Radix (gān cǎo) .1.5g

Prepare as a decoction by boiling with Zingiberis Rhizoma recens (shēng jiāng). Directs the qi downward to promote the clarifying functions of the Lungs and transforms phlegm to stop the coughing. For wheezing due to phlegm, and wheezing accompanied by audible phlegm obstructing the airways. Although this is a Ming-dynasty formula, its use has become popular only in contemporary practice. Compared to the principal formula, this one focuses more on smoothing the flow of the qi and directing the Lung qi downward, rather than on resolving the exterior.

Section 7

FORMULAS THAT INDUCE VOMITING

Induction of vomiting is one of the earliest strategies used in Chinese medicine, and the vomiting method (吐法 tù fǎ) is one of the eight basic methods of treatment. It is also alluded to in the *Inner Classic*, where, in Chapter 74 of *Basic Questions*, it is observed: "When it is at the upper [levels], lead it up and out." While it had a prominent place in Chinese herbal medicine in the past, its use is less widespread today. In part, this is due to lack of patient acceptance, and in part to having been supplanted by biomedical approaches in many situations. Traditionally, it was used for a variety of problems, including harbored food stagnation and ingestion of poisons, but because it is primarily thought to treat phlegm, we have placed the one formula that induces vomiting in this chapter. Note that there are other substances that are used by themselves to induce vomiting, the most important of which is the 'neck' of the ginseng plant, Ginseng Rhizoma (rén shēn lú).

Formulas that induce vomiting have significant side effects and should always be used with caution and stopped immediately when their effect is achieved. Relative contraindications include pregnancy, debility, and very young age. Dosage should be tightly controlled and, whenever possible, slowly built up. If the formula does not have its desired effect, mechanical means (such as tickling the throat with a feather) or the administration of extra warm water can be used. If the effect is too strong, substances should be administered to reduce vomiting, such as a small amount of ginger juice, congee, or cold water.

瓜蒂散

Melon Pedicle Powder

guā dì sǎn

Source *Discussion of Cold Damage* (c. 220)

Melo Pedicellus (guā dì)
Phaseoli Semen (chì xiǎo dòu)

Method of Preparation Grind equal amounts of the herbs into a paste and take 1-3g at a time with a warm decoction made from 9g of Sojae Semen praeparatum (dàn dòu chǐ). If vomiting does not ensue, slightly increase the dosage. If it still doesn't work, tickle the throat with a feather or cotton swab.

Actions Discharges phlegm or food stagnation through vomiting

Indications

Firm areas of focal distention in the chest, anguish and vexation (懊憹 ào náo), difficult breathing due to a sensation of qi rushing into the throat, and a slightly floating pulse at the distal position.

This condition is due to either phlegm clogging the chest and diaphragm, or stagnant food lodging in the upper epigastrium. Either factor may severely obstruct the flow of qi through this region and cause firm areas of focal distention in the chest, vexation, and difficult breathing due to a sensation of qi rushing into the throat. The upward-rushing of qi is also reflected in the slightly floating quality of the distal pulse.

Analysis of Formula

This type of obstruction in the chest cannot be treated with either diaphoretics or purgatives, but is only resolved through vomiting. Melo Pedicellus *(guā dì)* is a bitter substance that effectively induces vomiting to eliminate the phlegm or stagnant food. Phaseoli Semen *(chì xiǎo dòu),* another bitter substance, expels dampness and eliminates the irritability and fullness. Together, these herbs discharge the obstruction from the body through vomiting. The formula is often taken with a decoction of Sojae Semen praeparatum *(dàn dòu chǐ)*. This herb has a light, clear nature that unbinds the constraint in the chest and helps resolve problems in that area. Together with Phaseoli Semen *(chì xiǎo dòu),* it harmonizes the Stomach qi and helps ameliorate the injury to the normal qi caused by vomiting.

Cautions and Contraindications

Because Melo Pedicellus *(guā dì)* is a cold, bitter, and toxic substance that readily injures the Stomach qi and normal qi, this formula should be used with caution in weak patients. It is contraindicated when the phlegm is not lodged in the chest or when stagnant food has already passed into the intestines. If the formula causes unremitting vomiting, administer 0.3-0.6g of Caryophylli Flos *(dīng xiāng),* or one-tenth that amount of Moschus *(shè xiāng).*

Commentary

This is representative of the emetic class of formulas. Most patients suffering from this problem will have an urge to vomit, but are unable to do so. Although there is a tendency today to avoid the use of emetics whenever possible, there are no other appropriate methods for this type of problem. This formula is also often used in treating the very early stages of food poisoning, while the food is still in the stomach.

Biomedical Indications

With the appropriate presentation, this formula may be used to treat a variety of biomedically-defined disorders such as oral ingestion of poisons, acute gastritis, and some types of neuroses.

Variations

瓜蒂散

Melon Pedicle Powder from *Arcane Essentials from the Imperial Library*

guā dì sǎn

Source   *Arcane Essentials from the Imperial Library* (752)

Remove Sojae Semen praeparatum *(dàn dòu chǐ)* for acute jaundice with a hard, firm epigastrium, rough breathing, and extreme thirst.

瓜蒂散

Melon Pedicle Powder from *Systematic Differentiation of Warm Pathogen Diseases*

guā dì sǎn

Source   *Systematic Differentiation of Warm Pathogen Diseases* (1798)

Remove Sojae Semen praeparatum *(dàn dòu chǐ)* and add Gardeniae Fructus *(zhī zǐ)* for more irritability, focal distention in the chest, and an urge to vomit.

Associated Formula

三聖散 (三圣散)

Three-Sage Powder

sān shèng sǎn

Source   *Confucians' Duties to Their Parents* (1228)

Saposhnikoviae Radix *(fáng fēng)* 150g
Melo Pedicellus *(guā dì)* 150g
Veratri nigri Radix et Rhizoma *(lí lú)* 3-30g

Grind the ingredients into a coarse powder and take as a draft. Sip slowly, and stop when vomiting begins. May also be administered via nasogastric tube. Discharges wind-phlegm through vomiting. Also used for closed-type wind-stroke with aphasia or coma and the appearance of facial asymmetry, clenched jaw, hemiplegia, and a floating, excessive, and slippery pulse. Also used for seizures due to wind-phlegm, and can be used to treat ingestion of poisons. The dosage of Veratri nigri Radix et Rhizoma *(lí lú)* will vary depending on the strength of the patient and the severity of the condition.

This formula has a stronger emetic effect than the principal formula. It also focuses on the head and is used for wind-phlegm veiling the sensory orifices, while the principal formula focuses more on the chest and epigastrium. If this formula causes unremitting vomiting, administer a very concentrated decoction of scallions.

Comparative Tables of Principal Formulas

■ FORMULAS THAT DRY DAMPNESS AND TRANSFORM PHLEGM

Common symptoms: coughing with copious, clear, or white sputum that is easy to expectorate, focal distention, moist or greasy (usually white) tongue coating, slippery or wiry pulse

Formula Name	Diagnosis	Indications	Remarks
Two-Aged [Herb] Decoction (*èr chén tāng*)	Phlegm-dampness	Coughing with copious, white sputum that is easily expectorated, focal distention and a stifling sensation in the chest and diaphragm, palpitations, nausea or vomiting, dizziness, a white, moist or greasy tongue coating, and a slippery pulse	This is the representative formula for the treatment of phlegm via regulation of the qi dynamic.
Guide Out Phlegm Decoction (*dǎo tán tāng*)	Collapse due to phlegm, or wind-phlegm, or an accumulation of congested fluids	Fainting or vertigo with headache, stifling sensation and focal distention in the chest and diaphragm, reduced appetite, fullness in the hypochondria and flanks, restlessness, coughing and wheezing with copious sputum, thick nasal discharge and saliva, a white, greasy tongue coating, and a slippery pulse	For more severe phlegm obstructing the interior and preventing the proper expansion of the qi dynamic.
Scour Out Phlegm Decoction (*dí tán tāng*)	Internal obstruction due to severe phlegm that veils the Heart orifices	Stiffness of the tongue and speech impairment	Focuses the phlegm-dispersing actions on the Heart. Also for various patterns of phlegm pathology such as wheezing, dizziness, insomnia, or loss of motor function.
Poria Pill (*fú líng wán*)	Phlegm tarrying in the middle burner and overflowing into the channels and collaterals	Pain in both arms or shoulders with an inability to lift the hands (these symptoms are often more pronounced on one side), or numbness in both hands, or superficial edema in all four extremities, a white, greasy tongue coating, and a submerged and thin, or wiry and slippery pulse	Also for other patterns characterized by excess phlegm in the upper burner and Lungs, such as cough, plum-pit qi, or insomnia.
Warm Gallbladder Decoction (*wēn dǎn tāng*)	Disharmony between the Gallbladder and Stomach with phlegm-heat obstructing the qi dynamic	Dizziness, vertigo, nausea or vomiting, insomnia, dream-disturbed sleep, palpitations, anxiety, indeterminate gnawing hunger, or seizures accompanied by copious sputum, focal distention of the chest, a bitter taste in the mouth, slight thirst, a greasy, yellow tongue coating, and a rapid pulse that is either slippery or wiry	For deficiency irritability due to constraint by phlegm-heat. May also have feelings of apprehension, or hypersensitivity to noise, sounds, smells, etc.
Cyperus and Inula Decoction (*xiāng fù xuán fù huā tāng*)	Dampness leading to congested fluids that stagnate in the collaterals of the Liver	Hypochondriac pain with or without coughing, either afternoon fevers without chills or alternating chills and fever, a thickly-coated tongue with swollen edges, and a wiry pulse, especially in the middle position	This is propping thin mucus in the hypochondria following a lurking summerheat or damp-warmth disorder.

■ FORMULAS THAT CLEAR HEAT AND TRANSFORM PHLEGM

Common symptoms: focal distention and a stifling sensation in the chest, a greasy, yellow tongue coating, a slippery, rapid pulse

Formula Name	Diagnosis	Indications	Remarks
Clear the Qi and Transform Phlegm Pill *(qīng qì huà tán wán)*	Internal clumping of phlegm-heat	Coughing of yellow, viscous sputum that is difficult to expectorate, focal distention and a feeling of fullness in the chest and diaphragm, nausea, difficult breathing (severe cases), a red tongue with a greasy, yellow coating, and a slippery, rapid pulse	Also used for damp-heat obstructing the middle burner leading to nausea and vomiting, or phlegm-heat obstructing the Triple Burner causing insomnia and palpitations.
Minor Decoction [for Pathogens] Stuck in the Chest *(xiǎo xiàn xiōng tāng)*	Clumping in the chest	Focal distention (with or without nodules) in the chest and epigastrium that are painful when pressed, coughing up yellow and viscous sputum, constipation, bitter taste, a yellow, greasy tongue coating, and a slippery pulse that is either floating or rapid	For phlegm and heat in the epigastrium constraining the qi and disrupting the qi dynamic.
Flushing Away Roiling Phlegm Pill *(gǔn tán wán)*	Combination of excessive heat and chronic phlegm, or a long-term accumulation of phlegm-fire	Mania-withdrawal, anxiety, severe palpitations; or coughing and wheezing with thick sputum; or focal distention and a stifling sensation in the chest and epigastrium; or dizziness, vertigo, and tinnitus; all cases will have constipation, a yellow, thick, and greasy tongue coating, and a slippery, rapid, and forceful pulse	May also be facial tics, insomnia or strange dreams, sudden and deep pain in the joints, nodules in the neck, or a choking sensation. Focuses on driving out excess phlegm via the bowels.

■ FORMULAS THAT TRANSFORM PHLEGM AND DISPERSE CLUMPING

Common symptoms: firm masses near the surface of the body, usually in the neck region

Formula Name	Diagnosis	Indications	Remarks
Reduce Scrofula Pill *(xiāo luǒ wán)*	Phlegm nodules due to fire from constraint	Nodules on the neck that are firm and rubbery in consistency accompanied by a dry mouth and throat, a red tongue, and a rapid pulse that is slippery or wiry	For early-stage scrofula, that is, rubbery, mobile swellings that are not inflamed or ulcerating. Also used for a wide variety of nodular masses associated with phlegm-fire.
Sargassum Decoction for the Jade Flask *(hǎi zǎo yù hú tāng)*	Goiter due to stagnation of dampness, phlegm, qi, and blood	Masses in the center of the neck that are rock-like in hardness, immobile, cause no change in the color of the skin, and do not ulcerate, a thin, greasy tongue coating, and a wiry and slippery pulse	Also used for superficial tumors in other parts of the body. For relatively acute disorders that are excessive in nature.

■ FORMULAS THAT MOISTEN DRYNESS AND TRANSFORM PHLEGM

Formula Name	Diagnosis	Indications	Remarks
Fritillaria and Trichosanthes Fruit Powder *(bèi mǔ guā lóu sǎn)*	Dryness in the Lungs injuring the fluids and causing phlegm	Cough with deep-seated sputum that is difficult to expectorate, wheezing, a dry and sore throat, a red and dry tongue with white coating, and a rapid and thin but strong or slippery pulse	For patterns of phlegm-dryness. Focuses on moistening the Lungs to unblock constraint, transform phlegm, and clear heat.

■ FORMULAS THAT WARM AND TRANSFORM PHLEGM-COLD

Common symptoms: cough with copious sputum, discomfort in the chest, a white, greasy tongue coating, a slippery pulse

Formula Name	Diagnosis	Indications	Remarks
Poria, Licorice, Schisandra, Ginger, and Asarum Decoction (*líng gān wǔ wèi jiāng xīn tāng*)	Cold, thin mucus due to yang deficiency and ascendant yin	Coughing with profuse sputum that is thin, watery, and white accompanied by a feeling of discomfort in the chest and diaphragm, a white, slippery tongue coating, and a wiry, slippery pulse	For cold obstructing the movement of fluids within the Lungs.
Three-Seed Decoction to Nourish One's Parents (*sān zǐ yǎng qīn tāng*)	Phlegm clogging the Lungs with qi stagnation	Coughing and wheezing, copious sputum, focal distention in the chest, loss of appetite, digestive difficulties, a white, greasy tongue coating, and a slippery pulse	For phlegm and qi excess in the upper burner caused by a weak digestive system.

■ FORMULAS THAT TRANSFORM PHLEGM AND EXTINGUISH WIND

Common symptoms: greasy tongue coating, wiry or slippery pulse

Formula Name	Diagnosis	Indications	Remarks
Pinellia, White Atractylodes, and Gastrodia Decoction (*bàn xià bái zhú tiān má tāng*)	Upward disturbance of wind-phlegm	Dizziness or vertigo (possibly severe), headache, a stifling sensation in the chest, nausea or vomiting, copious sputum, a white, greasy tongue coating, and a wiry, slippery pulse	A distinctive feature of these head symptoms is that the head feels heavy and clouded.
Arrest Seizures Pill (*dìng xián wán*)	Seizure disorder arising from a combination of wind and phlegm	Sudden loss or clouding of consciousness accompanied by falling down, upward-rolling eyes, deviated mouth, spitting of mucus, and in severe cases, tonic-clonic convulsions, sudden shrieking, or incontinence, a white and greasy tongue coating, and a pulse that is usually wiry and slippery	Attacks may or may not have prodromal signs such as recurrent vertigo, weakness, and a stifling sensation in the chest. Also for withdrawal-mania with a similar presentation.
Stop Coughing Powder (*zhǐ sòu sǎn*)	Cough occurring as the sequela to externally-contracted wind-cold	Coughing with or without slight chills and fever, itchy throat, phlegm that is difficult to expectorate, a thin, white tongue coating, and a moderate, floating pulse	Effective, well-balanced formula for a lingering cough due to an externally-contracted disorder.

■ FORMULAS THAT INDUCE VOMITING

Formula Name	Diagnosis	Indications	Remarks
Melon Pedicle Powder (*guā dì sǎn*)	Phlegm clogging the chest and diaphragm, or stagnant food lodging in the upper epigastrium	Firm areas of focal distention in the chest, vexation, difficult breathing due to a sensation of qi rushing into the throat, and a slightly floating pulse at the distal position	Also for the very early stages of food poisoning, while the food is still in the stomach.

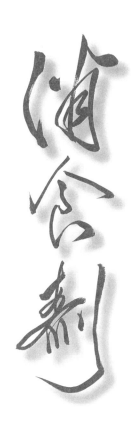

Chapter 18 Contents

Formulas that Reduce Food Stagnation

Formulas that Reduce Food Stagnation

AMONG THE EIGHT strategies of treatment, the formulas in this chapter rely on reducing (消 xiāo) and guiding out (導 dǎo) to relieve disorders caused by the stagnation or accumulation of food. Food stagnation (食滞 shí zhì) refers to the accumulation and stagnation of food in the digestive system, primarily the middle burner. This is characterized by epigastric and abdominal focal distention and fullness, an aversion to food, rotten-smelling belching, abdominal pain, and sometimes diarrhea. It also refers specifically to acute disorders that result from episodes of gross overeating. By contrast, food accumulation (食積 shí jī) is a more chronic condition that results from long-term overindulgence in food and drink and causes qi, dampness, phlegm, and even blood to accumulate. It, too, is characterized predominantly by abdominal distention and pain.

The notion that overeating can cause disease was first mentioned in *Basic Questions* (Chapter 43): "Drinking and eating to twice one's capacity injures the Intestines and Stomach." When food stagnation or accumulation occurs in the upper burner, the appropriate strategy is to induce vomiting; when it occurs in the lower burner, it should be purged; and when it occurs in the middle burner (by far the most common type of food stagnation), a moderate reducing strategy is most effective.

Because the middle burner is the fulcrum of the qi dynamic, food stagnation obstructing the ascent and descent of qi can have repercussions on the circulation of qi and dis-tribution of fluids throughout the body. If the ascent of yang qi becomes constrained, chills and fevers may result, as is often seen in cases of acute food poisoning. If the clarifying and descending functions of Lung qi are inhibited, there will be rebellious qi leading to asthma and coughing. Constraint of the coursing and dredging functions of the Liver qi may cause the generation of accumulations and masses. Even clouding of consciousness may result from food stagnation when the spirit dynamic becomes blocked.

Food stagnation is often subdivided into hot and cold types. The principal manifestations of the hot type are severe bad breath, a feeling of distention in the abdomen, a preference for cold food and beverages and an aversion to hot ones, a yellow, greasy tongue coating, and a forceful, slippery pulse. This condition usually arises with either externally-contracted diseases or heat from constraint. The cold type of food stagnation is due to Spleen or Stomach deficiency, or ingesting too much cold food. Major symptoms include a brackish feeling in the throat, nausea, spitting up clear fluids, a feeling of distention in the abdomen, preference for hot food and beverages and an aversion to cold ones, a white, greasy tongue coating, and a weak, thin pulse.

Food stagnation is, by definition, a condition of excess, even though it can occur against a background of Stomach and Spleen deficiency. Depending on which aspect dominates, the formulas in this chapter can be divided into two groups: those that focus primarily on excess by reducing accumulation of food and transforming stagnation, and those that reduce food stagnation but also tonify. No matter what the cause and precise constellation of excess and deficiency, food stagnation itself is treated by reducing, in accordance with the adage, "Eliminate what lodges [where it should not] (客者除之 *kè zhě chū zhī*)." The main herbs used for this purpose are those that relieve food stagnation such as Crataegi Fructus *(shān zhā)*, Massa medicata fermentata *(shén qū)*, Hordei Fructus germinatus *(mài yá)*, Setariae Fructus germinatus *(gǔ yá)*, Raphani Semen *(lái fú zǐ)*, and Gigeriae galli Endothelium corneum *(jī nèi jīn)*. However, because food stagnation is often a symptom rather than a cause, these herbs are not necessarily the chief ingredients of the formulas discussed in this section. These may be drawn from many different categories, including those that move the qi and break up stagnation, drive the qi downward, promote the draining of damp-heat, or tonify the Spleen and Stomach.

In selecting the formulas in this chapter, physicians must be clear about the difference between reducing food stagnation and purging internal accumulations. Reducing and purging (Chapter 2) are similar strategies in that both address conditions in which the pathogenic influence or stasis has accumulated and taken form. Clinically, however, the two strategies are quite distinct. Reducing is a relatively mild method that dissolves and disperses abdominal accumulation with focal distention, while purging is rather harsh and is used primarily for acute, substantial accumulation of stool with clumping in the intestines. In addition, all of the reducing formulas have a transforming aspect, while purgatives do not. This principle is summarized in *Essential Teachings of [Zhu] Dan-Xi*: "In accumulation disorders, one cannot use purgatives."

Although less harsh than purgatives, formulas that reduce food stagnation are nonetheless dispersing in nature. For patients with constitutional Spleen deficiency, or in whom a long-term condition of food stagnation has injured the normal qi, formulas that emphasize the functions of supporting the normal qi and strengthening the Spleen are used. For more severe disorders, purgatives should be added.

Section 1

FORMULAS THAT REDUCE FOOD ACCUMULATION AND TRANSFORM STAGNATION

The formulas in this section treat patterns of excess caused by food stagnating in the interior, leading to various forms of accumulation. The main symptoms of such disorders are focal distention in the chest and upper abdomen, acid regurgitation, belching, nausea, vomiting, abdominal pain, diarrhea, a greasy tongue coating, and a slippery, excessive pulse. The pulse, in particular, is an important sign for distinguishing these patterns from those of deficiency outlined below. The main treatment strategy for these conditions is to reduce accumulation and transform food stagnation. Depending on the precise nature of the pathology, these formulas combine herbs that specifically reduce food stagnation with others drawn from one or more of the following categories:

- Herbs that move the qi and break up stagnation such as Aurantii Fructus immaturus *(zhǐ shí)*, Magnoliae officinalis Cortex *(hòu pò)*, Citri reticulatae Pericarpium *(chén pí)*, Aucklandiae Radix *(mù xiāng)*, Arecae Semen *(bīng láng)*, and Sparganii Rhizoma *(sān léng)*. These herbs are important because fullness, distention, and pain are key symptoms of food stagnation patterns.

- Herbs that drive the qi downward such as Rhei Radix et Rhizoma *(dà huáng)*, Natrii Sulfas *(máng xiāo)*, and Pharbitidis Semen *(qiān niú zǐ)*. These herbs are important because food stagnation obstructs the Stomach and Intestines, and the bowels constitute a natural exit route for removing such excess from the body

- Herbs that promote the draining of damp-heat such Poria *(fú líng)*, Alismatis Rhizoma *(zé xiè)*, Forsythiae Fructus *(lián qiáo)*, and Coptidis Rhizoma *(huáng lián)*. These herbs are important because food stagnation invariably leads to the buildup of dampness in the middle burner, which readily generates heat due to constraint.

- Herbs that kill parasites such as Arecae Semen *(bīng láng)* or Quisqualis Fructus *(shǐ jūn zǐ)*.

- Herbs that warm the interior such as Zingiberis Rhizoma *(gān jiāng)* and Evodiae Fructus *(wú zhū yú)*. This may be necessary when food stagnation constrains the dissemination of the body's yang qi.

保和丸

Preserve Harmony Pill

bǎo hé wán

This formula reduces food stagnation and preserves the proper functioning of the digestive organs. It is composed of relatively mild, harmonious herbs, hence the name.

Source   *Essential Teachings of [Zhu] Dan-Xi* (1481)

Crataegi Fructus *(shān zhā)*	180g (9-15g)
Massa medicata fermentata *(shén qū)*	60g (9-12g)
Raphani Semen *(lái fú zǐ)*	30g (6-9g)
Citri reticulatae Pericarpium *(chén pí)*	30g (6-9g)
Pinelliae Rhizoma praeparatum *(zhì bàn xià)*	90g (9-12g)
Poria *(fú líng)*	90g (9-12g)
Forsythiae Fructus *(lián qiáo)*	30g (3-6g)

Grind the ingredients into a powder and form into pills with water. The normal dosage is 6-9g taken twice a day with warm water or prepared as a decoction made with Hordei Fructus germinatus (*mài yá*). May also be prepared as a decoction with the dosages specified in parentheses.

Actions   Reduces food stagnation and harmonizes the Stomach

Indications

Focal distention and fullness in the chest and epigastrium, abdominal distention with occasional pain, rotten-smelling belching, acid regurgitation, nausea and vomiting, aversion to food, a yellow, greasy tongue coating, and a slippery pulse. There may also be diarrhea.

This is the typical presentation of food stagnation that occurs from eating contaminated food or from gross overeating and drinking. Excessive consumption of alcohol, meat, and fatty foods in particular may inhibit the ability of the Spleen and Stomach to properly receive, transform, and transport food. This results in stagnation and accumulation of undigested food that obstructs the qi mechanisms of the middle burner, leading to focal distention and fullness in the chest and epigastrium and abdominal distention. When it is severe, pain ensues.

Food stagnation also disrupts the ascending and descending functions of the Spleen and Stomach. When the turbid-yin products of digestion do not properly descend, there is foul-smelling belching, acid regurgitation, nausea, and vomiting. When the Spleen qi is unable to rise, there is diarrhea. When the Stomach takes in more food than it can digest, there is an aversion to food. Stagnation in the digestive system is reflected in the greasy tongue and slippery pulse. The yellow coating reflects the presence of heat in the interior caused by the constraint from food stagnation.

Analysis of Formula

Food accumulating and tarrying in the Stomach is treated by reducing stagnation and transforming accumulation. The chief ingredient is sour, sweet, and slightly warm Crataegi Fructus (*shān zhā*). It awakens the Spleen, unbinds the Stomach, promotes food intake, and assists digestion. It is particularly useful for problems due to overindulgence in meat and greasy foods. There are two deputies. Acrid, sweet, and warm Massa medicata fermentata (*shén qū*) is especially useful in reducing the stagnant accumulation of alcohol and food. It directs qi downward to transform phlegm, warms the Stomach to transform thin mucus, and strengthens the Spleen to alleviate diarrhea and distention. Acrid, sweet, and neutral Raphani Semen (*lái fú zǐ*) excels at reducing the accumulation of phlegm from stagnant grains and at facilitating the flow of qi. Together, the chief and deputy ingredients thus reduce the stagnation and accumulation caused by overindulgence in food or drink of all types.

Among the assistant ingredients, Pinelliae Rhizoma praeparatum (*zhì bàn xià*) and Citri reticulatae Pericarpium (*chén pí*), which are both acrid and warming, promote the movement of qi and transform stagnation, thereby harmonizing the Stomach to stop the nausea and vomiting. Bland and neutral Poria (*fú líng*) strengthens the Spleen and leaches out dampness, thereby harmonizing the middle burner to stop the diarrhea. The accumulation of food readily gives rise to heat from constraint; bitter, slightly acrid, and slightly cold Forsythiae Fructus (*lián qiáo*) is added to address this problem, but also because of its ability to disperse and penetrate, which makes it a valuable herb for treating phlegm-heat. Sweet and neutral Hordei Fructus germinatus (*mài yá*) raises and stimulates the Stomach qi in order to digest food stagnation, particularly that associated with starches and all types of fruit. When the formula is taken with a decoction made from this herb, its reducing action is strengthened.

Cautions and Contraindications

Unless modified, this formula is contraindicated in cases with Spleen deficiency.

Commentary

This is the most popular formula for reducing food stagnation in contemporary practice. Its composition profoundly influenced the treatment of food stagnation, as reflected in the associated formulas discussed below. Its use is most appropriate in the early stages of food stagnation, or for relatively mild disorders. It is commonly used for treating the diarrhea associated with this disorder in children, and for childhood nutritional impairment. Key clinical markers are abdominal pain accompanied by diarrhea, with the pain being relieved by the passing of stools; or no abdominal pain, but rotten-smelling belching.

In terms of its composition, the formula may be regarded as a variation of Two-Aged [Herb] Decoction (*èr chén tāng*) with the addition of ingredients that reduce food stagnation. This is appropriate because the main purpose of Two-Aged [Herb] Decoction (*èr chén tāng*) is to regulate the qi and direct rebellious qi downward.

Issue of Heat

Commentators disagree about the extent to which heat is present in this condition. One view, represented by the Qing-dynasty physician Zhang Bin-Cheng in *Convenient Reader of Established Formulas*, argues that "any place where there is focal distention and hardness will have [some constraint due to] lurking yang. Hence, [this formula] employs the bitter, cooling of Forsythiae Fructus (*lián qiáo*) to disperse the clumping and clear the heat." An opposing view was offered by Zhang's contemporary, Fei Bo-Xiong, who wrote in *Discussion of Medical Formulas* that "this is a balanced formula for harmonizing the middle by reducing and guiding out [accumulation]. But Forsythiae Fructus *(lián qiáo)* can be omitted." In practice, one can decide on the basis of the presenting symptoms which of the two interpretations to follow and even include other bitter and cooling herbs, such as Coptidis Rhizoma *(huáng lián),* if heat signs are more pronounced.

Long-Term Treatment

Although the formula's action is mild and its composition is balanced, it is intended to resolve acute problems and is not indicated for long-term use. However, because recurrent food stagnation may require longer term treatment, in *Comprehensive Medicine According to Master Zhang,* the Qing-dynasty physician Zhang Lu recommends the following alternative:

> If one adds 60g of fried Atractylodis macrocephalae Rhizoma *(bái zhú)* to this formula, [one obtains a new formula that is called] Great Tranquility Pill *(dà ān wán).* [However,] both Preserve Harmony Pill *(bǎo hé wán)* and Great Tranquility Pill *(dà ān wán)* contain Hordei Fructus germinatus *(mài yá),* which damages the Kidneys, and Raphani Semen *(lái fú zǐ),* which damages the Spleen and Stomach qi. I am afraid that even these pills are unsuitable for long-term use. [For that purpose] one should substitute Gardeniae Fructus *(zhī zǐ)* and Cyperi Rhizoma *(xiāng fù)* as they have the same action without damaging both the true prenatal and postnatal qi.

Comparisons

➤ Vs. STRENGTHEN THE SPLEEN PILL *(jiàn pí wán)*

Both formulas treat food stagnation with abdominal distention and diarrhea, often with undigested food particles. However, Preserve Harmony Pill *(bǎo hé wán)* is primarily for food accumulating in the middle burner and focuses on reducing food stagnation and harmonizing the Stomach, without any significant tonification. There is usually epigastric distention, nausea, an aversion to food, rotten-smelling belching, acid regurgitation, a slippery pulse, and a greasy tongue coating. Strengthen the Spleen Pill *(jiàn pí wán)* treats both food stagnation and Spleen deficiency, with stagnant dampness that has transformed to heat. There is usually a generalized sense of fullness and distention throughout the abdomen, reduced appetite, generalized fatigue, a deficient pulse, and a greasy, slightly yellow tongue coating.

➤ Vs. THREE-SEED DECOCTION TO NOURISH ONE'S PARENTS *(sān zǐ yǎng qīn tāng)*

Both of these formulas are primarily composed of ingredients that reduce food stagnation and transform phlegm and thin mucus, yet their range of action is substantially different. In both cases, Raphani Semen *(lái fú zǐ)* is an important ingredient. Preserve Harmony Pill *(bǎo hé wán)* adds two more herbs that reduce food stagnation as well as Two-Aged [Herb] Decoction *(èr chén tāng),* the main formula for transforming phlegm. As a result, the formula focuses on trans-

forming food stagnation and harmonizing the Stomach, with phlegm regarded as a secondary consequence of this stagnation. Symptoms indicating stagnation of the qi dynamic are thus prominent and include abdominal fullness and distention, acid reflux, and vomiting. In a patient with a strong constitution, such stagnation can readily transform into heat, which necessitates the addition of heat-clearing and -draining ingredients.

Three-Seed Decoction to Nourish One's Parents *(sān zǐ yǎng qīn tāng),* on the other hand, combines Raphani Semen *(lái fú zǐ)* with the acrid and warming herbs Sinapis Semen *(bái jiè zǐ)* and Perillae Fructus *(zǐ sū zǐ).* As a result, that formula focuses on thin mucus obstructing the downward directing of the Lungs and Stomach, manifesting in symptoms such as cough or wheezing accompanied by copious phlegm. This pattern occurs against a background of internal cold from deficiency, thus no heat symptoms are observed. Preserve Harmony Pill *(bǎo hé wán)* also can treat patterns characterized by coughing up of phlegm, but only where it is caused by food stagnation. Three-Seed Decoction to Nourish One's Parents *(sān zǐ yǎng qīn tāng)* treats patterns characterized by a lack of appetite and a reduced ability to digest food, resulting in the production of phlegm and thin mucus, but it is not strong enough to disperse actual food stagnation.

Biomedical Indications

With the appropriate presentation, this formula may be used to treat a variety of biomedically-defined disorders including acute gastroenteritis, acute exacerbation of chronic gastritis, hepatitis, acute pancreatitis, and acute or chronic cholecystitis.

Modifications

- For more severe abdominal distention, add Aurantii Fructus immaturus *(zhǐ shí)* and Magnoliae officinalis Cortex *(hòu pò).*
- For sweating from the head due to accumulation of food that has transformed into heat, add ginger Coptidis Rhizoma *(jiāng huáng lián).*
- For constipation, add Rhei Radix et Rhizoma *(dà huáng)* and Arecae Semen *(bīng láng).*
- For early-stage dysenteric disorder with concurrent food stagnation, remove Poria *(fú líng)* and Forsythiae Fructus *(lián qiáo)* and add Coptidis Rhizoma *(huáng lián),* Aurantii Fructus immaturus *(zhǐ shí),* and Arecae Semen *(bīng láng).*

Variation

保和丸

Preserve Harmony Pill from *Precious Mirror*
bǎo hé wán

Source *Precious Mirror for Advancement of Medicine* (1777)

Add Hordei Fructus germinatus (*mài yá*) to strengthen the effect of the formula.

Associated Formulas

大安丸

Great Tranquility Pill

dà ān wán

Source *Essential Teachings of [Zhu] Dan-Xi* (1481)

dry-fried Massa medicata fermentata (*chǎo shén qū*)

Add Atractylodis macrocephalae Rhizoma (*bái zhú*) to increase the Spleen-strengthening action of the formula, which is often especially useful in children.

楂曲平胃散

Hawthorn and Medicated Leaven Calm the Stomach Powder

zhā qū píng wèi sǎn

Source *Pathodynamics and Treatment Strategies in Chinese Medicine* (1988)

Atractylodis Rhizoma (*cāng zhú*) 9g
Magnoliae officinalis Cortex (*hòu pò*) 9g
Citri reticulatae Pericarpium (*chén pí*) 9g
Glycyrrhizae Radix (*gān cǎo*) 9g
Pinelliae Rhizoma (*bàn xià*) 9g
Poria (*fú líng*) 15g
Crataegi Fructus (*shān zhā*) 15g
Massa medicata fermentata (*shén qū*) 15g
Hordei Fructus germinatus (*mài yá*) 15g

Decoction. Dries dampness and promotes the transporting function of the Spleen, eliminates food stagnation, and transforms accumulations. For cold-dampness encumbering the Spleen characterized by lack of appetite and a desire to lie down with curled up limbs. Also treats food stagnation obstructing the qi dynamic of the middle burner characterized by abdominal fullness and distention, acid regurgitation, nausea, diarrhea, a pale tongue with a white coating, and a soft and relaxed pulse. This is a combination of Calm the Stomach Powder (*píng wèi sǎn*) and Two-Aged [Herb] Decoction (*èr chén tāng*) with the addition of herbs that resolve food stagnation. In contrast to the principal formula, this is more acrid and warming, and also breaks up qi stagnation. It can treat two different patterns because they are closely related in terms of their underlying pathodynamic. Cold-dampness encumbering the Spleen invariably involves the accumulation of food and fluids in the Stomach, which also occurs when excess food obstructs the qi dynamic.

大和中飲 （大和中饮）

Major Harmonize the Middle Drink

dà hé zhōng yǐn

Source *Collected Treatises of [Zhang] Jing-Yue* (1624)

Citri reticulatae Pericarpium (*chén pí*) 3-6g

Aurantii Fructus immaturus (*zhǐ shí*) 3g
Amomi Fructus (*shā rén*) 1.5g
Crataegi Fructus (*shān zhā*) 6g
Hordei Fructus germinatus (*mài yá*) 6g
Magnoliae officinalis Cortex (*hòu pò*) 4.5g
Alismatis Rhizoma (*zé xiè*) 4.5g

Decoction. For food stagnation and accumulation with more pronounced signs of distention and fullness than in the pattern treated by the principal formula.

小和中飲 （小和中饮）

Minor Harmonize the Middle Drink

xiǎo hé zhōng yǐn

Source *Collected Treatises of [Zhang] Jing-Yue* (1624)

Citri reticulatae Pericarpium (*chén pí*) 3-6g
Crataegi Fructus (*shān zhā*) 6g
Poria (*fú líng*) 4.5g
Magnoliae officinalis Cortex (*hòu pò*) 4.5g
Glycyrrhizae Radix (*gān cǎo*) 1.5g
Lablab Semen album (*biǎn dòu*) 6g

Prepared as a decoction by boiling the herbs with 3-5 slices of Zingiberis Rhizoma recens (*shēng jiāng*). Transforms dampness and eliminates accumulations. The source text prescribes this formula for various types of accumulation that cannot be attacked (i.e., purged) but must be treated by gradual reducing and guiding out. Besides a pattern of food stagnation characterized by fullness and distention caused by eating excessively cold foods, these include focal distention with malarial symptoms, recovery from illness where turbid qi or fire has not been entirely cleared, vomiting and focal distention in children, and pox and papular rashes accompanied by abdominal distention.

枳實導滯丸 （枳实导滞丸）

Unripe Bitter Orange Pill to Guide Out Stagnation

zhǐ shí dǎo zhì wán

Source *Clarifying Doubts about Damage from Internal and External Causes* (1247)

dry-fried Aurantii Fructus immaturus (*chǎo zhǐ shí*) . . . 15g
Rhei Radix et Rhizoma (*dà huáng*) 30g
dry-fried Massa medicata fermentata (*chǎo shén qū*) . . . 15g
Poria (*fú líng*) 9g
Scutellariae Radix (*huáng qín*) 9g
Coptidis Rhizoma (*huáng lián*) 9g
Atractylodis macrocephalae Rhizoma (*bái zhú*) 9g
Alismatis Rhizoma (*zé xiè*) 6g

Method of Preparation Grind the ingredients into a powder and steam to form into small pills. The normal dosage is 6-9g twice a day with warm water. May also be prepared as a decoction.

Actions Reduces and guides out stagnation and accumulation, drains heat, and dispels dampness

Indications

Pain (that increases with pressure) and distention in the epigastrium and abdomen, dysenteric disorders or constipation (depending on the degree of obstruction), scanty, dark urine, a red tongue with a greasy or slippery, yellow coating, and a submerged, forceful pulse.

This is accumulation of food that transforms into damp-heat and obstructs the Stomach and Intestines. Alternatively, damp-heat already present in the body may combine with harbored food to clump in the Stomach and Intestines. Accumulation of food and damp-heat obstructs the qi dynamic, causing pain that increases with pressure (indicating excess), and distention in the epigastrium and abdomen. Initially, the body tries to expel the pathogenic accumulation via the bowels, which manifests as dysenteric disorder. If the damp-heat accumulation obstructs the movement of qi in the bowels, it manifests as constipation. Scanty, dark urine, a red tongue with a greasy or slippery, yellow coating, and a submerged, forceful pulse are all symptoms of damp-heat excess.

Analysis of Formula

Treating damp-heat and food accumulation simultaneously requires a strategy of reducing and guiding out stagnation and accumulation, draining heat, and dispelling dampness. The chief herb, therefore, is Rhei Radix et Rhizoma (dà huáng), which is used with a very high dosage. Bitter, cooling, and with a strong downward-directing action, it strongly mobilizes the Stomach and Intestines to flush away accumulated obstruction due to heat from excess. Bitter, draining, sinking, and downward-directing, Aurantii Fructus immaturus (zhǐ shí) serves as one of the two deputies in this formula to break up stagnant qi and reduce accumulation. *Transforming the Significance of Medicinal Substances* notes that without it, "one cannot treat excess fullness around the navel and abdomen, reduce phlegm clumps, expel water that has tarried, drive out harbored food stagnation, break up clumping in the chest, or unblock constipation." The other deputy is acrid, sweet, and warming Massa medicata fermentata (shén qū). It is especially useful in reducing the stagnant accumulation of alcohol, one of the main causes of damp-heat, but also directs qi downward to transform phlegm, warms the Stomach to transform thin mucus, and strengthens the Spleen to alleviate diarrhea and distention.

The remaining ingredients all serve as assistants. Bitter and cooling Coptidis Rhizoma (huáng lián) and Scutellariae Radix (huáng qín) drain heat, dry dampness, and stop dysenteric disorders. Poria (fú líng) and Alismatis Rhizoma (zé xiè) both promote water metabolism to facilitate the draining of damp-heat via the urine and provide a second exit route for the pathogen. Their downward-directing action on the qi dynamic supports that of the chief and deputy ingredients. Warming and tonifying Atractylodis macrocephalae Rhizoma (bái zhú) strengthens the Spleen and augments the qi to balance the draining action of the other ingredients and protect the normal qi.

Cautions and Contraindications

This formula is indicated only for excess patterns. It is contraindicated for dysenteric disorders in the absence of qi stagnation.

Commentary

This formula can be viewed as a combination of Unripe Bitter Orange and Atractylodes Pill (zhǐ zhú wán), discussed below, and Drain the Epigastrium Decoction (xiè xīn tāng), discussed in Chapter 4. Its original indication in the source text was "damage due to damp and heating things that are not being transformed and cause focal distention, fullness, a stifling sensation, confusion, or restlessness." Constipation is a common symptom of such stagnation. Later generations of physicians further extended its indications to dysenteric disorders due to damp-heat characterized by stools that contain pus or blood, and tenesmus.

Changing the Focus of the Formula

In each of these patterns the chief herb, Rhei Radix et Rhizoma (dà huáng), provides a slightly different action. In treating food accumulation obstructing the qi dynamic, the formula's author, Li Gao, followed very closely the original indications of this herb in *Divine Husbandman's Classic of the Materia Medica*. There it says that the herb "pushes out the old to create the new, regulates the middle to transform food, and quiets the five yin organs." Its use in the treatment of constipation is a straightforward purging of accumulations in the Intestines. When used in treating such disorders, it guides the entire formula toward the Intestines, a strategy known as 'facilitating the flow to treat disorders with too much flow' (通因通用 tōng yīn tōng yòng). Many modern textbooks thus identify Rhei Radix et Rhizoma (dà huáng) as the chief herb, irrespective of the condition treated.

A somewhat different interpretation is advanced by Chen Chao-Zu in *Treatment Strategies and Formulas in Chinese Medicine*. Chen suggests that the composition of the formula should be viewed differently (and, if necessary, also adjusted) depending on which pattern it treats:

> When a given formula treats different patterns, the strategy changes in line with those patterns. This formula provides an example [of this]. When food accumulates and tarries in the Stomach to generate damp-heat, one should guide out accumulation, dispel stagnation, clear heat, and promote the resolution of dampness. In this formula, Aurantii Fructus immaturus (zhǐ shí) drives the qi downward to eliminate focal distention; Rhei Radix et Rhizoma (dà huáng) drains downward to flush out accumulation; and Massa medicata fermentata (shén qū) reduces

food [stagnation] and transforms stagnation. [In this context, these ingredients] are really those that guide out accumulation. Coptidis Rhizoma *(huáng lián)* and Scutellariae Radix *(huáng qín)*—bitter, cooling, and drying dampness—are there to clear heat. Atractylodis macrocephalae Rhizoma *(bái zhú)* moves the Spleen, [while] Poria *(fú líng)* and Alismatis Rhizoma *(zé xiè)* leach out to eliminate dampness. Combining [these three actions] constitutes the formula. It is effective because it is able to eliminate accumulation, guide out stagnation, and eliminate dampness.

If one uses this formula to treating dysentery, this is no longer the case, as it is now necessary to urgently clear heat and resolve toxicity. Scutellariae Radix *(huáng qín)* and Coptidis Rhizoma *(huáng lián)* are now the chief herbs, able to effect removal of the cause of the disease. They combine with downward-draining and purging Rhei Radix et Rhizoma *(dà huáng)* to eliminate pestilential toxicity. Aurantii Fructus immaturus *(zhǐ shí)* moves the qi and guides out stagnation, which [now] resolves tenesmus. Massa medicata fermentata *(shén qū)*, Atractylodis macrocephalae Rhizoma *(bái zhú)*, Poria *(fú líng)*, and Alismatis Rhizoma *(zé xiè)* promote movement by the Spleen and eliminate dampness. Adjusting the functioning [of the formula in this manner] step by step transforms it from one that reduces accumulation and guides out stagnation into a strategy for clearing heat and stopping dysentery.

If, instead, one employs this formula to treat constipation, then Rhei Radix et Rhizoma *(dà huáng)* becomes the chief herb. The remaining herbs now also have the simultaneous function of eliminating. Once again, this changes [the original formula] into one that is designed to drain downward and unblock the Intestines, while also clearing heat and facilitating the resolution of dampness. If students focus intensely on the principle of how the formula is changed in accordance with the [required treatment] strategy and how the strategy follows the change in patterns, they will gain insight. With regard to the hackneyed practice that every formula must be analyzed in terms of chief, deputy, assistant, and envoy [ingredients], turning living formulas into dead ones, I am afraid that I dare not negligently agree.

In practice, the formula can thus be further adjusted to achieve an even better effect, and also used for other patterns due to damp-heat obstructing the qi dynamic. The case history literature gives examples of its use in the treatment of sciatica, vaginal wind, acute appendicitis, and colitis. The main diagnostic markers, in each case, are a greasy tongue coating, reduced urination, and dark urine.

Comparison

➤ Vs. Aucklandia and Betel Nut Pill *(mù xiāng bīng láng wán)*; see page 833

Modifications

- For dysenteric disorders with damp-heat in the Intestines, add Sophorae flavescentis Radix *(kǔ shēn)* and Sanguisorbae Radix *(dì yú)*.
- For fullness and distention, add Aucklandiae Radix *(mù xiāng)* and Arecae Semen *(bīng láng)*.

- For loss of appetite, add Crataegi Fructus *(shān zhā)* and Gigeriae galli Endothelium corneum *(jī nèi jīn)*.
- For abdominal pain, add Paeoniae Radix alba *(bái sháo)* and Glycyrrhizae Radix *(gān cǎo)*.

木香檳榔丸 （木香槟榔丸）
Aucklandia and Betel Nut Pill
mù xiāng bīng láng wán

Source   *Confucians' Duties to Their Parents* (1228)

Aucklandiae Radix *(mù xiāng)* 30g
Arecae Semen *(bīng láng)* 30g
Rhei Radix et Rhizoma *(dà huáng)* 90g
Pharbitidis Semen *(qiān niú zǐ)* .120g
Citri reticulatae viride Pericarpium *(qīng pí)* 30g
Citri reticulatae Pericarpium *(chén pí)* 30g
dry-fried Cyperi Rhizoma *(chǎo xiāng fù)* 120g
dry-fried Curcumae Rhizoma *(chǎo é zhú)* 30g
bran-fried Aurantii Fructus *(fū chǎo zhǐ ké)* 30g
Coptidis Rhizoma *(huáng lián)* 30g
Phellodendri Cortex *(huáng bǎi)* .90g

Method of Preparation   Grind the ingredients into a powder and form into pills with water. Take in 3-6g doses 2-3 times daily with warm water or a decoction of Zingiberis Rhizoma recens *(shēng jiāng)*. May also be prepared as a decoction with a proportionate reduction in dosage.

Actions   Promotes the movement of qi, guides out stagnation, purges accumulation, and drains heat

Indications

Focal and generalized distention, fullness, and pain in the epigastrium and abdomen accompanied by constipation; or red-and-white dysenteric diarrhea with tenesmus. In all cases, there will be a yellow, greasy tongue coating, and a submerged and excessive pulse.

This formula treats two patterns: accumulation of food obstructing the middle burner and dysenteric diarrhea. When harbored food accumulates and blocks the qi dynamic of the digestive organs, the obstruction of yang qi transforms into heat from constraint, which, together with the dampness caused by stagnation of food, becomes damp-heat. The obstruction of the qi dynamic produces focal and generalized distention and pain in the epigastrium and abdomen. When severe, the patient will experience a feeling of fullness, which is stronger than mere distention. The internal accumulation of damp-heat usually combines with the stagnant accumulation of food to obstruct the flow of qi in the yang organs. This results in constipation.

The second pattern is produced when epidemic toxin enters the Stomach and Intestines where it constrains the body's protective yang, leading to the accumulation of damp-heat. The steaming of damp-heat in the interior leads to the formation of pus that forces its way downward as red-and-white dysenteric diarrhea. Tenesmus indicates the stagnation of qi that accompanies the condition. In both cases, the yellow, greasy tongue coating and submerged, excessive pulse reflect the presence of stagnation and damp-heat.

Analysis of Formula

This formula treats patterns where the accumulation of food and stagnation of qi transforms into damp-heat, which in turn aggravates the stagnation and accumulation. To break this vicious cycle, it is important to focus on unblocking the qi dynamic while also guiding out accumulation and draining damp-heat. The chief herbs, Aucklandiae Radix *(mù xiāng)* and Arecae Semen *(bīng láng),* are both bitter, acrid, and warming, and promote the movement of qi and transform stagnation, thereby unblocking and facilitating the flow of qi in all the burners. Aucklandiae Radix *(mù xiāng)* warms the middle to promote transportation, and dries dampness, while Arecae Semen *(bīng láng)* reduces accumulation and guides out stagnation. This combination is thus not only very effective in treating focal and generalized distention and pain in the epigastrium and abdomen, but also treats tenesmus and facilitates the passage of mucus in dysenteric disorders. One group of deputies, consisting of Rhei Radix et Rhizoma *(dà huáng)* and Pharbitidis Semen *(qiān niú zǐ),* strongly purges accumulation, guides out stagnation, drains heat, and unblocks the bowels. The other group, Citri reticulatae viride Pericarpium *(qīng pí)* and Citri reticulatae Pericarpium *(chén pí),* helps the chief herbs to promote the movement of qi and transform accumulation.

Among the assistants are Cyperi Rhizoma *(xiāng fù)* and Curcumae Rhizoma *(é zhú),* which relieve Liver constraint and disperse stagnation in the qi aspect of the blood, thereby preventing the progression of this problem into the blood. Coptidis Rhizoma *(huáng lián)* and Phellodendri Cortex *(huáng bǎi)* clear heat and dry dampness in the digestive system, which stops the diarrhea. When Zingiberis Rhizoma recens *(shēng jiāng)* is used, it serves as the envoy by harmonizing the middle qi and reviving the Spleen.

Cautions and Contraindications

Contraindicated in cases with deficiency, since the formula may further injure the normal qi and thereby aggravate the condition.

Commentary

This formula was composed by Zhang Zi-He, one of the four masters of the Jin-Yuan era, famous for focusing on the elimination of pathogenic qi from the body. In the source text, he gives a far wider range of indications than is commonly noted today:

> [This formula treats the following patterns:] any kind of cooling foods that have not been digested, harbored food that is

not dispersed, cold-damage like [symptoms] such as severe shivering, headache, and stiffness of the entire back; any kind of deep accumulations that may be accompanied by edema and inability to eat that causes lightheadedness, vertigo, and an inability to stay lucid and calm; and any kind of damage due to bugs or beasts. It also [treats] ulcerated toxic swellings and sores on the back whether due to being hit with a stick, burned, or penetrating into the interior; [as well as] swollen bleeding toxic hemorrhoids.

Over the centuries, the indications were narrowed and more clearly specified, although their range still remained wider than it is today. For example, *Formulary of the Imperial Pharmacy* says that it treats "any kind of qi stagnation [characterized by] fullness or a stifling sensation in the epigastrium or abdomen, drum distention of the flanks, clumping and stagnation of urination and bowels with difficult voiding." *Collection of Versatility* states that it can be used for "Lung phlegm with cough and wheezing, [the qi dynamic] of chest and diaphragm not affording passage, and damp-heat jaundice."

In *Medical Formulas Collected and Analyzed,* the Qing-dynasty commentator Wang Ang attempted to summarize these various indications by defining them as damp-heat obstructing the qi dynamic of the Triple Burner. This accords well with the original indication, as it emphasizes obstruction of fluid metabolism as much as that of digestion and bowel movement. It also explains why the herbs that treat stagnant accumulation are regarded as the chief ingredients in the formula, even though they are prescribed in a smaller dosage than some of the other ingredients. Wang Ang further recommended adding Angelicae sinensis Radix *(dāng guī),* Sparganii Rhizoma *(sān léng),* and Natrii Sulfas *(máng xiāo).*

The formula is thus extremely effective for treating conditions of accumulation, obstruction, and damp-heat but should be reserved for patients without deficiency of normal qi, as explained by Fei Bo-Xiong (a staunch critic of Wang Ang) in *Discussion of Medical Formulas:*

> The formula contains many harshly-acting substances. One might therefore ask how much normal qi remains once the [acute manifestations] of the disorder have disappeared. Furthermore, what benefit is derived from adding Angelicae sinensis Radix *(dāng guī)* [resulting in a formula composed of] one moistening and eleven attacking [ingredients]? One must furthermore pay attention to the fact that formulas like this [and their attacking] strategies were originally published [to treat] strong, excessive people. Actually, strong, excessive people suffering from these patterns are extremely rare, while those with Spleen deficiency and feeble qi are common. It is absolutely inappropriate to prescribe formulas [that embody someone's] experience without paying proper attention [to the patients and disease dynamic that they treat].

Fei Bo-Xiong was famous for treating deficiency disorders in a clientele consisting mainly of upper class patients who were unaccustomed to exercise or physical labor and who were plagued by worries. Some contemporary practitioners believe that Zhang Zi-He's emphasis on elimination of excess may be more appropriate for patients in the West, while physicians in China use formulas such as this in the treatment of accumulations and masses such as cysts or fibroids.

Comparison

➤ Vs. Unripe Bitter Orange Pill to Guide Out Stagnation (zhǐ shí dǎo zhì wán)

Both formulas treat patterns where the accumulation of food and stagnation of qi transforms into damp-heat characterized by abdominal distention and pain, constipation, and dysenteric diarrhea. Both formulas combine herbs that open the qi dynamic with those that flush out accumulations from the Stomach and Intestines, and those that drain damp-heat. Moreover, when used for dysenteric disorders, both formulas apply a strategy known as 'facilitating the flow to treat disorders with too much flow.' However, Unripe Bitter Orange Pill to Guide Out Stagnation (zhǐ shí dǎo zhì wán) is stronger than this formula at eliminating dampness, but weaker at eliminating accumulation (i.e., the patient experiences distention without the feeling of fullness).

Modifications

- For dysenteric disorders, remove Citri reticulatae Pericarpium (chén pí), Curcumae Rhizoma (é zhú), and Pharbitidis Semen (qiān niú zǐ) and add Pulsatillae Radix (bái tóu wēng), Sophorae flavescentis Radix (kǔ shēn), and Paeoniae Radix alba (bái sháo).
- For harbored food, add Massa medicata fermentata (shén qū), Crataegi Fructus (shān zhā), and Raphani Semen (lái fú zǐ).
- For a thick, greasy tongue coating, add Atractylodis Rhizoma (cāng zhú).

Variations

木香檳榔丸 （木香槟榔丸）

Aucklandia and Betel Nut Pill from *Medical Formulas Collected and Analyzed*

mù xiāng bīng láng wán

Source *Medical Formulas Collected and Analyzed* (1682)

Add Angelicae sinensis Radix (dāng guī), Sparganii Rhizoma (sān léng), and Natrii Sulfas (máng xiāo) for severe obstruction with abdominal masses.

———————

木香檳榔丸 （木香槟榔丸）

Aucklandia and Betel Nut Pill from Zhu Dan-Xi

mù xiāng bīng láng wán

Source *Essential Teachings of [Zhu] Dan-Xi* (1481)

Add Aurantii Fructus (zhǐ ké) for more distention.

肥兒丸 （肥儿丸）

Fat Baby Pill

féi ér wán

This formula treats parasites in children that cause malnourishment and emaciation. When the problem is cured, the child becomes fat (a traditional sign of health), hence the name.

Source *Comprehensive and Subtle Discussion of Children's Health* (1156)

dry-fried Massa medicata fermentata (chǎo shén qū) 30g
Coptidis Rhizoma (huáng lián) 30g
roasted Myristicae Semen (wēi ròu dòu kòu) 15g
Quisqualis Fructus (shǐ jūn zǐ) 15g
dry-fried Hordei Fructus germinatus (chǎo mài yá) 15g
Arecae Semen (bīng láng) .12g
Aucklandiae Radix (mù xiāng) 6g

Method of Preparation Grind the ingredients into a powder and form into pills with pig gall. Take in 3g doses with warm water on an empty stomach. Reduce the dosage by half for infants under the age of one year.

Actions Kills parasites, reduces accumulation, strengthens the Spleen, and clears heat

Indications

Parasitic infestations with intermittent attacks of abdominal pain, indigestion, emaciation, loose stools, feverishness, foul-smelling breath, a sallow complexion, and a large, distended abdomen.

This is childhood nutritional impairment that develops from an accumulation of parasites. The accumulation injures the Spleen and gives rise to heat, which affects the Stomach. The movement of the parasites results in intermittent attacks of abdominal pain. Spleen deficiency is reflected in the indigestion, emaciation, and loose stools. Heat in the Stomach is manifested in the feverishness and foul-smelling breath. The combination of Spleen deficiency and heat in the Stomach results in a sallow complexion, emaciation, and a large, distended abdomen.

Analysis of Formula

This formula treats parasitic infestation by focusing on attacking the root, that is, the parasites themselves, while also clearing heat and strengthening the Spleen. The chief ingredients, Quisqualis Fructus (shǐ jūn zǐ) and Arecae Semen (bīng láng), have a strong antiparasitic effect. The deputies are Coptidis Rhizoma (huáng lián), which clears heat, and Myristicae Semen (ròu dòu kòu), which strengthens the Spleen. Together, they are an effective combination for treating Spleen deficiency due to accumulation with accompanying heat. In addition, the bitterness of Coptidis Rhizoma (huáng lián) assists the chief ingredients in directing the parasites downward. The assistants help reduce the stagnation in the middle burner: Aucklandiae Radix (mù xiāng) promotes the movement of qi in the middle burner; dry-fried Hordei Fructus germinatus (chǎo mài yá) and dry-fried Massa medicata fermentata (chǎo shén qū) directly reduce food stagnation. The pig gall used in making the pills serves as the envoy. When combined with Coptidis Rhizoma (huáng lián), it drains heat and accumulation from the Stomach, and conducts the actions of the other ingredients into the Stomach.

Cautions and Contraindications

This formula should be used only for primarily excessive types of childhood nutritional impairment, as it has no significant tonifying actions. Its name should not mislead one into using it as a general tonic or everyday supplement.

Commentary

Many different versions of this formula have been passed down, and the ingredients listed in different texts are not always the same (see ASSOCIATED FORMULA below). Furthermore, while its origin is widely traced to *Formulary of the Pharmacy Service for Benefiting the People in the Taiping Era*, the version that includes this formula was actually printed after the source text shown above. Most importantly, the name of this formula has led to considerable confusion and misuse over the centuries. Rather than employing it as a treatment for parasitic infection, physicians and patients have widely used it as a remedy to fatten up babies. In the early 17th century, already the Suzhou physician Zhang Lu commented on such malpractice:

> The [various versions] of this formula that have been transmitted through recent generations mainly contain [herbs such as] Picrorhizae Rhizoma (hú huáng lián), Omphalia (léi wán), and Ulmi macrocarpae Fructus preparatus (wú yí), which are very bitter and very cooling and greatly damage the original qi, but because of [the formula's] name, are utilized incorrectly. It is assumed that [its use] benefits infants and accordingly has been given happily by generations of physicians. If one understands the composition of this formula, [it is clear, however,] that its original [intention is the treatment] of hot-type nutritional impairment with a distended abdomen [despite general] emaciation. Therefore, one employs a formula that eliminates heat and curtails the Liver. By dispersing nutritional impairment accumulation, the original qi is able to return and the infant becomes fat again. However, if one prescribes it for cases without hot-type nutritional impairment, how does that differ from inviting a bandit in to ruin one's family?

Over two-hundred years later, the modern physician Xie Guan repeated the same warning in his *Great Encyclopedia of Chinese Medicine*. For this reason, perhaps, many contemporary textbooks list the formula as primarily antiparasitic in action. In clinical practice, it is important not to mistake signs such as lack of appetite, sallow complexion, fatigue, and weakness as signs of deficiency. Distinguishing signs are the distended abdomen, which in cases of qi deficiency would tend to be soft or, even if distended, relieved by pressure; constant low-grade fever, which in cases of qi deficiency would only occur after exertion; and bad breath, which would not be present in cases without heat.

Comparison

➢ Vs. CLOTH SACK PILL (bù dài wán); *see* PAGE 855

Biomedical Indications

With the appropriate presentation, this formula may be used to treat a variety of biomedically-defined disorders including ascariasis, hookworm, and chronic indigestion in children.

....

Alternate names

Seven Ingredient Fat Baby Pill (qī wèi féi ér wán) in *Collected Treatises of [Zhang] Jing-Yue*; Fat Baby Pill for Those Who Are Greatly Debilitated (dà wú féi ér wán) in *Collection of Versatility*

....

Modifications

• For severe qi deficiency accompanying the above presentation, add Codonopsis Radix (dǎng shēn) and Atractylodis macrocephalae Rhizoma (bái zhú).

• For cases with little or no internal heat, remove Coptidis Rhizoma (huáng lián).

• For constipation, add Rhei Radix et Rhizoma (dà huáng) and Aurantii Fructus immaturus (zhǐ shí).

• For firm masses in the abdomen, add Sparganii Rhizoma (sān léng) and Curcumae Rhizoma (é zhú).

Associated Formulas

金鑒肥兒丸 (金鉴肥儿丸)

Fat Baby Pill from *Golden Mirror*

Jīn jiàn féi ér wán

SOURCE   *Golden Mirror of the Medical Tradition* (1742)

Ginseng Radix (rén shēn)	12g
Atractylodis macrocephalae Rhizoma (bái zhú)	12g
Poria (fú líng)	1g
Coptidis Rhizoma (huáng lián)	12g
Picrorhizae Rhizoma (hú huáng lián)	12g
Quisqualis Fructus (shǐ jūn zǐ)	12g
dry-fried Massa medicata fermentata (chǎo shén qū)	12g
dry-fried Hordei Fructus germinatus (chǎo mài yá)	12g
Crataegi Fructus (shān zhā)	12g
Glycyrrhizae Radix praeparata (zhì gān cǎo)	6g
Aloe (lú huì)	12g

Grind the ingredients, mix with rice water, and form into millet-sized pills; 20-30 pills are taken per dose. Note that the dosage above comes from *Restoration of Health from the Myriad Diseases*.

This formula kills parasites, reduces accumulation, strengthens the Spleen, and clears heat. Compared to the principal formula, it has a much stronger ability to strengthen the Spleen and clear heat, making it suitable for longer-standing disorders or more severely deficient patients.

Comparision

➤ Vs. Open the Spleen Pill *(qǐ pí wán)*

Fat Baby Pill from *Golden Mirror (Jīn jiàn féi ér wán)* and Open the Spleen Pill *(qǐ pí wán)* both treat childhood nutritional impairment by dispersing accumulation and supplementing the middle burner. The first concentrates on dispersing food accumulations and clearing the heat that arises from accumulation of food and damp-heat in the digestive tract. In addition, it expels parasites. This inclusive approach makes the formula a good one for entrenched cases of childhood nutritional impairment, but leaves it with much less ability to supplement the middle than Open the Spleen Pill *(qǐ pí wán)*. That formula, on the other hand, is far less able to disperse stagnation than Fat Baby Pill from *Golden Mirror (Jīn jiàn féi ér wán)*. It also contains no agents to clear heat or expel parasites. Open the Spleen Pill *(qǐ pí wán)* is best suited for mild, initial cases of childhood nutritional impairment. When administering Fat Baby Pill from *Golden Mirror (Jīn jiàn féi ér wán)* to patients who are significantly deficient, it is useful to alternate it with doses of Open the Spleen Pill *(qǐ pí wán)* to ensure that middle burner qi is not depleted by the bitter and dispersing nature of Fat Baby Pill from *Golden Mirror (Jīn jiàn féi ér wán)*.

消乳丸

Reduce Infantile Stagnation Pill

xiāo rǔ wán

Source *Indispensable Tools for Pattern Treatment* (1602)

dry-fried Cyperi Rhizoma *(chǎo xiāng fù)*	60g
Glycyrrhizae Radix praeparata *(zhì gān cǎo)*	15g
Citri reticulatae Pericarpium *(chén pí)*	15g
Amomi Fructus *(shā rén)*	30g
dry-fried Massa medicata fermentata *(chǎo shén qū)*	30g
dry-fried Hordei Fructus germinatus *(chǎo mài yá)*	30g

Grind the ingredients into a powder and form into millet-sized pills with glutinous rice. Take after meals with a tea made from Zingiberis Rhizoma recens *(shēng jiāng)*. Reduces infantile stagnation and stops vomiting. For abdominal distention, vomiting, indigestion, and a submerged pulse in infants, usually associated with problems in nursing.

Section 2

FORMULAS THAT REDUCE FOOD STAGNATION BUT ALSO TONIFY

Food stagnation can readily lead to deficiency because it taxes the transporting and transforming functions of the middle burner. Likewise, patients with Spleen and Stomach deficiency are prone to food stagnation when they eat too much or when they eat food that they find difficult to digest. This leads to complex patterns that combine excess and deficiency in various degrees, characterized by such symptoms as lack of appetite, digestive difficulty, focal distention of the abdomen, loose stools, fatigue, a pale tongue with a white coating, and a deficient, frail pulse.

The formulas in this section are indicated for patterns where the symptoms of food stagnation are primary. They combine herbs that reduce food stagnation, move the qi, and drain heat with those that tonify the Spleen and Stomach such as Atractylodis macrocephalae Rhizoma *(bái zhú)*, Ginseng Radix *(rén shēn)*, Dioscoreae Rhizoma *(shān yào)*, Nelumbinis Semen *(lián zǐ)*, and Glycyrrhizae Radix *(gān cǎo)*. Once the main symptoms of food stagnation have been relieved, it is appropriate to switch to tonifying formulas to which qi-regulating and reducing ingredients have been added.

健脾丸

Strengthen the Spleen Pill

jiàn pí wán

This formula strengthens the Spleen while also reducing food stagnation that would further weaken that organ. Its principal ingredients are those of Four-Gentlemen Decoction *(sì jūn zǐ tāng)*, discussed in Chapter 8. This is one of the main formulas for tonifying the Spleen qi.

Source *Indispensable Tools for Pattern Treatment* (1602)

dry-fried Atractylodis macrocephalae Rhizoma *(chǎo bái zhú)*	75g
Poria *(fú líng)*	60g
Ginseng Radix *(rén shēn)*	45g
Dioscoreae Rhizoma *(shān yào)*	30g
roasted Myristicae Semen *(wēi ròu dòu kòu)*	30g
Crataegi Fructus *(shān zhā)*	30g
dry-fried Massa medicata fermentata *(chǎo shén qū)*	30g
dry-fried Hordei Fructus germinatus *(chǎo mài yá)*	30g
Aucklandiae Radix *(mù xiāng)*	22.5g
Citri reticulatae Pericarpium *(chén pí)*	30g
Amomi Fructus *(shā rén)*	30g
wine-fried Coptidis Rhizoma *(jiǔ chǎo huáng lián)*	22.5g
Glycyrrhizae Radix *(gān cǎo)*	22.5g

Method of Preparation Grind the ingredients into a powder and form into pills with water. Take 6-9g twice a day with warm water. At present, Codonopsis Radix *(dǎng shēn)* is usually substituted for Ginseng Radix *(rén shēn)* at 2-3 times its dosage. May also be prepared as a decoction with a proportionate reduction in dosage.

Actions Strengthens the Spleen, reduces food stagnation, and stops diarrhea

Indications

Reduced appetite with difficulty in digestion, bloating and focal distention of the epigastrium and abdomen, loose and watery diarrhea, a greasy, slightly yellow tongue coating, and a deficient, frail pulse.

This disorder occurs when Spleen and Stomach deficiency is complicated by food accumulation that has begun to transform into heat. When the Spleen and Stomach are weak and their transforming and transporting functions lose strength, there will be a loss of appetite and difficulty in digesting food. Bloating and focal distention in the epigastrium and abdomen are caused by food stagnation obstructing the qi mechanisms of the middle burner. The deficient Spleen is unable to send its qi upward and also gives rise to dampness, manifested as loose and watery diarrhea and a deficient, frail pulse. Because the accumulation of food has begun to transform into heat, the tongue coating is greasy and slightly yellow.

Analysis of Formula

In this pattern, the deficient aspects are more significant than those of excess. The primary focus of the formula is therefore on tonifying the Spleen, while reducing food stagnation is the secondary strategy.

The chief herbs are Atractylodis macrocephalae Rhizoma (bái zhú) and Poria (fú líng), used in a large dosage to strengthen the Spleen, leach out dampness, and stop the diarrhea. The deputies are Crataegi Fructus (shān zhā), dry-fried Massa medicata fermentata (chǎo shén qū) , and dry-fried Hordei Fructus germinatus (chǎo mài yá), which reduce food stagnation and harmonize the Stomach. Most of the other ingredients serve as assistants. Ginseng Radix (rén shēn) and Dioscoreae Rhizoma (shān yào) tonify the Spleen and Stomach and help the chief herbs in stopping the diarrhea. Myristicae Semen (ròu dòu kòu), Aucklandiae Radix (mù xiāng), Citri reticulatae Pericarpium (chén pí), and Amomi Fructus (shā rén) are acrid and aromatic herbs that regulate the qi and open the Stomach, awaken the Spleen, and transform dampness. Eliminating bloating and focal distention, they also ensure that the tonifying ingredients do not further obstruct the qi dynamic. In combination, Myristicae Semen (ròu dòu kòu) and Dioscoreae Rhizoma (shān yào) also warm the middle burner and bind up the Intestines. Wine-fried Coptidis Rhizoma (jiǔ chǎo huáng lián) drains heat and dries dampness. The envoy is Glycyrrhizae Radix (gān cǎo), which harmonizes the actions of the other herbs and helps the chief herbs tonify the middle burner.

Cautions and Contraindications

Contraindicated in acute cases of food stagnation from contaminated food or from overconsumption of food and drink. This is because the tonifying strategy underlying the formula may increase the stagnation and thereby aggravate such conditions.

Commentary

The original indications for this formula merely read "any situation of Spleen and Stomach not being harmonized [leading to] digestive overwork and fatigue." This implies that the formula is primarily tonifying in nature, as explained by Fei Bo-Xiong in *Discussion of Medical Formulas*:

> Although the strategy [here] is to use reducing within tonification, it principally excels when used for the purposes of tonification. Unless stagnant turbid qi has been cleared, a tonifying prescription [used on its own] will be rejected and thus does not enter.

However, the literature contains many variations of this formula, some of which reverse the relative dosage and number of reducing and tonifying ingredients. These formulas, such as Strengthen the Spleen Pill from *Medical Formulas Collected and Analyzed* (jiàn pí wán), listed below, can be used to treat acute food stagnation in patients with constitutional Spleen deficiency.

In clinical practice, abdominal distention and lack of appetite are key markers for the use of this formula. It should be modified according to the actual presentation, following the suggestions below.

Comparisons

➤ Vs. Unripe Bitter Orange and Atractylodes Pill (zhǐ zhú wán); see PAGE 838

➤ Vs. Preserve Harmony Pill (bǎo hé wán); see PAGE 828

➤ Vs. Unripe Bitter Orange Pill to Reduce Focal Distention (zhǐ shí xiāo pǐ wán); see PAGE 840

Biomedical Indications

With the appropriate presentation, this formula may be used to treat a variety of biomedically-defined disorders including chronic gastritis, chronic colitis, and indigestion.

Alternate name

Greatly Strengthen the Spleen Pill (dà jiàn pí wán) in *Collection of Versatility*

Modifications

- For cases with no symptoms of heat, remove wine-fried Coptidis Rhizoma (jiǔ chǎo huáng lián); if there are signs of cold, add Zingiberis Rhizoma (gān jiāng).

- For nausea and vomiting, add Pinelliae Rhizoma praeparatum (zhì bàn xià) and Zingiberis Rhizoma recens (shēng jiāng).

- For cases without diarrhea, replace Myristicae Semen (ròu dòu kòu) with Pinelliae Rhizoma (bàn xià).

- For diarrhea as the main symptom, add Coicis Semen (yì yǐ rén), Lablab Semen album (biǎn dòu), and Alismatis Rhizoma (zé xiè).

- For daybreak diarrhea with symptoms of food stagnation, take with Aconite Accessory Root Pill to Regulate the Middle (*fù zǐ lǐ zhōng wán*).

Associated Formula

健脾丸

Strengthen the Spleen Pill from *Medical Formulas Collected and Analyzed*

jiàn pí wán

Source *Medical Formulas Collected and Analyzed* (1682)

Ginseng Radix (*rén shēn*) 60g
dry-fried Atractylodis macrocephalae Rhizoma
  (*chǎo bái zhú*) 60g
Citri reticulatae Pericarpium (*chén pí*) 60g
dry-fried Hordei Fructus germinatus (*chǎo mài yá*) 60g
Crataegi Fructus (*shān zhā*) 45g
Aurantii Fructus immaturus (*zhǐ shí*) 90g

Compared to the principal formula, this is more strongly weighted toward reducing food stagnation, as explained by Zhang Bin-Cheng in *Convenient Reader of Established Formulas:*

> [This formula] treats Spleen deficiency [complicated by] food that has not been digested. This occurs when food accumulation, phlegm stagnation, and stasis in the interior [combine with] Spleen and Stomach deficiency. Spleen and Stomach deficiency occur gradually, and thus are the root of this disorder. Food accumulation tarrying [in the middle burner to cause] stagnation occurs suddenly, and thus is the manifestation of this disorder. In treating any disorder, one should be clear about root and manifestations, slow and urgent [pathological processes]. In urgent processes, one treats the manifestation; in slow processes, one treats the root. Thus, [this formula] employs bitter and cooling Aurantii Fructus immaturus (*zhǐ shí*) as chief to break up qi [stagnation], move the blood, and reduce food and phlegm [stagnation because] it is an important herb for wearing down accumulation. Secondarily, one employs Ginseng Radix (*rén shēn*) and Atractylodis macrocephalae Rhizoma (*bái zhú*) to control its excess and prevent it from damaging the normal qi.

A comparison of this analysis with that of Fei Bo-Xiong for the principal formula clearly reveals their differences.

枳术丸 (枳术丸)
Unripe Bitter Orange and Atractylodes Pill

zhǐ zhú wán

Source *Clarifying Doubts about Damage from Internal and External Causes* (1247)

Atractylodis macrocephalae Rhizoma (*bái zhú*) . . . 60g (12-18g)
dry-fried Aurantii Fructus immaturus (*chǎo zhǐ shí*) . . 30g (6-9g)

Method of Preparation Grind the ingredients into a powder and form into pills with rice fried in Nelumbinis Folium (*hé yè*).

Take 6-9g with water twice a day. (Many formulations omit the fried rice.) May also be prepared as a decoction with the dosage specified in parentheses.

Actions Tonifies the Spleen and reduces focal distention

Indications

Loss of appetite, focal distention in the epigastrium and abdomen, a white tongue coating, and a deficient pulse.

When the Spleen and Stomach are deficient, the transforming and transporting functions of these organs are diminished, and food is more likely to stagnate in the digestive system. The combination of Spleen and Stomach deficiency and food stagnation leads to a loss of appetite. It also obstructs the qi mechanism of the middle burner and causes focal distention in the epigastrium. The white tongue coating and deficient pulse reflect the underlying deficiency of the Spleen.

Analysis of Formula

Tonification is required to treat the deficient Spleen, and promotion of the movement of qi is required to treat the stagnation. The chief herb, Atractylodis macrocephalae Rhizoma (*bái zhú*), strengthens the Spleen and eliminates dampness to help the transforming and transporting functions of the Spleen. The deputy, Aurantii Fructus immaturus (*zhǐ shí*), effectively reduces epigastric focal distention by transforming stagnation and directing the qi downward. The fact that the dosage of the chief herb is twice that of the deputy reflects the precedence of tonification over the reduction of stagnation in this formula. Nelumbinis Folium (*hé yè*), used in the preparation of the pill, raises the clear yang of the Spleen and helps the chief herb strengthen the Spleen. When matched with the deputy, which causes the turbid to descend, it makes an effective combination for harmonizing the directional tendencies of the Spleen and Stomach.

Commentary

This is a variation of a formula found in *Essentials from the Golden Cabinet* called Unripe Bitter Orange and Atractylodes Decoction (*zhǐ zhú tāng*), which is discussed below. Because it is mentioned in all of Li Dong-Yuan's major works, his earliest-published book is listed as the source text. There the formula is clearly attributed to Li's own teacher, Zhang Yuan-Su, and introduced as the major formula for internal damage due to overeating in the course of internal damage disorders (see the discussion of Tonify the Middle to Augment the Qi Decoction (*bǔ zhōng yì qì tāng*) in Chapter 8 for a more detailed discussion of these disorders). In *Discussion of the Spleen and Stomach*, Li observes: "This formula is not designed to rapidly transform food stagnation, but to strengthen the Stomach qi so that injury does not recur." The idea here is that the body's nutritive and protective qi depend for their generation on the harmonious functioning of the middle burner. Lack of appetite thus indicates an inability to generate qi, including the qi that might be generated from herbs. *Clarifying Doubts about Injury from Internal and External Causes* explains how this formula facilitates digestion:

> Atractylodis macrocephalae Rhizoma (*bái zhú*) is bitter, sweet, and warming. Its sweet and warming [nature] tonifies the original qi of the Spleen and Stomach. Its bitter flavor eliminates damp-heat from the Stomach and facilitates [the physiological dynamic] of blood [in the area] between the waist and navel. In order to focus on tonifying a debilitated Spleen and Stomach, its dosage is double that of the digestion-promoting herb Aurantii Fructus immaturus (*zhǐ shí*). Aurantii Fructus immaturus (*zhǐ shí*) has a bitter taste and is cooling. It drains focal distention in the epigastrium and damage to digestion of the Stomach. This one herb drives the Stomach [qi] downward [to eliminate that which] a damaged [digestion] cannot itself eliminate. But one must only use 3g at a time and that which is eaten will be digested. Because one has first tonified the deficiency and then transformed that which was damaged, [this does not constitute] a harsh facilitation.

The ability of this formula to reduce food stagnation is not particularly strong, and it is therefore usually combined with other ingredients (see MODIFICATIONS below). Today, it is most often used as an additive to other formulas for food stagnation. Nevertheless, as Fei Bo-Xiong noted in *Discussion of Medical Formulas*, "[This formula composed of] one [herb] that tonifies the Spleen and one that eliminates excess is convenient, yet has a method. Do not dismiss it lightly just because it is simple and unassuming."

Comparisons

➤ Vs. STRENGTHEN THE SPLEEN PILL (*jiàn pí wán*)

Both of these formulas are frequently used for patterns characterized by food stagnation in the context of deficiency and digestive weakness, with deficiency being more prominent than stagnation. Unripe Bitter Orange and Atractylodes Pill (*zhǐ zhú wán*) is very simple in its composition, focusing mainly on middle burner deficiency accompanied by distention. This provides it with a wide range of applications, especially if it is further modified in accordance with the presenting signs and symptoms. Although Aurantii Fructus immaturus (*zhǐ shí*) is somewhat cooling, the formula is not indicated for patterns with significant heat, and a white tongue coating is a distinguishing sign. By contrast, the design of Strengthen the Spleen Pill from *Medical Formulas Collected and Analyzed* (*jiàn pí wán*) is more complex, encompassing herbs that tonify deficiency, disperse food stagnation, drain heat, resolve dampness, and warm the middle. While more tonifying in nature than Unripe Bitter Orange and Atractylodes Pill (*zhǐ zhú wán*), it is nevertheless able to drain heat from stasis. It is thus specifically indicated for patterns characterized by soft or loose stools on the one hand, and a thin, yellow tongue coating on the other.

➤ Vs. UNRIPE BITTER ORANGE PILL TO REDUCE FOCAL DISTENTION (*zhǐ shí xiāo pǐ wán*); see PAGE 840

Biomedical Indications

With the appropriate presentation, this formula may be used to treat a variety of biomedically-defined disorders including chronic gastritis, chronic colitis, and peptic ulcers.

Modifications

- For general debility, add Codonopsis Radix (*dǎng shēn*) and Poria (*fú líng*).
- For prolapse or ptosis, combine with Raise the Sunken Decoction (*shēng xiàn tāng*). For gastric ptosis, also add Amomi Fructus (*shā rén*) and Salviae miltiorrhizae Radix (*dān shēn*); for uterine prolapse, also add Leonuri Herba (*yì mǔ cǎo*) and Angelicae sinensis Radix (*dāng guī*); for rectal prolapse, also add Granati Pericarpium (*shí liú pí*).
- For diarrhea, add Poria (*fú líng*) and Coicis Semen (*yì yǐ rén*).
- For more pronounced food stagnation, add Massa medicata fermentata (*shén qū*), Crataegi Fructus (*shān zhā*), and Hordei Fructus germinatus (*mài yá*).

Variations

曲麥枳朮丸 (曲麦枳术丸)

Medicated Leaven, Barley Sprout, Unripe Bitter Orange, and Atractylodes Pill

qū mài zhǐ zhú wán

SOURCE *Indispensable Tools for Pattern Treatment* (1602)

Add Massa medicata fermentata (*shén qū*) and Hordei Fructus germinatus (*mài yá*) for severe food stagnation.

香砂枳朮丸 (香砂枳术丸)

Aucklandia, Amomum, Unripe Bitter Orange, and Atractylodes Pill

xiāng shā zhǐ zhú wán

SOURCE *Collected Treatises of [Zhang] Jing-Yue* (1624)

Add Aucklandiae Radix (*mù xiāng*) and Amomi Fructus (*shā rén*) for gastric pain.

Associated Formula

枳朮湯 (枳术汤)

Unripe Bitter Orange and Atractylodes Decoction

zhǐ zhú tāng

SOURCE *Essentials from the Golden Cabinet* (c. 220)

Aurantii Fructus immaturus (*zhǐ shí*). 12g
Atractylodis macrocephalae Rhizoma (*bái zhú*) 6g

Promotes the movement of qi, dissipates clumping, strengthens the Spleen, and reduces food stagnation. For hard, broad focal distention in the epigastrium due to thin mucus with reduced appetite, belching, a white, greasy tongue coating, and a submerged, wiry pulse. The relative dosage of the two herbs is reversed from that in the principal formula, as here the emphasis is on reducing focal distention by promoting the movement of qi, with tonification being of secondary importance. This difference is also reflected in the method of preparation: a decoction is taken for a relatively acute disorder, while a pill is more likely to be taken long-term.

枳實消痞丸（枳实消痞丸）
Unripe Bitter Orange Pill to Reduce Focal Distention

zhǐ shí xiāo pǐ wán

Source   *Secrets from the Orchid Chamber* (1336)

Aurantii Fructus immaturus (*zhǐ shí*). 15g
prepared Magnoliae officinalis Cortex (*zhì hòu pò*) 12g
Coptidis Rhizoma (*huáng lián*) 15g
Pinelliae Rhizoma praeparatum (*zhì bàn xià*) 9g
Ginseng Radix (*rén shēn*) 9g
Atractylodis macrocephalae Rhizoma (*bái zhú*) 6g
Poria (*fú líng*) 6g
Hordei Fructus germinatus (*mài yá*) 6g
Zingiberis Rhizoma (*gān jiāng*) 6g
Glycyrrhizae Radix praeparata (*zhì gān cǎo*). 6g

Method of Preparation   Grind the ingredients into a powder and form into small pills. Take 6-9g twice daily with warm water apart from meals. At present, Codonopsis Radix (*dǎng shēn*) is usually substituted for Ginseng Radix (*rén shēn*) at 2-3 times its dosage. May also be prepared as a decoction with a proportionate adjustment in dosage.

Actions   Reduces focal distention, eliminates fullness, strengthens the Spleen, and harmonizes the Stomach

Indications

Focal distention and fullness in the upper epigastrium, lack of thirst or appetite, fatigue, and weakness. There may also be focal distention in the chest and abdomen, a wan complexion, poor digestion, irregular bowel movements (sometimes loose, sometimes hard), and a wiry pulse at the right, middle position. The tongue coating is greasy and may be yellow in color.

This is a complex mixed pattern of deficiency and excess characterized by Spleen deficiency and qi stagnation with mutual clumping of heat and cold. This type of condition arises when a weak and deficient Spleen and Stomach lose control over the ascending and descending functions of the middle burner. The obstruction of these functions, together with the accumulation of dampness, results in focal distention and fullness in the upper epigastrium and a lack of thirst or appetite. The Spleen deficiency is reflected in the reduced appetite,

wan complexion, weakness, and fatigue. Lack of thirst and appetite indicate that, despite the presence of a yellow tongue coating, the yang qi is deficient and the yin is excessive. Yin excess here implies the presence of fluids, phlegm, and undigested food. This leads to constraint, as reflected in the wiry pulse, and consequently to the generation of heat. Weakness in the transporting functions of the Spleen, together with the internal cold-heat complex, disturb the movement of the bowels, leading to irregularity.

Analysis of Formula

Although this is a combined pattern of deficiency and excess, the excess is more pronounced than the deficiency, and the heat is more severe than the cold. Therefore, in this formula, more emphasis is placed on those herbs that reduce the focal distention and fullness than on those that strengthen the Spleen and harmonize the Stomach. The chief herb, Aurantii Fructus immaturus (*zhǐ shí*), promotes the movement of qi and is one of the principal substances used for treating focal distention in the epigastrium. One of the deputies, prepared Magnoliae officinalis Cortex (*zhì hòu pò*), promotes the movement of qi and eliminates fullness. It acts synergistically with the chief herb. Two other deputies, Coptidis Rhizoma (*huáng lián*) and Pinelliae Rhizoma praeparatum (*zhì bàn xià*), have complementary functions. The former has a bitter, cooling nature; it drains heat and dries dampness. The latter has an acrid, warming nature; it causes rebellious qi to descend and dissipates clumping. Together, they open up the middle burner to reduce focal distention and thereby assist the chief herb. The final deputy, Ginseng Radix (*rén shēn*), is used here to support the normal qi and prevent it from being harmed by the cold, dispersing ingredients in the formula. It also strengthens the Spleen, which is the root of this disorder.

Among the assistant herbs are Atractylodis macrocephalae Rhizoma (*bái zhú*) and Poria (*fú líng*), which strengthen the Spleen and dry dampness. They serve as adjuncts to Ginseng Radix (*rén shēn*). Hordei Fructus germinatus (*mài yá*) reduces food stagnation and harmonizes the Stomach, while Zingiberis Rhizoma (*gān jiāng*) promotes the movement of yang in the middle burner to disperse the cold. Together, they treat the obstructive combination of yin excess and food stagnation, an aspect not addressed by other herbs in the formula. The envoy, Glycyrrhizae Radix praeparata (*zhì gān cǎo*), primarily harmonizes the actions of the other herbs and also augments the middle qi.

Commentary

This formula is a variation of Pinellia Decoction to Drain the Epigastrium (*bàn xià xiè xīn tāng*), discussed in Chapter 3, which is combined here with Unripe Bitter Orange and Atractylodes Pill (*zhǐ zhú wán*), discussed above, and Four-

Gentlemen Decoction *(sì jūn zǐ tāng)*, discussed in Chapter 8. Key markers to the pattern for which this formula is indicated are the focal distention in the epigastrium and its related digestive weakness. The focal distention manifests as a subjective feeling of fullness, which on palpation is experienced as resistance, but can sometimes become a harder, palpable mass. The palpation does not, however, elicit pain. Digestive weakness is reflected in the occurrence of the symptoms in direct relation to eating. The patient may also present with one other symptom that is regarded by some as a sign of excess: a very strong aversion to a particular food, usually one in which they have overindulged.

Pathodynamic

Although the etiology of this pattern is often described in terms of a heat-cold complex, in which the aspects of heat and excess predominate, there are often no signs of heat or cold at all. As explained in the entry for Pinellia Decoction to Drain the Epigastrium *(bàn xià xiè xīn tāng)* in Chapter 3, some commentators have suggested that we view the warming and cooling herbs in this formula as promoting the ascent of clear yang and the downward draining of turbid yin, rather than as treating symptoms of heat or cold. Zhang Bin-Cheng's analysis of this formula in *Convenient Reader of Established Formulas* is representative of this view:

> Focal distention is fullness without pain. Focal distention pertains to the pathogens that have no form. Entering [the organism] from the outside, it lodges in the area between the chest and Stomach. It does not yet [lead to] a formed, mutual clumping of phlegm, blood, and food but is rather an illness contracted because the normal qi contending [with the pathogen] clusters in one place. Therefore, Coptidis Rhizoma *(huáng lián)* and Zingiberis Rhizoma *(gān jiāng)* are used synergistically. One is acrid, the other bitter; one disperses, the other directs downward. Regardless of whether pathogenic cold or heat are present, they open [the constraint] and drain [the excess]. These two herbs are truly important in treating focal distention.
>
> Naturally, when focal distention clumps in the middle [burner] the qi clogs up and dampness collects, which of necessity will gradually lead to combined obstruction by phlegm and food. Therefore, [the formula] employs Aurantii Fructus immaturus *(zhǐ shí)* to break up qi [stagnation], Magnoliae officinalis Cortex *(hòu pò)* to disperse dampness, Hordei Fructus germinatus *(mài yá)* to transform food [stagnation], and Pinelliae Rhizoma *(bàn xià)* to move phlegm and [thereby] obtain a momentum that does not make this a stubborn and difficult illness. However, in order for a pathogen to collect, a patient's qi must be deficient. Thus, one must use Four-Gentlemen Decoction *(sì jūn zǐ tāng)*, which takes command of the middle region, dispels pathogenic [qi] while supporting the normal [qi so that both aspects of treatment] remain aligned with each other. Accordingly, this formula is able to treat focal distention irrespective of whether it is due to excess or deficiency.

Pulse

Another important clinical marker for this pattern is a wiry pulse in the right middle pulse position, which corresponds to the Spleen and Stomach. This pulse reflects constraint in the ascent of the clear yang (governed by Liver wood) by phlegm and accumulated food, as explained by Fei Bo-Xiong in *Discussion of Medical Formulas*:

> The beauty of this formula rests entirely in [its combination] of Zingiberis Rhizoma *(gān jiāng)* and Coptidis Rhizoma *(huáng lián)* [because] bitter, acrid [herbs employed synergistically] are able to balance wood. Unless [this combination] addressed itself entirely to the Liver channel, would the indications speak of a wiry pulse in the right middle position?

Biomedical Indications

With the appropriate presentation, this formula may be used to treat a variety of biomedically-defined disorders including chronic gastritis and functional gastrointestinal disorders.

Comparisons

> ➢ Vs. Unripe Bitter Orange and Atractylodes Pill *(zhǐ zhú wán)* and Strengthen the Spleen Pill *(jiàn pí wán)*

All of these formulas treat food stagnation in the context of mixed patterns of excess and deficiency. However, while the principal formula focuses on the treatment of excess, the other two are more suitable for deficiency.

> ➢ Vs. Pinellia Decoction to Drain the Epigastrium *(bàn xià xiè xīn tāng)*

Both of these formulas treat focal distention in the epigastrium. Indeed, Unripe Bitter Orange Pill to Reduce Focal Distention *(zhǐ shí xiāo pǐ wán)* can be seen as a modification of Pinellia Decoction to Drain the Epigastrium *(bàn xià xiè xīn tāng)*. However, the former focuses more strongly on breaking up qi stagnation, which is reflected in the dosages of Aurantii Fructus immaturus *(zhǐ shí)* and Magnoliae officinalis Cortex *(hòu pò)*, which are the largest in the formula. This underscores the importance of promoting the movement of qi in treating food stagnation. Pinellia Decoction to Drain the Epigastrium *(bàn xià xiè xīn tāng)*, on the other hand, contains Scutellariae Radix *(huáng qín)*, reflecting its focus on draining, because the pathogen in that pattern was originally cold that has transformed into heat.

Alternate name

Sudden Smile Pill *(shī xiào wán)* in *Secrets from the Orchid Chamber*

Modifications

- For severe cold and pain, reduce the dosage of Coptidis Rhizoma *(huáng lián)* and increase that of Zingiberis Rhizoma *(gān jiāng)*; also add Alpiniae officinarum Rhizoma *(gāo liáng jiāng)* and Cinnamomi Cortex *(ròu guì)*.

- For a chronic, productive cough with wheezing and a sensation of fullness and focal distention in the chest and diaphragm, remove Coptidis Rhizoma *(huáng lián)* and add Citri reticulatae Pericarpium *(chén pí)* and Amomi Fructus *(shā rén)*.

- For accumulation due to parasites, add Quisqualis Fructus *(shǐ jūn zǐ)* and Arecae Semen *(bīng láng)*.

- For more pronounced qi stagnation with pain, add Aucklandiae Radix *(mù xiāng)* and Citri reticulatae Pericarpium *(chén pí)*.

- For more pronounced symptoms of food stagnation, add Crataegi Fructus *(shān zhā)* and Massa medicata fermentata *(shén qū)*.

- For more pronounced dampness, add Atractylodis Rhizoma *(cāng zhú)*.

葛花解醒散
Kudzu Flower Powder to Relieve Hangovers

gé huā jiě chéng sǎn

Source *Discussion of the Spleen and Stomach* (13th century)

Amomi Fructus rotundus *(bái dòu kòu)* 15g
Amomi Fructus *(shā rén)* 15g
Puerariae Flos *(gé huā)* 15g
Zingiberis Rhizoma *(gān jiāng)* 6.0g
dry-fried Massa medicata fermentata *(chǎo shén qū)* 6.0g
Alismatis Rhizoma *(zé xiè)* 6.0g
Atractylodis macrocephalae Rhizoma *(bái zhú)* 6.0g
Citri reticulatae Pericarpium *(chén pí)* 4.5g
Ginseng Radix *(rén shēn)* 4.5g
Polyporus *(zhū líng)* 4.5g
Poria *(fú líng)* 4.5g
Aucklandiae Radix *(mù xiāng)* 1.5g
Citri reticulatae viride Pericarpium *(qīng pí)* 0.9g

Method of Preparation The source text suggests grinding the ingredients into a powder and taking about 9g per dose with warm water. A slight sweat is produced that indicates that the disease from alcohol has been dispelled. At present, the formula is also prepared as a decoction, with the dosage of Citri reticulatae viride Pericarpium *(qīng pí)* and Aucklandiae Radix *(mù xiāng)* increased slightly.

Actions Separates and reduces alcohol-dampness, warms the middle, and strengthens the Spleen

Indications

Vomiting, headache, Heart irritability, trembling of the hands and feet, focal distention in the chest and diaphragm, re-

duced appetite, fatigue, diarrhea, inhibited urination, a greasy tongue coating, and a slippery pulse. These symptoms may occur after a single drinking bout or as the result of habitual overindulgence in alcohol.

Alcohol is derived from the essence of grain; in small amounts it moves the qi and blood, strengthens the Spleen and Stomach, and aids digestion. Excessive consumption, however, damages the same organs. Subsequently, a weakened Spleen is readily encumbered by dampness, which collects internally and gives rise to dizziness, vomiting, reduced appetite, fatigue, focal distention in the chest and diaphragm, and diarrhea.

Alcohol is extremely hot in nature, and excessive intake, combined with the impaired ability of the middle burner to transform and transport, gives rise to the accumulation of damp-heat in the yang-brightness channels. This can cause headache and irritability. The tongue and pulse reflect the presence of dampness.

Analysis of Formula

The chief ingredient, Puerariae Flos *(gé huā)*, enters the yang brightness, resolves alcohol toxicity, rouses the Spleen, and resolves damp-heat through gentle sweating. Its use in the treatment of the side effects of alcohol consumption goes back at least to the 6th-century text, *Miscellaneous Records of Famous Physicians*. The deputy ingredients focus on the stagnation in the middle burner. Amomi Fructus *(shā rén)*, Amomi Fructus rotundus *(bái dòu kòu)*, Citri reticulatae viride Pericarpium *(qīng pí)*, Aucklandiae Radix *(mù xiāng)*, and Zingiberis Rhizoma *(gān jiāng)* warm the middle, strengthen the Spleen, harmonize the Stomach, and regulate the qi dynamic. Thus, the Spleen gains control over the accumulation of dampness. Massa medicata fermentata *(shén qū)* resolves alcohol toxicity and assists the Spleen in transforming and transporting the stagnant, partially-digested food. This is necessary because a Spleen burdened with damp-heat accumulation is unable to move food along, and the stagnant food combines with the alcohol toxin to produce symptoms such as headache and nausea. Qi-moving agents, such as Amomi Fructus *(shā rén)* and Aucklandiae Radix *(mù xiāng)*, support Massa medicata fermentata *(shén qū)* in this function.

One group of assistants, Ginseng Radix *(rén shēn)* and Atractylodis macrocephalae Rhizoma *(bái zhú)*, tonifies the middle and strengthens the Spleen and Stomach, thus helping those organs to recuperate from the damage caused by excessive alcohol consumption. The other group, Poria *(fú líng)*, Polyporus *(zhū líng)* and Alismatis Rhizoma *(zé xiè)*, dispel damp-heat by promoting urination.

Li Dong-Yuan observed that the accumulation of damp-heat alcohol toxin is best resolved by dispersing it through mild sweating above and urination below. This formula accomplishes those goals while at the same time regulating the middle burner qi and dispersing accumulations of damp-heat and partially-digested food.

Cautions and Contraindications

This formula is suited for those with Spleen deficiency and accumulation of damp-heat, but should not be taken long-term as it can deplete the qi and injure the fluids. *Medical Formulas Collected and Analyzed* notes that the formula should not be given to patients who are very thirsty.

Commentary

Alternate Analyses of Formula

There are some who regard this formula as a modification of Six-Gentlemen Decoction with Aucklandia and Amomum *(xiāng shā liù jūn zǐ tāng)* in that its primary functions are to rectify and tonify the qi of the middle burner. In this analysis, Atractylodis macrocephalae Rhizoma *(bái zhú)* and Ginseng Radix *(rén shēn)* serve as the chief herbs. Another view, overlapping with that in the ANALYSIS OF FORMULA above, is that Puerariae Flos *(gé huā)* is the chief ingredient, the urine-promoting herbs are the deputies, and the qi-regulating and qi-tonifying herbs of Six-Gentlemen Decoction with Aucklandia and Amomum *(xiāng shā liù jūn zǐ tāng)* are the assistants. This debate underscores that the formula treats both root and branch. Which of these is emphasized in treatment depends on how entrenched the condition is, how extreme the symptoms are, and how depleted the patient is as a result of this illness.

Historical Context

In the source text, this formula appears in the context of a discussion on the correct manner of treating alcohol toxicity. At that time, the common method for treating this disorder was to purge, using either hot or cold, downward-draining herbs such as Rhei Radix et Rhizoma *(dà huáng)* or Pharbitidis Semen *(qiān niú zǐ)*. Li Gao suggested that this was ill-advised and could lead to such dire results as a disorder called 'alcohol jaundice' (酒疸 *jiǔ dǎn*). Instead, he suggested that gentle sweating and mild promotion of urination, coupled with regulation and tonification of middle burner qi, was the best way to treat this condition, and he cited this formula as an exemplar. Note that the adverse consequences of purging patients weakened by alcohol is also mentioned in *Essentials from the Golden Cabinet*: "If alcohol jaundice is purged, it will eventually lead to black jaundice."

Usage

This formula is listed as the primary choice for treatment of uncomplicated alcohol toxicity from the Yuan dynasty onward. The texts never say whether it is intended for a single bout of overindulgence and the resulting hangover, or for the accumulation of damp-heat toxin in one for whom the immoderate use of alcohol is a lifestyle. Certainly, most of the symptoms listed in the source text, and the name of the formula itself, would lead one to believe that hangovers are the intended target. Suffice to say that, at present, the formula is thought to be appropriate for both types of problems, as reflected in the unambiguous statement of the prominent contemporary physician, Zhu Liang-Chun: "Regardless of whether there is a single instance of excessive alcohol consumption giving rise to drunken toxicity, or if frequent alcohol excess has damaged the Spleen and Stomach, the use of this formula is appropriate."

Li Gao cautions those who might misuse this formula that, although it is designed to relieve alcohol toxicity and reduce the aftereffects of drinking alcohol, it does not prevent alcohol's damage to the source qi.

Biomedical Indications

With the appropriate presentation, this formula may be used to treat a variety of biomedically-defined disorders including hangovers and alcoholism.

Alternate names

Kudzu Flower Decoction to Relieve Hangovers *(gé huā jiě jiǔ tāng)* in *Great Compendium of Medical Formulas*; Decoction to Relieve Hangovers *(jiě chéng tāng)* in *Pulse, Causes, Symptoms, and Treatment*; Kudzu Flower Decoction *(gé huā tāng)* in *Essentials for Those Who Do Not Know Medicine*

Modifications

- For significant vomiting, add Pinelliae Rhizoma praeparatum *(zhì bàn xià)* and Zingiberis Rhizoma recens *(shēng jiāng)*.
- For extreme abdominal distention, add Aurantii Fructus immaturus *(zhǐ shí)* and Arecae Pericarpium *(dà fù pí)*.
- If food accumulation is present marked by distention and a lack of appetite, add Raphani Semen *(lái fú zǐ)* and Crataegi Fructus *(shān zhā)*.
- For more signs of cold, add Evodiae Fructus *(wú zhū yú)*.
- For more signs of damp-heat, add Coptidis Rhizoma *(huáng lián)* and Scutellariae Radix *(huáng qín)*.

Comparative Tables of Principal Formulas

■ FORMULAS THAT REDUCE FOOD ACCUMULATION AND TRANSFORM STAGNATION

Common symptoms: focal distention and pain in the epigastrium and abdomen, constipation or diarrhea, yellow, greasy tongue coating, slippery or submerged and excessive pulse

Formula Name	Diagnosis	Indications	Remarks
Preserve Harmony Pill (*bǎo hé wán*)	Food stagnation	Focal distention and fullness in the chest and epigastrium, abdominal distention with occasional pain, rotten-smelling belching, acid regurgitation, nausea and vomiting, aversion to food, possibly diarrhea, a yellow, greasy tongue coating, and a slippery pulse	For the early stages of food stagnation, or for relatively mild disorders.
Unripe Bitter Orange Pill to Guide Out Stagnation (*zhǐ shí dǎo zhì wán*)	Accumulation of food that transforms into damp-heat and obstructs the Stomach and Intestines	Pain (that increases with pressure) and distention in the epigastrium and abdomen, dysenteric disorders or constipation, scanty, dark urine, a red tongue with a greasy or slippery, yellow coating, and a submerged, forceful pulse	For excess-type patterns.
Aucklandia and Betel Nut Pill (*mù xiāng bīng láng wán*)	Accumulation of food obstructing the middle burner or dysenteric diarrhea	Focal and generalized distention, fullness, and pain in the epigastrium and abdomen accompanied by constipation; or red-and-white dysenteric diarrhea with tenesmus; yellow, greasy tongue coating, and a submerged and excessive pulse	Also for various patterns of damp-heat obstructing the qi dynamic of the Triple Burner.
Fat Baby Pill (*féi ér wán*)	Childhood nutritional impairment that develops from an accumulation of parasites	Parasitic infestations with intermittent attacks of abdominal pain, indigestion, emaciation, loose stools, feverishness, foul-smelling breath, a sallow complexion, and a large, distended abdomen	Focuses on killing parasites while also clearing heat and strengthening the Spleen.

■ FORMULAS THAT REDUCE FOOD STAGNATION BUT ALSO TONIFY

Common symptoms: reduced appetite, focal distention of the epigastrium and abdomen

Formula Name	Diagnosis	Indications	Remarks
Strengthen the Spleen Pill (*jiàn pí wán*)	Spleen and Stomach deficiency with food accumulation that has begun to transform into heat	Reduced appetite with difficulty in digestion, bloating and focal distention of the epigastrium and abdomen, loose and watery diarrhea, a greasy, slightly yellow tongue coating, and a deficient, frail pulse	In this pattern, the deficient aspects are more significant than those of excess.
Unripe Bitter Orange and Atractylodes Pill (*zhǐ zhú wán*)	Spleen and Stomach deficiency with food stagnation	Loss of appetite, focal distention in the epigastrium and abdomen, a white tongue coating, and a deficient pulse	Often used as an additive to other formulas for food stagnation.
Unripe Bitter Orange Pill to Reduce Focal Distention (*zhǐ shí xiāo pǐ wán*)	Spleen deficiency and qi stagnation with mutual clumping of heat and cold	Focal distention and fullness in the upper epigastrium, lack of thirst or appetite, fatigue, weakness; may also be focal distention in the chest and abdomen, a wan complexion, poor digestion, irregular bowel movements, and a wiry pulse at the right, middle position; greasy, possibly yellow tongue coating	This is a complex, mixed pattern of deficiency and excess in which excess predominates.
Kudzu Flower Powder to Relieve Hangovers (*gé huā jiě chéng sǎn*)	Accumulation of damp-heat alcohol toxin	Vomiting, headache, Heart irritability, trembling of the hands and feet, focal distention in the chest and diaphragm, reduced appetite, fatigue, diarrhea, inhibited urination, a greasy tongue coating, and a slippery pulse	These symptoms may occur after a single bout of drinking or as the result of habitual overindulgence in alcohol.

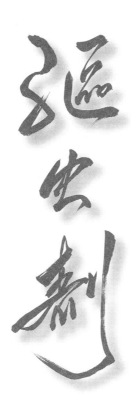

Chapter 19 Contents

Formulas that Expel Parasites

Formulas that Expel Parasites

19

THE FORMULAS IN this chapter are used to expel parasites from the digestive tract. While individual formulas are used for different types of parasites, similarities in their presentations include intermittent periumbilical pain, the ability to eat even when there is pain, and a change in the complexion (usually wan, pale, or dark). There are often white spots in the malar region, nighttime grinding of teeth, indeterminate gnawing hunger, vomiting of clear fluids, a peeled tongue coating, and a pulse that abruptly changes from large to small. If the condition is treated improperly and persists long-term, the patient will become emaciated and listless, lose interest in eating, and develop poor vision and hearing, dry hair, and a large, distended abdomen. Infestation by parasites is a common cause of childhood nutritional impairment.

Symptoms that are peculiar to specific parasites include itchy ears and nose and raised red and white spots on the inside of the lips for roundworms; itchy anus for pinworms; white segments of worms in the stools for tapeworms; and pica, an extremely wan complexion, and floating edema for hookworms.

Before treatment begins, one should examine the stools to determine which parasites are present. Remember that, in general, these formulas are not as potent as their modern pharmaceutical counterparts. They are, however, less toxic and cause fewer side effects. As such, they are very useful for treating parasites in the digestive tract.

Greasy and rich foods should be avoided during treatment for parasites. These formulas are most effective when taken on an empty stomach. Many of the substances that expel parasites have toxic properties. The dosage should be carefully monitored, and the formulas always used with caution. If the dosage is too small, the formula will have no effect; if too large, toxic side effects will develop and the normal qi will be injured. In any case, the formulas should be used with caution or avoided altogether in treating aged, weak, or pregnant patients. After the parasites have been successfully expelled, one should tonify the Spleen and Stomach, as these organs are usually weakened by the infestation.

烏梅丸 (乌梅丸)

Mume Pill

wū méi wán

Source *Discussion of Cold Damage* (c. 220)

Mume Fructus *(wū méi)* . . . . .300 pieces [480g] (24-30g)
Zanthoxyli Pericarpium *(huā jiāo)*. . . . . .12g [120g] (1.5-3g)
Asari Radix et Rhizoma *(xì xīn)* . . . . 18g [180g] (1.5-3g)
Coptidis Rhizoma *(huáng lián)* . . . . .48g [480g] (9-12g)
Phellodendri Cortex *(huáng bǎi)* . . . . .18g [180g] (6-9g)
Zingiberis Rhizoma *(gān jiāng)* . . . . .30g [300g] (6-9g)
Aconiti Radix lateralis praeparata *(zhì fù zǐ)* . . .18g [180g] (3-6g)
Cinnamomi Ramulus *(guì zhī)* . . . . .18g [180g] (3-6g)
Ginseng Radix *(rén shēn)* . . . . .18g [180g] (6-9g)
Angelicae sinensis Radix *(dāng guī)*. . . . . . . .12g [120g] (3-9g)

Method of Preparation   Steep the Mume Fructus *(wū méi)* overnight in vinegar, pit and mash, and cook with rice until the rice is done. Add the remaining ingredients, grind into a powder, and add refined honey to form into small pills the size of parasol tree seeds. Take 10 pills three times a day before meals. At present, Mume Fructus *(wū méi)* are soaked overnight in a solution that is 50 percent vinegar, pitted, and mashed. The remaining herbs are then added, and the mixture is dried, powdered, and made into pills with honey. It is taken in 9g doses with warm water, 1-3 times a day, on an empty stomach.

Codonopsis Radix *(dǎng shēn)* is often substituted for Ginseng Radix *(rén shēn)* at 2-3 times its dosage. The commonly-used dosages for pills are listed in brackets above, while the range for decoctions is listed in parentheses.

Actions   Warms the organs, drains heat, calms roundworms, drains the Liver, and calms the Stomach

Indications

At least since the time when the source text was published in the 3rd century, this formula has been used to treat three interrelated patterns. The first is inversion from roundworms (蛔厥 *huí jué*), which is characterized by intermittent attacks of abdominal pain, a stifling sensation, irritability, and warmth in the chest and epigastrium accompanied by vomiting after eating, and cold hands and feet. There may also be vomiting of roundworms.

The second pattern, which may or may not present together with the first, is the core pattern associated with terminal yin-warp disorders. This is characterized by unquenchable thirst, qi rushing upward toward the Heart, pain and heat in the Stomach, hunger with no desire to eat or vomiting immediately after eating, and cold extremities.

The third pattern is chronic diarrhea or dysentery characterized by incessant diarrhea, the discharge of small amounts of pus, and abdominal pain that responds favorably to pressure and the application of heat, borborygmus, and a red tongue with a white coating.

Inversion from roundworms is caused by heat in the chest and epigastrium (Stomach), and cold in the organs (Intestines). The intermittent attacks of abdominal pain and vomiting after eating reflect the presence of cold in the organs and the migration of the worms from a cold to a warmer part of the body. The stifling sensation, irritability, and warmth in the chest and epigastrium reflect the presence of heat in the chest. The roundworm infestation causes inversion, manifesting as cold hands and feet, and sometimes as vomiting of roundworms. Roundworms have an aversion to cold and an attraction to warmth. Here they migrate from the intestines toward the chest, the movement of which causes the major symptoms. The root of this disorder is poor communication between the yin and yang, which renders the patient more susceptible to infestation, and in turn is aggravated by the presence of the roundworms. Note that the Chinese character

厥 *jué*, translated here as inversion, also appears in the name of the terminal yin warp and the Liver channel, whose full name is the leg terminal yin (足厥陰 *zú jué yīn*) channel.

The manifestations of a terminal yin disorder reflect the particular physiology of this warp. The terminal yin represents the transformation of yin into yang within the body. As described by the Qing-dynasty physician Shen Jin-Ao in *Wondrous Lantern for Peering into the Origin and Development of Miscellaneous Diseases,* "All generated yang qi arises in the terminal yin, and there is nowhere in the entire body, high or low, that does not avail itself of this qi." This yang qi is the ministerial fire produced in the gate of vitality. Thus, it is also said that the Liver, the organ most closely associated with the terminal yin, "carries the ministerial fire inside." The Liver is able to manage the distribution of yang qi because it stores the blood, and it is the blood that carries warmth and yang qi to all the organs in the body. If the blood is strong, it can control the innate power of the yang. Here, the relationship between the blood (yin) and ministerial fire (yang) becomes disordered by the penetration of wind-cold into the terminal yin warp. The cold inhibits the yin and agitates the yang, leading to their separation. The ensuing pattern, often referred to as 'cold below, heat above' (下寒上熱 *xià hán shàng rè*), is characterized by the upward-rushing of hot ministerial fire (yang) via the Penetrating vessel and Stomach into the chest and Pericardium on the one hand, and by cold in the yin and yang organs because they are no longer supplied by the now pathological yang qi. This manifests as cold extremities, incessant diarrhea, and abdominal pain that is relieved by warmth.

Chronic diarrhea or dysentery with the discharge of small amounts of pus, abdominal pain that responds favorably to pressure and the application of heat, and a red tongue with a white coating also reflect the simultaneous presence of heat and cold that is characteristic of terminal yin disorders. Cold results in the inability of yang to transform yin, hence diarrhea, abdominal pain relieved by warmth, and white tongue coating. The presence of pathogenic heat becomes visible in the discharge of pus, and in the red tongue coating.

In contemporary Chinese medicine textbooks, which focus on organ-based pattern differentiation, the pathology addressed by this formula is commonly referred to as 'Liver heat attacking the Stomach with Spleen deficiency and cold in the Intestines' (肝熱犯胃，脾虛腸寒 *gān rè fàn wèi, pí xū cháng hán*).

Analysis of Formula

To treat a pattern characterized by the simultaneous presence of pathogenic heat and cold, this formula employs a complex strategy of directing heat downward with bitter, cooling herbs, opening the obstruction from yin cold with acrid, warming herbs, and calming the roundworms, irritability, and disorder with sour herbs. The chief herb is Mume Fructus *(wū méi),* a very sour substance that is quite effective in calming roundworms. According to Zhang Bing-Cheng in *Convenient Reader of Materia Medica:*

> Its flavor is sour, its nature is warming, and it specifically enters the blood level in Liver patients, while also indirectly influencing the Spleen, Lungs, and Large Intestine. Its functions are specifically to restrain, inhibit, stop, and bind up, thus it can be used for all chronic coughs, chronic dysenteric disorders, deficiency sweating, and devastated blood. Its ability to quiet parasites is because parasites hide when encountering sour [flavors].

Used with a very high dosage, Mume Fructus *(wū méi)* thus treats all of the major manifestations, but also guides the entire formula into the terminal yin. Moreover, by resonating with the sourness preferred by Liver wood, it is able to contain the warming and cooling properties of the formula.

The deputies are divided into two groups. The first, consisting of Zanthoxyli Pericarpium *(huā jiāo)* and Asari Radix et Rhizoma *(xì xīn),* are acrid and warming in nature. They expel parasites and warm the organs. The second group, consisting of Coptidis Rhizoma *(huáng lián)* and Phellodendri Cortex *(huáng bǎi),* are cooling and bitter in nature and make the worms move downward.

Among the assistants are Zingiberis Rhizoma *(gān jiāng),* Aconiti Radix lateralis praeparata *(zhì fù zǐ),* and Cinnamomi Ramulus *(guì zhī).* They warm the interior and are very useful in dispersing internal cold. Cinnamomi Ramulus *(guì zhī)* and Asari Radix et Rhizoma *(xì xīn)* facilitate the flow of yang qi and thereby help scatter the cold. Ginseng Radix *(rén shēn)* and Angelicae sinensis Radix *(dāng guī)* are the other assistants. They tonify the qi and nourish the blood to prevent further injury to the normal qi.

Cautions and Contraindications

This formula is contraindicated for explosive diarrhea or damp-heat dysenteric disorders.

Commentary

Function

This formula is distinctive for its use of both cooling and warming substances, and for addressing both the pathogenic influence and the normal qi. In *Golden Mirror of the Medical Tradition,* the 17th-century physician Ke Qin succinctly described the effect of this formula on roundworms: "When roundworms encounter sourness, they are calmed; when they encounter acridity, they are subdued; when they encounter bitterness, they are purged." This has become the standard formula for treating roundworm infestation. Other formulas used in treating this disorder are basically variations of this formula.

It should be noted, however, that the formula does not so much seek to expel the worms as to contain their activity, which is experienced by the host as unpleasant. This can be interpreted as an acceptance of the fact that symbiosis between host (the human organism) and parasites (roundworms, but also bacteria, etc.) is a normal fact of life. By adjusting the internal environment, this formula establishes a more physiological balance. Based on this perspective, Mume Pill *(wū méi wán)* has recently been used to treat food intolerance and food allergies.

Variety of Interpretations

Given its complex composition, the formula is interpreted differently depending on which pattern a particular commentator focuses. When used for chronic diarrhea or dysenteric disorders, for instance, the pathodynamic and thus the hierarchy and actions of the ingredients are often understood in a different manner. Thus, in *A Stick to Awaken Physicians,* the Qing-dynasty physician Zhang Nan redefined the formula as essentially treating a Liver-Spleen disharmony:

> Mume Pill *(wū méi wán)* is the formula that governs orthodox treatment of the terminal yin. When Liver [qi turns into] an unbridled pathogen, it invariably encumbers the middle earth. Accordingly, one employs acrid, heating and sweet, warming herbs to assist the yang of the Spleen and Stomach, while pacifying the Liver with sour [herbs] used with a high dosage and assisted by bitter, cooling [herbs] that drain fire. This is because Liver wood contains the ministerial fire.

Viewed from this perspective, the chief herbs are those which warm the middle and disperse cold, namely, Zingiberis Rhizoma *(gān jiāng),* Aconiti Radix lateralis praeparata *(zhì fù zǐ),* Cinnamomi Ramulus *(guì zhī),* and Asari Radix et Rhizoma *(xì xīn).* The deputies are Ginseng Radix *(rén shēn)* and Angelicae sinensis Radix *(dāng guī),* which tonify and nourish the qi and blood, and thereby enhance the functions of the middle burner. The assistants are Coptidis Rhizoma *(huáng lián)* and Phellodendri Cortex *(huáng bǎi),* which expel the pathogenic influence and resolve toxicity, together with sour, astringent Mume Fructus *(wū méi),* also used to help stop the diarrhea.

The contemporary physician Qin Bo-Wei took precisely the opposite view to Zhang Nan (who focused on Liver wood overcontrolling Spleen earth) by interpreting the formula as one for treating patterns of Liver deficiency:

> This formula treats deficiency and weakness of the normal qi of the Liver organ along with patterns of mixed heat and cold. It employs Ginseng Radix *(rén shēn)* and Angelica sinensis radix *(dāng guī)* to tonify the qi and blood; Asari Radix et Rhizoma *(xì xīn),* Zingiberis Rhizoma *(gān jiāng),* Aconiti Radix lateralis praeparata *(zhì fù zǐ),* Cinnamomi Ramulus *(guì zhī),* and Zanthoxyli Pericarpium *(huā jiāo)* to warm and unblock the blood vessels; and Coptidis Rhizoma *(huáng lián)* and Phellodendri Cortex *(huáng bǎi)* to clear fire. Furthermore, it uses Mume

Fructus (*wū méi*) with its sour flavor and [ability] to enter into the Liver as chief herb to gather the power of the various ingredients in one single channel. It is capable of treating chronic disorders characterized by symptoms such as abdominal pain, vomiting, diarrhea, and inversion from roundworms.

Yet another interpretation is provided by Qin's contemporary, Cheng Men-Xue, who focused on drug synergisms:

> Including vinegar, this formula contains eleven ingredients. Mume Fructus (*wū méi*) and Zanthoxyli Pericarpium (*huā jiāo*) constitute one synergistic pairing; Zingiberis Rhizoma (*gān jiāng*) and Coptidis Rhizoma (*huáng lián*) another one; and Asari Radix et Rhizoma (*xì xīn*) and Phellodendri Cortex (*huáng bǎi*) a third. This strategy of combining [herbs] to transform their [effects] by matching them in every detail is most exquisite. It can be modified to treat terminal yin Liver and Kidney and similar disorders. … Ye Tian-Shi went furthest in utilizing the subtlety of this strategy. The multiple ways in which he adopted it can be seen in his case records.
>
> Cinnamomi Ramulus (*guì zhī*) and Angelica sinensis radix (*dāng guī*) are used to warm and unblock the nutritive [qi and] blood. Ginseng Radix (*rén shēn*) and Aconiti Radix lateralis praeparata (*zhì fù zǐ*) are used to warm and unblock the nutritive and protective qi. Together, [these pairings] build up resistance to disease and attend to the qi and blood. [The combination of] Angelica sinensis radix (*dāng guī*), Cinnamomi Ramulus (*guì zhī*), and Asari Radix et Rhizoma (*xì xīn*), furthermore, embodies the intent of Tangkuei Decoction for Frigid Extremities (*dāng guī sì nì tāng*); while that of Ginseng Radix (*rén shēn*), Aconiti Radix lateralis praeparata (*zhì fù zǐ*), and Zingiberis Rhizoma (*gān jiāng*) embodies the intent of Frigid Extremities Decoction (*sì nì tāng*). Combining the strategies of these two different Frigid Extremities Decoctions in one treatment, which is then linked to the [synergisms] between the six ingredients analyzed previously, produces a complex [remedy] that has the power to support the normal qi [even as] it drains the Liver. This is what I call the ingenuity of complex remedies.
>
> Furthermore, combining Mume Fructus (*wū méi*) and Coptidis Rhizoma (*huáng lián*) with Zanthoxyli Pericarpium (*huā jiāo*), and Phellodendri Cortex (*huáng bǎi*) with Zingiberis Rhizoma (*gān jiāng*) and Coptidis Rhizoma (*huáng lián*) [represents the use of] salty, bitter, and acrid [flavors] to open [obstruction] and drain [downward, and of] sour and bitter [flavors] to drain heat. With [this method,] one can obtain excellent results in treating the Liver. Finally, because roundworms are calmed by sour and bitter [flavors,] the combination of bitter, acrid, and sour flavors is the method for treating parasites. Using sour [flavors] to bind, bitter [flavors] to drain, and acrid [flavors] to open are the basic rules for treating the Liver. Without going beyond these three [basic strategies] while adopting them to the complex [realities of clinical practice,] there truly are no limits to the uses of [Mume Pill (*wū méi wán*)].

Ye Tian-Shi's Approach

As Cheng Men-Xue emphasizes, the therapeutic power of this formula goes far beyond the treatment of roundworms, and no one understood that potential better than the Qing-dynasty physician Ye Tian-Shi. Drawing on the treatment principles outlined by Cheng Men-Xue, Ye Tian-Shi used modifications of Mume Pill (*wū méi wán*) to treat a wide variety of inter-nal medicine disorders extending from vomiting, abdominal pain, focal distention, diarrhea, and dysentery to chronic malarial and warm pathogen disorders. The following is a brief synopsis of Ye Tian-Shi's approach intended to help practitioners extend the formula's usage in contemporary practice:

- For patterns of rebellious Liver qi invading the Stomach characterized by such symptoms as vomiting, acid reflux, spitting up of saliva, subjective sensations of qi ascending into the throat; or alternatively for stuporous conditions with hunger but no desire to eat, soft stools or incomplete bowel movements, and a wiry pulse, Ye focused on the combination of sour, acrid, and bitter flavors. He removed Phellodendri Cortex (*huáng bǎi*), Cinnamomi Ramulus (*guì zhī*), Aconiti Radix lateralis praeparata (*zhì fù zǐ*), Asari Radix et Rhizoma (*xì xīn*), and Ginseng Radix (*rén shēn*) and combined Toosendan Fructus (*chuān liàn zǐ*) and Paeoniae Radix alba (*bái sháo*) with Coptidis Rhizoma (*huáng lián*), Mume Fructus (*wū méi*), Zanthoxyli Pericarpium (*huā jiāo*) and Zingiberis Rhizoma (*gān jiāng*) to emphasize draining the Liver and calming the Stomach.

- For patterns of debilitated Stomach yang and upward-rebellion of qi with such symptoms as vomiting of phlegm or clear fluids, sweating accompanied by shivers, edema, abdominal pain, borborygmi, and in severe cases stupor, Ye focused on the combination of sour, acrid, and sweet flavors. He removed the bitter herbs and combined Poria (*fú líng*), Citri reticulatae Pericarpium (*chén pí*), and Paeoniae Radix alba (*bái sháo*) with Ginseng Radix (*rén shēn*), Zanthoxyli Pericarpium (*huā jiāo*), Mume Fructus (*wū méi*), and Zingiberis Rhizoma (*gān jiāng*) to warm the middle and calm the Stomach.

- For patterns of internal stirring of Liver wind and heat from deficiency with such symptoms as unquenchable thirst, dry retching, rebellious Stomach qi with inability to eat, irritability and restlessness, chills and fever, diarrhea, and a shiny red tongue, Ye focused on the combination of sour, sweet, and bitter flavors. He removed the acrid, warming herbs and combined Asini Corii Colla (*ē jiāo*), Rehmanniae Radix (*shēng dì huáng*), and Ophiopogonis Radix (*mài mén dōng*) with Ginseng Radix (*rén shēn*), Coptidis Rhizoma (*huáng lián*), and Mume Fructus (*wū méi*) to transform the yin and clear heat. The resulting formula, known as Coptis and Mume Decoction (連梅湯 *lián méi tāng*), was also used by Ye to treat summerheat plundering the yin and attacking the lesser yin warp with such symptoms as disorientation, unquenchable thirst, irritability and restlessness, chills and fevers, spasms leading to collapse, and numbness.

- For summerheat plundering the yin and attacking the terminal yin warp with such symptoms as nausea, vomiting of roundworms, chills and fever, dysenteric diarrhea, unquenchable thirst, and a grey tongue coating, Ye combined

Coptidis Rhizoma (huáng lián), Scutellariae Radix (huáng qín), Zanthoxyli Pericarpium (huā jiāo), Mume Fructus (wū méi), Paeoniae Radix alba (bái sháo), Ginseng Radix (rén shēn), and Aurantii Fructus immaturus (zhǐ shí). This is known as Zanthoxylum and Mume Decoction (椒梅湯 jiāo méi tāng).

Usage

In contemporary practice, this formula is used to treat a wide variety of problems that manifest with terminal yin-warp symptoms extending from Heart problems such as angina and loss of consciousness; many types of digestive problems involving Stomach heat and Spleen cold; menstrual disorders such as dysmenorrhea and discharge; as well as skin disorders, diabetes, headaches, hypertension, and many more. In the treatment of parasites, it is often used as a setup prescription, which is then followed by a stronger purgative to expel them from the body.

Given the complex pathophysiology for which this formula is indicated, and the many ways that it can be modified to match ensuing patterns, allows for a multitude of presenting signs and symptoms. Its use may be considered in patients who present with a conjunction of the following:

- Signs of cold such as cold hands and feet, a generalized aversion to cold, cold sweats, diarrhea, or loose stools
- Signs of heat such as irritability and restlessness, red eyes, a bitter taste in the mouth, dark urine, thirst, or hunger
- Periods of calm that alternate with periods of irritability, or a temperament characterized by the need for quiet, withdrawal or solitude, yet also marked by restlessness, extroversion, and bouts of agitation and irritability.

Comparisons

➤ Vs. Coptis Decoction (huáng lián tāng)

Both formulas combine Cinnamomi Ramulus (guì zhī), Zingiberis Rhizoma (gān jiāng), Coptidis Rhizoma (huáng lián), and Ginseng Radix (rén shēn) to treat patterns characterized by heat above and cold below marked by abdominal pain, irritability, and vomiting. Their combination of bitter, cooling, and downward-directing ingredients with those that are acrid and warming facilitates the interconnection and interpenetration of yin and yang, a condition for which Cinnamomi Ramulus (guì zhī) is specifically useful. Coptis Decoction (huáng lián tāng) also contains Pinelliae Rhizoma praeparatum (zhì bàn xià) and thus focuses on the middle burner, specifically the Stomach, and so addresses patterns where cold congeals in the middle burner, leading to abdominal pain, nausea, and vomiting. Mume Pill (wū méi wán), on the other hand, includes ingredients such as Mume Fructus (wū méi) and Angelicae sinensis Radix (dāng guī) that direct the formula into the terminal yin warp as well as the strongly heating

herbs Aconiti Radix lateralis praeparata (zhì fù zǐ), Zanthoxyli Pericarpium (huā jiāo), and Asari Radix et Rhizoma (xì xīn), and the bitter, cooling Phellodendri Cortex (huáng bǎi), all of which direct its action into the lower burner. Besides parasites, patterns for which Mume Pill (wū méi wán) is indicated are also characterized by terminal yin-warp symptoms such as very cold extremities, alternating chills and fevers, bouts of quietude interspersed with irritability, and diarrhea, while abdominal pain need not be present.

➤ Vs. Regulate the Middle Pill (lǐ zhōng wán) and Frigid Extremities Decoction (sì nì tāng)

These are the three main formulas for treating cold from deficiency in the interior according to the six stages system of pattern differentiation outlined in Discussion of Cold Damage. The core symptoms of cold from deficiency shared by all these patterns are aversion to cold, abdominal pain, loose stools or diarrhea, and vomiting. The one ingredient shared by all three formulas is Zingiberis Rhizoma (gān jiāng), which suggests that warming the middle burner is central to treating these patterns. Given that Aconiti Radix lateralis praeparata (zhì fù zǐ) is often added to Regulate the Middle Pill (lǐ zhōng wán), this then becomes the second ingredient present in all three formulas. This adds the function of unblocking and dispersion of lower burner yang qi to facilitate a more complete warming action throughout the interior. The difference among the three formulas is the place/function to which they direct this yang qi, a difference that is mediated by the addition of the other ingredients in each formula.

Regulate the Middle Pill (lǐ zhōng wán) adds Atractylodis macrocephalae Rhizoma (bái zhú), Ginseng Radix (rén shēn), and Glycyrrhizae Radix praeparata (zhì gān cǎo) to warm the middle burner, strengthen the Spleen, and dry dampness. It is the formula of choice for cold-dampness obstructing the middle burner yang. Frigid Extremities Decoction (sì nì tāng) uses a relatively high dosage of Aconiti Radix lateralis praeparata (zhì fù zǐ) and Glycyrrhizae Radix praeparata (zhì gān cǎo) to strongly support diffusion of the yang qi throughout the body, while moderating any potential side effects. Mume Pill (wū méi wán) adds acrid, warming herbs such as Zanthoxyli Pericarpium (huā jiāo) and Asari Radix et Rhizoma (xì xīn), bitter, cooling herbs such as Coptidis Rhizoma (huáng lián) and Phellodendri Cortex (huáng bǎi), and Mume Fructus (wū méi) and Angelicae sinensis Radix (dāng guī), which together guide the entire formula into the terminal yin warp, to treat patterns characterized by heat above and cold below.

It follows that, while false heat due to floating yang may be present in patterns treated by both Regulate the Middle Pill (lǐ zhōng wán) and Frigid Extremities Decoction (sì nì tāng), the heat in Mume Pill (wū méi wán) patterns is excessive in nature. In clinical practice, one of the primary markers for the use of Mume Pill (wū méi wán) is that the false heat from floating yang tends to be continuous. This is because true cold in the interior is constant and simply pushes the remaining yang to the exterior. In terminal yin patterns, on the other hand, cold and heat tend to alternate. This is similar to lesser yang patterns, with the difference being that in those patterns, cold is merely a sign of constraint, while in terminal yin patterns, it is due to deficiency and is thus accompanied by the symptoms listed above.

Biomedical Indications

With the appropriate presentation, this formula may be used to treat a very wide variety of biomedically-defined disorders. These can be divided into the following groups:

- Parasitic infestations including ascariasis, biliary ascariasis, and hookworm

- Digestive diseases marked by diarrhea including chronic bacillary dysentery, ulcerative colitis, and irritable bowel syndrome

- Other digestive diseases including cholelithiasis, cholecystitis, peptic ulcers, functional gastric disorders, and neurogenic vomiting

- EENT diseases including keratitis, corneal ulcers, glaucoma, apthous ulcers, chronic suppurative otitis media, and Ménière's disease

- Gynecological disorders including morning sickness, chronic pelvic inflammatory disease, dysfunctional uterine bleeding, and primary dysmenorrhea.

This formula has also been used for treating hypertension, neurogenic headache, the sequelae of meningitis or encephalitis, autonomic dystonia, hysterical psychosis, vertiligo, sick sinus syndrome, asthma, pneumonia, diabetes, as well as recalcitrant hiccups or insomnia.

Alternate names

Mume Elixir (wū méi dān) in *Prescriptions of Universal Benefit*; Mume Stomach Pacifying Pill (wū méi ān wèi wán) in *Collected Formulas from the Crane Feeding Pavilion*; Antiparasitic Mume Pill (shā chóng wū méi wán) and Stomach Pacifying Pill (ān wèi wán) in *Nationwide Collection of TCM Patent Formulas*

Modifications

- In the absence of cold symptoms, remove Aconiti Radix lateralis praeparata (zhì fù zǐ) and Cinnamomi Ramulus (guì zhī).

- If the normal qi is not yet deficient, remove Ginseng Radix (rén shēn) and Angelicae sinensis Radix (dāng guī).

- For severe abdominal pain, add Toosendan Fructus (chuān liàn zǐ) and Aucklandiae Radix (mù xiāng).

- For constipation, add Arecae Semen (bīng láng) and Aurantii Fructus immaturus (zhǐ shí).

- For severe vomiting, add Evodiae Fructus (wú zhū yú) and Pinelliae Rhizoma praeparatum (zhì bàn xià).

- For chronic, unremitting dysenteric diarrhea, remove Phellodendri Cortex (huáng bǎi) and Ginseng Radix (rén shēn) and substitute Cinnamomi Cortex (ròu guì) for Cinnamomi Ramulus (guì zhī).

- For roundworms in the bile duct, add Quisqualis Fructus (shǐ jūn zǐ) and Meliae Cortex (kǔ liàn gēn pí).

- For chronic dysentery, add Aucklandiae Radix (mù xiāng) and Paeoniae Radix alba (bái sháo).

Associated Formulas

理中安蛔湯 （理中安蛔汤）

Regulate the Middle and Calm Roundworms Decoction

lǐ zhōng ān huí tāng

SOURCE   *Restoration of Health from the Myriad Diseases* (1587)

Ginseng Radix (rén shēn)	2.1g
Atractylodis macrocephalae Rhizoma (bái zhú)	3g
Poria (fú líng)	3g
Zanthoxyli Pericarpium (huā jiāo)	0.3g
Mume Fructus (wū méi)	3 pieces
Zingiberis Rhizoma (gān jiāng)	1.5g

Warms the middle burner and calms roundworms. For cold from deficiency of the Spleen and Stomach with vomiting of roundworms or passing them in very loose stools, clear and profuse urine, abdominal pain, borborygmus, cold limbs, a thin, white tongue coating, and a moderate, deficient pulse. At present, the dosage of Zanthoxyli Pericarpium (huā jiāo) is 6g and 3 pieces of Mume Fructus (wū méi) is usually 9g. *Note*: In the source text, this formula is simply called Calm Roundword Decoction (ān huí tāng); it is much more commonly known as Regulate the Middle and Calm Roundworm Decoction (lǐ zhōng ān huí tāng), which is drawn from *Treatment Decisions Categorized According to Pattern*.

連梅安蛔湯 （连梅安蛔汤）

Picrorhiza and Mume Decoction to Calm Roundworms

lián méi ān huí tāng

SOURCE   *Revised Popular Guide to the Discussion of Cold Damage* (Qing era)

Picrorhizae Rhizoma (hú huáng lián)	3g
Zanthoxyli Pericarpium (huā jiāo)	1.5g
Omphalia (léi wán)	9g
Mume Fructus (wū méi)	2 pieces (6-9g)
Phellodendri Cortex (huáng bǎi)	2.4g
Arecae Semen (bīng láng)	2 pieces (9-12g)

Clears heat and calms roundworms. For accumulation of roundworms with vigorous heat in the Liver and Stomach causing abdominal pain, loss of appetite, vomiting of roundworms after eating, irritability, and in severe cases, inversion. Accompanying signs and symptoms include a flushed face, dry mouth, fever, a red tongue, and a rapid pulse. Used for relatively mild cases of roundworm infestation accompanied by heat.

化蟲丸（化虫丸）

Dissolve Parasites Pill

huà chóng wán

Source *Formulary of the Pharmacy Service for Benefiting the People in the Taiping Era* (1148)

Carpesii abrotanoidis Fructus *(hè shī)* 1500g

Arecae Semen *(bīng láng)* 1500g

Meliae Cortex *(kǔ liàn gēn pí)* 1500g

Minium *(qiān dān)* 1500g

Alumen *(míng fán)* 375g

Method of Preparation Grind the ingredients into a powder and form into pills with wheat dough. Take 6g once daily on an empty stomach with rice soup. Children under the age of three should only take 1.5g at a time. Note that Minium *(qiān dān)* is toxic and should not be used and that Alumen *(míng fán)* also has significant side effects.

Actions Kills intestinal parasites

Indications

Intestinal parasites with intermittent attacks of abdominal pain that moves around and is worse in the periumbilical region. When severe, the pain leads to vomiting of clear fluids or parasites.

Intestinal parasites usually arise from improper or unsanitary eating habits, most commonly in people with cold, deficient constitutions. The pain is caused by movement of the parasites in the abdomen. As they move about the Small Intestine, the pain moves with them and is worse in the periumbilical region. If they disturb the Stomach, the qi of that organ loses its ability to properly descend, which causes vomiting of clear fluids or parasites.

Analysis of Formula

To treat a pattern caused by a variety of parasitic infestations, this formula utilizes a number of substances that attack an assortment of intestinal parasites. Carpesii abrotanoidis Fructus *(hè shī)*, an important ingredient for expelling many types of parasites, especially roundworms, is the chief ingredient. The deputies include Meliae Cortex *(kǔ liàn gēn pí)*, which kills roundworms and pinworms, and Arecae Semen *(bīng láng)*, which kills tapeworms and fasciolopsis. The source text calls for Minium *(qiān dān)*, which kills many types of intestinal parasites, but because it is extremely toxic, it should no longer be used. Arecae Semen *(bīng láng)* also has a downward-draining effect, which is helpful in expelling intestinal parasties. The assistant is Alumen *(míng fán)*, which resolves toxicity, dries dampness, and helps eliminate the parasites. The envoy, wheat dough, harmonizes the actions of the other ingredients. This is a relatively powerful formula that is used in treating a variety of intestinal parasites.

Cautions and Contraindications

This formula contains mostly toxic substances. While this will affect many tissues, its greatest effect is upon the neurological and hematological systems. For this reason, the formula should never be used by pregnant women, nor should it be used long-term or in greater than the prescribed dosage. It is often modified for children. In all cases, after the parasites are expelled, one should harmonize and tonify the Spleen and Stomach.

Commentary

Source

The source text, *Formulary of the Pharmacy Service for Benefiting the People in the Taiping Era*, describes the indications for this formula as follows:

> Childhood diseases often involve parasites. These parasites may become perturbed when the organs are deficient and weak, or after eating sweet or fatty foods. When they are perturbed, there is abdominal pain, with swellings when they gather and go back and forth, up and down [in the abdomen] so that the pain is continuous. They can also attack with Heart [epigastric] pain [such that the child] shouts and cries, scrunching up their eyes, arching their body, and pounding their fists. They will feel oppressed and confused, and spit up saliva or vomit clear fluids. The limbs will be emaciated and fatigued, the complexion a dark greenish-yellow, and while they will be able to get food down, it does not end up generating flesh. They may be chilled or feverish and subdued and downcast.
>
> If one does not know a way to get rid of this disease and the parasites are not treated, then a vicious cycle will develop and the [problem] will go on without a break. Once the parasites become a foot long, they will harm people.

Historical Influence

This formula has had a signifiant impact on the treatment of intestinal parasites in Chinese medicine up to the present, particularly the combination of antiparasitic medicinals with those that promote the movement of qi and drain downward. There have been at least 24 formulas by this name over the centuries, all combining the same strategies to a greater or lesser extent. For example, Dissolve Parasites Pill *(huà chóng wán)*, which appeared in the 18th-century work *Six Texts Summarizing the Medicine of Xu Ling-Tai*, added Ulmi macrocarpae Fructus preparatus *(wú yí)*, Quisqualis Fructus *(shǐ jūn zǐ)*, and Ginseng Radix *(rén shēn)* to simultaneously attack and tonify for those with parasites who are somewhat weak, but without a deficient pulse.

Most modern formulations remove the Alumen *(míng fán)* and Minium *(qiān dān)*, but add other ingredients that kill parasites as well as those that increase the downward-draining effects of the formula. An example from *Nationwide Collection of TCM Patent Formulas* makes these deletions, but nevertheless makes the formula stronger and harsher by adding Ulmi macrocarpae Fructus preparatus *(wú yí)*, Quisqualis Fructus *(shǐ jūn zǐ)*, Omphalia *(léi wán)*, Natrii Sulfas siccatus *(xuán míng fěn)*, Pharbitidis Semen *(qiān niú zǐ)*, and Rhei Radix et Rhizoma *(dà huáng)*.

Biomedical Indications

With the appropriate presentation, this formula may be used to treat a variety of biomedically-defined disorders including roundworms (ascariasis), tapeworms, pinworms, or fasciolopsis infestations.

....

Alternate name

Dissolve Parasites Special Pill *(huà chóng dān)* in *New Treatise on Children*

....

Modifications

- To increase the formula's ability to kill parasites, add Quisqualis Fructus *(shǐ jūn zǐ)* and Omphalia *(léi wán)*.

- For robust patients, add Rhei Radix et Rhizoma *(dà huáng)*.

- For children and weak patients, add Atractylodis macrocephalae Rhizoma *(bái zhú)* and Codonopsis Radix *(dǎng shēn)*.

- For concurrent food stagnation, add Crataegi Fructus *(shān zhā)*, Hordei Fructus germinatus *(mài yá)*, and Massa medicata fermentata *(shén qū)*.

Variation

化蟲丸 （化虫丸）

Dissolve Parasites Pill from *Medical Formulas Collected and Analyzed*

huà chóng wán

SOURCE   *Medical Formulas Collected and Analyzed* (1682)

Add Quisqualis Fructus *(shǐ jūn zǐ)* and Ulmi macrocarpae Fructus preparatus *(wú yí)* for a stronger effect.

Associated Formula

膽道驅蛔湯 （胆道驱蛔汤）

Drive Roundworms from the Biliary Tract Decoction

dǎn dào qū huí tāng

SOURCE   *New [Text on the] Acute Abdomen* (1978)

Aucklandiae Radix *(mù xiāng)* 9g
Aurantii Fructus *(zhǐ ké)* 6g
Arecae Semen *(bīng láng)* 30g
Meliae Cortex *(kǔ liàn gēn pí)* 15g
Quisqualis Fructus *(shǐ jūn zǐ)* 15g

Promotes the movement of qi, dissipates clumps, expels parasites, and alleviates pain. For parasitic infestations with severe abdominal

pain and a mass in the abdomen (usually the right upper quadrant). Originally designed for roundworms in the biliary tract, it can be effectively used for treating a wide variety of parasites including roundworms, pinworms, tapeworms, and fasciolopsis.

布袋丸
Cloth Sack Pill

bù dài wán

According to the source text, the pills are placed in a cloth sack before cooking with pork, hence the name.

Source   *Supplement to the Pocket-Sized Discussion of Formulas for Children* (late Ming)

Vespertilionis Faecesi *(yè míng shā)* 60g
Ulmi macrocarpae Fructus preparatus *(wú yí)* 60g
Quisqualis Fructus *(shǐ jūn zǐ)* 60g
Poria *(fú líng)* 15g
Atractylodis macrocephalae Rhizoma *(bái zhú)* 15g
Ginseng Radix *(rén shēn)* 15g
Glycyrrhizae Radix *(gān cǎo)* 15g
Aloe *(lú huì)* 15g

Method of Preparation   The source text advises to grind the ingredients into a powder and form into pills approximately 9g in weight. The pill is placed in a cloth sack and cooked with 60g of pork until the pork is thoroughly done, and then the juice is given to the child. At present, the ingredients are usually ground into a powder and taken in the morning on an empty stomach in 3g doses mixed with pork soup.

Actions   Expels roundworms, reduces childhood nutritional impairment, and tonifies the Spleen and Stomach

Indications

Sallow complexion, emaciated limbs and a large, distended abdomen, feverishness, dry and coarse hair, dull eyes, a pale tongue, and a frail pulse

This is childhood nutritional impairment due to parasites. Chronic infestation by parasites causes stagnation in the middle burner and injures the Spleen and Stomach. Food stagnates in the middle burner, and there is consequently a loss of nutrition to the head and limbs. This manifests as a sallow complexion and emaciated limbs with a large, distended abdomen. Over time, Spleen deficiency gives rise to heat from deficiency, which, in addition to the internal heat generated by the accumulation itself, results in feverishness.

The long-term disturbance caused by the parasites, combined with the reduced food intake and assimilation by the Spleen and Stomach, leads to blood deficiency, which manifests as dry and coarse hair. This deficiency primarily affects the Liver, causing dullness of the eyes and diminished acuity of vision. If the parasite is viewed as a pathogenic influence, this is a case in which the normal qi is weak and the pathogenic influence is strong. The pale tongue and frail pulse reflect the deficiency of the Spleen qi and Liver blood.

Analysis of Formula

Treatment of a condition where the effects of parasites have led to an underlying deficiency requires a formula that both directly attacks the parasites while simultaneously supporting the normal qi. The chief ingredients are the acrid, bitter, and warm Ulmi macrocarpae Fructus preparatus *(wú yí)* and the sweet and warm Quisqualis Fructus *(shǐ jūn zǐ)*, both of which are very effective in expelling roundworms and treating childhood nutritional impairment. The deputy is Aloe *(lú huì)*, which expels roundworms and is also a purgative that drains heat. These three herbs have a strong antiparasitic effect and eliminate the parasites via the stool. One of the assistants, Vespertilionis Faecesi *(yè míng shā)*, improves the acuity of vision while also dispersing accumulations and reducing childhood nutritional impairment. The other assistants are the constituents of Four-Gentlemen Decoction *(sì jūn zǐ tāng)* (see Chapter 8), and are used to benefit the Spleen and fortify the qi of the middle burner. The unusual method of administration has a similar effect because of the nutrients in the meat or soup. This indirect method also makes it easier for children to take this medicine, particularly because some of the ingredients have a bad taste.

Commentary

This formula is useful for anyone suffering from parasites (usually roundworms) accompanied by Spleen and Stomach deficiency, and is not limited to children. It has both purgative and tonifying aspects, which enables it to expel the parasites without harming the Spleen and Stomach.

Comparison

➢ Vs. Fat Baby Pill *(féi ér wán)*

Both formulas kill parasites and treat childhood nutritional impairment in patients with a sallow complexion, emaciation, and bloated abdomen. Fat Baby Pill *(féi ér wán)* focuses more on reducing accumulations and killing the parasites, and is therefore used primarily for patterns of excess. Cloth Sack Pill *(bù dài wán)*, on the other hand, is indicated when there is more significant Spleen deficiency.

Biomedical Indications

With the appropriate presentation, this formula may be used to treat a variety of biomedically-defined disorders including ascariasis, other parasitic infestations, and malnutrition.

Modifications

- For signs of severe internal heat, add Picrorhizae Rhizoma *(hú huáng lián)*.
- For concurrent food stagnation, add Massa medicata fermentata *(shén qū)* and Gigeriae galli Endothelium corneum *(jī nèi jīn)*.

Comparative Table of Principal Formulas

■ FORMULAS THAT EXPEL PARASITES

Common symptoms (first two formulas): intermittent abdominal pain, vomiting

Formula Name	Diagnosis	Indications	Remarks
Mume Pill *(wū méi wán)*	1. Inversion from roundworms; 2. terminal yin-warp disorder; 3. chronic diarrhea or dysentery	1. Intermittent abdominal pain, a stifling sensation, irritability, and warmth in the chest and epigastrium, vomiting after eating, cold hands and feet, and possibly vomiting of roundworms; 2. unquenchable thirst, qi rushing upward toward the Heart, pain and heat in the Stomach, hunger with no desire to eat, or vomiting immediately after eating, and cold extremities; 3. incessant diarrhea, discharge of small amounts of pus, abdominal pain that responds favorably to pressure and the application of heat, borborygmus, and a red tongue with a white coating	Treats patterns characterized by the simultaneous presence of pathogenic heat and cold by directing heat downward, opening obstruction due to yin cold, and calming roundworms. Recently used to treat food intolerance and food allergies.
Dissolve Parasites Pill *(huà chóng wán)*	Intestinal parasites	Intermittent attacks of abdominal pain that moves around and is worse in the periumbilical region; when severe, the pain leads to vomiting of clear fluids or parasites	A relatively powerful formula that is used in treating a variety of intestinal parasites.
Cloth Sack Pill *(bù dài wán)*	Childhood nutritional impairment due to parasites	Sallow complexion, emaciated limbs and a large, distended abdomen, feverishness, dry and coarse hair, dull eyes, a pale tongue, and a frail pulse	Focuses on both directly attacking the parasites and simultaneously supporting the normal qi.

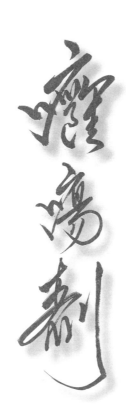

Chapter 20 Contents

Formulas that Treat Abscesses and Sores

Formulas that Treat Abscesses and Sores 20

ABSCESSES AND SORES, both external and internal, have been a focus of Chinese medicine since its very beginnings. Many types of treatment for these conditions were recorded in the early 2nd-century B.C.E. manuscript *Prescriptions for Fifty-Two Ailments*, discovered in the 1970s. The disease dynamic underlying the formation of yang sores was first described in *Basic Questions*, (Chapter 3): "If the nutritive and qi do not follow each other, they rebel into the interior of the flesh where they produce abscesses and swellings." *Divine Pivot* (Chapter 81) analyzed the formation of pus in similar terms:

> If the nutritive and protective qi linger within the channels, the blood stagnates and does not move. If it does not move, the protective qi follows suit and [no longer] connects [with it]. It becomes clogged and contained, thereby generating heat. If severe heat does not end, it eventually rots the flesh. This then becomes pus.

Because the site of toxic swellings in the body can vary and the etiology and progression can be both complex and dangerous, this topic can be quite involved. Treatment of toxic swellings requires that the practitioner carefully assess the state of the patient's normal qi and determine the underlying cause of the lesion. Formulas can then be chosen by observing the stage of the swelling, its nature, and its location.

Note that not all formulas used in the treatment of sores are found in this chapter. For example, the initial stages of hot toxic sores are frequently treated with Coptis Decoction to Resolve Toxicity *(huáng lián jiě dú tāng)*, described in Chapter 4; and Sage-Like Healing Decoction *(shèng yù tāng)*, in Chapter 8, is frequently used to treat sores whose slow healing is attributed to deficiency.

For patients with yang-type external or internal toxic sores, alcohol, spicy foods (especially garlic and hot peppers), greasy foods, and shellfish can all aggravate the condition. They should be avoided.

Section 1

FORMULAS THAT TREAT EXTERNAL ABSCESSES AND SORES

The term 'external abscesses and sores' (癰瘍 *yōng yáng*) is a general one that covers a large group of swollen, scabbing, open, oozing, and purulent lesions. These include toxic swellings such as abscesses (癰 *yōng*), flat abscesses (疽 *jū*), boils (癤 *jiē*), rooted sores (疔 *dīng*), scrofula (瘰癧 *luǒ lì*), rock tumors (岩 *yán*), as well as other lesions such as knife wounds, nonclosing sores, insect bites, and burns. The largest subset of this category are the toxic swellings (literally, 'abscesses and flat abscesses' 癰疽 *yōng jū*), a term that includes numerous manifestations of accumulation of toxins such as boils, rooted sores, rock swellings, and scrofula, and not just different types of abscesses.

The long history of Chinese medicine has resulted in a very well-developed approach to treating toxic swellings based on theories that go back at least as far as the *Inner Classic.* Chapter 81 of *Divine Pivot*, "Toxic Swellings," describes their etiology and formation, as discussed on the previous page of the present work. Similarly, Chapter 18 of the Western Han work *Essentials from the Golden Cabinet* is devoted to understanding the pathogenesis and treatment of different types of sores and abscesses, both external and internal.

Over time, a theoretical system was developed that posited a natural progression for the proper healing of toxic swellings, and a method of treatment was then devised to encourage that progression and to follow its natural course. The formation, development, dissipation, and ultimate healing of a toxic swelling is thought to have four stages:

1. *Initial stage:* The swelling gradually grows larger, slightly red, warm, painful, and hard to the touch. If the lesion is pale, barely protruding and producing a dull pain, it is a flat abscess and is thought to be more difficult to treat.

2. *Pus formation stage:* As the flesh rots and becomes pus, the swelling rises up and becomes redder and more painful. Palpating the sore will reveal a soft, liquid interior. Should the swelling turn dark and refuse to soften, this is regarded as an inauspicious sign that requires vigilant treatment.

3. *Bursting stage:* The sore opens and pus exudes. This is sometimes called the 'ulceration stage.' In the ideal situation, the pus is not too thick or foul-smelling, the swelling quickly recedes, and, when the sore is cleaned, the rotted flesh is easily removed. Symptoms of pain and fever should resolve once the swelling has burst. However, it is more problematic if, once the sore bursts, the pus has a foul odor, the flesh in the cavity is dull and lifeless, and the pain, swelling, and fever persist.

4. *Closing stage:* When the inner sore reveals healthy flesh that shows signs of new growth and the skin surrounding the sore is of a normal color, the sore will close quickly. It is important for the sore to remain open and heal from the inside out. If the flesh inside the sore is dull, leaks clear or turbid liquid, is slow to produce new flesh and there is abnormal color surrounding the wound, measures must be taken to aid the body to heal the wound.

When searching for the underlying cause of the stagnation in the channels that gives rise to toxic accumulation, one should examine the condition and flow of qi and blood, the functioning of the organs, and the site in the channels themselves where there is lack of flow. Treatment is based on the dishar-

mony that is identified in this search and analysis of the stage of the toxic swelling.

To address the various stages of toxic swellings, Chinese medicine has developed a number of different treatment principles. These can be sorted into three primary methods known as the 'dissipating method' (消法 *xiāo fǎ*), the 'supporting method' (托法 *tuō fǎ*), and the 'tonifying method' (補法 *bǔ fǎ*). The dissipating method is used in treating the initial stage of toxic swellings; formulas that dissipate encourage the toxic swellings to form pus and suppurate. Careful analysis of the cause of the toxic accumulation leads to proper treatment. For example, if initial stage boils or abscesses can be attributed to an exterior pattern that disrupts the flow of qi and blood in the channels, one can apply Immortals' Formula for Sustaining Life *(xiān fāng huó mìng yǐn)* or Schizonepeta and Saposhnikovia Powder to Overcome Pathogenic Influences *(jīng fáng bài dú sǎn)*, discussed in Chapter 1. If, on the other hand, the initial stage toxic swelling arises from internal disharmonies that create excess heat, formulas to clear heat and purge fire are chosen, includeing Internal Flow [-Promoting] Decoction with Coptis *(nèi liú huáng lián tāng)* or Cool the Diaphragm Powder *(liáng gé sǎn)*, discussed in Chapter 4. Successful treatment at this stage will result in either dissipation of the swelling or the formation of pus.

Careful analysis of the underlying pattern is extremely important to achieve proper results. Exterior pathogens must be resolved; interior excess calls for unblocking the obstruction; overabundant heat-toxin must be cleared; congealed interior cold stagnation must be warmly unblocked; congealed phlegm must be transformed and expelled; movement through areas of damp obstruction must be facilitated; and qi and blood stasis require moving the qi and blood. All of these strategies fall under the rubric of the dissipating method.

If, after appropriate time and treatment, the body is unable to encourage the swelling to produce or vent pus, then the supporting method is applied. This method aims to tonify the qi and blood and to harmonize the protective and nutritive aspects with the goal of supporting the normal qi and drawing out toxins. Support the Interior and Eliminate Toxin Drink *(tuō lǐ xiāo dú yǐn)* is the model formula for this method. If the patient suffers from a pattern of cold from deficiency, Powder to Support the Interior Worth a Thousand Gold Pieces *(qiān jīn nèi tuō sǎn)* should be considered. Formulas that facilitate the supporting method often combine tonifying agents, such as Ginseng Radix *(rén shēn)* and Angelicae sinensis Radix *(dāng guī)*, with herbs that vent pus, such as Gleditsiae Spina *(zào jiǎo cì)*, Platycodi Radix *(jié gěng)*, and Angelicae dahuricae Radix *(bái zhǐ)*, that support the body while helping it to draw out toxin.

The supplementing method is applied to lingering sores in deficient patients. Often, herbs that secure the exterior, generate flesh, and close sores such as Astragali Radix *(huáng qí*) are included in this category. All-Inclusive Great Tonifying Decoction (*shí quán dà bǔ tāng*), described in Chapter 8, is an example of a supplementing formula.

仙方活命飲 (仙方活命饮)
Immortals' Formula for Sustaining Life
xiān fāng huó mìng yǐn

This is one of the most important and influential formulas in the history of Chinese external medicine and is revered as if it had been passed on by the immortal sages. Its efficacy is said to bring a patient back from the edge of death and to sustain their life.

Source   *Fine Formulas for Women with Annotations and Commentary* (16th century)

Lonicerae Flos (*jīn yín huā*) .9g
Glycyrrhizae Radix (*gān cǎo*) .3g
Fritillariae thunbergii Bulbus (*zhè bèi mǔ*) 3g
Trichosanthis Radix (*tiān huā fěn*) 3g
Angelicae sinensis radicis Cauda (*dāng guī wěi*) 6-12g
Paeoniae Radix rubra (*chì sháo*) 3g
Olibanum (*rǔ xiāng*) 3g
Myrrha (*mò yào*) 3g
Saposhnikoviae Radix (*fáng fēng*) 3g
Angelicae dahuricae Radix (*bái zhǐ*) 3g
Manitis Squama (*chuān shān jiǎ*) 3g
Gleditsiae Spina (*zào jiǎo cì*) .3g
Citri reticulatae Pericarpium (*chén pí*) 9g

Method of Preparation   Cook the herbs in one part water and one part wine to strengthen the blood-invigorating action of the formula. The dregs may be applied topically.

Because of its endangered status, Manitis Squama (*chuān shān jiǎ*) is no longer used; Vaccariae Semen (*wáng bù liú xíng*) is often substituted. The dosages of both Fritillariae thunbergii Bulbus (*zhè bèi mǔ*) and Gleditsiae Spina (*zào jiǎo cì*) are usually increased.

Actions   Clears heat and resolves fire toxin, reduces swelling and promotes the discharge of pus, invigorates the blood, and alleviates pain

Indications

Early-stage sores and carbuncles with red, swollen, hot, and painful skin lesions, usually accompanied by fever, mild chills, headache, a thin tongue coating (either white or slightly yellow), and a rapid, forceful pulse.

This is a fire toxin or phlegm-fire of various origins, including the transformation of a pathogenic influence in the channels, overindulgence in rich or greasy foods, or trauma with transmission of toxic qi. Fire toxin or phlegm-fire causes the clumping of stagnant qi and blood in the relatively superficial levels of the body, which in turn causes the fluids to 'simmer.' The clumping in the channels between the levels of the skin and flesh forms sores or carbuncles that are characterized by inflammation and pus. The battle between heat and the normal qi in the exterior gives rise to fever, mild chills, headache, and a thin tongue coating. At first, the tongue coating will be white, but as the disorder progresses, it will turn yellow. The battle between the strong pathogenic influence and the strong normal qi produces a rapid, forceful pulse.

Analysis of Formula

The strategy for treating sores and carbuncles from fire toxin is primarily to clear the heat and resolve the toxicity and secondarily to invigorate the blood, regulate the qi, transform the phlegm, and dissipate the clumping. The chief ingredient, sweet and cool Lonicerae Flos (*jīn yín huā*), is very effective in resolving toxicity. It is regarded as a 'sage-like' herb in treating sores and carbuncles because it not only relieves the toxic heat in both the qi and blood levels, but also dissipates the clumping. One of the deputies, Citri reticulatae Pericarpium (*chén pí*), promotes the movement of qi. This directly affects the stagnant qi, and indirectly reinforces the actions of the other ingredients in treating this condition. Another group of deputies works on the blood. Angelicae sinensis Radix (*dāng guī*) and Paeoniae Radix rubra (*chì sháo*) invigorate and strengthen the flow of blood in the channels, and Olibanum (*rǔ xiāng*) and Myrrha (*mò yào*) eliminate blood stasis and alleviate pain.

Two of the assistant ingredients, Saposhnikoviae Radix (*fáng fēng*) and Angelicae dahuricae Radix (*bái zhǐ*), dispel wind and reduce superficial swelling. The other assistants, Fritillariae thunbergii Bulbus (*zhè bèi mǔ*) and Trichosanthis Radix (*tiān huā fěn*), clear heat and transform phlegm. Trichosanthis Radix (*tiān huā fěn*) also enters the blood where it reduces the swelling from blood stasis. Two of the envoys, Manitis Squama (*chuān shān jiǎ*) and Gleditsiae Spina (*zào jiǎo cì*), open and vent stagnation in the channels to expel the pus and thereby accelerate the healing process. They also serve to focus the actions of the other ingredients on the sores. The remaining envoy, Glycyrrhizae Radix (*gān cǎo*), harmonizes the actions of the other ingredients and assists in resolving toxicity.

Cautions and Contraindications

Side effects are rare and generally limited to nausea and vomiting, or, with long-term use, injury to the Spleen and Stomach qi. It should not be prescribed in cases of carbuncles that are already discharging pus and have become ulcerated, or for yin sores. It should be modified where there is Spleen deficiency.

Commentary

This formula is used for early-stage yang sores that develop rapidly. *Golden Mirror of Medicine* describes it as an "exalted medicine for sores, and a premier formula for external disorders." In the source text, Xue Ji wrote that "It treats all kind of sores and carbuncles. It disperses those that have not yet formed and [causes] those that have already formed to burst. … It is an effective prescription for stopping pain and discharging toxins." Its composition and efficacy thus make it the flagship formula for what is known as the 'dissipating method' (消法 *xiāo fǎ*), one of the three basic treatment strategies in Chinese external medicine (see chapter introduction). 'Dissipating' here implies dispersion of internal stagnation in order to treat problems in the exterior, as explained by Ye Tian-Shi in *Case Records as a Guide to Clinical Practice*:

> Generally, although external medicine patterns manifest in the exterior, the root of the disorder is located in the interior. If one is clear about yin and yang, excess and deficiency, heat and cold, and the channels, collateral, and every single acupuncture point, one is able to change serious patterns into minor ones, and make minor ones disappear. Those who excel at reducing and dissipating are superior craftsmen.

As noted in the chapter introduction, the initial cause of abscesses and sores was identified in Chapter 81 of *Divine Pivot* as stagnant nutritive qi and blood. This understanding was utilized by later physicians. Zhang Bing-Cheng, for example, wrote in *Convenient Reader of Established Formulas*:

> The initial stages of toxic swellings are always caused by the stagnation of nutritive qi and blood. The ensuing constraint [of protective qi] becomes heat. As nutritive and protective qi lose their regular [interconnection,] the disorder acquires form on the outside, hence exterior patterns will be apparent on the outside.

Given the close connection between nutritive qi and digestion, an improper diet and the invasion of pathogens via the Spleen and Stomach are the main cause of toxic swellings treated by this formula. This opens up a wide range of conditions beyond the narrow domain of external medicine. Chinese practitioners have thus expanded its application to the treatment of many types of inflammatory disorders that present with blood stasis, phlegm, and heat toxin. When considering the use of this formula in such cases, it is important, first, to ascertain whether the presenting pattern is one of excess. Then, because the formula is strongly cooling, there should also be clear signs indicating the presence of heat toxin such as localized redness and swelling, heat sensations, painful inflammation, a slightly yellow tongue coating, or a rapid pulse.

Name

A commonly used alternative name for this formula is True Person's Formula for Sustaining Life (*zhēn rén huó mìng yǐn*). In Daoism, 'true person' is another name for an immortal.

Comparisons

➤ Vs. Universal Benefit Drink to Eliminate Toxin (*pǔ jì xiāo dú yǐn*)

Both formulas clear heat and resolve toxicity. However, in the case of massive epidemic disorders of heat treated by Univer-

sal Benefit Drink to Eliminate Toxin (*pǔ jì xiāo dú yǐn*), wind-heat epidemic pathogens enter the body via the exterior and upper burner, and toxic heat is located entirely in the upper part of the body. Thus, the secondary principle of treatment for this formula is to disperse wind-heat from the exterior by enabling the ascent of yang qi. By contrast, Immortals' Formula for Sustaining Life (*xiān fāng huó mìng yǐn*) treats toxic heat caused by stasis of blood and stagnation of qi, with heat arising as a secondary consequence. Thus, it focuses on moving the qi, invigorating the blood, transforming phlegm, and reducing swelling.

➤ Vs. Five-Ingredient Drink to Eliminate Toxin (*wǔ wèi xiāo dú yǐn*); see PAGE 864

➤ Vs. Support the Interior and Eliminate Toxin Drink (*tuō lǐ xiāo dú yǐn*); see PAGE 868

➤ Vs. Ten-Ingredient Powder to Overcome Toxicity (*shí wèi bài dú sǎn*); see PAGE 872

Biomedical Indications

With the appropriate presentation, this formula may be used to treat a variety of biomedically-defined disorders including acute mastitis, multiple carbuncles, acute appendicitis, ulcerative colitis, tonsillitis, sinusitis, herpes zoster, infected wounds, psoriasis, osteomyelitis, pneumonia, and other localized, purulent lesions such as pelvic inflammatory disease as well as for purposes of postoperative care.

Alternate names

Secret Formula for Seizing Life (*mì fāng duó mìng sǎn*) in *Pocket Prescriptions*; True Man Powder for Sustaining Life (*zhēn rén huó mìng sǎn*) in *Mysteriously Effective Formulas for Abscesses*; True Man Drink for Sustaining Life (*zhēn rén huó mìng yǐn*) in *Multitude of Marvelous Formulas for Sustaining Life*; Divine Effect Decoction for Sustaining Life (*shén gòng huó mìng tāng*) in *Complete Treatise on Experience with Sores*; Thirteen-Ingredient Powder to Overcome Toxicity (*shí sān wèi bài dú sǎn*) in *Investigations of Medical Formulas*; True Man Drink for Seizing Life (*zhēn rén duó mìng yǐn*) in *Empirical Formulas from the Hall of Benevolent Righteousness*; Tangkuei Drink to Eliminate Toxin (*dāng guī xiāo dú yǐn*) in *Collectanea of Investigations from the Realm of Medicine*

Modifications

- To strengthen the ability of the formula to clear heat and resolve toxicity, add Taraxaci Herba (*pú gōng yīng*), Violae Herba (*zǐ huā dì dīng*), and Forsythiae Fructus (*lián qiáo*) and reduce the dosage of Citri reticulatae Pericarpium (*chén pí*) so that the formula is not too drying.

- If the sores are small and superficial, remove Manitis Squama (*chuān shān jiǎ*) and Gleditsiae Spina (*zào jiǎo cì*).

- For heat in the blood, add Moutan Cortex (*mǔ dān pí*).

- For high fever and severe thirst due to injury to the fluids, remove Angelicae dahuricae Radix (*bái zhǐ*) and Citri reticulatae Pericarpium (*chén pí*), increase the dosage of

Trichosanthis Radix (*tiān huā fěn*), and add Scrophulariae Radix (*xuán shēn*)

- For qi deficiency, add Astragali Radix (*huáng qí*).
- For bleeding, add Notoginseng Radix (*sān qī*).
- For constipation, add Rhei Radix et Rhizoma (*dà huáng*) and Cannabis Semen (*huǒ má rén*).
- For urinary difficulty, add Foeniculi Fructus (*xiǎo huí xiāng*) and Plantaginis Semen (*chē qián zǐ*).
- For sores and carbuncles, add the following herbs to direct the actions of the formula to particular parts of the body:

  HEAD: Chuanxiong Rhizoma (*chuān xiōng*)

  NECK: Platycodi Radix (*jié gěng*)

  CHEST: Trichosanthis Pericarpium (*guā lóu pí*)

  FLANKS: Bupleuri Radix (*chái hú*)

  BACK: Gentianae macrophyllae Radix (*qín jiāo*)

  UPPER EXTREMITIES: Curcumae longae Rhizoma (*jiāng huáng*)

  LOWER EXTREMITIES: Achyranthis bidentatae Radix (*niú xī*)

Associated Formulas

沖和湯（冲和汤）

Flush and Harmonize Decoction

chōng hé tāng

SOURCE *Indispensable Tools for Pattern Treatment* (1602)

Lonicerae Flos (*jīn yín huā*) 9g
Glycyrrhizae Radix (*gān cǎo*) 3g
Fritillariae thunbergii Bulbus (*zhè bèi mǔ*) 3g
branch roots of Angelicae sinensis Radix (*dāng guī wěi*) 3g
Paeoniae Radix rubra (*chì sháo*) 3g
Olibanum (*rǔ xiāng*) 3g
Angelicae dahuricae Radix (*bái zhǐ*) 3g
Gleditsiae Spina (*zào jiǎo cì*) 3g
Codonopsis Radix (*dǎng shēn*) 9g
Astragali Radix (*huáng qí*) 9g
Atractylodis macrocephalae Rhizoma (*bái zhú*) 9g
Poria (*fú líng*) 9g
Citri reticulatae Pericarpium (*chén pí*) 9g

Clears heat, resolves toxicity, reduces swelling, expels pus, invigorates the blood, and tonifies the qi. For qi deficiency with yin-yang sores (i.e., half-yin and half-yang sores characterized by swellings with no head, slight heat, redness and pain, and uncertain ulceration).

內流黃連湯（内流黄连汤）

Internal Flow[-Promoting] Decoction with Coptis

nèi liú huáng lián tāng

SOURCE *Collection of Writings on the Mechanism of Disease, Suitability of Qi, and the Safeguarding of Life as Discussed in Basic Questions* (1186)

Coptidis Rhizoma (*huáng lián*) 30g (9g)
Paeoniae Radix (*sháo yào*) 30g (9g)
Angelicae sinensis Radix (*dāng guī*) 30g (9g)
Arecae Semen (*bīng láng*) 30g (6g)

Aucklandiae Radix (*mù xiāng*) 30g (6g)
Scutellariae Radix (*huáng qín*) 30g (9g)
Menthae haplocalycis Herba (*bò hé*) 30g
Gardeniae Fructus (*zhī zǐ*) 30g (9g)
Platycodi Radix (*jié gěng*) 30g (6g)
Glycyrrhizae Radix (*gān cǎo*) 30g (6g)
Forsythiae Fructus (*lián qiáo*) 60g (18g)
Rhei Radix et Rhizoma (*dà huáng*) 3-6g (6-9g)

Powder. With the exception of Aucklandiae Radix (*mù xiāng*) and Arecae Semen (*bīng láng*), which are used as a fine powder, the other herbs are ground together. Decoct 30g of the powder in 1.5 cups of water until 1 cup remains, which is taken in one or two doses. The first time the prescription is taken, 3g of Rhei Radix et Rhizoma (*dà huáng*) are added, and then 6g. This should produce loose stools. At present, the formula is prepared as a decoction with the dosages indicated in parentheses.

Clears heat, resolves toxicity, reduces swelling, and dissipates knotting. For hard sores and carbuncles with a deep and large root and base but no change in color. Accompanying symptoms are nausea, belching, irritability, constipation, and a deep and excessive pulse. Compared to the principal formula, this prescription focuses more strongly on clearing heat and draining clumping from the interior of the body that, as a consequence of internal accumulation, transforms into toxins that seek to discharge through the skin. Immortals' Formula for Sustaining Life (*xiān fāng huó mìng yǐn*), on the other hand, is better for promoting the flow of nutritive and protective qi in the channels that has become blocked and causes sores or inflammatory conditions.

五味消毒飲（五味消毒饮）

Five-Ingredient Drink to Eliminate Toxin

wǔ wèi xiāo dú yǐn

SOURCE *Golden Mirror of the Medical Tradition* (1742)

Lonicerae Flos (*jīn yín huā*) 9g
Taraxaci Herba (*pú gōng yīng*) 3.6g
Violae Herba (*zǐ huā dì dīng*) 3.6g
Chrysanthemi indici Flos (*yě jú huā*) 3.6g
Semiaquilegiae Radix (*tiān kuí zǐ*) 3.6g

Method of Preparation Decoction. Add 2-3 tablespoons of rice wine before cooking. The decoction should be taken warm and the patient should bundle up with a few blankets to promote sweating. The dregs may be applied topically. At present, the dosage is generally increased 3-4 times.

Actions Clears heat, resolves toxicity, cools the blood, and reduces swelling

Indications

All types of boils and carbuncles with localized erythema, swelling, heat, and pain accompanied by fever, chills, a red tongue with a yellow coating, and a rapid pulse. Especially useful for deep-rooted and hard lesions, which are said to resemble nails or chestnuts.

This is fire toxin, which can arise from a variety of causes: externally-contracted heat from a warm pathogen disease, seasonal pathogenic influences accumulating in the organs or channels, overindulgence in rich or spicy foods, or heat that accumulates because of disharmony in any of the internal organs. Heat causes stagnation, which produces more accumulation, in turn generating more heat. As this cycle continues, the fire toxin deepens and gradually forms a very hard, rooted sore (疔瘡 *dīng chuāng*). At first, such sores tend to be hard and painful. However, because of the accumulating toxin, they turn increasingly red and become hot and more painful. Fever and chills, if present, reflect the battle between the pathogenic influence and the normal qi in the superficial levels of the body. The red tongue with a yellow coating and the rapid pulse indicate that there is more heat than stagnation of qi and blood.

Analysis of Formula

This formula focuses on treating the root of the disorder by resolving toxicity and reducing swelling, doing so by combining a number of cooling herbs that are specific for resolving toxicity. Lonicerae Flos *(jīn yín huā)*, the chief herb, clears heat and resolves toxicity from both the qi and blood levels and dissipates swellings. It is one of the principal substances in the materia medica for treating sores. According to the contemporary physician Yue Mei-Zhong, it is also sweet and thus has the particular advantage of not damaging the Stomach. The four deputies, Violae Herba *(zǐ huā dì dīng)*, Semiaquilegia Semen *(tiān kuí zǐ)*, Taraxaci Herba *(pú gōng yīng)*, and Chrysanthemi indici Flos *(yě jú huā)*, all have a relatively strong ability to resolve toxicity as well as cool the blood, reduce swellings, and disperse clumps. For this reason, they are commonly used to treat various types of purulent lesions.

The small amount of wine invigorates the blood, which helps reduce this type of swelling; it is viewed as the envoy in this formula. If the patient is also covered with a blanket, the alcohol will help to open the pores and produce a very light sweat. This is thought to facilitate the drawing out of toxins toward the exterior.

Cautions and Contraindications

Contraindicated for yin-type boils. Use with caution in cases with Spleen deficiency.

Commentary

This formula serves as the foundation for many formulas that are used in treating localized, superficial, purulent infections. Even though the formula is cold, clears heat, and resolves toxicity, it is nevertheless intended to induce sweating. This is in apparent contradiction to the therapeutic principle formulated by Zhang Zhong-Jing, who said that "It is forbidden to use sweating in patients with sores." The rationale underlying this principle is that sweating damages the qi and fluids and thereby aggravates the heat and stagnation that are the root

of the disorder. On the other hand, *Basic Questions* (Chapter 70) states that "Once [a patient] sweats, sores go away." This contradiction can be resolved by noting that the sweating induced by this formula is intended to be extremely light, while all of the herbs in the formula are cooling without being excessively bitter or drying. Thus, the qi dynamic is enabled without damaging the qi or blood.

The source text notes that the occurrence of the type of hard sores treated by this formula is a serious condition that can readily result in death from what at present is known as blood poisoning. This formula is thus designed not only to treat the manifestations, but also to stop the accumulation and dissemination of toxin. In the clinic, it can be used whenever the four key signs of an inflammatory response—heat, redness, pain, and swelling—are present. This expands the therapeutic scope of the formula to a very wide spectrum of conditions.

Comparisons

➣ Vs. Immortals' Formula for Sustaining Life *(xiān fāng huó mìng yǐn)*

While Immortals' Formula for Sustaining Life *(xiān fāng huó mìng yǐn)* focuses on invigorating the blood and reducing swelling, the emphasis of Five-Ingredient Drink to Eliminate Toxin *(wǔ wèi xiāo dú yǐn)* is on clearing heat and resolving toxicity. For this reason, it is most useful in treating abscesses and inflammatory swellings before pus has formed. Immortals' Formula for Sustaining Life *(xiān fāng huó mìng yǐn)*, on the other hand, treats abscesses and swellings where pus has already formed but has not yet been discharged or formed ulcerations.

➣ Vs. Support the Interior and Eliminate Toxin Drink *(tuō lǐ xiāo dú yǐn)*; see PAGE 869

Biomedical Indications

With the appropriate presentation, this formula may be used to treat a variety of biomedically-defined disorders including multiple furuncles, carbuncles, erysipelas, cellulitis, mastitis, appendicitis, conjunctivitis, bartholinitis, urinary tract infection, acute pyelonephritis, and acute hepatitis.

Alternate names

Five-Ingredient Decoction to Eliminate Toxin *(wǔ wèi xiāo dú tāng)* in *Investigations into External Medicine*; Eliminate Toxin Drink *(xiāo dú yǐn)* in *[Zhou] Ji-Ren's Collected Empirical Formulas*

Modifications

- For high fever and other signs of severe heat, add Coptidis Rhizoma *(huáng lián)* and Forsythiae Fructus *(lián qiáo)*.
- For severe swelling, add Saposhnikoviae Radix *(fáng fēng)* and Cicadae Periostracum *(chán tuì)*.

- For dark red and painful sores, add Moutan Cortex (mǔ dān pí) and Paeoniae Radix rubra (chì sháo).

- For concurrent damp-heat rash, add Dictamni Cortex (bái xiān pí), Kochiae Fructus (dì fū zǐ), and Zaocys (wū shāo shé).

- For breast abscess, add Trichosanthis Fructus (guā lóu), Fritillariae thunbergii Bulbus (zhè bèi mǔ), and Citri reticulatae viride Pericarpium (qīng pí).

- For septicemia, traditionally known as 'sores turning yellow,' add a large dosage of Isatidis Folium (dà qīng yè) and Scutellariae barbatae Herba (bàn zhī lián).

- For acute pyelonephritis, add Imperatae Rhizoma (bái máo gēn) and Maydis Stigma (yù mǐ xū).

- For use in deficient patients, add Ginseng Radix (rén shēn) or combine with Tangkuei Decoction to Tonify the Blood (dāng guī bǔ xuè tāng).

Associated Formulas

消炎解毒丸

Reduce Inflammation and Resolve Toxicity Pill

xiāo yán jiě dú wán

SOURCE *Medical Mirror of Past and Present* (Ming era)

Taraxaci Herba (pú gōng yīng)	15-30g
Lonicerae Flos (jīn yín huā)	15-30g
Forsythiae Fructus (lián qiáo)	12-24g
Saposhnikoviae Radix (fáng fēng)	9-12g
Glycyrrhizae Radix (gān cǎo)	3-6g

The source text does not specify dosage. Clears heat, resolves toxicity, and releases the exterior. For sores and carbuncles (such as mastitis) with obvious exterior symptoms.

銀花解毒湯 （银花解毒汤）

Honeysuckle Decoction to Resolve Toxicity

yín huā jiě dú tāng

SOURCE *Collected Experiences on Treating Sores* (1806)

Lonicerae Flos (jīn yín huā)	15-30g
Violae Herba (zǐ huā dì dīng)	15-30g
Bubali Cornu (shuǐ niú jiǎo)	15-30g
Poria rubra (chì fú líng)	9-12g
Forsythiae Fructus (lián qiáo)	12-24g
Moutan Cortex (mǔ dān pí)	9-12g
Coptidis Rhizoma (huáng lián)	6-9g
Prunellae Spica (xià kū cǎo)	12-24g

The source text does not specify dosage. Note that the original text specifies Rhinocerotis Cornu (xī jiǎo), which is no longer used, primarily because of the endangered status of the rhinoceros. Clears heat, resolves toxicity, drains fire, and cools the blood. For purulent skin lesions with signs of intense fire toxin due to wind-damp-heat. The focus is on cooling the blood.

連翹金貝煎 （连翘金贝煎）

Lonicera, Honeysuckle, and Bolbostemma Decoction

lián qiáo jīn bèi jiān

SOURCE *Collected Treatises of [Zhang] Jing-Yue* (1624)

Lonicerae Flos (jīn yín huā)	9g
Bolbostematis rhizoma (tǔ bèi mǔ)*	9g
Taraxaci Herba (pú gōng yīng)	9g
Prunellae Spica (xià kū cǎo)	9g
Carthami Flos (hóng huā)	24g
Forsythiae Fructus (lián qiáo)	30g

Decoction. The source text advises to decoct with 2 cups of mature wine until 1 cup remains, and then to huddle up in bed after drinking. Add Trichosanthis Radix (tiān huā fěn) for cases with overabundant heat, thirst, or mastitis. Decoction in water is recommended for yang toxicity with internal heat or for sores from the neck upward. Clears heat, resolves toxicity, softens swellings, and invigorates the blood. This formula is especially indicated for yang toxin abscesses in the Lungs, breast, or other internal organs.

清肝飲 （清肝饮）

Clear the Liver Drink

qīng gān yǐn

SOURCE *Selected and Compiled Clinical Experiences of Wei Chang-Chun* (1974)

Lonicerae Flos (jīn yín huā)	10g
Violae Herba (zǐ huā dì dīng)	15g
Taraxaci Herba (pú gōng yīng)	15g
Chrysanthemi indici Flos (yě jú huā)	15g
Prunellae Spica (xià kū cǎo)	10g
Artemisiae annuae Herba (qīng hāo)	10g
Mori Ramulus (sāng zhī)	12g
Imperatae Rhizoma (bái máo gēn)	15

Decoction. The source text does not specify dosage. Clears heat, cools the blood, resolves toxicity, vents lurking heat, and thrusts out dampness. For chronic or subacute cases of hepatitis. Formulated for cases where heat toxins lurk in the interior and are not vented to the exterior. This manifests as fatigue, right-sided flank pain or discomfort, irritability, poor temper, low-grade fever, and abnormal liver function studies. The author of this formula argues that although the four main herbs in this formula are cold, they are also flowers and thus have a light nature. Moreover, they are also acrid and sweet and are thus able to expel heat without form without plundering the yin or affecting the Stomach. The remaining herbs are included to unblock the Liver collaterals, vent pathogenic heat, and disperse the clumping of Liver qi.

四妙勇安湯 （四妙勇安汤）

Four-Valiant Decoction for Well-Being

sì miào yǒng ān tāng

---

* Bolbostematis rhizoma (土貝母 *tǔ bèi mǔ*) is slightly cold and bitter. It enters the Lung and Spleen channels and disperses clumps, reduces swellings, and resolves toxicity. The normal dosage is 9-15g.

Although there are only four herbs in this formula, their dosage is large and the effect is so distinct that patients experience a strong sense of well-being once the condition is relieved. The Chinese word for 'valiant' is a homonym for everlasting (yǒng), which expresses faith in this formula's ability to relieve the condition and prevent relapse.

Source   *New Compilation of Empirical Formulas* (1846)

Lonicerae Flos (*jīn yín huā*) 90g
Scrophulariae Radix (*xuán shēn*) 90g
Angelicae sinensis Radix (*dāng guī*) 60g
Glycyrrhizae Radix (*gān cǎo*) 30g

Method of Preparation   Decoction. A reduction in dosage will reduce its effectiveness. The source text prescribes a minimum 10-day course of treatment.

Actions   Clears heat, resolves toxicity, nourishes the yin, invigorates the blood, and alleviates pain

Indications

Ulcerated sores that do not heal on a limb that is dark red, slightly swollen and warm to the touch, and extremely painful. There may be a rotten smell to the lesion together with copious discharge. Accompanying symptoms include fever, thirst, a red tongue, and a rapid pulse.

This is sloughing ulcer (脫疽 *tuō jū*), which is due to obstruction by fire toxin leading to stasis of blood in the sinews and blood vessels. This condition may be attributed to long-standing Kidney deficiency, externally-contracted damp-cold painful obstruction, overindulgence in rich, greasy, or spicy foods, or the improper use of yang tonics. With chronic Kidney deficiency, the bones become malnourished and stagnation develops. Externally-contracted damp-cold painful obstruction impedes the circulation of blood; if left untreated, this will lead to constraint, which generates heat.

More than one factor is usually involved. Heat and toxin combine to produce hot, red, swollen, and painful lesions. Severe obstruction and the ensuing lack of nourishment leads to a darkening of the skin color, a moderation of the swelling, warmth (due to restricted local circulation), and increased pain. Toxin and stasis together produce putrefaction. The fever, thirst, red tongue, and rapid pulse are indicative of heat.

Analysis of Formula

To treat heat toxin developing at the level of the blood and sinews, this formula combines a strategy of clearing heat and resolving toxicity while also nourishing the yin fluids and invigorating the blood. Lonicerae Flos (*jīn yín huā*) is the chief herb in the formula because of its ability to clear heat, resolve toxicity, and reduce swelling. It is reinforced by the deputy, Scrophulariae Radix (*xuán shēn*), which drains fire, resolves toxicity, and nourishes the yin. The assistant herb, Angelicae sinensis Radix (*dāng guī*), invigorates the blood and breaks up stasis. The envoy, Glycyrrhizae Radix (*gān cǎo*), harmo-

nizes the actions of the other herbs and strengthens the formula's ability to resolve toxicity.

Cautions and Contraindications

Contraindicated in cases with cold, qi deficiency, or blood deficiency.

Commentary

The source text describes the pattern for which this formula is indicated as being able to erupt on the digits of both hands and feet, where "the skin looks [a brownish-reddish color] like that of a very well-cooked red date, or black, without subsiding. If it [is allowed to become] chronic, it will ulcerate with steady sloughing off, resulting in putrid, blackish, cave-like ulcerations on the backs of the hands and feet and pain that is difficult to endure." This is interpreted today as obstruction of the vessels and collaterals leading to gangrene associated with biomedical disorders such as thrombangitis obliterans, thrombophlebitis, or ateriosclerosis. Its use has been expanded to include other conditions associated with inflammation and stasis such as chronic hepatitis, gastritis, and gout, as well as sciatica and carpal tunnel syndrome.

The efficacy of the formula requires strict adherence to the prescribed dosage. At the same time, it can be adjusted to treat the root of the disorder by adding herbs such as Carthami Flos (*hóng huā*), Persicae Semen (*táo rén*), Paeoniae Radix rubra (*chì sháo*), Myrrha (*mò yào*), Olibanum (*rǔ xiāng*), Cinnamomi Ramulus (*guì zhī*), Aconiti Radix lateralis praeparata (*fù zǐ*), Astragali Radix (*huáng qí*), Codonopsis Radix (*dǎng shēn*), Rehmanniae Radix praeparata (*shú dì huáng*), or Cervi Cornus Colla (*lù jiǎo jiāo*). However, the emphasis must always be on clearing heat and resolving toxicity, and this emphasis should be reflected in the dosage.

Biomedical Indications

With the appropriate presentation, this formula may be used to treat a variety of biomedically-defined disorders including thromboangiitis obliterans, other disorders with thrombosis in the limbs, and gangrene (in conjunction with surgical debridement).

Modifications

- To strengthen the actions in opening up the channels and invigorating the blood, add 60g of Salviae miltiorrhizae Radix (*dān shēn*) and Ilicis pubescentis Radix (*máo dōng qīng*).
- For extreme pain, add Olibanum (*rǔ xiāng*) and Myrrha (*mò yào*).
- For severe heat, add Moutan Cortex (*mǔ dān pí*) and Rehmanniae Radix (*shēng dì huáng*).
- For pronounced blood stasis and obstruction, add Persicae Semen (*táo rén*) and Carthami Flos (*hóng huā*).

- For pronounced swelling, add Phellodendri Cortex *(huáng bǎi),* Alismatis Rhizoma *(zé xiè),* and Stephaniae tetrandrae Radix *(hàn fáng jǐ).*

Associated Formulas

神效托裡散 (神效托里散)

Miraculous Powder for Supporting the Interior

shén xiào tuō lǐ sǎn

SOURCE *Formulary of the Pharmacy Service for Benefiting the People in the Taiping Era* (1107)

Lonicerae Herba *(rěn dōng cǎo)* 150g
Astragali Radix *(huáng qí)* 150g
Angelicae sinensis Radix *(dāng guī)* 37.5g
Glycyrrhizae Radix *(gān cǎo)* 240g

Grind into a powder and take 6g as a draft cooked in 1.5 cups of wine until reduced to 0.5 cup. Take in the evening. Tonifies and augments the qi and blood, generates flesh, and resolves toxicity. For abscess (including mastitis and Intestinal abscess) with strong fever and chills in patients with qi and blood deficiency. This formula can be viewed as a modification of Tangkuei Decoction to Tonify the Blood *(dāng guī bǔ xuè tāng)*. The large dosage of Astragali Radix *(huáng qí)* and Glycyrrhizae Radix *(gān cǎo)* underscores this formula's suitability for the treatment of toxic swellings that fail to resolve owing to the body's qi deficiency.

五神湯 (五神汤)

Five-Miracle Decoction

wǔ shén tāng

SOURCE *Records of Pattern Discrimination* (1687)

Poria *(fú líng)* 30g
Plantaginis Semen *(chē qián zǐ)* 30g
Lonicerae Flos *(jīn yín huā)* 90g
Achyranthis bidentatae Radix *(niú xī)* 15g
Violae Herba *(zǐ huā dì dīng)* 30g

Grind the ingredients into a powder and take 6g twice a day as a draft. Clears heat, resolves toxicity, and separates and drains out damp-heat. This formula treats damp-heat accumulation in the lower body that may sink into the bones. The pattern manifests as disorders ranging from erysipelas and toxic rashes to bone abscess. Because damp-heat obstructing the qi dynamic of the Bladder is the hallmark of this pattern, dark, painful urination is often a part of the presentation. In modern times, this observation has led to the formula being used to treat hot, painful urinary dribbling disorder.

通塞片

Unblock Obstruction Pill

tōng sāi piàn

SOURCE *Journal of the Nanjing College of Chinese Medicine* (1984)

Astragali Radix *(huáng qí)* 15g
Codonopsis Radix *(dǎng shēn)* 12g
Angelicae sinensis Radix *(dāng guī)* 12g

Dendrobii Herba *(shí hú)* 12g
Scrophulariae Radix *(xuán shēn)* 18g
Lonicerae Flos *(jīn yín huā)* 18g
Achyranthis bidentatae Radix *(niú xī)* 12g
Glycyrrhizae Radix *(gān cǎo)* 12g

Grind the ingredients into a powder and make into tablets (the dosages above are those commonly used, as the source did not provide that detail). Take 8-12g twice a day. Clears heat, resolves toxicity, tonifies the qi, nourishes the yin, invigorates the blood, and transforms stasis. This is a modern formula developed for the treatment of thromboangiitis obliterans, arterial obstruction, and microvascular pathologies in the course of diabetes mellitus, myocardial infarctions, and similar disorders. In contrast to the principal formula, Unblock Obstruction Pill *(tōng sāi piàn)* also tonifies the body's qi and yin. The disorders treated by this formula involve deficiency of the Kidneys, Heart, Spleen, and the Penetrating vessel.

托裡消毒飲 (托里消毒饮)

Support the Interior and Eliminate Toxin Drink

tuō lǐ xiāo dú yǐn

Source *Orthodox Lineage of External Medicine* (1617)

Ginseng Radix *(rén shēn)* 3g
Chuanxiong Rhizoma *(chuān xiōng)* 3g
Paeoniae Radix alba *(bái sháo)* 3g
Astragali Radix *(huáng qí)* 3g
Angelicae dahuricae Radix *(bái zhǐ)* 2g
Gleditsiae Spina *(zào jiǎo cì)* 2g
Angelicae sinensis Radix *(dāng guī)* 3g
Atractylodis macrocephalae Rhizoma *(bái zhú)* 3g
Poria *(fú líng)* 3g
Lonicerae Flos *(jīn yín huā)* 3g
Glycyrrhizae Radix *(gān cǎo)* 2g
Platycodi Radix *(jié gěng)* 2g

Method of Preparation Decoction

Actions Tonifies the qi and blood, expels pus from the interior, and draws out toxicity

Indications

Treats toxic sores in patients with deficient constitutions. The sores either do not suppurate, or if they do, only leak pus slowly and fail to heal. Accompanying symptoms include fever, lassitude, lack of luster, and a rapid pulse with no strength.

These symptoms reflect a situation where either the toxic sore pathogen has existed long enough to deplete the qi, or the patient originally had qi and blood deficiency. The weakened qi and blood are unable to 'brew' the toxin from the toxic swellings into pus and push it out from the interior, so it collects, festers, and gives rise to the type of sores described above. The hot internal toxin also affects the entire body, causing fever and a rapid, though deficient, pulse.

Analysis of Formula

Treatment aims to tonify the qi and blood, expel the toxin, and dissipate the toxic swelling. To this end, Astragali Radix (huáng qí), Ginseng Radix (rén shēn), Atractylodis macrocephalae Rhizoma (bái zhú), Poria (fú líng), and Glycyrrhizae Radix (gān cǎo) fortify the Spleen and tonify the qi to expel toxin and thrust out pus. This is Four-Gentlemen Decoction (sì jūn zǐ tāng) plus Astragali Radix (huáng qí). In the case of nonhealing sores, the ability of Astragali Radix (huáng qí) to secure the exterior and generate flesh is invaluable.

Angelicae sinensis Radix (dāng guī), Chuanxiong Rhizoma (chuān xiōng), and Paeoniae Radix alba (bái sháo) nourish and harmonize the blood. Together with the five herbs above, they provide dual tonification of qi and blood, support the normal qi, and help it resolve toxicity, thrust out pus, and generate flesh. These eight herbs form the primary group. Their function of tonifying the qi and blood is reflected in the group's resemblance to Eight-Treasure Decoction (bā zhēn tāng), discussed in Chapter 8.

Gleditsiae Spina (zào jiǎo cì), Platycodi Radix (jié gěng), and Angelicae dahuricae Radix (bái zhǐ) thrust out pus and break up area of hardness. Lonicerae Flos (jīn yín huā) clears heat and resolves toxicity, and, with the other three herbs in this group, causes the pus to exit and the toxin to drain. This group of herbs dissipates the toxic swellings; they are, however, viewed as secondary to the first group.

Cautions and Contraindications

Because this formula contains Gleditsiae Spina (zào jiǎo cì), it is contraindicated during pregnancy.

Commentary

Toxic sores such as dermal abscesses are usually attributed to damp-heat and fire toxin blocking the channels and causing stagnation of qi and blood. The underlying cause can be any stagnating influence such as a diet too heavy in rich, sweet, or greasy foods. Alternatively, the toxin can enter the body through an open wound. The kind of toxic sore referred to in the literature regarding this formula is a dermal abscess. This is described as a red, painful swelling with a distinct border that feels soft when pressed, reflecting the presence of a pus-filled center. Attendant symptoms such as fever, thirst, a yellow tongue coating, and a rapid pulse display evidence of the body's battle with an internal heat toxin. The ideal outcome is for the swelling to either dissipate without suppurating or come to a head, perforate, suppurate, and close.

When the toxic sore pathogen is abundant and the normal qi is too deficient to push out the toxin, the dermal swelling becomes flat and broad and transforms very slowly into a pus-filled sore. Alternatively, if it does suppurate, it only leaks pus slowly from the sore. The rotted flesh within the sore remains and hinders the production of new flesh to close the sore. The sore may continue to suppurate scant, thin, watery pus with no reduction in the swelling.

While one generally thinks of using powerful dissipating and draining herbs to treat toxic dermal swellings, that approach is inappropriate for sores that are slow to ripen or heal. Chen Shi-Gong, the author of the source text, observed:

> It is suitable to take [this formula] to support the normal [qi]. Those [swellings] that have not yet formed [a head] will dissipate; those that have formed [a head] will ulcerate. The rotting flesh will be dispelled and new flesh generated. At this stage, one should not employ cold or cool agents that internally drain or disperse qi for that would cause damage to the Spleen and Stomach.

The Chinese medical literature contains a great many formulas for treating various aspects and stages of toxic sores. This formula is intended for the patient who has had a swelling for several days and it either is not suppurating at all or suppurates continuously with only a thin, watery pus. The formula aims to promote healing by supporting the body's ability to resolve the internal toxin and thrust out the pus, while at the same time employing herbs to dissipate the toxic swelling.

In practice, treatment of dermal abscesses, boils, or other toxic swellings will be greatly enhanced by application of herbal compresses or plasters such as Golden-Yellow Plaster (jīn huáng gāo) to reduce the swelling, clear the heat, and resolve the toxicity at the site of the lesion.

Comparisons

➤ Vs. Discharge Pus Powder (tòu nóng sǎn)

Both formulas tonify the normal while simultaneously discharging toxin. Support the Interior and Eliminate Toxin Drink (tuō lǐ xiāo dú yǐn) has more tonifying agents and includes one herb, Lonicerae Flos (jīn yín huā), to clear heat and resolve toxicity. In addition, it does not contain Manitis Squama (chuān shān jiǎ), which, because it is derived from an endangered animal, is unsuitable for modern use. Either formula is appropriate for patients who require simultaneous tonification of qi and blood and expelling of internal toxin.

➤ Vs. Other Formulas Commonly Used to Treat Dermal Abscesses

Among other formulas that are commonly used to treat dermal abscesses, Ten-Ingredient Powder to Overcome Toxicity (shí wèi bài dú sǎn), Schizonepeta and Saposhnikovia Powder to Overcome Pathogenic Influences (jīng fáng bài dú sǎn), and Immortals' Formula for Sustaining Life (xiān fāng huó mìng yǐn) have no tonifying actions and are used for the initial stage of dermal swellings in those with strong constitutions. If there are hot, deeply-rooted swellings, particularly if heat signs predominate (with a red tongue and rapid pulse) and there are no signs of dampness or cold, Five-Ingredient Drink to Eliminate Toxin *(wŭ wèi xiāo dú yĭn)* is indicated. Support the Interior and Eliminate Toxin Drink *(tuō lĭ xiāo dú yĭn)* is for toxic swellings that fail to suppurate. It is commonly used for later stage disorders where the qi has been damaged or for those whose qi is too debilitated to thrust out pus.

Since the patient rarely fits exactly one of the above situations, it is not uncommon to mix formulas by adding the key ingredients from one to those of another. For example, an initial-stage outbreak of toxic sores that present as damp-heat, but with the emphasis on heat, might be addressed by combining Ten-Ingredient Powder to Overcome Toxicity *(shí wèi bài dú sǎn)* with a few herbs from Five-Ingredient Drink to Eliminate Toxin *(wŭ wèi xiāo dú yĭn)* such as Taraxaci Herba *(pú gōng yīng)*, Lonicerae Flos *(jīn yín huā),* and Violae Herba *(zĭ huā dì dīng).*

Biomedical Indications

With the appropriate presentation, this formula may be used to treat a variety of biomedically-defined disorders including carbuncles, boils, abscesses, or inflamed cysts.

Modifications

- For breast abscesses, add Vaccariae Semen *(wáng bù liú xíng)*, Taraxaci Herba *(pú gōng yīng)*, and Liquidambaris Fructus *(lù lù tōng)* to unblock the breast and thrust out the pus.
- For patients who are decidedly Spleen deficient, remove the pungent, qi-dispersing Angelicae dahuricae Radix *(bái zhĭ)* and double the dose of Ginseng Radix *(rén shēn).* (source text)
- When middle burner yang is not invigorated and the patient presents with flat, broad swellings, reduced food intake, bland taste, vomiting, nausea or diarrhea, add Aconiti Radix lateralis praeparata *(zhì fù zĭ)* and Zingiberis Rhizoma praeparatum *(páo jiāng)* to warm the middle and expel the toxin.
- When a patient who suffers from yang qi deficiency presents with sores that are slowly oozing watery pus, add Cinnamomi Cortex *(ròu guì)* to warm, tonify the normal qi, and expel the toxin.
- If, after the sore has perforated, the patient suffers from stagnation and deficiency of the nutritive-blood and is in a great deal of pain, add Rehmanniae Radix *(shēng dì huáng)*, Olibanum *(rŭ xiāng)*, and Myrrha *(mò yào)* to tonify the blood, harmonize the nutritive, relieve the pain, and expel the toxin.

Associated Formula

六神丸

Six-Divine Pill

liù shén wán

SOURCE *Lei Yun-Shang's Song-Fen Pharmacy* (founded 1734)

Bovis Calculus *(niú huáng)* .4.5g
Margarita *(zhēn zhū)* 4.5g
Bufonis Venenum *(chán sū)* 3g
Realgar *(xióng huáng)* 3g
Borneolum *(bīng piàn)* 3g
Moschus *(shè xiāng)* 4.5g

Grind the ingredients into a fine powder, mix with wine, and form into millet-size or smaller pills. Adult dosage is 5-10 pills. Resolves fire toxin, reduces swelling, and alleviates pain. This formula was originally for unilateral or bilateral pustular tonsillitis with severe sore throat and difficulty in swallowing. Classical texts refer to this condition as 'milk moth' (乳蛾 *rŭ é*), a serious condition caused by phlegm and severe fire toxin rising to the throat. It is common in patients with chronic heat in the Spleen and Stomach when the throat is invaded by wind-heat. In such cases, the internally-generated heat rises and mixes with the externally-contracted heat. This causes the flesh and membranes of the throat to 'scorch and stew,' producing a pustular lesion of the throat accompanied by swelling and pain, which makes swallowing difficult. This formula is very effective in treating sore throat. Its use has been expanded to include many other conditions due to toxin, including carbuncles, acute localized infection, and lymphangitis. Recently, it has also been used in treating hepatitis and asthma. It is contraindicated during pregnancy.

We include this formula for completeness and to reflect its prominent place in contemporary China. In the West, however, the presence of toxic substances prohibits its use. These include Realgar *(xióng huáng)*, an arsenic compound; Bovis Calculus *(niú huáng)*, which is either very expensive or artificial, with the artificial product being of unknown safety; Bufonis Venenum *(chán sū)*, which is toxic and illegal in most Western countries; the artificial variety of Borneolum *(bīng piàn)*, which can contain chemical contaminants; and Moschus *(shè xiāng)*, which is drawn from the musk deer, a vulnerable species, and from which the musk is often unethically extracted. Lastly, the pills contain unacceptable levels of heavy metals.

陽和湯 (阳和汤)

Balmy Yang Decoction

yáng hé tāng

The term *yáng hé* refers to the warm qi of spring that manifests from the middle of spring onward. It is based on a passage in *Records of the Grand Historian:* "At twenty-nine years [Qin] Shi Huang toured the east … ascending it, he carved a stone. Its words read: Twenty-nine years is the time [that corresponds to the] middle of spring, the time when the yang qi is set free and takes off." This formula treats yin-type localized swellings by promoting the generation and dispersion of the body's yang qi, which heals just like the balmy qi of spring warms the earth to stimulate growth.

Source *Complete Collection of Patterns and Treatments in External Medicine* (1740)

Rehmanniae Radix praeparata *(shú dì huáng)* 30g
Cervi Cornus Colla *(lù jiǎo jiāo)* 9g
Cinnamomi Cortex *(ròu guì)* 3g
Zingiberis Rhizoma praeparatum *(páo jiāng)* 1.5g
Sinapis Semen *(bái jiè zĭ)* 6g

Ephedrae Herba *(má huáng)* 1.5g
Glycyrrhizae Radix *(gān cǎo)* 3g

Method of Preparation   Decoction. Cervi Cornu degelatinatum *(lù jiǎo shuāng)* may be substituted for Cervi Cornus Colla *(lù jiǎo jiāo)*, and Cinnamomi Ramulus *(guì zhī)* for Cinnamomi Cortex *(ròu guì)*.

Actions   Warms the yang, tonifies the blood, disperses cold, and unblocks areas of stagnation

Indications

Localized, painful swellings without a head that blend into the surrounding tissue and do not affect the texture or color of the skin, and are not hot to the touch. There is no thirst, the tongue is very pale, and the pulse is submerged, thin, and forceless.

This formula treats various manifestations of so-called 'yin-type flat abscess' (陰疽 *yīn jū*). These include not only problems in the flesh and muscles, but also in the joints, as in some types of crane's knee wind (鶴膝風 *hè xī fēng*), which is a swollen and painful knee joint accompanied by wasting of the muscles of the thigh and calf. Yin-type localized swelling commonly occurs in those with blood deficiency when cold or phlegm (or both) congeal in a discrete area of the muscles, sinews, bones, or blood vessels, and the yang qi is too weak to disperse them. The cold or yin nature of the swellings is evidenced by their blending into the surrounding tissue, the absence of heat signs, as well as more generalized signs of yang and blood deficiency that include a pale tongue with a white coating, and a deep and thin, or a slow and thin pulse.

Analysis of Formula

The composition of this formula is based on three treatment strategies listed in Chapter 74 of *Basic Questions*: "Heat what is cold," "Tonify what is deficient," and "Disperse what has clumped." Accordingly, it aims to warm the yang, tonify the blood, disperse the cold, and unblock areas of stagnation. Furthermore, in order to heal any type of swelling, treating the branch manifestations is more important than treating the root. For this reason, acrid and warming Cinnamomi Cortex *(ròu guì)* and Zingiberis Rhizoma praeparatum *(páo jiāng)* are regarded as the chief herbs. They enter the nutritive qi to warm the channels, unblock the blood vessels, disperse cold, and eliminate pathogenic qi. Two tonifying herbs serve as deputies to treat the root of the disorder. Rehmanniae Radix praeparata *(shú dì huáng)*, in a large dosage, tonifies the blood. It is supported in this role by Cervi Cornus Colla *(lù jiǎo jiāo)*, which tonifies the blood and assists the yang. One of the assistants, Sinapis Semen *(bái jiè zǐ)*, specifically expels phlegm lodged just beneath the skin. Combined with the heavy deputy herbs, its dispersing action unfolds at deeper levels of the body, such as the muscles and bones. The other assistant, Ephedrae Herba *(má huáng)*, opens up the inter-

stices and pores and helps lead out the cold. Moreover, the acrid nature of the two assistants counteracts the cloying nature of the deputies, preventing their tonifying nature from strengthening and retaining the pathogenic qi. Conversely, the herbs that promote movement are prevented from injuring the normal qi because of the presence of the chief ingredients. The envoy, Glycyrrhizae Radix *(gān cǎo)*, harmonizes the actions of the other ingredients in the formula.

Overall, this formula is a good example of the interrelationship between treating the branch (swelling) and the root (blood deficiency). It also illustrates the method of 'finding the yang within the yin.'

Cautions and Contraindications

This formula is contraindicated in patients with yang-type localized swellings, yin deficiency, or with swellings (even of the yin type) that have ulcerated for a long time. If the formula is modified, the ratio of Rehmanniae Radix praeparata *(shú dì huáng)* to Ephedrae Herba *(má huáng)* specified in the source text must be followed. If the relative dosage of Ephedrae Herba *(má huáng)* is too high, the deficiency will worsen and aggravate the condition.

Commentary

This formula was composed by the famous external medicine specialist of the Qing dynasty, Wang Wei-De, to treat crane's knee wind and all kinds of yin-type localized swellings. Its scope was later expanded to encompass yin-type sores, and it thus acquired the alternative name Life-Sustaining Special Pill for Yin-Type Flat-Abscesses (陰疽活命丹 *yīn jū huó mìng dān*). The characteristic symptoms of these lesions are the absence of redness or heat, the gradual appearance only of swellings, soreness, and aching rather than acute pain, and a thin pulse. In his critical commentary, *Complete Collection of Patterns and Treatments in External Medicine*, the famous 19th-century physician Ma Pei-Zhi gave this formula his highest rating: "This formula is without peer in treating yin-type patterns. Used appropriately, it delivers its effects without a hitch."

Expanded Usage

Interpreting Ma Pei-Zhi's analysis very liberally, physicians in contemporary China have expanded the range of application of this formula to include internal medical, gynecological, and pediatric disorders characterized by yang deficiency where cold leads to a congealing of fluids and stagnation of qi and blood. The key symptoms in such patterns are a pale and lusterless complexion along with lethargy. The wide range of clinical presentations can be seen under BIOMEDICAL INDICATIONS below.

Debates about the Chief Ingredients

There has been some debate in the literature regarding the

chief ingredient and, by implication, the main pathodynamic treated by this formula. The Qing-dynasty physician Zhang Bing-Cheng noted in *Convenient Reader of Established Formulas*: "The cause of this disorder lies in the blood aspect. Accordingly, one must seek to [treat] it from within the blood and therefore use Rehmanniae Radix praeparata *(shú dì huáng)*, an herb that strongly tonifies the yin blood, as chief." This interpretation is supported by the fact that this substance is prescribed in the largest dosage. Many modern textbooks follow Zhang Bing-Cheng's lead and designate Rehmanniae Radix praeparata *(shú dì huáng)* and Cervi Cornu *(lù jiǎo)*, an animal-derived substance that also affects the blood, as the chief ingredients.

Another method of looking at this issue is to examine Wang Wei-De's own approach to the treatment of yin-type toxic swellings and sores. As Li Fei shows in *Formulas,* the three herbs Cinnamomi Cortex *(ròu guì)*, Ephedrae Herba *(má huáng)*, and Zingiberis Rhizoma praeparatum *(páo jiāng)* appear in all of Yang's formulas for yin-type flat abscesses. He also composed a formula that he named Balmy Yang Pills *(yáng hé wán)* that simply combines these three herbs. From this perspective, this combination would be the core around which the rest of the formula is built. Several later external medicine specialists, such as the Qing-dynasty physician Zhang Zheng-Shen, followed Wang's lead and composed variations of this formula that contain Cinnamomi Cortex *(ròu guì)*, Zingiberis Rhizoma praeparatum *(páo jiāng)*, Ephedrae Herba *(má huáng)*, and Glycyrrhizae Radix *(gān cǎo)*, but do not always add tonifying herbs.

The contemporary formula expert Chen Zhao-Zu makes the following additional recommendations. He suggests replacing Cervi Cornus Colla *(lù jiǎo jiāo)* with Cervi Cornu degelatinatum *(lù jiǎo shuāng)* in order to make the formula more moving, without diminishing its tonifying properties; and to replace Cinnamomi Cortex *(ròu guì)* with Cinnamomi Ramulus *(guì zhī)* to focus the formula more strongly on unblocking the blood vessels.

Biomedical Indications

With the appropriate presentation, this formula may be used to treat a wide variety of biomedically-defined disorders. These can be divided into the following groups:

- Rheumatic and vascular diseases such as thromboangiitis obliterans, rheumatoid arthritis, Raynaud's disease, polyarthritis, idiopathic bone hyperplasia, and scleroderma
- Inflammatory diseases such as aseptic suppuration, lymphatic tuberculosis, tubercular joint disease, chronic osteomyelitis, chronic erysipelas, and chronic ulcerative colitis
- Neuromusculoskeletal disorders such as peripheral neuritis, sciatica, and intervertebral disc disease
- Women's diseases such as early-stage endometriosis, mastitis, and fibrocystic breasts

- Respiratory conditions such as chronic bronchitis, bronchial asthma, and emphysema.

This formula has also been used for treating sick sinus syndrome, urticaria, benign prostatic hypertrophy, epilepsy, and frostbite.

Modifications

- For general signs of cold, add Aconiti Radix lateralis praeparata *(zhì fù zǐ)*.
- For severe qi deficiency, add Astragali Radix *(huáng qí)* and Ginseng Radix *(rén shēn)*.
- For fibrocystic breasts, add Cyperi Rhizoma *(xiāng fù)*, Citri reticulatae Pericarpium *(chén pí)*, and Curcumae Radix *(yù jīn)*.
- For more severe pain, add blood-moving herbs like Myrrha *(mò yào)* and Olibanum *(rǔ xiāng)*.

Associated Formula

中和湯 （中和汤）

Even-Handed Decoction

zhōng hé tāng

SOURCE *Indispensable Tools for Pattern Treatment* (1602)

Ginseng Radix *(rén shēn)*	6g
Citri reticulatae Pericarpium *(chén pí)*	6g
Astragali Radix *(huáng qí)*	4.5g
Atractylodis macrocephalae Rhizoma *(bái zhú)*	4.5g
Angelicae sinensis Radix *(dāng guī)*	4.5g
Angelicae dahuricae Radix *(bái zhǐ)*	4.5g
Poria *(fú líng)*	3g
Chuanxiong Rhizoma *(chuān xiōng)*	3g
Gleditsiae Spina *(zào jiǎo cì)*	3g
Olibanum *(rǔ xiāng)*	3g
Myrrha *(mò yào)*	3g
Lonicerae Flos *(jīn yín huā)*	3g
Glycyrrhizae Radix *(gān cǎo)*	3g

Prepare as a decoction using one part water and one part wine. Tonifies the qi, invigorates the blood, reduces swelling, and alleviates pain. This formula has an even-handed approach to treating half-yin, half-yang localized swellings that look as if they are about to ulcerate, but do not. The swellings are just slightly delineated, mildly painful, pale red, slightly warm but not hot, and the patient shows signs of underlying qi deficiency. Although the Chinese name of this formula resembles that of the primary formula, its composition is much closer to that of Immortals' Formula for Sustaining Life *(xiān fāng huó mìng yǐn)*, discussed earlier in the chapter. This is because deficiency of qi leads, in the first instance, to stagnation and clumping of qi and blood in the vessels, which is directly addressed in both formulas. Yang deficiency, on the other hand, leads more directly to stagnation of fluids and the formation of phlegm, problems that are addressed in Balmy Yang Decoction *(yáng hé tāng)*.

十味敗毒散 (十味败毒散)

Ten-Ingredient Powder to Overcome Toxicity

shí wèi bài dú sǎn

Source   Experiential formula by Hanaoka Seshū (1760-1835)

Bupleuri Radix *(chái hú)* 3g
Angelicae pubescentis Radix *(dú huó)* 3g
Cerasi Cortex *(yīng pí)* * 3g
Saposhnikoviae Radix *(fáng fēng)* 3g
Platycodi Radix *(jié gěng)* 3g
Chuanxiong Rhizoma *(chuān xiōng)* 3g
Poria *(fú líng)* 4g
Schizonepetae Herba *(jīng jiè)* 1g
Glycyrrhizae Radix *(gān cǎo)* 1g
Zingiberis Rhizoma *(gān jiāng)* .1g

Method of Preparation   Decoction. Most practitioners in Taiwan, where the formula is popular, double the above dosages.

Actions   Dispels wind and transforms dampness, clears heat, and resolves toxicity

Indications

For heat toxin flushing through the exterior aspects of the body. Originally indicated for the initial stages of painful and hot toxic sores such as carbuncles and dermal abscesses; in modern times, the range of disorders has expanded to include all kinds of pus-filled sores and even acute episodes of eczema and hives. The list of disorders for which this formula is indicated includes acne, boils, dermal abscesses, eczema, hives, mastitis, inflamed lymph nodes, internal or external ear infections, and sties.

Analysis of Formula

For complex dermatological disorders, this formula follows the path of using mild herbs in small doses to resolve toxicity, dissipate the exterior, thrust pus out, clear heat, and dispel dampness. Modeled after Schizonepeta and Saposhnikovia Powder to Overcome Pathogenic Influences *(jīng fáng bài dú sǎn)*, the author of this formula replaced Peucedani Radix *(qián hú)*, Notopterygii Rhizoma seu Radix *(qiāng huó)*, Menthae haplocalycis Herba *(bò hé)*, Forsythiae Fructus *(lián qiáo)*, Aurantii Fructus *(zhǐ ké)*, and Lonicerae Flos *(jīn yín huā)* with the single herb Cerasi Cortex *(yīng pí)*, which is an herb used in Japan to collect and then and resolve toxicity. Its inclusion narrows the formula's function to the treatment of toxic swellings. Difficult to find nowadays in the West, Rosae

---

* Cerasi Cortex (櫻皮 *yīng pí*) is a Japanese medicinal that is derived from the bark of the Japanese cherry tree. The botanical name is *Prunus cerasus* or *Cerasus pseudocerasus*. It relieves toxicity, stops coughing, thrusts out pus, and relieves fevers. Traditionally, it was particularly used for food poisoning (especially from fish), urticaria, and for skin diseases marked by swelling. [Kenji Watanabe, personal communication]

laevigatae Fructus *(jīn yīng zǐ)* is frequently used as a substitute.

The other ingredients work together for a complete approach to this condition. Platycodi Radix *(jié gěng)* aids Cerasi Cortex *(yīng pí)* in resolving toxicity and also, with the help of Chuanxiong Rhizoma *(chuān xiōng)*, thrusting out the pus. Saposhnikoviae Radix *(fáng fēng)* and Angelicae pubescentis Radix *(dú huó)* dispel wind-dampness. Poria *(fú líng)* helps rid the body of dampness and at the same time enhances the body's ability to expel heat toxin through urination. Chuanxiong Rhizoma *(chuān xiōng)* moves blood and thrusts out pus. Schizonepetae Herba *(jīng jiè)* combines with Saposhnikoviae Radix *(fáng fēng)* and Angelicae pubescentis Radix *(dú huó)* to resolve the exterior and dissipate the accumulation of heat toxin in the exterior of the body. Bupleuri Radix *(chái hú)* resolves toxicity, releases pathogens from the exterior, and clears blood heat from both the interior and exterior. Zingiberis Rhizoma *(gān jiāng)* harmonizes the Stomach. Glycyrrhizae Radix *(gān cǎo)* harmonizes the formula and also resolves toxicity.

Cautions and Contraindications

This formula should not be used for toxic sores that have already suppurated.

Commentary

The formula's ability to treat pus-filled sores makes it a good candidate for acute outbreaks of boils or carbuncles, inflamed lymph nodes, mastitis, inner ear infections, and sties. It is only appropriate for the initial stage of these disorders. If they have persisted for more than 4-5 days, one should use stronger medicinals, such as Support the Interior and Eliminate Toxin Drink *(tuō lǐ xiāo dú yǐn)*, or stronger herbs that clear heat and thrust out pus, such as Coptidis Rhizoma *(huáng lián)* and Gleditsiae Spina *(zào jiǎo cì)*.

Aside from Cerasi Cortex *(yīng pí)*, the formula contains several other herbs that are frequently found in the dermatologist's arsenal. Schizonepetae Herba *(jīng jiè)* and Saposhnikoviae Radix *(fáng fēng)* are both light herbs that float to the surface to treat skin disorders, and Chuanxiong Rhizoma *(chuān xiōng)* and Platycodi Radix *(jié gěng)* are both regularly used to help toxic sores to suppurate.

In modern times, especially in Japan, this formula is often applied to allergic skin disorders. These include hives that present as exterior wind-cold trapping damp-heat with chills, red-hot swellings and the absence of sweating; or chronic, episodic eczema that is dry and red with moderate itching.

Comparison

➤ Vs. IMMORTALS' FORMULA FOR SUSTAINING LIFE *(xiān fāng huó mìng yǐn)*

While both of these formulas thrust out pus, resolve toxicity, and dissipate swelling, and are appropriate for those with strong constitutions, Immortals' Formula for Sustaining Life *(xiān fāng huó mìng yǐn)* is a more powerful formula. If, however, the condition is in its initial stage in a patient with a lesser yang constitution and signs of damp-heat, Ten-Ingredient Powder to Overcome Toxicity *(shí wèi bài dú sǎn)* may be the better choice. Also, this formula has the additional function of treating urticaria and eczema.

Biomedical Indications

With the appropriate presentation, this formula may be used to treat a variety of biomedically defined disorders including acne, boils, carbuncles, abscesses, cysts, eczema, seborrheic dermatitis, hives, mastitis, lymphadenitis, otitis media, and sties.

Modifications

- Forsythiae Fructus *(lián qiáo)* is often included to increase the formula's capacity to clear heat and resolve toxicity. If the sores are especially hot, add Coptidis Rhizoma *(huáng lián)*, Scutellariae Radix *(huáng qín),* and Gardeniae Fructus *(zhī zǐ).*
- For damp skin disorders, add Coicis Semen *(yì yǐ rén).*
- If itching is severe, add Tribuli Fructus *(cì jí lí).*
- To increase the formula's ability to thrust out pus, add Gleditsiae Spina *(zào jiǎo cì).*
- For constipation, add Rhei Radix et Rhizoma *(dà huáng).*
- For hives, combine with Cimicifuga and Kudzu Decoction *(shēng má gé gēn tāng).*
- For sties, add Forsythiae Fructus *(lián qiáo)*, Lonicerae Flos *(jīn yín huā),* and Taraxaci Herba *(pú gōng yīng).*
- For ear infections, add Scutellariae Radix *(huáng qín)*, Forsythiae Fructus *(lián qiáo)*, Paeoniae Radix rubra *(chì sháo)*, Ilicis latifoliae Folium *(kǔ dīng chá),* and Puerariae Radix *(gé gēn).*

千金內托散
Powder to Support the Interior Worth a Thousand Gold Pieces

qiān jīn nèi tuō sǎn

Source   *Restoration of Health from the Myriad Diseases* (1587)

The name of this formula reminds one that it supports the body's interior to help it heal lingering dermal and subdermal lesions. 'Thousand gold pieces' refers to the value of the formula.

Astragali Radix *(huáng qí)* 6g
Ginseng Radix *(rén shēn)* 6g
Angelicae sinensis Radix *(dāng guī)* 6g
Chuanxiong Rhizoma *(chuān xiōng)* 3g

Saposhnikoviae Radix *(fáng fēng)* 3g
Platycodi Radix *(jié gěng)* 3g
Angelicae dahuricae Radix *(bái zhǐ)* 3g
Magnoliae officinalis Cortex *(hòu pò)* 3g
Glycyrrhizae Radix *(gān cǎo)* 3g
Cinnamomi Cortex *(ròu guì)* .3g

Method of Preparation   The source text advises that the best effect is achieved by cooking the ingredients in wine. Alternatively, the ingredients can be ground into a powder and taken with yellow rice or millet wine, with 9g per dose. For those who do not drink alcohol, the text suggests that the powder be taken with a tea made from Aucklandiae Radix *(mù xiāng).*

Actions   Invigorates the blood, tonifies deficiency, expels foulness, and generates new flesh

Indications

This formula was originally intended to treat toxic swellings, both yang (癰 *yōng)* and yin (疽 *jū),* in patients with deficient constitutions.

Analysis of Formula

Because the formula treats conditions of deficiency, its main goal is to tonify. Secondarily, it addresses the branch symptoms of lingering abscesses and other swellings or lesions by moving the blood, dispelling foulness and pus, and generating flesh. It employs Astragali Radix *(huáng qí)* and Ginseng Radix *(rén shēn)* to tonify the qi and secure the exterior. They tonify the Spleen to help the body discharge toxin. Angelicae sinensis Radix *(dāng guī)* and Chuanxiong Rhizoma *(chuān xiōng)* tonify and invigorate the blood. Saposhnikoviae Radix *(fáng fēng)* brings the effect of the formula to the body's surface and prevents wind pathogens from disturbing the flow of qi in the area of the lesion. Platycodi Radix *(jié gěng)* and Angelicae dahuricae Radix *(bái zhǐ)* thrust pus out and reduce abscesses. Magnoliae officinalis Cortex *(hòu pò)* improves the Spleen's transporting function, dries dampness, and moves stagnation in the qi aspect. Cinnamomi Cortex *(ròu guì)* is included in many formulas that treat sores and abscesses that have some cold aspects in order to help warm and support the interior. By warming the middle and tonifying the yang, Cinnamomi Cortex *(ròu guì)* enhances the body's natural ability to heal lingering lesions. Glycyrrhizae Radix *(gān cǎo)* resolves toxicity and harmonizes the actions of the other ingredients in the formula.

This formula focuses on tonifying the root deficiency and therefore selects herbs that are not overly dispersing or draining to address the branch symptoms. A good analysis is provided in *Medical Formulas Collected and Analyzed:*

> Ginseng Radix *(rén shēn)* and Astragali Radix *(huáng qí)* tonify the qi; Chuanxiong Rhizoma *(chuān xiōng)* and Angelicae sinensis Radix *(dāng guī)* invigorate the blood; Glycyrrhizae Radix *(gān cǎo)* resolves toxicity; Cinnamomi Cortex *(ròu guì)*, Angelicae dahuricae Radix *(bái zhǐ)*, and Platycodi Radix *(jié*

gĕng) [work together to] push out pus; Magnoliae officinalis Cortex *(hòu pò)* drains excess and fullness; [and] Saposhnikoviae Radix *(fáng fēng)* disperses pathogenic wind. These external and internal qi and blood herbs work to aid [the body's] yang in supporting the interior.

Cautions and Contraindications

This formula is for patterns of cold and deficiency and is inappropriate for heat patterns. It is contraindicated for toxic swellings that are red, hot, and painful.

Commentary

The source text outlines two conditions for which this formula is indicated: first, toxic swellings that linger after suppurating and continue to leak pus, and second, toxic swellings that remain without producing pus and suppurating. Both of these conditions are attributed to a constitution that is too weak to thrust out pus and complete the healing process. The principle of treatment is to tonify the interior and help the body dissipate the accumulation at the site of the lesion and thrust pus and turbidity out. In the case of lingering open sores, the additional functions of generating flesh and closing the sores are also required.

History

This formula dates to the Song-dynasty text *Formulary of the Pharmacy Service for Benefiting the People in the Taiping Era,* where it was called Powder to Transform and Push out Pus, Tonify the Interior, and Completely Disseminate (化膿排膿 內補十宣散 *huà nóng pái nóng nèi bǔ shí xuān sǎn).* There it is said that the formula addresses all manner of abscesses, swellings, sores, and boils. It claims that when the formula is used to treat dermal sores, "those that have not come to a head will quickly dissipate and those that have already come to a head will quickly suppurate without the need for squeezing, and the noxious flesh will spontaneously heal without the need for a knife."

In *Medical Formulas Collected and Analyzed,* Wang Ang recommended the formula for toxic sores in thin patients or in those with a weak pulse. He pointed out that the formula works well for sores as long as they are not due to heat conditions such as alcohol toxicity, erysipelas Stomach deficiency, or consumption-qi constraint. This underscored the role of the formula in the treatment of pure deficiency patterns and pointed out that the herbs are too tonifying and hot to use where there is heat toxin or qi constraint. It is noteworthy that this formula is positioned next to the classic tonifying formula All-Inclusive Great Tonifying Decoction *(shí quán dà bǔ tāng)* in the section on abscesses and swellings in *Restoration of Health from the Myriad Diseases;* this suggests that that it treats toxic swellings by tonifying the body and augmenting its ability to expel toxin and dissipate swellings.

Usage

The modern application of this formula to such conditions as inner and outer ear infections and swollen lymph nodes is derived from Japanese texts. This may stem from a passage in the Japanese text *Formulary & Mnemonics from 'No Mistake' Pharmacy* that implies that the formula can be used for other conditions where deficiency limits the body's ability to thrust out pathogens: "This formula is a principal one for tonifying and supporting [the interior in the treatment of] toxic swellings, and the rash of pox … but it is not limited [to treating] toxic swellings."

In summary, the formula treats chronic sores that fail to come to a head or those that have already suppurated but continue to exude watery pus. By extension, it has also come to be used to treat chronic inner ear infections and other localized infections that linger and subsequently drain the body's qi.

Variations

Zhu Dan-Xi, Li Dong-Yuan, and others authored many variations of this formula. Most commonly, they used the same foundation as this formula, but added Myrrha *(mò yào),* Olibanum *(rǔ xiāng),* and Forsythiae Fructus *(lián qiáo)* to move the blood and qi and disperse accumulations. These acrid, dispersing agents increase the pus-expelling and swelling-dissipating functions of the formula, but reduce its capacity to tonify. Note that some versions contain Cinnamomi Ramulus *(guì zhī)* in place of Cinnamomi Cortex *(ròu guì).*

Comparisons

➤ Vs. Support the Interior and Eliminate Toxin Drink *(tuō lǐ xiāo dú yǐn)* and Tangkuei and Astragalus Decoction to Construct the Middle *(guī qí jiàn zhōng tāng)*

All three formulas treat deficient patients with toxic swelling that have been incompletely dissipated or not reduced at all:

- Support the Interior and Eliminate Toxin Drink *(tuō lǐ xiāo dú yǐn)* is for a very early stage where the swelling toxin is abundant and the body is slightly weakened.
- Powder to Support the Interior Worth a Thousand Gold Pieces *(qiān jīn nèi tuō sǎn)* is for a slightly later stage when the deficiency is more significant than the toxic pathogen.
- Tangkuei and Astragalus Decoction to Construct the Middle *(guī qí jiàn zhōng tāng)* is for a similar condition as the principal formula here, but in patients who are even more severely deficient.

Biomedical Indications

With the appropriate presentation, this formula may be used to treat a variety of biomedically-defined disorders includ-

ing lymphadenitis, tubercular osteomyelitis, boils, carbuncles, suppurative mastitis, otitis media, and otitis externa.

Alternate name

Powder to Support the Interior and Completely Tonify *(tuō lǐ shí bǔ sǎn)* in *Medical Formulas Collected and Analyzed*

Modifications

- For painful toxic swellings, increase the dosage of Angelicae dahuricae Radix *(bái zhǐ)*. (source text)
- If the swellings are not painful, increase the dosage of Cinnamomi Cortex *(ròu guì)*. (source text)
- For loss of appetite, add Amomi Fructus *(shā rén)* and Cyperi Rhizoma *(xiāng fù)*. (source text)
- If the pain is severe, add Olibanum *(rǔ xiāng)* and Myrrha *(mò yào)*. (source text)
- For sores that continue to exude fluid, add Anemarrhenae Rhizoma *(zhī mǔ)* and Fritillariae thunbergii Bulbus *(zhè bèi mǔ)*. (source text)
- For sores that hesitate to burst, add Gleditsiae Spina *(zào jiǎo cì)*. (source text)
- For constipation, add Rhei Radix et Rhizoma *(dà huáng)* and Aurantii Fructus *(zhǐ ké)*. (source text)
- For inhibited urination, add Ophiopogonis Radix *(mài mén dōng)* and Plantaginis Semen *(chē qián zǐ)*. (source text)
- For inner ear infections, add Paeoniae Radix rubra *(chì sháo)*, Puerariae Radix *(gé gēn)*, and Xanthii Fructus *(cāng ěr zǐ)*.
- For swollen lymph nodes, add Scrophulariae Radix *(xuán shēn)*, Moutan Cortex *(mǔ dān pí)*, and Prunellae Spica *(xià kū cǎo)*.

Associated Formulas

透膿散 （透脓散）

Discharge Pus Powder

tòu nóng sǎn

SOURCE *Orthodox Lineage of External Medicine* (1617)

Astragali Radix *(huáng qí)*	12g
Angelicae sinensis Radix *(dāng guī)*	6g
Chuanxiong Rhizoma *(chuān xiōng)*	9g
Manitis Squama *(chuān shān jiǎ)*	3g
Gleditsiae Spina *(zào jiǎo cì)*	4.5g

Pushes toxin outward and expels pus. For chronic abscesses without heads that produce pus but do not readily perforate to discharge the pus. Usually accompanied by localized pain, swelling, and heat. The normal qi in these patients is deficient, leaving it unable to push out the toxin. Chronic abscesses then form due to the inability of the normal qi to expel the pus that gathers below the skin. The retention of toxin creates pain, swelling, and heat. Because it contains Gleditsiae Spina *(zào jiǎo cì)*, the use of this formula is contraindicated during pregnancy.

內補黃耆湯 （内补黄芪汤）

Internally Tonifying Decoction with Astragalus

nèi bǔ huáng qí tāng

SOURCE *Formulas Bequeathed by the Unorthodox Genius Liu Juan-Zi* (499)

dry-fried Astragali Radix *(chǎo huáng qí)*	3g
Ophiopogonis Radix *(mài mén dōng)*	3g
Rehmanniae Radix praeparata *(shú dì huáng)*	3g
Poria *(fú líng)*	3g
Glycyrrhizae Radix praeparata *(zhì gān cǎo)*	1.5g
dry-fried Paeoniae Radix alba *(chǎo bái sháo)*	1.5g
dry-fried Polygalae Radix *(chǎo yuǎn zhì)*	1.5g
Chuanxiong Rhizoma *(chuān xiōng)*	1.5g
Cinnamomi Cortex *(ròu guì)*	1.5g
wine-fried Angelicae sinensis Radix *(jiǔ chǎo dāng guī)*	1.5g

Decoct with 3 pieces of Zingiberis Rhizoma recens *(shēng jiāng)* and 1 piece of Jujubae Fructus *(dà zǎo)*. At present, the dosage of the listed ingredients is usually tripled. Tonifies and augments the qi and blood, generates flesh, and closes wounds. It is used to treat toxic swellings after they have burst in patients with qi and blood deficiency marked by pain at the site of the ulceration, fatigue, laconic speech, difficulty sleeping, spontaneous sweating, dry mouth, and sometimes fever that does not recede even after a long time. The tongue is pale with a thin coating and the pulse is thin and weak.

Comparison

➤ Vs. All-Inclusive Great Tonifying Decoction *(shí quán dà bǔ tāng)*

Both formulas strongly tonify both the qi and blood, and both can be used for treating nonhealing ulcers. Internally Tonifying Decoction with Astragalus *(nèi bǔ huáng qí tāng)* has Ophiopogonis Radix *(mài mén dōng)* and Polygalae Radix *(yuǎn zhì)* to nourish the yin, clear heat, and calm the spirit and is specifically indicated for the treatment of ulcerated sores that do not heal in deficient patients who also have signs of heat, such as dry mouth and difficulty sleeping. By contrast, All-Inclusive Great Tonifying Decoction *(shí quán dà bǔ tāng)* has Atractylodis macrocephalae Rhizoma *(bái zhú)*, which allows it to better tonify the Spleen and strengthen that organ's transporting and transforming functions. This gives it a much wider scope of action.

散腫潰堅湯 （散肿溃坚汤）

Decoction to Disperse Swelling and Ulcerate What is Hard

sàn zhǒng kuì jiān tāng

Source *Secrets from the Orchid Chamber* (1336)

Eckloniae Thallus *(kūn bù)*	15g (12g)
wine-fried Phellodendri Cortex *(jiǔ chǎo huáng bǎi)*	15g (9g)

wine-fried Anemarrhenae Rhizoma (jiǔ chǎo zhī mǔ) 15g (9g)
Trichosanthis Radix (tiān huā fěn) 15g (12g)
Platycodi Radix (jié gěng) 15g (9g)
wine-fried Sparganii Rhizoma (jiǔ chǎo sān léng) 9g (9g)
wine-fried Curcumae Rhizoma (jiǔ chǎo é zhú) 9g (9g)
wine-fried Gentianae Radix (jiǔ chǎo lóng dǎn cǎo) 15g (6g)
Coptidis Rhizoma (huáng lián) 3g (3g)
Scutellariae Radix (huáng qín)
    [half wine-fried and half untreated] 24 (9g)
Puerariae Radix (gé gēn) 6g (9g)
Paeoniae Radix alba (bái sháo) 6g (6g)
Forsythiae Fructus (lián qiáo) 9g (9g)
Cimicifugae Rhizoma (shēng má) .9g (9g)
Bupleuri Radix (chái hú) 12g (9g)
Glycyrrhizae Radix praeparata (zhì gān cǎo) 15g (9g)
Angelicae sinensis radicis Cauda (dāng guī wěi) 6g (6g)

Method of Preparation   The source text instructs to grind half
the ingredients into a coarse powder and take 24-27g for each
dose. Soak in 2.8 cups of water for half a day, decoct down to
1 cup, remove the dregs, and drink warm. It is best to imbibe
the liquid slowly (ten swallows for each mouthful) and to lay
down so that the head is lower than the legs. Swallowing slowly
allows the herbs to temporarily remain in the area above the diaphragm. Lastly, grind half of the ingredients into a fine powder
and form into mung bean-sized honey pills. Take 100-150 pills
per day washed down with mouthfuls of the decocted herbs. At
present, the formula is simply taken as a decoction prepared in
the usual manner, typically with the amounts listed in parentheses.

Actions   Clears heat, resolves toxicity, reduces swelling, induces
ulceration, moves the blood, and dispels stasis

Indications

Saber sores (馬刀瘡 mǎ dāo chuāng, lit. 'horse-knife sores')
that are knotted and hard lumps, as hard as stones. These
may be located on the neck or shoulders and down to the
armpit, usually along the path of the hand and foot lesser
yang channels or the foot yang brightness channel. It also addresses scrofula, goiter, and other neck tumors.

Saber sores are also called 'saber lumps,' 'saber nodules,'
and 'pearl-string lumps.' These are attributed to fire rising
in the body, causing the fluids to congeal into phlegm. The
phlegm and fire accumulate in the neck area and form lumps
that cause further accumulation by obstructing the pathways
in the area. The main sources of the offending fire are disharmonies of the Liver, Stomach, Lungs, or Kidneys.

Analysis of Formula

Treating these types of swellings requires a formula to attack the problem on multiple fronts simultaneously: soften
hardness, disperse accumulations and swellings, move the
blood, clear heat, and resolve toxicity in order to cause hard
swellings in the neck region to soften and disperse. Eckloniae

Thallus (kūn bù) transforms phlegm and, being salty, softens
hardness. Sparganii Rhizoma (sān léng) and Curcumae Rhizoma (é zhú) move the blood and dispel stasis and thus aid
in dispersal of the hard swellings. Of these, Li Dong-Yuan
observed: "Use Sparganii Rhizoma (sān léng) and Curcumae
Rhizoma (é zhú) if the sores are very hard; if not, do not use
them." Angelicae sinensis radicis Cauda (dāng guī wěi) has
a similar function, although it is less dispersing than those
two herbs and can safely be used with softer swellings and
weaker patients. It also harmonizes and nourishes the blood.
The latter function is crucial to preventing the long-standing
heat disorder and bitter, drying herbs from wearing away the
yin-blood.

Phellodendri Cortex (huáng bǎi), Coptidis Rhizoma
(huáng lián), Gentianae Radix (lóng dǎn cǎo), and Scutellariae Radix (huáng qín) clear heat and resolve toxicity. These
herbs address the heat accumulation that occurs at the site
of the tumor and also the heat of specific organs that are
the root cause of the tumor. Anemarrhenae Rhizoma (zhī
mǔ), especially when combined with Puerariae Radix (gé gēn)
and Trichosanthis Radix (tiān huā fěn), clears heat while also
protecting yin that is susceptible to damage from the heat
accumulation and the bitter, drying herbs in the formula. In
addition, Anemarrhenae Rhizoma (zhī mǔ), together with the
other bitter, downward-homing herbs, causes fire to descend
and cease its attack on the upper body, and sweeps phlegm-
heat downward. Both Trichosanthis Radix (tiān huā fěn) and
Forsythiae Fructus (lián qiáo) clear heat and resolve toxicity,
while Trichosanthis Radix (tiān huā fěn) also thrusts pus out.
The acrid, dispersing nature of Forsythiae Fructus (lián qiáo)
aids in the dissipation of heat accumulation. Li Dong-Yuan
credits Trichosanthis Radix (tiān huā fěn) with the ability to
guide out the qi of swellings. Paeoniae Radix alba (bái sháo)
softens the Liver and nourishes the blood, thus helping Angelicae sinensis Radix (dāng guī) to protect the body's blood-
yin. By softening the Liver, it also addresses Liver fire, which
is often a contributing factor or main cause of the types of
swellings this formula treats.

Li Dong-Yuan notes that Glycyrrhizae Radix praeparata
(zhì gān cǎo) "harmonizes the formula, drains fire, augments
the Stomach qi, and also dispels sore toxins." Cimicifugae
Rhizoma (shēng má) and Puerariae Radix (gé gēn) guide the
herbs to the upper body and pertain to the foot yang brightness channel. Bupleuri Radix (chái hú) guides herbs to the
lesser yang channels and dredges the Liver. In *Secrets from the
Orchid Chamber,* in the course of discussing herbs in a similar formula, Li Dong-Yuan observed that Cimicifugae Rhizoma (shēng má) and Puerariae Radix (gé gēn) are for sores on
the yang brightness channel, and that Bupleuri Radix (chái
hú) can be omitted if the sores are not along the lesser yang
channels. Insight into Li Dong-Yuan's use of Platycodi Radix
(jié gěng) can be found in his entry for this herb in *Essential*

Teachings on Utilizing Medicinal: "[It] facilitates the flow of qi through the throat, chest, and diaphragm. … Platycodi Radix (*jié gěng*) can disperse."

In sum, the formula softens hardness, dissipates accumulations and swellings, moves the blood, clears heat, and resolves toxicity to cause hard swellings in the neck region to soften and dissipate.

Cautions and Contraindications

This formula contains several bitter, drying, and dispersing herbs. Care must be taken to protect the patient's yin fluids and qi. Elderly and debilitated patients may require simultaneous or intermittent tonification when this formula is used.

Commentary

This formula does what the name implies: disperses swelling and induces ulceration of hardness. In effect, it encourages hard swellings to behave like normal toxic swellings and thus to soften and burst open. The source text elaborates:

> Decoction to Disperse Swelling and Ulcerate What is Hard (*sàn zhǒng kuì jiān tāng*) treats saber lumps and nodules that are hard as stone [located] below the ear, to [the area around] ST-12 (*quē pén*) or on the shoulder or under the arm; these belong to the hand or foot lesser yang channels. [The formula] also [treats] scrofulous swellings below the cheek down to [the area around] ST-6 (*jiá chē*) that are firm and do not burst open [and are on the] foot yang brightness channel. Also, these two types of lesions [when they] have already broken open and expressed fluid. [This formula] treats all of these.

In more familiar terms, the formula can be used for treating accumulation of heat toxin that gives rise to hard swellings in the upper body, or to upper-body sores that have suppurated but maintain a hard inner core.

Since this formula primarily addresses the branch symptom, concurrent or follow-up treatment must consider the root cause. If Liver fire is paramount, the patient must be assessed to determine if Liver qi constraint or Liver yin-blood deficiency is the cause. Furthermore, Stomach heat or heat from deficiency of the Kidneys or Lungs must be kept in mind as potential sources of pathogenic fire. Over the course of treatment, the state of the patient's yin-fluids should be monitored carefully to obviate depletion by the heat pathogen and the bitter, drying herbs that are used in this formula.

Variant

This formula is also found in *Restoration of Health from the Myriad Diseases*. While the text appears to be copied directly from *Secrets from the Orchid Chamber*, what is probably a mistake in transcription led to Atractylodis macrocephalae Rhizoma (*bái zhú*) being inserted for Paeoniae Radix alba (*bái sháo*). In addition, that text adds Sargassum (*hǎi zǎo*) to the formula.

Biomedical Indications

With the appropriate presentation, this formula may be used to treat a variety of biomedically-defined disorders including goiter, scrofula, lymphadenitis, tubercular lymph nodes and other tumors of the neck, shoulders, or underarms, as well as goiter or hyperthyroidism.

Modifications

- If the swellings are on the lesser yang channels only, remove Cimicifugae Rhizoma (*shēng má*) and Puerariae Radix (*gé gēn*). (source text)
- If the swellings are squarely on the yang brightness channel, remove Bupleuri Radix (*chái hú*). (source text)
- Adding Lonicerae Flos (*jīn yín huā*) and Aurantii Fructus immaturus (*zhǐ shí*) will help the formula to bring swellings to a head. If fever accompanies the pattern, add Gypsum fibrosum (*shí gāo*) and Gardeniae Fructus (*zhī zǐ*).
- For qi deficiency, add Astragali Radix (*huáng qí*) and Ginseng Radix (*rén shēn*).
- For excess-type constipation, add Rhei Radix et Rhizoma (*dà huáng*). For constipation from blood dryness, also add Persicae Semen (*táo rén*).
- For enlarged thyroid, add Fritillariae thunbergii Bulbus (*zhè bèi mǔ*) and Prunellae Spica (*xià kū cǎo*). For hyperactive thyroid, also include Gardeniae Fructus (*zhī zǐ*) and Scrophulariae Radix (*xuán shēn*).

Associated Formula

紫根牡蠣湯 （紫根牡蛎汤）

Arenebia/Lithospermum and Oyster Shell Decoction

zǐ gēn mǔ lì tāng (shikon borei tō)

SOURCE *New Book on Syphilis and Leprosy* (1787)

Angelicae sinensis Radix (*dāng guī*)	9-12g
Paeoniae Radix alba (*bái sháo*)	6-9g
Arnebiae/Lithospermi Radix (*zǐ cǎo*)	6-9g
Rhei Radix et Rhizoma (*dà huáng*)	1-3g
Lonicerae Caulis (*rěn dōng téng*)	6-9g
Cimicifugae Rhizoma (*shēng má*)	1-3g
Astragali Radix (*huáng qí*)	6-9g
Ostreae Concha (*mǔ lì*)	6-9g
Glycyrrhizae Radix (*gān cǎo*)	1-3g

Decoction. The source text does not specify dosage; the above is the normal range used at present. Clears heat, resolves toxicity, dissipates swellings, and dispels noxious sores; also moderately tonifies the qi and blood. This formula was designed to treat chronic and deep red bayberry sore toxin (楊梅瘡毒 *yáng méi chuāng dú*), which overlaps roughly with the sores of secondary syphilis of biomedicine. At present, the formula is used in the treatment of breast cancer, chronic, stubborn skin lesions, mastitis, enlarged lymph nodes in the neck, appendicitis, impetigo, systemic lymph carcinoma, and red, itching skin disorders of unknown origin as well as painful hemorrhoids.

The formula's strength is in clearing heat toxin from the blood level. In most cases, it is applied to chronic, deep-lying disorders of the skin or lymph system. Because these disorders have existed long enough to whittle away the qi and blood, the formula also includes agents to tonify the qi and blood.

Modifications

- For deficient patients, remove Rhei Radix et Rhizoma (dà huáng). (source text)
- For patients with more excess-type conditions, remove Astragali Radix (huáng qí). (source text)
- For breast disorders, add Vaccariae Semen (wáng bù liú xíng) and Liquidambaris Fructus (lù lù tōng).
- For painful conditions, add Olibanum (rǔ xiāng) and Myrrha (mò yào).
- For Lung abscesses, add Houttuyniae Herba (yú xīng cǎo).
- For impetigo, add Taraxaci Herba (pú gōng yīng) and Forsythiae Fructus (lián qiáo).

Section 2

FORMULAS THAT TREAT INTERNAL ABSCESSES

In Chinese medicine, internal abscesses generally affect the Lungs and Intestines. Similar to external abscesses, they are attributed to heat and constraint that allows the formation of toxins. This secondarily leads to the formation of pus. The appropriate strategy is to discharge the toxin, eliminate the phlegm, clear the heat, and open the constraint.

Typical herbs for resolving toxicity in the treatment of internal abscesses include Phragmitis Caulis (wěi jīng), Lonicerae Flos (jīn yín huā), Scutellariae Radix (huáng qín), and Patriniae Herba (bài jiàng cǎo). These are combined with herbs that transform turbidity and move stasis such as Coicis Semen (yì yǐ rén), Benincasae Semen (dōng guā zǐ), and Persicae Semen (táo rén).

- If there is also clumping of heat with stasis and stagnation, add herbs such as Rhei Radix et Rhizoma (dà huáng) and Moutan Cortex (mǔ dān pí) to drain heat and dispel stasis.
- If heat toxins damage the yin fluids and blood, add herbs such as Scrophulariae Radix (xuán shēn), Ophiopogonis Radix (mài mén dōng), and Angelicae sinensis Radix (dāng guī) to enrich the fluids and nourish the blood.
- If the disorder has damaged the body's yang qi, thus exacerbating stagnation even in the presence of abscess formation, one can add warming herbs such as Aconiti Radix lateralis praeparata (zhì fù zǐ).

葦莖湯 (苇茎汤)
Reed Decoction
wěi jīng tāng

Source *Records of Proven Formulas Past and Present* (627), cited in *Arcane Essentials from the Imperial Library* (752)

Phragmitis Caulis (wěi jīng) 60g
Coicis Semen (yì yǐ rén) 30g
Benincasae Semen (dōng guā zǐ) 24g
Persicae Semen (táo rén) 9g

Method of Preparation Decoction. The source text advises to decoct Phragmitis Caulis (wěi jīng) in 20 cups of water until 5 cups remain, remove the dregs, and then add the other herbs before boiling down to 2 cups. At present, this formula is prepared as a decoction in the normal manner. *Note:* The source text merely specifies melon seed (瓜瓣 guā bàn); see COMMENTARY for more discussion of this identification issue.

Actions Clears heat from the Lungs, transforms phlegm, drives out blood stasis, and discharges pus

Indications

Cough with foul-smelling sputum (which may be streaked with blood), slight fever, mild chest pain, dry, scaly skin, a red tongue with a greasy, yellow coating, and a slippery, rapid pulse.

This is Lung abscess due to wind-heat toxin entering the Lungs accompanied by phlegm and blood stasis. Wind-heat obstructing the dissemination of protective yang in the exterior produces a slight fever that may at times be accompanied by cold shivers. The combination of heat, phlegm, and blood stasis produces Lung abscess. Heat toxin obstructs the dissemination of Lung qi, which leads to the coughing up of foul-smelling, yellow sputum. Heat injures the collaterals of the Lungs and produces blood-streaked sputum and mild chest pain. The stasis of blood prevents nourishment and moisture from reaching the skin, which becomes dry and scaly. The combination of heat and phlegm produces a red tongue with a greasy, yellow coating and a slippery, rapid pulse.

Analysis of Formula

This formula is designed for Lung abscess when heat toxin clogs the Lungs leading to clumping of phlegm and static blood. Thus, it clears the Lungs, transforms phlegm, drives out stasis, and expels pus. The chief herb, Phragmitis Caulis (wěi jīng), is sweet and cold, light and floating. These qualities allow it to clear heat from the Lungs. In *Encountering the Sources of the Classic of Materia Medica*, the 17th-century physician Zhang Lu wrote that it "specializes in facilitating passage through the orifices and thus is good at treating Lung abscess." One of the deputies, Benincasae Semen (dōng guā zǐ), clears and transforms phlegm-heat, resolves dampness, and eliminates pus. The other deputy, Coicis Semen (*yì yǐ rén*), clears heat from the Lungs and disperses pus from the upper parts of the body. It also leaches out dampness and helps restore proper function to the Intestines, thereby providing an outlet for dampness and heat through the urine. The assistant, Persicae Semen (*táo rén*), invigorates the blood and eliminates blood stasis, which reduces the clumping and thereby breaks up the abscess. Both Persicae Semen (*táo rén*) and Benincasae Semen (*dōng guā zǐ*) have a mild laxative effect, which provides another outlet for the phlegm through the stool.

Cautions and Contraindications

Because of the descending actions of Persicae Semen (*táo rén*) and Coicis Semen (*yì yǐ rén*), this formula is contraindicated during pregnancy.

Commentary

Functions

The expulsion of phlegm and pus is especially important in treating Lung abscess. Simply clearing the heat and regulating the qi is not enough. This formula can be used in treating both early-stage (without pus) and advanced-stage (with pus) Lung abscess. Other applications include Lung heat with coughing, fever, thirst, and red rashes (such as measles). It is also used during recuperation from a febrile disease when the patient has a slight fever and cough with thick sputum that is difficult to expectorate. Some modern practitioners use it for eye disorders due to upward-blazing of heat toxin. Yu Jing-He, one of the most famous external medicine physicians of the late Qing era, noted that according to the experience of his teacher Ma Pei-Zhi, the formula is not limited to the Lungs alone, but can be used in the treatment of all types of internal abscesses. With appropriate modifications, contemporary physicians have extended its usage even further to the treatment of acute upper respiratory infections, including lobar pneumonia, childhood pneumonia, and acute and chronic bronchitis with the formation of pus or thick yellow sputum.

The source text states that, after application of the formula, "one should observe the vomiting up of pus and blood." Some commentators have therefore classified the formula as an emetic. Emetic treatment strategies are used to eliminate pathogens located in the interior but above the diaphragm, which is the case with Lung abscesses. However, this formula does not contain herbs that induce vomiting. Rather, the expectoration of pus and blood-streaked sputum induced by this formula, which is similar in nature to the lancing of a boil, follows from its opening of the qi dynamic.

Identification of Ingredients

Commentators have also debated the precise identity of two of the substances used in the formula that are not clearly identified in the source text. The first is Phragmitis Caulis (*wěi jīng*), which is sometimes replaced today by Phragmitis Rhizoma (*lú gēn*). While 葦 *wěi* is another name for *lú* 蘆, referring to the reed *Phragmites communis*, the term *jīng* 莖 is taken by some physicians as referring to the aerial stem or stalk of the plant and by others to the rhizomatous roots. In *Extension of the Important Formulas Worth a Thousand Gold Pieces*, the Qing-dynasty commentator Zhang Lu supported the first interpretation:

> Phragmitis Caulis (*wěi jīng*) is a special [herb] for unblocking the Lungs and Stomach [if these have become obstructed] by clumped qi. It is able to eliminate heat toxin by draining it through the urine. It relies on its own core emptiness to excel at thrusting out [obstructions] from all orifices. [In clinical practice,] one uses the stems and not the root because their essential nature corresponds to heaven. [Like the Lungs,] they are intimately related to the upper [regions].

The opposing view—advocating use of the rhizomatous root stalks rather than the stems—is exemplified by Zhang Xi-Chun in *Essays on Medicine Esteeming the Chinese and Respecting the Western*:

> Some commentators say that one should use the stems and not the root of Phragmititis (*wěi*) but I disagree. The roots [of this plant] stay deep in the water, hence their nature is cooling and they excel at ascending. For patients [suffering from] massive head pestilential [qi] (大頭瘟 *dà tóu wēn*), it is often used as a guiding herb because its upwardly ascending power is able to reach the brain. Does this not also apply to the Lungs? Furthermore, its cooling nature is able to clear Lung heat, [and because its stem is empty like the Lungs,] it is able to regulate the Lung qi. Finally, it is also sweet and rich in yin fluids and thus excels at enriching the yin and nourishing the Lungs. Therefore, do not the roots clearly win out over the stalks?

If both sides defend their choice on the basis of presumed therapeutic properties, modern textual research demonstrates that Tang dynasty source texts like *Arcane Essentials from the Imperial Library* and *Important Formulas Worth a Thousand Gold Pieces* clearly distinguish between the use of the stem Phragmitis Caulis (*wěi jīng*) and the rhizomatous root Phragmitis Rhizoma (*lú gēn*). In the absence of clinical research that would demonstrate differences in clinical efficacy between the two parts of the plant, it may therefore be advisable to follow traditional usage and prescribe the stems wherever possible. However, Phragmitis Caulis (*wěi jīng*) is difficult to obtain.

The second substance that is not clearly identifiable from the source texts is the 'melon seeds' (瓜瓣 *guā bàn*). Most modern textbooks, following the Qing-dynasty physician Wang Shi-Xiong, define these as the seeds of the white gourd, or Benincasae Semen (*dōng guā zǐ*). However, Zhang Lu, cited above, thought that the source text referred to the seeds of the musk melon, or Melonis Semen *(tián guā zǐ)*.* And Wang Zi-Jie recommended the use of luffa seeds, or Luffae Fructus Semen *(sī guā zǐ)*.† The first two substances are both commonly used in the treatment of abscesses owing to their ability to drain phlegm from the Lungs and Intestines. Luffa seeds, however, were not in common use before the Tang and Song dynasties, and it is thus unlikely that they were referred to in the source text.

Origin

This formula was first listed under its present name in the official Song version of *Essentials from the Golden Cabinet,* published in 1065. The editor, Lin Yi, took the formula from an unnamed prescription in *Important Formulas Worth a Thousand Gold Pieces,* published in 650. However, *Arcane Essentials from the Imperial Library* contains a "formula for Lung abscess" (肺癰方 *fèi yōng fāng*) with the same ingredients, which it attributes to the no longer extant *Records of Proven Formulas Past and Present,* published in 627. This text must therefore be considered as the source text for this formula. Furthermore, textual evidence suggests that the formula or a variant may already have been included in the Han-dynasty work, *Discussion of Cold Damage,* but was omitted from extant versions of the text.

Comparison

➤ Vs. Drain the White Powder *(xiè bái sǎn)*

Both formulas can be used to treat Lung fire owing to their ability to drain heat from the Lungs. However, Drain the White Powder *(xiè bái sǎn)* focuses on heat constraint within the Lungs that causes coughing and wheezing. By contrast, the principal formula focuses on transforming phlegm and expelling pus, in addition to clearing heat. For this reason, it is indicated for the treatment of Lung abscess as well as other cases of phlegm-heat obstructing the Lungs.

Biomedical Indications

With the appropriate presentation, this formula may be used to treat a variety of biomedically-defined disorders including bronchitis, bronchiectasis, pneumonia, pertussis, and asthmatic bronchitis.

Modifications

• For pronounced heat in the Lungs, add Lonicerae Flos *(jīn yín huā)* and Houttuyniae Herba *(yú xīng cǎo)*.

• For marked pus in the sputum, add Platycodi Radix *(jié gěng)*, Fritillariae cirrhosae Bulbus *(chuān bèi mǔ)*, and Glycyrrhizae Radix *(gān cǎo)*.

• For excessive sputum, add Lepidii/ Descurainiae Semen *(tíng lì zǐ)*.

• For lingering heat and persistent cough with copious sputum during recuperation from a febrile disease, add Luffae Fructus Retinervus *(sī guā luò)*, Trichosanthis Pericarpium *(guā lóu pí)*, and Eriobotryae Folium *(pí pá yè)*.

• For measles with coughing, fever, thirst, and red rashes, add Scutellariae Radix *(huáng qín)*, Mori Cortex *(sāng bái pí)*, and Fritillariae cirrhosae Bulbus *(chuān bèi mǔ)*.

• For pronounced Lung heat with formation of pus or yellow sputum in disorders such as pneumonia or acute bronchitis, remove Coicis Semen *(yì yǐ rén)* and add Platycodi Radix *(jié gěng)*, Bupleuri Radix *(chái hú)*, Houttuyniae Herba *(yú xīng cǎo)*, and Lonicerae Flos *(jīn yín huā)*.

大黃牡丹湯 (大黄牡丹汤)
Rhubarb and Moutan Decoction
dà huáng mǔ dān tāng

Source *Essentials from the Golden Cabinet* (c. 220)

Rhei Radix et Rhizoma *(dà huáng)* .12g
Natrii Sulfas *(máng xiāo)*
 [dissolve in strained decoction] 9-12g
Moutan Cortex *(mǔ dān pí)* 3g
Persicae Semen *(táo rén)* 9-15g
Benincasae Semen *(dōng guā zǐ)* 15-30g

Method of Preparation Cook Rhei Radix et Rhizoma *(dà huáng)* with the other herbs, which tends to enhance its blood-moving action. Dosage is based on the source text. At present, 12-18g of Rhei Radix et Rhizoma *(dà huáng)* and 9g of Moutan Cortex *(mǔ dān pí)* are used.

Actions Drains heat, breaks up blood stasis, disperses clumping, and reduces swelling

Indications

Lower abdominal distention and pain (usually on the right) that increases on pressure with rebound tenderness, guarding of the abdominal musculature, a thin, yellow, and greasy tongue coating, and a slippery, rapid pulse. There may also be pain in the groin (resembling painful urinary dysfunction without urinary difficulty) that is relieved by flexing the hip and knee (usually on the right) and increases when extending the hip. In addition, there may be a mass in the lower right quadrant of the abdomen and irregular, intermittent fever followed by chills and sweating.

This pattern is one of early-stage Intestinal abscess, a condition of excess with interior clumping of heat and blood. As early as the *Divine Pivot* (Chapter 68), this was linked to poor

---

* Melonis Semen (甜瓜子 *tián guā zǐ*) is sweet, cold, and enters the Lung, Stomach, and Small Intestine channels. It clears the Lungs, moistens the Intestines, disperses clumps, and reduces stasis. The normal dose is 9-15g. It should not be used in patients with diarrhea from Spleen and Stomach deficiency.

† Luffae Fructus Semen (絲瓜子 *sī guā zǐ*) is bitter and cold. It promotes urination, unblocks the stool, and expels parasites. The normal dose is 6-9g.

dietary habits. Bingeing or overeating in general, or a diet that is high in greasy, rich, raw, or cold foods in particular, can lead to stagnation and obstruction of the Stomach and Intestines. Obstruction of any kind constrains the flow of qi and blood; constraint gives rise to heat, which putrefies the qi and blood in the Intestines and eventually forms an abscess. This condition is also commonly attributed to damp-heat accumulating in the Intestines, which similarly obstructs the flow of qi and blood.

The clumping of heat and stasis of blood in the Intestines manifests as pain (usually in the lower right quadrant of the abdomen) that increases on pressure, with rebound tenderness. Although the pain may extend to the genitals, it can be differentiated from painful urinary dysfunction because urination is normal. Gradually, as the qi and blood continue to putrefy, the abscess will form a palpable mass. The ebb and flow of the struggle between the body's normal qi and the pathogenic influences disturbs the nutritive and protective qi, which manifests as irregular, intermittent fever followed by chills and sweating. The yellow, greasy tongue coating and the slippery, rapid pulse reflect the clogging of the Intestines by heat.

Analysis of Formula

The pain associated with early-stage abscess is attributed to an interruption in the normal flow through the Intestines caused by accumulation of heat and stasis of blood. To restore normal flow, the heat must be drained and the stasis of blood broken up. The chief ingredient, Rhei Radix et Rhizoma (*dà huáng*), performs both actions quite well. One of the deputies, Natrii Sulfas (*máng xiāo*), softens the stool and aids in draining heat downward, thereby unclogging the Intestines. The other deputy, Moutan Cortex (*mǔ dān pí*), cools the blood and eliminates masses due to blood stasis. Persicae Semen (*táo rén*), an assistant ingredient, breaks up the stasis of blood and has a mild moistening and laxative effect. The other assistant, Benincasae Semen (*dōng guā zǐ*), expels pus, eliminates heat, and reduces abscesses, especially in the Intestines.

Cautions and Contraindications

This formula is unsuitable for necrotic appendicitis, appendicitis with peritonitis, appendicitis in infants, appendicitis during pregnancy, or appendicitis due to parasites. It should be used with extreme caution in the weak and elderly.

Commentary

In early-stage Intestinal abscess (before pus has formed), the pain is quite severe, there is localized hardness and heat, and the pulse is either slippery and rapid or tight. In fully-formed abscess (after pus has formed), there is a diminution in heat and pain, the tissues are more relaxed, and the pulse is tight.

The source text prohibits the use of purgatives in treating Intestinal abscesses with pus and a flooding, rapid pulse. What, exactly, this means has been the subject of debate for centuries. Some physicians interpret this to be an absolute contraindication of this formula when pus has formed. Others, however, use this formula, with modifications, for conditions with pus.

Original and Contemporary Usage

The original use of this formula corresponds primarily to acute stages of appendicitis. However, with the wide availability of surgery, the formula is no longer commonly used for this purpose today. Its range of applications has, however, been considerably extended—particularly by Japanese Kampo physicians—to include many acute and chronic inflammatory processes, particularly in the lower burner. The 19th-century text *Categorized Collected Formulas* notes:

> [This formula] treats all types of abscesses, deep-set toxic sores, lower [body] progressive sores (下疳 *xià gān*), bowel toxins, painful urinary dribbling hemorrhoids, organ toxins, scrofula, spreading sores (流注 *liú zhù*), long-term sores, toxic clumps, chronic pimples, nameless odious sores, incessant pus and bleeding, congealing obstructions or lumps in the abdomen, as well as difficult urination and defecation.

It is therefore used in modern Japan to treat skin problems and infections of the mucous membranes in the mouth and throat, infections in the lower digestive and urogenital systems, dysentery, severe abdominal pain, as well as a range of gynecological disorders including endometriosis, infertility, dysmenorrhea, and postpartum lower abdominal problems. A key clinical marker is the lower abdominal pain that is accompanied by rebound tenderness, which tends to be more pronounced on the right side. Secondary symptoms include constipation, blood in the stools, and a tendency toward infections, a thin, yellow, and slightly greasy tongue coating, and a slippery, rapid pulse.

Debate over Ingredients

Commentators disagree about the nature of the 'melon seeds' (*guā zǐ* 瓜子) prescribed in the source text. Some physicians, like the 17th-century writer Xu Bin in *Discussion and Annotation of the Essentials from the Golden Cabinet,* recommend the use of Benincasae Semen (*dōng guā zǐ*). Others, like his contemporary Cheng Lin in *True Explanation of the Essentials of the Golden Cabinet,* argue for the use of Melonis Semen (*tián guā zǐ*). Benincasae Semen (*dōng guā zǐ*) are sweet and cold, clear the Lungs, transform phlegm, and expel pus. Melonis Semen (*tián guā zǐ*) are also sweet and cold, but have the function of reducing stasis, dispersing clumping, clearing the Lungs, and moistening the Intestines. Taking these differences into account, one should choose Benincasae Semen (*dōng guā zǐ*) in cases of pronounced phlegm-dampness, while Melonis Semen (tián guā zǐ) are more suitable for cases with pronounced stasis, clumping, and pus formation.

Comparisons

➤ Vs. Major Order the Qi Decoction (dà chéng qì tāng) and Major Decoction [for Pathogens] Stuck in the Chest (dà xiàn xiōng tāng)

All three formulas use the combination of Rhei Radix et Rhizoma (dà huáng) and Natrii Sulfas (máng xiāo) for the purpose of draining downward the clumping heat that occurs in patterns of interior heat excess stagnation. Major Order the Qi Decoction (dà chéng qì tāng) treats clumping of heat and dry feces in the Intestines that is accompanied by qi stagnation. Abdominal fullness and distention in patients with other signs of heat at the yang brightness-organ level are key markers for the use of this formula. Major Decoction [for Pathogens] Stuck in the Chest (dà xiàn xiōng tāng) treats clumping of heat and fluids in the Stomach. Abdominal pain that extends from the epigastrium to the lower abdomen and is accompanied by signs indicating a breakdown of the water metabolism are key markers for the use of this formula. By contrast, Rhubarb and Moutan Decoction (dà huáng mǔ dān tāng) treats clumping of damp-heat in the interior leading to the formation of abscesses in the Intestines. The key markers for use of this formula are acute lower abdominal pain (indicating blood stasis in the lower burner) accompanied by signs of damp-heat clumping such as fever and a flooding, rapid pulse.

Biomedical Indications

With the appropriate presentation, this formula may be used to treat a wide variety of biomedically-defined disorders. These can be divided into the following groups:

- Encapsulated inflammatory diseases of the pelvis such as appendicitis, acute pelvic inflammatory disease, iliac fossa abscess, and diverticulitis
- Other types of abscesses such as subdermal abscess, renal abscess, hepatic abscess, and pulmonary abscess
- Other infectious diseases such as bacillary dysentery, pyelonephritis, mastitis, osteomyelitis, conjunctivitis, abdominal or lower extremity folliculitis, and postvasectomy infections.

This formula has also been used for treating blocked uterine tubes, cerebral thrombosis, primary dysmenorrhea, amenorrhea, hemorrhoids, benign prostatic hypertrophy, and eczema.

Modifications

- For high fever, add Coptidis Rhizoma (huáng lián).
- For rough dysenteric diarrhea, a red tongue, and a thin, rapid pulse, remove Natrii Sulfas (máng xiāo) and add

Scrophulariae Radix (xuán shēn) and Rehmanniae Radix (shēng dì huáng).

- For a palpable mass in the lower abdomen, add Angelicae sinensis Radix (dāng guī), Paeoniae Radix rubra (chì sháo), and Violae Herba (zǐ huā dì dīng).
- For more severe pain, add Corydalis Rhizoma (yán hú suǒ), Toosendan Fructus (chuān liàn zǐ), and Aucklandiae Radix (mù xiāng).
- For Intestinal abscess with pus, add Lonicerae Flos (jīn yín huā), Taraxaci Herba (pú gōng yīng), and Hedyotis diffusae Herba (bái huā shé shé cǎo).
- For qi deficiency, add Pseudostellariae Radix (tài zǐ shēn).
- For blood deficiency, add Angelicae sinensis Radix (dāng guī) and Salviae miltiorrhizae Radix (dān shēn).

Associated Formula

錦紅湯 （锦红汤）

Brocade Red Decoction

jǐn hóng tāng

Source　*Practical Chinese External Medicine*

Sargentodoxae Caulis (hóng téng) 60g
Taraxaci Herba (pú gōng yīng) 30g
Rhei Radix et Rhizoma (dà huáng) . . . . [add at end of decocting] 18g
Magnoliae officinalis Cortex (hòu pò) 12g

Decoction. Note that no dosage is listed in the source text. This formula can also be prepared as pills by grinding the first three ingredients into a powder and mixing it with the liquid extract of Magnoliae officinalis Cortex (hòu pò). Clears heat, resolves toxicity, moves the qi, opens the bowels, invigorates the blood, and reduces swelling. This formula was developed by the modern Shanghai physician Gu Bo-Hua, who belonged to a well-known lineage of external medicine specialists, for the treatment of acute appendicitis.

清腸飲 （清肠饮）

Clear the Intestines Drink

qīng cháng yǐn

Source　*Records of Pattern Discrimination* (1687)

Lonicerae Flos (jīn yín huā) 90g
Angelicae sinensis Radix (dāng guī) 60g
Sanguisorbae Radix (dì yú) 30g
Scrophulariae Radix (xuán shēn) 30g
Ophiopogonis Radix (mài mén dōng) 30g
Glycyrrhizae Radix (gān cǎo) 9g
Coicis Semen (yì yǐ rén) 15g
Scutellariae Radix (huáng qín) 6g

Method of Preparation　Decoction. The source text indicates that three doses of the decoction should bring a significant amelioration of the symptoms.

Actions　Drains fire excess, enriches the yin, resolves toxicity

Indications

For early-stage Intestinal abscess with severe abdominal pain (usually on the right) that increases on pressure with rebound tenderness. There may also be pain in the groin that is relieved by flexing the hip and knee (usually on the right) and is aggravated by extending the hip. The abdominal symptoms are accompanied by chills and fever, aversion to wind, spontaneous sweating, and dry, scaly skin. The mouth is dry, and the tongue is red with little moisture.

The etiology and disease dynamic is the same as that outlined for Rhubarb and Moutan Decoction *(dà huáng mǔ dān tāng)* above. However, the presence of such symptoms as a dry mouth and a red tongue with little moisture indicate that the yin fluids have been damaged.

Analysis of Formula

This formula combines strategies for invigorating the blood and resolving toxicity with those that enrich the yin and drain fire. The chief ingredients are Lonicerae Flos *(jīn yín huā)* and Glycyrrhizae Radix *(gān cǎo)*, a combination also found in Immortals' Formula for Sustaining Life *(xiān fāng huó mìng yǐn)*, discussed above. Lonicerae Flos *(jīn yín huā)* clears heat from both the qi and blood levels and disperses swelling. It is light in nature and thus does not damage the qi. Glycyrrhizae Radix *(gān cǎo)* also resolves toxicity and clears heat. In addition, it tonifies the middle and thus helps to secure the fetus. It also serves as the envoy and thus harmonizes the other herbs in the formula.

The deputies are Angelicae sinensis Radix *(dāng guī)* and Sanguisorbae Radix *(dì yú)*. Each focuses on one of the two different goals that the formula seeks to achieve and is supported, in turn, by a range of assistants. Angelicae sinensis Radix *(dāng guī)* tonifies the blood to moisten the Intestines, but is also acrid and warm to provide invigoration and movement. It is assisted by Scrophulariae Radix *(xuán shēn)*, which clears fire and resolves toxicity, and by Ophiopogonis Radix *(mài mén dōng)*, which calms irritability and restlessness. Both substances also enrich the yin fluids to open the blood vessels and facilitate bowel movements.

Sanguisorbae Radix *(dì yú)* is heavy and sinking in nature, directing the action of the entire formula on the lower burner. While it resolves toxicity, its ability to clear heat is not excessively draining, and while it is sour and restrains, it is not overly astringent. It is therefore regarded as one of the finest cooling-astringent hemostatic herbs. Its action is assisted by Coicis Semen *(yì yǐ rén)* and Scutellariae Radix *(huáng qín)*, both of which enter the Large Intestine, drain damp-heat, disperse pus, and thus assist in restoring the normal function of the Intestines.

Cautions and Contraindications

The use of this formula is inappropriate in cases without damage to the yin and blood. It is also not indicated for late-stage appendicitis where heat symptoms are not pronounced.

Commentary

This formula treats Intestinal abscess with yin deficiency and hyperactivity of fire, which is often a sequelae of damp-heat brewing in the interior for a long time, depleting the yin fluids and blood, while the heat itself increases. As noted in the source text, this formula should stop the pain after one dose. After three to four doses, the problem should be resolved. It is thus a formula for emergencies and not for the treatment of the underlying root disorder.

Intestinal abscesses combining stagnation of damp-heat, blood stasis, and heat toxin require the use of formulas that focus on draining heat, resolving toxicity, and eliminating stasis. However, during pregnancy, when strategies like downward draining, invigorating the blood, and moving the qi may induce a miscarriage, this approach is contraindicated. Chen Shi-Duo's formula solves this impasse with the help of herbs that moisten the Intestines and enrich the yin. These facilitate the reduction of stasis while simultaneously providing yin substance that prevents the downward movement from endangering the fetus. For this reason, the formula has been used in contemporary China for treating appendicitis during pregnancy. In a 1987 article in *Zhejiang Journal of Chinese Medicine,* the modern physician Zhang De-Wen notes:

> This formula relies mainly on substances that moisten the Intestines. By way of moistening, it moves stagnation. If the passages of the Intestines are moist, feces will naturally move. If the blood vessels are moist, the qi and blood do not clump. It combines [these herbs] with substances that cool the blood and resolve toxicity. They all mutually assist each other and enhance each others' efficacy so that results are very quickly achieved. This formula thus represents an effective strategy in the treatment of appendicitis, which [allows us] to see the magical contained within the ordinary.

The use of this formula is not limited to pregnancy but may be considered in any patient presenting with Intestinal abscess and severe damage to the yin and blood.

Biomedical Indications

With the appropriate presentation, this formula may be used to treat a variety of biomedically-defined disorders including both acute and chronic appendicitis.

Modifications

- To increase the effectiveness of the formula in reducing inflammation, add Taraxaci Herba *(pú gōng yīng)* and Violae Herba *(zǐ huā dì dīng)*. (Zhang De-Wen)

- For reduced urination, add Poria *(fú líng)* and Forsythiae Fructus *(lián qiáo)*. (Zhang De-Wen)

- For dryness of the stools, add Persicae Semen *(táo rén)*, Cannabis Semen *(huǒ má rén)*, and Rhei Radix et Rhizoma *(dà huáng)*. (Zhang De-Wen)
- For cases with severe fever, add Moutan Cortex *(mǔ dān pí)*. (Zhang De-Wen)

薏苡附子敗醬散 (薏苡附子败酱散)
Coix, Aconite Accessory Root, and Patrinia Powder
yì yǐ fù zǐ bài jiàng sǎn

Source   *Essentials from the Golden Cabinet* (c. 220)

Coicis Semen *(yì yǐ rén)* 24-30g
Aconiti Radix lateralis praeparata *(zhì fù zǐ)* 6-9g
Patriniae Herba *(bài jiàng cǎo)* 15-18g

Method of Preparation   The source text specifies to grind the herbs into a powder and then prepare as a draft by decocting a spoonful (about 4g) with 2 cups of water until half the liquid has evaporated. Administration of the draft is expected to increase urination. At present, it is usually prepared as a decoction. Also note that nowadays, when Patriniae Herba *(bài jiàng cǎo)* is prescribed, Thlaspi Herba *(sū bài jiàng)* is dispensed.

Actions   Expels pus, reduces abscesses, warms the yang, and disperses clumping

Indications

Distention of the abdomen with scaly, dry skin, tightness, and a mass-like appearance, but softness on palpation, and a rapid pulse despite the absence of fever.

This is Intestinal abscess where pus has already formed. This condition is commonly due to cold-dampness and static blood or, alternatively, damp-heat constraint steaming the fluids and causing long-term blood stasis. Pus has already formed, but the accumulation has not been reduced. This indicates that the body's yang qi has been impaired. Formation of pus in the course of Intestinal abscess depletes the blood and nutritive qi, which causes the skin to lose its nourishment. As a result, it becomes dry and desiccated, taking on the appearance of fish scales.

Clumping of phlegm in the Intestines indicates that their qi is not free flowing. This is reflected in tightness of the abdominal tissues with a mass-like appearance. However, because the Intestines are not obstructed by dry feces, the abdomen is soft when palpated without any of the guarding or rebound tenderness characteristic of an acute abdomen.

Chronic production of pus that is not being resolved indicates that the body's yang qi has been impaired. This is reflected in the absence of fever. Nevertheless, the body is still attempting to fight the pus-producing toxins accumulating in the Intestines, leading to a state of heightened physiological activity that is reflected in the rapid pulse.

Analysis of Formula

An Intestinal abscess that cannot be resolved presents as a pattern of mixed excess and deficiency. Although the accumulation of pus and heat toxins in the Intestines causes stasis of blood, the body's yang qi is insufficiently strong to overcome this blockage. Treatment must adapt to this condition by combining the clearing of toxins with the warming of yang to successfully expel the pus and reduce the abscess. The formula achieves these goals with a combination of three simple substances.

The chief ingredient is bland, sweet, and slightly cold Coicis Semen *(yì yǐ rén)*. Its combination of heat-clearing, dampness-resolving, and pus-expelling properties make it one of the most frequently used substances for the treatment of Lung and Intestinal abscesses in the Chinese materia medica. Patriniae Herba *(bài jiàng cǎo)* is acrid and slightly cold and is able to reduce blood stasis and abscesses from the bowels and lower burner. As deputy, it focuses the action of the chief ingredient on the Intestines, the resolution of abscesses, and the draining of pus.

If the action of these herbs is straightforward, the distinguishing feature of the formula is its use of a small amount of Aconiti Radix lateralis praeparata *(zhì fù zǐ)* as assistant herb. Its function is to stimulate the yang. Of all the substances that can fulfill this function, Aconiti Radix lateralis praeparata *(zhì fù zǐ)* is the only one that, in the words of the *Divine Husbandman's Classic of the Materia Medica*, "governs warming of the middle [and focuses on] metal inflicted wounds, on breaking up abdominal masses and hard accumulations." It assists Coicis Semen *(yì yǐ rén)* in dispersing cold-dampness and prevents the cooling nature of Patriniae Herba *(bài jiàng cǎo)* from causing further harm to the body's yang qi, even as it accentuates its ability to disperse abscesses, open areas of constraint, and unblock the movement of qi and blood in the Intestines.

Cautions and Contraindications

The use of this formula is contraindicated in cases characterized by high fever, a flooding and slippery pulse, severe abdominal pain, and constipation.

Commentary

Original Usage

This is an excellent formula for resolving Intestinal abscesses where pus has already formed. Although this is its classical indication, it can also be used to treat abscesses that fail to resolve, even if pus is not a main symptom, provided that the underlying disease dynamic indicates that the body's yang qi is insufficiently developed to resolve the condition. Key signs and symptoms of such deficiency include:

- A condition that does not improve
- A right-sided (usually) abdominal swelling that is soft when touched and not very painful
- General symptoms of insufficient yang such as cold extremities, a gray or pale complexion, a pale tongue with thin, white coating, absence of thirst as a symptom or even an aversion to drinks, and a pulse that is empty or weak, even though it may be rapid.

Expanded Usage

In its description of the pattern's presentation, the source text lists as the first symptom that "the [skin of patient's] body is scaly (甲錯 *jiǎ cuò*)." Given that it is customary to list the most important symptoms first, this has been interpreted to mean that the formula can be used to treat skin disorders in the absence of Intestinal abscess. The formula is thus used for eczema, neurodermatitis, pemphigus, psoriasis, scleroderma, and many other skin disorders characterized by dryness and inflammation, provided that the overall presentation matches that of the formula's core pattern. In particular, there will usually be some tenderness on palpation of the lower abdomen, even though the abdominal wall itself is soft and weak, and the pulse will be rapid but deficient and without force, even as the patient himself presents without fever or other obvious signs of heat.

Often these signs indicate deep-seated or chronic inflammation in the interior. This need not be centered on the Intestines, but may include pelvic inflammatory disorders such as endometritis, metritis, and prostatitis. The patient's general condition will be deficient, leading to a generalized lack of energy or aversion to cold.

Controversy

The precise meaning of the passage in the source text that administration of the formula "should [lead to] draining downward of urine" (小便當下 *xiǎo biàn dāng xià*) has been intensely debated among commentators. Some suggest that this must be a mistaken addition to the text. The early 17th-century scholar-physician Wei Nian-Ting, on the other hand, is representative of those who view the passage as possessing a deeper significance. In *Original Meaning of Formulas Discussed in Essentials from the Golden Cabinet*, Wei observed:

> Urination following the taking of this formula is the measure [of success]. Urination stands for qi transformation. If the qi is moving freely, the abscess with its clumping of pus can be opened up. That which has stagnated can be moved and the stools will drain out filth, pus, and [static] blood to resolve the abscess.

If, as Wei Nian-Ting thinks, the passage "should [lead to] draining downward of urine" can be read as "should lead to

the opening of the qi dynamic," then an increase in urination is not the only desirable consequence of administering this formula. Sweating has the same significance and is thus an equally important indicator of the formula's efficacy.

Comparison

➤ Vs. Rhubarb and Moutan Decoction (*dà huáng mǔ dān tāng*)

These are the two chief formulas for Intestinal abscess discussed in *Essentials from the Golden Cabinet*. The text commonly provides pairs of opposing formulas for the treatment of the same condition, where one formula treats a pattern characterized by heat (or yang) excess and the other by cold (or yin) deficiency.

Rhubarb and Moutan Decoction (*dà huáng mǔ dān tāng*) is a cold formula that focuses on draining excess heat from the Intestines. It is indicated for abscesses due to damp-heat and blood stasis with clumping of heat and feces in the Intestines. Key signs and symptoms suggesting its use are (right-sided) abdominal pain that increases on pressure, rebound tenderness, a thin, greasy, yellow tongue coating, and a slippery, rapid pulse. In contemporary practice, the formula is most often used for the early stages of acute appendicitis when pus has not yet formed.

Coix, Aconite Accessory Root, and Patrinia Powder (*yì yǐ fù zǐ bài jiàng sǎn*) is a balanced formula that combines clearing of heat and dispelling of dampness with warm dispersion in order to reduce abscesses and expel pus. It is indicated for abscesses due to cold-dampness and blood stasis, or damp-heat constraint steaming the body fluids that are not being resolved, indicating that the body's yang qi has been harmed. Key signs and symptoms for the use of this formula are a dry, scaly skin, abdominal distention and tightness that is soft when palpated, and a rapid pulse in the absence of fever. In contemporary practice, the formula is most often used for acute appendicitis when pus has already formed or for chronic appendicitis characterized by an ashen complexion, little or no pain, dampness that is more pronounced than heat, and a weak constitution.

Biomedical Indications

With the appropriate presentation, this formula may be used to treat a variety of biomedically-defined disorders including acute and chronic appendicitis, pelvic inflammatory disease, acute and chronic cholecystitis, keloids, eczema, neurodermatitis, pemphigus, psoriasis, scleroderma, and chronic osteomyelitis.

Alternate names

Aconite Decoction (*fù zǐ tāng*) in *Comprehensive Recording of Sagely Beneficence*; Patrinia Powder (*bài jiàng sǎn*) in *Fine Formulas for*

Women with Annotations and Commentary; Coicis and Aconite Accessory Root Powder *(yì yǐ fù zǐ sǎn)* in *Indispensable Tools for Pattern Treatment*; Coicis and Patrinia Decoction *(yì yǐ bài jiàng tāng)* in *Comprehensive Medicine According to Master Zhang*

Modifications

- For cases with more severe constraint and blood stasis indicated by abdominal swellings and lumps, add Persicae Semen *(táo rén)*, Moutan Cortex *(mǔ dān pí)*, and Angelicae sinensis Radix *(dāng guī)* to invigorate the blood and transform stasis, and Aurantii Fructus *(zhǐ ké)* and Citri reticulatae Pericarpium *(chén pí)* to move the qi and disperse clumping.

- For fatigue, lack of appetite, a pale tongue, and a weak pulse indicating Spleen qi deficiency, add Codonopsis Radix *(dǎng shēn)*, Astragali Radix *(huáng qí)*, Atractylodis macrocephalae Rhizoma *(bái zhú)*, and Poria *(fú líng)*.

- For fever indicating heat in the exterior, add Lonicerae Flos *(jīn yín huā)*, Forsythiae Fructus *(lián qiáo)*, and Taraxaci Herba *(pú gōng yīng)*.

- For more pronounced abdominal pain, add Paeoniae Radix alba *(bái sháo)* and Corydalis Rhizoma *(yán hú suǒ)*.

- For occasional burning pain in the lower abdomen indicating damp-heat and blood stasis, add Coptidis Rhizoma *(huáng lián)*, Scutellariae Radix *(huáng qín)*, Paeoniae Radix rubra *(chì sháo)*, Angelicae sinensis Radix *(dāng guī)*, and Moutan Cortex *(mǔ dān pí)*, and increase the dosage of Patriniae Herba *(bài jiàng cǎo)*.

Associated Formula

薏苡仁湯（薏苡仁汤）

Coix Decoction from *Indispensable Tools for Pattern Treatment*

yì yǐ rén tāng

SOURCE *Indispensable Tools for Pattern Treatment* (1602)

Coicis Semen *(yì yǐ rén)* 9g
Trichosanthis Semen *(guā lóu rén)* 9g
Moutan Cortex *(mǔ dān pí)* 6g
Persicae Semen *(táo rén)* 6g

Benefits dampness, moistens the Intestines, invigorates the blood, and relieves pain. For early-stage Intestinal abscess with stagnation of dampness and stasis of blood characterized by colicky abdominal pain or abdominal fullness with loss of appetite, and urinary difficulty. Also for postpartum abdominal pain or postmenstrual pain with the same etiology. In contrast to the principal formula, this one does not stimulate the yang, and in contrast to Rhubarb and Moutan Decoction *(dà huáng mǔ dān tāng)*, it does not focus on draining heat clumping in the Intestines.

清心利膈湯（清心利膈汤）
Clear the Heart and Enable the Diaphragm Decoction

qīng xīn lì gé tāng

Source *Indispensable Tools for Pattern Treatment* (1602)

Saposhnikoviae Radix *(fáng fēng)* 4.5g
Schizonepetae Herba *(jīng jiè)* 4.5g
Menthae haplocalycis Herba *(bò hé)* 4.5g
Platycodi Radix *(jié gěng)* 4.5g
Scutellariae Radix *(huáng qín)* 4.5g
Coptidis Rhizoma *(huáng lián)* 4.5g
Gardeniae Fructus *(zhī zǐ)* 2.5g
Forsythiae Fructus *(lián qiáo)* 2.5g
Scrophulariae Radix *(xuán shēn)* 2.5g
Rhei Radix et Rhizoma *(dà huáng)* 2.5g
impure Natrii Sulfas *(pò xiāo)* 2.5g
Arctii Fructus *(niú bàng zǐ)*
 . . . . [dry-fried and ground to a powder] 2.5g
Glycyrrhizae Radix *(gān cǎo)* 2.5g

Method of Preparation Decoction

Actions Clears heat, resolves toxicity, unblocks the stool, and benefits the throat

Indications

Red, swollen, and painful throat with difficulty swallowing, perhaps with small pustules on the tonsils, high fever, thirst with desire to drink cold liquids, bad breath, irritability, phlegm in the throat, constipation, a red tongue with a yellow coating, and a rapid, flooding pulse. The use of this formula has expanded in recent times to include sores in the mouth or tongue that present as part of a Lung or Stomach heat accumulation pattern.

The throat is the gate of the Lung and Stomach. If heat accumulates in these organs, heat toxin flares upward to the throat. Qi and blood gather and stagnate, and the flesh and membranes are damaged. This results in fever and a red, painful, swollen throat. It may also give rise to pustules on the membranes. The heat condensing the yang fluids produces constrained and clumped phlegm-fire in the form of painful, swollen nodules. Pathogenic heat flourishes internally and clumps in the Stomach where it causes high fever, thirst, constipation, and meager, dark urine.

Analysis of Formula

This problem has a complex etiology and requires an approach that uses multiple treatment strategies. In this case, the formula must clear heat, unblock the stool, resolve toxicity, and especially benefit the throat.

Coptidis Rhizoma *(huáng lián)*, Scutellariae Radix *(huáng qín)*, and Gardeniae Fructus *(zhī zǐ)* clear heat and resolve toxicity. Forsythiae Fructus *(lián qiáo)*, Menthae haplocalycis

Herba *(bò hé)*, Schizonepetae Herba *(jīng jiè)*, and Saposhnikoviae Radix *(fáng fēng)* are acrid and cool. They disperse clumped heat and clear pathogenic heat. Scrophulariae Radix *(xuán shēn)*, Platycodi Radix *(jié gěng)*, Arctii Fructus *(niú bàng zǐ)*, and Glycyrrhizae Radix *(gān cǎo)* work with Menthae haplocalycis Herba *(bò hé)* to resolve toxicity and disperse clumps, and to clear the throat. Rhei Radix et Rhizoma *(dà huáng)* and impure Natrii Sulfas *(pò xiāo)* drain fire by unblocking the stool. In this way, pathogenic heat is dredged from the exterior and cleared from the interior, the clumped heat is dispersed and drained, and the throat is cleared.

Cautions and Contraindications

This formula is intended for short-term use only. Do not use during pregnancy or for nursing mothers and use cautiously in young children, the debilitated, the elderly, or those with loose stools.

Commentary

In various premodern texts this formula is listed as treating painful obstruction of the throat, throat wind, throat abscess, swollen and immobile tongue, and the 'suckling moth' (乳蛾 *rǔ é*), which is suckling akin to tonsillitis. The early Qing-dynasty text *Great Compendium of External Medicine* adds that the pattern may also present with inhibition of the chest and diaphragm. These applications evolved from a simple sentence in the source text's section on painful obstruction of the throat, which says that the formula "treats swelling and pain in the throat [with] accumulation of phlegm and oral mucus."

Usage

There are many formulas available to treat disorders like sore throat, tonsillitis, and throat abscesses. Clear the Heart and Enable the Diaphragm Decoction *(qīng xīn lì gé tāng)* treats internal accumulation of excess heat. This internal heat can result from a direct attack of heat toxin to the interior or can be an attack on the exterior by cold that transforms to heat as it enters the interior. Alternatively, the condition can stem from internally-generated heat accumulation that combines with an external wind attack. Treatment differs depending on the stages and manifestations of the disorder.

Modern ear, nose, and throat texts generally recommend a variation of Honeysuckle and Forsythia Powder *(yín qiáo sǎn)* for treating wind-heat exterior patterns; Clear the Heart and Enable the Diaphragm Decoction *(qīng xīn lì gé tāng)* or a variation for Lung-heat accumulation patterns; Clear the Stomach Powder *(qīng wèi sǎn)* for cases where Stomach-heat accumulation is paramount; and a formula such as Anemarrhena, Phellodendron, and Rehmannia Pill *(zhī bǎi dì huáng wán)* for patterns of fire from yin deficiency.

Comparisons

➤ Vs. Universal Benefit Drink to Eliminate Toxin *(pǔ jì xiāo dú yǐn)* and Cool the Diaphragm Powder *(liáng gé sǎn)*

All three formulas treat throat disorders involving the accumulation of heat. Cool the Diaphragm Powder *(liáng gé sǎn)* and Clear the Heart and Enable the Diaphragm Decoction *(qīng xīn lì gé tāng)* both drain heat through the stool and are thus most appropriate for cases that present with constipation. The origin of the heat in the patterns that these two formulas treat may be from external invasion or internal disharmony. Because it has a stronger ability to drain heat, Cool the Diaphragm Powder *(liáng gé sǎn)* is best for more severe internal accumulation of heat. Clear the Heart and Enable the Diaphragm Decoction *(qīng xīn lì gé tāng)* is better for dredging the exterior and is thus suited for an acute condition where remnants of an exterior pathogen persist. Universal Benefit Drink to Eliminate Toxin *(pǔ jì xiāo dú yǐn)* is specifically for heat accumulation throat disorders that result from invasion from the exterior; it is unsuitable for internally-generated disorders. Moreover, it lacks any stool-moving agents and thus is best for patients whose bowels are moving normally.

Biomedical Indications

With the appropriate presentation, this formula may be used to treat a variety of biomedically-defined disorders including tonsillitis, peritonsillar abscess, or epiglottitis.

Modifications

- For expectoration of thick, yellow phlegm, add Belamcandae Rhizoma *(shè gān)*, Fritillariae thunbergii Bulbus *(zhè bèi mǔ)*, and Trichosanthis Pericarpium *(guā lóu pí)*.
- If the throat is especially swollen and painful or there are pustules on throat membranes, add Lasiosphaera/Calvatia *(mǎ bó)* and Sophorae tonkinensis Radix *(shān dòu gēn)*.
- If constipation is absent, remove Rhei Radix et Rhizoma *(dà huáng)* and impure Natrii Sulfas *(pò xiāo)*.
- For tonsillitis, add Paridis Rhizoma *(chóng lóu)* and Taraxaci Herba *(pú gōng yīng)*.

Variation

清咽利膈湯 （清咽利膈汤）

Clear the Throat and Enable the Diaphragm Decoction
qīng yān lì gé tāng

SOURCE *Precious Collection for Throat Diseases* (Qing dynasty)

Add Lonicerae Flos *(jīn yín huā)* to increase the formula's ability to clear heat and resolve toxicity.

十六味流氣飲 (十六味流气饮)
Sixteen-Ingredient Drink for Qi Flow
shí liù wèi liú qì yǐn

Source   *Introduction to Medicine* (1575)

Angelicae sinensis Radix (*dāng guī*)
Chuanxiong Rhizoma (*chuān xiōng*)
Paeoniae Radix alba (*bái sháo*)
Astragali Radix (*huáng qí*)
Ginseng Radix (*rén shēn*)
Cinnamomi Cortex (*ròu guì*)
Magnoliae officinalis Cortex (*hòu pò*)
Platycodi Radix (*jié gěng*)
Aurantii Fructus (*zhǐ ké*)
Linderae Radix (*wū yào*)
Aucklandiae Radix (*mù xiāng*)
Angelicae dahuricae Radix (*bái zhǐ*)
Arecae Semen (*bīng láng*)
Saposhnikoviae Radix (*fáng fēng*)
Perillae Folium (*zǐ sū yè*)
Glycyrrhizae Radix (*gān cǎo*)

Method of Preparation   The source text recommends that equal amounts of every herb be decocted and that the decoction be taken warm. *Restoration of Health from the Myriad Diseases* adds that the formula is best taken frequently, away from meals. *Note:* One version of the formula contains Gleditsiae Spina (*zào jiǎo cì*).

Actions   Tonifies the qi, nourishes the blood, promotes movement of qi, thrusts pus out, and dissipates swelling

Indications

According to *Introduction to Medicine*, this formula "treats unnamed noxious swellings, abscesses, flat abscesses, and such … if the pulse is not flooding, moderate, submerged, slow, tight, or thin, [this formula] is inappropriate." It also mentions treatment of the initial stage of neck tumors. In addition, *Restoration of Health from the Myriad Diseases* recommends the formula for treatment of 'breast rocks' (乳岩 *rǔ yán*), which it describes:

> Initially, a kernel, swollen [to a shape] like a tortoise the size of a chess piece * with no pain or itching. After five or six years, it transforms into a sore. … It most often occurs in depressed, middle-aged women who hold in their anger.

The text also recommends the formula for breast abscesses or for the toxic abscesses and tumors of pox disorders. What most all of these disorders share is a combination of external and internal disharmonies; the primary internal ones are of deficiency, and the external ones, either dermal or deeper, appear as excess in the form of heat and/or stagnation of qi and blood.

---

* Chinese chess uses small, disc-like markers.

Analysis of Formula

This is a complex formula that is designed for the treatment of a complex pattern with apparent excess (toxic swelling) in the midst of both interior and exterior deficiency. Angelicae sinensis Radix (*dāng guī*), Paeoniae Radix alba (*bái sháo*), and Chuanxiong Rhizoma (*chuān xiōng*) work together to harmonize and tonify the blood. Ginseng Radix (*rén shēn*) and Astragali Radix (*huáng qí*) tonify the qi. These five herbs provide support for the interior and aid the body's efforts to heal chronic lesions. The warm quality of Cinnamomi Cortex (*ròu guì*) assists the yang qi, and its acrid quality works with Angelicae sinensis Radix (*dāng guī*) and Chuanxiong Rhizoma (*chuān xiōng*) to break up blood stasis. Angelicae dahuricae Radix (*bái zhǐ*) and Platycodi Radix (*jié gěng*) thrust out the pus. Aucklandiae Radix (*mù xiāng*), Linderae Radix (*wū yào*), Arecae Semen (*bīng láng*), Aurantii Fructus (*zhǐ ké*), and Magnoliae officinalis Cortex (*hòu pò*) disperse qi stagnation. Perillae Folium (*zǐ sū yè*) and Saposhnikoviae Radix (*fáng fēng*) course the exterior to move the qi. Glycyrrhizae Radix (*gān cǎo*) works with Ginseng Radix (*rén shēn*) and Astragali Radix (*huáng qí*) to tonify the qi; it also harmonizes the formula. In the words of Zhu Dan Xi, this formula contains herbs that address "the interior and exterior, and the qi and blood, along with herbs that dredge wind and assist the yang." Thus, it can be used in treating the internal-external, deficiency-excess pattern in which these dermal lesions present.

Commentary

Although the Ming-dynasty text *Introduction to Medicine* is the source of record for this formula, it probably existed many years before that text was written. Books from the Ming and Qing dynasties record that the formula was in common use for the treatment of toxic swellings during Zhu Dan-Xi's time several hundred years earlier. Zhu's comments on the formula survive in the writings of later authors who quoted him. One such commentary discusses the simultaneous treatment of root and branch, saying that when practitioners treat toxic swellings, they:

> [O]ften do not differentiate channels, pulses, or patterns. [Nor do they] pay heed to the season. They [simply] say to eliminate and transform toxin. Others say [if the sore does] not abate, [then] add agents to tonify the qi and blood. This [type of thinking] causes people to doubt [the efficacy of the strategy embraced by this formula].

From this passage we can see that Zhu Dan-Xi felt that the formula was underutilized owing to the approach of most practitioners to first treat the branch symptom by clearing heat and resolving toxicity, and only if that is ineffective to treat the root and support the interior. In addition, it is clear that Zhu lamented the habit of some practitioners of his day to treat only the disorder and not the individual person and circumstance.

Place in Treatment

The reluctance to treat toxic sores without clearing heat and resolving toxicity is understandable when the practitioner is faced with a lesion that appears hot and toxic. When heat symptoms are present, it is counterintuitive to prescribe a formula that has no heat-clearing or toxicity-resolving herbs and is built on a foundation of tonifying herbs. Nonetheless, if the constitution is weak or the condition is chronic, that is often the proper approach.

Even so, it should be pointed out that some physicians, both past and present, suggest that this formula is best used as a follow-up after a more aggressive initial approach using cold and bitter, toxicity-resolving herbs. In contrast to this are many sources that suggest using the formula at the very beginning, when swellings appear as small lumps or nodules. Others suggest that, when used to treat hot, toxic sores, the formula should be modified to make it better able to clear heat, resolve toxicity, and thrust pus out. Each practitioner must weigh the degree of deficiency of the patient, the severity, stage, and toxicity of the lesion or swelling, and the current seasonal conditions to determine the best approach. Some of the modifications listed below are intended to help adjust the formula to meet these conditions.

Usage

In the classical literature, there are three primary categories of lesions addressed by this formula: breast disorders such as breast abscess, breast cancer, and breast nodules; swellings of the neck such as goiter, saber sores, and enlarged thyroid; and widespread or localized swelling such as pox sores.

In modern times, this formula has been used to treat a variety of breast, thyroid, skin, and lymphatic problems. In Japan, use of the formula has been expanded to ophthalmology; it is used for chronic, painful eye disorders such as chronic conjunctivitis.

Comparisons

➤ Vs. Support the Interior and Eliminate Toxin Drink *(tuō lǐ xiāo dú yǐn)*

Both Support the Interior and Eliminate Toxin Drink *(tuō lǐ xiāo dú yǐn)* and Sixteen-Ingredient Drink for Qi Flow *(shí liù wèi liú qì yǐn)* treat toxic swellings in patients suffering from internal deficiency. In *Introduction to Medicine*, the difference between the two formulas is discussed in the context of treating toxic swellings attributed to overwork or consumption (勞 *láo*) injury and qi constraint with the pathogen lodged in the channels and the nutritive and protective levels.

> [Lesions] owing to toxin from internal deficiency impairment [brought on by] by excessive sexual activity or constrained anger, although they appear swollen and painful, regarding the exterior, there are no signs of six-warp patterns, and regarding the interior, there is no impeding blockage, [one thus] knows

that the pathogen is in the channels and one must not blindly cause sweating or purging. It is suitable to tonify the body's qi, adjust the channels and vessels, harmonize the nutritive and protective levels, or focus on tonifying the Spleen and Stomach. [In cases of] constrained anger [use] Sixteen-Ingredient Drink for Qi Flow *(shí liù wèi liú qì yǐn)*. Deficiency consumption [calls for] Support the Interior and Eliminate Toxin Drink *(tuō lǐ xiāo dú yǐn)*.

This statement is based on the fact that Sixteen-Ingredient Drink for Qi Flow *(shí liù wèi liú qì yǐn)* contains more qi-moving herbs than Support the Interior and Eliminate Toxin Drink *(tuō lǐ xiāo dú yǐn)* and is thus better suited for cases with qi constraint. Another difference is that Support the Interior and Eliminate Toxin Drink *(tuō lǐ xiāo dú yǐn)* contains Lonicerae Flos *(jīn yín huā)* and thus, to a small degree, addresses the heat toxin associated with toxic swellings.

➤ Vs. Powder to Support the Interior Worth a Thousand Gold Pieces *(qiān jīn nèi tuō sǎn)*

These two formulas are very similar in their approach, scope of treatment, and constituent herbs. However, Powder to Support the Interior Worth a Thousand Gold Pieces *(qiān jīn nèi tuō sǎn)* contains fewer herbs to move the qi and dredge the exterior. This makes it less dispersing and more tonifying, and thus centered more on pure support of the interior. For this reason, it is mostly used for chronic conditions and is seldom applied to initial-stage disorders.

Toxic swellings such as abscesses and boils progress through various stages before they resolve. Sixteen-Ingredient Drink for Qi Flow *(shí liù wèi liú qì yǐn)* is most commonly applied to the initial stage, when the swelling refuses to dissipate or come to a head, or to the end-stage when, after suppurating, the sore does not close but continues to weep fluid.

Biomedical Indications

With the appropriate presentation, this formula may be used to treat a variety of biomedically-defined disorders including breast abscess, breast cancer, fibrocystic breast, enlarged thyroid, cervical lymphadenopathy, chronic skin abscess, and chronic conjunctivitis.

Modifications

* For stubborn sores, add Poria *(fú líng)*, Atractylodis macrocephalae Rhizoma *(bái zhú)*, and Rehmanniae Radix praeparata *(shú dì huáng)*.
* For lack of appetite, add Amomi Fructus *(shā rén)* and Cyperi Rhizoma *(xiāng fù)*.
* For pain, add Olibanum *(rǔ xiāng)* and Myrrha *(mò yào)*.
* For leaking sores that fail to dry, add Fritillariae thunbergii Bulbus *(zhè bèi mǔ)* and Anemarrhenae Rhizoma *(zhī mǔ)*.
* For swellings that are slow to come to a head and burst, add Gleditsiae Spina *(zào jiǎo cì)*.

- For breast abscesses, add Vaccariae Semen (*wáng bù liú xíng*) and Taraxaci Herba (*pú gōng yīng*).

- For cancerous breast tumors, add Cremastrae/Pleiones Pseudobulbus (*shān cí gū*), Solani lyrati Herba (*bái máo téng*),* Scutellariae barbatae Herba (*bàn zhī lián*), Citri re-

ticulatae viride Pericarpium (*qīng pí*), and Hedyotis diffusae Herba (*bái huā shé shé cǎo*).

- For swollen lymph nodes, add Prunellae Spica (*xià kū cǎo*), Scutellariae Radix (*huáng qín*), and Scrophulariae Radix (*xuán shēn*).

- For enlarged thyroid, add Prunellae Spica (*xià kū cǎo*), Scrophulariae Radix (*xuán shēn*), Fritillariae thunbergii Bulbus (*zhè bèi mǔ*), and Eckloniae Thallus (*kūn bù*).

---

* Solani lyrati Herba (白毛藤 *bái máo téng*) is sweet, bitter, cold, and slightly toxic. It enters the Gallbladder and Kidney channels and clears heat, resolves dampness, resolves toxicity, and reduces swellings. The normal dosage in decoctions is 15-30g.

Comparative Tables of Principal Formulas

■ FORMULAS THAT TREAT EXTERNAL ABSCESSES AND SORES

Common symptoms: soft or hard external swellings

Formula Name	Diagnosis	Indications	Remarks
Immortals' Formula for Sustaining Life (*xiān fāng huó mìng yǐn*)	Fire toxin or phlegm-fire	Early-stage sores and carbuncles with red, swollen, hot, and painful skin lesions, usually accompanied by fever, mild chills, headache, a thin tongue coating (either white or slightly yellow), and a rapid, forceful pulse	For early-stage yang sores that develop rapidly. Also used to treat various inflammatory disorders that present with blood stasis, phlegm, and heat toxin.
Five-Ingredient Drink to Eliminate Toxin (*wǔ wèi xiāo dú yǐn*)	Fire toxin	All types of boils and carbuncles with localized erythema, swelling, heat, and pain accompanied by fever, chills, a red tongue with a yellow coating, and a rapid pulse	Especially useful for deep-rooted and hard lesions that are said to resemble nails or chestnuts. A foundation for many formulas used to treat localized, superficial, purulent infections.
Four-Valiant Decoction for Well-Being (*sì miào yǒng ān tāng*)	Sloughing ulcer due to obstruction by fire toxin leading to stasis of blood in the sinews and blood vessels	Ulcerated, nonhealing sores (which may have a rotten smell and copious discharge) on a dark red, slightly swollen limb that is warm to the touch and extremely painful, along with fever, thirst, a red tongue, and a rapid pulse	Combines a strategy of clearing heat and resolving toxicity with nourishing the yin fluids and invigorating the blood.
Support the Interior and Eliminate Toxin Drink (*tuō lǐ xiāo dú yǐn*)	Toxic sores with qi and blood deficiency	Nonsuppurating toxic sores or ones that only slowly leak thin, watery pus and fail to heal, along with fever, lassitude, lack of luster, and a rapid pulse with no strength	For dermal abscesses described as red, painful swellings with distinct borders that feel soft when pressed, reflecting the presence of a pus-filled center.
Balmy Yang Decoction (*yáng hé tāng*)	Various manifestations of yin-type flat abscesses or yin-type localized swellings	Localized, painful swellings without a head that blend into the surrounding tissue and do not affect the texture or color of the skin, and are not hot to the touch, no thirst, a very pale tongue, and a pulse that is submerged, thin, and forceless	Also used for joint problems as well as internal medical, gynecological, and pediatric disorders characterized by yang deficiency where cold leads to a congealing of fluids and stagnation of qi and blood.
Ten-Ingredient Powder to Overcome Toxicity (*shí wèi bài dú sǎn*)	Heat toxin flushing through the exterior aspects of the body	For the initial stages of various types of pus-filled sores including acne, boils, dermal abscesses, eczema, hives, mastitis, inflamed lymph nodes, internal or external ear infections, and sties	In modern times, especially in Japan, this formula is often used for allergic skin disorders.

cont. ↘

Formula Name	Diagnosis	Indications	Remarks
Powder to Support the Interior Worth a Thousand Gold Pieces (*qiān jīn nèi tuō sǎn*)	Toxic swellings in patients with deficient constitutions	Chronic sores that fail to come to a head or those that have already suppurated but continue to exude watery pus	Also used to treat chronic inner ear infections and other localized infections that linger and subsequently drain the body's qi.
Decoction to Disperse Swelling and Ulcerate What Is Hard (*sàn zhǒng kuì jiān tāng*)	Saber sores owing to fire rising in the body causing fluids to congeal into phlegm	Knotted and hard lumps as hard as stones that may be located on the neck or shoulders and down to the armpit, usually along the paths of the hand and foot lesser yang channels or the foot yang brightness channel	Also for scrofula, goiter, and other neck tumors. Effectively disperses swelling and induces ulceration of hardness.

■ FORMULAS THAT TREAT INTERNAL ABSCESSES

Common symptoms: initial or late stage internal abscess, often associated with pain

Formula Name	Diagnosis	Indications	Remarks
Reed Decoction (*wěi jīng tāng*)	Lung abscess due to wind-heat toxin entering the Lungs accompanied by phlegm and blood stasis	Cough with foul-smelling sputum (may be streaked with blood), slight fever, mild chest pain, dry, scaly skin, a red tongue with a greasy, yellow coating, and a slippery, rapid pulse	Also used during recuperation from a febrile disease when the patient has a slight fever and cough with thick sputum that is difficult to expectorate.
Rhubarb and Moutan Decoction (*dà huáng mǔ dān tāng*)	Early-stage Intestinal abscess, a condition of excess with interior clumping of heat and blood	Lower abdominal distention and pain (usually on the right) that increases upon pressure with rebound tenderness, guarding of the abdominal musculature, a thin, yellow, and greasy tongue coating, and a slippery, rapid pulse	May also be groin pain, or lower right quadrant abdominal masses, with irregular, intermittent fever followed by chills and sweating.
Clear the Intestines Drink (*qīng cháng yǐn*)	Early-stage Intestinal abscess with yin deficiency and hyperactivity of fire	Severe abdominal pain (usually on the right) that increases on pressure with rebound tenderness, chills and fever, aversion to wind, spontaneous sweating, dry, scaly skin, dry mouth, and a red tongue with little moisture	May also be groin pain that is relieved by flexing the hip and knee (usually on the right) and intensified by extending the hip. For more severe damage to the yin and blood.
Coix , Aconite Accessory Root, and Patrinia Powder (*yì yǐ fù zǐ bài jiàng sǎn*)	Intestinal abscess where pus has already formed	Distention of the abdomen with scaly, dry skin, tightness, and a mass-like appearance, but softness on palpation, and a rapid pulse despite the absence of fever	Focuses on clearing toxins while warming the yang to successfully expel pus and reduce the abscess. Also for skin disorders.
Clear the Heart and Enable the Diaphragm Decoction (*qīng xīn lì gé tāng*)	Sore throat with internal accumulation of excess heat	Red, swollen, and painful throat with difficulty swallowing, perhaps with small pustules on the tonsils, high fever, thirst with desire to drink cold liquids, bad breath, irritability, phlegm in the throat, constipation, a red tongue with yellow coating, and a rapid, flooding pulse	The usage of this formula has expanded in recent times to include sores in the mouth or tongue that present as part of a pattern of Lung or Stomach heat accumulation.
Sixteen-Ingredient Drink for Qi Flow (*shí liù wèi liú qì yǐn*)	A complex pattern with apparent excess (toxic swelling) in the midst of both interior and exterior deficiency	Noxious swellings and abscesses, including those of the breast and neck, and widespread or localized swelling such as pox sores, with a flooding, moderate, submerged, slow, tight, or thin pulse	Modern usage extends to thyroid, skin, lymphatic, and eye disorders.

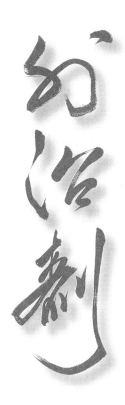

Chapter 21 Contents

Formulas for External Application

....

Formulas for External Application

THIS CHAPTER DIFFERS from others in this book by focusing its discussion on the method of application rather than on the treatment principle. For that reason, its nature and format do not strictly conform to that used in the other chapters. For example, the formula discussions in this chapter emphasize the method of preparation and application of the formulas to highlight and explain the often unique methods involved in external applications. Furthermore, analyses of the ingredients in the formulas are brief because formulators of external applications seldom disclose the basis for their compositions. Though extremely brief, it is our hope that this presentation helps the reader gain a basic understanding of the clinical use of externally-applied formulas.

While external application (外治法 *wài zhì fǎ*) is a broad category that embraces all treatment methods that do not involve the ingestion of herbs, including acupuncture, massage, moxibustion, and other nonherb-based treatments, we will limit our commentary here to applications of medicinal agents to the exterior of the body. Because we do not have sufficient space to cover all methods of topical application, we will focus on a few of the most commonly-used ones and give examples of each. Our goal is to introduce a few common methods along with a handful of formulas for each method presented. Both historically and at the present time, the majority of external applications are used in the context of the traditional specialties of external medicine (外科 *wài kē*) and trauma (傷科 *shāng kē*). We will focus on these uses

in our presentation, but will also present a few external treatments that address internal disorders.

Section 1

HISTORICAL ASPECTS

External applications of medicinals are found in the earliest extant medical works, including *Prescriptions for Fifty-Two Ailments* (probably from the early 2nd century B.C.E.) and *Han Dynasty Medical Bamboo Strips from Wuwei* (from the early part of the 1st century C.E.). These included plasters, soaks, powders, herbs placed in the ear, as well as adhering herbs. The majority of external applications in these texts were designed for treatment of skin disorders or traumatic injury, and this continues to be the case for external applications down to the present time.

The core texts of the Chinese medical tradition, the *Inner Classic* and *Discussion of Cold Damage*, both mentioned external applications of herbs, and the famous late-Han physician Hua Tuo described steaming, hot pressing, and washing as important methods of treatment. The Tang-dynasty physician Sun Si-Miao included numerous external applications in his 7th-century work, *Important Formulas Worth a Thousand Gold Pieces*. In the 16th century, when Li Shi-Zhen traveled around China collecting information about herbs for his *Comprehensive Outline of the Materia Medica*, he assembled a large number of external applications in use at the time. The most comprehensive collection of externally-used formulas was assembled in the 19th-century work, *Rhymed Prose on [Medical] Principles and Applications,* by Wu Shi-Ji. Wu, a member of a family with many generations of physicians, observed that there were shortcomings to internal herbal therapy such as the unavailability or expense of certain herbs, the ineffectiveness of internal treatment for certain disorders, and patients who were unable to take herbs. He thus dedicated himself to the study of external applications. For over twenty years, he scoured the classical texts for references to external applications and also collected folk remedies. His book is now regarded as the masterpiece on external applications (外治之宗 *wài zhì zhī zōng*).

Modern times have brought many new ingredients, adjuvants and actives, to the world of external applications. Steroids, salicylic acid, isopropyl alcohol, petroleum jelly, DMSO, and glycerin are just a few of the common modern substances now found in creams, ointments, and other external applications. New forms, such as lotions and gels, are also part of the modern evolution. In our discussion, we will focus on traditional methods and materials, mentioning modern developments only when they arise in the context of that discussion. There are many types of external applications. For a brief discussion, see the Introduction to this book.

Considerations Regarding the Use of External Applications

In *Rhymed Prose on [Medical] Principles and Applications,* Wu compared the use of external and internal therapies: "The principles (理 *lǐ*) of external treatment are the same as those applied to internal treatment; the herbs used for external treatment are the same as those used for internal treatment; the sole difference is method." This difference in method requires attention to some aspects of treatment that do not enter into consideration for internal methods of treatment. The following guidelines highlight some of the aspects that require attention and suggest means of ameliorating associated problems:

1. *Apply external applications to a small area first to test for sensitivity.*

   Although rare, patients can have reactions or sensitivities to certain applications. It may be an allergy to a specific herb or adjuvant, or to the combination. In any case, by applying a small amount to a sensitive area of the body, such as the inner surface of the forearm, one can test for any reaction. It is best to wait a few hours after the test to make sure the patient does not develop redness, itching, blisters, or pain.

2. *When first applying an external application, do so early in the day.*

   If a patient is to have an unfavorable reaction to an application, it is best that this happen early in the day so that by bed time, the irritation does not interfere with sleep.

3. *If toxic materials are in the application, be sure that they are properly labeled.*

   Labels should be attached to the jar and not the lid to prevent any confusion. Also, for toxic items, dispense only as much as needed so that the jar is not left around to be used improperly.

4. *Avoid bringing herbs in contact with eyes, mouth, open sores, and mucous membranes.*

   Except where specifically indicated, it is best to keep herbal preparations away from the eyes, mouth, and mucous membranes. Although it is common in China to put herbal preparations into open sores, the chance (albeit very low) that this may cause infection is reason enough to avoid this practice.

5. *Advise patients to stop using the application, and notify you if irritation or itching develops.*

   In addition to the first cautionary statement above, patients should be made aware that itching or redness is not normal. An exception to this rule is during the treatment of scabies, where itching typically worsens initially.

Section 2

....

EXTERNAL FORMULAS FOR EXTERNAL DISORDERS

冰硼散
Borneal and Borax Powder
bīng péng sǎn

Source   *Orthodox Lineage of External Medicine* (1617)

Borneolum (*bīng piàn*) 1.5g
Natrii Sulfas siccatus (*xuán míng fěn*) 15g
Cinnabaris (*zhū shā*) 1.8g
Borax (*péng shā*) 15g

Method of Preparation   Grind the above ingredients (adding Borneolum (*bīng piàn*) at the end of the grinding process) into a fine powder and store in an airtight container. Due to its unacceptably high levels of heavy metals, Cinnabaris (*zhū shā*) is generally omitted from the formula.

Method of Application Traditionally, the powder was blown into the throat or ear or applied directly to the mouth. The use of plastic, squeezable spray bottles are common in modern times for application to the throat, ears, or nose. A moist cotton ball or cotton-tipped swab can be used to apply the powder to sores in the mouth. It is recommended that a 0.03-0.1g/dose be applied 4-6 times a day.

Actions Clears heat and resolves toxicity, dispels putrescence, reduces swelling, and relieves pain

Indications

Sore, swollen throat, swelling or pain in the gums, mouth sores, and external ear infections. The source text notes that this formula is indicated for chronic or acute disorders of the throat or mouth, and for the sore throat and hoarseness associated with long-term phlegm-fire cough.

Analysis of Formula

Borneolum (*bīng piàn*) reduces swelling and alleviates pain. Natrii Sulfas siccatus (*xuán míng fěn*) softens hardness and drains fire. Borax (*péng shā*) clears heat, reduces swelling, and disperses clumps. Originally, Cinnabaris (*zhū shā*) was used to unblock the vessels and resolve toxicity.

Cautions and Contraindications

Application to the throat and oral cavity results in ingestion of small amounts of the formula. For this reason, it is important that natural Borneolum (*bīng piàn*) be used. The chemically-produced item is unsuitable for internal use. In addition, some action should be taken to ensure that the powder is not contaminated with bacteria or other pathogens if it is to be applied to mucous membranes or to open sores.

Biomedical Indications

With the appropriate presentation, this formula may be used to treat a variety of biomedically-defined disorders including thrush, gingivitis, mandibular osteomyelitis, acute and chronic middle ear infections, acute or chronic rhinitis, impetigo, mumps, and dermatitis bullosa.

Modifications

- If swelling and heat are prominent, add Coptidis Rhizoma (*huáng lián*) and Indigo naturalis (*qīng dài*)

- For open sores, add Catechu (*ér chá*) and powdered Margarita (*zhēn zhū fěn*).

- For swelling and pain in the throat due to wind-heat, add Bombyx batryticatus (*bái jiāng cán*) and Citrulli Praeparatio (*xī guā shuāng*).

- For bleeding, add charred Typhae Pollen (*pú huáng tàn*).

Associated Formulas

綠袍散 （绿袍散）

Green Robe Powder

lǜ páo sǎn

SOURCE *Formulas to Protect Life and the Most Treasured Family Possession* (1184)

Phellodendri Cortex (*huáng bǎi*)	120g
Glycyrrhizae Radix praeparata (*zhì gān cǎo*)	60g
Indigo naturalis (*qīng dài*)	30g

The ingredients are ground into a fine powder and applied to the gums or tongue 4-6 times a day using a gauze pad or cotton ball. Clears heat, resolves toxicity, dries dampness, and helps close sores. This formula treats sores of the mouth and gums and is frequently used to treat bleeding gums. It treats disorders that are treated internally by such formulas as Cool the Diaphragm Powder (*liáng gé sǎn*), Anemarrhena, Phellodendron, and Rehmannia Pill (*zhī bǎi dì huáng wán*), and Drain the Yellow Powder (*xiè huáng sǎn*) if the cause is internal disharmony; and by Honeysuckle and Forsythia Powder (*yín qiáo sǎn*) or Mulberry Leaf and Chrysanthemum Drink (*sāng jú yǐn*) when the cause is an external wind-heat pathogen.

月石散

Moon Stone Powder

yuè shí sǎn

SOURCE *Rhymed Prose on [Medical] Principles and Applications* (1870)

Natrii Sulfas siccatus (*xuán míng fěn*)	60g
Borax (*péng shā*)	60g
Menthae haplocalycis Herba (*bò hé*)	8g
dry-fried Typhae Pollen (*chǎo pú huáng*)	24g
Coptidis Rhizoma (*huáng lián*)	24g
Phellodendri Cortex (*huáng bǎi*)	24g
Borneolum (*bīng piàn*)	6g

Grind the first six ingredients into a fine powder and pass through a fine sieve (about 100 holes per inch), then grind in the Borneolum (*bīng piàn*). Store in an airtight container. Resolves toxicity, disperses swelling, generates flesh, and relieves pain. For acute or chronic redness, pain and swelling in the throat, oral cavity, or tonsils. A small amount is blown onto the affected area 3-4 times a day. For intensely painful situations, apply every two hours. *Note:* Moon stone (月石 *yuè shí*) is an another name for Borax (*péng shā*).

金黃散 / 金黃膏

Golden-Yellow Powder/ Golden-Yellow Plaster

jīn huáng sǎn/jīn huáng gāo

This formula is named for its color.

Source *Orthodox Lineage of External Medicine* (1617)

Trichosanthis Radix (*tiān huā fěn*)	500g
Phellodendri Cortex (*huáng bǎi*)	250g

Rhei Radix et Rhizoma (dà huáng) 250g
Curcumae longae Rhizoma (jiāng huáng) 250g
Angelicae dahuricae Radix (bái zhǐ) 250g
Magnoliae officinalis Cortex (hòu pò) 100g
Citri reticulatae Pericarpium (chén pí) 100g
Glycyrrhizae Radix (gān cǎo) 100g
Atractylodis Rhizoma (cāng zhú) 100g
Arisaematis Rhizoma praeparatum (zhì tiān nán xīng) 100g

Method of Preparation The ingredients are ground into a fine powder. If a plaster is desired, the powder can be mixed with honey, tea water, or sesame oil, among other media.

Method of Application Most sores and swellings require that the paste be spread on gauze. The gauze pad then is secured over the affected site. Change once a day, cleaning the site during each change. Small sores can be daubed with powder (if the sores are wet) or paste and can be left uncovered or covered with just a small bandage. At present, the powder is frequently mixed with petroleum jelly to make a plaster, in which case it is called Golden-Yellow Plaster (jīn huáng gāo).

Actions Clears heat, resolve toxicity, disperses stasis, reduces swelling, dispels dampness, and transforms phlegm

Indications

This formula is intended for red, hot swellings that have not yet come to a head. For example, *Golden Mirror of the Medical Tradition* lists a very wide range of disorders for which this formula is appropriate including abscesses, flat-headed abscesses on the back, deep-set toxic sores, swelling from trauma, damp-phlegm spreading sores, massive head febrile disorder, lacquer sores, erisipelas, wind-heat heaven-borne blisters (天皰瘡 tiān pào chuāng—white vesicles that appear in the upper body and eventually burst to exude a yellowish discharge; often associated with biomedically-defined impetigo), redness and swelling of the skin, burns, dry or damp leg qi, breast abscesses, and any type of stubborn malign, hot sore.

Analysis of Formula

Rhei Radix et Rhizoma (dà huáng) and Curcumae longae Rhizoma (jiāng huáng) move the blood; Rhei Radix et Rhizoma (dà huáng) and Phellodendri Cortex (huáng bǎi) clear heat and resolve toxicity; and Trichosanthis Radix (tiān huā fěn) thrusts out pus, reduces swelling, and unblocks the channels. Citri reticulatae Pericarpium (chén pí), Arisaematis Rhizoma praeparatum (zhì tiān nán xīng), Magnoliae officinalis Cortex (hòu pò), Angelicae dahuricae Radix (bái zhǐ), and Atractylodis Rhizoma (cāng zhú) dry dampness, transform phlegm, regulate the qi, and alleviate pain.

Cautions and Contraindications

With the exception of superficial blisters, such as impetigo and herpes, this formula should not be applied to open wounds.

Commentary

This formula, as a plaster, is found in almost every hospital of Chinese medicine in China. While originally designed to treat specific toxic swellings, it is now applied to a wide range of disorders in dermatology, trauma, and internal medicine.

Biomedical Indications

With the appropriate presentation, this formula may be used to treat a variety of biomedically-defined disorders including boils, carbuncles, abscesses, inflamed subdermal cysts, inflamed lymph nodes, inflamed or infected insect bites, burns, trauma such as sprains and contusions with redness and swelling, impetigo, cellulitis, herpes zoster, acute breast abscesses or mastitis, mumps, contact dermatitis (specifically lacquer irritations), and folliculitis.

Alternate name

This formula is often known as 'As You Desire' Golden-Yellow Powder (如意金黄散 rú yì jīn huáng sǎn). This name underscores one's good fortune in using the formula. When prepared as a soft plaster, it is called Golden-Yellow Plaster (jīn huáng gāo).

Modifications

- The powder can be sprinkled on wet sores directly.
- Add the liquid of green tea (honey can be added as well) to make a paste that can be used to treat hot swellings. (*Golden Mirror of the Medical Tradition*)
- Tea made from Chinese scallions (honey can be added as well), mixed in to make a paste, is best for encouraging the thrusting out of pus. (*Golden Mirror of the Medical Tradition*)
- Mix with sesame oil to treat burns or lacquer sores or, in modern times, to daub onto herpes sores. Cellulitis, lacquer sores, and impetigo are best treated by adding the fresh-squeezed juice of Isatis roots and leaves; a tea made from these herbs or fresh dandelion juice can be substituted for this. (*Golden Mirror of the Medical Tradition*)

紫當膏 (紫当膏)
Lithospermum/Arnebia and Tangkuei Ointment

zǐ dāng gāo

Source *Complete Book of Patterns and Treatments in External Medicine* (1831)

Arnebiae/Lithospermi Radix (zǐ cǎo) 30g
Angelicae sinensis Radix (dāng guī) 30g
sesame oil 350g
beeswax 50-100g

Method of Preparation Soak the Arnebiae/Lithospermi Radix (zǐ cǎo) and the Angelicae sinensis Radix (dāng guī) in sesame oil for one week. Heat the herbs and oil gently until it begins to slowly bubble. Lower the heat and cook until the Angelicae sinensis Radix (dāng guī) begins to slightly brown on the edges. Turn off the heat, and when the mixture cools to the point that it will not burn the skin, strain out the herbs. Reheat the liquid over a low flame. When it is warm enough to melt the beeswax, add it in. Stir the mixture until the beeswax is completely melted, and then spoon the mixture into glass containers to cool and harden into an ointment. The amount of beeswax needed depends on the type of beeswax used, the season of the year, and the consistency desired for the ointment. To achieve the proper consistency of ointment, more beeswax is needed in the summer and less in the winter.

When cooling the oil after it is boiled with the herbs, it is traditional in China to place the pot with the hot oil inside a pot with cool water, in a setup resembling a double boiler. This method of cooling the oil is thought to remove the fire toxin that the high heat has imparted to the oil.

Note: The source text does not specify the quantity of sesame oil or beeswax. The suggested quantities are estimates based on those used in similar ointments.

Method of Application   Gently rub a small amount of ointment into the affected area 3-4 times a day. For acute cases or to avoid staining fabric such as sheets or clothing, the ointment may be spread onto a gauze pad that is then secured over the affected site. In the latter case, the dressing should be changed once a day.

Actions   Clears heat, cools the blood, resolves toxicity, moistens dryness, and relieves pain and itching

Indications

Originally, the source text recommended this formula for various lip sores, but the ointment soon came to be used for all manner of skin rashes that present as heat toxin, dry, itching, or painful lesions. Also used for calluses, and dry, cracked skin.

Analysis of Formula

Angelicae sinensis Radix (dāng guī) moistens the skin and moves the blood and Arnebiae/Lithospermi Radix (zǐ cǎo) clears heat, cools the blood, and resolves toxicity. When the heat and toxicity are resolved and the damaged skin is moistened, the pain and itching will cease.

Cautions and Contraindications

None noted.

Comparison

➤ Vs. Double-Dark Plaster (èr qīng gāo); see page 900

Biomedical Indications

With the appropriate presentation, this formula can be used to treat a variety of biomedically-defined disorders including lip sores, eczema, psoriasis, seborrheic dermatitis, chilblains minor burns, and sunburn.

Modifications

- This ointment makes an excellent base for soft plasters used to treat skin rashes. Adding various powdered herbs to the ointment can alter its functions for specific circumstances. Generally, the added powder equals no more than one-fifth of the weight of the final plaster.

- For blood stasis rashes, add powdered Olibanum (rǔ xiāng) and Myrrha (mò yào).

- To increase the heat-clearing properties of the ointment, add powdered Phellodendri Cortex (huáng bǎi), Coptidis Rhizoma (huáng lián), or Hibisci mutabilis Folium (fú róng yè). Alternatively, Phellodendri Cortex (huáng bǎi) or Coptidis Rhizoma (huáng lián) may be cooked in the original oil.

- Mixing Indigo Powder (qīng dài sǎn) into the ointment makes a soft plaster suitable for treatment of acute, hot, eczema-like rashes.

Variation

潤肌膏 （润肌膏）

Skin-Moistening Ointment

rùn jī gāo

SOURCE   *Orthodox Lineage of External Medicine* (1617)

In this formula, the ratio of the ingredients is Arnebiae/Lithospermi Radix (zǐ cǎo) 3g, Angelicae sinensis Radix (dāng guī) 15g, sesame oil 120g, and beeswax 15g. This is a much softer ointment that is better suited to dryer skin rashes than Lithospermum/Arnebia and Tangkuei Ointment (zǐ dāng gāo). It is recommended in the source text for the treatment of white scaling wind (白屑風 bái xiè fēng), a traditional disease name that is thought to overlap with the biomedically-defined diseases psoriasis and seborrheic dermatitis.

二青膏

Double-Dark Plaster

èr qīng gāo

This formula is named for two of its ingredients, Indigo naturalis (qīng dài) and 青露 qīng lù, which is another name for Hibisci mutabilis Folium (fú róng yè). Both of these have a dark purple color and include the character 青 qīng in their names, hence the name of the formula.

Source   *Orthodox Lineage of External Medicine* (1617)

Indigo naturalis (qīng dài)	30g
Hibisci mutabilis Folium (fú róng yè) *	30g
impure Natrii Sulfas (pò xiāo)	30g
Rhei Radix et Rhizoma (dà huáng)	120g
Trichosanthis Radix (tiān huā fěn)	90g

* Hibisci mutabilis Folium (芙蓉葉 fú róng yè) is cool and slightly acrid. It clears the Lungs, cools the blood, reduces swelling, and expels pus.

Fossilia Ossis Mastodi (*lóng gǔ*) 30g
Phellodendri Cortex (*huáng bǎi*) 30g
Ampelopsis Radix (*bái liàn*) 30g
Cynanchi atrati Radix (*bái wēi*) 30g
Bletillae Rhizoma (*bái jí*) 30g
Angelicae dahuricae Radix (*bái zhǐ*) 30g
Dictamni Cortex (*bái xiān pí*) .30g

Method of Preparation   The ingredients are ground into a powder and mixed with an adjuvant to make a soft plaster. For treatment of yang-toxin swellings, mix with honey and vinegar to make a paste. For treatment of trauma, mix with rice wine and honey or with sesame oil. In modern China, petroleum jelly or a glycerin-based cream is often used as an adjuvant. Most swellings require that the paste be spread on gauze. The gauze pad is then secured over the affected site. Change once daily, cleaning the site during each change.

Actions   Clears heat, resolves toxicity, disperses swelling, and relieves pain

Indications

This formula is intended for red, hot swellings. If the swelling has come to a head, the ointment is put directly on the head; if no head is apparent, the ointment should encircle and cover the swelling. The formula is also suitable for treatment of first-stage trauma. It can be applied to strains, sprains, relocated dislocations, bruises, and bumps.

Analysis of Formula

Indigo naturalis (*qīng dài*), Hibisci mutabilis Folium (*fú róng yè*), Phellodendri Cortex (*huáng bǎi*), Cynanchi atrati Radix (*bái wēi*), Dictamni Cortex (*bái xiān pí*), Rhei Radix et Rhizoma (*dà huáng*), and impure Natrii Sulfas (*pò xiāo*) are bitter, cold, fire-draining, toxicity-resolving, swelling-dispersing, and pain-relieving medicinals. They treat internal clumping of heat toxin. Bletillae Rhizoma (*bái jí*), Angelicae dahuricae Radix (*bái zhǐ*), Trichosanthis Radix (*tiān huā fěn*), and Fossilia Ossis Mastodi (*lóng gǔ*) treat abscesses by dispersing clumping and swelling and thrusting out pus. Thus, stasis, clumps, swelling, and pain are all addressed and the heat is cleared, the toxicity resolved, the swelling dispersed, and the pain relieved.

Cautions and Contraindications

Do not apply to open wounds.

Comparison

> Vs. Golden-Yellow Plaster (*jīn huáng gāo*)

The source text mentions Double-Dark Plaster (*èr qīng gāo*) for two distinct situations. The first is red, hot, toxic yang swellings, whether or not they have come to a head. The ingredients aim to disperse and clear the accumulation of heat toxin. It has a stronger action than Golden-Yellow Plaster (*jīn huáng gāo*) for dispersing the accumulation but is less effective at bringing a swelling to a head quickly. Thus, for heat-toxin swellings that have not yet come to a head, but appear ready to do so, one should first think of that formula. For other stages of swellings, especially when heat clumping is characterized by a firm swelling, Double-Dark Plaster (*èr qīng gāo*) is a better choice.

The second situation mentioned for this ointment is what modern physicians refer to as first-stage trauma. Just as Double-Dark Plaster (*èr qīng gāo*) disperses the heat toxin associated with abscesses and other heat-toxin lesions, it can also disperse and clear the heat and toxin related to first-stage sprains, bruises, and other trauma. When the heat and toxin are cleared from the site of the injury, the body can attend to healing at a faster pace. For this purpose, it is a better choice than Golden-Yellow Plaster (*jīn huáng gāo*).

Biomedical Indications

With the appropriate presentation, this formula can be used to treat a variety of biomedically-defined disorders including boils, carbuncles, abscesses, inflamed subdermal cysts, inflamed lymph nodes, inflamed or infected insect bites, trauma such as sprains and contusions with redness and swelling, acute breast abscesses, or mastitis.

Modifications

- For treatment of first-stage trauma, mix with rice wine and honey or sesame oil and rice wine.

- For the presence of both stasis and heat as a traumatic injury approaches the second stage, add Olibanum (*rǔ xiāng*) and Myrrha (*mò yào*).

- To increase its efficacy for either trauma or heat-toxin swellings, add fresh Taraxaci Herba (*pú gōng yīng*) or Portulacae Herba (*mǎ chǐ xiàn*).

青黛散

Indigo Powder

qīng dài sǎn

Source   *Shanghai Municipal Medicine Standards* (1974)

Indigo naturalis (*qīng dài*) 60g
Gypsum fibrosum (*shí gāo*) 120g
Talcum (*huá shí*) 120g
Phellodendri Cortex (*huáng bǎi*) 60g

Method of Preparation   Grind the ingredients into a fine powder. Store in an air-tight container. This formula forms a paste when mixed with tea water and a salve when combined with sesame oil. It can form a soft plaster if mixed with petroleum jelly or an oil and beeswax salve such as Lithospermum/Arnebia and Tangkuei Ointment (*zǐ dāng gāo*).

Actions   Gathers in dampness, relieves itching, clears heat, and resolves toxicity

Indications

Treats all types of skin disorders that present with weeping, erosion, heat, swelling, itching, and pain. This often equates to acute eczema, contact dermatitis, or allergic dermatitis, including plant-based contact dermatitis such as poison ivy.

Analysis of Formula

Gypsum fibrosum (shí gāo), Indigo naturalis (qīng dài), and Phellodendri Cortex (huáng bǎi) clear heat, resolve toxicity, and dry dampness. Talcum (huá shí) dries dampness and relieves itching. As a powder or tea-water paste, the formula is especially able to dry dampness.

Commentary

This formula and its variations are very popular among modern practitioners in China. For damp, weeping lesions, the powder can be patted on with a cotton ball or sprinkled on the affected area. Alternatively, it can be mixed with tea water and made into a paste to be daubed onto sores. In either case, the powder can be brushed off once it is dried and a new measure applied.

It is sometimes more convenient to use the formula as a plaster. This is done by mixing one part of the powder with four parts (by weight) of the petroleum jelly and applying the paste to a gauze. The gauze should then be placed on the affected area, and the dressing changed once daily. It is important to clean the area well between dressings.

When making a plaster, a natural alternative medium such as Lithospermum/Arnebia and Tangkuei Ointment (zǐ dāng gāo) can be substituted for petroleum jelly. Amounts should be adjusted to obtain the proper consistency. Some practitioners pound fresh herbs, such as Taraxaci Herba (pú gōng yīng) and Portulacae Herba (mǎ chǐ xiàn), mix the moist poundings with Indigo Powder (qīng dài sǎn), and apply as a moist plaster.

Associated Formula

青蛤散

Indigo and Clam Shell Powder

qīng gé sǎn

SOURCE *Great Compendium of External Medicine* (1665)

powdered calcined Meretricis/Cyclinae Concha (gé qiào fěn) 30g
Gypsum praeparatum (duàn shí gāo) 30g
Calomelas (qīng fěn) 15g
Phellodendri Cortex (huáng bǎi) 15g
Indigo naturalis (qīng dài) 9g

Grind into a fine powder and mix with sesame oil to form a paste, adding cool water to achieve the desired consistency. Clears heat, gathers in dampness, dispels putrefaction, and helps close sores. As Meretricis/Cyclinae Concha (gé qiào) is more astringent than Talcum (huá shí), this formula is better than the principal formula when weeping is prominent. *Note:* At present, toxicity concerns preclude the use of Calomelas (qīng fěn).

苦参湯 (苦参汤)

Sophora Root Wash

kǔ shēn tāng

Source *Collected Experiences on Treating Sores* (1806)

Sophorae flavescentis Radix (kǔ shēn) 60g
Cnidii Fructus (shé chuáng zǐ) 30g
Angelicae dahuricae Radix (bái zhǐ) 15g
Lonicerae Flos (jīn yín huā) 30g
Chrysanthemi Flos (jú huā) 30g
Phellodendri Cortex (huáng bǎi) 15g
Kochiae Fructus (dì fū zǐ) 15g
Acori tatarinowii Rhizoma (shí chāng pǔ) 9g

Method of Preparation   The source text recommends decocting the ingredients, strain off the liquid, and mix in 4-5 pig gallbladders. At present, the last step is usually omitted.

It is common to start with about 6 cups of water for the amount of herbs listed above. For washes, a single boiling is usually done. Wash the affected area with the liquid and allow it to dry. The formula can also be applied as a compress by soaking a washcloth in the liquid and applying the moist cloth to the affected area for 10-20 minutes, keeping the compress warm by redipping it in the heated liquid.

Actions   Dispels wind, dries dampness, kills parasites, and relieves itching

Indications

A variety of scabbing skin disorders; leprosy and leprosy-like sores; red, itching swellings; and dry, scaling, itchy rashes. These are stubborn sores and rashes that scab or scale and do not respond to other treatment. Traditionally, this formula is indicated for the following lesions:

* Scab-sores (疥 jiè), which are small, scabbing sores as seen in scabies, but also in other conditions
* Leprous disorders (癩 lài) are, in the specific sense, the sores of leprosy, and in a general sense include the lesions of other serious contagious skin diseases
* Chronic ulcerating sores (瘋 fēng) are those that are similar to or synonymous with red bayberry sores, a lesion thought to be equivalent to second-stage syphilitic sores
* Lichenous rash (癬 xuǎn) are dry, scaly, and itchy sores of many varieties often symptomatic of what Western medicine views as fungal disorders, such as tinea.

Cautions and Contraindications

None noted.

Commentary

This formula treats a wide variety of damp skin disorders that present with itching. See the MODIFICATIONS below for suggestions on specific disorders. Generally, this formula is applied 2-3 three times daily. The affected area is moistened and the liquid is allowed to dry each time. If soaking is possible (fingers, toes, and other accessible areas), this is preferred. If, after 3-4 days, there is no improvement, this treatment should be discontinued.

Scabies

Treatment of scabies is an exception to the above procedure because the patient's itching will generally worsen when the treatment begins, and may continue for a week or so owing to the irritation caused by the parasites' corpses. For scabies, treatment should continue for 2 weeks even though the symptoms will have ceased before that time. This will ensure that newly-hatching parasites are killed before they mature and lay eggs.

For scabies, internal treatment is usually unnecessary, but for other skin diseases, internal herbs treat the root while the wash addresses the branch. See the discussion of internal treatment of skin disorders under the entry for Eliminate Wind Powder from the *Orthodox Lineage (xiāo fēng sǎn)* and its variations as well as Tangkuei Drink *(dāng guī yǐn zi)*, in Chapter 14.

Variant

Wondrous Lantern for Peering into the Origin and Development of Miscellaneous Diseases mentions a version of Sophora Root Wash *(kǔ shēn tāng)* with only two ingredients: Sophorae flavescentis Radix *(kǔ shēn)* and Acori tatarinowii Rhizoma *(shí chāng pú)*. As above, it is cooked with pig bile. This variant is applied to heat rash, especially in children.

Biomedical Indications

With the appropriate presentation, this formula may be used to treat a variety of biomedically-defined disorders including eczematous rashes such as atopic dermatitis and seborrheic dermatitis, or other disorders such as scabies, lichen planus, leprosy, and various fungal infections.

Modifications

- For scabies, add Sulfur *(liú huáng)* 15g and Toosendan Fructus *(chuān liàn zǐ)* 25g. In addition, apply Sulfur Plaster *(liú huáng gāo)* * to affected areas once daily.

- For seborrheic dermatitis, add Alumen *(míng fán)* 15g and Vaccariae Semen *(wáng bù liú xíng)* 10g.

- For extreme itching, add Artemisiae argyi Folium *(ài yè)* 10g.

- For heat, add Dictamni Cortex *(bái xiān pí)* 12g.

- For fungal infections such as athlete's foot or ringworm, add Meliae Cortex *(kǔ liàn gēn pí)*, Sulfur *(liú huáng)*, and

---

* Sulfur Plaster *(liú huáng gāo)* is made by combining Sulfur *(liú huáng)*, 10 percent by weight, in a salve of petroleum jelly (90 percent) or equivalent adjuvant.

Hydnocarpi Semen *(dà fēng zǐ)* 15g each. Cook the herbs in one-third rice vinegar, one-third rice wine, and one-third water. Soak (or apply compress to) the affected area for at least twenty minutes, 1-2 times a day.

海桐皮湯 (海桐皮汤)
Erythrina Wash
hǎi tóng pí tāng

Source   *Golden Mirror of the Medical Tradition* (1742)

Erythrinae Cortex *(hǎi tóng pí)* 6g
Speranskiae Herba seu Impatientis Caulis *(tòu gǔ cǎo)* † 6g
Olibanum *(rǔ xiāng)* 6g
Myrrha *(mò yào)* 6g
Angelicae sinensis Radix *(dāng guī)* 4.5g
Zanthoxyli Pericarpium *(huā jiāo)* 9g
Chuanxiong Rhizoma *(chuān xiōng)* 3g
Carthami Flos *(hóng huā)* 3g
Clematidis Radix *(wēi líng xiān)* 2.5g
Angelicae dahuricae Radix *(bái zhǐ)* 2.5g
Glycyrrhizae Radix *(gān cǎo)* 2.5g
Saposhnikoviae Radix *(fáng fēng)* .2.5g

Method of Preparation   The source text recommends grinding the herbs into a coarse powder, sewing them into a white cloth sack, and boiling them like a decoction. At present, the herbs are cooked in 2-3 cups of water. The liquid is brought to a boil and the herbs are simmered for 20-30 minutes in a loosely covered pot. The herb bag is removed from the decoction and the liquid is used to steam and then wash the affected area.

Alternatively, the bag of herbs can be used as a compress and placed on the affected area. If this method is used, covering the compress with a hot water bottle will obviate the need to continually redip the compress in the hot liquid. To increase the blood-moving properties of the steam-wash compress, a cup of rice wine is sometimes added toward the end of the cooking process.

Actions   Invigorates the blood, disperses swelling, dispels wind, dampness and cold, unblocks the collaterals, and relieves pain

Indications

Treats painful second- and third-stage trauma to sinews and bones that presents with aching, inhibited range of motion, and numbness.

Analysis of Formula

Erythrinae Cortex *(hǎi tóng pí)*, Speranskiae Herba seu Impatientis Caulis *(tòu gǔ cǎo)*, Clematidis Radix *(wēi líng xiān)*, Angelicae dahuricae Radix *(bái zhǐ)*, Saposhnikoviae Radix

---

† Speranskiae Herba (透骨草 *tòu gǔ cǎo*) is acrid, warm, and enters the Lung and Liver channels. It dispels wind and dampness and invigorates the blood with a normal oral dosage of 9-15g. Impatientis Caulis (鳳仙透骨草 *fèng xiān tòu gǔ cǎo*) is bitter, acrid, warm, and slightly toxic. It dispels wind-dampness, invigorates the blood, and resolves toxicity with a normal oral dosage of 3-9g. While these two medicinals have their differences, both are commonly dispensed when 透骨草 *tòu gǔ cǎo* is prescribed.

(fáng fēng), and Zanthoxyli Pericarpium *(huā jiāo)* unblock the channels, invigorate the collaterals, dispel dampness, and relieve pain. Combining these herbs with the blood-moving herbs Carthami Flos *(hóng huā),* Chuanxiong Rhizoma *(chuān xiōng),* Olibanum *(rǔ xiāng),* and Myrrha *(mò yào)* produces a formula that effectively clears stasis from the channels and collaterals, reduces swelling, dispels wind and dampness, and promotes an environment where healing is less obstructed by the pathogens of wind, dampness, cold, and stasis. Glycyrrhizae Radix *(gān cǎo)* both moderates the pain and harmonizes the actions of the other ingredients.

Commentary

This formula is found in the section on trauma in *Golden Mirror of the Medical Tradition.* It is first mentioned as a treatment for trauma to the cheekbone and subsequently as part of the suggested protocol for trauma to several other areas including the ribs, tailbone, heel, and occiput. The text frequently combines Erythrina Wash *(hǎi tóng pí tāng)* with internal treatment using Bonesetter's Purple-Gold Special Pill *(zhèng gǔ zǐ jīn dān),* discussed in Chapter 14.

Steam-soak compresses are typically applied to second- and third-stage trauma. Second-stage trauma is characterized by blood stasis (yellow-purple bruising), aching, pain, stiffness, and aversion to exposing the affected area to wind and cold. Although heat and swelling (inflammation) may still be present, they are almost completely resolved, and certainly greatly reduced, from their presentation in first-stage conditions. Any remaining swelling is hard and painful. Generally, treatment of second-stage trauma focuses on dispersing blood stasis, dispelling wind, dampness, and cold, and relieving pain. Third-stage trauma is equivalent to painful obstruction pattern and is treated by dispelling wind, dampness, and cold, moving the blood, and unblocking the collaterals. The difference in treatment of second- and third-stage trauma is one of emphasis. Where treatment of second stage centers on moving the blood, that for third stage places more importance on dispelling wind, cold, and dampness, and supplementing the body's qi and blood. In the clinic, these stages present as a continuum and are treated accordingly.

Erythrina Wash *(hǎi tóng pí tāng)* contains decidedly warm herbs, and, like most compresses, is unsuitable for first-stage trauma where the application of warm and hot herbs would aggravate the inflammation and swelling. For second- and third-stage trauma, however, soak compresses bring immediate comfort. Erythrina Wash *(hǎi tóng pí tāng)* is the model for this type of treatment.

Modifications

- For extreme blood stasis with purple, hard, and painful swelling, add Sparganii Rhizoma *(sān léng)* and Curcumae Rhizoma *(é zhú)* and add one cup of rice wine during cooking near the end.

- For cold stasis where the local area is cold to the touch and feels better with warmth, add Cinnamomi Cortex *(ròu guì)* and Aconiti kusnezoffii Radix praeparata *(zhì cǎo wū).*

- If some heat signs remain from the first stage of trauma, add Rhei Radix et Rhizoma *(dà huáng)* and Gardeniae Fructus *(zhī zǐ).*

Associated Formula

散瘀和傷湯（散瘀和伤汤）

Wash to Mollify Trauma by Dispersing Stasis

sàn yū hé shāng tāng

SOURCE *Golden Mirror of the Medical Tradition* (1742)

processed Strychni Semen *(zhì mǎ qián zǐ)*	15g
Carthami Flos *(hóng huā)*	15g
Pinelliae Rhizoma *(shēng bàn xià)*	15g
Drynariae Rhizoma *(gǔ suì bǔ)*	9g
Glycyrrhizae Radix *(gān cǎo)*	9g
Allii fistulosi Bulbus *(cōng bái)*	30g

Heat the herbs in 5 cups of water. After the liquid boils, simmer for 20 minutes. Add 60g of rice vinegar, and turn up the heat. Cook for approximately 5 minutes and allow the decoction to boil briefly. Steam and soak or apply a soak compress to the affected area 4-5 times daily.

This formula invigorates the blood, dispels stasis, and relieves pain. It treats bumps and bruises with accumulation of blood stasis, swelling, and severe pain. This may include the postinflammatory stage of soft tissue injuries, broken bones, and joint dislocations. This is not first-stage trauma, but the hard, entrenched swelling that consists of blood stasis and clumping of qi and blood during second- and third-stage trauma. The steam-soak compress can also be used to treat painful obstruction.

This formula is less able to move the blood and dispel stasis than the principal formula, but is more adept at dispersing clumping and unblocking the channels and collaterals. When hard swellings are palpable at the site of the trauma and create an impediment to healing, Wash to Mollify Trauma by Dispersing Stasis *(sàn yū hé shāng tāng)* is the soak compress of choice.

Note: Even in its prepared form, Strychni Semen *(mǎ qián zǐ)* is extremely toxic. Be sure to keep the herb itself and any resultant liquid away from pets and children, and to use only the prepared herb. It is not appropriate for pregnant or nursing women. A slightly safer and equally effective alternative to Strychni Semen *(mǎ qián zǐ)* is Momordicae Semen *(mù biē zǐ).*

Modifications

- To increase the formula's capacity to invigorate the blood and dispel stasis, add Paeoniae Radix rubra *(chì sháo)* and Chuanxiong Rhizoma *(chuān xiōng).*

- To increase the formula's function of dispersing stasis and relieving pain, add Olibanum *(rǔ xiāng)* and Myrrha *(mò yào).*

- For particularly hard swellings, add Sparganii Rhizoma *(sān léng)* and Curcumae Rhizoma *(é zhú).*

Section 3

. . . .

EXTERNAL FORMULAS
FOR INTERNAL DISORDERS

In Chinese medicine, there are a vast number of external applications of herbs for the treatment of internal disorders. Here, we present just a few examples that are representative of those in common use today.

吳茱萸膏 (吴茱萸膏)

Evodia Plaster

wú zhū yú gāo

Source   *Seeking Accuracy in the Materia Medica* (1769)

Evodiae Fructus *(wú zhū yú)*
rice vinegar

Method of Preparation   Grind Evodiae Fructus *(wú zhū yú)* into a fine powder and store in an airtight container. When needed, mix the powder with rice vinegar to make a paste. Use enough vinegar to make a paste that is moist but not runny.

Place a small amount of the paste (1/4 to 1/2 teaspoon) on the acupuncture point KI-1 *(yǒng quán)* on both feet and cover with cloth tape. Leave on overnight.

Actions   Guides heat downward

Indications

Sores of the throat, mouth, or tongue.

Commentary

This plaster treats heat-induced sores in the mouth and throat. Generally, it is used for treating heat from internal disharmonies and not for external heat pathogens. It guides the heat downward to relieve the symptoms but does not address the root cause of the heat, which must be ascertained and treated with internal herbs. This plaster is sometimes used for acute hypertension and for headaches associated with ascending fire.

The Ming-dynasty text *Prescriptions of Universal Benefit* includes a similar plaster that uses Arisaematis Rhizoma *(tiān nán xīng)* instead of Evodiae Fructus *(wú zhū yú)* to treat incessant vomiting and diarrhea.

蓽茇餅 (荜茇饼)

Long Pepper Cake

bì bá bǐng

Source   *Introduction to Medicine* (1575)

Piperis longi Fructus *(bì bá)*
Cyperi Rhizoma *(xiāng fù)*
garlic

Method of preparation   Grind equal amounts of Piperis longi Fructus *(bì bá)* and Cyperi Rhizoma *(xiāng fù)* together into a coarse powder. Store the powder in an airtight container. When ready to make cakes, pound the powder with enough fresh garlic to make a flat, round cake about 2cm in diameter and 1cm thick. Heat the cake and place it on the acupuncture point GV-22 *(xìn huì)* and burn moxa on top of the cake to keep it warm. Lift the cake if it gets too hot and to avoid burning the hair or skin. Note that the source text suggests using an iron to keep the cake warm, but nowadays, moxa is generally used.

Actions   Warms the exterior, dispels cold, and opens the nose

Indications

Nasal congestion with copious clear nasal discharge associated with a wind-cold exterior pattern.

This method of using herb cakes is also employed to treat disorders such as painful menstruation, abdominal pain, and painful obstruction. The herbs used to make the cakes, and the site on which the cake is placed, will differ according to the disorder being treated.

三棱洗乳方

Sparganium Breast Wash

sān léng xǐ rǔ fāng

Source   *Arcane Essentials from the Imperial Library* (752)

Sparganii Rhizoma *(sān léng)* 60g

Method of Preparation   Decoct the herb in 4 cups of water until 2 cups remain. Wash the breasts with the warm liquid.

Actions   Unblocks the channels and collaterals and promotes the flow of breast milk

Indications

Blocked or inhibited flow of breast milk.

安胎主膏

Fetus-Quieting Plaster

ān tāi zhǔ gāo

Source   *Rhymed Prose on [Medical] Principles and Applications* (1870)

Codonopsis Radix *(dǎng shēn)* .64g
Angelicae sinensis Radix *(dāng guī)* 64g
Rehmanniae Radix praeparata *(shú dì huáng)* 96g
wine-fried Scutellariae Radix *(jiǔ chǎo huáng qín)* 48g
Dioscoreae Rhizoma *(shān yào)* 48g
Atractylodis macrocephalae Rhizoma *(bái zhú)* 48g
Chuanxiong Rhizoma *(chuān xiōng)* 15g
wine-fried Paeoniae Radix alba *(jiǔ chǎo bái sháo)* 15g
Citri reticulatae Pericarpium *(chén pí)* 15g
Perillae Caulis *(zǐ sū gěng)* 15g
Cyperi Rhizoma *(xiāng fù)* 15g

Eucommiae Cortex (*dù zhòng*) 15g
Dipsaci Radix (*xù duàn*) 15g
Fritillariae thunbergii Bulbus (*zhè bèi mǔ*). 15g

Method of Preparation   Soak the herbs in sesame oil (about 800g) and cook over a low heat until they are slightly browned. The herbs are removed and about 400g of Minium (*qiān dān*) is added while the oil is still warm.

Note: Minium (*qiān dān*) is toxic and releases toxic smoke when added to hot oil. Thus, if it is made in the traditional manner, it should be done in an appropriately ventilated setting. At present, it is suggested to substitute 250g of beeswax, which will produce an ointment instead of a hard plaster. Usually, the plaster is applied bilaterally to the acupuncture point KI-23 (*shèn shū*), and secured in place with hypoallergenic tape that will not cause irritation. The source text does not mention it, but this type of plaster is generally changed once every 4-5 days.

Actions   Augments the qi and blood, tonifies the Liver and Kidneys, and quiets the fetus

Indications

For restless fetus owing to deficiency of qi or blood or insufficiency of the Liver or Kidneys.

Modifications

* For spotting, add Taxilli Herba (*sāng jì shēng*) and Asini Corii Colla (*ē jiāo*) 15g each. (source text)
* For pain, add Saposhnikoviae Radix (*fáng fēng*) and Angelicae pubescentis Radix (*dú huó*). (source text)
* For water swelling, grind Zingiberis Rhizomatis Cortex (*shēng jiāng pí*), Poriae Cutis (*fú líng pí*), Arecae Pericarpium (*dà fù pí*), and Citri reticulatae Pericarpium (*chén pí*) into a fine powder and mix into the plaster. (source text)
* For blood-heat induced blood in the urine, add Bupleuri Radix (*chái hú*) and Gardeniae Fructus (*zhī zǐ*). (source text)

Comparative Tables of Principal Formulas

■ FORMULAS FOR EXTERNAL HERBAL TREATMENT OF EXTERNAL DISORDERS

Common symptoms: external application only

Formula Name	Diagnosis	Indications	Remarks
Borneal and Borax Powder (*bīng péng sǎn*)	Chronic or acute disorders of the throat or mouth	Sore, swollen throat, swelling or pain in the gums, mouth sores, and external ear infections	Also for sore throat and hoarseness associated with long-term phlegm-fire cough.
Golden-Yellow Powder/Golden-Yellow Plaster (*jīn huáng sǎn/jīn huáng gāo*)	Hot sores or swellings	Various types of red, hot swellings that have not yet come to a head, abscesses, deep-set toxic sores, swelling from trauma, damp-phlegm spreading sores, redness and swelling of the skin, burns, dry or damp leg qi	Now applied to a wide range of disorders in dermatology, trauma, and internal medicine.
Lithospermum/ Arnebia and Tangkuei Ointment (*zǐ dāng gāo*)	Lip sores or skin rashes	All manner of skin rashes that present as heat toxin, dry, itching, or painful lesions	Also used for calluses, and dry, cracked skin.
Double-Dark Plaster (*èr qīng gāo*)	Yang toxic swellings	Red, hot yang-type swellings with or without the formation of a head	Also for first-stage trauma conditions such as strains, sprains, relocated dislocations, bruises and bumps.
Indigo Powder (*qīng dài sǎn*)	Damp-heat type lesions or sores	Various skin disorders that present with weeping, erosion, heat, swelling, itching, and pain	Often used for acute eczema, allergic dermatitis, or contact dermatitis such as poison ivy.
Sophora Root Wash (*kǔ shēn tāng*)	Damp skin disorders with itching	A variety of scabbing skin disorders, leprosy and leprosy-like sores, red, itching swellings, and dry, scaling, itchy rashes	Also for various types of dermatitis and fungal infections.
Erythrina Wash (*hǎi tóng pí tāng*)	Painful second and third stage trauma to sinews and bones	Depending on the stage of injury, symptoms may include yellow-purple bruising, aching, pain, stiffness, inhibited range of motion, numbness, and/or aversion to exposing the affected area to wind and cold	A warming compress suitable for the later stages of trauma when heat and swelling (inflammation) are resolved or greatly reduced.

■ FORMULAS FOR EXTERNAL HERBAL TREATMENT OF INTERNAL DISORDERS

Common symptoms: external application only

Formula Name	Diagnosis	Indications	Remarks
Evodia Plaster *(wú zhū yú gāo)*	Heat from internal disharmonies	Sores of the throat, mouth, or tongue	Also used for hypertension and headaches caused by ascending fire.
Long Pepper Cake *(bì bá bǐng)*	Nasal congestion due to external wind-cold invasion	Nasal congestion with copious, clear nasal discharge	A warming method often coupled with moxibustion.
Sparganium Breast Wash *(sān léng xǐ rú fāng)*	Obstruction of the channels and collaterals of the breast	Blocked or inhibited flow of breast milk	Focuses on unblocking the channels and collaterals and promoting the flow of breast milk.
Fetus-Quieting Plaster *(ān tāi zhǔ gāo)*	Restless fetus disorder with deficiency of the qi and blood, or Liver and Kidneys	Restless fetus	Focuses on augmenting the qi and blood, tonifying the Liver and Kidneys, and quieting the fetus.

Guide to *Pinyin* Pronunciation

Consonants

b-	like *b-* in *obstinate*
c-	like *-ts* in *its*
ch-	like *ch-* in *chair* but with the tongue on the palate
d-	as in English but not as voiced
f-	as in English
g-	as in English but not as voiced
h-	between the *h-* in *how* and the *ch-* in *chutzpah*
j-	as in English but with the tip of the tongue on the lower teeth
k-	as in English but more strongly aspirated
l-	as in English
m-	as in English
n-	as in English
p-	as in English but more strongly aspirated
q-	like *ch-* in *chair* but with the tip of the tongue on the lower teeth
r-	something like *r-* in *rapid* but with the tongue on the palate
s-	as in English
sh-	as in English but with the tongue on the palate
t-	as in English but more strongly aspirated
w-	as in English but softer
x-	something like *sh-* in *she* but with the tip of the tongue on the lower teeth
y-	as in English but softer
z-	like *-ds* in *pads*
zh-	like *j-* in *jar* but with the tongue on the palate

Vᴏᴡᴇʟs, Dɪᴘʜᴛʜᴏɴɢs ᴀɴᴅ Fɪɴᴀʟs[1]

a or *-a*	like *-a in father*
-ai	like *-ye* in *rye*
-an	like *-ohn* in *John*
-ang	something like *-ang* in the German *angst;* *ng* has both a nasalizing and gutteralizing action on the vowel
-ao	like *-ow* in *cow* but less fused
-e	like *-a* in *sofa*
-ei	like *-ay* in *bay*
-en	like *-un* in *fun*
-eng	like *-eng* in *lung*
er or *-er*	like *-ar* in *far*
-i	after *c-, ch-, s-, sh-, z-, zh-* something like the *-urr* in *burr* but shorter and with the tongue on the palate; after any other letter, like *-e* in *be*
-in	like *-een* in *sheen*
-ing	like *-ing* in *ring*
-iu	like *yo* in *yo-yo*
-o	like *-au* in *maudlin*
-ong	like *-ung* in *hung*
-ou	like *-ow* in *mow* but less fused
-u	after *j-, q-, x-, y-, l-,* or *n-* something like *-ew* in *knew* but with lips more pursed; after any other letter, like *-oo* in *boo*
-ua	like *-ua* in *Guam*
-uai	like *-ui* in *quiet*
-uan	like *-uan* in *quantity*
-uang	similar to *-uan* above but with a gutteral ending
-ui	like *-uay* in *quay* but slightly shorter
-un	after *j-, q-, x-, y-, l-,* or *n-* something like the *-une* in *June* but with lips more pursed; after any other letter, between the *-one* of *done* and the *-win* of *twin*
-uo	something like the *wa-* in *war*

Tᴏɴᴇs[2]

The four tones of Mandarin Chinese are as follows:

ꜰɪʀsᴛ ᴛᴏɴᴇ	*ō*	begins high and is held steady
sᴇᴄᴏɴᴅ ᴛᴏɴᴇ	*ó*	begins in the midrange and rises
ᴛʜɪʀᴅ ᴛᴏɴᴇ	*ǒ*	begins in the lower middle range and drops down before rising
ꜰᴏᴜʀᴛʜ ᴛᴏɴᴇ	*ò*	begins high and drops down sharply

1. Diphthongs that are pronounced as expected from the respective vowels are not further discussed.

2. We have included the tone markings in the main text to enable the reader to pronounce the names of the formulas as accurately as possible. Tone markings are also used in reference to technical terms that may be unfamiliar to the reader.

Pinyin-English Formula Cross Reference

ài fǔ nuǎn gōng wán	Mugwort and Cyperus Pill to Warm the Palace (*ài fǔ nuǎn gōng wán*), 581
ān gōng niú huáng wán	Calm the Palace Pill with Cattle Gallstone (*ān gōng niú huáng wán*), 488-490
ān tāi zhǔ gāo	Fetus-Quieting Plaster (*ān tāi zhǔ gāo*), 904-905
ān zhōng sǎn	Calm the Middle Powder (*ān zhōng sǎn*), 268
bā wèi dài xià fāng	Eight-Ingredient Formula for Vaginal Discharge (*bā wèi dài xià fāng*), 697-698
bā wèi dì huáng wán	Eight-Ingredient Pill with Rehmannia (*bā wèi dì huáng wán*), 369
bā xiān cháng shōu wán	Eight-Immortal Pill for Longevity (*bā xiān cháng shōu wán*), 369
bā zhēn tāng	Eight-Treasure Decoction (*bā zhēn tāng*), 346-348
bā zhēn yì mǔ wán	Eight-Treasure Pill to Benefit Mothers (*bā zhēn yì mǔ wán*), 348
bā zhèng sǎn	Eight-Herb Powder for Rectification (*bā zhèng sǎn*), 713-715
bǎi hé dì huáng tāng	Lily Bulb and Rehmannia Decoction (*bǎi hé dì huáng tāng*), 220-222
bǎi hé gù jīn tāng	Lily Bulb Decoction to Preserve the Metal (*bǎi hé gù jīn tāng*), 384-386
bǎi hé huá shí sǎn	Lily Bulb and Talcum Powder (*bǎi hé huá shí sǎn*), 223
bǎi hé jī zi huáng tāng	Lily Bulb and Egg Yolk Decoction (*bǎi hé jī zi huáng tāng*), 222
bǎi hé zhī mǔ tāng	Lily Bulb and Anemarrhena Decoction (*bǎi hé zhī mǔ tāng*), 222
bái hǔ chéng qì tāng	White Tiger and Order the Qi Decoction (*bái hǔ chéng qì tāng*), 155
bái hǔ jiā cāng zhú tāng	White Tiger plus Atractylodes Decoction (*bái hǔ jiā cāng zhú tāng*), 154-155
bái hǔ jiā guì zhī tāng	White Tiger plus Cinnamon Twig Decoction (*bái hǔ jiā guì zhī tāng*), 154
bái hǔ jiā rén shēn tāng	White Tiger plus Ginseng Decoction (*bái hǔ jiā rén shēn tāng*), 154

bái hǔ tāng	White Tiger Decoction (*bái hǔ tāng*), 150-154
bái sǎn	White Powder (*bái sǎn*), 76
bái tōng tāng	White Penetrating Decoction (*bái tōng tāng*), 277-278
bái tóu wēng jiā gān cǎo ē jiāo tāng	Pulsatilla Decoction plus Licorice and Ass-Hide Gelatin (*bái tóu wēng jiā gān cǎo ē jiāo tāng*), 211
bái tóu wēng tāng	Pulsatilla Decoction (*bái tóu wēng tāng*), 210-211
bǎi yè tāng	Arborvitae Twig Decoction (*bǎi yè tāng*), 607-608
baí zhú fù zǐ tāng	White Atractylodes and Aconite Accessory Root Decoction (*baí zhú fù zǐ tāng*), 270-271
baí zhú fù zǐ tāng	Atractylodes Macrocephalae and Aconite Accessory Root Decoction from *Arcane Essentials* (*baí zhú fù zǐ tāng*), 273
bái zǐ rén wán	Arborvitae Seed Pill (*bái zǐ rén wán*), 422
bái zǐ yǎng xīn wán	Arborvitae Seed Pill to Nourish the Heart (*bái zǐ yǎng xīn wán*), 462
bàn liú wán)	Pinellia and Sulphur Pill (*bàn liú wán*), 76-78
bàn xià bái zhú tiān má tāng	Pinellia, White Atractylodes, and Gastrodia Decoction (*bàn xià bái zhú tiān má tāng*), 811-812
bàn xià bái zhú tiān má tāng	Pinellia, White Atractylodes, and Gastrodia Decoction from *Discussion of the Spleen and Stomach* (*bàn xià bái zhú tiān má tāng*),
bàn xià hòu pò tāng	Pinellia and Magnolia Bark Decoction (*bàn xià hòu pò tāng*), 516-519
bàn xià shú mǐ tāng	Pinellia and Millet Decoction (*bàn xià shú mǐ tāng*), 474
bàn xià xiè xīn tāng	Pinellia Decoction to Drain the Epigastrium (*bàn xià xiè xīn tāng*), 127-130
bǎo chǎn wú yōu fāng	Worry-Free Formula to Protect Birth (*bǎo chǎn wú yōu fāng*), 360-362
bǎo hé wán	Preserve Harmony Pill from the *Precious Mirror* (*bǎo hé wán*), 828-829
bǎo hé wán	Preserve Harmony Pill (*bǎo hé wán*), 826-828
bào lóng wán	Embrace the Dragon Pill (*bào lóng wán*), 497
bǎo tāi zī shēng wán	Protect the Fetus and Aid Life Pill (*bǎo tāi zī shēng wán*), 317
baǒ yuán tāng	Preserve the Primal Decoction (*baǒ yuán tāng*), 313-314
bèi mǔ guā lóu sǎn	Fritillaria and Trichosanthes Fruit Powder (*bèi mǔ guā lóu sǎn*), 802-804
bēn tún wán	Running Piglet Pill (*bēn tún wán*), 524
bì bá bǐng	Long Pepper Cake (*bì bá bǐng*), 904
bì xiè fēn qīng yǐn	Tokoro Drink to Separate the Clear (*bì xiè fēn qīng yǐn*), 751-752
bì xiè fēn qīng yǐn	Tokoro Drink to Separate the Clear from *Awakening of the Mind in Medical Studies* (*bì xiè fēn qīng yǐn*), 753
bì yù sǎn	Jasper Powder (*bì yù sǎn*), 240
biàn zhì xīn qì yǐn	Modified Formulation of Heart Qi Drink (*biàn zhì xīn qì yǐn*), 741-742

bīng péng sǎn	Borneal and Borax Powder *(bīng péng sǎn)*, 896-897
bù dài wán	Cloth Sack Pill *(bù dài wán)*, 854-855
bǔ fèi ē jiāo tāng	Tonify the Lungs Decoction with Ass-Hide Gelatin *(bǔ fèi ē jiāo tāng)*, 386-387
bǔ fèi tāng	Tonify the Lungs Decoction *(bǔ fèi tāng)*, 331
bǔ gān tāng	Tonify the Liver Decoction *(bǔ gān tāng)*, 337
bù huàn jīn zhèng qì sǎn	Rectify the Qi Powder Worth More than Gold *(bù huàn jīn zhèng qì sǎn)*, 689-691
bǔ pí wèi xiè yīn huǒ shēng yáng tāng	Tonify Spleen-Stomach, Drain Yin Fire, and Raise Yang Decoction *(bǔ pí wèi xiè yīn huǒ shēng yáng tāng)*, 322-323
bǔ yáng huán wǔ tāng	Tonify the Yang to Restore Five [-Tenths] Decoction *(bǔ yáng huán wǔ tāng)*, 568-571
bǔ zhōng yì qì tāng	Tonify the Middle to Augment the Qi Decoction *(bǔ zhōng yì qì tāng)*, 317-322
cán shǐ tāng	Silkworm Droppings Decoction *(cán shǐ tāng)*, 707
cāng ěr zǐ sǎn	Xanthium Powder *(cāng ěr zǐ sǎn)*, 628-629
chái gé jiě jī tāng	Bupleurum and Kudzu Decoction to Release the Muscle Layer *(chái gé jiě jī tāng)*, 39-41
chái gé jiě jī tāng	Bupleurum and Kudzu Decoction to Release the Muscle Layer from *Awakening of the Mind in Medical Studies (chái gé jiě jī tāng)*, 41
chái hǔ bái hǔ tāng	Bupleurum White Tiger Decoction *(chái hǔ bái hǔ tāng)*, 155
chái hú dá yuán yǐn	Bupleurum Drink to Reach the Source *(chái hú dá yuán yǐn)*, 140
chái hú guì jiāng tāng	Bupleurum, Cinnamon Twig, and Ginger Decoction *(chái hú guì jiāng tāng)*, 140-142
chái hú guì zhī tāng	Bupleurum and Cinnamon Twig Decoction *(chái hú guì zhī tāng)*, 109-110
chái hú jiā lóng gǔ mǔ lì tāng	Bupleurum plus Dragon Bone and Oyster Shell Decoction *(chái hú jiā lóng gǔ mǔ lì tāng)*, 113-116
chái hú jiā máng xiāo tāng	Bupleurum Decoction plus Mirabilite *(chái hú jiā máng xiāo tāng)*, 110
chái hú qīng gān tāng	Bupleurum Decoction to Clear the Liver *(chái hú qīng gān tāng)*, 202-203
chái hú qīng zào tāng	Bupleurum Decoction to Clear Dryness *(chái hú qīng zào tāng)*, 111
chái hú shū gān sǎn	Bupleurum Powder to Dredge the Liver *(chái hú shū gān sǎn)*, 512-513
chái hú sì wù tāng	Bupleurum and Four Substance Decoction *(chái hú sì wù tāng)*, 110
chái hú xì xīn tāng	Bupleurum and Asarum Decoction *(chái hú xì xīn tāng)*, 573
chái hú xiàn xiōng tāng	Bupleurum Decoction [for Pathogens] Stuck in the Chest *(chái hú xiàn xiōng tāng)*, 794-795
chái hú zhǐ jié tāng	Bupleurum, Bitter Orange, and Platycodon Decoction *(chái hú zhǐ jié tāng)*, 110
chái píng tāng	Bupleurum and Calm the Stomach Decoction *(chái píng tāng)*, 110
cháng níng tāng	Intestinal Serenity Decoction *(cháng níng tāng)*, 350
cháng shān yǐn	Dichroa Drink *(cháng shān yǐn)*, 135
chéng qì yǎng róng tāng	Order the Qi and Nourish the Nutritive Decoction *(chéng qì yǎng róng tāng)*, 89

chì shí zhī yǔ yú liáng tāng	Halloysite and Limonite Decoction (*chì shí zhī yǔ yú liáng tāng*), 429
chōng hé tāng	Flush and Harmonize Decoction (*chōng hé tāng*), 863
chōng hé tāng	Penetrating and Harmonizing Decoction (*chōng hé tāng*), 26-27
chú shī weì líng tāng	Eliminate Dampness Decoction by Combining Calm the Stomach and Five-Ingredient Powder with Poria (*chú shī weì líng tāng*), 689
chuān xiōng chá tiáo sǎn	Chuanxiong Powder to be Taken with Green Tea from *Awakening of the Mind* (*chuān xiōng chá tiáo sǎn*), 628
chuān xiōng chá tiáo sǎn	Chuanxiong Powder to be Taken with Green Tea (*chuān xiōng chá tiáo sǎn*), 625-627
chūn zé tāng	Spring Marsh Decoction (*chūn zé tāng*), 729
cí zhū wán	Magnetite and Cinnabar Pill (*cí zhū wán*), 476-478
cōng bái qī wèi yǐn	Scallion Drink with Seven Ingredients (*cōng bái qī wèi yǐn*), 53-55
cōng chǐ jié gěng tāng	Scallion, Prepared Soybean and Platycodon Decoction (*cōng chǐ jié gěng tāng*), 6
cōng chǐ tāng	Scallion and Prepared Soybean Decoction (*cōng chǐ tāng*), 5-6
dà ān wán	Great Tranquility Pill (*dà ān wán*), 829
dà bàn xià tāng	Major Pinellia Decoction (*dà bàn xià tāng*), 549-551
dà bǔ yīn wán	Great Tonify the Yin Pill (*dà bǔ yīn wán*), 372-375
dà bǔ yuán jiān	Great Tonify the Primal Decoction (*dà bǔ yuán jiān*), 372
dà chái hú tāng	Major Bupleurum Decoction (*dà chái hú tāng*), 286-289
dà chéng qì tāng	Major Order the Qi Decoction (*dà chéng qì tāng*), 63-66
dà dìng fēng zhū	Major Arrest Wind Pearls (*dà dìng fēng zhū*), 651-653
dà fáng fēng tāng	Major Saposhnikovia Decoction (*dà fáng fēng tāng*), 760
dà hé zhōng yǐn	Major Harmonize the Middle Drink (*dà hé zhōng yǐn*), 829
dà huáng fù zǐ tāng	Rhubarb and Aconite Accessory Root Decoction (*dà huáng fù zǐ tāng*), 71-73
dà huáng gān cǎo tāng	Rhubarb and Licorice Decoction (*dà huáng gān cǎo tāng*), 67
dà huáng huáng lián xiè xīn tāng	Rhubarb and Coptis Infusion to Drain the Epigastrium (*dà huáng huáng lián xiè xīn tāng*), 173
dà huáng lián bǎi tāng	Rhubarb, Coptis, and Phellodendron Decoction (*dà huáng lián bǎi tāng*), 169-170
dà huáng mǔ dān tāng	Rhubarb and Moutan Decoction (*dà huáng mǔ dān tāng*), 880-882
dà huáng zhè chóng wán	Rhubarb and Ground Beetle Pill (*dà huáng zhè chóng wán*), 595-597
dà jiàn zhōng tāng	Major Construct the Middle Decoction (*dà jiàn zhōng tāng*), 268-270
dà qī qì tāng	Major Seven-Emotions Decoction (*dà qī qì tāng*), 519
dà qiāng huó tāng	Major Notopterygium Decoction (*dà qiāng huó tāng*), 27
dà qín jiāo tāng	Major Large Gentian Decoction (*dà qín jiāo tāng*), 629-631
dà qīng lóng tāng	Major Bluegreen Dragon Decoction (*dà qīng lóng tāng*), 11-13

dà tóu wēn tāng	Massive Febrile Disorder of the Head Decoction (*dà tóu wēn tāng*), 175-176
dà xiàn xiōng tāng	Major Decoction [for Pathogens] Stuck in the Chest (*dà xiàn xiōng tāng*), 69-71
dà xiàn xiōng wán	Major Pill [for Pathogens] Stuck in the Chest (*dà xiàn xiōng wán*), 71
dá yù tāng	Thrust Out Constraint Decoction (*dá yù tāng*), 511
dá yuán yǐn	Reach the Source Drink (*dá yuán yǐn*), 137-139
dà zào wán	Great Creation Pill (*dà zào wán*), 379-380
dǎn dào qū huí tāng	Drive Roundworms from the Biliary Tract Decoction (*dǎn dào qū huí tāng*), 854
dān huáng sì nì sǎn	Moutan and Phellodendron Powder for Frigid Extremities (*dān huáng sì nì sǎn*), 120
dàn liáo sì shén wán	Four-Miracle Pill from the Tranquil Hut (*dàn liáo sì shén wán*), 431-432
dān shēn yǐn	Salvia Drink (*dān shēn yǐn*), 594
dāng guī bèi mǔ kǔ shēn wán	Tangkuei, Fritillaria, and Sophora Decoction (*dāng guī bèi mǔ kǔ shēn wán*), 732
dāng guī bǔ xuè tāng	Tangkuei Decoction to Tonify the Blood (*dāng guī bǔ xuè tāng*), 338-341
dāng guī dì huáng yǐn	Tangkuei and Rehmannia Decoction (*dāng guī dì huáng yǐn*), 369
dāng guī jī xùe téng tāng	Tangkuei and Spatholobus Decoction (*dāng guī jī xùe téng tāng*), 338
dāng guī liù huáng tāng	Tangkuei and Six-Yellow Decoction (*dāng guī liù huáng tāng*), 218-220
dāng guī lóng huì wán	Tangkuei, Gentian, and Aloe Pill (*dāng guī lóng huì wán*), 203-205
dāng guī niān tòng tāng	Tangkuei Decoction to Pry Out Pain (*dāng guī niān tòng tāng*), 707-710
dāng guī sǎn	Tangkuei Powder (*dāng guī sǎn*), 590
dāng guī sháo yào sǎn	Tangkuei and Peony Powder (*dāng guī sháo yào sǎn*), 587-590
dāng guī shēng jiāng yáng ròu tāng	Mutton Stew with Tangkuei and Fresh Ginger (*dāng guī shēng jiāng yáng ròu tāng*), 346
dāng guī sì nì jiā wú zhū yú shēng jiāng tāng	Tangkuei Decoction for Frigid Extremities plus Evodia and Fresh Ginger (*dāng guī sì nì jiā wú zhū yú shēng jiāng tāng*), 255
dāng guī sì nì tāng	Tangkuei Decoction for Frigid Extremities (*dāng guī sì nì tāng*), 252-255
dāng guī yǐn zi	Tangkuei Drink (*dāng guī yǐn zi*), 639
dǎo chì chéng qì tāng	Guide Out the Red and Order the Qi Decoction (*dǎo chì chéng qì tāng*), 68-69
dǎo chì sǎn	Guide Out the Red Powder (*dǎo chì sǎn*), 195-196
dǎo qì tāng	Conduct the Qi Decoction (*dǎo qì tāng*), 529
dǎo shuǐ wán	Guide Out Water Pill (*dǎo shuǐ wán*), 94
dǎo tán tāng	Guide Out Phlegm Decoction (*dǎo tán tāng*), 780-781
dǐ dàng tāng	Appropriate Decoction (*dǐ dàng tāng*), 562-564
dì gǔ pí yǐn	Lycium Root Bark Drink (*dì gǔ pí yǐn*), 216
dì huáng yǐn zi	Rehmannia Drink from *A Simple Book* (*dì huáng yǐn zi*), 363-364

dì huáng yǐn zi	Rehmannia Drink (*dì huáng yǐn zi*), 405-407
dí tán tāng	Scour Out Phlegm Decoction (*dí tán tāng*), 782-783
dì yú sǎn	Sanguisorba Powder (*dì yú sǎn*), 606-607
diān kuáng mèng xǐng tāng	Decoction to Wake from the Nightmare of Insanity (*diān kuáng mèng xǐng tāng*), 568
diē dǎ wán	Trauma Pill (*diē dǎ wán*), 574-575
dìng chuǎn tāng	Arrest Wheezing Decoction (*dìng chuǎn tāng*), 540-542
dìng xián wán	Arrest Seizures Pill (*dìng xián wán*), 813-815
dīng xiāng jiāo ài tāng	Clove, Ass-Hide Gelatin, and Mugwort Decoction (*dīng xiāng jiāo ài tāng*), 612
dīng xiāng shì dì tāng	Clove and Persimmon Calyx Decoction (*dīng xiāng shì dì tāng*), 547-549
dīng yú lǐ zhōng tāng	Clove and Evodia Decoction to Regulate the Middle (*dīng yú lǐ zhōng tāng*), 260
dìng zhì wán	Settle the Emotions Pill (*dìng zhì wán*), 465-467
dìng zhì wán	Settle the Emotions Pill from *Wondrous Lantern* (*dìng zhì wán*), 467
dìng zhì wán	Settle the Emotions Pill from the Yang Family (*dìng zhì wán*), 467
dú huó jì shēng tāng	Pubescent Angelica and Taxillus Decoction (*dú huó jì shēng tāng*), 758-759
dū qì wán	Capital Qi Pill (*dū qì wán*), 368
dú shēn tāng	Unaccompanied Ginseng Decoction (*dú shēn tāng*), 281
ē jiāo jī zi huáng tāng	Ass-Hide Gelatin and Egg Yolk Decoction (*ē jiāo jī zi huáng tāng*), 653-655
èr chén tāng	Two-Aged [Herb] Decoction (*èr chén tāng*), 775-779
èr jiǎ fù mài tāng	Two-Shell Decoction to Restore the Pulse (*èr jiǎ fù mài tāng*), 651
èr jiā jiǎn zhèng qì sǎn	Second Modification of Rectify the Qi Powder (*èr jiā jiǎn zhèng qì sǎn*), 694
ěr lóng zuǒ cí wán	Pill for Deafness that is Kind to the Left [Kidney] (*ěr lóng zuǒ cí wán*), 369
èr miào sǎn	Two-Marvel Powder (*èr miào sǎn*), 720-721
èr mǔ sǎn	Fritillaria and Anemarrhena Powder (*èr mǔ sǎn*), 804
èr qīng gāo	Double-Dark Plaster (*èr qīng gāo*), 899-900
èr rén wán	Two-Seed Pill (*èr rén wán*), 79
èr xiān tāng	Two-Immortal Decoction (*èr xiān tāng*), 410-411
èr zhì wán	Two-Solstice Pill (*èr zhì wán*), 383-384
èr zhú tāng	Dual Atractylodes Decoction (*èr zhú tāng*), 785-786
fáng fēng tōng shèng sǎn	Saposhnikovia Powder that Sagely Unblocks (*fáng fēng tōng shèng sǎn*), 290-292
fáng jǐ fú líng tāng	Stephania and Poria Decoction (*fáng jǐ fú líng tāng*), 737-738
fáng jǐ huáng qí tāng	Stephania and Astragalus Decoction (*fáng jǐ huáng qí tāng*), 735-737
féi ér wán	Fat Baby Pill (*féi ér wán*), 833-834

fēn xiāo tāng	Separate and Reduce Decoction *(fēn xiāo tāng)*, 689
fēng yǐn tāng	Wind-Drawing Decoction *(fēng yǐn tāng)*, 639-641
fù fāng dà chéng qì tāng	Revised Major Order the Qi Decoction *(fù fāng dà chéng qì tāng)*, 69
fù líng gān cǎo tāng	Poria and Licorice Decoction *(fù líng gān cǎo tāng)*, 729
fú líng wán	Poria Pill *(fú líng wán)*, 783-785
fú tù dān	Poria and Cuscuta Special Pill *(fú tù dān)*, 438
fù yuán huó xuè tāng	Revive Health by Invigorating the Blood Decoction *(fù yuán huó xuè tāng)*, 571-573
fù zǐ jīng mǐ tāng	Aconite Accessory Root and Glutinous Rice Decoction *(fù zǐ jīng mǐ tāng)*, 270
fù zǐ lǐ zhōng wán	Aconite Accessory Root Pill to Regulate the Middle *(fù zǐ lǐ zhōng wán)*, 261
fù zǐ tāng	Aconite Accessory Root Decoction *(fù zǐ tāng)*, 747-749
fù zǐ xiè xīn tāng	Aconite Accessory Root Infusion to Drain the Epigastrium *(fù zǐ xiè xīn tāng)*, 173
gān cǎo fù zǐ tāng	Licorice and Aconite Accessory Root Decoction *(gān cǎo fù zǐ tāng)*, 749
gān cǎo gān jiāng fú líng bái zhú tāng	Licorice, Ginger, Poria and White Atractylodes Decoction *(gān cǎo gān jiāng fú líng bái zhú tāng)*, 742-743
gān cǎo gān jiāng tāng	Licorice and Ginger Decoction *(gān cǎo gān jiāng tāng)*, 270-272
gān cǎo xiè xīn tāng	Licorice Decoction to Drain the Epigastrium *(gān cǎo xiè xīn tāng)*, 130
gān jiāng huáng lián huáng qín rén shēn tāng	Ginger, Coptis, Scutellaria, and Ginseng Decoction *(gān jiāng huáng lián huáng qín rén shēn tāng)*, 133
gān jiāng rén shēn bàn xià wán	Ginger, Ginseng, and Pinellia Pill *(gān jiāng rén shēn bàn xià wán)*, 552
gān lù xiāo dú dān	Sweet Dew Special Pill to Eliminate Toxin *(gān lù xiāo dú dān)*, 702-705
gān lù yǐn	Sweet Dew Drink *(gān lù yǐn)*, 394-395
gān mài dà zǎo tāng	Licorice, Wheat, and Jujube Decoction *(gān mài dà zǎo tāng)*, 471-474
gān suì bàn xià tāng	Kansui and Pinellia Decoction *(gān suì bàn xià tāng)*, 91
gé gēn huáng qín huáng lián tāng	Kudzu, Scutellaria, and Coptis Decoction *(gé gēn huáng qín huáng lián tāng)*, 292-294
gé gēn jiā bàn xià tāng	Kudzu Decoction plus Pinellia *(gé gēn jiā bàn xià tāng)*, 21
gé gēn tāng	Kudzu Decoction *(gé gēn tāng)*, 19-21
gé huā jiě chéng sǎn	Kudzu Flower Powder to Relieve Hangovers *(gé huā jiě chéng sǎn)*, 841-842
gé xià zhú yū tāng	Drive Out Stasis Below the Diaphragm Decoction *(gé xià zhú yū tāng)*, 567
gēng yī wán	Pill Requiring a Change of Clothing *(gēng yī wán)*, 83
gōu téng sǎn	Uncaria Powder *(gōu téng sǎn)*, 813
gōu téng yǐn	Uncaria Decoction *(gōu téng yǐn)*, 644
gù běn zhǐ bēng tāng	Stabilize the Root and Stop Excessive Uterine Bleeding Decoction *(gù běn zhǐ bēng tāng)*, 355
gù biǎo zhǐ hàn tāng	Stabilize the Exterior and Stop Sweating Decoction *(gù biǎo zhǐ hàn tāng)*, 422

gù chōng tāng	Stabilize Gushing Decoction (*gù chōng tāng*), 443-444
gù jīng wán	Stabilize the Menses Pill (*gù jīng wán*), 445-446
gù yīn jiān	Stabilize the Yin Decoction (*gù yīn jiān*), 372
gù zhēn tāng	Stabilize the True Decoction (*gù zhēn tāng*), 313
guā dì sǎn	Melon Pedicle Powder (*guā dì sǎn*), 817-818
gūa dì sǎn	Melon Pedicle Powder from *Arcane Essentials from the Imperial Library* (*gūa dì sǎn*), 818
gūa dì sǎn	Melon Pedicle Powder from *Systematic Differentiation of Warm Pathogen Diseases* (*gūa dì sǎn*), 818
gūa lǒu xiè bái bái jiǔ tāng	Trichosanthes Fruit, Chinese Garlic, and Wine Decoction (*gūa lǒu xiè bái bái jiǔ tāng*), 515
gūa lǒu xiè bái bàn xià tāng	Trichosanthes Fruit, Chinese Garlic, and Pinellia Decoction (*gūa lǒu xiè bái bàn xià tāng*), 516
guā lóu zhǐ shí tāng	Trichosanthes Fruit and Unripe Bitter Orange Decoction (*guā lóu zhǐ shí tāng*), 792
guì fù lǐ zhōng tāng	Cinnamon and Prepared Aconite Accessory Root Decoction to Regulate the Middle (*guì fù lǐ zhōng tāng*), 260-261
guì líng gān lù yǐn	Cinnamon and Poria Sweet Dew Drink (*guì líng gān lù yǐn*), 241-242
guì líng gān lù yǐn	Cinnamon and Poria Sweet Dew Drink from *Confucians' Duties* (*guì líng gān lù yǐn*), 242
guì líng wǔ wèi gān cǎo tāng	Cinnamon Twig, Poria, Schisandra, and Licorice Decoction (*guì líng wǔ wèi gān cǎo tāng*), 808
guī lù èr xiān jiāo	Tortoise Shell and Deer Antler Two-Immortal Syrup (*guī lù èr xiān jiāo*), 407-408
guī pí tāng	Restore the Spleen Decoction (*guī pí tāng*), 353-355
guī qì jiàn zhōng tāng	Tangkuei and Astragalus Decoction to Construct the Middle (*guī qì jiàn zhōng tāng*), 267
guì zhī èr yuè bì yī tāng	Two-Parts Cinnamon Twig Decoction with One-Part Maidservant from Yue's Decoction (*guì zhī èr yuè bì yī tāng*), 19
guì zhī fú líng wán	Cinnamon Twig and Poria Pill (*guì zhī fú líng wán*), 583-586
guì zhī gān cǎo lóng gǔ mǔ lì tāng	Cinnamon Twig, Licorice, Dragon Bone, and Oyster Shell Decoction (*guì zhī gān cǎo lóng gǔ mǔ lì tāng*), 441
guì zhī jiā fù zǐ tāng	Cinnamon Twig plus Aconite Accessory Root Decoction (*guì zhī jiā fù zǐ tāng*), 19
guì zhī jiā gé gēn tāng	Cinnamon Twig Decoction plus Kudzu (*guì zhī jiā gé gēn tāng*), 19
guì zhī jiā guì tāng	Cinnamon Twig Decoction plus Cinnamon (*guì zhī jiā guì tāng*), 18
guì zhī jiā hòu pò xìng zǐ tāng	Cinnamon Twig Decoction plus Magnolia Bark and Apricot Kernel (*guì zhī jiā hòu pò xìng zǐ tāng*), 18-19
guì zhī jiā lóng gǔ mǔ lì tāng	Cinnamon Twig Decoction plus Dragon Bone and Oyster Shell (*guì zhī jiā lóng gǔ mǔ lì tāng*), 439-441
guì zhī jiā sháo yào tāng	Cinnamon Twig Decoction plus Peony (*guì zhī jiā sháo yào tāng*), 18
guì zhī má huáng gè bàn tāng	Half Cinnamon Twig and Half Ephedra Decoction (*guì zhī má huáng gè bàn tāng*), 19

guì zhī qù sháo yào tāng	Cinnamon Twig Decoction minus Peony (*guì zhī qù sháo yào tāng*), 18
guì zhī rén shēn tāng	Cinnamon Twig and Ginseng Decoction (*guì zhī rén shēn tāng*), 298-300
guì zhī sháo yào zhī mǔ tāng	Cinnamon Twig, Peony, and Anemarrhena Decoction (*guì zhī sháo yào zhī mǔ tāng*), 760-762
guì zhī tāng	Cinnamon Twig Decoction (*guì zhī tāng*), 13-18
gǔn tán wán	Flushing Away Roiling Phlegm Pill (*gǔn tán wán*), 795-797
guò qī yǐn	Delayed Menstruation Drink (*guò qī yǐn*), 341-342
hǎi tóng pí tāng	Erythrina Wash (*hǎi tóng pí tāng*), 902-903
hǎi zǎo yù hú tāng	Sargassum Decoction for the Jade Flask (*hǎi zǎo yù hú tāng*), 800-801
hāo qín qīng dǎn tāng	Sweet Wormwood and Scutellaria Decoction to Clear the Gallbladder (*hāo qín qīng dǎn tāng*), 111-113
hé rén yǐn	Fleeceflower Root and Ginseng Drink (*hé rén yǐn*), 362-363
hēi xiāo yáo sǎn	Black Rambling Powder (*hēi xiāo yáo sǎn*), 124
hòu pò qī wù tāng	Seven-Substance Decoction with Magnolia Bark (*hòu pò qī wù tāng*), 289
hòu pò sān wù tāng	Three-Substance Decoction with Magnolia Bark (*hòu pò sān wù tāng*), 67-68
hòu pò wēn zhōng tāng	Magnolia Bark Decoction for Warming the Middle (*hòu pò wēn zhōng tāng*), 519-521
hǔ pò duō mèi wán	Succinum Pill For Promoting Sleep (*hǔ pò duō mèi wán*), 468
hǔ qián wán	Hidden Tiger Pill from *Medical Formulas Collected and Analyzed* (*hǔ qián wán*), 379
hǔ qián wán	Hidden Tiger Pill (*hǔ qián wán*), 377-379
huà bān tāng	Transform Maculae Decoction (*huà bān tāng*), 181-182
huà chóng wán	Dissolve Parasites Pill (*huà chóng wán*), 853-854
huà chóng wán	Dissolve Parasites Pill from *Medical Formulas Collected and Analyzed* (*huà chóng wán*), 854
huá gài sǎn	Canopy Powder (*huá gài sǎn*), 10
huá shí dài zhě tāng	Talcum and Hematite Decoction (*huá shí dài zhě tāng*), 222
huà tán xiāo hé wán	Transform Phlegm and Reduce Nodules Pill (*huà tán xiāo hé wán*), 801
huái huā sǎn	Sophora Japonica Flower Powder (*huái huā sǎn*), 605-606
huái jiǎo wán	Sophora Japonica Fruit Pill (*huái jiǎo wán*), 606
huán shào dān	Rejuvenation Special Pill (*huán shào dān*), 404-405
huáng lián ē jiāo tāng	Coptis and Ass-Hide Gelatin Decoction (*huáng lián ē jiāo tāng*), 469-470
huáng lián jiě dú tāng	Coptis Decoction to Resolve Toxicity (*huáng lián jiě dú tāng*), 167-169
huáng lián shàng qīng wán	Coptis Pill to Clear the Upper [Burner] (*huáng lián shàng qīng wán*), 170
huáng lián tāng	Coptis Decoction (*huáng lián tāng*), 131-133
huáng lián wēn dǎn tāng	Warm Gallbladder Decoction with Coptis (*huáng lián wēn dǎn tāng*), 789

huáng lián xiāng rú yǐn	Coptis and Mosla Drink (*huáng lián xiāng rú yǐn*), 236
huáng lóng tāng	Yellow Dragon Decoction (*huáng lóng tāng*), 86-87
huáng qí guì zhī wǔ wù tāng	Astragalus and Cinnamon Twig Five-Substance Decoction (*huáng qí guì zhī wǔ wù tāng*), 255-257
huáng qí jiàn zhōng tāng	Astragalus Decoction to Construct the Middle (*huáng qí jiàn zhōng tāng*), 267
huáng qín huá shí tāng	Scutellaria and Talcum Decoction (*huáng qín huá shí tāng*), 702
huáng qín tāng	Scutellaria Decoction (*huáng qín tāng*), 208-210
huáng tǔ tāng	Yellow Earth Decoction (*huáng tǔ tāng*), 608-610
huí chūn dān	Special Pill to Restore Life (*huí chūn dān*), 495-497
huí yáng jiù jí tāng	Restore and Revive the Yang Decoction from *Revised Popular Guide* (*huí yáng jiù jí tāng*), 279
huí yáng jiù jí tāng	Restore and Revive the Yang Decoction (*huí yáng jiù jí tāng*), 278-279
huó luò xiào líng dān	Fantastically Effective Pill to Invigorate the Collaterals (*huó luò xiào líng dān*), 592-594
huò pò xià líng tāng	Patchouli/Agastache, Magnolia Bark, Pinellia, and Poria Decoction (*huò pò xià líng tāng*), 701-702
huó rén cóng chǐ tāng	Scallion and Prepared Soybean Decoction from *Book to Safeguard Life* (*huó rén cóng chǐ tāng*), 6
huò xiāng zhèng qì sǎn	Patchouli/Agastache Powder to Rectify the Qi (*huò xiāng zhèng qì sǎn*), 691-694
ián zhū yǐn	String of Pearls Drink (*lián zhū yǐn*), 590
jì chuān jiān	Benefit the River [Flow] Decoction (*jì chuān jiān*), 84-85
jǐ jiāo lì huáng wán	Stephania, Zanthoxylum, Tingli Seed, and Rhubarb Pill (*jǐ jiāo lì huáng wán*), 94-95
jī míng sǎn	Powder to Take at Cock's Crow (*jī míng sǎn*), 753-754
jī sū sǎn	Peppermint Powder (*jī sū sǎn*), 240
jiā jiǎn bǔ zhōng yì qì tāng	Modified Tonify the Middle to Augment the Qi Decoction (*jiā jiǎn bǔ zhōng yì qì tāng*), 322
jiā jiǎn dá yuán yǐn	Modified Reach the Source Drink (*jiā jiǎn dá yuán yǐn*), 139
jiā jiǎn dǎo chì xiè xīn tāng	Modified Guide Out the Red and Drain the Epigastrium Decoction (*jiā jiǎn dǎo chì xiè xīn tāng*), 197
jiā jiǎn fù mài tāng	Modified Restore the Pulse Decoction (*jiā jiǎn fù mài tāng*), 359
jiǎ jiǎn liáng gé sǎn	Modified Cool the Diaphragm Powder (*jiǎ jiǎn liáng gé sǎn*), 178
jiā jiǎn shēng mài sǎn	Modified Generate the Pulse Powder (*jiā jiǎn shēng mài sǎn*), 330
jiā jiǎn wēi ruí tāng	Modified Solomon's Seal Decoction (*jiā jiǎn wēi ruí tāng*), 55-56
jiā jiǎn xiǎo chái hú tāng	Modified Minor Bupleurum Decoction (*jiā jiǎn xiǎo chái hú tāng*), 111
jiā jiǎn zhú yè shí gāo tāng	Modified Lophatherum and Gypsum Decoction (*jiā jiǎn zhú yè shí gāo tāng*), 157-158
jiā wèi bā zhèng sǎn	Augmented Eight-Herb Powder for Rectification (*jiā wèi bā zhèng sǎn*), 715

jiā wèi bái tóu wēng tāng	Augmented Pulsatilla Decoction (*jiā wèi bái tóu wēng tāng*), 211-212
jiā wèi dà chái hú tāng	Augmented Major Bupleurum Decoction (*jiā wèi dà chái hú tāng*), 289
jiā wèi èr chén tāng	Augmented Two-Aged [Herb] Decoction (*jiā wèi èr chén tāng*), 780
jiā wèi èr miào wán	Augmented Two-Marvel Pill (*jiā wèi èr miào wán*), 721-722
jiā wèi liù wèi dì huáng wán	Augmented Six-Ingredient Pill with Rehmannia (*jiā wèi liù wèi dì huáng wán*), 369
jiā wèi mài mén dōng tāng	Augmented Ophiopogonis Decoction (*jiā wèi mài mén dōng tāng*), 673
jiā weì shèn qì wán	Augmented Kidney Qi Pill (*jiā weì shèn qì wán*), 400
jiā wèi sì wù tāng	Augmented Four-Substance Decoction (*jiā wèi sì wù tāng*), 338
jiā wèi wǔ lín sǎn	Augmented Powder for Five Types of Painful Urinary Dribbling (*jiā wèi wǔ lín sǎn*), 717
jiā wèi wū yào tāng	Augmented Lindera Decoction (*jiā wèi wū yào tāng*), 535-536
jiā wèi xiāng sū sǎn	Augmented Cyperus and Perilla Leaf Powder (*jiā wèi xiāng sū sǎn*), 27-29
jiā wèi xiǎo xiàn xiōng tāng	Augmented Minor Decoction [for Pathogens] Stuck in the Chest (*jiā weì xiǎo xiàn xiōng tāng*), 794
jiā wèi xiāo yáo sǎn	Augmented Rambling Powder (*jiā wèi xiāo yáo sǎn*), 124
jiàn líng tāng	Construct Roof Tiles Decoction (*jiàn líng tāng*), 647
jiàn pí wán	Strengthen the Spleen Pill (*jiàn pí wán*), 835-837
jiàn pí wán	Strengthen the Spleen Pill from *Medical Formulas Collected and Analyzed* (*jiàn pí wán*), 837
jiàng dàn tāng	Direct Nitrogen Downward Decoction (*jiàng dàn tāng*), 75
jiàng qì huà tán tāng	Direct Qi Downward and Transform Phlegm Decoction (*jiàng qì huà tán tāng*), 817
jiāo ài tāng	Ass-Hide Gelatin and Mugwort Decoction (*jiāo ài tāng*), 610-612
jiāo tài wán	Grand Communication Pill (*jiāo tài wán*), 470-471
jiě gān jiān	Resolve the Liver Decoction (*jiě gān jiān*), 533
jié nuè qī bǎo yǐn	Seven-Treasure Drink to Check Malarial Disorders (*jié nuè qī bǎo yǐn*), 134-135
jīn fèi cǎo sǎn	Inula Powder (*jīn fèi cǎo sǎn*), 32-34
jīn fèi cǎo sǎn	Inula Powder from *Book to Safeguard Life* (*jīn fèi cǎo sǎn*), 34
jǐn hóng tāng	Brocade Red Decoction (*jǐn hóng tāng*), 882
jīn huáng gāo	Golden-Yellow Plaster (*jīn huáng gāo*), 897-898
jīn huáng sǎn	Golden-Yellow Powder (*jīn huáng sǎn*), 897-898
Jīn jiàn féi ér wán	Fat Baby Pill from *Golden Mirror* (*Jīn jiàn féi ér wán*), 834
jīn líng zǐ sǎn	Melia Toosendan Powder (*jīn líng zǐ sǎn*), 522-524
jīn shuǐ liù jūn jiān	Six-Gentlemen of Metal and Water Decoction (*jīn shuǐ liù jūn jiān*), 779
jīn suǒ gù jīng wán	Metal Lock Pill to Stabilize the Essence (*jīn suǒ gù jīng wán*), 435-436

jīng fáng bài dú sǎn	Schizonepeta and Saposhnikovia Powder to Overcome Pathogenic Influences (*jīng fáng bài dú sǎn*), 49-50
jīng jiè lián qiáo tāng	Schizonepeta and Forsythia Decoction (*jīng jiè lián qiáo tāng*), 45-46
jiǔ wèi qiāng huó tāng	Nine-Herb Decoction with Notopterygium (*jiǔ wèi qiāng huó tāng*), 24-26
jiǔ xiān sǎn	Nine-Immortal Powder (*jiǔ xiān sǎn*), 423-424
jú hé wán	Tangerine Seed Pill (*jú hé wán*), 529-531
jú huā chá tiáo sǎn	Chrysanthemum Powder to be Taken with Green Tea (*jú huā chá tiáo sǎn*), 627
jú pí tāng	Tangerine Peel Decoction (*jú pí tāng*), 546-547
jú pí zhú rú tāng	Tangerine Peel and Bamboo Shavings Decoction (*jú pí zhú rú tāng*), 544-546
jú pí zhú rú tāng	Tangerine Peel and Bamboo Shavings Decoction from *Formulas to Aid the Living* (*jú pí zhú rú tāng*), 547
jú xìng wán	Tangerine and Apricot Pill (*jú xìng wán*), 79
jǔ yuán jiān	Lift the Source Decoction (*jǔ yuán jiān*), 323
juān bì tāng	Remove Painful Obstruction Decoction (*juān bì tāng*), 756-757
juān bì tāng	Remove Painful Obstruction Decoction from *Awakening of the Mind in Medical Studies* (*juān bì tāng*), 757-758
ké xuè fāng	Coughing of Blood Formula (*ké xuè fāng*), 601-603
kòng xián dān	Control Mucus Special Pill (*kòng xián dān*), 91
Kǒng zi zhěn zhōng dān	Special Pill from Confucius' Pillow (*Kǒng zi zhěn zhōng dān*), 468
kǔ shēn tāng	Sophora Root Wash (*kǔ shēn tāng*), 901-902
Léi shì qīng liǎng dì shǔ fǎ	Master Lei's Method for Clearing, Cooling and Scouring Out Summerheat (*Léi shì qīng liǎng dì shǔ fǎ*), 240-241
Léi shì qīng liáng dí shǔ tāng	Master Lei's Decoction to Clear, Cool, and Remove Summerheat (*Léi shì qīng liáng dí shǔ tāng*), 245
Léi shì xuān tòu mó yuán fǎ	Lei's Method for Disseminating and Venting [Dampness and Heat from] the Membrane Source (*Léi shì xuān tòu mó yuán fǎ*), 139
lěng xiào wán	Cold Asthma Pill (*lěng xiào wán*), 808
lǐ zhōng ān huí tāng	Regulate the Middle and Calm Roundworms Decoction (*lǐ zhōng ān huí tāng*), 852
lǐ zhōng huà tán wán	Regulate the Middle and Transform Phlegm Pill (*lǐ zhōng huà tán wán*), 779-780
lǐ zhōng wán	Regulate the Middle Pill (*lǐ zhōng wán*), 257-260
lián lǐ tāng	Regulating Decoction with Coptis (*lián lǐ tāng*), 260
lián méi ān huí tāng	Picrorhiza and Mume Decoction to Calm Roundworms (*lián méi ān huí tāng*), 852
lián pò yǐn	Coptis and Magnolia Bark Drink (*lián pò yǐn*), 705-707
lián qiào jīn bèi jiān	Lonicera, Honeysuckle, and Bolbostemma Decoction (*lián qiào jīn bèi jiān*), 865
liáng fù wán	Galangal and Cyperus Pill (*liáng fù wán*), 521-522

liáng gé sǎn	Cool the Diaphragm Powder *(liáng gé sǎn)*, 176-178
líng gān wǔ wèi jiā jiāng xīn bàn xià xìng rén tāng	Poria, Licorice, and Schisandra plus Ginger, Asarum, Pinellia, and Apricot Kernel Decoction *(líng gān wǔ wèi jiā jiāng xīn bàn xià xìng rén tāng)*, 808
líng gān wǔ wèi jiāng xīn tāng	Poria, Licorice, Schisandra, Ginger, and Asarum Decoction *(líng gān wǔ wèi jiāng xīn tāng)*, 806-808
líng guì zhú gān tāng	Poria, Cinnamon Twig, Atractylodes, and Licorice Decoction *(líng guì zhú gān tāng)*, 738-741
líng jiǎo gōu téng tāng	Antelope Horn and Uncaria Decoction *(líng jiǎo gōu téng tāng)*, 642-644
líng xī bái hǔ tāng	White Tiger with Antelope and Rhinoceros Horn Decoction *(líng xī bái hǔ tāng)*, 155
liù ān jiān	Six-Serenity Decoction *(liù ān jiān)*, 780
liù hé tāng	Harmonize the Six Decoction *(liù hé tāng)*, 695-697
liù jūn zǐ tāng	Six-Gentlemen Decoction *(liù jūn zǐ tāng)*, 311-312
liù mò tāng	Six Milled-Herb Decoction *(liù mò tāng)*, 526
liù shén sǎn	Six-Miracle Powder from *Indispensable Tools for Pattern Treatment (liù shén sǎn)*, 312
liu shén tōng jiě sǎn	Six-Miracle Powder to Unblock and Release *(liu shén tōng jiě sǎn)*, 296
liù shén wán	Six-Divine Pill *(liù shén wán)*, 869
liù wèi dì huáng wán	Six-Ingredient Pill with Rehmannia *(liù wèi dì huáng wán)*, 365-368
liù wèi xiāng rú yǐn	Six-Ingredient Drink with Mosla *(liù wèi xiāng rú yǐn)*, 236
liù yī sǎn	Six-to-One Powder *(liù yī sǎn)*, 238-240
lù páo sǎn	Green Robe Powder *(lù páo sǎn)*, 897
lóng chǐ qīng hún sǎn	Dragon Tooth Powder to Clear the Ethereal Soul *(lóng chǐ qīng hún sǎn)*, 468
lóng dǎn xiè gān tāng	Gentian Decoction to Drain the Liver from *Precious Mirror (lóng dǎn xiè gān tāng)*, 201
lóng dǎn xiè gān tāng	Gentian Decoction to Drain the Liver *(lóng dǎn xiè gān tāng)*, 199-200
loú xiè liù rén tāng	Six-Seed Decoction with Trichosanthis and Chinese Garlic *(loú xiè liù rén tāng)*, 664-665
má huáng deng shí wèi wán	Ephedra Pill with Ten Ingredients *(má huáng deng shí wèi wán)*, 24
má huáng fù zǐ gān cǎo tāng	Ephedra, Aconite Accessory Root, and Licorice Decoction *(má huáng fù zǐ gān cǎo tāng)*, 52
má huáng jiā zhú tāng	Ephedra Decoction plus Atractylodes *(má huáng jiā zhú tāng)*, 10
má huáng tāng	Ephedra Decoction *(má huáng tāng)*, 7-9
má huáng xì xīn fù zǐ tāng	Ephedra, Asarum, and Aconite Accessory Root Decoction *(má huáng xì xīn fù zǐ tāng)*, 50-52
má huáng xìng rén yì yǐ gān cǎo tāng	Ephedra, Apricot Kernel, Coicis, and Licorice Decoction *(má huáng xìng rén yì yǐ gān cǎo tāng)*, 10-11
má xìng shí gān tāng	Ephedra, Apricot Kernel, Gypsum, and Licorice Decoction *(má xìng shí gān tāng)*, 183-185

má zǐ rén wán	Hemp Seed Pill (*má zǐ rén wán*), 81-83
mài mén dōng tāng	Ophiopogonis Decoction (*mài mén dōng tāng*), 670-673
miào xiāng sǎn	Marvelously Fragrant Powder (*miào xiāng sǎn*), 468-469
míng mù dì huáng wán	Improve Vision Pill with Rehmannia (*míng mù dì huáng wán*), 369-370
mǔ lì sǎn	Oyster Shell Powder (*mǔ lì sǎn*), 420-422
mù xiāng bīng láng wán	Aucklandia and Betel Nut Pill from Zhu Dan-Xi (*mù xiāng bīng láng wán*), 833
mù xiāng bīng láng wán	Aucklandia and Betel Nut Pill from *Medical Formulas Collected and Analyzed* (*mù xiāng bīng láng wán*), 833
mù xiāng bīng láng wán	Aucklandia and Betel Nut Pill (*mù xiāng bīng láng wán*), 831-833
nǚ shén sǎn	Goddess Powder (*nǚ shén sǎn*), 511-512
nèi bù dāng guī jiàn zhōng tāng	Internally Tonifying Tangkuei Decoction to Construct the Middle (*nèi bù dāng guī jiàn zhōng tāng*), 267-268
nèi bǔ huáng qí tāng	Internally Astragalus (*nèi bǔ huáng qí tāng*), 350
nèi liú huáng lián tāng	Internal Flow [Promoting] Decoction with Coptis (*nèi liú huáng lián tāng*), 863
nèi shū huáng lián tāng	Internal Dispersing Decoction with Coptis (*nèi shū huáng lián tāng*), 173
níng sòu sǎn	Calm Coughing Pill (*níng sòu sǎn*), 28
níng xuè tāng	Quiet the Blood Decoction (*níng xuè tāng*), 601
niú huáng chéng qì tāng	Cattle Gallstone Decoction to Order the Qi (*niú huáng chéng qì tāng*), 490
niú huáng shàng qīng wán	Cattle Gallstone Pill to Clear the Upper [Burner] (*niú huáng shàng qīng wán*), 170
niú xī sǎn	Achyranthes Powder (*niú xī sǎn*), 587
nǚ kē bái zǐ rén wán	Arborvitae Seed Pill for Women's Disorders (*nǚ kē bái zǐ rén wán*), 342-344
nuǎn gān jiān	Warm the Liver Decoction (*nuǎn gān jiān*), 531-533
pái qì yǐn	Discharge Gas Drink (*pái qì yǐn*), 511
píng wèi sǎn	Calm the Stomach Powder (*píng wèi sǎn*), 687-688
pǔ jì xiāo dú yǐn	Universal Benefit Drink to Eliminate Toxin (*pǔ jì xiāo dú yǐn*), 173-175
qī bǎo měi rán dān	Seven-Treasure Special Pill for Beautiful Whiskers (*qī bǎo měi rán dān*), 409-410
qǐ gé sǎn	Open Up the Diaphragm Powder (*qǐ gé sǎn*), 533-535
qǐ jú dì huáng wán	Lycium Fruit, Chrysanthemum, and Rehmannia Pill (*qǐ jú dì huáng wán*), 368
qī lí sǎn	Seven-Thousandths of a Tael Powder (*qī lí sǎn*), 573-575
qǐ pí wán	Open the Spleen Pill (*qǐ pí wán*), 313
qī pí yǐn	Seven-Peel Drink (*qī pí yǐn*), 734
qī wèi bái zhú sǎn	Seven-Ingredient Powder with White Atractylodes (*qī wèi bái zhú sǎn*), 316
qī wù jiàng xià tāng	Seven-Substance Decoction for Directing Downward (*qī wù jiàng xià tāng*), 338

qiān jīn nèi tuō sǎn	Powder to Support the Interior Worth a Thousand Gold Pieces *(qiān jīn nèi tuō sǎn)*, 873-875
qiān zhèng sǎn	Lead to Symmetry Powder *(qiān zhèng sǎn)*, 633-634
qiāng huó shèng shī tāng	Notopterygium Decoction to Overcome Dampness *(qiāng huó shèng shī tāng)*, 755-756
qín jiāo biē jiǎ sǎn	Large Gentian and Soft-Shelled Turtle Shell Powder *(qín jiāo biē jiǎ sǎn)*, 216-218
qín lián sì wù tāng	Four-Substance Decoction with Scutellaria and Coptis *(qín lián sì wù tāng)*, 337
qīng bí tāng	Clear the Nose Decoction *(qīng bí tāng)*, 21
qīng cháng yǐn	Clear the Intestines Drink *(qīng cháng yǐn)*, 882-884
qīng dài sǎn	Indigo Powder *(qīng dài sǎn)*, 900-901
qīng dài tāng	Clear Discharge Decoction *(qīng dài tāng)*, 450
qīng dǎn xiè huǒ tāng	Clear the Gallbladder and Drain Fire Decoction *(qīng dǎn xiè huǒ tāng)*, 201
qīng é wán	Young Maiden Pill *(qīng é wán)*, 402
qīng fèi tāng	Clear the Lungs Decoction *(qīng fèi tāng)*, 804-805
qīng fèi yǐn	Clear the Lungs Drink *(qīng fèi yǐn)*, 805
qīng fèi yǐn zi	Clear the Lungs Drink *(qīng fèi yǐn zi)*, 715
qīng gān dá yù tāng	Clear the Liver and Thrust Out Constraint Decoction *(qīng gān dá yù tāng)*, 125
qīng gān yǐn	Clear the Liver Drink *(qīng gān yǐn)*, 865
qīng gé sǎn	Indigo and Clam Shell Powder *(qīng gé sǎn)*, 901
qīng gōng tāng	Clear the Palace Decoction *(qīng gōng tāng)*, 163-165
qīng gǔ sǎn	Cool the Bones Powder *(qīng gǔ sǎn)*, 214-216
qīng hāo biē jiǎ tāng	Sweet Wormwood and Soft-shelled Turtle Shell Decoction [Version 1] *(qīng hāo biē jiǎ tāng)*, 212-214
qīng hāo biē jiǎ tāng	Sweet Wormwood and Soft-shelled Turtle Shell Decoction [Version 2] *(qīng hāo biē jiǎ tāng)*, 214
qīng jīn huà tán wán	Clear Metal and Transform Phlegm Pill *(qīng jīn huà tán wán)*, 792
qīng jīng sǎn	Clear the Menses Powder *(qīng jīng sǎn)*, 216
qīng liáng yǐn zi	Clearing and Cooling Drink *(qīng liáng yǐn zi)*, 171
qīng luò yǐn	Clear the Collaterals Drink *(qīng luò yǐn)*, 232-233
qīng pí tāng	Clear the Spleen Decoction *(qīng pí tāng)*, 137-138
qīng qì huà tán wán	Clear the Qi and Transform Phlegm Pill *(qīng qì huà tán wán)*, 790-792
qīng shàng fáng fēng tāng	Clear the Upper [Burner] Decoction with Saposhnikovia *(qīng shàng fáng fēng tāng)*, 171
qīng shī huà tán tāng	Clear Dampness and Transform Phlegm Decoction *(qīng shī huà tán tāng)*, 785
qīng shǔ yì qì tāng	Clear Summerheat and Augment the Qi Decoction *(qīng shǔ yì qì tāng)*, 243-245

qīng shǔ yì qì tāng	Clear Summerheat and Augment the Qi Decoction from *Clarifying Doubts* (*qīng shǔ yì qì tāng*), 244-245
qīng wèi sǎn	Clear the Stomach Powder (*qīng wèi sǎn*), 191-192
qīng wèi tāng	Clear the Stomach Decoction (*qīng wèi tāng*), 193
qīng wēn bài dú yǐn	Clear Epidemics and Overcome Toxicity Drink (*qīng wēn bài dú yǐn*), 179-181
qīng xīn lì gé tāng	Clear the Heart and Enable the Diaphragm Decoction (*qīng xīn lì gé tāng*), 886-887
qīng xīn lián zǐ yǐn	Clear the Heart Drink with Lotus Seed (*qīng xīn lián zǐ yǐn*), 197-199
qīng xīn liáng gé sǎn	Clear the Heart and Cool the Diaphragm Powder (*qīng xīn liáng gé sǎn*), 178
qīng yān lì gé tāng	Clear the Throat and Enable the Diaphragm Decoction (*qīng yān lì gé tāng*), 887
qīng yí tāng	Clear the Pancreas Decoction (*qīng yí tāng*), 289
qīng yíng tāng	Clear the Nutritive Level Decoction (*qīng yíng tāng*), 161-163
qīng zào jiù fèi tāng	Clear Dryness and Rescue the Lungs Decoction (*qīng zào jiù fèi tāng*), 667-669
qióng yù gāo	Precious Jade Syrup (*qióng yù gāo*), 389-391
qū fēng zhì bǎo dān	Greatest Treasure Special Pill to Dispel Wind (*qū fēng zhì bǎo dān*), 291-292
qū mài zhǐ zhú wán	Medicated Leaven, Barley Sprout, Unripe Bitter Orange, and Atractylodes Pill (*qū mài zhǐ zhú wán*), 838
rén shēn bài dú sǎn	Ginseng Powder to Overcome Pathogenic Influences (*rén shēn bài dú sǎn*), 47-49
rén shēn gé jiè sǎn	Ginseng and Gecko Powder (*rén shēn gé jiè sǎn*), 331-333
rén shēn hú táo tāng	Ginseng and Walnut Decoction (*rén shēn hú táo tāng*), 333
rén shēn huà bān tāng	Ginseng Transform Maculae Decoction (*rén shēn huà bān tāng*), 182
rén shēn huáng qí sǎn	Ginseng and Astragalus Powder (*rén shēn huáng qí sǎn*), 214
rén shēn wū méi tāng	Ginseng and Mume Decoction (*rén shēn wū méi tāng*), 246-247
rén shēn xiè fèi tāng	Ginseng Decoction to Drain the Lungs (*rén shēn xiè fèi tāng*), 178
rén shén xiè xīn tāng	Ginseng Decoction to Drain the Epigastrium (*rén shén xiè xīn tāng*), 131
rén shēn yǎng róng tāng	Ginseng Decoction to Nourish Luxuriance (*rén shēn yǎng róng tāng*), 350-352
rú xìng tāng	Mosla and Apricot Kernel Decoction (*rú xìng tāng*), 234
rùn cháng wán	Moisten the Intestines Pill from *Discussion of the Spleen and Stomach* (*rùn cháng wán*), 80
rùn cháng wán	Moisten the Intestines Pill from Master Shen's Book (*rùn cháng wán*), 80
rùn jī gāo	Skin-Moistening Ointment (*rùn jī gāo*), 899
rùn zào shēn shī tāng	Moisten Dryness and Leach Out Dampness Decoction (*rùn zào shēn shī tāng*), 665
sān ǎo tāng	Three-Unbinding Decoction (*sān ǎo tāng*), 10
sān bì tāng	Three Painful Obstruction Decoction (*sān bì tāng*), 759-760
sān caí tāng	Three-Talents Decoction (*sān caí tāng*), 391

sān huà tāng	Three-Transformation Decoction *(sān huà tāng)*, 68
sān huáng shí gāo tāng	Three-Yellow and Gypsum Decoction *(sān huáng shí gāo tāng)*, 169
sān jiǎ fù mài tāng	Three-Shell Decoction to Restore the Pulse *(sān jiǎ fù mài tāng)*, 649-651
sān jiā jiǎn zhèng qì sǎn	Third Modification of Rectify the Qi Powder *(sān jiā jiǎn zhèng qì sǎn)*, 694
sān jīn tāng	Three-Gold Decoction *(sān jīn tāng)*, 716
sān léng xǐ rú fāng	Sparganium Breast Wash *(sān léng xǐ rú fāng)*, 904
sān miào wán	Three-Marvel Pill *(sān miào wán)*, 721
sān rén tāng	Three-Seed Decoction *(sān rén tāng)*, 699-701
sān rén wán	Three-Seed Pill *(sān rén wán)*, 79
sān shèng sǎn	Three-Sage Powder *(sān shèng sǎn)*, 818
sān shēng yǐn	Drink from Three Unprepared Ingredients *(sān shēng yǐn)*, 624-625
sān shí tāng	Three-Minerals Decoction *(sān shí tāng)*, 242-243
sān wù bèi jí wán	Three-Substance Pill Prepared for Emergencies *(sān wù bèi jí wán)*, 75-76
sàn yū hé shāng tāng	Wash to Mollify Trauma by Dispersing Stasis *(sàn yū hé shāng tāng)*, 903
sàn zhǒng kuì jiān tāng	Decoction to Disperse Swelling and Ulcerate What is Hard *(sàn zhǒng kuì jiān tāng)*, 875-877
sān zǐ yǎng qīn tāng	Three-Seed Decoction to Nourish One's Parents *(sān zǐ yǎng qīn tāng)*, 808-810
sāng dān xiè bái tāng	Mulberry Leaf and Moutan Decoction to Drain the White *(sāng dān xiè bái tāng)*, 188
sāng jú yǐn	Mulberry Leaf and Chrysanthemum Drink *(sāng jú yǐn)*, 35-36
sāng má wán	Mulberry Leaf and Sesame Seed Pill *(sāng má wán)*, 384
sāng piāo xiāo sǎn	Mantis Egg-Case Powder *(sāng piāo xiāo sǎn)*, 436-438
sāng xìng tāng	Mulberry Leaf and Apricot Kernel Decoction *(sāng xìng tāng)*, 665-667
shā shēn mài mén dōng tāng	Glehnia and Ophiopogonis Decoction *(shā shēn mài mén dōng tāng)*, 669-670
shàng zhōng xià tōng yòng tòng fēng wán	Pill to Treat Painful Wind Anywhere *(shàng zhōng xià tōng yòng tòng fēng wán)*, 763-765
shào fù zhú yū tāng	Drive Out Stasis from the Lower Abdomen Decoction *(shào fù zhú yū tāng)*, 567-568
sháo yào gān cǎo fù zǐ tāng	Peony, Licorice, and Aconite Accessory Root Decoction *(sháo yào gān cǎo fù zǐ tāng)*, 345
sháo yào gān cǎo tāng	Peony and Licorice Decoction *(sháo yào gān cǎo tāng)*, 344-345
sháo yào tāng	Peony Decoction *(sháo yào tāng)*, 207-208
shè gān má huáng tāng	Belamcanda and Ephedra Decoction *(shè gān má huáng tāng)*, 24
shēn fù tāng	Ginseng and Aconite Accessory Root Decoction *(shēn fù tāng)*, 279-281
shēn líng bái zhú sǎn	Ginseng, Poria, and White Atractylodes Powder *(shēn líng bái zhú sǎn)*, 314-316
shēn líng bái zhú sǎn	Ginseng, Poria, and White Atractylodes Powder from *Medical Formulas Collected and Analyzed* *(shēn líng bái zhú sǎn)*, 316

shēn líng dān	Pregnancy Panacea (*shēn líng dān*), 446-447
shén mì tāng	Mysterious Decoction (*shén mì tāng*), 542
shèn qì wán	Kidney Qi Pill (*shèn qì wán*), 395-400
Shěn shì zhū líng tāng	Polyporus Decoction from Master Shen (*Shěn shì zhū líng tāng*), 731
shēn sū yǐn	Ginseng and Perilla Leaf Drink (*shēn sū yǐn*), 50
shēn tōng zhú yū tāng	Drive Out Stasis from a Painful Body Decoction (*shēn tōng zhú yū tāng*), 568
shén xī dān	Magical Rhinoceros Special Pill (*shén xī dān*), 167
shén xiào tuō lǐ sǎn	Miraculous Powder for Supporting the Interior (*shén xiào tuō lǐ sǎn*), 867
shēng huà tāng	Generating and Transforming Decoction (*shēng huà tāng*), 581-583
shēng jiāng gān cǎo tāng	Fresh Ginger and Licorice Decoction (*shēng jiāng gān cǎo tāng*), 272
shēng jiāng xiè xīn tāng	Fresh Ginger Decoction to Drain the Epigastrium (*shēng jiāng xiè xīn tāng*), 130
shēng má gé gēn tāng	Cimicifuga and Kudzu Decoction (*shēng má gé gēn tāng*), 41-43
shēng mài sǎn	Generate the Pulse Powder (*shēng mài sǎn*), 328-330
shēng tiě luò yǐn	Iron Filings Drink (*shēng tiě luò yǐn*), 478-480
shēng xiàn tāng	Raise the Sunken Decoction (*shēng xiàn tāng*), 323-324
shēng yáng sàn huǒ tāng	Raise the Yang and Disperse Fire Decoction (*shēng yáng sàn huǒ tāng*), 326
shēng yáng yì wèi tāng	Raise the Yang and Augment the Stomach Decoction (*shēng yáng yì wèi tāng*), 324-326
shèng yù tāng	Sage-like Healing Decoction (*shèng yù tāng*), 337
shí bǔ wán	Ten-Tonic Pill (*shí bǔ wán*), 400
shì dì tāng	Persimmon Calyx Decoction (*shì dì tāng*), 549
shí gāo tāng	Gypsum Decoction (*shí gāo tāng*), 294-295
shí gāo tāng	Gypsum Decoction from *Six Texts* (*shí gāo tāng*), 295
shí hú yè guāng wán	Dendrobium Pill for Night Vision (*shí hú yè guāng wán*), 393
shí huī sǎn	Ten Partially-charred Substances Powder (*shí huī sǎn*), 598-600
shí liù wèi liú qì yǐn	Sixteen-Ingredient Drink for Qi Flow (*shí liù wèi liú qì yǐn*), 888-890
shí pí yǐn	Bolster the Spleen Drink (*shí pí yǐn*), 749-750
shí quán dà bǔ tāng	All-Inclusive Great Tonifying Decoction (*shí quán dà bǔ tāng*), 348-350
shí quán yù zhēn tāng	All-Inclusive Decoction for Fostering the True (*shí quán yù zhēn tāng*), 597
shí shén tāng	Ten-Miracle Decoction (*shí shén tāng*), 30-32
shí wèi bài dú sǎn	Ten-Ingredient Powder to Overcome Toxicity (*shí wèi bài dú sǎn*), 872-873
shí wéi sǎn	Pyrrosiae Powder (*shí wéi sǎn*), 717
shí wèi wēn dǎn tāng	Ten-Ingredient Warm Gallbladder Decoction (*shí wèi wēn dǎn tāng*), 789
shí wèi xiāng rú yǐn	Ten-Ingredient Drink with Mosla (*shí wèi xiāng rú yǐn*), 236

shī xiào sǎn	Sudden Smile Powder *(shī xiào sǎn)*, 591-592
shí zǎo tāng	Ten-Jujube Decoction *(shí zǎo tāng)*, 90-91
shǒu niān sǎn	Pinch Powder *(shǒu niān sǎn)*, 592
shòu tāi wán	Fetus Longevity Pill *(shòu tāi wán)*, 441-442
shū fēng huó xuè tāng	Dredge the Wind and Invigorate the Blood Decoction *(shū fēng huó xuè tāng)*, 760
shū gān lǐ pí tāng	Dredge the Liver and Regulate the Spleen Decoction *(shū gān lǐ pí tāng)*, 125
shū gān tāng	Dredge the Liver Decoction *(shū gān tāng)*, 513-514
shū jīng huó xuè tāng	Relax the Channels and Invigorate the Blood Decoction *(shū jīng huó xuè tāng)*, 571
shū záo yǐn zi	Dredging and Cutting Drink *(shū záo yǐn zi)*, 95-97
shuǎng jiě jiā cóng chǐ tāng	Double Releasing Decoction with Spring Onions and Prepared Soybeans *(shuǎng jiě jiā cóng chǐ tāng)*, 295-296
shuāng jiě tōng shèng sǎn	Double Releasing Powder that Sagely Unblocks *(shuāng jiě tōng shèng sǎn)*, 291
shuǐ lù èr xiān dān	Water and Earth Immortals Special Pill *(shuǐ lù èr xiān dān)*, 436
shùn jīng tāng	Smooth the Menses Decoction *(shùn jīng tāng)*, 601
sì jiā jiǎn zhèng qì sǎn	Fourth Modification of Rectify the Qi Powder *(sì jiā jiǎn zhèng qì sǎn)* 694
sì jūn zǐ tāng	Four-Gentlemen Decoction *(sì jūn zǐ tāng)*, 309-311
sì líng sǎn	Four-Ingredient Powder with Poria *(sì líng sǎn)*, 728
sì miào wán	Four-Marvel Pill *(sì miào wán)*, 721
sì miào yǒng ān tāng	Four-Valiant Decoction for Well-being *(sì miào yǒng ān tāng)*, 865-867
sì mò tāng	Four Milled-Herb Decoction *(sì mò tāng)*, 525-526
sì nì jiā rén shēn tāng	Frigid Extremities Decoction plus Ginseng *(sì nì jiā rén shēn tāng)*, 277
sì nì sǎn	Frigid Extremities Powder *(sì nì sǎn)*, 116-120
sì nì tāng	Frigid Extremities Decoction *(sì nì tāng)*, 274-277
sì qì tāng	Minor Seven-Emotions Decoction *(sì qì tāng)*, 519
sì qī tāng	Four-Ingredient Decoction for the Seven Emotions *(sì qī tāng)*, 519
sì shén wán	Four-Miracle Pill *(sì shén wán)*, 429-431
sì shēng wán	Four-Fresh Pill *(sì shēng wán)*, 600-601
sì wèi xiāng rú yǐn	Four-Ingredient Drink with Mosla *(sì wèi xiāng rú yǐn)*, 236
sì wù tāng	Four-Substance Decoction *(sì wù tāng)*, 333-336
sì wù xiāo fēng yǐn	Eliminate Wind Drink with the Four Substances *(sì wù xiāo fēng yǐn)*, 638
sì yīn jiān	Four-Yin Decoction *(sì yīn jiān)*, 675
sōu fēng shùn qì wán	Track Down Wind and Smooth the Flow of Qi Pill *(sōu fēng shùn qì wán)*, 83
sū hé xiāng wán	Liquid Styrax Pill *(sū hé xiāng wán)*, 498-500

wēn jīng tāng	Flow-Warming Decoction from *Fine Formulas for Women* (*wēn jīng tāng*), 589-581
wēn pí tāng	Warm the Spleen Decoction from *Formulas of Universal Benefit* (*wēn pí tāng*), 75
wēn pí tāng	Warm the Spleen Decoction (*wēn pí tāng*), 73-75
wēn qīng yǐn	Warming and Clearing Drink (*wēn qīng yǐn*), 337
wú bǐ shān yào wǎn	Incomparable Dioscorea Pill (*wú bǐ shān yào wǎn*), 400-401
wǔ hǔ tāng	Five-Tiger Decoction (*wǔ hǔ tāng*), 186
wǔ hǔ zhuī fēng sǎn	Five-Tiger Powder to Pursue Wind (*wǔ hǔ zhuī fēng sǎn*), 636
wǔ jī sǎn	Five-Accumulation Powder (*wǔ jī sǎn*), 296-298
wù jǐ wán	Fifth and Sixth Heavenly Stem Pill (*wù jǐ wán*), 206
wǔ jiā jiǎn zhèng qì sǎn	Fifth Modification of Rectify the Qi Powder (*wǔ jiā jiǎn zhèng qì sǎn*), 694-695
wǔ lín sǎn	Powder for Five Types of Painful Urinary Dribbling (*wǔ lín sǎn*), 716-717
wǔ líng sǎn	Five-Ingredient Powder with Poria (*wǔ líng sǎn*), 724-728
wǔ líng tōng guān tāng	Five Ingredients with Poria Decoction to Open the Gate (*wǔ líng tōng guān tāng*), 731-732
wū méi wán	Mume Pill (*wū méi wán*), 847-852
wǔ mò yǐn zi	Five Milled-Herb Drink (*wǔ mò yǐn zi*), 526-527
wǔ pí sǎn	Five-Peel Powder (*wǔ pí sǎn*), 732-734
wǔ pí yǐn	Five-Peel Drink (*wǔ pí yǐn*), 734
wǔ rén wán	Five-Seed Pill (*wǔ rén wán*), 78-79
wǔ shén tāng	Five-Miracle Decoction (*wǔ shén tāng*), 867
Wú shì lián méi tāng	Master Wu's Coptis and Mume Decoction (*Wú shì lián méi tāng*), 246
wū tóu guì zhī tāng	Aconite and Cinnamon Twig Decoction (*wū tóu guì zhī tāng*), 19
wū tóu tāng	Aconite Decoction (*wū tóu tāng*), 624
wǔ wèi xiāo dú yǐn	Five-Ingredient Drink to Eliminate Toxin (*wǔ wèi xiāo dú yǐn*), 863-865
wǔ wù xiāng rú yǐn	Five-Substance Drink with Mosla (*wǔ wù xiāng rú yǐn*), 236
wū yào shùn qì sǎn	Lindera Powder to Smooth the Flow of Qi (*wū yào shùn qì sǎn*), 623-624
wǔ yè lú gēn tāng	Reed Decoction with Five Leaves (*wǔ yè lú gēn tāng*), 233
wǔ zhī yǐn	Five-Juice Drink (*wǔ zhī yǐn*), 677
wú zhū yú gāo	Evodia Plaster (*wú zhū yú gāo*), 904
wú zhū yú tāng	Evodia Decoction from *Comprehensive Recording* (*wú zhū yú tāng*), 264
wú zhū yú tāng	Evodia Decoction (*wú zhū yú tāng*), 261-264
wǔ zǐ tāng	Five-Seed Decoction (*wǔ zǐ tāng*), 80-81

xī dì toù yíng tāng	Rhinoceros and Rhemannia Decoction for Venting the Nutritive Level *(xī dì toù yíng tāng)*, 163
xǐ gān míng mù sǎn	Wash the Liver to Clear the Eyes Powder *(xǐ gān míng mù sǎn)*, 203
xǐ gān sǎn	Liver-Washing Powder *(xǐ gān sǎn)*, 203
xī jiǎo dì huáng tāng	Rhinoceros Horn and Rehmannia Decoction *(xī jiǎo dì huáng tāng)*, 165-166
xià kū cǎo gāo	Prunella Syrup *(xià kū cǎo gāo)*, 799-800
xià yū xuè tāng	Purge Static Blood Decoction *(xià yū xuè tāng)*, 562
xiān fāng huó mìng yǐn	Immortals' Formula for Sustaining Life *(xiān fāng huó mìng yǐn)*, 861-863
xiāng bèi yǎng róng tāng	Cyperus and Fritillaria Decoction to Nourish Luxuriance *(xiāng bèi yǎng róng tāng)*, 352
xiāng fù xuán fù huā tāng	Cyperus and Inula Decoction *(xiāng fù xuán fù huā tāng)*, 789-790
xiāng lián wán	Aucklandia and Coptis Pill *(xiāng lián wán)*, 206
xiāng rú sǎn	Mosla Powder *(xiāng rú sǎn)*, 234-235
xiāng shā liù jūn zǐ tāng	Six-Gentlemen Decoction with Aucklandia and Amomum *(xiāng shā liù jūn zǐ tāng)*, 312
xiāng shā píng wèi sǎn	Aucklandia and Amomum Calm the Stomach Powder *(xiāng shā píng wèi sǎn)*, 688-689
xiāng shā píng wèi sǎn	Cyperus and Amomum Calm the Stomach Powder *(xiāng shā píng wèi sǎn)*, 688
xiāng shā yǎng wèi tāng	Nourish the Stomach Decoction with Aucklandia and Amomum *(xiāng shā yǎng wèi tāng)*, 312
xiāng shā zhǐ zhú wán	Aucklandia, Amomum, Unripe Bitter Orange, and Atractylodes Pill *(xiāng shā zhǐ zhú wán)*, 838
xiǎng shēng pò dí wán	Pill for Restoring Sound to a Broken Flute *(xiǎng shēng pò dí wán)*, 795
xiāng sū cóng chǐ tāng	Cyperus, Perilla Leaf, Scallion, and Prepared Soybean Decoction *(xiāng sū cóng chǐ tāng)*, 29
xiāng sū sǎn	Cyperus and Perilla Leaf Powder *(xiāng sū sǎn)*, 29
xiǎo bàn xià jiā fú líng tāng	Minor Pinellia plus Poria Decoction *(xiǎo bàn xià jiā fú líng tāng)*, 551-552
xiǎo bàn xià tāng	Minor Pinellia Decoction *(xiǎo bàn xià tāng)*, 551
xiǎo chái hú tāng	Minor Bupleurum Decoction *(xiǎo chái hú tāng)*, 104-109
xiǎo chéng qì tāng	Minor Order the Qi Decoction *(xiǎo chéng qì tāng)*, 66-67
xiǎo dìng fēng zhū	Minor Arrest Wind Pearls *(xiǎo dìng fēng zhū)*, 653
xiāo fēng sǎn	Eliminate Wind Powder from *Orthodox Lineage (xiāo fēng sǎn)*, 636-638
xiāo fēng sǎn	Eliminate Wind Powder from *Formulary of the Pharmacy Service (xiāo fēng sǎn)*, 638
xiāo fēng sǎn	Eliminate Wind Powder from *Effective Formulas (xiāo fēng sǎn)*, 638
xiǎo hé zhōng yǐn	Minor Harmonize the Middle Drink *(xiǎo hé zhōng yǐn)*, 829
xiǎo huó luò dān	Minor Invigorate the Collaterals Special Pill *(xiǎo huó luò dān)*, 631-632
xiǎo jì yǐn zi	Small Thistle Drink *(xiǎo jì yǐn zi)*, 603-605

xiǎo jiàn zhōng tāng	Minor Construct the Middle Decoction *(xiǎo jiàn zhōng tāng)*, 264-267
xiāo luǒ wán	Reduce Scrofula Pill *(xiāo luǒ wán)*, 798-799
xiǎo qīng lóng jiā shí gāo tāng	Minor Bluegreen Dragon Decoction plus Gypsum *(xiǎo qīng lóng jiā shí gāo tāng)*, 24
xiǎo qīng lóng tāng	Minor Bluegreen Dragon Decoction *(xiǎo qīng lóng tāng)*, 21-24
xiāo rǔ wán	Reduce Infantile Stagnation Pill *(xiāo rǔ wán)*, 835
xiǎo xiàn xiōng tāng	Minor Decoction [for Pathogens] Stuck in the Chest *(xiǎo xiàn xiōng tāng)*, 793-794
xiǎo xù mìng tāng	Minor Extend Life Decoction *(xiǎo xù mìng tāng)*, 621-623
xiāo yán jiě dú wán	Reduce Inflammation and Resolve Pill *(xiāo yán jiě dú wán)*, 865
xiāo yáo sǎn	Rambling Powder *(xiāo yáo sǎn)*, 120-123
xiè bái sǎn	Drain the White Powder from *Wondrous Lantern (xiè bái sǎn)*, 188
xiè bái sǎn	Drain the White Powder *(xiè bái sǎn)*, 186-188
xiè bái sǎn	Drain the White Powder from *Indispensable Tools for Pattern Treatment (xiè bái sǎn)*, 188
xiè gān tāng	Drain the Liver Decoction *(xiè gān tāng)*, 170
xiè huáng sǎn	Drain the Yellow Powder *(xiè huáng sǎn)*, 190-191
xiè qīng wán	Drain the Green Pill *(xiè qīng wán)*, 201-202
xiè xīn dǎo chì tāng	Drain the Epigastrium and Guide Out the Red Decoction *(xiè xīn dǎo chì tāng)*, 197
xiè xīn tāng	Drain the Epigastrium Decoction *(xiè xīn tāng)*, 171-173
xīn jiā huáng lóng tāng	Newly Augmented Yellow Dragon Decoction *(xīn jiā huáng lóng tāng)*, 87-88
xīn jiā sān ǎo tāng	Newly Augmented Three-Unbinding Decoction *(xīn jiā sān ǎo tāng)*, 10
xīn jiā xiāng rú yǐn	Newly Augmented Mosla Drink *(xīn jiā xiāng rú yǐn)*, 237-238
xīn jiā yù nǚ jiān	Newly Augmented Jade Woman Decoction *(xīn jiā yù nǚ jiān)*, 195
xīn yí qīng fèi yǐn	Magnolia Flower Drink to Clear the Lungs *(xīn yí qīng fèi yǐn)*, 188-190
xīn yí sǎn	Magnolia Flower Powder *(xīn yí sǎn)*, 629
xīn zhì jú pí zhú rú tāng	Newly-Formulated Tangerine Peel and Bamboo Shavings Decoction *(xīn zhì jú pí zhú rú tāng)*, 547
xìng qián cōng chǐ tāng	Apricot Kernel, Peucedanum, Scallion, and Prepared Soybean Decoction *(xìng qián cōng chǐ tāng)*, 6, 664
xìng rén huá shí tāng	Apricot Kernel and Talcum Decoction *(xìng rén huá shí tāng)*, 702
xìng sū sǎn	Apricot Kernel and Perilla Leaf Powder *(xìng sū sǎn)*, 663-664
xìng sū yǐn	Apricot Kernel and Perilla Drink *(xìng sū yǐn)*, 29-30
xìng sū yǐn [yòu kē]	Apricot Kernel and Perilla Drink [pediatric version] *(xìng sū yǐn) [yòu kē]*, 34
xiōng guī tiáo xuè yǐn	Chuanxiong and Tangkuei Drink to Regulate the Blood *(xiōng guī tiáo xuè yǐn)*, 583
xù mìng tāng	Major Extend Life Decoction *(xù mìng tāng)*, 623

xuān baí chéng qì tāng	Disseminate the White and Order the Qi Decoction (*xuān baí chéng qì tāng*), 68
xuān bì tāng	Disband Painful Obstruction Decoction (*xuān bì tāng*), 762-763
xuān dú fā biǎo tāng	Dissipate Toxin and Release the Exterior Decoction (*xuān dú fā biǎo tāng*), 43
xuān fèi rùn cháng tāng	Disseminate the Lungs and Moisten the Intestines Decoction (*xuān fèi rùn cháng tāng*), 81
xuán fù dài zhě tāng	Inula and Hematite Decoction (*xuán fù dài zhě tāng*), 542-544
xuán fù huā tāng	Inula Decoction (*xuán fù huā tāng*), 575-577
xuān yù tōng jīng tāng	Diffuse Constraint and Unblock the Channels Decoction (*xuān yù tōng jīng tāng*), 590-591
xuè fǔ zhú yū tāng	Drive Out Stasis from the Mansion of Blood Decoction (*xuè fǔ zhú yū tāng*), 564-567
yán hú suǒ tāng	Corydalis Decoction (*yán hú suǒ tāng*), 524-525
yán nián bàn xià tāng	Pinellia Decoction to Extend Life (*yán nián bàn xià tāng*), 264
yáng hé tāng	Balmy Yang Decoction (*yáng hé tāng*), 869-871
yǎng xīn tāng	Nourish the Heart Decoction from *Comprehensive Collection* (*yǎng xīn tāng*), 461
yǎng xīn tāng	Nourish the Heart Decoction from *Indispensable Tools* (*yǎng xīn tāng*), 462
yǎng yīn qīng fèi tāng	Nourish the Yin and Clear the Lungs Decoction (*yǎng yīn qīng fèi tāng*), 673-675
yǎng zhēng tōng yōu tāng	Nourish the Normal and Unblock the Pylorus Decoction (*yǎng zhēng tōng yōu tāng*), 86
yì gān sǎn	Restrain the Liver Powder (*yì gān sǎn*), 124
yì gōng sǎn	Extraordinary Merit Powder (*yì gōng sǎn*), 311
yī guàn jiān	Linking Decoction (*yī guàn jiān*), 381-383
yì huáng sǎn	Benefit the Yellow Powder (*yì huáng sǎn*), 433-434
yì huáng tāng	Change Yellow [Discharge] Decoction (*yì huáng tāng*), 450-452
yī jiǎ fù mài tāng	One-Shell Decoction to Restore the Pulse (*yī jiǎ fù mài tāng*), 651
yī jiā jiǎn zhèng qì sǎn	First Modification of Rectify the Qi Powder (*yī jiā jiǎn zhèng qì sǎn*), 694
yì qì cōng míng tāng	Augment the Qi and Increase Acuity Decoction (*yì qì cōng míng tāng*), 323
yì qì qīng jīn tāng	Augment Qi and Clear the Metal Decoction (*yì qì qīng jīn tāng*), 386
yì wèi tāng	Benefit the Stomach Decoction (*yì wèi tāng*), 393-394
yì yǐ fù zǐ bài jiàng sǎn	Coix, Aconite Accessory Root, and Patrinia Powder (*yì yǐ fù zǐ bài jiàng sǎn*), 884-886
yì yǐ rén tāng	Coix Decoction from *Indispensable Tools for Pattern Treatment* (*yì yǐ rén tāng*), 886
yì yǐ rén tāng	Coicis Decoction from *Enlightened Physicians* (*yì yǐ rén tāng*), 762
yì yuán sǎn	Augment the Primal Powder (*yì yuán sǎn*), 240
yǐ zì tāng	Decoction "B" (*yǐ zì tāng*), 607
yīn chén fù zǐ gān jiāng tāng	Virgate Wormwood, Aconite Accessory Root, and Ginger Decoction (*yīn chén fù zǐ gān jiāng tāng*), 274

yīn chén hāo tāng	Virgate Wormwood Decoction (*yīn chén hāo tāng*), 710-712
yīn chén sì nì tāng	Virgate Wormwood Decoction for Frigid Extremities (*yīn chén sì nì tāng*), 712
yīn chén wǔ líng sǎn	Virgate Wormwood and Five-Ingredient Powder with Poria (*yīn chén wǔ líng sǎn*), 729
yīn chén zhú fù tāng	Virgate Wormwood, Atractylodes, and Aconite Accessory Root Decoction (*yīn chén zhú fù tāng*), 712-713
yín huā jiě dú tāng	Honeysuckle Decoction to Resolve Toxicity (*yín huā jiě dú tāng*), 865
yín qiáo bài dú sǎn	Honeysuckle and Forsythia Powder to Overcome Pathogenic Influences (*yín qiáo bài dú sǎn*), 49
yín qiáo mǎ bó sǎn	Honeysuckle, Forsythia, and Puffball Powder (*yín qiáo mǎ bó sǎn*), 39
yín qiáo sǎn	Honeysuckle and Forsythia Powder (*yín qiáo sǎn*), 36-39
yín qiáo tāng	Honeysuckle and Forsythia Decoction (*yín qiáo tāng*), 39
yòu guī wán	Restore the Right [Kidney] Pill (*yòu guī wán*), 401-402
yòu guī yǐn	Restore the Right [Kidney] Drink (*yòu guī yǐn*), 402
yù dài wán	Cure Discharge Pill (*yù dài wán*), 722
Yǔ gōng sǎn	Yu's Achievement Powder (*Yǔ gōng sǎn*), 93-94
yù nǚ jiān	Jade Woman Decoction (*yù nǚ jiān*), 193-194
yù píng fēng sǎn	Jade Windscreen Powder (*yù píng fēng sǎn*), 326-328
yù quán wán	Jade Spring Pill (*yù quán wán*), 375-377
yù yè tāng	Jade Fluid Decoction (*yù yè tāng*), 675-677
yù zhēn sǎn	True Jade Powder (*yù zhēn sǎn*), 635-636
yù zhú sǎn	Jade Candle Powder (*yù zhú sǎn*), 338
yuè bì jiā bàn xià tāng	Maidservant from Yue's Decoction plus Pinellia (*yuè bì jiā bàn xià tāng*), 185-186
yuè bì jiā zhú tāng	Maidservant from Yue's Decoction plus Atractylodes (*yuè bì jiā zhú tāng*), 185
yuè bì tāng	Maidservant from Yue's Decoction (*yuè bì tāng*), 185
yuè huá wán	Moonlight Pill (*yuè huá wán*), 387
yuè jū wán	Escape Restraint Pill (*yuè jū wán*), 507-510
yuè shí sǎn	Moon Stone Powder (*yuè shí sǎn*), 897
zài zào sǎn	Renewal Powder (*zài zào sǎn*), 52-53
zàn yù dān	Special Pill to Aid Fertility (*zàn yù dān*), 403-404
zēng yè chéng qì tāng	Increase the Fluids and Order the Qi Decoction (*zēng yè chéng qì tāng*), 88-89
zēng yè tāng	Increase the Fluids Decoction (*zēng yè tāng*), 677-679
zhā qu píng wèi sǎn	Hawthorn and Medicated Leaven Calm the Stomach Powder (*zhā qu píng wèi sǎn*), 829
zhé chòng yǐn	Drink to Turn Back the Penetrating [Vessel] (*zhé chòng yǐn*), 586

zhèn gān xī fēng tāng	Sedate the Liver and Extinguish Wind Decoction *(zhèn gān xī fēng tāng)*, 644-647
zhèn nì bái hǔ tāng	White Tiger Decoction to Suppress Rebellion *(zhèn nì bái hǔ tāng)*, 155
zhēn rén yǎng zàng tāng	True Man's Decoction to Nourish the Organs *(zhēn rén yǎng zàng tāng)*, 425-427
zhēn wǔ tāng	True Warrior Decoction *(zhēn wǔ tāng)*, 744-747
zhēn zhū mǔ wán	Mother-of-Pearl Pill *(zhēn zhū mǔ wán)*, 480-481
zhèng gǔ zǐ jīn dān	Bone-Setter's Purple-Gold Special Pill *(zhèng gǔ zǐ jīn dān)*, 575
zhī bǎi dì huáng wán	Anemarrhena, Phellodendron, and Rehmannia Pill *(zhī bǎi dì huáng wán)*, 369
zhì bǎo dān	Greatest Treasure Special Pill *(zhì bǎo dān)*, 493-495
zhì gān cǎo tāng	Prepared Licorice Decoction *(zhì gān cǎo tāng)*, 356-359
zhǐ jìng sǎn	Stop Spasms Powder *(zhǐ jìng sǎn)*, 634
zhǐ shí dǎo zhì wán	Unripe Bitter Orange Pill to Guide Out Stagnation *(zhǐ shí dǎo zhì wán)*, 829-830
zhǐ shí lǐ zhōng wán	Unripe Bitter Orange Pill to Regulate the Middle *(zhǐ shí lǐ zhōng wán)*, 261
zhǐ shí sháo yào sǎn	Unripe Bitter Orange and Peony Powder *(zhǐ shí sháo yào sǎn)*, 120
zhǐ shí xiāo pǐ wán	Unripe Bitter Orange Pill to Reduce Focal Distention *(zhǐ shí xiāo pǐ wán)*, 839-840
zhǐ shí xiè bái guì zhī tāng	Unripe Bitter Orange, Chinese Garlic, and Cinnamon Twig Decoction *(zhǐ shí xiè bái guì zhī tāng)*, 514-515
zhǐ shí zhī zǐ chǐ tāng	Bitter Orange, Gardenia, and Prepared Soybean Decoction *(zhǐ shí zhī zǐ chǐ tāng)*, 160
zhǐ sòu sǎn	Stop Coughing Powder *(zhǐ sòu sǎn)*, 815-817
zhì zhōng wán	Treat the Middle Pill *(zhì zhōng wán)*, 261
zhǐ zhú tāng	Unripe Bitter Orange and Atractylodes Decoction *(zhǐ zhú tāng)*, 838-839
zhǐ zhú wán	Unripe Bitter Orange and Atractylodes Pill *(zhǐ zhú wán)*, 837-838
zhī zǐ bǎi pí tāng	Gardenia and Phellodendron Decoction *(zhī zǐ bǎi pí tāng)*, 713
zhī zǐ chǐ tāng	Gardenia and Prepared Soybean Decoction *(zhī zǐ chǐ tāng)*, 158-160
zhī zǐ dà huáng tāng	Gardenia and Rhubarb Decoction *(zhī zǐ dà huáng tāng)*, 161
zhī zǐ gān cǎo chǐ tāng	Gardenia, Licorice, and Prepared Soybean Decoction *(zhī zǐ gān cǎo chǐ tāng)*, 160
zhī zǐ gān jiāng tāng	Gardenia and Ginger Decoction *(zhī zǐ gān jiāng tāng)*, 160
zhī zǐ hòu pò tāng	Gardenia and Magnolia Bark Decoction *(zhī zǐ hòu pò tāng)*, 160-161
zhī zǐ qín gé tāng	Gardenia, Scutellaria, and Kudzu Decoction *(zhī zǐ qín gé tāng)*, 161
zhī zǐ shēng jiāng chǐ tāng	Gardenia, Fresh Ginger, and Prepared Soybean Decoction *(zhī zǐ shēng jiāng chǐ tāng)*, 160
zhōng hé tāng	Even-Handed Decoction *(zhōng hé tāng)*, 871
zhōng mǎn fēn xiāo tāng	Separate and Reduce Fullness in the Middle Decoction *(zhōng mǎn fēn xiāo tāng)*, 724
zhōng mǎn fēn xiāo wán	Separate and Reduce Fullness in the Middle Pill *(zhōng mǎn fēn xiāo wán)*, 722-724

zhōng hé tāng	Even-Handed Decoction (*zhōng hé tāng*), 871
zhōu chē wán	Vessel and Vehicle Pill (*zhōu chē wán*), 91-92
zhù chē wán	Halt the Carts Pill (*zhù chē wán*), 432-433
zhù jǐng wán	Preserve Vistas Pill (*zhù jǐng wán*), 391-392
zhù jǐng wán jiā jiǎn fāng	Formula Modified from Preserve Vistas Pill (*zhù jǐng wán jiā jiǎn fāng*), 492-493
zhú lì dá tán wán	Bamboo Sap Pill to Thrust Out Phlegm (*zhú lì dá tán wán*), 797-798
zhū líng tāng	Polyporus Decoction from *Comprehensive Recording* (*zhū líng tāng*), 731
zhū líng tāng	Polyporus Decoction (*zhū líng tāng*), 729-731
zhū shā ān shén wán	Cinnabar Pill to Calm the Spirit (*zhū shā ān shén wán*), 475-476
zhú yè chēng liǔ tāng	Lophatherum and Tamarisk Decoction (*zhú yè chēng liǔ tāng*), 43-45
zhú yè shí gāo tāng	Lophatherum and Gypsum Decoction (*zhú yè shí gāo tāng*), 155-157
zhú yè yù nǚ jiān	Lophatherum Jade Woman Decoction (*zhú yè yù nǚ jiān*), 194-195
zǐ dāng gāo	Lithospermum/Arnebia and Tangkuei Ointment (*zǐ dāng gāo*), 898-899
zǐ gēn mǔ lì tāng	Arnebia/Lithospermum and Oyster Shell Decoction (*zǐ gēn mǔ lì tāng*), 877-878
zī shèn míng mù tāng	Enrich the Kidneys and Improve Vision Decoction (*zī shèn míng mù tāng*), 370
zī shuǐ qīng gān yǐn	Enrich Water and Clear the Liver Drink (*zī shuǐ qīng gān yǐn*), 383
zǐ xuě dān	Purple Snow Special Pill (*zǐ xuě dān*), 490-493
zī yīn jiàng huǒ tāng	Decoction to Enrich Yin and Direct Fire Downward (*zī yīn jiàng huǒ tāng*), 388-389
zuǒ guī wán	Restore the Left [Kidney] Pill (*zuǒ guī wán*), 370-372
zuǒ guī yǐn	Restore the Left [Kidney] Drink (*zuǒ guī yǐn*), 372
zuǒ jīn wán	Left Metal Pill (*zuǒ jīn wán*), 205-206

List of Cited Sources

THIS IS A list of all books and other sources cited in our text arranged by title corresponding to how we have acknowledged sources in the text. Following the English translation of the title, we give the name in Chinese characters, the transliteration of the name, the transliterated name of the putative author, and the date of first publication to the best of our knowledge.

Note that the actual authorship for premodern titles is frequently disputed or unclear. The very oldest texts, like the *Inner Classic*, are compilations by multiple unknown authors. Later on in the history of Chinese medicine, texts are sometimes published under a physician's name by their students or family members based on manuscripts, fragments of writings, or case records. Authors also sometimes published their ideas using the name of a well-known physician rather than their own. The text then comes to be associated with the more famous physician, even though he was clearly not the author. Sometimes these relationships can be easily traced, and sometimes not. Because this book is not a historical study, we list the authors as they are recorded in the *National Union Catalog of Primary Sources for Chinese Medicine* or the *Encyclopedia of Traditional Chinese Medicine*.

We have consulted premodern texts through a variety of both primary and secondary sources such as modern Chinese editions of the source texts, the digital collection of Chinese medical texts published under the name *Medical Classics of Chinese Medicine,* and extracts of primary sources reprinted in modern Chinese secondary sources. A full list of the modern editions of the source texts is available online in the *"Formulas and Strategies* Bibliography of Sources for Premodern Texts"* posted on the Resources page of our publisher's website, *www.eastlandpress.com.*

Wherever we encountered difficulties in a textual passage we have checked different versions of the source text against each other. However, the present volume is not a sinological work. This means that we have relied, in the main, on the accuracy of the sources we have consulted. Anything else would have made the compilation of our text untenable. For the same reason, we do limit ourselves to referencing our translations to the name of the source text, rather than providing full bibliographic details. However, using the sources and bibliographic sources we have listed, it should be possible to trace the original passages with relative ease.

English Title	Chinese Title	Pinyin Title	Author (English)	Author (Chinese)	Date/Dynasty
A Stick to Awaken Physicians	醫門棒喝	*Yī mén bàng hè*	Zhāng Nán / Zhāng Xū-Gǔ	章楠 / 章虛穀	1825
Accounts of Formulas and Symptoms	方症會要	*Fāng zhèng huì yào*	Wú Mài	吳邁	1756
Achievements Regarding Epidemic Rashes	疫疹一得	*Yì zhěn yī dé*	Yú Lín / Yú Shī-Yú	余霖 / 余師愚	1794
Achieving Longevity by Guarding the Source	壽世保元	*Shòu shì bǎo yuán*	Gōng Tíng-Xián	龔廷賢	1615
Additions to the Essential Teachings of [Zhu] Dan-Xi	丹溪心法附餘	*Dān-xī xīn fǎ fù yú*	Fāng Guǎng-Lèi	方廣類	1536
Annotated and Corrected Craft of Medicines and Patterns for Children	小兒藥證直訣箋正	*Xiǎo ér yào zhèng zhí jué qiān zhèng*	Zhāng Shān-Léi / Zhāng Shòu-Yí	張山雷 / 張壽頤	1922
Annotated and Corrected Master Yan's Discussion of Formulas for Children	閻氏小兒方論箋正	*Yàn shì xiǎo ér fāng lùn jiān zhèng*	Zhāng Shān-Léi / Zhāng Shòu-Yí	張山雷 / 張壽頤	1922
Annotated and Corrected Synopsis of Shen's Women's Disorders	沈氏女科輯要箋正	*Shén shì nǚ kē jí yào jiān zhèng*	Zhāng Shān-Léi / Zhāng Shòu-Yí	張山雷 / 張壽頤	1933
Annotated Fine Formulas from Generations of Famous Physicians	歷代名醫良方註釋	*Lì dài míng yī liáng fāng zhù shì*	Rǎn Xuě-Fēng	冉雪峰	1983
Annotation and Explanation of the Discussion of Cold Damage	注解傷寒論	*Zhù jiě shāng hán lùn*	Chéng Wú-Jǐ	成無己	1144
Appendices to the Classified Classic	類經附翼	*Lèi jīng fù yì*	Zhāng Jiè-Bīn / Zhāng Jǐng-Yuè	張介賓 / 張景岳	1624
Appendices to the Golden Cabinet	金匱翼	*Jīn guì yì*	Yóu Zài-Jīng	尤在涇	1768
Applications of Chinese Medical Prescriptions	中藥處方的應用	*Zhōng yào chù fāng de yìng yòng*	Wáng Zhàn-Xǐ	王占璽	1980
Arcane Essentials from the Imperial Library	外台秘要	*Wài tái mì yào*	Wáng Tāo	王燾	752
Assorted Works from Enlightened Physicians	明醫雜著	*Míng yī zá zhù*	Wáng Lún; annotated by Xuē Jǐ	王綸; 薛己	1549
Awakening of the Mind in Medical Studies	醫學心悟	*Yī xué xīn wù*	Chéng Guó-Péng	程國彭	1732
Awakening to the Real	真悟篇	*Zhēn wù piān*	Zhāng Bó-Duān	張伯端	1075
Bases of Medicine	醫原	*Yī yuán*	Shí Shòu-Táng / Shí Fú-Nán	石壽棠 / 石芾南	1861
Basic Questions	素問	*Sù wèn*	Anonymous		Primarily later Han
Book on Nourishing the Elderly and Serving One's Parents	養老奉親書	*Yǎng lǎo fèng qīn shū*	Chén Zhí	陳直	1085
Book to Safeguard Life Arranged According to Pattern	類證活人書	*Lèi zhèng huó rén shū*	Zhū Gōng	朱肱	1108
Building Efficacious Formulas on the Eight Methods	八法效方舉隅	*Bā fǎ xiào fāng jǔ yú*	Rǎn Xuě-Fēng	冉雪峰	1959

English Title	Chinese Title	Pinyin Title	Author (English)	Author (Chinese)	Date/Dynasty
Careful Deliberations on Wind Stroke	中風斠詮	*Zhòng fēng jiào quán*	Zhāng Shān-Léi / Zhāng Shòu-Yí	張山雷 / 張壽頤	1922
Case Histories of Cheng Men-Xue	程門雪醫案	*Chéng Mén-Xuě yī àn*	Shanghai College of Chinese Medicine	上海中醫學院	2002
Case Histories of Ding Gan-Ren	丁甘仁醫案	*Dīng gān rén yī àn*	Dīng Gān-Rén / Zé Zhōu	丁甘仁 / 澤周	1927
Case Histories of Huang Wen-Dong	黃文東醫案	*Huáng Wén-Dōng yī àn*	Huáng Wén-Dōng	黃文東	2001
Case Records as a Guide to Clinical Practice	臨證指南醫案	*Lín zhèng zhǐ nán yī àn*	Yè Guì / Yè Tiān-Shì / Yè Xiāng-Yán	葉桂 / 葉天士 / 葉香岩	1746
Casual Notes on Medicine	醫醫偶錄	*Yī yī ǒu lù*	Chén Niàn-Zǔ / Chén Xiū-Yuán	陳念祖 / 陳修園	1802
Categorization of Formulas from the Discussion of Cold Damage	傷寒論類方	*Shāng hán lùn lèi fāng*	Xú Dà-Chūn / Xú Líng-Tái	徐大椿 / 徐靈台	1759
Categorized Collected Formulas	類聚方	*Ruijuhō*	Yoshimasu Todō	吉益東洞	1853
Categorized Essentials for Normalizing the Structure	正體類要	*Zhèng tǐ lèi yào*	Xuē Jǐ	薛己	1529
Chinese Medical Formulas	中醫方劑學	*Zhōng yī fang jì xué*	Nanjing College of Traditional Chinese Medicine	南京中醫學院	1959
Chinese Medical Treatment for Epidemic Encephalitis B	流行性乙型腦炎中醫治療法	*Liú xíng xìng yǐ xíng nǎo yán zhōng yī zhì liáo fǎ*	Hebei Provincial Health Workers Association	河北省衛生工作者協會	1955
Clarifying Doubts about Damage from Internal and External Causes	內外傷辨惑論	*Nèi wài shāng biàn huò lùn*	Lǐ Gǎo / Lǐ Dōng-Yuán	李杲 / 李東垣	1247
Classic of Difficulties	難經	*Nán jīng*	Anonymous; traditionally attributed to Qín Yuè-Rén	秦越人	Probably Eastern Han
Classified Compilation of Medical Prescriptions	醫方類聚	*Uibang yuchwi*	Kim Yemong	金禮蒙	1445
Clear Explanations to the Discussion of Cold Damage and Later Systematic Differentiations	傷寒論後條辨直解	*Shāng hán lùn jīhòu tiáo biàn zhí jiě*	Chéng Yīng-Máo / Chéng Jiān-Qiàn	程應旄 / 程郊倩	1670
Cold Damage Revelations	傷寒大白	*Shāng hán dà bái*	Qín Zhī-Zhēn / Qín Huáng-Shì	秦之楨 / 秦皇士	1714
Collectanea of Investigations from the Realm of Medicine	醫林纂要探源	*Yī lín zuān yaò tàn yuán*	Wāng Fú	汪紱	1758
Collected Annotations on the Discussion of Cold Damage	傷寒論集注	*Shāng hán lùn jí zhù*	Zhāng Zhì-Cōng / Zhāng Yǐn-Ān	張志聰 / 張隱庵	1683
Collected Experiences of Zhu Liang-Chun in Using Medicines	朱良春用藥經驗集	*Zhū Liáng-Chūn yòng yào jīng yàn jí*	Zhū Bù-Xiān / Hé Shào-Qí, eds.	朱步先 / 何紹奇　整理	1999
Collected Experiences on Treating Sores	瘍科心得集	*Yáng kē xīn dé jí*	Gāo Bǐng-Jūn	高秉鈞	1806
Collected Formulas from the Crane-Feeding Pavilion	飼鶴亭集方	*Sì hè tíng jí fāng*	Líng Huàn	凌奐	1892

English Title	Chinese Title	Pinyin Title	Author (English)	Author (Chinese)	Date/Dynasty
Collected Medical Writings of Jiang Chun-Hua	姜春華醫論集	*Jiāng Chūn-Huá yī lùn jí*	Jiāng Chūn-Huá	姜春華	1986
Collected Medical Writings of Li Ke-Shao	李克紹醫學文集	*Lǐ Kè-Shào yī xué wén jí*	Lǐ Kè-Shào	李克紹	2006
Collected Treatises of [Zhang] Jing-Yue	景岳全書	*Jǐng-Yuè quán shū*	Zhāng Jiè-Bīn / Zhāng Jǐng-Yuè	張介賓 / 張景岳	1624
Collected Writings on Renewal of the Discussion of Cold Damage	傷寒來蘇集	*Shāng hán lái sū jí*	Kē Qín / Kē Yùn-Bó	柯琴 / 柯韻伯	Qing
Collection for the Common Pursuit of Longevity	同壽錄	*Tōng shòu lù*	Xiāng Tiān-Ruì	項天瑞	1762
Collection of Empirical Formulas	集驗良方	*Jí yàn liáng fāng*	Nián Xī-Yáo	年希堯	1724
Collection of Excellent, Efficacious Formulas	靈驗良方匯編	*Líng yàn liáng fāng huì biān*	Tián Jiān-Lái / Tián-Shì-Ān	田间来 / 田是庵	1729
Collection of Experiential and Secret Chinese Medical Formulas from Shanxi Province	山西省中醫驗方秘方匯集	*Shān xī shěng zhōng yī yàn fāng mì fāng huì jí*	Shanxi Provincial Health Bureau	山西省衛生廳	1956
Collection of Medical Writings Following the Work of Others	醫學從眾錄	*Yī xué cóng zhòng lù*	Chén Niàn-Zǔ / Chén Xiū-Yuán	陳念祖 / 陳修園	1820
Collection of Orally Transmitted Explanations of Medical Formulas	醫方口訣集	*Ihō kuketsu shū*	Tosa Dōju	土佐 道壽	1687
Collection of Treasured Essentials	寶精集	JAPANESE 200807 Unknown	Yakazu Dōmei	矢數道明	Unknown
Collection of Versatility	不居集	*Bù jū jí*	Wú Chéng / Wú Jiàn-Quán / Wú Shī-Lǎng	吳澄 / 吳鑒泉 / 吳師朗	1739
Collection of Writings on the Mechanisms of Disease, Suitability of Qi, and the Safeguarding of Life as Discussed in Basic Questions	素問病機宜保名集	*Sù wèn bìng jī yí bǎo míng jí*	Liú Wán-Sù	劉完素	1186
Collection on External Medicine to be Kept Close at Hand	外科集腋	*Wài kē jí yè*	Zhāng Jǐng-Yán	張景顏	1814
Collection on the Discussion of Cold Damage	傷寒論集成	*Shōkanron shūsei / Shāng hán lùn jí chéng*	Yamada Seichin	山田正珍	1789
Collection Picked by Immortals	仙拈集	*Xiān nián jí*	Lǐ Wén-Bǐng / Lǐ Huàn Zhāng	李文炳 / 李煥章	1754
Commentary on the Classic of Materia Medica	本經疏証	*Běn jīng shū zhèng*	Zōu Shù / Zōu Rùn-Ān	鄒澍 / 鄒潤安	c. 1837, pub. 1849
Compendium of China's Medicine and Medicinals	中國醫藥匯海	*Zhōng guó yī yào huì hǎi*	Cài Lù-Xiān	蔡陸仙	1937
Compendium of Secrets for Women's Diseases	女科秘訣大全	*Nǚ kē mì jué dà quán*	Chén Lián-Fǎng	陳蓮舫	1909
Compendium of Songs on Modern Formulas	時方歌括	*Shí fāng gē kuò*	Chén Niàn-Zǔ / Chén Xiū-Yuán	陳念祖 / 陳修園	1801
Compendium of the Rules of Conduct for Physicians	醫林繩墨大全	*Yī lín shéng mò dà quán*	Fāng Yú-Jí	方隅集	1584
Compilation of Materials of Benevolence for the Body	體仁彙編	*Tǐ rén huì biān*	Péng Yòng-Guāng	彭用光	1549

English Title	Chinese Title	Pinyin Title	Author (English)	Author (Chinese)	Date/Dynasty
Complete Book of Patterns and Treatments in External Medicine	外科證治全書	*Wài kē zhèng zhì quán shū*	Xǔ Kè-Chāng	許克昌	1831
Complete Collection of Charts and Texts Past and Present	古今圖書集成	*Gǔ jīn tú shū jí chéng*	Jiǎng Tíng-Xī / Yáng Sūn / Yǒu Jūn / Xī Gǔ / Nán shā	蔣廷錫 / 揚孫 / 酉君 / 西谷 / 南沙	1726
Complete Compendium of Cold Damage	傷寒全生集	*Shāng hán quán shēng jí*	Anonymous		1445
Complete Compendium of Patterns and Treatments in External Medicine	外科證治全生集	*Wài kē zhèng zhì quán shēng jí*	Wáng Wéi-Dé	王維德	1740
Complete Treatise for Benefiting Society	濟世全書	*Jì shì quán shū*	Wāng Qǐ-Shèng	汪啓聖	1696
Complete Treatise on Experience with Sores	瘡瘍經驗全書	*Chuāng yáng jīng yàn quán shū*	Dòu Mò (Jié) / Dòu Zǐ-Shēng	竇默(又名傑) / 竇子聲	1569
Complete Treatise on Measles	麻疹全書	*Má zhěn quán shū*	Huá Shòu [attributed]	滑壽	Yuan
Complete Treatise on Respecting Life from the Lofty Precipice	嵩崖尊生全書	*Sōng yá zūn shēng quán shū*	Jǐng Rì-Zhěn / Jǐng Dōng Yáng / Jǐng Sōng Yá	景日昣 / 景東陽 / 景嵩崖	1696
Comprehensive and Subtle Discussion on Children's Health	小兒衛生總微論	*Xiǎo ér wèi shēng zǒng wēi lùn*	Unknown		1156
Comprehensive Medicine According to Master Han	韓氏醫通	*Hán shì yī tōng*	Hán Mào	韓懋	1522
Comprehensive Medicine According to Master Zhang	張氏醫通	*Zhāng shì yī tōng*	Zhāng Lù / Zhāng Lù-Yù / Zhāng Shí-Wán	張璐 / 張路玉 / 張石頑	1695
Comprehensive Outline of Medicine	醫學網目	*Yī xué gāng mù*	Lóu Yīng	樓英	1565
Comprehensive Outline of the Materia Medica	本草網目	*Běn cǎo gāng mù*	Lǐ Shí-Zhēn / Lǐ Dōng-Bì	李時珍 / 李東璧	1590
Comprehensive Outline on Benefiting Yang	濟陽網目	*Jì yáng gāng mù*	Wǔ Zhī-Wàng / Shū-Qīng / Yáng-Yū	武之望 / 叔卿 / 陽紆	1626
Comprehensive Outline on Benefiting Yin	濟陰網目	*Jì yīn gāng mù*	Wǔ Zhī-Wàng / Shū Qīng / Yáng-Yū	武之望 / 叔卿 / 陽紆	1620
Comprehensive Recording of Sagely Beneficence	聖濟總錄	*Shèng jì zǒng lù*	[Short form of *Comprehensive Recording of Sagely Beneficence from the Zhenghe Era*]		
Comprehensive Recording of Sagely Beneficence from the Zhenghe Era	政和聖濟總錄	*Zhèng hé shèng jì zǒng lù*	Song imperial court		1117
Concise Formulas to Aid the Multitudes	簡要濟眾方	*Jiǎn yào jì zhòng fāng*	Zhōu Yìng	周應	1051
Concise Medical Guidelines	簡明醫殼	*Jiǎn míng yī gòu*	Sūn Zhì-Hóng / Sūn Kè-Róng / Sūn Tái-Shí	孫志宏 / 孫克容 / 孫台石	1629
Concise Medicine	醫便	*Yī biàn*	Wáng Sān-Cái	王三才	1587

English Title	Chinese Title	Pinyin Title	Author (English)	Author (Chinese)	Date/Dynasty
Confucians' Duties to Their Parents	儒門事親	*Rú mén shì qīn*	Zhāng Cóng-Zhèng / Zhāng Zǐ-Hé	張從正 / 張子和	1228
Contemporary Explanations of Ancient Formulas	古方今釋	*Gǔ fāng jīn shì*	Dīng Xué-Píng	丁學屏	2002
Continuation of Classified Case Histories by Renowned Physicians	續名醫類案	*Xù míng yī lèi àn*	Wèi Zhī-Xiù	魏之琇	1770
Continuing Discussing Cold Damage	傷寒纘論	*Shāng hán zuǎn lùn*	Zhāng Lù / Zhāng Lù-Yù / Zhāng Shí-Wán	張璐 / 張路玉 / 張石頑	1667
Convenient Reader of Established Formulas	成方便讀	*Chéng fāng biàn dú*	Zhāng Bǐng-Chéng	張秉成	1904
Convenient Reader of Materia Medica	本草便讀	*Běn cǎo biàn dú*	Zhāng Bǐng-Chéng	張秉成	1887
Correct Transmission of Medicine	醫學正傳	*Yī xué zhèng chuán*	Yú Tuán	虞搏	1515
Correction of Errors Among Physicians	醫林改錯	*Yī lín gǎi cuò*	Wáng Qīng-Rèn	王清任	1830
Craft of Medicines and Patterns for Children	小兒藥證真訣	*Xiǎo ér yào zhèng zhí jué*	Qián Yǐ	錢乙	1119
Delving into the Mysteries of the Golden Cabinet	金匱鉤玄	*Jīn guī gōu xuán*	Zhū Zhèn-Hēng / Zhū Dān-Xī / Zhū Yàn-Xiū	朱震亨 / 朱丹溪 / 朱彥修	Yuan
Deriving New Treatments for Patterns of Miscellaneous Disorders in Chinese Internal Medicine	中醫內科雜病證治新義	*Zhōng yī nèi kē zá bìng zhèng zhì xīn yì*	Hú Guāng-Cí	胡光慈	1958
Detailed Explanation of Versified Prescriptions	湯頭歌訣詳解	*Tāng tóu gē jué xiáng jiě*	Zhū Liáng-Chūn, Xuē Bàn-Dīng	朱良春, 薛半丁	1963
Detailed Materia Medica	本草詳節	*Běn cǎo xiáng jié*	Mǐn Yuè	閩鉞	1681
Differential Diagnosis in Traditional Chinese Medicine	中醫症狀鑑別診斷學	*Zhōng yī zhèng zhuàng jiàn bié zhěn duàn xué*	China Academy of Traditional Chinese Medicine, Zhào Jīn-Duó	中國中醫研究院, 趙金鐸	1984
Differentiating Lurking Pathogens and Externally-Contracted Diseases during Three Seasons	三時伏氣外感篇	*Sān shí fú qì wài gǎn piàn*	Yè Guì / Yè Tiān-Shì / Yè Xiāng-Yán	葉桂 / 葉天士 / 葉香岩	Early 18th century
Discourse on Tracing Back to the Medical Classics	醫經溯迴集	*Yī jīng sù huí jí*	Wáng Lǚ	王履	1368
Discourse on Tracing Back to the Source of [the Discussion] of Cold Damage	傷寒溯源集	*Shāng hán sù yuán jí*	Qián Huáng	錢潢	1707
Discussing Medicinal Substances	論藥物	*Lùn yào wù*	Zhāng Cì-Gōng / Zhāng Chéng-Zhī	章次公 / 章成之	1930's
Discussing the Remainders of the [Discussion of] Cold Damage	傷寒緒論	*Shāng hán xù lùn*	Zhāng Lù / Zhāng Lù-Yù / Zhāng Shí-Wán	張璐 / 張路玉 / 張石頑	1678
Discussion and Annotation of the Essentials from the Golden Cabinet	金匱要略論注	*Jīn guì yào lüè lùn zhù*	Xú Bīn	徐彬	1671
Discussion Illuminating the Principles of Cold Damage	傷寒明理論	*Shāng hán míng lǐ lùn*	Chéng Wú-Jǐ	成無己	1156

English Title	Chinese Title	Pinyin Title	Author (English)	Author (Chinese)	Date/Dynasty
Discussion of Blood Patterns	血證論	*Xuè zhèng lùn*	Táng Zōng-Hǎi / Táng Róng-Chūan	唐宗海 / 唐容川	1884
Discussion of Cold Damage Edited for Meaning	傷寒論輯義	*Shōkanron shugi*	Tamba Motoyasu	丹波元簡	1801
Discussion of Cold Damage	傷寒論	*Shāng hán lùn*	Zhāng Jī / Zhāng Zhòng-Jǐng	張機 / 張仲景	c. 220
Discussion of Emergency Formulas for Pediatric Macules	小兒斑疹備急方論	*Xiǎo ér bān zhěn bèi jí fāng lùn*	Dǒng Jí	董汲	Late 11th century
Discussion of Famous Physicians' Formulas [alternate name for *Discussion of Famous Physicians' Formulas Past and Present*]	名醫方論	*Míng yī fāng lùn*	Luó Měi	羅美	1675
Discussion of Famous Physicians' Formulas Past and Present	古今名醫方論	*Gǔ jīn míng yī fāng lùn*	Luó Měi	羅美	1675
Discussion of Formulas for Pediatric Pox and Rashes	小兒痘疹方論	*Xiǎo ér dòu zhěn fāng lùn*	Chén Wén-Zhōng	陳文中	13th century
Discussion of Illnesses, Patterns, and Formulas Related to the Unification of the Three Etiologies	三因極一病證方論	*Sān yīn jí yī bìng zhèng fāng lùn*	Chén Yán	陳言	1174
Discussion of Medical Formulas	醫方論	*Yī fāng lùn*	Fèi Bó-Xióng	費伯雄	1865
Discussion of Medicinal Properties	藥性論	*Yào xìng lùn*	Chén Zhōu	陳周	19th century
Discussion of Seasonal Diseases	時病論	*Shí bìng lùn*	Léi Fēng	雷豐	1882
Discussion of Sudden Turmoil Disorders	霍亂論	*Huò luàn lùn*	Wáng Shì-Xióng	王士雄	1862
Discussion of the Origins of the Symptoms of Disease	諸病源侯論	*Zhū bìng yuán hòu lùn*	Cháo Yuán-Fāng	巢元方	610
Discussion of the Spleen and Stomach	脾胃論	*Pí wèi lùn*	Lǐ Gǎo / Lǐ Dōng-Yuán	李杲 / 李東垣	13th century
Discussion of Warm Epidemics	溫疫論	*Wēn yì lùn*	Wú Yǒu-Xìng / Wú Yòu-Kě	吳有性 / 吳又可	1642
Discussion of Warm-Heat Pathogen [Disorders]	溫熱論	*Wēn rè lun*	Yè Guì / Yè Tiān-Shì / Yè Xiāng-Yán	葉桂 / 葉天士 / 葉香岩	Early 18th century
Displays of Enlightened Physicians	明醫指掌	*Míng yī zhǐ zhǎng*	Huáng-Fǔ Zhōng	皇甫中	Ming
Dissecting the Secrets of Sustaining Life	攝生秘剖	*Shè shēng mì pōu*	Hóng Jī / Hóng Jiǔ-Yǒu	洪基 / 洪九有	1638
Diverse Collection of Famous Formulas	雜類名方	*Zá lèi míng fāng*	Dù Sī-Jìng	杜思敬	Yuan
Divine Husbandman's Classic of the Materia Medica	神農本草經	*Shén nóng běn cǎo jīng*	Anonymous		Probably later Han
Divine Pivot	靈樞	*Líng shū*	Anonymous		Probably later Han
Divinely Ingenious Surefire Formulas	神巧萬全方	*Shén qiǎo wàn quán fāng*	Liú Yuán-Bīn / Liú Zǐ-Yí / Tōng Zhēn Zǐ	劉元賓 / 劉子儀 / 通真子	Song

English Title	Chinese Title	Pinyin Title	Author (English)	Author (Chinese)	Date/Dynasty
Dong-Yuan's Tried and Tested Formulas	東垣試效方	Dōng-Yuán shì xiào fāng	Lǐ Gǎo / Lǐ Dōng-Yuán; edited by Luó Tiān-Yì	李杲 / 李東垣；羅天益 整理	1202
Dream Creek Essays	夢溪筆談	Mèng xī bǐ tán	Shěn Kuò / Shěn Cún-Zhōng	沈括 / 沈存中	11th century
Effective Formulas from Generations of Physicians	世醫得效方	Shì yī dé xiào fāng	Wēi Yì-Lín	危亦林	1345
Effective Formulas from the Hall of Literature	文堂集驗方	Wén táng jí yàn fāng	Hé Jīng / Hé Huì Chuān	何京 / 何惠川	1775
Effective Medical Formulas Arranged by Category by Master Zhu	類編朱氏集驗醫方	Lèi biān Zhū shì jí yàn yī fāng	Zhū Zuǒ	朱佐	1266
Elaborating on the Subtleties of Cold Damage	傷寒發微	Shāng hán fā wēi	Cáo Jiā-Dá / Cáo Yǐng-Fú	曹穎甫 / 曹家達	1933
Elaborating on the Subtleties of the Golden Cabinet	金匱發微	Jīn guì fā wēi	Cáo Jiā-Dá / Cáo Yǐng-Fú	曹穎甫 / 曹家達	1936
Elucidating the Meaning of Discussion of Formulas from the Golden Cabinet	金匱方論衍義	Jīn guì fāng lùn yǎn yì	Zhào Liáng-Rén / Zhào Yǐ-Dé	趙良仁 / 趙以德	1368
Elucidations of the Signs and Explications of the Graphs	說文解字	Shuō wén jiě zì	Xǔ Shèn	許慎	100
Emergency Formulas to Keep Up One's Sleeve	肘後備急方	Zhǒu hòu bèi jí fāng	Gě Hóng	葛洪	3rd century
Encountering the Sources of the Classic of Materia Medica	本經逢原	Běn jīng féng yuán	Zhāng Lù / Zhāng Lù-Yù / Zhāng Shí-Wán	張璐 / 張路玉 / 張石頑	c. 1670
Encountering the Sources of Warm-Heat Pathogen Diseases	溫熱逢原	Wēn rè féng yuán	Liǔ Bǎo-Yí / Liǔ Gǔ-Sūn / Liǔ Guān-Qún	柳寶詒 / 柳谷孫 / 柳冠群	Late Qing
Encyclopedia of Chinese Medical Formulas	中醫方劑大辭典	Zhōng yī fang jì dà cí diǎn	Péng Huái-Rén	彭懷仁	1999
Encyclopedia of Chinese Medicine	中醫大辭典	Zhōng yī dà cí diǎn	China Academy of Traditional Chinese Medicine, Guangzhou College of Traditional Chinese Medicine	中國中醫研究院，廣州中醫學院	1995
Encyclopedia of the Medicine of China	中國醫學大辭典	Zhōng guó yī xué dà cí diǎn	Xiè Guān	謝觀	1936
Enumeration of Formulas Omitted from the Inner Classic	內經拾遺方論	Nèi jīng shí yí fāng lùn	Luò Lóng-Jí	駱龍吉	Song
Essays on Medicine Esteeming the Chinese and Respecting the Western	醫學衷中參西錄	Yī xué zhōng zhōng cān xī lù	Zhāng Xī-Chún / Zhāng Shòu-Fǔ	張錫純 / 張壽甫	1918-1934
Essential Formulas to Support Longevity	扶壽精方	Fú shòu jīng fāng	Wú Mín / Wú Jìn Shān	吳旻 / 吳近山	1534
Essential Meaning of the Medical Classics [Approached] through the Convergence and Assimilation of Chinese and Western [Knowledge]	中西匯通醫經精義	Zhōng xī huì tōng yī jīng jīng yì	Táng Zōng-Hǎi / Táng Róng Chuān	唐宗海 / 唐容川	1892

English Title	Chinese Title	Pinyin Title	Author (English)	Author (Chinese)	Date/Dynasty
Essential Subtleties on the Silver Sea	銀海精微	*Yín hǎi jīng wēi*	Sūn Sī-Miǎo [attributed]	孫思邈	Prob. compiled late 16th century
Essential Teachings about Pox and Rashes Passed Down in Medical Lineages	痘疹世醫心法	*Dòu zhěn shì yī xīn fǎ*	Wàn Quán	萬泉	1568
Essential Teachings of [Zhu] Dan-Xi	丹溪心法	*Dān Xī xīn fǎ*	Zhū Zhèn-Hēng / Zhū Dān-Xī / Zhū Yàn-Xiū	朱震亨 / 朱丹溪 / 朱彥修	1481
Essential Teachings on External Medicine	外科心法	*Wài kē xīn fǎ*	Xuē Jǐ	薛己	16th century
Essential Teachings on Pregnancy and Childbirth	胎產心法	*Tāi chǎn xīn fǎ*	Yán Chún-Xǐ / Chéng Zhāi	閻純璽 / 誠齋	1730
Essentials for Those Who Do Not Know Medicine	不知醫必要	*Bù zhī yī bì yào*	Liáng Lián-Fū / Zǐ Cūn	梁廉夫 / 子村	1880
Essentials from the Golden Cabinet	金匱要略	*Jīn guì yào lüè*	Zhāng Jī / Zhāng Zhòng-Jǐng	張機 / 張仲景	c. 220
Essentials of [Zhu] Dan-Xi's Treatment Methods	丹溪治法心要	*Dān-Xī zhì fǎ xīn yào*	Gāo Shū-Yuán	高叔原	1543
Essentials of the Materia Medica	本草備要	*Běn cǎo bèi yào*	Wāng Áng / Wāng Rèn-Ān	汪昂 / 汪訒庵	1664
Everlasting Categorization of Inscribed Formulas	永類鈐方	*Yǒng lèi qián fāng*	Lǐ Zhòng-Nán	李仲南	1331
Exemplars for Applying the Principles of External Medicine	外科理例	*Wài kē lǐ lìè*	Wāng Jī	汪機	Ming
Expansion of the Categorized Collected Formulas	類聚方廣義	*Ruijuhō kōgi*	Odai Yōdō	尾台榕堂	1853
Experiential Formulas from the Auspicious Bamboo Hall	瑞竹堂經驗方	*Ruì Zhú-Táng jīng yàn fāng*	Shā-Tú Mù-Sū	沙圖穆蘇	1326
Explaining [Zhang Zhong-Jing's] 113 Strategies	百一三方解	*Bǎi yī sān fāng jiě*	Wén Mèng-Xiāng	文夢香	Qing
Explanation of the Classic of Materia Medica	本草經解	*Běn cǎo jīng jiě*	Yè Guì / Yè Tiān-Shì / Yè Xiāng-Yán	葉桂 / 葉天士 / 葉香岩	1724
Explanation of the Discussion of Cold Damage	傷寒論講解	*Shāng hán lùn jiǎng jiě*	Wáng Qí	王琦	1988
Explicating the Discussion of Cold Damage	傷寒釋義	*Shāng hán lùn shì yì*	Nánjīng College of Traditional Chinese Medicine	南京中醫學院	1958
Expounding on the [Essentials from] the Golden Cabinet	金匱詮釋	*Jīn guì quán shì*	Jīn Shòu-Shān	金壽山	1986
Expounding on the Origins of Medicine	醫學啟源	*Yī xué qǐ yuán*	Zhāng Yuán-Sù / Zhāng Jié-Gǔ	張元素 / 張潔古	Yuan
Extension of the Important Formulas Worth a Thousand Gold Pieces	千金方衍義	*Qiān jīn fāng yǎn yì*	Zhāng Lù / Zhāng Lù-Yù / Shí wán lǎo rén	張璐 / 字路玉 / 石頑老人	1698
Extension of the Materia Medica	本草衍義	*Běn cǎo yǎn yì*	Kòu Zōng-Shì	寇宗奭	1116

English Title	Chinese Title	Pinyin Title	Author (English)	Author (Chinese)	Date/Dynasty
Extensive Essentials of Miscellaneous Diseases	雜病廣要	*Zatsubyō Kōyō*	Tamba Motoyasu	丹波元簡	1856
Extensive Notes on Medicine [from the First-awakened Studio]	【先醒齋】醫學廣筆記	*[Xiān xǐng zhāi] Yī xué guǎng bǐ jì*	Miào Xī-Yōng / Miào Zhòng-Chún / Miào Mù-Tái	繆希雍 / 繆仲醇 / 繆慕台	1613
Externally-Contracted Patterns from Xitang	西塘感證	*Xī táng gǎn zhèng*	Dǒng Fèi-Wēng	董廢翁	1725
Extraordinarily Correct Formulas	奇正方	*Kishō hō*	Kako Kakushū	賀古角洲	1831
Family Secrets for Nursing Infants	育嬰家秘	*Yù yīng jiā mì*	Wàn Quán / Wàn Mì-Zhāi	萬全 / 萬密齋	1549
Fang's Orthodox Lineage of Pulse and Symptoms	方氏脈證正宗 / 醫學正宗	*Fāng shì mài zhèng zhèng zōng also known as Yī xué zhèng zōng*	Fāng Zhào-Quán	方肇權	1749
Feng's Secret Records from the Brocade Purse	馮氏錦囊秘錄	*Féng shì jǐn náng mì lù*	Féng Zhào-Zhāng	馮兆張	1702
Fine Formulas by Su and Shen	蘇沈良方	*Sū Shěn liáng fāng*	Sū Shì / Sū Zǐ-Zhān / Sū Dōng-Pō and Shěn Kuò / Shěn Cún-Zhōng	蘇軾 / 蘇子瞻 / 蘇東坡; 沈括 / 沈存中	1075
Fine Formulas for Women	婦人良方	*Fù rén liáng fāng*	Chén Zì-Míng	陳自明	1237
Fine Formulas for Women with Annotations and Commentary	校注婦人良方	*Jiào zhù fù rén liáng fāng*	Chén Zì-Míng; edited by Xuē Jǐ	陳自明; 薛己	Ming [16th century]
Fine Formulas of Wonderful Efficacy	奇效良方	*Qí xiào liáng fāng*	Dǒng Sù / Fāng Xián	董宿 / 方賢	1470
Five Texts by [Hu] Shen-Rou	慎柔五書	*Shèn-Róu wǔ shū*	Hú Shèn-Róu	胡慎柔	1636
Formula Appearances from the Inner Platform of the Golden Mirror	金鏡內台方儀	*Jīn jìng nèi tái fāng yí*	Xǔ Hóng / Xǔ Zōng Dào	許宏 / 許宗道	1422
Formulary and Mnemonics from 'No Mistake' Pharmacy	勿誤藥室方函口訣	*Futsugo yakushitsu hōkan kuketsu*	Asada Sōhaku	淺田宗伯	1956
Formulary of the Imperial Pharmacy	御藥院方	*Yù yào yuàn fāng*	Xǔ Guó-Zhēn	許國楨	1267
Formulary of the Pharmacy Service for Benefiting the People in the Taiping Era	太平惠民和劑局方	*Tài píng huì mín hé jì jú fāng*	Imperial Medical Bureau	太醫局	1107
Formulas	方劑學	*Fāng jì xué*	Lǐ Fēi, ed.	李飛(編)	2002
Formulas Bequeathed by the Unorthodox Genius Liu Juan-Zi	劉涓子鬼遺方	*Liú Juān-Zǐ guǐ yí fāng*	Liú Juān-Zǐ	劉涓子	499
Formulas Categorized by the Stratagems of Pattern Treatment	證治要訣類方	*Zhèng zhì yào jué lèi fāng*	Dài Yuán-Lǐ / Dài Sī-Gōng / Dài Fù Yǎn	戴原禮 / 戴思恭 / 戴復厓	1405
Formulas from Benevolent Sages Compiled during the Taiping Era	太平聖惠方	*Tài píng shèng huì fāng*	Wáng Huái-Yǐn, et. al.	王懷隱	992
Formulas from the Hall of Benevolent Righteousness	惠直堂經驗方	*Huì zhí táng jīng yàn fāng*	Táo Chén-Xī / Táo Dōng-Táo / Qīng Shān xué shì	陶承熹 / 陶東亭 / 青山學士	1734

English Title	Chinese Title	Pinyin Title	Author (English)	Author (Chinese)	Date/Dynasty
Formulas from the Discussion Illuminating the Yellow Emperor's Basic Questions	黃帝素問宣明論方	Huáng Dì sù wèn xuān míng lùn fāng	Liú Wán-Sù	劉完素	1172
Formulas from the Discussion on Women's Precious Delivery	婦寶產論方	Fuhosan ronhō	Kagawa Shigen	賀川子玄	1851
Formulas in Verse from the Scholar's Studio in Two Volumes	書種室歌訣二種	Shū Zhǒng Shì gē jué èr zhǒng	Chéng Mén-Xué [edited by Zhāng Jìn-Rén, et. al.]	程門學 [張鏡人等整理]	1985
Formulas Kept by the Wei Family	魏氏家藏方	Wèi shì jiā cáng fāng	Wèi Xiàn	魏峴	1227
Formulas of Broad Benefit	博濟方	Bó jì fāng	Wáng Gǔn, ed.	王袞,編	1047
Formulas of Universal Benefit from My Practice	普濟本事方	Pǔ jì běn shì fāng	Xǔ Shū-Wēi	許叔微	1132
Formulas to Aid the Living	濟生方	Jì shēng fāng	Yán Yòng-Hé	嚴用和	1253
Formulas to Protect Life and the Most Treasured Family Possession	衛生家寶方	Wèi shēng jiā bǎo fāng	Zhū Duān-Zhāng	朱端章	1184
Formulas with Short Articles	小品方	Xiǎo pǐn fāng	Chén Yán-Zhī	陳延之	Eastern Jin [4th century]
Fu Qing-Zhu's Women's Disorders	傅青主女科	Fù Qīng-Zhǔ nǔ kē	Fù Qīng-Zhǔ	傅青主	17th century [published in 1826]
Further Appendices to the Discussion of Cold Damage	傷寒附翼	Shāng hán fù yì	Kē Qín / Kē Yùn-Bó	柯琴 / 柯韻伯	Qing
Gathering of Songs for Golden Cabinet Formulas	金匱方歌括	Jīn guì fāng gē kuò	Chén Yuán-Xī	陳元犀	1811
General Discussion of the Disease of Cold Damage	傷寒總病論	Shāng hán zǒng bìng lùn	Páng Ān-Shí	龐安時	1100
Golden Mirror of the Medical Tradition	醫宗金鑑	Yī zōng jīn jiàn	Wú Qiān / Wú – Liù-Jí	吳謙 / 吳六吉	1742
Golden Mirror Record of Pox and Rashes	痘疹金鏡錄	Dòu zhěn jīn jìng lù	Wēng Zhòng-Rén / Wēng Jiā-Dé	翁仲仁 / 翁嘉德	1519
Good Friend Compilation	良朋匯集	Liāng péng huì jí	Sūn Wěi / Wáng Lín	孫偉 / 望林	1711
Grandfather Lei's Discussion of Herb Preparation	雷公炮炙論	Léi Gōng páo zhì lùn	Léi Xiào	雷斅	5th century
Great Compendium of External Medicine	外科大承	Wài kē dà chéng	Qí Kūn	祁坤	1665
Great Compendium of Medical Formulas	醫方大成	Yī fāng dà chéng	Sūn Yǔn-Xián	孫允賢	Yuan
Great Compendium of Medicine for Sores	瘍醫大全	Yáng yī dà quán	Gù Shì-Chéng	顧世澄	1760
Guide to Clinical Usage of Classical Formulas	經方臨證指南	Jīng fāng lín zhèng zhǐ nán	Liú Dù-Zhōu	劉渡舟	1993
Guide to Pediatrics	幼科指南	Yòu kē zhǐ nán	Zhōu Shèn-Qí	周慎齊	1789
Guide to Pregnancy and Childbirth	胎產指南	Tāi chǎn zhǐ nán	Shàn Nán-Shān	單南山	Qing
Guide to the Silver Sea	銀海指南	Yín hǎi zhǐ nán	Gù Xī	顧錫	1807

English Title	Chinese Title	Pinyin Title	Author (English)	Author (Chinese)	Date/Dynasty
Hanaoka Seshū	華岡青州				1760-1835
Handbook of Chinese Medical Formulas	中醫方劑臨床手冊	*Zhōng yī fāng jì lín chuáng shǒu cè*	Unknown		1950s
Handbook of Chinese Medicinal Pharmaceutics	中藥制劑手冊	*Zhōng yào zhì jì shǒu cè*	China Academy of Chinese Medical Sciences, Institute of Chinese Materia Medica	中醫研究院中藥研究所	1974
Handed-Down Rare and Treasured Formulas	傳家秘寶方	*Chuán jiā mì bǎo fāng*	Sūn Yòng-Hé	孫用和	Song
Handouts on Chinese Medical Formulas	中醫方劑學講義	*Zhōng yī fāng jì xué jiǎng yì*	Nanjing College of TCM Formula Teaching and Research	南京中醫學院方劑教研	1960
Hard-Won Knowledge	此事難知	*Cǐ shì nán zhī*	Wáng Hào-Gǔ / Wáng Jìn-Zhī / Wáng Hǎi-Cáng	王好古 / 王進之 / 王海藏	1308
Hidden Aspects of the Materia Medica	本草蒙荃	*Běn cǎo méng quán*	Chén Jiā-Mó / Chén Yán-Cǎi / Chén Yuè-Míng	陳嘉謨 / 陳延采 / 陳月明	1525
Hong's Collection of Experiential Formulas	洪氏集驗方	*Hóng shì jí yàn fāng*	Hóng Zūn / Hóng Jǐng-Píng	洪遵 / 洪景平	1170
Illumination of Medicine	醫學發明	*Yī xué fā míng*	Lǐ Gǎo / Lǐ Dōng-Yuán	李杲 / 李東垣	Jin
Illustrated Classic of the Materia Medica	本草圖經	*Běn cǎo tú jīng*	Sū Sòng / Sū Zǐ-Róng	蘇頌 / 蘇子容	1061
Imperial Han Medicine	皇漢醫學	*Kōkan igaku*	Yumoto Kyushin	湯本求眞	1930
Important Formulas Worth a Thousand Gold Pieces	千金要方	*Qiān jīn yào fāng*	Sūn Sī-Miǎo	孫思邈	650
Indispensable Tools for Pattern Treatment	證治准繩	*Zhèng zhì zhǔn shéng*	Wáng Kěn-Tāng	王肯堂	1602
Inner Classic	內經	*Nèi jīng*	See Yellow Emperor's Inner Classic		
Integrated Chinese and Western Medical Treatment of the Acute Abdomen	中西醫結合治療急腹症	*Zhōng xī yī jié hé zhì liáo jí fù zhèng*	Nankai Hospital of Tianjin	天津南開醫院	1973
Introduction to Medicine	醫學入門	*Yī xué rù mén*	Lǐ Chān / Lǐ Jiàn-Zhāi	李梴 / 李健齋	1575
Investigations into External Medicine	外科探源	*Wài kē tàn yuán*	Yú Yīng-Tài / Yú Xīng-Jiē	俞應泰 / 俞星階	Qing
Investigations of Medical Formulas	醫方考	*Yī fāng kǎo*	Wú Kūn	吳崑	1584
Invoking Blessings for Healthy Children	活幼口儀	*Huó yòu kǒu yí*	Zēng Shì-Róng	曾世榮	1294
Jade Key to Layered Stories	重樓玉鑰	*Chóng lóu yù yào*	Zhèng Méi-Jiàn	鄭梅澗	18th century
Ji-Feng's Formulas of Universal Benefit	雞峰普濟方	*Jī-Fēng pǔ jì fāng*	Zhāng Ruì / Zhāng Zǐ Gāng / Zhāng Jī-Fēng	張銳 / 張子剛 / 張雞峰	1133
Jottings from Repeated Celebration Hall	重慶堂隨筆	*Chóng qìng táng suí bǐ*	Wáng Xué-Quán	王學權	1852 (written c. 1810)

English Title	Chinese Title	Pinyin Title	Author (English)	Author (Chinese)	Date/Dynasty
Lecture Notes on Traditional Chinese Traumatology	中醫傷科學講義	*Zhōng yī shāng kē xué jiǎng yì*	Traumatology Teaching Group of the Shanghai College of Traditional Chinese Medicine	上海中醫學院傷科教研	1963
Lectures on Warm Pathogen Diseases	溫病學講義	*Wēn bìng xué jiǎng yì*	Chén Rèn-Méi	陳任枚	1924
Lei Yun-Shang's Song-Fen Pharmacy	雷允上誦芬堂	*Léi Yǔn-Shàng Sòng-Fēn Táng*	Herb shop in Suzhou		founded 1734
Li's Mirror of Medicine	李氏醫鑒	*Lǐ shì yī jiàn*	Lǐ Wén-Lái / Lǐ Chāng-Qí	李文來 / 李昌期	Qing
Lingnan Formulas for Preserving Health	嶺南衛生方	*Lǐng nán wèi shēng fāng*	Shì Jì-Hóng / Shì Dàn-Liáo	釋繼洪 / 釋澹寮	Jin
Manual of the Art of Benevolence	仁術便覽	*Rén shù biàn lǎn*	Zhāng Hào-Zhuàn	张浩撰	1585
Marvelous Formulas for Traumatic Injuries	跌損妙方	*Diē sǔn miào fāng*	Yì-Yuǎn Zhēn-Rén / Sūn Yìng-Kē [revised]	異遠真人 / 孫應科 [校訂]	Ming / 1836
Master Fu's Formulas for Reviving Infants	傅氏活嬰方	*Fù shì huó yīng fāng*	Unknown		Unknown
Master Luo's Distillation of Medical Knowledge	羅氏會約醫鏡	*Luó shì huì yuē yī jìng*	Luó Guó-Gāng / Zhèn Zhào / Zhěng Zhāi	羅國綱 / 振召 / 整齋	1789
Master Wan's Family Compilation of Songs for Protecting Life	萬氏家傳保命歌括	*Wàn shì jiā chuán bǎo mìng gē kuò*	Wàn Quán / Wàn Mì-Zhāi	萬全 / 萬密齋	Ming
Master Xue's Case Records	薛氏醫案	*Xuē shì yī àn*	Xuē Jǐ; Wú Guǎn [ed.]	薛己; 吳琯輯 [編]	Ming
Master Ye's Patterns and Treatments in Women's Diseases	葉氏女科證治	*Yè shì nǔ kē zhèng zhì*	Yè Guì / Yè Tiān-Shì / Yè Xiāng-Yán	葉桂 / 葉天士 / 葉香岩	Unknown
Mastery of Pox and Rashes	痘疹會通	*Dòu zhěn huì tōng*	Zēng Dǐng / Yì Yì / Xiāng Tián	曾鼎 / 亦帝 / 香田	1786
Materia Medica Arranged According to Pattern	證類本草	*Zhèng lèi běn cǎo*	Táng Shèn-Wēi / Táng Shěn-Yuán	唐慎微 / 唐審元	1108
Materia Medica for Decoctions	湯液本草	*Tāng yè běn cǎo*	Wáng Hào-Gǔ / Wáng Jìn-Zhī / Wáng Hǎi-Cáng	王好古 / 王進之 / 王海藏	1306
Materia Medica of Combinations	得配本草	*Dé pèi běn cǎo*	Yán Jié, Shī Wén, Hóng Wěi	嚴潔, 施雯, 洪煒	1761
Materia Medica of Ri Hua-Zi	日華子本草	*Rì Huá-Zǐ běn cǎo*	Rì Huá-Zǐ	日華子	713
Medical Collectanea of Kong Bo-Hua	孔伯華醫集	*Kǒng Bó-Huá yī jí*	Beijing Traditional Chinese Medical Assocation	北京中醫學會	1988
Medical Directives on Warmth and Summerheat	溫暑醫旨	*Wēn shǔ yī zhǐ*	Zhāng Wǎn-Xiāng	張畹香	1776-1870

English Title	Chinese Title	Pinyin Title	Author (English)	Author (Chinese)	Date/Dynasty
Medical Formulas Collected and Analyzed	醫方集解	*Yī fāng jí jiě*	Wāng Áng Wāng Rèn-Ān	汪昂 汪訒庵	1682
Medical Mirror of Past and Present	古今醫鑒	*Gǔ jīn yī jiàn*	Gōng Xìn [compiler]; Gōng Yán Xián [later editor]; Wáng Kěn-Táng [supplementary notes]	龔信纂輯; 龔廷賢續編; 王肯堂訂補	Ming
Medical Records	醫錄	*Yī lù*	Liú Zuò-Lín / Yuán Quán	劉作霖 / 元銓	Qing
Medical Texts from the Bettering the World Studio	世補齋醫書	*Shì bǔ zhāi yī shū*	Lù Maò–Xiū / Lù Jiǔ-Zhī	陸懋修 / 陸九芝	1884
Medicinal Teachings from the Respectfully Decorated Hall	敬修堂藥説	*Jìng xiū táng yào shuō*	Qián Shù-Tián	錢澍田	Late 18th century
Medicine Bag of Classic Formulas	古方藥囊	*Kohō Yakunō*	Araki Shō	荒木性次	1954
Medicine is Truly Easy	醫學實在易	*Yī xué shí zài yì*	Chén Niàn-Zǔ / Xiū-Yuán / Liáng-Yǒu / Shèn-Xiū	陳念祖 / 修園 / 良友 / 慎修	1808
Medicine Path of Song-Ya	松崕醫徑	*Sōng-Yá yī jìng*	Chéng Jiè / Chéng Wén-Yù / Sōng-Yá	程玠 / 程文玉 / 松崕	1600
Methodology for Using the Six Warps in Ophthalmology	眼科六經法要	*Yǎn kē liù jīng fǎ yào*	Chén Dá-Fū	陳達夫	1979
Miraculous Book of Ten Remedies for Consumption	勞症十藥神書	*Láo zhèng shí yào shén shū*	Gé Qián–Sūn	葛乾孫	1348
Miscellaneous Records of Famous Physicians	名醫別錄	*Míng yī bié lù*	Táo Hóng-Jǐng / Táo Tōng-Míng	陶弘景 / 陶通明	c. 500
Miscellaneous Records of the Materia Medica [4]	本草別錄	*Běn cǎo bié lù*	Unknown		Unknown
Miscellaneous Writings of Enlightened Physicians	明醫雜著	*Míng yī zá zhù*	Wáng Lùn	王綸	1549
Modern Explanation of the Golden Cabinet	金匱要略今釋	*Jīn guì yào lüè jīn shì*	Lù Yuān-Léi	陸淵雷	1935
Modern Explanations of Ancient Formulas	古方今解	*Gǔ fang jīn jiě*	Dīng Xué-Píng	丁學屏	2002
Monthly Ordinances Worth a Thousand Gold Pieces	千金月令	*Qiān jīn yuè lǐng*	Sūn Sī-Miǎo	孫思邈	7th century
Multitude of Marvelous Formulas for Sustaining Life	攝生眾妙方	*Shè shēng zhòng miào fāng*	Zhāng Shí-Chè / Zhāng Wéi Jìng / Zhāng Dōng Shā	張時徹 / 張維靜 / 張東沙	1550
My Humble Complete Collection of Fine Formulas	管見大全良方	*Guǎn jiàn dà quán liáng fāng*	Chén Zì-Míng / Chén Liáng -Fǔ / Chén Liáng-Fù	陳自明 / 陳良甫 / 陳良父	1271
Mysteriously Effective Formulas for Abscesses	癰疽神秘驗方	*Yōng jū shén mì yàn fāng*	Táo Huá / Táo Shàng-Wén / Táo Jié-Ān	陶華 / 陶尚文 / 陶節庵	1445

English Title	Chinese Title	Pinyin Title	Author (English)	Author (Chinese)	Date/Dynasty
Nationwide Collection of TCM Patent Formulas	全國中藥成藥處方集	*Quán guó zhōng yào chéng yào chù fāng jí*	Traditional Chinese Medicine Research Institute of the China Academy of Traditional Chinese Medicine	中國中醫研究院中醫研究所	1962
Necessities for Women's Diseases	女科切要	*Nǚ kē qiè yào*	Wú Dào-Yuán / Wú Běn-Lì	吳道源 / 吳本立	1738
New [Text on the] Acute Abdomen	新急腹症學	*Xīn jí fù zhèng xué*	Nankai Hospital of Tianjin, Zunyi Medical School	天津南開醫院, 遵義醫學院	1978
New Book on Syphilis and Leprosy	黴癩新書	*Bai rai shinsho*	Katakura Kakuryo	片倉鶴陵	1787
New Compilation of Empirical Formulas	驗方新編	*Yàn fāng xīn biān*	Bào Xiàng-Áo	鮑相璈	1846
New Compilation of Materia Medica	本草新編	*Běn cǎo xīn biān*	Chén Shì-Duó / Chén Yuǎn-Gōng / Zhū Huá Zǐ	陳士鐸 / 陳遠公 / 朱華子	1694
New Discussion of Epidemic Diarrheal Diseases	瀉疫新論	*Shaekishinron*	Takashima Hisatsuru	高島久貫	1867
New Edition of Mei's Empirical Formulas	梅氏驗方新編	*Méi shì yàn fāng xīn biān*	Méi Qǐ-Zhào	梅啟照	1878
New Explanations of Medical Formulas	醫方新解	*Yī fāng xīn jiě*	Mǎ Yǒu-Dù	馬有度	1980
New Treatise on Children	幼幼新書	*Yòu yòu xīn shū*	Liú Fǎng	劉昉	Song
Newly Compiled Book of Empirical Formulas	验方新编	*Yàn fāng xīn biān*	Bào Xiang-Áo / Bào Yún-Sháo	鮑相璈 / 鮑云韶	Qing
Nie's Study of Cold Damage	聶氏傷寒學	*Niè shì shāng hán xué*	Niè Huì-Mín	聶惠民	2002
Notated Discussion of Cold Damage Editied for Meaning	傷寒論輯義按	*Shāng háng lùn jí yì àn*	Yùn Tiě-Qiáo	惲鐵樵	1929
Notes on the Discussion of Cold Damage Edited for Meaning	傷寒論輯義按	*Shāng hán lùn jí yì àn*	Yùn Tiě-Qiáo [annotator] / Tamba Motoyasu [original author]	惲鐵樵 / 丹波元簡	1929 / 1810
Omissions from the [Classic of the] Materia Medica	本草拾遺	*Běn cǎo shí yí*	Chén Cáng-Qì	陳藏器	720
On the Origins and Development of Medicine	醫學源流論	*Yī xúe yuán liú lùn*	Xú Dà-Chūn / Xú Líng-Tái	徐大椿 / 徐靈台	1757
On the Origins and Development of Medicine in China	中國醫學源流論	*Zhōng guó yī xué yuán liú lùn*	Xiè Guān / Xiè Lì-Héng	謝觀 / 謝利恒	1935
One-Hundred Questions on Women's Disorders	女科百問	*Nǚ kē bǎi wèn*	Qí Zhòng-Fǔ	齊仲甫	1220
One-Hundred Supremely Effective Medicinals	百藥效用奇觀	*Bǎi yào xiào yòng qí guān*	Zhāng Shù-Shēng	張樹生	1987
One-Hundred Classic Formulas	經方100首	*Jīng fāng 100 shǒu*	Huáng Huáng	黃煌	2006
Original Meaning of Formulas Discussed in Essentials from the Golden Cabinet	金匱要略方論本義	*Jīn guì yào lüè fāng lùn běn yì*	Wèi Lì-Tóng / Wèi Niàn-Tíng	魏荔彤 / 魏念庭	1720

English Title	Chinese Title	Pinyin Title	Author (English)	Author (Chinese)	Date/Dynasty
Orthodox Lineage of External Medicine	外科正宗	Wài kē zhèng zōng	Chén Shí-Gōng / Chén Yù-Rén / Chén Ruò-Xū	陳實功 / 陳毓仁 / 陳若虛	1617
Outline of Medical Formulas	醫方概要	Yī fāng gài yào	Lǐ Chóu-Rén	李疇人	1935
Pathodynamics and Treatment Strategies in Chinese Medicine	中醫病機治法學	Zhōng yī bìng jī zhì fǎ xué	Chén Cháo-Zǔ	陳潮組	1988
Pattern Differentiation and Treatment for Women's Disorders [from the] Zhulin [Monastery]	竹林女科証治	Zhúlín nǔ kē zhèng zhì	Annonymous		Qing
Patterns and Treatment of Miscellaneous Disorders	雜病證治	Zá bìng zhèng zhì	Xú Dà-Chūn / Xú Líng-Tái	徐大椿 / 徐靈台	1759
Pediatrics: Categorized and Brought Together	幼科類萃	Yòu kē lèi cuì	Wáng Luán / Wén Róng / Róng Hú	王鑾 / 文融 / 容湖	1521
Personal Standards for Internal Medicine	内科心典	Nèi kē xīn diǎn	Xú Shí-Jìn	徐時進	1777
Personal Standards for the Essentials from the Golden Cabinet	金匱要略心典	Jīn guì yào lüè xīn diǎn	Yóu Yí	尤怡	1729
Pocket Prescriptions	袖珍方	Xiù zhēn fāng	Lǐ Héng / Zhū Shào	李恒 / 朱櫹	1391
Popular Guide to the Discussion of Cold Damage	通俗傷寒論	Tōng sú shāng hán lùn	Yú Gēn-Chū	俞根初	Qing
Posthumous Manuscript from [Bian Que in] Handan	邯鄲遺稿	Hándān yí gǎo	Zhào Xiàn-Kě	趙獻可	17th century
Pouch of Pearls	珍珠囊	Zhēn zhū náng	Zhāng Yuán-Sù / Zhāng Jié-Gǔ	張元素 / 張潔古	1186
Practical Chinese External Medicine	實用中醫外科學	Shí yòng zhōng yī wài kē xué	Gù Bó-Huá	顧伯華	1985
Practical Established Formulas	成方切用	Chéng fāng qiè yòng	Wú Yì-Luó	吳儀洛	1761
Practice of Syndrome Treatment in Kampo	症候による漢方治療の実際	Shoko ni yoru Kampo chiryo no jissai	Otsuka Yoshinori	大塚敬節	1963
Precepts for Physicians	醫門法律	Yī mén fǎ lǜ	Yù Chāng / Yù Jiā-Yán	喻昌 / 喻嘉言	1658
Precious Collection for Throat Diseases	喉科紫珍集	Hóu kē zǐ zhēn jí	Unknown		Qing
Precious Mirror for Advancement of Medicine	醫級寶鑑	Yī jí bǎo jiàn	Dǒng Xī-Yuán	董西園	1777
Precious Mirror of Eastern Medicine	東醫寶鑑	Dongui bogam	Heo Jun [Xǔ Jùn]	許浚	1613
Precious Mirror of Health	衛生寶鑑	Wèi shēng bǎo jiàn	Luó Tiān-Yì	羅天益	Yuan
Precious Mirror of Patterns and Treatments	證治寶鑑	Zhèng zhì bǎo jiàn	Pān Qià	潘楫	Qing
Precise Usage of Herbs Based on their Nature	藥性切用	Yào xìng qiè yòng	Xú Dà-Chūn / Xú Líng-Tái	徐大椿 / 徐靈台	1741
Prescriptions of Universal Benefit	普濟方	Pǔ jì fāng	Zhū Dì	朱棣	Early 15th century
[Qin] Qian-Zhai's Lecture Notes on Medicine	謙齋醫學講稿	Qiān-Zhāi yī xué jiǎng gǎo	Qín Bó-Wèi / Qín Zhī-Jì / Qín Qiān-Zhāi	秦伯未 / 秦之濟 / 秦謙齋	1964

English Title	Chinese Title	Pinyin Title	Author (English)	Author (Chinese)	Date/Dynasty
Random Notes while Reading about Medicine	讀醫隨筆	*Dú yī suí bǐ*	Zhōu Xué-Hǎi / Zhōu Chéng-Zhī	周學海 / 周澄之	1898
Readings from the Discussion of Cold Damage	傷寒論選讀	*Shāng hán lùn xuǎn dú*	Hubei College of Traditional Chinese Medicine	湖北中醫學院	1979
Record of Challenges [to the Classics]	質疑錄	*Zhì yí lù*	Zhāng Jiè-Bīn / Zhāng Jǐng-Yuè	張介賓 / 張景岳	1624
Records of Experiences with Classic Formulas	經方實驗錄	*Jīng fāng shí yàn lù*	Cáo Jiā-Dá / Cáo Yǐng-Fǔ	曹穎甫 / 曹家達	1937
Records of Pattern Discrimination	辯證錄	*Biàn zhèng lù*	Chén Shì-Duó / Chén Yuǎn-Gōng / Zhū Huá Zǐ	陳士鐸 / 陳遠公 / 朱華子	1687
Records of Proven Formulas Past and Present	古今錄驗方	*Gǔ jīn lù yàn fāng*	Zhēn Lì-Yán	甄立言	627
Records of the Grand Historian	史記	*Shǐ jì*	Sī-Mǎ Qiān	司馬遷	91 B.C.E.
Records of Thoughtful Differentiation of Materia Medica	本草思辨錄	*Běn cǎo sī biàn lù*	Zhōu Yán / Zhōu Bó-Dù	周岩 / 周伯度	1904
Rectification of the Meaning of Materia Medica	本草正義	*Běn cǎo zhèng yì*	Zhāng Shān-Léi / Zhāng Shòu-Yí	張山雷 / 張壽頤	1914
Red Water and Dark Pearls	赤水玄珠	*Chì shuǐ xuán zhū*	Sūn Yī-Kuí	孫一奎	1584
Renewed Materia Medica	本草再新	*Běn cǎo zài xīn*	Yè Guì / Yè Xiǎo-Fēng	葉桂 / 葉小峰	1820
Required Readings from the Medical Tradition	醫宗必讀	*Yī zōng bì dú*	Lǐ Zhōng-Zǐ / Lǐ Shì-Cái / Lǐ Niàn-É	李中梓 / 李士材 / 李念莪	1637
Resolving Uncertainties about the [Discussion] of Cold Damage	傷寒析疑	*Shāng hán xī yí*	Jiāng Jiàn-Guó	姜建國	1993
Restoration of Health from the Myriad Diseases	萬病回春	*Wàn bìng huí chūn*	Gōng Tíng-Xián	龔廷賢	1587
Restoration of Life from the Groves of Medicine	杏苑生春	*Xìng yuàn shēng chūn*	Ruì Jīng, Jì Mèng-Dé	芮經, 紀夢德	1610
Revised and Expanded Discussion of Warm-Heat Pathogen Diseases	重訂廣溫熱論	*Chóng dìng guǎng wēn rè lùn*	Hé Bǐng-Yuán / Hé Lián-Chén	何炳元 / 何廉臣	1907
Revised Popular Guide to the Discussion of Cold Damage	重定通俗傷寒論	*Chóng dìng Tōng sú shāng hán lùn*	Reviser: Hé Bǐng-Yuán / Hé Lián-Chén, original author: Yú Gēn-Chū	重訂者: 何炳元 / 何廉臣, 原作: 俞根初	Qing
Revision of the Subtle Discussions on Caring for Life	刪補頤生微論	*Shān bǔ yí shēng wēi lùn*	Lǐ Zhōng-Zǐ / Lǐ Shì-Cái / Lǐ Niàn-É	李中梓 / 李士材 / 李念莪	1642
Rhymed Prose on [Medical] Principles and Applications	理瀹駢文	*Lǐ yuè pián wén*	Wú Shàng-Xiān	吳尚先	1870
Scrutiny of the Precious Jade Case	審視瑤函	*Shěn shì yáo hán*	Fù Rén-Yǔ	傅仁宇	1642
Secret Empirical Formulas	經驗秘方	*Jīng yàn mì fāng*	Yáng Shū-Hé / Fù Jiāo	楊舒和 / 馥蕉	1888
Secret Essentials of Main Indications	主治秘要	*Zhǔ zhì mì yào*	Unknown	Unknown	Quoted in *Expounding on the Origins of Medicine*
Secret Formulas from the Court of Lu	魯府禁方	*Lǔ fǔ jìn fāng*	Gōng Tíng-Xián / Gōng Zǐ-Cái / Gōng Yún-Lín	龔廷賢 / 龔子才 / 龔云林	1594

English Title	Chinese Title	Pinyin Title	Author (English)	Author (Chinese)	Date/Dynasty
Secret Formulas to Manage Trauma and Reconnect Fractures Received from an Immortal	仙授理傷續斷秘方	*Xiān shòu lǐ shāng xù duàn mì fāng*	Daoist priest Lìn	藺道人	c. 846
Secretly Transmitted Effective Medicine	醫效秘傳	*Yī xiào mì chuán*	Yè Guì / Yè Tiān-Shì / Yè Xiāng-Yán; ed. & annotated by Wú Jīn-Shòu	葉桂 / 葉天士 / 葉香岩; 吳金壽校	1831
Secrets from the Orchid Chamber	蘭室秘藏	*Lán shì mì cáng*	Lǐ Gǎo / Lǐ Dōng-Yuán	李杲 / 李東垣	1336
Seeking Accuracy in the Materia Medica	本草求真	*Běn cǎo qiú zhēn*	Huáng Gōng-Xiù	黃宮繡	1769
Select Treatments for Sores	瘍科選粹	*Yáng kē xuǎn cuì*	Chén Wén-Zhì	陳文治	1628
Selected and Compiled Clinical Exprinces of Wei Chang-Chun	魏長春臨床經驗選輯	*Wèi Cháng-Chūn lín chuáng jīng yàn xuǎn jí*	Jiangsu Provincial Chinese Medicine Hospital	江蘇省中醫院	1974
Selected Annotations to Ancient Formulas from the Garden of Crimson Snow	絳雪園古方選注	*Jiàng xuě yuán gǔ fāng xuǎn zhù*	Wáng Zǐ-Jiē / Wáng Jìn-Sān	王子接 / 王晋三	1732
Selected Chinese Patent Medicines	中國國藥固有成方選輯	*Zhōng guó guó yào gù yǒu chéng fāng xuǎn jí*	Drug Administration of China	藥品管理處	1994
Selected Clinical Experiences of Wei Wen-gui in Ophthalmology	韋文貴眼科臨床經驗選	*Wéi Wén-Guì yǎn kē lín chuáng jīng yàn xuǎn*	Wéi Wén-Guì	韋文貴	1980
Selected Formulas [aka Selected Formulas from the Praiseworthy Studio]	百一選方 [是齋百一選方]	*Bǎi yī xuǎn fāng [Shì zhāi bǎi yī xuǎn fāng]*	Wáng Qiú	王璆	1196
Selected Formulas for Warm-Heat Pathogen Diseases	溫熱病方匯選	*Wēn rè bìng fāng huì xuǎn*	Hé Bǐng-Yuán / Hé Lián-Chén	何炳元 / 何廉臣	c. 1900
Selected Formulas of Famous Physicians	名家方選	*Maikehosen*	Yamada Yasunari	山田元倫	1781
Selections from the Clinical Experience of Guan You-Po	關幼澯臨床經驗選	*Guān Yòu-Pō lín chuáng jīng yàn xuǎn*	Guān Yòu-Pō	關幼澯	2006
Selections of Formulas and Cases from the Hall of Longevity	眉壽堂方案選存	*Méi shòu táng fāng ān xuǎn cún*	Yè Guì / Yè Tiān-Shì / Yè Xiāng-Yán; ed. Guō Wéi-Jùn	葉桂 / 葉天士 / 葉香岩; 郭維浚編	1746
Shaanxi New Medicine	陝西新醫藥	*Shǎnxī xīn yī yào*	Shaanxi Provincial Chinese Medicine Research Institute	陝西省中醫研究所	1972
Shanghai Municipal Medicine Standards	上海市藥品標準	*Shánghǎi shì yào pǐn biāo zhǔn*	Shanghai Municipal Department of Health	上海市衛生局	1974
Shen's Book for Revering Life	沈氏尊生書	*Shěn shì zūn shēng shū*	Shěn Jīn-Ào	沈金鰲	1773
Shen's Annotated Essentials from the Golden Cabinet	沈氏注金櫃要略	*Shěn shì zhù jīn guì yào lüè*	Shěn Míng-Zōng / Mù-Nán	沈明宗 / 目南	1692
Simple and Applicable Medical Formulas	醫方簡義	*Yī fāng jiǎn yì*	Wáng Qīng-Yuán	王清源	1883
Simple Annotation of the Discussion of Cold Damage	傷寒論淺注	*Shāng hán lùn qiǎn zhù*	Chén Niàn-Zǔ / Chén Xiū-Yuán	陳念祖 / 陳修園	1803
Simple Annotation of the Essentials from the Golden Cabinet	金匱要略淺注	*Jīn guì yào lüè qiǎn zhù*	Chén Niàn-Zǔ / Chén Xiū-Yuán	陳念祖 / 陳修園	1803

English Title	Chinese Title	Pinyin Title	Author (English)	Author (Chinese)	Date/Dynasty
Simple Book of Formulas	易簡方	*Yì jiǎn fāng*	Wáng Shuò	王碩	1191
Simple Explications of Han Formulas	漢方簡義	*Hàn fāng jiǎn yì*	Wáng Miǎo-Dá	王邈達	1956
Simple Formulas for Health	衛生易簡方	*Wēi shēng yì jiǎn fāng*	Zhōu Jǐng	周憬	1905
Six Texts on Cold Damage	傷寒六書	*Shāng hán liù shū*	Táo Huá	陶華	1445
Six Texts on Medicine by Wang Xu-Gao	王旭高醫書六種	*Wáng Xù-Gāo yī shū liù zhǒng*	Wáng Tài-Lín / Wáng Xù-Gāo	王泰林 / 王旭高	1897
Six Texts Summarizing the Medicine of Xu Ling-Tai	徐靈胎醫略六書	*Xú Líng-Tāi yī lüè liù shū*	Xú Dà-Chūn / Xú Líng-Tāi	徐大椿 / 徐靈胎	1727
Small Collection of Fine Formulas	良方集腋	*Liáng fáng jí yè*	Xiè Yuán-Qìng	謝元慶	1842
Song Family Secret Texts on Women's Disorders	宋氏女科秘書	*Sòng shì nǚ kē mì shū*	Sòng Lín-Gāo	宋林皋	1612
Speaking of Studying the Classics	研經言	*Yán jīng yán*	Mò Wén-Quán / Mò Mù-Shì	莫文泉 / 莫牧士	1879
Standards from the Imperial Archives	蘭臺軌範	*Lán tái guǐ fàn*	Xú Dà-Chūn / Xú Líng-Tāi	徐大椿 / 徐靈胎	1764
Straight Directions from [Yang] Ren-Zhai aka Discussion of Formulas from Straight Directions from [Yang] Ren-Zhai	仁齋直指 [仁齋直指方論]	*Rén-zhāi zhí zhǐ [Rén-zhāi zhí zhǐ fāng lùn]*	Yáng Shì-Yíng / Yáng Rén-Zhāi	楊士瀛 / 楊仁齋	1264
String of Pearls from the [Discussion] of Cold Damage	傷寒貫珠集	*Shāng hán guàn zhū jí*	Yōu Yí	尤怡	1810
Subtle Import of the Jade Key	玉機微義	*Yù jī wēi yì*	Xú Yàn-Chún / Xú Yòng-Chéng	徐彥純 / 徐用誠	1396
Summary of Internal Medicine	內科摘要	*Nèi kē zhāi yào*	Xuē Jǐ	薛己	Ming
Summary Songs for Formulas from Changsha	長沙方歌括	*Chángshā fāng gē kuò*	Chén Niàn-Zǔ / Chén Xiū-Yuán	陳念祖 / 陳修園	1803
Supplement to Important Formulas Worth a Thousand Gold Pieces	千金翼方	*Qiān jīn yì fāng*	Sūn Sī-Miǎo	孫思邈	7th century
Supplement to the Elegant Lexicon of Itinerant Physicians	串雅補	*Chuàn yǎ bǔ*	Lǔ Zhào	魯照	1759
Supplement to the Pocket-sized Discussion of Formulas for Children	補要袖珍小兒方論	*Bǔ yào xiù zhēn xiǎo ér fāng lùn*	Zhuāng Yīng-Qí	莊應祺	Late Ming
Supplemental Critical Annotations to the Systematic Discussion of Warm Pathogen Diseases	增補評註溫病條辨	*Zēng bǔ píng zhù Wēn bìng tiáo biàn*	Wáng Shì-Xióng / Yè Lín / Zhèng Xuě-Táng	王士雄 / 葉霖 / 鄭雪堂	Mid-19th century
Supplemental Formulas Omitted from the Inner Classic	增補內經拾遺方論	*Zēng bǔ nèi jīng shí yí fāng lùn*	Luò Lóng-Jí	駱龍吉	Song
Supplemented Collections on Patterns and Treatments	證治匯補	*Zhèng zhì huì bǔ*	Lǐ Yòng-Cuì	李用粹	1687
Supreme Commanders of the Medical Ramparts	醫壘元戎	*Yī lěi yuán róng*	Wáng Hào-Gǔ	王好古	1291
Symptom, Cause, Pulse, and Treatment	症因脈治	*Zhèng yīn mài zhì*	Qín Jǐng-Míng	秦景明	1706

English Title	Chinese Title	Pinyin Title	Author (English)	Author (Chinese)	Date/Dynasty
Synopsis for Protecting Infants	保嬰撮要	*Bǎo yīng cuō yào*	Xuē Kǎi / Liáng Wǔ	薛鎧 / 良武	1555
Systematic Differentiation of the Discussion of Cold Damage	傷寒論條辨	*Shāng hán lùn tiáo biàn*	Fāng Yǒu-Zhí / Fāng Zhōng-Xíng	方有執 / 方仲行	1592
Systematic Differentiation of Warm Pathogen Diseases	温病條辨	*Wēn bìng tiáo biàn*	Wú Táng / Wú Jū-Tōng	吳瑭 / 吳鞠通	1798
Systematic Great Compendium of Medicine Past and Present	古今醫統大全	*Gǔ jīn yī tǒng dà quán*	Xú Chūn-Fǔ	徐春甫	1556
Systematic Instructions on Medicine	醫學統旨	*Yī xué tǒng zhǐ*	Yè Wén-Líng	葉文齡	1534
Teachings on the Manifestation and Root of Cold Damage, Categorized and Gathered	傷寒標本心法類萃	*Shāng hán biāo běn xīn fǎ lèi cuì*	Liú Wán-Sù / Liú Shǒu Zhēn / Tōng Xuán Chǔ Shì / Hé Jiān Jū Shì	劉完素 / 劉守真 / 通玄處士 / 河間居士	1186
Ten Lectures on Personal Experiences with Formulas	方劑心得十講	*Fāng jì xīn dé shí jiǎng*	Jiāo Shù-Dé	焦樹德	1995
The Refined in Medicine Remembered	醫醇賸義	*Yī chún shèng yì*	Fèi Bó-Xióng	費伯雄	1863
Therapeutic Experiences of Pu Fu-Zhou	蒲輔周醫療經驗	*Pú Fǔ-Zhōu yī liáo jīng yàn*	Chinese Academy of Traditional Chinese Medicine	中醫研究院	1976
Thorough Investigations of the Materia Medica	藥性通考	*Yào xìng tōng kǎo*	Liú Hàn-Jī	劉漢基	19th century
Thorough Understanding of Cold Damage	傷寒指掌	*Shāng hán zhǐ zhǎng*	Wú Kūn-Ān	吳坤安	1796
Thorough Understanding of Cold Damage with Charts and Songs to Safeguard Life	傷寒圖歌活人指掌	*Shāng hán tú gē huó rén zhǐ zhǎng*	Wú Shù / Rǔ Xīn / Méng Zhāi	吳恕 / 如心 / 蒙齋	1338
Thread Through Medicine	醫貫	*Yī guàn*	Zhào Xiàn-Kě / Zhào Yǎng-Kuí	趙獻可 / 趙養葵	1687
Three Works on the Discussion of Cold Damage by Xu Shu-Wei	許叔微傷寒論著三種	*Xǔ Shū-Wēi Shāng hán lùn zhù sān zhòng*	Xǔ Shū-Wēi	許叔微	Song
Traditional Chinese Internal Medicine	中醫內科	*Zhōng yī nèi kē*	Shanghai College of TCM	上海中醫學院	c. 1970
Traditional Chinese Ophthalmology	中醫眼科學	*Zhōng yī yǎn kē xué*	Unknown		c. 1970
Traditional Chinese Traumatology	中醫傷科學	*Zhōng yī shāng kē xué*	Unknown		c. 1970
Tranquil Hut Collection of Experiential Secret Formulas	澹寮集驗秘方	*Dàn liáo jí yàn mì fāng*	Shì Jì-Hóng	釋繼洪	Song-Yuan
Transforming the Significance of Medicinal Substances	藥品化義	*Yào pǐn huà yì*	Jiǎ Jiǔ-Rú / Jiǎ Suǒ-Xué	賈九如 / 賈所學	1644
Transmitted Trustworthy and Suitable Formulas	傳信適用方	*Chuán xìn shì yòng fāng*	Wú Yàn-Kuí	吳彥夔	1180
Treasury Classic	中藏經	*Zhōng cáng jīng*	Huá Tuó	華佗	Prob. 4th century
Treatment Decisions Categorized According to Pattern	類證治裁	*Lèi zhèng zhì cái*	Lín Pèi-Qín	林珮琴	1839

English Title	Chinese Title	Pinyin Title	Author (English)	Author (Chinese)	Date/Dynasty
Treatment Methods for Damp-Warm Seasonal Epidemics	濕溫時疫治療法	*Shī wēn shí yì zhì liáo fǎ*	Shaoxing Medical Society	紹興醫學會	1912
Treatment Strategies and Formulas in Chinese Medicine	中醫治法與方劑	*Zhōng yī zhì fǎ yǔ fāng jì*	Chén Cháo-Zǔ	陳潮祖	1995 [1st edition 1975]
Trivial Comments on Medical Matters	証治摘要	*Sōkeitei ijishōgen*	Hara Nanyō	原南陽	1820
True Explanation of the Essentials of the Golden Cabinet	金匱要略真解	*Jīn guì yào lüè zhēn jiě*	Chéng Lín	程林	1673
Two Commentaries on the Classic of the Golden Cabinet and Jade Coffer	金匱玉函經二注	*Jīn guì yù hán jīn èr zhù*	Zhōu Yáng-Jùn	周揚俊	1687
Understanding in an Instant	紅爐點雪	*Hóng lú diǎn xuě*	Gōng Jū-Zhōng	龔居中	1630
Unusually Effective Empirical Formulas	經驗奇方	*Jīng yàn qí fāng*	Liú Yī-Míng	刘一明	Qing
Unwilting Formulas	不謝方	*Bù xiè fāng*	Lù Maò–Xiū	陸懋修	Qing
Versified Prescriptions	湯頭歌訣	*Tāng tóu gē jué*	Wāng Áng / Wāng Rèn-Ān	汪昂 / 汪訒庵	1694
Wan Family Tradition Jade Tablets on Pox and Rashes	萬氏家傳片玉痘疹	*Wàn shì jiā chuán piàn yù dòu zhěn*	Wàn Quán / Wàn Mì-Zhāi	萬全 / 萬密齋	1549
Warp and Woof of Warm-Heat Diseases	溫熱經緯	*Wēn rè jīng wěi*	Wáng Shì-Xióng / Wáng Mèng-Yīng	王士雄 / 王孟英	1852
Wondrous Lantern for Peering into the Origin and Development of Miscellaneous Diseases	雜病源流犀燭	*Zá bìng yuán liú xī zhú*	Shěn Jīn-Ào	沈金鰲	1773
Writings for Posterity of [Zhou] Shen-Zhai	慎齋遺書	*Shèn-Zhāi yí shū*	Zhōu Zhī-Gān / Zhōu Shèn-Zhāi	周之干 / 周慎齋	1573
Writings on Damp-Heat Pathogen Diseases	濕熱病篇	*Shī rè bìng piān*	Xuē Xuě / Xuē Shēng-Bái; ed. by Wáng Shì-Xióng / Wáng Mèng-Yīng	薛雪, 王士雄 / 王孟英補(訂)	1852
Writings on the Esteemed Discussion	尚論篇	*Shàng lùn piān*	Yù Chāng / Yù Jiā-Yán	喻昌 / 喻嘉言	1648
Writings Taking Personal Responsiblity for the Medical Tradition	醫宗己任編	*Yī zōng jǐ rèn piān*	Gāo Gǔ-Fēng	高鼓峰	Qing
Xu Ren-Ze's Formulas	許仁則方	*Xǔ rén zé fāng*	Xǔ Rén-Zé	許仁則	Tang
Yang Family Formulas	楊氏家藏方	*Yáng shì jiā zàng fāng*	Yáng Tán	楊倓	1178
Ye Xi-Chun's Case Histories	葉熙春醫案	*Yè xī chūn yī àn*	Zhejiang Provincial Health Department	浙江省衛生廳	1954
Yellow Emperor's Inner Classic	黃帝內經	*Huáng Dì nèi jīng*	Anonymous		Probably Later Han
Yun Qi-Zi's Collection for Safeguarding Life	雲岐子保命集	*Yún qí zǐ bǎo mìng jí*	Zhāng Bì / Yún Qí Zǐ	張璧 / 雲岐子	Yuan, before 1315
Yun Qi-Zi's Notes on Pulse in Verse with Formulas	雲岐子注脈訣並方	*Yún qí zǐ zhù mài jué bìng fāng*	Zhāng Bì / Yún Qí Zǐ	張璧 / 雲岐子	Yuan

English Title	Chinese Title	Pinyin Title	Author (English)	Author (Chinese)	Date/Dynasty
Zhejiang Journal of Chinese Medicine	浙江中醫雜誌	*Zhéjiāng zhōng yī zá zhì ["Learning from treating 100 Cases of Appendicitis with Clear the Intestines Decoction"* 清腸飲治療闌尾炎100例體會]	Zhāng Dé-Wén	張德文	1987 (4)
Zheng Family Formulas for Women's Diseases Worth Ten Thousand in Gold	鄭氏家傳女科萬金方	*Zhèng shì jiā chuán nǚ kē wàn jīn fāng*	Zhèng Yuán-Liáng	鄭元良	Qing
Zheng Family Secret Formulas for Women's Diseases	鄭氏女科家傳祕方	*Zhèng shì nǚ kē jiā chuán mì fāng*	Zhèng Yān-Shān	鄭燕山	1697
[Zhou] Ji-Ren's Collected Empirical Formulas	吉人集驗方	*Jí rén jí yàn fāng*	Zhōu Jí-Rén	周吉人	1924

Bibliography of Modern Sources

Academy of Traditional Chinese Medicine 中國中醫研究院 et al. *Encyclopedia of Traditional Chinese Medicine: Formulas* (中醫大辭典 *Zhōng yī dà cí diǎn*), 2nd edition. Beijing: People's Medical Publishing House, 2005.

Academy of Traditional Chinese Medicine 中國中醫研究院, 朱仁康 et al. *Traditional Chinese External Medicine* (中醫外科學 *Zhōng yī wài kē xué*). Beijing: China Press of Traditional Chinese Medicine, 1987.

Bā Kūn-Jié 巴坤傑. *Difficult Questions about Formulas* (方劑問難 *Fāng jì wèn nán*). Hefei: Anhui Science and Technology Press, 1986.

Cháng Shì-Ān 常世安. *Modern Reflections on Ancient Formulas* (古方今鑒 *Gǔ fāng jīn jiàn*). Xi'an: Shaanxi Science and Technology Press, 1983.

Chén Áo-Zhōng 陳敖忠 (ed.) *One Thousand Formulas to Treat a Hundred Diseases* (千方治百病 *Qiān fāng zhì bǎi bìng*). Beijing: People's Military Medical Press, 1994.

Chén Cháo-Zǔ 陳潮祖. *Pathodynamics and Treatment Strategies in Chinese Medicine* (中醫病機治法學 *Zhōng yī bìng jī zhì fǎ xué*). Chengdu: Sichuan Science and Technology Press, 1988.

— (ed.) *Chinese Medicine Treatment Strategies and Formulas*, 4th edition (中醫治法與方劑 *Zhōng yī zhì fǎ yǔ fāng jì*). Beijing: People's Medical Publishing House, 2005.

Chén Míng 陳明, Zhāng Yìn-Shēng 張印生. *Selected Experiences and Cases of Famous Doctors on Cold Damage* (傷寒名醫驗案精選 *Shāng hán míng yī yàn àn jīng xuǎn*). Beijing: Xueyuan Publishing House, 1998.

Chéng Mén-Xué [ed. Zhāng Jìn-Rén et al.] 程門學 [張鏡人等整理]. *Formulas in Verse from the Scholar's Studio in Two Volumes* (書種室歌訣二種 *Shū Zhǒng Shì gē jué èr zhǒng*). Beijing: People's Medical Publishing House, 1985.

Chengdu College of Traditional Chinese Medicine 成都中醫學院. *Traditional Chinese Ophthalmology* (中醫眼科學 *Zhōng yī yǎn kē xué*). Beijing: People's Medical Publishing House, 1985.

Cuī Měi-Qí 崔美琪, Gāo Zé-Míng 高澤明, Gāo Xiǎo-Yǎ 高曉雅 (eds.). *Compendium of Differentiation and Usage of Similar Forumlas in Chinese Medicine* (中醫類似方劑鑑別運用大全 *Zhōng yī lèi sì fāng jì jiàn bié yùn yòng dà quán*). Beijing: People's Military Medical Press, 2001.

Dīng Xué-Píng 丁學屏. *Contemporary Interpretations to Ancient Formulas* (古方今釋 *Gǔ fāng jīn shì*). Beijing: China Press of Traditional Chinese Medicine, 2002.

— (ed.) *Collected Scholarship and Experience of Zhang Yao-Qing* (張耀卿學術經驗集 *Zhāng Yào-Qīng xué shú jīng yàn jí*). Beijing: People's Medical Publishing House, 2007.

Duàn Kǔ-Hán 段苦寒 (ed.) *Dictionary of Chinese Medicine Formulas Grouped by Categories* (中醫類方辭典 *Zhōng yī lèi fāng cí diǎn*). Tianjin: Tianjin University Press, 1995.

Duàn Kǔ-Hán 段苦寒. *Distinguishing the Uses of Famous Traditional Medical Formulas* (中醫名方鑑別運用 *Zhōng yī míng fāng jiàn bié yùn yòng*). Tianjin: Tianjin Science and Technology Press, 1987.

Ellis, Andrew. *Notes from South Mountain*. Berkeley: Thin Moon Publishing, 2003.

Fán Qiǎo-Líng 樊巧玲. *Formulas (方劑學 Fāng jì xué)*. Shanghai: Shanghai University of Traditional Chinese Medicine, 2002.

Fāng Wén-Xián ed. 方文賢. *Secret Clinical Uses of Famous Formulas in Chinese Medicine (中醫名方臨證秘用 Zhōng yī míng fāng lín zhèng mì yòng)*. Beijing: China Press of Traditional Chinese Medicine, 1993.

Fù Yǎn-Kuí 傅衍魁, Yóu Róng-Jí 尤榮輯. *Elaboration of Medical Formulas (醫方發揮 Yī fāng fā huī)*. Shenyang: Liaoning Science and Technology Press, 1984.

Gàn Zǔ-Wàng 幹祖望. *Master Gan's Eye, Ear, Nose and Throat Diseases (幹氏耳鼻咽喉口腔科學 Gàn shì ěr bí yān hóu kǒu qiāng kē xué)*. Nanjing: Jiangsu Science and Technology Publishing House, 1999.

Gōng Shì-Chéng 龔士澄, Gōng Xiǎo-Lín 龔曉林 (eds.) *Formulas and Herbs According to Clinical Patterns (臨證方藥 Lín zhèng fāng yào)*. Beijing: People's Medical Publishing House, 2002.

Gù Bó-Huá 顧伯華. *Practical Chinese External Medicine (實用中醫外科學 Shí yòng zhōng yī wài kē xué)*. Shanghai: Shanghai Science and Technology Press, 1985.

Guān Yòu-Bō 關幼波. *Selections from the Clinical Experience of Guan You-Bo (關幼波臨床經驗選 Guān Yòu-Bō lín chuáng jīng yàn xuǎn)*. Beijing: People's Medical Publishing House, 2006.

Guangzhou College of Traditional Chinese Medicine 廣州中医学院. *Formulas (方劑學 Fāng jì xué)*. Beijing: People's Medical Publishing House, 1983.

Guō Shì-Róng 郭世榮 (trans.) *Detailed Explanations of the Clinical Uses of Kanpo Formulas (臨床漢方處方詳解 Lín chuáng hàn fāng chǔ fāng xiáng jiě)*. Tainan: Zhengyan Publishing House, 1990

Hán Chéng-Rén 韓成仁. et al. (eds.) *Encyclopedia of Chinese Medical Patterns and Disease Names (中醫證病名大辭典 Zhōng yī zhèng bìng míng dà cí diǎn)*. Beijing: Publishing House of Ancient Chinese Medical Books, 2000.

Hóng Wén-Xù 洪文旭, Sū Lǐ 蘇禮 (eds.) *Explanation of Formula Names (方名釋 Fāng míng shì)*. Beijing: China Medical and Pharmacological Technology Press, 1987.

Huáng Huáng 黃煌. *Ten Key Chinese Medical Formula Families (中醫十大類方 Zhōng yī shí dà lèi fāng)*. Nanjing: Jiangsu Science and Technology Press, 1995.

— (ed.) *Awakening the Mind in Understanding Formulas and Herbs (方藥心悟 Fāng yào xīn wù)*. Nanjing: Jiangsu Science and Technology Press, 1999.

— (ed.) *One-Hundred Classic Formulas (經方100首 Jīng fāng 100 shǒu)*. Nanjing: Jiangsu Science and Technology Press, 2006.

Huáng Huáng 黃煌, Shǐ Xīn-Dé 史欣德 (eds.) *Famous Chinese Physicians' Discourse on Formulas and Herbs (名中醫論方藥 Míng zhōng yī lùn fāng yào)*. Nanjing: Phoenix Publishing and Media Network, 2005.

Huáng Róng-Zōng 黃榮宗 (ed.) *Formulas for Orthopedics and Trauma (骨傷方劑學 Gǔ shāng fāng jì xué)*. Beijing: People's Medical Publishing House, 1989.

— (ed.) *Vernacular Explanations of Songs on Orthopedic and Trauma Formulas (骨傷方歌白話解 Gǔ shāng fāng gē bái huà jiě)*. Beijing: Publishing House of Ancient Chinese Medical Books, 1989.

Huáng Róng-Zōng 黃榮宗, Chén Huàn-Hóng 陳煥泓, Wǔ Dà-Zhēn 吳大真 (eds.) *Guide to Medical Formulas for Clinical Patterns (醫方臨證指南 Yī fāng lín zhèng zhǐ nán)*. Beijing: China Press of Traditional Chinese Medicine, 1998.

Hubei College of Traditional Chinese Medicine — Formulas Research Group 湖北中醫學院方劑教研室. *Elaboration of Famous Ancient and Contemporary Formulas (古今名方發微 Gǔ jīn míng fāng fā wēi)*. Changsha: Hubei Science and Technology Press, 1986.

Japan Ministry of Health, Labour and Welfare Bureau of Medicines 日本厚生省藥物局監修, trans. by Chén Qín 陳琴. *Handbook of Kanpo Formulas in Common Use (常用漢方處方手冊 Cháng yòng hàn fāng chǔ fāng shǒu cè)*. Taipei: Lide Publishing Company, 1991.

Jì Zhì-Huá 冀志華. "Brief summary of Zhang Hui-Wu's use of Minor Extend Life Decoction to treat 88 cases of post-stroke hemiplegia" (張惠五用小續命湯治療中風偏枯88例小結 Zhāng Huī-Wǔ yòng xiǎo xù mìng tāng zhì liǎo zhòng fēng piān kū 88 lì xiǎo jié) in *Forum on Traditional Chinese Medicine* (國醫論壇 Guó yī lùn tán) 1989, 4(6): 22.

Jiǎ Dà-Míng 賈大明 (ed.) *Analysis of the Essence of Experiential Formulas by Chinese Physicians through the Ages (中國歷代名醫驗方析要 Zhōng guó lì dài míng yī yàn fāng xī yào)*. Shanxi: Shanxi Science and Technology Press, 1994.

Jiǎ Dé-Dào 賈德道. *Concise History of Medicine in China* (中國醫學史略 *Zhōng guó yī xué shǐ lüè*). Taoyuan: Shanxi People's Press, 1979.

Jiāng Chūn-Huá 姜春華. *Collected Medical Writings of Jiang Chun-Hua* (姜春華論醫集 *Jiāng Chūn-Huá yī lùn jí*). Fuzhou: Fuzhou Science and Technology Press, 1986.

Jiāng Kè-Míng 江克明, Bāo Míng-Huī 包明蕙 (eds.) *Concise Dictionary of Formulas* (簡明方劑辭典 *Jiǎn míng fāng jì cí diǎn*). Shanghai: Shanghai Science and Technology Press, 1987.

Jiangsu Provincial Chinese Medicine Hospital 江蘇省中醫院. *Selected and Compiled Clinical Experiences of Wei Chang-Chun* (魏長春臨床經驗選輯 *Wèi Cháng-Chūn lín chuáng jīng yàn xuǎn jí*). Nanjing: Jiangsu Science and Technology Press, 1974.

Jiāo Shù-Dé 焦樹德. *Ten Lectures on Experiences with Formulas* (方劑心得十講 *Fāng jì xīn dé shí jiǎng*). Beijing: People's Medical Publishing House, 1995.

Jīn Jiā-Jùn 金家浚, Jiǎng Wéi-Yǔ 蔣維宇 (eds.) *Compendium to the Various Schools of Chinese Medicine Physicians' Discourse on Formulas* (中醫百家方論薈萃 *Zhōng yī bǎi jiā fāng lùn huì cuì*). Chongqing: Chongqing Publishing House, 1994.

Jīn Shòu-Shān 金壽山. *Interpretation of the Golden Cabinet* (金匱詮釋 *Jīn guī quán shì*). Shanghai: Shanghai Science and Technology Press, 1986.

Kobe Traditional Chinese Medicine Research Group. *Explanation of Traditional Chinese Medical Formulas* (中醫處方解釋 *Chū i shohō kaisetsu*). Tokyo: Ishiyaku shuppan kabushikikaisha, 1982.

Lǐ Bǎo-Shùn 李寶順 (ed.) *A Collection of Famous Formulas by Famous Physicians* (名醫名方錄 *Míng yī míng fāng lù*), vol. 1-3. Beijing: Chinese Medicine Ancient Literature Publishing House, 1993.

Lǐ Fēi 李飛 (ed.) *A Selection of Essential Discussions on Chinese Medicine Formulas through the Ages* (中醫歷代方論精選 *Zhōng yī lì dài fāng lùn jīng xuǎn*). Nanjing: Jiangsu Science and Technology Press, 1998.

— (ed.) *Formulas* (方劑學 *Fāng jì xué*). Beijing: People's Medical Publishing House, 2002.

Lǐ Fēi 李飛, Chái Ruì-Jì 柴瑞霽, Fán Qiǎo-Líng 樊巧玲. *Methodology of Combining Herbs in Formulas* (方劑的配伍方法 *Fāng jì de pèi wǔ fāng fǎ*). Beijing: People's Medical Publishing House, 2001.

Lǐ Kè-Shào 李克紹. *Collected Medical Writings of Li Ke-Shao* (李克紹醫學文集 *Lǐ Kè-Shào yī xué wén jí*). Ji'nan: Shandong Science and Technology Press, 2006.

Lǐ Péi-Shēng 李陪生 et al. *Lectures on the Discussion of Cold Damage* (傷寒論講義 *Shāng hán lùn jiǎng yì*). Shanghai: Shanghai Science and Technology Press, 1985.

Lǐ Qìng-Yè 李慶業 (ed.) *Differentiation of the Clinical Uses of Commonly Used Formulas and Herbs – Formula Volume* (臨床常用方藥應用鑒別 – 方劑分冊 *Lín chuáng cháng yòng fāng yào yìng yòng jiàn bié – fāng jì fēn cè*). Beijing: People's Medical Publishing House, 2003.

Lǐ Qìng-Yè 李慶業, Yáng Bīn 楊斌 (eds.) *Formulas with Graphical Explanations* (方劑學圖表解 *Fāng jì xué tú biǎo jiě*). Beijing: People's Medical Publishing House, 2004.

Lǐ Shì-Cāng ed. 李世滄. *Handbook on the Clinical Use of Commonly Used Chinese Formulas* (臨床常用中藥方劑手冊 *Lín chuáng cháng yòng zhōng yào fāng jì shǒu cè*). Taizhong: Hongxiang Publishing Company, 1991.

Lǐ Wén-Ruì 李文瑞, Lǐ Qiū-Guì 李秋貴. *Discussion and Treatment of the Formulas and Patterns of Essentials of the Golden Cabinet* (金櫃要略湯證論治 *Jīn guì yào lüè tāng zhèng lùn zhì*). Beijing: China Science and Technology Press, 2000.

Lǐ Xiào-Rán 李笑然 (ed.) *Formulas* (方劑學 *Fāng jì xué*). Suzhou: Suzhou University Press, 2004.

Lǐ Xīn-Jī 李心機. *Explanations of Difficulties in the Discussion of Cold Damage* (《傷寒論》疑難解讀 *Shāng hán lùn yí nán jiě dú*). Beijing: People's Medical Publishing House, 1999.

Lǐ Yè 李業 (ed.) *The Craft of Composition in Famous Chinese Medicine Formulas* (中醫名方配伍技巧 *Zhōng yī míng fāng pèi wǔ jì qiǎo*). Beijing: Beijing Science and Technology Press, 1998.

Lǐ Yì 李義 (ed.) *Frequently Used Formulas* (常用方劑 *Cháng yòng fāng jì*). Taiyuan: Shanxi Science and Technology Press, 1991.

Liáng Yǒng-Cái 梁勇才 (ed.) *Quick Reference Handbook of Formulas and Herbs for External Treatment* (外治方藥速查手冊 *Wài zhì fāng yào sù chá shǒu cè*). Beijing: People's Military Medical Publisher, 2002.

Lide Chinese Medical Research Department 立得中醫研究室. *Study of Chinese Formulas and Patterns* (漢方方證學 *Hàn fāng fāng zhèng xué*). Taipei: Lide Publishing Company, 1991.

Liú Dù-Zhōu 劉渡舟. *Guide to Clinical Usage of Classical Formulas* (經方臨證指南 *Jīng fāng lín zhèng zhǐ nán*). Tianjin: Tianjin Science and Technology Press, 1993.

Liú Gōng-Wàng 劉公望 (ed.) *Famous Formulas Transmitted through the Ages* (傳世名方 *Chuán shì míng fāng*). Beijing: Huaxia Publishing Company, 2007.

Lǚ Zhì-Jié 呂志傑 (ed.) *Zhang Zhong-Jing's Formulas* (張仲景方劑學 *Zhāng Zhōng-Jǐng fāng jì xué*). Beijing: China Medical and Pharmacological Technology Press, 2004.

Mǎ Dà-Zhèng 馬大正. *Developmental History of Obstetrics and Gynecology in China* (中國婦產科發展史 *Zhōng guó fù chǎn kē fā zhǎn shǐ*). Taiyuan: Shanxi Science and Technology Press, 1992.

Mǎ Yǒu-Dù 馬有度. *New Explanations of Medical Formulas* (醫方新解 *Yī fāng xīn jiě*). Shanghai: Shanghai Science and Technology Press, 1980.

— . *The Marvelous Use of Formulas and Medicines* (方藥妙用 *Fāng yào miào yòng*). Beijing: People's Medical Publishing House, 2003.

Mǎ Zhì-Wén 馬志文 (ed.) *New Songs for Memorizing Formulas* (湯頭新歌 *Tāng tóu xīn gē*). Xi'an: Shaanxi Science and Technology Press, 1986.

Mò Méi-Shì 莫枚士 (ed.) *Explanation of Classical Formulas with Examples* (經方例釋 *Jīng fāng lì shì*). Beijing: China Press of Traditional Chinese Medicine, 1996.

Nakamura Kensuke 中村謙介. *Encyclopedic Explanation of Kampo Formulas* (和漢藥方意辭典 *Wakanyaku hōi jiten*). Tokyo: Midori shohō, 2004.

Nánjīng College of Traditional Chinese Medicine 南京中醫學院. *Chinese Medical Formulas* (中醫方劑學 *Zhōng yī fāng jì xué*). Shanghai: Shanghai Science and Technology Press, 1959.

—. *Explicating the Discussion of Cold Damage* (傷寒論釋義 *Shāng hán lùn shì yì*). Shanghai: Shanghai Science and Technology Press, 1964.

Ní Chéng 倪誠 (ed.) *A New Edition of Formulas* (新編方劑學 *Xīn biān fāng jì xué*). Beijing: People's Medical Publishing House, 2006.

Niè Huì-Mín 聶惠民. *Key Formula Discussions of Classic Formulas* (經方方論薈要 *Jīng fāng fāng lùn huì yào*). Changsha: Hunan Science and Technology Publishing House, 1999.

— . *Nie's Study of Cold Damage* (聶氏傷寒學 *Niè shì shāng hán xué*). Beijing: Xueyuan Publishing House, 2002.

Péng Huái-Rén 彭懷仁. *Encyclopedia of Chinese Medical Formulas* (中醫方劑大辭典 *Zhōng yī fāng jì dà cí diǎn*). Beijing: People's Medical Publishing House, 1999.

Qín Bó-Wèi 秦伯未. *Essential Case Records by Famous Qing Dynasty Physicians* (清代名醫醫案精華 *Qīng dài míng yī yī àn jīng huá*). Shanghai: Shanghai Chinese Medicine Publishing House, 1927.

Qiū Dé-Wén 邱德文 (ed.) *Formulas* (方劑學 *Fāng jì xué*). Guiyang: Guizhou People's Press, 1989.

Qiú Pèi-Rán 裘沛然 (ed.) *Collection of Famous Chinese Medical Formulas through the Ages* (中醫歷代名方集成 *Zhōng yī lì dài míng fāng jí chéng*). Shanghai: Shanghai Lexicographical Publishing House, 1994.

Shaanxi College of Traditional Chinese Medicine 陝西中醫學院 (ed.) *Annotated and Explained Corrections of Errors Among Physicians* (醫林改錯注釋 *Yī lín gǎi cuò zhù shì*). Beijing: People's Medical Publishing House, 1976.

Sivin, Nathan. *Traditional Medicine in Contemporary China.* Ann Arbor: University of Michigan Center for Chinese Studies, 1987.

Sūn Shì-Fā 孫世發 (ed.) *An Analysis of the Composition and Usage of Famous Formulas* (名方配伍分析及應用 *Míng fāng pèi wǔ fēn xī jí yìng yòng*). Beijing: People's Medical Publishing House, 2002.

Takayama Kōsei 高山宏世 (ed.) *Analysis of Commonly Used Kampo Formulas According to Pattern with Graphical Explanations* (臨證圖解漢方常用處方解說 *Rinkai kanpo jōyō hōkai*). Tokyo: 三考塾叢刊, 2005.

Tán Xìng-Guì 譚興貴, Liào Chuán-Qīng 廖泉清. *Problems with Traditional Chinese Medical Formulas* (中醫方劑問題 *Zhōng yī fāng jì wèn tí*). Changsha: Hunan Science and Technology Press, 1988.

Taylor, K. "Cholera and the Composition of the *Wenre Jingwei* (Complementing the Classics on Warmth and Heat) (1852). In Jiāng Xiǎo-Yuán 江曉原 (ed.), *A Multicultural History of Science: An Anthology of Essays from the 10th International Conference on East Asian History of Science.* Shanghai: Jiao Tong University Press, 2005.

Wáng Jūn-Níng 王均宁 (ed.) *Formulas* (方劑學 *Fāng jì xué*). Beijing: Science Press, 2005.

Wáng Mián-Zhī 王綿之. *Lecture Notes on Formulas* (方劑學講稿 *Fāng jì xué jiǎng gǎo*). Beijing: People's Medical Publishing House, 2005.

Wáng Qí 王琦. *Explanation of the Discussion of Cold Damage* (傷寒論講解 *Shāng hán lùn jiǎng jiě*). Xinxiang: Henan Science and Technology Press, 1988.

Wáng Qìng-Guó 王慶國, Jiǎ Chūn-Huá 賈春華 (eds.) *A Selection of Famous Japanese Kampo Formulas* (日本漢醫名方選 *Rìběn hàn yī míng fāng xuǎn*). Beijing: China Science and Technology Press, 1992.

Wáng Shū-Zhēn 王淑珍. *Unusual Formulas for Difficult Disorders: A Series of Reference Books* (難病奇方系列從書 *Nán bìng qí fāng xì liè cóng shū*). Beijing: China Press of Traditional Chinese Medicine, 2006.

Wáng Yǒng-Yán 王永炎, Zhāng Bó-Lǐ 張伯禮 (eds.) *Combining Formulas According to Qi and Flavor* (方劑氣味配伍 *Fāng jì qì wèi pèi wǔ*). Beijing: China Press of Traditional Chinese Medicine, 2006.

Wáng Zhàn-Xǐ 王佔璽. *Studies on the Medicinal Strategies of Zhang Zhong-Jing* (張仲景藥法研究 *Zhāng Zhōng-Jǐng yào fǎ yán jiū*). Beijing: Science and Technology Press, 1984.

Wiseman, Nigel. *A Practical Dictionary of Chinese Medicine.* Brookline: Paradigm Publications, 1997.

Wú Jiè-Chéng 吳介誠 (ed.) *Collected Experience with Sores* (瘡瘍經驗錄 *Chuāng yáng jīng yàn lù*). Beijing: People's Medical Publishing House, 1988.

Xiè Míng 謝鳴 (ed.) *Modern Studies of the Medical Formulas in Traditional Chinese Medicine* (中醫方劑現代研究 *Zhōng yī fāng jì xiàn dài yán jiū*). Beijing: Xue Yuan Press, 1997.

Xǔ Jì-Qún 許濟群, Wáng Mián-Zhī 王綿之 (eds.) *Formulas* 方濟學. Beijing: People's Medical Publishing House, 1995.

Xú Zhì-Hé 徐智和 (ed.) *Formulas* (方劑學 *Fāng jì xué*). Beijing: China Medical and Pharmacological Technology Press, 1999.

Xuē Qīng-Lù 薛清錄 et al. (eds.) *National Union Catalog of Primary Sources for Chinese Medicine* (全國中醫圖書聯合目錄 *Quán guó zhōng yī tú shū lián hé mù lù*). Beijing: Chinese Medicine Ancient Literature Publishing House, 1990.

Xuē Yú 薛愚. *Historical Materials of Traditional Chinese Medicinal Studies* (中國藥學史料 *Zhōng guó yào xué shǐ liào*). Beijing: People's Medical Publishing House, 1984.

Yakazu Dōmei 矢数道明, trans. by Lǐ Wén-Ruì 李文瑞 et al. *Clinically Practical Explanations of Kanpo Formulas* (臨床應用漢方處方解說 *Lín chuáng yìng yòng hàn fāng jiě shuō*). Beijing: People's Medical Publishing House, 1983.

Yán Rùn-Hóng 閆潤紅. *Formulas* (方劑學 *Fáng jì xué*). Beijing: Science Press, 2002.

Yáng Jí-Xiàng 楊吉相 (ed.) *Secret Collection of Patterns and Treatments for Sores* (瘡瘍證治秘錄 *Chuāng yáng zhèng zhì mì lù*). Shenyang: Liaoning Science and Technology Press, 1990.

Yóu Róng-Jí 游榮輯, Liú Xué-Wén 劉學文 (eds.) *New Contemporary Formulas* (現代新方劑學 *Xiàn dài xīn fāng jì xué*). Shanghai: Shanghai University of Traditional Chinese Medicine, 1991.

Yú Shèn-Chū 俞慎初. *Basic History of Medicine in China* (中國醫學簡史 *Zhōng guó yī xué jiǎn shǐ*). Fuzhou: Fujian Science and Technology Press, 1983.

Yuè Měi-Zhōng 岳美中. *Collected Medical Cases of Yue Mei-Zhong* (岳美中醫案集 *Yuè Měi-Zhōng yī àn jí*). Beijing: People's Medical Publishing House, 1978.

Zhāng Gǔ-Cái 張谷才 (ed.) *[Zhang] Zhong-Jing's Formulas* (仲景方劑學 *Zhōng-Jǐng fāng jì xué*). Shanghai: Shanghai University of Traditional Chinese Medicine, 2008.

Zhāng Hào-Liáng 張浩良 (ed.) *Essential Dictionary of Formulas* (方劑精華辭典 *Fāng jì jīng huá cí diǎn*). Tianjin: Tianjin Science and Technology Publishing House, 1996.

Zhāng Mín-Qìng 張民慶 (ed.) *Formulas in Contemporary Clinical Practice* (現代臨床方劑學 *Xiàn dài lín chuáng fāng jì xué*). Beijing: People's Medical Publishing House, 2004.

Zhāng Shù-Shēng 張樹生. *One Hundred Supremely Effective Medicinals* (百藥效用奇觀 *Bǎi yào xiào yòng qí guān*). Beijing: Chinese Medicine Ancient Literature Publishing House, 1987.

Zhào Cún-Yì 趙存義. *Study of the Formula Names of Ancient Formulas in Chinese Medicine* (中醫古方方名考 *Zhōng yī gǔ fāng fāng míng kǎo*). Beijing: China Press of Traditional Chinese Medicine, 1994.

Zhongshan Hospital 中山醫學院 (ed.) *Lectures on Selected Formulas in Traditional Chinese Medicine* (中醫方劑選講 *Zhōng yī fāng jì xuǎn jiǎng*). Guangdong: Guangdong Science and Technology Press, 1981.

Zhōu Fēng-Wú 周風梧. *Formulary Studies of Zhou Feng-Wu* (周風梧方劑學 *Zhōu Fēng-Wú fāng jì xué*). Ji'nan: Shandong Science and Technology Publishing House, 2005.

Zhōu Wén-Cǎi 周文采 (ed.) *An Essential Selection of Medical Formulas* (醫方選要 *yī fāng xuǎn yào*). Beijing: China Press of Traditional Chinese Medicine, 1993.

Zhū Liáng-Chūn 朱良春 (ed.) *Zhang Ci-Gong's Medical Craft and Experience: A Collection* (章次公醫術經驗集 *Zhāng Cì-Gōng yī shú jīng yàn jí*). Changsha: Hunan Science and Technology Press, 2000.

Zhuāng Guó-Kāng 莊國康, Wáng Guǎng-Jīn 王廣津 (eds.) *Materia Medica for External Treatment of Sores* (瘡瘍外用本草 *Chuāng yáng wài yòng běn cǎo*). Beijing: People's Medical Publishing House, 1982.

Zhuó Yǔ-Nóng 卓雨農. *Traditional Chinese Medical Therapeutics for Women's Diseases* (中醫婦科治療學 *Zhōng yī fù kē zhì liáo xué*). Chengdu: Sichuan Science and Technology Press, 1980.

Basic Formulary for Symptoms and Disorders

APPENDIX **5**

NE OF THE prominent features of traditional Chinese medicine is its focus on treating the cause of disease, instead of the symptom or disorder. For this reason, any symptom or disorder can have a multitude of possible treatments, depending on the nature of the underlying pathodynamics. In this appendix we present, in tabular form, some of the mechanisms involved in producing different symptoms and traditionally-defined disorders, together with the appropriate formulas for treatment from the book.

This list is by no means exhaustive, nor is it intended as a substitute for a firm grounding in internal medicine. Rather, it is hoped that it will spur the reader on to more in-depth study. We have omitted those disorders which are essentially covered in one of the chapters of the book. For example, because all of the exterior disorders are basically discussed in Chapter 1 (see page 1) colds are not included here. Similarly, as abscesses and sores are covered in detail in Chapter 20 (see page 857), they are not presented in these tables.

Abdominal and/or Epigastric Pain		
Food stagnation producing damp-heat	Fullness and pain in the epigastrium and abdomen accompanied by constipation, a yellow, greasy tongue coating, and an excessive pulse	Aucklandia ad Betel Nut Pill (*mù xiāng bīng láng wán*), 831
Heat in the Stomach and cold in the Intestines	Intermittent attacks of abdominal pain, a stifling sensation, irritability, and warmth in the chest and epigastrium accompanied by vomiting after eating, and cold hands and feet	Mume Pill (*wū méi wán*), 847
Liver qi stagnation with cold in the Stomach	Epigastric pain that responds favorably to warmth, a stifling sensation in the chest, hypochondriac pain, painful menstruation, and a white tongue coating	Galangal and Cyperus Pill (*liáng fù wán*), 521
Blood stasis and qi stagnation in the middle burner	Abdominal or epigastric pain which may radiate upward accompanied by signs and symptoms of blood stasis and qi stagnation	Salvia Drink (*dān shēn yǐn*), 594
Blood buildup in the lower burner	Acute lower abdominal pain, smooth urination, night fevers, delirious speech, irritability, restlessness and thirst, and a submerged, full, or choppy pulse	Peach Pit Decoction to Order the Qi (*táo hé chéng qì tāng*), 559
Cold from deficiency with qi stagnation and blood stasis	Spasmodic pain that occurs when the stomach is empty, a moist tongue with a white coating, and a large, frail pulse	Calm the Middle Powder (*ān zhōng sǎn*), 268

Consumptive deficiency	Intermittent, spasmodic pain that responds favorably to warmth and pressure, a lusterless complexion, reduced appetite, a pale tongue with a white coating, and a thin, wiry, and moderate pulse	Minor Construct the Middle Decoction *(xiǎo jiàn zhōng tāng)*, 264
Stomach yin deficiency	Faint or indistinct pain or burning in the epigastric region, hunger but no desire to actually eat, a dry mouth and throat, constipation, retching, hiccup, a dry, red tongue with scanty coating, and a thin, rapid pulse	Benefit the Stomach Decoction *(yì wèi tāng)*, 393
Middle burner yang deficiency with internal cold	Excruciating epigastric and abdominal pain, a strong sensation of cold in the epigastrium, vomiting to the point of being unable to eat, a white, slippery tongue coating, and a thin, tight or slow, wiry pulse	Major Construct the Middle Decoction *(dà jiàn zhōng tāng)*, 268

Bulging Disorders

Cold causing stagnation in the Liver channel	Lower abdominal pain radiating to the testicles, a pale tongue with a white coating, and either a submerged and slow or a wiry pulse	Top-Quality Lindera Powder *(tiān tái wū yào sǎn)*, 527
Deficient yang with wind-cold	Abdominal pain, cold extremities, numb hands and feet, generalized body aches	Aconite and Cinnamon Twig Decoction *(wū tóu guì zhī tāng)*, 19
Cold from deficiency	Lower abdominal pain that is sharp, localized, and is aggravated by the local application of cold, a pale tongue, and a submerged, tight pulse	Warm the Liver Decoction *(nuǎn nuǎn gān jiān)*, 531
Damp-cold invading the Liver channel	Unilateral testicular swelling with colicky pain reaching to the umbilicus, or a rock-like hardness and swelling of the scrotum, or oozing of a yellow fluid from the scrotum	Tangerine Seed Pill *(jú hé wán)*, 529

Chest Pain

Lack of arousal of the chest yang	Deep aching in the chest, wheezing, cough with copious sputum, shortness of breath, a thick, greasy tongue coating, and a tight or submerged, wiry pulse	Trichosanthes Fruit, Chinese Garlic, and Wine Decoction *(guā lóu xiè bái bái jiǔ tāng)*, 515
Congealing due to cold and turbid phlegm	Fullness, pain, and a sensation of cold in the chest and abdomen	Liquid Styrax Pill *(sū hé xiāng wán)*, 498
Clumping of phlegm in the chest	Pain in the chest and diaphragm such that the patient is unable to rotate the trunk, sputum that is difficult to expectorate, a stifling sensation and fullness in the chest, fever and chills, and labored breathing	Trichosanthes Fruit and Unripe Bitter Orange Decoction *(guā lóu zhǐ shí tāng)*, 792
Blood stasis in the chest	Chronic pain in the chest, hypochondria, and head, incessant hiccup, palpitations, insomnia, a dark-red tongue, dark spots on the sides of the tongue, and a choppy or wiry, tight pulse	Drive out Stasis from the Mansion of Blood Decoction *(xuè fǔ zhú yū tāng)*, 564

Constipation

Yang brightness organ warp	Frequent passing of gas, general feeling of fullness and tension in the abdomen, abdominal pain that increases with pressure, a dry, yellow or black, prickled tongue coating, and a deep, excessive pulse	Major Order the Qi Decoction (*dà chéng qì tāng*), 63
Yang brightness organ-warp pattern with severe depletion of body fluids	Dry stools that do not respond to purgatives, distention and fullness of the epigastrium and abdomen, dry mouth and lips, a dry tongue with a thin, yellow or burnt yellow coating, and a rapid, thin pulse	Increase the Fluids and Order the Qi Decoction (*zēng yè chéng qì tāng*), 88
Cold accumulation in the interior	Abdominal and hypochondriac pain, chills, low-grade feverishness, cold hands and feet, a white, greasy tongue coating, and a submerged, tight, and wiry pulsecoating, and a submerged, tight, and wiry pulse	Rhubarb and Aconite Accessory Root Decoction (*dà huáng fù zǐ tāng*), 71
Heat drying the Stomach and Intestines	Hard stool that is difficult to expel, urinary frequency, a dry, yellow tongue coating, and a submerged and rapid or floating and choppy pulse	Hemp Seed Pill (*má zǐ rén wán*), 81
Constraint and clumping of the Liver qi	Constipation, belching, and abdominal distention and pain	Six Milled-Herb Decoction (*liù mò tāng*), 526
Desiccated Intestines	Lusterless skin and nails, parched mouth with an unquenchable thirst, a dry tongue, and a thin pulse	Moisten the Intestines Pill from Master Shen's Book (*rùn cháng wán*), 80
Dry Intestines from injured fluids	Thirst, a dry, red tongue, and a thin and slightly rapid pulse, or one that is weak and without strength	Increase the Fluids Decoction (*zēng yè tāng*), 677
Deficient Kidney yang and qi	Clear and copious urination, lower backache, and a cold sensation in the back	Benefit the River [Flow] Decoction (*jì chuān jiān*), 84

Cough

Wind-cold attacking the Lungs	Cough with copious sputum and a constricted sensation in the chest	Canopy Powder (*huá gài sǎn*) or Three-Unbinding Decoction (*sān ǎo tāng*), 10
Wind-heat	Slight fever and thirst, and a rapid, floating pulse	Mulberry Leaf and Chrysanthemum Drink (*sāng jú yǐn*), 35
Wind-cold with thin mucus (weak constitution)	Fever and chills, headache, nasal congestion, a stifling sensation in the chest, a white tongue coating, and a weak pulse	Ginseng and Perilla Leaf Drink (*shēn sū yǐn*), 50
Cold and thin mucus lingering in the chest	Marked coughing and wheezing with a rattling sound	Belamcanda and Ephedra Decoction (*shè gān má huáng tāng*), 24
Cool-dryness	Watery sputum, slight headache, chills without sweating, a dry throat, a dry, white tongue coating, and a wiry pulse	Apricot Kernel and Perilla Leaf Powder (*xìng sū sǎn*), 663

Warm-dryness	Scanty, sticky sputum or a dry, hacking cough, moderate fever, headache, thirst, a red tongue with a dry, white coating, and a floating, rapid pulse	Mulberry Leaf and Apricot Kernel Decoction (*sāng xìng tāng*), 665
Wind attacking the Lungs with remnants of an exterior disorder	Slight chills and fever, an itchy throat, a thin, white tongue coating, and a moderate, floating pulse	Stop Coughing Powder (*zhǐ sòu sǎn*), 815
Dryness attacking the Lungs	Hacking cough, fever, wheezing, parched throat, dry nasal passages, a sensation of fullness in the chest, hypochondriac pain, irritability, a dry tongue with no coating, and a deficient, big, rapid pulse	Clear Dryness and Rescue the Lungs Decoction (*qīng zào jiù fèi tāng*), 667
Internal dryness of the Lungs (Lung and Kidney yin deficiency)	Blood-streaked sputum, wheezing, dry and hot palms and soles, night sweats, a red tongue with little coating, and a thin, rapid pulse	Lily Bulb Decoction to Preserve the Metal (*bǎi hé gù jīn tāng*), 384
Heat lodged in the Lungs	Viscous and difficult-to-expectorate sputum, fever with or without sweating, thirst, wheezing, labored breathing, nasal flaring and pain, a yellow tongue coating, and a slippery, rapid pulse	Ephedra, Apricot Kernel, Gypsum, and Licorice Decoction (*má xìng shí gān tāng*), 183
Lurking heat in the Lungs	High, clear-sounding cough that is nonproductive, fever, skin that feels hot to the touch, dry mouth, a thin, rapid pulse, and a red tongue with a yellow coating	Drain the White Powder (*xiè bái sǎn*), 186
Liver fire scorching the Lungs	Coughing that causes pain in the chest and flanks, an inability to rotate or bend the trunk, and in severe cases, blood-streaked sputum	Mulberry Leaf and Moutan Decoction to Drain the White (*sāng dān xiè bái tāng*), 188
Damp-phlegm from Spleen deficiency	Copious, white sputum that is easy to expectorate, a stifling sensation in the chest and diaphragm, nausea or vomiting, dizziness, a swollen tongue with a white, thick, greasy coating, and a slippery pulse	Two-Aged [Herb] Decoction (*èr chén tāng*), 775
Lung qi deficiency	Shortness of breath, spontaneous sweating, occasional chills and feverishness, coughing, wheezing, a pale tongue, and a frail or deficient and large pulse	Tonify the Lungs Decoction (*bǔ fèi tāng*), 331
Lung qi deficiency with heat in the Lungs	Thick, yellow sputum often with pus and blood, a sensation of heat and irritability in the chest, facial edema, gradual emaciation, a purple tongue with a thin coating, and a floating, deficient pulse	Ginseng and Gecko Powder (*rén shēn gé jiè sǎn*), 331
Lung qi and yin deficiency	Sparse sputum that is difficult to expectorate, shortness of breath, spontaneous sweating, dry mouth and tongue, a pale red tongue with a dry, thin coating, and a deficient pulse that is rapid or thin	Generate the Pulse Powder (*shēng mài sǎn*), 328
Lung and Kidney yin deficiency	Dry cough (may have blood-streaked sputum), tidal fever, heat in the five centers, emaciation, dry throat, reduced appetite, shortness of breath, scanty urine, a red, dry tongue, and a thin, rapid pulse	Moonlight Pill (*yuè huá wán*), 387

Yin deficiency consumptive disorder	Dry cough with little sputum accompanied by a dry throat or spitting of blood, muscle wasting, shortness of breath, weakness, a red tongue with little coating, and a thin, rapid pulse	Precious Jade Syrup *(qióng yù gāo)*, 389
Lung qi and yin exhaustion	Chronic, unremitting cough with wheezing, a shiny-white complexion, shortness of breath, spontaneous sweating, and a deficient, rapid pulse	Nine-Immortal Powder *(jiu xiān sǎn)*, 423

Diarrhea

Deficient Spleen with internally-generated dampness	Reduced appetite, weakness of the extremities, weight loss, distention in the chest and epigastrium, pallid and wan complexion, a pale tongue with a white coating, and a moderate pulse that is thin or deficient	Ginseng, Poria, and White Atractylodes Powder *(shēn líng bái zhú sǎn)*, 314
Middle burner cold from deficiency	Watery stool, nausea and vomiting, loss of appetite, abdominal pain, a pale tongue with a white coating, and a submerged, thin pulse	Regulate the Middle Pill *(lǐ zhōng wán)*, 257
Greater yang disorder with cold obstructing the greater yin	Fever, chills, headache, and joint pains accompanied by severe diarrhea and hard focal distention in the epigastrium	Cinnamon Twig and Ginseng Decoction *(guì zhī rén shēn tāng)*, 298
Severe cold from deficiency of the Spleen, Stomach, and Kidneys	Undigested food in the stool or daybreak diarrhea, aversion to cold, cold extremities, back pain, reduced appetite, a pale tongue with a white coating, and a submerged, slow, and deficient pulse	Cinnamon and Prepared Aconite Accessory Root Decoction to Regulate the Middle *(guì fù lǐ zhōng tāng)*, 260
Deficient Spleen with over-controlling Liver	Recurrent problems of borborygmus, abdominal pain, and diarrhea with pain accompanying each urge to have a bowel movement that is relieved upon completion, a thin, white tongue coating, and a wiry, thin pulse	Important Formula for Painful Diarrhea *(tòng xiè yào fāng)*, 125
Deficient Spleen and Kidney yang	Diarrhea that occurs daily just before sunrise, lack of appetite, soreness of the lower back with cold limbs, fatigue, a pale tongue with a thin, white coating, and a submerged, slow, and forceless pulse	Four-Miracle Pill *(sì shén wán)*, 429

Dizziness

Wind-phlegm	Headache, a stifling sensation in the chest, nausea or vomiting, copious sputum, a white, greasy tongue coating, and a wiry, slippery pulse	Pinellia, White Atractylodes, and Gastrodia Decoction *(bàn xià bái zhú tiān má tāng)*, 811
Heat excess in the Liver and/or Gallbladder channels	Headache, red and sore eyes, hearing loss, swelling in the ears, a bitter taste in the mouth, irritability, hypochondriac pain, short temper, a wiry, rapid, and forceful pulse, and a red tongue with a yellow coating	Gentian Decoction to Drain the Liver *(lóng dǎn xiè gān tāng)*, 199
Gallbladder and Stomach disharmony with phlegm-heat	Nausea or vomiting, insomnia, anxiety, copious sputum, focal distention of the chest, a bitter taste in the mouth, slight thirst, a greasy, yellow tongue coating, and a rapid pulse that is slippery or wiry	Warm Gallbladder Decoction *(wēn dǎn tāng)*, 786

Liver and Kidney yin deficiency with ascendant Liver yang	A feeling of distention in the eyes, tinnitus, feverish sensation in the head, headache, irritability, flushed face (as if intoxicated), and a wiry, long, and forceful pulse	Sedate the Liver and Extinguish Wind Decoction *(zhèn gān xī fēng tāng)*, 644
Ascendant Liver yang with internal Liver wind	Headache, tinnitus, blurred vision, a sensation of heat rushing to the head, insomnia with dream-disturbed sleep, a red tongue, and a wiry, rapid pulse	Gastrodia and Uncaria Drink *(tiān má gōu téng yǐn)*, 647
Yin deficiency and ascendant yang (often in a warm-febrile disease)	Tinnitus, dry throat, palpitations, bleeding symptoms, a dry, glossy, peeled tongue, and a thin, wiry pulse	Three-Shell Decoction to Restore the Pulse *(sān jiǎ fù mài tāng)*, 649
Blood deficiency	Blurred vision, lusterless complexion and nails, generalized muscle tension, irregular menstruation with little flow, lower abdominal pain, a pale tongue, and a thin and wiry or choppy pulse	Four-Substance Decoction *(sì wù tāng)*, 333
Blood and yin deficiency	Headache, tinnitus, dry eyes, photophobia, blurred vision, irritability, bad temper, numbness, muscle twitches, malar flush, a red, dry tongue, and a wiry, thin, and rapid pulse	Tonify the Liver Decoction *(bǔ gān tāng)*, 337
Liver and Kidney yin deficiency	Blurred vision, weakness and soreness of the lower back and knees, dry and parched mouth and throat, insomnia, spontaneous emissions, premature graying or loss of hair, and a red, dry tongue	Two-Solstice Pill *(èr zhì wán)*, 383
Yin deficiency, dried blood, and wind-dampness	Blurred vision, chronic cough, constipation with very dry stools, dry, flaky skin, numbness, and painful obstruction	Mulberry Leaf and Sesame Seed Pill *(sāng má wán)*, 384

Dysenteric Disorders

Wind-cold-dampness (early stages)	Chills, fever, lack of sweating, head pain and distention, generalized body pain, and a floating and tight or rapid pulse	Ginseng Powder to Overcome Pathogenic Influences *(rén shēn bài dú sǎn)*, 47
Wind-heat (early stages)	Fever, foul-smelling stools, burning sensation in the anus, a red tongue with a yellow coating, and a rapid pulse	Kudzu, Scutellaria, and Coptis Decoction *(gé gēn huáng qín huáng lián tāng)*, 292
Heat toxin searing the Stomach and Intestines	Abdominal pain, burning sensation around the anus, diarrhea that contains more blood than pus, thirst, a red tongue with a yellow coating, and a wiry, rapid pulse	Pulsatilla Decoction *(bái tóu wēng tāng)*, 210
Damp-heat lodging in the Intestines	Abdominal pain, difficulty with defecation, diarrhea with equal amounts of pus and blood, a burning sensation around the anus, scanty and dark urine, a greasy, slightly yellow tongue coating, and a rapid pulse	Peony Decoction *(sháo yào tāng)*, 207
Chronic damp-heat damaging the yin and yang	Intermittent discharge of blood and pus from the bowels, tenesmus, continuous abdominal pain, irritability of the chest, a red tongue with little coating, and a thin rapid pulse	Halt the Carts Pill *(zhù chē wán)*, 432
Spleen and Kidney cold from deficiency	Unremitting diarrhea to the point of incontinence or prolapsed rectum, abdominal pain that responds favorably to warmth or pressure, a pale tongue with a white coating, and a slow, thin pulse	True Man's Decoction to Nourish the Organs *(zhēn rén yǎng zàng tāng)*, 425

Cold from deficiency with internal obstruction of damp-cold	Chronic conditions with dark blood and pus in the stool, abdominal pain that responds favorably to local pressure or warmth, a pale tongue, and a pulse that is slow and frail or faint and thin	Peach Blossom Decoction (*táo huā tāng*), 427

Edema

External wind-cold with internal thin mucus	Floating edema, fever and chills without sweating, cough, wheezing, sputum that is copious, white, and stringy, a stifling sensation in the chest, body aches, a moist tongue coating, and a floating, tight pulse	Minor Bluegreen Dragon Decoction (*xiǎo qīng lóng tāng*), 21
Wind-edema	Aversion to drafts, generalized edema that begins in the face, slight fever, slight but continuous sweating, and a floating pulse	Maidservant from Yue's Decoction (*Yuè bì tāng*), 185; or for more severe cases, Maidservant from Yue's Decoction plus Atractylodes (*Yuè bì jiā zhú tāng*), 185
Exterior deficiency with wind-dampness	Superficial edema, sweating, a heavy sensation in the body, urinary difficulty, a pale tongue with a white coating, and a floating pulse	Stephania and Astragalus Decoction (*fáng jǐ huáng qí tāng*), 735
Exterior wind-cold with interior heat	Acute superficial edema, severe chills and fever without sweating, body aches, irritability, and a floating, tight pulse	Major Bluegreen Dragon Decoction (*dà qīng lóng tāng*), 11
Obstruction due to accumulation of thin mucus	Edema that is worse below the waist, abdominal distention, wheezing, fullness in the chest, and difficult urination and defecation	Ten-Jujube Decoction (*shí zǎo tāng*), 90
Internal accumulation of water and dampness	Generalized sensation of heaviness, diarrhea, urinary difficulty, and possibly vomiting and diarrhea	Five-Ingredient Powder with Poria (*wǔ líng sǎn*), 724
Yang edema from invasion of water dampness	Generalized floating edema, abdominal distention, wheezing and fullness, constipation, urinary difficulty, and a submerged and forceful pulse	Yu's Achievement Powder (*Yǔ gōng sǎn*), 93
Spleen deficiency with dampness and qi stagnation	Generalized edema with a sensation of heaviness, distention in the epigastrium and abdomen, labored and heavy breathing, urinary difficulty, a white, greasy tongue coating, and a submerged, moderate pulse	Five-Peel Powder (*wǔ pí sǎn*), 732
Spleen and Kidney yang deficiency	Edema that is worse below the waist, cold extremities, chest and abdominal distention, loss of appetite, scanty urine, semi-liquid stools, a thick, greasy tongue coating, and a submerged pulse that is slow or thin	Bolster the Spleen Drink (*shí pí yǐn*), 749
Kidney yang deficiency	Edema of the legs, aversion to cold, cold extremities, scanty urination, soreness of the lower back, a pale, swollen, tooth-marked tongue with a white, slippery coating, and a submerged, wiry pulse	Augmented Kidney Qi Pill (*jiā wèi shèn qì wán*), 400

Headache

Externally-contracted wind	Chills and fever, nasal congestion, and a floating pulse	Chuanxiong Powder to be Taken with Green Tea (*chuān xiōng chá tiáo săn*), 625
Externally-contracted wind-heat	Fever, dizziness, yellow sputum, and a floating, rapid pulse	Chrysanthemum Powder to be Taken with Green Tea (*jú huā chá tiáo săn*), 627
Severe fire in the qi and blood levels	Intense fever, strong thirst, dry heaves, severe and stabbing headache, extreme irritability, a dark-red tongue, and a rapid pulse that is either submerged and thin or floating and large	Clear Epidemics and Overcome Toxicity Drink (*qīng wēn bài dú yǐn*), 179
Lesser yang-warp disorder with qi constraint	Lateral forehead pain, diminished hearing, vertigo, chest and hypochondriac pain, alternating fever and chills, a white tongue coating, and a wiry pulse that is slippery on the right and floating and large on the left	Bupleurum, Bitter Orange, and Platycodon Decoction (*chái hú zhǐ jié tāng*), 110
Phlegm-fire agitating the Heart	Severe, throbbing pain, restless agitation, bad temper, insomnia, extreme emotional instability, manic behavior, a scarlet tongue with a yellow, greasy coating, and a wiry, rapid pulse	Iron Filings Drink (*shēng tiě luò yǐn*), 478
Blood stasis in the upper part of the body	Vertigo, chronic tinnitus, hair loss, dark-purple complexion, darkness around the eyes, and 'brandy' nose	Unblock the Orifices and Invigorate the Blood Decoction (*tōng qiào huó xuè tāng*), 567
Wind-dampness in the channels	Dizziness, vertigo, nasal congestion, numbness of the skin, itchiness, and rashes	Eliminate Wind Powder from *Formulary of the Pharmacy Service* (*xiāo fēng săn*), 638
Ascendant Liver yang with internal Liver wind	Dizziness, tinnitus, blurred vision, a sensation of heat rushing to the head, insomnia with dream-disturbed sleep, a red tongue, and a wiry, rapid pulse	Gastrodia and Uncaria Drink (*tiān má gōu téng yǐn*), 647
Cold from deficiency	Dull ache, sore throat and raspy voice, chronic cough and/or wheezing	Ephedra, Asarum, and Aconite Accessory Root Decoction (*má huáng xì xīn fù zǐ tāng*), 50

Hypochondriac Pain

Thin mucus fluids stagnating in the collaterals of the Liver	Coughing (sometimes), either afternoon fevers without chills or alternating chills and fever, a thickly-coated tongue with swollen edges, and a wiry pulse, especially in the middle position	Cyperus and Inula Decoction (*xiāng fù xuán fù huā tāng*), 789
Heat excess in the Liver and/or Gallbladder channels	Dizziness, headache, red and sore eyes, hearing loss, swelling in the ears, a bitter taste in the mouth, irritability, short temper, a wiry, rapid, and forceful pulse, and a red tongue with a yellow coating	Gentian Decoction to Drain the Liver (*lóng dăn xiè gān tāng*), 199

Fire and dampness in the Liver and Gallbladder	Unremitting pain, a bitter taste in the mouth, dry mouth, alternating fever and chills, abdominal distention, a red or dark-red tongue with a yellow, dry coating, and a wiry, slippery, and rapid or a flooding, rapid pulse	Clear the Gallbladder and Drain Fire Decoction (*qīng dǎn xiè huǒ tāng*), 201
Liver and Stomach disharmony due to heat in the Liver	Indeterminate gnawing hunger, epigastric focal distention, vomiting, acid regurgitation, belching, a bitter taste in the mouth, dry mouth, a red tongue with a yellow coating, and a wiry, rapid pulse	Left Metal Pill (*zuǒ jīn wán*), 205
Liver-Spleen disharmony	Distention (sometimes with epigastric pain and fullness), a bitter taste in the mouth, belching, reduced appetite, and a wiry, forceful pulse	Frigid Extremities Powder (*sì nì sǎn*), 116
Liver constraint with heat	Intermittent pain that is aggravated by the ingestion of hot food or beverage, irritability, a red tongue with a yellow coating, and a wiry or rapid pulse	Melia Toosendan Powder (*jīn líng zǐ sǎn*), 522
Trauma to the Liver and Gallbladder channels	Excruciating pain associated with traumatic injury	Revive Health by Invigorating the Blood Decoction (*fù yuán huó xuè tāng*), 571
Liver constraint with blood deficiency	Headache, vertigo, a bitter taste in the mouth, dry mouth and throat, fatigue, reduced appetite, a pale-red tongue, and a wiry, deficient pulse	Rambling Powder (*xiāo yáo sǎn*), 120
Liver and Kidney yin deficiency with qi stagnation	Chest pain, epigastric and abdominal distention, a dry, parched mouth and throat, acid regurgitation, a red, dry tongue, and a thin, frail or deficient, wiry pulse	Linking Decoction (*yī guàn jiān*), 381

Inversion/collapse (厥 *jué*)

Early-stage heat inversion	Fever, cold extremities, thirst, sweating from the head, constipation, scanty and dark urine, disorientation, delirious speech, a hot sensation in the sternum and epigastrium, and an excessive pulse	Major Order the Qi Decoction (*dà chéng qì tāng*), 63
Cold or yin-type inversion (Kidney yang deficiency with internal cold)	Extremely cold extremities, aversion to cold, a constant desire to sleep, abdominal pain and cold, a pale tongue with a white, slippery coating, and a submerged pulse that is thin or faint	Frigid Extremities Decoction (*sì nì tāng*), 274
Cold or yin-type inversion (sudden collapse of the yang qi)	Cold extremities, sweating, shortness of breath, dizziness, extremely pale complexion, a pale tongue, and a faint pulse that is almost imperceptible	Ginseng and Aconite Accessory Root Decoction (*shēn fù tāng*), 279
Qi and yin deficiency inversion	Shortness of breath, spontaneous sweating, a dry mouth and tongue, a pale, red tongue with a dry, thin coating, and a deficient pulse that is either rapid or thin	Generate the Pulse Powder (*shēng mài sǎn*), 328
Hot or yang-type inversion	Frigid fingers and toes, a warm body (sometimes with a sensation of irritability and fullness in the chest and hypochondria), a red tongue with a yellow coating, and a wiry pulse	Frigid Extremities Powder (*sì nì sǎn*), 116
Phlegm-heat in the Pericardium (limb collapse)	High fever, irritability and restlessness, delirious speech, impaired consciousness, a red or deep-red tongue, and a rapid pulse	Calm the Palace Pill with Cattle Gallstone (*ān gōng niú huáng wán*), 488

Sudden attack of turbid qi (comatose collapse)	Loss of consciousness, clenched jaw, extreme difficulty in breathing, foaming at the mouth, and a pale, ashen complexion	Open the Gate Powder (*tōng guān sǎn*), 500
Tetanic collapse (heat sinking into the Pericardium)	High fever, irritability and restlessness, delirious speech, impaired consciousness, muscle twitches, spasms, convulsions, thirst, parched lips, dark urine, and severe constipation	Purple Snow Special Pill (*zǐ xuě dān*), 490; or Stop Spasms Powder (*zhǐ jìng sǎn*), 634
Inversion due to roundworms	Intermittent attacks of abdominal pain, a stifling sensation, irritability, and warmth in the chest and epigastrium accompanied by vomiting after eating, and cold hands and feet	Mume Pill (*wū méi wán*), 847
Inversion due to phlegm	Fainting, a stifling sensation and focal distention in the chest and diaphragm, reduced appetite, coughing and wheezing with copious sputum, a white, greasy tongue coating, and a slippery pulse	Guide Out Phlegm Decoction (*dǎo tán tāng*), 780

Joint Pain

Wind in the joints	Crackling sensation in the joints	Bupleurum and Cinnamon Twig Decoction (*chái hú guì zhī tāng*), 109
Wind-heat-dampness	High fever, sweating, irritability, thirst, pain and swelling of the joints, a white tongue coating, and a wiry, rapid pulse	White Tiger plus Cinnamon Twig Decoction (*bái hǔ jiā guì zhī tāng*), 154
Damp painful obstruction which has transformed into heat	Fever, epigastric distention, profuse sweating, a generalized sensation of heaviness, pain in the joints, cold feet, and a red, greasy tongue	White Tiger plus Atractylodes Decoction (*bái hǔ jiā cāng zhú tāng*), 154
Wind attacking the extremities	Numbness, headache, and dizziness	Lindera Powder to Smooth the Flow of Qi (*wū yào shùn qì sǎn*), 623
Relatively early-stage wind-cold-dampness painful obstruction	Pain that increases with cold and diminishes with warmth, possibly accompanied by a sensation of heaviness, and a slow, possibly slippery pulse	Remove Painful Obstruction Decoction (*juān bì tāng*), 756
Wind-cold-dampness painful obstruction	Fixed or migrating pain with reduced range of motion aggravated by cold, and a white, moist tongue coating	Minor Invigorate the Collaterals Special Pill (*xiǎo huó luò dān*), 631
Wind-cold-dampness with qi deficiency	Generalized sensation of heaviness in the body, stiffness in the neck, shoulders, and upper back, numbness in the extremities, difficulty in moving, a white tongue coating, and a moderate pulse	Remove Painful Obstruction Decoction (*juān bì tāng*), 756
Recurrent wind-cold-dampness with heat from constraint	Swollen and painful joints (especially of the lower extremities) that are warm to the touch and worsen at night, chills, absence of sweating, weight loss, headache, a white, greasy tongue coating, and a wiry, slippery pulse	Cinnamon Twig, Peony, and Anemarrhena Decoction (*guì zhī sháo yào zhī mǔ tāng*), 760
Damp-heat in the channels	Heat in the joints, reduced mobility, fever and shaking chills, a lusterless, yellow complexion, scanty, dark urine, and a gray or yellow, greasy tongue coating	Disband Painful Obstruction Decoction (*xuān bì tāng*), 762

Long-term invasion of the channels by wind-dampness	Intense pain and severely restricted motion in the joints, particularly those of the hands and feet	Aconite Decoction (*wū tóu tāng*), 624
Blood stasis and qi stagnation	Shoulder pain, arm pain, lower back pain, leg pain, or other chronic aches and pains of the body with signs of blood stasis	Drive Out Stasis from a Painful Body Decoction (*shēn tōng zhú yū tāng*), 568
Liver and Kidney deficiency	Fixed pain in the lower back and lower extremities, weakness and stiffness, an aversion to cold and attraction to warmth, shortness of breath, a pale tongue with a white coating, and a thin, weak, slow pulse	Pubescent Angelica and Taxillus Decoction (*dú huó jì shēng tāng*), 758

Malarial Disorders

Dampness	Chills predominant, generalized body aches, a sensation of heaviness in the limbs, loss of appetite, and a soggy pulse	Bupleurum and Calm the Stomach Decoction (*chái píng tāng*), 110
Damp-heat	Intermittent, strong fevers and chills, a stifling sensation in the chest, nausea and/or vomiting, headache, irritability, a tongue with deep red edges and a thick, foul, pasty coating, and a rapid, wiry pulse	Reach the Source Drink (*dá yuán yǐn*), 137
Damp-phlegm	Intense, unremitting attacks of alternating fever and chills, abdominal distention, a greasy, white tongue coating, and a wiry, slippery, floating, and big pulse at the distal position	Seven-Treasure Drink to Check Malarial Disorders (*jié nuè qī bǎo yǐn*), 134
Qi and blood deficiency	Chronic, unremitting malarial disorder with emaciation, a pale tongue and a moderate, big pulse that is deficient. The slightest amount of exertion will exacerbate the condition.	Fleeceflower Root and Ginseng Drink (*hé rén yǐn*), 362

Painful Urinary Dribbling

Heat excess in the Liver and/or Gallbladder channels	Sensation of heat in the urethra, headache, bitter taste in the mouth, irritability, short temper, a wiry, rapid, and forceful pulse, and a red tongue with a yellow coating	Gentian Decoction to Drain the Liver (*lóng dǎn xiè gān tāng*), 199
Heat in the Heart and Small Intestine channels	Dark, scanty urination, irritability with a sensation of heat in the chest, thirst with a desire to drink cold beverages, red face, possibly sores around the mouth, a red tongue, and a rapid pulse	Guide Out the Red Powder (*dǎo chì sǎn*), 195
Damp-heat clumping in the lower burner	Dark, turbid, and scanty urination, a dry mouth and throat, a yellow, greasy tongue coating, and a slippery, rapid pulse	Eight-Herb Powder for Rectification (*bā zhèng sǎn*), 713
Heat in the blood (stony or bloody)	Rough, painful urination that is red or the color of red bean juice (or cola), or with multiple tiny stones	Powder for Five Types of Painful Urinary Dribbling (*wǔ lín sǎn*), 716
Painful urinary dribbling during pregnancy	Dirty-yellow complexion, dry mouth with no desire to drink, stifling sensation in the chest, reduced appetite, a red tongue with a yellow coating, and a slippery, rapid pulse	Augmented Powder for Five Types of Painful Urinary Dribbling (*jiā wèi wǔ lín sǎn*), 717

Damp-heat in the lower burner (stony)	Urinary urgency with burning, anuria, or oliguria due to stones in the urinary tract	Three-Gold Decoction *(sān jīn tāng)*, 716
Static heat accumulating in the lower burner (bloody)	Blood in the urine, thirst, irritability, a red tongue with a thin, yellow coating, and a rapid, forceful pulse	Small Thistle Drink *(xiǎo jì yǐn zi)*, 603
Cold from deficiency in the lower burner (cloudy)	Frequent urination with cloudy, dense, milky (resembling rice water) or greasy urine	Tokoro Drink to Separate the Clear *(bì xiè fēn qīng yǐn)*, 757
Damp-heat seeping into the Bladder (cloudy)	Cloudy urine that continues to drip after completion, and a yellow, greasy tongue coating	Tokoro Drink to Separate the Clear from *Awakening of the Mind in Medical Studies (bì xiè fēn qīng yǐn)*, 753

Sudden Turmoil Disorders

Externally-contracted sudden turmoil disorder	Fever and chills, abdominal distention and fullness	Rectify the Qi Powder Worth More than Gold *(bù huàn jīn zhèng qì sǎn)*, 689
External wind-cold with internal damp turbidity	Chills and fever, headache, sensation of fullness and stifling oppression in the chest, pain in the epigastrium and abdomen, borborygmus, an inability to taste food, a white, greasy tongue coating, and a moderate, soggy pulse	Patchouli/Agastache Powder to Rectify the Qi *(huò xiāng zhèng qì sǎn)*, 691
Dampness injuring the Spleen in the summer	Sensation of fullness and distention in the diaphragmatic region, and a white, slippery tongue coating	Harmonize the Six Decoction *(liù hé tāng)*, 695
Accumulation of damp-heat	Focal distention and a stifling sensation in the chest and epigastrium, dark, scanty urine, and a yellow, greasy tongue coating	Coptis and Magnolia Bark Drink *(lián pò yǐn)*, 705
Summerheat with internal stagnation of water and dampness	Fever, headache, irritability, thirst, urinary difficulty with scanty urine	Cinnamon and Poria Sweet Dew Drink *(guì líng gān lù yǐn)*, 241
Internal accumulation of water and dampness	Edema, sensation of heaviness, urinary difficulty	Five-Ingredient Powder with Poria *(wǔ líng sǎn)*, 724

Vomiting or Belching

Simultaneous greater yang and yang brightness disorder	Fever and chills (chills predominant), absence of sweating, headache, body aches, a thin, white tongue coating, and a floating, tight pulse	Kudzu Decoction plus Pinellia *(gé gēn jiā bàn xià tāng)*, 21
Simultaneous lesser yang and yang brightness disorder	Continuous vomiting, alternating chills and fever, fullness in the chest and hypochondria, a bitter taste in the mouth, either burning diarrhea or no bowel movements, a yellow tongue coating, and a wiry, forceful pulse	Major Bupleurum Decoction *(dà chái hú tāng)*, 286
Phlegm turbidity obstructing the interior	Unremitting belching, hiccup, regurgitation, nausea or vomiting, hard epigastric focal distention, a white, slippery tongue coating, and a wiry, deficient pulse	Inula and Haematite Decoction *(xuán fù dài zhě tāng)*, 542

Heat in the Stomach with qi deficiency	Hiccup, vomiting, or retching accompanied by a tender, red tongue and a deficient, rapid pulse	Tangerine Peel and Bamboo Shavings Decoction (*jú pí zhú rú tāng*), 547
Heat in the Stomach without qi deficiency	Hiccup, vomiting, or retching accompanied by a red tongue and a rapid pulse	Newly-Formulated Tangerine Peel and Bamboo Shavings Decoction (*xīn zhì jú pí zhú rú tāng*), 547
Cold from deficiency of the Stomach	Hiccup, belching, or vomiting with a stifling sensation in the epigastrium, focal distention of the chest, a pale tongue with a white coating, and a submerged, slow pulse	Clove and Persimmon Calyx Decoction (*dīng xiāng shì dì tāng*), 547
Cold from deficiency of the Stomach and Liver	Vomiting immediately after eating, indeterminate gnawing hunger, and acid regurgitation with or without epigastric pain, a white, slippery tongue coating, and a thin, slow or thin, wiry pulse	Evodia Decoction (*wú zhū yú tāng*), 261
Stomach cold in children	Vomiting in the evening what was eaten in the morning, undigested particles of food in the stool, cold extremities, and a pale complexion and lips	Clove and Evodia Decoction to Regulate the Middle (*dīng yú lǐ zhōng tāng*), 260

Wheezing		
Exterior wind-cold	Simultaneous fever and chills without sweating	Ephedra Decoction (*má huáng tāng*), 7
Exterior wind-cold with interior thin mucus	Simultaneous fever and chills (chills predominant) without sweating, coughing of sputum that is copious, clear, white, stringy, and difficult to expectorate, and a stifling sensation in the chest	Minor Bluegreen Dragon Decoction (*xiǎo qīng lóng tāng*), 21
Wind-cold in the exterior with phlegm-heat in the interior	Coughing with copious, thick, and yellow sputum, labored breathing, a greasy, yellow tongue coating, and a slippery, rapid pulse	Arrest Wheezing Decoction (*dìng chuǎn tāng*), 540
Wind-cold in the exterior with Liver qi constraint	Nonproductive cough with an uncomfortable sensation in the chest and hypochondria, difficult breathing (especially when lying down), and a rough sound in the throat	Mysterious Decoction (*shén mì tāng*), 542
Phlegm-dryness	Cough with deep-seated sputum that is difficult to expectorate, wheezing, a dry and sore throat, a red and dry tongue with little coating, and a rapid and thin but strong pulse	Fritillaria and Trichosanthes Fruit Powder (*bèi mǔ guā lóu sǎn*), 802
Cold in the Lungs with food stagnation	Cough with copious sputum, focal distention in the chest, loss of appetite, digestive difficulties, a white, greasy tongue coating, and a slippery pulse	Three-Seed Decoction to Nourish One's Parents (*sān zǐ yǎng qīn tāng*), 808
Internal clumping of phlegm-heat	Coughing of yellow, viscous sputum that is difficult to expectorate, focal distention and a feeling of fullness in the chest and diaphragm, nausea, a red tongue with a greasy, yellow coating, and a slippery, rapid pulse	Clear the Qi and Transform Phlegm Pill (*qīng qì huà tán wán*), 790

Lung and Kidney yin deficiency with rising phlegm	Wheezing, copious, white sputum that is difficult to expectorate, nausea, and a peeled tongue	Six-Gentlemen of Metal and Water Decoction (*jīn shuǐ liù jūn jiān*), 779
Phlegm-cold obstructing the Lungs with Kidney deficiency	Cough with watery, copious sputum, a stifling sensation in the chest and diaphragm, shortness of breath marked by relatively labored inhalation and smooth exhalation, and a white, greasy tongue coating	Perilla Fruit Decoction for Directing Qi Downward (*sū zǐ jiàng qì tāng*), 537
Cold, thin mucus due to yang deficiency and ascendant yin	Cough with profuse sputum that is thin, watery, and white accompanied by a feeling of discomfort in the chest and diaphragm, a white, slippery tongue coating, and a wiry, slippery pulse	Poria, Licorice, Schisandra, Ginger, and Asarum Decoction (*líng gān wǔ wèi jiāng xīn tāng*), 806
Constraint and clumping of the Liver qi	Labored breathing, an irritable, stifling sensation in the chest and diaphragm, epigastric focal distention and fullness, and a loss of appetite	Four Milled-Herb Decoction (*sì mò tāng*), 525
Lung yin deficiency with vigorous heat	Cough with a dry and parched throat, scanty or blood-streaked sputum, a red tongue with little coating, and a floating, thin, and rapid pulse	Tonify the Lungs Decoction with Ass-Hide Gelatin (*bǔ fèi ē jiāo tāng*), 386

Wind-stroke

Invasion by wind-cold	Hemiplegia, facial asymmetry, slow and slurred speech. Usually accompanied by fever and chills, a pale tongue with a thin, white coating, and a deficient, floating pulse	Minor Extend Life Decoction (*xiǎo xù mìng tāng*), 621
Damp-cold and turbid phlegm (closed disorder)	Sudden collapse, clenched jaw, a pale complexion, purple lips, excessive mucus and saliva, cold extremities, a pale tongue with a slippery, greasy coating, and a submerged, slippery pulse	Liquid Styrax Pill (*sū hé xiāng wán*), 498
Phlegm-heat (closed disorder)	Fever, restlessness, delirious speech, impaired consciousness, copious sputum with labored and raspy breathing, spasms, a red or deep-red tongue with a foul, greasy, yellow coating, and a slippery, rapid pulse	Greatest Treasure Special Pill (*zhì bǎo dān*), 493
Internally-generated wind and heat	Facial asymmetry, paraplegia or hemiplegia, raving and/or sudden loss of consciousness with severe heat symptoms	Greatest Treasure Special Pill to Dispel Wind (*qū fēng zhì bǎo dān*), 291
Channel obstruction after wind-stroke	Chronic pain, weakness, and numbness (especially in the lower extremities) that is aggravated by cold, and a white, moist tongue coating	Minor Invigorate the Collaterals Special Pill (*xiǎo huó luò dān*), 631
Deficiency of the normal and yang qi with blood stasis in the channels	Sequelae of wind-stroke including hemiplegia, facial paralysis, and slurred speech accompanied by dry stools, frequent urination or urinary incontinence, a white tongue coating, and a moderate pulse	Tonify the Yang to Restore Five [-Tenths] Decoction (*bǔ yáng huán wǔ tāng*), 568

Formula Index

B

U

V

General Index

D

Downward-draining method (下法 *xià fǎ*), xxii, xxvi, 61
    formula comparisons, 97–99
    for seasonal epidemic disorders, 62

Drafts (煮散 *zhǔ sǎn*), xxxv

Draining, within fortification, 88

Draining as substitute for clearing (以瀉代清 *yǐ xiè dài qīng*), 172

Draining fire (泄火 *xiè huǒ*), *vs.* clearing heat, 149

Draining out water (瀉水 *xiè shuǐ*), 93

Dredging (决 *jué*), 558

Dredging and cutting strategy, 06, 95

Dried blood below the umbilicus, 562

Drum-like abdominal distention (鼓脹 *gǔ zhàng*), 722, 724

Dry blood (干血 *gān xuè*), 595

Dry dampness and transform phlegm formulas, 774–775
    formula comparisons, 819

Dry leg qi, 754

Dry stools, 65

Dry sudden turmoil disorder (乾霍亂 *gān huò luàn*), 706

Dry-type sudden turmoil disorder, 499

Dryness (燥 *zào*), 63, 661
    injury to Lungs, Stomach, and fluids from, 669
    internal *vs.* external, 661
    moistening by enriching yin, 670
    in three burners, 662

Dryness-dispersing and -moistening formulas, 662
    formula comparisons, 679

Dryness-treating formulas, 661–662
    dryness-dispersing and -moistening formulas, 662
    formula comparisons, 679–680
    yin-enriching and dryness-moistening formulas, 670

Dysenteric disorders, 424
    causing leaking abandonment, 425
    chronic/intermittent due to damp-heat leading to qi stagnation/blood stasis, 432
    due to cold from deficiency, 427
    in food stagnation formulas, 831

Dysenteric disorders (痢疾 *lì jí*), viii

Dysenteric wind (痢風 *lì fēng*), 760

Dysmenorrhea, due to qi stagnation, 535

Dysphagia-occlusion (噎嗝 *yē gé*), 534

E

Early-stage dysenteric disorders, 293

Early-stage exterior disorders, 4–5
    formula comparisons, 56–57

Early-stage measles, 3
    warm pathogen perspective, 44

Early-stage sores and carbuncles, 861

Earth failing to transport water, 725

Earth-tonifying current (補土派 *bǔ tǔ pài*), xx

Edema, 726
    constraining Kidney qi, 734
    due to constraint of protective qi, 51
    as thin mucus, 726
    treatment strategies, 96
    yin-type, 750

Eight battle arrays (八陣 *bā zhèn*), xxx

Eight parameters of diagnosis (八綱 *bā gāng*), xxv

Eight treatment methods (八法 *bā fǎ*), xxv, 4
    clearing method (清法 *qīng fǎ*), xxvi, 149
    downward-draining method (下法 *xià fǎ*), xxvi, 61
    harmonizing method (和法 *hé fǎ*), xxvi, 103
    reducing method (消法 *xuē*), xxviii
    releasing pathogens from exterior, 3
    sweating method (汗法 *hàn fǎ*), xxvi
    tonifying method (補法 *bǔ fǎ*), xxviii, 307
    vomiting method (吐法 *tù fǎ*), xxvi
    warming method (溫法 *wēn fǎ*), xxvi, 251

Elixers. *See* Special pills

Emetic formulas, 817–818. *See also* Vomiting method

Emotional disorders
    and constraint, 510
    disease due to, 104
    non-Liver origins of, 518
    phlegm-heat in, 790
    and plum-pit qi, 517

Endemic infectious disorders (鄉土流行疾病 *xiāng tǔ liú xíng jí bìng*), 703

Environment, adapting treatments to, xxv

Envoy ingredients, xxxi

Epidemic infectious disorders, 149
    miasmatic malarial disorder, 692
    venting pathogens from membrane source in, 13

Epidemic pox disorders, 31

Epidemic toxin (疫毒 *yì dú*), 674

Epigastric focal distention, 128, 511, 527, 543, 825

Epigastric pain, 521
    intermittent, 522

Epigastric softness, 129

Eructation and rebellion (噦逆 *yuě nì*), 545

Essence
    augmenting in Kidney harm, 307
    deer cart and, 433

Ethereal soul, 334
    loss of mooring, 471

Excess above and deficiency below, 539, 540

Excess heat, accumulating in Stomach and Intestines, 62

Excess phlegm, downward-draining strategy for, 62

Excess water
    formula comparisons, 99
    formulas driving out, 89

Excessive deliberation, 353

Exterior (表 *biǎo*), 3

Exterior cold
    with heat from constraint in the interior, 11
    with interior dampness contracted in summer, 234
    with preexisting yang deficiency, 50

Exterior deficiency, 15
    with weak and unstable protective qi, 326

Exterior disorders, 3. *See also* Exterior wind-cold disorders; Exterior wind-heat disorders
    early-stage, 4–5
    improper treatment with purgatives, 292
    with interior deficiency, 46–47, 58

Exterior-interior excess releasing formulas, 285–286, 300–301
    releasing exterior and clearing interior, 292
    releasing exterior and purging interior formulas, 286
    releasing exterior and warming interior, 296

Exterior wind-cold disorders
    formula comparisons, 56–57
    sequelae with persistence of dryness, 665
    with simultaneous blood/yin deficiency due to long-term illness, 54

Exterior wind-heat disorders, 34–35
    formula comparisons, 57–58

External abscesses and sores (癰瘍 *yōng yáng*), 859
    formula comparisons, 890–891
    formulas treating, 859–861

External application formulas, xxxix–xli, 895
    for external disorders, 896
    formula comparisons, 905–906
    historical aspects, 895–896
    for internal disorders, 904
    labeling of toxic materials, 896
    liquids and gases, xl
    miscellaneous topical applications, xl–xli
    skin irritation or itching precautions, 896
    testing for sensitivity, 896
    time of application, 896

External applications (外治法 *wài zhì fǎ*), 895

External disorders
    external formulas for, 896
    formula comparisons, 905

External dryness, 661
    vs. internal dryness, 670

External medicine (外科 *wài kē*), 895

External wind, 619
    damage to blood from, 639
    formula comparisons, 655–656
    formulas to dredge and disperse, 620–621
    headache from, 625
    mutual production with internal wind, 619
    with preexisting qi deficiency, 621
    with qi and blood deficiency, 623

External wind-cold, with internal damp turbidity, 691

Yin clumping (陰結 *yīn jié*), 76

Yin collaterals, damage to, 597, 609

Yin deficiency
  with deficiency fire, 388
  and dryness, 662
  externally-contracted wind-heat with
    underlying, 55
  fire of deficiency and concurrent phlegm
    in, 367
  of Liver, Heart, and Kidney channels
    generating internal heat, 376
  role in phlegm-dryness formulas, 802
  in scrofula, 799
  steaming bone disorder in, 373
  with vigorous fire, 374

Yin deficiency consumptive disorder, 390
  with blazing of ministerial fire, 675

Yin-enriching and dryness-moistening
  formulas, 670
    formula comparisons, 679–680

Yin-enriching current (滋陰派 *zī yīn pài*), xxi

Yin fire (陰火 *yīn huǒ*), 373–374
  in context of yin deficiency, 374
  from Lung and Stomach yin deficiency, 671
  treatment of, 319

Yin fluids, storage by Kidney, 398

Yin fluids damage, 364
  in nutritive-/blood-level disorders, 42

Yin summerheat, 235

Yin tonifying and nourishing formulas, 364–365
  formula comparisons, 414–415

Yin-type agitation (陰躁 *yīn zào*), 724

Yin-type edema, 750

Yin-type flat abscess (陰疽 *yīn jū*), 870

Yin-type inversion, 117

Yin-type localized swellings, 869

Yin-yang sores, 863, 871

Yishui (易水 *Yì shuǐ*) current, 25

Yuan dynasty, xx–xxi

ABOUT THE AUTHORS

Dr. Volker Scheid is a scholar physician who engages with East Asian medicine as a clinician, researcher, and teacher. He is a principal research fellow at the University of Westminster, London (UK), where he directs EAST*medicine* (East Asian Sciences & Traditions in Medicine), an innovative trans-disciplinary research center dedicated to the integration of East Asian medicines into contemporary health care. He has published widely in academic and professional journals, including two previous books: *Chinese Medicine in Contemporary China: Plurality and Synthesis* and *Currents of Tradition in Chinese Medicine, 1626-2006*. He maintains a private medical practice in London and lectures internationally.

Dan Bensky is a graduate of the Macau Institute of Chinese Medicine (Oriental Medicine Diploma, 1975), University of Michigan (B.A. in Chinese Language and Literature, 1978), Michigan State University College of Osteopathic Medicine (Doctor of Osteopathy, 1982), University of Washington (M.A. in Classical Chinese, 1996), and Chinese Academy of Traditional Chinese Medical Sciences (Ph.D. in *Discussion of Cold Damage*, 2006). He contributed to the translation and editing of *Acupuncture: A Comprehensive Text*, and to the compilation and translation of *Chinese Herbal Medicine: Materia Medica*, and *Chinese Herbal Medicine: Formulas & Strategies*. Dr. Bensky is a founder of the Seattle Institute of Oriental Medicine. In 2008, he was awarded the Wang Dingyi Cup International Prize for contributions to Chinese Medicine.

Andrew Ellis first studied Chinese medicine with Dr. James Tin Yau So at the New England School of Acupuncture. He left New England in 1983 to study Chinese language in Taiwan and apprenticed with Chinese herbalist Xu Fu-Su there for several years. Later he studied internal medicine and gynecology at the Xiamen Hospital of Chinese medicine. While there, he also specialized in the study of acupuncture with Dr. Shi Neng-Yun and dermatology with Dr. Zhang Guang-Cai. Andy is the founding owner of Spring Wind Herbs in Berkeley, California and has authored, translated, or co-translated several books on Chinese medicine including *Grasping the Wind*, *The Clinical Experience of Dr. Shi Neng-Yun*, *Notes from South Mountain*, and *Fundamentals of Chinese Medicine*.

Randall Barolet is a graduate of Cornell University (B.S. in Environmental Engineering, 1972), New England School of Acupuncture (Diploma, 1978), Nanjing College of TCM Advanced International Acupuncture Course (Certificate, 1983), California Acupuncture College (Doctor of Oriental Medicine, 1986), and the Professional Course of the National Center for Homeopathy (1989). He apprenticed as a homeopath and dowser (1986-90), studied and worked as a writer at the School of Energy Mastery (1993-94), and professionally trained in vedic astrology with Hart de Fouw (1999-2001). He is currently co-editor of *B-Alive International Magazine* for the B-Society.org in Copenhagen, and practices and teaches integrative healing arts in the United States and Scandinavia.